The 5-Minute Pediatric Consult Premium

7th EDITION

The 5-Minute Pediatric Consult Premium

7th EDITION

Editor

Michael D. Cabana, MD, MPH
Professor of Pediatrics, Epidemiology & Biostatistics
Chief, UCSF Division of General Pediatrics
University of California, San Francisco
UCSF Benioff Children's Hospital San Francisco
Philip R. Lee Institute for Health Policy Studies
San Francisco, California

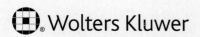

Wolters Kluwer

Philadelphia • Baltimore • New York • London
Buenos Aires • Hong Kong • Sydney • Tokyo

5MinuteConsult™

ASSOCIATE EDITORS

Paul Brakeman, MD, PhD
Associate Professor of Pediatrics
Medical Director, Pediatric Dialysis Unit
UCSF Benioff Children's Hospital San Francisco
Department of Pediatrics
University of California, San Francisco
San Francisco, California

Megan L. Curran, MD
Assistant Professor of Pediatrics
Department of Pediatrics
Northwestern University Feinberg School of Medicine
Attending Physician
Division of Rheumatology
Ann & Robert H. Lurie Children's Hospital of Chicago
Chicago, Illinois

Linda A. DiMeglio, MD, MPH
Professor of Pediatrics
Department of Pediatrics, Section of Pediatric Endocrinology and Diabetology
Indiana University School of Medicine
Riley Hospital for Children at Indiana University Health
Indianapolis, Indiana

W. Christopher Golden, MD
Assistant Professor of Pediatrics
Eudowood Neonatal Pulmonary Division
The Johns Hopkins University School of Medicine
Neonatologist and Medical Director
Full-Term Nursery
The Johns Hopkins Hospital
Baltimore, Maryland

Robert E. Goldsby, MD
Professor of Clinical Pediatrics
Divisions of Pediatric Hematology/Oncology/BMT
UCSF Benioff Children's Hospital San Francisco
Department of Pediatrics
University of California, San Francisco
San Francisco, California

Adam L. Hartman, MD
Associate Professor
Department of Neurology & Pediatrics
The Johns Hopkins University School of Medicine
Attending Physician
Department of Neurology
The Johns Hopkins Hospital
Baltimore, Maryland

Terry Kind, MD, MPH
Associate Professor of Pediatrics
Assistant Dean for Clinical Education
The George Washington University
Children's National Health System
Washington, DC

Carlton K.K. Lee, PharmD, MPH
Clinical Pharmacy Specialist, Pediatrics
PGY-2 Pediatric Pharmacy Residency Program Director
Department of Pharmacy
The Johns Hopkins Hospital
Associate Professor, Pediatrics
The Johns Hopkins University School of Medicine
Baltimore, Maryland

Jenifer R. Lightdale, MD, MPH
Professor of Pediatrics
Department of Pediatrics
University of Massachusetts Medical School
Division Chief, Pediatric Gastroenterology, Hepatology and Nutrition
Chief Quality Officer
UMass Memorial Children's Medical Center
Worcester, Massachusetts

Camille Sabella, MD
Associate Professor of Pediatrics
Vice-Chair for Education, Pediatric Institute
Director, Center for Pediatric Infectious Diseases
Cleveland Clinic Children's
Cleveland, Ohio

Ronn E. Tanel, MD
Professor of Clinical Pediatrics
Director, Pediatric Arrhythmia Service
UCSF Benioff Children's Hospital San Francisco
Department of Pediatrics
University of California, San Francisco
San Francisco, California

Acquisitions Editor: Jamie M. Elfrank
Product Development Editor: Ashley Fischer
Editorial Assistant: Brian Convery
Marketing Manager: Stephanie Kindlick
Production Project Manager: Priscilla Crater
Design Coordinator: Teresa Mallon
Manufacturing Coordinator: Beth Welsh
Prepress Vendor: Absolute Service, Inc.

7th Edition

9 8 7 6 5 4 3 2 1

Printed in China

Library of Congress Cataloging-in-Publication data available on request from publisher.

ISBN: 978-1-4511-9103-5

LWW.com

CCS0515

To Cewin, Alexandra, Abigail, Annie, Binko, and Tarquin

–MICHAEL D. CABANA, MD, MPH

To my parents Donald J. Curran, DO, and Victoria Renz for instilling in me the value of education, to my patients for teaching me on a daily basis, and to Adam for supporting me unconditionally

–MEGAN L. CURRAN, MD

To my patients, colleagues, friends, and family (especially Bob, Richard, Luke, and Max) who infuse my life with purpose and joy

–LINDA A. DIMEGLIO, MD, MPH

To my Golden family–Sherita, Andrew, Anne (Mom), Stacey, G. Bernard, and William (Dad, in memory)–and to my teachers, mentors, and patients. Thank you for love, support, and education

–W. CHRISTOPHER GOLDEN, MD

To my family and all of the patients who have allowed me to be part of their lives

–ROBERT E. GOLDSBY, MD

To my family, teachers, colleagues, and patients–thank you

–ADAM L. HARTMAN, MD

Thanks to my pediatric and medical education colleagues, my patients, and my Kind-Simon family, all of whom inspire me. Let's grow together

–TERRY KIND, MD, MPH

To Wayne, Isobel, and Nathan, as well as everyone at BCH and UMass

–JENIFER R. LIGHTDALE, MD, MPH

To Paula, Carmen, Julia, Annmarie, and my parents for all their love and support

–CAMILLE SABELLA, MD

To Sarah, Meghan, and Lauren

–RONN E. TANEL, MD

PREFACE

On the last Friday of the nursery rotation at UCSF Benioff Children's Hospital, the third-year medical students are given an assignment which seems simple at first. For this final task, the students are asked to present a talk on any pediatric newborn topic of their choice. One of the parameters is that the presentation can *only* be 3 minutes in length, at most. Surely, one would think that the brevity of the talk might make the presentation that much easier and quicker to prepare. However, as many students eventually discover, it is actually *much* more challenging to teach something of substance with so little time. For a short presentation, there is limited time to discuss the key concepts or pathophysiology about the condition as well as the most important diagnostic or therapeutic issues. From large heaps of information, students need to select only the most important information to present on Friday morning. Choices need to be made, and students learn to become connoisseurs of which clinical facts are worthy of presentation. This assignment highlights the difficulty in keeping our explanations concise as well as the art and skill of efficient clinical teaching. Although Mark Twain was not an academic pediatrician, I think he recognized this irony of efficient communication when he once quipped, "I didn't have time to write a short letter, so I wrote a long one instead."

I have always been impressed by my teachers and colleagues who could so easily and so efficiently teach with so little time. These colleagues could punctuate rounds with the most wonderful few minutes of teaching and their consultations have always been the most valuable over time. This book, *The 5-Minute Pediatric Consult*, can be thought of as a collection of all those insightful and efficient consultations all placed into one book. The authors of each chapter strive to provide a comprehensive, but efficient, 5-minute consult for a busy clinician.

It is an honor to continue this tradition of *The 5-Minute Pediatric Consult* with this new seventh edition. M. William Schwartz, MD, at the University of Pennsylvania, Perelman School of Medicine, edited the initial editions of the book and established a comprehensive and indispensable resource for health care professionals who care for children. The first edition was published in 1997. Throughout the last two decades, the continuing popularity of *The 5-Minute Pediatric Consult* is a testimony to the outstanding work of the previous authors and editors as well as the production staff.

Once again, the seventh edition continues to innovate and build on previous editions. For this new edition, our editorial review now includes an additional pharmacologic review by Carlton K.K. Lee, PharmD, MPH. We have also expanded the content for several topics with additional chapters, including pediatric dental health issues (e.g., Dental Caries, Dental Health and Prevention, Dental Infections) and psychiatric conditions (e.g., Depression, Separation Anxiety Disorder, Trichotillomania) as well as new chapters for a variety of conditions (e.g., Cyclic Vomiting Syndrome; Ankyloglossia; Diabetes Mellitus, Type 2). Some chapters have been reorganized to reflect broader clinical situations that a clinician may face (e.g., Hypercalcemia, Hypocalcemia, Hyperleukocytosis), and other topics reflect new therapies available to clinicians (e.g., Prebiotics).

Several new topics reflect the changing epidemiology of childhood illness and pediatric care, in general. With the growing success of pediatric cancer treatment, four of five children with childhood cancer now achieve long-term survival. In addition, nearly two thirds of survivors develop chronic health issues related to their previous diagnosis and treatment. As a result, we have added a topic on Cancer Therapy Late Effects for primary care and subspecialty clinicians who care for these children. In addition, the care of former premature infants is quite common in pediatric practice. We have added topics such as Meconium Aspiration Syndrome, Neonatal Encephalopathy, Respiratory Distress Syndrome, and Retinopathy of Prematurity. Although these are clinical topics primarily addressed in the neonatal intensive care unit (NICU), many primary care clinicians who care for former "NICU-graduates" may appreciate information and clinical pearls on issues associated with the disease prognosis, follow-up, or ongoing care.

Finally, we realize that many clinicians who use this book also play a key role in the clinical teaching and instruction of trainees at all levels. With this issue in mind, Terry Kind, MD, MPH, has created and developed "The 5-Minute Educator," which is also included in this book. The four topics (Precepting, Direct Observation, Feedback, and Clinical Reasoning) are authored by seasoned educators who provide efficient, practical and accessible consultation on how to be a more effective clinical educator in a busy clinical setting.

With all these changes, this edition now includes more than 500 topics and features a group of new as well as returning authors. These authors have demonstrated great skill in distilling large amounts of information into an easily accessible 5-minute synopsis or "consult" on a plethora of clinical topics. Although the topics are a short two pages, each topic represents years of clinical experience as well as countless hours of research, writing, and editing.

To organize this effort, I am also fortunate to have a wonderfully diverse, distinguished, and talented team of associate editors, who have recruited such accomplished authors for each topic. Ronn E. Tanel, MD, has the distinction of serving as an associate editor on previous editions of this book and has provided wonderful continuity for this project. The new associate editors include Paul Brakeman, MD, PhD; Megan L. Curran, MD; Linda A. DiMeglio, MD, MPH; W. Christopher Golden, MD; Robert E. Goldsby, MD; Adam L. Hartman, MD; Terry Kind, MD, MPH; Carlton K.K. Lee, PharmD, MPH; Jenifer R. Lightdale, MD, MPH; and Camille Sabella, MD. This group is a "dream" team of clinicians, educators, editors, and scholars. They have already taught me so much with each comment on each draft of each chapter they edited and reviewed. Finally, I would also like to thank the staff at Absolute Service, Inc., and Wolters Kluwer including Rodel Fariñas, Rebecca Gaertner, Ashley Fischer, and Jamie Elfrank, who have organized and presented this work so beautifully.

In the preface to the sixth edition of *The 5-Minute Pediatric Consult*, Dr. Schwartz wrote,

"Being involved in many ways with educating medical students . . . and visiting many hospitals, I was able to see firsthand how this book was helpful to trainees, primary care pediatricians, and nurses, and thus, justifying the name of *The 5-Minute Pediatric Consult*."

As one of the many trainees and primary care pediatricians who benefited from the previous editions of *The 5-Minute Pediatric Consult*, I hope that this new edition will continue to be a useful clinical companion and continue to help another generation of trainees and health care providers who care for children.

MICHAEL D. CABANA, MD, MPH
San Francisco, 2015

CONTRIBUTING AUTHORS

Fizan Abdullah, MD, PhD
Associate Professor of International Health
Bloomberg School of Public Health
Associate Professor of Surgery
Division of General Pediatric Surgery
The Johns Hopkins Hospital
Baltimore, Maryland

Bethlehem Abebe-Wolpaw, MD
Assistant Clinical Professor of Pediatrics
Department of Pediatrics
University of California, San Francisco
UCSF Benioff Children's Hospital San Francisco
San Francisco, California

Erika Abramson, MD, MS
Assistant Professor
Pediatrics & Public Health
Weill Cornell Medical College
Attending Physician
Pediatrics
New York-Presbyterian Hospital
New York, New York

Jennifer A. Accardo, MD, MSCE
Assistant Professor
Department of Neurology and Pediatrics
The Johns Hopkins University School of Medicine
Director, Sleep Disorders Clinic and Laboratory
Department of Neurology and Developmental Medicine
Kennedy Krieger Institute
Baltimore, Maryland

Dewesh Agrawal, MD
Associate Professor
Department of Pediatrics and Emergency Medicine
The George Washington University School of Medicine & Health Sciences
Director
Pediatric Residency Program
Children's National Medical Center
Washington, DC

Allison Agwu, MD, ScM
Associate Professor
Department of Pediatrics
Division of Infectious Diseases
The Johns Hopkins University School of Medicine
The Johns Hopkins Hospital
Baltimore, Maryland

Syed I. Ahmed, MD
Chief
Orthopedic Surgery Service
Landstuhl Regional Medical Center
Germany

Jeremy T. Aidlen, MD
Assistant Professor
Department of Surgery and Pediatrics
University of Massachusetts Medical School
Department of Surgery, Division of Pediatric Surgery
UMass Memorial Children's Medical Center
Worcester, Massachusetts

Akinyemi O. Ajayi, MD
Pediatric Pulmonologist
Winter Park, Florida

Stamatia Alexiou, MD
Pediatric Pulmonology Fellow
Department of Pulmonary Medicine
The Children's Hospital of Philadelphia
Philadelphia, Pennsylvania

Craig A. Alter, MD
Professor of Clinical Pediatrics
Division of Endocrinology and Diabetes
The Children's Hospital of Philadelphia
Philadelphia, Pennsylvania

Lusine Ambartsumyan, MD
Assistant Professor of Pediatrics
Director, Gastrointestinal Motility
Seattle Children's Hospital
Seattle, Washington

Mansi D. Amin, MD
Department of Pediatric Medicine and Emergency Medicine
Texas Children's Hospital
Houston, Texas

Prina P. Amin, MD
Assistant Professor
Department of Pediatrics
Weill Cornell Medical College
Attending Physician
Pediatrics
New York-Presbyterian Hospital
New York, New York

Evan J. Anderson, MD
Assistant Professor
Departments of Pediatrics and Medicine
Emory University School of Medicine
Children's Healthcare of Atlanta at Egleston Hospital
Atlanta, Georgia

John S. Andrews, MD
Associate Professor
Department of Pediatrics
Associate Dean
Graduate Medical Education
University of Minnesota
Minneapolis, Minnesota

Garrick A. Applebee, MD
Associate Professor
Department of Neurological Sciences
Department of Pediatrics
University of Vermont College of Medicine
Burlington, Vermont

Ravit Arav-Boger, MD
Associate Professor
Division of Pediatric Infectious Diseases
The Johns Hopkins Hospital
Johns Hopkins Children's Center
Baltimore, Maryland

John Arnold, MD
Assistant Professor
Department of Pediatrics
Uniformed Services University of the Health Sciences
Chairman
Department of Pediatrics
Naval Medical Center, San Diego
San Diego, California

Stephen S. Arnon, MD, MPH
Chief, Infant Botulism Treatment and Prevention Program
Division of Communicable Disease Control
California Department of Public Health
Richmond, California

Allison Ast, MD
Pediatrician
Gainesville, Florida

Darlene Atkins, PhD
Associate Clinical Professor of Pediatrics
Department of Pediatrics
The George Washington University School of Medicine & Health Sciences
Director, Eating Disorders Clinic
Adolescent and Young Adult Medicine
Children's National Medical Center
Washington, DC

Susan W. Aucott, MD
Associate Professor
Department of Pediatrics
The Johns Hopkins University School of Medicine
Medical Director, NICU
Department of Pediatrics
The Johns Hopkins Hospital
Baltimore, Maryland

J. Christopher Austin, MD
Associate Professor of Urology
Department of Pediatric Urology
Oregon Health & Science University
Portland, Oregon

Philippe F. Backeljauw, MD
Professor of Clinical Pediatrics
University of Cincinnati College of Medicine
Director, Pediatric Endocrinology Fellowship Program
Cincinnati Children's Hospital Medical Center
Cincinnati, Ohio

Oluwakemi B. Badaki-Makun, MD, CM
Assistant Professor
Department of Pediatrics
The Johns Hopkins University School of Medicine
Attending Physician
Division of Pediatric Emergency Medicine
Johns Hopkins Children's Center
Baltimore, Maryland

Charles Bailey, MD, PhD
Assistant Professor of Clinical Pediatrics
Department of Pediatrics
Perelman School of Medicine at the University of Pennsylvania
Attending Physician
Department of Pediatrics
The Children's Hospital of Philadelphia
Philadelphia, Pennsylvania

Fran Balamuth, MD, PhD
Assistant Professor
Department of Pediatrics
Perelman School of Medicine at the University of Pennsylvania
Attending Physician
Division of Emergency Medicine
The Children's Hospital of Philadelphia
Philadelphia, Pennsylvania

Christina Bales, MD
Assistant Professor of Clinical Pediatrics
Department of Pediatrics
Perelman School of Medicine at the University of Pennsylvania
Philadelphia, Pennsylvania

Kristin W. Barañano, MD, PhD
Clinical Associate
Department of Neurology
The Johns Hopkins University School of Medicine
Baltimore, Maryland

Jennifer M. Barker, MD
Associate Professor
Department of Pediatrics
University of Colorado School of Medicine
Program Director
Pediatric Director
Pediatric Endocrinology
Children's Hospital Colorado
Aurora, Colorado

Laurence Baskin, MD
Professor of Urology
Department of Urology
University of California, San Francisco
Chief of Pediatric Urology
UCSF Benioff Children's Hospital San Francisco
San Francisco, California

Anne S. Bassett, MD, FRCPC
Canada Research Chair in Schizophrenia Genetics and Genomic Disorders
Dalglish Chair in 22q11.2 Deletion Syndrome
Professor of Psychiatry, University of Toronto
Associate Staff, Division of Cardiology, University Health Network
Associate Member, Canadian College of Medical Geneticists
Director, Clinical Genetics Research Program
Centre for Addiction & Mental Health
Toronto, Ontario, Canada

Hamid Bassiri, MD, PhD
Assistant Professor of Pediatrics
Perelman School of Medicine at the University of Pennsylvania
Attending Physician
Division of Infectious Diseases
The Children's Hospital of Philadelphia
Philadelphia, Pennsylvania

Suzanne E. Beck, MD
Professor of Clinical Pediatrics
Department of Pediatrics
Division of Pulmonary Medicine and Cystic Fibrosis Center
Perelman School of Medicine at the University of Pennsylvania
Attending Physician
Department of Pediatrics
The Children's Hospital of Philadelphia
Philadelphia, Pennsylvania

David Becker, MD, MPH, MA
Associate Clinical Professor
Department of Pediatrics
University of California, San Francisco
San Francisco, California

Julia Belkowitz, MD
Assistant Professor
Department of Pediatrics
University of Miami Miller School of Medicine
Miami, Florida

Kelly A. Benedict, MD
Fellow
Department of Pediatrics, Division of Nephrology
University of California, San Francisco
San Francisco, California

Daniel K. Benjamin, Jr., MD, PhD, MPH
Professor
Department of Pediatrics
Duke Clinical Research Institute
Duke University
Durham, North Carolina

Amanda K. Berry, MSN, CRNP, PhD
Pediatric Nurse Practitioner
Division of Urology
The Children's Hospital of Philadelphia
Philadelphia, Pennsylvania

Anita Bhandari, MD
Associate Professor
Pediatrics
University of Connecticut School of Medicine
Farmington, Connecticut
Associate Professor
Pediatric Pulmonology
Connecticut Children's Medical Center
Hartford, Connecticut

Vineet Bhandari, MD, DM
Associate Professor
Pediatrics-Obstetrics, Gynecology and Reproductive Sciences
Yale University
Attending Neonatologist
Pediatrics
Yale-New Haven Children's Hospital
New Haven, Connecticut

Sumit Bhargava, MD
Clinical Associate Professor
Department of Pediatrics
Stanford University
Pediatric Pulmonologist & Sleep Medicine
Department of Pediatrics
Lucile Packard Children's Hospital Stanford
Palo Alto, California

Diana X. Bharucha-Goebel, MD
Neurophysiologist
Departments of Epilepsy, Neurophysiology, and Critical Care Neurology
Children's National Health System
Washington, DC

Cara L. Biddle, MD, MPH
Assistant Clinical Professor
Department of Pediatrics
The George Washington University
Medical Director, Children's Health Center
Department of General Pediatrics
Children's National Medical Center
Washington, DC

Mercedes M. Blackstone, MD
Assistant Professor of Clinical Pediatrics
Department of Pediatrics
Perelman School of Medicine at the University of Pennsylvania
Attending Physician
Division of Emergency Medicine
The Children's Hospital of Philadelphia
Philadelphia, Pennsylvania

Seth J. Bokser, MD, MPH
Associate Clinical Professor of Pediatrics
University of California, San Francisco
Pediatric Hospitalist
UCSF Benioff Children's Hospital San Francisco
San Francisco, California

Jeffrey Bolton, MD
Instructor
Department of Neurology
Harvard Medical School
Staff Physician
Department of Pediatric Neurology
Boston Children's Hospital, Harvard
Boston, Massachusetts

Emily C. Borman-Shoap, MD
Assistant Professor
Department of Pediatrics
University of Minnesota
Minneapolis, Minnesota

John Bower, MD
Associate Professor
Department of Pediatrics
Northeast Ohio Medical University
Rootstown, Ohio
Infectious Diseases
Department of Pediatrics
Akron Children's Hospital
Akron, Ohio

Alison M. Boyce, MD
Assistant Professor
Department of Pediatrics
The George Washington University School of Medicine & Health Sciences
Division of Endocrinology & Diabetes
Children's National Medical Center
Washington, DC

Paul Brakeman, MD, PhD
Associate Professor of Pediatrics
Medical Director, Pediatric Dialysis Unit
UCSF Benioff Children's Hospital San Francisco
Department of Pediatrics
University of California, San Francisco
San Francisco, California

Wendy J. Brickman, MD
Associate Professor
Department of Pediatrics
Northwestern University Feinberg School of Medicine
Attending Physician
Department of Pediatrics; Division of Pediatric Endocrinology
Ann & Robert H. Lurie Children's Hospital of Chicago
Chicago, Illinois

Lee J. Brooks, MD
Professor
Department of Pediatrics
Perelman School of Medicine at the University of Pennsylvania
Attending Physician
Pediatric Pulmonary Division
The Children's Hospital of Philadelphia
Philadelphia, Pennsylvania

Jeffrey P. Brosco, MD, PhD
Professor of Clinical Pediatrics
University of Miami Miller School of Medicine
Associate Director
Mailman Center for Child Development
Miami, Florida

Laura H. Brower, MD
Clinical Fellow
Hospital Medicine
Cincinnati Children's Hospital Medical Center
Cincinnati, Ohio

Valerie I. Brown, MD, PhD
Associate Professor
Division of Pediatric Hematology/Oncology
Department of Pediatrics
Penn State College of Medicine
Director of Experimental Therapeutics
Associate Professor
Division of Pediatrics Hematology/Oncology
Penn State Milton S. Hershey Medical Center
Hershey, Pennsylvania

Terri Brown-Whitehorn, MD
Associate Professor of Clinical Pediatrics
Department of Pediatrics
Perelman School of Medicine at the University of Pennsylvania
Attending Physician
Allergy & Immunology
The Children's Hospital of Philadelphia
Philadelphia, Pennsylvania

Ann B. Bruner, MD
Adolescent Medicine Physician
Mountain Manor Treatment Center
Baltimore, Maryland

Sara M. Buckelew, MD, MPH
Associate Professor of Pediatrics
Director, Eating Disorders Program
Department of Pediatrics
University of California, San Francisco
San Francisco, California

Jennifer C. Burnsed, MD, MS
Assistant Professor of Pediatrics
Division of Neonatology
University of Virginia School of Medicine
Charlottesville, Virginia

Melissa A. Buryk, MD
Assistant Professor
Department of Pediatrics
Uniformed Services University of the Health Sciences
Bethesda, Maryland
Pediatric Endocrinology Fellow
Departments of Pediatrics
Children's Hospital of Pittsburgh of UPMC
Pittsburgh, Pennsylvania

Amaya L. Bustinduy, MD, MPH
Clinical Research Fellow
Paediatric Infectious Diseases Research Group
Infection and Immunity Institute
St George's University of London
London, United Kingdom

Lavjay Butani, MD
Professor of Pediatrics
University of California, Davis
Sacramento, California

Francesca A. Byrne, MD
Pediatric Cardiologist
Department of Pediatrics
Miller Children's Hospital
Long Beach, California

Susanne M. Cabrera, MD
Assistant Professor
Department of Pediatrics
Medical College of Wisconsin
Faculty
Department of Pediatrics
Children's Hospital of Wisconsin
Milwaukee, Wisconsin

Mark P. Cain, MD
Department of Urology - Pediatric Urology
Indiana School of Medicine
Riley Hospital for Children
Indianapolis, Indiana

Andrew C. Calabria, MD
Assistant Professor
Department of Pediatrics
Perelman School of Medicine at the University of Pennsylvania
Attending Physician
Division of Endocrinology and Diabetes
The Children's Hospital of Philadelphia
Philadelphia, Pennsylvania

Robert Campbell, MD
Professor of Orthopaedic Surgery
University of Pennsylvania School of Medicine
Director, Center of Thoracic Insufficient Syndrome
Division of Orthopaedics
Children's Hospital of Philadelphia
Philadelphia, Pennsylvania

Joseph B. Cantey, MD
Fellow
Division of Pediatrics
University of Texas Southwestern Medical Center
Dallas, Texas

Vanessa S. Carlo, MD
Assistant Professor
Department of Pediatrics
Thomas Jefferson University
Philadelphia, Pennsylvania

Michael C. Carr, MD, PhD
Associate Professor of Urology in Surgery
Division of Urology
The Children's Hospital of Philadelphia
Philadelphia, Pennsylvania

Leslie Castelo-Soccio, MD, PhD
Assistant Professor
Department of Pediatrics & Dermatology
University of Pennsylvania School of Medicine
Attending Physician
Department of Pediatrics & Dermatology
The Children's Hospital of Philadelphia
Philadelphia, Pennsylvania

Elizabeth Candell Chalom, MD
Assistant Professor
Department of Pediatrics
University of Medicine and Dentistry of New Jersey
Newark, New Jersey
Director, Pediatric Rheumatology
Pediatrics
Saint Barnabas Medical Center
Livingston, New Jersey

Anthony Chan, MBBS
Division of Paediatric Hematology/Oncology
Department of Paediatrics
McMaster Children's Hospital, McMaster University
Hamilton, Ontario

Tiffany Chang, MD
Fellow
Department of Pediatric Oncology/Hematology
University of California, San Francisco
San Francisco, California

Michael F. Chiang, MD
Knowles Professor
Department of Ophthalmology
Oregon Health & Science University
Portland, Oregon

Eric H. Chiou, MD
Assistant Professor
Department of Pediatrics
Baylor College of Medicine
Attending Faculty
Department of Pediatrics
Texas Children's Hospital
Houston, Texas

Peter Chira, MD, MS
Assistant Professor of Clinical Pediatrics
Department of Pediatrics, Section of Pediatric Rheumatology
Indiana University School of Medicine
Staff Pediatric Rheumatologist
Department of Pediatrics, Section of Pediatric Rheumatology
Riley Hospital for Children at Indiana University Health
Indianapolis, Indiana

Maribeth Chitkara, MD
Associate Professor of Pediatrics
Department of Pediatrics
Stony Brook Long Island Children's Hospital
Stony Brook, New York

Christine S. Cho, MD, MPH, MEd
Assistant Professor
Department of Emergency Medicine and Pediatrics
University of California, San Francisco
UCSF Benioff Children's Hospital San Francisco
San Francisco, California

Esther K. Chung, MD, MPH
Professor
Department of Pediatrics
Sidney Kimmel Medical College of Thomas Jefferson University
Jefferson Pediatrics/Nemours-Philadelphia
Philadelphia, Pennsylvania
Nemours Alfred I. duPont Hospital for Children
Wilmington, Delaware

Melissa G. Chung, MD
Assistant Professor
Department of Pediatrics
The Ohio State University
Director of Critical Care Neurology
Division of Neurology and Critical Care Medicine
Nationwide Children's Hospital
Columbus, Ohio

Gwynne D. Church, MD
Assistant Professor
Department of Pediatrics
University of California, San Francisco
UCSF Benioff Children's Hospital San Francisco
San Francisco, California

Danielle N. Clark, DO
Pediatric Rheumatology Fellow
Department of Pediatrics
Section of Pediatric Rheumatology
Indiana University School of Medicine
Riley Hospital for Children at Indiana University Health
Indianapolis, Indiana

Stephanie Clark, MD, MPH
Fellow Physician
Department of Pediatrics
University of Pennsylvania
Fellow Physician
Department of Nephrology
The Children's Hospital of Philadelphia
Philadelphia, Pennsylvania

Jessica P. Clarke-Pounder, MD
Assistant Professor
Department of Pediatrics
University of North Carolina, Charlotte
Neonatologist
Department of Pediatrics
Levine Children's Hospital
Charlotte, North Carolina

Meryl S. Cohen, MD
Professor of Pediatrics
University of Pennsylvania School of Medicine
Program Director, Cardiology Fellowship
Medical Director, Echocardiography Laboratory
The Children's Hospital of Philadelphia
Philadelphia, Pennsylvania

Ronald D. Cohn, MD, FACMG
Associate Professor
Department of Pediatrics and Molecular Genetics
University of Toronto
Chief, Clinical and Metabolic Genetics
Department of Pediatrics
The Hospital for Sick Children
Toronto, Ontario, Canada

Nailah Coleman, MD, FAAP, FACSM
Pediatrician
Pediatrics, Adolescent Medicine, and Obesity Institute
Children's National Medical Center
The George Washington University
Washington, DC

Kara J. Connelly, MD
Assistant Professor
Department of Pediatrics
Oregon Health & Science University
Pediatric Endocrinologist
Department of Pediatrics
Doernbecher Children's Hospital
Portland, Oregon

Stephen Contompasis, MD
Professor
Department of Pediatrics
University of Vermont College of Medicine
Burlington, Vermont

Hillary L. Copp, MD, MS
Assistant Professor
Pediatric Urologist
Department of Urology
University of California, San Francisco
San Francisco, California

Kelly M. Cordoro, MD
Associate Professor of Dermatology and Pediatrics
Department of Dermatology
University of California, San Francisco
UCSF Benioff Children's Hospital San Francisco
San Francisco, California

Thomas O. Crawford, MD
Professor of Neurology and Pediatrics
Division of Pediatric Neurology
The Johns Hopkins Hospital
Baltimore, Maryland

Randy Q. Cron, MD, PhD
Professor
Department of Pediatrics
University of Alabama at Birmingham
Director
Pediatric Rheumatology
Children's of Alabama
Birmingham, Alabama

Megan L. Curran, MD
Assistant Professor of Pediatrics
Department of Pediatrics
Northwestern University Feinberg School of Medicine
Attending Physician
Division of Rheumatology
Ann & Robert H. Lurie Children's Hospital of Chicago
Chicago, Illinois

Sandra Cuzzi, MD
Assistant Professor
Department of Pediatrics
The George Washington University School of Medicine & Health Sciences
Associate Residency Program Director
Hospitalist Division
Children's National Medical Center
Washington, DC

Aarti Dalal, DO
Fellow
Department of Pediatric Cardiology
Emory University
Fellow
Department of Cardiology
Children's Healthcare of Atlanta
Atlanta, Georgia

Richard S. Davidson, MD
Clinical Professor of Orthopaedic Surgery
Department of Orthopaedic Surgery
University of Pennsylvania School of Medicine
Staff Physician
Children's Orthopaedics, Department of Surgery
The Children's Hospital of Philadelphia
Philadelphia, Pennsylvania

Peter de Blank, MD, MSCE
Assistant Professor
Department of Pediatrics
Case Western Reserve University
Assistant Professor
Division of Pediatric Hematology/Oncology
Rainbow Babies & Children's Hospital
Cleveland, Ohio

Marissa Janel Defreitas, MD
Pediatric Nephrology Fellow
Department of Pediatric Nephrology
University of Miami/Holtz Children's Hospital
Miami, Florida

Diva D. De León, MD, MSCE
Associate Professor
Department of Pediatrics
Perelman School of Medicine at the University of Pennsylvania
Director, Congenital Hyperinsulinism Center
Division of Pediatric Endocrinology
The Children's Hospital of Philadelphia
Philadelphia, Pennsylvania

Jeannine Del Pizzo, MD
Assistant Professor of Clinical Pediatrics
Department of Pediatrics
Perelman School of Medicine at the University of Pennsylvania
Division of Emergency Medicine
The Children's Hospital of Philadelphia
Philadelphia, Pennsylvania

Sophia D. Delpe, MD
Resident
Department of Urology
Yale–New Haven Hospital
New Haven, Connecticut

Michelle Denburg, MD, MSCE
Professor of Pediatrics
Department of Pediatrics
Division of Nephrology
The Children's Hospital of Philadelphia
Philadelphia, Pennsylvania

Craig DeWolfe, MD, MEd
Assistant Professor
Department of Pediatrics
The George Washington University School of Medicine & Health Sciences
Medical Unit Director, Main Pediatric Hospitalist Division
Children's National Health System
Washington, DC

Katherine Deye, MD
Assistant Professor
Department of Pediatrics
The George Washington University School of Medicine & Health Sciences
Pediatrician
Freddie Mac Child and Adolescent Protection Center
Children's National Medical Center
Washington, DC

Jennifer DiPace, MD
Assistant Professor
Director, Pediatric Graduate Medical Education
Department of Pediatrics
New York-Presbyterian/Weill Cornell
New York, New York

Michael DiSandro, MD
Professor
Department of Urology
University of California, San Francisco
Staff
Department of Urology
UCSF Medical Center
San Francisco, California

Mark F. Ditmar, MD
Clinical Associate Professor of Pediatrics
Jefferson Medical College
Philadelphia, Pennsylvania
Department of Pediatrics
Southern Ocean Medical Center
Manahawkin, New Jersey

Stacy E. Dodt, MD
Pediatric Endocrinology Fellow
Division of Endocrinology and Diabetes
The Children's Hospital of Philadelphia
Philadelphia, Pennsylvania

John P. Dormans, MD
Professor
Department of Orthopaedic Surgery
Perelman School of Medicine at the University of Pennsylvania
Chief
Division of Orthopedic Surgery
The Children's Hospital of Philadelphia
Philadelphia, Pennsylvania

Morna J. Dorsey, MD, MMSc
Associate Professor
Department of Pediatrics
University of California, San Francisco
Clinical Director, Allergy & Immunology
Department of Pediatrics
UCSF Benioff Children's Hospital San Francisco
San Francisco, California

Monica D. Dowling, PhD
Assistant Professor of Clinical Pediatrics
Department of Pediatrics
University of Miami Miller School of Medicine
Miami, Florida

Colleen A. Hughes Driscoll, MD
Assistant Professor
Department of Pediatrics
University of Maryland School of Medicine
Baltimore, Maryland

Nancy Drucker, MD
Associate Professor
Department of Pediatrics
University of Vermont
Pediatric Cardiologist
Department of Pediatrics
Fletcher Allen Health Care
Burlington, Vermont

Steven G. DuBois, MD, MS
Associate Professor
Department of Pediatrics
University of California, San Francisco
Attending Physician
Department of Pediatrics
UCSF Benioff Children's Hospital San Francisco
San Francisco, California

Alcia Edwards-Richards, MD
Fellow
Department of Pediatric
Division of Pediatric Nephrology
University of Miami Miller School of Medicine
Miami, Florida

Deborah B. Ehrenthal, MD, MPH, FACP
Lifecourse Initiative for Healthy Families Endowed Chair
Visiting Associate Professor
Departments of Obstetrics & Gynecology, Population Health Sciences, and Medicine
School of Medicine and Public Health
University of Wisconsin-Madison
Madison, Wisconsin

Jorina Elbers, MD
Assistant Professor
Departments of Neurology and Neurological Sciences
Stanford University
Stanford, California
Assistant Professor
Child Neurology
Lucile Packard Children's Hospital Stanford
Palo Alto, California

Scott Elisofon, MD
Instructor
Department of Pediatrics
Harvard Medical School
Attending Physician
Division of Gastroenterology, Hepatology, and Nutrition
Boston Children's Hospital
Boston, Massachusetts

Gary A. Emmett, MD
Professor
Director of Hospital
Department of Pediatrics
Thomas Jefferson University Hospital
Philadelphia, Pennsylvania

Heidi Engel, DPT, PT
Assistant Clinical Professor
Department of Physical Health and Science
University of California, San Francisco
Physical Therapist
UCSF Rehabilitative Services
UCSF Medical Center
San Francisco, California

Jessica E. Ericson, MD
Pediatric Infectious Diseases Fellow
Department of Pediatrics
Duke University
Duke Children's Hospital
Durham, North Carolina

Erica A. Eugster, MD
Professor of Pediatrics
Department of Pediatrics
Indiana University School of Medicine
Director, Section of Pediatric Endocrinology
Riley Hospital for Children at Indiana University Health
Indianapolis, Indiana

Stephen J. Falchek, MD
Division Chief
Division of Pediatric Neurology
Department of Pediatrics
Nemours Alfred I. duPont Hospital for Children
Wilmington, Delaware

Marni J. Falk, MD
Assistant Professor of Pediatrics
Department of Pediatrics
The Children's Hospital of Philadelphia
Philadelphia, Pennsylvania

Rima Fawaz, MD
Instructor in Pediatrics
Harvard Medical School
Attending Physician
Medical Director, Intestine and Multivisceral Transplant
Division of Gastroenterology, Hepatology & Nutrition
Boston Children's Hospital
Boston, Massachusetts

Kristen A. Feemster, MD
Assistant Professor
Department of Pediatrics
Perelman School of Medicine at the University of Pennsylvania
Attending Physician
Division of Infectious diseases
The Children's Hospital of Philadelphia
Philadelphia, Pennsylvania

Daniel E. Felten, MD, MPH
Assistant Professor
Department of Pediatrics
Washington University Medical School
Pediatrician
Department of General Pediatrics
Children's National Medical Center
Washington, DC

James Feusner, MD
Medical Director, Oncology
Department of Hematology-Oncology
UCSF Benioff Children's Hospital Oakland
Oakland, California

Amy G. Filbrun, MD, MS
Associate Professor of Pediatrics
Department of Pediatrics, Pulmonary Division
University of Michigan
Attending Faculty
Pediatrics
C.S. Mott Children's Hospital
Ann Arbor, Michigan

Anna B. Fishbein, MD, MS
Assistant Professor
Department of Pediatrics
Northwestern University
Division of Allergy & Immunology
Ann & Robert H. Lurie Children's Hospital of Chicago
Chicago, Illinois

Michael J. Fisher, MD
Associate Professor
Department of Pediatrics
Perelman School of Medicine at the University of Pennsylvania
Attending Physician
Division of Oncology
The Children's Hospital of Philadelphia
Philadelphia, Pennsylvania

Laurie N. Fishman, MD
Assistant Professor
Department of Pediatrics
Harvard Medical School
Director of Medical Education
Department of Pediatric Gastroenterology
Boston Children's Hospital
Boston, Massachusetts

Jonathan Fleenor, MD
Assistant Professor
Department of Pediatrics
Eastern Virginia Medical School
Pediatric Cardiologist
Cardiology
Children's Hospital of King's Daughters
Norfolk, Virginia

Leah Fleming, MD
Medical Genetics Fellow
National Human Genome Research Institute
National Institutes of Health
Bethesda, Maryland

Jay Fong, MD
Assistant Professor of Pediatrics
Department of Pediatrics
University of Massachusetts Medical School
UMass Memorial Medical Center
Boston, Massachusetts

Michelle Forcier, MD, MPH
Associate Professor, Clinical
Department of Pediatrics
The Warren Alpert Medical School of Brown University
Adolescent, Young Adult
Pediatrics
Hasbro Children's Hospital
Providence, Rhode Island

Craig M. Forester, MD, PhD
Fellow
Department of Pediatric Hematology/Oncology
University of California, San Francisco
San Francisco, California

Sara F. Forman, MD
Assistant Professor
Department of Pediatrics
Harvard Medical School
Clinical Director
Division of Adolescent/Young Adult Medicine
Boston Children's Hospital
Boston, Massachusetts

Karen R. Fratantoni, MD, MPH
Children's National Medical Center
Washington, DC

Melissa B. Freizinger, PhD
Instructor
Department of Psychiatry
Harvard Medical School
Associate Director, Eating Order Program
Adolescent Medicine
Boston Children's Hospital
Boston, Massachusetts

Ilona Frieden, MD
Professor
Department of Dermatology
University of California, San Francisco
Chief, Pediatric Dermatology
Vice-Chair, Department of Dermatology
University of California, San Francisco
San Francisco, California

Joel Aaron Friedlander, DO, MA
Assistant Professor
Departments of Pediatrics, Pediatric Gastroenterology
University of Colorado School of Medicine
Assistant Professor
Digestive Health Institute
Children's Hospital Colorado
Aurora, Colorado

Linda Fu, MD, MS
Assistant Professor of Pediatrics
Department of Pediatrics
The George Washington University
Pediatrician
Department of Pediatrics
Children's National Medical Center
Washington, DC

Ramsay L. Fuleihan, MD
Associate Professor of Pediatrics
Division of Allergy & Immunology
Department of Pediatrics
Northwestern University Feinberg School of Medicine
Attending Physician
Division of Allergy & Immunology
Department of Pediatrics
Ann & Robert H. Lurie Children's Hospital of Chicago
Chicago, Illinois

Nora M. Fullington, MD
Resident
Department of Surgery
University of Massachusetts Medical School
UMass Memorial Medical Center
Worchester, Massachusetts

John S. Fuqua, MD
Professor of Clinical Pediatrics
Section of Pediatric Endocrinology
Indiana University School of Medicine
Riley Hospital for Children at Indiana University Health
Indianapolis, Indiana

Susan L. Furth, MD, PhD
Professor
Departments of Pediatrics & Epidemiology
Perelman School of Medicine at the University of Pennsylvania
Chief, Division of Nephrology
Pediatrics
The Children's Hospital of Philadelphia
Philadelphia, Pennsylvania

Payal K. Gala, MD
Assistant Professor of Clinical Pediatrics
Department of Pediatrics
Perelman School of Medicine at the University of Pennsylvania
Attending Physician
Division of Emergency Medicine
The Children's Hospital of Philadelphia
Philadelphia, Pennsylvania

Theodore J. Ganley, MD
Associate Professor of Orthopaedic Surgery
Division of Orthopaedic Surgery
The Children's Hospital of Philadelphia
Philadelphia, Pennsylvania

Matthew Grady, MD
Assistant Professor
Department of Pediatrics
University of Pennsylvania School of Medicine
Primary Core Sports Medicine Fellowship Director
Department of Surgery, Division of Orthopedic
The Children's Hospital of Philadelphia
Philadelphia, Pennsylvania

George D. Gantsoudes, MD
Assistant Clinical Professor
Orthopaedic Surgery
Indiana University School of Medicine
Riley Hospital for Children at Indiana University Health
Indianapolis, Indiana

Ana Catarina Garnecho, MD
Pediatrician
Children's Hospital of Rhode Island
Pawtucket, Rhode Island

Jackie P-D. Garrett, MD
Attending Physician
Pediatrics
University of Pennsylvania
Attending Physician
Allergy and Immunology
Children's Hospital of Philadelphia
Philadelphia, Pennsylvania

Estelle B. Gauda, MD
Professor
Department of Pediatrics
Division of Neonatology
The Johns Hopkins University School of Medicine
Baltimore, Maryland

John P. Gearhart, MD
Robert D. Jeffs Professor of Pediatric Urology
The Johns Hopkins University School of Medicine
Director of Pediatric Urology
The Johns Hopkins Hospital
Baltimore, Maryland

Jeffrey S. Gerber, MD, PhD, MSCE
Assistant Professor of Pediatrics
Department of Pediatrics
The Children's Hospital of Philadelphia
Philadelphia, Pennsylvania

Saskia Gex, MD
Senior Clinical Associate
Chief Resident
Department of Pediatrics
New York-Presbyterian/Weill Cornell
New York, New York

Maureen M. Gilmore, MD
Assistant Professor
Department of Pediatrics
The Johns Hopkins University School of Medicine
Director of Neonatology
Pediatrics
Johns Hopkins Bayview Medical Center
Baltimore, Maryland

Janet Gingold, MD, MPH
Quality Improvement Coach
Goldberg Center for Community Pediatric Health
Children's National Medical Center
Washington, DC

Nicole S. Glaser, MD
Professor
Department of Pediatrics
University of California, Davis School of Medicine
Sacramento, California

Jenifer A. Glatz, MD
Assistant Professor
Department of Pediatrics
Dartmouth College
Lebanon, New Hampshire
Active Clinical Staff
Department of Pediatrics
Mary Hitchcock Memorial Hospital
Manchester, New Hampshire

W. Christopher Golden, MD
Assistant Professor of Pediatrics
Eudowood Neonatal Pulmonary Division
The Johns Hopkins University School of Medicine
Neonatologist and Medical Director
Full-Term Nursery
The Johns Hopkins Hospital
Baltimore, Maryland

Samuel B. Goldfarb, MD
Associate Professor of Clinical Pediatrics
Department of Pediatrics
University of Pennsylvania
Medical Director, Lung and Heart/Lung Transplant Programs
Department of Pediatrics
The Children's Hospital of Philadelphia
Philadelphia, Pennsylvania

Mitchell A. Goldstein, MD, MBA
Assistant Professor
Department of Pediatrics
The Johns Hopkins University School of Medicine
Child Protection Team Medical Director
Department of Pediatrics
Johns Hopkins Children's Center
Baltimore, Maryland

Stuart Goldstein, MD
Professor
Department of Pediatrics
University of Cincinnati College of Medicine
Director
Center for Acute Care Nephrology
Cincinnati Children's Hospital Medical Center
Cincinnati, Ohio

Esteban I. Gomez, MD
Hematology/Oncology Fellow
UCSF Benioff Children's Hospital - Oakland
Oakland, California

Blanca E. Gonzalez, MD
Assistant Professor
Center for Pediatric Infectious Diseases
Cleveland Clinic Lerner College of Medicine of Case Western University
Cleveland Clinic Children's Hospital
Cleveland, Ohio

Zoe M. Gonzalez-Garcia, MD
Pediatric Endocrinology Fellow
Department of Endocrinology
Phoenix Children's Hospital
Phoenix, Arizona

Vani V. Gopalareddy, MD
Associate Professor
Division of Pediatric GI/Hepatology
Department of Pediatrics
Levine Children's Hospital
Charlotte, North Carolina

Marc H. Gorelick, MD, MSCE
President and CEO, Children's Specialty Group
Professor of Pediatrics, Emergency Medicine
Sr. Associate Dean for Clinical Affairs (CSG)
Executive VP, Children's Hospital and Health System
The Medical College of Wisconsin
Children's Specialty Group, Children's Corporate Center
Milwaukee, Wisconsin

Jayaprakash A. Gosalakkal, MD
Pediatrician
Children's Medical Center
St. Rita's Medical Center
Dayton, Ohio

Craig H. Gosdin, MD, MSHA
Assistant Professor of Pediatrics
Hospital Medicine
Cincinnati Children's Hospital Medical Center
Cincinnati, Ohio

Swathi Gowtham, MD
Pediatric Infectious Disease Specialist
Geisinger Health System
Janet Weis Children's Hospital
Danville, Pennsylvania

Rose C. Graham, MD, MSCE
Pediatric Gastroenterology
Durham, North Carolina

Cori Green, MD, MSc
Assistant Professor
General Academic Pediatrics
Weill Cornell Medical College
New York-Presbyterian
New York, New York

Adda Grimberg, MD
Associate Professor
Department of Pediatrics
Perelman School of Medicine at the University of Pennsylvania
Scientific Director
Diagnostic and Research Growth Center
The Children's Hospital of Philadelphia
Philadelphia, Pennsylvania

Andrew B. Grossman, MD
Assistant Professor of Clinical Pediatrics
Perelman School of Medicine at the University of Pennsylvania
Attending Physician
Co-Director, Center for Pediatric Inflammatory Bowel Disease
The Children's Hospital of Philadelphia
Philadelphia, Pennsylvania

Amit S. Grover, MD
Clinical Fellow in Pediatrics
Department of Pediatrics
Harvard Medical School
Boston Children's Hospital
Boston, Massachusetts

Roberto Gugig, MD
Gastroenterologist
Department of Gastroenterology
Valley Children's Hospital
Madera, California

Deepti Gupta, MD
Pediatric Dermatology Fellow
Department of Dermatology
University of California, San Francisco
San Francisco, California

Natasha Gupta, BS
Medical Student
Department of Pediatrics
The Johns Hopkins University School of Medicine
Baltimore, Maryland

Blaze Robert Gusic, MD
Pediatrician
West Chester, Pennsylvania

Kathleen Gutierrez, MD
Associate Professor
Pediatrics
Stanford University School of Medicine
Physician
Pediatrics-Infectious Disease
Lucile Packard Children's Hospital, Stanford University Hospital
Stanford, California

Maha N. Haddad, MD
Director of Pediatric Dialysis
Associate Professor
Pediatric Nephrologist
UC Davis Medical Center
University of California, Davis
Sacramento, California

Elizabeth J. Hait, MD, MPH
Instructor
Department of Pediatrics
Harvard Medical School
Attending Physician
Department of Gastroenterology and Nutrition
Boston Children's Hospital
Boston, Massachusetts

Chad R. Haldeman-Englert, MD
Assistant Professor
Department of Pediatrics-Genetics
Wake Forest School of Medicine
Winston-Salem, North Carolina

Mark E. Halstead, MD
Assistant Professor
Pediatrics and Orthopedics
Washington University School of Medicine
Assistant Professor
Pediatrics and Orthopedics
St. Louis Children's Hospital
St. Louis, Missouri

J. Nina Ham, MD
Assistant Professor
Department of Pediatrics
Emory University
Children's Healthcare of Atlanta
Atlanta, Georgia

Ada Hamosh, MD, MPH
Professor
Department of Pediatrics
McKusick-Nathans Institute of Genetic Medicine
Professor
Department of Epidemiology, Bloomberg School of Public Health
The Johns Hopkins University School of Medicine
Baltimore, Maryland

Brian D. Hanna, MD, PhD
Clinical Professor of Pediatrics
University of Pennsylvania School of Medicine
Director, Section of Pulmonary Hypertension
The Children's Hospital of Philadelphia
Philadelphia, Pennsylvania

Zeev Harel, MD
Pediatrician
Division of Adolescent Medicine
Hasbro Children's Hospital
Providence, Rhode Island

Daphne M. Hasbani, MD, PhD
Clinical Neurophysiology and Epilepsy Fellow
Division of Neurology, Department of Pediatrics
The Children's Hospital of Philadelphia
Philadelphia, Pennsylvania

Caroline Hastings, MD
Fellowship Director
Pediatric Hematology/Oncology
Children's Hospital and Research Center Oakland
Oakland, California

Sarah Z. Hatab, MD
Pediatric Endocrinology Fellow
Department of Pediatric, Division of Endocrinology & Metabolism
Emory University School of Medicine
Children's Healthcare of Atlanta
Atlanta, Georgia

David Hehir, MD, MS
Associate Professor
Department of Pediatrics
Sidney Kimmel Medical College of Thomas Jefferson University
Philadelphia, Pennsylvania
Chief
Division of Cardiac Critical Care
Nemours Alfred I. duPont Hospital for Children
Wilmington, Delaware

Mayada A. Helal, MD
Fellow
Department of Pediatrics
The Hospital for Sick Children
Toronto, Ontario, Canada

Michelle L. Hermiston, MD, PhD
Associate Professor
Department of Pediatrics
University of California, San Francisco
UCSF Benioff Children's Hospital San Francisco
San Francisco, California

Eugene R. Hershorin, MD
Professor
Department of Pediatrics
University of Miami Miller School of Medicine
Miami, Florida

Kathryn Hillenbrand, MD, CCC-SLP
Master Clinical Specialist
Department of Speech Pathology and Audiology
Western Michigan University
Kalamazoo, Michigan

Bernadette A. Hillman, MD
Assistant Professor
Department of Pediatrics
University of Connecticut
Farmington, Connecticut
Attending Clinical Instructor
Department of Pediatrics
Yale University
New Haven, Connecticut
Neonatologist
Department of Pediatrics
The Hospital of Central Connecticut
New Britain, Connecticut

Tanya Hinds, MD, MS, FAAP
Assistant Professor
Department of Pediatrics
The George Washington University
Child Abuse Pediatrician
Child and Adolescent Protection Center
Children's National Medical Center
Washington, DC

Gurumurthy Hiremath, MD, MBBS
Pediatric Cardiology Fellow
Department of Pediatrics
University of California, San Francisco
UCSF Benioff Children's Hospital San Francisco
San Francisco, California

Michael P. Hirsh, MD
Professor of Surgery and Pediatrics
University of Massachusetts Medical School
Associate Director
Pediatric Intensive Care Unit
Worchester, Massachusetts

Hiwot Hiruy, MD
Postdoctoral Fellow
Department of Pediatrics
The Johns Hopkins University School of Medicine
Postdoctoral Fellow
Department of Pediatrics
The Johns Hopkins Hospital
Baltimore, Maryland

Adam B. Hittelman, MD, PhD
Assistant Professor
Department of Urology
Yale School of Medicine
Pediatric Urology
Department of Urology
Yale–New Haven Hospital
New Haven, Connecticut

Janice E. Hobbs, MD, MPH
Postdoctoral Fellow
Department of Pediatrics
The Johns Hopkins University School of Medicine
Neonatology Fellow
Pediatrics
The Johns Hopkins Hospital
Baltimore, Maryland

Robert J. Hoffman, MD, MS
Director, Clinical Toxicology
Emergency Medicine
Sidra Medical and Research Center
Doha, Qatar

Paul Hofman, MD
Professor Pediatric Endocrinology
Liggins Institute
University of Auckland
Auckland, New Zealand

David K. Hong, MD
Clinical Assistant Professor, Pediatrics-Infectious Disease
Department of Pediatrics
Stanford University
Palo Alto, California

Stefany B. Honigbaum, MD
Pediatric Gastroenterology and Nutrition Fellow
Department of Pediatrics
The Johns Hopkins University School of Medicine
Division of Pediatric Gastroenterology and Nutrition
Johns Hopkins Children's Center
Baltimore, Maryland

Biljana N. Horn, MD
Clinical Professor
Medical Director Pediatric BMT
Department of Pediatrics
UCSF Benioff Children's Hospital San Francisco
San Francisco, California

Arvind Hoskoppal, MD, MHS
Assistant Professor of Pediatrics and Internal Medicine
University of Utah
Salt Lake City, Utah

Renee Howard, MD
Associate Professor
Department of Dermatology
University of California, San Francisco
San Francisco, California

Jessica Howlett, MD
Neonatologist
Sunflower Neonatology Associates
Overland Park, Kansas

Michael H. Hsieh, MD, PhD
Assistant Professor
Department of Urology
Stanford University School of Medicine
Lucile Packard Children's Hospital Stanford
Stanford, California

Benjamin J. Huang, MD
Clinical Fellow
Department of Pediatrics
Division of Hematology/Oncology
University of California, San Francisco
Clinical Fellow
Department of Pediatrics
Division of Hematology/Oncology
UCSF Benioff Children's Hospital San Francisco
San Francisco, California

James N. Huang, MD
Professor
Department of Pediatrics
University of California, San Francisco
Director of Hematology
Department of Pediatrics
UCSF Benioff Children's Hospital San Francisco
San Francisco, California

Tannie Huang, MD
Assistant Adjunct Professor
Department of Pediatric Hematology Oncology
University of California, San Francisco
San Francisco, California

Jennifer Huffman, MD
Pediatric Neurologist
Department of Pediatrics
Randall Children's Hospital
Portland, Oregon

Erik A. Imel, MD
Assistant Professor of Medicine and Pediatrics
Department of Medicine & Department of Pediatrics
Indiana University School of Medicine
Department of Pediatrics, Section of Pediatric Endocrinology
Riley Hospital for Children at Indiana University Health
Indianapolis, Indiana

Allison M. Jackson, MD, MPH, FAAP
Associate Professor of Pediatrics
School of Medicine and Health Sciences
The George Washington University
Division Chief
The Freddie Mac Foundation Child and Adolescent Protection Center
Children's National Medical Center
Washington, DC

Oksana A. Jackson, MD
Assistant Professor
Division of Plastic Surgery
Perelman School of Medicine at the University of Pennsylvania
Attending Surgeon
Division of Plastic Surgery
The Children's Hospital of Philadelphia
Philadelphia, Pennsylvania

Shonul A. Jain, MD
Assistant Professor
Department of Pediatrics
University of California, San Francisco
Medical Director, Children's Health Center
Department of Pediatrics
San Francisco General Hospital
San Francisco, California

John L. Jefferies, MD, MPH, FACC
Associate Professor, Pediatric Cardiology and Adult Cardiovascular Diseases
The Heart Institute
Director, Advanced Heart Failure Pediatrics
Cincinnati Children's Hospital Medical Center
Cincinnati, Ohio

Karen E. Jerardi, MD, MEd
Assistant Professor
Department of Pediatrics
University of Cincinnati School of Medicine
Attending Physician
Division of Hospital Medicine
Cincinnati Children's Hospital Medical Center
Cincinnati, Ohio

Chandy C. John, MD, MS
Professor
Departments of Pediatrics and Medicine
University of Minnesota
Director, Division of Global Pediatrics
Department of Pediatrics
University of Minnesota Amplatz Children's Hospital
Minneapolis, Minnesota

Ray J. Jurado, DDS
Pediatric Dentist
Ann & Robert H. Lurie Children's Hospital of Chicago
Chicago, Illinois

Dylan Kann, MD
Clinical Fellow
Department of Pediatrics
Stanford University School of Medicine
Clinical Fellow
Department of Pediatric Infectious Diseases
Lucile Packard Children's Hospital Stanford
Stanford, California

Chirag R. Kapadia, MD
Clinical Assistant Professor
Department of Pediatrics
University of Arizona College of Medicine Phoenix
Faculty
Endocrinology
Phoenix Children's Hospital
Phoenix, Arizona

Robert D. Karch, MD, MPH
Nutrition Section
Division of Gastroenterology, Hepatology and Nutrition
Nemours Children's Hospital
Assistant Professor of Pediatrics
University of Central Florida College of Medicine
Orlando, Florida

Erin E. Karski, MD
Clinical Instructor
Department of Pediatrics
UCSF Benioff Children's Hospital San Francisco
San Francisco, California

Himala Kashmiri, DO
Clinical Instructor, Fellow
Department of Pediatrics, Division of Endocrinology
Medical College of Wisconsin/Children's Hospital of Wisconsin
Milwaukee, Wisconsin

Jennifer C. Kelley, MD
Pediatric Endocrinology Fellow
Department of Pediatric Endocrinology
The Children's Hospital of Philadelphia
Philadelphia, Pennsylvania

Judith Kelsen, MD
Assistant Professor of Pediatrics
Perelman School of Medicine at the University of Pennsylvania
Pediatric Gastroenterologist
Division of Gastroenterology, Hepatology and Nutrition
The Children's Hospital of Philadelphia
Philadelphia, Pennsylvania

Shellie M. Kendall, MD, FAAP
Staff Pediatric Cardiologist
Department of the Navy
Naval Medical Center San Diego
San Diego, California

Sadiqa Edmonds Kendi, MD
Assistant Professor
Department of Emergency Medicine
The Warren Alpert Medical School Brown University
Hasbro Children's Hospital
Providence, Rhode Island

Kalpashri Kesavan, MBBS
Neonatologist
Mattel Children's Hospital UCLA
Los Angeles, California

Jessica M. Khouri, MD
Senior Medical Officer
Infant Botulism Treatment and Prevention Program
California Department of Public Health
Richmond, California

Monica Khurana, MD
Fellow
Department of Hematology, Oncology
Children's Hospital and Research Center Oakland
Oakland, California

Harry K. W. Kim, MD, MS
Associate Professor
Orthopaedic Surgery
University of Texas Southwestern Medical Center
Director
Center of Excellence in Hip Disorders
Texas Scottish Rite Hospital for Children
Dallas, Texas

Jason Y. Kim, MD, MSCE
Assistant Professor of Clinical Pediatrics
Department of Pediatrics
The Children's Hospital of Philadelphia
Philadelphia, Pennsylvania

Sivan Kinberg, MD, MS
Postdoctoral Fellow
Department of Pediatric Gastroenterology, Hepatology and Nutrition
Columbia University Medical Center
Morgan Stanley Children's Hospital of New York-Presbyterian
New York, New York

Terry Kind, MD, MPH
Associate Professor of Pediatrics
Assistant Dean for Clinical Education
The George Washington University
Children's National Health System
Washington, DC

Eric S. Kirkendall, MD, MBI
Assistant Professor
Department of Pediatrics
University of Cincinnati
Medical Director, Clinical Decision Support
Pediatrics, Division of Hospital Medicine
Cincinnati Children's Hospital Medical Center
Cincinnati, Ohio

Kirsten Kloepfer, MD, MS
Assistant Professor
Department of Pediatrics
Indiana University School of Medicine
Indianapolis, Indiana

Kelly G. Knupp, MD
Assistant Professor
Pediatrics and Neurology
University of Colorado
Division of Pediatric Neurology
Children's Hospital Colorado
Aurora, Colorado

Chawkaew Kongkanka, MD
Department of Pediatrics
Samitivej Srinakarin Hospital
Suanluang, Bangkok

Aaron E. Kornblith, MD
Associate Physician
Department of Emergency Medicine
University of California, San Francisco
Fellow Physician
Division of Pediatric Emergency Medicine
UCSF Benioff Children's Hospital Oakland
Oakland, California

Renee K. Kottenhahn, MD
Clinical Associate Professor of Pediatrics
Department of Pediatrics
Sidney Kimmel Medical College of Thomas Jefferson University
Philadelphia, Pennsylvania
Associate Director, Wilmington Hospital Pediatric Practice Program
Department of Pediatrics
Christiana Care Health System
Wilmington, Delaware

Courtney L. Kraus, MD
Instructor of Ophthalmology
Ophthalmology
Storm Eye Institute
Medical University of South Carolina
Charleston, South Carolina

Richard M. Kravitz, MD
Associate Professor of Pediatrics
Department of Pediatrics
Duke University Medical Center
Medical Director, Pediatric Sleep Lab
Department of Pediatrics
Duke Children's Hospital
Durham, North Carolina

Matthew P. Kronman, MD, MSCE
Assistant Professor
Department of Pediatrics
Division of Infectious Diseases
University of Washington
Seattle Children's Hospital
Seattle, Washington

Elaine Ku, MD
Clinical Fellow
Department of Pediatrics
University of California, San Francisco
San Francisco, California

Johnny I. Kuttab, DDS
Attending Physician
Division of Dentistry
Ann & Robert H. Lurie Children's Hospital of Chicago
Chicago, Illinois

Michele P. Lambert, MD, MTR
Assistant Professor
Department of Pediatrics
Perelman School of Medicine at the University of Pennsylvania
Attending Physician
Division of Hematology
The Children's Hospital of Philadelphia
Philadelphia, Pennsylvania

Judith Brylinski Larkin, MD
Instructor in Pediatrics
Department of Pediatrics
Sidney Kimmel Medical College of Thomas Jefferson University
Active Staff
Department of Pediatrics
Thomas Jefferson University Hospital
Philadelphia, Pennsylvania

Greggy D. Laroche, MD
Fellow
Division of Pediatric Gastroenterology, Hepatology, and Nutrition
The Johns Hopkins Hospital
Johns Hopkins Children's Center
Baltimore, Maryland

Ilse A. Larson, MD
Assistant Clinical Professor
Department of Pediatrics
University of California, San Francisco
San Francisco, California

Howard M. Lederman, MD, PhD
Professor of Pediatrics, Medicine and Pathology
The Johns Hopkins University School of Medicine
Director, Immune Deficiency Clinic
Pediatrics
The Johns Hopkins Hospital
Baltimore, Maryland

Christine K. Lee, MD
Instructor in Pediatrics
Harvard Medical School
Boston Children's Hospital
Boston, Massachusetts

Lara Wine Lee, MD
Pediatrician
Charleston, South Carolina

Marsha Lee, MD
Assistant Clinical Professor
Department of Pediatrics, Division of Nephrology
University of California, San Francisco
UCSF Benioff Children's Hospital San Francisco
San Francisco, California

Paul R. Lee, MD, PhD
Clinical Fellow
National Institute of Neurological Disorders and Stroke
National Institutes of Health
Bethesda, Maryland

Rebecca K. Lehman, MD
Assistant Professor
Department of Neurosciences
Medical University of South Carolina
Charleston, South Carolina

Kevin V. Lemley, MD, PhD
Professor of Pediatrics (Clinical Scholar)
Department of Pediatrics
Keck School of Medicine of USC
Division of Nephrology
Children's Hospital of Los Angeles
Los Angeles, California

Eric B. Levey, MD
Associate Professor
Pediatrics
The Johns Hopkins University School of Medicine
Medical Director, Feeding Disorders Program
Neurology and Developmental Medicine
Kennedy Krieger Institute
Baltimore, Maryland

Leonard J. Levine, MD
Associate Professor
Department of Pediatrics
Drexel University College of Medicine
Attending Physician
Division of Adolescent Medicine
St. Christopher's Hospital for Children
Philadelphia, Pennsylvania

Cara Lichtenstein, MD, MPH
Assistant Professor of Pediatrics
Department of Pediatrics
The George Washington University School of Medicine & Health Sciences
Attending Pediatrician
General & Community Pediatrics
Children's National Medical Center
Washington, DC

Richard Lirio, MD
Assistant Professor
Department of Pediatrics
University of Massachusetts Medical School
Attending Physician
Department of Pediatric Gastroenterology, Hepatology, and Nutrition
UMass Memorial Children's Medical Center
Worcester, Massachusetts

Robert Listernick, MD
Professor of Pediatrics
Northwestern University Feinberg School of Medicine
Director, Diagnostic and Consultation Services
Ann & Robert H. Lurie Children's Hospital of Chicago
Chicago, Illinois

Steven Liu, MD
Pediatric Gastroenterologist
GI Care for Kids
Atlanta, Georgia

Warren Lo, MD
Clinical Professor
Department of Pediatrics and Neurology
The Ohio State University
Pediatric Neurologist
Division of Neurology
Nationwide Children's Hospital
Columbus, Ohio

Tobias Loddenkemper, MD
Associate Professor of Neurology
Harvard Medical School
Epileptologist/Pediatric Neurologist
Department of Neurology, Division of Epilepsy and Clinical Neurophysiology
Boston Children's Hospital
Boston, Massachusetts

Maya B. Lodish, MD, MHSCR
Clinical Investigator
Staff Clinician
Eunice Kennedy Shriver National Institute of Child Health and Human Development
National Institutes of Health
Bethesda, Maryland

Richard Loffhagen, MD
Emergency Consultant
Program Director
Residency Training
Sheikh Khalifa Medical City
Abu Dhabi, United Arab Emirates

Melissa Long, MD
Assistant Clinical Professor
Department of Pediatrics
The George Washington University School of Medicine & Health Sciences
Attending Physician
General Pediatrics and Community Health
Children's National Medical Center
Washington, DC

Sahira Long, MD, IBCLC
Assistant Professor
The George Washington University
Medical Director, Children's Health Centers of SE
Goldberg Center for Community Pediatric Health
Children's National Health System
Washington, DC

Kathleen M. Loomes, MD
Associate Professor of Pediatrics
Perelman School of Medicine at the University of Pennsylvania
Division of Gastroenterology, Hepatology and Nutrition
The Children's Hospital of Philadelphia
Philadelphia, Pennsylvania

Katherine Lord, MD
Assistant Professor
Department of Pediatrics
Perelman School Medicine at the University of Pennsylvania
Attending Physician
Department of Pediatrics
The Children's Hospital of Philadelphia
Philadelphia, Pennsylvania

Alexander Lowenthal, MD
Pediatric Cardiologist
Department of Pediatric Cardiology
Schneider Children's Medical Center of Israel
Petach Tikvah, Israel

Jeffrey R. Lukish, MD, FACS
Associate Professor
Department of Surgery
The Johns Hopkins University School of Medicine
Baltimore, Maryland

Kimberly M. Lumpkins, MD
Assistant Professor of Pediatric Surgery and Urology
Department of Surgery
University of Maryland School of Medicine
Baltimore, Maryland

Sarah S. Lusman, MD, PhD
Assistant Professor of Pediatrics
Departments of Pediatric Gastroenterology, Hepatology and Nutrition
Columbia University Medical Center
Assistant Attending Pediatrician
Pediatric Gastroenterology, Hepatology and Nutrition
Morgan Stanley Children's Hospital of New York-Presbyterian
New York, New York

Minnelly Luu, MD
Assistant Professor of Dermatology
Department of Dermatology
University of Southern California
Children's Hospital Los Angeles
Los Angeles, California

Ngoc P. Ly, MD, MPH
Associate Professor
Department of Pediatrics
University of California, San Francisco
Pediatric Pulmonologist
Pediatrics
UCSF Benioff Children's Hospital San Francisco
San Francisco, California

Brian M. Inouye, MD
Department of Urology
Division of Pediatric Urology
The Johns Hopkins University School of Medicine
The Johns Hopkins Hospital
Baltimore, Maryland

Sheela N. Magge, MD, MSCE
Assistant Professor of Pediatrics
Department of Pediatrics
The Children's Hospital of Philadelphia
Philadelphia, Pennsylvania

Melanie M. Makhija, MD, MS
Assistant Professor of Pediatrics
Pediatrics
Northwestern University Feinberg School of Medicine
Attending Physician
Allergy & Immunology
Ann & Robert H Lurie Children's Hospital of Chicago
Chicago, Illinois

Michael A. Manfredi, MD
Instructor in Pediatrics
Harvard Medical School
Associate Director, Esophageal Atresia Treatment Program
Associate Director, Gastrointestinal Procedure Unit
Attending Physician
Division of Gastroenterology, Hepatology & Nutrition
Boston Children's Hospital
Boston, Massachusetts

Melissa L. Mannion, MD
Fellow, Pediatric Rheumatology
Department of Pediatrics
University of Alabama at Birmingham
Birmingham, Alabama

Bradley S. Marino, MD, MPP, MSCE
Associate Professor of Pediatrics
Department of Pediatrics
University of Cincinnati College of Medicine
Director, Heart Institute Research Core
Attending Cardiac Intensivist, Cardiac Intensive Care Unit
Divisions of Cardiology and Critical Care Medicine
Cincinnati Children's Hospital Medical Center
Cincinnati, Ohio

Fiona Marion, MB, BCh, BAO
Fellow
Division of Pediatric Pulmonary Medicine
UCSF Benioff Children's Hospital San Francisco
San Francisco, California

Jennifer A. Markowitz, MD
Instructor in Neurology
Department of Pediatric Neurology
Harvard Medical School
Attending in Neurology
Department of Pediatric Neurology
Boston Children's Hospital
Boston, Massachusetts

Andrea Marmor, MD
Associates Professor, Pediatrics
Department of Pediatrics
University of California, San Francisco
San Francisco General Hospital
San Francisco, California

Renée Marquardt, MD
Child & Adolescent Psychiatry
University of California, San Francisco
San Francisco, California

Anne M. Marsh, MD
Associate Hematologist-Oncologist
Department of Pediatric Hematology & Oncology
Children's Hospital & Research Center Oakland
Oakland, California

Holly H. Martin, MD
Assistant Professor
Department of Pediatrics
University of California, San Francisco
San Francisco, California

Zankhana Master, MD
Neonatology Fellow
Department of Pediatrics, Division of Neonatology
The Johns Hopkins University School of Medicine
Baltimore, Maryland

Lucy D. Mastrandrea
Assistant Professor
Department of Pediatrics
University at Buffalo, School of Medicine and Biomedical Sciences
Physician
Division of Pediatric Endocrinology
Women and Children's Hospital of Buffalo
Buffalo, New York

Erin Mathes, MD
Assistant Professor of Dermatology and Pediatrics
Department of Dermatology
University of California, San Francisco
San Francisco, California

Carol A. Mathews, MD
Langley Porter Psychiatric Institute
Associate Professor
Department of Psychiatry
University of California, San Francisco
San Francisco, California

Anubhav Mathur, MD, PhD
Assistant Clinical Professor
Department of Dermatology
University of California, San Francisco
UCSF Benioff Children's Hospital San Francisco
San Francisco, California

Alison T. Matsunaga, MD
Assistant Clinical Instructor
Department of Pediatric Hematology Oncology
University of California, San Francisco
Hematologist/Oncologist
Department of Hematology Oncology
Children's Hospital and Research Institute Oakland
Oakland, California

Oscar H. Mayer, MD
Associate Professor of Clinical Pediatrics
Department of Pediatrics
Perelman School of Medicine at the University of Pennsylvania
Division of Pulmonary Medicine
The Children's Hospital of Philadelphia
Philadelphia, Pennsylvania

Angela Mazur, MD
Department of Pediatric Medicine, Academic Medicine
Texas Children's Hospital
Houston, Texas

Donna M. McDonald-McGinn, MS, CGC
Division of Human Genetics
The Children's Hospital of Philadelphia
Philadelphia, Pennsylvania

Scott McKay, MD
Assistant Professor of Orthopedics
Baylor College of Medicine
Attending Physician
Department of Surgery, Orthopedics
Texas Children's Hospital
Houston, Texas

Tracey A. McLean, MD
Clinical Instructor
Departments of Obstetrics, Gynecology and Reproductive Sciences
University of California, San Francisco
San Francisco, California

Maureen C. McMahon, MD
Assistant Professor
Department of Pediatrics
Jefferson Medical College
Philadelphia, Pennsylvania
General Pediatrician
General Pediatrics
Nemours duPont Pediatrics, Lankenau
Wynnewood, Pennsylvania

Margaret M. McNamara, MD
Associate Clinical Professor of Pediatrics
Department of Pediatrics
Director of Preceptor Outreach, UCSF Office of Medical Education
Co-Director Foundations of Patient Care
University of California, San Francisco
San Francisco, California

Maireade E. McSweeney, MD, MPH
Instructor
Harvard Medical School
Attending Physician
Division of Gastroenterology, Hepatology & Nutrition
Boston Children's Hospital
Boston, Massachusetts

Heather L. Meluskey, CRNP-AC
Pediatric Nurse Practitioner
Section of Pulmonary Hypertension
Division of Cardiology
The Children's Hospital of Philadelphia
Philadelphia, Pennsylvania

Shina Menon, MD
Fellow
Center for Acute Care Nephrology
Cincinnati Children's Hospital Medical Center
Cincinnati, Ohio

Jondavid Menteer, MD
Assistant Professor
Department of Pediatrics
Keck School of Medicine of USC
Director
Heart Failure Program
Division of Cardiology
Children's Hospital Los Angeles
Los Angeles, California

Laura Mercer-Rosa, MD, MSCE
Assistant Professor
Department Pediatrics
University of Pennsylvania
Cardiologist
Pediatrics
The Children's Hospital of Philadelphia
Philadelphia, Pennsylvania

Dan Merenstein, MD
Director, Research Division
Georgetown University Medical Center
Washington, DC

Caitlin Messner, MD
Pediatrician
Cleveland, Ohio

Michele Mietus-Snyder, MD
Associate Professor
Department of Pediatrics
The George Washington University
Co-Director Children's National Obesity Institute
Department of Cardiology
Children's National Health System
Washington, DC

Jane E. Minturn, MD, PhD
Assistant Professor
Department of Pediatrics
Perelman School of Medicine at the University of Pennsylvania
Attending Physician
Division of Oncology
The Children's Hospital of Philadelphia
Philadelphia, Pennsylvania

Hussnain S. Mirza, MD
Assistant Professor
Pediatrics
University of Central Florida College of Medicine
Attending Neonatologist
Neonatal ICU/Pediatrics
Florida Hospital for Children
Orlando, Florida

Nazrat Mirza, MD, ScD
Associate Professor
Department of General Pediatrics and Adolescent Medicine
The George Washington University
Attending Physician
General Pediatrics and Adolescent Medicine
Children's National Medical Center
Washington, DC

Douglas B. Mogul, MD, MPH
Assistant Professor
Department of Pediatrics
The Johns Hopkins University School of Medicine
Baltimore, Maryland

Angela P. Mojica, MD
Pediatric Endocrinologist
Department of Pediatrics
Marshfield Clinic
Marshfield, Wisconsin

Kimberly Molina, MD
Assistant Professor
Department of Pediatrics
University of Utah
Salt Lake City, Utah

Bradley J. Monash, MD
Assistant Clinical Professor
Department of Medicine
Academic Hospitalist
Department of Medicine and Pediatrics
University of California, San Francisco
San Francisco, California

Rachel Moon, MD
Professor
Department of Pediatrics
The George Washington University School of Medicine & Health Sciences
Director of Academic Development
Goldberg Center for Community Pediatric Health
Children's National Medical Center
Washington, DC

Craig Munns, MBBS, PhD, FRACP
Associate Professor
Department of Pediatrics and Child Health
University of Sydney
Senior Staff Specialist
Department of Endocrinology and Diabetes
The Children's Hospital at Westmead
Sydney, Australia

Krupa R. Mysore, MD
Fellow
Division of Pediatric Gastroenterology and Hepatology
Texas Children's Hospital
Baylor College of Medicine
Houston, Texas

John R. Mytinger, MD
Assistant Professor
Department of Pediatrics
Division of Pediatric Neurology
Ohio State University
Nationwide Children's Hospital
Columbus, Ohio

Zeina M. Nabhan, MD
Associate Professor of Clinical Pediatrics
Department of Pediatric Endocrinology
Indiana University School of Medicine
Associate Professor
Department of Pediatrics
Riley Hospital for Children at Indiana University Health
Indianapolis, Indiana

Frances M. Nadel, MD, MSCE
Professor of Clinic Pediatrics
Department of Pediatrics
Perelman School of Medicine at the University of Pennsylvania
Attending Physician
Division of Emergency Medicine
Children's Hospital of Philadelphia
Philadelphia, Pennsylvania

Jessica Rose Nance, MD, MS
Assistant Professor
Department of Neurology
The Johns Hopkins University School of Medicine
The Johns Hopkins Hospital
Baltimore, Maryland

Jessica Nash, MD
Associate Professor
Department of Pediatrics
The George Washington University
General Pediatrics & Community Health
Children's National Medical Center
Washington, DC

Luz Natal-Hernandez, MD
Pediatric Cardiologist
Pediatric Specialties
Roseville Medical Center
Roseville, California

Avindra Nath, MD
Clinical Director
National Institute of Neurological Disorders and Stroke
National Institutes of Health
Bethesda, Maryland

Pradeep P. Nazarey, MD
Assistant Professor of Surgery
University of Massachusetts Medical School
UMass Memorial Medical Center
Boston, Massachusetts

Kelly L. Neale, RN, MS, CPNP
Pediatric Nurse Practitioner
Department of Pediatric Oncology/Hematology
University of California, San Francisco
San Francisco, California

Todd D. Nebesio, MD
Associate Professor of Clinical Pediatrics
Department of Pediatrics
Indiana University School of Medicine
Riley Hospital for Children at Indiana University Health
Indianapolis, Indiana

Bettina Neumann, PT, LLCC
Consultant
Department of Rehab Services
University of San Francisco
Physical Therapist, CEO
Outpatient Physical Therapy in Private Practice
Rising Sun Physical Therapy
San Francisco, California

Jason Newland, MD, MEd
Associate Professor
Department of Pediatrics
University of Missouri-Kansas City School of Medicine
Faculty
Department of Pediatrics
The Children's Mercy Hospital
Kansas City, Missouri

Jessica Newman, DO
Assistant Professor
Division of Infectious Diseases, Department of Internal Medicine
University of Kansas Medical Center
Kansas City, Kansas

Ross Newman, DO
Associate Program Director, Pediatrics
University of Missouri-Kansas City School of Medicine
Kansas City, Missouri

Peter D. Ngo, MD
Attending Gastroenterologist
Division of Gastroenterology, Hepatology & Nutrition
Boston Children's Hospital
Boston, Massachusetts

Stephanie Nguyen, MD, MAS
Assistant Professor
Department of Pediatrics
Division of Nephrology
University of California, Davis
Assistant Professor
Department of Pediatrics
UC Davis Medical Center
Sacramento, California

Julie M. Nogee, MD
Associate Physician
Department of Pediatrics
University of California, San Francisco
San Francisco, California

Lawrence M. Nogee, MD
Professor
Department of Pediatrics, Eudowood Neonatal Respiratory Division
The Johns Hopkins University School of Medicine
Attending Neonatologist
Department of Pediatrics
Johns Hopkins Children's Center
Baltimore, Maryland

Frances J. Northington, MD
Professor of Neonatal-Perinatal Medicine
The Johns Hopkins University School of Medicine
Department of Pediatrics
Johns Hopkins Children's Center
Baltimore, Maryland

D. David O'Banion, MD
Fellow in Developmental-Behavioral Pediatrics
Department of Pediatrics
University of Oklahoma Health Sciences Center
Oklahoma City, Oklahoma

Christopher B. Oakley, MD
Assistant Professor-Clinical Educator
Neurology
The Johns Hopkins University School of Medicine
The Johns Hopkins Hospital
Baltimore, Maryland

Julie O'Brien, MD, MS
Assistant Clinical Professor
Department of Pediatrics
University of California, San Francisco
San Francisco, California

Heather Olson, MD
Fellow in Epilepsy/Neurogenetics
Department of Neurology, Division of Epilepsy and Clinical Neurophysiology
Boston Children's Hospital
Boston, Massachusetts

Kent Olson, MD
Clinical Professor, Medicine & Pharmacy
University of California, San Francisco
Medical Director
San Francisco Division
California Poison Control System
Department of Clinical Pharmacy
University of California, San Francisco
San Francisco, California

Oluwakemi B. Badaki-Makun, MD, CM
Assistant Professor
Department of Pediatrics
The Johns Hopkins University School of Medicine
Attending Physician
Division of Pediatric Emergency Medicine
Johns Hopkins Children's Center
Baltimore, Maryland

Bruce A. Ong, MD, MPH
Pediatric Pulmonologist
Department of Pediatrics
Tripler Army Medical Center
Honolulu, Hawaii

Anna E. Ordóñez, MD
Assistant Professor
Department of Psychiatry
University of California, San Francisco
Medical Director
Infant Child and Adolescent Psychiatry
Department of Psychiatry
San Francisco General Hospital
San Francisco, California

Kevin C. Osterhoudt, MD, MS
Professor
Department of Pediatrics
Perelman School of Medicine at the University of Pennsylvania
Medical Director
The Poison Control Center
The Children's Hospital of Philadelphia
Philadelphia, Pennsylvania

Mary Ottolini, MPH
Professor of Pediatrics
Pediatrics
The George Washington University School of Medicine & Health Sciences
Vice-Chair of Education
Designated Institutional Official
Children's National Medical Center
Washington, DC

Vikash S. Oza, MD
Fellow
Department of Pediatric Dermatology
University of California, San Francisco
San Francisco, California

Erica S. Pan, MD, MPH, FAAP
Associate Clinical Professor
Department of Pediatrics, Division of Infectious Diseases
University of California, San Francisco
San Francisco, California
Deputy Health Officer
Director
Division of Communicable Disease Control & Prevention
Alameda County Public Health Department
Oakland, California

Rita Panoscha, MD
Pediatrician
Oregon Health & Sciences University
Portland, Oregon

Helen Pappa, MD
Assistant Professor of Pediatrics
Cardinal Glennon Children's Medical Center
St. Louis, Missouri

Carolyn A. Paris, MD
Associate Professor
Department of Emergency Medicine
Seattle Children's Hospital
Seattle, Washington

Hee-Jung Park, MD, MPH
Pediatric Ophthalmologist
Virginia Mason Hospital and Seattle Medical Center
Seattle, Washington

Kristen L. Park, MD
Assistant Professor
Departments of Pediatrics and Neurology
University of Colorado
Division of Pediatric Neurology
Children's Hospital Colorado
Aurora, Colorado

Michelle W. Parker, MD
Assistant Professor
University of Cincinnati Department of Pediatrics
Attending Physician
Division of Hospital Medicine
Cincinnati, Ohio

Kiran Patel, MD, MS
Allergy & Immunology Fellow
Department of Pediatrics
University of California, San Francisco
San Francisco Medical Center
San Francisco, California

Irina Pateva, MD
Fellow
Department of Pediatrics
Case Western Reserve University
Fellow
Division of Pediatrics Hematology/Oncology
Rainbow Babies & Children's Hospital
Cleveland, Ohio

Barry Pelz, MD
Allergy-Immunology Fellow
Northwestern University Feinberg School of Medicine
Chicago, Illinois

Elena Elizabeth Perez, MD, PhD
Associate Professor
Department of Pediatrics
University of Miami
Associate Professor
Department of Pediatrics
University of Miami, Jackson Memorial Hospital
Miami, Florida

Farzana Perwad, MD
Assistant Adjunct Professor of Pediatrics
University of California, San Francisco
Department of Nephrology
UCSF Benioff Children's Hospital San Francisco
San Francisco, California

Christopher Petit, MD
Assistant Professor of Pediatrics
Department of Pediatrics
Emory University School of Medicine
Attending Physician
Sibley Heart Center
Children's Healthcare of Atlanta
Atlanta, Georgia

Shabnam Peyvandi, MD
Assistant Professor of Clinical Pediatrics
Department of Pediatrics, Division of Cariology
University of California, San Francisco
UCSF Benioff Children's Hospital San Francisco
San Francisco, California

Joseph A. Picoraro, MD
Postdoctoral Fellow
Department of Pediatric Gastroenterology, Hepatology and Nutrition
Columbia University Medical Center
Morgan Stanley Children's Hospital of New York-Presbyterian
New York, New York

Nelangi Pinto, MD
Associate Professor
Division of Pediatric Cariology
Department of Pediatrics
University of Utah
Salt Lake City, Utah

Pisit Pitukcheewanont, MD
Assistant Professor of Clinical Pediatrics
Department of Pediatrics
Keck School of Medicine of USC
Los Angeles, California

Jonathan R. Pletcher, MD
Associate Professor
Department of Pediatrics
University of Pittsburgh School of Medicine
Clinical Director
Department of Adolescent Medicine
Children's Hospital of Pittsburgh of UPMC
Pittsburgh, Pennsylvania

Annapurna Poduri, MD, MPH
Assistant Professor
Department of Neurology
Harvard Medical School
Attending in Epilepsy
Director, Epilepsy Genetics
Department of Neurology
Boston Children's Hospital
Boston, Massachusetts

Charles A. Pohl, MD
Professor
Department of Pediatrics
Sidney Kimmel Medical Center
Department of Pediatrics
Thomas Jefferson University/Nemours
Philadelphia, Pennsylvania

Anthony A. Portale, MD
Professor in Residence, Pediatrics
Chief, Division of Pediatric Nephrology
Medical Director, Pediatric Renal Transplant Program
Program Director, Pediatric Nephrology Fellowship Training Program
Department of Pediatrics
University of California, San Francisco
San Francisco, California

Evelyn Porter, MD, MS
Assistant Professor
Departments of Emergency Medicine and Pediatrics
University of California, San Francisco
San Francisco, California

Jill C. Posner, MD, MSCE
Associate Professor of Clinical Practice
Department of Pediatrics, Division of Pediatric Emergency Medicine
Perelman School of Medicine at the University of Pennsylvania
Attending Physician
Department of Pediatrics, Division of Pediatric Emergency Medicine
The Children's Hospital of Philadelphia
Philadelphia, Pennsylvania

Madhura Pradhan, MD, DCH
Associate Professor of Clinical Pediatrics
Department of Pediatrics
Perelman School of Medicine at the University of Pennsylvania
The Children's Hospital of Philadelphia
Philadelphia, Pennsylvania

Victoria E. Price
Division of Hematology/Oncology
Department of Pediatrics
IWK Health Centre
Halifax, Nova Scotia, Canada

Benjamin T. Prince, MD
Fellow
Department of Pediatrics
Northwestern University Feinberg School of Medicine
Division of Allergy and Immunology
Ann & Robert H. Lurie Children's Hospital of Chicago
Chicago, Illinois

Manisha Punwani, MD
Director, Child and Adolescent Psychiatry Training
Associate Professor
Department of Psychiatry
University of California, San Francisco
San Francisco, California

Latika Puri, MD
Fellow
Pediatric Hematology/ Oncology
Children's Hospital and Research Center Oakland
Oakland, California

Katherine B. Püttgen, MD
Assistant Professor
Department of Dermatology, Division of Pediatric Dermatology
The Johns Hopkins University School of Medicine
Baltimore, Maryland

Nashmia Qamar, DO
Fellow
Department of Pediatrics, Division of Allergy & Immunology
Northwestern University Feinberg School of Medicine
Ann & Robert H. Lurie Children's Hospital of Chicago
Chicago, Illinois

Keith Quirolo, MD
Clinical Instructor
Department of Pediatrics
UCSF Benioff Children's Hospital San Francisco
San Francisco, California
Director, Apheresis
Hematology
UCSF Benioff Children's Hospital Oakland
Oakland, California

Christopher P. Raab, MD
Assistant Professor
Department of Pediatrics
Sidney Kimmel Medical College of Thomas Jefferson University
Philadelphia, Pennsylvania
Staff Pediatrician
Department of Pediatrics
Nemours Alfred I. duPont Hospital for Children
Wilmington, Delaware

Kacy A. Ramirez, MD
Assistant Professor
Department of Pediatrics
Wake Forest School of Medicine
Assistant Professor
Department of Pediatrics
Brenner Children's Hospital/Wake Forest Baptist Medical Center
Winston-Salem, North Carolina

Daniel Ranch, MD
Assistant Professor
Department of Pediatrics
University of Texas Health Science Center, San Antonio
San Antonio, Texas

Sergio E. Recuenco
Epidemiologist
NCEZID/HCPP/PRB/Rabies Program
U.S. Centers for Disease Control and Prevention
Atlanta, Georgia

Richard J. Redett, MD
Associate Professor
Department of Plastic and Reconstructive Surgery
The Johns Hopkins University School of Medicine
Baltimore, Maryland

Rebecca Reindel, MD
Pediatrician
Children's Memorial Hospital
Chicago, Illinois

Michael X. Repka, MD, MBA
Professor
Wilmer Eye Institute
The Johns Hopkins University School of Medicine
Active Staff
Wilmer Eye Institute
Baltimore, Maryland

David C. Rettew, MD
Associate Professor
Department of Psychiatry
Department of Pediatrics
The University of Vermont School of Medicine
Burlington, Vermont

Leah G. Reznick, MD
Assistant Professor
Department of Ophthalmology
Casey Eye Institute
Oregon Health & Sciences University
Portland, Oregon

Hope Rhodes, MD
General Pediatrician
Assistant Professor
Department of Pediatrics
The George Washington University School of Medicine & Health Sciences
General Pediatrician
General and Community Pediatrics
Children's National Medical Center
Washington, DC

Alisson Richards, MD
Child Psychiatrist
Department of Psychiatry
Department of Pediatrics
The University of Vermont Medical Center
Burlington, Vermont

Richard C. Rink, MD
Robert A. Garrett Professor of Pediatric Urologic Research
Professor
Indiana University School of Medicine
Department of Urology
Indianapolis, Indiana

Elizabeth Robbins, MD
Clinical Professor
Department of Pediatrics
University of California, San Francisco
Clinical Professor
Department of Pediatrics
UCSF Benioff Children's Hospital San Francisco
San Francisco, California

Laura Robertson, MD
Associate Clinical Professor
Department of Pediatrics
University of California, San Francisco
UCSF Benioff Children's Hospital San Francisco
San Francisco, California

Rachel G. Robison, MD
Assistant Professor
Department of Pediatrics
Northwestern University Feinberg School of Medicine
Attending Physician
Pediatrics, Division of Allergy & Immunology
Ann & Robert H. Lurie Children's Hospital of Chicago
Chicago, Illinois

Rohini Coorg, MD
Fellow, Pediatric Epilepsy
Department of Neurology
Washington University School of Medicine
St. Louis Children's Hospital
St. Louis, Missouri

Kristina W. Rosbe, MD, FAAP, FACS
Professor
Departments of Otolaryngology and Pediatrics
University of California, San Francisco
Chief of Pediatric Otolaryngology
UCSF Benioff Children's Hospital San Francisco
San Francisco, California

Rebecca Ruebner, MD, MSCE
Assistant Professor
Department of Pediatrics
University of Pennsylvania
Assistant Professor
Department of Pediatrics, Division of Nephrology
The Children's Hospital of Philadelphia
Philadelphia, Pennsylvania

Matthew J. Ryan, MD
Assistant Professor of Pediatrics
Department of Pediatrics
Perelman School of Medicine at the University of Pennsylvania
Attending Physician
Pediatrics
The Children's Hospital of Philadelphia
Philadelphia, Pennsylvania

Thomas G. Saba, MD
Fellow
Department of Pediatrics, Pulmonary Division
University of Michigan
C.S. Mott Children's Hospital
Ann Arbor, Michigan

Camille Sabella, MD
Associate Professor of Pediatrics
Vice-Chair for Education, Pediatric Institute
Director, Center for Pediatric Infectious Diseases
Cleveland Clinic Children's
Cleveland, Ohio

Sabina Sabharwal, MD, MPH
Instructor
Department of Pediatrics
Harvard Medical School
Attending Staff Physician
Department of Pediatric Gastroenterology and Nutrition
Boston Children's Hospital
Boston, Massachusetts

Amit J. Sabnis, MD
Instructor
Department of Hematology-Oncology
UCSF Benioff Children's Hospital San Francisco
San Francisco, California

Denise A. Salerno, MD
Professor of Clinical Pediatrics
Department of Pediatrics
Temple University School of Medicine
Philadelphia, Pennsylvania

Kara N. Saperston, MD
Pediatric Urology Clinical Fellow
Department of Urology
University of California, San Francisco
San Francisco, California

Julia Shaklee Sammons, MD, MSCE
Assistant Professor
Department of Pediatrics, Division of Infectious Diseases
Perelman School of Medicine at the University of Pennsylvania
Medical Director and Hospital Epidemiologist
Department of Infection Prevention and Control
The Children's Hospital of Philadelphia
Philadelphia, Pennsylvania

Pablo J. Sanchez, MD
Professor of Pediatrics
The Ohio State University College of Medicine
Director of Clinical and Translational Research in Neonatology
Nationwide Children's Hospital
Columbus, Ohio

Melissa T. Sanford, MD
Resident Physician
Department of Urology
University of California, San Francisco
San Francisco, California

Emily M. Schaaf, MD
Pediatric Infectious Disease Fellow
Department of Pediatric Infectious Disease
University of Minnesota Amplatz Children's Hospital
Minneapolis, Minnesota

Adrienne M. Scheich, MD
Health Systems Clinician
Department of Pediatrics
Northwestern University Feinberg School of Medicine
Attending Physician
Department of Pediatric Gastroenterology
Ann & Robert H. Lurie Children's Hospital of Chicago
Chicago, Illinois

Rebecca Schein, MD
Assistant Professor
Department of Pediatrics
Case Western Reserve University
Physician-Infectious Disease
Department of Pediatrics
MetroHealth Medical Center
Cleveland, Ohio

Angela Scheuerle, MD
Professor
Department of Pediatrics, Division of Genetics and Metabolism
University of Texas Southwestern Medical Center
Dallas, Texas

Jocelyn H. Schiller, MD
Associate Professor
Department of Pediatrics and Communicable Diseases
University of Michigan Medical School
Pediatric Hospitalist
Department of Pediatrics and Communicable diseases
University of Michigan Health System
Ann Arbor, Michigan

Amanda C. Schondelmeyer, MD
Division of Hospital Medicine
Cincinnati Children's Hospital Medical Center
Cincinnati, Ohio

Alan R. Schroeder, MD
Clinical Assistant Professor
Department of Pediatrics
Stanford University
Palo Alto, California
Director, PICU and Chief of Pediatric Inpatient Services
Department of Pediatrics
Santa Clara Valley Medical Center
San Jose, California

Gordon E. Schutze, MD, FAAP
Professor of Pediatrics
Executive Vice-Chairman
Department of Pediatrics
Baylor College of Medicine
Martin I. Lorin, MD, Chair in Medical Education
Texas Children's Hospital
Houston, Texas

Kathleen B. Schwarz, MD
Professor
Department of Pediatric Gastroenterology
The Johns Hopkins University
Baltimore, Maryland

Steven M. Selbst, MD
Professor
Department of Pediatrics
Sidney Kimmel Medical Center
Philadelphia, Pennsylvania
Vice-Chair for Education, Residency Program Director
Department of Pediatrics
Nemours Alfred I. duPont Hospital for Children
Wilmington, Delaware

Samir S. Shah, MS, MSCE
Professor
Department of Pediatrics
University of Cincinnati College of Medicine
Director and Cincinnati Children's Research Foundation Endowed Chair
Division of Hospital Medicine
Cincinnati Children's Hospital Medical Center
Cincinnati, Ohio

Sonal Shah, MD
Fellow
Department of Pediatric Dermatology
University of California at San Francisco
San Francisco, California

Pirouz Shamszad, MD
Assistant Professor of Pediatrics
Department of Pediatrics
University of Cincinnati College of Medicine
Assistant Professor of Pediatrics
The Heart Institute, Division of Cardiology
Cincinnati Children's Hospital Medical Center
Cincinnati, Ohio

Andi L. Shane, MD, MPH, MSc
Associate Professor
Department of Pediatrics
Division of Infectious Diseases
Emory University School of Medicine
Marcus Professor, Hospital Epidemiology and Infection Control
Children's Healthcare of Atlanta
Atlanta, Georgia

Hemant P. Sharma, MD
Associate Division Chief, Allergy and Immunology
Children's National Medical Center
Washington, DC

Helen M. Sharp, PhD, CCC-SLP
Associate Professor
Department of Speech Pathology and Audiology
Western Michigan University
Kalamazoo, Michigan

Erin E. Shaughnessy, MD
Assistant Professor
Department of Pediatrics
University of Cincinnati
Medical Director, Hospital Medicine Surgical Service
Division of Hospital Medicine
Cincinnati Children's Hospital Medical Center
Cincinnati, Ohio

David D. Sherry, MD
Professor
Department of Pediatrics
Perelman School of Medicine at The University of Pennsylvania
Chief, Rheumatology Section
Department of Pediatrics
The Children's Hospital of Philadelphia
Philadelphia, Pennsylvania

T. Matthew Shields, MD
Assistant Professor of Pediatrics
Division of Pediatric Gastroenterology
UMass Memorial Medical Center
Worcester, Massachusetts

Rhonique Shields-Harris, MD, MHA
Assistant Professor
Department of General Pediatrics
The George Washington University
Executive Director, Public Sector
Child Health Advocacy Institute
Children's National Medical Center
Washington, DC

Kristin A. Shimano, MD
Assistant Professor of Clinical Pediatrics
Department of Pediatrics
University of California, San Francisco
San Francisco, California

Timothy R. Shope, MD, MPH
Associate Professor
Department of Pediatrics
University of Pittsburgh School of Medicine
General Academic Pediatrics
Department of Pediatrics
Children's Hospital of Pittsburgh of UPMC
Pittsburgh, Pennsylvania

Stanford Shulman
Virginia Rogers Professor of Pediatric Infectious Diseases
Northwestern University Feinberg School of Medicine
Chief
Division of Infectious diseases (Pediatric)
Ann & Robert H. Lurie Children's Hospital of Chicago
Chicago, Illinois

Stephan Siebel, MD, PhD
Clinical Fellow
Eunice Kennedy Shriver National Institute of Child Health and Human Development
Bethesda, Maryland

Brooke I. Siegel, MD
Senior Clinical Associate
Chief Resident
Department of Pediatrics
New York-Presbyterian/Weill Cornell
New York, New York

Melissa A. Simon, MD
Fellow
Department of Pediatric Ophthalmology
Oregon Health & Science University Casey Eye Institute
Portland, Oregon

Anne Marie Singh, MD
Assistant Professor
Departments of Pediatrics-Allergy and Immunology, Medicine-Allergy-Immunology
Northwestern University Feinberg School of Medicine
Ann & Robert H. Lurie Children's Hospital of Chicago
Chicago, Illinois

William B. Slayton, MD
Division Chief
Department of Pediatric Hematology
University of Florida
Gainesville, Florida

Sabrina E. Smith, MD, PhD
Adjunct Assistant Professor
Department of Neurology
Perelman School of Medicine at the University of Pennsylvania
Philadelphia, Pennsylvania
Attending Physician
Department of Pediatrics, Division of Neurology
Kaiser Permanente Oakland Medical Center
Oakland, California

Michael J. Smith, MD, MSCE
Associate Professor
Department of Pediatrics
University of Louisville
Attending Physician
Kosair Children's Hospital
Louisville, Kentucky

Lauren G. Solan, MD
Hospital Medicine Attending
Division of Hospital Medicine
Cincinnati Children's Hospital Medical Center
Cincinnati, Ohio

Patrick B. Solari, MD
Clinical Assistant Professor
Department of Pediatrics
University of Washington
Attending Physician
Emergency Medicine
Seattle Children's Hospital
Seattle, Washington

Danielle Soranno, MD
Assistant Professor
Children's Hospital Colorado
Aurora, Colorado

Angela M. Statile, MD, MEd
Assistant Professor of Pediatrics
University of Cincinnati College of Medicine
University of Cincinnati
Cincinnati Children's Hospital Medical Center
Cincinnati, Ohio

Andrew A. Stec, MD
Assistant Professor
Department of Urology
Medical University of South Carolina
Director of Pediatric Urology
Department of Urology
Medical University of South Carolina
Charleston, South Carolina

Andrew P. Steenhoff, MBBCh, DCH (UK), FCPaed (SA), FAAP
Assistant Professor
Department of Pediatrics
Perelman School of Medicine at the University of Pennsylvania
Attending Physician
Division of Infectious Diseases
The Children's Hospital of Philadelphia
Philadelphia, Pennsylvania

Robert D. Steiner, MD
Executive Director
Marshfield Clinic Research Foundation
Marshfield, Wisconsin
Visiting Professor
Department of Pediatrics
University of Wisconsin School of Medicine and Public Health
Madison, Wisconsin

Julie W. Stern, MD
Clinical Associate Professor
Pediatrics, Division of Hematology & Oncology
Perelman School of Medicine at the University of Pennsylvania
Philadelphia, Pennsylvania

C. Matt Stewart, MD, PhD
Assistant Professor
Otolaryngology, Head and Neck Surgery
The Johns Hopkins University School of Medicine
Baltimore, Maryland

F. Dylan Stewart, MD
Assistant Professor
Director of Pediatric Trauma
Division of Pediatric Surgery
Director of Pediatric Burn Unit
Johns Hopkins Children's Center
The Johns Hopkins Hospital
Baltimore, Maryland

Paul Stewart, MD
Ophthalmologist
UCSF Medical Center
San Francisco, California

Rosalyn W. Stewart, MD, MS, MBA
Associate Professor
Internal Medicine and Pediatrics
The Johns Hopkins University School of Medicine
Baltimore, Maryland

John Stirling, MD
Director, Center for Child Protection
Santa Clara Valley Medical Center
San Jose, California

Constantine A. Stratakis, MD, DSc
Senior Investigator
Eunice Kennedy Shriver National Institute of Child Health and Human Development
National Institutes of Health
Bethesda, Maryland

Paul K. Sue, MD, CM
Assistant Professor of Pediatrics
Division of Pediatric Infectious Disease
University of Texas Southwestern Medical Center
Dallas, Texas

Kathleen E. Sullivan, MD, PhD
Professor of Pediatrics
Perelman School of Medicine at the University of Pennsylvania
Division of Allergy and Immunology
The Children's Hospital of Philadelphia
Philadelphia, Pennsylvania

John I. Takayama, MD, MPH
Professor of Clinical Pediatrics
Site Director, Pediatric Resident Continuity Clinic
Associate Director, General Pediatrics Fellowship Program
Department of Pediatrics
University of California, San Francisco
San Francisco, California

Jennifer A. Talarico, MS
Clinical Research Coordinator
Division of Orthopaedic Surgery
The Children's Hospital of Philadelphia
Philadelphia, Pennsylvania

Ronn E. Tanel, MD
Professor of Clinical Pediatrics
Director, Pediatric Arrhythmia Service
UCSF Benioff Children's Hospital San Francisco
Department of Pediatrics
University of California, San Francisco
San Francisco, California

Carl Tapia, MD
Assistant Professor
Division of Pediatrics
Baylor College of Medicine
Houston, Texas

Anupama R. Tate, DMD, MHP
Associate Professor
Department of Pediatrics
The George Washington University School of Medicine & Health Sciences
Director, Advocacy & Research
Division of Oral Care
Children's National Medical Center
Washington, DC

Danna Tauber, MD, MPH
Assistant Professor
Department of Pediatrics
Drexel University College of Medicine
Attending Physician
Section of Pulmonology
St. Christopher's Hospital for Children
Philadelphia, Pennsylvania

Jesse A. Taylor, MD
Assistant Professor
Department of Surgery
Perelman School of Medicine at the University of Pennsylvania
Plastic Surgeon
Department of Plastic Surgery
The Children's Hospital of Philadelphia
Philadelphia, Pennsylvania

David T. Teachey, MD
Assistant Professor
Department of Pediatrics
Perelman School of Medicine at the University of Pennsylvania
Attending Physician
Department of Pediatrics
The Children's Hospital of Philadelphia
Philadelphia, Pennsylvania

Peter J. Tebben, MD
Assistant Professor
Departments of Internal Medicine and Pediatrics
Mayo Clinic
Rochester, Minnesota

Jennifer A. F. Tender, MD, IBCLC
Assistant Professor
Department of General Pediatrics
The George Washington University School of Medicine & Health Services
Attending Physician
General Pediatrics
The Children's National Health System
Washington, DC

M. Elizabeth Tessier, MD
Pediatric GI, Hepatology & Nutrition Fellow
Division of Pediatrics
Baylor College of Medicine
Texas Children's Hospital
Houston, Texas

Sheila Thampi, MD
Clinical Fellow-Hematology & Oncology
Department of Pediatrics
University of California, San Francisco
San Francisco, California

Liu Lin Thio, MD, PhD
Associate Professor of Neurology, Pediatrics and Anatomy & Neurobiology
Director, Pediatric Epilepsy Center
Washington University School of Medicine
St. Louis Children's Hospital
St. Louis, Missouri

Joanna E. Thomson, MD
Attending Physician
Division of Hospital Medicine
Cincinnati Children's Hospital Medical Center
Cincinnati, Ohio

Shannon Thyne, MD
Professor of Clinical Pediatrics
Department of Pediatrics
University of California, San Francisco
Chief of Medical Staff
San Francisco General Hospital
San Francisco, California

John E. Tis, MD
Assistant Professor
Department of Orthopedic Surgery
The Johns Hopkins Hospital
Baltimore, Maryland

Laura L. Tosi, MD
Orthopaedic Surgeon
Children's National Health System
Washington, DC

James R. Treat, MD
Pediatric Dermatologist
Division of Dermatology
The Children's Hospital of Philadelphia
Philadelphia, Pennsylvania

Maria E. Trent, MD, MPH
Associate Professor
Department of Pediatrics
The Johns Hopkins University School of Medicine
Faculty
Pediatrics
Johns Hopkins Children's Center
Baltimore, Maryland

Nicholas Tsarouhas, MD
Professor of Clinical Pediatrics
Department of Pediatrics
Perelman School of Medicine at the University of Pennsylvania
Medical Director, Emergency Transport Team
Associate Medical Director, Emergency Department
Division of Emergency Medicine
The Children's Hospital of Philadelphia
Philadelphia, Pennsylvania

Shamir Tuchman, MD, MPH
Assistant Professor of Pediatrics
Division of Pediatric Nephrology
The George Washington University School of Medicine & Health Sciences
Attending Nephrologist
Division of Pediatric Nephrology
Children's National Medical Center
Washington, DC

Krishna K. Upadhya, MD, MPH
Assistant Professor
Department of Pediatrics
The Johns Hopkins University School of Medicine
Baltimore, Maryland

Susma Vaidya, MD, MPH
Assistant Professor of Pediatrics
Department of General Pediatrics
The George Washington University School of Medicine & Health Sciences
Children's National Medical Center
Washington, DC

Kristin L. Van Buren, MD
Assistant Professor of Pediatrics
Division of Pediatrics, Gastroenterology, Hepatology & Nutrition
Baylor College of Medicine
Assistant Professor of Pediatrics
Division of Pediatrics, Gastroenterology, Hepatology & Nutrition
Texas Children's Hospital
Houston, Texas

Gigi Veereman, MD, PhD
Professor
Department of Pediatrics
Free University of Brussels (VUB)
Consultant
Department of Pediatric Gastroenterology and Nutrition
University Hospital Brussels
Belgium

Hilary Vernon, MD, PhD
Assistant Professor
McKusick-Nathans Institute of Genetic Medicine and Department of Medicine
Division of Pediatrics
McKusick-Nathans Institute of Genetic Medicine
The Johns Hopkins University School of Medicine
Baltimore, Maryland

Elliott Vichinsky, MD
Medical Director, CHO Hematology/Oncology Programs
UCSF Benioff Children's Hospital Oakland
Oakland, California

Kieuhoa T. Vo, MD
Clinical Fellow
Department of Pediatrics
University of California, San Francisco
UCSF Benioff Children's Hospital San Francisco
San Francisco, California

Patricia Vuguin, MD, MSc
Associate Professor of Pediatrics
Department of Pediatrics
School of Medicine at Hofstra University
Hempstead, New York
Pediatric Endocrinology Fellowship Director
Pediatric Endocrinology
Cohen Children's Medical Center
New Hyde Park, New York

R. Paul Wadwa, MD
Associate Professor of Pediatrics
Barbara Davis Center for Childhood Diabetes
University of Colorado School of Medicine
Aurora, Colorado

Lars M. Wagner, MD
Professor of Pediatrics
Division of Pediatric Hematology/Oncology
University of Kentucky
Chief, Pediatric Hematology/Oncology
Department of Pediatrics
Kentucky Children's Hospital
Lexington, Kentucky

Waqar Waheed, MD
Assistant Professor
Department of Neurological Sciences
University of Vermont
Burlington, Vermont

Justin T. Wahlstrom, MD
Assistant Professor
Department of Pediatrics
University of California, San Francisco
UCSF Children's Hospital
San Francisco, California

Elizabeth M. Wallis, MD
Assistant Professor
Department of Pediatrics
Medical University of South Carolina
Charleston, South Carolina

Daniel Walmsley, DO
Clinical Assistant Professor of Pediatrics
Pediatric Clerkship Site Director
Jefferson Medical College/ Nemours
Pediatrician
Nemours Pediatrics, Thomas Jefferson University Hospital
Philadelphia, Pennsylvania

Ming-Hsien Wang, MD
Assistant Professor
Department of Urology
The Johns Hopkins University School of Medicine
Assistant Professor
Department of Pediatric Urology
The Johns Hopkins Hospital
Baltimore, Maryland

Dascha C. Weir, MD
Instructor in Pediatrics
Harvard Medical School
Associate Director
The Celiac Disease Program
Attending Physician
Division of Gastroenterology, Hepatology & Nutrition
Boston Children's Hospital
Boston, Massachusetts

Peter Weiser, MD
Assistant Professor
Division of Rheumatology, Department of Pediatrics
The University of Alabama at Birmingham
Children's of Alabama
Birmingham, Alabama

Marceé J. White, MD
Assistant Professor
Department of General Pediatrics
The George Washington University
Medical Director
Mobile Health Programs
Children's National Medical Center
Washington, DC

Benjamin M. Whittam, MD, MS
Assistant Professor
Department of Urology-Pediatric Urology
Indiana University School of Medicine
Riley Hospital for Children at Indiana University Health
Indianapolis, Indiana

M. Edward Wilson, MD
N. Edgar Miles Professor of Ophthalmology and Pediatrics
Department of Ophthalmology
Storm Eye Institute
Medical University of South Carolina
Charleston, South Carolina

Erica Winnicki, MD
Assistant Professor
Department of Pediatrics
Section of Nephrology
University of California, Davis
Department of Pediatrics,
Section of Nephrology
UC Davis Medical Center
Sacramento, California

Sarah E. Winters, MD
Clinical Assistant Professor of Pediatrics
Department of Pediatrics
Perelman School of Medicine at the University of Pennsylvania
Philadelphia, Pennsylvania

Elaine C. Wirrell, MD
Director of Pediatric Epilepsy
Consultant
Child and Adolescent Neurology and Epilepsy
Mayo Clinic
Rochester, Minnesota

Thomas E. Wiswell, MD
Professor
Department of Pediatrics
University of Central Florida
Attending Neonatologist
Department of Pediatrics
Florida Hospital for Children
Orlando, Florida

Selma Feldman Witchel, MD
Associate Professor of Pediatrics
Department of Pediatrics
University of Pittsburgh
Fellowship Director
Pediatrics
Children's Hospital of Pittsburgh of UPMC
Pittsburgh, Pennsylvania

Char Witmer, MD, MSCE
Assistant Professor
Department of Pediatrics
Perelman School of Medicine at the University of Pennsylvania
Philadelphia, Pennsylvania

Margaret Wolff, MD
Assistant Professor
Departments of Emergency Medicine and Pediatrics
University of Michigan
Faculty
Department of Emergency Medicine
University of Michigan, C.S. Mott Children's Hospital
Ann Arbor, Michigan

Mark Wolraich, MD
Shaun Walters Professor of Pediatrics
Chief of Section of Developmental and Behavioral Pediatrics
Department of Pediatrics
University of Oklahoma Health Sciences Center
Oklahoma City, Oklahoma

Lily C. Wong-Kisiel, MD
Assistant Professor
Department of Neurology
Mayo Clinic
Rochester, Minnesota

George Anthony Woodward, MD, MBA
Professor
Department of Pediatrics
University of Washington School of Medicine
Chief, Medical Director
Pediatric Emergency Medicine
Seattle Children's Hospital
Seattle, Washington

Hsi-Yang Wu, MD
Associate Professor
Department of Urology
Stanford University
Stanford, California
Fellowship Program Director
Pediatric Urology
Lucile Packard Children's Hospital Stanford
Palo Alto, California

Menno Verhave, MD
Lecturer
Harvard Medical School
Attending Physician
Clinical Director, Gastroenterology
Division of Gastroenterology, Hepatology & Nutrition
Boston Children's Hospital
Boston, Massachusetts

Desalegn Yacob, MD
Assistant Professor
Department of Pediatrics
The Ohio State University
Attending Pediatric Gastroenterologist
Pediatric Gastroenterology
Nationwide Children's Hospital
Columbus, Ohio

Jennifer Yang, MD
Assistant Professor
Department of Urology
University of California, Davis
Sacramento, California

Michael Yaron, MD
Professor of Emergency Medicine
Department of Emergency Medicine
University of Colorado School of Medicine
Attending Physician
Emergency Department
University of Colorado Hospital
Aurora, Colorado

Yvette E. Yatchmink, MD, PhD
Associate Professor (Clinical)
Division of Developmental Behavioral Pediatrics
The Warren Alpert Medical School of Brown University
Departmental-Behavioral Pediatrician
Children's NeuroDevelopment Center
Hasbro Children's, Rhode Island Hospital
Providence, Rhode Island

Robert F. Yellon, MD
Professor of Otolaryngology
Department of Otolaryngology
University of Pittsburgh School of Medicine
Director of Clinical Services, and Co-Director
Department of Pediatric Otolaryngology
Children's Hospital of Pittsburgh of UPMC
Pittsburgh, Pennsylvania

Elizabeth H. Yen, MD
Assistant Professor
UCSF Benioff Children's Hospital San Francisco
Department of Pediatrics
Division of Gastroenterology, Hepatology and Nutrition
San Francisco, California

M. Elizabeth M. Younger, CRND, PhD
Assistant Professor
Department of Pediatric Allergy & Immunology
The Johns Hopkins University School of Medicine
Program Coordinator
Department of Pediatric Immunology
The Johns Hopkins Hospital
Baltimore, Maryland

Jenny Yu, MD
Assistant Professor
Division of Neonatology
The Johns Hopkins University School of Medicine
Neonatologist
Department of Pediatrics
Johns Hopkins Children's Center
Baltimore, Maryland

Jonathan A. Zelken, MD
Resident
Department of Plastic and Reconstructive Surgery
The Johns Hopkins University School of Medicine
Baltimore, Maryland

Karen P. Zimmer, MD, MPH, FAAP
Assistant Professor
Department of Pediatrics
The Johns Hopkins University School of Medicine
Baltimore, Maryland
Attending Physician Pediatrics
Alfred I. duPont Hospital for Children
Wilmington, Delaware

Raezelle Zinman, MD
Clinical Professor
Department of Pediatrics
Perelman School of Medicine at the University of Pennsylvania
The Children's Hospital of Philadelphia
Philadelphia, Pennsylvania

Naamah Zitomersky, MD
Instructor in Pediatrics
Harvard Medical School
Staff Physician and Physician Scientist
Department of Pediatric Gastroenterology
Boston Children's Hospital
Boston, Massachusetts

SIXTH EDITION AUTHOR ACKNOWLEDGMENTS

The editors and authors of the seventh edition gratefully acknowledge the past contributions of the following previous edition authors:

Ali Al-Omari
Lindsay Abenberg
Robert Baldassano
Diane Barsky
Timothy Beukelman
James Boyd
Laura K. Brennan
Genevieve L. Buser
Carla Campbell
Joy L. Collins
Kristin E. D'Aco
Dennis J. Dlugos
Naomi Dreisinger
C. Pace Duckett
Joel A. Fein
Brian T. Fisher
Brian J. Forbes
David F. Friedman
Scott M. Goldstein
Andres J. Greco
Marleine Ishak
Douglas Jacobstein
Anne K. Jensen
Peter B. Kang
Andrea Kelly
Jeremy King
Matthew P. Kirschen
Thomas F. Kolon
Sanjeev V. Kothare
Wendy J. Kowalski
David R. Langdon
Jerry Larrabee
Javier J. Lasa
Petar Mamula
Maria R. Mascarenhas
Kiran P. Maski
Hugh J. McMillan
William G. McNett
Kevin E. C. Meyers
Monte D. Mills
Divya Moodalbail
Sogol Mostoufi-Moab
Jane Nathanson
Seth L. Ness
Thomas Nguyen
Cynthia F. Norris
Juliann M. Paolicchi
Nadja Peter
Virginia M. Pierce
Jennifer R. Reid
Anne F. Reilly
Michelle T. Rook
Ann Salerno
Matthew G. Sampson
Samantha A. Schrier
Mitchell R. M. Schwartz
Teena Sebastian
Daniel Shumer
Jessica Wen
Alexis Weymann
Albert Yan
Andrew F. Zigman

CONTENTS

ABDOMINAL MASS

Maireade E. McSweeney • Rose C. Graham

BASICS

DESCRIPTION

A palpable lesion or fullness in the abdominal cavity which may or may not be related to abdominal viscera; the mass may be abdominal or retroperitoneal in origin

EPIDEMIOLOGY

- Etiologies for abdominal masses are varied and the differential depends on age and anatomic location.
- Majority are nonsurgical in nature; many are associated with constipation.
- Approximately 57% of abdominal masses in children are due to organomegaly (hepatomegaly or splenomegaly).

DIAGNOSIS

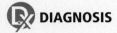

- Stomach
  - Gastric distension or gastroparesis
  - Duplication
  - Foreign body or bezoar
  - Gastric torsion
  - Gastric tumor (lymphoma, sarcoma)
- Intestine
  - Feces (constipation)
  - Intestinal distension or toxic megacolon
  - Foreign body
  - Meconium ileus
  - Duplication
  - Volvulus
  - Intussusception
  - Intestinal atresia or stenosis
  - Malrotation
  - Complications of inflammatory bowel disease (abscess, phlegmon)
  - Appendiceal inflammation
  - Meckel diverticulum or abscess
  - Duodenal hematoma (trauma)
  - Lymphoma, adenocarcinoma, GI stromal tumor
  - Carcinoid (appendiceal)
- Liver
  - Hepatomegaly due to intrinsic liver disease
    - Hepatitis (e.g., infectious, autoimmune)
    - Metabolic or storage disorders (e.g., Wilson disease, glycogen storage disease)
    - Infiltration of liver (cyst, tumors)
    - Biliary obstruction
    - Vascular obstruction/impaired venous congestion (Budd-Chiari syndrome, congestive heart failure)
  - Cystic disease (e.g., Caroli disease)
  - Solid tumor (hepatoblastoma; hepatocellular carcinoma; hepatic adenoma; or other diffuse, systemic, neoplastic process)
  - Vascular tumor (hemangioma or hemangioendothelioma)
  - Other: hamartomas, focal nodular hyperplasia
- Gallbladder/biliary tract
  - Choledochal cyst
  - Hydrops of gallbladder
  - Obstruction (stone, stricture, trauma)
- Spleen
  - Congenital cysts
  - Storage disease (e.g., Gaucher, Niemann-Pick)
  - Langerhans cell histiocytosis
  - Leukemia
  - Hematologic (hemolytic disease [e.g., sickle cell] or other RBC disorders [e.g., hereditary spherocytosis])
  - Portal hypertension
  - Wandering spleen
- Pancreas
  - Congenital cysts
  - Pseudocyst (trauma, pancreatitis)
  - Pancreatoblastoma
  - Neuroendocrine tumors (insulinomas, gastrinomas)
  - Solid and papillary epithelial neoplasms
- Kidney
  - Hydronephrosis or ureteropelvic obstruction
  - Multicystic dysplastic kidney
  - Polycystic disease
  - Tumor (mesoblastic nephroma, Wilms tumor, renal cell carcinoma)
  - Renal vein thrombosis
  - Cystic nephroma
- Bladder
  - Bladder distension
  - Neurogenic bladder
- Adrenal
  - Adrenal hemorrhage
  - Adrenal abscess
  - Neuroblastoma
  - Pheochromocytoma
- Uterus
  - Pregnancy
  - Hematocolpos
  - Hydrocolpos or hydrometrocolpos
- Ovary
  - Cysts (dermoid, follicular)
  - Torsion
  - Germ cell tumor
- Peritoneal
  - Ascites
  - Teratoma
- Abdominal wall
  - Umbilical/inguinal/ventral hernia
  - Omphalocele/gastroschisis
  - Urachal cyst
  - Trauma (rectus hematoma)
  - Tumor (fibroma, lipoma, rhabdomyosarcoma)
- Omentum/mesentery
  - Cysts
  - Mesenteric fibromatosis
  - Mesenteric adenitis
- Other
  - Tumors (liposarcoma, leiomyosarcoma, fibrosarcoma, mesothelioma)
  - Intra-abdominal testicle (torsion)
  - Lymphangioma
  - Fetus in fetu
  - Sacrococcygeal teratoma

APPROACH TO PATIENT

When evaluating a pediatric abdominal mass, an organized approach is critical:

- **Phase 1:** Perform a careful clinical history and abdominal examination in order to help assess clinical symptoms, duration of symptoms, and approximate anatomic location of the mass.
- **Phase 2:** Perform diagnostic tests:
  - Obtain abdominal x-ray to assess for bowel obstruction, fecal load, or mass effect; obtain ultrasound to identify organ of origin and tissue components (e.g., cystic, hemorrhage, etc.).
  - Laboratory testing as indicated
- **Hints for screening problems**
  - Constipation and fecal impaction can present as a large, hard mass extending from the pubis.
  - In neonates, a palpable liver edge can be normal; assess the total liver span.
  - In infants, a full bladder is often mistaken for an abdominal mass.
  - Certain genetic disorders/syndromes are associated with increased risk of tumor development (e.g., Beckwith-Wiedemann syndrome and Wilms tumor).
  - Gastric distention should be considered in all children who present with a tympanitic epigastric mass.

HISTORY

- **Question:** Weight loss?
- *Significance:* Malignancy, inflammatory bowel disease
- **Question:** Fever?
- *Significance:* Infection, malignancy
- **Question:** Jaundice?
- *Significance:* Hepatobiliary or hematologic disease
- **Question:** Hematuria or dysuria?
- *Significance:* Renal disease
- **Question:** Vomiting, bilious vomiting, or early satiety?
- *Significance:* Intestinal obstruction
- **Question:** Abdominal pain?
- *Significance:* Appendicitis, intussusception, intestinal obstruction
- **Question:** Frequency and quality of bowel movements?
- *Significance:* Constipation, intussusception, compression of bowel by mass
- **Question:** Bleeding or bruising?
- *Significance:* Liver disease, coagulopathy
- **Question:** Pallor or weakness?
- *Significance:* Sign of anemia or blood loss
- **Question:** History of abdominal trauma?
- *Significance:* Pancreatic pseudocyst, duodenal hematoma
- **Question:** Sexual activity?
- *Significance:* Pregnancy

- **Question:** Age of patient?
- *Significance*:
  - In neonates, the most common origin of abdominal masses are genitourinary (cystic kidney disease, hydronephrosis).
  - In adolescent-aged girls, ovarian disorders, hematocolpos, and pregnancy should be considered.
  - Most common *malignant* abdominal tumors by age: (1) infants: neuroblastoma, Wilms tumor; (2) children: Wilms tumor, sarcomas, germ cell tumors, (3) children >10 years of age: sarcomas, germ cell tumors, and abdominal lymphomas

PHYSICAL EXAM

- **Finding:** General appearance?
- *Significance*: Ill appearance or cachexia point toward infection or malignancy.
- **Finding:** Location of abdominal mass?
- *Significance*:
  - Left lower quadrant: feces, ovarian process, ectopic pregnancy
  - Left upper quadrant: splenomegaly, anomaly of the kidney
  - Right lower quadrant: abscess (inflammatory bowel disease), intestinal phlegmon, appendicitis, intussusception, ovarian process, ectopic pregnancy
  - Right upper quadrant: liver, gallbladder, biliary tree, or intestine
  - Epigastric: abnormality of the stomach (bezoar, torsion), pancreas (pseudocyst), or enlarged liver
  - Suprapubic: pregnancy, hydrometrocolpos, hematocolpos, posterior urethral valves
  - Flank: renal disease (cystic kidney, hydronephrosis, Wilms tumor)
- **Finding:** Characteristics of abdominal mass?
- *Significance:* Mobility, tenderness, firmness, smoothness, and/or irregularity of the surface of the mass can provide clues to its significance.
- **Finding:** Hard and immobile mass?
- *Significance:* Tumor
- **Finding:** Extension of mass across midline or into pelvis?
- *Significance:* Tumor, hepatomegaly, splenomegaly
- **Finding:** Percussion of mass?
- *Significance:* Dullness indicates a solid mass; tympany indicates a hollow organ.
- **Finding:** Shifting dullness, fluid wave?
- *Significance:* Ascites
- **Finding:** Skin exam?
- *Significance:* Bruising and petechiae may occur with coagulopathy related to liver disease and malignant infiltration of bone marrow; café au lait spots are associated with neurofibromas.
- **Finding:** Lymphadenopathy or lymphadenitis?
- *Significance:* Systemic process either malignant or infectious
- **Finding:** Peritoneal signs?
- *Significance:* Appendicitis, bowel obstruction or perforation; indication for urgent surgical consultation
- **Finding:** Rectal bleeding?
- *Significance:* Intestinal inflammation, polyp, or other bleeding lesion

DIAGNOSTIC TESTS & INTERPRETATION

- **Test:** CBC with differential
- *Significance*: Anemia, hemolysis
- **Test:** Chemistry panel
- *Significance*:
  - Renal disease: BUN and creatinine levels
  - Liver disease (bilirubin, ALT, AST, alkaline phosphatase, GGT, albumin, PT/PTT)
  - Gallbladder disease (bilirubin, GGT)
  - Pancreatic disease: amylase/lipase levels
  - Intestinal disease: hypoalbuminemia
- **Test:** Uric acid and lactate dehydrogenase levels
- *Significance*: Elevated in the setting of rapid cell turnover of solid tumors
- **Test:** Serum quantitative beta-human chorionic gonadotropin (hCG)
- *Significance:* Pregnancy, germ cell tumor

Imaging

- Plain radiographs
  - Evaluate for intestinal obstruction (dilated bowel loops, air fluid levels), bowel gas pattern, calcifications, or fecal impaction; urinary retention
- Ultrasound
  - Can identify the origin of the mass and differentiate between solid and cystic tissue; Doppler ability can help assess vascularity. Disadvantage is operator variability, and visualization may be limited by overlying bowel gas.
- CT scan
  - Can provide more detail when there is overlying gas or bone; if malignancy is suspected, should also do chest in addition to abdomen and pelvis
- MRI
  - Vascular lesions of liver, major vessels, and tumors
- Nuclear medicine
  - Radioisotope cholescintigraphy (HIDA) scan of liver, gallbladder/biliary tree
  - Meckel scan: can identify gastric mucosa contained within a Meckel diverticulum or intestinal duplication
  - Intravenous urography to assess renal system
- Fluoroscopy
  - Upper GI studies and barium enema studies: may be of benefit when the mass involves the intestine
  - Voiding cystourethrography (VCUG) to assess renal system

TREATMENT

GENERAL MEASURES

- Immediate hospitalization for patients who present with an abdominal mass and/or signs of dehydration, intestinal obstruction, bleeding, feeding intolerance, or clinical decompensation
- In addition to initial diagnostic and laboratory testing, a pediatric surgical or oncologic consultation should be obtained as indicated.
- The remaining causes of abdominal masses require urgent care and timely evaluation and referral to appropriate specialists.

ISSUES FOR REFERRAL

Except for the diagnosis of constipation, the presence of an abdominal mass in children requires immediate attention, and diagnostic studies should be performed expeditiously at a pediatric health care facility.

Admission Criteria

- Immediate hospitalization for patients who present with an abdominal mass and signs and/or symptoms of intestinal obstruction, distension, or peritoneal symptoms (intussusception, volvulus, gastric torsion, bezoar, foreign body, appendicitis)
  - Toxic megacolon
  - Ovarian torsion
  - Ectopic pregnancy
  - Biliary obstruction (stone, hydrops)
  - Fever
  - Anemia, coagulopathy
  - Pancreatitis (pseudocyst)
- The remaining causes of abdominal masses require urgent care and timely evaluation and referral to appropriate specialists.

ADDITIONAL READING

- Chandler JC, Gauderer MWL. The neonate with an abdominal mass. *Pediatr Clin North Am*. 2004;51(4):979–997.
- Golden CB, Feusner JH. Malignant abdominal masses in children: quick guide to evaluation and diagnosis. *Pediatr Clin North Am*. 2002;49(6):1369–1392.
- Ladino-Torres MF, Strouse PJ. Gastrointestinal tumors in children. *Radiol Clin North Am*. 2011;49(4): 665–677.
- Stevenson RJ. Abdominal masses. *Surg Clin North Am*. 1985;65(6):1481–1504.

CODES

ICD10

- R19.00 Intra-abd and pelvic swelling, mass and lump, unsp site
- R16.0 Hepatomegaly, not elsewhere classified
- R16.1 Splenomegaly, not elsewhere classified

ABDOMINAL MIGRAINE

Desalegn Yacob

BASICS

DESCRIPTION

Paroxysmal disorder of an acute onset, severe, noncolicky, periumbilical abdominal pain accompanied variably with nausea, vomiting, anorexia, headache, and pallor

EPIDEMIOLOGY

Incidence

- Occurs mostly in children; mean onset at age 7 years (3–10 years)
- Peak symptoms 10–12 years of age
- More common in girls (3:2)

Prevalence

- May affect as many as 1–4% of children at some point in their lives
- Declining frequency toward adulthood

RISK FACTORS

Genetics

Parents of affected children often have history of migraine headaches and motion sickness.

ETIOLOGY

- May involve neuronal activity originating in the hypothalamus with involvement of the cortex and autonomic nervous system
- Serotonin is implicated, and blockade of serotonin receptors may prevent abdominal migraine.
- Recent studies suggest involvement of local intestinal vasomotor factors

DIAGNOSIS

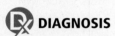

Rome III criteria—2 episodes within 12 months meeting all of the following criteria:

- Paroxysmal intense periumbilical pain that lasts >1 hour
- Intervening episodes of health between episodes
- Pain that interferes with activity
- Pain associated with ≥2 of the following: anorexia, nausea, vomiting, headache, photophobia, or pallor
- No evidence of inflammatory, anatomic, metabolic, or neoplastic process
- No evidence of elevated intracranial pressure (tumor, hydrocephalus)

HISTORY

- Ask about a family history of migraine headache or unexplained bouts of abdominal pain as children.
- Pain typically lasts <6 hours.
- Generalized abdominal pain; can often be localized to upper quadrants
- No abdominal pain between episodes
- Repetition of identical abdominal crises, anywhere from 1 time per week to several times a year
- Migraine in the history of patient or relatives
- Occasionally, other migraine phenomena such as nausea, vomiting, perspiration, body temperature changes, focal paresthesias, radiation of pain to a limb, visual disturbances, or general malaise
- Associated fatigue, lethargy, or impairment of consciousness

PHYSICAL EXAM

- Physical exam, including complete neurologic and abdominal exam, is usually unremarkable.
- Complete eye exam including funduscopic exam should be done to evaluate for papilledema (elevated intracranial pressure).

DIAGNOSTIC TESTS & INTERPRETATION

- Abdominal migraine is a diagnosis of exclusion.
- Even if a patient meets most or all diagnostic criteria for abdominal migraine, studies as outlined below should be strongly considered to ensure that another serious disorder does not exist.

Lab

- CBC with differential
- ESR and CRP
- Urinalysis
- Pregnancy test
- Amylase and lipase
- Stool Hemoccult
- Stool culture
- Lactose breath test for lactose intolerance
- Lead level
- Evaluation for porphyria or familial Mediterranean fever
- Metabolic evaluation (obtain during symptomatic episode, not during quiescence): urine organic acids, plasma amino acids, ammonia, lactate, blood gas, acylcarnitine profile, imaging

Diagnostic Procedures/Other

- Obstruction series to assess for intermittent or partial bowel obstruction
- Upper GI to rule out anatomic abnormalities
- US or CT scan to rule out mass lesion or chronic appendicitis
- Renal US during episodes to rule out ureteropelvic junction (UPJ) obstruction
- Barium enema (during painful crisis) to rule out intussusception
- EEG may help differentiate between abdominal migraine and epilepsy.
- Visual evoked response (VER) to red and white flashlight: Children with abdominal migraine may display a specific fast-wave activity response.
- Rarely, brain imaging with CT or MRI may be useful for evaluating causes of intermittent hydrocephalus.

DIFFERENTIAL DIAGNOSIS

- Infection
  - Giardia
- Environmental
  - Lead intoxication
- Tumors
- Metabolic
  - Porphyria, lactose intolerance, female carriers of (X-linked) ornithine transcarbamylase (OTC) gene mutation, organic acidemias
- Psychosocial
  - Functional abdominal pain/irritable bowel syndrome
- Surgical
  - Appendicitis, intussusception, biliary colic
- Inflammation
  - Inflammatory bowel disease, peptic ulcer disease, mesenteric adenitis
- GI
  - Irritable bowel syndrome, gastroesophageal reflux, wandering spleen, cyclical vomiting syndrome, recurrent abdominal pain, functional abdominal pain, constipation, superior mesenteric artery (SMA) syndrome, recurrent pancreatitis
- Anatomic
  - Meckel diverticulum, UPJ obstruction
- Neurologic
  - Abdominal epilepsy—but has a shorter duration of pain (minutes), altered consciousness during event, abrupt onset, abnormal discharges in EEG in 80%
  - Temporal lobe epilepsy
  - Intermittent hydrocephalus (possibly secondary to a 3rd ventricle colloid cyst)

ALERT

Because it is usually a diagnosis of exclusion, many patients go through a large workup to rule out other causes of pain, sometimes including laparotomy.

TREATMENT

MEDICATION

- Medications can be used to abort acute attacks or be taken as daily prophylaxis.
- For most patients, risks of side effects and complications from the use of these medications may outweigh the relief of pain, especially in children who are experiencing infrequent episodes.
- Limited data exist on abortive agents for abdominal migraines; however, several agents have shown benefit in specialty-based clinical practice, including metoclopramide, steroids, intranasal sumatriptan, and NSAIDs (although the latter may be avoided if there are clinical concerns for gastritis or peptic ulcer disease). Consider benzodiazepines (i.e., lorazepam) and antiemetics (i.e., ondansetron) for vomiting-predominant symptoms.
- Suggested prophylactic treatments are similar to those for migraine headaches and include tricyclic antidepressants (e.g., amitriptyline), topiramate, propranolol, cyproheptadine, and valproic acid. If EEG or other data point to possible epilepsy, empiric treatment with anticonvulsants may be considered.

ADDITIONAL TREATMENT

General Measures

- Trigger avoidance
  - An event diary should be kept to identify possible migraine triggers.
  - Avoiding triggers is the most optimal strategy for preventing recurrent attacks:
    - Common triggers include caffeine, nitrites, amines, emotional arousal, travel, prolonged fasting, altered sleep, exercise, and/or flickering lights.
- Cognitive therapies
  - Behavioral therapies and lifestyle modification (regular sleep, hydration, and exercise) may also be of benefit. Biofeedback in conjunction with other cognitive therapies and/or relaxation programs may be helpful. Assistance from a trained pediatric mental health professional may be useful.

ONGOING CARE

FOLLOW-UP RECOMMENDATIONS

- Most children outgrow abdominal migraine symptoms (~60%) by early adolescence.
- A substantial percentage of patients (~70%) may develop more typical migraine headaches during adulthood.
- Although nonspecific EEG changes are seen more commonly in this condition, very few children go on to develop epilepsy.
- 10% of children who have a diagnosis of migraine headaches have previously suffered from unexplained recurrent abdominal pain.
- Adult migraine headache sufferers experience abdominal pain more frequently than do tension headache sufferers.

PATIENT EDUCATION

- To help child during bouts of pain, allow the child to do whatever makes him or her comfortable—rest, positioning, being quiet.
- Whether the patient should be excused from school depends on various factors:
  - Frequency, severity, and duration of pain
  - Age, maturity, and coping skills of the child

ADDITIONAL READING

- Catto-Smith AG, Ranuh R. Abdominal migraine and cyclical vomiting. *Semin Pediatr Surg*. 2003;12(4):254–258.
- Cuvellier JC, Lépine A. Childhood periodic syndromes. *Pediatr Neurol*. 2010;42(1):1–11.
- Lewis DW. Pediatric migraine. *Neurol Clin*. 2009;27(2):481–501.
- Li BU, Balint JP. Cyclic vomiting syndrome: evolution in our understanding of a brain-gut disorder. *Adv Pediatr*. 2000;47:117–160.
- Popovich DM, Schentrup DM, McAlhany AL. Recognizing and diagnosing abdominal migraines. *J Pediatr Health Care*. 2010;24(6):372–377.
- Rasquin A, Di Lorenzo C, Forbes D, et al. Childhood functional gastrointestinal disorders: child/adolescent. *Gastroenterology*. 2006;130(5):1527–1537.
- Russell G, Abu-Arafehl, Symon DN. Abdominal migraine: evidence for existence and treatment options. *Paediatr Drugs*. 2002;4(1):1–8.
- Tan V, Sahami AR, Peebes R, et al. Abdominal migraine and treatment with intravenous valproic acid. *Psychosomatics*. 2006;47(4):353–355.
- Weydert JA, Ball TM, Davis MF. Systematic review of treatments for recurrent abdominal pain. *Pediatrics*. 2003;111(1):e1–e11.

CODES

ICD10

- G43.D0 Abdominal migraine, not intractable
- G43.D1 Abdominal migraine, intractable

FAQ

- Q: Does this diagnosis mean my child will develop migraine headaches?
- A: There is no accurate way to predict whether your child will develop migraine headaches.
- Q: I have 2 younger children. What chance do they have of developing abdominal migraines?
- A: Although migraine headaches do tend to run in families, there is no known mendelian inheritance pattern.
- Q: What can I do to help my child during bouts of pain?
- A: First, allow the child to do whatever makes him or her comfortable. This may mean resting, positioning, or being quiet. Acetaminophen or NSAID-based pain relievers may help to a certain degree. Whether the patient should be excused from school depends on various factors such as the frequency, severity, and duration of the pain as well as the age, maturity, and coping skills of the child.
- Q: My child is having frequent episodes that are affecting his/her quality of life. What can we do?
- A: It may be appropriate to trial him/her on prophylactic daily medications.

ABDOMINAL PAIN

Adrienne M. Scheich

BASICS

DESCRIPTION

- Abdominal pain is a subjective symptom that can originate from any intra-abdominal organ but also be secondary to non-abdominal sources (e.g., peridiaphragmatic conditions [e.g., pneumonia], referred pain, systemic infection [e.g., strep A or viral pharyngitis], depression).
- Acute abdominal pain is often due to benign and self-limited etiologies but may also be due to potentially life-threatening conditions.
- Chronic abdominal pain, defined as present >2 months, can either be of organic origin (anatomic, infectious, inflammatory, or metabolic) or, more frequently, part of a functional gastrointestinal disorder (FGID) based on specific diagnostic criteria (Rome III).

EPIDEMIOLOGY

- Abdominal pain is one of the most common complaints in pediatric patients.
- Chronic abdominal pain represents 2–4% of general pediatrics office visits and more than 50% of pediatric gastroenterology visits and can be associated with significant morbidity. Thus, chronic pain also warrants careful consideration and management.

PATHOPHYSIOLOGY

- The nature of abdominal pain is multifactorial and may evolve in nature over time (i.e., in acute appendicitis, pain typically migrates from periumbilical to right lower quadrant).
- Visceral pain (particularly from small intestine) is often poorly localized and is described as dull, diffuse, cramping, or burning. Visceral pain may be associated with autonomic reflex responses (diaphoresis, pallor, nausea, and/ or vomiting).
- More localized, sharp somatoparietal pain typically indicates peritoneal involvement (appendicitis, cholecystitis).
- Referred pain is related to the level of spinal cord entry of visceral afferent nerves (e.g., scapular pain in cholecystitis).

ETIOLOGY

- Right upper quadrant
  - Cholelithiasis/cholecystitis
  - Hepatitis/perihepatitis
  - Nephrolithiasis
  - Ureteropelvic junction obstruction
  - Right lower lobe pneumonia
- Epigastric area
  - Gastroesophageal reflux disease (GERD)
  - Esophagitis (GERD, eosinophilic)
  - Gastritis (NSAID, allergic, *Helicobacter pylori*, Crohn disease)
  - Functional dyspepsia
  - Ulcer disease (NSAID, *H. pylori*)
  - Pancreatitis
  - Cholecystitis
  - Gastric/small intestinal volvulus
- Left upper quadrant
  - Splenic hematoma
  - Renal disease (see above)
  - Left lower lobe pneumonia
  - Constipation
- Right lower quadrant
  - Appendicitis/perforation/psoas abscess
  - Mesenteric adenitis
  - Intussusception
  - Inflammatory bowel disease (IBD)
  - Infection (tuberculosis, *Yersinia*)
  - Ovarian/testicular torsion
  - Ectopic pregnancy
  - Inguinal hernia
- Left lower quadrant
  - Constipation
  - Colitis (inflammatory/infectious)
  - Sigmoid volvulus
  - Genitourinary disease (see above)
- Hypogastric area
  - Constipation
  - Colitis
  - Cystitis
  - Dysmenorrhea/uterine disease
  - Pelvic inflammatory disease
- Periumbilical area
  - FGID
  - Constipation
  - Gastroenteritis (infectious/eosinophilic)
  - Pancreatitis
  - Gastric/small bowel volvulus
  - Appendicitis (early)
  - Incarcerated umbilical hernia
- Diffuse
  - Constipation
  - FGID
  - Giardiasis
  - Carbohydrate malabsorption
  - Celiac disease
  - Streptococcal/viral pharyngitis
  - IBD
  - Allergic/eosinophilic gastroenteritis
  - Ischemic necrotizing enterocolitis (NEC)
  - Perforation/peritonitis
  - Malrotation with volvulus
  - Lead/iron poisoning/pica syndrome
  - Cyclic vomiting syndrome
  - Porphyria
  - Sickle cell crisis
  - Familial Mediterranean fever
  - Diabetic ketoacidosis
  - Henoch-Schönlein purpura (HSP)
  - Tumor
  - Trauma
  - Hemolytic uremic syndrome (HUS)

DIAGNOSIS

APPROACH TO PATIENT

Initial step is to establish the acuity and severity of symptoms and to rule out a potentially life-threatening emergency (e.g., appendicitis, perforation, bowel obstruction associated with volvulus, adhesions, or intussusception).

HISTORY

- Onset and duration of symptoms
  - Acute versus chronic
- Age of patient may be indicative of certain etiologies particularly in acute presentation.
  - NEC (newborn/prematurity), malrotation/volvulus (80% present in first month of life), intussusception (more frequent in infants/ toddlers), foreign body ingestion in young child
- Localization and radiation of pain
  - May point to specific organ—see etiologies
- Triggering or relieving factors
  - Meals/spices, specific foods (lactose, sucrose)
  - General position with knees bent can be relieving in acute appendicitis.
  - Pain relieved by defecation (constipation) versus pain worsened by defecation (colitis)
- Bowel pattern and stool appearance
  - Stool frequency and consistency: diarrhea versus constipation
  - Urgency or nocturnal diarrhea (colitis)
  - Presence of bloating and excessive flatulence (giardiasis, carbohydrate malabsorption)
  - Presence of mucus (may be normal but can be associated with colitis)
  - Hematochezia (fissure, hemorrhoid, polyp, colitis, HSP); if bright red "currant jelly" appearance, suspect intussusception
  - Melena (upper gastrointestinal bleeding/ulcer)
  - Pale/acholic stools (hepatic or biliary disease)
  - Perirectal disease (IBD)
- Anorexia/nausea/vomiting
  - If postprandial, indicative of upper gastrointestinal condition; nausea may be functional.
  - May indicate extraintestinal disease (urinary tract infection, UPJ obstruction, or pneumonia)
  - Hematemesis suggests esophagitis/gastritis; more significant blood volume suggests ulcer disease, Mallory-Weiss tear (lower esophagus)
  - Bilious emesis indicates intestinal obstruction (volvulus, intussusception, NEC in newborns)
- Dysphagia/food impaction
  - In older children, suspect eosinophilic esophagitis
  - GERD
- Fever
  - Acute infection, acute appendicitis, chronic inflammatory process
- Weight loss/growth failure/delayed puberty
  - Chronic inflammatory process, celiac disease
- Extraintestinal symptoms
  - Dysuria
  - Skin rash (atopy may point to eosinophilic process; purpura: abdominal pain may be first symptom of HSP)
  - Respiratory symptoms (pneumonia)
  - Arthralgias (IBD, HSP)
- Preexisting conditions (infectious diarrhea preceding HUS; hemoglobinopathy or cystic fibrosis risk factors for cholecystitis)
- Exposures
  - Lead/iron in young children
  - Travel/well water/pets (giardiasis)
  - Insect bite (HSP)
  - NSAID use (gastritis)
  - Tetracycline (pill esophagitis)
- Dietary history to assess fiber and fluid intake; excessive use of sugar-free gum (sorbitol malabsorption); intake of sucrose-, fructose-, or lactose-containing foods (various disaccharidase deficiencies, most commonly lactose intolerance)
- Prior abdominal surgical history (adhesions)
- Family history of IBD, *H. pylori*, celiac disease, atopy, migraine
- Social history and identification of stressors, school attendance, signs of mood disorder

PHYSICAL EXAM

- In an acute setting, an abdominal exam may need to be serially performed, as location of pain may change over time.
- Signs of acute appendicitis:
  - Exquisite pain at McBurney point on percussion or palpation
  - Involuntary guarding
  - Rovsing sign (palpation LLQ), psoas sign, obturator sign
  - Rebound tenderness (peritoneal inflammation)
  - Pain on movement (walking, jumping)
  - Pain may be relieved temporarily if the appendix ruptures followed by signs of peritonitis.
  - Right upper quadrant pain on inspiration (cholecystitis)
  - Flank tenderness (renal pathology)
  - Perianal examination may reveal skin tags/ fissures (constipation, IBD), perianal abscess (IBD), hemorrhoids
- Rectal examination done carefully can be indicative of
  - Peritoneal irritation (appendicitis/peritonitis)
  - Hematochezia (IBD, HSP), perianal disease
  - Fecal retention/abnormal sphincter tone (anal stricture, absent relaxation of IAS suggesting anal achalasia)
- Skin rashes (eczema, purpura)
- Other signs of chronic disease include pallor, clubbing, edema

DIAGNOSTIC TESTS & INTERPRETATION

- Laboratory testing, if any, should be carefully guided by the history and clinical picture.
  - If a benign acute condition such as acute viral gastroenteritis is suspected, any further testing can be delayed with close follow-up (in absence of clinical evidence of dehydration).
  - In the presence of "red flags" (see "Referral"), blood and stool testing should be performed
- CBC/differential
  - Leukocytosis (appendicitis/abscess, acute infectious process); normal white blood cell count may indicate low risk for acute appendicitis
  - Anemia (gastrointestinal blood loss)
  - Microcytosis (chronic inflammation, IBD, celiac disease)
- Elevated ESR or CRP (acute infection, chronic inflammation)
- Hypoalbuminemia and low ferritin (IBD, celiac disease); diarrhea may be absent
- Pancreatic enzymes, hepatic enzymes
- Fecal cultures in the presence of bloody diarrhea (colitis); ova and parasites (giardiasis)
- Fecal calprotectin and lactoferrin (inflammation or infection)
- Urinalysis to rule out urinary tract infection (leukocyturia may be present in acute appendicitis)
- Celiac screening (anti-tissue transglutaminase IgA or anti-endomysial IgA in presence of normal total IgA levels) should be considered if abdominal pain and/or constipation do not respond to bowel regimen or if unexplained diarrhea, weight loss/growth failure; also at risk: type 1 diabetes, autoimmune thyroiditis, Down/Turner syndrome
- Thyroid screen if abdominal pain/chronic constipation unresponsive to therapy

ALERT
H. pylori testing is NOT indicated in the evaluation of chronic abdominal pain, nonulcer dyspepsia, or newly diagnosed GERD unless the patient has endoscopically documented peptic ulcer disease, a family history of gastric cancer, documented mucosa-associated lymphoid tissue (MALT) lymphoma, or unexplained iron deficiency anemia.

- Radiologic evaluation (abdominal decubitus and upright films)
  - Dilatation or air–fluid levels: acute obstruction
  - "Double bubble" sign and airless abdomen: midgut volvulus/malrotation
  - Air–fluid level or fecalith in right lower quadrant: acute appendicitis if suspected
  - Radiopaque renal stones or dilated ureters
- Upper gastrointestinal contrast study to document anatomic anomalies (i.e., malrotation)
- Ultrasound/CT scan in the evaluation of trauma, acute appendicitis, intussusception, suspected abscess in IBD, tumors, pancreatitis/ pseudocyst, cholecystitis
- Use of CT scan in suspected acute appendicitis should be carefully considered, as it can both lead to unnecessary appendectomies or be falsely negative. In patients identified as "low risk" for appendicitis (absent leukocytosis with left shift), ultrasound and/or close observation should be considered as alternative to CT scan.

TREATMENT

GENERAL MEASURES

- In the acute setting of abdominal pain suggesting a potential life-threatening condition (acute appendicitis, acute obstruction, volvulus), the patient should be stabilized and referred appropriately for further management including surgery if indicated.
- In the setting of extraintestinal conditions (i.e., pneumonia, pharyngitis, or urinary tract infection), antibiotic therapy should be initiated if indicated.
- In the setting of chronic pain and in the absence of red flags (see "Referral"), the most likely diagnoses can be categorized as abdominal pain–related FGIDs. These include functional dyspepsia, IBS, abdominal migraine, and functional abdominal pain syndrome. The diagnosis of these entities is based on specific symptom based criteria (Rome III).

SURGERY/OTHER PROCEDURES

- Functional dyspepsia: trial of proton pump inhibitor (PPI) therapy for 4 weeks to rule out postviral dyspepsia. Avoid use of NSAIDs, spicy and fatty foods, and caffeine. If no response or unable to tolerate progressive taper of PPIs, refer to a gastroenterologist for endoscopic evaluation.
- Irritable bowel syndrome: address bowel pattern: diarrhea (antidiarrheals); constipation (nonstimulating laxatives); peppermint oil or antispasmodics may alleviate pain; probiotics
- Functional abdominal pain syndrome: Use biopsychosocial approach; behavioral treatment with or without trial of tricyclic antidepressants (particularly in presence of anxiety)

ALERT
Psychological comorbidities should be addressed in all FGIDs.

REFERRAL

- The presence of clinical red flags, in the setting of acute or chronic abdominal pain, may indicate an underlying mucosal pathology of the gastrointestinal tract (other than infectious), warranting referral to a gastroenterologist for further endoscopic evaluation and management. These include the following:
  - Nocturnal pain: pain that wakes from sleep
  - Persistent vomiting and/or dysphagia
  - GERD non responsive to PPI trial
  - Hematemesis
  - Nocturnal diarrhea
  - Hematochezia
  - Perianal disease
  - Weight loss/delayed growth and/or puberty
  - Family history of PUD or IBD

ADDITIONAL-READING

- Chitkara DK, Rawat DJ, Talley NJ. The epidemiology of childhood recurrent abdominal pain in Western countries: a systematic review. *Am J Gastroenterol*. 2005;100(8):1868–1875.
- Kharbanda AB, Dudley NC, Bajaj L, et al. Validation and refinement of a prediction rule to identify children at low risk for acute appendicitis. *Arch Pediatr Adolesc Med*. 2012;166(8):738–744.
- Koletzko S, Jones NL, Goodman KJ, et al. Evidence-based guidelines from ESPGHAN and NASPGHAN for Helicobacter pylori infection in children. *J Pediatr Gastroenterol Nutr*. 2011;53(2):230–243.
- Korterink JJ, Ockeloen L, Benninga MA, et al. Probiotics for functional gastrointestinal disorders: a systematic review and meta-analysis. *Acta Paediatr*. 2014;103(4):365–372.
- McCollough M, Sharieff GQ. Abdominal pain in children. *Pediatr Clin North Am*. 2006;53(1):107–137, vi.
- Nurko S, Di Lorenzo C. Functional abdominal pain: time to get together and move forward. *J Pediatr Gastroenterol Nutr*. 2008;47(5):679–680.
- Rasquin A, Di Lorenzo C, Forbes D, et al. Childhood functional gastrointestinal disorders: child/ adolescent. *Gastroenterology*. 2006;130(5): 1527–1537.
- Ross A, LeLeiko NS. Acute abdominal pain. *Pediatr Rev*. 2010;31(4):135–144.
- Saps M, Youssef N, Miranda A, et al. Multicenter, randomized, placebo-controlled trial of amitriptyline in children with functional abdominal gastrointestinal disorders. *Gastroenterology*. 2009;137(4): 1261–1269.

CODES

ICD10

- R10.9 Unspecified abdominal pain
- R10.0 Acute abdomen
- R10.31 Right lower quadrant pain

ABNORMAL BLEEDING

Char Witmer

BASICS

DESCRIPTION

Abnormal bleeding may present as

- Frequent or significant mucocutaneous bleeding (epistaxis, bruising, gum bleeding, or menorrhagia)
- Bleeding in unusual sites such as muscles, joints, or internal organs
- Excessive postsurgical bleeding

ETIOLOGY

Abnormal bleeding can be the result of a coagulation factor deficiency, an acquired or congenital disorder of platelet number or function, or inherited or acquired collagen vascular disorders.

DIAGNOSIS

DIFFERENTIAL DIAGNOSIS

Platelet disorders may be quantitative or qualitative, collagen vascular disorders can be acquired or inherited, and disorders of coagulation factors can be congenital or acquired.

- Thrombocytopenia: defective production
  - Congenital/genetic
    - Thrombocytopenia with absent radii syndrome
    - Amegakaryocytic thrombocytopenia
    - Fanconi anemia
    - Metabolic disorders
    - Wiskott-Aldrich syndrome
    - Bernard-Soulier syndrome
    - Other rare familial syndromes (e.g., MYH9-related disorders, RUNX1 mutations)
  - Acquired
    - Aplastic anemia
    - Drug-associated marrow suppression
    - Virus-associated marrow suppression
    - Chemotherapy
    - Radiation injury
    - Nutritional deficiencies (e.g., vitamin B_{12} and folate)
  - Marrow infiltration
    - Neoplasia (e.g., leukemia, solid tumor)
    - Histiocytosis
    - Osteopetrosis
    - Myelofibrosis
    - Hemophagocytic syndromes
    - Storage diseases
- Thrombocytopenia: increased destruction
  - Idiopathic thrombocytopenia
  - Neonatal alloimmune thrombocytopenia
  - Maternal autoimmune thrombocytopenia
  - Drug-induced (heparin, sulfonamides, digoxin, chloroquine)
  - Disseminated intravascular coagulation
  - Infection: viral, bacterial, fungal, rickettsial
  - Microangiopathic process (e.g., thrombotic thrombocytopenic purpura or hemolytic uremic syndrome)
  - Kasabach-Merritt syndrome
- Thrombocytopenia: sequestration
  - Hypersplenism
  - Hypothermia
- Platelet function disorders
  - Storage pool disorders (e.g., dense granule deficiency, Hermansky-Pudlak or Chediak-Higashi syndrome)
  - Platelet receptor abnormalities (e.g., Glanzmann thrombasthenia, adenosine 5′-diphosphate receptor defect)
  - Drugs (e.g., aspirin, NSAIDs, guaifenesin, antihistamines, phenothiazines, anticonvulsants)
  - Uremia
  - Paraproteinemia
- Coagulation disorders
  - Prolongation of activated partial thromboplastin time (aPTT)
    - Deficiency of factors VIII, IX, XI, or XII; prekallikrein; or high-molecular-weight kininogen
    - Acquired inhibitor or lupus anticoagulant
  - Prolongation of prothrombin time (PT)
    - Deficiency of factor VII
    - Mild vitamin K deficiency
    - Liver disease, mild to moderate
  - Prolongation of PT and aPTT
    - Liver disease, severe
    - Disseminated intravascular coagulation
    - Severe vitamin K deficiency
    - Hemorrhagic disease of the newborn
    - Deficiency of factors II, V, or X or fibrinogen
    - Dysfibrinogenemia
    - Hypoprothrombinemia associated with a lupus anticoagulant
  - Normal screening (PT, aPTT) laboratory tests
    - Von Willebrand disease
    - Factor XIII deficiency
    - Alpha-2-antiplasmin deficiency
    - Plasminogen activator inhibitor-I deficiency
- Vessel wall disorders
  - Congenital
    - Hereditary hemorrhagic telangiectasia
    - Ehlers-Danlos syndrome
    - Marfan syndrome
  - Acquired
    - Vasculitis (systemic lupus erythematosus, Henoch-Schönlein purpura, and others)
    - Scurvy (vitamin C deficiency)

ALERT

Always consider nonaccidental injury as a cause of increased bruising.

APPROACH TO PATIENT

- **Phase 1**
  - Includes a thorough history and physical exam
  - Familial history specifically of bleeding or consanguinity
  - Standard screening laboratory tests include PT, aPTT, and platelet count.
- **Phase 2**
  - If a bleeding disorder is suspected but the initial screening tests are negative, testing for von Willebrand disease, qualitative platelet disorders, dysfibrinogenemia, or factor XIII deficiency is warranted.
- **Phase 3**
  - Any abnormal screening tests need further evaluation with additional testing to define the specific disorder (e.g., factor assays).

HISTORY

By taking into account the patient's age, sex, clinical presentation, past medical history, and family history, the most likely cause of bleeding can be usually determined.

- Hemophilia is X-linked, most common in males.
- A family history of bleeding suggests an inherited bleeding disorder.
- Bleeding in unusual places without significant trauma (intracranial, joints) indicates a significant bleeding disorder.
- Persistent palpable bruising is highly suggestive of a bleeding disorder.
- Several surgeries without bleeding makes an inherited bleeding disorder less likely.
- Mucocutaneous bleeding (gum bleeding, bruises, epistaxis, recurrent petechiae, menorrhagia) may indicate thrombocytopenia, a platelet disorder, or von Willebrand disease.
- The use of aspirin and NSAIDs (e.g., ibuprofen) negatively affect platelet function and result in an acquired bleeding disorder.

PHYSICAL EXAM

- Children with bleeding disorders are more likely to have large bruises (>5 cm), palpable bruises, and bruises on more than one body part.
- Uncommon sites for bruising for all ages include the back, buttocks, arms, and abdomen.
- **Finding:** Petechiae in skin and mucous membranes?
- *Significance*: Disorder of platelet number or function, von Willebrand disease, or vasculitis
- **Finding:** Bruises in unusual places?
- *Significance*: Possible platelet disorder or von Willebrand disease
- **Finding:** Large bruises or palpable bruises?
- *Significance*: Coagulation deficiencies, severe platelet disorders, or von Willebrand disease
- **Finding:** Delayed wound healing?
- *Significance*: Factor XIII deficiency or dysfibrinogenemia
- **Finding:** Purpura localized to lower body (buttocks, legs, ankles)?
- *Significance*: Henoch-Schönlein purpura

DIAGNOSTIC TESTS & INTERPRETATION

- The aPTT may be extremely prolonged in patients with deficiencies of the contact factors (prekallikrein, high molecular weight kininogen, factor XII). These deficiencies do not result in bleeding.
- Improper specimen collection including heparin contamination or underfilling of the specimen tube can result in artificially prolonged clotting times.
- **Test:** Phase 1: initial laboratory screening
  - Platelet count
  - PT and aPTT
- **Test:** Phase 2
- Test for von Willebrand disease
  - Factor VIII:C
  - Von Willebrand factor antigen (VIIIR:Ag)
  - Von Willebrand factor activity (ristocetin cofactor)
  - Von Willebrand factor multimeric analysis—only send after the diagnosis of von Willebrand disease has been established
  - Thrombin time and fibrinogen assay to screen for afibrinogenemia and dysfibrinogenemia
  - Definitive platelet testing includes platelet aggregation and secretion studies with specific agonists.
  - Factor XIII deficiency suspected: factor XIII assay (Urea clot lysis study is a screening test.)
- **Test:** Phase 3: discriminating laboratory studies for abnormal phase 1 or 2 tests
- When thrombocytopenia is present:
  - Inspection of blood smear
  - Mean platelet volume (may be normal or elevated in destructive causes, elevated in congenital macrothrombocytopenias, low in Wiskott-Aldrich syndrome)
  - Bone marrow aspiration (rarely necessary)
- Prolonged aPTT
  - Inhibitor screen (50:50 mixing study of patient's and normal plasma)
  - If aPTT fully corrects with mixing, this is consistent with a factor deficiency:
    - Assess for specific factor deficiencies: factors VIII, IX, XI, or XII; prekallikrein; and high-molecular-weight kininogen
  - If partial or no correction after mixing study:
    - Inhibitor is present.
    - Confirmatory test for the presence of a lupus anticoagulant with a platelet-neutralizing procedure or dilute Russel viper venom time (DRVVT)
- Prolonged PT
  - Inhibitor screen should also be considered for prolonged PT.
  - Specific factor level (VII)
- Prolonged PT and aPTT
  - Factor assays: II (prothrombin), V, X, and fibrinogen
  - Potential other causes: disseminated intravascular coagulation, liver disease, and fibrinogen disorders, as described previously
  - Vitamin K deficiency, moderate to severe

ALERT

Pitfalls of testing:

- **PFA-100**
  - Low specificity and sensitivity
  - Affected by medications (NSAIDs)
  - Not recommended as a screening test
- **Bleeding time**
  - Prolonged when platelets $<100{,}000/\text{mm}^3$
  - Affected by medications such as aspirin, NSAIDs, antihistamines
  - Does not correlate with bleeding risk
  - Highly operator dependent
  - Not recommended as a screening test
- **PT and aPTT**
  - Normal ranges are age-dependent.
  - Polycythemia (hematocrit 65%) or underfilling of the specimen tube may result in a spuriously prolonged result.
  - Heparin contamination results in a spuriously prolonged result.
- **Von Willebrand disease studies**
  - Values fluctuate over time and may be periodically normal in affected individuals.
  - May require repeated testing to make diagnosis

EMERGENCY CARE

- Pressure, elevation, and ice are generally helpful for most bleeding disorders when active bleeding is present.
- More definitive care is dictated by the nature of the underlying hemostatic defect:
  - Platelet transfusions are useful in disorders of thrombocytopenia owing to decreased production and for intrinsic qualitative platelet disorders but not for immune platelet disorders.
  - Frozen plasma should be used only in severe cases when the exact diagnosis is not readily available but a defect in coagulation is suspected.
- Head injuries in patients with thrombocytopenia or hemophilia require immediate medical attention.

TREATMENT

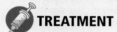

GENERAL MEASURES

- Pressure on wound
- Elevation
- Topical application of thrombin
- Topical application of clot-activating polymers

ADDITIONAL READING

- Buchanan GR. Bleeding signs in children with idiopathic thrombocytopenic purpura. *J Pediatr Hematol Oncol*. 2003;25(Suppl 1):S42–S46.
- Khair K, Liesner R. Bruising and bleeding in infants and children: a practical approach. *Br J Haematol*. 2006;133(3):221–231.
- Koreth R, Weinert C, Weisdorf DJ, et al. Measurement of bleeding severity: a critical review. *Transfusion*. 2004;44(4):605–617.
- Lillicrap D, Nair SC, Srivastava A, et al. Laboratory issues in bleeding disorders. *Haemophilia*. 2006;12(Suppl 3):68–75.
- Sarnaik A, Kamat D, Kannikeswaran N. Diagnosis and management of bleeding disorder in a child. *Clin Pediatr*. 2010;49(5):422–431.

CODES

ICD10

- D68.9 Coagulation defect, unspecified
- R04.0 Epistaxis
- T14.8 Other injury of unspecified body region

FAQ

- Q: What are the proper preoperative screening tests for bleeding disorders prior to elective surgery such as tonsillectomy?
- A: A thorough personal history, familial history, and physical exam are by far the most important screening tests. A bleeding time or PFA-100 is not recommended. A CBC, PT, and aPTT are often requested by the surgeon, but normal results do not ensure that a bleeding complication will not occur. Overall, the sensitivity and specificity of these screening tests is poor.
- Q: Bruising is a normal part of childhood. How does one know when bruising is "too much"?
- A: Small bruises on boney prominences on the front of the body are common in children and probably reflect trauma rather than a bleeding disorder. Children with bleeding disorders are more likely to have large bruises (>5 cm), palpable (raised) bruises, and bruises on more than one body part. Uncommon sites for bruising for all ages include the back, buttocks, arms, and abdomen

ACETAMINOPHEN POISONING

Kevin C. Osterhoudt

BASICS

DESCRIPTION

- Acetaminophen poisoning may occur after acute or chronic overdose.
- Acetaminophen is sold under many brand names and is often an ingredient in combination pain reliever preparations.
- Acetaminophen poisoning may be clinically occult until frank hepatic or renal injury become evident.
- After acute overdose, a serum acetaminophen level above the treatment line of the Rumack-Matthew acetaminophen poisoning nomogram should be considered possibly hepatotoxic.
- Serious hepatotoxicity after a single acute exploratory ingestion by young children is rare compared with that from intentional overdose by adolescents.
- Most toddlers with acetaminophen hepatotoxicity suffer repeated supratherapeutic dosing.

EPIDEMIOLOGY

- Analgesics are the most common drugs implicated in poisoning exposures reported to U.S. poison control centers.
- Acetaminophen preparations make up ~45% of all analgesic poisoning exposures reported to poison control centers.

Incidence

Acetaminophen poisoning is the most common cause of acute liver failure in the United States.

RISK FACTORS

- Depression
- Pain syndromes
- Glutathione depletion: prolonged vomiting, alcoholism, etc.
- CYP2E1 induction: alcoholism, isoniazid therapy, etc.

GENERAL PREVENTION

- Acetaminophen should be stored with child-resistant caps, out of sight of young children.
- Proper use of acetaminophen products should be taught to patients with pain or fever.

PATHOPHYSIOLOGY

- Most absorbed acetaminophen is metabolized through formation of hepatic glucuronide and sulfate conjugates.
- Some acetaminophen is metabolized by the CYP450 mixed-function oxidase system, leading to the formation of the toxic *N*-acetyl-p-benzoquinoneimine (NAPQI).
- NAPQI is quickly detoxified by glutathione under usual circumstances.
- After overdose, metabolic detoxification can become saturated:
  - Drug elimination half-life becomes prolonged.
  - Proportionately more NAPQI is produced.
  - Glutathione supply cannot meet detoxification demand.
  - Hepatic or renal toxicity may ensue.

ETIOLOGY

- Single acute overdose of >150 mg/kg or 10 g
- Repeated overdose of >100 mg/kg/day or 6 g/day, for >2 days

COMMONLY ASSOCIATED CONDITIONS

- Acetaminophen is often marketed in combination with other pharmaceuticals, which may complicate a drug overdose situation.
- Adolescents frequently overdose on more than 1 drug preparation.

DIAGNOSIS

HISTORY

- Medical history of pain or fever
  - Acetaminophen ingestion should be explored in any patient being treated for pain or fever.
- Amount of acetaminophen ingested
  - A single, acute ingestion of <150 mg/kg (≤10 g in adolescents) is unlikely to cause significant toxicity among otherwise healthy individuals.
- Timing of ingestion
  - Allows application of the Rumack-Matthew nomogram
- Sustained-release preparation
  - Acetaminophen is now available in sustained-release form.
- Medication list
  - Use of isoniazid or other CYP2E1 hepatic enzyme inducers may increase risk for toxicity.
- Signs and symptoms
  - Initially may be clinically silent
  - Vomiting
  - Anorexia

PHYSICAL EXAM

Right upper quadrant tenderness may suggest acetaminophen-induced hepatitis.

DIAGNOSTIC TESTS & INTERPRETATION

Lab

- Serum acetaminophen level
  - Allows application of the Rumack-Matthew nomogram after acute overdose
  - Rumack-Matthew nomogram applies only to single, acute acetaminophen overdose scenarios.
- Hepatic transaminases
  - Aspartate aminotransferase (AST) is the most sensitive of the widely available measures to assess acetaminophen hepatotoxicity and begins to rise 12–24 hours after significant overdose.
- Liver and kidney function tests
  - As the AST rises, it is important to follow liver and kidney function with tests such as serum glucose, prothrombin (PT) and partial thromboplastin (PTT) times, serum creatinine, plasma pH, and serum albumin.
  - The PT and PTT may be slightly elevated owing to direct effect of elevated blood acetaminophen concentrations or *N*-acetylcysteine therapy, without signifying liver injury.
  - The decline of an elevated serum AST may indicate either liver recovery or profound liver failure and must be interpreted in context.
- Salicylate level
  - May be a coingestant in the setting of analgesic drug overdose

Pathologic Findings

Hepatic zone III (centrilobular) necrosis

DIFFERENTIAL DIAGNOSIS

- Infectious hepatitis
- Other drug-induced hepatitis

TREATMENT

MEDICATION

First Line

- Single acute overdose
  - Activated charcoal, 1–2 g/kg (maximum 75 g), may be administered if acetaminophen is judged to be present in the stomach or proximal intestine (usually within 1 hour of ingestion).
  - *N*-acetylcysteine should be administered if a serum acetaminophen level obtained >4 hours after overdose falls above the treatment line of the Rumack-Matthew nomogram (see Appendix, Figure 4).
  - Patients presenting to medical care >7 hours after overdose should be given a loading dose of *N*-acetylcysteine while waiting for the serum acetaminophen level result.
  - Oral *N*-acetylcysteine dose: 140 mg/kg loading dose, followed by 70 mg/kg maintenance doses q4h (see "FAQ")
  - Intravenous *N*-acetylcysteine dose: 150 mg/kg loading dose over 1 hour, then 12.5 mg/kg/h for 4 hours, then 6.25 mg/kg/h (see "FAQ ")

ALERT

Some toxicologists suggest higher dosing for very large acetaminophen overdoses.

- Repeated supratherapeutic ingestion
  - Consider *N*-acetylcysteine therapy if
    - Ingestion of >100 mg/kg or 6 g/day for consecutive days
    - Patient is symptomatic
    - AST level is elevated
    - Acetaminophen level is higher than would be expected given dosing, and AST level is normal
- Once started, *N*-acetylcysteine therapy should be continued until
  - The serum acetaminophen level is nondetectable
  - A simultaneous serum AST has not risen or, if elevated, liver enzymes and liver function are clearly improving

Second Line

- Acetaminophen poisoning and oral *N*-acetylcysteine therapy are emetogenic: chill and cover the *N*-acetylcysteine. Consider antiemetic therapy with drugs such as metoclopramide and/or ondansetron. Enteral *N*-acetylcysteine may be given slowly via nasogastric or nasoduodenal tube.
- Intravenous *N*-acetylcysteine has been associated with anaphylactoid reactions, which may require cessation or slowing of infusion, antihistamines, corticosteroids, and/or epinephrine.

ADDITIONAL TREATMENT

General Measures

Evaluate for possible polypharmacy overdose.

ISSUES FOR REFERRAL

- Patients with AST approaching 1,000 IU/L should be considered for transfer to a liver transplant center.
- Mental health services should be provided to victims of intentional overdose.

SURGERY/OTHER PROCEDURES

Liver transplant should be considered per transplant center protocols. The King's College Hospital Criteria include the following:

- pH <7.30 after resuscitation, or
- PT >1.8 times control, plus
- Serum creatinine >3.3 mg/dL, plus
- Encephalopathy

INPATIENT CONSIDERATIONS

Admission Criteria

- *N*-acetylcysteine therapy
- Psychiatric evaluation warranted

Discharge Criteria

- *N*-acetylcysteine therapy concluded
- No concern for developing liver injury

ONGOING CARE

FOLLOW-UP RECOMMENDATIONS

Patient Monitoring

- Cardiorespiratory monitoring is warranted during intravenous *N*-acetylcysteine therapy.
- Intensive care monitoring is warranted during fulminant hepatic failure.

PATIENT EDUCATION

- Drug administration education should be offered to victims of chronic overdose.
- Home safety education should be provided after pediatric exploratory ingestions.

PROGNOSIS

- Among previously healthy children, hepatotoxicity is rare with single doses <150–200 mg/kg.
- After single acute acetaminophen overdose, likelihood of hepatotoxicity may be determined by using the Rumack-Matthew nomogram.
- *N*-acetylcysteine therapy prevents hepatic failure in >99% of acetaminophen-poisoned patients if administered within 8 hours of overdose.
- *N*-acetylcysteine therapy is less efficacious when administered >8 hours after overdose but should still be offered.
- Repetitive dosing of acetaminophen >75 mg/kg/day should be evaluated cautiously, especially in the presence of the following:
  - Febrile illness
  - Vomiting or malnourishment
  - Anticonvulsant or isoniazid therapy

COMPLICATIONS

- Hepatic failure
- Renal insufficiency
- Anaphylactoid shock may complicate intravenous *N*-acetylcysteine therapy.

ADDITIONAL READING

- Betten DP, Cantrell FL, Thomas SC, et al. A prospective evaluation of shortened course oral N-acetylcysteine for the treatment of acute acetaminophen poisoning. *Ann Emerg Med*. 2007;50(3):272–279.
- Bronstein AC, Spyker DA, Cantilena LR, et al. 2011 annual report of the American Association of Poison Control Centers' National Poison Data System. *Clin Toxicol*. 2012;50(10):911–1164.
- Chun LJ, Tong MJ, Busuttil RW, et al. Acetaminophen hepatotoxicity and acute liver failure. *J Clin Gastroenterol*. 2009;43(4):342–349.
- Dart RC, Erdman AR, Olson KR, et al. Acetaminophen poisoning: an evidence-based consensus guideline for out-of-hospital management. *Clin Toxicol*. 2006;44(1):1–18.
- Heard KJ. Acetylcysteine for acetaminophen poisoning. *New Engl J Med*. 2008;359(3):285–292.
- Rumack BH, Bateman DN. Acetaminophen and acetylcysteine dose and duration: past, present and future. *Clin Toxicol*. 2012;50(2): 91–98.

CODES

ICD10

- T39.1X4A Poisoning by 4-Aminophenol derivatives, undetermined, init
- K71.9 Toxic liver disease, unspecified
- T39.1X1A Poisoning by 4-Aminophenol derivatives, accidental, init

FAQ

- Q: What is "patient-tailored" *N*-acetylcysteine (NAC) therapy?
- A: The duration of *N*-acetylcysteine therapy used to depend on the pharmaceutical form administered but is now tailored to the patient based on serum acetaminophen level and liver function.
- Q: Should NAC be given PO or IV?
- A: Both seem to be similarly efficacious. Oral administration of NAC is complicated by taste aversion and vomiting. IV NAC may lead to anaphylactoid shock. Few cost–benefit studies are available for direct comparison of patient-tailored courses of oral NAC and IV NAC.

ACNE

Deepti Gupta • Renee Howard

BASICS

DESCRIPTION

Acne vulgaris is one of the most common skin conditions in children and adolescents. It is a disorder of pilosebaceous units (PSUs). PSUs are found predominantly on the face, chest, back, and upper arms. Acne presents as comedonal or inflammatory lesions and can cause depressed scars and hyperpigmentation. Presentation, treatment, and associated systemic manifestations differ by age of presentation, pubertal status, and severity of disease.

- Classification of acne by age:
  - Neonatal (birth to 6 weeks): affects up to 20% of neonates. Also known as neonatal cephalic pustulosis. Presents with a papulopustular eruption predominantly on face. Thought to be due to *Malassezia* colonization. No treatment necessary. For severe cases can use ketoconazole cream 2%.
  - Infantile acne (6 weeks to 1 year): presents with comedonal and inflammatory lesions on face. Some evidence that it may predispose to severe adolescent acne. Often, no underlying endocrine abnormality. Self-limited but in severe cases can use topical acne treatments
  - Midchildhood acne (1–6 years): uncommon. Presents with comedonal and inflammatory lesions on face. Suspect an underlying endocrinopathy.
  - Preadolescent (7–11 years): presents with predominantly comedonal lesions in "T-zone," central face. Can be first sign of onset of puberty
  - Adolescent (12–19 years): very common presentation, affects 85% of adolescents

RISK FACTORS

Genetics

Familial patterns exist, but no inheritance pattern has been demonstrated.

GENERAL PREVENTION

- Effective and early treatment limits scarring, postinflammatory pigment alteration, and minimizes psychosocial impact.
- Use of noncomedogenic moisturizers and sunscreens

PATHOPHYSIOLOGY

Pathogenesis of acne is multifactorial and involves 4 different components:

- Increased sebum production: stimulated by an increase in androgen levels. The adrenal gland is active during the 1st year of life and then reawakens in preadolescent time period. Production peaks in teens and decreases in the 20s.
- Alteration in follicular growth and differentiation leading to the creation of a microcomedone, a precursor of inflammatory and comedonal acne lesions
- Follicular colonization with *Propionibacterium acnes*, an anaerobic, gram-positive diphtheroid bacteria. *P. acnes* produces free fatty acids (FFAs) leading to inflammation.
  - Inflammation and immune response through the innate immune system

ETIOLOGY

- Androgen excess (physiologic vs. pathologic)
- Medication-induced (corticosteroids, anticonvulsants, lithium, etc.)
- Occlusion (from topical- or oil-based products)
- Friction from athletic helmets, shoulder pads, chin straps, or bra straps may worsen acne.

COMMONLY ASSOCIATED CONDITIONS

- Polycystic ovarian syndrome (PCOS)
- SAPHO syndrome: synovitis, acne, pustulosis, hyperostosis, and osteitis
- Adrenal or gonadal/ovarian tumors
- Late-onset congenital adrenal hyperplasia

DIAGNOSIS

HISTORY

- Age of onset: Early or late onset of acne may indicate androgen excess.
- Medications and supplement use (including some OCPs, progestin implants, depot medroxyprogesterone, steroids (topical, inhaled, or oral), anticonvulsants, lithium, isoniazid, nicotine products) may worsen acne.
- Menstrual history: Premenstrual flares may occur due to androgenic effects of progesterone.
- Androgen excess (history of or current)
  - Prepubertal: early-onset acne or body odor, increased linear growth, axillary or pubic hair, genital maturation, or clitoromegaly
  - Postpubertal: alopecia, hirsutism, truncal obesity, acanthosis nigricans, irregular menses, increased muscle mass
- Previous treatments tried and reason failed (cost, adherence, tolerability, ease of use).

ALERT

Psychological impact: Ask patients about self-esteem, depression, and suicidal ideations.

PHYSICAL EXAM

- Skin
  - Distribution of lesions
  - Type of acne lesions: comedonal (open: blackhead, due to oxidation of lipids and not dirt; closed: whitehead), inflammatory (erythematous papule, pustule, nodule, pseudocyst)
  - Scarring and hyperpigmentation
- Global assessment of acne severity (number, size, extent, and scarring)
- Note signs of androgen excess (see "History").
- Height, weight, growth curve
- Blood pressure

DIAGNOSTIC TESTS & INTERPRETATION

Lab/Imaging

- Consider for patients with signs of androgen excess, midchildhood acne, or acne unresponsive to traditional therapy.
  - Serologic testing (LH, FSH, testosterone total and free, DHEA-S, androstenedione prolactin, 17-hydroxyprogesterone)
  - Bone age
  - Referral to pediatric endocrinology
  - Imaging for adrenal or gonadal tumor
- Lab monitoring while using isotretinoin should include baseline and monthly complete blood count, fasting lipid panel (triglycerides and cholesterol), transaminases, and pregnancy test for females. Prior to starting females need two negative pregnancy tests 1 month apart.

DIFFERENTIAL DIAGNOSIS

- Adenoma sebaceum (facial angiofibromas)
- Keratosis pilaris
- Flat warts
- Molluscum contagiosum
- Periorificial dermatitis
- Milia
- Miliaria
- Syringomas
- *Demodex* folliculitis
- *Malassezia* (*Pityrosporum*) folliculitis
- Gram-negative folliculitis
- Staphylococcal folliculitis
- Chloracne (exposure to chlorinated aromatic hydrocarbons)
- Papular sarcoidosis

TREATMENT

- Choose regimen based on previous therapies, cost, vehicle selection, regimen complexity, active scarring, and psychosocial impact.
- Vehicle selection:
  - Creams and lotions less drying than gels and solutions
  - Creams better for sensitive skin/eczema
  - Gels and solutions may be better for oily skin or for make-up application.
- Manage patient expectations.
- Treatment may take 2–3 months to be effective.
- Acne may initially flare prior to improving.
- Counsel about medication side effects.

GENERAL APPROACH

Categorized by acne severity and age of patient.

- Mild acne: comedonal, inflammatory, or mixed
  - Initial:
    - Topical monotherapy:
      - Benzoyl peroxide (BP)
      - Topical retinoid
    - Topical combination therapy:
      - BP + antibiotic
      - Retinoid +BP
      - Retinoid + BP + antibiotic

- Inadequate response:
  - Assess adherence.
  - Add BP or retinoid if not already prescribed.
  - Change:
    - Topical retinoid concentration, type, or formulation
    - Change topical combination therapy.
- Moderate acne: comedonal, inflammatory, or mixed
  - Initial:
    - Topical combination therapy:
      - Retinoid + BP
      - Retinoid + BP + antibiotic
    - Oral antibiotic + topical retinoid + BP
  - Inadequate response:
    - Assess adherence.
    - Change topical retinoid concentration, type, or formulation.
    - Add or change oral antibiotic.
    - Females: consider hormonal therapy
    - Consider oral isotretinoin.
    - Consider dermatology referral.
- Severe acne: inflammatory, mixed, and/or nodular lesions. Extensive involvement often with significant scarring
  - Initial:
    - Oral antibiotic + topical retinoid + BP ± topical antibiotic
    - Consider dermatology referral.
  - Inadequate response:
    - Assess adherence.
    - Change topical retinoid concentration, type, or formulation.
    - Change oral antibiotic
    - Females: Consider hormonal therapy.
    - Consider oral isotretinoin.
    - Scars warrant aggressive treatment targeting inflammation.

MEDICATION (DRUGS)

- Topical agents/over the counter
  - Gentle cleansers:
    - Use gentle soap free, pH-balanced cleansers are recommended for everyday washing.
  - Benzoyl peroxide (BP):
    - Bactericidal, mild comedolytic, and anti-inflammatory properties.
    - Limits antibiotic resistance and provides increased efficacy in combination with retinoids
    - Available as lotion, cream, wash, and gel in 2.5–10%
    - Increased concentration does not increase efficacy but can cause more irritation.
    - 5% concentration generally effective. Can start with lower concentration or decrease number of days of use if too irritating
    - Side effects: drying, erythema, burning, peeling, stinging, and rarely contact dermatitis
    - Cautions: can cause bleaching of hair, clothing, and linen; increased risk of photosensitivity. Rare but serious and potentially life-threatening allergic reactions or severe irritation have been reported.
  - Salicylic acid (SA):
    - Promotes comedolysis with drying and peeling
    - Not as effective as BP
  - Sulfur/sulfacetamide:
    - Mild antibacterial and keratolytic properties
    - Very well-tolerated
    - Distinctive odor

ALERT
Avoid vigorous cleansing of the skin or harsh facial astringents and toners that may irritate the skin.

- Prescription topical medications
  - Topical antibiotics (erythromycin, clindamycin):
    - Reduce *P. acnes* concentration and inflammatory mediators
    - Available in combination products to increase compliance, but these products are often more expensive
    - Combine with BP to decrease antibiotic resistance.
    - Combine with retinoids to help yield faster results.
    - Side effects: well-tolerated but may include drying or irritation
  - Topical retinoids:
    - Prevent formation of microcomedones, clear existing microcomedones, anti-inflammatory
    - Available in 3 forms
    - Adapalene
      - Available as cream, gel, lotion. Also as a combination product with BP
      - Pregnancy class C (see Appendix 4; Table 10)
      - Photostable
      - Better tolerability than tretinoin
    - Tretinoin
      - Available as cream, gel, microsphere gel of various strengths
      - Pregnancy class C (see Appendix 4; Table 10)
      - Apply to dry skin.
      - Can be very irritating and drying
      - Start with 0.025%, low strength only a few times a week, and titrate up.
      - Inactivated by sunlight, use at nighttime.

ALERT
BP inactivates tretinoin when used together. Apply BP in the morning and tretinoin at night.

    - Tazarotene
      - Available in cream and gel
      - Pregnancy class X; contraindicated in pregnancy
      - Apply to dry skin.
      - More irritating than other retinoids
      - Inactivated by sunlight, use at nighttime.
    - 1st-line therapy for most patients
    - Side effects: erythema, dryness, irritation, initially acne flares, and photosensitivity (advise use of daily noncomedogenic sunscreen with SPF 30+ and facial moisturizer applied *before* tazarotene).
    - Apply at night, as medication is inactivated by sunlight.
    - Apply pea-sized amount to entire face.
    - Start with lowest strength three times a week, and increase frequency slowly to every night as tolerated. Some patients may not tolerate medication every night. Increase concentration of medication if patient still with oily skin or getting new acne lesions.
  - Azelaic acid:
    - Comedolytic and antibacterial; decreases hyperpigmentation
    - 15% gel or 20% cream, applied twice daily.
    - Pregnancy class B (see Appendix 4; Table 10)
    - Side effects include itching, burning, tingling, stinging, and erythema.
    - Consider for patients with comedonal acne who cannot use retinoids.
  - Topical dapsone:
    - Synthetic sulfone has antimicrobial and anti-inflammatory effects.
    - Available in 5% gel, twice daily application recommended
    - Most effective against inflammatory acne lesions
    - Safe in patients with G6PD deficiency and with sulfonamide allergy
    - Enhanced efficacy when combined with retinoids
    - Side effects: erythema and dryness
    - Caution: When used with BP, a temporary orange staining of skin can occur.

ALERT
Do not use antibiotics as monotherapy due to slow onset of action and development of antibiotic resistance. Use with BP.

- Oral antibiotics: reduce *P. acnes* concentration and inflammatory mediators
  - Tetracyclines (doxycycline, minocycline, tetracycline): pregnancy class D. Must be >8 years of age due to staining of tooth enamel
    - Doxycycline and minocycline are preferred due to 1–2×/day dosing and greater follicular penetration.
      - Dosing: 50–100 mg daily or b.i.d.
    - Tetracycline is cheap but has least efficacy.
    - Increasing antibiotic resistance. Limit treatment length and do not use as monotherapy. Use with BP or topical retinoid.
    - Taper or switch to topical retinoid monotherapy after 12 weeks and when patient is no longer getting new acne lesions.
    - Systemic side effects and cautions:
      - Doxycycline: GI upset, vaginal candidiasis, pill esophagitis, photosensitivity (phototoxicity), benign intracranial hypertension. Take with food and large glass of water, stay upright 1 hour after taking medication, photoprotection, can use enteric-coated form.
      - Minocycline: acute vestibular reaction (vertigo, dizziness), vaginal candidiasis, hyperpigmentation, drug hypersensitivity reaction 2–8 weeks after starting medication, lupuslike syndrome, Stevens-Johnson syndrome (SJS), benign intracranial hypertension

- Sulfa (trimethoprim-sulfamethoxazole):
  - Dosing: 160–800 mg PO b.i.d.
  - Used judiciously, refractory cases
  - Systemic side effects: severe cutaneous reactions (SJS, toxic epidermal necrolysis, drug hypersensitivity reaction, fixed drug eruption), bone marrow suppression
  - Check baseline CBC and periodically thereafter.
- Cephalosporins (cephalexin, cefadroxil):
  - Dosing: 500 mg PO b.i.d.
  - Well-tolerated
  - Systemic side effects: GI upset
- Penicillins (amoxicillin):
  - Well-tolerated
  - Systemic side effects: GI upset
- Macrolides (erythromycin, azithromycin)
  - High prevalence of *P. acnes* resistance to erythromycin
  - Systemic side effects: erythromycin: GI upset, drug–drug interaction

- Oral retinoids (isotretinoin): decreases sebum production, is anti-inflammatory, and reduces *P. acnes*.
  - Used as monotherapy
  - Used for recalcitrant acne or with significant scarring, given side effects
  - Dosing:
    - Start with 0.5 mg/kg/day for first 4 weeks and then advance to 1 mg/kg/day.
    - Goal cumulative treatment course is 120–150 mg/kg.
    - For patients with severely inflamed acne, start at lower dose to prevent initial acne flares or pretreat with oral corticosteroids.
  - Need baseline and monthly labs (see "Lab/Imaging")
  - Side effects:
    - Common: dry skin, dry eyes, cheilitis, myalgias
    - Teratogen
      - 2 forms of birth control need to be used while on medication.
      - FDA-mandated registry (iPledge: see https://www.ipledgeprogram.com/). Prescribed only by registered users
    - Depression and suicide have been reported in patients on isotretinoin (causality not established, but counsel about this risk).
    - IBD: conflicting data. Association may exist, but rare, and there are many confounding factors.
    - Bone effects: conflicting data regarding increased risk of fractures and demineralization. Hyperostoses and premature epiphyseal closure are rare and uncommon side effects.
    - Rare, sporadic reports of serious skin infections including erythema multiforme, Stevens-Johnson syndrome, and toxic epidermal necrolysis

ALERT

Do not use tetracycline antibiotics with oral retinoids due to risk of pseudotumor cerebri.

- Hormonal therapy: 2nd-line therapy for women. Usually used in combination with other acne treatments
  - OCPs (for women): Suppress ovarian androgen production.
  - Can be used as an adjunct for females with moderate to severe acne not responding to topical retinoids
  - 3 OCPs are FDA-approved for acne:
    - Ethinyl estradiol (35 mcg) and norgestimate (≥15 years of age)
    - Ethinyl estradiol (20–30–35 mcg) and norethindrone (≥15 years of age)
    - Ethinyl estradiol (30 mcg) and drospirenone (3 mg) (≥14 years of age)
  - Screen for personal tobacco use and family history of thromboembolic event.
    - Use caution in girls who smoke tobacco.
  - May need 3–6 months to see improvement
  - Side effects include nausea, breast tenderness, headache, weight gain, breakthrough menstrual bleeding, myocardial infarction, ischemic stroke, and DVTs.
  - Controversial effect on bone density and growth. Recommendation to start at least 1 year after onset of menstruation
- Spironolactone (for women): Blocks androgen receptor in sebaceous gland
  - Give 50–150 mg daily.
  - Off-label use can be used in combination with OCP.
  - Teratogenic effect must be on oral contraceptive.

COMPLEMENTARY & ALTERNATIVE THERAPIES

- Limited empiric studies on CAM and acne.
- RCTs of the following showed that they were not as effective as 5% BP but resulted in less skin irritation:
  - Tea tree oil: a mixture of terpenes and alcohols with antibiotic and antifungal properties; 5% solution may be effective in treating comedonal and inflammatory acne; may be associated with male gynecomastia
  - Gluconolactone 14% solution may be effective on comedonal and inflammatory acne.

ONGOING CARE

PATIENT EDUCATION

- http://www.aad.org/dermatology-a-to-z/diseases-and-treatments/a–d/acne
- http://www.nlm.nih.gov/medlineplus/acne.html (handout in Spanish also available)

COMPLICATIONS

- Scarring may be permanent.
- Hyperpigmentation: occurs more in dark-skinned individuals. Self resolves but may take months to years
- Self-esteem: Acne severity correlated to social variables including embarrassment and lack of enjoyment in social activities among teenagers.
- Patients with mild to moderate acne showed clinical depression and >5% suicidal ideation. Depression scores improve in correlation with response to acne treatment.

ADDITIONAL READING

- Eichenfield LF, Krakowski AC, Piggott C, et al. Evidence-based recommendations for the diagnosis and treatment of pediatric acne. *Pediatrics*. 2013;131(Suppl 3):163–186.
- Friedlander SF, Eichenfield LF, Fowler JF Jr, et al. Acne epidemiology and pathophysiology. *Semin Cutan Med Surg*. 2010;29(2)(Suppl 1):2–4.
- Sawni A, Singh A. Complementary, holistic, and integrative medicine: acne. *Pediatr Rev*. 2013;34(2):91–93.
- U.S. Food and Drug Administration. Over-the-counter topical acne products: drug safety communication—rare but serious hypersensitivity reactions. http://www.fda.gov/Safety/MedWatch/SafetyInformation/SafetyAlertsforHumanMedicalProducts/ucm402722.htm. Accessed February 5, 2015.
- Yan AC, Baldwin HE, Eichenfield LF, et al. Approach to pediatric acne treatment: an update. *Semin Cutan Med Surg*. 2011;30(3)(Suppl):S16–S21.

CODES

ICD10

- L70.9 Acne, unspecified
- L70.4 Infantile acne
- L70.0 Acne vulgaris

FAQ

- Q: Can I modify my diet to improve my acne?
- A: No. Specific dietary modifications are recommended, but there has been limited data that low glycemic diets may be correlated with improvement in acne.
- Q: Does poor hygiene cause acne?
- A: No. Use of harsh astringents, exfoliating scrubs, and vigorous scrubbing can worsen acne by causing more inflammation and scarring. They also can be more irritating and drying, decreasing tolerability of acne treatments. Recommend use of a gentle, soap free, pH-balanced cleanser for daily use in addition to noncomedogenic moisturizers and sunscreen in conjunction with acne treatments.
- Q: Do cosmetics worsen acne?
- A: Recommend use of oil free, noncomedogenic make-up, which have been proven not to delay treatment response or worsen acne severity.

ACQUIRED HYPOTHYROIDISM

Adda Grimberg

BASICS

DESCRIPTION

Hypothyroidism that occurs after the neonatal period

EPIDEMIOLOGY

- May develop at any age
- Autoimmune thyroid disorders occur more frequently in children and adolescents with type 1 diabetes and other autoimmune conditions.
- Chronic lymphocytic thyroiditis prevalence correlates with iodine intake; countries with the highest dietary iodine also have the highest prevalence.

RISK FACTORS

Genetics

- Family history of thyroid disease or other autoimmune endocrinopathies increases risk.
- Genetic predisposition in patients with chronic lymphocytic thyroiditis; 30–40% of patients have a family history of thyroid disease, and up to 50% of their 1st-degree relatives have thyroid antibodies.
- Weak associations of chronic lymphocytic thyroiditis with certain human leukocyte antigen haplotypes; also associated with genotypes of cytotoxic T lymphocyte–associated 4 (*CTLA4*) and interleukin-18 (*IL-18*) genes.
- Autoimmune thyroid disease may be part of Schmidt syndrome (type II polyglandular autoimmune disease).
- Genetic syndromes associated with higher incidence of autoimmune thyroiditis:
  - Down syndrome
  - Turner syndrome (especially those with isochromosome Xq)

ETIOLOGY

- Myriad causes (see "Differential Diagnosis")
- Can result from thyroid gland dysfunction (primary hypothyroidism) or from pituitary/hypothalamic dysfunction leading to understimulation of the thyroid gland (secondary and tertiary hypothyroidism)

COMMONLY ASSOCIATED CONDITIONS

- Vitiligo
- Alopecia areata
- Pernicious anemia
- Other autoimmune conditions

DIAGNOSIS

HISTORY

- Linear growth failure can be the first sign of thyroid dysfunction.
- Declining school performance is a sensitive marker for lethargy and reduced focus.
- Radiation exposure, history of type 1 diabetes, family history of other autoimmune disorders
- Signs and symptoms:
  - Early primary hypothyroidism can be asymptomatic.
  - Hypothyroid-related symptoms indicate progression from compensated to uncompensated hypothyroidism.
  - Hypothyroidism may be preceded in some cases by temporary hyperthyroidism (Hashitoxicosis).
  - Goiter may be the presenting sign of acquired hypothyroidism; tenderness suggests an infectious process.

PHYSICAL EXAM

- Bradycardia: Thyroid hormone has cardiac effects.
- Short stature (or fall-off on growth curve) and increased upper/lower segment ratio: Euthyroidism is required to maintain normal growth.
- Goiter: Note consistency, symmetry, nodularity, signs of inflammation:
  - May give a clue regarding cause of hypothyroidism
  - May provide a clinical marker to follow during therapy
- Myxedema (water retention) is not limited to subcutaneous tissue; it may also lead to cardiac failure, pleural effusions, and coma.
- Muscle hypertrophy, yet muscle weakness
  - Most obvious in arms, legs, and tongue
  - Hypothyroidism causes disordered muscle function.
- Delayed relaxation phase of deep tendon reflexes due to slowed muscle contraction
- Pale, cool, dry, carotenemic (yellow-colored) skin due to decreased cell turnover
- Increase in lanugo hair in children; can be reversed with treatment
- Sexual development is an important factor. Hypothyroidism may be associated with either
  - Delayed puberty (due to low thyroid hormone level)
  - Precocious puberty and galactorrhea (due to elevated TSH

DIAGNOSTIC TESTS & INTERPRETATION

Lab

- T_4 (low) and TSH (elevated): Elevated TSH with normal T_4 indicates compensated (subclinical) primary hypothyroidism.
- Free T_4: The most sensitive marker for secondary/tertiary hypothyroidism (TSH elevation lost; total T_4 may still be low normal)
- Thyroglobulin antibodies and thyroid peroxidase (microsomal) antibodies are markers for chronic lymphocytic thyroiditis.
- The following conditions may test false-positive for acquired hypothyroidism:
  - Thyroid-binding globulin deficiency: low total T_4 but normal free T_4 and TSH
  - Peripheral resistance to thyroid hormone: normal/high total T_4
  - "Euthyroid sick" syndrome: low T_4 and T_3; normal/low TSH; increased shunting to reverse T_3
- The following tests may be affected in acquired hypothyroidism:
  - Serum creatinine: elevated due to reduced glomerular filtration rate
  - LDL cholesterol level: elevated due to decreased LDL receptor expression
  - Creatine kinase: increased; hypothyroidism is a rare cause of rhabdomyolysis.

Imaging

Head MRI for cases of suspected secondary/tertiary hypothyroidism or pituitary or hypothalamic lesion

DIFFERENTIAL DIAGNOSIS

- Immunologic
  - Chronic lymphocytic thyroiditis (Hashimoto thyroiditis)
  - Polyglandular autoimmune syndrome (Schmidt syndrome)
- Infectious
  - Postviral subacute thyroiditis
  - Associated with congenital infections
    - Rubella
    - Toxoplasmosis
- Environmental
  - Goitrogen ingestion
    - Iodides
    - Expectorants
    - Thioureas
- Iatrogenic
  - Following surgical thyroidectomy for thyroid cancer, hyperthyroidism, or extensive neck tumors
  - Following radioiodine ablative therapy for hyperthyroidism or thyroid cancer
  - Following head or neck irradiation for cancer treatment
  - Medications: lithium, amiodarone, iodine contrast dyes, tiratricol (an OTC fat-loss supplement)
- Metabolic
  - Cystinosis
  - Histiocytosis X
- Congenital
  - Late-onset congenital, large ectopic gland
- Genetic syndromes
  - Down syndrome
  - Turner syndrome
- Secondary or tertiary hypothyroidism
  - Hypothalamic or pituitary disease
- Consumptive hypothyroidism
  - Due to increased type 3 iodothyronine deiodinase activity in hemangiomas

TREATMENT

MEDICATION

L-Thyroxine (synthetic thyroid hormone) replacement

- Indicated for the treatment of overt or compensated hypothyroidism
- 2–5 mcg/kg PO once daily
- Monitor T_4 and TSH and titrate dose to maintain normalized thyroid function tests.
- Duration of therapy:
  - Lifetime
  - In 30% of the cases, children with chronic lymphocytic thyroiditis will undergo spontaneous remission.
  - Need for treatment can be reassessed after growth is completed.

ONGOING CARE

FOLLOW-UP RECOMMENDATIONS

Patient Monitoring

- Whenever starting medication or adjusting dose, check T_4 and TSH at 4–6-week intervals to assess adequacy of the new dose.
- Once dose established, 6-monthly monitoring until linear growth completed
- Monitor response to treatment by measuring T_4 and TSH levels to ensure compliance.

PATIENT EDUCATION

Pharmacies in recent years have been recommending that L-thyroxine be administered on an empty stomach. The Drugs and Therapeutics Committee of the Pediatric Endocrine Society recommended that consistency in administration, coupled with regular dose titration based on thyroid function laboratory tests, is more important than improving absorption by restricting intake to only times of empty stomach.

PROGNOSIS

- If patients are adherent, prognosis is excellent.
- Treated patients often resume growth at a rate greater than normal (catch-up growth).
- In children in whom treatment has been delayed, catch-up growth may not fully normalize height to predicted values.
- Other signs and symptoms resolve at a variable rate.
- Goiters in chronic lymphocytic thyroiditis may not completely regress with treatment (enlargement due to persistent inflammation does not correct, although TSH-mediated hypertrophy will).

COMPLICATIONS

- Most significant complication is impaired linear growth.
- Puberty can also be affected.
- Myxedema coma may occur.
- Encephalopathy of varied clinical presentation has been associated with high titers of thyroid antibodies, especially antimicrosomal; this condition responds well to corticosteroid treatment.

ADDITIONAL READING

- Ai J, Leonhardt JM, Heymann WR. Autoimmune thyroid diseases: etiology, pathogenesis, and dermatologic manifestations. *J Am Acad Dermatol*. 2003;48(5):641–659.
- Ban Y, Tomer Y. Genetic susceptibility in thyroid autoimmunity. *Pediatr Endocrinol Rev*. 2005;3(1):20–32.
- Haugen BR. Drugs that suppress TSH or cause central hypothyroidism. *Best Pract Res Clin Endocrinol Metab*. 2009;23(6):793–800.
- Monzani A, Prodam F, Rapa A, et al. Endocrine disorders in childhood and adolescence. Natural history of subclinical hypothyroidism in children and adolescents and potential effects of replacement therapy: a review. *Eur J Endocrinol*. 2012;168(1):R1–R11.
- Nabhan ZM, Kreher NC, Eugster EA. Hashitoxicosis in children: Clinical features and natural history. *J Pediatr*. 2005;146(4):533–536.
- Nebesio TD, Wise MD, Perkins SM, et al. Does clinical management impact height potential in children with severe acquired hypothyroidism? *J Pediatr Endocrinol Metab*. 2011;24(11–12):893–896.
- Pearce EN, Farwell AP, Braverman LE. Thyroiditis. *N Engl J Med*. 2003;348(26):2646–2655.
- Radetti G, Maselli M, Buzi F, et al. The natural history of the normal/mild elevated TSH serum levels in children and adolescents with Hashimoto's thyroiditis and isolated hyperthyrotropinaemia: a 3-year follow-up. *Clin Endocrinol (Oxf)*. 2012;76(3):394–398.
- Stathatos N, Wartofsky L. Perioperative management of patients with hypothyroidism. *Endocrinol Metab Clin North Am*. 2003;32(2):503–518.
- Wasniewska M, Corrias A, Salerno M, et al. Thyroid function patterns at Hashimoto's thyroiditis presentation in childhood and adolescence are mainly conditioned by patients' age. *Horm Res Paediatr*. 2012;78(4):232–236.
- Weber G, Vigone MC, Stroppa L, et al. Thyroid function and puberty. *J Pediatr Endocrinol Metab*. 2003;16(Suppl 2):S253–S257.
- Zeitler P, Solberg P; Pharmacy and Therapeutics Committee of the Lawson Wilkins Pediatric Endocrine Society. Food and levothyroxine administration in infants and children. *J Pediatr*. 2010;157(1):13.e1–14.e1.

CODES

ICD10

- E03.9 Hypothyroidism, unspecified
- E03.8 Other specified hypothyroidism
- E06.3 Autoimmune thyroiditis

FAQ

- Q: What happens if my child forgets a dose?
- A: Give the dose as soon as you remember. If it is the next day, give 2 doses.
- Q: How long will my child have to take these pills?
- A: Probably for life.
- Q: Are there any side effects from the medication?
- A: No. The medication contains only the hormone that your child's thyroid gland is not making. The hormone is made synthetically, so there is also no infectious risk.
- Q: If my child takes twice the dose, will his or her growth catch up faster?
- A: Your child may grow a little faster but will also have adverse effects from having too much thyroid hormone.
- Q: Does the medication have to be taken at any particular time of day?
- A: No, but consistently choosing the same time of day helps to remember to take it. Do not take simultaneously with soy products, iron-containing medication, calcium supplements, or raloxifene (an antiestrogen medication) because they can cause malabsorption of levothyroxine.
- Q: What if my child needs surgery?
- A: Treatment of hypothyroidism such that the patient is euthyroid (normal thyroid status) prior to surgery is preferable whenever possible (only exception is ischemic heart disease requiring surgery). Euthyroid sick syndrome, which is common in very ill patients, should not be treated.

ACUTE DRUG WITHDRAWAL

Robert J. Hoffman

BASICS

DESCRIPTION
- Drug withdrawal is a physiologic response to an effectively lowered drug concentration in a patient with tolerance to that drug.
- Withdrawal results in a predictable pattern of symptoms that are reversible if the drug in question or another appropriate substitute is reintroduced.
- Sedative-hypnotic withdrawal is the most common life-threatening withdrawal syndrome in children. This includes withdrawal from barbiturates, benzodiazepines, as well as gamma-hydroxybutyrate and similar substances.
- Other substances that are associated with withdrawal syndromes include opioids, selective serotonin reuptake inhibitors (SSRIs), and caffeine.

EPIDEMIOLOGY
- The most common life-threatening withdrawal syndrome, alcohol withdrawal, rarely occurs in children.
- Neonates born to alcohol-dependent mothers are at risk.

RISK FACTORS
Patients receiving sedatives or analgesics capable of causing tolerance are at risk. This is particularly true with infusions or high doses of such substances in previously naïve patients.

GENERAL PREVENTION
- Clinician familiarity with tolerance and withdrawal associated with prescribed medications allows appropriate drug tapering.
- Drug abuse prevention is appropriate for all children.

PATHOPHYSIOLOGY
- Altered CNS neurochemistry is the most important and clinically relevant aspect of withdrawal pathophysiology.
- Under normal conditions, the CNS maintains a balance between excitation and inhibition. Although there are several ways to achieve this balance, excitation is constant and actions occur through removal of inhibitory tone.
- Relative to adults and younger children, adolescents are more prone to develop dependence and withdrawal syndrome due to immaturity of their prefrontal cortex.

ETIOLOGY
- Neonates
  - Maternal alcohol, caffeine, opioid, sedative-hypnotic, or SSRI use may result in a neonatal abstinence syndrome.
  - Treatment with caffeine, opioids, or sedative-hypnotics may result in subsequent development of an abstinence syndrome.
- Older children
  - Subsequent to treatment with opioids, or sedative-hypnotics, an abstinence syndrome may result.
  - Substance abuse, particularly opioids, gamma-hydroxybutyrate, or other sedative-hypnotics, may result in an abstinence syndrome.
  - Frequent caffeine or nicotine use may lead to an abstinence syndrome.
- Use of opioid antagonists such as naloxone, naltrexone, and nalmefene is associated with opioid withdrawal.

DIAGNOSIS

- Drug withdrawal is a clinical diagnosis.
- Patients should be evaluated for associated diagnoses such as traumatic injury, pneumonia, etc.

HISTORY
- Typically, a history of substance exposure, either direct exposure or maternal use, will be elicited.
  - Exposure may be to prescribed medication or abusable substances.
  - Substance use by the mother or child might intentionally be concealed.
- The timing of withdrawal varies depending on the half-life of the substance involved.
  - The shorter the half-life, the sooner the onset of withdrawal and typically the more severe withdrawal symptoms.
- Alcohol or sedative-hypnotics
  - Withdrawal from these may result in tremulousness, diaphoresis, agitation, insomnia, altered mental status, or withdrawal seizures.
  - Baclofen withdrawal is more frequently severe or life threatening relative to benzodiazepine withdrawal. History of pump manipulation or malfunction should be sought.
- Caffeine
  - Withdrawal may result in dysphoria, headache, behavioral changes, or agitation.
- Opioids
  - Nausea, vomiting, diarrhea, irritability, yawning, sleeplessness, diaphoresis, lacrimation, tremor, and hypertonicity may result.
  - Neonates can also have seizures, a high-pitched cry, skin mottling, and excoriation. These latter signs and symptoms are more typical of opioid withdrawal and rarely occur with neonatal alcohol withdrawal.
- Nicotine
  - Dysphoria, agitation, behavioral changes, and increased appetite may all occur.
- SSRIs
  - Neonatal withdrawal from SSRIs may result in jitteriness, agitation, crying, shivering, increased muscle tone, breathing and sucking problems, as well as seizure.
  - Children withdrawing from SSRIs may have jitteriness, agitation, dysphoria, behavioral changes, shivering, increased muscle tone, and seizure.

PHYSICAL EXAM
- Vital signs including temperature should be evaluated regularly. Vital sign changes such as tachycardia and hypertension may occur concomitantly with acute drug withdrawal.
- Technology-dependent patients, such as children with an intrathecal baclofen pump, should have evaluation of the machine to determine if it is working properly.
- Most cases of substance withdrawal only result in behavioral changes.
- Opioid withdrawal may be accompanied by diaphoresis, mydriasis, yawning, and lacrimation.
- Sedative-hypnotic withdrawal may result in hypertension, tachycardia, hyperthermia, agitation, hallucinations, and seizure.

DIAGNOSTIC TESTS & INTERPRETATION

Imaging
Neuroimaging to rule out intracranial pathology may rarely be indicated.

Diagnostic Procedures/Other
- No routine lab tests are indicated for patients with substance withdrawal.
- Tests necessary to rule out differential diagnoses should be obtained when appropriate.

DIFFERENTIAL DIAGNOSIS
- Hypoglycemia
- Intoxication with sympathomimetics, anticholinergics, theophylline, caffeine, aspirin, or lithium
- Thyroid storm
- Serotonin syndrome
- Neuroleptic malignant syndrome
- Encephalitis
- Meningitis
- Sepsis

TREATMENT

MEDICATION
- Symptom-triggered treatment has been demonstrated to be superior to fixed-regimen treatment in terms of patient outcome as well as length of stay.
- Patients experiencing withdrawal from benzodiazepines or barbiturates after treatment in a chronic or intensive care setting may be treated by reinstituting the drug and then tapering.
- Iatrogenic withdrawal induced by use of opioid antagonists should not be treated by opioid administration.
  - Withdrawal induced by naloxone should abate rapidly due to the brief half-life of naloxone.
  - Withdrawal induced by naltrexone or nalmefene will be much longer lasting. Symptomatic treatment may be indicated.

- There is no fixed quantity of drug to use for any withdrawal syndrome. Each patient requires a unique quantity of drug.
  - Repeated dosing should continue until the symptoms are controlled, at which point maintenance and then tapering can occur.
- Sedative-hypnotic withdrawal
  - Ideally, withdrawal is treated with the same class of substance, such as benzodiazepine or barbiturate, if not the precise same drug.
  - Benzodiazepines are particularly useful due to the rapid onset of effect.
  - Diazepam has active metabolites that assist in tapering the drug.
  - Propofol is an outstanding medication for treatment of severe alcohol or sedative-hypnotic withdrawal in adults.
    - Propofol may be used in pediatric cases refractory to benzodiazepines and barbiturates.
    - Use is associated with respiratory depression.
    - Clinicians must be capable of airway management and expect airway support to be necessary when propofol is used.
    - Propofol use is safe in children, but rare cases of metabolic acidemia have occurred when prolonged infusions are used. Prolonged use of propofol infusion should be accompanied by close observation for acidemia.
- Opioid withdrawal
  - Heroin (as well as other opioids) withdrawal is best treated with an opioid of similar potency and equal or longer duration of action.
  - Methadone is a preferred treatment for withdrawal in adolescents and adults, but most neonatologists have limited or no experience with this drug.
  - Patients who experience opioid withdrawal in the setting of chronic or intensive care may be treated by reinstituting infusion or dosing of the drug they were on before withdrawal symptoms and then tapering this, typically by 10% daily.
- Caffeine withdrawal
  - Caffeine as soft drink or tea taken to treat headache or agitation
  - Neonatal caffeine abstinence symptoms may be treated by reinstituting 75–100% of the caffeine dosage that was discontinued. This amount is then tapered, typically by 10% daily.
- Nicotine withdrawal is not typically treated in children.
- Use of nicotine patch, gum, or other delivery methods is used to increase success rate of abstinence rather than for medical management of the withdrawal syndrome.

ADDITIONAL TREATMENT

General Measures

- Initial stabilization
  - Initial management is aimed at evaluating and supporting airway, breathing, circulation, serum glucose, and ECG ("A, B, C, D, E").
- Supportive care is the most important general principle.
- The illness is managed with intent of close monitoring and addressing issues as they arise.

ISSUES FOR REFERRAL

- Any patient with substance abuse issues should be referred for appropriate psychiatric or drug counseling.
- Most cases of substance withdrawal are best handled by an addiction specialist, medical toxicologist, intensivist, or other clinician experienced with management of withdrawal.

INPATIENT CONSIDERATIONS

Admission Criteria

- Inpatient treatment for alcohol or sedative-hypnotic withdrawal is mandatory.
- Although withdrawal from opioids and SSRIs is not life threatening, admission with initial management as an inpatient is preferable.

IV Fluids

- Maintenance IV fluid may be required in patients who are unable to take PO.
- Dehydration was once a leading cause of death among patients with alcohol withdrawal.

Discharge Criteria

- Inpatients who have been converted from parenteral to oral medications and are controlled with oral medications may be discharged for home tapering.
- Patients who never require parenteral therapy may be discharged with oral replacement medication after consultation with the appropriate specialist.

ONGOING CARE

FOLLOW-UP RECOMMENDATIONS

- If disposition will be discharge, it is crucial to ensure that the patient's condition is stable before discharge.
- If there is any question regarding whether the patient can be appropriately managed as an outpatient, initial inpatient management is preferable.

Patient Monitoring

- Sedative-hypnotic withdrawal or any other withdrawal syndrome with severe symptoms is best cared for with initial cardiopulmonary monitoring until vital sign abnormalities are controlled with appropriate replacement therapy.
- Patients should be closely monitored until vital signs are within acceptable limits.
- Vigilance for agitation or delirium with sedative-hypnotic withdrawal is necessary.
- Vigilance to detect oversedation and respiratory depression is necessary.

PATIENT EDUCATION

Patients or parents should be aware of withdrawal symptoms to be vigilant for detecting future events.

PROGNOSIS

- With appropriate therapy, withdrawal is well tolerated.
- Poor prognostic factors are primarily related to comorbidities.

COMPLICATIONS

Complications of hypertension, tachycardia, hyperthermia, and CNS agitation or seizure may occur with sedative-hypnotic withdrawal.

ADDITIONAL READING

- Anand KJS, Willson DF, Berger J, et al. Tolerance and withdrawal from prolonged opioid use in critically ill children. *Pediatrics*. 2010;125(5):e1208–e1225.
- Dyer JE, Roth B, Hyma BA. Gamma-hydroxybutyrate withdrawal syndrome. *Ann Emerg Med*. 2001;37(2):147–153.
- Galinkin J, Koh JL. Recognition of and management of iatrogenically induced opioid dependence and withdrawal in children. *Pediatrics*. 2014;133(1):152–155.
- Hudak ML, Tan RC. Neonatal drug withdrawal. *Pediatrics*. 2012;129(2):e540–e560.
- Neonatal complications after intrauterine exposure to SSRI antidepressants. *Prescrire Int*. 2004;13(71):103–104.
- Nordeng H, Lindeman R, Perminov KV, et al. Neowithdrawal syndrome after in utero exposure to selective serotonin reuptake inhibitors. *Acta Paediatr*. 2001;90(3):288–291.
- Robe LB, Gromisch DS, Iosub S. Symptoms of neonatal ethanol withdrawal. *Curr Alcohol*. 1981;8:485–493.
- Tobias JD. Tolerance, withdrawal, and physical dependency after long-term sedation and analgesia of children in the pediatric intensive care unit. *Crit Care Med*. 2000;28(6):2122–2132.

CODES

ICD10

- P96.1 Neonatal w/drawal symp from matern use of drugs of addiction
- P96.2 Withdrawal symptoms from therapeutic use of drugs in newborn
- F13.939 Sedatv/hyp/anxiolytc use, unsp w withdrawal, unsp

ACUTE KIDNEY INJURY

Shina Menon • Stuart Goldstein

BASICS

DESCRIPTION

- Acute kidney injury (AKI) is defined as an abrupt (within 48 hours) reduction in kidney function with an absolute increase in serum creatinine of more than or equal to 0.3 mg/dL, or a 1.5-fold increase from baseline or a reduction in urine output (documented oliguria of less than 0.5 mL/kg per hour for more than 6 hours).
- The pediatric modified RIFLE (risk, injury, failure, loss, and end-stage renal disease) system classifies the degree of renal insult by changes in serum creatinine and/or the duration of oliguria.
- In AKI, the urine output is variable: anuria, oliguria and, in some cases, polyuria can all be observed at presentation.

EPIDEMIOLOGY

- The epidemiology of AKI has changed over the recent years from primary kidney disease to a syndrome secondary to other systemic illness.
- AKI may be seen in up to 10% of all hospitalized children. The incidence is higher in ICU admissions and with increasing multiorgan disease severity.

PATHOPHYSIOLOGY

The pathogenesis of AKI is multifactorial. It may be initiated by ischemia or toxins, and the subsequent injury involves a complex interplay between vasoconstriction, leukostasis, vascular congestion, cell death, and abnormal immune modulators.

ETIOLOGY

Previously, AKI was subcategorized into 3 groups: prerenal, renal, and postrenal. The differentiation between "prerenal" and "renal" causes can be difficult because renal hypoperfusion may coexist with any stage of AKI.

- Prerenal azotemia (functional)
  - Decreased glomerular filtration rate (GFR) resulting from renal hypoperfusion in a structurally intact kidney
  - Often rapidly reversible when the underlying cause is corrected
- Intrinsic (structural)
  - Disorders that directly affect the kidney
  - Acute tubular necrosis (ATN) was used in the past to describe a form of intrinsic AKI from severe and persistent hypoperfusion of the kidneys. However, the histologic diagnosis of tubular necrosis is rarely confirmed by biopsy.
  - Glomerular disorders include the various forms of acute glomerulonephritis (AGN) (e.g., postinfectious, rapidly progressive [crescentic]).
  - Vascular lesions compromise glomerular blood flow. Hemolytic uremic syndrome (HUS) is the most common vascular disorder that causes intrinsic AKI in children.
  - Acute interstitial nephritis (AIN) most often occurs as a result of exposure to medications such as NSAIDs. It may also be associated with infections (e.g., pyelonephritis), systemic diseases, or tumor infiltrates.
- Postrenal
  - Obstructive process (either structural or functional)
  - Obstruction can be in the lower tract or bilaterally in the upper tracts (unless the patient has a single kidney).
  - More common in newborns

DIAGNOSIS

HISTORY

- Previous infection, neurogenic bladder, single kidney
- Exposure to nonsteroidal anti-inflammatory agents, β-lactam antibiotics, acyclovir, aminoglycosides, amphotericin B, cisplatin
- Gross hematuria: AGN (tea colored), renal calculi (bright red blood)
- Trauma: crush injury
- Signs and symptoms: fever, rash bloody diarrhea, pallor, severe vomiting or diarrhea, abdominal pain hemorrhage, shock, anuria, polyuria

PHYSICAL EXAM

- General: weight and hydration status; shock, edema (calculation of percent fluid overload), jaundice
- Lungs: rales
- Heart: gallop
- Abdomen/pelvis: mass
- Skin: rash, petechiae
- Joints: arthritis

DIAGNOSTIC TESTS & INTERPRETATION

Lab

- All patients with AKI should have a urinalysis with microscopic exam, serum chemistries, and a CBC:
  - Urinalysis: specific gravity (>1.020 suggests prerenal AKI), proteinuria (>3+ intrinsic, glomerular AKI), eosinophiluria (AIN), pyuria (pyelonephritis), granular casts (prerenal, ATN), pigmenturia (ATN), erythrocyte casts (glomerulonephritis, AIN, ATN)
  - Serum chemistries: hyponatremia, acidosis, hyperkalemia, hypocalcemia, hyperphosphatemia
  - CBC: microangiopathic hemolytic anemia, thrombocytopenia (i.e., HUS), eosinophilia (i.e., AIN)
  - Selected patients require further studies, including serologies, urine electrolytes, imaging, and renal biopsy:
    - Serologies: hypocomplementemia, antineutrophil cytoplasmic antibodies, antinuclear antibodies (AGN)
- The fractional excretion of sodium (FENa)
  - Can be useful to assess tubular function. FENa = [(UNa/PNa)/(Ucreat/Pcreat)] × 100.
  - The FENa should not be obtained after diuretics are administered. FENa >2: ATN; FENa <1: AGN, prerenal
  - FENa can be <1% despite ATN in case of radiocontrast nephropathy or pigment nephropathy.
- Fractional excretion of urea (FEUrea)
  - Less affected by diuretics
  - FEUrea = [(UUrea/PUrea)/(Ucreat/Pcreat)] × 100
  - FEUrea <35: prerenal AKI; FEUrea >50: ATN

Imaging

- Chest radiograph: cardiomegaly or pulmonary edema (fluid overload)
- Renal US: hydronephrosis, trabeculated bladder (i.e., obstruction), increased echogenicity (i.e., ATN, AIN, AGN, HUS), abnormal Doppler study (renal venous thrombosis)

Diagnostic Procedures/Other

Renal biopsy: indicated in patients with prolonged, unexplained AKI or suspicion for crescentic glomerulonephritis

DIFFERENTIAL DIAGNOSIS

- Chronic kidney disease: insidious, associated with poor growth, normocytic anemia, hyperparathyroidism
- Azotemia (elevated BUN): hypercatabolic states including corticosteroid therapy or upper GI bleeding
- Elevated creatinine: caused by rhabdomyolysis, drugs (trimethoprim-sulfamethoxazole, cimetidine)

TREATMENT

MEDICATION

- Clearance of many medications is impaired in AKI. Careful monitoring of drug dosing and levels can minimize toxicity.
- Low-dose (renal dose) dopamine is ineffective in improving kidney function in AKI. Loop diuretics (furosemide) and osmotic diuretics (mannitol) do not affect the progression or outcome of AKI and may be harmful.
- Bicarbonate may be useful to treat AKI in rhabdomyolysis.
- *N*-acetylcysteine and bicarbonate, used prophylactically, may prevent contrast nephropathy.

ADDITIONAL THERAPIES

- Supportive
  - Avoid nephrotoxic medications when possible.
  - Monitor electrolytes closely. Avoid drugs, fluids, or foods containing potassium in patients with oliguria or anuria.
  - Hyponatremia is usually due to free water excess and should be managed with fluid restriction. Hypertonic saline should be used only if CNS symptoms are present.
- Fluid management
  - Can be divided into 3 phases based on the clinical status
  - Fluid resuscitation/repletion: The goal is to restore end-organ perfusion.
  - Fluid balance maintenance: After initial resuscitation, the patient's ongoing fluid needs (blood products, medications, nutrition) should be balanced with the output (urine and insensible losses). Fluid restriction may be needed to avoid worsening fluid overload. Increasing degrees of fluid overload (%FO) at initiation of renal replacement therapy (RRT) are independently associated with mortality.
  - Fluid overload may be calculated as:
    - %FO = (Fluid Input [L] − Fluid Output [L])/ Patient ICU admission weight (kg) × 100
  - Fluid removal/recovery: If the fluid conservative strategy does not work, RRT may be needed to remove the volumes associated with patient needs.
- RRT is indicated for fluid overload, refractory acidosis, severe hyperkalemia, and uremic symptoms (e.g., pericarditis, lethargy, bleeding diathesis). The modality of RRT (hemodialysis or continuous RRT) depends on the hemodynamic status of the patient.
- Provision of adequate nutrition is essential due to the high prevalence of malnutrition in this group and the associated morbidity and mortality. Protein restriction with the aim of delaying RRT is not recommended.
- Specific treatment based on etiology: Each cause of AKI may necessitate specific treatment, such as fluid resuscitation (i.e., prerenal), urologic intervention (i.e., obstruction), and corticosteroids (i.e., AIN, some forms of AGN).

INPATIENT CONSIDERATIONS

Initial Stabilization

- If hypovolemic, rapidly establish euvolemia with 0.9% NS or balanced solution boluses.
- If urine output remains low after euvolemia is established, begin fluid restriction (insensible losses and urine output).
- In severe hyperkalemia (>6.5 mEq/L), consider the following:
  - Calcium gluconate (100 mg Ca gluconate salt/kg IV) over 5–10 minutes if symptomatic
  - Glucose (0.5 g/kg) and insulin (0.1 U/kg) IV over 30 minutes
  - Sodium bicarbonate (1–2 mEq/kg) IV over 10–30 minutes if acidotic
  - When administering sodium bicarbonate, monitor serum calcium carefully because the hypocalcemia may worsen.
  - Kayexalate (1 g/kg) PO or PR in sorbitol
  - Furosemide (1–2 mg/kg) if renal function is adequate
  - RRT

ONGOING CARE

FOLLOW-UP RECOMMENDATIONS

- The likelihood of recovery from AKI depends on the underlying cause.
- AKI may result in full recovery or incomplete recovery leading to chronic kidney disease. In severe cases, nonrecovery may lead to end-stage renal disease.
- Long-term follow-up to monitor renal function is recommended.

PROGNOSIS

The mortality rate increases in patients with multisystem organ failure despite good supportive care. AKI is independently associated with increased mortality in ICU patients.

COMPLICATIONS

- A significant postobstructive diuresis can be seen after treatment for obstructive AKI.
- Fluid overload, resulting in congestive heart failure, hypertension, or hyponatremia
- Hyperkalemia, affecting cardiac function by causing arrhythmias
- Uremia, manifest by mental status changes, increased risk of bleeding, and infection
- Metabolic acidosis
- Hypocalcemia, causing tetany

ADDITIONAL READING

- Fortenberry JD, Paden ML, Goldstein SL. Acute kidney injury in children: an update on diagnosis and treatment. *Pediatr Clin North Am*. 2013;60(3): 669–688.
- KDIGO AKI Work Group. KDIGO clinical practice guideline for acute kidney injury. *Kidney Int Suppl*. 2012;2(1):1–138.
- Singri N, Ahya SN, Levin ML. Acute renal failure. *JAMA*. 2003;289(6):747–751.
- Zappitelli M. Epidemiology and diagnosis of acute kidney injury. *Semin Nephrol*. 2008;28(5):436–446.

CODES

ICD10

- N17.9 Acute kidney failure, unspecified
- N17.0 Acute kidney failure with tubular necrosis
- N00.9 Acute nephritic syndrome with unsp morphologic changes

FAQ

- Q: What is the expected recovery time in patients with AKI who present with anuria?
- A: Recovery time depends on the etiology of the AKI. Children with HUS may recover in days to weeks. In severe HUS or AKI requiring RRT, ongoing recovery to new, baseline renal function occurs over several months. Those with ATN recover days after treatment for the cause. Children with AKI secondary to an obstructive process usually recover as soon as the obstruction is removed.
- Q: When should renal function return to normal?
- A: Renal function may never return to normal in patients with long-standing anuria. In other cases, after recovery occurs, serum creatinine levels return to normal within weeks.
- Q: Which indices should be observed after a patient recovers from AKI?
- A: Patients recovering from AKI should have renal function (serum creatinine and cystatin C), BP, and urinalysis for proteinuria monitored regularly.

ACUTE LIVER FAILURE

Krupa R. Mysore • Kristin L. Van Buren • Eric H. Chiou

BASICS

DESCRIPTION

- A set of criteria has been proposed to diagnose pediatric acute liver failure (ALF).
  - Biochemical evidence of liver injury due to rapid loss of hepatocyte function
  - No previous history of chronic liver disease
  - Coagulopathy not responsive to vitamin K administration
  - International normalized ratio (INR) >1.5 in presence of encephalopathy or INR >2 without encephalopathy
- In older children, in whom hepatic encephalopathy can be more easily assessed, ALF may more simply be defined as follows:
  - Onset of encephalopathy <8 weeks after the onset of symptoms referable to liver dysfunction in a patient without preexisting liver disease

EPIDEMIOLOGY

- Exact frequency of ALF in children is unknown but accounts for 10–15% of pediatric liver transplants in the United States annually.
- In infants and children <3 years of age, indeterminate and metabolic etiologies predominate.
- In older children, drug-induced toxicity (especially acetaminophen), autoimmune hepatitis become more common.
- Infectious etiologies, (e.g., viral hepatitis) vary in prevalence based on geographic region.

PATHOPHYSIOLOGY

- Hepatocellular necrosis leads to release of growth factors that promote hepatic regeneration.
- Hepatic failure may become irreversible if:
  - The initial insult overcomes the liver's regenerative capacity.
  - The offending agent or derangement is not eliminated or corrected.
  - Secondary complications, such as shock or disseminated intravascular coagulation, lead to further injury.

ETIOLOGY

The major causes of ALF can be grouped into the following broad categories:

- Indeterminate
- Drug-induced/toxin
- Metabolic/genetic
- Infectious
- Vascular/ischemic
- Malignancy
- Immune dysregulation

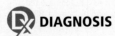

DIAGNOSIS

HISTORY

- Age: may suggest possible etiologic subgroup
- Toxin exposure: prescription, over-the-counter, herbal, or supplemental medications
- Symptoms of viral prodrome
- Travel history, exposure history
- Length of symptoms, acuity of onset
- Associated symptoms/ROS:
  - Jaundice, bleeding, bruising
  - Weakness, fatigue
  - Abdominal distension, pain, diarrhea
  - Pruritus secondary to cholestasis

PHYSICAL EXAM

- Skin: jaundice, bruising
- Eyes: scleral icterus
- Abdomen: hepatomegaly, ascites with dullness to percussion or fluid wave, splenomegaly
- Neurologic
  - Sequential mental status exams are paramount to monitor for change and should include age-appropriate questions.
  - Assess for presence of encephalopathy:
    - Grade I: confused, altered sleep; reflexes normal, may have tremor or apraxia
    - Grade II: drowsy, inappropriate behavior; hyperreflexic or asterixis; dysarthria or ataxia
    - Grade III: stupor but may obey simple commands, sleepy; hyperreflexic, asterixis, Babinski-positive; increased general tone
    - Grade IV: comatose; reflexes absent; decerebrate or decorticate posturing

DIAGNOSTIC TESTS & INTERPRETATION

Imaging

- Abdominal ultrasound with Doppler: visualization of both hepatic parenchyma and vasculature (direction of portal flow, presence of thrombosis)
- Head CT scan without IV contrast in presence of encephalopathy or neurologic signs to rule out intracranial hemorrhage or cerebral edema

Diagnostic Procedures/Other

- Initial laboratory testing
  - Hepatocellular injury: aminotransferases (AST, ALT) often markedly elevated; degree of elevation may depend on mechanism and time frame of injury.
  - Biliary injury/obstruction: elevated alkaline phosphatase, γ-glutamyl transpeptidase (GGT), total/conjugated bilirubin
  - General labs: CBC with differential, electrolytes, glucose, blood urea nitrogen and creatinine, amylase/lipase
- Assessment of synthetic function
  - Prolonged PT/INR (with adequate supply of vitamin K)
  - Depressed factors V, VII levels
  - Hypoalbuminemia
  - Hypoglycemia: Frequent glucose measurements should be followed during initial evaluation and with any mental status or neurologic change.
- Encephalopathy: ammonia level (has not been proven to correlate directly to presence or grade of encephalopathy)
- Tests to determine etiology
  - Testing priority should be guided by the age group and population, and for conditions amenable to specific therapies.
  - Toxin: urine or serum drug screen, serum acetaminophen and aspirin levels
  - Infectious: hepatitis virus serologic testing, comprehensive viral cultures; PCR testing for EBV, CMV, HSV, and other viruses; antibody tests
  - Autoimmune hepatitis: antinuclear, anti–smooth muscle/F-actin, anti-LKM antibodies, total IgG
  - Wilson disease: decreased serum ceruloplasmin (may not be reliable in setting of ALF), increased serum or urinary copper, Coombs-negative hemolytic anemia
  - Pregnancy test in adolescent females
  - Metabolic: urine succinylacetone, reducing substances, and organic acids; plasma amino acids, acylcarnitine profile, lactate/pyruvate, creatinine kinase; newborn screen
  - Hemophagocytic lymphohistiocytosis: ≥2 cytopenias, elevated ferritin, elevated triglycerides, and low fibrinogen
  - Gestational alloimmune liver disease (neonatal hemochromatosis): severe hypoglycemia and coagulopathy, elevated ferritin with near-normal aminotransferase. Evidence of iron deposition on buccal biopsy or abdominal MRI
- Liver biopsy: Generally, not considered critical for management or diagnosis due to substantial risks of hemorrhage. Transjugular approach may reduce risks. May be appropriate to attempt to identify a specific etiology that may influence treatment strategy (e.g., Wilson disease). Severity of necrosis may not predict potential liver recovery.

DIFFERENTIAL DIAGNOSIS

The cause of ALF can be indeterminate in up to 50% of cases across all age groups. Etiologic subgroups include the following:

- Drug-induced/toxin
  - Acetaminophen: most common in older children and adolescents
  - Salicylates, iron compounds, anticonvulsants, antibiotics
  - Recreational drugs
  - *Amanita* species (mushrooms)
- Metabolic/genetic/misc: early infancy
  - Galactosemia, tyrosinemia
  - Gestational alloimmune liver disease
  - Storage diseases
  - Mitochondrial disorders
  - Fatty acid oxidation disorders
  - Hereditary fructose intolerance
- Metabolic/genetic/misc: older children
  - Autoimmune hepatitis
  - Wilson disease
  - Pregnancy (HELLP syndrome, AFL)
  - Reye syndrome
- Infectious
  - Hepatitis virus: A, B, E; less commonly C
  - Herpes virus: HSV, EBV, CMV, VZV, HHV6
  - Echovirus, especially in neonates
  - Parvovirus, adenovirus
- Vascular/ischemic
  - Congestive heart failure
  - Hypotensive shock
  - Budd-Chiari syndrome: hepatic venous outflow obstruction
  - Veno-occlusive disease: Nonthrombotic occlusion of hepatic venules, typically occurs following stem cell transplantation.
- Malignancy
  - Primary: hepatoblastoma, hepatocellular carcinoma
  - Other: leukemia, lymphoma, hemophagocytic lymphohistiocytosis
- Heatstroke, hyperthermia, rhabdomyolysis

TREATMENT

MEDICATION

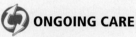

- Hematologic
  - Vitamin K: Administer IV or SQ/IM for prolonged PT/INR, and monitor response with repeat PT/INR 4–6 hours afterward.
  - FFP and cryoprecipitate should be reserved for acute severe bleeding or prior to invasive procedure; their use prohibits subsequent monitoring of PT/INR or specific factor levels.
  - Recombinant factor VIIa can be used in cases of acute severe bleeding.
- Neurologic/hepatic encephalopathy
  - Sedatives, especially benzodiazepines, should be avoided, as they may worsen encephalopathy.
  - Lactulose (oral, enema forms) should be used if encephalopathy present; goal is to acidify stool (pH <6) and increase frequency of stool but not cause diarrhea.
  - Oral or rectal administration of antibiotics (neomycin, rifaximin) may be effective by reducing ammonia production in the gut.
  - Elevated arterial ammonia levels may help predict development of encephalopathy and intracranial hypertension.
- Infectious disease
  - Prophylactic antibiotics and antifungal medications if febrile, after obtaining cultures from any central venous access or catheterization.
- Renal
  - Nephrotoxic drugs should be avoided when possible. Diuretics should be used with caution; renal dose medications if renal compromise present
  - Renal replacement therapy as indicated
- Other:
  - *N*-acetylcysteine is the treatment for acetaminophen-induced hepatic toxicity.
  - IV acid suppression should be considered.
  - Removal of offending agent when identified

ADDITIONAL TREATMENT

General Measures

- Close monitoring, preferably in an ICU setting with a liver transplant program
- General supportive care
  - Fluid restriction: 75–95% of maintenance requirements to prevent worsening of portal hypertension, ascites, and pulmonary edema
  - Sodium restriction: Patients should typically not receive >0.25 NS as maintenance fluids. A total sodium intake of 1 mEq/kg/24 h is usually adequate. Hyponatremia should not be corrected with hypertonic saline, as this can worsen fluid overload and encephalopathy.
  - Glucose infusion: Maintenance fluid typically should include 10% dextrose; glucose infusion may need to be increased, as patients are at risk for hypoglycemia.
  - Nutrition: Adequate nutrition should be maintained either via enteral route or TPN.
  - Blood products should be given slowly to avoid rapid expansion of intravascular space.
  - Minimize invasive catheterization when possible due to infection risk.

SURGERY/OTHER PROCEDURES

- Those more likely to require liver transplantation include children with ALF secondary to indeterminate cause, idiosyncratic drug toxicity, hepatic vein thrombosis, or Wilson disease.
- Transplant-free survival >50% for ALF due to acetaminophen, hepatitis A, shock liver or pregnancy-related disease, whereas all other etiologies have <25% transplant free survival.
- Currently, available liver support systems are not recommended outside of clinical trials.

INPATIENT CONSIDERATIONS

Initial Stabilization

- Initial evaluation should include assessment of neurologic status.
- Elective intubation as well as ICP monitoring should be considered in grade III or IV encephalopathy with somnolence.
- Aggressive initial fluid resuscitation should be avoided unless there is evidence of hemodynamic compromise.
- Central venous access should be considered to allow for higher glucose infusion rates and for central nutrition.

ONGOING CARE

PROGNOSIS

- Etiology of ALF provides good indicator of prognosis and also dictates management.
- Existing liver failure scoring systems based on biochemical markers (e.g., INR) and/or clinical features, including the Kings College Hospital Criteria, have not been shown to be useful for predicting survival or death in pediatric ALF.
- Decisions for liver transplantation in pediatric ALF often challenging due to uncertainty of diagnosis and possibility of spontaneous recovery, potential morbidity/mortality of the transplant procedure itself, and the limited number of organs available.
- Overall 1-year survival following liver transplant is lower in patients transplanted for ALF compared to chronic liver failure; however, after the 1st year this trend is reversed and ALF patients have better long-term survival.

COMPLICATIONS

- Complications are a direct consequence of loss of hepatic metabolic function:
  - Hepatic encephalopathy: decreased elimination of neurotoxins or depressants
  - Cerebral edema: pathogenesis incompletely understood
  - Coagulopathy: failure of hepatic synthesis of clotting and fibrinolytic factors
  - Hypoglycemia: impaired glucose synthesis and release, decreased degradation of insulin
  - Acidosis: failure to eliminate lactic acid or free fatty acids
  - Hepatorenal syndrome: typically low urine sodium and no improvement with volume expansion; continuous venovenous hemofiltration or dialysis may be necessary.
- In cases of suspected hepatic encephalopathy, consider other etiologies of neurologic change including hypoglycemia, intracranial hemorrhage, acute infection, or sepsis.
- There is often rapid progression through the stages of encephalopathy. Increased intracranial pressure can develop quickly and can lead to irreversible neurologic sequelae.

ADDITIONAL READING

- Bass NM, Mullen KD, Sanyal A, et al. Rifaximin treatment in hepatic encephalopathy. *N Engl J Med*. 2010;362(12):1071–1081.
- Bucuvalas J, Yazigi N, Squires RH Jr. Acute liver failure in children. *Clin Liver Dis*. 2006;10(1):149–168.
- Kortsalioudaki C, Taylor RM, Cheeseman P, et al. Safety and efficacy of N-acetylcysteine in children with non-acetaminophen-induced acute liver failure. *Liver Transpl*. 2008;14(1):25–30.
- Lee WM, Stravitz RT, Larson AM. Introduction to the revised American Association for the Study of Liver Diseases Position Paper on acute liver failure 2011. *Hepatology*. 2012;55(3):965–967.
- Miyake Y, Sakaguchi K, Iwasaki Y, et al. New prognostic scoring model for liver transplantation in patients with non-acetaminophen-related fulminant hepatic failure. *Transplantation*. 2005;80(7): 930–936.
- Squires RH Jr, Shneider BL, Bucuvalas J, et al. Acute liver failure in children: the first 348 patients in the pediatric acute liver failure study group. *J Pediatr*. 2006;148(5):652–658.
- Sundaram SS, Alonso EM, Narkewicz MR, et al. Characterization and outcomes of young infants with acute liver failure. *J Pediatr*. 2011;159(5):813–818.

CODES

ICD10

- K72.00 Acute and subacute hepatic failure without coma
- K71.10 Toxic liver disease with hepatic necrosis, without coma

FAQ

- Q: What are the most common causes of ALF in infants?
- A: Up to 40–50% of cases are indeterminate, followed by neonatal hemochromatosis, viral infection, and metabolic disorders.
- Q: What is the risk of bleeding in ALF-associated coagulopathy?
- A: Spontaneous, clinically significant bleeding in ALF is generally rare, despite abnormal INR. Thromboelastography (TEG), which assesses overall hemostasis including the cumulative effects of procoagulant and anticoagulant proteins, fibrinogen, platelets, and red blood cells, may be a better guide for administration of blood products in ALF than INR.
- Q: Is the initial level of elevation of transaminases is directly correlated to the prognosis of patient?
- A: False. In viral hepatitis and acetaminophen toxicity, initial transaminases can be in 1,000s, but patients can have complete recovery.

ACUTE LYMPHOBLASTIC LEUKEMIA

Latika Puri • Caroline Hastings

BASICS

DESCRIPTION

- Acute lymphoblastic leukemia (ALL) is a hematopoietic malignancy that results from malignant proliferation of immature WBC (B cells and T cells).
- Risk group classification:
  - Infant ALL: age less than 1 year
  - Standard risk ALL: age 1 to younger than 10 years; initial WBC count $<50{,}000/\mu L$
  - High risk ALL: age 10 years or older; WBC $\geq 50{,}000/\mu L$
- Further risk stratification done based on multiple factors including National Cancer Institute (NCI) criteria (age and WBC count), biologic, cytogenetic characteristics, and response to initial therapy. This classification determines the intensity of therapy and prognosis.
  - Low-risk ALL: NCI standard risk group
    - Favorable cytogenetic changes (hyperdiploidy, trisomies of 4, 10, and 17; t[12;21]);
    - Pre B lymphoblasts and negative minimal residual disease (MRD) at end of induction
  - Average risk ALL: NCI standard risk group
    - Noncontributory cytogenetics
    - Negative MRD at end of induction
    - No extramedullary (CNS or testicular) involvement
    - Negative MRD at end of induction
  - High-risk ALL: NCI high-risk group
    - Age >10 years regardless of WBC count, extramedullary (CNS or testicular) involvement
    - T-cell phenotype
    - No or very low MRD at end of induction
  - Very high-risk ALL
    - Unfavorable cytogenetics (t[9;22] Philadelphia positive ALL)
    - Hypodiploidy
    - *MLL* gene rearrangement
    - Induction failure (>25% lymphoblasts in bone marrow at end of induction)
    - Positive MRD at the end of induction

EPIDEMIOLOGY

- ALL is the most common childhood malignancy.
- Accounts for approximately 30% of cancer diagnosis in children younger than 15 years of age
- More common in Caucasians and males
- ALL incidence: 3–4 cases per 100,000 per year
- Peak incidence is between ages 2 and 5 years.

RISK FACTORS

- Prior cancer therapy (chemotherapy or radiation)
- Twin with ALL
- Genetic syndrome listed in the following sections

Genetics

- Increased risk of leukemia, higher with monozygotic twin
- Associated genetic syndromes
  - Trisomy 21 (Down syndrome)
  - Fanconi anemia
  - Bloom syndrome
  - Shwachman-Diamond syndrome
  - Ataxia telangiectasia
- Neurofibromatosis type 1
- Li-Fraumeni syndrome p53 (familial cancer syndrome)
- Congenital immunodeficiencies (Wiskott-Aldrich syndrome)

PATHOPHYSIOLOGY

Leukemia arises from lymphoid progenitor cells that have sustained multiple specific genetic damages that lead to malignant transformation and proliferation, lack of cell maturation, and resistance to normal cell death processes (apoptosis). This lymphoblastic proliferation replaces the normal bone marrow precursor cells, causing ineffective hematopoiesis and infiltration of lymphatic tissue and end organs.

DIAGNOSIS

- Clinical features due to direct invasion of the bone marrow:
  - Pancytopenia: anemia, thrombocytopenia, leukopenia, or neutropenia
  - Anemia: irritability, fatigue, anorexia, headache, pallor
  - Thrombocytopenia: bleeding is usually mild and manifests as petechiae, bruising, gingival oozing, epistaxis
- Fever: may be a sign of presumed cytokine release or underlying infection due to neutropenia and immunosuppression
- Bone pain
  - Typically long bones
  - Could be due to direct leukemic infiltration of the periosteum or expansion of marrow cavity by leukemic cells
  - Pathologic fractures, leukemic lines on plain radiographs, or T2-weighted changes on MRI
- Testicular involvement (2–5 % of the boys), unilateral or bilateral painless testicular enlargement
- CNS involvement (2–5% of patients on presentation for B cell, 10–15% for T-cell ALL)
  - Increased intracranial pressure (morning headache, vomiting, lethargy, visual changes, seizures, CN VI palsy, diplopia, and esotropia)
- Superior vena cava (SVC) syndrome (due to a mediastinal mass)
  - Swelling of the face, neck, chest, and, rarely, upper arms with or without visual venous distension, cough, dyspnea, dysphagia
- Leukostasis (large number of deformable blasts plugging the microcirculation)
  - Respiratory symptoms: dyspnea, hypoxia
  - Neurologic symptoms: visual changes, headache, dizziness, tinnitus, lethargy
  - Rare symptoms including renal insufficiency, priapism, acute limb ischemia
- Spinal cord compression (due to a chloroma, an extramedullary collection of lymphoblasts): extremity weakness, numbness, and tingling

PHYSICAL EXAM

- Pallor (anemia)
- Tachycardia/murmurs (anemia)
- Lymphadenopathy (leukemic infiltration)
- Hepatosplenomegaly (leukemic infiltration)
- Testicular enlargement (leukemic infiltration)
- Bone: tenderness, fracture (marrow infiltration)
- Skin: bruises, petechiae, rash in form of subcutaneous nodules (leukemia cutis, most commonly seen in infants)
- Papilledema (CNS involvement)
- Focal neurologic signs (CNS involvement, chloroma)

DIAGNOSTIC TESTS & INTERPRETATION

- CBC
  - Increased or decreased WBC (50% present with WBC $<10{,}000/\mu L$ and 20% present with WBC $\geq 50{,}000/\mu L$)
  - Anemia: Hgb <10 g/dL (80% of cases)
  - Thrombocytopenia (platelets $<100{,}000/\mu L$ in 75% at presentation)
  - Peripheral smear: may see circulating lymphoblasts, especially with high WBC
- Serum chemistry
  - Signs of tumor lysis: elevated uric acid, hyperkalemia, hyperphosphatemia (with secondary hypocalcemia), elevated lactate dehydrogenase (LDH)
  - Elevated liver enzymes (leukemic infiltrate)
  - Elevated creatinine (due to uric acid/calcium phosphate crystal deposition in renal tubules or leukemic infiltrates)

Imaging

- CXR: mediastinal mass (5–10% of cases)
- Plain films of long bones in case of bone pain/ tenderness may show leukemic lines.

Diagnostic Procedures/Other

- Bone marrow aspirate and biopsy (presence of more than 25% blasts consistent with diagnosis of leukemia). Immunophenotyping and cytochemistry is then used to differentiate ALL from acute myeloid leukemia (AML) and identify T-cell or B-cell phenotype.
- Lumbar puncture is also performed for CSF analysis for lymphoblasts.
- Immunophenotyping
  - B cell: CD 10+, 19+, 20+, 22+, TdT+
  - Pre T cell: CD 3+. 5+, 7+, TdT+
  - Myeloid markers: CD 13+, 33+, 34+ (in minority)
  - CNS I: No detectable blasts
  - CNS 2: <5 WBC/μL, blasts present
  - CNS 3: ≥ 5 WBC/μL, and blasts or symptoms of CNS leukemia)

DIFFERENTIAL DIAGNOSIS

- Infectious: infectious mononucleosis, Epstein-Barr virus (EBV), pertussis, parapertussis, parvovirus; cytomegalovirus (CMV), acute infectious lymphocytosis
- Juvenile rheumatoid arthritis
- Hematologic: immune thrombocytopenic purpura (ITP), aplastic anemia, Evans syndrome (ITP and autoimmune hemolytic anemia)
- Malignant disorders: round blue cell tumors with bone marrow involvement (neuroblastoma, rhabdomyosarcoma, Langerhans cell histiocytosis, lymphoma, retinoblastoma), myelodysplastic syndrome, AML, chronic myeloid leukemia (CML)

TREATMENT

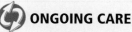

- Patient suspected with ALL must be referred to a pediatric oncologist as soon as possible for further evaluation and management.
- Initial emergent stabilization may be required in case of
  - Hyperleukocytosis, defined as a WBC ≥100,000/μL
  - Tumor lysis syndrome with renal insufficiency
  - Spinal cord compression
- Mediastinal mass causing SVC syndrome
- Therapy is aimed at inducing permanent biologic and clinical remission and is divided into various phases. Many children and adolescents are enrolled on clinical trials through the Children's Oncology Group or local institution. Treatment is standardized by prognostic indicators and provided by highly specialized teams with expertise in childhood cancer.
  - Induction (first 28–35 days). Typically includes the following drugs:
    - A glucocorticoid (prednisone or dexamethasone)
    - Vincristine
    - L-asparaginase
    - Anthracycline (in high-risk patients only)
    - Intrathecal chemotherapy (initial dose of cytarabine; subsequent treatment with methotrexate)
  - Consolidation: focuses on CNS prophylaxis; weekly intrathecal chemotherapy with
    - Low/average-risk patients: weekly vincristine, oral 6-mercaptopurine (6-MP), L-asparaginase, intensified with cyclophosphamide and cytarabine in certain subsets of patients
    - High-risk patients: more intensive systemic therapy with cyclophosphamide, cytarabine, methotrexate, vincristine, and L-asparaginase
    - Patients with initial involvement of the CNS or testes may receive radiation during this phase.
  - Interim maintenance: similar to maintenance therapy but more intensified
    - Vincristine, methotrexate, L-asparaginase
    - Intrathecal methotrexate
  - Delayed intensification: (reintensification and reconsolidation)
    - Combination of intensive therapy similar to induction and consolidation
  - Maintenance: continuation of therapy (lasts for 2–3 years)
    - Daily 6-MP, weekly oral methotrexate, pulse glucocorticoids, and vincristine with periodic intrathecal chemotherapy
- Ph+ patients t(9;21) receive continuous tyrosine kinase inhibitors (imatinib or dasatinib)
- Patients with CNS and testicular involvement get prophylactic and therapeutic radiation therapy.
- Patients with Down syndrome and ALL have increased treatment-related morbidity and mortality and require some treatment modifications.
- Very high-risk patients may be treated with bone marrow transplant, following remission induction.
- Length of treatment from 2 to 3.25 years, depending on protocol and gender

ONGOING CARE

FOLLOW-UP RECOMMENDATIONS

Early intensification has led to an increase in relapse-free survival.

Patient Monitoring

After completion of therapy:

- CBC, complete metabolic panel with LDH, liver and renal function tests every month for the 1st year, every 2 months for the 2nd year, then every 3 months for the 3rd year, every 6 months for the 4th year, and yearly thereafter
- Cardiac evaluation every year, dependent on cumulative dose of anthracycline and possible radiation scatter
- Endocrine evaluation close to puberty, especially in children who have received cranial or testicular radiation
- Monitor for late effects in cancer survivors clinic.

PROGNOSIS

- Long-term survival
  - Overall: approaches 90%
  - Low-risk patients: 90–95%
  - Standard risk group: 85%
  - High-risk group: 60–75%
  - Very high-risk group: ~20–50%
  - Infant group: 50%

COMPLICATIONS

- Bone marrow suppression (anemia and thrombocytopenia requiring transfusion support, possible transfusion-related infection or iron overload)
- Neutropenia leading to increased risk of infection
- L-asparaginase: anaphylaxis, pancreatitis, thrombosis, stroke
- Anthracyclines (daunorubicin and doxorubicin): cardiac toxicity, secondary AML
- Intrathecal methotrexate: neurotoxicity (frequently reversible)
- Steroids: avascular necrosis of bone, decreased bone density
- Cranial radiation: secondary brain tumors, growth retardation, learning difficulties and/or cognitive impairment
- Testicular radiation: lack of pubertal development, sterility
- Relapse
  - Approximately 10–30% of children and adolescents with ALL will relapse, usually within 5 years of diagnosis.
  - If relapse occurs while the patient is receiving therapy, outcomes are poor (<20%) even with systemic retreatment and possible bone marrow transplant (BMT).
  - If relapse occurs >36 months from diagnosis or is isolated to an extramedullary site such as the CNS or testis, survival is improved to 40–70% with systemic chemotherapy and possible focal radiation therapy.

ADDITIONAL READING

- Borowitz MJ, Devidas M, Hunger SP, et al. Clinical significance of minimal residual disease in childhood acute lymphoblastic leukemia and its relationship to other prognostic factors: a Children's Oncology Group study. *Blood*. 2008;111(12):5477–5485.
- Hunger SP, Loh ML, Whitlock JA, et al. Children's Oncology Group's 2013 blueprint for research: acute lymphoblastic leukemia. *Pediatr Blood Cancer*. 2013;60(6):957–963.
- Hunger SP, Lu X, Devidas M, et al. Improved survival for children and adolescents with acute lymphoblastic leukemia between 1990 and 2005: a report from the children's oncology group. *J Clin Oncol*. 2012;30(14):1663–1669.
- Lo Nigro L. Biology of childhood acute lymphoblastic leukemia. *J Pediatr Hematol Oncol*. 2013;35(4): 245–252.
- Pui CH, Robison LL, Look AT. Acute lymphoblastic leukaemia. *Lancet*. 2008;371(9617):1030–1043.

CODES

ICD10

- C91.00 Acute lymphoblastic leukemia not having achieved remission
- C91.01 Acute lymphoblastic leukemia, in remission
- C91.02 Acute lymphoblastic leukemia, in relapse

FAQ

- Q: Can a child on treatment for ALL go to school or leave the house?
- A: Yes. Most centers encourage the child to live a normal life, including school, activities, and travel.
- Q: Will hair fall out and will the child be sick for ALL 3 years on chemotherapy?
- A: The hair usually falls out within a few weeks of initiating therapy and grows back when maintenance therapy begins (6–8 months). Most children feel relatively well during therapy, especially maintenance chemotherapy, and can resume a lot of normal activities.
- Q: Does the child need to be isolated from other children?
- A: The most serious infections a child on chemotherapy gets come from bacteria that the child is already colonized with, not community-acquired viruses. That being said, the child should be isolated from any child who has varicella or other known symptomatic infection.

ACUTE MYELOID LEUKEMIA

Allison Ast • William B. Slayton • David T. Teachey

BASICS

DESCRIPTION

- Acute myeloid leukemia (AML) results from a block in differentiation and unregulated proliferation of myeloid progenitor cells.
- AML is classified according to the World Health Organization (WHO) classification (2008).
- Formerly classified by French-American-British (FAB) classification
- WHO classification is based on genetic alterations, whereas FAB is based on morphology.

EPIDEMIOLOGY

- AML is the 7th most common pediatric malignancy.
- Leukemia that occurs in first 4 weeks of life is usually AML.
- Ratio of AML to acute lymphoblastic leukemia (ALL) throughout childhood is 1:5.
- Boys and girls are equally affected.
- Rates are highest in Asian and Pacific Islanders followed by Hispanics, Caucasians, and African Americans.

Incidence

- AML incidence peaks in infants younger than 1 year of age and again in children 10–14 years of age.
- Around 500 children/year in the United States

RISK FACTORS

Genetics

- 20–30% of pediatric blasts have normal karyotype versus 40–50% in adults.
- 60% of abnormal karyotypes fall into known subgroups.
- Translocations or duplications of the *MLL* gene at 11q23 or monosomy 7 carry a poor prognosis.
- These genetic abnormalities are found in many cases of therapy-induced AML.
- FLT3-ITD with high allelic ratio, a drug targetable lesion, has been recently shown to carry a poor prognosis.
- Translocations t(8;21), t(15;17), and inv(16), as well as *NPM* and *CEPB*α mutations carry a good prognosis.
- AML associated with Down syndrome has an excellent prognosis.
- Certain congenital syndromes that carry an increased risk of AML:
  - Fanconi anemia
  - Bloom syndrome
  - Neurofibromatosis type I
  - Down syndrome
  - Severe congenital anemia (i.e., Kostmann disease treated with granulocyte colony-stimulating factor)
  - Diamond-Blackfan anemia
  - Paroxysmal nocturnal hemoglobinemia
  - Li-Fraumeni syndrome
  - Shwachman-Diamond syndrome
  - Dyskeratosis congenita
  - Noonan syndrome (RASopathies)

PATHOPHYSIOLOGY

- Principal defect is a block in the differentiation of primitive myeloid precursor cells.
- 2 mechanisms predominate:
  - Defect at the level of transcriptional activation
  - Defects in the signaling pathway of hematopoietic growth factors. For example, the proto-oncogene *Ras* is mutated in up to 1/3 of patients with AML.

ETIOLOGY

- Exact cause unknown in most cases.
- Acquired risk factors include the following:
  - Exposure to benzene
  - Exposure to ionizing radiation
  - Therapy induced, from chemotherapy for a prior malignancy
  - Alkylating agents such as cyclophosphamide, nitrogen mustard, chlorambucil, and melphalan (typically presents several years after therapy)
  - Epipodophyllotoxins such as VP16, VM26 (typically occurs within 2 years after therapy and is characterized by rearrangements involving 11q23)

DIAGNOSIS

HISTORY

Children with AML can present with very few symptoms or with life-threatening sepsis or hemorrhage. Common symptoms include the following:

- Fever: 30–40%
- Pallor: 25%
- Weight loss/anorexia: 22%
- Fatigue: 19%
- Bleeding (i.e., cutaneous, mucosal, menorrhagia): 33%
- Bone or joint pain: 18%

PHYSICAL EXAM

- Signs of anemia:
  - Pallor
  - Fatigue
  - Headache
  - Dyspnea
  - Systolic flow murmur
- Signs of thrombocytopenia:
  - Petechiae
  - Bruising
  - Epistaxis
  - Gingival bleeding
- Signs of infection:
  - Fever
  - Bacterial infections of lung, sinuses, gingiva, perirectal area, skin
- Other exam findings:
  - Hepatomegaly
  - Splenomegaly
  - Lymphadenopathy
  - Gingival hyperplasia
  - Papilledema, cranial nerve palsies (rare)
  - Colorless or slightly purple subcutaneous nodules: "blueberry muffin" lesions of leukemia cutis (more commonly seen in neonates)
  - Chloroma is an extramedullary collection of leukemic cells that can present as a mass

DIAGNOSTIC TESTS & INTERPRETATION

Techniques such as fluorescence in situ hybridization, flow cytometry Southern blotting, and reverse transcriptase-polymerase chain reaction are used to diagnose and classify AML.

Lab

- CBC
  - Anemia, thrombocytopenia, elevated or low total WBC peripheral smear
  - Circulating myeloblasts may be seen.
- Prothrombin time (PT)/partial thromboplastin time (PTT), fibrin spit products
  - Elevated in some cases, especially with acute promyelocytic leukemia (M3)
  - Can have severe, life-threatening disseminated intravascular coagulation (DIC)
- Electrolytes (abnormalities associated with tumor lysis syndrome)
  - Hyperkalemia
  - Hypocalcemia
  - Hyperphosphatemia
  - Hyperuricemia
- CSF analysis for cell count and cytology:
  - >5 WBC/μL is suggestive of CNS disease.
  - 5–15% of cases have CNS involvement at diagnosis.

Diagnostic Procedures/Other

Bone marrow aspirate:

- $>20\%$ myeloblasts is typically seen.
- To differentiate between AML with low blast count and myelodysplastic syndrome, serial bone marrow aspirates and biopsies are required as well as detailed cytogenetic analysis.
- At diagnosis, morphology, cytochemistry, immunophenotyping, and molecular and cytogenetics of the bone marrow aspirate are required.

Pathologic Findings

- Immunophenotyping
  - Precursor stage: CD34, CD117
  - Myelomonocytic markers: CD11B, CD11C, CD13, CD14, CD15, CD33, CD64, CD65, i-lysozyme
  - Lymphoid markers: T and B cell markers may be present on 30–60% of pediatric blasts.
  - CD41, CD42, and CD61 (megakaryocytic): particularly prevalent in patients with Down syndrome
- Morphology
  - Large blasts with low nuclear/cytoplasmic ratio
  - Multiple nucleoli and cytoplasmic granules
- Cytochemistry
  - Blasts are positive for myeloperoxidase and Sudan Black and usually negative for periodic acid–Schiff (PAS) and terminal deoxynucleotide transferase (TdT).

DIFFERENTIAL DIAGNOSIS
- Myeloid blast crisis of chronic myeloid leukemia (Philadelphia chromosome positive)
- Transient myeloproliferative disorder of the newborn (in Down syndrome)
- ALL
- Leukemoid reaction
- Exaggerated leukocytosis
- Myelodysplastic syndrome

TREATMENT

MEDICATION
- Patients are treated with 6–9 months of intensive chemotherapy given in cycles.
- The most effective drugs for remission induction in AML combine anthracyclines (e.g., doxorubicin, daunorubicin, daunomycin, and mitoxantrone) and cytarabine (Ara-C).
- Other agents sometimes used in combination chemotherapy include etoposide (VP-16), gemtuzumab (anti-CD33 monoclonal antibody), fludarabine, dexamethasone, L-asparaginase, and 6-thioguanine.
- Patients with acute promyelocytic leukemia can be cured with all-*trans*-retinoic acid and arsenic.
- Intrathecal Ara-C for CNS prophylaxis
- FLT3 inhibitors including sorafenib are being used in some patients with FLT3-ITD.
- Hematopoietic stem cell transplant is recommended for patients with high-risk cytogenetics (monosomy 7, monosomy 5, 5q-, FLT3-ITD) or those whom not in remission following 2 courses of induction therapy

ADDITIONAL TREATMENT
General Measures
- Hydration, alkalization, and allopurinol during induction
- Consider rasburicase in patients with marked elevations in uric acid and renal compromise (contraindicated in patients with G6PD deficiency).
- Blood product support
  - Avoid products from family members as sensitization can lead to poor engraftment after allogeneic bone marrow transplant.
- Broad-spectrum antibiotics and antifungal therapy for fever and neutropenia
- Prophylactic trimethoprim-sulfamethoxazole for *Pneumocystis* infection

ADDITIONAL THERAPIES
Allogeneic bone marrow transplant is recommended for high-risk AML in first remission.

INPATIENT CONSIDERATIONS
Initial Stabilization
Children with suspected AML should have immediate evaluation with physical exam, history, and laboratory data including CBC, PT/PTT, electrolytes, calcium, phosphorus, uric acid, and creatinine.

ONGOING CARE

FOLLOW-UP RECOMMENDATIONS
Patient Monitoring
- Blood counts monthly for 1st year, every 4 months for the 2nd year, and every 6 months thereafter
- Liver and kidney function tests every 3–6 months
- Cardiac function every 12 months.
- Endocrine function should be tested in pubertal children.

PROGNOSIS
- 85% achieve remission with intensive chemotherapy.
- ~60–70% achieve long-term survival (>5 years after diagnosis).
- Factors associated with poor prognosis:
  - WBC count >100,000/μL
  - Monosomy 7, monosomy 5 or del(5q)
  - Secondary AML or prior myelodysplastic syndrome
  - FLT3-ITD
  - Presence of multiple other genetic translocation events or mutations
  - Poor initial response to therapy (induction failure or presence of >0.1% minimal residual disease [MRD] in the bone marrow at the end of induction)
  - MRD testing measures quantities of residual leukemia not seen on morphologic exam using flow cytometry or standard cytogenetics.

COMPLICATIONS
- Bleeding (usually secondary to thrombocytopenia)
- DIC occurs in some types of AML, including acute promyelocytic leukemia (M3).
- Treat bleeding aggressively with fresh frozen plasma and platelets.
- Other cytopenias require blood product support.
- Infection
  - 40% of patients are febrile at diagnosis.
  - Empiric antibiotic therapy must be started after blood cultures are obtained.
- Leukostasis
  - Intravascular clumping of blasts causing hypoxia, infarction, and hemorrhage
  - Usually occurs when WBC >200,000/μL
  - Brain and lung are commonly affected.
  - Leukapheresis or exchange transfusion may be indicated for patients who are symptomatic with extremely high blast counts.
- Tumor lysis syndrome
  - Refers to the metabolic consequences from the release of cellular contents of dying leukemic cells
  - Hyperuricemia can lead to renal failure.
  - Hyperkalemia, hyperphosphatemia, and secondary hypocalcemia can be life threatening.
  - Patients should be hydrated with fluid containing bicarbonate and given allopurinol.

ADDITIONAL READING

- Creutzig U, van den Heuvel-Eibrink M, Gibson B, et al. Diagnosis and management of acute myeloid leukemia in children and adolescents: recommendations from an international expert panel. *Blood*. 2012;120(16):3187–3205.
- Kersey JH. Fifty years of studies of biology and therapy of childhood leukemia. *Blood*. 1997;90(11): 4243–4251.
- Pui CH, Carroll WL, Meshinchi S, et al. Biology, risk stratification, and therapy or pediatric acute leukemias: an update. *J Clin Oncol*. 2011;29(5):551–565.
- Puumala S, Ross J, Aplenc R, et al. Epidemiology of childhood acute myeloid leukemia. *Pediatr Blood Cancer* 2013;60(5):728–733.
- Rubnitz JE, Gibson B, Smith FO. Acute myeloid leukemia. *Hematol Oncol Clin North Am*. 2010;24(1): 35–63.
- Vardiman JW, Thiele J, Arber DA, et al. The 2008 revision of the World Health Organization (WHO) classification of myeloid and acute leukemia: rationale and important changes. *Blood*. 2009;114(5): 937–951.

CODES

ICD10
- C92.00 Acute myeloblastic leukemia, not having achieved remission
- C92.01 Acute myeloblastic leukemia, in remission
- C92.02 Acute myeloblastic leukemia, in relapse

FAQ
- Q: Is an indwelling line required for therapy?
- A: Always
- Q: Are repeated hospitalizations likely?
- A: Repeated hospitalizations are needed for chemotherapy and infectious complications.

ADENOVIRUS INFECTION

Jason Newland • Jessica Newman

BASICS

DESCRIPTION

Adenoviruses are ubiquitous, nonenveloped, double-stranded DNA viruses capable of causing respiratory tract disease and gastroenteritis.

EPIDEMIOLOGY

- Primary infection usually occurs early in life (by age 5 years) and is, most often, characterized by upper respiratory symptoms.
- Military trainees are especially susceptible to infection, probably due to crowded living conditions.
- Respiratory and enteric infections may occur at any time of year. In temperate climates, peaks tend to occur in winter months.
- Cause approximately 5% of all pediatric respiratory tract infections and 5–10% of pneumonias
- Transmission of respiratory disease occurs via infected droplets.
  - Transmission of enteric adenoviruses is via the fecal–oral route.
  - Transmission can less commonly occur via contact with infected conjunctiva.
- Outbreaks of pharyngoconjunctival fever have been associated with inadequately chlorinated swimming pools and shared towels.
- One of the most common causes of viral myocarditis in children and adults

Incidence

Peaks in the first 2 years of life

RISK FACTORS

Exposure to adenovirus

GENERAL PREVENTION

Precautions for hospitalized patients

Symptoms	Type of precautions
Respiratory disease	Contact and droplet
Gastrointestinal	Contact
Conjunctivitis	Contact

A live oral vaccine for prevention of acute respiratory tract disease is used in military personnel.

PATHOPHYSIOLOGY

Adenoviruses may cause a lytic infection or a chronic/latent infection. In addition, they are capable of inducing oncogenic transformation of cells, although the clinical significance of this observation remains unclear.

ETIOLOGY

There are at least 57 identified human serotypes classified into 7 species (species A to G).

COMMONLY ASSOCIATED CONDITIONS

- Respiratory infections
  - Upper respiratory tract infections: otitis media, common cold, pharyngitis
  - Lower respiratory tract infection: pneumonia, pertussis-like syndrome, croup, necrotizing bronchitis, bronchiolitis (serotypes 3, 7, and 21 predominant in pneumonia epidemics)
- Pharyngoconjunctival fever
  - Low-grade fever associated with conjunctivitis, pharyngitis, rhinitis, and cervical adenitis
  - 15% of patients may have meningismus.
  - Increased incidence in summer months
  - Common source outbreaks most often associated with type 3
- Epidemic keratoconjunctivitis
  - Bilateral conjunctivitis with preauricular adenopathy
  - May persist for up to 4 weeks
  - Corneal opacities may persist for several months.
  - Associated with types 8, 19, and 37
- Myocarditis preceding viral illness
  - Present with cardiovascular collapse, congestive heart failure, respiratory distress, or ventricular tachycardia
  - Prognosis is poor.
  - High mortality; a large number require transplant, and a portion develop dilated cardiomyopathy.
- Hemorrhagic cystitis may cause microscopic or gross hematuria.
  - If present, gross hematuria persists on average for 3 days.
  - Often associated with dysuria and urinary frequency
  - More common in males than females
  - Associated with types 11 and 21
  - Can occur in both immunocompetent and immunocompromised hosts
- Infantile diarrhea
  - Watery diarrhea associated with fever
  - Symptoms may persist for 1–2 weeks
  - Associated with types 40, 41, and less often 31
- CNS infection epidemics (associated with outbreaks of respiratory disease) and sporadic cases of encephalitis and meningitis have been observed; often associated with pneumonia
- Immunocompromised hosts
  - Can cause disseminated disease including pneumonia, hepatitis, and gastroenteritis
  - Frequently observed in transplanted patients; up to 40% of pediatric human stem cell transplant recipients and in 5–10% of solid organ transplant recipients
  - Fatality rates much higher, up to 30–75% in hematopoietic stem cell transplant patients
- Miscellaneous: associated with intussusception (isolated in up to 40% of cases) and fatal congenital infection

DIAGNOSIS

HISTORY

- Fever
  - Nonspecific
- Rhinitis
  - Upper respiratory infection (URI)
- Laryngitis, sore throat
  - URI
- Nonproductive or croupy cough
  - Respiratory infection
- Headache, myalgias
  - CNS infection
- Hematuria (gross or microscopic), dysuria, urinary frequency
  - Hemorrhagic cystitis
- Watery diarrhea
  - Enteric adenovirus
- Conjunctivitis, rhinitis, exudative pharyngitis, and meningismus
  - Typical findings of adenovirus

PHYSICAL EXAM

- Pulmonary tachypnea, wheezing, rales
  - Pneumonia
- Tachycardia, tachypnea, gallop rhythm, hepatomegaly
  - Myocarditis
- Abdominal tenderness, distention
  - Gastroenteritis

DIAGNOSTIC TESTS & INTERPRETATION

Lab

- CBC
  - Leukocytosis or leukopenia, often with left shift in the differential counts
- Erythrocyte sedimentation rate (ESR)
  - Often elevated
- Viral isolation
  - From nasopharyngeal secretions, urine, conjunctivae, or stool
- Viral identification
  - Observe viral antigen in infected cells by immunofluorescence, amplify genome by polymerase chain reaction.
  - Stool antigen enzyme immunoassay (EIA) test
  - Highest yield from nasopharyngeal swab or stool
  - Adenovirus polymerase chain reaction (PCR) may be helpful in narrowing differential diagnosis, especially regarding the immunocompromised host, and can be used for prognostic purposes.
- ECG
  - Low-voltage QRS
  - Low-amplitude or inverted T waves
  - Small or absent Q wave in V_5 and V_6

Imaging
- Echocardiogram for suspected myocarditis
  - Poor ejection fraction
- Chest x-ray
  - Bilateral patchy interstitial infiltrates (lower lobes) or enlarged heart
  - Cardiomegaly

DIFFERENTIAL DIAGNOSIS
- Respiratory infection
  - Influenza
  - Parainfluenza
  - Human metapneumovirus
  - Pertussis
  - Mycoplasma pneumonia
  - Bacterial pneumonia
  - Bocavirus
- Pharyngoconjunctival fever
  - Group A *Streptococcus*
  - Epstein-Barr virus
  - Parainfluenza
  - Enterovirus
  - Measles
  - Kawasaki disease
- Epidemic keratoconjunctivitis
  - Herpes simplex
  - Chlamydia
  - Enterovirus
- Myocarditis
  - Enteroviruses
  - Herpes simplex
  - Epstein-Barr virus
  - Influenza
  - Bacterial myocarditis
- Hemorrhagic cystitis
  - Glomerulonephritis
  - Vasculitis
  - Renal tuberculosis
- Infantile diarrhea
  - Rotavirus
  - Calicivirus (including norovirus)
  - Astrovirus
  - Salmonella
  - Shigella
  - Campylobacter
- CNS infection
  - Enterovirus
  - Herpes simplex virus
  - Mycoplasma
  - Bacterial meningitis

TREATMENT

GENERAL MEASURES
- Supportive care
- Monitor for secondary bacterial infections.
- Avoid steroid-containing ophthalmic ointments.

MEDICATION
First Line
- Cidofovir
  - Has been shown to have benefit in immunocompromised patients with disseminated disease, specifically in hematopoietic stem cell transplant (HSCT) patients, where a reduction in adenovirus-related mortality compared with historical controls has been reported
  - However, a risk of developing a dose-limiting nephrotoxicity exists and optimal dosing is not known.
  - Reducing immunosuppression in transplanted patients should be considered for those with adenovirus disease.
- Infusion of AdV-specific cytotoxic T cells or intravenous immunoglobulin (IVIG) may have some benefit in immunocompromised patients, particularly HSCT patients.

ONGOING CARE

PROGNOSIS
Most syndromes are self-limited in the immunocompetent host.

COMPLICATIONS
- Bronchiolitis obliterans (rare)
- Corneal opacities with visual disturbance (usually resolves spontaneously)
- Congestive heart failure
- Dilated cardiomyopathy

ADDITIONAL READING

- Bowles NE, Ni J, Kearney KL, et al. Detection of viruses in myocardial tissues by polymerase chain reaction: evidence of adenovirus as a common cause of myocarditis in children and adults. *J Amer Coll Cardiol*. 2003;42(3):466–472.
- Hammond S, Chenever E, Durbin JE. Respiratory virus infection in infants and children. *Pediatr Dev Pathol*. 2007;10(3):172–180.
- Leruez-Ville M, Midard V, Lacaille F, et al. Real-time blood plasma polymerase chain reaction for management of disseminated adenovirus infection. *Clin Infect Dis*. 2004;38(1):45–52.
- Lindemans CA, Leen AM, Boelens JJ. How I treat adenovirus in hematopoietic stem cell transplant recipients. *Blood*. 2010;116(25):5476–5485.
- Tebruegge M, Curtis N. Adenovirus: an overview for pediatric infectious diseases specialists. *Pediatr Infect Dis J*. 2012;31(6):626–627.

CODES

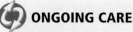

ICD10
- B34.0 Adenovirus infection, unspecified
- A08.2 Adenoviral enteritis
- B97.0 Adenovirus as the cause of diseases classified elsewhere

FAQ
- Q: Is there anything one can do to prevent these infections?
- A: Washing hands and avoiding contact with ill persons will help slow the spread of these infections.

ALCOHOL (ETHANOL) INTOXICATION

Ann B. Bruner

BASICS

DESCRIPTION

- Acute ingestion (accidental or intended) of alcohol, resulting in loss of inhibition, often associated with unruly/violent behavior, impaired judgment and/or coordination, diminished alertness/responsiveness, and sedation or coma
- Accidental ingestion is more common in toddlers and younger children.
- Frequency of intentional alcohol use increases with age.
- Alcohol–drug interactions are common because acute intoxication reduces hepatic clearance for other drugs, thereby increasing their serum concentrations.

EPIDEMIOLOGY

Alcohol is the most used drug by young people: 30% of 8th graders, 69% of 12th graders, and 81% of college students have consumed alcohol.

Prevalence

- 71% of high school students have consumed alcohol in their lifetime; 21% had their first drink before age 13 years; 39% had one drink in past 30 days; 54% of 12th graders and 13% of 8th graders have been drunk at least once.
- Underage (12–20 years old) drinkers are 3 times more likely than adults to use illicit drugs with alcohol.
- Over 90% of alcohol is consumed through binge drinking; prevalence of binge alcohol use (>5 drinks once in past 2 weeks) in 2012 was 5% of 8th graders, 16% of 10th graders, 24% of 12th graders, 37% of college students, and 36% of young adults.
- 24% of high school students have ridden in a car driven by someone who had been drinking alcohol; 8% had driven a car when they had been drinking.
- 56% of college students mixed energy drinks with alcohol in the past month.
- Household products (medicinal, cosmetic, cleaning, hygiene) can contain up to 100% ethanol; rates of accidental exposure to and intentional intoxication from hand sanitizers are increasing.

RISK FACTORS

Patients with psychiatric conditions are at an increased risk for abuse of alcohol and other drugs.

GENERAL PREVENTION

- Promote family discussions about alcohol use and abuse.
- Provide safety recommendations to prevent accidental ingestions.

PATHOPHYSIOLOGY

- Effects of alcohol ingestion are related to dose, the time in which alcohol was consumed and then absorbed, and the patient's history of alcohol exposure; peak serum concentrations occur 30–60 minutes after ingestion.
- Alcohol absorption, decreased by the presence of food in the stomach and increased if liquid is carbonated, occurs rapidly and largely in the small intestine.
- Minimal quantities of alcohol are excreted in urine, sweat, and breath.
- >90% of alcohol oxidized in liver follows zero-order kinetics, primarily by alcohol dehydrogenase (ADH) and then acetaldehyde dehydrogenase (ALDH); rate of metabolism is fixed (not related to dose or time) and is proportional to body weight. Ethnic/racial and gender variabilities exist on quantity and efficacy of ADH.
- Ethanol is metabolized by ADH to acetaldehyde, then to acetate, and finally to ketones, fatty acids, or acetone; ketosis and, infrequently, metabolic acidosis can occur.
- Respiratory acidosis can occur secondary to carbon dioxide retention from respiratory depression due to ethanol intoxication.
- Hypoglycemia occurs during acute ethanol intoxication due to impaired gluconeogenesis resulting from changes in the NADH/NAD+ ratio associated with ethanol metabolism.
- Alcohol affects the CNS primarily through the γ-aminobutyric acid (GABA) and glutamate neurotransmitter systems.

ETIOLOGY

Alcohol is produced from fermentation/distillation of sugar from grapes (wine), grains/corn (beer/whiskey), potatoes (vodka), or sugar cane (rum) then mixed into solution to make specific beverages; products are marketed according to alcohol content or proof (twice the percent). Alcohol content ranges from 3–6% (6–12 proof) in beer to 40–75% (80–150 proof) in vodka/rum/whiskey. Alcohol is often consumed concurrently with other substances (licit and illicit), presenting a mixed clinical picture of intoxication.

COMMONLY ASSOCIATED CONDITIONS

- Alcohol is involved in 30% of all drug overdoses.
- A significant percentage of adolescent trauma patients, especially victims of gunshot wounds, have positive toxicology screens for alcohol and other drugs. Ethanol use increases trauma risk by 3- to 7-fold.

DIAGNOSIS

HISTORY

- Medical: Baseline health will affect patient's response to alcohol; diabetics, for example, may have worse hypoglycemia.
- Type and dose of other drugs ingested:
  - Clinical effects of and treatment for other ingestions can vary depending on substance.
  - Polysubstance ingestion is very common.
- Psychiatric history: Evaluate for possible suicidal ideation.
- Gathering details regarding the alcohol consumed (type, amount, and over what time period) may help predict clinical course. For example, blood alcohol concentration (BAC) may continue rising if ingestion occurred recently.
- Intoxication presents clinically with signs ranging from lack of coordination, slurred speech, and confusion (BAC of 20–200 mg/dL) to ataxia and nausea/vomiting (BAC 200–300 mg/dL) to amnesia, seizures, or coma (BAC >300 mg/dL).

PHYSICAL EXAM

- Bruises, lacerations, and fractures may suggest trauma and raise concern about CNS injury.
- Neurologic exam, including mental status, will assess degree of intoxication and consciousness, including patient's ability to protect his or her airway, and risk for aspiration.
- Tachycardia and hypotension may indicate dehydration.
- Fever may suggest infection.
- Average time for normalization of mental status in intoxicated adults is 3–3.5 hours; patients without clinical improvement in 3 hours should be evaluated for other causes of altered mental status.

DIAGNOSTIC TESTS & INTERPRETATION

Lab

- BAC
  - Generally correlates with clinical picture
  - In children, signs of intoxication may be present at levels of 50 mg/dL.
  - Serum levels of 600–800 mg/dL can be fatal.
- Blood and/or urine toxicology screen
  - Most urine toxicology screens do not test for alcohol.
  - Concurrent ingestions are common.
- Acetaminophen level
  - Usually not part of the general serum toxicology screen
  - Consider if polysubstance ingestion suspected and/or if patient has suicidal ideation
- Serum electrolytes
  - Alcohol is a diuretic. The associated nausea and vomiting seen with intoxication may result in severe dehydration.
  - Ketosis and, infrequently, metabolic acidosis can occur.
- Serum glucose level: Ethanol inhibits gluconeogenesis and can be associated with hypoglycemia.
- Blood gas can show both respiratory and metabolic acidosis.

DIFFERENTIAL DIAGNOSIS

- Environmental
  - Other ingestions (overdose of sedatives or illicit drugs, such as benzodiazepines, marijuana, narcotics, lysergic acid diethylamide [LSD], and phencyclidine [PCP])
  - Toxic exposures (ethylene glycol, methanol, carbon monoxide)
  - Head trauma
- Infection
  - Meningitis
  - Encephalitis
  - Sepsis
- Tumor: brain tumor
- Metabolic
  - Hypoglycemia
  - Ketoacidosis
  - Hyperammonemia
  - Electrolyte imbalances (hyponatremia, hypernatremia)
- Miscellaneous
  - Increased intracranial pressure from hydrocephalus, mass, other
  - Stroke

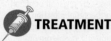

TREATMENT

MEDICATION

IV dextrose as needed for hypoglycemia

ADDITIONAL TREATMENT

General Measures

- Assess airway, breathing, and circulation (ABC).
- Protect airway: The patient may require intubation and mechanical ventilation.
- Mainstay is supportive therapy as no specific ethanol antidote exists.
- Appropriate trauma management as needed
- Because alcohol is absorbed rapidly, gastric lavage is indicated only if the patient is seen immediately after ingestion (within minutes).

ISSUES FOR REFERRAL

- Refer to substance abuse specialist (addiction medicine, psychiatrist, or certified addictions counselor) for detailed evaluation and treatment.
- Refer for psychiatric evaluation if depression, anxiety, suicidal ideation, or any other mental health condition is suspected.
- Assess for other risk-taking behaviors—including other substance use, sexual activity, use of motor vehicles while intoxicated, weapon carrying, and delinquency—and their sequelae, including pregnancy, sexually transmitted infections, and violence.

INPATIENT CONSIDERATIONS

Initial Stabilization

Keep patient awake; watch for vomiting as patients are at risk for choking owing to depressed gag reflex.

Admission Criteria

- Unstable vital signs (hypotension)
- Persistent CNS depression/impaired mental status
- Potential severity of comorbid psychiatric conditions (depression/suicidality)
- Inability to contact a parent/guardian

IV Fluids

IV fluids for dehydration and hypotension

Nursing

Observe and monitor vital signs and neurologic status.

Discharge Criteria

- Stable vital signs
- Patient awake, alert, responsive, and oriented
- Decreasing BAC
- Parent/guardian fully informed about patient's alcohol use

DIET

NPO secondary to depressed gag reflex

PROGNOSIS

BAC serum levels of 600–800 mg/dL can be fatal.

COMPLICATIONS

- Diuresis and dehydration
- Vasodilation and hypotension
- Vomiting, aspiration, potential respiratory arrest
- Hypoglycemia
- Metabolic acidosis
- Impaired mental status
- Engagement in risk-taking behaviors (e.g., other drug use, unprotected intercourse) while intoxicated
- CNS depression
- Gastritis
- GI bleeding
- Acute pancreatitis
- Motor vehicle collisions associated with driving while intoxicated
- Alcoholism
- Alcohol withdrawal following a period of intoxication in chronic users (symptoms include tachycardia, elevated blood pressure, irritability, nausea, vomiting, and tremor)

ADDITIONAL READING

- Centers for Disease Control and Prevention. 2011 Youth Risk Behavior Survey. www.cdc.gov/yrbs. Accessed September 1, 2013.
- Howland J, Rohsenow DJ. Risks of energy drinks mixed with alcohol. *JAMA*. 2013:309(31):245–246.
- Johnston LD, O'Malley PM, Bachman JG, et al. *Monitoring the Future National Results on Drug Use: 2012 Overview, Key Findings on Adolescent Drug Use*. Ann Arbor, MI: Institute for Social Research, The University of Michigan; 2013.
- Rayar P, Ratnapalan S. Pediatric ingestions of household products containing ethanol: a review. *Clin Pediatr*. 2013;52(3):203–209.
- The Center on Alcohol Marketing and Youth. Prevalence of underage drinking. http://www.camy.org/factsheets/sheets/Prevalence_of_Underage_Drinking.html. Accessed September 1, 2013.

CODES

ICD10

- F10.929 Alcohol use, unspecified with intoxication, unspecified
- T51.0X4A Toxic effect of ethanol, undetermined, initial encounter
- F10.920 Alcohol use, unspecified with intoxication, uncomplicated

FAQ

- Q: How quickly is alcohol metabolized?
- A: The liver metabolizes ~10 g of ethanol per hour, which corresponds to a decline in BAC of 18–20 mg/dL/h.
- Q: What is binge drinking in youth?
- A: For children 9–13 years old and girls 14–17 years old, 3 or more drinks; for boys 14–15 years old, 4 or more
- Q: Are younger children at any increased risk from alcohol poisoning?
- A: Ethanol inhibits gluconeogenesis; younger children have an increased risk of hypoglycemia because they have relatively smaller hepatic glycogen stores; however, children tend to have more rapid clearance rates (up to 30 mg/dL/h).

ALLERGIC CHILD

Barry Pelz • Anne Marie Singh

BASICS

Allergic diseases include atopic dermatitis, food allergy, asthma, and allergic rhinitis. Atopic or allergic diseases are becoming more and more prevalent in the population.

- Food allergy in its most severe form may manifest as anaphylaxis.
- The conditions may present in a variety of ways as described below.

DESCRIPTION

- Atopic dermatitis
  - Atopic dermatitis (or eczema) is characterized by chronic, relapsing, pruritic inflamed skin which is often erythematous, xerotic, and/or excoriated.
  - Atopic dermatitis may occur in isolation without other atopic diseases.
  - Atopic dermatitis may also be the beginning of the "atopic march" in which atopic dermatitis precedes the onset of other atopic conditions which may include food allergy, asthma, and allergic rhinitis.
- Urticaria
  - Refers to hives or the erythematous wheals that occur when histamine is released from mast cells
  - May be caused by a number of triggers
  - Viral infection is the most common cause of urticaria in children.
  - The allergic child may develop urticaria when an antigen such as a food or animal dander causes IgE-mediated release of mast cell mediators.
- Food allergy
  - Presents with an IgE-mediated reaction after exposure to a food to which the child is sensitized
  - Reactions may present with any number of symptoms, including urticaria, lip or tongue swelling, closing of the throat, wheezing, shortness of breath, repeated vomiting after allergen ingestion, diarrhea, or any combination of the above.
  - The most common food allergens include cow's milk, egg white, peanut, tree nuts, wheat, soy, fish, and shellfish.
  - Food allergy should be distinguished from food intolerance which has a nonimmunologic basis and does not carry a risk of anaphylaxis.
- Asthma
  - An obstructive airway disease characterized by recurrent wheezing, bronchoconstriction, increased mucous production, and airway inflammation
  - Asthma is one of many potential causes of wheezing in children.
  - Wheezing with RSV and human rhinovirus infection are risk factors for the development of asthma.
- Allergic rhinitis
  - A condition in which children are sensitized to perennial allergens, seasonal allergens, or both
  - Perennial allergens include dust mite, molds, cockroach, and animal dander.
  - Seasonal allergens include tree pollens, grass pollens, or ragweed.
  - Rhinitis symptoms may include watery eyes, itchy eyes, rhinorrhea, nasal discharge, itchy nose, postnasal drip, headache, sinus pressure, nasal obstruction, mouth breathing, or snoring.
  - Symptoms may be seasonal, year-round, or triggered by exposure to specific allergens (such as cats or dogs).

RISK FACTORS

Genetics

- Children who do not have a family history of atopy have approximately 25% chance of being atopic.
- For children with at least one parent who is atopic, the risk of atopy approximately doubles compared to the general population.

PATHOPHYSIOLOGY

Most of these allergic conditions are IgE mediated, and all of them result from a complex interaction between multiple genetic and environmental factors.

DIAGNOSIS

A thorough history and physical examination are the keys to diagnosing the allergic child.

HISTORY

- History should elicit signs and symptoms of allergic diseases while at the same time exploring other potential etiologies for the child's symptoms.
- The allergic child should have symptoms of atopic dermatitis, urticaria, wheezing, reactions to foods, or symptoms of rhinitis such as sneezing, itchy eyes, watery eyes, itchy nose, runny nose, or itchy throat.
- The practitioner should also review the family history as atopic disease often runs in families.

PHYSICAL EXAM

A complete physical exam is essential to rule out systemic diseases that can mimic allergic disease.

- **Finding:** Ocular signs may include the following:
  - Dark circles under the eyes or the so-called "allergic shiners" which result from venous stasis secondary to passive congestion in the nose, impeding venous return to the vessels under the eyes
  - Cobblestoning of the conjunctiva
  - Erythematous injection of the conjunctiva
  - Dennie-Morgan lines or infraorbital folds associated with suborbital edema secondary to chronic inflammation from atopic dermatitis
  - Clear stringy ocular discharge
- **Finding:** Nasal allergic signs may include the following:
  - Pale edematous nasal mucosa
  - Clear nasal discharge with or without occlusion
  - Nasal crease across the bridge of nose secondary to repeated upward rubbing of the nose from "the allergic salute"
  - Nasal polyps may be present, although they are much more common in adults and should prompt consideration of diseases such as cystic fibrosis when seen in children.
- **Finding:** Ear allergic signs may include the following:
  - Fluid in the middle ear or retracted tympanic membranes
  - Eustachian tube dysfunction associated with allergic inflammation
- **Finding:** Throat allergic signs may include the following:
  - Cobblestoning of the posterior pharynx secondary to submucosal lymphoid hyperplasia
- **Finding:** Lung allergic signs may include the following:
  - Wheezes, rhonchi, decreased air entry, prolonged expiration, and chronic obstruction secondary to allergic responses
- **Finding:** Skin allergic signs may include the following:
  - Eczema, hives, angioedema, and dermatographism

DIFFERENTIAL DIAGNOSIS

The differential for allergic diseases is extensive and should focus on considering other etiologies for the symptoms.

- Ear/nose symptoms
  - Eye findings may be caused by physical or chemical irritants or by viral or bacterial infection.
  - Allergic rhinitis symptoms may resemble upper respiratory infections, sinusitis, nasal foreign bodies, or nonallergic rhinitis.
  - A number of medications can also lead to rhinitis medicamentosa, or symptoms of nasal congestion due to medication use.
  - Systemic diseases such as cystic fibrosis, immotile cilia syndrome, Kartagener syndrome, or immunodeficiencies may present with recurrent nasal symptoms and/or with lung symptoms.
  - Lung symptoms may be caused by physical or chemical irritants including tobacco smoke, environmental pollution, and inhalants.
- Chest symptoms
  - Lung symptoms may also result from gastroesophageal reflux leading to (nocturnal) cough.
  - Foreign body aspiration may produce lung symptoms and auscultatory signs, although typically, foreign bodies create more focal lung findings.
  - Anatomic defects in the airway may also result in symptoms that are similar to allergic symptoms.
- Skin symptoms
  - Skin findings may be caused by a number of etiologies including irritant dermatitis, viral exanthems, autoimmune disorders, bacterial, fungal, or parasitic infections.
- Multisystem
  - Anaphylaxis may sometimes be confused with angioedema, vocal cord dysfunction, globus hystericus, or with other causes of shock (sepsis, hypovolemia, cardiogenic).
  - Food allergy may sometimes be confused with food intolerance, but food intolerances present with abdominal discomfort, bloating, flatulence, or nonspecific malaise, whereas food allergy presents with true IgE-mediated reactions.

DIAGNOSTIC TESTS & INTERPRETATION

The diagnosis of allergic diseases can be strongly suggested based on history and physical alone. Specific tests can be done by a specialist in allergy and immunology in order to be properly interpreted. Often, initial therapy can be initiated without definitive tests.

Once the allergic child is referred to the allergist, testing may include the following:

- Immediate hypersensitivity testing
  - Skin prick tests to suspected allergens based on history may demonstrate IgE sensitization if positive.
  - Intradermal skin tests for patients who have a negative skin prick test and a suspicious history pose a greater risk of systemic reactions but can be done for environmental allergens, not for foods.
- Blood-specific IgE testing
  - ImmunoCAP tests measure free serum IgE to a specific antigen to which a particular patient may be sensitized.
  - Although panels are available, these tests are best done for targeted potential allergens that are suggested by the history and should be interpreted by an allergist with experience in interpreting and guiding therapy.
  - Incorrect use or interpretation of ImmunoCAP testing may result in inappropriate dietary restrictions, nutritional deficits, and undue anxiety.
  - ImmunoCAP levels may be trended over time to help monitor for the development of tolerance.
- Eosinophilia
  - Eosinophils in the blood (on a CBC) or in respiratory secretions or nasal samples may be indicative of an allergic diathesis.
- Pulmonary function tests (PFTs)
  - PFTs or spirometry should be obtained on asthmatic children or in children with respiratory allergic histories to evaluate for obstructive diseases.

TREATMENT

GENERAL MEASURES

- The main principle of therapy for allergic diseases is avoidance of allergic triggers.
- For atopic dermatitis, general treatment measures include measures to help lock moisture into skin, treat inflammation when present, control pruritus, minimize skin irritants, and treat infection when present.
- For food allergy, the most important therapeutic measure is strict avoidance of the food that causes the allergy in order to prevent an allergic reaction.
  - Children at risk for a reaction to a food allergen should be prescribed an epinephrine autoinjector to use in the event of systemic symptoms or anaphylaxis.
  - An emergency action plan should be provided, reviewing the signs and symptoms of a reaction and the doses and medications that should be used in the event that an accidental ingestion occurs.
- For allergic rhinitis, systemic antihistamines may be helpful in controlling symptoms. Many patients also benefit from intranasal corticosteroids when indicated.
  - Specific environmental control measures may be indicated based on specific skin testing results.
  - Pets should be kept out of the bedroom if a child has allergic stigmata due to animal dander.
  - To minimize exposure to dust mite allergen, the bedding should be encased in dust mite encasements and washed in hot water at least once every 2 weeks.
  - Immunotherapy may be indicated for patients with allergic rhinitis or venom allergy.
- For patients with asthma, treatment should follow the latest National Heart, Lung and Blood Institute (NHLBI) of the National Institutes of Health (NIH) asthma guidelines with consideration to the child's symptomatology, impairment, and risk. Therapies may include use of rescue inhalers, controller medications such as inhaled corticosteroids, leukotriene antagonists, and others (see Appendix, Figure 5). Control of comorbidities such as allergic rhinitis and GERD are also important therapeutic steps.

ISSUES FOR REFERRAL

- Any child with allergic symptoms may benefit from referral to an allergist-immunologist.
- A patient failing medical management of upper respiratory or ocular allergies with routine antihistamine/decongestant medications may be referred to an allergist who can help identify triggers contributing to the problem.
- Poorly controlled asthma not responding to intermittent inhaled β-agonists or an asthmatic child who is symptomatic between exacerbations or has an atypical pattern of exacerbations should be referred.
- Asthma patients with frequent hospitalizations or steroid dependence should be referred.
- Patients who are absent from school frequently because of allergic or asthmatic symptoms should be referred.
- Patients with food allergy, drug allergy, latex allergy, or difficult-to-manage atopic dermatitis should also be referred to an allergist.

ONGOING CARE

PROGNOSIS

- In general, environmental allergies that cause rhinitis and asthma persist into adulthood.
- About 50% of milk-allergic children may outgrow their allergy by school age and about 80% by age 16 years. Those who tolerate baked milk seem to have a higher likelihood of outgrowing the allergy.
- About 60–80% of egg-allergic children may outgrow their egg allergy. Children who tolerate baked egg seem more likely to outgrow the allergy.
- Children may occasionally outgrow peanut, tree nut, or shellfish allergy.
- Allergic diseases may have a significant impact on the patient and family's quality of life and may lead to issues with anxiety and mental health.

ADDITIONAL READING

- Adkinson NF, Bochner BS, Busse WW, et al. *Middleton's Allergy Principles and Practice*. 7th ed. Philadelphia, PA: Mosby; 2009.
- Hatzler L, Hofmaier S, Papadopoulos NG. Allergic airway diseases in childhood—marching from epidemiology to novel concepts of prevention. *Pediatr Allergy Immunol*. 2012;23(7):616–622.
- Langley EW, Gigante J. Anaphylaxis, urticaria and angioedema. *Pediatr Rev*. 2013;34(6):247–257.
- Papadopoulos NG, Arakawa H, Carlsen KH, et al. International consensus on (ICON) pediatric asthma. *Allergy*. 2012;67(8):976–997.
- Wood RA, Sicherer SH, Vickery BP, et al. The natural history of milk allergy in an observational cohort. *J Allergy Clin Immunol*. 2013;131(3):805–812.

CODES

ICD10

- L20.9 Atopic dermatitis, unspecified
- L27.2 Dermatitis due to ingested food
- J45.909 Unspecified asthma, uncomplicated

FAQ

- Q: Do children outgrow allergies?
- A: In general, environmental allergies that cause rhinitis and asthma persist into adulthood. However, most children outgrow food allergies to milk, egg, soy, and wheat. Children may occasionally outgrow peanut, tree nut, or shellfish allergies.
- Q: If a parent is allergic to a specific allergen, can the child inherit this allergy?
- A: Children inherit the tendency to be allergic, but they do not inherit specific allergies.
- Q: How can allergies be prevented?
- A: Allergy prevention is currently not possible, but research in this field is ongoing.

ALOPECIA (HAIR LOSS)

Hope Rhodes • Terry Kind

BASICS

DESCRIPTION
- Absence of hair where it normally grows
- Categorized as acquired or congenital
  - Most cases are acquired: Tinea capitis is most common, followed by traumatic alopecia and alopecia areata.
- Also categorized as diffuse or localized
  - Most cases of alopecia are localized and, of these, tinea capitis is the most common.
- Many normal healthy newborns lose their hair in the first few months of life.
  - Hair loss may be exacerbated by friction from bedding/sleep surface, especially in atopic infants.
- Normally, about 50–100 hairs are shed and simultaneously replaced every day.
- 90% of alopecia cases are due to the following disorders:
  - Tinea capitis
  - Alopecia areata
  - Traction alopecia
  - Telogen effluvium
    - Alopecia is preceded by a psychologically or physically stressful event 6–16 weeks prior to the onset of hair loss.
    - Growing hairs convert rapidly to resting hairs.

RISK FACTORS
Genetics
- Alopecia areata
  - Polygenic with variety of triggering factors
  - Family history in 10–42% of cases
  - Males and females equally affected
  - Onset usually before age 30 years
- Monilethrix (also called beaded hair)
  - A rare autosomal dominant disorder

DIAGNOSIS

DIFFERENTIAL DIAGNOSIS
Consider the most likely diagnoses first.
- Infectious
  - Tinea capitis
  - Varicella
  - Syphilis
- Congenital
  - Aplasia cutis congenita
  - Incontinentia pigmenti
  - Oculomandibulofacial syndrome (sparse hair, hypoplastic teeth, cataracts, short stature)
  - Goltz syndrome (alopecia, focal dermal hypoplasia, strabismus, nail dystrophy)
  - Triangular alopecia of the frontal scalp
  - Focal dermal hypoplasia
  - Hair-shaft defects (trichodystrophies)
  - Ectodermal dysplasias
  - Nevi
  - Progeria
- Nutritional
  - Zinc deficiency
  - Marasmus
  - Kwashiorkor
  - Anorexia or bulimia
  - Hypervitaminosis A
  - Celiac disease
- Endocrinologic
  - Androgenetic alopecia
  - Hypothyroidism
  - Hyperthyroidism
  - Hypoparathyroidism
  - Hypopituitarism
  - Diabetes mellitus
- Autoimmune
  - Alopecia areata
  - Systemic lupus erythematosus
  - Scleroderma
- Trauma
  - Traction alopecia
  - Trichotillomania
  - Scalp electrode scar from in utero monitoring
- Toxic exposures:
  - Antimetabolites
  - Anticoagulants
  - Antithyroid medications
  - Heavy metals (e.g., arsenic, lead)
  - Radiation
- Stress
  - Trichotillomania
- Miscellaneous:
  - Telogen effluvium
  - Darier disease (keratotic crusted papules, keratosis follicularis)
  - Lichen planus
  - Burn
  - Stress

COMMONLY ASSOCIATED CONDITIONS
- May be associated with a genetic, endocrine, or toxin-mediated condition
- Look for nail, skin, teeth, or gland involvement.
- Trichotillomania is frequently associated with a finger-sucking habit.

APPROACH TO PATIENT
- Treatment of alopecia is guided by underlying etiology.
- Systemic treatment is needed for tinea capitis; topical antifungals alone are not adequate. Selenium sulfide or ketoconazole shampoo is recommended for tinea capitis to decrease fungal shedding and risk of spread to others.
- Other than reassurance and waiting, there is no proven effective long-term therapy for alopecia areata. Topical steroids may show short-term benefit. There are no randomized clinical trials on the use of topical immunotherapy or intralesional steroids.
- Caution regarding side effects of all potential treatments.

HISTORY
- Attempt to classify the alopecia. This will guide the diagnosis and treatment plan.
- **Question:** Is the loss acquired or congenital? Is the alopecia treatable? Is it likely to be self-limited?
- *Significance*: Consider most likely diagnoses, including tinea capitis, traumatic alopecia, and alopecia areata.
- **Question:** Associated abnormalities?
- *Significance*: may be part of a syndrome
- **Question:** Is there an endocrine abnormality or a toxin/medication effect?
- *Significance*: Some of these would require prompt attention.
- **Question:** Assess extent of hair loss.
- *Significance*:
  - Increased amount of hair in the brush or in the shower/tub drain?
  - Does hair appear or feel thinner?
  - Patches of hair loss or broken hairs noted?
- **Question**: Considering trichotillomania?
- *Significance*: Note that patients often deny hair-pulling. Direct confrontation is rarely helpful.

PHYSICAL EXAM
- Assess localized versus diffuse hair loss.
- **Finding:** appearance of the scalp
- *Significance*:
  - Alopecia areata: Except for well-demarcated hair loss, scalp appears normal with smooth surface.
  - Tinea capitis: Scalp is often scaly and may be erythematous; areas of hair loss with broken hair stubs, referred to as *black-dot* alopecia.
- **Finding:** bizarre configuration and irregular border; hairs of varying lengths
- *Significance*: distinguishes traction/traumatic alopecia from alopecia areata
- **Finding:** short broken hairs but not black dots
- *Significance*: Short hairs are usually associated with trichotillomania, whereas black dot alopecia is seen with tinea capitis.
- **Finding:** frontal, vertex, or bitemporal decreased hair density in adolescents
- *Significance*: may be adolescent-onset, androgenetic alopecia
- **Finding:** Hair shaft varies in thickness, with small node-like deformities (like beads), increased breakage, and partial alopecia.
- *Significance*:
  - Monilethrix
  - Other hair-shaft abnormalities with increased fragility include pseudomonilethrix, trichorrhexis, pili torti, pili bifurcati, Menkes kinky hair syndrome, and trichothiodystrophy.
- **Finding:** associated systemic signs or any nonscalp findings
- *Significance*: may signify a genetic syndrome or endocrine abnormality

- **Finding:** nail defects such as dystrophic changes and fine stippling
- *Significance*:
  - Nail defects are seen in 10–20% of cases of alopecia areata.
  - Nail defects accompanying localized alopecia along with syndactyly, strabismus, and dermal hypoplasia may be found in Goltz syndrome.
  - In ectodermal dysplasias, nails, hair, teeth, or glands may be affected.
- **Finding:** pubic hair and eyebrow hair loss
- *Significance*:
  - Found in a form of alopecia areata called *alopecia universalis*, where nearly all body hair is lost (alopecia totalis involves the loss of all scalp hair)
  - Body hair loss such as pubic hair or eyebrow hair may also occur in trichotillomania.

DIAGNOSTIC TESTS & INTERPRETATION

- **Test:** fungal culture
- *Significance*:
  - Recommended when assessing for tinea capitis as a cause of alopecia
  - Definitive results may take up to several weeks; may treat while awaiting results
  - Using a cotton-tipped applicator, culturette, toothbrush, or direct plating on Sabouraud dextrose agar, culture will be positive for *Trichophyton tonsurans* in >90% of cases in North America.
  - Less common are *Microsporum canis*, *Microsporum audouinii*, *Trichophyton mentagrophytes*, and *Trichophyton schoenleinii*.
- **Test:** dermatophyte-testing medium (DTM)
- *Significance*:
  - Assessing for tinea capitis
  - Definitive results may take from days to weeks. If dermatophyte colonies grow on the medium, the phenol red indicator in the agar will turn from yellow to red.
- **Test:** Wood's light (lamp) examination
- *Significance*:
  - *M. canis*, *M. audouinii*, or *T. schoenleinii* fluoresces green.
  - *T. tonsurans* does not fluoresce.
- **Test:** potassium hydroxide (KOH) exam
- *Significance*:
  - The KOH exam is another way to assess for tinea capitis.
  - Hyphae and spores within hair shaft indicate tinea capitis.
  - With *Microsporum*, spores surround the hair shaft.
- **Test**: endocrine testing
- *Significance*:
  - Alopecia areata or diffuse alopecia is associated with several endocrine disorders (e.g., hyperthyroidism, diabetes).
  - Based on history of physical exam, consider relevant screening tests or referral to an endocrinologist or dermatologist for further evaluation.
  - Routine screening for autoimmune disorders is generally not indicated.
- **Test:** hair-pluck test
- *Significance*:
  - Used to determine the ratio of telogen (resting) to anagen (growing) hairs
  - ~50 hairs are plucked (with 1 firm tug using a hemostat clamped around the hair ~1 cm from the scalp) and examined under the low-power lens of a microscope to determine the percentage of hairs that are telogen and anagen hairs.
  - >25% telogen hairs are indicative of telogen effluvium.
- **Test:** scalp biopsy
- *Significance*:
  - Can help to distinguish alopecia areata and trichotillomania
  - In alopecia areata, hair follicles become small but continue to produce fine hairs; there is mitotic activity in the matrix and often inflammation is present.
  - In trichotillomania, follicles are not small. They are usually in a transitional (catagen) phase and no longer produce normal hair shafts. Keratinous debris, fibrosis, and clumps of dark melanin pigment are present. Significant inflammation is absent.
  - In telogen effluvium, follicles remain intact without inflammation.

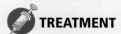

TREATMENT

MEDICATION

First Line

- For tinea capitis: microsize griseofulvin 20–25 mg/kg/24 h (maximum 1 g) or ultramicrosize griseofulvin 10–15 mg/kg/24 h (maximum 750 mg) orally once per day for 4–6 weeks; approved for children >2 years of age
- For alopecia areata requiring treatment: Topical corticosteroids may be used for isolated patches for short-term benefit.

Second Line

- For tinea capitis: Terbinafine, itraconazole, or fluconazole may be effective, although only terbinafine is FDA-approved for this condition.
- For alopecia areata: There is limited evidence for long-term effectiveness of any treatment. For trial of other therapies (intralesional steroid, topical immunotherapy), seek consultation with a dermatologist.

General Measures

- Treatment of alopecia is guided by the underlying cause.
- If alopecia signifies a toxic exposure or an endocrine abnormality, the underlying condition may require prompt diagnosis and treatment.
- Infectious causes of alopecia (such as with tinea capitis) should be treated promptly.
- Most patients with alopecia areata do not need treatment, as regrowth will occur spontaneously.
- Complementary and alternative medicine (CAM):
  - Hypnotherapy, massage, acupuncture, and onion juice are among the complementary therapies that have been tried for conditions like alopecia areata and trichotillomania. Of note, although many patients try CAM for alopecia, more research is needed.

ONGOING CARE

PROGNOSIS

- Tinea capitis, alopecia areata, and traction alopecia
  - Hair will regrow, may take months.
  - There is a poorer prognosis with alopecia universalis. <10% have full recovery.
- Telogen effluvium
  - Spontaneous regrowth is expected unless the stressful event continues/recurs.
- Alopecia areata may spontaneously remit and then recur.

ADDITIONAL READING

- Alkhalifah A, Alsantali A, Wang E, et al. Alopecia areata update. *J Am Acad Dermatol*. 2010;62(2):177–188, 191–202.
- Food and Drug Administration. Consumer updates: Lamisil approved to treat scalp ringworm in children. http://www.fda.gov/forconsumers/consumerupdates/ucm048710.htm. March 19, 2015.
- Haynes JW, Persons R, Jamieson B. Clinical inquiries: childhood alopecia areata: what treatment works best? *J Fam Pract*. 2011;60(1):45–52.
- Hunt N, McHale S. The psychological impact of alopecia. *BMJ*. 2005;331(7522):951–953.
- Sardesai V, Prasad S, Agarwal T. A Study to evaluate the efficacy of various topical treatment modalities for alopecia areata. *Int J Trichology*. 2012;4(4):265–270.
- Swanson A, Canty K. Common pediatric skin conditions with protracted courses: a therapeutic update. *Dermatol Clin*. 2013;31(2):239–249.
- National Alopecia Areata Foundation: http://www.naaf.org
- van den Biggelaar FJ, Smolders J, Jansen JF. Complementary and alternative medicine in alopecia areata. *Am J Clin Dermatol*. 2010;11(1):11–20.

CODES

ICD10

- L65.9 Nonscarring hair loss, unspecified
- B35.0 Tinea barbae and tinea capitis
- L63.9 Alopecia areata, unspecified

FAQ

- Q: When can children with tinea capitis return to school?
- A: Once treatment with a systemic antifungal has begun, the child may return to school. A topical shampoo such as selenium sulfide or ketoconazole is recommended to decrease fungal shedding and the risk of spread.
- Q: Will the hair grow back?
- A: For the 3 most common causes of childhood alopecia—accounting for 90% of cases; tinea capitis, alopecia areata, and traction alopecia—hair will regrow, but may take months to do so.

ALPHA-1 ANTITRYPSIN DEFICIENCY

Christine K. Lee

BASICS

DESCRIPTION

- Alpha-1 antitrypsin (AAT) is a serine protease inhibitor and a 55-kd glycoprotein which is primarily synthesized in the liver and released into the circulation.
- AAT is the main inhibitor of neutrophil proteases, which can cause host tissue damage.
- AAT deficiency is an autosomal codominant genetic disorder that causes lung, liver, and skin disease.
- Classic PiZZ AAT deficiency is caused by homozygosity for Z mutant allele of AAT.
- Lung disease in AAT deficiency can develop after the 3rd decade of life and progress to emphysema.
- Liver disease may present as jaundice in infants or as elevated liver enzymes, portal hypertension, or cirrhosis in older patients.
- Skin disease is more rare and presents as necrotizing panniculitis in adults (mean age of onset is 40 years).

EPIDEMIOLOGY

Most common genetic cause of liver disease in children and of emphysema in adults

Incidence

- Incidence of the PiZZ genotype is highest in Caucasians in North America, Australia, and Europe, particularly in Scandinavia, British Isles, Northern France, and the Tyrol region of Italy.
- In the United States, the PiZ allele is found in ~14.5 per 1,000 people, with higher frequency in Caucasians and lower frequency in Asians, blacks, and Hispanics.
- The incidence of classic AAT deficiency (PiZZ) is 1 in 1,800–2,000 live births.

Prevalence

- It has been estimated that approximately 70,000–100,000 individuals are affected in the United States.
- Of these genetically affected individuals, fewer than 10% are estimated to have been diagnosed with AAT deficiency
- Approximately 25 million people in the United States are thought to be carriers of a mutant allele.

RISK FACTORS

Genetics

- AAT is a serine protease inhibitor encoded by the *SERPINA1* gene, which is located on the long arm of chromosome 14.
- The normal allele is M, with over 100 variant alleles identified.
- The classic PiZZ genotype is the result of a point mutation at position 342 in the AAT gene, which encodes a substitution of lysine for glutamate
- The S allele (2nd most common mutation) occurs from a substitution of valine for glutamate at position 246.
- Patients with PiZZ alleles have serum AAT levels, which are less than 15% of normal.
- Heterozygous carriers of the Z allele are found in 1.5–3% of the population. In and of itself, this genetic mutation is not a cause of liver disease, but it may contribute to pathophysiology of other liver diseases.
- PiMS, PiMZ, and PiSS are also not directly associated with liver disease, although referral center data reports patients with chronic liver disease having a higher frequency of PiMZ than would be predicted by chance.
- The mutant S protein, when coexpressed with Z-protein, can form abnormal polymers leading to liver disease, which is identical to PiZZ patients.
- Because ~10% of affected PiZZ or PiSZ individuals have clinically significant liver disease, there may be other genetic or environmental factors which are important modifiers of AAT.

PATHOPHYSIOLOGY

- Lung disease in patients with PiZZ results from inadequate levels of AAT to protect the lungs from destructive enzymes, such as elastase, leading to early emphysema. This process is further worsened by exposure to cigarette smoke and environmental pollutants.
- Liver disease occurs from accumulation of the abnormal Z mutant protein within liver cells.
  - The mutant Z gene is transcribed, translated, and then translocated into the endoplasmic reticulum (ER).
  - Some molecules undergo proteolytic degradation, others aggregate to form large protein polymers, and few are secreted, leading to intrahepatocyte accumulation and thereby resulting in low AAT serum levels.
  - ER-associated degradation of mutant Z-protein is less efficient, leading to a great burden of protein in the liver and increased liver injury.
  - Autophagy degradation has also been proposed as an important route for degradation of the AAT mutant Z polymers.
- Panniculitis involves inflammation of the fat underneath the skin, causing hardening in lumps and patches, likely due to the unrestrained, destructive action of neutrophil elastase.

ETIOLOGY

Mutations in the *SERPINA1* gene result in lung disease through unopposed protease activity and in liver disease by intracellular retention of mutant AAT.

DIAGNOSIS

HISTORY

- Highly variable presentation in neonates and young children
- Most infants develop cholestatic jaundice, hepatosplenomegaly, poor feeding, and poor weight gain.
- Jaundice typically improves around 1 year of age and can then lead to either a continuation of liver disease, progression to cirrhosis, or normal liver function.
- Older children can present as asymptomatic chronic hepatitis, poor feeding, failure to thrive, hepatosplenomegaly, or complications of portal hypertension and cirrhosis.
- Risk of hepatocellular carcinoma in AAT may be independent of cirrhosis.
- Fulminant hepatic failure is rare but has been reported.

PHYSICAL EXAM

There may be signs of jaundice, hepatosplenomegaly, abdominal distention, and other stigmata of chronic liver disease.

DIAGNOSTIC TESTS & INTERPRETATION

Lab

- Elevated total and conjugated bilirubin, elevated serum transaminases, hypoalbuminemia, or coagulopathy
- Gold standard assessment is protein electrophoresis to determine the protease inhibitor (Pi) phenotype.
- Serum levels of AAT can be helpful to guide workup before phenotype results are available.
- Quantitative serum AAT levels
  - PiMM: 80–200 mg/dL
  - PiZZ: ≤20–45 mg/dL
  - Pi null/null phenotype: 0 mg/dL
  - As an acute-phase reactant, AAT levels can be falsely negative, as they may rise into the normal range in an ill patient.

Imaging

Abdominal ultrasound with Doppler can be useful to assess for portal hypertension and/or for pretransplantation evaluation in the setting of end-stage liver disease.

Diagnostic Procedures/Other

Diagnosis is determined by identification of the AAT phenotype by serum protein electrophoresis. Liver biopsy is not required for diagnosis but can help to support it.

Pathologic Findings

- Liver biopsy findings can be variable in infants and may include giant cell transformation, lobular hepatitis, steatosis, fibrosis, hepatocellular necrosis, bile duct paucity, or bile duct proliferation.
- Globular eosinophilic inclusions in some hepatocytes can be seen under H&E stain, which represent dilated ER membranes with polymerized mutant protein.
- Staining with periodic acid–Schiff (PAS) followed by digestion with diastase to stain glycoproteins can be performed to highlight these globules.
- These findings are sometimes seen in other liver diseases, are not visible in all hepatocytes, and may even be absent in neonates.

DIFFERENTIAL DIAGNOSIS

- The differential diagnosis varies with age at presentation.
- Infants generally present with jaundice; the differential diagnosis in infants should include biliary atresia, anatomic biliary abnormalities, congenital infections, galactosemia, and tyrosinemia. (See "Neonatal Cholestasis" and "Jaundice" for complete listing.)
- In older children, viral (hepatitis viruses, EBV, and CMV), toxic (ethanol, acetaminophen), metabolic (Wilson disease), and obstructive causes should be considered.

TREATMENT

- There is no specific treatment for the liver disease associated with AAT deficiency.
- Management involves supportive care to try to prevent complications of chronic liver disease.
- Patients with advanced liver disease should avoid alcohol and other hepatotoxins.
- Liver transplantation can be considered for end-stage liver disease. When transplanted, the graft will secrete normal AAT and stop further progression of lung disease.
- Due to increased risk of hepatocellular carcinoma, surveillance imaging and/or α-fetoprotein levels should be considered.
- Patients should be cautioned to avoid smoking, secondhand smoking, and other agents of inhalation injury.
- Although enzyme replacement therapy can be used in adults to prevent progression of lung disease, it has no effect on liver disease.
- Vaccination against hepatitis A and B

MEDICATION

- Ursodeoxycholic acid, a choleretic agent, can be used to manage cholestasis and pruritus in patients with liver disease.
- Augmentation therapy
  - Pooled human plasma–derived AAT (alpha-1 antiprotease) is the most efficient way to increase the circulating levels of AAT in the plasma and lung.
  - Therapy has been reported to decrease the rate of decline in 1-second forced expiratory volume (FEV_1) and mortality rate during the period of study

SURGERY/OTHER PROCEDURES

- There is no primary therapeutic surgical intervention for AAT deficiency aside from liver transplantation.
- Surgery in patients with native livers can be used to treat complications of portal hypertension.
- Orthotopic liver transplantation should be considered in patients with end-stage liver disease.
- Following transplantation, serum phenotype and AAT level return to donor levels. Lung damage will not progress but is unlikely to be reversed after liver transplantation.
- For lung disease, volume reduction surgery or lung transplantation may be considered.

ONGOING CARE

FOLLOW-UP RECOMMENDATIONS

Patient Monitoring

- Annual liver and pulmonary function testing
- Surveillance for hepatocellular carcinoma in Pi ZZ patients is suggested, but consensus on frequency and methodology is lacking.

PROGNOSIS

Approximately 10% of PiZZ and PiSZ individuals will have clinically significant liver disease during childhood; ~50% of the remaining individuals will have mildly elevated aminotransferases. Further significant liver disease may develop later in life.

COMPLICATIONS

- Patients with liver disease may develop complications of chronic liver disease including portal hypertension, cirrhosis, and/or hepatocellular carcinoma.
- Lung disease may progress to early-onset lower lobe emphysema.

ADDITIONAL READING

- Miranda E, Pérez J, Ekeowa UI, et al. A novel monoclonal antibody to characterize pathogenic polymers in liver disease associated with α1-antitrypsin deficiency. *Hepatology*. 2010;52(3):1078–1088.
- Perlmutter DH. Alpha-1-antitrypsin deficiency: diagnosis and treatment. *Clin Liver Dis*. 2004;8(4):839–859.
- Perlmutter DH. Pathogenesis of chronic liver injury and hepatocellular carcinoma in alpha-1-antitrypsin deficiency. *Pediatr Res*. 2006;60(2):233–238.
- Steiner SJ, Gupta SK, Croffie JM, et al. Serum levels of alpha1-antitrypsin predict phenotype expression of the alpha1-antitrypsin gene. *Dig Dis Sci*. 2003;48(9):1793–1796.
- Stoller JK, Brantly M. The challenge of detecting alpha-1 antitrypsin deficiency. *COPD*. 2013;10(Suppl 1):26–34.
- Teckman J. Alpha1-antitrypsin deficiency in childhood. *Semin Liver Dis*. 2007;27(3):274–281.
- Teckman J. Liver disease in alpha-1 antitrypsin deficiency: current understanding and future therapy. *COPD*. 2013;10(Suppl 1):35–43.
- Teckman J, Jain A. Advances in alpha-1-antitrypsin deficiency liver disease. *Curr Gastroenterol Rep*. 2014;16(1):367.

CODES

ICD10

E88.01 Alpha-1-antitrypsin deficiency

FAQ

- Q: Do all patients with presumed AAT require liver biopsy for diagnosis?
- A: No. A liver biopsy is not required for diagnosis but may help be performed to support it.
- Q: Are PAS-positive, diastase-resistant globules on liver biopsy diagnostic for AAT deficiency?
- A: No. Diagnosis is made by identification of the AAT phenotype by serum protein electrophoresis. Evidence of these globules on liver biopsy can support the diagnosis but may be absent in PiZZ neonates.
- Q: Will liver transplantation for AAT deficiency have any effect on the lungs?
- A: Yes. When a patient with AAT deficiency gets an orthotopic liver transplant, serum levels of AAT usually return to normal. This halts further progression of lung disease but does not reverse lung damage, which has already occurred.

ALTITUDE ILLNESS

Michael Yaron

BASICS

DESCRIPTION

High-altitude illness represents a spectrum of clinical entities with neurologic and pulmonary manifestations that overlap presentations and share elements of pathophysiology. Acute mountain sickness (AMS) is the relatively benign and self-limited presentation, whereas high-altitude pulmonary edema (HAPE) and high-altitude cerebral edema (HACE) represent the potentially life-threatening manifestations.

EPIDEMIOLOGY

- Altitude illness common with rapid ascent to *moderate altitude* (8,000–11,500 feet); most serious cases occur at *very high altitude* (11,500–18,000 feet).
- Children risk developing altitude illness when travelling to high locations with their families.

Incidence

- Children have the same incidence of altitude illness as adults.
- The rapid ascent profile associated with air travel to high-altitude locations results in higher AMS rates. Among skiers who fly or drive to resorts in the western United States, the frequency is approximately 25%.
- HACE is extremely rare in children primarily occurring after prolonged stays at very high altitudes; a place most children should not be.
- HAPE frequency is 1–2% with primary ascent, but reentry HAPE may occur in 6–17% of children who are permanent altitude residents.

RISK FACTORS

- Incidence depends on rate of ascent, sleeping altitude, and previous altitude exposure.
- Individual (genetic) susceptibility plays a key role in risk assessment. Most children with a previous history of AMS or HAPE are likely to experience similar symptoms with similar ascent profiles.
- Underlying medical conditions resulting in hypoxia sensitivity or pulmonary hypertension: incomplete postnatal circulatory transition, viral respiratory infection, atrial or ventricular septal defects, PFO, PDA, pulmonary vein stenosis, congenital absence of pulmonary artery, obstructive sleep apnea, Down syndrome, hypoplastic lung, and sickle cell disease

GENERAL PREVENTION

- Assess risk factors and plan rate of ascent:
  - Slow ascent is the best prevention strategy; sleeping altitude: ideally first night no higher than 9,200 feet, then 2–3 nights at 8,200–9,800 feet, with subsequent increases limited to 1,500 feet each night and 1 extra day without ascent for every 3,000 feet gained
- Formulation of emergency communication and evacuation plan
  - Difficult descent situations (i.e., further ascent needed before descent possible) should be avoided.
  - Cell or satellite communication may fail.
- Prompt recognition of symptoms
  - Train parents in symptom recognition and treatment principles.

PATHOPHYSIOLOGY

- AMS/HACE: rising intracranial volume and pressure with ascent ultimately resulting in vasogenic edema (HACE). A "tight-fitting" CNS within the skull and spine has less ability to buffer edema and may be more susceptible.
- HAPE: elevated pulmonary artery pressure, uneven vasoconstriction, pulmonary overperfusion injury and leakage, inflammation, and impaired alveolar fluid clearance

DIAGNOSIS

HISTORY

Previous altitude illness suggests similar symptoms in future with similar ascent profiles, rapid rate of ascent to high sleeping altitudes; increased exertion, preexisting medical conditions with hypoxia sensitivity or pulmonary hypertension, use of prophylaxis medication or respiratory depressants.

- Acute mountain sickness (AMS):
  - All symptoms may range from mild to severe and incapacitating. The diagnosis requires recent altitude gain, a headache, and at least one of the following: anorexia, nausea or vomiting, general weakness or fatigue, dizziness or light-headedness, or difficulty sleeping. These symptoms comprise the adult criteria for AMS and may be used in older children who are able to verbally express headache or hunger. Headache can be assessed by asking if the "head hurts" and GI symptoms by asking the child if they are "hungry" rather than evaluating appetite. Sleep disturbance is common in all visitors to high altitudes but is exacerbated in the setting of AMS.
  - Among infants and older preverbal children (up to 3 years of age), AMS is diagnosed using nonverbal criteria. AMS is manifested by increased fussiness (headache equivalent), decreased playfulness, decreased appetite, and sleep disturbance. In most cases, all of these symptoms are present. Fussiness is a state of irritability that is not easily explained by a cause, such as tiredness, wet diaper, hunger, teething, or pain from an injury. Fussy behavior includes crying, restlessness, or muscular tension. Decreased playfulness may be profound, vomiting may occur, and sleep disturbance is most often manifest as decreased sleep and the inability to nap.
  - Parents can learn to recognize AMS in preverbal children using the Children's Lake Louise Score.
    - To calculate score, combine the fussiness score with the symptom score.
    - Children's LLS score ≥ 7 with fussiness score ≥ 4 + symptom score ≥ 3 is considered diagnostic of AMS.

Fussiness score	0	1	2	3	4	5	6
Amount	None		Intermittent			Constant	
Intensity	Not fussy		Moderately fussy			Extremely fussy	

Symptom score	0	1	2	3
Eating	Norm	Slightly less	Much less	Not eating; vomiting
Playing	Norm	Slightly less	Much less	Not playing
Sleeping	Norm	Slightly less or more	Much less or more	Not able to sleep

  - Symptoms develop within a few hours after ascent and generally reach maximum severity between 24 and 48 hours, followed by gradual resolution over 1–3 days. The vague nature of AMS presentation has resulted misdiagnoses and morbidity. These symptoms warrant a presumptive diagnosis of AMS and limitation of further ascent, until proven otherwise.
- High-altitude cerebral edema (HACE):
  - Rare in children but rapidly fatal if unrecognized. Develops 2–4 days after ascent.
  - Differentiated from AMS by the presence of neurologic signs. Most common are ataxia, and altered mental status including confusion, progressive unresponsiveness, and coma. Less common are focal cranial nerve palsies, motor and sensory deficits, and seizures.
- High-altitude pulmonary edema (HAPE):
  - Develops over 24–96 hours and may be associated with concurrent viral illness.
  - Although all children have dyspnea on exertion at altitude, dyspnea at rest is an early indicator of HAPE. AMS precedes HAPE development in approximately 1/2 of cases. General malaise progresses to a more specific signs of dyspnea at rest, then cardiopulmonary distress.
  - Young children may show agitation and general debility. Older children may complain of headache, and all ages frequently experience nausea and vomiting. Cough is common.
  - Dyspnea at rest, orthopnea, cyanosis, chest pain, and tachycardia, herald worsening compromise leading within hours to production of pink-tinged sputum, increasing hypoxia with eventual coma, and death.

PHYSICAL EXAM

- There are no diagnostic physical signs in cases of mild AMS. Any evidence of CNS dysfunction, such as mild ataxia or altered mentation is early evidence of HACE.
- Similarly, although dyspnea on exertion is universal at high altitudes, dyspnea at rest is an early indicator of HAPE.
- HAPE exam findings are often less severe than a patient's chest radiograph and the hypoxemia on pulse oximetry would predict. Children appear pale, with or without visible cyanosis. Low-grade fever (<38.5°C) and tachypnea are common. Auscultation reveals rales, usually greater in the right lung.

DIAGNOSTIC TESTS & INTERPRETATION

- ECG: HAPE: may reveal RV strain
- Pulse oximetry: HAPE: Arterial oxygen desaturation is a consistent finding, with saturations frequently less than 75%.

Lab

Evaluate arterial blood gas, carbon monoxide level, and CBC (often reveals a leukocytosis with a left shift of the granulocyte series).

Imaging

- Chest x-ray
  - Pulmonary edema pattern variable, from patchy/peripheral to homogeneous in severe cases. Right lung shows more radiographic changes of edema than left. Peribronchial and perivascular cuffing and enlargement of pulmonary artery are common.
- Pulmonary ultrasonography
  - Comet tail microreflection artifacts within interlobular septae thickened by interstitial/alveolar edema
- Brain CT/MR imaging
  - CT imaging consistent with edema and increased intracranial pressure. MRI: high T2 signal in the white matter, specifically in the splenium of the corpus callosum, with diffusion-weighted technique

DIFFERENTIAL DIAGNOSIS

Differential of HAPE includes pneumonia, bronchitis/bronchiolitis, asthma, other pulmonary edema, and pulmonary embolism. HAPE is most frequently misdiagnosed as pneumonia. With AMS, a differential of viral illness, sepsis, alcohol/drug intoxication, hypothermia, carbon monoxide poisoning, and dehydration should be considered.

TREATMENT

MEDICATION

- Oxygen relieves AMS symptoms (1–2 L/min), easily available in most resorts, reserved for severe cases in remote settings. Hyperbaric therapy also effective, as it simulates descent
- Acetazolamide (carbonic anhydrase inhibitor)
  - Prevention of AMS: 2.5 mg/kg PO q12h, max 125 mg/dose; not routinely used in children. Indicated with unavoidable rapid ascent profile or previous history with similar ascent planned
  - AMS treatment: 2.5 mg/kg PO q8–12h, max 250 mg/dose; **caution if patient has a sulfa allergy**.
  - Paresthesia and taste alterations common
- Dexamethasone (steroid)
  - Prevention of AMS: risk of adverse effects; use not warranted, use slow ascent or acetazolamide.
  - AMS/HACE treatment: 0.15 mg/kg PO/IM/IV q6h, max 4 mg/dose. Oxygen/descent are treatment of choice for severe AMS; if patient has a sulfa allergy, dexamethasone may be used; oxygen, descent, and dexamethasone for HACE
- Nifedipine (calcium channel blocker)
  - Prevention and treatment of HAPE: small children: immediate-release 0.5 mg/kg/dose q4–8h, max 20 mg/dose. If >60 kg, 30 mg sustained-release (SR) PO q12h or 20 mg SR PO q8h. Indicated for treatment in emergency setting where oxygen and descent are not an option. (Oxygen alone provides maximal treatment, no advantage adding nifedipine) May cause hypotension
- Sildenafil (phosphodiesterase inhibitor)
  - Prevention/treatment of HAPE: 0.5 mg/kg/dose PO q8h, max 50 mg/dose q8h. For treatment, only indicated in emergency setting where oxygen and descent are not an option, if nifedipine not well-tolerated, this medication is an alternative. (FDA warns against use in children.)

General Measures

- Descent (of 1,600–3,300 feet) from altitude of illness onset is effective treatment for all forms of altitude illness.
- Mild AMS
  - Usually self-limited not requiring treatment. Stop ascent and rest until symptoms improve.
  - May be treated without descent if monitoring by reliable caregiver available.
- Moderate to severe AMS
  - Symptomatic treatment with analgesics and antiemetics: ibuprofen, acetaminophen, ondansetron; oxygen if available, give acetazolamide; descend if persistent or severe.
- HACE
  - Descend immediately.
  - Supplemental oxygen to keep Spo_2 >90%, bed rest, dexamethasone, portable hyperbaric chamber while awaiting descent
- HAPE
  - Without medical expertise, descend immediately. Otherwise, if mild may treat by stopping ascent, rest, and oxygen to keep Spo_2 >90%. Use nifedipine in severe cases if descent is delayed or oxygen unavailable.

ONGOING CARE

FOLLOW-UP RECOMMENDATIONS

Refer to primary care physician for education of prevention strategies and consideration of prophylaxis with future ascent. History of HAPE or severe hypoxemia warrants cardiopulmonary evaluation including echocardiography.

PROGNOSIS

- Excellent if recognized quickly, ascent stopped, and descent and/or therapy initiated
- Can be poor if symptoms go unrecognized or noted without appropriate descent and therapy

ADDITIONAL READING

- Imray C, Wright A, Subudhi A, et al. Acute mountain sickness: pathophysiology, prevention, and treatment. *Prog Cardiovasc Dis*. 2010;52(6):467–484.
- Luks AM, McIntosh SE, Grissom CK, et al. Wilderness Medical Society consensus guidelines for the prevention and treatment of acute altitude illness. *Wilderness Environ Med*. 2010;21(2):146–155.
- Niermeyer S. Going to high altitude with a newborn infant. *High Alt Med Biol*. 2007;8(2):117–123.
- Yaron M, Niermeyer S. Travel to high altitude with young children: an approach for clinicians. *High Alt Med Biol*. 2008;9(4):265–269.

CODES

ICD10

- T70.20XA Unspecified effects of high altitude, initial encounter
- T70.29XA Other effects of high altitude, initial encounter
- R09.02 Hypoxemia

FAQ

- Q: Can one develop AMS at moderate altitudes, such as during a ski vacation?
- A: Yes. 25% of visitors from sea level will get AMS symptoms, although the altitudes encountered rarely lead to the development of severe symptoms.
- Q: When can we bring our newborn baby to our mountain house at 9,000 feet?
- A: The postnatal cardiopulmonary transition is nearly complete by 6 weeks and then most babies can safely ascend to moderate altitudes.
- Q: Should I give prophylaxis to my child to prevent AMS?
- A: Not usually. Only children with a significant history of AMS or unavoidable rapid ascent should be given prophylaxis.
- Q: Is it safe to take my child on a 3-week trek crossing several mountain passes in Nepal?
- A: Not necessarily. Balance the benefits against the risks of being in a remote environment with exposure to environmental dangers (altitude, weather, infectious disease), without easy medical care, evacuation, or communication.

AMBIGUOUS GENITALIA

Sarah Z. Hatab • J. Nina Ham

BASICS

DESCRIPTION

- Genitalia can be defined as ambiguous when it is not possible to categorize the gender of the child based on outward genital appearance.
- Ambiguous genitalia result from various disorders of sexual development (DSD), a generic term defined as a congenital condition in which development of chromosomal, gonadal, or phenotypic sex is atypical.
  - General DSD categories are sex chromosome DSD; 46,XX DSD; 46,XY DSD; ovotesticular DSD; 46,XX testicular DSD; and 46,XY complete gonadal dysgenesis.
  - Specific diagnoses (when available) are preferable to these broad categories.
  - Previous terms such as "intersex," "pseudohermaphroditism," or "sex reversal" should be avoided.
- Criteria that suggest DSD include the following:
  - Bilateral nonpalpable testes
  - Micropenis (stretched length <2.5 cm)
  - Perineal hypospadias or mild hypospadias with a unilateral undescended testis
  - Clitoromegaly (width >6 mm or length >9 mm), posterior labial fusion
  - An inguinal/labial mass
  - Family history of a DSD
  - Discordance between genital appearance and prenatal karyotype
- DSDs also comprise sex chromosome disorders including Turner (45,X) and Klinefelter syndromes (47,XXY), which usually do not present as ambiguous genitalia.

EPIDEMIOLOGY

- Genital anomalies at birth may have a prevalence as high as 1 in 300.
- External genitalia ambiguity has a prevalence of approximately 1 in 5,000 births.
- Congenital adrenal hyperplasia (CAH) is the most common cause of DSD (classified as a 46,XX DSD) and is discussed in detail in a separate chapter.
- Partial androgen insensitivity syndrome (PAIS) is the next most common cause of DSD (classified as a 46,XY DSD).
- Disorders causing sexual ambiguity are congenital and usually present in the newborn period.
- Later presentations in older children and young adults can occur. Examples:
  - 46,XY individuals with complete 17α-hydroxylase/17,20-lyase deficiency may present in adolescence with hypertension and delayed puberty.
  - Women with complete androgen insensitivity syndrome (CAIS) may present during adolescence with primary amenorrhea.
  - Children with 5α-reductase deficiency may become virilized during puberty.

GENETICS

- Several single-gene disorders causing gonadal dysgenesis have been described. However, only 15–20% of patients with DSDs are diagnosed at the molecular level.
- 46,XY DSD may be associated with mutations in the following genes:
  - Genes involved in testicular development: sex-determining region on Y (*SRY*), *SOX9*, steroidogenic factor 1 (*SF-1*), Wilms tumor suppressor gene (*WT1*), *WNT4* duplication, and *DAX1* duplication.
  - Genes involved in steroid hormone action or synthesis (autosomal recessive, except for the androgen receptor)
    - LH/choriogonadotropin receptor (*LHCGR*) gene leading to Leydig cell hypoplasia and decreased testosterone
    - Genes encoding adrenal steroidogenic enzymes: 17α-hydroxylase (*CYP17A1*), 3β-hydroxysteroid dehydrogenase, (*HSD3B2*), P450 oxidoreductase, and StAR protein (lipoid hyperplasia)
    - Gene encoding 5α-reductase (*SRD5A2*), leading to defective conversion of testosterone (T) to dihydrotestosterone (DHT). DHT is necessary for the development of male external genitalia in utero.
    - Androgen receptor (*AR*) gene located on the X chromosome (X-linked recessive), leading to impaired androgen action
- 46,XX DSD may be associated with mutations in the following genes:
  - Genes involved in ovarian development and leading to gonadal dysgenesis: FSH receptor (*FSHR*), *SF-1*
  - Genes involved in testicular development: presence of *SRY*, *SOX9* duplication
  - Genes encoding steroidogenic enzymes, involved in cortisol biosynthesis, leading to virilizing CAH: 21-hydroxylase (*CYP21A*), the most common form; 11β-hydroxylase (*CYP11B1*); 3β-hydroxysteroid dehydrogenase (*HSD3B2*)
  - Aromatase gene (*CYP19A1*), leading to impaired placental conversion of fetal adrenal androgens to estrogens
- Sex chromosome DSD (45,X; 47,XXY; 45,X/46,XY; and 46,XX/46,XY) are caused by meiotic or mitotic nondisjunction.

PATHOPHYSIOLOGY

- 46,XX DSD
  - Masculinization of the female fetus is caused by androgens produced by the fetus or transferred across the placenta. The most common cause is CAH in which the fetal adrenal glands overproduce androgens in an attempt to correct cortisol deficiency.
  - The ovaries and müllerian derivatives are normal, and the sexual ambiguity is limited to masculinization of the external genitalia.
- 46,XY DSD
  - Incomplete masculinization of the male fetus can be caused by enzyme disorders of testosterone synthesis (e.g., CAH, 5α-reductase deficiency), unresponsiveness to testosterone action (androgen insensitivity syndromes), or defects in testicular development (complete or partial gonadal dysgenesis).
- Ovotesticular DSD
  - Includes patients with both ovarian and testicular elements. Combinations include one ovary and one testis, two ovotestes, or one ovotestis with either an ovary or a testis. Often, differentiation of internal and external genitalia coincides with the gonad on the ipsilateral side.
  - Karyotypes are 46,XX most commonly; the molecular basis of this disorder may not be known; 46,XX/46,XY and 46,XX/47,XXY reported.
- Gonadal dysgenesis
  - Mixed gonadal dysgenesis (classically 45,X/46,XY) involves a streak gonad on one side and a testis, often dysgenetic, on the other side. The clinical phenotype is highly variable and ranges from female external genitalia through all stages of ambiguous genitalia to a normal male.
  - Pure (complete) gonadal dysgenesis (46,XX, 46,XY, or a Turner syndrome karyotype) involves replacement of gonads by streak gonads. Neonates look female at birth and often present later in life with delayed puberty and primary amenorrhea.

DIAGNOSIS

- Ambiguous genitalia in the neonate should be treated as an emergency, and diagnostic evaluation undertaken as soon as possible.
- CAH, the most common cause of DSD, can be life threatening when accompanied by salt wasting. Also, DSD is disturbing for families and calls for immediate investigation, counseling, and support.

HISTORY

Obtain a careful pregnancy and family history addressing the following:

- Drug ingestions
- Teratogen exposures
- Infections during the pregnancy
- Androgenic changes in the mother
- Family history suggestive of CAH or androgen insensitivity
- History of consanguinity

PHYSICAL EXAM

Notable features include phallic size, symmetry of external genitalia, presence and location of palpable gonads, and presence of additional anomalies.

- Palpable gonads: imply the presence of Y-chromosome material
- Labial fusion: measurement of the anogenital ratio (distance from anus to posterior fourchette divided by distance from anus to base of phallus). If >0.5, this suggests virilization with posterior labial fusion.
- Presence of a vagina
- Position of the urethra
- Length and diameter of penis/clitoris: stretched penile length at term usually ≥2.5 cm; clitoral length is usually ≤1 cm.
- Development of the scrotum
- Asymmetry of external genitalia: suggests ovotesticular or 45,X/46,XY DSDs
- Other dysmorphic features

- Hypertension is seen with 17α-hydroxylase and 11-hydroxylase deficiencies.
- Features of the classic disorders of adrenal steroidogenesis

DIAGNOSTIC TESTS & INTERPRETATION

Lab

Initial evaluation should be targeted to help with sex assignment and assessment of gonadal and adrenal steroids. A 1st-line investigation includes the following:

- Karyotype, or fluorescence in situ hybridization (FISH) (X- and Y-specific probes)
- Measurement of 17α-hydroxyprogesterone (17-OHP), testosterone, anti–müllerian hormone (AMH) (reliable indicator of testicular tissue), and serum electrolytes

Second-line investigations depend on the karyotype, the presence of palpable gonads, and the 17-OHP levels. These can be ordered after the 1st-line tests or ordered simultaneously, depending on the clinical situation.

- Karyotype is 46,XX and nonpalpable gonads:
  - Most commonly due to CAH
- Karyotype is 47,XY: Investigations include tests to determine if testes are present and capable of producing normal levels of androgens:
  - LH, FSH, müllerian-inhibiting substance (MIS), T, and DHT
  - hCG stimulation test will help differentiate disorders of abnormal response to androgen from disorders of androgen synthesis.

Imaging

- Ultrasonography of the abdomen and pelvis
  - Part of the 1st-line investigation
  - Can help determine the presence of gonads, uterus, and/or vagina
  - Only 50% accurate in showing intraabdominal testes
- Retrograde urethrogram can help evaluate the urogenital sinus.
- MRI can further delineate the internal anatomy.

Diagnostic Procedures/Other

- Cystoscopy/vaginoscopy is gold standard method to assess the urethral and vaginal anatomy.
- Laparoscopy +/− gonadal biopsy may be required for definitive evaluation of the reproductive structures.

DIFFERENTIAL DIAGNOSIS

- Gonadal dysgenesis
- Ovotesticular DSD
- 46,XX DSD
  - CAH causing virilization in female
  - Maternal androgen exposure
  - Exogenous androgens or endogenous production (e.g., maternal virilizing tumor)
- 46,XY DSD
  - CAH causing undervirilization of boys
  - 5α-Reductase deficiency prevents in utero formation of male external genitalia.
  - Syndromes of androgen resistance due to abnormalities in androgen receptor or postreceptor defects.
- Multiple congenital anomalies: Ambiguous genitalia can be a part of a spectrum of congenital anomalies involving the rectum and urologic system.
- Idiopathic

TREATMENT

- Counsel family to not make announcements describing gender until gender assignment is determined.
- Medical staff should use terms such as "your child" or "the baby" rather than "he" or "she."
- Parents should be counseled that the diagnostic information as well as surgical factors, prediction of hormone function, and potential for fertility will be taken together as a whole.
- Gender assignment should be made through a multidisciplinary team approach with consultations from endocrinology, urology, neonatology, genetics, psychiatry/psychology, and social work. If these services are not available, the child and family may benefit from transfer to a pediatric tertiary care facility that can provide this multidisciplinary approach.

MEDICATION

- With the exception of CAH, most DSD conditions do not require specific medical treatment until puberty.
- At the time of expected puberty, hormonal therapy is usually started in patients with hypogonadism: between 10.5 and 12 years for females and 12.5 and 14 years for males.

ADDITIONAL TREATMENT

General Measures

- Surgical management
  - If the gender assignment is female, delaying clitoral surgery should be considered given the potential risk for disturbance of sensation. Vaginoplasty may be acceptable in infancy given the potential for improved functional outcome.
  - If gender assignment is male, phallic reconstruction can be done when the team and parents are comfortable with the timing. Urethral reconstruction for hypospadias is usually scheduled between 6 and 24 months of age.
  - Gonadectomy or repositioning may be recommended in patients at risk of gonadal malignancy (gonads bearing the Y chromosome). Tumor risk is heterogeneous among DSDs (e.g., high in mixed gonadal dysgenesis [MGD] and low in AR), and the optimal age and type of surgery can vary substantially.
- Psychosocial management
  - Long-term counseling for the child and parents by mental health staff with expertise in DSDs is critical to promote psychosocial adaption at all stages of cognitive and psychological development.
  - The team can facilitate decision-making processes involving gender assignment/reassignment, timing of surgery, and hormonal replacement.

ONGOING CARE

FOLLOW-UP RECOMMENDATIONS

- Long-term follow-up may involve monitoring hormone levels, linear growth, and sexual and psychological development.
- Follow-up also involves monitoring for gonadal malignancy. Surveillance imaging and testicular palpation should be performed in all DSD patients with abdominal or scrotal testes respectively.

PROGNOSIS

The cosmetic outcome from surgery is usually good. The potential for age-appropriate sexual function is usually good with therapy. The potential for reproductive function depends on the diagnosis. Long-term studies of psychological adjustment are underway.

ADDITIONAL READING

- Barbaro M, Wedell A, Nordenström A. Disorders of sex development. *Semin Fetal Neonatal Med*. 2011;16(2):119–127.
- Lambert SM, Vilain EJ, Kolon TF. A practical approach to ambiguous genitalia in the newborn. *Urol Clin North Am*. 2010;37(2):195–205.
- Lee PA, Houk CP, Ahmed SF, et al. Consensus statement on management of intersex disorders. *Pediatrics*. 2006;118(2):e488–e500.
- MacLaughlin DT, Donahoe PK. Sex determination and differentiation. *N Engl J Med*. 2004;350(4):367–378.
- Murphy C, Allen L, Jamieson MA. Ambiguous genitalia in the newborn: an overview and teaching tool. *J Pediatr Adolesc Gynecol*. 2011;24(5): 236–250.
- Romao RL, Salle JL, Wherrett DK. Update on the management of disorders of sex development. *Pediatr Clin North Am*. 2012;59(4):853–869.

CODES

ICD10

- Q56.4 Indeterminate sex, unspecified
- E25.0 Congenital adrenogenital disorders assoc w enzyme deficiency
- Q56.3 Pseudohermaphroditism, unspecified

FAQ

- Q: Should a child's sex assignment be consistent with the karyotype?
- A: This is a major decision that should involve the family and the treatment team. Future potential for sexual, hormonal, and reproductive function, in addition to genetics, are all important factors.
- Q: What clues can the physical exam give to the timing of in utero events causing sexual ambiguity?
- A: In the virilized female, labioscrotal fusion results from androgen exposure prior to 12 weeks' gestation. Thereafter, androgen exposure can cause only clitoromegaly.

AMBLYOPIA

Melissa A. Simon • Michael F. Chiang

BASICS

DESCRIPTION

Amblyopia is a decrease in best corrected visual acuity in an otherwise anatomically normal eye. It is generally classified by cause, with 3 primary types:

- Refractive amblyopia: resulting from uncorrected refractive error (improper focusing of light by the eye which generally requires correction by eyeglasses or contact lenses), with the following subtypes:
  - Anisometropic amblyopia: resulting from asymmetric refractive error and resultant unilateral blurring. This condition is the most common cause of refractive amblyopia. One specific example is meridional amblyopia, which results from large uncorrected astigmatism in one or both eyes.
  - Ametropic amblyopia: resulting from significant refractive error in both eyes
- Strabismic amblyopia: resulting from strabismus (misalignment of the eyes) and subsequent lack of an image that can be "fused" or integrated into a single image in the brain. This condition is most likely with early-onset, constant strabismus. Approximately 50% of patients with strabismus will also have amblyopia.
- Deprivation amblyopia: resulting from optical or anatomic pathology (e.g., cataract, ptosis, corneal opacity, prolonged patching), which prevents the formation of a clear image in one or both eyes. Deprivation, especially if it begins early in life, is associated with the most severe amblyopia.

EPIDEMIOLOGY

Amblyopia is the most common cause of unilateral vision loss in children and young adults.

Prevalence

Large population-based studies indicate that 0.8–3.3% of the adult population has amblyopia.

PATHOPHYSIOLOGY

- Asymmetric input between the 2 eyes (e.g., unilateral cataract, anisometropia, etc.) is more likely to cause amblyopia than symmetrically poor images due to competitive influences between the 2 eyes. As a result, amblyopia is usually unilateral.
- Bilateral amblyopia may result from severe, symmetric bilateral image degradation such as bilateral cataract, bilateral high ametropia (high refractive error), etc.
- Visual acuity in amblyopic eyes varies from minimal impairment (20/25) to legal blindness (<20/200) or worse. Other significant impairments in amblyopic eyes may include reduced contrast sensitivity, reduced or absent binocularity and depth perception, and impaired or distorted spatial perception. Peripheral visual fields are preserved, and vision is never completely lost (no light perception) from amblyopia alone.

DIAGNOSIS

SIGNS & SYMPTOMS

Poor vision

HISTORY

- Age of onset of vision loss
- Eye trauma, injury, or surgery
- Refractive error or glasses
- Ptosis or ocular occlusion (because amblyopia related to ptosis is often due to resultant astigmatism, this can occur even if the affected eye is not completely occluded)
- Family history of strabismus, anisometropia, or amblyopia
- History of prematurity or developmental delay

PHYSICAL EXAM

- Visual acuity is the single most significant sign in detection of amblyopia. Vision must be tested in each eye separately with reliable occlusion (ideally an adhesive patch). Because most amblyopia is monocular, testing vision with both eyes open is inadequate as a screening tool.
- Binocularity tests such as Titmus stereopsis (3D fly) will detect suppression, which is frequently associated with amblyopia.

DIAGNOSTIC TESTS & INTERPRETATION

- Vision testing in young children is difficult and, sometimes, unreliable.
- Children must be tested with each eye separately.
- Repeating the tests and adjunctive tests including the Titmus test, cover testing, photoscreening, and Brückner red reflex test will increase the sensitivity of screening.

Imaging

Imaging studies of the optic nerves and posterior visual pathways may be useful in selected cases to exclude other causes of vision loss.

DIFFERENTIAL DIAGNOSIS

- Amblyopia is diagnosed by exclusion: Conditions that cause vision loss without easily recognized pathology might be mistaken for amblyopia.
- In children, the differential diagnosis of vision loss in eyes that appear normal by penlight includes the following:
  - Uncorrected refractive error (hyperopia, myopia, astigmatism)
  - Optic nerve hypoplasia
  - Optic atrophy
  - Compressive, toxic, or hereditary optic neuropathies
  - Retinopathies, including Leber congenital amaurosis, Stargardt disease, retinitis pigmentosa, and others
  - Central visual impairment (cortical blindness)
  - Glaucoma
  - Factitious or functional causes (hysterical blindness)

TREATMENT

GENERAL MEASURES

- Refractive correction, when needed, is critical and can improve amblyopia before additional treatment.
- Unilateral amblyopia
  - Treat underlying cause of vision loss (strabismus, anisometropia, optical opacity) and force preferential use of the amblyopic eye.
  - The classic and most common treatment is occlusion with an adhesive patch worn over the opposite (unaffected) eye for hours daily.
  - The amount of time of occlusion necessary to reverse amblyopia depends on variables including the severity of amblyopia, cause of amblyopia, age, and other associated ocular conditions. Research studies have not identified an optimal time of occlusion.
  - Typical duration of treatment is from a few weeks to months but can be longer in some cases.
  - Infants and very young children require closer observation to prevent reversing the amblyopia to the previously preferred eye (occlusion amblyopia) from excessive patching.
  - Optical penalization of the opposite (unaffected) eye using topical cycloplegic eyedrops, such as atropine 1%. Recent studies suggest that atropine penalization may be as effective as patching to treat mild or moderate amblyopia.
  - Treatment should be attempted in amblyopic children within the "sensitive period" of birth to 8 years of age. Successful outcomes are far more likely when treatment is initiated early. However, recent research suggests that treatment can still be effective in teenagers, especially those who have not been previously treated. Treatment is usually continued until visual acuity is equal to the opposite eye or no further improvement is seen over several examinations with treatment.
  - The primary risk of treatment is overcorrection, with iatrogenic amblyopia in the occluded opposite eye.
- In strabismic amblyopia, initiation of treatment for amblyopia need not wait for correction of the strabismus. Moreover, the stability of the surgical strabismus correction is improved if amblyopia therapy is initiated before surgery.
  - Treatment is usually continued until visual acuity in both eyes is equal or until vision in the amblyopic eye shows no further improvement after several examinations over a period of time.

ISSUES FOR REFERRAL

Prompt referral of failures and children suspected of poor vision for complete ophthalmic examination is essential for successful amblyopia screening programs.

ONGOING CARE

FOLLOW-UP RECOMMENDATIONS

- In general, the younger the patient, the more intensive the patching therapy, and the milder the amblyopia, the more frequent vision testing is necessary to ensure that vision in the opposite, occluded eye is not harmed.
- Children are clever at finding ways to avoid the temporary vision impairment from patching and will peek or remove patches frequently.
- In younger children, amblyopia may recur after successful treatment.

Patient Monitoring

- Children should be retested frequently and retreated if vision drops after finishing successful initial treatment.
- Approximately 1/4 of children treated for amblyopia experience a recurrence in the 1st year after treatment.
- Testing should continue at least annually until the child is at least 8 years old, and recent trials suggest there may be benefit to monitoring through adolescence.

PATIENT EDUCATION

Because the outcome of amblyopia depends entirely on early detection and treatment within the first few years of life, all children should be screened by monocular recognition visual acuity as early as possible, and testing has traditionally been recommended to be repeated annually until 8 years of age (although evidence now suggests potential benefits of screening through adolescence). The U.S. Preventive Services Task Force recommends screening beginning at age 3 years. Ongoing research is investigating potential benefits of screening children as early as age 1 year. In general, children who are not capable of accurate visual acuity testing by 4 years of age should be referred for complete evaluation.

PROGNOSIS

- After treatment, amblyopia may recur, and vision should be retested regularly.
- Patients with strabismus, even if previously treated with glasses or surgery, must be followed for amblyopia.
- Vision loss from amblyopia will persist even after the condition that originally caused the amblyopia has resolved. In some cases, when there is no obvious cause, a history of episodes of anisometropia, occlusion, or strabismus must be considered.

COMPLICATIONS

- Left untreated, amblyopia results in irreversible, uncorrectable vision loss after visual maturity (8–10 years of age).
- Usually, the vision loss is unilateral, and the functional effects may be minimal if vision in the remaining eye is normal.
- In bilateral cases, or if other diseases or injury affects the remaining eye, the outcome can be significant functional impairment, including legal blindness.

ADDITIONAL READING

- American Academy of Ophthalmology. *Preferred Practice Pattern: Amblyopia*. San Francisco, CA: American Academy of Ophthalmology; 2012.
- American Academy of Ophthalmology. *Preferred Practice Pattern: Pediatric Eye Examination*. San Francisco, CA: American Academy of Ophthalmology; 2012.
- Demirkilinc BE, Uretmen O, Kose S. The effect of optical correction on refractive development in children with accommodative esotropia. *J AAPOS*. 2010;14(4):305–310.
- Gunton KB. Advances in amblyopia: what have we learned from PEDIG trials? *Pediatrics*. 2013;131(3):540–547.
- Longmuir SQ, Boese EA, Pfeifer W, et al. Practical community photoscreening in very young children. *Pediatrics*. 2013;131(3):e764–e769.

CODES

ICD10

- H53.009 Unspecified amblyopia, unspecified eye
- H53.029 Refractive amblyopia, unspecified eye
- H53.039 Strabismic amblyopia, unspecified eye

FAQ

- Q: My child refuses to wear a patch. Are there alternatives to patching?
- A: Yes. Optical penalization with glasses, atropine cycloplegic penalization, and even contact lens occlusion can be effective. Research shows that patching and atropine can be similarly effective depending on severity of amblyopia and refractive error. Parental support, encouragement, and reward are essential for treatment compliance.
- Q: How long will patching or atropine be necessary?
- A: It is not possible to predict exactly how long treatment will be necessary to restore vision. In general, the younger the patient, the milder the impairment, and the more intensive the patching, the more quickly vision is restored. In general, patching is usually continued for 1–6 months in most cases of anisometropic or strabismic amblyopia. Normalization of vision or lack of further improvement is usually the treatment end point.
- Q: Will vision be normal after treatment?
- A: The degree of recovery with amblyopia therapy depends on the density of the amblyopia, the cause, and the age at which treatment is initiated. In almost all children younger than 6–8 years of age, some visual improvement can be expected with amblyopia treatment, although not all patients will improve to 20/20 vision.
- Q: Will patching eliminate the need for glasses?
- A: No. Patching does not influence the outcome of refractive errors (power of glasses, refractive error). Glasses may still be needed after patching or atropine is completed. In fact, glasses can improve amblyopia before additional treatment is introduced.
- Q: Will treatment for amblyopia improve the strabismus?
- A: No. In most cases, patching for amblyopia will not eliminate strabismus or the need for strabismus surgery. However, in most cases, it is best to begin amblyopia treatment before surgery to improve the surgical outcome.
- Q: Is "vision therapy" without patching an effective treatment for strabismus?
- A: Although eye exercises, pleoptics, and other vision therapies have been used to treat amblyopia, none is as effective as patching or other occlusive therapy. Current vision therapy techniques have not been proven to improve amblyopia.

AMEBIASIS

Jason Y. Kim

BASICS

DESCRIPTION

Clinical syndromes associated with *Entamoeba histolytica* infection

EPIDEMIOLOGY

- Fecal–oral transmission
- Transmission also via contaminated water and food
- The incubation period is typically 1–3 weeks but can range from a few days to months or years.

Incidence

- Amebiasis accounts for 40–50 million cases of colitis worldwide.
- 40,000–110,000 deaths annually

Prevalence

- The estimated prevalence in the United States is 4%, although there have been no recent serosurvey in developed countries.
- Worldwide distribution involving an estimated 10% or more of the world's population
  – Most common in tropical areas, with infection rates as high as 20–50%
  – Highest morbidity and mortality are seen in developing countries in Central America, South America, Africa, and Asia.

GENERAL PREVENTION

- Treatment of drinking water
- Hand washing
- Appropriate disposal of human fecal waste
- Use of condoms
- Infection-control measures: Standard precautions are recommended for the hospitalized patient.

RISK FACTORS

- The very young, the elderly, and patients with underlying immunosuppression or malnutrition are at highest risk for severe disease.
- Patients in whom the diagnosis should be considered include the following:
  – Immigrants from or travelers to endemic areas
  – Children with bloody stools or mucus in stools
  – Children with hepatic abscess
  – The febrile child with right upper quadrant pain and tenderness, abdominal pain, or discomfort
  – The child with hepatomegaly, typically without jaundice

PATHOPHYSIOLOGY

- *E. histolytica* is excreted as cysts or trophozoites in the stool of infected patients.
- Ingested cysts are unaffected by gastric acid and become trophozoites that colonize and invade the colon.
  – Amebae attach to epithelial cells via a galactose/*N*-acetylgalactosamine (Gal/GalNac)–binding lectin.
  – The parasite has the ability to lyse human epithelial cells or kill by inducing apoptosis.
  – Then cytokines and chemokines released attract neutrophils, macrophages, and lymphocytes. The host immune response contributes significantly to the reduction of epithelial integrity.
  – Amebae then use cysteine protease to cleave extracellular matrix proteins to invade the submucosal layers.
  – The EhCPDH112 complex interacts with mucosal tight junction proteins to produce mucosal damage.
- Amebae can then disseminate directly from the intestine to the liver in up to 10% of patients. Dissemination from the liver to the lung, heart, brain, and spleen has been described.

ETIOLOGY

- *E. histolytica* is a nonflagellated protozoan parasite.
- Other species of the *Entamoeba* family are nonpathogenic, including the morphologically identical *Entamoeba dispar*.

DIAGNOSIS

HISTORY

- Intestinal disease may be asymptomatic or have mild symptoms such as abdominal discomfort, flatulence, constipation, and occasionally diarrhea.
- Nondysenteric colitis is characterized by intermittent diarrhea and abdominal pain.
- Acute amebic colitis (dysenteric) is associated with grossly bloody stools with mucus, abdominal pain, and tenesmus.

PHYSICAL EXAM

- Fever may be present
- Abdominal tenderness, abdominal rigidity, and rebound are variably present.
- Right upper quadrant tenderness and jaundice may be present in cases of liver abscess.

DIAGNOSTIC TESTS & INTERPRETATION

The diagnosis of amebiasis depends on the recognition of typical symptoms and routine laboratory tests.

Lab

- CBC typically reveals a leukocytosis.
- Transaminases are often not elevated.
- Occult blood is detected in stool.
- Stool samples
  – Isolation and visualization
    ○ Serial stool samples, usually 3, are recommended.
    ○ Samples obtained within 1–2 hours of passage should be examined by wet mount and fixed in formalin and polyvinyl alcohol.
    ○ Serial stool samples are necessary because cysts may be shed intermittently. 3 serial stool samples will detect up to 70% of patients with amebic colitis and 50% of patients with hepatic abscess.
    ○ Stool samples should not be contaminated by urine, water, barium, enema substances, laxatives, or antibiotics because these substances may destroy or interfere with identification of the trophozoites.
    ○ Microscopy has a sensitivity of <60% and specificity of 10–50% on a single sample.
  – 2nd-generation stool antigen testing kits (commercially available) also have demonstrated excellent sensitivity and specificity comparable to real time PCR.
  – Molecular testing to differentiate *E. histolytica* from nonpathogenic *Entamoeba* species is in the research phase.
- Serology
  – Serum antiamebic antibodies are considered an adjunct to diagnosis.
  – ~85% of patients with amebic dysentery and 99% of patients with liver amebiasis will have positive serology.

Imaging

- US, CT, or MRI of the liver may reveal liver abscess.
- In patients with hepatic amebiasis, chest x-ray may reveal elevation of the right hemidiaphragm.

Diagnostic Procedures/Other

- Note: Amebae are difficult to visualize in abscess aspirates, and substantial risk is associated with CT- or US-guided procedures, including bleeding, peritonitis secondary to spillage of amebae, or rupture of echinococcal cysts.
- Colonoscopy

Pathologic Findings

- Identification of trophozoites or cysts in the stool
- Colonic or rectal mucosa visualized by colonoscopy reveals ulcerations, and amebae can often be found around these lesions.

DIFFERENTIAL DIAGNOSIS

The diagnosis is often missed in children because the diagnosis is not considered in the differential. Because it is not common in the United States, amebiasis may initially be misdiagnosed as bacterial dysentery. Differential diagnosis includes the following:

- Infection
  – *Salmonella* species
  – *Shigella* species
  – *Campylobacter* species
  – *Yersinia* species
  – *Clostridium difficile*
  – *Escherichia coli* (enteroinvasive and enterohemorrhagic)
- Pyogenic abscess
- Echinococcal cyst
- Inflammatory bowel disease
  – Crohn disease
  – Ulcerative colitis
- Ischemic colitis
- Diverticulitis
- Arteriovenous malformations
- Hepatoma

TREATMENT

MEDICATION

First Line

- Asymptomatic intestinal amebiasis: intraluminal agents
  - Iodoquinol is the drug of choice. The recommended dosage is 30–40 mg/kg/24 h (max, 1,950 mg) PO in 3 divided doses for 20 days.
- Acute amebic colitis or extraintestinal amebiasis
  - Metronidazole (a tissue-active agent) 35–50 mg/kg/24 h PO in 3 divided doses for 10 days (max, 2,250 mg/24 hr) **plus** a course of treatment with an intraluminal-active agent (as the preceding)
  - ~1/3 of patients treated with metronidazole alone will relapse.

Second Line

- Asymptomatic intestinal amebiasis
  - Diloxanide furoate (Furamide) at doses of 20 mg/kg/24 h (max, 1,500 mg/24 h) PO in 3 divided doses or paromomycin, 25–35 mg/kg/24 h PO in 3 divided doses for 7 days
- Acute amebic colitis or extraintestinal amebiasis
  - 1 study has reported good efficacy using nitazoxanide in children; however, the sample size was small and the analyses combined *E. histolytica* and *E. dispar* into 1 stratum.
  - However, nitazoxanide shows good activity in vitro against *E. histolytica*.

General Measures

- The goal of treatment is the elimination of tissue-invading trophozoites and intestinal cysts.
- The choice of treatment regimens depends on the clinical presentation.
- Agents that are active against *E. histolytica* are divided into 2 categories: drugs with activity against intraluminal amebae and drugs with activity against extraintestinal and invasive amebiasis.

SURGERY/OTHER PROCEDURES

Patients with large liver abscesses or who have failed medical therapy should be considered candidates for surgical or percutaneous drainage.

ONGOING CARE

FOLLOW-UP RECOMMENDATIONS

Patient Monitoring

- Follow-up stool examination is always necessary to ensure eradication of intestinal amebae.
- For amebic abscesses, drainage should be considered if response to medical therapy has not occurred in 4–5 days.

PROGNOSIS

Clinical improvement is expected within 72 hours of initiation of therapy.

COMPLICATIONS

- Amebic liver abscess
  - 2nd most common presentation of amebiasis, often not associated with amebic dysentery
- Ameboma
  - Abdominal mass representing granulation tissue in the colon
- Extraintestinal manifestations of amebiasis are presumed to be a result of direct extension from liver abscesses. These include the following:
  - Pericarditis
  - Pleuropulmonary abscess or empyema
  - Bronchohepatic fistula
  - Genitourinary tract abscess
  - Cerebral abscess
  - Cutaneous amebiasis
    - This is a rare finding in children, with ~6,510 cases reported in the literature.
    - Shallow painful cutaneous ulcers in the diaper area, usually found in association with amebic colitis or dysentery.
  - Epidemiologic studies from countries with high prevalence of amebiasis show an association between amebic diarrhea and poor growth. The negative effect on growth was significantly more deleterious than diarrhea caused either by *Giardia* or *Cryptosporidium*.

ADDITIONAL READING

- Bercu TE, Petri WA, Behm JW. Amebic colitis: new insights into pathogenesis and treatment. *Curr Gastroenterol Rep.* 2007;9(5):429–423.
- Haque R, Huston CD, Hughes M, et al. Amebiasis. *N Engl J Med.* 2003;348(16):1565–1573.
- Mangaña ML, Fernández-Díez, Mangaña M. Cutaneous amebiasis in pediatrics. *Arch Dermatol.* 2008;144(10):1369–1372.
- Mondal D, Petri WA, Sack RB, et al. *Entamoeba histolytica*-associated diarrheal illness is negatively associated with the growth of preschool children: evidence from a prospective study. *Trans R Soc Trop Med Hyg.* 2006;100(11):1032–1038.
- Ravdin JI, Stauffer WM. Entamoeba histolytica (amebiasis). In: Mandell GL, Bennett JE, Dolin R, eds. *Principles and Practice of Infectious Diseases*, Vol 2. 6th ed. Philadelphia: Churchill Livingstone; 2005: 3097–3111.
- Stauffer W, Ravdin JI. *Entamoeba histolytica*: an update. *Curr Opin Infect Dis.* 2003;16(5):479–485.
- Tanyukse IM, Petri WA. Laboratory diagnosis of amebiasis. *Clin Microbiol Rev.* 2003;16(4):713–729.

CODES

ICD10

- A06.9 Amebiasis, unspecified
- A06.0 Acute amebic dysentery
- A06.4 Amebic liver abscess

FAQ

- Q: How often does a liver abscess complicate intestinal amebiasis?
- A: About 10% of children with intestinal amebiasis will develop a liver abscess.
- Q: What is the best diagnostic study for a suspected amebic liver abscess?
- A: Serology is the best way to diagnose amebiasis as the cause of a liver abscess. Stool studies are usually negative at the time that a liver abscess has complicated intestinal amebiasis; thus, the yield of stool studies is low.

AMENORRHEA

Renee K. Kottenhahn • Deborah B. Ehrenthal

BASICS

DESCRIPTION

Amenorrhea is the absence of menstruation. It is divided into 2 categories:

- Primary amenorrhea is the failure to begin menstruation by 16 years of age in girls with otherwise appropriate pubertal development or by age 14 years in the absence of secondary sexual characteristics. This diagnosis should also be considered if a girl has not menstruated within 2 years of obtaining Tanner IV breast development regardless of her age.
- Secondary amenorrhea is the cessation of menstruation for 3 cycles or 6 months in girls and women with previously established regular cycles:
  - Should not be used when referring to girls who are within 2 years of menarche because regular ovulatory cycles have not yet been established; their periods are unpredictable.

A regular menstrual cycle is a sign of good health. The absence of menses or disruption of regular cycles once they have been established can result from systemic disease, genetic or anatomic abnormalities, physical or emotional stress, or unrecognized pregnancy. The goal of the evaluation is to identify the underlying cause.

EPIDEMIOLOGY

There is insufficient information about the incidence of amenorrhea in contemporary pediatric populations.

- Primary amenorrhea
  - Approximately 5% of girls in North America fail to reach menarche by 14.5 years of age.
  - The most common chromosomal abnormality associated with primary amenorrhea is Turner syndrome, occurring in 1 to 2,500 female live births.
- Secondary amenorrhea
  - Excluding pregnancy, anovulation is the most common cause of secondary amenorrhea.
  - Amenorrhea associated with obesity or polycystic ovary syndrome (PCOS) is becoming a common cause of both primary and secondary amenorrhea among adolescents in developing countries.

GENERAL PREVENTION

- Healthy lifestyle avoiding excess weight gain or weight reduction
- Avoidance of excessive athletic activity or training
- Management of emotional stress
- Adherence with chronic disease management (adequate glycemic control for persons with diabetes) and avoidance of additional physiologic stressors

ETIOLOGY

Menstruation requires the presence of functional female internal genitalia with an intact and patent outflow tract and appropriate stimulation and regulation of the endometrial lining by the hypothalamic–pituitary–ovarian axis. Genetic disorders, anatomic abnormalities, or disruption at any level of the hormonal axis can each lead to amenorrhea.

DIAGNOSIS

GENERAL APPROACH

A stepwise approach to the evaluation, guided by the history and physical exam, is recommended.

- Phase 1: Exclude pregnancy by urine or serum β-hCG testing.
- Phase 2: Obtain a complete menstrual history to differentiate between primary and secondary amenorrhea to help identify the underlying cause.
- Phase 3: Perform a directed physical exam.
- Phase 4: Initiate stepwise diagnostic testing to assess for causes of amenorrhea.

HISTORY

- Age of patient
  - Genetic abnormalities should be a consideration in younger patients with primary amenorrhea.
  - Premature ovarian failure is a stronger consideration with increasing patient age.
- Past and current medical history
  - Prior/current/chronic illness including autoimmune, renal, thyroid, or liver disease; diabetes; or cancer (radiation or chemotherapy), which may be the underlying cause of amenorrhea
- Stressful life events
  - Stress can lead to amenorrhea but should be considered a diagnosis of exclusion.
- Growth and weight changes
  - Consider endocrinopathy, genetic disease, PCOS, rapid weight gain, eating disorder, or other chronic disease.
- Behavioral
  - Eating disorder and/or excessive exercise
- Headaches
  - Assess for visual field defects, dizziness (suggesting pituitary tumor or other intracranial process)
- Reproductive and menstrual history
  - Age at menarche
  - Menstrual cycle history: regularity, flow, duration; characteristics of last menstrual period (normal or abnormal)
  - Sexual history: sexual activity, prior pregnancy, current or prior contraceptive use (Depo-Provera can cause amenorrhea for up to 18 months)
  - A history of symptoms of pre/perimenstrual molimina (breast tenderness, fluid retention, cramping) suggests prior ovulatory cycles.
  - Risk factors for uterine scarring, such as prior gynecologic surgery
- Galactorrhea
  - Spontaneous milky discharge from the breast suggests elevated prolactin or thyroid abnormality or may be due to manual stimulation, medications, pituitary tumor, or illicit drug use (cannabis, opiates, amphetamines).
- Abdominal or pelvic pain
  - Cyclic or intermittent severe abdominal/pelvic pain suggests a uterine anomaly or obstruction.
- Skin and hair
  - Excess hair growth (inquire about shaving, plucking, or waxing), acne, balding, and acanthosis nigricans are symptoms of androgen excess and suggest PCOS, congenital adrenal hyperplasia (rare), or a tumor (rare).
  - Easy bruising or violaceous striae suggest Cushing syndrome.
- Medications
  - Hormonal medications (e.g., Depo-Provera or hormonal contraceptives), cytotoxic medications, illicit drugs, antidepressant drugs, antipsychotic drugs (e.g., risperidone), and other medications including opiates

PHYSICAL EXAM

- General appearance, height, and weight with calculation of body mass index (BMI, in kg/m^2):
  - Obesity raises suspicion of PCOS or possible Cushing syndrome.
  - Athleticism or underweight suggests female athlete triad or eating disorder, respectively.
  - Stigmata of Turner syndrome (short stature, webbed neck, etc.) or other genetic syndromes
  - Abnormal growth pattern suggests endocrinopathy, dietary restriction, chronic disease, or genetic disorder.

- Skin exam
  - Acne, hirsutism (increased facial hair, midline hair over sternum and lower abdomen), acanthosis nigricans, and balding are suggestive of virilization or PCOS.
  - Bruises or pigmented striae suggest Cushing syndrome.
- Tanner staging and breast exam
  - Abnormal Tanner stage for chronologic age suggests an endocrine, metabolic, or genetic abnormality.
  - Galactorrhea suggests abnormalities in prolactin or thyroid.
- Thyroid nodule or enlargement
  - Evaluate for hyperthyroidism or hypothyroidism.
- Abdominal mass
  - Evaluate for uterine obstruction, tumor
- Genitourinary exam
  - Abnormal external genitalia suggest outflow tract abnormalities.
  - Clitoral enlargement is a sign of virilization and raises suspicion for an androgen-secreting tumor or congenital adrenal hyperplasia.
  - The decision to do a digital or speculum pelvic exam should be based on the patient's age/maturity/gynecologic history/and ability to tolerate the exam. When presented with primary amenorrhea, an ultrasound should be used to evaluate anatomy (see the following discussion). An ultrasound may be needed as an adjunct to laboratory testing when evaluating secondary amenorrhea.

DIAGNOSTIC TESTS & INTERPRETATION

Lab

- Standard initial testing: pregnancy test, FSH/LH, estradiol, TSH, free T_4, prolactin (8 a.m.)
- For primary amenorrhea, include genetic testing by checking a karyotype for sex chromosome abnormalities.
- If PCOS is suspected or virilization is identified, also include total and free testosterone, dehydroepiandrosterone-sulfate (DHEA-S), and 17-hydroxyprogesterone.
- If Cushing syndrome is suspected, consider an overnight dexamethasone suppression test or 24-hour urinary free cortisol excretion.

Imaging

- Imaging should be used selectively.
- Transvaginal or pelvic ultrasound
  - Confirm presence of normal müllerian structures (uterus and ovaries) for patients with primary amenorrhea.
  - Exclude ovarian mass and renal abnormalities based on abnormal physical exam or laboratory results.
- MRI of the pituitary gland if indicated based on neurologic symptoms, galactorrhea, and/or laboratory results (elevated prolactin)

DIFFERENTIAL DIAGNOSIS

- Pregnancy
- Outflow tract abnormalities
  - Imperforate hymen, transverse vaginal septum, müllerian agenesis, androgen insensitivity syndrome
- Ovarian failure
  - Chromosomal abnormalities and other inherited defects such as Turner syndrome and androgen insensitivity syndrome
  - Radiation- or chemotherapy-induced ovarian failure, autoimmune premature ovarian failure, idiopathic premature ovarian failure
- Chronic anovulation
  - Androgen excess: PCOS (common), congenital adrenal hyperplasia, ovarian or adrenal tumor
  - Elevated prolactin: prolactinoma, medications, hypothyroidism, others. Remember that stress can cause mild elevations in serum prolactin that are not pathologic.
  - Low or normal LH/FSH: chronic or systemic illness, eating disorders, extreme obesity, excessive exercise, psychological stress, hypopituitarism
  - Thyroid disease
  - Cortisol excess: Cushing syndrome
- Medications:
  - Cytotoxic, hormonal contraception, opiates, psychiatric medications, and others

TREATMENT

- Identification and management depends on the underlying disorder.
- Estrogen/progestin hormonal therapy may have a role but should not be initiated prior to completing a full evaluation.
- Premature use of hormonal therapy may alter subsequent testing.
- Contraindications to hormone therapy must be ruled out (refer to World Health Organization [WHO] *Medical Eligibility Criteria* at http://www.who.int/reproductivehealth/publications/family_planning/en/).

ADDITIONAL THERAPIES

Behavioral interventions: An interdisciplinary team may be required to effectively manage eating disorders, complex behavior problems, or emotional symptoms.

ADDITIONAL READING

- Domine F, Dadoumont C, Bourguignon JP. Eating disorders throughout female adolescence. *Endocr Dev*. 2012;22:271–286.
- Gray SH. Menstrual disorders. *Pediatr Rev*. 2013;34(1):6–17.
- Roupas ND, Georgopoulos NA. Menstrual function in sports. *Hormones*. 2011;10(2):104–116.
- Santoro N. Update in hyper- and hypogonadotropic amenorrhea. *J Clin Endocrinol Metab*. 2011;96(11):3281–3288.
- Slap GB. Menstrual disorders in adolescence. *Best Pract Res Clin Obstet Gynaecol*. 2003;17(1):75–92.
- Viswanathan V, Eugster EA. Etiology and treatment of hypogonadism in adolescents. *Pediatr Clin North Am*. 2011;58(5):1181–1200.

CODES

ICD10

- N91.2 Amenorrhea, unspecified
- N91.0 Primary amenorrhea
- N91.1 Secondary amenorrhea

FAQ

- Q: What are the normal benchmarks for evaluating pubertal development in girls?
- A: Normal benchmarks for evaluating pubertal development in girls: breast development by age 12–13 years, menarche ~2 years after breast development (by age 14 years), or menarche within 2 years of achieving Tanner IV breast stage
- Q: Does a patient who says she has never had sex still need a pregnancy test?
- A: Yes.

ANAEROBIC INFECTIONS

Hamid Bassiri

BASICS

DESCRIPTION

- Anaerobic bacteria are organisms capable of growing in a reduced oxygen environment, either exclusively (obligate anaerobes) or in addition to growing in air (facultative anaerobes).
- Anaerobic bacteria can cause invasive and serious diseases.
- Anaerobic bacteria tend to participate in polymicrobial infections with other anaerobic and aerobic flora.

EPIDEMIOLOGY

- Although anaerobic bacteremia is less frequent in children than in adults, other anaerobic infections such as chronic sinusitis or chronic otitis media are common in children.
- Because of their fastidious nature, the ability of microbiology laboratories to identify anaerobic bacteria is highly dependent on proper collection and transport of culture specimens; hence, anaerobic bacteria are often missed and likely underreported.

RISK FACTORS

- Impaired host immunity
  - Malignancy
  - Splenic dysfunction
  - Hypogammaglobulinemia
- Presence of devitalized tissue
- Surgery, trauma
- Vascular insufficiency
- Poorly controlled diabetes
- Presence of foreign bodies
- Colitis

PATHOPHYSIOLOGY

- Anaerobic infections commonly derive from the normal flora of the oropharynx, skin, intestines, or the female genital tract; thus, anaerobic infections occur when there is a loss of integrity of anatomic or epithelial barriers at these sites.
- Virulence factors include production of exotoxins (e.g., *Clostridia* spp.), endotoxins (e.g., *Fusobacterium* spp.), and presence of phagocyte-inhibiting capsules (e.g., *Bacteroides* spp.).

ETIOLOGY

- The most common clinically-relevant anaerobes include the following:
  - Gram-negative rods (*Bacteroides*, *Prevotella*, *Porphyromonas*, *Fusobacterium*)
  - Gram-positive cocci (*Peptostreptococcus*, *Peptococcus*)
  - Spore-forming gram-positive bacilli (*Clostridia*)
  - Non–spore-forming gram-positive bacilli (*Eubacterium*, *Bifidobacterium*, *Propionibacterium*, *Actinomyces*, *Lactobacillus*)
  - Gram-negative cocci (*Veillonella*, *Acidaminococcus*)
  - Spirochetes (many of which are anaerobic)

COMMONLY ASSOCIATED CONDITIONS

- CNS infections:
  - Brain abscess due to bacteremia
  - Subdural empyema
  - Epidural abscess (most commonly due to complications from sinusitis)
- Head and neck infections:
  - Sinusitis (generally polymicrobial)
  - Chronic otitis media
  - Ludwig angina (infection of the submandibular space)
  - Cervical adenitis
  - Peritonsillar abscess
  - Dental abscess
  - Gingivitis
  - Actinomycosis of jaw
  - Lemierre disease (septic thrombophlebitis of the internal jugular vein owing to anaerobic bacteremia, most commonly with *Fusobacterium* spp., often resulting in pulmonary abscess formation)
- Pleuropulmonary infections:
  - Aspiration of infected amniotic or vaginal secretions in neonates
  - Aspiration of oral or gastrointestinal fluids in children (severe gingival or periodontal may be a risk factor)
  - Pneumonia, abscess formation due to aspirated foreign bodies
  - Actinomycosis
- Peritonitis/peritoneal abscess:
  - Appendiceal abscess
  - Perforated viscus
  - Postoperative complication
  - Trauma-related
  - Actinomycosis
- Cholangitis
  - Ascending infection may occur following biliary tract surgery (e.g., Kasai procedure)
- Soft tissue infections:
  - Paronychia
  - Pilonidal cyst
  - Hidradenitis suppurativa
  - Crepitant cellulitis
  - Necrotizing fasciitis
  - Gas gangrene (*Clostridium* spp.)
  - Infected decubitus ulcers (may result in contiguous osteomyelitis)
  - Penetrating wounds (may lead to tetanus)
- Infections of the female genital tract:
  - Endometritis
  - Salpingitis
  - Tubo-ovarian or adnexal abscess
  - Pelvic inflammatory diseases
  - Pelvic abscess
  - Bartholin gland, vulvar, or perineal abscess
  - Bacterial vaginosis
- Infected bite wounds
  - Anaerobes isolated from 50% of human or animal bites
- Bacteremia
  - Often associated with focal primary site of involvement (gastrointestinal disease, abscess)
- Neonatal infections:
  - Cellulitis at fetal monitoring sites
  - Aspiration pneumonia
  - Omphalitis
  - Conjunctivitis
  - Infant botulism

DIAGNOSIS

Involvement of anaerobic bacteria should be suspected in infections with suppuration or foul smell, abscess formation, tissue necrosis, or in hosts with systemic disease or defective immunity.

HISTORY

- Impaired mental status
  - Increased risk of aspiration
- History of thumb sucking
  - Anaerobes frequently isolated from paronychia
- History of animal or human bites
- Recent surgery or trauma
  - Poor drainage or devitalized tissue associated with anaerobic infection
- Underlying immunodeficiency or chronic illness
  - Impaired phagocytic function
- History of pus that is "sterile" (no growth on routine cultures).

PHYSICAL EXAM

- Location of infection
  - See "Commonly Associated Conditions."
- Poor dentition
  - Increased colonization of oropharynx with anaerobic organisms
- Necrotic tissue
- Crepitus with gas gangrene
- "Dishwater" pus or discharge with foul odor
  - Characteristic of anaerobic infections
- Lateral neck pain in association with respiratory distress:
  - Lemierre disease results in septic thrombophlebitis of the internal jugular vein and formation of lung abscesses; untreated or undiagnosed Lemierre disease carries a significant mortality rate.

DIAGNOSTIC TESTS & INTERPRETATION

Lab

- Certain anaerobic bacteria have unique morphology on Gram stains:
  - *Bacteroides* spp.: small, pleomorphic gram-negative bacilli
  - *Clostridium* spp.: large gram-positive organisms with "boxcar" morphology
- Anaerobic cultures
  - Should be performed on tissue or aspirated fluid obtained directly from the infected sites in a sterile fashion
  - Anaerobically collected specimens should be transported to the laboratory promptly.
  - Swabs should not be sent for anaerobic cultures.

Imaging

- Radiographs may show the following:
  – Air–fluid levels
  – Cavity formation
  – Gas in tissue
- CT and/or MRI scans
  – Often important to define anatomic location and extent of disease, and to determine surgical approaches to drainage or debridement

TREATMENT

MEDICATIONS

Empiric antibiotics for anaerobic infections include the following:

- Metronidazole
- Carbapenems (e.g. meropenem or imipenem)
- Chloramphenicol (supplies in the United States may be limited)
- β-Lactam/β-lactamase inhibitor combinations (e.g., amoxicillin-clavulanate, ampicillin-sulbactam, ticarcillin-clavulanate, or piperacillin-tazobactam)
- Clindamycin
- Cephamycins (e.g., cefoxitin or cefotetan)
- Vancomycin has activity against gram-positive but not gram-negative anaerobes.
- Penicillins, cephalosporins, tetracyclines, macrolides, aminoglycosides, trimethoprim-sulfamethoxazole, and monobactams have either variable or poor activity against anaerobes and should not be used empirically.
- Most fluoroquinolones also have variable activity, but exceptions exist (e.g., moxifloxacin).
- Antibiotic resistance is increasing in certain anaerobes, especially *Bacteroides* spp.; not all microbiology laboratories routinely test anaerobes for antibiotic susceptibility.
  – If a patient with a documented anaerobic infection does not appear to be responding to empiric therapy, it is advisable to consult with a infectious diseases specialist for further recommendations.

Empiric drug therapy reflects the polymicrobial nature of infections in which anaerobic bacteria are predominantly found:

- CNS infections
  – Vancomycin + 3rd or 4th generation cephalosporin (e.g., ceftriaxone) + metronidazole
  – Avoid using β-lactam-/β-lactamase inhibitor combinations for brain abscesses, as β-lactamase penetration across blood–brain barrier may be suboptimal.
- Head and neck infections
  – Ampicillin-sulbactam, amoxicillin-clavulanate, or clindamycin alone if gram-negative aerobic bacteria are of little concern
- Pleuropulmonary infections due to aspiration
  – Ampicillin-sulbactam, amoxicillin-clavulanate, or clindamycin
- Peritonitis/peritoneal abscess
  – Ampicillin-sulbactam, ticarcillin-clavulanate, piperacillin-tazobactam, cefoxitin, meropenem, or imipenem
- Cholangitis
  – Piperacillin-tazobactam, meropenem, or imipenem
- Soft tissue infection
  – Clindamycin, ampicillin-clavulanate
- Infections of the female genital tract
  – Ampicillin-sulbactam, ticarcillin-clavulanate, piperacillin-tazobactam, cefoxitin, meropenem, or imipenem
- Infected bite wounds
  – Ampicillin-sulbactam, piperacillin-tazobactam, amoxicillin-clavulanate
- Bacteremia
  – Isolate-dependent, but it may be reasonable to start with vancomycin + 3rd or 4th generation cephalosporin (e.g., ceftriaxone) + metronidazole until isolate speciated and bacteremia confirmed to be due to anaerobic bacteria

COMPLEMENTARY & ALTERNATIVE THERAPIES

- Neutralization of toxins, especially in the case of botulism or tetanus, is critical.
- Hyperbaric oxygen, although still sometimes used (especially in clostridial infections), has not been shown to be of proven benefit, although it may help define and demarcate the borders of devitalized tissues.

SURGERY/OTHER PROCEDURES

- Effective drainage of abscesses and debridement of devitalized tissue is essential.
- Cultures should be obtained by aspirating fluids into sterile syringes, capping them, and transporting these to the laboratory promptly.
- Cultures can also be obtained from intact tissues that are transported to the laboratory promptly.
- Swabs should not be sent for anaerobic cultures.

ONGOING CARE

PROGNOSIS

- Determined by speed with which infection is appropriately treated with antibiotics and/or drainage
- High rates of morbidity and mortality associated with untreated anaerobic bacteremia
- Specific prognosis depends on the bacterial species involved and the status of the patient's immune system.
- Soft tissue infections, necrotizing fasciitis, or gas gangrene caused by *Clostridium* spp. may cause up to 20% mortality despite aggressive therapy.

COMPLICATIONS

- Vary with nature of infection, but can include extension of infection to adjacent structures
- Development of bacteremia

ADDITIONAL READING

- Brook I. Anaerobic infections in children. *Adv Exp Med Biol*. 2011;697:117–152.
- Brook I. Clinical review: bacteremia caused by anaerobic bacteria in children. *Crit Care*. 2002;6(3):205–211.
- Japanese Society of Chemotherapy Committee on Guidelines for Treatment of Anaerobic Infections; Japanese Association for Anaerobic Infections Research. Chapter 1-1. Anaerobic infections (General): epidemiology of anaerobic infections. *J Infect Chemother*. 2011;17(Suppl 1):4–12.
- Nagy E. Anaerobic infections: update on treatment considerations. *Drugs*. 2010;70(7):841–858.

CODES

ICD10

- A49.9 Bacterial infection, unspecified
- A49.8 Other bacterial infections of unspecified site
- J32.9 Chronic sinusitis, unspecified

ANAPHYLAXIS

Benjamin T. Prince • Rachel G. Robison

BASICS

DESCRIPTION

- Anaphylaxis is a serious, life-threatening, systemic allergic reaction that is rapid in onset, and is a result of mast cell and basophil activation and degranulation.
- Skin and mucosal symptoms such as flushing, itching, urticaria, or angioedema are present in 80–90% of patients with anaphylaxis. Yet, absence of skin findings does not exclude anaphylaxis.
- In fatal anaphylaxis, initial signs and symptoms may include respiratory distress without urticaria resulting in delayed diagnosis and treatment.

EPIDEMIOLOGY

- 0.05–2% lifetime prevalence
- Rate of occurrence appears to be increasing.
- Estimated to be fatal in 0.7–2% of cases

RISK FACTORS

Genetics

There are few studies of genetic factors in human anaphylaxis; however, individuals with a previous history of anaphylaxis or a history of atopy are at increased risk for future anaphylaxis episodes.

PATHOPHYSIOLOGY

- In anaphylaxis, mast cells and basophils are activated via an IgE-mediated (most common) or non–IgE-mediated mechanism releasing preformed and newly generated mediators of inflammation.
  - Mediators include histamine, tryptase, proteoglycans, leukotrienes, prostaglandins, platelet-activating factor, and cytokines.
  - Local or systemic effects can include increased vascular permeability, vasodilation, smooth muscle contraction, complement activation, and coagulation.
- IgE-mediated anaphylaxis occurs when IgE is synthesized in response to allergen exposure (sensitization) and becomes fixed to high-affinity IgE receptors located on the surface of mast cells and basophils. Subsequent allergen exposure results in receptor-bound IgE aggregation and cell activation.
- Non–IgE-mediated anaphylaxis generally results from nonimmune stimulation of mast cells or basophils. Rarely, IgG and complement can be implicated.

ETIOLOGY

- IgE-mediated:
  - Foods (peanut, tree nuts, fish, shellfish, milk, egg, wheat, soy)
  - Medications (antibiotics, especially, β-lactams, NSAIDs, biologic products)
  - Venoms (usually from stinging insects including fire ants)
  - Latex (direct exposure to natural rubber or ingestion of cross-reacting foods)
  - Other (vaccines, occupational allergens, and rarely inhaled allergens)
- Non–IgE-mediated:
  - Radiocontrast media (can also trigger IgE-dependent anaphylaxis)
  - Medications (opiates, NSAIDs, dextrans, vancomycin, polymyxin B)
  - Physical stimuli (exercise, cold, heat, sunlight/UV radiation)
  - Ethanol

DIAGNOSIS

Anaphylaxis is a clinical diagnosis that is considered highly likely when any one of the following three criteria is met:

- Acute onset of illness (minutes to hours) with involvement of skin, mucosa, or both and at least one of the following: (a) respiratory compromise or (b) reduced blood pressure or associated symptoms of organ dysfunction.
- Two or more of the following occurring acutely (minutes to hours) after exposure to a likely allergen: (a) involvement of skin-mucosal tissue (b) respiratory compromise (dyspnea, wheezing, stridor, hypoxemia), (c) reduced blood pressure or associated symptoms of organ dysfunction, (d) persistent gastrointestinal symptoms (abdominal cramping, vomiting).
- Reduced systolic blood pressure acutely (minutes to hours) after exposure to known allergen for that patient. Defined by age-specific normals or $>30\%$ decrease from patient's baseline

HISTORY

- A detailed history of exposures and events in minutes to hours prior to onset should be obtained after treatment is initiated.
- Any previous history of anaphylaxis?
  - Can help direct history and patient education, especially if epinephrine was indicated but not given or if a known allergen was not recognized
- Food triggers
  - Most common: peanut, tree nuts, fish, shellfish, milk, egg, wheat, soy, sesame, additives (spices, colorants, contaminants)
  - Foods need to be ingested for a reaction to occur, but rarely anaphylaxis can be caused by inhalation of aerosolized vapors from cooking or processing (fish and shellfish).
  - Gastrointestinal symptoms tend to be more prominent than in other etiologies.
- Medication triggers
  - Specifically inquire about NSAIDs, supplements, and herbal treatments.
  - β-Blockers and ACE inhibitors can increase severity and/or make treatment of anaphylaxis more difficult.

ALERT

For patients with anaphylaxis who are taking β-blockers or ACE inhibitors and have persistent hypotension and bradycardia despite epinephrine, consider giving glucagon.

- Insect stings
  - If possible, attempt to identify the insect (honeybees leave stinger at sting site).
  - All patients should be referred to an allergist, as immunotherapy is effective in preventing 98% of future anaphylactic reactions.
- Natural rubber latex
  - Latex-allergic patients can develop anaphylaxis after ingestion of cross-reactive foods including banana, kiwi, papaya, avocado, potato, and tomato.

PHYSICAL EXAM

- Skin and mucosa
  - Flushing, itching, conjunctival erythema, urticaria, angioedema
- Respiratory
  - Upper airway: nasal itching, congestion, rhinorrhea, sneezing, dysphonia, hoarseness, stridor, drooling (can be a sign of angioedema or obstruction)
  - Lower airway: tachypnea, cough, wheezing/bronchospasm, decreased peak expiratory flow
  - Cyanosis, respiratory arrest
- Cardiovascular system
  - Tachycardia or bradycardia (less common), hypotension, arrhythmias, shock, urinary or fecal incontinence, cardiac arrest
- Gastrointestinal
  - Abdominal pain/cramping, vomiting, diarrhea, dysphagia
- Central nervous system
  - Patients may appear uneasy or describe a sense of impending doom.
  - Altered mental status, confusion, tunnel vision

DIAGNOSTIC TESTS & INTERPRETATION

Anaphylaxis is a clinical diagnosis; however, certain tests can aid in confirming the diagnosis. Treatment of anaphylaxis should be initiated immediately if a patient presents with a clinical picture that is consistent with anaphylaxis.

Lab

- Serum total tryptase
  - Elevated 15 minutes to 3 hours after onset of anaphylaxis
  - Elevated in patients with anaphylaxis due to injected medications, insect stings, and when hypotension is present
  - Can be normal in anaphylaxis due to foods or in those who are normotensive
  - Normal serum tryptase does not rule out anaphylaxis.
  - Laboratory test that is routinely used in practice
- Plasma histamine
  - Elevated if measured 15–60 minutes after onset of anaphylaxis due to its short half-life
  - Blood sample requires special handling.
  - Normal level does not rule out anaphylaxis.
- Urine histamine and *N*-methylhistamine
  - 24-hour urine histamine and *N*-methylhistamine (metabolite) can be elevated in the context of anaphylaxis.

Imaging

Chest radiograph: may be useful to rule out foreign body aspiration, or congenital malformations of the respiratory or gastrointestinal tract

DIFFERENTIAL DIAGNOSIS

- Allergic/atopic
  - Acute urticaria
  - Acute asthma
  - Pollen-food syndrome
- Cardiovascular
  - Myocardial infarction
  - Pulmonary embolus

- Genetic/metabolic
  - Hereditary or acquired angioedema
- Infectious
  - Septic shock
- Neoplastic
  - Mastocytosis/clonal mast cell disorders
  - Carcinoid
  - Basophilic leukemia
  - Pheochromocytoma
- Neurologic
  - Syncope
  - Seizure
- Nonorganic disease
  - Panic attack
  - Vocal cord dysfunction
  - Munchausen syndrome
- Other:
  - Foreign body aspiration
  - Scombroidosis (ingestion of fish containing high levels of histamine)
  - Red Man syndrome

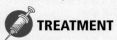

TREATMENT

MEDICATION

First Line

- IM epinephrine 1:1,000 (1 mg/mL) solution
  - 0.01 mg/kg, maximum of 0.3 mg (child) or 0.5 mg (adult), repeated q5–15min as needed (most respond to 1 or 2 doses)
  - Many deaths from anaphylaxis are associated with delayed administration of epinephrine.

Second Line

- Diphenhydramine IV or PO (or equivalent H_1-antihistamine)
  - 1 mg/kg, maximum of 50 mg, q4–6h
- Albuterol 2.5 mg/3 mL solution
  - Nebulized and inhaled via face mask
- Ranitidine IV
  - 1 mg/kg, maximum 50 mg
- Methylprednisolone IV (or equivalent glucocorticoid)
  - 1–2 mg/kg, maximum of 60 mg (may be continued PO once daily for 1- to 3-day course)
  - Thought to prevent biphasic or protracted anaphylaxis, but unlikely to provide benefit in initial minutes of anaphylaxis

ADDITIONAL TREATMENT

General Measures

- Maintain airway:
  - Supplemental oxygen
  - Bag mask or intubation if necessary
- Maintain circulation:
  - Place patient supine and elevate lower extremities if possible.
  - Volume resuscitation with 0.9% saline
  - IV vasopressors may be necessary in patients with refractory hypotension or shock.

ONGOING CARE

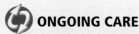

FOLLOW-UP RECOMMENDATIONS

Most patients who are diagnosed with anaphylaxis will benefit from a referral to an allergist/immunologist for further evaluation, recommendations, and management.

Patient Monitoring

Biphasic anaphylaxis, in which symptoms recur within 1–72 hours (usually 8–10 hours) after resolution of initial symptoms, occurs in up to 23% of adults and up to 11% of children with anaphylaxis.

- A prescription for autoinjectable epinephrine should be provided on discharge in any patient diagnosed with anaphylaxis.
- A 1- to 3-day course of oral steroids may prevent or limit biphasic or protracted anaphylaxis.
- Medical monitoring after return to baseline should be individualized and depend on degree of symptoms and other risk factors.
  - Patients with moderate respiratory compromise should be monitored for a minimum of 4 hours or longer if indicated (especially young patients or patients with comorbidities).

PATIENT EDUCATION

All patients should be instructed on allergen avoidance measures and provided with a written personalized emergency plan detailing appropriate management of future anaphylactic episodes.

PROGNOSIS

Good with trigger identification and avoidance

COMPLICATIONS

- Laryngeal edema and airway obstruction
- Pulmonary edema, pulmonary hemorrhage, and pneumothorax
- Myocardial ischemia and infarction
- End-organ ischemia and damage
- Death secondary to airway obstruction (asphyxiation) and/or shock

ADDITIONAL READING

- Greenberger PA, Rotskoff BD, Lifschultz B. Fatal anaphylaxis: postmortem findings and associated comorbid diseases. *Ann Allergy Asthma Immunol*. 2007;98(3):252–257.
- Simons FE. Anaphylaxis. *J Allergy Clin Immunol*. 2010;125(2)(Suppl 2):S161–S181.
- Simons FE, Ardusso LR, Bilò MB, et al. World Allergy Organization guidelines for the assessment and management of anaphylaxis. *World Allergy Organ J*. 2011;4(2):13–37.
- Webb LM, Lieberman P. Anaphylaxis: a review of 601 cases. *Ann Allergy Asthma Immunol*. 2006;97(1):39–43.

CODES

ICD10

- T78.2XXA Anaphylactic shock, unspecified, initial encounter
- T78.00XA Anaphylactic reaction due to unspecified food, init encntr
- T63.891A Toxic effect of contact with other venomous animals, accidental (unintentional), initial encounter

FAQ

- Q: Can a patient have an anaphylactic reaction on first exposure to an allergen?
- A: In IgE-mediated anaphylaxis, a patient must have been previously exposed to the offending allergen for sensitization to occur with a subsequent exposure potentially resulting in anaphylaxis. Remember, however, that the absence of a previous exposure on history does *not* exclude an allergen as causal because sensitization may have previously occurred unknowingly (through skin contact, in breast milk, in utero). Non–IgE-mediated anaphylaxis can occur on first exposure to the offending allergen.
- Q: Should patients with a history of anaphylaxis carry more than one autoinjectable epinephrine device?
- A: Yes, up to 20% of patients with anaphylaxis are reported to require a second dose of epinephrine either because of ongoing symptoms or because of biphasic anaphylaxis.
- Q: Can a patient develop anaphylaxis to an allergen that they have tolerated previously?
- A: Yes, this often occurs with medications or foods (particularly peanut, tree nuts, fish, and shellfish) especially if there is a long period of time between exposures.

ANEMIA OF CHRONIC DISEASE (ANEMIA OF INFLAMMATION)

Michele P. Lambert

BASICS

DESCRIPTION

Anemia that accompanies a variety of systemic diseases, with the common features of chronicity and inflammation. Anemia of chronic disease is more properly called anemia of inflammation (AI) and is the combined result of mildly increased destruction of RBCs, relative erythropoietin resistance, and iron-restricted erythropoiesis.

PATHOPHYSIOLOGY

Typically mild to moderate anemia (Hgb 7–12 g/dL); develops in the setting of infection, inflammatory disorders, and some malignancies

- Deficient cellular iron in the setting of hepcidin excess (functionally inaccessible iron)
- Typically normochromic, normocytic but, if long-standing, can be hypochromic, microcytic (especially in children)
- Main mechanism appears to be
  - Iron restriction (limited iron supply to erythropoiesis)
  - Hepcidin is increased by interleukin 6 (IL-6) and causes depletion of the only known membrane iron transporter (ferroportin).
  - These changes result in cellular inability to release stored iron and enterocyte inability to absorb iron because of inability to transport iron over cell membrane into bloodstream.
- Other factors contributing to anemia in various degrees include the following:
  - Increased red cell destruction
  - Diagnostic phlebotomy or other blood loss
  - Cytokine-mediated interference with erythropoietin signaling
  - Cytokine-mediated suppression of erythropoiesis
  - Cytokines such as interleukin-1 (IL-1) and IL-6 can activate ferritin synthesis. The ferritin can lead to sequestration of iron, which eventually is converted into hemosiderin.

ETIOLOGY

Underlying disease process

COMMONLY ASSOCIATED CONDITIONS

- Underlying disease process
  - Infections, both acute and chronic
  - Inflammatory disease
  - Collagen vascular diseases
  - Malignancies
  - Renal failure
- Anemia of chronic disease often coexists with other causes of anemia, including occult blood loss, hemolysis, dietary iron deficiency, and drug-related marrow suppression.

DIAGNOSIS

SIGNS AND SYMPTOMS

- Various abnormal physical findings may be present, depending on the underlying chronic disease process.
- May have mild pallor but will not have signs of circulatory collapse
- Similar disease can be seen more acutely in the setting of anemia of critical illness (also part of AI).

HISTORY

Anemia develops over the 1st month of the underlying disease process and then remains fairly stable over time.

PHYSICAL EXAM

- Mild pallor
- Mild tachycardia, may be inapparent at rest
- Very rarely more overt signs of anemia such as flow murmur, gallop, or hepatomegaly
- Physical findings of the underlying disease

DIAGNOSTIC TESTS & INTERPRETATION

If only the serum iron is obtained, without other iron studies, the child may be inappropriately diagnosed with iron deficiency.

Lab

- CBC with indices
  - Normocytic, normochromic (can be microcytic, hypochromic when very long-standing) anemia with hematocrit rarely $<20\%$
  - Reticulocyte count usually in the normal range, but low for the level of anemia.
- Iron studies
  - Low plasma iron, with low total iron-binding capacity
  - Low transferrin saturation by iron
  - Normal or high ferritin level
- Elevated free erythrocyte protoporphyrin
- Hemosiderin in bone marrow macrophages is increased if bone marrow aspiration is done and the aspirate is viewed with iron stains.
- Albumin and transferrin are both low.
- Acute-phase reactants such as C-reactive protein may be elevated.
- Hepcidin levels will be elevated.

Diagnostic Procedures/Other

Bone marrow aspiration is generally not indicated.

DIFFERENTIAL DIAGNOSIS

Anemia of chronic disease is often confused with iron deficiency anemia.

- In anemia of chronic disease:
  - Mild to moderate anemia
  - Mild anisocytosis
  - Usually normochromic, normocytic but can be hypochromic with microcytosis
  - Decreased plasma iron
  - Decreased iron-binding capacity
  - Normal or slightly low transferrin saturation
  - Decreased marrow sideroblasts
  - Normal or elevated reticuloendothelial iron
  - Elevated free erythrocyte protoporphyrin
  - Normal or elevated ferritin
  - Increased hepcidin
- In iron deficiency:
  - Decreased plasma iron
  - Increased iron-binding capacity
  - Decreased transferrin saturation
  - Decreased marrow sideroblasts
  - Decreased reticuloendothelial iron
  - Increased free erythrocyte protoporphyrin
  - Decreased serum ferritin
  - Decreased hepcidin
- In both iron deficiency and anemia of chronic disease:
  - Decreased plasma iron
  - Decreased transferrin saturation
  - Decreased marrow sideroblasts
  - Elevated free erythrocyte protoporphyrin
  - Decreased reticulocyte count
- Tests that help differentiate iron deficiency from anemia of chronic disease:
  - Iron-binding capacity
  - Serum ferritin
  - Reticuloendothelial iron stain in marrow
  - Hepcidin level (although not available everywhere)

TREATMENT

GENERAL MEASURES

- Iron
  - Generally, no role for iron therapy unless there is coexisting iron deficiency anemia. However, recent studies in patients with renal disease have shown improved response to erythropoietin with coadministration of parenteral iron.
- Recombinant human erythropoietin
  - Effective, but indications for use are still not universally accepted
  - Often used in chronic renal failure
  - Has been used in inflammatory bowel disease, with good results
  - Should be used for more severe and symptomatic anemia in which the underlying disease is likely to be prolonged and difficult to treat
- Treatment should be directed at the underlying disease process.

SPECIAL THERAPY

Transfusion of packed RBCs is sometimes indicated intermittently in severe anemia with hemodynamic compromise.

ONGOING CARE

FOLLOW-UP RECOMMENDATIONS

Patient Monitoring

Treatment of underlying disease process may promote slow resolution of associated anemia. Hematocrit increases ~6–8 weeks after start of recombinant human erythropoietin therapy; continues to rise over 6 months.

COMPLICATIONS

If severe, patients may be transfusion dependent and, thus, be at risk for complications associated with packed RBC transfusions.

ADDITIONAL READING

- Cullis J. Anaemia of chronic disease. *Clin Med*. 2013;13(2):193–196.
- Ganz T. Molecular pathogenesis of anemia of chronic disease. *Pediatr Blood Cancer*. 2006;46(5):554–557.
- Ganz T, Nemeth E. Iron sequestration and anemia of inflammation. *Semin Hematol*. 2009;46(4):387–393.
- Goodnough LT, Skikne B, Brugnara C. Erythropoietin, iron, and erythropoiesis. *Blood*. 2000;96(3):823–833.

CODES

ICD10

- D63.8 Anemia in other chronic diseases classified elsewhere
- D63.1 Anemia in chronic kidney disease
- D63.0 Anemia in neoplastic disease

FAQ

- Q: Does anemia that is associated with a chronic disease require further evaluation?
- A: If the anemia fits within the usual expectations for the patient's diagnosis, there is no need to pursue further investigation, except in specific cases. If there is an associated malignancy for which marrow metastasis is possible, a bone marrow aspirate and biopsy should be done. In conditions with malabsorption, nutritional deficiencies and blood loss should be ruled out.

ANKYLOGLOSSIA

Timothy R. Shope • Robert F. Yellon • Melissa A. Buryk

BASICS

DESCRIPTION

Anatomic variation of the tongue in which the lingual frenulum is unusually tight and short. Also known as tongue-tie. This condition may result in impaired tongue mobility with early breastfeeding problems, maternal nipple pain, and, later, speech problems.

EPIDEMIOLOGY

- Incidence ranges from 1.7 to 5% of newborns in various studies.
- About half of breastfeeding infants with ankyloglossia will have difficulty feeding or cause maternal nipple pain during feeds.
- Incidence of speech articulation disorders due to ankyloglossia is unknown.
- Male-to-female ratio of 3:1.

RISK FACTORS

- Pedigree analysis suggests significant hereditary component, possibly X-linked.
- Studies show 40–50% of patients with ankyloglossia had a relative with the same condition and an inheritance rate of about 21%.
- Rarely, mutations in the T-box transcription factor TBX22 may lead to heritable ankyloglossia with or without cleft lip, cleft palate, or hypodontia.
- Rarely, may be associated with Opitz syndrome or orodigital facial syndrome
- No known environmental risk factors

PATHOPHYSIOLOGY

- Newborns with ankyloglossia
  - Are often asymptomatic but problems can occur with breastfeeding
  - May have poor or ineffective latch or may cause maternal nipple pain due to poor tongue mobility and prolonged feeding times
- Later in childhood, the effect of ankyloglossia is controversial.
  - May cause problems with articulation of certain sounds that require tongue to reach teeth, palate, and lips (e.g., "t," "d," "z," "s," "th," "n," "l")
  - Not a cause of speech delay
  - May also result in mechanical problems including difficulty with oral hygiene (inability to lick lips), inability to lick ice cream cone, play wind instruments, or French kiss

DIAGNOSIS

Diagnosis based on physical appearance and functional impairment of breastfeeding or speech

HISTORY

- Maternal report of difficulty with infant latch or nipple pain while breastfeeding
- Report of inability of infant/child to extrude tongue beyond alveolus/teeth
- Ankyloglossia varies in severity. Some children can protrude tongue past alveolus/teeth but not past lower lip and still have difficulties.

PHYSICAL EXAM

- Commonly missed finding on newborn exam because the mouth is usually not open.
- Examiner should pass the small finger, pad-side down, under the infant's tongue to feel for resistance at the site of the lingual frenulum.
- Examiner should also visualize the floor of mouth and lingual frenulum using tongue depressors, Q-tips, or fingers to open the mouth or by observation of the infant crying.
- Visualization of the tongue will show
  - Abnormally short frenulum, inserting at or near the tip of the tongue
  - Difficulty lifting tongue to upper alveolus/palate
  - Inability to protrude tongue beyond lower alveolus/teeth
  - Notching or heart shape of tip of tongue when protruded
  - Note: Some children can protrude tongue past alveolus/teeth but not past lower lip and still have difficulties.

DIAGNOSTIC TESTS & INTERPRETATION

Imaging

- No imaging indicated
- Functional ultrasound of tongue movement during breastfeeding has been used experimentally to quantify milk transfer.

Diagnostic Procedures/Other

- Mothers of infants with ankyloglossia and difficulty breastfeeding should meet with lactation consultant to rule out other potential causative factors,
- Children with speech articulation difficulty should meet with speech therapist for therapy and to assess for other causes.

DIFFERENTIAL DIAGNOSIS

- Consider other causes of poor breastfeeding including inexperience, poor positioning, or poor suck.
- Consider other causes of speech articulation difficulties including incoordination and neuromuscular disease.

TREATMENT

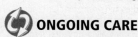

GENERAL MEASURES

- Observation if there is no functional impairment of breastfeeding or speech
- Surgical treatment if functional impairment is present
- Treatment is frenotomy—incision of lingual frenulum.
  - For most healthy newborns, this may be performed in an outpatient setting. Topical lidocaine and oxymetazoline on a cotton ball are applied before and after incision with sterile scissors. Infants with a thick frenulum should have the procedure performed in the operating room setting to avoid bleeding.
  - For older children unlikely to cooperate, and any patient with medical comorbidities or coagulopathy, the procedure should be performed in the operating room under general anesthesia.
- Frenotomy has been shown to be effective for improving infant breastfeeding problems and weight gain and maternal nipple pain while breastfeeding. There are 5 randomized controlled trials with similar positive results.
- Breastfeeding rates in infants treated with frenotomy for ankyloglossia appear similar to healthy infants (approximately 40–45% at 6 months and 25% at 12 months).
- There is anecdotal clinical evidence that frenotomy improves speech articulation problems. However, studies evaluating this are of low quality, with lack of randomization and small sample sizes. Further studies are needed.
- Complications have rarely been reported including severe infection or severe bleeding. Severe bleeding was associated with untrained individuals performing the surgery.

ONGOING CARE

FOLLOW-UP RECOMMENDATIONS

- Infants should be seen about one week after frenotomy to assess feeding and weight gain.
- Older children should be seen about 6 weeks after surgery to assess function and to determine whether a revision procedure for scar formation is needed.

PROGNOSIS

- Infants treated for tongue-tie have an excellent prognosis.
- <1% require repeat frenotomy and local flaps may be required.

ADDITIONAL READING

- Buryk M, Bloom D, Shope T. Efficacy of neonatal release of ankyloglossia: a randomized trial. *Pediatrics*. 2011;128(2):280–288.
- Dollberg S, Botzer E, Grunis E, et al. Immediate nipple pain relief after frenotomy in breast-fed infants with ankyloglossia: a randomized, prospective study. *J Pediatr Surg*. 2006;41(9):1598–1600.
- Han SH, Kim MC, Choi YS, et al. A study on the genetic inheritance of ankyloglossia based on pedigree analysis. *Arch Plast Surg*. 2012;39(4):329–332.
- Opara PI, Gabriel-Job N, Opara KO. Neonates presenting with severe complications of frenotomy: a case series. *J Med Case Rep*. 2012;6:77.
- Webb A, Hao W, Hong P. The effect of tongue-tie division on breastfeeding and speech articulation: a systematic review. *Int J Pediatr Otorhinolaryngol*. 2013;77(5):635–646.

CODES

ICD10

- Q38.1 Ankyloglossia
- P92.8 Other feeding problems of newborn

FAQ

- Q: What is the appropriate time to perform frenotomy in breastfeeding newborns with ankyloglossia?
- A: Optimal timing is not known. A reasonable approach is to allow enough time to establish that there is a problem with breastfeeding caused by the ankyloglossia. Some infants with ankyloglossia will not have problems. Usually, this issue is evident in the first 2 days of life. Newborns with identified breastfeeding difficulty should have frenotomy performed quickly to allow for continued breastfeeding. Delay may cause some mothers to abandon breastfeeding due to pain or difficulty. Optimal timing is probably between 2 and 7 days of life.
- Q: In infants with ankyloglossia who are either bottlefeeding or breastfeeding with no difficulty, should frenotomy be performed to help "prevent" future problems with speech or functional difficulties?
- A: Data regarding speech/functional outcome in these children are not known at present.
- Q: Who does frenotomies?
- A: ENT or oral surgeons most commonly perform the procedure. In areas where access to these specialists is difficult, general pediatricians, family practitioners, neonatologists, or newbornists may perform the procedure after sufficient training and appropriate credentialing. The procedure is not difficult. It can be done in the inpatient or outpatient setting. It is billed under the CPT Code 41010 (frenotomy).
- Q: What are the postoperative instructions after frenotomy?
- A: For all patients after frenotomy: acetaminophen for pain. Although complications are rare, patients should go to an emergency department if bleeding, infection, or swelling occurs. For older children, avoid citrus; spicy; or hard, scratchy foods for 1 week after the procedure.

ANOMALOUS LEFT CORONARY ARTERY FROM THE PULMONARY ARTERY (ALCAPA)

Shellie M. Kendall

BASICS

DESCRIPTION

The anomalous coronary artery arises from the pulmonary artery rather than the aorta. Most commonly, the anomalous left coronary artery arises from the pulmonary artery in a condition known as ALCAPA or Bland-White-Garland syndrome.

EPIDEMIOLOGY

Incidence

Very rare anomaly, occurring in 0.25% of congenital heart disease

Prevalence

The majority of patients present in infancy at approximately 2 months of age (when pulmonary vascular resistance is falling). There are case reports of patients presenting as late as the 4th–7th decades of life.

PATHOPHYSIOLOGY

- In the fetal and neonatal period, pulmonary artery pressure is increased owing to elevated pulmonary vascular resistance. This elevated pulmonary artery pressure provides antegrade flow from the pulmonary artery through the anomalous coronary artery.
- As pulmonary vascular resistance drops, pulmonary arterial pressure drops. When the diastolic blood pressure in the pulmonary artery decreases below myocardial perfusion pressure (or diastolic aortic pressure), pulmonary run-off "steals" blood from the myocardium, resulting in myocardial ischemia of the anterolateral left ventricular wall and mitral valve papillary muscle dysfunction.
- The fact that the left ventricle is perfused with desaturated blood plays a less important role than the overall perfusion-related imbalance between myocardial oxygen demand and supply.

ETIOLOGY

- Abnormal septation of the conotruncus into the aorta and pulmonary artery
- Persistence of the pulmonary buds and involution of the aortic buds that usually eventually form the coronary arteries
- As-yet-unspecified genetic predisposition

DIAGNOSIS

HISTORY

- Typically presents with paroxysms of poor feeding, pallor, tachypnea, respiratory distress, and diaphoresis
- Irritability, crying, appearance of being in pain (especially after meals)
- Can be asymptomatic
- Can be symptomatic in infancy and then gradually improve (with the development of adequate coronary collateralization)
- Older children and adults may have dyspnea, syncope, or angina pectoris.
- Sudden death

PHYSICAL EXAM

- Signs of congestive heart failure (CHF) such as cachexia, tachycardia, tachypnea, lethargy, diaphoresis
- Signs of low cardiac output such as pallor, diminished peripheral pulses and perfusion
- Gallop rhythm
- Loud P_2 component of S_2 (if left ventricular heart failure raises pulmonary arterial pressure)
- Murmur of mitral regurgitation or a continuous murmur reminiscent of a coronary arteriovenous fistula
- Diagnosis should be entertained in any infant presenting with cardiomegaly or perplexing cardiorespiratory symptoms.

DIAGNOSTIC TESTS & INTERPRETATION

Imaging

- Chest radiograph: cardiomegaly, pulmonary edema
- Electrocardiography: anterolateral infarct pattern in an infant (Q in I, aVL, V_4–V_6), abnormal R-wave progression in precordial leads
- Echocardiogram: attachment of coronary artery to pulmonary artery by 2-dimensional imaging. Doppler interrogation shows flow passing from coronary artery to great artery rather than vice versa (if pulmonary vascular resistance has fallen).
  - Dilation of the right coronary artery
  - Left ventricular function impairment, wall motion abnormalities, and dilation
  - Mitral regurgitation
  - Echogenic papillary muscles
- Coronary CT angiography
  - Excellent diagnostic modality for older patients with slower heart rates, allowing better resolution
  - Emerging CT technology is allowing this technique to be used in infancy with lower radiation doses and excellent resolution.
- Nuclear imaging: Thallium myocardial perfusion imaging shows reduced uptake in ischemic regions.
- Cardiac catheterization: Angiographic and hemodynamic parameters may correlate with degree of cardiovascular dysfunction.
  - Low cardiac output
  - High left atrial filling pressures
  - Pulmonary arterial hypertension
  - Aortic root angiography shows passage of contrast medium from normally connected right coronary artery to the left coronary arterial system to the pulmonary artery.
  - Pulmonary artery angiogram shows reflux of contrast medium into the left coronary artery and/or a "negative wash-in" of unopacified blood flowing from left coronary to pulmonary artery.

DIFFERENTIAL DIAGNOSIS
- Cardiomyopathy
- Myocarditis
- Coronary artery fistula
- Left ventricular failure from other causes
- Mitral valve regurgitation
- Respiratory distress from other causes
- Colic

TREATMENT

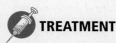

GENERAL MEASURES
The first priority is to safely institute supportive care measures while expeditiously planning for surgical intervention.

SURGERY/OTHER PROCEDURES
- Direct reimplantation of the left coronary artery into the aorta using a button of pulmonary arterial tissue and/or an extension-tube graft of anterior and posterior pulmonary arterial wall tissue sewn into a narrow cylinder to avoid tension, distortion, and stenosis of the coronary
- Creation of an aortopulmonary window and tunnel that directs blood from aorta to the left coronary ostium (Takeuchi procedure).
- Ligation of the origin of the left coronary artery and reconstitution of flow with saphenous or internal mammary graft rarely used in the current era.
- Ligation of the origin of the left coronary artery (to prevent flow runoff into the pulmonary artery or "steal") is rarely ever used, even in very ill infants.

INPATIENT CONSIDERATIONS
Initial Stabilization
- Attention to basic life support measures (airway, breathing, and circulation) and prompt referral to a pediatric cardiac center are indicated immediately on presentation.
- As myocardial ischemia can be worsened with traditional heart failure treatments such as oxygen administration, afterload reduction, and inotropic support, these therapies should be administered in consultation with a pediatric cardiac care center.
- An excess of procedures, interventions, and manipulation is poorly tolerated by this group of critically ill patients.

ONGOING CARE

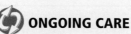

PROGNOSIS
- Untreated, 90% of those who present in infancy will die before the age of 1 year, usually at 1 to 2 months of age (when pulmonary vascular resistance falls).
- Very few of those who present early improve spontaneously.
- Late results after surgery are excellent in many centers. Hospital mortality in larger selected series of these frequently moribund patients is ≤5%, with very little subsequent attrition.
- Mitral regurgitation usually improves after surgery establishes a patent dual-coronary system, but this may take 6–12 months to be fully realized. Follow-up evaluation is warranted, as mitral regurgitation may progress despite surgery, and valve repair may be required later.

ADDITIONAL READING

- Azakie A, Russell JL, McCrindle BW, et al. Anatomic repair of anomalous left coronary artery from the pulmonary artery by aortic re-implantation: early survival, patterns of ventricular recovery and late outcome. *Ann Thorac Surg*. 2003;75(5):1535–1541.
- Bland E, White P, Garland J. Congenital anomalies of the coronary arteries: report of an unusual case associated with cardiac hypertrophy. *Am Heart J*. 1933;8:787–801.
- Dodge-Khatami A, Mavroudis C, Backer CL. Anomalous origin of the left coronary artery from the pulmonary artery: collective review of surgical therapy. *Ann Thorac Surg*. 2002;74(3):946–955.
- Ginde S, Earing M, Bartz P, et al. Late complications after Takeuchi repair of anomalous left coronary artery from the pulmonary artery: case series and review of literature. *Pediatr Cardiol*. 2012;33(7):1115–1123.
- Keane JF, Lock JE, Fyler DC, eds. *Nadas' Pediatric Cardiology*. Philadelphia, PA: WB Saunders; 2006.
- Lange R, Vogt M, Horer J, et al. Long-term results of repair of anomalous origin of the left coronary artery from the pulmonary artery. *Ann Thorac Surg*. 2007;83(4):1463–1471.
- Michielon G, Di Carlo D, Brancaccio G, et al. Anomalous coronary artery origin from the pulmonary artery: correlation between surgical timing and left ventricular function recovery. *Ann Thorac Surg*. 2003;76(2):581–588, discussion 588.
- Pelliccia A. Congenital coronary artery anomalies in young patients: new perspectives for timely identification. *J Am Coll Cardiol*. 2001;37(2):598–600.

CODES

ICD10
Q24.5 Malformation of coronary vessels

FAQ
- Q: How do you differentiate crying from the symptoms of myocardial ischemia from crying from colic?
- A: This is not easy, but clinical assessment should manifest the signs of CHF, shock, and low cardiac output, which are decidedly atypical for the usual patient with colic. If the patient is still feeding, the crying in patients with this lesion classically occurs after meals, when blood is shunted to the liver and intestines. This is not a highly sensitive finding, and concern should lead to further objective evaluation.

ANOREXIA NERVOSA

Darlene Atkins • Sara M. Buckelew

BASICS

DESCRIPTION

Anorexia nervosa (AN) is a complex biopsychosocial illness.

- *Diagnostic and Statistical Manual of Mental Disorders* 5th edition (*DSM-5*) criteria:
  - Restriction of energy intake relative to requirements, leading to a significantly low body weight in the context of age, sex, developmental trajectory, and physical health. Significantly low weight is defined as weight that is less than minimally normal or, for children and adolescents, less than minimally expected.
  - Intense fear of gaining weight or becoming fat, or persistent behavior that interferes with weight gain, even though at a significantly low weight
  - Disturbance in the way in which one's body weight or shape is experienced, undue influence of body weight or shape on self-evaluation, or persistent lack of recognition of the seriousness of current low body weight
- Types: Restricting (no binge eating or purging) or binge eating/purging (purging includes vomiting, laxatives and/or diuretic use)
- Reprinted with permission from the American Psychiatric Association. *Diagnostic and Statistical Manual of Mental Disorders*. 5th ed. American Psychiatric Association; 2013:171.

EPIDEMIOLOGY

Prevalence

- Approximately 0.5% of adolescent girls in the United States have AN.
- 10% of all patients with eating disorders are males.
- In younger patients, approximately equal numbers of females and males
- Increasing prevalence of eating disorders is seen in preadolescents, in males, and in minority populations within the United States.

RISK FACTORS

- Early physical/pubertal development
- Personality traits such as perfectionism and eagerness to please
- Family history of eating disorders, alcoholism, or mood disorders
- Involvement in sports or activities that emphasize shape/weight
- "Dieting" itself is a risk factor for developing an eating disorder.

Genetics

Family studies demonstrate that 1st-degree relatives have a 10-fold increased lifetime risk of developing AN. Twin studies also support role of genetics and familial concordance of AN.

GENERAL PREVENTION

- Assess height, weight, and BMI at every preventive visit at a minimum; evaluate for deviations.
- Discourage "dieting" behavior. Instead, focus on promoting healthy eating behaviors and lifestyle change.
- Strongly encourage regular family meals. Research supports this as a protective factor for all types of eating disorders and obesity.

PATHOPHYSIOLOGY

- Physical manifestations are primarily the result of caloric restriction and consequences of malnutrition, which can affect all organ symptoms. The degree of symptoms seen may be due in part to the duration and severity of caloric restriction.
- Associated changes may also be due to purging, including vomiting, laxative use, or diet pill use.
- Bradycardia and hypothermia may result from significantly decreased metabolic rate due to malnutrition and caloric restriction.
- Hormonal changes due to starvation include resumption of prepubertal gonadotropin secretion.

ETIOLOGY

Evidence for specific etiology is not definitive; most likely multifactorial, including genetic risk factors, environmental triggers, and individual and family life experiences

COMMONLY ASSOCIATED CONDITIONS

- Amenorrhea
- Osteopenia/osteoporosis
- Female athlete triad (disordered eating, amenorrhea, osteoporosis)
- Depression
- Anxiety disorders including obsessive-compulsive disorder
- Substance abuse

DIAGNOSIS

Diagnosis is made using *DSM-5* criteria. However, many patients exhibit marked symptoms but do not meet the full criteria for AN; for example, despite drastic weight loss, the patient's weight remains in the normal range. These patients may be diagnosed with other specified feeding or eating disorder, also called subclinical or atypical anorexia nervosa. These patients likely still require close monitoring and potential intervention.

HISTORY

- Weight history: highest and lowest weight in last year; patient's "target weight" they were attempting to reach with restriction. Ask, "How often do you weigh yourself? What is the most you have weighed in past year? The least? What do you think of as your own ideal weight?"
- Psychological assessment: interviews with patient and parents, detailed history of body image concerns, obsession with weight and/or shape, developmental and family history, social and academic history, cognitive and personality traits, and premorbid and current level of functioning. Critical in establishing a diagnosis and developing a treatment plan.
- Other psychological symptoms: Assess mood and anxiety symptoms, suicidal ideation, substance use, and other risky or self-injurious behaviors.
- Diet and nutrition history: 24-hour dietary recall, history of binge eating, purging (including use of diuretics, laxatives, diet pills, or emetics), food restrictions, or calorie counting
- Exercise history: type, how much and intensity.
- Menstrual history: last menstrual period (LMP), weight at LMP, history of skipped periods

PHYSICAL EXAM

- Vital signs, specifically orthostatic heart rates (HR) and blood pressures (to evaluate for vital sign instability that may be an indicator of severity and need for inpatient management), and temperature
- Weight, height, and BMI plotted in comparison to historical growth curve.
- HEENT: evaluate for signs of dehydration, dental exam for erosion due to purging
- CV: cardiac status
- GI: evaluate for pain, tenderness, organomegaly
- Derm: lanugo, Russell sign (callousing of the finger from self-induced purging), evidence of self-injurious behavior
- GU: Tanner staging for pubertal development
- Neurologic: complete exam including funduscopic exam to rule out brain tumor

DIAGNOSTIC TESTS & INTERPRETATION

Lab

- Serum electrolytes, BUN/creatinine, glucose: typically normal if patient is not purging
- Serum calcium, magnesium, phosphorous: May all be low. If hospitalized, follow phosphorous daily to assess for refeeding syndrome.
- TSH; if indicated, free T_4, T_3: to rule out thyroid disease. If abnormal, may be due solely to starvation.
- CBC with differential: Anemia may be present due to iron deficiency or chronic disease but may be falsely normal if patient is dehydrated; low WBC count is seen with malnutrition.
- ESR: generally low due to malnutrition
- AST, ALT: occasionally abnormal due to fatty liver
- β-hCG): Rule out pregnancy if amenorrheic.
- Urinalysis: Evaluate specific gravity to assess for dehydration or may have dilute urine if patients water load to falsely increase their weight.
- Consider EKG: may demonstrate bradycardia, prolonged QTc
- Patients amenorrheic for >6 months:
  - Dual-energy x-ray absorptiometry (DEXA) scan: Evaluate bone density, risk of compression fracture, and bone loss. May be helpful motivator for treatment as may not be reversible.
  - Serum LH, FSH, prolactin, if persistent amenorrhea with normal weight: LH and FSH will generally be low.

DIFFERENTIAL DIAGNOSIS

- Medical conditions such as
  - Pregnancy
  - Oncologic: brain tumor, other cancers
  - GI: inflammatory bowel disease (including Crohn and ulcerative colitis), celiac disease
  - Endocrinologic: diabetes mellitus, thyroid disease, hypopituitarism, Addison disease
  - HIV or other chronic infections
- Psychiatric or psychological conditions such as
  - Psychiatric: depression, obsessive-compulsive disorder, substance abuse, psychotic symptoms
  - *DSM-5* avoidant/restrictive food intake disorder: food aversions/hypersensitivity, extreme picky eating, decreased intake due to fears of swallowing/choking

TREATMENT

- Multidisciplinary team approach is considered the state of the art standard of care and includes medical monitoring, nutritional counseling, and psychological treatments.
- Family-based treatment (FBT) is the only evidence-based psychological treatment for pediatric and adolescent AN. Parents/caregivers are viewed as an integral part of the treatment team.
- Initially, all meals and snacks are prepared by and supervised by the parents. Gradually, age appropriate autonomy regarding eating is returned to the child/adolescent as physical and psychological progress is made.

MEDICATION

- Medications are not the primary mechanism for treating AN but may be helpful in the treatment of co-occurring illnesses such as depression and anxiety.
- Medications to treat constipation may be necessary but should be used with caution.
- Supplements such as multivitamin, calcium, and vitamin D should be considered.
- Refeeding is the treatment of choice for amenorrhea rather than starting oral contraceptive pills (OCPs).

ISSUES FOR REFERRAL

Depending on severity and availability, refer to an adolescent medicine specialist or other eating disorder specialist.

INPATIENT CONSIDERATIONS

Admission Criteria

- Criteria for inpatient hospitalization:
  - Severe malnutrition with weight <75% ideal body weight or weight loss despite treatment
  - Bradycardia including daytime HR <50 bpm
  - Nighttime HR <45 bpm
  - Systolic blood pressure <90 mm Hg
  - Orthostatic hypotension or significant orthostatic changes in pulse
  - Severe hypothermia (temperature <96°F)
  - Arrhythmia
  - Acute food refusal
  - Severe electrolyte abnormalities.
- Suicidality may require psychiatric hospitalization.

Discharge Criteria

Once a patient is medically stable and no longer meets admission criteria, insurance companies may limit lengths of hospital stays. Most patients are treated solely as outpatients.

ONGOING CARE

- Ongoing medical monitoring with emphasis placed on overall vital signs and not on weight alone
- Goals are set for nutritional rehabilitation. Meal plans are established and reassessed at each subsequent visit.
- Referral to a family therapist with this expertise is advised. Individual psychotherapy may be useful for many patients also particularly given the anxiety that is typically generated by the refeeding process.
- Group psychotherapy can be a useful adjunct particularly for some older adolescent patients.
- More intensive services include intensive outpatient, day, or residential treatment.
- Other adjunctive therapies include mindfulness training, expressive arts, etc.

PROGNOSIS

- Most adolescent patients recover fully but generally not without a long course of treatment. Overall, children and adolescents have better outcomes than adults.
- Better outcomes are associated with shorter duration of symptoms, earlier diagnosis, absence of purging behaviors, and less severity of psychiatric comorbidity. However, outcome findings vary depending on factors such as length of follow-up and definitions of recovery.
- Mortality rates for adolescents with AN are reported to be 1.8%, primarily from effects of starvation or from suicide.

COMPLICATIONS

- Majority of complications may be reversed with improved nutrition.
- Refeeding syndrome: As the patient is refed, the body may shift from a catabolic state to an anabolic state, resulting in a release of insulin which may drive phosphorous and potassium intercellularly and drop extracellular levels resulting in delirium, coma, arrhythmias, cardiac failure, and death.
- CV: arrhythmias, pericardial effusions
- GI: delayed gastric emptying, slowed intestinal motility and constipation, pancreatitis; elevated cholesterol
- Endocrine: amenorrhea, osteoporosis, sick euthyroid syndrome, growth delay
- Complications related to purging include Mallory-Weiss tears, esophagitis, electrolyte and fluid imbalances (particularly hypokalemia)
- Neuropsychological: anxiety, poor concentration, depressed mood, cognitive impairment, cortical atrophy

ADDITIONAL READING

- Academy for Eating Disorders. Eating disorders. AED Report 2012. 2nd ed. www.aedweb.org. Accessed March 11, 2015.
- American Psychiatric Association. Guideline Watch (August 2012): Practice Guideline for the *Treatment of Patients with Eating Disorders*. 3rd ed. http://psychiatryonline.org. Accessed March 11, 2015.
- Rosen DS; American Academy of Pediatrics Committee on Adolescence. Identification and management of eating disorders in children and adolescents. *Pediatrics*. 2010;126(6):1240–1253.
- Silber T. Anorexia nervosa in children and adolescents: diagnosis, treatment and the role of the pediatrician. *Minerva Pediatrica*. 2013;65(1):1–17.
- Trace E, Baker JH, Peñas-Lledó E, et al. Genetics of eating disorders. *Annu Rev Clin*. 2013;9:589–620.

SEE ALSO

- National Eating Disorders Association (www.nationaleatingdisorders.org)
- Maudsleyparents.org; FEASTED.org
- Bulimia chapter

CODES

ICD10

- F50.00 Anorexia nervosa, unspecified
- F50.01 Anorexia nervosa, restricting type
- F50.02 Anorexia nervosa, binge eating/purging type

FAQ

- Q: If the patient presents with severe low mood, why not start them on an antidepressant right away?
- A: Many of their depressive symptoms may be secondary to the effects of their malnourished state. It's best to begin nutritional rehabilitation and reassess as intake improves.
- Q: Can patients have AN if they do not report feeling fat or intentionally dieting?
- A: Yes. Denial is very often associated with AN. Rely on behavioral signs and parental report.
- Q: Can AN be diagnosed in preadolescents?
- A: Yes. The age of onset of AN has continued to decrease. If they present with weight preoccupation, pursuit of thinness, and other diagnostic criteria, their diagnosis is AN.

ANTHRAX

Andrew P. Steenhoff

BASICS

DESCRIPTION

Bacillus anthracis is a spore-forming, gram-positive rod that can cause acute infection (anthrax) in humans and animals.

EPIDEMIOLOGY

- Anthrax is primarily zoonotic. Most naturally acquired anthrax infections are cutaneous (95%). Inhalational (5%) and GI (<1%) forms are particularly rare.
- Prior to October 2001, only 18 cases of inhalational anthrax were reported in the United States during the 20th century.
- No human-to-human spread of inhalational anthrax has been reported.
- Rare cases of human-to-human transmission of cutaneous anthrax have been reported after direct contact with infected skin lesions.
- Anthrax has been used as an agent of bioterrorism.

GENERAL PREVENTION

- Antibiotics are effective against germinating *B. anthracis* but not against the spores. Therefore, if prophylactic antibiotics are stopped prematurely, remaining spores can cause disease when they germinate. This phenomenon of delayed-onset disease does not occur with cutaneous or GI exposures.
- Where the threat of transmission of *B. anthracis* spores is deemed credible, decontamination of skin and potential fomites (e.g., clothing) may be considered to reduce the risk for cutaneous and GI forms of the disease.
- Anthrax vaccine absorbed (AVA) is the only licensed human anthrax vaccine in the United States. Primary vaccination consists of subcutaneous injections at 0, 2, and 4 weeks and 3 booster vaccinations at 6, 12, and 18 months. Annual booster injections are required to maintain immunity. The most common adverse event is injection-site discomfort (e.g., edema, pain, local hypersensitivity).
- Infection control
  - Immediately notify the hospital epidemiologist, infection control department, or local health department of suspected cases.
  - No data suggest that patient-to-patient transmission of inhalational anthrax occurs. Standard barrier isolation precautions are recommended for all hospitalized patients with all forms of anthrax infection. High-efficiency particulate air-filter masks or other measures for airborne precautions are not indicated.
  - There is no need to immunize or provide prophylaxis to patient contacts unless they, like the patient, were exposed to the aerosol.
  - If anthrax is used as a bioweapon, spores may be detected on environmental surfaces. Inhalational anthrax is unlikely to be caused by secondary aerosolization of these spores.

ALERT

Pulmonary disease caused by anthrax is a hemorrhagic mediastinitis with pleural effusions and *not* a bronchopneumonia.

PATHOPHYSIOLOGY

- After inhalation, wound inoculation, or ingestion, *B. anthracis* spores infect macrophages, germinate, and proliferate.
  - Proliferation occurs at the site of infection and in regional lymph nodes.
  - Replicating bacteria release toxins, leading to edema, hemorrhage, and necrosis.
- Incubation period depends on the route of transmission.
  - Inhalational anthrax: Infection requires inhalation of >8,000 spores; incubation period is 2–60 days.
  - Cutaneous anthrax: Spores enter a cut or abrasion in the skin; incubation period is 1–12 days.
  - GI anthrax: Spores are ingested in undercooked, infected meat; incubation period is 1–7 days; infection occurs in the upper (oropharyngeal lesions) or lower (intestinal lesions) GI tract.
- Hematogenous spread of the bacteria causes infection at other sites, including the CNS, liver, spleen, and kidney.

COMMONLY ASSOCIATED CONDITIONS

If anthrax is intentionally released, physicians must be alert for diseases caused by other potential biologic warfare agents (e.g., plague, tularemia, Q fever, smallpox, and botulism).

DIAGNOSIS

HISTORY

- Inhalational anthrax
  - Clinical presentation is a 2-stage illness.
  - Initial symptoms are nonspecific and last 1–3 days. They include low-grade fever, dry cough, headache, vomiting, chills, weakness, abdominal pain, and substernal discomfort. This stage may be followed by a brief period of apparent recovery.
  - 2nd-stage symptoms develop abruptly 2–5 days later: fever, hemoptysis, dyspnea, chest pain, and profuse diaphoresis. Death may occur within 1–2 days.
- Cutaneous anthrax
  - Painless lesions develop on affected areas soon after exposure.
  - Systemic symptoms of fever, malaise, and headache may occur.
- GI anthrax
  - Oropharyngeal form causes sore throat, dysphagia, and fever.
  - Intestinal form also causes nausea, vomiting, anorexia, severe abdominal pain, and bloody diarrhea.

PHYSICAL EXAM

- Clinical presentation of anthrax in children is varied; rapid diagnosis and effective treatment require recognition of the broad spectrum of clinical presentations.
- Inhalational anthrax
  - Tachypnea, hypoxia, cyanosis
  - Stridor, rales, signs of pleural effusion
  - Hemoptysis, hematemesis, melena
- Cutaneous anthrax
  - Initial painless, pruritic macule or papule enlarges into a 1–3-cm round ulcer by the second day.
  - 1–3-mm vesicles with clear or serosanguineous fluid surround the ulcer.
  - A painless, depressed, black eschar follows, often with extensive local edema.
  - Over 1–2 weeks, the eschar dries, loosens, and falls off, occasionally with scarring.
  - Painful, regional lymphadenopathy may occur.
- GI anthrax
  - Unilateral oral or esophageal ulcers, cervical lymphadenopathy
  - Cecal or terminal ileal ulcers (Intestinal anthrax progresses to massive ascites and acute abdomen.)
- Disseminated anthrax (potential complication of any of the above forms of anthrax):
  - Sepsis syndrome: tachycardia, hypotension, septic shock
  - Meningitis: meningismus, delirium, obtundation

DIAGNOSTIC TESTS & INTERPRETATION

Lab

- Gram stain smear and culture from vesicular fluid
  - Diagnose cutaneous anthrax
  - Gram stain reveals large, gram-positive, boxcar-shaped bacilli.
  - Capsule is visible on polychrome methylene blue stain.
  - *B. anthracis* grows readily on blood agar.
- Anthraxin skin test
  - Measures anthrax cell-mediated immunity
  - It is positive in 80% of patients within 72 hours of infection and in >95% of cases within 3 weeks.
  - The test was positive in 72% of patients >16 years after recovery.
- Serologic enzyme-linked immunosorbent assay (ELISA):
  - Measures antibodies to the lethal and edema toxins of *B. anthracis*
  - Positive if a single acute-phase titer is >1:32 or if there is a 4-fold or greater rise between acute and convalescent titers collected 4 weeks apart
- Polymerase chain reaction, immunohistochemical staining
- Nasopharyngeal swab or induced respiratory secretion culture
  - Used for epidemiologic investigation
  - The sensitivity, specificity, and predictive value of nasal swab testing are unknown; therefore, this test should not be used to guide the use of postexposure prophylactic antibiotics.

- Blood culture: Patients with cutaneous anthrax may have bacteremia with *B. anthracis* even without significant signs of systemic disease.
- CBC
- Serum electrolytes, glucose, and calcium
  – Hypokalemia, acidosis, hypoglycemia, and hypocalcemia occurred during experimental anthrax infection in animals.
  – Hemorrhagic meningitis

Imaging

Chest x-ray (or chest CT scan)

- Inhalational anthrax causes a hemorrhagic mediastinitis.
- May show a widened mediastinum and pleural effusions
- No infiltrates are present.

DIFFERENTIAL DIAGNOSIS

- The prodromal illness of inhalational anthrax may resemble a lower respiratory tract infection, although upper respiratory infection symptoms are characteristically absent.
- Patients with inhalational anthrax may have a widened mediastinum on chest radiograph which may resemble an aortic aneurysm or bacterial mediastinitis.
- Necrotic skin lesions may resemble plague, tularemia, ecthyma gangrenosum, and brown recluse spider bite.
- GI anthrax may be confused with other infectious enteritides (e.g., *Shigella*, *Salmonella*, *Yersinia*, *Campylobacter*, enterohemorrhagic *Escherichia coli*, *Clostridium difficile*, colitis), intussusception, Meckel diverticulum, and inflammatory bowel disease.

TREATMENT

MEDICATION

- Postexposure prophylaxis
  – Ciprofloxacin 15 mg/kg (up to 500 mg) *or* doxycycline 2.2 mg/kg (up to 100 mg) or levofloxacin 8 mg/kg (up to 250 mg) PO b.i.d. for 60 days.
  – Pediatric: Use ciprofloxacin for initial prophylaxis. Switch to amoxicillin or penicillin if susceptibility testing permits.
- Treatment
  – For all forms of anthrax, begin with IV therapy and switch to oral therapy when clinically appropriate. Treat for 60 days (IV and PO combined).
  – Inhalational or GI anthrax: ciprofloxacin 15 mg/kg (up to 400 mg) *or* doxycycline 2.2 mg/kg (up to 100 mg) IV q12h *plus* clindamycin or rifampin
  – Cutaneous anthrax: ciprofloxacin or doxycycline IV. (Pediatric: Begin therapy with ciprofloxacin [plus clindamycin or rifampin for inhalational/GI anthrax] and convert to penicillin G IV if susceptibility testing permits and when clinical improvement is documented.)

GENERAL MEASURES

Direct physical contact with a substance alleged to be anthrax:

- Wash exposed skin and articles of clothing with soap and water.
- Administer postexposure prophylaxis until the substance is proved not to be anthrax.
- Contact the public health department or the Centers for Disease Control and Prevention (CDC).
- For severe anthrax, anthrax-specific hyperimmune globulin 5% should be considered in consultation with CDC.

ONGOING CARE

PROGNOSIS

- Inhalational anthrax
  – Case fatality rates were previously estimated to be >85% after symptoms develop. However, early use of appropriate antibiotic therapy appears to improve survival.
  – Survival rate is higher if symptoms develop >30 days after exposure.
- Cutaneous anthrax
  – Case fatality rate is 20% without antibiotic treatment and <1% with antibiotic treatment.
- GI anthrax: Case fatality rate is 25–60%.

COMPLICATIONS

- Antibiotic therapy of cutaneous anthrax limits the likelihood of developing systemic symptoms but does not change the course of the eschar formation.
- Systemic dissemination of inhalational, cutaneous, or GI anthrax may lead to sepsis, meningitis, and death.

ADDITIONAL READING

- Akbayram S, Dogan M, Akgun C, et al. Clinical findings in children with cutaneous anthrax in Eastern Turkey. *Pediatr Dermatol*. 2010;27(6):600–606.
- Alexander JJ, Colangelo PM, Cooper CK, et al. Amoxicillin for postexposure inhalational anthrax in pediatrics: rationale for dosing recommendations. *Pediatr Infect Dis J*. 2008;27(11):955–957.
- Bravata DM, Holty JE, Wang E, et al. Inhalational, gastrointestinal, and cutaneous anthrax in children: a systematic review of cases: 1900 to 2005. *Arch Pediatr Adolesc Med*. 2007;161(9):896–905.
- Centers for Disease Control and Prevention. Use of anthrax vaccine in the United States: recommendations of the Advisory Committee on Immunization Practices (ACIP). *MMWR* 2000;49(RR-15):1–20. *MMWR*. 2001;50(42):909–919. Erratum in: *MMWR*. 2001;50(43):962.
- Hendricks KA, Wright ME, Shadomy SV, et al. Centers for Disease Control and Prevention expert panel meetings on prevention and treatment of anthrax in adults. *Emerg Infect Dis*. 2014;20(2).
- Kyriacou DN, Adamski A, Khardori N. Anthrax: from antiquity and obscurity to a front-runner in bioterrorism. *Infect Dis Clin North Am*. 2006;20(2):227–251.
- Li F, Nandy P, Chien S, et al. Pharmacometrics-based dose selection of levofloxacin as a treatment for postexposure inhalational anthrax in children. *Antimicrob Agents Chemother*. 2010;54(1):375–379.
- Scorpio A, Blank TE, Day WA, et al. Anthrax vaccines: Pasteur to the present. *Cell Mol Life Sci*. 2006;63:2237–2248.
- Stocker JT. Clinical and pathological differential diagnosis of selected potential bioterrorism agents of interest to pediatric health care providers. *Clin Lab Med*. 2006;26(2):329–344.

CODES

ICD10

- A22.9 Anthrax, unspecified
- A22.0 Cutaneous anthrax
- A22.1 Pulmonary anthrax

FAQ

- Q: Does the government have a plan in place if there were mass exposure to anthrax?
- A: Yes. Under emergency plans, the federal government would ship appropriate antibiotics from its stockpile to wherever they are needed.
- Q: Should individuals ask their physicians to write a prescription for ciprofloxacin (or other antibiotic) so they have prophylaxis available?
- A: No. Ciprofloxacin and other antibiotics should not be prescribed unless there is a clearly indicated need. In addition, indiscriminate prescribing and widespread use of ciprofloxacin could hasten the development of drug-resistant organisms.
- Q: Can a person get screened or tested for anthrax?
- A: No screening test is available to determine whether anthrax exposure has occurred. The only way exposure can be determined is through a public health investigation.
- Q: What are the clues to differentiate pulmonary or inhalational anthrax from RSV in children?
- A: Children with pulmonary anthrax display a high WBC count with left shift compared to the relatively normal WBC of those with RSV. Blood O_2 levels may be severely depressed in inhalational anthrax.

APLASTIC ANEMIA

Craig M. Forester • James N. Huang

BASICS

DESCRIPTION

Aplastic anemia represents a heterogenous group of disorders characterized by peripheral pancytopenia and bone marrow hypocellularity.

EPIDEMIOLOGY

Incidence

- Estimated incidence of 2:1,000,000 per year in Western Hemisphere and Europe with increased incidence of 5–7:1,000,000 per year in Far East and those of Asian descent
- In the pediatric population, most commonly presents between ages 15 and 25 years

RISK FACTORS

Genetics

Patients with a number of inherited bone marrow failure syndromes are at increased risk of developing aplastic anemia, but there is no known genetic mutation associated with acquired aplastic anemia.

GENERAL PREVENTION

There are no preventive measures for acquired aplastic anemia.

PATHOPHYSIOLOGY

- Most instances of acquired aplastic anemia are thought to occur through a T-cell dependent autoimmune process leading to apoptosis of hematopoietic stem or progenitor cells.
- Additionally, exposure to certain toxins, chemicals, medications (classically chloramphenicol), and high doses of radiation can also lead to marrow aplasia.

ETIOLOGY

- Acquired
  - Idiopathic (70% of cases)
  - Toxin: exposure to arsenic, benzene, radiation, organophosphates, organochlorines
  - Drugs: chloramphenicol, numerous chemotherapeutic agents
  - Radiation
  - Paroxysmal nocturnal hemoglobinuria (PNH)
  - Seronegative hepatitis (non-A, non-B, and non-C)
  - HIV-1, Epstein-Barr virus (EBV), human herpes virus-6, cytomegalovirus (CMV)
  - Malnutrition
  - Pregnancy

COMMONLY ASSOCIATED CONDITIONS

- Congenital or inherited bone marrow failure syndromes
  - Fanconi anemia, Shwachman-Diamond syndrome, Diamond-Blackfan anemia, dyskeratosis congenita, congenital amegakaryocytic thrombocytopenia, Pearson syndrome
- Acquired
  - Differentiating aplastic anemia from refractory cytopenia of childhood (RCC), defined by thrombocytopenia/neutropenia with impaired maturation of erythroid lineage and increased proerythroblasts in bone marrow, is crucial.
  - Differentiating RCC from aplastic anemia can be difficult but important as RCC should be considered a form of myelodysplastic syndrome (MDS) and evaluated for hematopoietic stem cell transplantation (HSCT).

DIAGNOSIS

HISTORY

- Detailed history including birth history, growth trajectory, antecedent illnesses, infections, environmental exposures
- Comprehensive review of systems with emphasis on neurologic (including developmental delay and learning disabilities), dermatologic, cardiac, pulmonary, endocrine (hypogonadism, growth delay), and hematologic systems
- Family history of cancer predisposition, excessive toxicity to chemotherapy, unexplained fetal loss, anemia/cytopenias, or congenital anomalies

PHYSICAL EXAM

- Thorough physical exam combined with plotting of growth curves
- Head: evaluate for eye, epicanthal folds, jaw, palate abnormalities, oral mucosal lesions/bleeding, thrush
- Cardiopulmonary: auscultation for cardiac anomalies, dyspnea, diminished aeration, asymmetry
- GI: hepatosplenomegaly, palpation for masses
- GU: renal/urinary/ureter abnormalities, gonadal abnormalities, or undescended testes
- Skeletal: dysmorphisms, forearms, thumbs, vertebral anomalies, osteopenia
- Skin: pigmentation changes, eczematous rash, nail abnormalities, bruising, petechiae, pallor
- Lymphadenopathy

DIAGNOSTIC TESTS & INTERPRETATION

Lab

To confirm the diagnosis:

- Diagnosis requires exclusion of other disease processes associated with pancytopenia (see "Etiology" and "Differential Diagnosis" sections) as well as the following:
  - Empty or hypoplastic bone marrow
  - 2 out of 3 of the following: absolute neutrophil count (ANC) $<1,500 \times 10^6$/L, platelets $<50,000 \times 10^6$/L, hemoglobin (Hgb) <10 g/dL
- Severe aplastic anemia (sAA)
  - Bone marrow cellularity <25%
  - 2 out of 3 of the following: ANC $<500 \times 10^6$/L, platelets $<20,000 \times 10^6$/L, absolute reticulocyte count $<20 \times 10^9$/L
- Very severe aplastic anemia: the criteria are the same as for sAA, except for ANC $<200 \times 10^6$/L.

To exclude other causes:

- Complete blood count, + reticulocyte count
- Peripheral blood smear
- Hgb F %
- Liver function tests, lactate dehydrogenase (LDH), uric acid
- Direct and indirect Coombs assay
- Baseline serum iron, ferritin, total iron-binding capacity (TIBC)
- Flow cytometry for glycosylphosphatidylinositol (GPI)-anchored proteins CD55/CD59
- Vitamin B_{12}, folate, copper levels
- Viral studies: hepatitis A, B, and C; EBV, CMV, HIV, human herpesvirus 6 (HHV-6), varicella-zoster virus (VZV), parvovirus
- Antinuclear antibody (ANA), anti-double stranded DNA (dsDNA)
- Acid-fast bacillus (AFB) staining of bone marrow aspirate
- Human leukocyte antigen (HLA) typing of patient and family members
- Ruling out inherited bone marrow failure syndromes:
  - Chromosomal breakage (mitomycin C or diepoxybutane): Fanconi anemia
  - Telomere length: dyskeratosis congenita
  - Exocrine pancreatic testing: serum trypsinogen and pancreatic isoamylase: Shwachman-Diamond syndrome
  - Erythrocyte adenosine deaminase: Diamond-Blackfan anemia
  - c-MPL mutation: congenital amegakaryocytic thrombocytopenia

Imaging

- Chest x-ray
- Abdominal ultrasound (US)
- Echocardiogram

Diagnostic Procedures/Other

- Bone marrow aspirate and biopsy
- Cytogenetics of bone marrow with fluorescence in situ hybridization (FISH) for monosomy 5, 7, 8

Pathologic Findings

Bone marrow fragments are hypocellular with prominent fat spaces and reduced erythropoiesis, megakaryocytes, and granulocytes. Lymphocytes, macrophages, plasma cells, or mast cells may be prominent. Appearance of dysplasia in megakaryocyte or granulocytic lineage, blasts, hypercellularity, or increased reticulin staining are not consistent with aplastic anemia.

DIFFERENTIAL DIAGNOSIS

- Myelosuppression secondary to ongoing infection (viral, tuberculosis)
- MDS (including RCC)
- Hematologic malignancy
- Nutritional deficiency: vitamin, mineral, or starvation/anorexia
- Autoimmune disease: systemic lupus erythematosus (SLE), thyroid disease, rheumatoid arthritis
- PNH
- Metastatic disease
- Hemophagocytic histiocytosis

TREATMENT

Treatment for aplastic anemia that does not meet the severe or very severe criteria is individualized and controversial as some patients do spontaneously improve. However, patients with severe or very severe aplastic anemia should be promptly treated because of their high risk of infection.

MEDICATION

First Line

In all patients with sAA who are younger than the age of 40 years and without significant comorbidities, the treatment of choice is HSCT with a matched sibling donor (MSD). Superior and durable outcomes for MSD transplants conditioned with cyclophosphamide/antithymocyte globulin (ATG) as 1st-line therapy stresses importance of timely workup and HLA typing.

Second Line

For patients without an MSD or with significant comorbidities:

- Immunosuppressive therapy (IST) with combination horse ATG and cyclosporine (ATG/CsA) followed by prolonged taper of cyclosporine.
- If patients do not show clinical improvement within 3–6 months, consider an alternative donor HSCT such as with a matched unrelated donor (MUD) HSCT, if available, or repeat trial of IST.

Supportive Therapy:

Patients should be transfused when symptomatic with leukocyte-reduced, irradiated PRBCs and platelets. Transfusions are weighed against the risk of alloimmunization and graft rejection with allogeneic bone marrow transplant (BMT), but most institutions will transfuse to keep Hgb >7–8 g/dL and platelets above $10{,}000/mm^3$. Transfusions should be with CMV-negative blood (if patient is CMV seronegative) if patient is likely to undergo transplant.

ISSUES FOR REFERRAL

Pediatric hematology/oncology/BMT: As a rare disorder, patients are typically managed by centers with hematologic experience and transplant capabilities.

ADDITIONAL THERAPIES

- Use of *Pneumocystis carinii* (*jiroveci*) pneumonia (PCP) prophylaxis prior to BMT is institution-dependent but some recommend use of pentamidine (with atovaquone or dapsone as second line), avoiding sulfamethoxazole/trimethoprim due to its myelosuppressive properties.
- Antifungal prophylaxis is also used by many institutions.
- Granulocyte colony-stimulating factor (G-CSF) support may be used in setting of acute infection but has not been shown to improve overall survival or remission rates.
- Supportive care, androgens, cyclosporine, or growth factors alone are not definitive therapies. Corticosteroids alone are also not proven to be effective and lead to increased susceptibility to fungal infections.

INPATIENT CONSIDERATIONS

Initial Stabilization

- Patients should be transfused slowly initially with PRBC 5 cc/kg over 4 hours to avoid pulmonary overcirculation.
- Platelet transfusions for symptomatic bleeding
- Cultures of blood and urine should be obtained with all fevers, and empiric broad-spectrum antibiotics coverage should be started while awaiting culture results.

Admission Criteria

Symptomatic anemia, fever, severe thrombocytopenia, or any evidence of clinical bleeding must be admitted for supportive care and monitoring.

IV Fluids

Unless the patient has had a recent history of inadequate intake or losses, IV fluids are not usually necessary at the outset. Bear in mind that the patient will likely be receiving additional volume due to transfusions.

Nursing

Patients should be roomed in isolation if possible.

ONGOING CARE

FOLLOW-UP RECOMMENDATIONS

Regardless of whether IST or BMT is chosen for treatment modality, follow-up should be lifelong given risk of recurrence of aplastic anemia or transformation to MDS or malignancy. Long-term retrospective studies have demonstrated rates of relapse of up to 38%, with incidence of clonal transformation in 10–25% of patients who undergo IST.

Patient Monitoring

Those who undergo HSCT are expected to have hematopoietic reconstitution as they engraft. Hematologic recovery in those who undergo IST may take several months: 90% of patients who respond will do so by 3 months, but some patients may take up to 6 months from ATG to recover marrow function.

Parameters of Recovery

- Improve overall hematopoiesis to reduce transfusion dependency and no longer fulfill criteria for sAA by 6 months. Neutrophil recovery may be the first cytopenia to improve.
- Relapse or clonal evolution commonly occurs at 2–4 years from time of IST. Some centers recommend monitoring bone marrow aspirates with biopsy at 6-month intervals for 1st year after IST, then annually.

PATIENT EDUCATION

- NIH site: http://www.nhlbi.nih.gov/health/health-topics/topics/aplastic/
- Aplastic Anemia & MDS International Foundation: http://www.aamds.org/about/aplastic-anemia

DIET

Recommend low bacterial content diet.

PROGNOSIS

- Aplastic anemia has a high rate of mortality if left untreated. Death is predominantly from infection and hemorrhage. If patients are treated with antibiotics and transfusions alone, mortality is 80% in 2 years.
- First line
  - MSD: HSCT with MSD from bone marrow source has a predicted 6-year outcome of 80–91% in children younger than 20 years of age.
- Second line
  - IST: Response rate of IST in children is 75%.
- Relapse/salvage: aplastic anemia refractory to IST at 6 months should be considered for salvage therapy: MUD-HSCT for younger patients; repeat IST for older patients and those with significant comorbidities.
- MUD: Recent trials have shown improved survival of >60% and as high as 94% in children who have undergone MUD-HSCT for sAA.
- Repeat IST: Patients refractory to the initial course of IST had a response rate of 30–40% at 6 months to ATG/CsA.

COMPLICATIONS

- Infection
- Hemorrhage
- Iron overload requiring phlebotomy or chelation therapy
- Allosensitization to transfusion products

ADDITIONAL READING

- Bacigalupo A, Passweg J. Diagnosis and treatment of acquired aplastic anemia. *Hematol Oncol Clin North Am*. 2009;23(2):159–170.
- Marsh JC, Ball SE, Cavenagh J, et al. Guidelines for the diagnosis and management of aplastic anemia. *Br J Haematol*. 2009;147(1):43–70.
- Niemeyer CM, Baumann I. Classification of childhood aplastic anemia and myelodysplastic syndrome. *Hematology Am Soc Hematol Educ Program*. 2011;2011:84–89.
- Scheinberg P, Nunez O, Weinstein B, et al. Horse versus rabbit antithymocyte globulin in acquired aplastic anemia. *N Engl J Med*. 2011;365(5):430–438.
- Scheinberg P, Young NS. How I treat acquired aplastic anemia. *Blood*. 2012;120(6):1185–1196.
- Shimamura A. Clinical approach to marrow failure. *Hematology Am Soc Hematol Educ Program*. 2009;1:329–337.
- Young NS, Scheinberg P, Calado RT. Aplastic anemia. *Curr Opin Hematol*. 2008;15:162–168.

CODES

ICD10

- D61.9 Aplastic anemia, unspecified
- D61.89 Oth aplastic anemias and other bone marrow failure syndromes
- D61.3 Idiopathic aplastic anemia

FAQ

- Q: When starting IST, should I choose horse ATG or rabbit ATG as part of the ATG/cyclosporine/prednisone regimen?
- A: A head to head comparison of horse ATG (hATG) versus rabbit ATG (rATG) in immunosuppressive regimens showed inferiority of rATG in 1st-time treatment for sAA (Scheinberg, NEJM 2011).
- Q: When should patient and family members be HLA typed when considering aplastic anemia?
- A: HLA typing should be performed on patient and family members once peripheral pancytopenia and bone marrow hypocellularity is confirmed.
- Q: What are common side effects of the IST regimen?
- A: ATG may cause hypersensitivity reactions, whereas cyclosporine A may cause hypertension, electrolyte abnormalities, nephropathy, and hirsutism.

APPARENT LIFE-THREATENING EVENT

Craig DeWolfe

BASICS

DESCRIPTION

- Apparent life-threatening event (ALTE) is an episode that is frightening to the observer and is characterized by some combination of the following:
  - Apnea: central or occasionally obstructive
  - Color change: usually cyanotic or pallid but occasionally erythematous or plethoric
  - Marked change in muscle tone: usually limp
  - Choking or gagging
- ALTE describes a presentation rather than a diagnosis and should therefore trigger a pursuit of an etiology.

EPIDEMIOLOGY

- 43% of healthy term infants have at least one 20-second apneic episode over a 3-month period.
- 5.3% of parents recall seeing apnea.
- 0.2–0.9% of infants have an episode of apnea that results in an admission to the hospital.

RISK FACTORS

- Preterm infants born less than 34 weeks post–conceptual age have higher rates of apnea.
  - Differences resolve by 43 weeks post–conceptual age.
- Prematurity, multiple ALTEs, and suspected child maltreatment confer a greater risk for a future adverse event and/or serious underlying diagnosis.

PATHOPHYSIOLOGY

- No unifying pathophysiology because of the numerous potential presentations and underlying diagnoses
  - Central apnea: disrupted propagation of respiratory signals from the brainstem along the descending neuromuscular pathways. Examples include the following:
    - Head trauma
    - Congenital central hypoventilation syndrome
  - Obstructive apnea: neuromuscular respiratory effort disrupted by an occluded airway. Examples include the following:
    - Upper respiratory infection
    - Pierre Robin
  - Mixed apnea: combination of central and obstructive apnea. Examples include the following:
    - Laryngomalacia with a sedating ingestion
    - Prematurity with superimposed viral infection
  - Color change from decreased oxygenation or differential blood flow. Examples include the following:
    - Cyanotic heart disease
    - Acrocyanosis
  - Altered muscle tone from central or autonomic nervous system disruption. Examples include the following:
    - Seizure
    - Breath-holding spell
  - Choking or gagging: protective response to a stimulation of the airway

DIAGNOSIS

ALERT

ALTE is a symptom complex rather than a diagnosis. The practitioner should therefore attempt to identify an underlying diagnosis to explain the presentation.

HISTORY

A full, uninterrupted description of the event by a witness may answer or prompt the need to explore the following features:

- Presence of apnea
  - Type suggests different causes.
    - Obstructive symptoms
    - Central symptoms
  - Duration may suggest severity: <20-second central apnea is physiologic if not associated with other symptoms such as cyanosis.
- Presence of color change and distribution
  - Perioral and peripheral cyanosis are not suggestive of hypoxia unless accompanied by central cyanosis.
  - Blue/purple discoloration of face, lips, or core body indicates central cyanosis.
- Change in tone, rhythmic shaking, and/or eye deviation may suggest a seizure.
- Relationship to feeds and/or milk in the mouth may suggest aspiration.
- Fatigue or diaphoresis with feeds may suggest a cardiac condition.
- Coryza may suggest an upper or lower respiratory infection.
- Fever may suggest an infectious etiology.
- History of trauma may suggest an intracranial bleed.
- State of alertness prior to ALTE may suggest sleep apnea.
- Discrepancies among witnesses may suggest nonaccidental trauma.
- Type of resuscitation needed may provide a sense of severity or an opportunity for anticipatory guidance.
- Current condition of child and/or time required to reach baseline: may suggest an ongoing, evolving condition and/or postictal period
- Location of event and position of child (i.e., supine/prone)
- Medications dosed or taken by a breastfeeding mother
- Prematurity
- Prior history of ALTE
- Family history of ALTE, SIDS, or sudden unexpected death

PHYSICAL EXAM

- Ongoing abnormal symptoms may suggest an evolving and/or underlying condition and should be approached differently than if the patient had a normal exam.
  - Arousal
  - Vital signs
  - Signs of trauma
    - Irritability
    - Full fontanelle
    - Pupil reactivity, conjunctival/retinal hemorrhage
    - Bruising or bleeding
  - Persisting signs of disordered breathing
  - Heart rhythm/murmurs suggestive of an arrhythmia or cyanotic heart disease
  - Neurologic exam
- Consider observing a feeding.

ALERT

Recurrent ALTEs; historical discrepancies; a family history of ALTE, SIDS, or unexplained death; parents calling emergency services; unexplained facial bruising or bleeding; and the presence or irritability at the time of presentation would warrant a thorough assessment for possible child maltreatment.

DIAGNOSTIC TESTS & INTERPRETATION

- Routine testing is unlikely to be helpful in patients who are well-appearing and have no other findings suggestive of a particular diagnosis.
- In addition to discomfort, inconvenience, risk, and costs of various tests, an indiscriminate number of screening tests may affect the reliability of the results and initiate an inappropriate and unnecessary testing cascade.

Lab

- If indicated by the history and/or physical
  - Basic metabolic panel
  - Blood culture
  - Cerebral spinal fluid analysis +/− culture
  - Complete blood count
  - Lactate level
  - Newborn metabolic screen
  - Urine analysis +/− culture
  - Venous blood gas
  - Viral studies

Imaging

- If indicated by the history and/or physical
  - Airway imaging
  - Contrast study of the gastrointestinal tract
  - Chest x-ray
  - Head CT
  - Isotope-labeled milk scan

Additional Testing

- In one study, even though 89% of patients presenting with ALTE had radiographic evidence of GER, half had another diagnosis that was thought to be more consistent with the presentation.
- If indicated by the history and/or physical
  - Airway visualization
  - Dilated funduscopic examination
  - Electrocardiography
  - Electroencephalography
  - Four-extremity blood pressure
  - pH probe
  - Sleep study

DIFFERENTIAL DIAGNOSIS

Estimated frequency of the involved system given as a percentage

- Gastrointestinal: 34%
  - Colic
  - Dysphagia
  - Esophageal dysfunction
  - Gastroenteritis
  - GER
  - Surgical abdomen
- Neurologic: 17%
  - Apnea of prematurity
  - Brain tumor
  - Central hypoventilation syndrome (Ondine's curse)
  - Congenital malformation of the brainstem
  - Head injury (intraventricular hemorrhage, subarachnoid hemorrhage)
  - Hydrocephalus
  - Meningitis/encephalitis
  - Neuromuscular disorders
  - Seizure
  - Vasovagal reaction
- Respiratory: 11%
  - Aspiration pneumonia
  - Foreign body
  - Other lower or upper respiratory tract infection
  - Reactive airway disease
  - Respiratory syncytial virus
  - Pertussis
- Otolaryngologic: 4%
  - Laryngomalacia or tracheomalacia
  - Anatomic airway stenosis or obstruction
  - Obstructive sleep apnea
- Child maltreatment syndrome: 1–2%
  - Intentional suffocation
  - Munchausen syndrome by proxy
  - Shaken baby syndrome
  - Head injury
  - Ingestion
- Cardiovascular: 1%
  - Cardiac arrhythmia/prolonged QTc
  - Cardiomyopathy
  - Congenital heart disease
  - Myocarditis
- Metabolic/endocrine: 1%
  - Electrolyte disturbance
  - Hypoglycemia
  - Inborn error of metabolism
- Other infections: 2%
  - Sepsis
  - Urinary tract infections
- Other: 6%
  - Anemia
  - Breath-holding spell
  - Choking
  - Drug or toxin reaction
  - Hypothermia
  - Physiologic event (periodic breathing, acrocyanosis)
  - Unintentional smothering
- Idiopathic/apnea of infancy: 23%

TREATMENT

INPATIENT CONSIDERATIONS

- Hospital admission is not necessary if the patient is well-appearing and has a self-limited diagnosis to explain the presentation. Admission criteria would include the following:
  - Premature patients less than 45 weeks post–gestational age
  - Patients with clusters or multiple episodes of ALTE
  - Suspected child maltreatment
- If admitted, place on a cardiorespiratory monitor with pulse oximetry.
- Manage patients with persistent symptoms based on the underlying working diagnosis.

ONGOING CARE

- All patients should be offered the following anticipatory guidance:
  - Safe sleep practices and other SIDS prevention techniques
  - CPR overview

FOLLOW-UP RECOMMENDATIONS

Return to medical attention for recurrence.

PROGNOSIS

- Studies on morbidity and mortality are generally incomplete and often contradictory. Differences in reported prognoses from such studies may reflect differences in study design (e.g., patient inclusion criteria, definitions, and follow-up periods, etc.).
  - Studies report mortality between 0 and 6%.
  - Insufficient data to quantify risk of subsequent event or underlying diagnosis in the asymptomatic patient
  - No developmental repercussions among patients who are discharged without a serious underlying diagnosis and have no subsequent events

ADDITIONAL READING

- DeWolfe CC. Apparent life-threatening event: a review. *Pediatr Clin North Am*. 2005;52(4):1127–1146.
- National Institutes of Health Consensus Development Conference on infantile apnea and home monitoring, Sept 29 to Oct 1, 1986. *Pediatrics*. 1987;79(2): 292–299.
- Ramanathan R, Corwin MJ, Hunt CE, et al. Cardiorespiratory events recorded on home monitors: comparison of healthy infants with those at increased risk for SIDS. *JAMA*. 2001;285(17):2199–21207.
- Tieder JS, Altman RL, Bonkowsky JL, et al. Management of apparent life-threatening events in infants: a systematic review. *J Pediatr*. 2013;163(1):94–99.

CODES

ICD10

- R68.13 Apparent life threatening event in infant (ALTE)
- P28.4 Other apnea of newborn
- R23.0 Cyanosis

FAQ

- Q: What is the relationship between ALTE and SIDS?
- A: There is no established relationship between ALTE and SIDS. The use of the terms "near-miss SIDS" and "aborted crib death" are discouraged. 4–13% of patients diagnosed with SIDS had a preceding history of apnea, a percentage only slightly higher than healthy controls. The "back to sleep" campaign, which has dramatically decreased the SIDS rate, has had no effect on ALTE presentations.
- Q: What is the role of home monitoring in ALTE?
- A: Home monitors are not efficacious in preventing mortality among patients with ALTE. In fact, there is evidence that caregivers may have increased anxiety, depression, and hostility, whereas patients may have worse developmental consequences. The American Academy of Pediatrics suggests that home monitors may have a role in certain situations such as a known unstable airway, abnormal respiratory control, or symptomatic and technologically dependent chronic lung disease.
- Q: Why aren't there established guidelines with respect to the evaluation and management of patients presenting with ALTE?
- A: No study has compared diagnostic or treatment strategies among first presenters with a sample size large enough to detect rare events in a prospective fashion. Future study of ALTE would be enhanced by applying definitions that could distinguish patient populations.

APPENDICITIS

Nora M. Fullington • Michael P. Hirsh

BASICS

DESCRIPTION

Acute inflammation or infection of the vermiform appendix

EPIDEMIOLOGY

- Most common surgical emergency of childhood
- Affects 5 of 100,000 persons in the United States
- 293,000 admissions in the United States in 2010
- 80,000 pediatric cases per year in United States
- Most commonly seen in ages 5–40 years, with peak age of incidence age 28 years

PATHOPHYSIOLOGY

- Acute inflammation of the appendiceal lumen is caused by obstruction (i.e., by a fecalith, calculi, parasites, hyperplastic lymphoid tissue, or tumor).
- Appendix is innervated by somatic afferent nerves of the 10th dermatome overlying the epigastrium and periumbilical areas.
- In the first phase of pain, occlusion causing increasing wall tension results in vague pain poorly referred to this area.
- Increasing wall tension and full-thickness serositis results in inflammation of surrounding tissues, and the second phase of pain is localized to the area in which the appendix is lying.
- In 85% of patients, this is at McBurney point, but pelvic, retrocecal, retroperitoneal, inguinoscrotal, or other orientations will result in variance of location and intensity of this pain.

DIAGNOSIS

Classic signs and symptoms include right lower quadrant pain, anorexia, nausea and vomiting, and fever.

HISTORY

- Abdominal pain is most common symptom.
- Pain usually begins in the periumbilical or epigastric regions prior to migrating to the right lower quadrant. Pain is followed by nausea and vomiting with fever.
- Leukocytosis occurs later.
- Timing of pain preceding nausea and vomiting and absence of diarrhea in most cases are distinguishing factors from gastroenteritis.
- Anorexia is present in the majority of cases but may not be a prominent symptom if the appendix is retrocecal or retroperitoneal.
- Perforation of the inflamed appendix may result in temporary relief of pain. These patients can proceed to develop distension, dehydration, diarrhea from perirectal irritation, and dysuria from perivesicular irritation.
- Delayed diagnosis and perforation occur more frequently in young children, presumably because they are less able to articulate their symptoms.

PHYSICAL EXAM

- Low-grade fever is common unless perforation has already occurred.
- Perforation can result in worsened fever, tachypnea, and tachycardia.
- Pain and tenderness at McBurney point (1/3 the distance from the anterior superior iliac spine [ASIS] in a line from the umbilicus to the ASIS)
- Findings may include abdominal rebound tenderness, guarding, and focal tenderness on rectal exam.
- Other signs:
  - Rovsing sign is pain in the right lower quadrant with palpation in the left lower quadrant.
  - Psoas sign is pain in the right lower quadrant with passive right hip extension and may be associated with a retrocecal appendix.
  - Obturator sign is pain in right lower quadrant with right hip and knee flexion followed by internal rotation and may be associated with a pelvic appendix.

DIAGNOSTIC TESTS & INTERPRETATION

Lab

- CBC, expect elevated WBC count (10,000–17,000 cells per μL range) with left shift
- Erythrocyte sedimentation rate is usually normal.
- C-reactive protein can be elevated but is nonspecific.

Imaging

Diagnosis can often be made with history, physical exam, and laboratory studies without imaging with a diagnostic accuracy of 80–90% in some studies.

- Abdominal radiograph
  - Often normal
  - May show fecalith, indistinct psoas margins, cecal wall thickening
  - Free air or pneumoperitoneum may indicate a perforation.
- Ultrasound
  - Currently considered the initial imaging study of choice for the diagnosis of appendicitis
  - Findings include edema, inflammation, or abscess formation.
  - Most specific finding is an appendiceal maximum outer diameter (MOD) of $\geq$7 mm (associated with a sensitivity of 98.7% and a specificity of 95.4% for the diagnosis).
- CT scan
  - Has a high diagnostic accuracy for appendicitis and may have a higher sensitivity than ultrasound; however, requires exposure to ionizing radiation and may be avoidable with careful history and physical exam, use of labs, and less invasive imaging
  - Findings include fat stranding, abscess or phlegmon, appendicolith when present, and focal cecal thickening.

DIFFERENTIAL DIAGNOSIS

- Infection
  - Gastroenteritis (e.g., *Yersinia*, *Campylobacter*)
  - Constipation
  - Right lower lobe pneumonia
  - Mesenteric adenitis
  - Typhlitis
  - Urinary tract infection
  - Pelvic inflammatory disease, tubo-ovarian abscess, or ectopic pregnancy
  - Parasitic infection (*Trichuris trichiura*, *Ascaris lumbricoides*)
- Inflammatory
  - Inflammatory bowel disease
  - Anaphylactic purpura
  - Cholecystitis
  - Pancreatitis
  - Diverticulitis
- Genetic/metabolic
  - Diabetes
  - Sickle cell disease
  - Renal stones
  - Hypernatremia
  - Crohn disease
- Miscellaneous
  - Functional abdominal pain
  - Torsion of testes or ovaries
  - Ovarian cyst
  - Endometriosis
  - Small bowel obstruction

TREATMENT

GENERAL MEASURES

- IV fluids to correct hypovolemia, electrolyte abnormalities
- Broad-spectrum antibiotics
- Pain medications

SURGERY/OTHER PROCEDURES

- Emergency appendectomy
  - Laparoscopic technique is now practiced by most surgeons in the United States.
  - It shows comparable results to open technique, allows wider exploration, and is associated with faster recovery in adults to daily activity.
  - Laparoscopic approaches now include single-port technology that limit the incision to the umbilical location.
- Given the relative risk and delay of care with CT prep, there is some evidence that immediate surgery may be preferential to radiologic investigation.
- Perforated appendicitis
  - Can also be treated via a laparoscopic approach and use of suction/irrigation devices to cleanse the abdomen of collections.
  - In many patients with perforated appendicitis, nonoperative management with percutaneous abscess drainage and broad-spectrum antibiotics followed by interval appendectomy may be preferable.

ONGOING CARE

PROGNOSIS

- Recovery is rapid.
- Prognosis is excellent.
- Overall current survival rate in United States is 98%.
- It is estimated that 35,000 people die yearly from appendicitis worldwide.

COMPLICATIONS

- Rate of wound complication post laparoscopic appendectomy is 3.1%.
- Rate of abscess formation post appendectomy is 0–4% for nonperforated appendicitis and 14–20% for perforated appendicitis.
- Perforated appendicitis may result in greater risk of postoperative ileus and small bowel obstruction or fertility issues longer term.

ADDITIONAL READING

- Bansal S, Banever GT, Kerrer FM, et al. Appendicitis in children less than 5 years old: influence of age on presentation and outcome. *Am J Surg*. 2012;204(6): 1031–1035.
- Gasior AC, St. Peter SD, Knott M, et al. National trends in approach and outcomes with appendicitis in children. *J Pediatr Surg*. 2012;47(12):2264–2267.
- Trout AT, Sanchez R, Ladino-Torres MF, et al. A critical evaluation of US for the diagnosis of pediatric acute appendicitis in a real-life setting: how can we improve the diagnostic value of sonography? *Pediatr Radiol*. 2012;42(7):813–822.

CODES

ICD10

- K37 Unspecified appendicitis
- K35.80 Unspecified acute appendicitis
- K35.89 Other acute appendicitis

FAQ

- Q: What were historical milestones in the treatment of appendicitis?
- A: In 1735, Dr. Claudius Amyand performed an appendectomy in a situation of an appendicitis within a right inguinal hernia (this is now referred to as Amyand hernia). In 1886, Dr. Reginald Heber Fitz first described what we recognize as appendicitis in his treatise "Diseases of the Vermiform Appendix." In 1887, Dr. Thomas Morton performed the first successful appendectomy under ether anesthesia. In 1889, Dr. Charles McBurney described the localization of pain from appendicitis.

ARTHRITIS, JUVENILE IDIOPATHIC (RHEUMATOID)

Elizabeth Candell Chalom

BASICS

DESCRIPTION

Chronic synovial inflammation of unknown etiology in at least 1 joint, for at least 6 weeks. Age of onset must be <16 years old.

Juvenile idiopathic arthritis (JIA) is classified as one of 7 subtypes:

- Oligoarticular arthritis affects <5 joints during the first 6 months of the disease. Tends to involve large joints, especially the knee. Peak age of onset is 1–6 years; 80% are antinuclear antibody (ANA)-positive:
  - Persistent oligoarticular JIA remains in <5 joints.
  - Extended oligoarticular JIA spreads to involve 5 or more joints. Has worse prognosis than persistent oligoarthritis.
- Polyarticular juvenile idiopathic arthritis affects ≥5 joints. Can occur at any age: Peak ages of onset are 1–4 years and 7–10 years.
  - Rheumatoid factor–positive (RF+) polyarticular juvenile idiopathic arthritis is like adult-onset idiopathic arthritis that occurs in a child. Often quite aggressive
  - Rheumatoid factor–negative (RF−) polyarticular juvenile idiopathic arthritis is usually less aggressive and easier to control.
- Systemic-onset idiopathic juvenile arthritis
  - Characterized by high, spiking quotidian or diquotidian fevers and an evanescent pink/salmon-colored macular rash
  - Affected children may also have lymphadenopathy, hepatosplenomegaly, pericarditis, or pleuritis.
  - Arthritis may not appear until weeks to months after the onset of the systemic symptoms.
  - Can occur at any age
- Enthesitis-related arthritis (ERA)
  - Entheses (e.g., osteotendinous junctions, osteoligamentous junctions) are sites where tendons or ligaments attach to bone.
  - ERA generally affects boys in late childhood or adolescence.
  - Many are human leukocyte antigen-B27–positive.
- Psoriatic arthritis is associated with psoriasis. It often begins in a few joints and then becomes polyarticular. It often involves small joints of hands and feet, as well as knees. Dactylitis is seen in nearly 50% of patients.

EPIDEMIOLOGY

Incidence

- Incidence ranges from 1 to 22/100,000/year.
- Affects ~70,000–100,000 children in the United States

Prevalence

- Prevalence ranges from 8 to 150/100,000; varies, but is thought to be ~1/1,000
- Girls are affected twice as often as boys, but boys are affected more frequently with ERA.
- ~50% of children with JIA have the oligoarticular type.
- 30% have the polyarticular type.
- 10% have systemic-onset JIA.

RISK FACTORS

Genetics

- Rare in siblings, but many studies have demonstrated increased frequencies of various human leukocyte antigen markers in JIA.
- Each marker may be associated with a different subtype of JIA:
  - Human leukocyte antigen-DR4: RF+ polyarticular JIA
  - Human leukocyte antigen-DR1: oligoarticular disease without uveitis
  - Human leukocyte antigen-DR5: oligoarticular JIA with uveitis
  - Human leukocyte antigen-B27: ERA
  - Human leukocyte antigen-A2: early-onset oligoarticular JIA

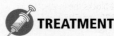

DIAGNOSIS

HISTORY

- Morning stiffness that improves after a warm shower/bath or with stretching and mild exercise is common in JIA. Many young children do not complain of pain, but walk with a limp or refuse to walk down stairs in the morning.
- Joints often become sore/painful again in the late afternoon or evening.
- Patients with JIA generally do not complain of severe pain, but rather they avoid using joints that are particularly affected.
  - If a child has severe pain in a joint, especially pain that seems out of proportion to the physical findings, diagnoses other than JIA should be entertained.
- In systemic JIA, the fever curve is important to document.
  - Between fever spikes, the child is often completely afebrile.
  - The rash is evanescent and patients often have a history of fatigue, malaise, and weight loss.

PHYSICAL EXAM

- Arthritis must be present, not just arthralgias:
  - In addition to swelling, warmth, and tenderness, there may be restricted range of motion in the affected joints and soft tissue contractures.
- Enthesitis and sacroiliac tenderness are often seen in ERA.
- In systemic JIA, the rash, if present, is very suggestive of this disease.
- Lymphadenopathy and hepatosplenomegaly may be seen in systemic JIA.
- A careful cardiac and pulmonary examination must be done to look for pericarditis and pleuritis.

ALERT

Arthritis must be present for at least 6 weeks before a patient can be diagnosed with JIA. Many viral illnesses can produce joint pain and swelling that mimics JIA, but resolves within 4–6 weeks.

DIAGNOSTIC TESTS & INTERPRETATION

Lab

- No laboratory finding is diagnostic for JIA.
- Many patients with JIA, especially the polyarticular and systemic types, have elevated sedimentation rates and anemia.
- Antinuclear antibody is a useful test in classifying patients with JIA and determining the risk of uveitis. Positive in the following:
  - 80% of oligoarticular
  - 40–60% of polyarticular
  - 15–20% of normal population
- Rheumatoid factor will be positive in 15–20% of patients with polyarticular arthritis and usually indicates a more aggressive form of arthritis.

Imaging

- Radiography is often normal early in JIA.
- Later, if arthritis persists, bone demineralization, loss of articular cartilage, erosions, and joint fusion may be seen.

DIFFERENTIAL DIAGNOSIS

- Monoarticular JIA
  - Septic joint
  - Toxic synovitis
  - Trauma
  - Hemarthrosis
  - Villonodular synovitis
- Monoarticular or oligoarticular JIA
  - Lyme disease
  - Acute rheumatic fever or poststreptococcal arthritis
  - Viral/postviral arthritis
  - Malignancies
  - Sarcoidosis
  - Inflammatory bowel disease
- Polyarticular JIA
  - Viral or postviral illness (especially parvovirus)
  - Lyme disease
  - Lupus
- Systemic-onset JIA
  - Infection
  - Oncologic process (leukemia, lymphoma)
  - Inflammatory bowel disease
  - Lupus

TREATMENT

MEDICATION

First Line

- Steroids (glucocorticoids):
  - Intra-articular steroids: Triamcinolone hexacetonide injections are often used when patients have only 1 or 2 active joints.
  - Systemic steroids
    - Systemic steroids are often needed to control flares or with the initial presentation of polyarticular or systemic JIA. Because of the many side effects, patients should be weaned off steroids as soon as possible.
    - Glucocorticoids can be given orally (daily or every other day) or as IV pulses (every 1–8 weeks).

- NSAIDs
  - 1st-line therapy for mild JIA
  - If there is no response to the initial NSAID after 4–6 weeks of an adequate dose, a different one should be tried. Patients will often respond differently to the various NSAIDs.
  - If patients experience GI upset or excessive bruising, COX-2 inhibitors may be used. If arthritis remains active after 2–3 months, a 2nd-line treatment should be added.

Second Line

- If NSAIDs are ineffective in controlling the disease, or the patient has moderate to severe arthritis, a 2nd-line agent should be used, such as methotrexate or sulfasalazine.
- Methotrexate
  - If the arthritis does not respond to NSAIDs, methotrexate is the most common 2nd-line agent for active arthritis in multiple joints.
  - Laboratory values must be monitored closely in these patients, looking for bone marrow suppression or elevation of transaminase levels.
- Sulfasalazine
  - Most often used in ERA

Third Line

- Biologic agents are often added when patients do not respond adequately to methotrexate or cannot tolerate its side effects, or when the arthritis is severe.
- Antitumor necrosis factor therapy is frequently used:
  - Etanercept is a receptor for tumor necrosis factor; given SC once or twice a week
  - Infliximab is a chimeric antibody to tumor necrosis factor; given IV every 4–8 weeks
  - Adalimumab is a fully humanized antibody to tumor necrosis factor; given SC every other week
- IL-1 inhibition may work better than TNF inhibition in systemic JIA.
  - Anakinra is a recombinant IL-1 receptor antagonist. Given as a daily SC injection
  - Canakinumab is given SC once monthly.
  - Rilonacept is an SC injection given weekly.
- Anti–IL-6 therapy (tocilizumab)
  - An IV medication given every other week.
  - It has been approved for children with systemic-onset and polyarticular JIA.
- Abatacept
  - Costimulation blocker. It blocks the interaction of CD28 on T cells with CD80 and CD86 receptors on antigen-presenting cells.
  - It is given IV every 4 weeks.
  - It is currently being tested as an SC injection in children (SC form is approved in adults).
- Rituximab
  - An antibody to CD20, which is present on all B cells
  - Approved for use in adult RA but not JIA
- Medications such as cyclophosphamide or thalidomide are sometimes necessary to control severe systemic-onset JIA.

ADDITIONAL TREATMENT

General Measures

- Responses to treatments for juvenile idiopathic arthritis vary tremendously:
  - Some patients may respond to NSAIDs within 1–2 weeks.
  - Others take 4–6 weeks to improve, and some may not respond at all.
  - Steroids usually start to relieve symptoms within a few days.
  - Methotrexate usually takes 4–8 weeks until a benefit is seen.
  - Antitumor necrosis factor therapy can start decreasing symptoms in as little as 1–2 weeks, or it may take up to 3 months.
  - Other 2nd-line agents can take up to 16 weeks until the maximum benefit is seen.
- The waxing and waning nature of JIA itself adds to the variability of response to treatment.

ADDITIONAL THERAPIES

- Physical and occupational therapy are important in the management of JIA.
- The goal is to maintain range of motion, muscle strength, and function.

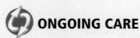

ONGOING CARE

PROGNOSIS

- Varies considerably
- Children with oligoarticular JIA usually do well and often go into remission within a few years of starting treatment. They may have flares, however, even up to 10 years after being symptom-free and off all medications.
- Patients with polyarticular JIA who are RF+ often develop a severe arthritis that may persist into adulthood.
- RF− polyarticular patients generally fare better, and many outgrow their disease.
- 50% of patients with systemic-onset JIA will develop severe chronic polyarticular arthritis.

COMPLICATIONS

- Joint degeneration with loss of articular cartilage
- Soft tissue contractures
- Leg length discrepancy
- Micrognathia
- Cervical spine dislocation
- Rheumatoid nodules
- Growth retardation
- Uveitis
  - Oligoarticular JIA, especially with a positive ANA test, is associated with chronic uveitis, which can lead to loss of vision if not detected early with routine slit-lamp eye examinations.
  - May be seen in polyarticular JIA but is less common
- Pericarditis, pleuritis, and severe anemia may develop in patients with systemic-onset JIA.
- Macrophage activation syndrome or hemophagocytic syndrome
  - Rare, but potentially lethal complication of systemic-onset JIA, resulting from an overproduction of inflammatory cytokines
  - May present as an acute febrile illness with pancytopenia and hepatosplenomegaly
  - Bone marrow aspiration can be diagnostic.
  - Treatment is often high-dose steroids and high-dose IL-1 inhibitors, or cyclosporine.

ADDITIONAL READING

- Andersson Gäre B. Juvenile arthritis—who gets it, where and when? A review of current data on incidence and prevalence. *Clin Exp Rheumatol*. 1999;17(3):367–374.
- Ilowite NT. Update on biologics in juvenile idiopathic arthritis. *Curr Opin Rheumatol*. 2008;20(5):613–618.
- Patel H, Goldstein D. Pediatric uveitis. *Pediatr Clin North Am*. 2003;50(1):125–136.
- Prakken B, Albani S, Martini A. Juvenile idiopathing arthritis. *Lancet*. 2011;377(9783):2138–2149.
- Ringold S, Weiss PF, Beukelman T, et al. 2013 update of the 2011 American College of Rheumatology recommendations for the treatment of juvenile idiopathic arthritis: recommendations for the medical therapy of children with systemic juvenile idiopathic arthritis and tuberculosis screening among children receiving biologic medications. *Arthritis Rheum*. 2013;65(10):2499–2512.
- Schneider R, Passo MH. Juvenile idiopathic arthritis. *Rheum Dis Clin North Am*. 2002;28(3):503–530.
- Weiss J, Ilowite N. Juvenile idiopathic arthritis. *Pediatr Clin North Am*. 2005;52(2):413–442.

CODES

ICD10

- M08.80 Other juvenile arthritis, unspecified site
- M08.849 Other juvenile arthritis, unspecified hand
- M08.879 Other juvenile arthritis, unspecified ankle and foot

FAQ

- Q: Will the patient outgrow JIA?
- A: Prognosis depends on the type of JIA. In some studies, up to 50% of patients with JIA still had active disease 10 years after diagnosis, but only 15% had loss of function.
- Q: Will siblings of patients with JIA develop the disease?
- A: Rarely, but it can occur.

ASCARIS LUMBRICOIDES (ASCARIASIS)

Amaya L. Bustinduy

BASICS

DESCRIPTION

Ascaris lumbricoides is a large parasitic nematode (roundworm), 15–40 cm in length, which infects humans via eggs found in soil.

EPIDEMIOLOGY

- Geographic distribution: South America, sub-Saharan Africa, China, and East Asia
- All ages may be affected; however, children are more frequent hosts owing to oral behavior and tend to have a higher worm burden.
- Ascariasis is more common where sanitation is poor and population is dense.
- Eggs are viable in the soil for more than 6 years in temperate climates.
- It is the most prevalent helminth infection in the world.
- ~1/6 of the world's population is infected.
- 8–15% of infections are symptomatic.
  - 120–220 million cases
  - Mostly moderate and heavy worm loads

GENERAL PREVENTION

Infection control

- Sanitary disposal of human excrement, not using human feces as fertilizer, and hand washing has the potential to eliminate this infection.
- In communities with high transmission of *Ascaris*, community-wide mass drug delivery of anthelmintics is effective in controlling morbidity.

PATHOPHYSIOLOGY

- Fertilized eggs are ingested from soil contaminated with human feces.
- Larvae hatch in the small intestine and migrate to cecum and colon.
- Larvae invade the mucosa into the venous system and travel to the portal circulation, inferior vena cava, and finally, pulmonary capillaries.
- During migration through the pulmonary vessels, an eosinophilic response is evoked.
- Larvae penetrate the alveoli, are expelled by coughing, and swallowed back (days 10–14).
- Larvae become adult worms in the small intestine (day 24).
- Female worms excrete up to 200,000 eggs per day.
- Ingestion to excretion takes 2–3 months.
- Once in soil, fertilized eggs require 2–3 weeks of incubation in soil to become infectious and restart cycle.

ETIOLOGY

Children commonly acquire this infection from playing in dirt contaminated with *Ascaris* eggs.

COMMONLY ASSOCIATED CONDITIONS

- This infection may be associated with other soil-transmitted helminths:
  - Hookworm (*Necator americanus*, *Ancylostoma duodenale*)
  - *Trichuris trichiura*
  - *Strongyloides stercoralis*
  - *Toxocara canis*

DIAGNOSIS

HISTORY

- Gastrointestinal symptoms include the following:
  - Abdominal distention
  - Pain
  - Nausea
  - Diarrhea
  - Decreased appetite
- In the chronic phase, ascariasis is associated with the following:
  - Growth stunting
  - Cognitive delays
- Severe respiratory symptoms during the pulmonary migratory stage, when larvae cause an inflammatory response (Löeffler syndrome), characterized by the following:
  - Dyspnea
  - Cough
  - Fever
  - Shifting pulmonary infiltrates
  - Eosinophilia
- Severe presentation during the intestinal phase, when symptoms are due to the presence of worms:
  - Pain
  - Obstruction (2 per 1,000)
  - Peritonitis from perforation
  - Biliary colic, hepatitis, or pancreatitis from blockages due to worms
- History of passage of large worms in the stool or vomitus is suggestive of ascariasis.
- History of wheezing may precede passage of worms by 2–3 months.

PHYSICAL EXAM

- Chest: may have rales or wheezing if *Ascaris* larvae are in the lungs
- Abdomen
  - Distended
  - Auscultate and palpate for signs of obstruction or perforation

DIAGNOSTIC TESTS & INTERPRETATION

Lab

- Microscopic examination of stool specimens will demonstrate the characteristic ascaris eggs (round with thick shell).
- During the pulmonary phase, may have peripheral eosinophilia and larvae in sputum, but negative stool examinations
- Serologic tests are unnecessary and are poorly specific to the diagnosis.

Imaging

- Chest radiograph, if cough is present
- Abdominal imaging, if abdominal signs or symptoms of obstruction or perforation

DIFFERENTIAL DIAGNOSIS

Ascariasis should be considered in the differential diagnosis when a patient presents with pneumonia, peripheral eosinophilia, and/or intestinal obstruction in returned traveler or resident from an endemic area.

TREATMENT

MEDICATION

First Line

- Oral
  - Albendazole
    - 400 mg, single dose
    - WHO recommends 200 mg single dose for children <1 year old.
  - Mebendazole
    - 100 mg, b.i.d. for 3 days or 500 mg once
  - Ivermectin
    - 150–200 mcg/kg, single dose
- Alternatives (oral):
  - Pyrantel pamoate
    - 11 mg/kg to max 1 g per day for 3 days
  - Piperazine citrate
    - 75 mg/kg/24 h for 2 days; maximum, 3.5 g
    - Has been used historically for cases of intestinal obstruction (causes worm paralysis), but it is no longer available in the United States

SURGERY/OTHER PROCEDURES

Surgery or endoscopic retrograde cholangiopancreatography may be required for severe intestinal or biliary tract obstruction.

ONGOING CARE

FOLLOW-UP RECOMMENDATIONS

- Treatment is highly effective.
- Reexamination of stool specimens 2 weeks after therapy can be considered but is not essential.
- Reinfection is common in endemic areas and has led to mass drug administration programs.

Patient Monitoring

Warn parents about passage of worms in stool with treatment.

PROGNOSIS

- Once intestinal infection is detected and treated, the prognosis is excellent.
- If obstructive or respiratory complications have occurred, the prognosis is less favorable.
- The case fatality rate in cases with complications is up to 5%, most from obstruction.

COMPLICATIONS

- Bronchopneumonia may be seen during the pulmonary migrational stage, producing fever, cough, dyspnea, wheeze, eosinophilia, and pulmonary infiltrates (Löeffler syndrome).
- Heavy infestations may cause abdominal pain, malabsorption, and growth failure.
- Children may experience obstruction (ileocecal), malabsorption, or intussusception.
- Perforation or migration into the appendix, biliary, or pancreatic ducts may rarely occur.
- Hepatitis, acute cholecystitis, or pancreatitis can occur. Liver abscess can occur if intrahepatic ducts are obstructed.

ADDITIONAL READING

- American Academy of Pediatrics. *Ascaris lumbricoides infections*. In: Pickering LK, Baker CJ, Kimberlin DW, et al, eds. *Red Book: 2012 Report of the Committee on Infectious Diseases*. 29th ed. Elk Grove Village, IL: American Academy of Pediatrics; 2012:239–240.
- Capello M, Hotez PJ. Intestinal nematodes. In: Long S, Pickering L, Prober C, eds. *Principles and Practice of Pediatric Infectious Diseases*. 3rd ed. Churchill Livingstone/Elsevier; 2008:1296–1298.
- Centers for Disease Control and Prevention. Parasites-ascariasis. http://www.cdc.gov/parasites/ascariasis/. Accessed November 24, 2013.
- Dold C, Holland CV. Ascaris and ascariasis. *Microbes Infect*. 2011;13(7):632–637.
- Hall A, Hewitt G, Tuffrey V, et al. A review and meta-analysis of the impact of intestinal worms on child growth and nutrition. *Matern Child Nutr*. 2008;4(Suppl 1):118–236.
- O'Lorcain P, Holland CV. The public health importance of *Ascaris lumbricoides*. *Parasitology*. 2000;121(Suppl):S51–S71.
- World Health Organization. Intestinal worms. http://www.who.int/intestinal_worms/en/. Accessed November 24, 2013.

CODES

ICD10

- B77.9 Ascariasis, unspecified
- B77.0 Ascariasis with intestinal complications
- B77.81 Ascariasis pneumonia

FAQ

- Q: What are the long term effects of untreated *Ascaris* infection in children?
- A: Growth stunting and cognitive delays are the most common long-term effects of untreated infections. Given the prevalence of this infection in the world, this is a major cause of morbidity in the world.

ASCITES

Rima Fawaz

BASICS

DESCRIPTION

- Ascites is defined as a pathologic accumulation of intraperitoneal fluid.
- Peritoneal fluid formation is a dynamic process of production and absorption.
- In children, ascites is usually the result of liver or renal disease.
- In adults, ascites is most often due to portal hypertension from cirrhosis.
- Ascites is the most common of the three major complications of cirrhosis; the other two complications of cirrhosis are hepatic encephalopathy and variceal hemorrhage.

PATHOPHYSIOLOGY

- Normal circulation
  - Blood enters the liver from the hepatic artery and portal vein, perfuses the hepatic sinusoids, and exits the liver via the hepatic veins.
  - Hepatic lymph, formed by the filtration of sinusoidal plasma into the space of Disse, drains from the liver via the transdiaphragmatic lymphatic vessels to the thoracic duct.
  - Hepatic lymph is isosmotic to plasma, as the sinusoidal endothelium is highly permeable to albumin.
  - In the intestine, the mesenteric capillary membrane is impermeable to albumin. The osmotic gradient favors the return of interstitial fluid/lymph into the capillary.
  - Intestinal lymph from regional lymphatics combines with hepatic lymph in the thoracic duct.
- Portal hypertension
  - Ascitic fluid production is due to a net transfer of fluid that exceeds the drainage capacity of the lymphatics.
- Cirrhotic ascites results from three pathophysiologic process:
  - Portal hypertension
  - Vasodilation: mediated predominantly by nitric oxide
  - Hyperaldosteronism: Decreased effective volume sensed by the kidneys stimulate the renin-angiotensin-aldosterone system, leading to increased sympathetic activity and antidiuretic hormone secretion.
- Noncirrhotic ascites can be the result of the following:
  - Proteinaceous material produced by malignant cells or by inflammation of visceral and/or parietal peritoneum: peritoneal carcinomatosis, tuberculous ascites
  - Obstruction of lymphatic flow by mass, tumor, or external pressure
  - Impaired portal flow: right-sided heart failure, Budd-Chiari syndrome, portal venous malformations
  - Decreased effective arterial blood volume: heart failure
  - Decreased oncotic pressure/ hypoalbuminemia: nephrotic syndrome, protein-losing enteropathy, severe malnutrition
  - Primary (congenital) abnormalities of the lymphatics, metabolic disorders (lysosomal storage diseases including sialidosis, Wolman disease, GM1 gangliosidosis, Gaucher disease, and Niemann-Pick type C)
  - Rupture of intra-abdominal viscus or peritoneal/mesenteric cyst, bowel perforation, ureteral rupture

ETIOLOGY

Accumulation of fluid occurs with the following:

- Inflammatory conditions (e.g., mesenteric adenitis, tuberculosis, pancreatitis, secondary to inflammation of visceral, and/or parietal peritoneum)
- Portal hypertension or obstruction of portal vein flow and/or lymphatic flow by mass, tumor, or external pressure; tumors of abdominal viscera, retroperitoneum, thorax, or mediastinum (often characterized by chylous ascites)
- Infectious processes: abscess, tuberculosis, *Chlamydia* infection, schistosomiasis
- Gastrointestinal: infarcted bowel/perforation, pancreatitis, ruptured pancreatic duct, parenchymal liver disease
- Gynecologic: ovarian tumors, torsion, or rupture
- Renal: nephrotic syndrome, obstructive uropathy, perforated urinary tract, peritoneal dialysis
- Cardiac: CHF, constrictive pericarditis, inferior vena cava web
- Neoplastic: lymphoma, neuroblastoma
- Miscellaneous: systemic lupus erythematous, eosinophilic ascites, chylous ascites, hypothyroidism, ventriculoperitoneal shunt

DIAGNOSIS

HISTORY

- The etiology for acute decompensation in hepatocellular function (e.g., massive bleeding, sepsis, superimposed infections) should be investigated.
- Weight gain
- Use of umbilical catheters in newborn period (increased risk of portal vein thrombosis)
- Evidence of chronic liver disease
- Respiratory distress
- Exposure to hepatotoxins
- Developmental delay or growth failure suggestive of metabolic disease

PHYSICAL EXAM

- Vital signs:
  - Increased heart rate (increased cardiac output)
  - Lower blood pressure seen in cirrhotics
- General appearance: cachexia
- Abdominal exam
  - Protuberant abdomen, bulging flanks (fluid wave or shifting dullness)
  - Caput medusae, umbilical hernia,
  - Dullness to percussion
  - Peritoneal signs
  - Abdominal pain
  - Splenomegaly
- Auscultation of the pericardium: pericardial friction rub (pericarditis), cor pulmonale
- Neurologic exam: hepatic encephalopathy
- Skin
  - Jaundice
  - Spider angioma
  - Palmar erythema
  - Scratch marks
  - Striae
  - Xanthomas
- Extremities
  - Clubbing
  - Edema

DIAGNOSTIC EVALUATION

Laboratory

- Complete blood count
- Electrolytes
- Liver test: transaminases, prothrombin time/international normalized ratio, total protein, albumin, total and fractionated bilirubin
- Amylase and lipase (to exclude pancreatitis)
- Creatinine and blood urea nitrogen
- Fluid cultures: blood, urine, ascitic fluid
- Urinalysis
- Specific testing for etiologies of ascites from chronic liver disease and other causes as deemed appropriate

Imaging

- Ultrasound of the abdomen with Doppler study
  - Study of choice to differentiate between free and loculated fluid collection and the presence of intra-abdominal masses
  - Can evaluate patency of hepatic and portal vasculature and directionality of flow
- Plain radiography (centralized bowel loops)
- Abdominal computed axial tomography
- Abdominal magnetic resonance imaging

Abdominal Paracentesis

- Ascitic fluid analysis is essential:
  - Cell count and differential
  - Albumin, total protein
  - Culture, Gram stain
  - Glucose (low in infection)
  - Lactate dehydrogenase concentration (high in infection, bowel perforation, or tumor)
  - Other optional tests include amylase (high in perforated viscus or pancreatitis), triglycerides (high in chylous ascites), and cytology (peritoneal carcinomatosis).
- Serum to ascites albumin gradient (SAAG)
  - (Serum albumin) – (ascites albumin)
  - Blood and ascitic fluid analysis should be obtained on same day.
  - SAAG $\geq$1.1 g/dL suggests presence of portal hypertension.
  - If SAAG $<$1.1 g/dL, suspect other causes.

DIFFERENTIAL DIAGNOSIS

- Organomegaly: enlarged liver or spleen
- Mesenteric cyst or ovarian cyst: does not have shifting dullness when position is changed
- Bowel obstruction
- Cancer
- Heart failure
- Nephrotic syndrome

TREATMENT

- The management of the ascites should be directed toward the underlying etiology.
- Benefits of treatment of ascites should always be weighed against risks and complications of treatment.
- Mobilization of cirrhotic ascitic fluid is best accomplished by creating a negative sodium balance and then maintaining the balance.
- In patients with cirrhosis, causes of decompensation should be sought, such as sodium and fluid overload, infection, esophageal hemorrhage, spontaneous bacterial peritonitis.

- In adults, dietary sodium intake is restricted to 44–88 mEq (1–2 g/24 h) or approximately 17–35 mEq (0.4–0.8 g) per thousand calories.
- In pediatrics, restricting dietary sodium intake is recommended: diet with no extra salt to a maximum 2 mEq/kg/24 h (to be balanced against palatability of food and nutritional needs).
- Water is only restricted in patients with profound hyponatremia (<125 mEq/L): 50–75% of maintenance requirements.
- Goal of diuretic therapy is reduction of bodyweight by 0.5–1% daily until ascites is resolved.
- Spironolactone (PO)
  – Most effective single diuretic, as it counteracts the hyperaldosteronism present in cirrhotic ascites
  – Acts on the distal collecting system, hence, inhibits reabsorption of 2% of filtered sodium
  – Bioactive metabolites have long half-lives, hence, need >5 days to achieve steady state.
  – Start at 2–3 mg/kg/24 h as a single morning (max 100 mg initial dose). In adults, typical starting dose is up to 100 mg/24 h and can be increased to max 400 mg/24 h.
  – Most effective in combination with furosemide
- Adequacy of spironolactone therapy can be monitored with urinary sodium excretion (desired >50 mEq/L). If no response, furosemide is added.
- Furosemide (PO)
  – Loop diuretic: can increase sodium excretion by 30%
  – Start at 1 mg/kg (max initial dose 40 mg), may increase every few days if needed.
  – Adults maintain ratio of 100 mg of spironolactone to 40 mg of furosemide to maintain eukalemia (max 400 mg spironolactone to 160 mg of furosemide daily)
- When diuretics are used, urine output and serum electrolytes should be closely monitored to prevent prerenal azotemia and decreased effective blood flow to the kidneys.
- Albumin: Supplementation may aid fluid mobilization if albumin is <2.5 g/dL (use 1 g/kg of 25% albumin until level >2.5 g/dL).
- Refractory ascites: Diuretic-refractory ascites derives from a lack of response to dietary sodium restriction and maximal diuretic therapy. Treatment options are the following:
  – Therapeutic abdominal paracentesis (large-volume paracentesis) is used in adults with refractory ascites.
  – In children, this approach is used to relieve respiratory distress or other sequelae of rapidly increasing intra-abdominal pressure.
  – Paracentesis of volumes >1 L should be accompanied by IV infusion of 25% albumin during the procedure.
  – Transjugular intrahepatic portosystemic shunting may be valuable in cases where portal hypertension is felt to be the underlying etiology of ascitic accumulation.
  – Orthotopic liver transplantation is the only curative therapy for refractory ascites from liver disease and the only definitive treatment that has been shown to improve survival.
- When diuretics are used, urine output and serum electrolytes should be closely monitored to prevent prerenal azotemia and decreased effective blood flow to the kidneys.

ALERT

- Ultrasonography should be the initial diagnostic imaging of choice for evaluation of ascites.
- With congenital ascites, evaluate for lysosomal storage diseases.
- Diagnostic paracentesis is crucial in the evaluation of new-onset ascites.
- Calculate SAAG to differentiate between portal hypertension and other causes.
- In patients with liver disease and new-onset ascites, evaluate for etiologies to explain acute decompensation.

PROGNOSIS

- Development of ascites in the setting of cirrhosis is a landmark in the natural history of cirrhosis: 15% of adult patients succumb in 1 year and 44% in 5 years.
- Liver transplantation dramatically improves survival.
- Prognosis depends on etiology of ascites: nephrotic syndrome (ascites will regress as proteinuria clears), infection, hepatic decompensation (prognosis improves if able to reverse cause of liver injury).

COMPLICATIONS

- Spontaneous bacterial peritonitis (SBP)
  – Spontaneous ascitic fluid infection: Infection of the peritoneal fluid may occur in the absence of secondary cause (e.g., bowel perforation or intra-abdominal abscess).
  – Fever, irritability, abdominal tenderness, and distention are common signs, vomiting and diarrhea may occur.
  – Abdominal paracentesis must be performed and ascitic fluid must be analyzed before a confident diagnosis of ascitic fluid infection can be made. The blood culture bottle should be injected with peritoneal fluid at the bedside in order to increase the culture yield.
  – Diagnosis: ascitic fluid absolute polymorphonuclear leukocytes ≥250 cells/mm^3 without evidence of an intra-abdominal process
  – Bacterial organisms commonly identified are the following: *Streptococcus pneumoniae*, *Escherichia coli*, *Klebsiella pneumoniae*, enterococci, and *Haemophilus influenzae*.
  – Broad-spectrum antibiotics with gram-negative coverage such as third generation cephalosporin can be used until identification of bacterial pathogen allows narrower coverage.
  – Prophylaxis for recurrent SBP has been recommended in certain situations.
- Other complications:
  – Respiratory distress from decreased lung volume and diaphragmatic limitation: hepatic hydrothorax (large symptomatic pleural effusion that occurs in a cirrhotic patient in the absence of primary cardiopulmonary disease), abdominal wall hernias with rupture, tense ascites with leakage (especially after paracentesis)
  – Conservative management consists of appropriate initial therapy for most of these except hernia rupture, which requires surgical reduction.

ADDITIONAL READING

- European Association for the Study of the Liver. EASL clinical practice guideline on the management of ascites, spontaneous bacterial peritonitis, and hepatorenal syndrome in cirrhosis. *J Hepatol*. 2010,53(3):397–417.
- Griefer MJ, Murray KF, Colleti RB. Pathophysiology, diagnosis, and management of pediatric ascites. *J Pediatr Gastroenterol Nutr*. 2011;52(5):503–513.
- Hou W, Sanyal AJ. Ascites: diagnosis and management. *Med Clin North Am*. 2009;93(4):801–817.
- Runyon BA. Management of adult patients with ascites due to cirrhosis: update 2012. *Hepatology*. 2013(6):2087–2107.

CODES

ICD10

- R18.8 Other ascites
- R18.0 Malignant ascites
- A18.31 Tuberculous peritonitis

FAQ

- Q: What etiologies are likely in cases of congenital ascites?
- A: Lysosomal storage disorders and/or other metabolic diseases should be excluded. If hepatic function is impaired, causes of neonatal liver failure should also be investigated.
- Q: What is the best test to discriminate the type of ascites?
- A: Analysis of the peritoneal fluid collected by abdominal paracentesis is required for this purpose. The SAAG is helpful to discriminate ascites due to portal hypertension from other etiologies.
- Q: Where does the word "ascites" come from?
- A: It is thought that the word ascites is derived from the Greek word "*askos*" which refers to a container of wine or a wineskin.

ASPERGILLOSIS

Jessica E. Ericson • Daniel K. Benjamin, Jr.

BASICS

DESCRIPTION

- Diseases caused by species of the mold *Aspergillus* include superficial, immune-mediated, and invasive conditions depending on host factors.
- Most human disease is caused by *Aspergillus fumigatus*, *Aspergillus flavus*, or *Aspergillus niger*; other *Aspergillus* spp. may occasionally cause disease.

EPIDEMIOLOGY

- *Aspergillus* spp. are common, ubiquitous environmental saprophytic molds that are found growing in soil, grain, dung, bird droppings, and decaying plant matter.
- Reproduce through conidia (spore) formation. Spores are hardy and become airborne when soil is disturbed.
- Conidia are inhaled and are typically eliminated by alveolar macrophages and neutrophils.
- Disease occurs when airborne spores are inhaled but not effectively cleared; person-to-person spread does not occur.
- The incubation period has not been defined.
- Nosocomial infections can occur when ventilation or water systems become contaminated or when large numbers of spores become airborne during nearby construction or renovation projects.

Incidence

Aspergillosis incidence varies by the population studied. It is not common in a normal host. Ten percent of patients needing sinus surgery have *Aspergillus*. Up to 5% of leukemia and bone marrow transplant patients may develop invasive aspergillosis.

RISK FACTORS

- Otomycosis, fungal sinusitis, and allergic bronchopulmonary aspergillosis (ABPA) can occur in otherwise healthy patients.
- Most patients infected with *Aspergillus* have some degree of immunocompromise.
- Patients receiving chemotherapy for malignancy or rheumatologic disorders, chronic steroid therapy, organ and bone marrow transplant recipients, and those with HIV or primary immunodeficiencies are at increased risk.

GENERAL PREVENTION

- Hospitalized, immunosuppressed patients are at risk for invasive aspergillosis.
- Careful control of airflow using filters and laminar flow systems especially aimed at limiting exposure to air from construction sites is important.
- Shower heads should be cleaned regularly to prevent aerosolization of mold particles.

PATHOPHYSIOLOGY

- *Aspergillus* most frequently enters the body through the respiratory tract; however, the ear canal and breaks in the skin (especially if acquired from contact with a soiled surface) can also allow infection to occur.
  - Progression to disease depends largely on its ability to evade host defenses.
  - Macrophages and neutrophils can typically eliminate *Aspergillus* without difficulty, explaining its rarity in normal hosts.
  - *Aspergillus* produces proteolytic enzymes and cytotoxins, which may contribute to its pathogenesis.
- Conditions that alter the normal immunologic mechanisms predispose to invasive aspergillosis. Examples include leukemia (neutropenia), corticosteroids (decreased neutrophil mobilization and macrophage killing), and chronic granulomatous disease (decreased oxidative-mediated killing).

ETIOLOGY

Aspergillus sp.: *A. fumigatus* is most common and can cause the whole spectrum of disease. *A. niger* causes sinus and otomycosis and *A. flavus* causes sinus disease.

COMMONLY ASSOCIATED CONDITIONS

- Cutaneous: typically follows trauma, can also occur in premature infants or due to embolism in disseminated disease
- Otomycosis: typically a localized infection, often a superinfection of bacterial otitis externa. More common in warm, moist climates. Host may be normal or have altered mucosal immunity (diabetes, eczema, steroid use).
- Sinusitis: occurs as an aspergilloma, acute or chronic sinus disease. Normal and immunocompromised patients can be affected. Associated with nasal polyps and aspirin allergy in normal hosts.
- ABPA: an IgE-mediated hypersensitivity response to inhaled spores. Most commonly occurs in settings of chronic lung disease (cystic fibrosis, asthma). Often have wheezing, productive cough with brown sputum. Diagnostic criteria include +skin test to *Aspergillus* antigens, serum IgE $>$1,000 ng/mL, transient infiltrates on chest x-ray, total eosinophil count $>$500 cells/microliter.
- Aspergilloma: fungus balls that grow in preexisting lung cavities (congenital, secondary to TB, sarcoid, chronic lung disease)
- Invasive pulmonary aspergillosis occurs in the immunocompromised host, most commonly following bone marrow or solid organ transplants, and patients with hematologic malignancy or primary immunodeficiency. Invasion of blood vessels by *Aspergillus* leads to infarction, necrosis, and hematogenous dissemination; resulting pulmonary hemorrhage is often fatal.
- Invasive aspergillosis in immunocompromised hosts can disseminate to the sinuses, brain, or skin. Rarer infections include endocarditis, meningitis, osteomyelitis, esophagitis, or infection of the eye.

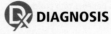

DIAGNOSIS

HISTORY

- Otomycosis: ear pain, pruritus, hearing loss
- Sinusitis: environmental allergies, chronic congestion, sinusitis unresponsive to antibiotics
- ABPA: unexplained worsening of asthma symptoms, cough productive of dark mucous plugs
- Lung disease: exposure to construction site or gardening (especially involving mulch or compost)
- Immunity: Is the patient immunocompromised?
  - Immunocompromised patients, especially those with prolonged neutropenia, are at highest risk for invasive aspergillosis.

PHYSICAL EXAM

- Cutaneous: necrotic-appearing painful ulcer
- Otomycosis: relapsing otorrhea with thick greasy exudate and pain on tragal movement. Black spores (*A. niger*) may be visible in the canal. Rarely invasive but may cause facial nerve palsy if it is.
- Sinusitis: Nasal obstruction, polyps, facial pain, and proptosis are typically seen. Invasive sinus aspergillosis may also cause monocular blindness and bony destruction on radiographic films, with erosion into the orbit or the cranial vault, or with widespread dissemination. The maxillary sinuses are most commonly involved.
- Lung disease: often indistinguishable from other causes of pneumonia on physical examination. Fever, tachypnea, rales, hypoxemia, and hemoptysis (due to angioinvasion) may be present.

DIAGNOSTIC TESTS & INTERPRETATION

Lab & Radiography

- *Aspergillus* can be isolated from nearly any body site including blood, cerebrospinal fluid, sputum, urine, bronchoalveolar lavage (BAL) fluid, and tissue biopsy specimens.
- Respiratory specimens growing *Aspergillus* spp. on culture (e.g., sputum and nasal cultures) may represent colonization in the immunocompetent host but may indicate invasive disease in certain hosts. The entire clinical picture including history and physical exam should be considered when interpreting culture results.
- Presence of branching, septate hyphae on stained biopsy specimens or a wet preparation performed with 10% potassium hydroxide (KOH) is suggestive of *Aspergillus* or other mold species.

- Cutaneous aspergillosis, otomycosis, and sinusitis: Suggestive lab findings include biopsy culture growing *Aspergillus* sp., pathology specimen with septate hyphae on KOH preparation in the setting of a consistent clinical picture.
- Sinusitis and ABPA: may also see elevated serum IgE, eosinophilia, *Aspergillus*-specific serum IgE, and an immediate-type skin test response to *Aspergillus* antigen which may support diagnosis
- Isolation of *Aspergillus* sp. by culture is ideal but often does not occur in pulmonary and disseminated disease.
- Radiographic studies may support the diagnosis but are not definitive.
  - ABPA: centrilobular nodules, "finger in glove," upper lobe infiltrate
  - Pulmonary disease: cavitations, nodules (seen in ~35%). Classic CT findings of "halo sign" (an area of low attenuation surrounding a nodule) initially and later the "crescent sign" (an air crescent near the periphery of a lung nodule, caused by contraction of infarcted tissue) are seen infrequently in children but may be present in adolescents.
- Adjunctive tests: Galactomannan is a polysaccharide of *Aspergillus* cell walls. Enzyme immunoassay (EIA) for galactomannan from serum or BAL fluid early in the course may aid diagnosis of aspergillosis in immunocompromised children.

DIFFERENTIAL DIAGNOSIS

- Bacterial sinusitis, otitis, or pneumonia
- Asthma, cystic fibrosis
- Nocardia, *Streptococcus pneumoniae*, and *Staphylococcus aureus* can cause similar-appearing pulmonary lesions.

TREATMENT

MEDICATION

First Line

Voriconazole is primary therapy for invasive aspergillosis. Treatment is generally at least 12 weeks. Therapeutic drug monitoring should be performed because of interpatient variability.

Second Line

- Echinocandins (micafungin, caspofungin)
- Amphotericin B and the lipid-based amphotericin products can be used for salvage therapy or empirically in cases when mold is suspected and zygomycetes cannot be ruled out. Lipid-based products tend to have less toxicity and may be better tolerated.
- Posaconazole: requires that patients tolerate a fatty diet for optimal absorption
- Itraconazole is occasionally used as step-down therapy for mild to moderate aspergillosis, but with newer agents, this is rarely necessary.

ADDITIONAL TREATMENT

General Measures

- Otomycosis: As it is often a coinfection with bacterial external otitis, treatment of the bacterial infection and debridement of canal debris is usually curative. Otic antifungal preparations or acetic acid may be considered if the tympanic membrane is intact.
- Sinusitis: If noninvasive, surgical drainage or debridement is usually curative.
- ABPA: First-line therapy is oral steroids. Addition of itraconazole or voriconazole may help refractory cases.
- Aspergilloma: Surgical excision is necessary as antifungals cannot penetrate cavitation well.

SURGERY/OTHER PROCEDURES

Surgical excision or localized debridement, in addition to antifungal medication, may be required for invasive disease. Mortality may be improved with surgical excision of lung lesions, but the procedure itself is often risky.

ONGOING CARE

FOLLOW-UP RECOMMENDATIONS

Patient Monitoring

Ongoing infections should be carefully monitored with serial radiographic studies as complications can be severe.

ALERT

- The classic radiographic findings of pulmonary aspergillosis are infrequently seen in children and their absence should NOT be used to eliminate *Aspergillus* as the causative agent.
- Evaluation for *Aspergillus* should be performed in immunocompromised patients with persistent fever who do not improve on broad-spectrum antibiotics; empiric antifungals should be considered.
- Aspergillosis in a normal host often does not require antifungal therapy.

PROGNOSIS

- Noninvasive disease (otomycosis, sinusitis) in the normal host usually resolves but may take several weeks.
- ABPA has variable outcomes: Resolution, steroid dependence, and ongoing lung destruction due to inflammatory dysregulation are all possible.
- Immunosuppressed or neutropenic patients may have rapid extension or dissemination of disease; prognosis is often very poor. Early recognition and aggressive treatment and debridement are necessary.

COMPLICATIONS

- Progression to invasive disseminated disease can occur as the initial manifestation if host factors are altered. Involvement of CNS, heart, or bones worsen prognosis.
- Otitis and sinusitis can erode through cranial bones to involve the orbits or CNS.
- Pulmonary disease can progress to pulmonary hemorrhage as angioinvasion occurs; respiratory failure or pneumothorax may develop as lung tissue is destroyed.

ADDITIONAL READING

- Burgos A, Zaoutis TE, Dvorak CC, et al. Pediatric invasive aspergillosis: a multicenter retrospective analysis of 139 contemporary cases. *Pediatrics*. 2008;121(5):e1286–e1294.
- Choi SH, Kang ES, Eo H, et al. *Aspergillus* galactomannan antigen assay and invasive aspergillosis in pediatric cancer patients and hematopoietic stem cell transplant recipients. *Pediatr Blood Cancer*. 2013;60(2):316–322.
- Huppmann MV, Monson M. Allergic bronchopulmonary aspergillosis: a unique presentation in a pediatric patient. *Pediatr Radiol*. 2008;38(8):879–883.
- Schubert MS. Allergic fungal sinusitis: pathophysiology, diagnosis and management. *Med Mycol*. 2009;47(Suppl 1):S324–S330.
- Stevens DA, Melikian GL. Aspergillosis in the "nonimmunocompromised" host. *Immunol Invest*. 2011;40(7–8):751–766.
- Vennewald I, Klemm E. Otomycosis: diagnosis and treatment. *Clin Dermatol*. 2010;28(2):202–211.
- Walsh TJ, Anaissie EJ, Denning DW, et al. Treatment of aspergillosis: clinical practice guidelines of the Infectious Diseases Society of America. *Clin Infect Dis*. 2008;46(3):327–360.

CODES

ICD10

- B44.9 Aspergillosis, unspecified
- B44.1 Other pulmonary aspergillosis
- B44.81 Allergic bronchopulmonary aspergillosis

FAQ

- Q: Is aspergillosis contagious?
- A: No. Disease is acquired by inhalation of airborne spores. People living or working in the same environment may be exposed to similar amounts of spores so clusters of infection are possible.

ASPLENIA/HYPOSPLENIA

Joseph A. Picoraro • Sarah S. Lusman

BASICS

DESCRIPTION

- Asplenia is the absence of the spleen due to either a congenital anomaly or a surgical procedure.
- Hyposplenia is the reduced or absent function of the spleen, impairing the capacity to prevent bacterial infections.

EPIDEMIOLOGY

- The exact incidence is not known.
- Asplenia is present in about 3% of neonates with structural heart disease.
- Isolated asplenia is most often recognized at autopsy.

PATHOPHYSIOLOGY

- The spleen is a major component of the reticuloendothelial system; it is important both for antibody synthesis and for clearance of opsonized organisms by phagocytosis.
- Antibody-mediated phagocytosis is the primary mechanism to destroy encapsulated microbes, such as pneumococcus, meningococcus, and *Haemophilus*.
- In the absence of the spleen's phagocytic pathway, the polysaccharide-rich capsules of these bacteria protect them from destruction and permit them to effect systemic bacterial infection that may lead to overwhelming sepsis.
- For patients <4 years of age in whom few alternate routes of bacterial clearance exist, significant pathology can result from impaired splenic function.

ETIOLOGY

- Surgical splenectomy
- Congenital asplenia
- In association with certain diseases or conditions (see "Differential Diagnosis")

COMMONLY ASSOCIATIED CONDITIONS

- Besides splenectomy, when asplenia is known, patients with certain diseases are at risk of asplenia or hyposplenia (see "Differential Diagnosis").
- Asplenia or hyposplenia should be suspected in any patient with overwhelming infection with an encapsulated organism.

DIAGNOSIS

HISTORY

- Any patient with a condition known to be associated with asplenia/hyposplenia (see "Differential Diagnosis") deserves evaluation for splenic function.
- In the apparently healthy child with no identified risk factors who presents with an overwhelming infection with an encapsulated organism, a blood smear should be examined for signs of hyposplenism (see "Lab").

PHYSICAL EXAM

- The spleen may be normal, large, or nonpalpable. Therefore, the size of the spleen cannot be used as an indicator of splenic function.
- The size is most closely linked to the underlying etiology.
  - Portal hypertension or complete splenic replacement by cysts, neoplasm, or amyloid can lead to splenomegaly.
  - Sequestration crises such as those associated with sickle cell disease and malaria clog the spleen with cellular debris, which may also result in increased spleen size.
  - Sickle cell disease patients typically have splenomegaly early in life, as the spleen tends to sequester the abnormal red cells. With time, the spleen slowly autoinfarcts and eventually becomes nonpalpable.

DIAGNOSTIC TESTS & INTERPRETATION

Lab

- The reduction or absence of splenic function can be determined by specific hematologic changes detectable on a blood smear.
  - The spleen normally removes intercellular debris such as Howell-Jolly bodies (nuclear remnants), Heinz bodies (denatured hemoglobin), and Pappenheimer bodies (iron granules).
  - Findings of target cells (red cells with a bull's eye center due to excessive membrane relative to the amount of iron and hemoglobin), Howell-Jolly bodies, Heinz bodies, Pappenheimer bodies, and pitted (or pocked) erythrocytes are indicative of hyposplenia or asplenia.
- Surface indentations, pits or "pocks," of the red cell surface when seen in >12% of red blood cells are the most sensitive indicator of hyposplenia. These are submembranous vacuoles that can be seen only in wet preparations of red cells fixed in 1% glutaraldehyde and viewed using direct interference-contrast microscopy.

Imaging

- US with Doppler: to assess spleen size and direction of flow in splenic vein and portal vessels
- CT/MRI: to detect polysplenia
- Radionucleotide (technetium-99m) liver/spleen scan: to detect functional reticuloendothelial cells

DIFFERENTIAL DIAGNOSIS

Diminished splenic function is associated with the following:

- Congenital
  - Isolated congenital asplenia
  - Heterotaxy syndrome
- Hematologic
  - Sequestration crises (e.g., sickle hemoglobinopathies, essential thrombocytosis, malaria)
  - Sickle cell disease
  - Hereditary hemoglobinopathies
- Autoimmune
  - Glomerulonephritis
  - Systemic lupus erythematosus
  - Rheumatoid arthritis
  - Sarcoidosis
  - Sjögren syndrome
  - Graves disease
  - Graft-versus-host disease
- GI/hepatic
  - Celiac disease
  - Inflammatory bowel disease
  - Chronic liver disease/portal hypertension
- Space-occupying lesions
  - Tumors, such as lymphoma
  - Amyloidosis
  - Cysts
- Postsplenectomy
  - Trauma
  - β-Thalassemia
  - Hereditary spherocytosis
- Vascular
  - Splenic artery occlusion
  - Splenic vein thrombosis
- Miscellaneous:
  - Normal infants
  - Elderly
  - Bone marrow transplant
  - HIV infection
- Splenic irradiation

TREATMENT

GENERAL MEASURES

- Immunization with pneumococcal, meningococcal and *Haemophilus* vaccines should be carried out in all patients with asplenia/hyposplenia.
- In those patients who will be undergoing a scheduled splenectomy, the pneumococcal, meningococcal, and *Haemophilus* vaccines should be given at least 14 days prior to the operation.
- All children between 6 weeks and 59 months of age should receive the 4-dose series of the 13-valent pneumococcal conjugate vaccine (PCV13).
  - In children 2–5 years of age with asplenia/hyposplenia, the 23-valent pneumococcal polysaccharide vaccine (PPSV23) should be administered following the 4-dose series of PCV13.
  - A repeat of the PPSV23 should be administered 5 years after the initial dose.
- Infants between 6 weeks and 18 months of age with asplenia/hyposplenia should receive the 4-dose series of the meningococcal groups C and Y and *Haemophilus influenzae* b tetanus toxoid conjugate vaccine (Hib-MenCY-TT).
  - Children older than 19 months should wait until 2 years of age and then receive the 2-dose series of the quadrivalent meningococcal conjugate vaccine (MenACWY).
  - Revaccination is recommended every 5 years.
- Children should also receive the *Haemophilus influenzae* type b vaccine if not completed, as above.
- Antimicrobial prophylaxis should be strongly considered in all children with asplenia/hyposplenia.
  - Penicillin or amoxicillin is most commonly used; however, with increasing penicillin resistance, it may be replaced by amoxicillin-clavulanic acid, fluoroquinolones, or cefuroxime.
- Sickle cell patients have impaired splenic function at all stages and should receive antimicrobial prophylaxis.

INPATIENT CONSIDERATIONS

Any patient with asplenia/hyposplenia with a febrile illness should be evaluated for systemic bacterial illness. Blood culture with broad-spectrum antibiotic coverage should be strongly considered.

ONGOING CARE

PATIENT EDUCATION

- Patients should be counseled regarding the risk of bacterial infection and considerations in setting of febrile illness.
- MedicAlert bracelets/necklaces can be used to indicate splenic function and risk of sepsis.

COMPLICATIONS

- Bacteremia
  - For asplenic or hyposplenic patients, risk of bacteremia is highest in younger children and in the years immediately following splenectomy.
  - The most common pathogens causing bacteremia are the encapsulated organisms, *Streptococcus pneumonia*, *Haemophilus influenzae*, and *Neisseria meningitidis*.
  - There is also an increased risk of infection with *Babesia microti* and *Plasmodium falciparum* (intraerythrocytic parasites) and *Capnocytophaga canimorsus* (via dog bites).

ALERT

Generally, for patients <4 years, splenectomy is contraindicated because of the risk of developing bacterial infection.

ADDITIONAL READING

- Centers for Disease Control and Prevention. Use of 13-valent pneumococcal conjugate vaccine and 23-valent pneumococcal polysaccharide vaccine among children aged 6-18 years with immunocompromising conditions: recommendations of the Advisory Committee on Immunization Practices (ACIP). *MMWR Morb Mortal Wkly Rep.* 2013;62(25):521–524.
- Cohn AC, MacNeil JR, Clark TA, et al; Centers for Disease Control and Prevention. Prevention and control of meningococcal disease: recommendations of the Advisory Committee on Immunization Practices (ACIP). *MMWR Recomm Rep.* 2013;62(RR-2):1–28.
- Melles DC, de Marie S. Prevention of infections in hyposplenic and asplenic patients: an update. *Neth J Med.* 2004;62(2):45–52.
- Rubin LG and, W Schaffner W. Clinical practice. Care of the asplenic patient. *N Engl J Med.* 2014;371(4):349–356.
- Spelman D, Buttery J, Daley A, et al. Guidelines for the prevention of sepsis in asplenic and hyposplenic patients. *Intern Med J.* 2008;38(5):349–356.

CODES

ICD10

- Q89.01 Asplenia (congenital)
- Z90.81 Acquired absence of spleen
- D73.89 Other diseases of spleen

FAQ

- Q: What should I do if my child has a fever?
- A: All patients with asplenia/hyposplenia should be evaluated for a serious bacterial infection and treated appropriately.
- Q: Are there any special times I need to worry about infections?
- A: Patients with asplenia/hyposplenia receiving dental work or GI endoscopy should be considered on a case-by-case basis. Antibiotic prophylaxis should be strongly considered in patients undergoing high-risk endoscopic procedures (i.e., sclerotherapy or stricture dilation).Rubin LG and, W Schaffner W. Clinical practice. Care of the asplenic patient. *N Engl J Med.* 2014;371(4):349–356.

ASTHMA

Lee J. Brooks

BASICS

DESCRIPTION

- Characterized by 3 components:
  - Reversible airway obstruction
  - Airway inflammation
  - Airway hyperresponsiveness to a variety of stimuli
- Diagnosis (the 3 "R"s)
  - Recurrence: Symptoms are recurrent.
  - Reactivity: Symptoms are brought on by a specific occurrence or exposure (trigger).
  - Responsive: Symptoms diminish in response to bronchodilator or anti-inflammatory agent.

ALERT

Pitfalls

- Not recognizing that asthma can manifest as chronic cough; wheezing may not be evident.
- Reluctance to "label" child with having asthma (using terms such as reactive airway disease or bronchitis)
- Frequent antibiotic or cough medicine use to treat asthma symptoms
- "Recurrent pneumonias" often are actually asthma exacerbations; subsegmental atelectasis on chest radiograph misdiagnosed as an infiltrate
- Underreporting of asthma symptoms; beware of the child who "doesn't like to play sports"; he/she may have learned that exercise causes dyspnea.
- Poor adherence with therapy when symptoms are controlled
- Failure to use inhaled medications properly: Inhaled medication use must be taught and reviewed at each visit. A fixed-volume holding chamber should always be used with a pressurized metered-dose inhaler (pMDI), regardless of patient age. pMDIs should be refilled based on the number of doses used, not by estimating contents by shaking or spraying. pMDIs with a built-in dose counter are preferred.

EPIDEMIOLOGY

Incidence

- Most common chronic illness in children
- About 20% of children are diagnosed with asthma at some point before age 20 years.
- Death from asthma in children more than tripled from 1979 to 1996 but has been decreasing since then, perhaps owing to better recognition and increased use of anti-inflammatory medications. The incidence of death from asthma does not seem to correlate with severity.

Prevalence

- Wheezing in children is extremely common in the industrialized world (cumulative prevalence, 30–60%).
- In younger children, most episodes occur following viral infections.
- >50% of children who wheeze in early childhood stop wheezing by age 6 years.
- 14% of all young children (40% of those who wheeze during infancy) continue to wheeze.

RISK FACTORS

Genetics

- Children of asthmatics have higher incidence of asthma.
  - 6–7% risk if neither parent has asthma
  - 20% risk if 1 parent has asthma
  - 60% risk if both parents have asthma
- Several genes are known to be associated with the development of atopy and bronchial muscle responsiveness.

GENERAL PREVENTION

- Patient and caregiver education is mandatory to establish provider/caregiver partnership and ensure adherence with treatment plan.
- Every patient/caregiver should be taught that asthma is a chronic, inflammatory condition that can be controlled with proper therapy.
- All medications should be explained and potential risks (side effects) and benefits reviewed.
- A written asthma management plan should be provided, outlining daily therapy and an "action plan" for managing exacerbations of asthma.
- Environmental counseling:
  - Avoid airborne irritants (tobacco smoke, wood stoves, noxious fumes).
  - Minimize dust-mite exposure.
  - Minimize stuffed animals, quilts, books, and clutter.
  - Use dust mite–proof coverings on mattresses, pillows, and box springs.
  - Wash pillows, blankets, and sheets in hot water.
  - Avoid molds by decreasing relative humidity to 50%.
  - Remove pets from child's bedroom and from house if patient is allergic to the animal.

PATHOPHYSIOLOGY

- Immune and inflammatory responses in the airways are triggered by an array of environmental antigens, irritants, or infectious organisms.
- Atopy and asthma are related.
  - Eosinophilia and the ability to make excess IgE in response to antigen are associated with increased airway reactivity.
  - Asthma is more common in children who have allergic rhinitis and eczema.
- Viral infections, particularly respiratory syncytial virus (RSV) during infancy, may play a role in the development of asthma or may modify the severity of asthma.
- Exposure to cigarette smoke and other airway irritants influences the development and severity of asthma.
- Airway is stimulated and primary inflammatory mediators released.
- Airway is invaded by inflammatory cells (mast cells, basophils, eosinophils, macrophages, neutrophils, B and T lymphocytes).
- Inflammatory cells respond to and produce various mediators (cytokines, leukotrienes, lymphokines), augmenting the inflammatory response.
- Airway epithelium is inflamed and becomes disrupted, and basal membrane is thickened.
- Airway smooth muscle is hyperresponsive, and bronchoconstriction ensues.
- Airway smooth muscle hypertrophy and airway epithelial hyperplasia are characteristic chronic changes resulting from poorly controlled asthma.

DIAGNOSIS

HISTORY

- Inquire about these symptoms: coughing, wheezing, shortness of breath, chest tightness:
  - Frequency of symptoms defines severity.
  - Precipitating factor (trigger)
  - Response to bronchodilator or anti-inflammatory medication
  - Family history of asthma or atopy
- Pattern of symptoms:
  - Perennial versus seasonal
  - Continuous versus acute
  - Duration and frequency of episodes
  - Diurnal variation/nocturnal symptoms

- Do any of the following set off the breathing difficulty?
  - Infections (upper respiratory, sinusitis)
  - Exposure to dust (mites), animal dander, pollen, mold
  - Cold air or weather changes
  - Exercise or play
  - Environmental stimulants (e.g., cigarette smoke, strong odors, pollutants)
  - Emotional factors (e.g., laughing, crying, fear)
  - Drug intake (aspirin, nonsteroidal anti-inflammatory drugs, β-blockers)
  - Food additives
  - Endocrine factors (e.g., menses, pregnancy, thyroid dysfunction)
- Review of systems:
  - Symptoms of complicating factors (gastroesophageal reflux, sinusitis, allergies)
  - Dyspepsia, sour taste (gastroesophageal reflux); throat clearing, purulent nasal discharge, halitosis, cephalalgia, or facial pain (sinusitis); nasal itching ("allergic salute"), eye rubbing, sneezing, watery nasal discharge (allergies)
- Impact of asthma:
  - Number of hospitalizations/intensive care unit admissions
  - Number of emergency room visits/doctor's office visits
  - Asthma attack frequency
  - Number of missed school days/parent workdays
  - Limitation on activity (may be subtle)
  - Number of courses of systemic steroids needed
- Environmental history:
  - Type of home
  - Location of home (urban, suburban, rural)
  - Heating system/air conditioning
  - Use of humidifier
  - Presence of molds, cockroaches, rodents
  - Fireplace/wood burning stove
  - Carpeting
  - Stuffed animals
  - Pets
  - Exposure to cigarette smoke

PHYSICAL EXAM

- Pulmonary exam may be normal when asymptomatic.
- Assess work of breathing:
  - Level of distress
  - Intercostal/supraclavicular muscle retractions
- Chest shape (i.e., normal vs. barrel-shaped)
- Lung auscultation:
  - Wheezing
  - End-expiratory involuntary cough
  - Prolonged expiratory phase
  - Crackles or coarse breath sounds
  - Stridor (indicates extrathoracic airway obstruction)
- Head, eyes, ears, nose, and throat exam: signs of allergies or sinusitis:
  - Watery or itchy eyes
  - Allergic shiners
  - Dennie lines
  - Nasal congestion
  - Boggy nasal turbinates
  - Nasal polyps
  - Postnasal drip
- General exam (vital signs):
  - Blood pressure (pulsus paradoxus)
  - Respiratory rate (tachypnea)
- Skin: evidence of eczema
- Extremities: digital clubbing (very rare in asthma; suggests alternative diagnosis)
- Physical exam pearl: forced-exhalation maneuver to observe for wheezes or for precipitating coughing

DIAGNOSTIC TESTS & INTERPRETATION

Lab

- Pulmonary function tests
  - Very sensitive; may show airway obstruction even when the physical exam is normal
  - Essential for the assessment and ongoing care of children with asthma
  - Spirometer measures the degree of airway obstruction and the response to bronchodilators.
  - Values obtained can measure absolute degree of airway obstruction.
  - Serial values can follow progress of disease and response to treatment.
  - Children as young as 4–5 years old can usually perform spirometry with practice.
- Provocational testing
  - Exercise challenge: determines effect of exercise on triggering airway obstruction
  - Cold-air challenge: indirect test of airway hyperresponsiveness
  - Methacholine challenge: A positive test supports the diagnosis of asthma (useful in cases for which history is equivocal and pulmonary function test is normal), measures the degree of airway hyperreactivity.
- Allergy evaluation:
  - Blood tests (eosinophil count, IgE level)
  - Skin testing (best test for assessing allergen sensitivity)
  - RAST testing (not as accurate as skin testing)
  - Sputum/nasal examination for presence of eosinophilia
- Exhaled nitric oxide
- Identifies Th2-mediated airway inflammation
- May identify/exclude steroid responsive airway inflammation
- Other studies:
  - Gastroesophageal reflux evaluation
  - pH probe
  - Milk scan
  - Barium swallow (confirms normal anatomy)
- Peak flow meter (home testing)
  - Measures peak flow rate (PEFR)
  - Effort-dependent
  - Assesses central, not peripheral, airway obstruction
  - Used with patients who have poor symptom recognition or labile asthma
  - Dips in peak flow rate precede onset of clinical asthmatic symptoms.
  - Peak flow rate should be performed at least once a day.
  - Peak flow rate values are divided into 3 zones:
    - Green: ≥80% of baseline
    - Yellow: 50–80% of baseline
    - Red: 50% of baseline
- Specific peak flow rate guidelines should be individualized for each patient based on the best measurement obtained during a 14-day period when the child is well.

Imaging

- Chest radiograph
  - Can be obtained if the diagnosis is uncertain or there is not the expected response to treatment, to rule out congenital lung malformations or obvious vascular malformations
    - Findings can be normal.
    - Common findings are peribronchial thickening, subsegmental atelectasis, and hyperinflation.
- Sinus CT is useful if symptoms suggest sinusitis.
- Chest CT should be performed if bronchiectasis or anatomic abnormality is suspected.

Diagnostic Procedures/Other

Bronchoscopy can rule out anatomic malformations, foreign bodies, mucous plugging, vocal cord dysfunction, and aspiration (lipid-laden macrophages).

DIFFERENTIAL DIAGNOSIS

- Infectious
  - Pneumonia
  - Bronchiolitis
  - *Chlamydia* infection
  - Laryngotracheobronchitis
  - Sinusitis
  - Immune deficiency
- Mechanical
  - Extrinsic airway compression
  - Vascular ring
  - Foreign body
  - Vocal cord dysfunction
  - Tracheobronchomalacia
- Miscellaneous:
  - Cystic fibrosis
  - Bronchopulmonary dysplasia
  - Pulmonary edema
  - Gastroesophageal reflux
  - Recurrent aspiration
  - Bronchiolitis obliterans

TREATMENT

MEDICATION

- Corticosteroids (anti-inflammatory agents)
  - Most effective anti-inflammatory agents
  - Inhaled: reduce airway inflammation and hyperresponsiveness more than any other inhaled agents; inhibit production and release of cytokines and arachidonic acid–associated metabolites; enhance β-adrenoreceptor responsiveness
    - Side effects include oral thrush; may minimally affect growth velocity at moderate or high doses
    - Dosage individualized to each patient (see Figure 5 in Appendix for Stepwise Approach for Managing Asthma Long Term). Agents vary in topical potency and systemic bioavailability; available as pMDIs, dry-powder inhalers (DPIs), or nebulized. Fluticasone (Flovent) 44, 110, 220 mcg/puff pMDI and 50, 100, 250 mcg DPI; budesonide (Pulmicort) 90, 180 mcg/puff DPI and 250, 500, and 1,000-mcg vials for nebulizer; beclomethasone (Qvar) 40, 80 mcg/puff; flunisolide (AeroBid) 80 mcg/puff; ciclesonide (Alvesco) 80, 160 mcg/puff; mometasone (Asmanex) 100 mcg/puff pMDI and 110, 220 mcg DPI (see Table 14 in Appendix for Comparative doses)
  - Oral: used for asthma exacerbations or for severe asthma that cannot be otherwise controlled.
    - Exacerbations: prednisone or prednisolone 1–2 mg/kg/24 hr for 3–7 days or longer; usually tapered if >7 days of therapy required or if systemic steroids are used frequently. Shorter 2-day courses of oral dexamethasone have also been described in clinical trials.
    - Ongoing therapy: 0.5–1 mg/kg/24 hr daily or every other day for patients with severe asthma
    - Undesirable side-effect profile. When used daily, assess bone density and for cataract formation at least yearly.
  - IV: Methylprednisolone (Solu-Medrol) 1–2 mg/kg/24 hr IV divided q6–12h until improved and able to take oral medication
- Leukotriene modifiers (anti-inflammatory agents)
  - Block the synthesis and/or action of leukotrienes
  - 5-lipoxygenase inhibitors, zileuton: may cause hepatic dysfunction
  - Leukotriene receptor antagonists: zafirlukast (10 mg; Accolate) and montelukast (4, 5, and 10 mg; Singulair)
  - Indicated as monotherapy for mild or exercise-induced asthma and in combination with an inhaled corticosteroid for more effective symptom control or using a lower dose of inhaled corticosteroid
- Mast-cell stabilizers
  - Weak anti-inflammatory agents
  - Preparations: cromolyn sodium; nedocromil sodium (Tilade, available in Canada)
  - Decrease bronchial hyperresponsiveness
  - Can be used prior to exercise for exercise-induced symptoms
  - No significant side effects
  - Inhaled: nebulizer; MDI
- β_2-Agonists (bronchodilators)
  - Indication is for relief of acute bronchoconstriction (quick-relief medicine); used as needed in people with asthma who have breakthrough symptoms; used prior to exercise in exercise-induced bronchospasm
  - Regular use or overuse associated with worsened control of asthma
  - Routes include metered-dose inhaler or nebulizer
  - Short-acting (4–6 hours) preparations include albuterol (Ventolin, Proventil, ProAir), terbutaline (Brethaire, Brethine), and metaproterenol (Alupent); a single-isomer preparation of albuterol (Xopenex) may have a slightly longer duration of action and perhaps fewer side effects.
  - Longer acting (up to 12 hours) preparations include salmeterol (Serevent) and formoterol (Foradil) available as pMDI, and DPI can be used daily in conjunction with anti-inflammatory agent for improved symptom control.
  - Fixed combination products of inhaled corticosteroid and a long-acting β-agonist (Advair, Dulera, Symbicort) are available as DPIs and pMDIs.
- There may be an increased risk of asthma-related deaths in patients using long-acting β-agonists (LABAs), and it is suggested that LABAs be prescribed only for patients not adequately controlled on other asthma-controller medications or whose disease severity warrants initiation of treatment with 2 maintenance therapies.
- Theophylline (bronchodilator)
  - 2nd-line agent used when more conventional therapies are unsuccessful
  - Indications are chronic, poorly controlled asthma and nocturnal asthma (if no gastroesophageal reflux); adjunctive therapy with β_2-drugs and steroids in hospitalized patients in selected cases; route (oral or IV); serum levels must be routinely monitored (therapeutic levels are 10–20 mg/mL).
  - Side effects are seen with increased levels.
  - Many factors affect theophylline levels. Increased levels are seen with erythromycin, ciprofloxacin, cimetidine, viral illnesses, fever. Decreased levels are seen with phenobarbital, phenytoin, rifampin.
  - Sustained-release tablets should not be crushed.
- Anticholinergic agents (bronchodilators): Adjunctive bronchodilators may be useful in patients who only partially respond to β-agonists; preparations include ipratropium bromide MDI or ampule for nebulization (Atrovent).
- Monoclonal antibodies against IgE (Xolair) can be given as a monthly SC injection in severe asthma patients with moderately high IgE levels.

ISSUES FOR REFERRAL

- A patient who requires hospitalization more than once a year, or who has required intensive care
- A patient who requires frequent bursts of systemic corticosteroids
- A patient whose airway obstruction is not easily reversible
- A patient who has clinical features suggesting another pulmonary process

COMPLEMENTARY & ALTERNATIVE THERAPIES

- Miscellaneous drugs used in severe cases
- Steroid-sparing agents:
  - Troleandomycin (TAO): Macrolide antibiotic decreases clearance of corticosteroids, thus prolonging the effects of corticosteroids on the lung; lower corticosteroid dosing required

– Methotrexate: Potent immunosuppressive drug needs further investigation in children.
– Cyclosporine: shown to have steroid-sparing effect in adult population with asthma; side effects are significant and may limit use.
– Magnesium sulfate ($MgSO_4$): used intravenously as a smooth muscle relaxer in severe acute asthma exacerbation

- Helium
  – May improve airflow in severe asthma
  – Can improve ventilation and potentially oxygenation
- Immunotherapy
  – Efficacy in asthma is controversial.
  – Most effective if a single antigen can be identified
  – Used only in select cases if medical management and environmental control measures are ineffective

ONGOING CARE

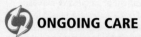

FOLLOW-UP RECOMMENDATIONS

Long-term follow-up is essential to maintain normal activity and pulmonary function. All patients should use a valved holding chamber with pMDIs, and technique for all inhaled medications should be reviewed regularly.

Patient Monitoring

Signs that may indicate problems: increased symptoms (cough day or night, wheeze), exercise limitations or symptoms during exercise, decrease in peak flow rate, increasing use of inhaled bronchodilators, subject not improving on enhanced home therapy. For patients requiring a daily controller medication, regularly assess level of asthma control based on a standard clinical instrument (e.g., pediatric asthma control test [P-ACT], the Asthma Therapy Assessment Questionnaire for children and adolescents [the pediatric ATAQ]). If asthma not well controlled, consider increasing level of daily controller medication.

DIET

- Avoid foods or food additives (if truly allergic).
- Food-induced asthma is uncommon.

PATIENT EDUCATION

Activity

- Most patients with asthma can participate fully in sports, even at a high level, with close follow-up. Extra medications such as albuterol and/or cromolyn may be required before vigorous exercise. All athletes should have their quick-relief medications on hand at all times.
- Athletes with asthma may need to report their medications to the governing bodies of their sport.

PROGNOSIS

With proper therapy and good adherence to treatment regimen: excellent

COMPLICATIONS

Morbidity: frequent hospitalizations and absence from school. Psychological impact of having a chronic illness. Decline in lung function over time

ADDITIONAL READING

- Allen JL, Bryant-Stephens T, Pawlowski NA. *The Children's Hospital of Philadelphia Guide to Asthma*. Philadelphia: Wiley-Liss; 2004.
- Bush A, Saglani S. Management of severe asthma in children. *Lancet*. 2010;376(9743):814–825.
- Ducharme FM, Ni Chroinin M, Greenstone I, et al. Addition of long-acting beta2-agonists to inhaled corticosteroids versus same dose inhaled corticosteroids for chronic asthma in adults and children. *Cochrane Database Syst Rev*. 2010;(5):CD005535.
- Halken S, Lau S, Valovirta E. New visions in specific immunotherapy in children: an iPAC summary and future trends. *Pediatr Allergy Immunol*. 2008;19(Suppl 19):60–70.
- Hedlin G, Konradsen J, Bush A. An update on paediatric asthma. *Eur Respir Rev*. 2012;21(125):175–185.
- Kercsmar CM. Current trends in management of pediatric asthma. *Respir Care*. 2003;48(3):194–205; discussion 205–208.
- Liu AH, Szefler SJ. Advances in childhood asthma: hygiene hypothesis, natural history, and management. *J Allergy Clin Immunol*. 2003;111(3)(Suppl):S785–S792.
- Mahr TA, Malka J, Spahn JD. Inflammometry in pediatric asthma: a review of fractional exhaled nitric oxide in clinical practice. *Allergy Asthma Proc*. 2013;34(3):210–219.
- National Asthma Education and Prevention Program. *Expert Panel Report 3: Guidelines for the diagnosis and management of asthma*. NIH-NHLBI publication. Washington, DC: U.S. Government Printing Office; August 2007.
- Reid MJ. Complicating features of asthma. *Pediatr Clin North Am*. 1992;39(6):1327–1341.
- Salvatoni A, Piantanida E, Nosetti L, et al. Inhaled corticosteroids in childhood asthma: long-term effects on growth and adrenocortical function. *Paediatr Drugs*. 2003;5(6):351–361.
- Silverstein MD, Mair JE, Katusic SK, et al. School attendance and school performance: a population-based study of children with asthma. *J Pediatr*. 2001;139(2):278–283.
- Stempel DA. The pharmacologic management of childhood asthma. *Pediatr Clin North Am*. 2003;50(3):609–629.

CODES

ICD10

- J45.909 Unspecified asthma, uncomplicated
- J45.901 Unspecified asthma with (acute) exacerbation
- J45.990 Exercise induced bronchospasm

FAQ

- Q: Will my child outgrow his or her asthma?
- A: Family history and allergies affect the ultimate outcome. Wheezing during the 1st 3 years of life is extremely common, with 40–50% of all children wheezing at some time. Many of these children do not develop asthma and "outgrow" their illness by school age. Some patients develop asthma again as young adults.
- Q: Can my child become dependent on asthma medications?
- A: Children do not become "dependent" on these medications as they would with narcotic agents. Daily asthma medications are required to maintain airway patency and to control airway inflammation.
- Q: Will my child be on medications for the rest of his or her life?
- A: This depends on the severity of the asthma. The types, doses, and frequency of asthma medications will change over a patient's lifetime.

ATAXIA

Kristin W. Barañano

BASICS

DESCRIPTION

- Ataxia refers to incoordination of movement out of proportion to weakness.
- Can be caused by dysfunction of cerebellum, proprioception, or vestibular system
- Careful history of timing of onset and antecedent events key in framing differential: acute, subacute, chronic/progressive, episodic

EPIDEMIOLOGY

- Acute cerebellar ataxia (ACA) was previously seen in 1 per 5,000 cases of varicella, accounting for 25% of total cases. The risk following varicella-zoster virus (VZV) vaccination is 1.5 per 1,000,000 doses.
- Most cases of ACA are still postviral, followed by ingestions, then Guillain-Barré syndrome (GBS) (combined account for 80% of total).
- Dominantly inherited spinocerebellar ataxias (SCAs) are 1–5 per 100,000 but tend to have a later age of onset.
- More likely to see autosomal recessive (AR) ataxias in childhood; most common is Friedreich (FRDA) at 1 in 30,000–50,000

PATHOPHYSIOLOGY

- The cerebellum does not generate motor commands; instead, it modifies them to make them accurate and adaptive.
- The cerebellum receives input from the vestibular apparatus, spinal cord, and the cerebral cortex (via the pons).
- Both input and output is ipsilateral (i.e., right-sided cerebellar lesions cause right-sided ataxia).
- Midline cerebellum (vermis) controls gait, head and trunk stability, eye movements; lesions of vermis result in wide-based ("drunken sailor") gait, truncal sway, and head titubation (bobbling movements).
- Cerebellar hemispheres control limb tone and coordination, motor learning, speech, eye movements; lesions of the cerebellar hemispheres cause limb dysmetria (trouble with finger nose finger testing).
- Function can be impaired by chemicals, autoimmune processes, genetic mutations; typical pathologic finding is loss of Purkinje cells and injury to their elaborate dendritic arbor.

ETIOLOGY

- Acute onset
  - Ingestions/intoxications: alcohol, anticonvulsants including phenytoin, benzodiazepines, antihistamines, heavy metals, carbon monoxide
  - Infections (e.g., *Bartonella*, *Mycoplasma*, Epstein-Barr virus)
  - Postinfectious
  - Postvaccination
  - Demyelinating events: multiple sclerosis, acute disseminated encephalomyelitis (ADEM) (can be associated with altered mental status and seizure), Miller Fisher variant of GBS (triad of ataxia, ophthalmoplegia, areflexia; look for eye movement abnormalities and areflexia)
  - Initial presentation of recurrent ataxia
- Subacute onset
  - Cerebellar hemorrhage
  - Ischemic stroke
  - Encephalitis or cerebellitis
  - Acute labyrinthitis/vestibular neuronitis (often prominent nausea/vomiting, hearing affected)
  - Posterior fossa tumors (e.g., medulloblastoma)
  - Paraneoplastic syndromes (opsoclonus-myoclonus syndrome, with multidirectional chaotic eye movements; evaluate for neuroblastoma)
- Chronic or progressive
  - Developmental defects: Dandy Walker, cerebellar agenesis, rhombencephalosynapsis, Chiari I malformation
  - Ataxic cerebral palsy
  - Tumors
  - Paraneoplastic
  - Metabolic/degenerative
    - With pathologic accumulation: hexosaminidase deficiency, Niemann-Pick type C, metachromatic leukodystrophy, Wilson disease
    - Hypomyelinating leukodystrophies (e.g., Pelizaeus-Merzbacher disease)
    - SCAs
    - AR ataxias including FRDA (associated pes cavus, cardiomyopathy, diabetes, polyneuropathy), ataxia telangiectasia (frequent infections, increased susceptibility to leukemia/lymphoma; telangiectasias are a late finding, check alpha fetoprotein [AFP] level, sensitive after 1 year of age)
- Recurrent
  - Migraine (vestibular migraine can present with ataxia and vertigo without headache)
  - Episodic ataxia (EA1 and EA2 best characterized, at least 6 loci identified)
  - Metabolic disorders: mitochondrial disorders, Hartnup disease, urea cycle defects, intermittent forms of maple syrup urine disease

DIAGNOSIS

HISTORY

- Focus on the time course of onset.
- Elicit possible ingestions, access to medications at homes of friends, family
- Antecedent infections or vaccinations (fever, especially upper respiratory infection [URI] and GI symptoms)
- Recent trauma (concussion, possible vertebral artery dissection)
- Past medical history: similar episodes, migraines, congenital heart defect, multiple organ system involvement suggestive of metabolic/mitochondrial disease, unusual susceptibility to infection
- Family history: recurrent or progressive ataxias, migraines
- Symptoms to elicit: altered mental status, headache, diplopia, vertigo (illusion of movement or dizziness), history of seizure, nausea/vomiting, diminished hearing, or tinnitus

PHYSICAL EXAM

- Vital signs: presence of fever
- General exam: presence of meningismus, otoscopic examination for otitis, assess for pharyngitis, lymphadenopathy, splenomegaly, rash, skin and eyes for telangiectasias
- Neurologic exam
  - Mental status: altered with ingestions, CNS infections, ADEM
  - Cranial nerves: funduscopic exam for papilledema, eye movement abnormalities, presence of nystagmus, head impulse (thrust) test for vestibular function, hearing with tuning fork (Weber and Rinne tests), dysarthria or scanning speech
  - Motor: presence of hypotonia or tremor, exclude weakness as cause of incoordination
  - Reflexes: absence suggestive of GBS
  - Sensory: assess for sensory ataxia due to lack of proprioceptive input
  - Coordination: presence of head titubation, truncal ataxia, intention tremor, and limb dysmetria with finger-nose-finger, overshoot with finger-chase, dysdiadochokinesia with rapid alternating movements, heel to shin test
  - Gait: ability to tandem walk, sway with Romberg test (either cerebellar or proprioceptive defect)

DIAGNOSTIC TESTS & INTERPRETATION

Labs

- Initial ER screening labs for acute presentation:
  - CBC, comprehensive metabolic panel (CMP)
  - Lactate, ammonia
  - Toxicology screen and drug levels for specific intoxications
- Additional investigations for chronic/progressive ataxias:
  - Rule out reversible/potentially treatable causes:
    - Exposures: heavy metals, zinc (chelates copper)
    - Autoimmune: celiac, anti-glutamic acid decarboxylase (GAD), paraneoplastic panel, urine homovanillic acid/vanillylmandelic acid (HVA/VMA) for neuroblastoma
    - Metabolic: TSH, vitamin E, coenzyme Q, B_{12} and B_1 levels, copper, ceruloplasmin, lactate, ammonia, plasma amino acids, urine organic acids, urine amino acids (for Hartnup disease), very-long-chain fatty acid (VLCFA) with phytanic acid (Refsum), paired CSF and serum glucose levels or *SLC2A1* sequencing for GLUT1 deficiency, cholestanol (cerebrotendinous xanthomatosis), lysosomal enzymes
  - Other potential screening laboratories: lipid panel, IgA levels, AFP
  - Ataxia panels for inherited cerebellar ataxias (e.g., SCAs); most not clinically distinguishable in early stages

Imaging

- Head CT in the acute setting for altered mental status or concern for hemorrhage
- MRI of brain more sensitive in assessing posterior fossa pathology; consider administration of contrast if concern for infection/demyelination; MRA of brain and neck if concern for stroke/dissection.

Diagnostic Procedures/Other

- Lumbar puncture
  - For infection or ADEM: cell counts, protein, glucose, bacterial culture and viral polymerase chain reactions (PCRs), IgG index, oligoclonal bands
  - For suspected metabolic disorders: glucose, protein, cell counts, lactate, pyruvate, 5-methyltetrahydrofolate (MTHF), amino acids; pair with serum glucose and amino acids
- Metaiodobenzylguanidine (MIBG) scan and body CT for potential neuroblastoma
- Nerve conduction studies: suspected GBS
- Electronystagmography (ENG) for potential vestibular involvement
- EEG for consideration of epileptic ataxia

DIFFERENTIAL DIAGNOSIS

- Movement disorders: tremor, chorea, athetosis may be mistaken for ataxia
- Weakness: incoordination in proportion to weakness (myasthenia gravis, GBS)
- Conversion disorder: variability, distractibility, lack of associated cerebellar signs, astasia-abasia (exaggerated factitious inability to walk or stand)
- Epileptic ataxia (pseudoataxia): episodic, associated alteration of awareness
- Optic ataxia: difficulty reaching for target due to lesions in posterior parietal lobe resulting in impaired visual input to cerebellum

TREATMENT

- Treatment of many of the acute ataxias (ingestions, postviral) is supportive.
- Specific therapies
  - ADEM: steroids
  - GBS: intravenous immunoglobulin (IVIG), plasmapheresis
  - Paraneoplastic: treatment of malignancy, immunosuppression
  - Migraine: avoidance of food triggers, preventive medications (e.g., calcium channel blockers, tricyclic antidepressants [TCAs])
  - Episodic ataxias: acetazolamide
  - Inherited ataxias: some evidence for use of medications such as amantadine, riluzole, varenicline
  - Possible role for treatment with specific vitamins and cofactors (carnitine, coenzyme Q, vitamin E, riboflavin, folinic acid) for mitochondrial disorders

ONGOING CARE

PROGNOSIS

- Most acute ataxias are ingestions and postviral and have a good prognosis. If recovery from a presumed postviral ataxia is delayed (more than 2 weeks), evaluation for neuroblastoma should be undertaken.
- Recovery from GBS is generally good but can be incomplete.
- Specific diagnosis of an inherited cerebellar ataxia is helpful in predicting clinical course (time to wheelchair, potential for cognitive decline, death).

COMPLICATIONS

- Risk of injury due to falls
- Risk of aspiration due to swallow dysfunction
- Autonomic instability can be associated with GBS.
- With inherited cerebellar ataxias: Some patients also develop neuropathy, spasticity, and cognitive decline.
- Risk of depression and cognitive impairment given increasingly recognized role of cerebellum in cognition and emotion

ADDITIONAL READING

- Poretti A, Benson JE, Huisman TA, et al. Acute ataxia in children: approach to clinical presentation and role of additional investigations. *Neuropediatrics*. 2013;44(3):127–141.
- Vedolin L, Gonzalez G, Souza CF, et al. Inherited cerebellar ataxia in childhood: a pattern-recognition approach using brain MRI. *AJNR Am J Neuroradiol*. 2013;34(5):925–934.
- Whelan HT, Verma S, Guo Y, et al. Evaluation of the child with acute ataxia: a systematic review. *Pediatr Neurol*. 2013;49(1):15–24.
- National Ataxia Foundation: www.ataxia.org
- Neuromuscular Disease Center of Washington University: http://neuromuscular.wustl.edu/ataxia/aindex.html

CODES

ICD10

- R27.0 Ataxia, unspecified
- G11.9 Hereditary ataxia, unspecified
- G11.1 Early-onset cerebellar ataxia

FAQ

- Q: Which ingestions are most likely to cause ataxia?
- A: Alcohol, anticonvulsants, antihistamines, benzodiazepines, TCAs
- Q: What is the typical time course of postinfectious ataxia?
- A: Typically, it will be maximal in onset in the first day or two, then improve within 2 weeks. Ataxia persisting beyond 2 weeks should prompt evaluation for neuroblastoma.
- Q: What is the role of physical therapy for cerebellar ataxia?
- A: Studies have demonstrated that intensive coordination training improves motor performance in progressive cerebellar disorders and translates into improved activities of daily living.
- Q: What is the risk of transmitting a hereditary cerebellar ataxia?
- A: It depends of the mode of inheritance: AR (25%), autosomal dominant (50%, with risk of anticipation for disorders with polyglutamine expansion), maternal (mitochondrial and X-linked disorders).

ATELECTASIS

Richard M. Kravitz

BASICS

DESCRIPTION
- State of collapsed and airless alveoli
- May be subsegmental, segmental, or lobar or may involve the entire lung
- A radiographic sign of an underlying disease and not a diagnosis unto itself

EPIDEMIOLOGY
- Depends on the underlying disease causing atelectasis
- Resorption atelectasis is the most common form.

RISK FACTORS
Genetics

Depends on the underlying disease causing atelectasis (i.e., cystic fibrosis, primary ciliary dyskinesia)

GENERAL PREVENTION
- Maintaining adequate cough
- Good airway clearance techniques in patients at risk for atelectasis

PATHOPHYSIOLOGY
- Reduced lung compliance
- Loss of alveoli (if extensive) may lead to hypoxia.
- Intrapulmonary shunting develops from hypoxia-induced pulmonary arterial vasoconstriction, which may lead to areas of ventilation–perfusion (V/Q) mismatch and further hypoxia.
- If atelectasis is extensive and long-term, pulmonary hypertension may develop.
- Atelectatic areas are prone to bacterial overgrowth and possible secondary infection.

ETIOLOGY
- Airway obstruction (resorption atelectasis)
  - Most common cause of atelectasis in children
  - Obstructed communication between alveoli and trachea
- Large airway obstruction
  - Intrinsic
    - Foreign body aspiration
    - Mucous plug
    - Tumor
    - Plastic bronchitis
  - Extrinsic
    - Hilar adenopathy
    - Mediastinal mass
    - Congenital lung malformations
- Small airway obstruction
  - Acute infection
    - Bronchiolitis
    - Pneumonia
    - Respiratory infections are the most common cause of acute atelectasis
  - Altered mucociliary clearance:
    - CNS depression
    - Smoke inhalation
    - Pain
- Mechanical compression of the pulmonary parenchyma or pleural space (compressive atelectasis)
  - Intrathoracic compression
    - Pneumothorax
    - Pleural effusion
    - Lobar emphysema
    - Intrathoracic tumors
    - Cardiomegaly
    - Diaphragmatic hernias
  - Abdominal distention
    - Large intra-abdominal tumors
    - Hepatosplenomegaly
    - Massive ascites
    - Morbid obesity
- Decreased surface tension in the small airways and alveoli (adhesive atelectasis)
  - Stems from surfactant deficiency
  - Diffuse surfactant deficiency
    - Hyaline membrane disease
    - Acute respiratory distress syndrome
    - Smoke inhalation
  - Localized surfactant deficiency
    - Acute radiation pneumonitis
    - Pulmonary embolism
- Neuromuscular weakness (hypoventilation)
  - Inherent weakness
    - Duchenne muscular dystrophy
    - Spinal muscular atrophy
    - Paralysis
  - Acquired weakness (e.g., postanesthesia hypoventilation)

DIAGNOSIS

HISTORY
- Depends on the underlying disease process
- May be asymptomatic
- Cough and/or wheeze can be present.
- Dyspnea
- Chest pain
- Special questions:
  - Is the atelectasis acute, recurrent, or chronic in terms of its duration?
  - Is there a history of asthma, chronic lung disease, or exposure to smoke or toxic fumes that would increase the risk for atelectasis?

PHYSICAL EXAM
- May be normal
- Tachypnea
- Rales or rhonchi
- The most specific sign is localized decrease or loss of breath sounds.
- Dullness to percussion if large area involved
- Tracheal deviation and shift of heart sounds toward atelectatic side
- Localized wheezes in cases of partial obstruction
- Cyanosis (seen when extensive atelectasis is present, causing impairment of oxygenation and areas of ventilation/perfusion mismatch)

DIAGNOSTIC TESTS & INTERPRETATION
Lab

Appropriate test depends on the underlying etiology:
- Asthma
  - Spirometry
  - Sweat test (if cystic fibrosis suspected)
- Infection
  - Cultures (sputum, blood, bronchoalveolar lavage fluid)
  - Nasal washing (especially for viruses)
  - PPD (when tuberculosis is suspected)
- Foreign body aspiration
  - Bronchoscopy (to remove the obstructing agent. Rigid bronchoscopy is indicated if the obstructing agent is a foreign body; flexible: can be used for mucous plugs, plastic bronchitis, or infectious etiology)
- Immunodeficiency
  - CBC with differential
  - Immunoglobulins (IgG, IgA, IgM)
  - HIV testing
- Congenital malformations
  - CT scan of the chest (for lung malformation)
  - Bronchoscopy (for H-type tracheoesophageal fistula [TEF] or bronchial stenosis)

Imaging
- Chest radiograph
  - Most important diagnostic tool
  - Radiographic signs of atelectasis:
    - Loss of lung volume from the affected lobe
    - Compensatory hyperexpansion of the remaining lobes on the affected side
    - Shift of interlobar fissures
    - Elevation of diaphragm
    - Mediastinal shift toward the affected side
    - Approximation of ribs on the affected side
- CT of chest
  - Confluence of bronchi and blood vessels converge toward the affected side.
  - Provides information regarding precise location and extent of any obstructing process

DIFFERENTIAL DIAGNOSIS
- Pneumonia
  - Viral pneumonia versus subsegmental atelectasis
  - Bacterial pneumonia versus segmental or lobar atelectasis
- Thymus (may often be mistaken for atelectasis in an upper lobe)
- Congenital malformations (e.g., sequestration, bronchogenic cyst)
- Pleural effusion
- Asthma (acute exacerbation or poorly controlled)

TREATMENT

GENERAL MEASURES
- Treat underlying disease (i.e., removal of aspirated foreign body, clearance of mucous plugs, treatment of any underlying infection)
- Chest physical therapy with bronchodilators (usually for at least 1 month)
- If no improvement with conservative therapy, a bronchoscopy with lavage to remove possible mucous plug is indicated (lavage may be with saline or, in select cases, with recombinant human DNase, *N*-acetylcysteine, or hypertonic saline).
- Consider surgery to remove the affected region:
  - Chronic or recurrent atelectasis
  - Unresponsive to therapy
  - Focal bronchiectasis has developed.
  - Significant morbidity is seen.
- Prevention of recurrent or future atelectasis: directed toward underlying cause, when applicable
- Airway clearance is important in clearing areas of atelectasis.
- Various techniques are available including the following:
  - Manuel chest physiotherapy
  - Mechanical chest physiotherapy (ThAIRapy vest)
  - Incentive spirometry
  - Acapella or Flutter devices
  - Intermittent positive pressure breathing (IPPB) or intrapulmonary percussive ventilator (IPV)
  - Mechanical insufflator–exsufflator (Cough Assist):
    - For patients with weakened cough (i.e., neuromuscular weakness)

ONGOING CARE

FOLLOW-UP RECOMMENDATIONS
Patient Monitoring
Expect improvement: 1–3 months in typical, uncomplicated cases

PROGNOSIS
- Depends on the underlying disease process
- In otherwise healthy individuals: excellent

COMPLICATIONS
- Recurrent infections
- Bronchiectasis
- Hemoptysis
- Abscess formation
- Fibrosis of the pulmonary parenchyma

ADDITIONAL READING

- Altunhan H, Annagür A, Pekcan S, et al. Comparing the efficacy of nebulizer recombinant human DNase and hypertonic saline as monotherapy and combined treatment in the treatment of persistent atelectasis in mechanically ventilated newborns. *Pediatr Int*. 2011;54(1):131–136.
- Birnkrant DJ, Pope JF, Eiben RM. Management of the respiratory complications of neuromuscular diseases in the pediatric intensive care unit. *J Child Neurol*. 1999;14(3):139–143.
- Hough JL, Flenady V, Johnston L, et al. Chest physiotherapy for reducing respiratory morbidity in infants requiring ventilator support. *Cochrane Database Syst Rev*. 2008;(3):CD006445.
- McCool FD, Rosen MJ. Nonpharmacologic airway clearance therapies: ACCP evidence-based clinical practical guidelines. *Chest*. 2006;129(1)(Suppl):250S–259S.
- Oermann CM, Moore RH. Foolers: things that look like pneumonia in children. *Semin Respir Infect*. 1996;11(3):204–213.
- Redding GJ. Atelectasis in childhood. *Pediatr Clin North Am*. 1984;31(4):891–905.
- Riethmueller J, Kumpf M, Borth-Bruhns T, et al. Clinical and in vitro effect of dornase alfa in mechanically ventilated pediatric non-cystic fibrosis patients with atelectasis. *Cell Physiol Biochem*. 2009;23(1–3):205–210.
- Slattery DM, Waltz DA, Denham B, et al. Bronchoscopically administered recombinant human DNase for lobar atelectasis in cystic fibrosis. *Pediatr Pulmonol*. 2001;31(5):383–388.

CODES

ICD10
- J98.11 Atelectasis
- P28.10 Unspecified atelectasis of newborn
- P28.0 Primary atelectasis of newborn

FAQ
- Q: What should be considered if atelectasis is recurrent in nature but in different segments?
- A: Asthma should always be considered if atelectasis is recurrent and in varying segments.
- Q: When is the optimal time for bronchoscopy?
- A: There are no established criteria for when a bronchoscopy should be performed. A bronchoscopy should be done early in the course of illness when:
  - There is a high suspicion of a foreign body
  - Significant respiratory distress is present
  - Cases of acute chest syndrome in patients with sickle cell disease
  - The atelectasis is extensive and conservative treatment is ineffective
  - Bronchoscopy is infrequently performed in patients with cystic fibrosis secondary to its recurrent nature.

ATOPIC DERMATITIS

Rhonique Shields-Harris • Marceé J. White

BASICS

DESCRIPTION

Atopic dermatitis or eczema is a chronic skin condition characterized by an acute, intermittent pruritic rash. It most commonly begins in infancy or early childhood with an age-specific pattern of skin involvement. Individuals with atopic dermatitis usually have a personal or family history of atopy (e.g., asthma, hay fever, or rhinitis).

EPIDEMIOLOGY

- Common, occurs in nearly 1 in 5 children
- 60% of affected children will develop atopic dermatitis in the 1st year of life and 85% by age 5 years.
- Higher prevalence in Nevada, Utah, Idaho, and East Coast states
- Higher prevalence in urban versus rural areas
- Usually worse in the winter, but flares can occur at any time of year

RISK FACTORS

Genetics

- Genetic predisposition in affected patients with 30–70% of family members having atopy (allergies, asthma, eczema)
- Mode of inheritance is not well defined and is likely multifactorial.
- Studies show that genetic mutations in the filaggrin gene (FLG) are associated with skin barrier defects and occur in early-onset atopic dermatitis.

PATHOPHYSIOLOGY

- Histologic findings depend on the stage of atopic dermatitis (i.e., acute or chronic).
- Atopic dermatitis is a disorder of immune dysregulation with increased T-cell activation and increased cytokine production of interleukin (IL)-4, IL-5, and IL-13, which lead to increased IgE production.
- Acute atopic dermatitis shows spongiosis, a manifestation of intercellular edema that can lead to vesicle formation.
- Mutations in the filaggrin gene (FLG) are associated with abnormal skin barrier function and cause increased transepidermal water loss and increased penetration of allergens.

ETIOLOGY

- Etiology of atopic dermatitis is multifactorial, with genetic, environmental, physiologic, and immunologic factors.
- Increased viral (warts and molluscum) and dermatophyte infections seen in atopic patients appear to be related to cytokine-induced suppression of endogenous antimicrobial peptides.
- Patients often have elevated IgE levels and decreased chemotaxis of neutrophils.

DIAGNOSIS

HISTORY

- Age of onset
- Location of skin findings
- Pruritus
- Prior treatment
- Bathing habits
- Family history of atopy (allergies)
- Asthma
- Allergic rhinitis
- Exposure to allergens (i.e., change in detergents/soaps, excessive dryness)

PHYSICAL EXAM

- Acute flares reveal erythematous and scaly maculopapular exudative patches.
- Chronic disease is characterized by hyperpigmentation or hypopigmentation, lichenification, and scaling.
- Age-specific patterns of skin involvement:
  - In infancy, atopic dermatitis is widespread, primarily affecting extensor surfaces and also involves the cheeks, forehead, and scalp.
  - In childhood, the disease affects the characteristic flexural sites with lichenification. The hands and face can also be involved.
  - From adolescence to adulthood, the flexures, neck, hands, and feet are primarily involved.
- Severe atopic dermatitis can present as exfoliative erythroderma with diffuse scaling and erythema.
- Other associated findings include Dennie-Morgan folds (infraorbital folds), pityriasis alba (dry white patches), hyperlinear palms, facial pallor, infraorbital darkening, follicular accentuation, keratosis pilaris (dry, rough hair follicles on extensor surfaces of upper arms and thighs), and ichthyosis.

DIAGNOSTIC TESTS & INTERPRETATION

Lab

- There are no diagnostic tests for atopic dermatitis.
- Biopsy can be helpful to rule out other skin disorders, such as psoriasis.
- IgE levels can be elevated but need not be checked.
- Bacterial cultures of skin can be obtained to rule out superinfections.
- Rapid fluorescent antibody studies, polymerase chain reaction studies, or viral cultures and Tzanck smear can identify the presence of eczema herpeticum.

DIFFERENTIAL DIAGNOSIS

- Tinea corporis
- Severe seborrheic dermatitis
- Contact dermatitis
- Allergic or irritant psoriasis
- Wiskott-Aldrich syndrome
- Langerhans cell histiocytosis
- Acrodermatitis enteropathica
- Scabies
- Xerosis
- Hyper-IgE syndrome
- Metabolic deficiencies
  - Carboxylase deficiencies
  - Prolidase deficiencies

TREATMENT

MEDICATION

- Topical steroids
  - Mainstay of therapy to control inflammation
  - Mid- to high-potency steroids are used during acute flares, with tapering to milder potency steroids when control is achieved.
  - Long-term use of steroids can lead to atrophy, telangiectasias, and tachyphylaxis
- Oral antihistamines, such as hydroxyzine or diphenhydramine, may help to decrease itching in selected patients.
- Oral antibiotics
  - Indicated when there is superinfection of lesions
- Oral antivirals are indicated in cases of eczema herpeticum.
- Topical calcineurin inhibitors (TCIs)
  - Include tacrolimus ointment and pimecrolimus cream
  - Approved for use in children 2 years of age and older
  - These topical agents act to suppress T-cell function.
  - Sun damage can be potentiated, so children who receive these medications should receive instructions for diligent sun protection and sunscreen use.
- Systemic steroids are generally not used because of the chronicity of atopic dermatitis. They are reserved for refractory atopic dermatitis, and if used, it should only be for a short duration.
- Phototherapy with UVB can be used in patients with extensive disease resistant to other therapies.
- Topical barrier repair agents including N-palmitoylethanolamine cream, MAS063DP cream, and various ceramide formulations may be useful adjuncts to therapy.

ADDITIONAL TREATMENT

General Measures

- There is no cure for atopic dermatitis.
- Parents must understand that this is a chronic disease with intermittent flares and that control is the aim of treatment.
- Good skin care is critical to maintenance and includes use of mild soaps, frequent use of emollients, and wet wraps.
- Dilute bleach baths (about 1/4 cup per full tub of water or about 1 tsp per gallon of water) can be used as a once- or twice-weekly 10-minute soak to help reduce bacterial skin colonization and risk for recurrent skin infection.
- Avoidance of environmental irritants is recommended. Nail trimming and protective clothing at night to avoid scratching while sleeping is also helpful.
- Vitamin D supplementation has been shown to decrease the severity of atopic dermatitis due to effects on immunomodulation

ONGOING CARE

FOLLOW-UP RECOMMENDATIONS

Patient Monitoring

- It should be emphasized to parents that atopic dermatitis is a chronic disease and that good skin care is necessary to control disease activity and enhance quality of life.
- To improve compliance with treatment, providers should use therapeutic patient education techniques so parents and patients can manage this chronic disease.
- Address parental concerns about the safety of topical steroids in order to reduce steroid phobia.

PROGNOSIS

Up to 40–50% of children will outgrow their atopic dermatitis after the age of 5 years.

COMPLICATIONS

- Skin infections
  - Decreased cell-mediated immunity, decreased chemotaxis, and decreased production of endogenous antimicrobial peptides can result in increased infection (e.g., viral, dermatophyte, bacterial).
  - Patients with atopic dermatitis have a high density of *Staphylococcus aureus* on their skin, and given the fissures and open excoriations, there is a risk of superinfection.
- Eczema herpeticum
  - The decreased integrity of the skin can result in widely spread cutaneous infections such as herpes simplex infection, known as Kaposi varicelliform eruption or eczema herpeticum.
  - Similar problems can also be seen with coxsackievirus or molluscum contagiosum and used to occur with vaccinia.
- Overuse of topical medications
  - Overuse of potent topical steroids can result in hypopigmentation, telangiectasias, atrophy, and striae as well as excess systemic absorption leading to hypothalamic–pituitary axis suppression and growth retardation.
  - Pigmentary changes may result from overuse of topical medications; however, the lesions of atopic dermatitis may themselves cause postinflammatory skin color changes independent of topical therapy.
- Early growth delay is not uncommon among children with atopic dermatitis, although later catch-up growth is generally seen. This may be related to various mechanisms including impaired growth hormone release. Growth delay can occur independent of topical steroid exposure.
- Increased prevalence of emotional, behavioral, and psychological issues secondary to sleep disturbance in patients with atopic dermatitis

ADDITIONAL READING

- Barbarot S, Bernier C, Deleuran M. Therapeutic patient education in children with atopic dermatitis: position paper on objectives and recommendations. *Pediatr Dermatol*. 2013;30(2):199–206.
- Batchelor JM, Grindlay DJ, Williams HC. What's new in atopic eczema? An analysis of systematic reviews published in 2008 and 2009. *Clin Exp Dermatol*. 2010;35(8):823–827.
- Bieber T. Mechanisms of disease: atopic dermatitis. *N Engl Med*. 2008;358(14):1483–1494.
- Garmhausen D, Hagemann T, Bieber T, et al. Characterization of different courses of atopic dermatitis in adolescent and adult patients. *Allergy*. 2013;68(4):498–506.
- Krakowski AC, Eichenfield LF, Dohil MA. Management of atopic dermatitis in the pediatric population. *Pediatrics*. 2008;122(4):812–824.
- Ong PY, Leung DYM. Immune dysregulation in atopic dermatitis. *Curr Allergy Asthma Rep*. 2006;6(5):384–389.
- O'Regan GM, Irvine AD. The role of filaggrin in the atopic diathesis. *Clin Exp Allergy*. 2010;40(7):965–972.
- Spergel JM. Epidemiology of atopic dermatitis and atopic march in children. *Immunol Allergy Clin North Am*. 2010;30(3):269–280.

CODES

ICD10

- L20.9 Atopic dermatitis, unspecified
- L20.83 Infantile (acute) (chronic) eczema
- L20.89 Other atopic dermatitis

FAQ

- Q: Will the child outgrow this?
- A: Up to 40–50% of children will outgrow their atopic dermatitis after age 5 years. In some patients, however, the disease will persist to varying degrees throughout adulthood.
- Q: Will the steroid treatment change my child's skin color?
- A: Skin pigment changes are caused primarily by the lesions of atopic dermatitis, which cause postinflammatory hyper- or hypopigmentation (darkening or lightening), independent of topical therapy. The discoloration will eventually fade but may take weeks or months.
- Q: When atopic dermatitis is controlled, is any treatment necessary?
- A: Excessive dryness can exacerbate or flare disease. Therefore, less frequent use of soaps and frequent use of emollients are recommended.
- Q: Do food hypersensitivities play a role in atopic dermatitis?
- A: This is a debated issue. In general, the majority of patients are probably not adversely affected by foods. However, some individuals, particularly those who are unresponsive to routine therapy, may benefit from screening for food hypersensitivity and a trial of avoidance to any foods that test positive. The most common foods associated with exacerbation when an association can be made are eggs, milk, wheat, soy, peanuts, and fish.

ATRIAL SEPTAL DEFECT

Jonathan Fleenor

BASICS

DESCRIPTION

- An opening in the atrial septum, other than a patent foramen ovale (PFO)
- 4 major types of atrial septal defects (ASDs)
  - Secundum ASD
  - Primum ASD
  - Sinus venosus ASD
  - Coronary sinus ASD
- A PFO usually does not cause a significant intracardiac shunt. A probe-patent PFO can be found in up to 15–25% of normal hearts at pathologic exam.
- Secundum defects make up 60–70% of all ASDs. Usually, there is a shunt from the left atrium to the right atrium.
- Primum defects occur in ~30% of all ASDs. They are usually associated with a cleft mitral valve. This defect is the result of an abnormality of the endocardial cushions and therefore is also referred to as an incomplete atrioventricular (AV) canal defect.
- Sinus venosus defects can be of the superior or inferior vena caval type and occur in ~5–10% of all ASDs. In ASDs of the superior vena caval type, the right pulmonary veins (usually right upper lobe) may drain anomalously to the superior vena cava or right atrium.
- Coronary sinus ASDs are rare and occur in <1% of all ASDs. They are often associated with absence of the coronary sinus and a persistent left superior vena cava that joins the roof of the left atrium (also known as an "unroofed coronary sinus").

EPIDEMIOLOGY

Females > males (2:1)

Incidence

- Difficult to determine
- Represents 6–10% of all cardiac anomalies encountered

PATHOPHYSIOLOGY

- A left-to-right shunt occurs through the ASD. For large defects, this results in right atrial and right ventricular volume overload.
- There is usually increased pulmonary blood flow.
- The left-to-right shunt generally increases with time as pulmonary resistance drops and right ventricular compliance normalizes.
- Moderate and large defects are associated with a Qp/Qs ratio of >2:1.
- The direction of atrial shunting is determined by the relative compliance of the right and left ventricles.

ETIOLOGY

- ASDs may be associated with partial or total anomalous pulmonary venous drainage, mitral valve anomalies, transposition of the great arteries, or tricuspid atresia.
- Although usually isolated, ASDs may occur as part of a syndrome (Holt-Oram [autosomal dominant]).

DIAGNOSIS

HISTORY

- Most infants are asymptomatic.
- Older children with moderate left-to-right shunts are often asymptomatic but may have mild fatigue or dyspnea, especially with exercise.
- Children with large left-to-right shunts may complain of fatigue and dyspnea, which may become noticeable as the child gets older.
- Growth failure is uncommon.
- Older patients with large atrial shunts may develop atrial arrhythmias.

PHYSICAL EXAM

- Inspection and palpation of the precordium are usually normal, although older children with a large ASD may have a hyperdynamic precordium, right ventricular heave, or precordial bulge.
- Auscultation reveals 3 important features:
  - Wide and "fixed" splitting of S_2. Splitting of S_2 (A_2 and P_2 components) is caused by a delay in emptying of a volume-loaded right ventricle.
  - A systolic ejection murmur at the upper left sternal border. This murmur is caused by an increase in blood flow across a normal pulmonary valve. It may be differentiated from the murmur of pulmonary stenosis because there is no click.
  - A diastolic murmur at the lower sternal border, indicating a Qp/Qs ratio of at least 2:1. This murmur is caused by increased flow across the tricuspid valve.

DIAGNOSTIC TESTS & INTERPRETATION

Lab

- ECG
  - Usually normal sinus rhythm with an rSR′ (incomplete right bundle branch block pattern) in leads V_1, V_3R, and V_4R, indicating right ventricular volume overload. For larger shunts, ECG may show evidence of right atrial enlargement as well as 1st-degree AV block. A late finding suggestive of pulmonary hypertension is right ventricular hypertrophy.
- Chest radiograph
  - Cardiomegaly (right atrium and right ventricle), increased pulmonary vascular markings, and a dilated pulmonary trunk are seen in patients with significant left-to-right shunts.
- Echocardiogram
  - A 2-D echo study is diagnostic; it reveals the location, size, and associated defects, if any. It may demonstrate dilated right heart structures. Color Doppler generally permits visualization of the direction of shunt flow. Older children and adolescents may require transesophageal echo to best define the ASD.
- Cardiac catheterization
  - Generally unnecessary. It is indicated when pulmonary vascular disease is suspected (determination of pulmonary vascular resistance) or for associated cardiac defects.

DIFFERENTIAL DIAGNOSIS

- Ventricular septal defect
- Patent ductus arteriosus
- AV canal defect
- Valvar pulmonary stenosis

TREATMENT

ADDITIONAL TREATMENT

General Measures

- Infants with congestive heart failure should be treated with diuretics.
- Elective closure is indicated for ASDs associated with large left-to-right shunts, cardiomegaly, or symptoms.
  - The timing of closure is usually deferred until 3–5 years of age.
  - For most secundum-type ASDs, device closure of the defect can be performed in the cardiac catheterization laboratory, thus avoiding surgery.
- Prevention of paradoxical emboli and cerebrovascular accidents is an uncommon but possible indication for closure of ASDs or PFO.
- Irreversible pulmonary hypertension from a long-term left-to-right shunt usually does not occur until adolescence or young adulthood.
- Sinus venosus, primum, and coronary sinus–type ASDs require surgical closure. The mortality of surgical repair for an uncomplicated ASD approaches 0%.
- There is some anecdotal evidence suggesting that PFOs are a cause of migraine headaches in certain populations. Prospective adult studies are currently ongoing to further investigate this question, but to date no study has found an indication for PFO closure in migraine patients.

ONGOING CARE

FOLLOW-UP RECOMMENDATIONS

Patient Monitoring

- Children with typical auscultation, chest radiograph, and ECG findings should undergo an echocardiographic evaluation to determine the location and size of the ASD.
- Children with ASDs should have regular follow-up to assess for signs of congestive heart failure or right ventricular volume overload. Restriction of activity is unnecessary. Subacute bacterial endocarditis (SBE) prophylaxis is not indicated for an isolated secundum ASD. Residual ASD after surgery is rare.
- SBE prophylaxis is indicated for the first 6 months (assuming no residual defect) after closure of a secundum defect.
- Complications related to surgery include the following:
  - Sinus node dysfunction
  - Venous obstruction (facial or pulmonary edema) may occur after a sinus venosus ASD repair.
  - Postpericardiotomy syndrome, which manifests with nausea, vomiting, chest pain, abdominal pain, or fever, may occur a few weeks after surgical repair. Although a friction rub may not be present, the chest radiograph may show cardiomegaly and the echocardiogram may reveal a pericardial effusion.

PROGNOSIS

- The prognosis for small ASDs seems excellent without specific therapy.
- Spontaneous closure of small secundum ASDs can occur in up to 80% of infants in the 1st year of life. Isolated secundum ASDs of moderate and large size do not typically cause symptoms in most infants and children.
- Pulmonary hypertension is rare in childhood.
- Atrial flutter and fibrillation occur in up to 13% of unoperated patients older than 40 years of age.
- Bacterial endocarditis is rare in children with isolated ASD.
- Paradoxical emboli may occur and should be considered in patients with cerebral or systemic emboli.

ADDITIONAL READING

- Horton SC, Bunch TJ. Patent foramen ovale and stroke. *Mayo Clin Proc*. 2004;79(1):79–88.
- Kharouf R, Luxenberg DM, Khalid O, et al. Atrial septal defect: spectrum of care. *Pediatr Cardiol*. 2008;29(2):271–280.
- Meijboom F, Roos-Hesselink J, Sievert H. The role of the atria in congenital heart disease. *Cardiol Clin*. 2002;20(3):351–366.
- Ohye RG, Bove EL. Advances in congenital heart surgery. *Curr Opin Pediatr*. 2001;13(5):473–481.
- Radzik D, Davignon A, van Doesburg N, et al. Predictive factors for spontaneous closure of atrial septal defect diagnosed in the first 3 months of life. *J Am Coll Cardiol*. 1993;22:851–853.
- Rocchini AP. Pediatric cardiac catheterization. *Curr Opin Cardiol*. 2002;17(3):283–288.
- Zanchetta M, Rigatelli G, Pedon L, et al. Role of intracardiac echocardiography in atrial septal abnormalities. *J Interv Cardiol*. 2003;16(1):63–77.

CODES

ICD10

- Q21.1 Atrial septal defect
- Q21.2 Atrioventricular septal defect

FAQ

- Q: When should a moderate secundum ASD be closed?
- A: This can generally be electively performed in children prior to their starting grade school.
- Q: What is the significance of a patient having gastrointestinal complaints (nausea and vomiting) 2–3 weeks after surgical closure of an ASD?
- A: This may represent a pericardial effusion (postpericardiotomy syndrome).

ATTENTION-DEFICIT/HYPERACTIVITY DISORDER

D. David O'Banion • Mark Wolraich

BASICS

DESCRIPTION

- Attention-deficit/hyperactivity disorder (ADHD) is a chronic condition that is characterized by a pattern of developmentally inappropriate behaviors of inattention and/or hyperactivity/impulsivity.
- *DSM-5* criteria for diagnosis:
  - At least 6 of 9 behaviors in inattention and/or 6 of 9 hyperactivity/impulsivity behaviors and
  - Maladaptive behaviors persisting for at least 6 months and
  - Impairment from symptoms present in 2 or more major settings (home, school, day care, after-school activities) and
  - Some symptoms existed before age 12 years.
- It can be classified into 3 subtypes:
  - Hyperactive/impulsive
  - Inattentive
  - Combined type
- Symptoms cannot be better explained by another mental health disorder. Autism spectrum disorder is no longer an exclusion criteria.

EPIDEMIOLOGY

- 2:1 males-to-female ratio
- 3–10% prevalence of school-age children
- Females more likely to have inattentive type

RISK FACTORS

Genetics

- Risk of ADHD in 1st-degree relatives is ~25%.
- Concordance in monozygotic twins: 59–81%; dizygotic twins: 33%

COMMONLY ASSOCIATED CONDITIONS

- Learning disorders
- Language disorders
- Anxiety disorder
- Mood disorders
- Sleep disorders
- Tic disorder (may affect treatment decisions)
- Oppositional defiant disorder and conduct disorder
- Poor social skills

DIAGNOSIS

- Primary care clinicians should consider an extended visit to evaluate any child, age 4–18 years, presenting with behavioral and/or academic problems related to ADHD symptoms.
- To make the diagnosis, the clinician should ensure *DSM-5* criteria are met and document impairments in >1 major setting (e.g., home, school, day care). Information should be gathered from more than one reporter, when possible (e.g., caregivers and teachers).
- Comorbid conditions may prompt a referral to a subspecialist.
- In general, the diagnosis does not require any specific psychological test, cardiac test, laboratory test, or referral.
- Watchful waiting is not recommended, as evidence-based treatments can make significant improvements even at a young age.

HISTORY

- A detailed history of the child's behavior at home, school, and with peers
- Onset and duration of noted behaviors—sudden onset should prompt consideration of other conditions (mood disorder, trauma, abuse, substance use, etc.).
- Timing of behaviors with respect to developmentally appropriate expectations placed on the child
- Frequent or excessive need of supervision and redirection in age-appropriate common tasks and routines
- Not following rules/requests—oppositional and/or "forgetful" (getting lost or side-tracked)
- Academic progress with particular attention to academic problems with specific subjects, and behaviors during specific subjects
- Disruption of peer relationships
- Developmental history (developmental delay is *not* characteristic of ADHD)
- Sleep history—adequate length, hygiene
- Participation in age-appropriate organized activities (e.g., scouts, camp, team sports)
- Family history of dropping out of school, ADHD, or learning disorders
- Family history of early cardiac disease including arrhythmias, hypertrophic cardiomyopathy, sudden cardiac death or unexpected death in children or young adults
- Social history: those who live with patient, recent family discord, separation, recent death in the family, recent change in schools
- Past medical history and medication history
- Adverse pregnancy or birth history

ALERT
Ability to concentrate for hours on video games is *not* reassuring but commonly reported.

PHYSICAL EXAM

- Comprehensive physical and neurologic examination with attention to specific systems based on the history
- Vital signs: weight, height, pulse, BP, visual and hearing acuity
- Note any dysmorphology.

DIAGNOSTIC TESTS & INTERPRETATION

- Validated rating scales of behavior help the clinician review *DSM-5* criteria. After the initial concern is raised, these can be distributed, collected, and reviewed prior to a scheduled evaluation.
  - Connor Rating Scales-Revised, Vanderbilt ADHD Rating Scales, SNAP, ADHD RS
  - Ideally, collect rating scales from parents and teachers.
  - Some assess only for ADHD; others include assessment of comorbidities such as anxiety, oppositional defiant disorder, and depression (Vanderbilt).
  - Most clinicians choose a single tool and gain familiarity with it.
  - Most scales are useful to measure change with treatment.
  - Some are proprietary (Conner), and some are freely distributed (Vanderbilt).
- IQ and achievement testing
  - Not required but should be guided by specific concerns for disabilities
  - An evaluation for an Individual Educational Program (IEP) or 504 plan may be obtained following parental written request to the child's school.

Lab

Not required except as guided by history and physical. Screening ECGs are not recommended or considered cost-effective.

DIFFERENTIAL DIAGNOSIS

- Developmental
  - Learning disabilities
  - Intellectual disability
  - Autism spectrum disorder
  - Language or speech disorder
- Psychiatric
  - Anxiety disorders
  - Depression
  - Obsessive-compulsive disorder
  - Oppositional defiant disorder or conduct disorder
  - Adjustment disorder
- Medical
  - Genetic disorder
  - Sleep disorder
  - Sensory impairment (vision, hearing)
  - Medication side effects
  - Toxins (lead)
  - Iron deficiency anemia
  - Postconcussion syndrome
- Educational
  - Inappropriate school environment
  - Developmentally inappropriate expectations
- Social
  - Disorganized/chaotic family environment
  - Child abuse and neglect or sexual abuse
  - Psychosocial stressors

TREATMENT

GENERAL MEASURES

- Treat ADHD as a chronic disease and use the medical home model. Partner and discuss treatment options with families. Include the school when possible.
- The family and patient choose target goals and actively participate in measuring/monitoring achievement of these goals.
- 3 treatment modalities:
  - Behavior therapy (evidence based)
  - Educational support
  - Medication

NONPHARMACOLOGIC

- Children 4–5 years: behavior therapy
- Reduces core symptoms of ADHD in multiple settings. Different from interpersonal talk/play therapy, which has not been efficacious in treatment. Parent education, parent training programs, and behavior therapies usually have a planned number of weeks (10–16 weeks). Their focus is increasing positive behavior through rewards and extinguishing negative behavior through ignoring and effective discipline.
- Cognitive behavioral therapy can be helpful for older children and adults.

- Educational support options:
  - Request a 504 Plan through patient's school to evaluate for possible accommodations (different from an IEP).
  - Small teacher-to-student ratio is ideal.
  - Good communication between school and home (e.g., a daily behavior report card)
  - Homework log monitored by teacher and parent
- Psychological support may be helpful for:
  - Patient who has poor peer relations, such as peer groups or social training groups
  - Patient with a comorbidity
  - Commonly, families have difficulty with parenting a child with ADHD.

MEDICATION

Consider family preferences, other family member's reaction to specific medications, duration of coverage (shorter school day in younger child), ability to swallow pills, and concern for divergence (or abuse).

First Line

- **Stimulants:** FDA-approved. All are either methylphenidate or amphetamine-class derivatives.
- **Efficacy:** extensive evidence supporting efficacy and safety. 80% of children with ADHD show significant improvement.
- **Pharmacokinetics:** Individual response is highly variable. Effectiveness and side effects can be seen within hours of starting medication. Duration varies by preparation. Younger children may metabolize stimulants slowly, giving a longer duration than expected for immediate-release preparations. Does not "build up" in the system, so no known permanent effects. Daily dosing therefore necessary for symptom relief
- **Dose:** Weight-based dosing is not appropriate due differences in metabolism and idiosyncratic responses. Start with smallest dose and titrate up in single-dose increments weekly as needed. Base titrations on changes in rating scales and achievement toward target goals, weighing improvements against side effects. Start with short-acting medication in children younger than 7 years. For some younger children, this may provide a sufficient duration of therapy for school. Consider long-acting/extended-release in older children. Start medication when the parents are available to watch for side effects and duration of action (typically over a weekend). Follow closely with the parents; ask them to get feedback from school on a weekly basis until dose is properly adjusted. This process may take 1–2 months to be completed. If at highest dose and still not having good effect, or having significant side effects at a lower dose, switch to the lowest dose of the other class of stimulants and repeat the titration process.
- **Side effects:** Side effects last less than 24 hours. Families should know that any unacceptable side effects will abate if the medication is stopped. Most side effects can be managed expectantly.
- Decreased appetite is common, although sustained weight loss is not.
- Abdominal pain, tics, headache, difficulty falling asleep, and jitteriness
- Difficulty shifting attention, overfocus (the "zombie effect") is from too high of a dose.
- Severe movement disorders, obsessive–compulsive thoughts, or psychotic symptoms are rare and cease when medication is stopped.
- Growth velocity may slow. Final adult height is minimally decreased, if at all affected.
- **Contraindications:** glaucoma, symptomatic cardiovascular disease (except with guidance by cardiology), hyperthyroidism, hypertension

Second Line

- Atomoxetine: selective norepinephrine uptake inhibitor. Once-a-day or b.i.d. dosing. Must be taken daily for 4 weeks before effects are at maximum. Similar side-effect profile as stimulants but with increased chance of suicidal thinking. Less evidence for use and less efficacious than stimulants. Start with 0.5 mg/kg/24 h for 1 week, and if no side effects (often GI upset), increase to 1.2 mg/kg/24 h, max 1.4 mg/kg/24 h or 100 mg/24 h if >70 kg.
- Adjuvants: extended-release α-adrenergic agonists (clonidine, guanfacine). Must take daily. Commonly causes sedation that may improve with time

ISSUES FOR REFERRAL

- When comorbidities are suspected, or when contraindications for treatment are present
- If patient is not responding to titration attempts of both stimulant classes
- If the patient is having difficulty tolerating different stimulants, or having unexpected or severe side effects

ONGOING CARE

FOLLOW-UP RECOMMENDATIONS

- Initially, follow-up by phone may be every 1–2 weeks until proper dosing is achieved. Follow up in clinic in 1 month. After successful titration, patients should be seen every 3–6 months specifically for ADHD visits.
- Consider mailing refills once titrated to prevent burden on families who'd otherwise pick up the paper prescription.
- Monitor weight, height, BP, and heart rate.
- Weight loss is not usually sustained.
- Encourage meals when patient is hungry, perhaps later than family's usual dinner.
- Assess for change in growth velocity.
- Assess family and peer relationship.
- Assess school performance.
- Assess for ongoing need for medication.

ADDITIONAL READING

- Collett BR, Ohan JL, Myers KM. Ten-year review of rating scales. V: scales assessing attention-deficit/hyperactivity disorder. *J Am Acad Child Adolesc Psychiatry*. 2003;42(9):1015–1037.
- A 14-month randomized clinical trial of treatment strategies for attention-deficit/hyperactivity disorder. *Arch Gen Psychiatry*. 1999;56(12):1073–1086.
- Graham J, Banaschewski T, Buitelaar J, et al., European Guidelines Group. European guidelines on managing adverse effects of medication for ADHD. *Eur Child Adolesc Psychiatry*. 2011;20(1):17–37.
- Perrin JM, Friedman RA, Knilans TK, et al. Cardiovascular monitoring and stimulant drugs for attention-deficit/hyperactivity disorder. *Pediatrics*. 2008;122(2):451–453.
- Weber W, Newmark S. Complementary and alternative medical therapies for attention-deficit/hyperactivity disorder and autism. *Pediatr Clin North Am*. 2007;54(6):983–1006.
- Wolraich M, Brown L, Brown RT, et al. Clinical practice guideline for the diagnosis, evaluation, and treatment of attention-deficit/hyperactivity disorder in children and adolescents. *Pediatrics*. 2011;128(5):1007–1022.

CODES

ICD10

- F90.9 Attention-deficit hyperactivity disorder, unspecified type
- F90.1 Attn-defct hyperactivity disorder, predom hyperactive type
- F90.0 Attn-defct hyperactivity disorder, predom inattentive type

FAQ

- Q: What is the role of diet or complementary and alternative medical (CAM) therapies?
- A: Although in the past, it has been thought that certain foods and additives caused ADHD, there are no studies that show changes in diet to be of benefit. Frequently, families will want to explore the use of CAM therapies either in conjunction with or instead of treatment with stimulant medication. If safety can be assured, it may be reasonable for patients to try for a finite period of time if it ultimately helps the patient. If CAM therapy fails, the parents may be more willing to try stimulant medication.
- Q: Is medication needed every day?
- A: This depends on the needs of the patient and type of medication. Some patients need medication daily in order to function successfully with peers or in structured environments, like team sports or weekend schools. Other patients who need help mainly with focusing attention do well with medication only during learning periods (school days). Some patients will not need medication during the summer holiday or during school breaks.
- Q: How long will my child be on medication?
- A: A large percentage of children with ADHD will continue to have symptoms as adults. Although every patient is different, some patients may need to continue medication through formal learning (high school and college). During this time, they should be able to learn coping strategies to minimize the effects of their symptoms. If treatment goals are being met, it is reasonable to have a trial off medications to see if performance off medications can be sustained (sometimes called a drug holiday).
- Q: Are there support groups available?
- A: An organization that is widely recognized as an advocacy and support group for families is Children and Adults with Attention Deficit/Hyperactivity Disorder (www.chadd.org). Use discretion when using online resources; there are many online Web sites that are sponsored by pharmaceutical companies and others that encourage alternatives to medication and actively discourage use of currently recommended treatments.

AUTISM SPECTRUM DISORDER

Alisson Richards • David C. Rettew

BASICS

DESCRIPTION

- Neurodevelopmental disorder characterized by the following:
  - Delays/impairments in development of social communication and social interaction
  - Restricted, repetitive patterns of behavior, interests, or activities
  - Symptoms present in early childhood
  - Significant impairment in functioning
- Diagnostic criteria changes since 2013:
  - The *Diagnostic and Statistical Manual of Mental Disorders* 4th edition (*DSM-IV*) previously included autistic disorder, Asperger disorder, Rett disorder, childhood disintegrative disorder, and pervasive developmental disorder, not otherwise specified within overall category.
  - *DSM-5* has eliminated these separate diagnoses due to insufficient evidence.
  - *DSM-5* added severity levels (1–3) based on the level of support required.
- Associated with specific and known genetic disorder (e.g., fragile X) in minority of cases
- Behaviors exist along continuum with unclear boundaries between trait and disorder.

EPIDEMIOLOGY

Prevalence

- Approximately 1% of population
- Rate rising over past decades
- 4 times more common in males than females
  - Females are more severely impaired with intellectual disability.

RISK FACTORS/ETIOLOGY

- Strong genetic influence
- Risk in 1st-degree relatives 2–10%
- Multiple genes involved
- Other risk factors: closer spacing of pregnancies, advanced maternal or paternal age, extreme premature birth (<26 weeks), possible maternal inflammation in utero
- Link to vaccinations not supported by scientific evidence
- Cause(s) unknown but may be associated with abnormalities in cortical laminar architecture during prenatal brain development

COMMONLY ASSOCIATED CONDITIONS

- Intellectual disabilities
- Gastrointestinal problems
- Seizure disorders
- Sleep disorders
- Attention problems, anxiety, depression, mood disturbances
- Aggression and self-injury

DIAGNOSIS

Typically, pediatricians are the first point of contact and play an important role in screening and early recognition, followed by more in-depth evaluation with a developmental pediatrician, psychologist, child psychiatrist, or neurologist where assessment and treatment plans can be coordinated with the schools.

HISTORY

- A detailed prenatal, developmental, medical, family, and social history are essential.
- Delays/impairments in social communication and social interaction
  - Delayed language development
  - Impairment in eye contact, facial expression, nonverbal social behaviors (pulling parents by hand but not looking at them)
  - Lack of pointing
  - Impaired social interactions and relationships
  - Lack of imaginary play appropriate to developmental level
  - Does not include others in play
- Stereotyped behaviors and restricted interests
  - Stereotypies (e.g., rocking, hand flapping)
  - Echolalia
  - Restricted range of interests/activities
  - Attachment to unusual objects, fascination with parts of objects
  - Behavioral rigidity, distress with changes in routine
  - Hyper- or hyporeactivity to sensory input or unusual sensory interests in objects or persons (smelling, touching, sensitivity to clothing)

PHYSICAL EXAM

- Evaluate for growth disturbance.
- 20–30% have macrocephaly: neurocutaneous disorder, storage disease, hydrocephalus, or no identifiable cause
- Signs of self-injurious behavior
- Stereotypical behavior, involuntary movements, motor coordination abnormalities, mirror/overflow movements
- Ophthalmologic/audiologic evaluations to rule out visual or hearing deficits
- Long, thin face; prominent ears: fragile X (macroorchidism may not be present until after puberty)
- Wood's lamp examination: Neurocutaneous syndromes and hypopigmented macules/fibromas suggest tuberous sclerosis.
- Microcephaly: toxoplasmosis, other viruses, rubella, cytomegalovirus, herpes virus (TORCH) infection; Angelman syndrome; Rett disorder
- Look for spasticity, visual loss, ataxia: leukodystrophy

DIAGNOSTIC TESTS & INTERPRETATION

Lab

- Electroencephalogram if epilepsy is suspected (~25%)
- Head MRI/CT: if intellectual or focal neurologic deficit is present or if suspected neurocutaneous disease
- Chromosome studies: if child is intellectually disabled
- Microarray analysis increasingly recommended
- Toxoplasma, other viruses, rubella, cytomegalovirus, herpes virus titers: setting of microcephaly
- CBC: evaluation of growth delay and/or pica
- Blood lead level: rule out lead intoxication
- Thyroid function tests: rule out hyper-/hypothyroidism
- Audiogram/brainstem auditory evoked response: for children with speech and language delay and to rule out hearing deficits
- Ophthalmologic evaluations to rule out visual deficits

Diagnostic Procedures/Other

- Screening tools
- Modified Checklist for Autism in Toddlers (M-CHAT) with new Revised with Follow-up Version downloadable at http://www2.gsu.edu/~psydlr/M-CHAT/Official_M-CHAT_Website.html
- Social Responsiveness Scale (SRS)
- Autism Diagnostic Observation Schedule (ADOS) and Autism Diagnostic Interview (ADI-R) are structured interviews and assessments usually performed by a psychologist, developmental pediatrician, psychiatrist, or neurologist: considered the gold standard

DIFFERENTIAL DIAGNOSIS

- Intellectual impairment: MAY not have autistic spectrum disorder if communication, behavior, play, and social skills appropriate to developmental age
- Social (pragmatic) communication disorder: lack of restricted, repetitive patterns of behavior or interests
- Rett syndrome: females; hand washing/hand-wringing movements, head growth deceleration before 48 months of age, MeCP2 gene
- Deafness: delayed/absent oral language acquisition; behavioral/social difficulties may relate to language delays.
- Language disorder: no deficits in social interactions or restricted range of interests
- Landau-Kleffner syndrome: distinct abnormal EEG, aphasia; children appear deaf
- Selective mutism: Early development is not disturbed.
- Anxiety, ADHD, obsessive-compulsive disorder, reactive attachment disorder or schizophrenia

TREATMENT

MEDICATION

- Pharmacotherapy treats associated symptoms of autism.
- Symptoms/medications to consider:
  - Self-injurious behavior: atypical/typical antipsychotics, guanfacine, clonidine
  - Sleep disturbances: melatonin, clonidine, trazodone
  - Seizures: newer anticonvulsants, carbamazepine, phenytoin, valproate, barbiturates (may worsen hyperactivity/irritability)
  - Hyperactivity/attention difficulties: psychostimulants, atomoxetine, bupropion, clonidine, guanfacine
  - Obsessive-compulsive disorder symptoms/perseveration: SSRIs, clomipramine
  - Tic disorders: guanfacine, clonidine, atypical/typical antipsychotics
  - Depression: SSRIs, bupropion, venlafaxine
  - Anxiety: SSRIs, buspirone, venlafaxine, benzodiazepines (may increase disorganization and agitation)
  - Aggression: atypical antipsychotics, SSRIs, anticonvulsants, guanfacine
- U.S. Food and Drug Administration (FDA)–approved medications include aripiprazole for ages 6–17 years and risperidone for ages 5–16 years
  - Important to monitor baseline glucose and lipids as atypical antipsychotics are associated with metabolic syndrome
  - Used for associated aggression and irritability

ALERT

- Autism spectrum disorders vary greatly in symptom presentation. Discordancy among clinicians' diagnoses and under- and overdiagnosis of these disorders are common.
- Symptom presentation differs at different stages of development.
- Medication often not helpful for core autistic features and patients often develop side effects
- Subclinical seizure types may be detected only on electroencephalogram.

ADDITIONAL TREATMENT

General Measures

Nonpharmacologic

- Psychoeducational assessment
  - Cognitive ability and adaptive skills
  - Speech language assessment with both receptive and expressive language measures
  - Occupational therapy may be needed for sensory or motor difficulties
- Early sustained structured behavioral intervention using applied behavior analysis (ABA) and behavior modification highly beneficial in many children
- Vocational training important for some adolescents and adults
- Social skills training especially for higher functioning patients is essential.
- Education and support for parents and siblings integral to treatment
- Conventional psychotherapy not indicated to address core features of autism and pervasive developmental disorder

COMPLEMENTARY & ALTERNATIVE THERAPIES

- Almost 1/3 of children with ASD have received some form of complementary and alternative medicine (CAM).
- Important to ask and understand what is being used

ONGOING CARE

FOLLOW-UP RECOMMENDATIONS

Patient Monitoring

- Prognosis linked to cognitive ability and acquisition of social/communication skills
- Early intervention and provision of services can improve prognosis.
- If no language by 5 years of age, substantial language development is unlikely.
- Children with autism/pervasive developmental disorder often require lifelong treatment and support.
- Physician should remain active in long-term treatment planning and individual and family support.

DIET

Little systematic evidence to support that gluten-free diets are helpful, but there are many claims of their effectiveness

ADDITIONAL READING

- Committee on Children with Disabilities. Technical report: the pediatrician's role in the diagnosis and management of autistic spectrum disorder in children. *Pediatrics*. 2001;107(5):E85.
- Greenspan SI, Brazelton TB, Cordero J, et al. Guidelines for early identification, screening, and clinical management of children with autism spectrum disorders. *Pediatrics*. 2008;121(4):828–830.
- Gutstein S, Sheely R. *Relationship Development Intervention Activities For Young Children*. London, United Kingdom: Jessica Kingsley Publications; 2002.
- Johnson CP, Myers SM; American Academy of Pediatrics Council on Children with Disabilities. Identification and evaluation of children with autism spectrum disorders. *Pediatrics*. 2007;120(5):1183–1215.
- Meyers MM, Johnson CP; American Academy of Pediatrics Council on Children with Disabilities. Clinical report: management of children with autism spectrum disorders. *Pediatrics*. 2007;120(5):1162–1182.
- Moeschler JB, Shevell M; American Academy of Pediatrics Committee on Genetics. Clinical genetic evaluation of the child with mental retardation or developmental delays. *Pediatrics*. 2006;117(6):2304–2316.
- Rogers SJ, Vismara LA. Evidence-based comprehensive treatments for early autism. *J Clin Child Adolesc Psychol*. 2008;37(1):8–38.
- Scahill L, Martin A. Psychopharmacology. In: Volkmarr FR, Klin A, Paul R, et al, eds. *Handbook of Autism and Pervasive Developmental Disorders*. Hoboken, NJ: Wiley; 2005:1102–1122.
- Stoner R, Chow ML, Boyle MP, et al. Patches of disorganization in the neocortex of children with autism. *New Engl J Med*. 2014;370(13):1209–1219.
- Volkmar F, Siegel M, Wodbury-Smith M, et al. Practice parameter for the assessment and treatment of children and adolescents with autism spectrum disorders. *Am Acad Child Adolesc Psychiatry*. 2013;53(2):237–257. www.aacap.org. Accessed November 30, 2014.

CODES

ICD10

- F84.0 Autistic disorder
- F84.2 Rett's syndrome
- F84.5 Asperger's syndrome

FAQ

- Q: What are the chances of having a 2nd child with autism?
- A: In families with 1 child with autism, the recurrence risk for subsequent children is 3–7%. This is in contrast to the risk in the general population, which is 0.1–0.2%.
- Q: What is the value of brain imaging in autism?
- A: MRI may help diagnose a heritable syndrome with genetic counseling implications (e.g., leukodystrophy, tuberous sclerosis) but is usually unhelpful in high-functioning cases without severe intellectual impairment and focal neurologic findings.
- Q: Does the MMR vaccine cause autism?
- A: There is no causal association between the MMR vaccine and autism.

AUTOIMMUNE HEMOLYTIC ANEMIA

Michele P. Lambert

BASICS

DESCRIPTION

- Autoimmune hemolytic anemia (AIHA) is characterized by shortened red cell survival that is caused by autoantibodies directed against RBCs, with or without the participation of complement on the red cell membrane.
- Natural history
  - Acute disease
    - Onset with rapid fall in hemoglobin level over hours to days
    - Usual course: complete resolution of disease within 3–6 months
    - Resolution more likely in children who present between 2 and 12 years of age
  - Chronic disease
    - Slower onset of anemia over weeks to months, with some having persistence of hemolysis or intermittent relapses
    - More likely to be associated with underlying chronic Illness
    - More common in adults and children <2 years or >12 years of age

EPIDEMIOLOGY

- Less common in children and adolescents than in adults
- No apparent racial or sexual predisposition (in childhood)

Incidence

- ~1–3:100,000 persons/year
- Peak incidence in childhood is in first 4 years of life with warm AIHA.

PATHOPHYSIOLOGY

- Warm autoantibodies (~80% cases)
  - Maximal activity of in vitro antibody RBC binding at 37°C
  - IgG-class antibody usually
  - IgG-coated RBCs cleared, predominantly in the spleen, by macrophages.
- Cold autoantibodies (cold agglutinins) (7–25%)
  - Maximal activity of in vitro RBC binding at temperatures between 0°C and 30°C
  - Almost always caused by IgM antibody with specificity for antigens of the i/I system on RBCs
  - Anti-I antibodies characteristic of *Mycoplasma pneumoniae*–associated hemolysis
  - Anti-I antibodies are usually found in infectious mononucleosis.
  - Hemolysis is complement-dependent.
- Paroxysmal cold hemoglobinuria
  - IgG autoantibody binds RBC at cooler areas of the body (i.e., extremities), causing irreversible binding of complement components (C3 and C4). When coated RBCs enter warmer areas of the body, IgG falls off and complement causes hemolysis (Donath–Landsteiner biphasic hemolysin).
  - Unusual IgG antibody with anti-P specificity
  - Most frequently found in children with viral infections (30%)

ETIOLOGY

- Idiopathic
- Passive transfer of maternal antibodies
- Secondary to an underlying disorder
  - Infection: viral (e.g., *Mycoplasma*, Epstein-Barr virus, cytomegalovirus, hepatitis, HIV) or bacterial (e.g., *Streptococcus*, typhoid fever, *Escherichia coli* septicemia)
  - Drugs: antimalarials, antipyretics, sulfonamides, penicillin, rifampin
  - Hematologic disorders: leukemia, lymphoma
  - Autoimmune disorders: lupus, mixed connective tissue disorders, Wiskott-Aldrich syndrome, ulcerative colitis, rheumatoid arthritis, common variable immunodeficiency, scleroderma, Evans syndrome, ALPS (autoimmune lymphoproliferative syndrome), 22q11.2 deletion syndrome
  - Tumors: ovarian, carcinomas, thymomas, dermoid cysts

DIAGNOSIS

HISTORY

- Pallor
- Jaundice
- Dark urine
- Fever
- Weakness
- Dizziness
- Syncope
- Exercise intolerance

PHYSICAL EXAM

- Pallor
- Jaundice
- Splenomegaly
- Hepatomegaly
- Tachycardia, systolic flow murmur, S_3 gallop
- Orthostasis in acute onset

DIAGNOSTIC TESTS & INTERPRETATION

Lab

CBC

- Hemoglobin level decreased (occasionally, thrombocytopenia seen in Evans syndrome).
- Mean corpuscular volume may be normal.
- Reticulocyte count increased (although may also be decreased if reticulocytes bear the target antigen).
- Peripheral smear: spherocytes, polychromasia, macrocytes, agglutination
- Direct antiglobulin test (Coombs)—positive (usually)
  - Single most important test
  - Warm AIHA will have IgG ± C3-positive.
  - Cold AIHA and paroxysmal cold hemoglobinuria will have C3-positive.
- Haptoglobin level decreased.
- Indirect hyperbilirubinemia
- Elevated lactate dehydrogenase
- Urinalysis: hemoglobinuria, increased urobilinogen
- Bone marrow aspiration: erythroid hyperplasia (to rule out leukemia or lymphoma associated with AIHA)
- Cold agglutinin titer: positive (usually >1:64)
- Donath–Landsteiner test should be performed in cases of suspected paroxysmal cold hemoglobinuria.

ALERT

- A negative Coombs test can occur when small numbers of IgG or C3 molecules are present on the red cell membrane or if most of the coated red cells are cleared from circulation (i.e., in cases of less severe hemolysis, low-affinity antibodies, or in cases of very severe, rapid clearance).
- Radiolabeled Coombs test or enzyme immunoassays are more sensitive diagnostic tests in these circumstances.
- Reticulocytopenia may occur in some cases where the antibody coats and removes reticulocytes.

DIFFERENTIAL DIAGNOSIS

- Defects intrinsic to RBC:
  - Membrane defects such as hereditary spherocytosis
  - Enzyme defects including hemolytic episode due to G6PD deficiency
  - Hemoglobin defects
  - Congenital dyserythropoietic anemias
  - Paroxysmal nocturnal hemoglobinuria
- Defects extrinsic to RBC:
  - Immune-mediated
    - Isoimmune: hemolytic disease of the newborn, blood group incompatibility
    - Autoimmune (see "Etiology")
    - Drug-dependent RBC antibodies
    - Hemolytic transfusion reaction
- Non–immune-mediated
  - Idiopathic
  - Secondary to an underlying disorder (i.e., hemolytic uremic syndrome, thrombotic thrombocytopenic purpura)
  - Mechanical: march hemoglobinuria, heart valves

TREATMENT

MEDICATION

First Line

Corticosteroids

- Indication:
  - In IgG-mediated disease, steroids have been shown to interfere with macrophage Fc and C3b receptors responsible for RBC destruction. In addition, they have been shown to elute IgG Ab from the RBC surface (improving survival).
  - In chronic, warm, AIHA, pulsed high-dose dexamethasone has been shown to be effective in some cases.
- Complications:
  - Both short- and long-term side effects
  - Generally not effective in cold agglutinin disease
- Dose:
  - Start prednisone PO/methylprednisolone IV at 2 mg/kg/24 h in divided doses.
  - Tapering of steroids should begin after a therapeutic response is achieved (may take several days to weeks).
- Goal:
  - Initially, to return to normal hemoglobin level with tolerable doses of steroid or off steroids entirely

- In some patients, goal may be achieving decreased hemolysis and a clinically asymptomatic state with minimal steroid side effects.
- Alternative treatments should be considered for patients unresponsive to steroids or who require high doses for maintenance of hemoglobin level.

Second Line

- IV immunoglobulin
  - Indication:
    - May be useful in selected cases of immune hemolytic anemia unresponsive to steroids
  - Mechanism of action is not entirely clear.
  - Effect is usually temporary; retreatment may be required every 3–4 weeks.
  - Complications:
    - Red cell antibodies in IVIG preparations may be a confounder.
    - Aseptic meningitis
    - Theoretical risk of transfusion-transmitted viral infection
  - Expensive
  - Dose: Up to 1 g/kg/24 h for 5 days has been required to achieve a beneficial effect.
  - Large doses of IVIG have been associated with causing hemolytic anemia.
- Plasmapheresis/exchange transfusion
  - Indication:
    - Will slow the rate of hemolysis in severe disease, especially if IgM-mediated
  - Indicated if thrombotic thrombocytopenic purpura cannot be excluded
  - Complications:
    - Only of short-term benefit
  - Expensive
- Rituximab: monoclonal anti-CD20 antibody likely works through depletion of B cells
  - Indicated in refractory AIHA (375 mg/m^2 weekly for 2–4 weeks)
  - Response 40–100%
  - Particularly useful in warm AIHA
  - Adverse effects: fever, chills, rigors, hypertension, bronchospasm; rare risk of viral infections
- Immunosuppressive agents (antimetabolites and alkylating agents)
  - Indication:
    - When there is a clinically unacceptable degree of hemolysis that is refractory to steroids and splenectomy
- Some have been effective in cold agglutinin disease.
  - Complications:
    - There are varying side effects dependent on the agent used. Therefore, clinical indications must be strong and exposure to drug should be limited.
  - Dose:
    - Adjusted to maintain WBC >2,000, absolute neutrophil count (ANC) >1,000, and platelet count at 50,000–100,000 cells/mm^3
- Alemtuzumab (anti-CD52): may be effective very refractory AIHA particularly secondary to B-cell chronic lymphocytic leukemia (B-CLL)

ADDITIONAL TREATMENT

General Measures

Blood transfusion: should only be used with great caution in this setting in patients with very low hemoglobin/brisk hemolysis because of difficulty with appropriate cross-matching

- Indication: physiologic compromise from the anemia (usually only in severe acute onset)
- Complications:
  - The blood bank may be unable to find compatible blood. In IgG-mediated disease, autoantibody is usually pan-reactive; therefore, you must use the least incompatible unit of blood.
  - In cold agglutinin disease, use a blood warmer for all infusions to decrease IgM binding, and monitor for acute hemolysis during transfusion.

SURGERY/OTHER PROCEDURES

Splenectomy

- Indication:
  - Patients unresponsive to medical management, who require moderate- to high-maintenance doses of steroids or who develop steroid intolerance may be candidates.
- Not effective in cold agglutinin disease
- Response rate is 50–70%, with many partial remissions.

ONGOING CARE

FOLLOW-UP RECOMMENDATIONS

Patient Monitoring

- Hemoglobin level q4h–q12h (depending on severity) until stable
- Reticulocyte count: daily
- Spleen size: daily
- Hemoglobinuria: daily
- Coombs: weekly

PROGNOSIS

- Dependent on age, underlying disorder (if any), and response to therapy. See also "Description" section (natural history).
- Mortality in pediatric series ranged from 9 to 19%.

COMPLICATIONS

- May be increased risk of venous thrombosis in patients with AIHA
- May be associated with a predisposition to lymphoproliferative disorders
- Gallstones related to chronic hemolysis

ADDITIONAL READING

- Barros MMO, Blajchman MA, Borde JO. Warm autoimmune hemolytic anemia: recent progress in understanding the immunobiology and treatment. *Transfus Med Rev*. 2010;24(3):195–210.
- Hoffman PC. Immune hemolytic anemia—select topics. *Hematology*. 2009:80–86.
- King K, Ness PM. Treatment of autoimmune hemolytic anemia. *Semin Hematol*. 2005;42(3):131–136.
- Petz LD. Cold antibody autoimmune hemolytic anemia. *Blood Rev*. 2008;22(1):1–15.

CODES

ICD10

- D59.1 Other autoimmune hemolytic anemias
- D59.0 Drug-induced autoimmune hemolytic anemia

FAQ

- Q: Will the anemia go away?
- A: Children with cold autoantibodies tend to have short-lived illness, whereas children with warm antibodies often have a chronic clinical course characterized by periods of remissions and relapses.
- Q: Is this contagious?
- A: No. Another child may acquire the same viral illness; however, the body's response to produce an autoantibody is dependent on the individual patient.

AVASCULAR (ASEPTIC) NECROSIS OF THE FEMORAL HEAD (HIP)

Craig Munns

BASICS

DESCRIPTION

- Avascular (aseptic) necrosis results from the interruption of the blood supply to bone (either traumatic or nontraumatic occlusion).
- The femoral head is the most common site.
- A particular type of self-limiting idiopathic avascular necrosis of the hip that occurs in children is known as Perthes disease (see the "Perthes Disease" chapter).

RISK FACTORS

Genetics

Variable, depending on cause

PATHOPHYSIOLOGY

- Death and necrosis of bone with gradual return of blood supply
- Necrotic bone gradually resorbed and replaced by new bone
- During bone resorption, structural integrity of femoral head may be reduced, leading to collapse.

ETIOLOGY

- Traumatic
  - Hip fracture
  - Hip dislocation
  - Slipped capital femoral epiphysis
  - Complication of casting, bracing, surgery
- Nontraumatic
  - Idiopathic (older, after physeal closure); similar to adult avascular necrosis
  - Idiopathic (younger, before physeal closure, Perthes disease)
  - Caisson disease
  - Sickle cell disease
  - Septic arthritis
  - Steroids or chemotherapy
  - Malignancy (leukemia)
  - Gaucher disease
  - Viral infection (HIV, CMV)
  - Radiation therapy
  - Hypercoagulable states

DIAGNOSIS

HISTORY

- Onset (gradual or after traumatic event)
- Association with the following:
  - Trauma
  - Medications (steroids or chemotherapy)
  - Casting, splinting, surgery (iatrogenic)
  - Pain, limping
  - Stiffness (decreased range of motion)
  - Perthes disease may occasionally be bilateral or occur in contralateral hip at a later time point.

PHYSICAL EXAM

- Gait
  - Limping
  - Antalgic ("against pain") gait (shortened stance phase relative to swing phase)
  - Trendelenburg gait
- Note range of motion:
  - Flexion and extension
  - Abduction and adduction
  - Internal and external rotation
- Hip joint irritability (short arc rotation)
- Signs of other disease processes associated with avascular necrosis (e.g., sickle cell disease)
- Physical examination pearl
  - Loss of internal rotation is usually the first and most affected loss of motion seen.

DIAGNOSTIC TESTS & INTERPRETATION

Lab

- Laboratory examinations should be normal in most forms of avascular necrosis of the femoral head.
- Exceptions:
  - Sickle cell disease
  - Septic arthritis
  - Chemotherapy

Imaging

- Radiographic findings:
  - Sclerosis
  - Subchondral fracture
  - Collapse
  - Reossification
  - Repair
- Magnetic resonance imaging (MRI)
  - Bone edema
  - If contrast medium used, area of reduce blood flow evident
- Bone scan
  - Reduced signal in affected hip
- Other potential findings:
  - Cysts
  - Physeal growth arrest (young)
  - Early osteoarthritis
  - Subluxation

DIFFERENTIAL DIAGNOSIS

- Trauma
  - Osteochondral fracture
  - Impaction fracture
  - Epiphyseal/physeal fracture
- Infection
  - Osteomyelitis
  - Septic arthritis
- Neoplastic process: epiphyseal tumors (chondroblastoma, Trevor disease, etc.)
- Rheumatologic processes
- Skeletal dysplasia, particular if bilateral hip involvement

TREATMENT

MEDICATION

- NSAIDs may reduce pain by decreasing associated inflammation but may also reduce new bone formation.
- If associated with corticosteroid use, discontinuation or elimination of steroids may be helpful if appropriate.
- Bisphosphonate therapy may help preserve joint shape.

ADDITIONAL TREATMENT

General Measures

- Maintain range of motion (physical therapy, traction, continuous passive motion).
- Contain the femoral head in the acetabulum (see treatment principles listed in "Perthes Disease" chapter).
- Duration of therapy variable, depending on cause
- Reduced weight bearing on affected hip may help prevent collapse.

SURGERY/OTHER PROCEDURES

Redirectional osteotomy

- Femoral or acetabular reorientation
- Core decompression to stimulate new blood supply

ONGOING CARE

DIET

- Thought not to alter disease process
- Recommend general balanced diet
- During immobilization, excessive weight gain may occur.

PROGNOSIS

- Depends on extent of femoral head collapse
- Good if mild involvement and patient is young
- When to expect improvement: variable, depending on cause
- Moderate to severe cases often have significant collapse and end up requiring a total hip replacement.

COMPLICATIONS

- Joint collapse with decreased range of motion, pain, limping
- Osteoarthritis
- Physeal arrest with growth disturbance

ALERT

Signs to watch for:

- Subluxation
- Early osteoarthritis
- Growth arrest

ADDITIONAL READING

- Lahdes-Vasama T, Lamminen A, Merikanto J, et al. The value of MRI in early Perthes' disease: an MRI study with a 2-year follow-up. *Pediatr Radiol*. 1997; 27(6):517–522.
- Mont MA, Jones LC, Hungerford DS. Nontraumatic osteonecrosis of the femoral head: ten years later. *J Bone Joint Surg Am*. 2006;88(5):1117–1132.
- Roposch A, Mayr J, Linhart WE. Age at onset, extent of necrosis, and containment in Perthes disease. Results at maturity. *Arch Orthop Trauma Surg*. 2003;123(2):68–73.
- Shipman SA, Helfand M, Moyer VA, et al. Screening for developmental dysplasia of the hip: a systematic literature review for the US Preventive Services Task Force. *Pediatrics*. 2006;117(3):e557–e576.
- Tokmakova KP, Stanton RP, Mason DE. Factors influencing the development of osteonecrosis in patients treated for slipped capital femoral epiphysis. *J Bone Joint Surg Am*. 2003;85-A(5):798–801.

CODES

ICD10

- M87.059 Idiopathic aseptic necrosis of unspecified femur
- M91.10 Juvenile osteochondrosis of head of femur, unspecified leg
- M87.052 Idiopathic aseptic necrosis of left femur

FAQ

- Q: What type of medication is most often associated with avascular necrosis of the hip?
- A: Corticosteroids
- Q: For avascular necrosis in children (Perthes disease of the hip, for example), is younger or older age associated with a better prognosis?
- A: Younger age (<8 years)

BABESIOSIS

Oluwakemi B. Badaki-Makun • Frances M. Nadel

BASICS

DESCRIPTION

- Human babesiosis is a tick-borne malaria-like illness characterized by fever, malaise, and hemolytic anemia.
- Most infected individuals are asymptomatic.

EPIDEMIOLOGY

- Human babesiosis is a protozoal illness caused by the intraerythrocytic parasite of the *Babesia* genus.
  - *Babesia microti* is responsible for most cases of babesiosis in the United States.
  - *Babesia divergens* is responsible for most European cases.
- The parasite is transmitted by the tick vector *Ixodes scapularis* (deer tick), the same vector responsible for transmission of *Borrelia burgdorferi* (the causative agent in Lyme disease)
- The white-footed mouse (*Peromyscus leucopus*) is the primary reservoir host of *Babesia*.
- Most cases in the United States occur in the Northeast and Upper Midwest.
  - 96% of reported cases in 2012 occurred in Connecticut, Massachusetts, New Jersey, New York, Rhode Island, Minnesota, and Wisconsin.
- Human infection most commonly occurs in the warm months—late spring to early fall.

Incidence

- In January 2011, babesiosis became a nationally notifiable disease monitored by the Centers for Disease Control and Prevention (CDC).
- According to the CDC, 937 cases were reported in the United States in the year 2012, more cases than meningococcal disease, streptococcal toxic shock syndrome, or botulism combined.

Prevalence

- Prevalence is difficult to ascertain as asymptomatic infection appears to be common in endemic areas. For instance, seroprevalence is as high as 9% in some endemic areas of Rhode Island.

RISK FACTORS

- Asplenia (functional or anatomic)
- Extremes of age, especially age >50 years
- HIV/AIDS
- Immunosuppressive medications
- Malignancy
- Primary immunodeficiency syndrome

Genetics

There is no known genetic predisposition.

GENERAL PREVENTION

- Prevention begins with avoidance of tick bites.
- Simple measures include wearing long-sleeved shirts and long pants, with pants tucked into the socks in tick-infested areas.
- Avoid endemic regions during the peak months of May to September.
- Light clothing will make ticks easier to see.
- Use DEET-containing insect repellents during outdoor activities.
- Spraying one's clothing with a permethrin tick repellent may be helpful.
- Children and dogs should be inspected daily for ticks after being outside.
- Prophylaxis is not recommended after a tick bite.
- No vaccine is currently available.
- There is currently no universal laboratory screening of blood products.

PATHOPHYSIOLOGY

- Babesial infection of the erythrocyte causes membrane damage and lysis, which promotes adherence to the endothelium and microvascular stasis.
- This process results in a hemolytic anemia.
- The spleen plays an important role in decreasing the protozoal load through antibody production and filtering of abnormally shaped infected red blood cells.

ETIOLOGY

- A bite from an infected tick transmits the protozoa.
- Incubation period
  - Usually 1–4 weeks for tick-transmitted disease
  - 1–9 weeks for transfusion-associated disease
- Human-to-human transmission is limited to infection through contaminated blood.
  - Babesiosis is currently the most common transfusion-transmitted infection in the United States.
  - Rare cases of transplacental and perinatal infection have been reported.

COMMONLY ASSOCIATED CONDITIONS

- 11–23% of patients have concurrent Lyme disease.
  - Coinfections with *Borrelia* account for 80% of tick-borne coinfections.

DIAGNOSIS

HISTORY

- Few patients recall a tick bite.
- Patients live in or have recently traveled to an endemic region.
- Initial symptoms begin 1–4 weeks after the tick bite and are vague. They may include progressive fatigue, malaise, headaches, and anorexia, accompanied by intermittent fevers as high as 40°C.
- Chills, myalgias, and arthralgias may follow these symptoms.
- Less common complaints include cough, sore throat, abdominal pain, and emotional lability.

PHYSICAL EXAM

- Fever and tachycardia are often the only findings.
- Mild conjunctival injection and pharyngeal erythema occasionally occur.
- Mild hepatomegaly and/or splenomegaly may be seen.
- Jaundice or hematuria may also be observed.
- Petechiae and ecchymosis occur in rare cases, most often in the presence of severe illness with associated shock and/or DIC.

DIAGNOSTIC TESTS & INTERPRETATION

Lab

- Giemsa- or Wright-stained thick and thin blood smears may demonstrate the intraerythrocytic ring form:
  - This is often confused with the ring form of *Plasmodium falciparum*, the etiologic agent of malaria.
  - Rarely, the pathognomonic "Maltese cross" forms of the *Babesia* parasite may be seen on the blood smear.
  - Multiple smears should be performed as initial smears may be falsely negative.
- Indirect immunofluorescent assay
  - Antigen-specific for *B. microti*
  - In endemic areas, the test has a sensitivity of 91% and a specificity of 99%.
  - Can be used when blood smears are negative
  - In general, a titer = 1:64 indicates exposure.
  - Titer = 1:256 suggests acute infection.
  - There is little correlation between titer levels and severity of disease.
  - Immunoglobulin levels decline rapidly within months of recovery.
- Polymerase chain reaction is highly sensitive and specific when available.
- Other tests: Most of the abnormal routine test results are the result of hemolysis.
- Urinalysis
  - Proteinuria
  - Hemoglobinuria
- CBC
  - Normal leukocyte count/leukopenia
  - Normocytic/normochromic anemia
  - Thrombocytopenia
  - Atypical lymphocytosis
  - Reticulocytosis
- Possible positive Coombs test
- Elevated ESR
- Liver function tests: elevated bilirubin, lactate dehydrogenase, and liver transaminases
- Elevated BUN and creatinine
- In asymptomatic patients, these tests are often normal.

ALERT

False negatives:

- Blood smears may not demonstrate the protozoa at low levels of parasitemia.
- Serologic false positives for *B. microti* include cross-reactivity with other *Babesia* sp. or malarial organisms

DIFFERENTIAL DIAGNOSIS

- Ehrlichiosis
- Influenza
- Lyme disease
- Malaria
- Nonspecific viral syndrome

TREATMENT

MEDICATION

- No treatment is required for asymptomatic patients who are otherwise healthy.
- For symptomatic patients, treatment is generally for 7–10 days regardless of regimen; more severely ill patients may require a longer duration of therapy.

First Line

- Clindamycin in combination with quinine
  - Standard therapy for asplenic, immunodeficient, or severely ill patients
- Pediatric dosing:
  - Clindamycin: 20–40 mg/kg/day IV/PO divided q6–8h (max 600 mg/dose)
  - Quinine: 30 mg/kg/day PO divided into 3 doses
- Adult dosing:
  - Clindamycin: 600 mg PO q8h or 300–600 mg IV q6h
  - Quinine: 650 mg PO q8h

Second Line

- Atovaquone in combination with azithromycin
  - Has similar treatment effectiveness with fewer side effects (such as vertigo, tinnitus, and GI upset) than clindamycin and quinine in adults
  - Use of atovaquone and azithromycin has not been studied in the pediatric population; clindamycin and quinine are the recommended treatment choice for symptomatic children.
- Pediatric dosing:
  - Atovaquone 40 mg/kg/day PO divided into 2 doses (max 750 mg q12h)
  - Azithromycin 10 mg/kg/day (max 500 mg) PO on day 1 and 5 mg/kg/day (max 250 mg) PO daily thereafter
- Adult dosing:
  - Atovaquone 750 mg PO q12h
  - Azithromycin 500–1,000 mg PO on day 1 and 250–1,000 mg PO daily thereafter
- In areas endemic for Lyme disease and ehrlichiosis, consider adding doxycycline to either regimen until lab confirmation of absence of either disease in the patient with babesiosis.

ADDITIONAL TREATMENT

General Measures

Those with mild clinical disease usually recover without treatment.

ADDITIONAL THERAPIES

- For life-threatening infections, exchange transfusion has been successful. Consider in patients with severe parasitemia (≥10%), severe hemolysis, or renal/hepatic/pulmonary compromise.
- Progressive respiratory distress may require mechanical ventilation.

ALERT

- Signs to watch for:
  - Respiratory distress, especially after treatment has begun
  - Pancytopenia and lymphadenopathy: may indicate the development of hemophagocytic syndrome
- Pitfalls
  - Children who are from endemic areas and have an acute febrile illness may be misdiagnosed with a nonspecific viral illness.
  - One should be suspicious for a coinfection with Lyme disease or ehrlichiosis in those who are not responding to standard therapy.
  - Delayed recognition of this uncommon disease may be life threatening in the immunocompromised patient.
  - In endemic areas, babesiosis should be considered in a posttransfusion febrile illness in at-risk populations.

ONGOING CARE

FOLLOW-UP RECOMMENDATIONS

When to expect improvement:

- Some improvement of symptoms should be noted within 24–48 hours of onset of therapy.
- Those who are only mildly affected usually have resolution of their symptoms over a few weeks.
- For severely affected and immunodeficient patients, the convalescent period may be as long as 18 months.
- In untreated asymptomatic individuals, parasitemia may persist for months to years.
- Long-term complications are rare.
- Recrudescence has been reported.

COMPLICATIONS

- Rarely fatal in the United States
- Pancytopenia and overwhelming secondary bacterial sepsis may occur.
- Serious and fulminant complications have been described:
  - Pulmonary edema and adult respiratory distress syndrome, often happening after treatment has begun.
  - CHF
  - Renal failure
  - Hemophagocytic syndrome/DIC
  - Seizures/coma
- Those coinfected with Lyme disease are susceptible to more severe disease and complications.

ADDITIONAL READING

- American Academy of Pediatrics. Babesiosis. In: Pickering LK, Baker CJ, Kimberlin DW, et al, eds. *Red Book: 2012 Report of the Committee on Infectious Diseases*. 29th ed. Elk Grove Village, IL: American Academy of Pediatrics; 2012:244–245.
- Centers for Disease Control and Prevention. Summary of notifiable diseases—United States, 2010. *MMWR Morb Mortal Wkly Rep*. 2012;59(53): 1–111.
- Vannier E, Gewurz BE, Krause PJ. Human babesiosis. *Infect Dis Clin North Am*. 2008;22(3):469–488, viii–ix.
- Vannier E, Krause PJ. Human babesiosis. *N Engl J Med*. 2012;366(25):2397–2407.
- Wormser GP, Dattwyler RJ, Shapiro ED, et al. The clinical assessment, treatment, and prevention of Lyme disease, human granulocytic anaplasmosis, and babesiosis: clinical practice guidelines by the Infectious Diseases Society of America. *Clin Infect Dis*. 2006;43(9):1089–1134.

CODES

ICD10

B60.0 Babesiosis

FAQ

- Q: How long does a tick have to be attached for infection to occur?
- A: In general, successful transmission requires at least 24 hours of attachment.
- Q: How should a tick be removed?
- A: The tick should be grasped with forceps as close to its head as possible and pulled straight up. If possible, it should be saved for identification.
- Q: Does infection confer lifetime immunity?
- A: Reinfection is possible.

BACK PAIN

Danielle N. Clark • Peter Chira

BASICS

DESCRIPTION

Any condition causing pain of the thoracic, lumbar, or sacral spine

EPIDEMIOLOGY

- 12-month period prevalence: 10–20% of children
- Lifetime prevalence: 12–50%

RISK FACTORS

- Poor conditioning or high athletic performance
- Joint hypermobility
- Role of backpack weight and style of wear undetermined
- Role of overweight or obesity yet to be determined

GENERAL PREVENTION

- Back muscle strengthening and hamstring stretching exercises may be helpful.
- Maximum backpack load: 10–15% body weight
- Weight loss and increased physical activity in overweight or obese children

PATHOPHYSIOLOGY

- Dependent on underlying cause
- Hyperextension with rotational spinal loading in the case of pars defects (e.g., spondylolysis or spondylolisthesis)
- Autoimmune or autoinflammatory processes as with juvenile idiopathic arthritis (JIA) or juvenile ankylosing spondylitis

ETIOLOGY

- Unidentified in 50% of cases
- 30% of chronic cases (back pain >3 years) without clear etiology despite workup

DIAGNOSIS

HISTORY

- History can be helpful with elucidating most likely cause.
- Musculoskeletal/trauma
  - Direct trauma
  - Worsening pain after activity
  - Repetitive movements causing microtrauma
- Inflammatory
  - Morning stiffness (variable pain)
  - Pain/stiffness improves with movement.
  - Family history of rheumatic disease
- Infectious
  - Fever
  - Recent exposure to infection or tuberculosis (TB)
- Malignancy
  - Night sweats, fever, weight loss, malaise, pain waking at night
  - Previous history of malignancy
- Neurologic
  - Radiating pain or foot drop
  - Loss of bowel or bladder function
- Endocrine/metabolic
  - Long-term steroid use
  - Vitamin D deficiency
- Psychosocial stressors (e.g., family coping mechanisms and response to pain and stress)

PHYSICAL EXAM

- **Finding:** observation: sacral dimple, vascular anomalies, posture, spinal curvature, anterior superior iliac spine (ASIS) height, limb length discrepancy, foot arch, lower limb alignment, rib rotation
  - *Significance*: occult problem; mechanical or musculoskeletal problem. Scoliosis is rarely painful. Increased fixed kyphosis of 40 degrees is indicative of Scheuermann disease.
- **Finding:** palpation: point or focal tenderness along spine; sacroiliac (SI) joint tenderness
  - *Significance*: If bony, consider fracture, vertebral osteomyelitis; if paraspinal, consider muscle strain. If SI tenderness, consider spondylitis.
- **Finding:** range of motion: pain with spinal extension (causing strain of anterior elements of spine)
  - *Significance*: Consider spondylolisthesis (forward vertebral displacement), spondylolysis (vertebral defect), fracture, vertebral osteomyelitis, or tumor.
- **Finding:** range of motion: forward spinal flexion limitation
  - *Significance*: If painful, consider diskitis, vertebral osteomyelitis, vertebral body tumor, and herniated disc if pain radiates.
  - *Significance*: If limited as noted by flattening of lumbosacral region with movement, consider spondylitis.
- **Finding:** range of motion: restriction of spine with pain (especially with neck extension) and other associated joint abnormalities (swelling or pain/tenderness with limitation)
  - *Significance*: Consider JIA.
- **Special Tests:** pain with straight-leg raise: Consider tight hamstrings, psoas strain, or disc herniation.
- **Special Tests:** pain with FABER (flexion, abduction, external rotation with foot on opposite knee) testing or direct palpation of SI joint: SI joint irritation or inflammation
- **Special Tests:** Assess reflexes, sensation, Babinski, pain, and proprioception; deficits may indicate neuronal involvement.
- Abdominal or pelvic exam may be helpful.

DIAGNOSTIC TESTS & INTERPRETATION

- **Tests:** CBC with differential, sedimentation rate, C-reactive protein (CRP), and comprehensive metabolic panel with uric acid and LDH
  - *Significance*: malignancy, infection, inflammatory
- Antinuclear antibody, rheumatoid factor, anticyclic citrullinated antibody, and HLA B27 only if obvious other associated joint abnormalities found
  - *Significance*: inflammatory/autoimmune disorders
- Cultures, PPD, or other TB study
  - Significance: infection
- 25-OH vitamin D, PTH, calcium, phosphorus, alkaline phosphorus
  - *Significance*: vitamin D deficiency or osteoporosis

Imaging

- Plain x-rays
  - AP and lateral; oblique and flexion/extension (if warranted) of the spine
  - Assess for fracture, spinal curvature, osteomyelitis, and masses.
  - Intra-articular pars defect commonly in L4/L5 indicates spondylolysis.
  - Bilateral pars defect with vertebral body displacement indicates spondylolisthesis.
- Bone scan
  - Occult/subtle bony lesions and spondylolysis and spondylolisthesis
- CT spine
  - Useful to categorize lesions seen on bone scan such as spondylosis/spondylolisthesis
- MRI
  - Tumor, infection, disk injuries, synovitis (including effusions or erosions), and neurologic findings

DIFFERENTIAL DIAGNOSIS

- Mechanical/trauma
  - Overuse injury
  - Disc herniation
- Direct trauma, contusion
  - Musculoskeletal strain in children with closed growth plates
  - Apophyseal ring fracture
- Structural
  - Pars defects: children usually >10 years of age
  - Spondylolysis/spondylolisthesis (anterior displacement/"slip" of vertebral body, evolution of bilateral spondylolysis)
  - Scheuermann kyphosis: deformity of thoracic spine associated with vertebral body wedging
- Inflammatory
  - JIA
  - Juvenile ankylosing spondylitis
  - Chronic recurrent multifocal osteomyelitis
- Neoplastic
  - Ewing sarcoma
  - Lymphoma, leukemia
- Infectious
  - Osteomyelitis
  - Epidural abscess
  - Pyelonephritis
  - Diskitis
- Endocrine/metabolic
  - Osteoporosis
  - Vitamin D deficiency
- Other
  - Pain amplification syndrome (fibromyalgia, myofascial pain)
  - Sickle cell crises, abdominal disease (pancreatitis, pyelonephritis)
- Age differentiation
  - <10 years: diskitis, tumor, epidural
  - >10 years: pars defects, inflammatory disorders

ALERT

- Warning signs of potentially serious causes of back pain in children include the following:
  - Young age: <7 years old
  - Duration of pain: >4 weeks
  - Acute trauma
  - Night pain, fever, weight loss, or malaise
  - Abdominal mass
  - Early morning stiffness
  - History of tumor
  - Exposure to TB
  - Limp
  - Chronic interference with normal activity (e.g., school, sports, play)
  - Postural changes causing scoliosis or kyphosis
  - Other associated joint abnormalities (swelling OR pain/tenderness with joint limitation)

TREATMENT

MEDICATION

- Nonsteroidal anti-inflammatory drugs (NSAIDs) for overuse or strains in adolescents and for patients with arthritis
- Additional medication may be necessary depending on underlying condition such as antibiotics for infection, chemotherapy for malignancy, immunosuppression for inflammatory/autoimmune, or vitamin D and calcium supplementation for vitamin D deficiency or osteoporosis.

ADDITIONAL TREATMENT

General Measures

- If no warning signs, conservative management with NSAIDs, physical therapy, and close follow-up are appropriate.
- Abnormal exam/history or focal symptoms warrant imaging.
- Spondylolysis/spondylolisthesis
  - <50% slip: conservative medical treatment
  - >50% slip/persistent back pain: surgical treatment
- Diskitis: antistaphylococcal coverage
- Bed rest/activity limitation: Adult data do not support this strategy.

ISSUES FOR REFERRAL

- Sports medicine or orthopedics appropriate with Scheuermann disease, spondylolysis or spondylolisthesis
- Concern for malignancy or long-standing inflammatory process such as JIA or juvenile ankylosing spondylitis warrants referral to hematology/oncology or rheumatology, respectively.
- Endocrinology referral for suspected osteoporosis

ADDITIONAL THERAPIES

- Physical therapy with focus on core strength and flexibility if cause is due to overuse or due to a sedentary lifestyle
- Removal from activity for overuse injuries with slow gradual return
- Structural problems such as spondylolysis, spondylolisthesis, and Scheuermann disease often respond to rest, ice, NSAIDs, and thoraco-lumbar-sacral orthosis bracing.
- A biopsychosocial approach is needed for patients with pain amplification syndromes in conjunction with physical and cognitive behavioral therapies and emphasis on functionality.

COMPLEMENTARY & ALTERNATIVE THERAPIES

- Yoga and Pilates emphasizing core strength and flexibility may be useful in the adolescent.
- Cochrane systematic review determined massage may be useful in the setting of acute or subacute back pain in adults.
- Acupuncture may be useful for dealing with pain.

SURGERY/OTHER PROCEDURES

Indicated in patients with spondylolisthesis slip of >50%

ONGOING CARE

FOLLOW-UP RECOMMENDATIONS

- Patients managed conservatively should be reevaluated within 2 weeks and then spaced further as their pain improves.
- If symptoms not improving with conservative measures, then consider workup as outlined and appropriate referral depending on results.

Patient Monitoring

No specific lab tests need to be routinely followed.

PATIENT EDUCATION

- Patients and families need to be aware that musculoskeletal and structural causes may take several weeks to heal.
- Pain in spondylolysis and spondylolisthesis does not always correlate with degree of involvement.
- Patients should be told to report changes in symptoms, especially any red flags.

PROGNOSIS

- Dependent on the underlying cause
- With proper diagnosis and treatment, the majority do well, without significant sequelae.
- Not possible to predict future course of spondylolysis, spondylolisthesis, or Scheuermann kyphosis

COMPLICATIONS

- Contractures and loss of function
- Paralysis, other permanent neuromuscular injury
- Chronic back pain or development of pain amplification syndrome

ADDITIONAL READING

- Davis PC, Williams HJ. The investigation and management of back pain in children. *Arch Dis Child Educ Pract Ed*. 2008;93(3):73–83.
- Furlan AD, Imamura M, Dryden T, et al. Massage for low-back pain: an updated systematic review within the framework of the Cochrane Back Review Group. *Spine (Phila Pa 1976)*. 2009;34(16):1669–1684.
- Houghton, K. Review for the generalist: evaluation of low back pain in children and adolescents. *Ped Rheum*. 2010;8:28.
- Jackson C, McLaughlin K, Teti B. Back pain in children: a holistic and diagnostic approach. *J Ped Health Care*. 2011;25(5):284–293.

CODES

ICD10

- M54.9 Dorsalgia, unspecified
- M54.6 Pain in thoracic spine
- M54.5 Low back pain

FAQ

- Q: Which children with back pain should have activity restriction?
- A: Children with spinal or bony abnormalities should avoid hyperextension and high-impact sports.
- Q: When can/should the child resume activities after an acute back injury?
- A: Children with a normal neurologic exam and diagnostic studies can resume activity or sports as tolerated.
- Q: Should a trial of steroids be used to rule out inflammatory back pain?
- A: Pain improvement with glucocorticoids may suggest an inflammatory condition but is not diagnostic. It is not recommended in children, as it can often complicate the clinical picture, as noninflammatory back pain will sometimes respond to treatment as well.

BAROTITIS

Judith Brylinski Larkin

BASICS

DESCRIPTION

- Barotrauma of the middle or inner ear, most commonly caused by flying in an airplane or scuba diving but also caused by elevators and high altitudes
- May also be seen in those who have used a hyperbaric oxygen chamber and in people involved in explosions—blast injuries
- Referred to as "middle ear squeeze" by scuba divers

EPIDEMIOLOGY

- Severe disease is uncommon in commercial aircraft because of pressurization.
- Significant disease is more common in scuba divers, in those who fly military aircraft, and during use of hyperbaric oxygen chambers.
- There is wide variation, with studies reporting an incidence of 8–55% for children after a single flight.
- Most studies agree that the incidence is ~20% in adults after a single flight.
- 40% frequency in scuba diving

RISK FACTORS

- Age: Infants or toddlers are at higher risk because of small eustachian tubes.
- Disease states that impede normal eustachian tube function: otitis media, upper respiratory tract infection (URI), allergic rhinitis
- Smoking
- Vigorous use of Valsalva maneuver

GENERAL PREVENTION

- Gradual descent during scuba diving—never rapid
- When ascending, divers should avoid rising more quickly than their air bubbles.
- Yawning, swallowing, chewing, or doing Valsalva maneuver during takeoff and landing in planes and during ascent and descent when scuba diving
- Gentle Valsalva—never vigorous
- Avoid flying or diving when you have a URI or allergic rhinitis.
- Avoid sleeping on plane during takeoff and landing.
- Break seal of wet suit hood to allow water to fill external canal before descent.
- Avoid use of earplugs.

PATHOPHYSIOLOGY

- Boyle's law states that as pressure of a gas decreases, volume increases, and as pressure of a gas increases, volume decreases.
- Ambient pressure decreases during airplane/scuba diving ascent and increases during descent.
- During ascent, the tympanic membrane (TM) bulges outward and the eustachian tube vents the excess middle ear pressure. Pressure is easily equalized.
- During descent, the TM bulges inward and the eustachian tube resists inward flow of air. Pressure equalization is difficult.
- At a pressure differential of 60 mm Hg (greater ambient to middle ear pressure), subjective discomfort is reported.
- At a pressure differential of 90 mm Hg, the eustachian tube collapses and becomes obstructed. Autoinflation is unsuccessful.
- TM can rupture at pressure differentials >100–400 mm Hg.
- Barotitis is sometimes classified using Teed classification of disease severity (see "Physical Exam").

ETIOLOGY

Differences in the atmospheric pressure between the inner ear, middle ear, and environment result in injury to the middle and/or inner ear.

DIAGNOSIS

HISTORY

- Ear pain, pressure sensation, diminished hearing
- Symptoms of inner ear damage may include vestibular and/or auditory complaints including tinnitus, vertigo, nausea, and vomiting.
- History of recent airplane flying, scuba diving, or hyperbaric oxygen chamber use

PHYSICAL EXAM

- Nystagmus
- Hearing loss
- Teed classification to describe appearance of the TM:
  - Grade 0: symptoms without physical signs
  - Grade 1: diffuse redness and retraction of TM
  - Grade 2: grade 1 plus slight hemorrhage into TM
  - Grade 3: grade 1 plus gross hemorrhage into TM
  - Grade 4: bulging TM with air–fluid level, blood in TM
  - Grade 5: free hemorrhage into TM and ear canal with perforation of TM

DIAGNOSTIC TESTS & INTERPRETATION

Imaging

CT of the inner ear may be indicated in patients with vestibular symptoms or hearing loss to rule out inner ear damage.

Diagnostic Procedures/Other

Hearing tests should be performed on all patients who have signs of barotrauma and on patients with normal physical exams but who are symptomatic.

DIFFERENTIAL DIAGNOSIS

- Otitis media with effusion
- Acute otitis media
- Otitis externa
- Blunt trauma to the TM
- Exposure to extremely loud noise

TREATMENT

MEDICATION

- Nasal decongestant sprays (oxymetazoline [Afrin])
  - Have been reported by some to be helpful, but a randomized clinical trial showed no advantage over placebo
  - Theory: By constricting mucosal arterioles, eustachian tube function is enhanced.
  - Topical decongestants are used 1 hour prior to plane travel/diving and 1/2 hour prior to plane descent.
  - 2 drops/sprays per nostril
  - Use in children older than 6 years of age.
- Oral decongestants
  - 2 randomized controlled trials suggest that oral decongestants may be effective, although a trial in children did not show a beneficial effect.
  - May be helpful through the same physiologic pathway as topical agents
  - Should be initiated 1–2 days prior to the expected pressure change
- Antihistamines
  - May also be helpful by reducing mucosal edema and enhancing the eustachian tube orifice
  - Can be used on the day of the expected pressure change
- Nasal surfactants may be useful but ongoing studies are needed.
- Pain relievers such as acetaminophen, ibuprofen, and naproxen may be useful for severe pain.

ADDITIONAL TREATMENT

General Measures

- Valsalva maneuver (blowing the nose while pinching the nostrils closed) may be helpful when diving or descending and will force air into the middle ear via the eustachian tube, thereby equalizing the pressure between the middle ear and the environment. This should be done gently.
- Swallowing, yawning, and chewing can help to release pressure through the eustachian tube when descending in an airplane or when returning to the water surface while scuba diving.
- Politzer bag: instrument used for clearing pressure disequilibrium that has not improved with Valsalva maneuvers and a trial of decongestants
- Otovent: Another instrument that may be used for treatment or prevention; usage can be taught to children as young as 2–6 years of age.
- Myringotomy with or without tubes may be required to relieve pressure in severe disease. It may also be used as a preventive measure in those with a history of barotitis.
- Myringotomy is effective for the patient with excruciating pain or unrelenting eustachian tube dysfunction; this is best performed by an otolaryngologist.

SURGERY/OTHER PROCEDURES

Rarely, myringotomy with or without tube insertion is required to relieve pressure and pain as well as prevent complications. Myringotomy is a surgical procedure where a small incision is made in the TM. This opens the middle ear space and equalizes the pressure on both sides of the TM. Myringotomy without tube insertion will relieve pressure, but the opening may close very quickly and may not allow time for the barotrauma to heal; on occasion, myringotomy with tube insertion is necessary. Tympanostomy tubes are not appropriate for scuba divers.

ONGOING CARE

FOLLOW-UP RECOMMENDATIONS

Patient Monitoring

Most patients with barotitis can be managed conservatively. Those with complications noted earlier require specialist referral.

PROGNOSIS

- Complete spontaneous resolution in mild cases
- Middle ear barotrauma is usually self-limited and correctable with the techniques described in the "General Measures" section. In rare instances, where there is severe pain or eustachian tube dysfunction, myringotomy with or without tube insertion will relieve the pressure differential.
- Pressure differential without damage to the middle or inner ear usually resolves within a few days of returning to normal atmospheric pressure.
- Barotitis that results in injury to the middle or inner ear has a variable rate of improvement; some damage may be permanent (e.g., that to the organ of Corti), whereas other injury is reversible (e.g., that involving the TM).
- Variable outcome for auditory and vestibular symptoms and injuries to the inner ear

COMPLICATIONS

- Vertigo
- Tinnitus
- Hearing loss
- TM rupture
- Oval or round window rupture
- Hemorrhage

ADDITIONAL READING

- Buchanan BJ, Hoagland J, Fischer PR. Pseudoephedrine and air travel-associated ear pain in children. *Arch Pediatr Adolesc Med*. 1999;153(5):466–468.
- Janvrin S. Middle ear pain and trauma during air travel. *Clin Evid*. 2002;7:466–468.
- Jones JS, Sheffeild W, White L, et al. A double-blind comparison between oral pseudoephedrine and topical oxymetazoline in the prevention of barotrauma during air travel. *Am J Emerg Med*. 1998;16(3):262–264.
- Mirza S, Richardson H. Otic barotraumas from air travel. *J Laryngol Otol*. 2005;119(5):366–370.
- Rosenkvist L, Klokker M, Katholm M. Upper respiratory infections and barotraumas in commercial pilots: a retrospective survey. *Aviat Space Environ Med*. 2008;79(10):960–963.
- Stangerup SE, Klokker M, Vesterhauge S, et al. Point prevalence of barotitis and its prevention and treatment with nasal balloon inflation: a prospective, controlled study. *Otol Neurotol*. 2004;25(2):89–94.
- Weiss MH, Frost JO. May children with otitis media with effusion safely fly? *Clin Pediatr (Phila)*. 1987;26(11):567–568.

CODES

ICD10

- T70.0XXA Otitic barotrauma, initial encounter
- H92.09 Otalgia, unspecified ear
- H93.19 Tinnitus, unspecified ear

FAQ

- Q: Is the Valsalva maneuver also effective on plane ascent?
- A: Yes. Creating even greater pressure in the middle ear by performing the Valsalva maneuver can overcome a resistant eustachian tube and result in sudden venting of increased middle ear pressure.
- Q: Can children with otitis media travel in airplanes?
- A: Yes. Weiss and Frost (1987) have shown that commercial air travel did not result in worsening of symptoms and, in fact, the presence of otitis media with effusion seemed to be protective against barotitis.
- Q: How can I minimize my child's ear pain when traveling in an airplane?
- A: For infants: Have them nurse, take a bottle, or suck on a pacifier during ascent and descent. Older children may eat or chew gum or suck on hard candies. This will result in pharyngeal movements that will repeatedly open the eustachian tube and equalize middle ear pressure to environmental pressure. Children can also be taught the Valsalva maneuver. If the child is currently experiencing a URI, use of decongestants prior to flight may be helpful.

BARTTER SYNDROME

Elaine Ku • Anthony A. Portale

BASICS

DESCRIPTION

- Bartter syndrome is a hereditary renal salt-wasting tubulopathy characterized by hypokalemic, hypochloremic metabolic alkalosis and normal or low blood pressure.
- The genetic defect is localized to the thick ascending limb of the loop of Henle.
- Timing and severity of presentation are variable depending on the type of genetic defect.
- Two phenotypes:
  - Antenatal (types I, II, and IV)
    - Associated with polyhydramnios and premature delivery
    - Presents in the first 4–6 weeks of life, often with polyuria and signs/symptoms of severe dehydration
    - Associated with hypercalciuria and nephrocalcinosis
    - Type IV is associated with sensorineural deafness.
  - Classic (type III)
    - Symptoms begin at age 2 years and diagnosis is usually made later in childhood or during adolescence.

EPIDEMIOLOGY

- Bartter syndrome is a very rare disorder.
  - Prevalence: 1 per million
  - Prevalence is higher in areas where consanguinity is common.

ETIOLOGY

- Mode of transmission: autosomal recessive except for type V which is autosomal dominant
- Five genetic subtypes and their various genetic defects:
  - Type I: sodium-potassium-chloride cotransporter (NKCC)
  - Type II: potassium channel (ROMK)
  - Type III: chloride channel (ClC-Kb)
  - Type IV: barttin protein
  - Type V: Calcium-sensing receptor associated with autosomal dominant hypocalcemia

PATHOPHYSIOLOGY

- Mutations in NKCC, ROMK, barttin, or ClC-Kb result in the Bartter syndrome phenotype of salt wasting and hypokalemia by disrupting the molecular pathways for electrolyte transport in the thick ascending limb as described below.
- In the thick ascending limb of the loop of Henle, approximately 25% of filtered sodium chloride is reabsorbed via the sodium-potassium-2-chloride cotransporter (NKCC2), which is the target of loop diuretics such as furosemide.
- Potassium exits the cell via potassium channels (ROMK) on the apical (lumen) side of the tubule and is recycled via the NKCC2, thus permitting continued sodium chloride reabsorption.
- Chloride exits the cell and enters the bloodstream via a basolateral chloride channel (ClC-Kb) that is anchored by an accessory protein, barttin.
- A calcium-sensing receptor on the blood (basolateral) side, when activated by calcium, inhibits ROMK activity, which interferes with NKCC activity. A gain-of-function mutation in the calcium-sensing receptor results in a Bartter-like syndrome (type V).
- Calcium and magnesium are normally reabsorbed paracellularly in the thick ascending limb, driven by the lumen-positive potential that is created by sodium chloride transport across NKCC.
  - Hypercalciuria, and sometimes hypermagnesuria, occurs due to decreased paracellular transport of calcium and magnesium in the setting of salt wasting.
- Renin and aldosterone levels are typically increased (triggered by volume depletion) and contribute to metabolic alkalosis and hypokalemia.
- A functional thick ascending limb is necessary for the function of the countercurrent multiplier that is responsible for renal concentrating ability; impaired function of the thick ascending limb results in impaired urinary concentration.
- Prostaglandin E levels are typically very elevated in Bartter syndrome.

DIAGNOSIS

HISTORY

- Dehydration
- Emesis
- Diarrhea
- Recurrent fevers
- Failure to thrive
- Polydipsia
- Polyuria
- Growth retardation
- Anorexia
- Symptoms of hypokalemia
  - Muscle weakness
  - Constipation
- Cognitive and developmental delay
- Salt craving
- Seizures
- Kidney stones (antenatal Bartter)
- History of hearing loss (antenatal Bartter)

PHYSICAL EXAM

- Constitutional: failure to thrive
- Head: large forehead
- Eyes: large eyes
- Ears: protuberant
- Face: triangular facies
- Neurologic: developmental and cognitive delay
- Skin: decreased turgor, prolonged capillary refill

DIAGNOSTIC TESTS & INTERPRETATION

Lab

- Serum electrolytes
  - To identify the presence of hypochloremic metabolic alkalosis and hypokalemia
  - Phosphorus level (can be low)
- Serum creatinine: to evaluate GFR
- Urine electrolytes
  - Urine chloride is typically >10 mEq/day.
  - Urine sodium and potassium are elevated.

- Urinalysis
  - Low specific gravity due to urinary concentrating defect
- Random urine for calcium/creatinine ratio
  - To detect hypercalciuria
  - Normal values are age-dependent.
- Renin level (typically elevated)
- 24-hour urine aldosterone excretion (typically elevated)

Imaging

Renal ultrasound: to determine presence of nephrocalcinosis and kidney stones

Diagnostic Procedures/Other

DIFFERENTIAL DIAGNOSIS

- Chronic or cyclical vomiting
- Chloride-losing diarrhea
- Pyloric stenosis
- Cystic fibrosis
- Diuretic abuse
- Gitelman syndrome
- Mineralocorticoid excess

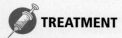

TREATMENT

MEDICATION

- Sodium chloride supplementation
- Potassium chloride supplementation
- Nonsteroidal anti-inflammatory drugs (NSAIDs) such as indomethacin
- Potassium-sparing diuretic such as spironolactone to help counter hypokalemia
- Angiotensin-converting enzyme inhibitors
- Growth hormone

ADDITIONAL TREATMENT

General Measures

- High-salt and high-potassium diet
- Adequate fluid intake to match urinary losses in the setting of salt wasting and polyuria

ONGOING CARE

FOLLOW-UP RECOMMENDATIONS

- Frequent monitoring of serum electrolytes
- Close follow-up of linear growth
- Monitor for signs of kidney stone.

PROGNOSIS

Can progress to chronic kidney disease or end-stage renal disease due to hypokalemia-induced interstitial disease and concurrent chronic NSAID use

ADDITIONAL READING

- Chadha V, Alon US. Hereditary renal tubular disorders. *Semin Nephrol*. 2009;29(4):399–411.
- Fremont OT, Chan JC. Understanding Bartter syndrome and Gitelman syndrome. *World J Pediatr*. 2012;8(1):25–30.
- Seyberth HW. An improved terminology and classification of Bartter-like syndromes. *Nat Clin Pract Nephrol*. 2008;4(10):560–567.

CODES

ICD10

E26.81 Bartter's syndrome

FAQ

- Q: Can Bartter syndrome be treated with renal transplantation?
- A: Yes. A few cases of renal transplantation in Bartter syndrome have been described for correction of severe electrolyte disorders, growth disturbances, or treatment of chronic kidney disease.
- Q: How can vomiting be distinguished from Bartter syndrome?
- A: In vomiting, urine chloride is typically <10 mEq/L, whereas in Bartter syndrome, the urine chloride is typically much higher (typically >40 mEq/L).
- Q: How does Bartter syndrome differ from Gitelman syndrome?
- A: Gitelman syndrome is a defect of the thiazide-sensitive sodium chloride cotransporter in the distal convoluted tubule. Patients with Gitelman syndrome also present with hypokalemic metabolic alkalosis but typically have hypocalciuria in contrast to normal or increased urinary calcium in patients with Bartter syndrome. Patients with Gitelman also typically have persistent hypomagnesemia and high urinary fractional excretion of magnesium. In addition, patients with Gitelman syndrome typically have a blunted thiazide response (manifested by an increase in the fractional excretion of chloride after thiazide administration), whereas patients with Bartter syndrome will respond to thiazide diuretics
- Q: How can Bartter syndrome be distinguished from diuretic abuse?
- A: Both Bartter syndrome and diuretic abuse will present with similar electrolyte abnormalities and an elevated urinary chloride. The best test for diuretic abuse is a urinary diuretic screen.
- Q: What is the role of genetic testing in Bartter syndrome?
- A: Genetic testing is available but is currently expensive and may not include all known or as yet unrecognized mutations, which limits its use.

BELL PALSY

Stephen J. Falchek

BASICS

DESCRIPTION

- This paralysis may involve all of the modalities affected by the 7th cranial nerve:
  - Mimetic facial movement
  - Taste
  - Cutaneous sensation
  - Hearing acuity
  - Lacrimation
  - Salivation
- The most important feature in diagnosis and management of Bell palsy is the distinction between a peripheral and a central 7th nerve palsy.

EPIDEMIOLOGY

Incidence

- Annually, incidence ranges from 3/100,000 in patients <10 years to 25/100,000 in adults.
- Only 1% of cases have bilateral involvement.

PATHOPHYSIOLOGY

Nearly all cases of true Bell palsy are believed to arise from a viral infection of the facial nerve and, in particular, the geniculate ganglion.

ETIOLOGY

- Idiopathic: pregnancy-related
- Infectious
  - Herpes simplex virus 1
  - Human herpesvirus 6
  - Herpes zoster (without Ramsay Hunt syndrome)

COMMONLY ASSOCIATED CONDITIONS

- Associated illnesses can cause or predispose to an isolated facial nerve palsy but are important to distinguish from a classic Bell palsy.
- Rubella
- Lyme disease (*Borrelia burgdorferi)*
- Epstein-Barr virus (EBV)
- Cytomegalovirus (CMV)
- Mumps
- HIV
- *Mycoplasma pneumoniae*
- Sarcoidosis

DIAGNOSIS

HISTORY

- Mastoid or retroauricular pain ipsilateral to the side of developing symptoms (40–50% of patients)
- 50% of patients will have no clear sensory prodrome.
- Bell palsy often follows some identifiable infectious illness, such as viral upper respiratory tract infection (URI) symptoms, *M. pneumoniae* infection, Lyme disease, or infectious mononucleosis. However, an identified antecedent illness is not requisite for the diagnosis.
- The onset is almost always rapid, with progression to a fairly constant state of unilateral paresis or paralysis within hours to 2–3 days.
- As the weakness progresses, the patient (and family members) may note the following:
  - Difficulty with oral motor tasks (e.g., eating and drinking) due to inability to maintain mouth closure
  - Inability to completely close the eye on the affected side (sometimes leading untrained observers to note an eyelid "droop" on the normal side due to the contrast with normal eyelid closure and movements)
  - Decreased lacrimation and eye itching and burning
  - Hyperacusis
  - Ipsilateral facial numbness (less commonly)
  - Distortion of the taste of foods (dysgeusia)
- Bilateral symptoms (<1%) are distinctly rare and suggest an alternative diagnosis, such as Guillain-Barré syndrome or other infectious, inflammatory, or metabolic disease.

PHYSICAL EXAM

- Weakness of all muscles of mimetic facial movement is noted on the affected side.
- A classic feature of peripheral facial nerve palsies is symmetric weakness or paralysis of the upper (frontalis), middle (orbicularis oculi), and lower (orbicularis oris) muscles on voluntary and involuntary mimetic movements. Having the patient wrinkle his or her forehead/raise his or her eyebrows, close his or her eyes tightly, and bare his or her teeth or smile, respectively, tests these muscles.
- Occasionally, slow or absent spontaneous blinking on the affected side
- The corneal reflex should be decreased or absent on the affected side, but the consensual response on the unaffected side should be preserved.
- The sensory division of the 7th cranial nerve is tested by examining taste perception on the anterior tongue:
  - This is done by applying, ipsilaterally, swabs soaked in a sugar solution and a salt solution to the anterolateral aspect of the tongue, without allowing for mouth closure and dispersion of the substances to the other side. Taste sensation should be ipsilaterally decreased.
  - Despite complaints of retroauricular pain and unilateral facial "numbness," abnormalities of cutaneous sensation typically are not verifiable by sensory testing in pure 7th nerve palsies. The presence of true diminution of sensation should raise the question of other cranial nerve involvement (e.g., 5th cranial nerve).
- Examination of the external auditory canal on both sides is crucial.
  - Vesicular lesions of the tympanic membrane indicate a zoster-associated palsy (i.e., Ramsay Hunt syndrome).
  - Purulent acute otitis media or evidence of trauma mandate aggressive antibiotic treatment and possibly urgent surgical subspecialty evaluation and imaging of the temporal bone.

DIAGNOSTIC TESTS & INTERPRETATION

Imaging

- The decision to defer medical imaging in the evaluation of a typical Bell palsy should be based on a sound clinical history and physical examination. Unusual features should provoke thoughtful review and broader investigation where indicated.
- MRI of the head with gadolinium enhancement: recommended in cases of unusual presentation or progression (e.g., bilateral involvement, slow progression [>1 week], or other cranial nerve findings). Several small series have proposed that gadolinium enhancement of the involved 7th nerve predicts a slower or less optimal recovery.

DIFFERENTIAL DIAGNOSIS

- Trauma
  - Birth (especially forceps pressure to lateral face)
  - Congenital facial palsies should not be regarded as Bell palsy but rather symptomatic of some other cause.
  - Temporal bone/petrous bone fractures
  - Deep lacerations or trauma to parotid region
- Infection
  - Purulent acute otitis media/mastoiditis
  - Basilar meningitis
  - Petrous apicitis (Gradenigo syndrome)
  - Varicella-zoster virus (VZV; Ramsay Hunt syndrome)
  - Syphilis
  - Trichinosis
  - Tuberculosis
  - Leprosy
- Inflammatory
  - Sarcoidosis
  - Behçet disease
  - Giant cell arteritis
  - Polyarteritis nodosa
  - Guillain-Barré syndrome
  - Melkersson-Rosenthal syndrome: rare neurologic disorder characterized by recurring facial paralysis, swelling of the face and lips (usually the upper lip), and the development of folds and furrows in the tongue
- Tumors
  - Cerebellopontine angle tumors, osteosarcomas, cholesteatomas, neurofibromas, lymphoma
  - Hyperostosis cranialis interna, osteopetrosis
- Metabolic
  - Diabetes (nerve ischemia)
  - Hyperparathyroidism
  - Hypothyroidism
  - Porphyria
- Congenital/genetic
  - Congenital absence or hypoplasia of depressor anguli oris muscle
  - Möbius syndrome
  - Chiari malformation
  - Syringobulbia

TREATMENT

Identifying treatable causes of 7th nerve palsy (e.g., Lyme borreliosis and Ramsay Hunt syndrome) is crucial for optimizing outcome and preventing comorbidities of these illnesses.

GENERAL MEASURES

- Eye protection and lubrication: A significant risk for corneal injury is best managed by applying artificial tear solutions at least 3–4 times daily and lubricating gels (e.g., Lacri-Lube) at night. Patching and protective eyewear, during active play and sleep, is usually prescribed based on the degree of remaining eyelid closure.
- Corticosteroids: prednisone, considered only within the first 72 hours of symptoms. Recommended dose: 1 mg/kg/24 h PO (maximum 80 mg) once daily for 5 days, with a taper over the following 5 days.

- Acyclovir: Most clearly indicated for the treatment of Ramsay Hunt syndrome. It is also used empirically by some practitioners in standard Bell palsy management, although evidence for its supplementary use to corticosteroids is relatively weak; see discussion in the following text. Recommended dose: 20 mg/kg/dose q.i.d. PO for 10 days; maximum 400 mg/dose. Generally, any evidence of vesicular eruption in the ear canal or face should be treated promptly with acyclovir, as outcomes from VZV-associated palsies are reported to be worse in general.

PHYSICAL THERAPY

The benefits of facial muscle physical therapy remain controversial. Despite an increasing number of studies, some with controls, and subsequent meta-analyses, the results are conflicting. At present, there is no incontrovertible evidence for benefit due to facial physical therapy. There is no evidence that facial physiotherapy is harmful. The decision to pursue physical therapy after Bell palsy is a matter of personal preference for the practitioner and family.

MEDICATION

- Corticosteroids: Recent large series and meta-analyses indicate that treatment with corticosteroids is effective in reducing the risk of incomplete recovery; however, this treatment seems to be only effective if initiated within the first 48 hours of symptoms. Furthermore, statistical significance in treatment versus placebo seems to be most evident only in patients older than 40 years. However, the occurrence of synkinesias does seem to be less likely in patients treated with steroids within 48 hours across all age groups.
- Antivirals: These same series suggest that there is little or no benefit to therapy with either acyclovir or valacyclovir alone and that there is at best a non–statistically significant enhancement of improvement when used in combination with corticosteroids. The best evidence for added efficacy of antivirals in combination with corticosteroids seems to be in cases with particularly severe degrees of paralysis or in cases with suspected herpes zoster infection.
- Antibiotics: In areas where Lyme disease is endemic, many practitioners will begin treatment with oral antibiotics presumptively, while awaiting serologies (recall that the IgM titer is the most useful in the acute setting). (See "Lyme Disease" chapter.)

First Line

- Prednisone, 60–80 mg/24 h PO once daily for 5 days, with a subsequent taper over 5 days; total treatment course 10 days; must be initiated in the first 48 hours for significant results
- Amoxicillin, 50 mg/kg/24 h PO divided in 3 doses for 21–28 days, when Lyme disease suspected

Second Line

- For presumed Lyme disease:
  - Patients >8 years: doxycycline, 100 mg PO b.i.d. for 21–28 days
  - Patients of all ages: cefuroxime, 30 mg/kg/24 h PO in 2 divided doses for 21–28 days
- In cases where zoster infection is suspected or with particularly severe paralysis at onset:
  - Valacyclovir, 20 mg/kg/dose (max 1 g/dose) divided t.i.d. for 5 days (as adjunct to corticosteroids; treatment guidelines not well-established)

SURGERY/OTHER PROCEDURES

Surgical decompression: Previously, surgical decompression of the 7th nerve had been proposed as a possible treatment in cases where recovery was delayed or the clinical course more severe. No clinical evidence to support the benefit of this strategy has emerged. Surgical decompression is best reserved for "other" cases of facial nerve palsy in which there is a definable syndrome of nerve compression due to extrinsic factors, such as exostoses, tumor, etc.

ISSUES FOR REFERRAL

Subspecialty consultation: In general, patients are referred if their recovery time is prolonged or if there is a relapsing pattern or other deviations from the expected course. However, the presence of other questionable cranial nerve involvement, recent trauma, meningeal symptoms, or neurologic findings (e.g., eye movement abnormalities, acute hemiparesis, etc.) should be viewed with great concern and evaluated in an urgent care setting.

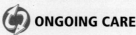

ONGOING CARE

DIET

There are no dietary restrictions that affect the outcome of Bell palsy.

PATIENT EDUCATION

Minimizing risk for injury to the cornea ipsilateral to the facial palsy may require either restricting some activities where debris or contusions to the eye are likely or wearing protective eyewear during such activities (e.g., beach activities and competitive sports). These restrictions only need to be in effect so long as there is inadequate closure of the eyelid on the affected side.

PROGNOSIS

- 60–70% full-recovery rate from isolated 7th nerve palsy
- Signs of recovering function (generally improving control of mimetic movement) are typically apparent by the 3rd week after onset.
- Prognosis for recovery seems to be worse with either a secondary deterioration in function after 2–4 days, no signs of recovery after 3 weeks, or demonstrated gadolinium enhancement of the affected facial nerve on MRI.
- Of patients with less than total recovery, many will experience at least partial return to normal function; cosmetic results vary in this group.
- Outcome of idiopathic facial palsy as a pregnancy complication seems to be less favorable (~55% full recovery).
- Up to 7% of patients may experience a 2nd occurrence at some point in the future.

COMPLICATIONS

- Corneal injury, due to decreased lacrimation and poor eye closure
- Several sequelae, generally related to aberrant reinnervation of affected end organs, are observed after an episode of Bell palsy.
  - Various synkinesias (abnormal involuntary movements that accompany a normally executed voluntary movement), including the Marin–Amat phenomenon (spontaneous eye closure with mouth opening, or its converse)
  - Blepharospasm, hemifacial spasm, facial contractures
  - The "crocodile tears" phenomenon (eating provokes ipsilateral tearing) results from crossed reinnervation between lacrimal and salivary parasympathetic fibers.

ADDITIONAL READING

- Axelsson S, Berg T, Jonsson L, et al. Prednisolone in Bell's palsy related to treatment start and age. *Otol Neurotol*. 2011;32(1):141–146.
- Gronseth GS, Paduga R. Evidence-based guideline update: steroids and antivirals for Bell palsy: report of the Guideline Development Subcommittee of the American Academy of Neurology. *Neurology*. 2012;79(22):2209–2213.
- Lee HY, Byun JY, Park MS, et al. Steroid-antiviral treatment improves the recovery rate in patients with severe Bell's palsy. *Am J Med*. 2013;126(4): 336–341.
- Numthavaj P, Thakkinstian A, Dejthevaporn C, et al. Corticosteroid and antiviral therapy for Bell's palsy: a network meta-analysis. *BMC Neurol*. 2011;11: 1–10.
- Pereira LM, Obara K, Dias JM, et al. Facial exercise therapy for facial palsy: systematic review and meta-analysis. *Clin Rehabil*. 2011;25(7):649–658.
- Teixeira LJ, Soares BG, Vieira VP, et al. Physical therapy for Bells' palsy (idiopathic facial paralysis). *Cochrane Database Syst Rev*. 2008;(3):CD006283.

CODES

ICD10

G51.0 Bell's palsy

FAQ

- Q: How does one differentiate between peripheral facial nerve palsy and a CNS lesion?
- A: A critical step in diagnosis is the differentiation of peripheral from central (upper motor neuron) lesions. With upper motor neuron lesions (above the level of the 7th nerve nucleus), there is preferential weakness of lower facial musculature and, sometimes, differential paresis of voluntary versus spontaneous emotional mimetic movements. Brainstem lesions, on the other hand, may produce a peripheral-appearing lesion but almost always have involvement of other pathways and cranial nerve nuclei, for example, ipsilateral lateral rectus palsy and contralateral somatic hemiplegia (Millard–Gubler syndrome).

BEZOARS

Andrew B. Grossman

BASICS

DESCRIPTION

- Accumulation of foreign material in the gastrointestinal (GI) tract
- Commonly divided into 3 categories based on the substances from which the bezoar is derived:
  - Phytobezoar (from vegetables/fruits)
  - Trichobezoar (hair)
  - Lactobezoar (milk/formula)
- Documented to occur in humans for more than 2 millennia, suggesting formation of bezoars may have been/still be culturally important for certain societies

EPIDEMIOLOGY

- Phytobezoars occur almost exclusively in adults.
- 90% of trichobezoars occur in female patients younger than 20 years of age.
- Lactobezoars occur mostly in premature, low-birth-weight infants.

PATHOPHYSIOLOGY

- Trichobezoars
  - Associated with mental retardation, pica, trichotillomania, and trichophagia; may ingest own hair but also rugs and animal or doll hair
  - Most cases of trichophagia do not result in bezoar formation (~1%).
  - History of trichophagia is obtained in only 50% of cases.
  - Retention and accumulation of hair strands in the gastric folds
  - Trichobezoars may become large and form a cast in the stomach leading to abdominal mass.
  - Bezoar may extend through the pylorus into the small bowel. This "tail" may obstruct the ampulla of Vater, leading to jaundice and pancreatitis. This phenomenon is commonly referred to as Rapunzel syndrome.
- Phytobezoars
  - Most common form among adults, rare in children
  - Associated with gastric dysmotility and poor gastric emptying (either primary or following gastric surgery) and hypochlorhydria
  - Composed primarily of cellulose, hemicellulose, lignins, and tannins
- Lactobezoars (milk)
  - Most often reported in premature, low-birth-weight infants being fed high-calorie premature formula (although there are reports in full-term infants and exclusively breastfed infants)
  - Factors contributing to lactobezoar formation include the following:
    - Formulas with high casein content
    - Early and rapid feeding advancement in small infants
    - High-caloric-density formulas
    - Formulas with high calcium/phosphate content
    - Continuous tube feedings
    - Altered gastric motility in low-birth-weight infants

ETIOLOGY

Classification of bezoars is dependent on the most prominent substance from which they are formed, including:

- Trichobezoars: hair, carpet
- Phytobezoars: indigestible fruit and vegetable matter
- Lactobezoars: milk
- Less common materials include the following:
  - Foreign bodies
  - Gallstones
  - Medications, including vitamins, antacids, psyllium, sucralfate, cimetidine, and nifedipine
- Can occur in cystic fibrosis (CF) patients after lung transplantation
- Colonic and rectal bezoars
  - Due to indigestible sunflower seeds, popcorn, and gum have been reported in children and adults
  - These usually present with obstruction, although encopresis and colitis-type symptoms have been described.

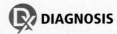

DIAGNOSIS

HISTORY

- Signs and symptoms of bezoar formation include the following:
  - Pain
  - Halitosis
  - Nausea
  - Vomiting
  - Diarrhea
  - Gastric ulceration
  - Upper GI bleeding and perforation
  - Left upper quadrant mass
- Trichobezoars
  - Unusual patterns of balding
  - Palpable left upper quadrant mass in the abdomen is often detected.
  - Hair found in the stool
- Phytobezoars
  - Abdominal mass is palpable in <50% of patients.
- Lactobezoars
  - Abdominal distention, diarrhea, emesis, and increased gastric residuals

DIAGNOSTIC TESTS & INTERPRETATION

Lab

- Iron deficiency anemia
- Presence of steatorrhea or protein-losing enteropathy

Imaging

- Plain abdominal x-ray
  - Heterogenous intragastric mass that could be mistaken for food-filled stomach
- Upper GI barium studies
  - May identify and outline the mass
- Ultrasound and CT can also be helpful.

Diagnostic Procedures/Other

Endoscopy allows for direct visualization and elucidation of composition of bezoar.

DIFFERENTIAL DIAGNOSIS

Any gastric foreign body can mimic a gastric mass and may present on palpation.

TREATMENT

GENERAL MEASURES

- Trichobezoars
  - Difficult to remove endoscopically, attempts to fragment may result in migration and small bowel obstruction
  - Treatment is usually surgical removal: Trichobezoars are normally large and hair is not dissolvable.
- Phytobezoars
  - Medications such as prokinetic agents to stimulate gastric motility
  - Enzyme therapy to help dissolve the material
  - *N*-acetylcysteine treatment via nasogastric tube has been documented in one case report.
  - Endoscopic fragmentation or extraction
  - Coca-Cola administration with or without endoscopic extraction has been reported to be effective.
  - Surgical extraction
  - Diet alteration
- Lactobezoars
  - Withholding feedings for 48 hours while the patient is sustained on intravenous (IV) fluids will resolve most lactobezoars.
  - Gentle gastric lavage may be helpful.

ADDITIONAL READING

- Chogle A, Bonilla S, Browne M, et al. Rapunzel syndrome: a rare cause of biliary obstruction. *J Pediatr Gastroenterol Nutr*. 201vw0;51(4):522–523.
- DuBose TM V, Southgate WM, Hill JG. Lactobezoars: a patient series and literature review. *Clin Pediatr*. 2001;40(11):603–606.
- Ladas SD, Kamberoglou D, Karamanolis G, et al. Systematic review: Coca-Cola can effectively dissolve gastric phytobezoars as a first-line treatment. *Aliment Pharmacol Ther*. 2013;37(2):169–173.
- Lynch KA, Feola PG, Guenther E. Gastric trichobezoar: an important cause of abdominal pain presenting to the pediatric emergency department. *Pediatr Emerg Care*. 2003;19(5):343–347.
- Taylor JR, Streetman DS, Castle SS. Medication bezoars: a literature review and report of a case. *Ann Pharmacother*. 1998;32(9):940–946.

CODES

ICD10

- T18.9XXA Foreign body of alimentary tract, part unspecified, initial encounter
- T18.2XXA Foreign body in stomach, initial encounter
- T18.3XXA Foreign body in small intestine, initial encounter

FAQ

- Q: What are some commonly used medications that can lead to bezoar formation?
- A: Vitamins, antacids, psyllium, sucralfate, cimetidine, and nifedipine
- Q: What may place an infant at risk for formation of a bezoar?
- A: The literature suggests that formulas with high casein content may be linked with lactobezoar formation. Other possible contributing factors include early and rapid feeding advancement in small infants, high-density formulas, formulas with a high calcium/phosphate content, continuous tube feedings, and altered gastric motility in low-birth-weight infants.

BILIARY ATRESIA

Greggy D. Laroche • Douglas B. Mogul

BASICS

DESCRIPTION

Biliary atresia (BA) is a congenital disease characterized by fibrosis, obstruction, and obliteration of the biliary system that is universally fatal without intervention.

EPIDEMIOLOGY

- BA accounts for approximately 30% of cases of neonatal cholestasis.
- BA is the most common cause of persistent cholestasis in infants and children and the most frequent indication for pediatric liver transplantation.
- The disease affects 1:8,000 to 1:18,000 live births.

RISK FACTORS

Genetics

- No single genetic mutation has been identified as the sole cause of BA, and there is no clear pattern of inheritance.
- Genes influencing morphogenesis may contribute to pathophysiology.

PATHOPHYSIOLOGY

- Biliary obstruction begins at, or near, the time of birth and progresses throughout early infancy, leading to damage and ultimately scarring of liver parenchyma.
- Approximately 20% of biliary patients have at least one other major congenital anomaly (i.e., embryonal form) including splenic malformation, interrupted inferior vena cava, midline liver, situs inversus, preduodenal portal vein, and intestinal malrotation.
- More common form is the perinatal form that is not associated with malformations.

ETIOLOGY

Etiology is not completely defined, but many different pathogenic mechanisms have been proposed, including the following:

- Perinatal infection of the liver and biliary tract with potential organisms including cytomegalovirus, rotavirus, and reovirus
- Immune dysregulation
- Defective morphogenesis
- Environmental toxin exposure
- Vascular insufficiency

DIAGNOSIS

HISTORY

- Newborns appear healthy at birth with good growth and development. However, jaundice of the skin and eyes persists beyond the 2-week interval of physiologic jaundice. Acholic stools and dark urine may be noted.
- In addition, infants with BA may present with poor weight gain, bleeding (due to vitamin K deficiency), and/or increased stool frequency.

PHYSICAL EXAM

- Jaundice can be seen in the eyes, skin, or buccal mucosa.
- Infants may have hepatomegaly and splenomegaly.
- Rectal exam, including digital exam, may reveal acholic stools.

SCREENING

- An infant stool color card that identifies acholic and normal stool has been used in Taiwan, where it was shown to decrease the time to diagnosis in BA and improve outcomes for children with BA.
- Infants with BA have elevated direct bilirubin at 24 hours of life, suggesting a potential role for screening with this blood test.

ALERT

- One of the most important factors determining outcomes in BA, including survival and need for transplantation, is the age at which a patient is referred for workup.
- The 10-year survival rate of patients diagnosed and treated prior to 60 days versus after 90 days is 73% and 11%, respectively.

DIAGNOSTIC TESTS & INTERPRETATION

Initial Lab Tests

- Conjugated hyperbilirubinemia (defined as a conjugated fraction >2 mg/dL or a conjugated bilirubin >20% of the total bilirubin) may be elevated *as early as the first 24 hours of life*.
- Additional laboratory findings may include mild to moderate elevations in AST, ALT, and alkaline phosphatase as well as significant elevations in γ-glutamyltransferase (GGT)
- Additional diagnostic testing should be done as clinically indicated.
- Bacterial cultures (blood, urine, stool), viral studies (hepatitis B, hepatitis C, Epstein-Barr virus, toxoplasmosis, other viruses, rubella, cytomegalovirus, herpes virus [TORCH] infections, HIV, adenovirus, enterovirus)
- Metabolic profiles (plasma amino acids, urine organic acids and urine succinylacetone, lactate/pyruvate ratio)
- Serum alpha-1-antitrypsin level and phenotype
- Thyroid function tests (TSH, free T_4)
- Urine-reducing substances to evaluate for galactosemia (if infant has taken breast milk or lactose-containing formula)
- CBC, coagulation studies (prothrombin time/international normalized ratio/partial thromboplastin time [PT/INR/PTT]), total protein, albumin, and fat-soluble vitamins

Imaging

- Abdominal ultrasound
  - Should be obtained to rule out choledochal cyst but has poor sensitivity and specificity for BA unless "triangular chord" sign seen (80% sensitive, 98% specific)
  - May also assist in defining embryonal versus perinatal form
- Hepatobiliary iminodiacetic acid (HIDA) scan/hepatobiliary scintigraphy can be obtained to evaluate biliary excretion.

Additional Testing

- Discussion with pediatric gastroenterologist should be obtained following evidence of persistent cholestasis.
- Liver biopsy: In BA, findings may include bile duct proliferation, bile stasis, periportal inflammation, and periportal fibrosis.
- Sweat chloride test (cystic fibrosis)
- Ophthalmology exam for Alagille syndrome (posterior embryotoxon) and congenital infections
- Spine film to evaluate butterfly vertebrae of Alagille syndrome
- Echo to evaluate cardiac anomalies in Alagille syndrome
- Urine bile acid analysis
- Intraoperative cholangiogram
  - Gold standard for diagnosis of BA but is an invasive test
  - Reserved for individuals with high suspicion of BA.

DIFFERENTIAL DIAGNOSIS

- Intrahepatic
  - Infection: sepsis, UTI, gastroenteritis, TORCH infections, HIV, viral hepatitis (A, B, C, D, E), Epstein-Barr virus, adenovirus, coxsackie B virus, echovirus, enterovirus

- Systemic disease: panhypopituitarism, congestive heart failure, ischemic hepatopathy, trauma
- Metabolic: galactosemia, tyrosinemia, alpha-1-antitrypsin, cystic fibrosis, citrin deficiency, respiratory chain disorders, hereditary fructose intolerance, disorders of bile acid synthesis, storage disorders, neonatal iron storage disease
- Genetic: Alagille syndrome, Zellweger syndrome, Down syndrome, Turner syndrome
- Progressive familial intrahepatic cholestasis (i.e., PFIC 1, 2, and 3)
- Toxins and drugs: total parenteral nutrition, antibiotics, and other medications
- Miscellaneous: neonatal hepatitis, neonatal lupus, congenital hepatic fibrosis, Caroli syndrome, inspissated bile syndrome, histiocytosis X

• Extrahepatic
  - Choledochal cyst
  - Choledocholithiasis
  - Neonatal sclerosing cholangitis
  - Tumor/mass compression
  - Spontaneous perforation of common bile duct

TREATMENT

SURGERY/OTHER PROCEDURES

- A hepatoportoenterostomy (Kasai procedure) is the only effective therapy for BA other than a liver transplant. The goal of the Kasai procedure is to restore bile flow from the liver to the intestine.
- Despite the Kasai procedure, 70–80% of patients with BA ultimately require liver transplantation.
  - At 3 months after Kasai procedure, a total serum bilirubin <2 mg/dL is associated with low likelihood of requiring hepatic transplant within 2 years.
  - A total serum bilirubin ≥ 6 mg/dL is associated with failure of adequate bile flow and higher likelihood of need for liver transplantation.
- Indications for transplantation include the following:
  - Synthetic dysfunction of the liver
  - Complications of portal hypertension (PHTN) such as life-threatening hemorrhage, ascites, and spontaneous bacterial peritonitis
  - Persistent cholestasis with impaired quality of life such as intractable pruritus
  - Recurrent cholangitis

ALERT

- Without surgical intervention, 50–80% of patients with BA will die from biliary cirrhosis by 1 year of age and 90–100% by 3 years of age.
- If diagnosed within the first 3 months of life, surgical therapy can successfully restore bile flow from liver into the intestinal tract in 30–80% of patients.

MEDICATION

- After the Kasai operation, patients receive
  - Ursodeoxycholic acid to promote bile flow
  - Supplemental fat-soluble vitamins
  - Oral prophylactic antibiotics to prevent ascending cholangitis
- Corticosteroids have not been shown to improve outcomes in patients with BA.

ONGOING CARE

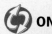

FOLLOW-UP RECOMMENDATIONS

In conjunction with a GI specialist, obtain routine serum biomarkers including CBC, liver function tests, and GGT to determine progression of disease. Physicians should also monitor closely fat-soluble vitamins as well as coagulation studies to evaluate liver function including production of clotting factors and absorption of vitamin K.

DIET

- Anthropometrics should be performed consistently and frequently to evaluate growth as patients tend to have decreased fat stores and decreased lean body mass.
- For individuals with poor weight gain on breast milk or receiving standard formula supplementation, patients should use formulas enriched with medium-chain triglycerides because these fats do not require bile for absorption.
- If patients exhibit poor weight gain on oral feedings, an enteric feeding tube for supplemental nutrition should be strongly considered.
- Due to decrease bile acid excretion, patients with BA malabsorb fat-soluble vitamins (A, D, E, and K) and likely need supplementation.

COMPLICATIONS

- Ascending bacterial cholangitis: Patients are predisposed to this infection after the portoenterostomy procedure given the absence of the ampulla of Vater and present with fever, elevated liver function tests, hypopigmented stools, increased pruritus, and/or increased GGT. Recurrent ascending cholangitis can lead to sclerosis and loss of remaining intrahepatic bile ducts. Antibiotic prophylaxis is helpful in preventing recurrent infections.
- Pruritus: Occurs frequently and is due to elevated circulating bile acid. Ursodeoxycholic acid, antihistamines, rifampin, naloxone, and cholestyramine may be used to alleviate itching.
- Ascites: Spironolactone, chlorothiazide, and furosemide are commonly used diuretics. However, their use should be monitored closely in order to avoid the development of hepatorenal syndrome.
- PHTN: Monitoring liver firmness, texture, and span along with splenomegaly will be helpful. Progressive thrombocytopenia suggests further splenomegaly. PHTN can also manifest as ascites, spontaneous bacterial peritonitis, portosystemic encephalopathy, portopulmonary syndrome, or GI hemorrhage from esophageal or gastric varices.

ADDITIONAL READING

- Chen SM, Chang MH, Du JC, et al. Screening for biliary atresia by infant stool color card in Taiwan. *Pediatrics*. 2006;117(4):1147–1154.
- Cowles RA, Lobritto SJ, Ventura KA, et al. Timing of liver transplantation in biliary atresia—results in 71 children managed by a multidisciplinary team. *J Pediatr Surg*. 2008;43(9):1605–1609.
- Davenport M, Tizzard SA, Underhill J, et al. The biliary atresia splenic malformation syndrome: a 28-year single-center retrospective study. *J Pediatr*. 2006;149(3):393–400.
- Hartley JL, Davenport M, Kelly DA. Biliary atresia. *Lancet*. 2009;374(9702):1704–1713.
- Karrer FM, Bensard DD. Neonatal cholestasis. *Semin Pediatr Surg*. 2000;9(4):166–169.
- Mack CL. The pathogenesis of biliary atresia: evidence for a virus-induced autoimmune disease. *Semin Liver Dis*. 2007;27(3):233–242.
- Shneider BL, Brown MB, Haber B, et al. A multicenter study of the outcome of biliary atresia in the United States, 1997 to 2000. *J Pediatr*. 2006;148(4):467–474.
- Sokol RJ, Mack C, Narkewicz MR, et al. Pathogenesis and outcome of biliary atresia: current concepts. *J Pediatr Gastroenterol Nutr*. 2003;37(1):4–21.

CODES

ICD10

- Q44.2 Atresia of bile ducts
- K83.1 Obstruction of bile duct
- R16.0 Hepatomegaly, not elsewhere classified

FAQ

- Q: How soon should parents contact their primary care provider when they see pale-colored stools?
- A: The first time they notice these stools are acholic.
- Q: What should a physician do if he or she is concerned about persistent jaundice?
- A: Obtain a thorough history, perform a thorough physical exam, and measure both total and direct bilirubin. If there is significant conjugated bilirubinemia, contact your local pediatric gastroenterologist and begin neonatal cholestasis diagnostic workup, ruling out the most immediately dangerous etiologies (including potentially fatal metabolic diseases and infections) as well as common etiologies such as BA.

BLASTOMYCOSIS

Evan J. Anderson

BASICS

DESCRIPTION

- Systemic infection caused by the dimorphic soil fungus *Blastomyces dermatitidis*
- Dimorphism is characterized by a mold phase (mycelial form) that grows at room temperature and a yeast form that grows at body temperature.
- Incubation period estimated at 30–45 days

EPIDEMIOLOGY

- Similar to other dimorphic fungi, *B. dermatitidis* is a soil saprophyte (mycelial form).
- Congenital infections occur rarely.
- Infection is endemic in the upper Midwest and Southern United States, particularly in the wooded Mississippi and Ohio River valleys and the Great Lakes. The highest incidence in the United States is in Wisconsin, Mississippi, and Tennessee followed by Minnesota, Illinois, North Dakota, Alabama, and Louisiana.
- Substantial disease occurs in the Canadian provinces of Manitoba and northwestern Ontario. Other reported areas of infection include Africa, India, and South America.
- Children account for 3–11% of all cases of blastomycosis.
- Blastomycosis is a very uncommon diagnosis even in endemic regions.

RISK FACTORS

- Blastomycosis is more common in males. This is thought to be due to occupational or recreational activities that increase risk of exposure.
- Underlying immunodeficiency is rarely observed among children with blastomycosis.

GENERAL PREVENTION

- No special precautions for hospitalized patients are indicated.
- The natural reservoir is undetermined.

PATHOPHYSIOLOGY

- Inhalation of the fungus into the lung is followed by an inflammatory response with neutrophils and macrophages.
- Blastomycosis most commonly presents as subacute pulmonary disease, but the clinical spectrum of the disease extends from asymptomatic to disseminated disease that can involve lung, skin, bone, and central nervous system (CNS).
- As many as 50% of infections are asymptomatic.

ETIOLOGY

- Infection is almost always caused by inhalation of spores from *B. dermatitidis*.
- Rarely, blastomycosis has occurred through accidental inoculation, dog bites, conjugal transmission, and intrauterine transmission.
- Point-source outbreaks have occurred with occupational and recreational activities that occur in areas with moist soil and decaying vegetation, such as along streams and rivers.
- Natural infection occurs in humans and dogs.

COMMONLY ASSOCIATED CONDITIONS

- Pulmonary blastomycosis
  - Most common form of infection by *Blastomyces* in children
  - Can be acute, subacute, or chronic
  - Illness severity can vary greatly, from asymptomatic to upper respiratory tract infection, bronchitis, pleuritis, pneumonia, or severe respiratory distress.
- Cutaneous blastomycosis
  - Skin manifestations are variable and include nodules, verrucous lesions, subcutaneous abscesses, or ulcerations.
  - Cutaneous disease usually occurs after pulmonary infection with dissemination to the skin, rarely by direction inoculation.
- Bone blastomycosis
  - Bone disease usually occurs after pulmonary infection with dissemination to the bone resulting in osteomyelitis and bone destruction.
- Disseminated blastomycosis
  - Recent series suggest that this occurs in less than 1/2 of children
  - Usually begins as pulmonary infection, with subsequent spread to involve skin, bone, genitourinary tract, and/or CNS.
  - Can disseminate to virtually any organ
  - The classic triad of lung, bone, and skin disease occurs in ≤15% of children.

DIAGNOSIS

HISTORY

- History of residence or travel to an endemic area is very important.
- For children with acute pulmonary blastomycosis, the most common presenting symptoms are the following:
  - Cough (may be productive)
  - Fever
  - Chest pain
  - Malaise
- Children with chronic pulmonary disease present with the following:
  - Chronic (>2 weeks) nonproductive cough
  - Pleuritic chest pain
  - Poor appetite
  - May also be a history of fever, chills, weight loss, fatigue, night sweats, or, rarely, hemoptysis

PHYSICAL EXAM

- Initial pulmonary infection may present with physical exam findings similar to those of bacterial pneumonia.
- Respiratory signs and symptoms often have resolved by the time cutaneous manifestations are apparent.
- Skin involvement appears as nodules, nodules with ulceration, or granulomatous lesions.
- Bone involvement usually presents with progressive focal pain and point tenderness.

DIAGNOSTIC TESTS & INTERPRETATION

Diagnostic Procedures/Other

- Definitive diagnosis requires the growth of *B. dermatitidis* from a clinical specimen. In the cooler temperature at which fungal culture is performed in the laboratory, *B. dermatitidis* usually switches back to the mold form.
- Direct visualization of the yeast form may be performed on samples of sputum, urine, cerebrospinal fluid, bronchoalveolar lavage sample, or tissue biopsy.
- Although the most accurate serologic test is the enzyme immunoassay, all serologic tests have poor sensitivity and specificity.
- An assay to detect *Blastomyces* antigen in urine is available and is about 93% sensitive. Cross-reactivity occurs in patients with histoplasmosis, paracoccidioidomycosis, and *Penicillium marneffei* infections.
- Chest radiography commonly reveals lobar consolidation. Cavitation, fibronodular patterns, mass, and mass effect may also be seen.

DIFFERENTIAL DIAGNOSIS

- Acute bacterial infection
- Neoplasm
- Tuberculosis
- Sarcoidosis
- Other fungal infections causing pneumonia (e.g., histoplasmosis)

TREATMENT

MEDICATION

- Although acute pulmonary infections may resolve without treatment, the high rate of progression to extrapulmonary disease leads many experts to recommend treatment for all cases of blastomycosis.
- Mild or moderate pulmonary or extrapulmonary disease
  - Oral itraconazole
  - Alternative agents include fluconazole or voriconazole.
- Severe pulmonary disease, other severe infection, or immunosuppression
  - IV amphotericin B: Many experts prefer a lipid formulation of amphotericin B over amphotericin B deoxycholate.
  - Therapy may be switched to oral itraconazole after clinical stabilization with amphotericin B.
- CNS blastomycosis
  - Lipid formulation of amphotericin B at 5 mg/kg/day over 4–6 weeks, followed by an oral azole
- During pregnancy
  - IV amphotericin B
  - Azoles should be avoided owing to potential teratogenicity.
- Length of therapy is site dependent:
  - ≥6 months or longer for pulmonary disease
  - ≥12 months or longer for bone or CNS disease
- Lifelong suppressive therapy with oral itraconazole may be required for immunosuppressed patients and in patients who experience relapse despite appropriate therapy.
- Voriconazole, a newer azole, has in vitro activity against *B. dermatitidis* and penetrates the CSF better than itraconazole. Anecdotal reports support its use as an option for step-down therapy for CNS infection.

SURGERY/OTHER PROCEDURES

Occasionally, drainage of abscesses and debridement of bone are necessary.

ONGOING CARE

FOLLOW-UP RECOMMENDATIONS

Patient Monitoring

- All azoles can cause hepatitis. Thus, hepatic enzymes should be measured before starting therapy, 2–4 weeks after therapy has begun, and every 3 months during therapy.
- All azoles interact with P450 enzymes. Consider drug–drug interactions when the patient is taking other medications.
- Itraconazole capsules are poorly absorbed; the oral solution is poorly tolerated due to taste. Monitoring adherence to therapy is important and many recommend following itraconazole levels.
- Amphotericin B commonly causes acute kidney injury and electrolyte wasting (particularly potassium and magnesium). Infusion-related toxicity is also common. Lipid formulations are typically better tolerated than the deoxycholate.

PROGNOSIS

- Before antifungal medications were available, the mortality associated with blastomycosis was up to 90%.
- Appropriate treatment with antifungal medications results in excellent cure rates and mortality rates of <10%.
- Worse outcomes tend to occur in association with a delay between onset of symptoms and establishment of a diagnosis.

COMPLICATIONS

- Dissemination is the main complication of the infection, occurring in less than 50% of children with blastomycosis.
- Residual orthopedic issues can persist in children with bone involvement.
- Systemic infection may be well advanced before symptoms are noted, requiring long-term therapy and follow-up.

ADDITIONAL READING

- Anderson EJ, Ahn PB, Yogev R, et al. Blastomycosis in children: a study of 14 cases. *J Ped Infect Dis Soc*. 2014;2:386–390.
- Baddley JW, Winthrop KL, Patkar NM, et al. Geographic distribution of endemic fungal infections among older persons, United States. *Emerg Infect Dis*. 2011;17:1664–1669.
- Chapman SW, Dismukes WE, Proia LA, et al. Clinical practice guidelines for the management of blastomycosis: 2008 update by the Infectious Diseases Society of America. *Clin Infect Dis*. 2008;46:1801–1812.
- Chu JH, Feudtner C, Heydon KH, et al. Hospitalizations for endemic mycoses: a population based national sample. *Clin Infect Dis*. 2006;42(6):822–825.
- Durkin M, Witt J, LeMonte A, et al. Antigen assay with the potential to aid in diagnosis of blastomycosis. *J Clin Micro*. 2004;42:4873–4875.
- Fanella S, Skinner S, Trepman E, et al. Blastomycosis in children and adolescents: a 30 year experience from Manitoba. *Med Mycol*. 2011;49(6):627–632.
- Montenegro BL, Arnold JC. North American dimorphic fungal infections in children. *Pediatr Rev*. 2010;31(6):e40–e48.

CODES

ICD10

- B40.9 Blastomycosis, unspecified
- B40.2 Pulmonary blastomycosis, unspecified
- B40.7 Disseminated blastomycosis

FAQ

- Q: When should I suspect blastomycosis?
- A: Consider blastomycosis in a child with exposure to an endemic blastomycosis area that is presenting with subacute to chronic pneumonia. Oftentimes, these children will have been treated with multiple prior antibiotics and have ongoing or progressive pneumonia or develop skin or bone lesions.
- Q: Blastomycosis is on my differential; how can I best test for it?
- A: The urine antigen test is the most sensitive test for the detection of blastomycosis but can be falsely positive. Usually, a clinical specimen is ultimately needed to establish a diagnosis.
- Q: I have a child hospitalized with blastomycosis; should I start with itraconazole or amphotericin B?
- A: If the child is not in the ICU, is not acutely worsening, and is able to take itraconazole by mouth, then it is reasonable to start with itraconazole. Itraconazole is generally much better tolerated than are amphotericin B formulations.

BLEPHARITIS

Prina P. Amin • Erika Abramson

BASICS

DESCRIPTION
- Inflammatory or infectious process of the eyelid margin, typically involving skin, lashes, and meibomian glands
  - Associated with itchiness, redness, flaking, and crusting of the eyelids
  - Usually chronic, intermittent with exacerbations and remissions
  - Typically bilateral
  - No universal classification system
- Historically classified according to location, anterior versus posterior
  - Anterior blepharitis: affects the base of the eyelashes and eyelash follicles
  - Posterior blepharitis: affects the meibomian glands
- Can also be classified by etiology
  - Inflammatory: seborrheic, meibomian gland dysfunction, allergic, associated with rosacea
  - Infectious: bacterial (most commonly *Staphylococcus aureus* or *Staphylococcus epidermidis*), viral, fungal, or parasitic

EPIDEMIOLOGY
- One of the most common ocular disorders
  - Presents in patients of all ages
  - Mean age of presentation is age 50 years.
  - No gender differences seen.

RISK FACTORS
- Presence of atopic, allergic, or seborrheic dermatitis
- Rosacea
- Tear deficiency and dysfunction
- Contact lens use
- Isotretinoin used to treat severe cystic acne
- Less common risk factors include underlying immunologic disorders such as lupus, eyelid tumors, trauma, and other dermatoses.

PATHOPHYSIOLOGY
- Complex and results from the interplay between abnormal lid margin secretions, lid margin organisms, and dysfunction of the tear film
- Infectious blepharitis: Bacteria such as *Staphylococcus* may cause direct infection of the eyelids, evoke reaction to the exotoxin, or provoke an allergic reaction to the staphylococcal antigens.
- Inflammatory blepharitis: Inflammation of the meibomian glands leads to impaired gland secretions and instability of the tear film.
- This condition can have a direct toxic effect and promote bacterial overgrowth.

COMMONLY ASSOCIATED CONDITIONS
- Seborrheic dermatitis
- Allergic or contact dermatitis
- Down syndrome (trisomy 21)
- Ocular rosacea
- Dry eye (keratoconjunctivitis sicca)
- Hordeolum
- Chalazion

DIAGNOSIS

SIGNS AND SYMPTOMS
- Redness of eyelid margin
- Irritation
- Burning
- Tearing
- Gritty sensation
- Dry or watery eyes
- Increased blinking
- Loss of eyelashes
- Photophobia
- Contact lens intolerance
- Eye discharge or crust, particularly along lashes
- Eyelid sticking, especially in the morning

HISTORY
- Duration of symptoms: Blepharitis is often chronic, with periods of exacerbation and remission.
- Symptoms and signs of systemic disease
- Current and previous systemic and topical medications (in particular: antihistamines, drugs with anticholinergic effects, and isotretinoin
- Contact lens use
- Exacerbating conditions such as eye makeup use, smoke, allergens
- Previous intraocular or eyelid surgery
- Trauma
- Past medical and family histories of atopy
- Recent exposure to lice

PHYSICAL EXAM
- Use a focused direct light source to carefully evaluate the eyelids for abnormal eyelid position, eyelash loss, hyperemia of the eyelid margins, abnormal deposits at the base of the eyelids, ulceration, vesicles, scaling, chalazion/hordeolums, and scarring.
- Examine the conjunctiva and sclera to look for signs of inflammation, which warrants a slit-lamp examination.
- Assess visual acuity.
- Perform a general exam looking for signs of systemic disease such as seborrhea, atopic dermatitis, rosacea, and lupus.

DIAGNOSTIC TESTS & INTERPRETATION
Lab
- Diagnosis is made clinically. There are no specific diagnostic tests to confirm the diagnosis of blepharitis.
- In refractory cases or cases of recurrent anterior blepharitis with severe inflammation, cultures of the eyelid margins may be useful.

DIFFERENTIAL DIAGNOSIS
- Acute conjunctivitis (bacteria, viral, or allergic)
- Atopic or contact dermatitis
- Keratitis
- Iritis
- Glaucoma
- Chemical burn
- Corneal abrasion
- Foreign body
- Hordeolum
- Chalazion
- Lice
- Trichotillomania

TREATMENT

GENERAL MEASURES
- Several treatments may be helpful and are generally used in combination.
- Treatments may provide symptomatic relief but usually do not result in cure for chronic cases.
- Treatments include the following:
  - Warm compresses
  - Eyelid hygiene
  - Antibiotics (topical and/or systemic)
  - Topical short course anti-inflammatory agents
- Warm compresses should be applied for 15 minutes at least twice daily to loosen crusts.
- Eyelid hygiene
  - Consists of massaging the eyelid margins daily and carefully removing the crusts using cotton swabs, cotton balls, commercial eyelid scrubs, and/or diluted baby shampoo
  - Children should be instructed to avoid rubbing their eyes if possible and to wash hands frequently.
- Wearing contact lens or eye makeup should be avoided during exacerbations.
- Activities that result in decreased blinking can dry out the eye and worsen exacerbations. Such activities may include television watching and use of computers or video games.

MEDICATION
- Warm compresses and eyelid hygiene are the traditional mainstay of therapy.
- Medications can be added in conjunction with conservative measures.
- A topical antibiotic ophthalmic ointment (such as bacitracin or erythromycin) may be applied 1–4 times daily until inflammation resolves.
- A brief course of topical corticosteroids are generally reserved for severe inflammation and in cases of severe conjunctival injection or marginal keratitis.
- The minimal effective dose of corticosteroid should be used and for as short a time as possible.
- Long-term use of oral antibiotics (such as erythromycin or tetracyclines) may be useful in severe cases.

ISSUES FOR REFERRAL
- Moderate or severe pain
- Vision loss
- Severe or chronic redness
- Corneal involvement
- Traumatic eye injury
- Recent ocular surgery
- Distorted pupil
- Recurrent episodes
- More severe eyelid inflammation with nodular mass, ulceration, or extensive scarring
- Lack of improvement with conservative measures and topical antibiotics

ONGOING CARE
- No additional care is needed if symptoms resolve completely.
- Patients should be educated about the potential for recurrence and chronicity with blepharitis.
- Warm compresses and eyelid hygiene treatment may be required long term.

ADDITIONAL READING

- American Academy of Ophthalmology Cornea/External Disease Panel. *Preferred Practice Pattern® Guidelines. Blepharitis: Limited Revision*. San Francisco, CA: American Academy of Ophthalmology; 2011. http://www.aao.org/ppp. Accessed July 17, 2013.
- Bernardes TF, Bonfioli AA. Blepharitis. *Semin Ophthalmol*. 2010;25(3):79–83.
- Jackson WB. Blepharitis: current strategies for diagnosis and management. *Can J Ophthalmol*. 2008;43(2):170–179.
- Lindsley K, Matsumura S, Hatef E, et al. Interventions for chronic blepharitis. *Cochrane Database Syst Rev*. 2012;(5):CD005556. doi:10.1002/14651858.CD005556.pub2.

CODES

ICD10
- H01.009 Unspecified blepharitis unspecified eye, unspecified eyelid
- H01.019 Ulcerative blepharitis unspecified eye, unspecified eyelid
- L21.8 Other seborrheic dermatitis

FAQ
- Q: Is blepharitis contagious?
- A: Blepharitis is not contagious. However, if blepharitis is due in part to bacterial infection, the bacteria can be transmitted to other family members and result in conjunctivitis. Thus, good hand hygiene is important.
- Q: Will the child outgrow this?
- A: Although some children may be cured, for many, blepharitis is a chronic condition in which symptomatic control is the goal.
- Q: Is blepharitis common in children?
- A: Although blepharitis can occur in patients of all ages, it tends to be seen much more frequently in adults.

BONE MARROW AND STEM CELL TRANSPLANT

Justin T. Wahlstrom • Biljana N. Horn

BASICS

DESCRIPTION

- Hematopoietic stem cell transplantation (HSCT) is the infusion of progenitor stem cells with the intention of restoring hematopoiesis and immunity. HSCT can be classified by
  - Donor type: syngeneic (derived from an identical twin), allogeneic (derived from a related or unrelated donor), or autologous (derived from the patient prior to stem cell-toxic therapy)
  - Product type
    - Bone marrow transplantation (BMT): Stem cells are obtained by harvesting bone marrow under anesthesia.
    - Peripheral blood stem cell transplantation (PBSCT): Stem cells are mobilized to the periphery with cytokines (GCSF) and collected by apheresis.
    - Umbilical cord blood transplantation (UCBT): Stem cells are collected from the umbilical cord and placenta following delivery.
- Stem cells are infused in the peripheral blood of the recipient using a central venous catheter, similar to a blood transfusion. They then home to the bone marrow niche and over the next 2–4 weeks differentiate into mature blood components.

EPIDEMIOLOGY

- In 2010, 1,479 pediatric allogeneic (and 782 autologous) HSCTs were performed in the United States. Approximately 40% of allogeneic transplants are from matched related donors.
- The use of unrelated PBSCT and unrelated UCBT has been gradually increasing since the late 1990s, whereas the use of related BMT/PBSCT has remained stable. The use of unrelated BMT has been steadily decreasing.

TREATMENT

INDICATIONS

- HSCT is typically used to provide stem cell rescue following myeloablative therapy (cancers), to provide new stem cells to correct an intrinsic cellular defect (inborn errors of metabolism, other stem cell defects), or to alter the immune system to improve or correct an immunologic defect (e.g., autoimmune disease).
- Examples of diseases for which HSCT can be beneficial include the following:
  - Leukemia (ALL, AML, JMML, and CML)
    - High-risk ALL (indications for transplant include lack of response to chemotherapy or early relapse)
    - High-risk AML (indication based on cytogenetic markers, response to therapy, or early relapse)
    - All JMML patients require HSCT for cure.
    - CML only if not well-controlled on tyrosine-kinase inhibitor therapy (imatinib, dasatinib)
- Solid tumors (lymphoma, neuroblastoma, brain tumors, some sarcomas)
- Severe primary immunodeficiencies (SCID, WAS, CGD, hyper IgM, XLP, Chediak-Higashi syndrome, Griscelli syndrome)
- Stem cell defects (aplastic anemia, myelofibrosis, Fanconi anemia, thalassemia major, sickle cell disease)
- Inborn errors of metabolism (Hurler syndrome, Hunter syndrome, adrenoleukodystrophy)
- Autoimmune disease (HLH, severe SLE)

DONOR SELECTION

- Optimal major histocompatibility antigen (HLA) matching of the donor to the recipient minimizes the risks of rejection and GVHD.
- HLA matching is important at the A, B, C, and DR loci (8/8 match is recommended in most cases).
- Additional HLA matching at the DQ and DP loci (12/12) may be important in some cases.
- For nonmalignant disease, donor preference is syngeneic > matched familial > unrelated.
- Matched unrelated donor: Over 18 million potential donors registered worldwide. Disadvantages include long search time (2–3 months), lower chance of finding an 8/8 match for minorities, increased risk of graft failure and GVHD, and slower immune reconstitution.
- Alternative donors include mismatched unrelated donor (match at ≥7/8 HLA Ag), umbilical cord blood (match at ≥4/6 HLA Ag), or haploidentical (parental) donor (4/8 matching requires ex vivo manipulation of the graft to deplete T cells in order to prevent fatal GVHD).
- Other donor characteristics to consider include age, gender, and CMV status. CMV reactivation risk is based on donor/recipient serologies:
  - D−/R−: very low risk
  - D+/R−: intermediate risk
  - R+: high risk; CMV+ donor is preferred.

CONDITIONING & TOXICITY

- 3 goals of conditioning (depending on disease):
  - Myeloablation (M): Clear space to allow stem cell engraftment.
  - Immunosuppression (I): Prevent rejection and GVHD.
  - Antineoplastic effect (N): Eradicate any remaining leukemia/tumor cells.
- Agents used during conditioning differ by their M/I/N effects and are used in combination to produce the desired outcome. Side effects of conditioning agents:
  - Total body irradiation (M/I/N): cognitive delay, poor growth, cataracts, abnormal dental development, pulmonary and cardiac dysfunction, pituitary dysfunction, infertility, 2nd malignancy
  - Busulfan (M/N): restrictive lung disease, seizures and possibly neurocognitive deficits, skin rash and hyperpigmentation, 2nd malignancy
  - Thiotepa (M/I/N): skin rash, hemorrhagic cystitis, 2nd malignancy
  - Melphalan (M/N): mucositis, cardiac dysfunction, 2nd malignancy
  - Cyclophosphamide (I/N): cardiac dysfunction, SIADH, hemorrhagic cystitis, 2nd malignancy
  - Etoposide (M/N): allergic reaction, hypotension, 2nd malignancy
  - Fludarabine (I/N): cerebellar syndrome, peripheral neuropathy
  - Carmustine (M/N): pulmonary toxicity, 2nd malignancy
  - Alemtuzumab (Campath) (I): anaphylaxis, fever, hypotension, hives, viral and fungal infection
  - Antithymocyte globulin (ATG) (I): anaphylaxis, fever, hypotension, hives, serum sickness, viral and fungal infection
- Nonmyeloablative or reduced toxicity regimens
  - Goal of reduced toxicity regimens is to allow partial donor stem cell engraftment, while limiting toxic effects of conditioning agents.
  - Indications include preexisting organ toxicity precluding full-dose chemotherapy; low performance status, often in the elderly; and primary DNA repair defects resulting in sensitivity to ionizing radiation and alkylating agents (Fanconi anemia, dyskeratosis congenita).
  - Uses lower doses of chemotherapy or lower dose of radiation.
  - Relies more heavily on the GVL effect of alloreactive donor T cells to control or eradicate any remaining neoplastic disease.

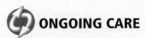

ONGOING CARE

COMPLICATIONS

Treatment-related mortality (TRM) has been declining over time (40% in 1987–1995 to 15% in 2003–2006) and is attributable to the following complications:

- Infection
  - Correlates with timing of immunologic defect (early or <100 days vs. late or >100 days from transplant)
  - Bacterial
    - Early bacterial infections are due to neutropenia, mucositis, or central line (*Staphylococcus* spp, gram-negative rods, *Clostridium difficile*, VRE, atypicals). Later, prolonged adaptive immunity defect and chronic GVHD are risks for mycobacteria and encapsulated bacteria.
    - Treat neutropenic fever empirically with broad-spectrum antibiotics.
    - Role of prophylactic antibiotics is under investigation.
  - Viral
    - Early viral infections are due to lymphopenia, T-cell depletion, cord blood source, and previous viral exposures. Common infections include RSV, rhinovirus, adenovirus, influenza, and herpes virus reactivation (HSV, CMV, HHV-6). Persistent defect in adaptive immunity contributes to later infections such as CMV, VZV, and EBV/PTLD.
    - Acyclovir prophylaxis to prevent HSV reactivation
    - At detection of CMV viremia, rule out CMV retinitis with funduscopic exam and begin preemptive therapy for CMV viremia with foscarnet or ganciclovir. For CMV organ involvement, consider Cytogam, IVIG, or intravitreal foscarnet for CMV retinitis. Continue maintenance therapy with ganciclovir or valganciclovir once viremia is cleared.

– Fungal
  ○ Combined innate and adaptive immunity defects (early) and persistent T-cell dysfunction (late) confer risk for *Candida*, *Aspergillus*, *Pneumocystis*, and other fungal infection (*Fusarium*, *Zygomycetes/Mucor*, *Cryptococcus*, *Histoplasma*, *Coccidioides*).
  ○ Prophylaxis: Fungal prophylaxis is with fluconazole (yeast coverage) or caspofungin; *Pneumocystis* prophylaxis is with cotrimoxazole before conditioning and after engraftment.
  ○ Treatment with voriconazole empirically for sustained fever without source (strong mold/*Aspergillus* coverage)
    ▪ Decrease calcineurin inhibitor/sirolimus dose when starting voriconazole due to inhibition of cytochrome P450 metabolism.
    ▪ Document infection (BAL) whenever possible.

- Mucositis
  – Grades 1–4 based on WHO classification (mild to severe).
  – Prevention: Reduced intensity protocols, glutamine, palifermin; consider holding posttransplant methotrexate if severe mucositis
  – Treatment: IV pain control, TPN, suction
- Veno-occlusive disease (VOD)/sinusoidal obstruction syndrome (SOS)
  – Due to hepatic accumulation of toxic metabolites leading to reduced hepatic venous outflow and postsinusoidal intrahepatic portal hypertension
  – Overall risk of VOD is 10–25%. Risk factors include mismatched or unrelated donor, previous hepatic tumor involvement or abdominal RT, pretransplant elevation of AST, and medications such as busulfan.
  – Diagnosis
    ○ Modified Seattle criteria: Any 2 of the following present by day +20: jaundice (bilirubin >2 mg/dL); painful hepatomegaly; or ascites ± weight gain of >2% from baseline
    ○ Baltimore criteria: bilirubin >2 mg/dL before day +21 and any 2 of the following: hepatomegaly, ascites, or weight gain (>5% from baseline)
    ○ Reversal of portal venous flow on ultrasound (US) is characteristic but not part of diagnostic criteria.
  – Prophylaxis may include ursodiol, *N*-acetylcysteine, or defibrotide (under investigation)
  – Treatment
    ○ Defibrotide: Porcine intestinal mucosal oligonucleotide. Anticoagulant with effects on endothelial cells, platelets, and fibrinolysis
    ○ Supportive care: restriction of sodium and fluid intake; diuresis to keep fluid balance even (spironolactone if able to take PO)
  – Complications of VOD include renal insufficiency, altered mental status, cardiac failure, and bleeding.
- Thrombotic microangiopathy
  – Diagnosis: RBC fragmentation, thrombocytopenia with increased need for frequent platelet transfusions, elevated LDH, concurrent renal and/or neurologic dysfunction
    ○ Calcineurin GVHD prophylaxis is a risk factor (CSA > tacrolimus). Combination with sirolimus triples the risk from 4.2% to 10.8%.
  – Treatment: Discontinue calcineurin inhibitors; supportive care. Limited data for plasmapheresis, eculizumab (anticomplement C5), infliximab, and defibrotide.
- Engraftment syndrome
  – Cytokine-mediated inflammation due to increasing neutrophil activity
  – Usually occurs by day +28 (earlier for autos, later for cord blood transplants)
  – Characterized by rash, fever, and pulmonary edema at the time of engraftment or before neutrophil recovery
  – Treatment: rule out infection, then methylprednisolone for 3–7 days.
- Interstitial pneumonitis
  – Complication of TBI, chemotherapy (busulfan, Cytoxan), or infection (fungal, CMV). Idiopathic pneumonia syndrome (IPS) if no etiology is found.
  – Diagnosis:
    ○ Cough, dyspnea, hypoxemia, fever
    ○ CXR/CT: diffuse versus focal consolidations, nodules or cavitary lesions suggestive of fungus
    ○ BAL: sensitive for CMV, RSV, PCP, other respiratory viruses. Less sensitive for fungus.
  – Treatment: early empiric broad-spectrum antibiotics and antifungals, respiratory support. Consider corticosteroids or TNF blockade for IPS.
- GVHD
  – See GVHD section

Immune Reconstitution

- Innate immunity recovers within 2–4 weeks posttransplant and includes monocytes, followed by granulocytes and NK cells.
- Adaptive immunity recovers over months to years, with peripheral expansion of donor memory T cells (1st wave) followed by thymic development of donor stem cells (2nd wave). Measurements of adaptive immune reconstitution include ALC, donor chimerism, lymphocyte phenotyping, T-cell function (proliferation to mitogen and antigen), B-cell function (serum IgA/IgM and isohemagglutinin titers), and vaccine titers before and after revaccination.
- Revaccination: Effects of conditioning require revaccination with killed vaccines when adaptive immunity has recovered (approximately 1 year posttransplant). If titers demonstrate an immunologic response, live-attenuated vaccines are administered after 2 years.

OUTCOMES

- Overall: 10–20% transplant-related mortality from rejection (<1–8%); toxicity (including infection, 5–20% mortality); and GVHD (5–15% mortality). Additional risk of relapse ranges from 15 to 40%. Risks are modified by several factors:
  – Rejection risks: disease, donor match, cell dose
  – Toxicity risks: infectious risks, conditioning, performance status/organ function.
  – GVHD risks: HLA match, number of donor T cells infused, GVHD prophylaxis.
  – Relapse risks: disease, disease status, conditioning regimen, donor type

LONG-TERM EFFECTS

- Risk is based on doses of chemotherapy and/or TBI received and presence/severity of GVHD.
- Incidence at 10 years (and etiologies):
  – Pulmonary: 20% (TBI, busulfan, GVHD/bronchiolitis obliterans)
  – Ophthalmologic: 44% (TBI, steroids, GVHD)
  – Hypothyroidism: 36% (TBI, busulfan)
  – Osteoarticular: 29% (steroids, GVHD)
  – Cardiac: 11% (TBI, Cytoxan, prior anthracyclines)
  – Hepatic: 16% (iron overload, GVHD)
  – Dental: 15% (TBI, GVHD)
  – Secondary malignancy: 5–10% (TBI, alkylators, VP16, immunodeficiency)
  – Infertility: >90% (TBI, alkylators)
  – Other effects include GH deficiency, hearing loss, hypogonadism, chronic renal insufficiency, neurocognitive defects.
  – Long-term follow-up should include evaluations of disease physical exam, immune status, cardiopulmonary function, endocrine function, hepatic function renal function, ophthalmologic exam, audiology, and neurocognitive evaluation.
  – Immunization strategy posttransplant

ADDITIONAL READING

- Dvorak CC, Cowan MJ. Hematopoietic stem cell transplantation for primary immunodeficiency disease. *Bone Marrow Transplant*. 2008;41(2):119–126.
- Fisher BT, Alexander S, Dvorak CC, et al. Epidemiology and potential preventative measures for viral infections in children with malignancy and those undergoing hematopoietic cell transplantation. *Pediatr Blood Cancer*. 2012;59(1):11–15.
- Pulsipher MA, Skinner R, McDonald GB, et al. National Cancer Institute, National Heart, Lung and Blood Institute/Pediatric Blood and Marrow Transplantation Consortium First International Consensus Conference on late effects after pediatric hematopoietic cell transplantation: the need for pediatric-specific long-term follow-up guidelines. *Biol Blood Marrow Transplant*. 2012;18(3):334–347.
- Spellman SR, Eapen M, Logan BR, et al. A perspective on the selection of unrelated donors and cord blood units for transplantation. *Blood*. 2012;120(2):259–265.

CODES

ICD10

- Z94.81 Bone marrow transplant status
- Z94.84 Stem cells transplant status
- Z52.3 Bone marrow donor

FAQ

- Q: Should friends and family of a patient needing a transplant be tested as a potential match?
- A: If family contacts are willing to donate for an unrelated patient in need of a stem cell transplant, they should join the National Marrow Donor Program (NMDP) registry. However, extended family members are very unlikely to be a match for a related patient.
- Q: Can transplant recipients meet their donors?
- A: The NMDP has guidelines for donor/recipient contact. If both parties agree, contact is allowed 1–2 years after the transplant.

BOTULISM AND INFANT BOTULISM

Jessica M. Khouri • Stephen S. Arnon

BASICS

DESCRIPTION

- An acute illness caused by neurotoxins produced by *Clostridium botulinum* or related neurotoxigenic species, which results in cranial nerve palsies and a symmetric, descending, flaccid paralysis
- The neurotoxin may be elaborated either in the large intestine of individuals temporarily colonized with the bacterium, or ingested, or absorbed from infected wounds.
- There are 3 main forms of the disease:
  - IB is the intestinal toxemia form in which swallowed spores germinate and colonize the infant's colon and elaborate toxin in situ.
  - Foodborne botulism in children and adults occurs when preformed toxin is ingested with improperly prepared or stored foods.
  - Wound botulism occurs when spores of the bacterium contaminate the wound, germinate, and produce toxin that is then absorbed.

EPIDEMIOLOGY

- Infant botulism (IB) is the most common form of human botulism in the United States.
- IB occurs in the 1st year of life, with ~90% of cases reported in the first 6 months of life.
- IB affects infants of all racial backgrounds and socioeconomic groups.
- Male to female ratio is 1:1.
- Toxin types A and B represent 95.7% of cases in United States (1976–2010), with dual toxin types (e.g., Ba, Bf) and more rare type E and type F comprising the remaining 4.3%.
- IB has been recognized in all 50 states, with a greater proportion of toxin type B cases east of the Mississippi River and toxin type A cases west of the Mississippi.
- Recognized on 5 of the 6 inhabited continents, Africa being the exception.
- Often, a history of a recent change in feeding practice is found.
- Honey is an identified food reservoir of *C. botulinum* spores. Honey consumption in U.S. IB patients from 1976 to 2010 was approximately 5.4%.
- For the majority of IB cases, spore acquisition likely occurs from the natural environment, that is, infants inhale and then swallow spores attached to airborne microscopic dust particles. Nearby soil disruption may play a role.
- Breastfed infants who acquire IB tend to be older at onset than are formula-fed infants.
- Foodborne cases are usually associated with home-processed, low acid foods—especially vegetables, fruits, and condiments. Restaurant-associated outbreaks have occurred. Recent outbreaks in U.S. prisons have been associated with fermented alcoholic beverage commonly referred to as *pruno*.
- Wound botulism has been associated with "black tar" heroin injection drug use and traumatic injuries in teenagers.

Incidence

- U.S. IB incidence: 2.2 cases per 100,000 live births (1976–2010). The states with the highest incidence in descending order include Delaware, Hawaii, Utah, Pennsylvania, and California.
- Approximately 80–130 IB cases annually in United States
- Since the disease was first recognized over 35 years ago, more than 3,700 cases of IB have been reported worldwide.
- Foodborne cases occur sporadically yet may result from a common exposure.
- Wound botulism is very rare.

RISK FACTORS

- Infants who have <1 bowel movement per day may be at increased risk of developing IB.
- Honey is an identified, avoidable food source of *C. botulinum* spores.
- Ingestion of improperly canned or preserved low-acid foods may result in foodborne botulism.

GENERAL PREVENTION

- Do not feed honey or raw honey–containing products to infants.
- Botulinum toxin is heat-labile; 5 minutes of boiling will destroy the toxin.
- Spores are heat-resistant.
- Proper food preservation, storage, and preparation will prevent foodborne botulism.

PATHOPHYSIOLOGY

- Neurotoxin is endocytosed at peripheral cholinergic nerve endings; it blocks release of acetylcholine at the neuromuscular junction.
- Cranial nerves are usually affected first and most severely, leading to ptosis, ophthalmoplegia, decreased facial expression, difficulty swallowing, and loss of airway-protective reflexes. Respiratory failure may ensue.
- Sensation and sensorium remain intact.
- Recovery occurs through regeneration of motor neuron axon terminals and the formation of new motor end plates.
- Infants are particularly prone to temporary colonic colonization by *C. botulinum*. When foods other than breast milk are introduced to breastfed infants, perturbation of the intestinal flora may predispose to illness.

ETIOLOGY

C. botulinum, the etiologic agent, is a gram-positive, spore-forming, obligate anaerobic bacterium that is found in dust, soil, and marine sediments worldwide. Rarely, neurotoxigenic *Clostridium butyricum* and *Clostridium baratii* may cause disease due to toxin type E and type F, respectively.

DIAGNOSIS

HISTORY

- IB
- Symptoms include constipation, poor feeding/poor latch, diminished facial expression, droopy eyelids, difficulty swallowing, and generalized weakness.
  - Fever is typically absent (barring concomitant infections).
  - Infants may appear lethargic (from ptosis and decreased facial expression).
  - Occasionally, rapid progression of symptoms may result in respiratory arrest or an apparent life-threatening event (ALTE).
- Foodborne botulism
  - ~50% of patients report emesis.
  - There may initially be complaints of diarrhea followed by constipation.
  - The incubation period from ingestion to the onset of symptoms is usually 18–36 hours (range, a few hours to several days).
  - Patients complain of weakness and dry mouth.
  - Visual complaints include blurry vision, loss of accommodation, and diplopia.
  - Patients may complain of difficulty swallowing or slurred speech.
  - Patients may have urinary retention.
  - Occasionally, progression may be quite rapid, and the abrupt onset of lethargy and weakness may suggest bacterial sepsis or meningitis.
- Wound botulism
  - Often history of IV drug use
  - Incubation period ranges from 4 to 14 days.
  - Fever may be present from wound infection not botulism.
  - Patients often report constipation but rarely nausea or vomiting.
  - Patients may complain of purulent discharge from the wound.

PHYSICAL EXAM

- IB
  - Patients are typically afebrile and appear lethargic.
  - Cranial nerve findings include ptosis, diminished facial expression, weak cry, poor latch/suck, drooling/dysphagia, weak gag, and poor head control.
  - Pupils
    - Often midposition initially. May be normal to sluggishly reactive but fatigue with repetitive stimulation
    - In some cases, pupils appear fixed and dilated for a period.
  - Frog-leg positioning due to weakness of hip girdle musculature
  - Generalized weakness and loss of motor milestones
  - Flaccid, descending paralysis, and hyporeflexia
  - The remainder of the physical examination is normal.
  - Helpful physical examination findings:
    - In infants, early in the course of the disease, pupillary and corneal reflexes may fatigue easily (refer to physical examination tools under "For Physicians—Clinical Diagnosis" tab at www.infantbotulism.org)
- Older children and adults
  - May appear alert and are afebrile
  - Ptosis, extraocular palsies, and dilated, sluggishly reactive pupils are often the 1st signs of descending paralysis.
  - Dysphagia, dysarthria, and hypoglossal weakness indicate lower cranial nerve involvement.
  - Respiratory failure may rapidly ensue from upper airway obstruction resulting from loss of pharyngeal tone, loss of airway-protective reflexes, and respiratory muscle weakness.
  - The triad of bulbar palsies, clear sensorium, and absence of fever should prompt immediate consideration of botulism.
  - Signs of autonomic instability may include unexpected fluctuations in skin color, BP and heart rate, and urinary retention.

DIAGNOSTIC TESTS & INTERPRETATION

Lab

- For IB, stool or enema is submitted for diagnostic testing to a state health department or the Centers for Disease Control and Prevention (CDC). Diagnosis is established by identification of toxin by mouse neutralization assay and/or isolation of a toxigenic organism. Serum testing is not routinely performed.

Clinicians should request specific instructions on specimen submission from their state health departments.
- In foodborne and wound botulism, tests for the presence of toxin or organisms can be conducted on patient samples (serum, gastric aspirates, feces, or wound exudate) or suspected foodstuffs.
- Anaerobic cultures of wound material may yield the organism.
- In infant and foodborne botulism, excretion of toxin and organisms in feces may persist for weeks to months after symptom onset.

Imaging
EEG, MRI, and CT are nonspecific and usually normal in the absence of complications.

Diagnostic Procedures/Other
- Most tests for toxin and organism are done by state health departments or the CDC.
- The most common test performed is an assay for botulinum toxin in stool.
- Specimens must be shipped in sealed, break-proof, and leak-proof containers. Even minute amounts of toxin, if inhaled or ingested, can lead to disease.
- Suspect foods should be shipped refrigerated and in their original containers if possible.
- Electromyography (EMG) may demonstrate a characteristic pattern of brief, small, overly abundant motor unit action potentials (BSAPs). EMG results may be normal or inconclusive in botulism patients. Nerve conduction velocities are normal.

DIFFERENTIAL DIAGNOSIS
- Top 2 clinical mimics of IB are spinal muscular atrophy (SMA) type I and metabolic disorders.
- Infections
  - In infants, sepsis, meningitis and polio-like enteroviruses may present in a similar way.
  - In older children and adults, bacterial sepsis, meningitis, poliomyelitis, tick paralysis, and diphtheric polyneuritis
  - Postinfectious demyelinating processes may mimic botulism but generally have asymmetric findings.
  - Absence of fever and a clear sensorium make sepsis and meningitis less likely.
- Neurologic
  - Myasthenia gravis spares the pupillary constrictor response, which in botulism is either fatigable, sluggish, or absent.
  - In Werdnig-Hoffmann disease (SMA type I), extraocular and sphincter muscles are spared.
- Metabolic/genetic
  - Certain metabolic or genetic conditions may closely mimic IB.
- Toxins: Drug ingestions may lead to weakness and lethargy.

TREATMENT

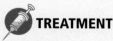

MEDICATION
- Prompt recognition of IB and early treatment with intravenous human botulism immune globulin (BabyBIG; BIG-IV) significantly shortens hospital stay, time in intensive care, and duration of respiratory and nutritional support. BabyBIG is available through the California Department of Public Health's Infant Botulism Treatment and Prevention Program (IBTPP).
- Treatment with BIG-IV should be promptly initiated based on clinical findings and *not* delayed for laboratory diagnostic studies.
- Antibiotics are not helpful in IB:
  - In suspected IB, avoid aminoglycoside antibiotics (e.g., gentamicin); an abrupt worsening of weakness and respiratory failure may result from potentiating effects at the neuromuscular junction.
- Equine-derived antitoxin is not recommended for the treatment of IB but has been used to treat type-F IB cases.
- Antibiotics are indicated only for documented complications such as pneumonia or urinary tract infections.
- Cathartics are not beneficial.
- Foodborne or wound botulism
  - Should be treated with the licensed, equine-derived heptavalent botulinum antitoxin (BAT), available from the CDC
  - Antitoxin should not be administered to asymptomatic individuals who have only eaten suspect foods.
- Wound botulism should be treated with IV penicillin G 250,000 U/kg/24 h or equivalent and BAT antitoxin.

ADDITIONAL TREATMENT
General Measures
- Patients with suspected botulism should be hospitalized and have continuous monitoring of heart rate, respiratory rate, and oxygenation, as well as frequent assessment of respiratory effort and airway-protective reflexes.
- The mainstay of therapy is meticulous supportive care. Particular attention should be paid to respiratory and nutritional needs.
- Endotracheal intubation is necessary for patients with respiratory failure or loss of airway-protective reflexes.
- Wounds should be explored and debrided and anaerobic cultures obtained.
- Cases of suspected toxin ingestion should be treated early with induced emesis and/or gastric lavage in an attempt to decrease toxin exposure.
- All suspect cases should be immediately reported to the state health department and the CDC.

INPATIENT CONSIDERATIONS
Initial Stabilization
Meticulous supportive care with particular emphasis on respiratory and nutritional needs is the most important consideration.

ONGOING CARE

PROGNOSIS
- IB has an estimated mortality rate of <1% in hospitalized patients. Complete recovery can be expected when the disease is recognized early and treated appropriately.
- The mortality rate of adult foodborne botulism is 20–25%. In patients <20 years old it is 10%.
- Patients with a shorter incubation period usually have more severe involvement and a worse prognosis, probably related to an increased amount of toxin ingested.
- If recognized early and treated aggressively, botulism has a favorable prognosis, and complete recovery can generally be expected. Fatigability may persist for up to 1 year.

COMPLICATIONS
- Fatal respiratory failure from paralysis of respiratory muscles is the most serious complication.
- Bulbar dysfunction in IB may lead to dehydration and starvation ketosis before presentation.
- Loss of airway-protective reflexes can lead to aspiration and pneumonia.
- Constipation and urinary retention may precede the onset of paralysis and may complicate later management. Cases of severe *Clostridium difficile* enterocolitis with hypovolemia, hypotension, and prolonged ICU stays have occurred in IB patients.
- Recurrent urinary tract infections and syndrome of inappropriate antidiuretic hormone secretion (SIADH) are rare complications of IB.

ADDITIONAL READING

- Arnon SS, Schechter R, Maslanka SE, et al. Human botulism immune globulin for the treatment of infant botulism. *N Engl J Med*. 2006;354(5):462–471.
- Francisco AM, Arnon SS. Clinical mimics of infant botulism. *Pediatrics*. 2007;119(4):826–828.
- Koepke R, Sobel J, Arnon SS. Global occurrence of infant botulism, 1976–2006. *Pediatrics*. 2008;122(1):e73–e82.
- Mitchell WG, Tseng-Ong L. Catastrophic presentation of infant botulism may obscure or delay diagnosis. *Pediatrics*. 2005;116(3):e436–e438.
- Passaro DJ, Werner SB, McGee J, et al. Wound botulism associated with black tar heroin among injecting drug users. *JAMA*. 1998;279(11):859–863.
- Vugia DJ, Mase SR, Cole B, et al. Botulism from drinking pruno. *Emerg Infect Dis*. 2009;15(1):69–71. doi:10.3201/eid1501.081024.

CODES

ICD10
- A05.1 Botulism food poisoning
- A48.51 Infant botulism
- A48.52 Wound botulism

FAQ
- Q: Can IB recur?
- A: True recurrence of IB has not been documented.
- Q: Should antitoxin be given to persons who have ingested food that they think might be contaminated with botulinum toxin (foodborne botulism)?
- A: Because the antitoxin carries a risk of serum sickness, it should be given only to persons exhibiting symptoms consistent with botulism.
- Q: Where is antitoxin obtained?
- A: For suspected IB cases human-derived antitoxin, BabyBIG (BIG-IV), may be obtained from the Infant Botulism Treatment and Prevention Program, California Department of Public Health, 24/7/365 Ph: 510-231-7600; www.infantbotulism.org.
- For non-IB patients, the licensed heptavalent (A–G) equine-derived antitoxin, BAT, may be obtained from the CDC, Atlanta, Georgia; 770-488-7100.
- Q: How is human-derived antitoxin, BabyBIG produced?
- A: BIG-IV; BabyBIG is produced from pooled human plasma from screened adult volunteers immunized against botulinum toxin for occupational protection.

BRAIN ABSCESS

Karen E. Jerardi • Samir S. Shah

BASICS

DESCRIPTION
- Suppurative infection involving the brain parenchyma
- May be a single or multiple lesions

EPIDEMIOLOGY
- Males more commonly affected (2:1 male-to-female predominance).
- Typical age of presentation is 4–7 years but varies according to predisposing factor.
- 85% of cases have a predisposing risk factor.

Incidence
~1,500–2,500 cases (adults and pediatric combined) occur per year with up to 25% being children.

RISK FACTORS
- Cyanotic congenital heart disease (tetralogy of Fallot is most common)
- Otorhinolaryngologic infections such as sinusitis, mastoiditis, and chronic otitis media
- Meningitis (especially in neonates)
- Penetrating head trauma
- Surgical manipulation of the brain (ventriculoperitoneal shunts, tumor removal)
- Congenital lesions of the head and neck
- Cystic fibrosis
- Dental infections
- Lung infections
- Patients who have traveled to endemic areas where neurocysticercosis (Latin America, parts of Africa, Asia, and the Indian subcontinent) is endemic
- Immunocompromised patients (congenital or acquired)

GENERAL PREVENTION
- During recreational activities, wearing helmets may prevent penetrating head trauma.
- Appropriate management of acute otitis media and acute sinusitis and timely recognition of treatment failure

PATHOPHYSIOLOGY
- Microorganisms enter the brain parenchyma by contiguous or hematogenous extension.
- Location of brain abscesses:
  – Cyanotic congenital heart disease patients tend to have abscesses within the middle meningeal artery distribution: frontal, parietal, and temporal lobes.
  – Frontal abscesses are commonly seen with sinus and dental infections.
  – Temporal, parietal, or cerebellar abscesses tend to occur with mastoiditis or otitis media.
  – Brain abscesses can occur anywhere in the brain parenchyma, regardless of a predisposing risk factor, secondary to hematogenous metastasis.

ETIOLOGY
- Bacteria are the most common causes.
- *Streptococcus milleri* group and *Staphylococcus* sp. are the most commonly cultured microorganisms.
- Neonates may develop brain abscesses as a complication of Gram-negative meningitis (*Proteus*, *Citrobacter*, *Enterobacter*, and *Cronobacter* species).
- Polymicrobial infections occur in 30–50% of cases.
- Anaerobic organisms are found with increasing incidence with improved laboratory and culture techniques. Common pathogens include *Bacteroides*, *Peptostreptococcus*, *Fusobacterium*, *Propionibacterium*, *Actinomyces*, *Veillonella*, and *Prevotella*.
- Neurocysticercosis is caused by the parasite, *Taenia solium*. Fungi and protozoa can cause brain abscess in immunocompromised patients.

DIAGNOSIS

HISTORY
The location of the brain abscess or abscesses will influence the clinical presentation.
- Classic triad of fever, headache, and focal neurologic findings occurs in <30% of cases.
- Fever, headache, and vomiting each occur in 60–70% of cases.
- Headache is the most common complaint.
- Vomiting and mental status changes can be the presenting chief complaints.
- Neonates will often have a history of meningitis before developing a brain abscess.
- Questions should focus on acute or chronic otolaryngologic infections.
- A history of cyanotic congenital heart disease should be obtained, as well as partially repaired cyanotic congenital heart disease.

PHYSICAL EXAM
- Neonates may present with a full fontanel, increasing head circumference, seizures, or vomiting.
- Older children may have signs of a focal neurologic deficit, hemiparesis, or even papilledema.
- Meningeal symptoms occur in 30% of patients.
- Ataxia may be found with cerebellar lesions.

DIAGNOSTIC TESTS & INTERPRETATION

Lab
- Routine lab tests are not helpful and cannot rule out the diagnosis.
- <10% of blood cultures are positive.
- Peripheral WBC may be mildly elevated, but <10% will show band forms.
- ESR is a poor indicator of brain abscesses.
- Electrolytes may show low sodium, indicating syndrome of inappropriate secretion of antidiuretic hormone (SIADH).
- A lumbar puncture is contraindicated if any intracranial mass lesion is suspected, but if CSF is obtained:
  – It may show a mild to moderate pleocytosis (20% of patients may have normal values).
  – Opening pressure may be elevated.
  – Glucose is decreased in 30% of patients.
  – Protein is elevated in 70% of cases.
  – CSF Gram stain and cultures are often negative.

Imaging
- CT with contrast and MRI scans are the studies of choice in diagnosing brain abscesses.
- Although CT can provide more rapid results, occult intracranial infections can be missed in up to 50% of cases.
- Cranial ultrasound may be useful in premature neonatal cases.

ALERT
- Not all patients with brain abscesses have fevers.
- Pitfalls
  – Failure to consider a brain abscess in a child with altered mental status, fevers, and meningismus or in a child with nonspecific symptoms but risk factors, such as cyanotic congenital heart disease
  – Failure to recognize symptoms not typically seen in sinusitis, such as vomiting

DIFFERENTIAL DIAGNOSIS
- Infectious
  – Meningitis
  – Encephalitis
  – Subdural empyema
  – Epidural abscess
- Vascular
  – Venous sinus thrombosis
  – Migraine
  – Cerebral infarct
  – Cerebral hemorrhage
- Miscellaneous
  – Primary or secondary tumor
  – Pseudotumor cerebri
  – Hydrocephalus

TREATMENT

MEDICATION

- Broad-spectrum antibiotics that penetrate the CNS should be given at the time of diagnosis directed at most likely pathogens. The combination of a third-generation cephalosporin, vancomycin, and metronidazole provide good empiric coverage.
- Culture-directed antimicrobial therapy is recommended whenever possible. Typical antibiotic courses are 4–6 weeks.
- Consider neurosurgical and/or otolaryngology consultation.
- MRI or CT-guided stereotactic aspiration is encouraged to obtain cultures and identify the causative organism(s).
- Some patients are managed successfully with antibiotics alone, especially if there is a single, small (<2 cm) abscess.
- Antiparasitic medications (albendazole) with or without corticosteroids should be considered for treatment of neurocysticercosis.
- Antifungals should be considered for immunocompromised patients.
- Evaluation by cardiology, dental, otorhinolaryngology, and/or immunology may help identify predisposing factors.

INPATIENT CONSIDERATIONS

Initial Stabilization

- If a patient is manifesting signs and symptoms of increased intracranial pressure (Cushing triad: bradycardia, hypertension, and abnormal respirations) or if the patient is unable to protect his or her airway, endotracheal intubation is indicated. Hyperventilation and mannitol should be considered.
- Electrolyte abnormalities such as SIADH may occur. Frequent monitoring of electrolytes is warranted.
- Seizures and focal neurologic deficits can occur early in presentation. They typically resolve with drainage of the lesion. Careful and frequent neurologic exams should be part of the hospital care.

Admission Criteria

All patients with concern for brain abscess should be admitted for clinical monitoring, diagnostic evaluation, and treatment.

Discharge Criteria

Generally, patients may be discharged home once their symptoms have resolved and antibiotic therapy is complete or can be completed at home.

ONGOING CARE

FOLLOW-UP RECOMMENDATIONS

- Follow-up with neurosurgical, rehabilitation, and neurology clinics is usually required.
- Repeat imaging prior to cessation of antibiotic therapy should be done to document resolution of the abscess.

COMPLICATIONS

- Long-term complications arise from the location, size, and number of intracranial abscesses.
- Multiple abscesses, coma on presentation, <2 years of age, and rupture of abscess into the ventricle carry a higher mortality rate.
- 30–40% of patients have some morbidity associated with brain abscess; seizures, hydrocephalus, focal neurologic deficits (motor and sensory dysfunction), and behavorial or personality changes are potential complications. Mortality rates have decreased because of advances in imaging to assist in rapid diagnosis and surgical management.

ADDITIONAL READING

- Goodkin HP, Harper MB, Pomeroy SL. Intracerebral abscess in children: Historical trends at Children's Hospital Boston. *Pediatrics*. 2004;113(6):1765–1770.
- Saez-Llorens X. Brain abscess in children. *Semin Pediatr Infect Dis*. 2003;14(2):108–114.
- Yogev R, Bar-Meir M. Management of brain abscess in children. *Pediatr Infect Dis J*. 2004;23(2):157–160.
- Herrmann BW, Chung JC, Eisenbeis JF, et al. Intracranial complications of pediatric frontal rhinosinusitis. *Am J Rhinol*. 2006;20(3):320–324.
- Seydoux C, Francioli P. Bacterial brain abscesses: factors influencing mortality and sequelae. *Clin Infect Dis*. 1992;15(3):394–401.

CODES

ICD10

G06.0 Intracranial abscess and granuloma

FAQ

- Q: Do all brain abscesses require surgery?
- A: No. Often times, brain abscesses will respond to intravenous antibiotics and will not require drainage. Close clinical and radiographic follow-up is imperative in these cases. Stereotactic aspiration of a brain abscess can be very helpful in identifying the microbiology of a brain abscess and help direct specific treatment.
- Q: What is the best imaging study to definitively diagnose a brain abscess?
- A: MRI

BRAIN INJURY, TRAUMATIC

Mark E. Halstead

BASICS

DESCRIPTION

Traumatic brain injury (TBI): damage to the brain from accidental or nonaccidental trauma

- Children >1 year: Glasgow Coma Scale (GCS) <14, amnesia >15 minutes for event, penetrating head injury (see Appendix, Table 5)
- Children <1 year: any LOC, protracted emesis, suspected abuse (see Appendix, Table 6)
- Mild brain injury : GCS >14
- Severe brain injury: usually initial GCS <9

EPIDEMIOLOGY

- Trauma, number 1 cause of death of children >1 year. Head injury most common contributor to morbidity and mortality
- Almost 500,000 emergency department visits each year for TBI for those aged 0–14 years. Males age 0–4 years highest rate of TBI emergency department visits
- 75% of TBIs each year are mild.
- <2 years old: Nonaccidental trauma is principal cause of TBI.
- >2 years old: Falls (~37%) are most common cause of trauma.
- For severe TBI, nonaccidental trauma remains principal cause in young children.
- Motor vehicle accidents in older children, although penetrating injuries becoming more common

PATHOPHYSIOLOGY

- Primary
  - Focally applied forces: lacerations, penetration injuries, skull fractures
  - Contusions, intracerebral hematomas uncommon. Epidurals, classic subdurals <10% in children
  - Acceleration–deceleration/shearing forces: cervical spine injuries, diffuse axonal injury (DAI), nonaneurysmal subarachnoid hemorrhage, subdural hematoma (SDH) from shear forces
- Secondary
  - Extension of injury to viable tissue/entire brain
  - Dysautoregulation of cerebral blood flow, neuroexcitotoxicity, and inflammatory mediators. In severe TBI, CT or MRI signs of edema may progress over 3–5 days (see "Treatment").
- Age-specific pathophysiology:
  - Infants/toddler
    - Shear forces on the brain due to acceleration/deceleration avulse axons from their cell bodies (DAI); often compounded by tearing and bleeding of dural veins
    - Unmyelinated infant brain absorbs rather than transfers impact. Immature, distensible skull renders brain less likely to contuse or herniated, but more likely to sustain diffuse secondary injuries, with swelling.
    - Subgaleal hematoma, cephalohematoma (below the periosteum), and caput succedaneum (confined to the superficial scalp) at birth do not predict brain injury.
    - More severe birth trauma can result in SDH.
    - Bilateral interhemispheric SDH suggests nonaccidental trauma.
    - Diffuse injuries secondary to shaken impact syndrome can lead to cerebral swelling with secondary infarction and/or decreased central respiratory control, leading to apnea, hypoxia, and cerebral edema.
    - Suspect nonaccidental trauma with growing skull fracture, if >1 cranial bone involved, or if other injuries are present.
  - Older children/adolescents
    - Mild TBI likely due to neuronal disruption, potassium efflux with release of glutamate. Increases demand of ATP and glucose.
    - Still more subject to DAI than adults due to incomplete myelination
    - Projectile injuries in adolescent population

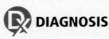

DIAGNOSIS

HISTORY

- Eyewitness accounts are invaluable.
- Details of who was caring for the child
- Falls: Did loss of consciousness precede fall? Height of fall, surface of impact
- History of epilepsy, cardiac problems
- History of previous concussions (consider "second impact syndrome") or trauma
- Intoxication (of child, caregiver, others in the environment)
- Prior physical abuse/neglect?
- Restrained motor vehicle passenger? Angle of impact
- How did patient act or change over time? Unresponsive? Confused? Headache? Visual changes? Vomiting? Seizure?
- Consider use of published concussion symptom checklists.

PHYSICAL EXAM

Rapid neurologic exam in trauma

- Can derive some of these by observation. Note presence of neuromuscular blockers/sedation:
  - Level of arousal: awake, lethargic, stuporous, unresponsive
  - Resting posture: spontaneous, restless, still normal, flexor, extensor
  - Respiration: in context of arousal and posture, hyperpnea, or Cheyne-Stokes respiration
  - Response to stimulation: voice, pain (of earlobe to avoid spinal withdrawal response); note localization, withdrawal, posturing.
  - Pupils: equal, anisocoria >1 mm, unequal/sluggish pupil, unequal/wide/fixed pupil
  - Extraocular movements: disconjugate gaze nonlocalizing with drugs/trauma, 3rd nerve palsy uncal herniation sign, 4th nerve palsy common in head injuries, 6th nerve palsy from trauma or increased ICP.
  - Brainstem reflexes: corneals (V & VII), oculocephalic if patient unable to cooperate with eye exam and cervical spine cleared. Avoid gag—raises ICP.
  - Muscle reflexes/motor exam: Lateralizing signs may indicate contralateral hemispheric lesion, with ipsilateral dilated pupil may indicate uncal herniation.
  - Sensory: brief for 4 limbs/spinal level if indicated
- This exam should be repeated often according to the patient's level of acuity. A more detailed exam tailored to degree of arousal can be done as the patient is stabilized.
- Mild TBI can be assessed with standard neurologic exam as outlined earlier. Balanced assessment and neurocognitive assessment (short-term memory, months of the year in reverse, digits in reverse) may be useful. Use of SCAT3 in sport concussion assessment may be beneficial on sideline or emergency department.

DIAGNOSTIC TESTS & INTERPRETATION

Lab

In all patients with suspected TBI, consider:

- CBC (infants can have a large amount of intracranial blood loss)
- PT/PTT (to evaluate a possible bleeding disorder as a possible preoperative laboratory test)
- Electrolytes
- Toxin screen
- Laboratory studies likely not necessary in mild TBI unless laboratory abnormality suspected as contributor to TBI.

Imaging

- In mild TBI, imaging most likely not needed. High risk for lesion includes GCS <15 at 2 hours post injury, suspicion of open skull fracture, worsening headache, and irritability. Medium risk for lesion includes large, boggy hematoma, signs of basal skull fracture, and dangerous mechanism of injury.
- Unenhanced CT scan of the brain is the imaging study of choice for initial evaluation of a patient with suspected TBI.
- Abnormal CT: lesion density, midline shift, compression of cisterns, bone fragments
- MRI: useful for DAI (with a negative head CT) as well as showing small lesions (e.g., punctate contusions)
- In suspected cervical spine injury where patient is unresponsive, CT scan initially with consideration for MRI of the spine to rule out noncontiguous unstable ligamentous injury.
- Long bone films if degree of injury is not consistent with history or history of fall from unclear height
- Consider EEG and lumbar puncture if a non-traumatic etiology for altered mental status is suspected, if CT normal.

DIFFERENTIAL DIAGNOSIS

Neurologic presentation varies in severity from a normal examination through coma similar to hypoxic-ischemic brain injuries (e.g., near-drowning), other causes of stupor/coma, seizure activity (postictal encephalopathy).

Distinction between simple concussion, DAI, and hypoxic-ischemic injury may be difficult at initial presentation, becoming clear as clinical picture/neuroimaging evolves.

TREATMENT

- Airway, breathing, circulation
- Cervical spine stabilization in unconscious patient with unclear mechanism of injury
- Prehospital stabilization: Avoid hypoxemia and hypotension (strong, possibly modifiable, independent predictors of outcome in TBI).

ADDITIONAL TREATMENT

General Measures

- For acute mild TBI, recommend physical rest and reducing cognitive stress while symptomatic.
- AAP guidelines set conditions for return to play depending on symptoms:
  - An AAP concussion statement outlines graduated return to activity if no return of symptoms and suggests (a) no same-day return; (b) and medical clearance needed before initiating return to activity progression.
- A rapid neurologic exam repeated over time is instrumental in directing the patient's care.
- For more severe trauma or in infants
- Secondary survey: external evidence of head injury/deformities, ecchymoses (periorbital-orbital roof fracture; mastoid-petrous temporal fracture), lacerations, penetrations. CSF leak nasal/otic
- Seizures: lorazepam 0.05–0.1 mg/kg IV at 2 mg/min or rectal Diastat 0.3–0.5 mg/kg if no IV access. Then load fosphenytoin 15–20 mg/kg IV. Important to treat to avoid increased ICP, neurotoxicity, hypoxia
- No evidence that seizure prophylaxis >1 week post trauma prevents late seizures
- No evidence that steroids improve outcome
- Hypothermia may be protective in severe TBI, no difference in long-term outcome.
- No evidence for prophylactic use of mannitol, although it is effective for control of increased ICP. Bolus doses 0.25 g/kg of body weight to 1 g/kg of body weight to goal ICP <20 mm Hg
- Hypertonic 3% saline IV for increased ICP as above under fluid resuscitation
- The postresuscitation GCS score should be recorded in all trauma patients.
- Involvement of neurosurgery with moderate GCS <13 injury, even if patient initially stable
- Survival for children with severe TBI is greater when treated in pediatric ICU.
- Decompressive craniectomy may be considered given the following conditions:
  - Diffuse cerebral swelling on cranial CT imaging
  - Within 48 hours of injury
  - No episodes of sustained ICP >40 mm Hg before surgery
  - GCS >3 at some point subsequent to injury
  - Secondary clinical deterioration
  - Evolving cerebral herniation syndrome

INPATIENT CONSIDERATIONS

Initial Stabilization

- Cervical spine stabilization and clearance; in severe TBI, entire spine is stabilized:
  - If necessary, orotracheal intubation with rapid sequence induction; avoid hypotension.
  - Hyperventilation may induce regional cerebral ischemia in children, especially in first 24 hours.
  - Increased ICP managed by bed elevation of 30 degrees, hypertonic fluids, sedation
- Hemodynamic stabilization (normal high systolic BP ~135) predictor of better outcome in TBI (median systolic BP = 90 mm Hg + [2 × age in years])
  - Hemodynamic instability indicative of systemic hemorrhage (abdomen, long bone fractures). Pericardial tamponade (narrow pulse pressure). Neurogenic shock
  - Hypotension late sign. early: ↑HR, ↓capillary refill, ↓urine output
  - Fluid resuscitation: Consider hypertonic saline. Mounting evidence of improved outcomes especially with hemorrhagic shock and TBI (titrate continuous 3% saline infusion 0.1–1 mL/kg/h).
  - Fluid bolus may worsen intracranial hypertension (ICP).
  - Consider monitoring ICP to maintain <20 mm Hg for abnormal admission CT scan, and GCS 3–8 after CPR, or normal CT and GCS 3–8, and posturing, or hypotension, or if serial neurologic exams precluded by sedation.

ONGOING CARE

PROGNOSIS

- Majority of mild TBI patients recovery without significant sequelae
- Presence of both hypoxemia and hypotension on arrival to ER bode poorly.
- 24-hour GCS better predictor of outcome than postresuscitation; PRISM score also helpful
- GCS <3 poor prognosis unless secondary to epidural hematoma; rapid evacuation can minimize permanent deficits.
- Diffuse white matter, subcortical gray, or brainstem lesions on MRI portend long periods of coma and poorer outcome.
- Somatosensory-evoked potentials (VEPS or BAEPs) are less sensitive but have high specificity in predicting neurologic outcome.
- Degree of injury on head CT can be predictive.
- Patients who have sustained moderate to severe head injury (GCS = 13) often have academic difficulties, memory abnormalities, and disinhibition.
- Monitoring for cognitive difficulties, hyperactivity, seizures, hydrocephalus, movement disorders, paralysis, visual/hearing disturbance, headache; psychologists, neurologists, neurosurgeons, ophthalmologists, audiologists, and physical therapists may be helpful.
- Refer any patient with known skull fracture who manifests a new swelling in area of old fracture to neurosurgery for 3-D CT imaging of the head.
- ~10% of patients with severe head injury will develop epilepsy.

ADDITIONAL READING

- Adelson PD, Bratton SL, Carney NA, et al. Critical pathway for the treatment of established intracranial hypertension in pediatric traumatic brain injury. *Pediatr Crit Care Med*. 2003;4(3)(Suppl):S65–S67.
- Centers for Disease Control and Prevention: www.cdc.gov/concussion/HeadsUp/high_school.html
- Halstead ME, Walter KD; Council on Sports Medicine and Fitness. Clinical report—sport-related concussion in children and adolescents. *Pediatrics*. 2010;126(3):597–615.
- Hymel KP, Makoroff KL, Laskey AL, et al. Mechanisms, clinical presentations, injuries, and outcomes from inflicted versus noninflicted head trauma during infancy: results of a prospective, multicentered, comparative study. *Pediatrics*. 2007;119(5):922–929.
- Jagannathan J, Okonkwo DO, Dumont AS, et al. Outcome following decompressive craniectomy in children with severe traumatic brain injury: a 10-year single-center experience with long-term follow-up. *J Neurosurg*. 2007;106(4)(Suppl):268–275.
- Osmond MH, Klassen TP, Wells GA, et al. CATCH: a clinical decision rule for the use of computed tomography in children with minor head injury. *CMAJ*. 2010;182(4):341–348.
- White JR, Farukhi Z, Bull C, et al. Predictors of outcome in severely head-injured children. *Crit Care Med*. 2001;29(3):534–540.

CODES

ICD10

- S06.9X0A Unsp intracranial injury w/o loss of consciousness, init
- S06.9X9A Unsp intracranial injury w LOC of unsp duration, init
- S06.9X1A Unspecified intracranial injury with loss of consciousness of 30 minutes or less, initial encounter

BRAIN TUMOR

Jane E. Minturn • Michael J. Fisher

BASICS

DESCRIPTION
A primary neoplasm arising in the CNS

EPIDEMIOLOGY
- Most common solid neoplasm of childhood (2nd to leukemia in overall incidence)
- Slight male predominance
- Majority arise infratentorially (within cerebellum or brainstem) in children 1–11 years of age.
- Majority arise supratentorially in children <1 year of age.

Incidence
- Incidence rising (>3,000 new cases/year)
- 4.5 cases/100,000 children/year
- Peak incidence in children ≤7 years of age

RISK FACTORS
Genetics
- Not a heritable condition
- Primary CNS tumors are associated with several familial syndromes:
  - Neurofibromatosis with optic pathway gliomas (NF1) and meningiomas (NF2)
  - Tuberous sclerosis with gliomas and rarely ependymomas
  - Li-Fraumeni syndrome with astrocytomas
  - Von Hippel-Lindau with cerebellar hemangioblastoma
  - Turcot syndrome with primitive neuroectodermal tumor

PATHOPHYSIOLOGY
The majority of tumors are classified based on their histology. The most common are the following:
- Glioma
  - Arises from glial cells (e.g., astrocytes most common)
  - >50% of childhood CNS tumors
  - Ranges from low-grade (often in the cerebellum or optic pathway) to high-grade (grade III–IV; in the cerebrum or brainstem)
  - Locally recurrent and invasive when high-grade
- Primitive neuroectodermal tumor/medulloblastoma
  - Malignant embryonal tumor arising from unknown cell type
  - Comprises ~20% of childhood CNS tumors
  - Most common malignant brain tumor in children
  - Majority arise in the midline of the cerebellum (referred to as medulloblastoma).
  - Predisposition for leptomeningeal dissemination
- Ependymoma
  - Arises from ependymal cells that line the ventricular system
  - 8–10% of childhood CNS tumors
  - Most commonly occurs in the 4th ventricle; may arise in the spinal cord
  - Locally recurrent and invasive; spinal metastases rare at initial diagnosis
- Germ cell tumor
  - Derived from totipotent germ cells
  - 3–5% of childhood CNS tumors
  - Majority are located in the pineal or suprasellar region.
- Atypical teratoid/rhabdoid tumor
  - Rare embryonal tumor arising from unknown cell type; often misdiagnosed as primitive neuroectodermal tumor
  - <3% of childhood CNS tumors
  - Majority arise in children <5 years of age.
  - Propensity to arise in the posterior fossa with frequent leptomeningeal dissemination; reported in association with malignant rhabdoid tumors of the kidney
- Craniopharyngioma: 6–9% of childhood CNS tumors
- Choroid plexus tumors (papilloma and carcinoma)
- Ganglioglioma
- Meningioma and hemangioblastoma, rare in children

ETIOLOGY
- No specific causative agents are known, but there is an association with radiation, chemical exposure, other malignancies, familial/heritable diseases, immunosuppression/immunodeficiency (CNS lymphoma).
- Molecular markers and variants of individual tumor types are being identified.

DIAGNOSIS

Tumor location dictates symptoms and signs.

HISTORY
- Headache and vomiting (particularly in the morning), irritability, and lethargy are associated with increased intracranial pressure.
- Difficulty swallowing, slurred speech, and diplopia may indicate brainstem tumor.
- Visual field deficits (bumps into things) could indicate optic pathway lesion.
- Focal weakness hints at pyramidal tract lesion.
- Ataxia may be a sign of cerebellar lesion.
- Changes in behavior or school performance, new-onset seizures, and weakness could be signs of supratentorial lesion.
- Polyuria/polydipsia may indicate hypothalamic/pituitary lesion.
- Failure to thrive, emaciation, euphoria, and increased appetite in an infant may indicate hypothalamic lesion (diencephalic syndrome).
- Back pain, extremity weakness, and bowel/bladder dysfunction could signify spinal cord metastases (often seen with primitive neuroectodermal tumor/medulloblastoma and germ cell tumors).

PHYSICAL EXAM
- Papilledema, impaired upgaze and/or lateral gaze, macrocephaly (infants), and bulging fontanelle are signs of increased intracranial pressure.
- Focal deficit on neurologic exam helps localize the mass lesion:
  - Isolated cranial nerve VI and VII palsies may indicate brainstem tumor.
  - Ataxia and dysmetria could indicate cerebellar mass.
  - Decreased visual acuity, visual field deficit, absent pupillary light response, and strabismus may all be signs of optic pathway tumor.
  - Changes in cognitive function, mood, and affect could indicate supratentorial lesion.
  - Impaired upgaze, convergence nystagmus, and pupils responding to accommodation but poorly to light are signs of pineal lesion (Parinaud or dorsal midbrain syndrome).
- Signs of neurocutaneous disease (e.g., café au lait spots, Lisch nodules) may indicate a syndrome such as neurofibromatosis type 1.

DIAGNOSTIC TESTS & INTERPRETATION
Imaging
- MRI with and without gadolinium enhancement is the "gold standard" for identification, localization, and characterization of tumors.
- CT can be used as an initial study, but if negative and a high index of suspicion, follow with MRI. Useful to evaluate for hydrocephalus and hemorrhage

Diagnostic Procedures/Other
Staging of tumor
- Postoperative head MRI within 24–48 hours to determine residual disease before postoperative inflammatory changes are prominent
- Spine MRI and CSF cytology required for neuraxis staging of tumors with high risk of leptomeningeal dissemination
- Elevated α-fetoprotein and quantitative β-human chorionic gonadotropin in CSF and serum are markers for germ cell tumors.

DIFFERENTIAL DIAGNOSIS
- Infection: cerebral abscess
- Tumors: metastatic tumor to brain, uncommon with childhood cancers
- Trauma: hemorrhage unlikely to be confused with tumor
- Congenital
  - Arteriovenous malformation
  - Hamartoma
  - Dysplastic brain
- Psychosocial: Some patients with nausea, vomiting, or behavior changes are first diagnosed with psychiatric disorders, GI disorders, failure to thrive, or anorexia nervosa prior to discovery of a brain tumor.

ALERT
New onset of psychoses should prompt imaging to rule out tumor.

TREATMENT

SURGERY/OTHER PROCEDURES

- Both for histology and to attempt maximal tumor debulking; should be performed by experienced pediatric neurosurgeon
- Rarely indicated in intrinsic pontine (brainstem) glioma; although biopsy for molecular profiling increasingly in use
- Ventriculoperitoneal shunt or endoscopic 3rd ventriculostomy when needed for obstructive hydrocephalus (risk of peritoneal seeding minimal)

ALERT
Patient should be referred to a pediatric brain tumor/oncology center at diagnosis (preoperatively).

Radiotherapy

- Volume and dose vary depending on histology.
- Radiation therapy to the tumor bed is used for most patients with brain tumors.
- Medulloblastoma/primitive neuroectodermal tumor patients need craniospinal radiation therapy. The one exception is infants and young children (<3 years of age) in whom cognitive deficits from radiation therapy are devastating.
- Duration of radiation therapy: usually 6 weeks
- Newer approaches to limit exposure of normal brain include intensity-modulated and proton radiotherapy.

MEDICATION

- Dexamethasone to control increased intracranial pressure (0.5 mg/kg/24 h IV/PO divided q6h)
- Chemotherapy
  - Drugs are most often used in combination:
    - Carboplatin, vincristine, or 6-thioguanine, procarbazine, CCNU, vincristine for low-grade glioma
    - Cisplatin, CCNU, vincristine, etoposide, and cyclophosphamide are active agents for primitive neuroectodermal tumor/medulloblastoma.
    - Temozolomide for high-grade glioma
  - New protocols currently being evaluated:
    - High-dose chemotherapy with autologous stem cell rescue for high-risk primitive neuroectodermal tumor/medulloblastoma
    - Targeted therapies, angiogenesis inhibitors
  - Duration of chemotherapy: 6 months to 2 years

ALERT
Possible conflict with other treatments: Chemotherapy can alter anticonvulsant levels.

ONGOING CARE

- Neurologic deficits can take months to improve or stabilize with permanent deficit.
- Any worsening or relapse of symptoms must be evaluated for tumor recurrence.
- MRI every 3 months the 1st year, every 6 months for the next 2 years, and annually thereafter. Benefit of routine surveillance imaging is controversial.

PROGNOSIS

- Dependent on histology of tumor, location, and extent of initial resection
- Glioma
  - Low-grade: ≥90% 5-year progression-free survival (PFS) following gross total resection; 45–65% for subtotal resection
  - High-grade: median survival 8–31 months; depends on grade and extent of resection
  - Intrinsic pontine: median overall survival of 9–13 months from diagnosis
- Medulloblastoma
  - 79–83% PFS at 5 years if localized, gross total resection achieved, and >3 years old at diagnosis
  - <50% PFS if disseminated
- Ependymoma
  - 50–70% survival at 5 years with total resection
  - <30% survival with subtotal resection
- Infants overall have a worse prognosis, possibly due to the limitations of therapy and/or the aggressiveness of the tumor.

ALERT
Even benign tumors may be life threatening if their location precludes resection.

COMPLICATIONS

- Secondary to disease
  - Increased intracranial pressure
    - Obstruction of CSF flow
    - Requires immediate neurosurgical evaluation
- Secondary to radiotherapy
  - Neurocognitive sequelae (age- and dose-related)
  - Endocrinopathy (growth hormone deficiency, hypothyroidism, gonadal dysfunction)
  - Risk of second malignancies (meningioma, glioma, sarcoma)
  - Increased risk of stroke
- Secondary to chemotherapy
  - Risks associated with bone marrow suppression (infection, bleeding, anemia)
  - Hearing loss
  - Risk of secondary leukemia

ADDITIONAL READING

- Abdullah S, Qaddoumi I, Bouffet E. Advances in the management of pediatric central nervous system tumors. *Ann N Y Acad Sci*. 2008;1138:22–31.
- Blaney SM, Haas-Kogan D, Poussaint TY, et al. Gliomas, ependymomas, and other nonembryonal tumors. In: Pizzo PA, Poplack DG, eds. *Principles and Practice of Pediatric Oncology*. 6th ed. Philadelphia: Lippincott Williams & Wilkins; 2010:717–824.
- Ostrom QT, Gittleman H, Liao P, et al. CBTRUS statistical report: primary brain and central nervous system tumors diagnosed in the United States in 2007–2011. *Neuro Oncol*. 2014;16(Suppl 4):iv1–iv63.
- Packer RJ. Brain tumors in children. *Arch Neurol*. 1999;56(4):421–425.
- Phillips PC, Grotzer MA. Brain tumors in children. In: Asbury AK, McKhann GM, McDonald WI, et al, eds. *Diseases of the Nervous System: Clinical Neuroscience and Therapeutic Principles*. 3rd ed. Cambridge, United Kingdom: Cambridge University Press; 2002:1448–1461.
- Sievert AJ, Fisher MJ. Pediatric low-grade gliomas. *J Child Neurol*. 2009;24(11):1397–1408.

CODES

ICD10

- D49.6 Neoplasm of unspecified behavior of brain
- C71.9 Malignant neoplasm of brain, unspecified
- D33.2 Benign neoplasm of brain, unspecified

FAQ

- Q: Are my other children at risk for getting a brain tumor?
- A: No (except in rare cases of certain familial syndromes).
- Q: Did something I do caused this?
- A: No. In addition, the claims made about high-power lines and cellular phones causing brain tumors or cancer are unproven.

BRANCHIAL CLEFT MALFORMATIONS

Anita Bhandari • Raezelle Zinman

BASICS

DESCRIPTION
- Phylogenetically, the branchial apparatus represents the "gills" seen in fish and amphibians.
- The fetal branchial apparatus is a foregut derivative and develops in the 2nd fetal week.
- Five paired pharyngeal arches are separated by four endodermal pouches internally and four ectodermal clefts externally.
- Overgrowth of the second through fourth cleft creates the cervical sinus and occurs during weeks 4 and 5.
- Persistence of the cervical sinus produces a spectrum of cysts, sinus tracts, and fistulae.
- Classification
  - First branchial cleft anomalies
    - Site: anywhere from external auditory canal to angle of mandible, usually superior to or within parotid
    - Fistula tract: external auditory canal
  - Second branchial cleft anomalies
    - Site: ventral to anterior border of sternocleidomastoid muscle, lateral to carotid sheath, and dorsal to submandibular gland
    - Fistula tract: palatine tonsil
  - Third branchial cleft anomalies
    - Site: posterior triangle in middle to lower left side of the neck near level of upper thyroid lobe
    - Fistula: upper lateral piriform sinus wall to lower lateral neck posterior to sternocleidomastoid muscle
  - Fourth branchial cleft anomalies
    - Site: close association to thyroid gland associated with clinical thyroiditis if cyst infected
    - Fistula: apex of piriform sinus to base of neck anterior to sternocleidomastoid muscle

EPIDEMIOLOGY
- Overwhelming majority of cysts in newborns and infants are developmental, whereas in children and adults, they are inflammatory or neoplastic.
- Branchial cleft cysts are the most common congenital neck lesion. Although congenital, usually present in older children and adults.
- Branchial fistula and sinuses are common in children but cysts are more commonly seen in adults.
- Midline malformations are most often thyroglossal duct cysts or dermoids.
- Cysts occurring in the laterocervical region are usually branchial cleft malformations; the most common of these are derivatives of the second cleft, followed by those of the first cleft, of the fourth pouch and thymic cysts.
- Third and fourth branchial cleft anomalies are rare, with most presenting as sinus tracts rather than cysts.
- Suspect congenital anomaly in the clinical setting of recurrent infection.

RISK FACTORS
Genetics
Familial history of branchial defects occasionally noted

DIAGNOSIS

HISTORY
- Present since birth
- Recurrent neck infections
- Intermittent discharge from neck
- Fever
- Tenderness

PHYSICAL EXAM
- Mass usually mobile
- Usually a single lesion
- Nonpulsatile
- Lesion usually nontender (unless actively infected)
- Assess for sites of drainage:
  - At the anterior or posterior border of the sternocleidomastoid muscle
  - In the posterior pharynx at the tonsillar fossa or piriform sinus

DIAGNOSTIC TESTS & INTERPRETATION
Lab
- Complete blood count with differential: Increased white blood cell count with left shift seen with infection.
- Tuberculin test and interferon-gamma release assays to rule out mycobacterial infection, including atypical mycobacteria
- Microbiology: Oral cavity flora in neck abscess is suspicious for a branchial pouch anomaly.

Imaging
- Chest radiography to assess for hilar adenopathy, suggesting a systemic process (such as tuberculosis or malignancy)
- Lateral neck radiography to assess for airway compromise (not usually seen)
- Ultrasound to help differentiate solid masses from cystic masses
- Fistulogram to inject contrast into the fistula to delineate its course
- Computed tomography (CT) scan of neck for superior spatial delineation and definition of anatomic compartment of the lesion
- Magnetic resonance imaging (MRI) for more detailed soft tissue characterization and recognition of solid components within cystic masses
- CT scans and MRI may be used for preoperative planning in patients with recurrent neck masses or clinically complex cases

DIFFERENTIAL DIAGNOSIS
- Congenital
  - Anterior triangle of neck
  - Thymic cyst
  - Midline and anterior triangle of neck
    - Ranula
    - Laryngocele
    - Sialocele
    - Thyroglossal cyst
    - Dermoid/teratomatous cyst
    - Bronchogenic cyst
  - Posterior triangle of neck
    - Lymphangioma
    - Hemangioma

- Inflammatory
  - Adenitis
  - Granulomatous disease (sarcoidosis, tuberculosis)
  - Lymphoepithelial cysts (HIV)
  - Otorrhea
  - Parotiditis
  - Retropharyngeal abscess
  - Thyroiditis
- Tumors
  - Lymphoma
  - Rhabdomyosarcoma
  - Cystic schwannoma (anterior triangle of neck)
  - Pilomatrixoma

TREATMENT

MEDICATION
Antibiotics are indicated if the lesion is infected.

SURGERY/OTHER PROCEDURES
- Excision of the entire lesion is the standard approach.
- Novel endoscopic and marsupialization approaches have been reported.
- Surgery should be delayed if infection is present.

ONGOING CARE

FOLLOW-UP RECOMMENDATIONS
- Postoperative follow-up as outpatient for wound inspection
- Observation for recurrence or reinfection

ALERT
- Lesion may recur if not completely excised.
- High incidence of reinfection if not properly treated.

PROGNOSIS
If lesion completely excised: excellent. Many patients require multiple procedures.

COMPLICATIONS
- Cysts, sinus tracts, and fistulas can become recurrently infected (especially with abscess formation).
- Surgery is more difficult if there has been previous infections or previous surgery.
- Damage to facial, hypoglossal, and glossopharyngeal nerves, internal jugular vein, or carotid artery can occur during surgical repair.
- Cyst, fistula, or sinus recurrence
- Thyroiditis
- Parotiditis (more common in first branchial arch malformation)

ADDITIONAL READING

- Acierno SP, Waldhausen JH. Congenital cervical cysts, sinuses and fistulae. *Otolaryngol Clin North Am*. 2007;40(1):161–176.
- Geddes G, Butterly MM, Patel SM, et al. Pediatric neck masses. *Pediatr Rev*. 2013;34(3):115–124.
- Goins MR, Beasley MS. Pediatric neck masses. *Oral Maxillofac Surg Clin North Am*. 2012;24(3):457–468.
- Graham A. Development of the pharyngeal arches. *Am J Mes Genet A*. 2003;119A(3):251–256.
- Mandell DL. Head and neck anomalies related to the branchial apparatus. *Otolaryngol Clin North Am*. 2000;33(6):1309–1332.
- Nicollas R, Guelfucci B, Roman S, et al. Congenital cysts and fistulas of the neck. *Int J Pediatr Otorhinolaryngol*. 2000;55(2):117–124.
- Nicoucar K, Giger R, Jaecklin T, et al. Management of congenital fourth branchial arch anomalies: a review and analysis of published cases. *J Pediatr Surg*. 2009;44(7):1432–1439.
- Nicoucar K, Giger R, Jaecklin T, et al. Management of congenital third branchial arch anomalies: a systematic review. *Otolaryngol Head Neck Surg*. 2010;142(1):21–28.
- Pahlavan S, Haque W, Pereira K, et al. Microbiology of third and fourth branchial pouch cysts. *Laryngoscope*. 2010;120:458–462.
- Prabhu V, Ingrams D. First branchial arch fistula: diagnostic dilemma and improvised surgical management. *Am J Otolaryngol*. 2011;32(6):617–619.

CODES

ICD10
- Q18.2 Other branchial cleft malformations
- Q18.0 Sinus, fistula and cyst of branchial cleft

FAQ
- Q: Can the cyst, fistula, or sinus recur?
- A: Only a 3% recurrence rate is seen if the lesion is completely excised. A higher rate of recurrence is seen in cases of incomplete excision or with previous surgeries.
- Q: Should the lesion be removed as soon as it is discovered?
- A: The lesion should not be removed if there is an active infection present; treat the infection first and then schedule elective surgery.
- Q: What is the likelihood that a pediatric neck mass is malignant?
- A: Most neck masses in childhood are either developmental or inflammatory but up to 15% may be neoplastic.

BREAST ABSCESS

Charles A. Pohl

BASICS

DESCRIPTION
- Breast abscess: infection of the breast bud or tissue associated with localized pus and inflammation
- Mastitis: infection of the breast tissue observed primarily during lactation

EPIDEMIOLOGY
- 5–11% of women with breastfeeding mastitis develop a breast abscess.
- Affects primarily infants (peak age 1–6 weeks) and adolescents
- Bilateral abscesses, seen among neonates, are rare.
- Male-to-female ratio is 1:2 in neonates.

RISK FACTORS
- In lactating teens, primiparity
- Gestational age >40 weeks
- Mastitis
- Obesity, black race, tobacco use

GENERAL PREVENTION
- Avoid breast manipulation (including piercing).
- In lactating teens, establish good breastfeeding techniques.
- Recognize and treat mastitis early.

PATHOPHYSIOLOGY
- Newborns
  - Trauma, breast hypertrophy from maternal estrogen, or compromised host defenses enable spread of bacteria that often colonize the nasopharynx and umbilicus.
  - The bacteria and/or its toxin, in turn, cause(s) subcutaneous destruction and loculated pus formation.
- Adolescents/adults: Trauma (e.g., sexual manipulation, nipple rings, tight-fitting bras, incorrect latching during breastfeeding), contiguous spread of a local infection (e.g., mastitis, acne), or underlying structural abnormalities (e.g., mammary duct ectasia, epidermal cysts) cause breast tissue edema and destruction by bacteria and/or its toxin.
- When mastitis is associated with breastfeeding, the inflammation inhibits milk release. The stasis of milk, in turn, may allow for bacterial proliferation.

ETIOLOGY
- Newborn infection: *Staphylococcus aureus* (most common), group A or B *Streptococcus*, *Bacteroides* species, and gram-negative enteric bacteria, including *Escherichia coli*, *Pseudomonas aeruginosa*, *Proteus mirabilis*, *Salmonella* species
- Adolescent/adult infection: *S. aureus* (most common) with up to 19% being methicillin-resistant, *E. coli*, *P. aeruginosa*, *Mycobacterium tuberculosis*, *Neisseria gonorrhoeae*, and *Treponema pallidum* are infrequent pathogens.

DIAGNOSIS

HISTORY
- Ask about history of breast trauma or manipulation, concomitant illness or infections, and patient's immunologic status.
- Constitutional symptoms including irritability and lethargy usually are absent unless the infection involves deeper tissue or the bloodstream (1/3 of cases).
- Low-grade fever
- *Salmonella* infections generally present with GI symptoms.

PHYSICAL EXAM
- Firm, tender breast mass with overlying erythema and warmth. Fluctuant mass may be present.
- Regional adenopathy
- Purulent nipple discharge (rare)
- Necrotizing fasciitis is distinguished from breast abscess by pain out of proportion to the cutaneous signs, crepitus, or presence of straw-colored bullae.

DIAGNOSTIC TESTS & INTERPRETATION

Lab
- Gram stain and culture of nipple discharge, needle aspirate, and/or surgical incision and drainage help(s) guide therapeutic decisions if a fluctuant mass or discharge is present.
- Blood culture
  - Useful in neonates
  - Consider full sepsis workup if patient is febrile and toxic-appearing, or < 28 days old.
- CBC: Leukocytosis (>15,000 cells/mm^3) is present in 1/2–2/3 of patients.
- Surveillance cultures of nasopharynx and umbilicus should be considered in neonates to rule out colonization with *S. aureus*.

Imaging
Ultrasound may be useful if fluctuant mass is suspected or if poor response to antimicrobial therapy.

Diagnostic Procedures/Other
If fluctuant, needle biopsy may be diagnostic and therapeutic.

DIFFERENTIAL DIAGNOSIS
- Physiologic conditions:
  - Breast engorgement (usually bilateral; absence of fever, erythema and tenderness)
  - Mastodynia (painful breast engorgement; associated with ovulatory cycles; cyclic pattern)
- Infectious: cellulitis including mastitis (absence of a loculated breast mass)
- Tumors (rare):
  - Fibroadenomas
  - Rhabdomyosarcoma
  - Non-Hodgkin lymphoma
  - Fibrocystic disease
  - Intraductal papilloma
  - Cystosarcoma phyllodes
  - Hemangioma
- Trauma:
  - Contusion (firm, tender, poorly defined mass)
  - Hematoma (sharply defined mass with ecchymosis)
  - Fat necrosis (firm, nontender, circumscribed, mobile mass)
- Miscellaneous: Mondor disease (thrombophlebitis of the subcutaneous veins in the breast)
  - Typically seen in adults
  - Presents with tenderness and pain
  - Associated with trauma
  - Spontaneously resolves
- Vascular malformation

ALERT
- Neonatal infections require prompt recognition, intervention, and identification of other involved sites to avoid widespread infection and poor outcome.
- Unrecognized fluctuant mass and its subsequent drainage will delay therapeutic response.
- Incidence of community-acquired methicillin-resistant *Staphylococcus aureus* (CA-MRSA) is increasing in many regions of the country.

TREATMENT

MEDICATION

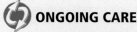

- Neonatal infection (specific dosage interval based on degree of prematurity)
  - Parenteral β-lactamase–resistant antistaphylococcal antibiotics (e.g., nafcillin 75–100 mg/kg/24 h) or cefotaxime 100–200 mg/kg/24 h)
  - Aminoglycosides (e.g., gentamicin) should be included if the infant appears ill or if the Gram stain reveals gram-negative bacilli.
  - Consider vancomycin (40 mg/kg/24 h) if MRSA suspected in neonate older than 1 month of age.
- Adolescent infection
  - Parenteral antistaphylococcal antibiotics (e.g., nafcillin 50–100 mg/kg/24 h; maximum 12 g/24 h)
  - Consider amoxicillin-clavulanic acid orally (45 mg/kg/24 h or 875 mg b.i.d.) or clindamycin (450–1,800 mg/24 h orally with max dose 1.8 g/24 h; 1,200–1,800 mg/24 h parenterally with max dose 4.8 g/24 h) in patients with penicillin allergies and those who are well-appearing and without systemic symptoms.
  - Consider adding aminoglycosides in situations as described earlier.
  - Consider vancomycin, clindamycin, or trimethoprim-sulfamethoxazole if MRSA suspected.
- Duration
  - Usually for 10–14 days
  - Length of parenteral treatment is based on isolate and the clinical response. Oral agents may be used after a few days if a good clinical response occurs.

ADDITIONAL TREATMENT

General Measures

- Warm compresses
- Nonsteroidal anti-inflammatory agents (NSAIDs) help control the inflammation and pain in older children.
- Continuation of breast milk expression helps prevent engorgement and further milk stasis.

ISSUES FOR REFERRAL

Consider referral to an infectious disease specialist if recurrent.

SURGERY/OTHER PROCEDURES

- Incision and drainage if a fluctuant mass is present
- Surgical exploration is necessary if necrotizing fasciitis is suspected.

INPATIENT CONSIDERATIONS

Admission Criteria

- Ill appearance
- Neonates
- Inability to tolerate oral medications
- Concern for medication nonadherence

ONGOING CARE

FOLLOW-UP RECOMMENDATIONS

Clinical improvement should be evident after 48 hours of parenteral antibiotics.

ALERT

Signs to watch for are the following:

- A poor or delayed clinical response to antibiotic therapy suggests a resistant organism, an unusual pathogen, or a different diagnosis.
- An evolving fluctuant mass warrants surgical intervention.
- Reaccumulation of fluctuant mass
- Toxic appearance, prolonged fever, purulent discharge, or progressive erythema postoperatively
- Crepitus associated with excessive pain and/or straw-colored bullae suggests necrotizing fasciitis.

PATIENT EDUCATION

- Continue breastfeeding.
- Establish good breastfeeding techniques.

PROGNOSIS

- Most children recover without any sequelae.
- Neonates are more likely to have bilateral abscesses (<5% cases).
- Neonates have higher morbidity and complications.

COMPLICATIONS

- Cellulitis (most common; 5–10%)
- Abscess rupture with disseminated infection (e.g., bacteremia, pneumonia)
- Septicemia
- Toxin syndromes (e.g., toxic shock syndrome)
- Necrotizing fasciitis
- Scar formation from mammary gland destruction (associated with a reduced breast size after puberty)
- Mammary duct fistula

ADDITIONAL READING

- Barbosa-Cesnik C, Schwartz K, Foxman B. Lactation mastitis. *JAMA*. 2003;289(13):1609–1612.
- Bharat A, Gao F, Aft RL, et al. Predictors of primary breast abscesses and recurrence. *World J Surg*. 2009;33(12):2582–2586.
- Fortunov RM, Hulten KG, Hammerman WA, et al. Community-acquired *Staphylococcus aureus* infections in term and near-term previously healthy neonates. *Pediatrics*. 2006;118(3):874–881.
- Moazzez A, Kelso RL, Towfigh S, et al. Breast abscess bacteriologic features in the era of community-acquired methicillin-resistant *Staphylococcus aureus* epidemics. *Arch Surg*. 2007;142(9):881–884.
- Strickler T, Navratil F, Foster I, et al. Nonpuerperal mastitis in adolescents. *J Ped*. 2006;148(2):278–281.
- Stricker T, Navratil F, Sennhauser FH. Mastitis in early infancy. *Acta Paediatr*. 2005;94(2):166–169.

CODES

ICD10

- N61 Inflammatory disorders of breast
- P39.0 Neonatal infective mastitis
- O91.219 Nonpurulent mastitis associated w pregnancy, unsp trimester

FAQ

- Q: How can you differentiate a breast abscess from mastitis?
- A: Although both illnesses involve signs of inflammation (i.e., warmth, erythema, swelling, tenderness), a breast abscess is distinguished from mastitis in that the former presents as a firm, well-defined mass (with or without fluctuant material).
- Q: Should a mother discontinue breastfeeding if she has a breast abscess?
- A: To avoid milk stasis, breastfeeding should be continued unless impeded by a surgical incision site or the overall clinical condition of the mother.
- Q: What is the role of homeopathic remedies (e.g., belladonna, *Phytolacca*) in the treatment of mastitis and breast abscess?
- A: Currently, there is insufficient scientific evidence to support their routine use.
- Q: Are anaerobic organisms common pathogens for breast abscesses?
- A: No. Although anaerobic pathogens are isolated in up to 40% of infections, their role is controversial, and therapy directed at them is unnecessary.

BREAST MILK AND BREASTFEEDING JAUNDICE

Jennifer A. F. Tender • Sahira Long

BASICS

DESCRIPTION

The 3 major categories of unconjugated hyperbilirubinemia associated with breastfeeding:

- Physiologic jaundice: occurs between 1 and 7 days of life and peaks at 3–5 days.
- Breastfeeding jaundice (BFJ): exaggerated physiologic jaundice associated with inadequate milk intake.
- Breast milk jaundice (BMJ): occurs between 1 and 12 weeks in thriving breast milk–fed infant.

EPIDEMIOLOGY

Prevalence

- Physiologic jaundice: 40–60% of infants
- BFJ: 10% of breastfed infants
- BMJ: 0.5–2% of breastfed infants

RISK FACTORS

- Jaundice in first 24 hours (pathologic)
- Predischarge elevated total serum bilirubin
- Blood type incompatibility
- Glucose-6-phosphate dehydrogenase (G6PD) deficiency
- Gestational age <36 weeks
- Previous sibling receiving phototherapy
- Cephalohematoma or significant bruising
- Exclusive breastfeeding
- Eastern Asian race

PATHOPHYSIOLOGY

- Normal physiology: Bilirubin is a breakdown product of hemoglobin. Unconjugated bilirubin is bound to albumin, transported to the liver, and conjugated by the hepatic enzyme uridine diphosphate glucuronosyl transferase (UGT1A1). Conjugated bilirubin is transported into the small intestines via the bile ducts, where it is modified and excreted in stool. If stooling is delayed, bilirubin is deconjugated by intestinal enzymes and returned to the liver via the portal circulation (enterohepatic circulation).
- Physiologic jaundice: bilirubin levels are elevated in newborns due to several factors:
  - Increased hematocrit and red blood cell volume
  - Increased red blood cell lysis due to shorter red blood cell lifespan.
  - Impaired bilirubin excretion because of an immature hepatic UGT1A1 enzyme and increased enterohepatic circulation.
- BFJ: Lack of effective breastfeeding causes inadequate milk and calorie intake and results in decreased stooling and increased enterohepatic circulation. Infants may also be dehydrated.
- BMJ: Mechanism unclear. Hypotheses include factors found in the milk that may inhibit hepatic UGT1A1. BMJ is associated with East Asian infants who are more likely to have a UGT1A1 mutation and weight loss.

DIAGNOSIS

HISTORY

- BFJ
  - Weight loss: Infants should not lose more than 8% of their birth weight. Infants should gain 15–30 g/day after maternal copious milk production (around day 4 or 5).
  - Frequency and duration of breastfeeding: Breastfed infants should suckle at least 8–12 times/24 hours.
  - Pain with breastfeeding may indicate poor latch and therefore decreased milk transfer.
  - Urination/24 hours: urinates 1 time for each day of life until copious milk production (around 4–5 days) then at least 6 urine/24 hours
  - Stooling: changed from meconium to transitional to yellow seedy by 4–5 days of life. Has at least 3–4 yellow stools/24 hours.
  - Maternal causes of decreased milk production: prior breast surgery, hypothyroidism, retained placenta, insufficient glandular tissue, few medications, obesity, and infertility
- BMJ
  - Infants should be in good health, gaining at least 15–30 g/day and nursing well.
  - Family history of neonatal jaundice? May indicate a genetic propensity for developing jaundice.
  - Screen for risk factors associated with pathologic jaundice:
    - Jaundice in the first 24 hours of life
    - Direct hyperbilirubinemia
    - Maternal blood type to screen for Rh or ABO incompatibility
    - Inherited hemolytic diseases (hereditary spherocytosis). Ask about family history of severe neonatal jaundice, anemia, or splenectomy.
    - Infection: maternal group B strep infection, maternal chorioamnionitis or intrapartum fever, prolonged rupture of membranes, infant fever ≥100.4°F rectally, decreased infant feeding, increased infant sleepiness or fussiness

PHYSICAL EXAM

- Infant
  - General: thin, not thriving infant in first week associated with BFJ. Well appearing, thriving older infant associated with BMJ. An ill-appearing, grunting, tachypneic, sleepy, or fussy infant not interested in nursing should be evaluated for infection. Sleepy infants may be or become dehydrated.
  - Mucous membranes: dry mucous membranes associated with dehydration
  - Skin: Jaundice (and bilirubin levels) generally progress from head to toe but bilirubin levels estimated visually may be inaccurate. Infants with dark skin tones are especially difficult to assess.
  - Cephalohematomas and bruising are associated with increased red blood cell breakdown.
  - Abdomen: Hepatosplenomegaly is associated with metabolic or hemolytic process or biliary obstruction. Abdominal distension may be a result of intestinal obstruction.
- Direct observation of a feeding is crucial:
  - Lips should be everted and mouth wide open approaching a 180-degree angle. As much of the areola as possible should be in the infant's mouth. The infant should have deep movement of the jaw and suck/swallow/breathe rhythmically with milk visible in infant's mouth.

DIAGNOSTIC TESTS & INTERPRETATION

Lab

- All mothers should be screened for blood and Rh type. Infants of mothers with blood type O or Rh negative need their cord blood tested for blood type and Coombs to identify risk for hemolytic anemia. These infants are at greater risk for kernicterus and need to be treated at lower total serum bilirubin levels.
- Infants should have a pre-discharge either total serum bilirubin or transcutaneous bilirubin level.
  - Bilirubin levels are interpreted based on age in hours/days and risk factors (blood incompatibility, preterm, illness). Use of a nomogram tool (such as www.bilitool.com) stratifies the infants' risk based on the American Academy of Pediatrics (AAP) bilirubin guidelines.
- Generally, minimal laboratory evaluation is needed in a healthy breastfed infant with mild jaundice in the absence of risk factors. However, BFJ and BMJ are diagnoses of exclusion. The following tests should be considered, depending on the clinical presentation:
  - Conjugated/unconjugated (direct/indirect) bilirubin level interpreted based on age and risk factors
    - May guide treatment
    - Must be measured in all infants with very early jaundice <24 hours of age
    - Recommended in all infants with persistent jaundice
  - Conjugated or direct serum bilirubin: Elevated level (>1 mg/dL or 10% of total serum bilirubin) may indicate infection, biliary obstructive disease, cholestasis, metabolic disease, or severe hemolysis.
  - CBC and smear:
    - Look for polycythemia or anemia
    - Smear may assist with diagnosing hemolysis.
    - Decreases in hematocrit over time may reflect ongoing hemorrhage or hemolysis.
    - A mean corpuscular hemoglobin concentration (MCHC) of >36.0 g/dL may suggest hereditary spherocytosis.
    - Abnormal white cell count may indicate infection.

- G6PD quantitative test
  - G6PD deficiency may cause an increase in bilirubin later than other hemolytic disease and has been associated with an increased risk of kernicterus.
  - Electrolytes (especially sodium) in infant, if concern for dehydration.

DIFFERENTIAL DIAGNOSIS

- Increased bilirubin production
  - Hematologic
    - ABO or Rh isoimmunization
    - Erythrocyte enzyme defects (e.g., G6PD deficiency)
    - Erythrocyte membrane defects (e.g., hereditary spherocytosis)
    - Polycythemia
- Impaired bilirubin conjugation
  - Gilbert syndrome
  - Crigler-Najjar syndrome
- Decreased bilirubin excretion
  - Biliary obstruction
  - Biliary atresia
  - Choledochal cyst
  - Dubin-Johnson syndrome
  - Rotor syndrome
- Intestinal obstruction
  - Meconium ileus
  - Hirschsprung disease
- Congenital: transient familial neonatal hyperbilirubinemia
- Metabolic
  - Hypothyroidism
  - Galactosemia
- Miscellaneous
  - Dehydration
  - Sepsis
  - Cephalohematoma
  - Maternal oxytocin use

TREATMENT

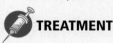

- BFJ
  - Evaluate and treat for insufficient milk intake. Assess latch, position, and milk transfer. Consult a lactation expert if needed.
  - Increase frequency of effective breastfeeding to 8–12 times/24 hours.
  - Supplement with formula, pumped breast milk, or donor breast milk if needed.
  - Phototherapy if serum bilirubin levels exceed the AAP recommended threshold levels for phototherapy for full-term healthy infants based on infant's age in hours, gestational age, and neurotoxicity risk factors
  - Phototherapy may contribute to dehydration; it is essential to monitor hydration status.
  - Consider partial exchange blood transfusion with phototherapy if indicated per the AAP hyperbilirubinemia guidelines.
    - Full-term healthy infants 25–48 hours old with total serum bilirubin $>$19–22 mg/dL and for infants $\geq$48 hours old with total serum bilirubin $>$22–25 mg/dL
    - Consider home phototherapy if bilirubin levels close to threshold. Home phototherapy poses less of an obstruction to breastfeeding.
    - Monitor serum bilirubin levels closely until they are acceptable. Check levels after stopping phototherapy.
- BMJ
  - Monitor clinically after excluding other causes of hyperbilirubinemia.
  - Encourage and support breastfeeding.
  - Consider stopping breastfeeding for 24 hours (with continued pumping to preserve supply) if bilirubin levels $\geq$20 mg/dL. Level should decrease 3 mg/dL in 24 hours.

ONGOING CARE

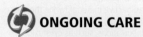

FOLLOW-UP RECOMMENDATIONS

- Follow up 2–3 days after discharge, earlier if infant at high risk for jaundice. Weight check, physical exam, assessment of hydration, and observation of feeding. Bilirubin level if clinically indicated.
- Close follow-up 1–2 days later if concern about milk intake or jaundice
- Patient education: Mother should be assisted with latch and positioning and be taught signs/symptoms of adequate milk intake, dehydration, illness, and jaundice.
- Late preterm/near-term infants need especially close follow-up as they have increased risk of poor milk intake.
- Visual assessment of jaundice may be inaccurate. Consider an objective measure of jaundice (e.g., total serum bilirubin or transcutaneous bilirubin level) for follow-up assessment.

INPATIENT CONSIDERATIONS

If a breastfed infant is hospitalized for jaundice, encourage continued breastfeeding if possible. For infants with BFJ, consult a lactation expert to evaluate cause for insufficient milk intake and provide assistance. The mother may need a hospital grade double electric pump to increase her milk supply.

COMPLICATIONS

- Kernicterus (bilirubin encephalopathy)
  - Acute symptoms: lethargy, hypotonia, opisthotonus, seizures, high-pitched cry
  - Chronic symptoms: hearing loss, upward gaze palsy, cerebral palsy, cognitive impairment
- Unnecessary cessation of breastfeeding
- Parental and health care provider anxiety

ADDITIONAL READING

- Academy of Breastfeeding Medicine. Clinical protocols. Guidelines for management of jaundice in the breastfeeding infant equal to or greater than 35 weeks' gestation. http://www.bfmed.org/Resources/Protocols.aspx. Accessed March 14, 2015.
- American Academy of Pediatrics Subcommittee on Hyperbilirubinemia. Management of hyperbilirubinemia in the newborn infant 35 or more weeks of gestation. *Pediatrics*. 2004;114(4):297–316.
- Christensen RD, Henry E. Hereditary spherocytosis in neonates with hyperbilirubinemia. *Pediatrics*. 2010;125(1):120–125.
- Maisels MJ, Bhutani VK, Bogen D, et al. Hyperbilirubinemia in the newborn infant $>$ or $=$ 35 weeks' gestation: An update with clarifications. *Pediatrics*. 2009;124(4):1193–1198.
- Lauer BJ, Nancy ND. Hyperbilirubinemia in the newborn. *Pediatr Rev*. 2011;32(8):341–349.

CODES

ICD10

- P59.3 Neonatal jaundice from breast milk inhibitor
- P59.8 Neonatal jaundice from other specified causes
- P59.9 Neonatal jaundice, unspecified

FAQ

- Q: Will jaundice cause my baby to have developmental or neurologic problems?
- A: If hyperbilirubinemia is appropriately monitored and treated, it should not cause any developmental problems.
- Q: What can be done to prevent BFJ?
- A: Early, frequent, and effective breastfeeding at least 8–12 times in 24 hours can decrease the risk of BFJ. Do not supplement unless recommended by a health care provider. Get help from a breastfeeding expert if you have pain or the infant is not latching on or nursing well.
- Q: Should I stop breastfeeding if my baby is jaundiced?
- A: The frequency and effectiveness of breastfeeding should be increased and appropriate lactation consultation obtained for BFJ. For BMJ, temporary cessation of breastfeeding will lower total serum bilirubin; however, this recommendation should only be considered (along with formula supplementation and phototherapy) if total serum bilirubin is $\geq$20 mg/dL.

BREASTFEEDING

Jennifer A. F. Tender • Sahira Long

BASICS

DESCRIPTION

Breast milk is recognized as the optimal nutrition for infants by the American Academy of Pediatrics (AAP), the World Health Organization (WHO), the Surgeon General, and all major medical groups.

PHYSIOLOGY

- Breast milk production
  - Lactogenesis I: Milk production begins around 16 weeks prenatally.
  - Lactogenesis II: onset of copious milk secretion around 2–3 days after vaginal delivery. Under hormonal control initiated by the expulsion of placenta and decrease in progesterone levels
  - Lactogenesis III: Mature milk production (maintenance) depends on autocrine (local) control. The amount of milk removed influences milk volume. If milk is not removed, a protein (feedback inhibitor of lactation) accumulates and inhibits prolactin release.
  - Prolactin is released from the anterior pituitary in response to nipple stimulation and triggers milk secretion into the lumen of breast alveoli.
  - Oxytocin is released from the posterior pituitary gland, causing ejection of milk into the breast ducts (milk ejection reflex).
  - Let-down can be triggered by physical stimulation of the breast or by mental stimulation such as hearing a baby cry.
- Composition
  - Largely independent of maternal diet, except for fatty acids and water-soluble vitamins
  - Colostrum contains high levels of secretory immunoglobulin A for immune protection. Lactoferrin stimulates meconium passage and promotes colonization with protective lactobacillus bifidus.
  - High whey-to-casein ratio
  - Milk changes within a feed and throughout the day. Hindmilk and milk at night contains higher fat and calories.
- Risks of *not* breastfeeding:
  - For child: increases risk of postneonatal death; gastroenteritis, necrotizing enterocolitis for preterm infants, lower respiratory infections, acute otitis media, bacterial meningitis, obesity, sudden infant death syndrome (SIDS), asthma, leukemia, and type II diabetes
  - For mother: increases risk of ovarian and breast cancer, cardiovascular disease, and postpartum hemorrhage. Loss of benefit of lactational amenorrhea and child spacing
  - For family: increased expenditures, more workdays lost to care for ill child
  - For society: increases environmental impact and costs at least $13 billion annually related to an increase in childhood diseases

EPIDEMIOLOGY

Prevalence

- 79% of infants in the United States initiate breastfeeding, according to 2013 data from the Centers for Disease Control and Prevention.
- At 3 months, 41% breastfed exclusively.
- At 6 months, 49% breastfed, 16% exclusively
- At 12 months, 27% breastfed.
- Racial and economic disparities in breastfeeding exist; lower rates among African American women and women living in poverty

RISK FACTORS

- Contraindications to breastfeeding:
  - Infant with classic galactosemia
  - Maternal conditions:
    - HIV (in industrialized countries)
    - Illicit drug use
    - Active, untreated tuberculosis
    - Herpes simplex virus lesions on breast
    - HTLV-I– or HTLV-II–positive
    - Exposure to radioactive material, while there is radioactivity in the milk
    - Use of some medications, such as cytotoxic drugs
- Infant conditions that may interfere with breastfeeding:
  - Prematurity
  - Low birth weight
  - Hypotonia
  - Cleft lip or palate
  - Ankyloglossia (tongue-tie)
- Maternal conditions that may interfere with breastfeeding:
  - History of breast surgery
  - Abnormal breast shape (glandular insufficiency)
  - Inverted nipples
  - Medications that inhibit lactation
  - Endocrine: infertility, hypothyroidism, polycystic ovary, retained placenta, Sheehan syndrome, obesity
- Common reasons cited for early termination of breastfeeding:
  - Perceived insufficient milk supply
  - Poor latch
  - Sore nipples
  - Returning to work or school

DIAGNOSIS

HISTORY

- Experience breastfeeding previous children
- Prior breast surgery
- Breast enlargement during pregnancy
- Frequency and duration of feedings
  - Feed >8–12 times a day in the 1st few weeks of life, with no more than 4 hours between feedings.
  - Newborns typically need >8–10 minutes of active suckling to "empty" a breast.
- Signs of adequate milk intake:
  - Adequate hydration: 1 wet diaper for each day of life until milk "comes in" around day 4 of life; then ≥6 wet diapers per 24 hours
  - Adequate nutrition: stool changes from meconium to transitional to yellow seedy by 4th day of life. Infant typically has >3–4 yellow stools/24 h in the first month. Stool pattern often changes at 1 month, and infant may only stool every 3–7 days.
- Infant may lose up to 8% of birth weight until milk "comes in" around day 4 or 5.
- Infant should gain 15–30 g/day and be back to birth weight by 10–14 days.
- The WHO growth charts better represent typical growth of breastfed infants.
- Breast/nipple pain: Women may experience discomfort at first, but breastfeeding should not hurt. The most common cause of pain is poor latch. Other causes include candidal infection of the nipple, or mastitis.

PHYSICAL EXAM

- Direct observation of a feeding is crucial:
  - Examine the infant's oropharynx for thrush, ankyloglossia, or anatomic abnormalities.
  - Examine the mother's breasts for scars (prior surgery), nipple inversion, erythema (possible candida), or cracking (poor latch).
  - Infant feeding cues: Rooting, lip smacking, and sucking are early signs of hunger; crying is a late sign.
  - The mother should be positioned comfortably and not have to bend down.
- Two types of infant positioning:
  - Infant-led: The mother is semireclined in bed with the infant's head at breast height. The infant initiates the latch.
  - Mother-led:
    - Cross-cradle: easy visualization of latch. Mother holds her baby with the arm opposite the breast she is using, holds the back of the baby's neck, and brings the baby to breast height. Her other hand supports and compresses her breast. The infant should be in a straight line with ear, shoulder, and hip aligned.
    - Other positions include cradle, football, and sidelying.
- For an effective latch, the mother touches the infant's nose or upper lip to her nipple and waits until the infant opens wide. She brings the infant to her breast. She may compress her breast with her thumb by the infant's nose parallel to upper lip.
- Evaluating the latch: Lips should be everted and mouth wide open approaching a 180 degrees angle. As much as possible of the areola is in the infant's mouth. More of the areola shows above the infant's mouth than below. The mother's nipple should not be distorted after the infant suckles.
- Signs of good milk transfer: Infant relaxed and breasts less full after nursing, infant has deep movement of the jaw and sucks/swallows/breathes rhythmically, milk visible in infant's mouth.

DIAGNOSTIC TESTS & INTERPRETATION

Lab

- Total/direct bilirubin level, if clinically indicated
- Electrolytes (especially sodium) in infant, if there is concern for dehydration

TREATMENT

MEDICATION

- Vitamin D, 400 IU/24 h orally for all infants starting at the first visit if not given at hospital discharge, even if supplementing with formula
- The AAP Section on Breastfeeding recommends starting iron-rich complementary foods at 6 months, whereas the AAP Committee on Nutrition recommends elemental iron, 1 mg/kg/day, from age 4 months until iron-rich food is introduced. Elemental iron at 2 mg/kg/day starting by age 1 month is recommended for preterm infants.
- Thrush or candidal infection of the nipples requires simultaneous treatment of both mother and infant with a topical antifungal agent and thorough washing of all artificial nipples. Treatment options include nystatin or oral fluconazole for resistant cases.
- Most maternal medications are compatible with breastfeeding. Mothers should not breastfeed if using illicit or cytotoxic drugs, or radioactive compounds until cleared from the mother's milk. Choose medications with short half-lives, high protein binding, low oral bioavailability, high molecular weight, and low lipid solubility. Refer to databases such as the National Library of Medicine's LactMed.

ADDITIONAL TREATMENT

General Measures

- Cracked nipples should be treated by correcting the latch. Women can apply breast milk or purified lanolin. Keep nipples dry.
- Engorgement can be relieved by frequent and effective feeding or pumping, breast massaging, and applying cool compresses.
- Clogged milk ducts may be treated with warm compresses, frequent emptying of the breast, massaging the area, and varying feeding positions.
- Pumping may help with inverted nipples. A nipple shield can be tried if inverted nipples cause trouble latching. Prolonged nipple shield use is controversial, as concerns exist regarding their impact on milk supply; thus their use should be limited to a short period of time (~1 month).
- Mastitis can be treated with antibiotics, frequent and effective feeding and maternal rest.
- Infants with ankyloglossia that affects latch or impedes milk transfer should be referred for frenotomy.

COMPLEMENTARY & ALTERNATIVE THERAPIES

- Herbs traditionally used to try to increase milk supply (galactagogues) include the following:
  - Fenugreek (*Trigonella foenum-graecum*): taken as tea or capsules. May be effective; probably safe in moderate doses
  - Milk thistle (*Silybum marianum*): usually taken as a tea; increased milk supply in one study (no available safety data support use)

INPATIENT CONSIDERATIONS

If a breastfed infant is hospitalized, encourage continued breastfeeding if possible. If the infant is not able to breastfeed, provide a hospital-grade double electric pump and encourage pumping at least 8 times/24 h.

FOLLOW-UP RECOMMENDATIONS

Patient Monitoring

- In general, 2–3 days after hospital discharge. Weight check, physical exam, and observation of feeding
- Close follow-up 1–2 days later if concern about milk intake or jaundice then as needed
- At age 2–3 weeks: weight check and breastfeeding support
- Patient education: Mother should be assisted with latch and positioning and should know signs/symptoms of adequate milk intake (urine output, stooling), dehydration, and illness.

DIET

- For the infant:
  - Except for vitamin D, no food or fluid other than breast milk is needed for the first 6 months of life.
  - After 6 months, iron-rich foods and other complementary foods may be introduced.
- For the mother:
  - ~500 kcal/day are used for breastfeeding.
  - Women should avoid breastfeeding for at least 2 hours after alcohol consumption.
  - If infant has G6PD deficiency, mother should avoid fava beans and certain medications.

COMPLICATIONS

- Infant
  - Hyperbilirubinemia
  - Dehydration/hypernatremia
- Mother
  - Engorgement
  - Clogged milk duct
  - Mastitis
  - Candidal nipple infection
  - Cracked nipples

ADDITIONAL READING

- The Academy of Breastfeeding Medicine protocols: http://www.bfmed.org/Resources/Protocols.aspx
- Bartick M, Reinhold A. The burden of suboptimal breastfeeding in the United States: a pediatric cost analysis. *Pediatrics*. 2010;125(5):e1048–e1056.
- Breastfeeding and the use of human milk. *Pediatrics*. 2012;129(3):e827–e841.
- Kramer MS, Kakuma R. Optimal duration of exclusive breastfeeding. Cochrane Database Syst Rev. 2009;(1).
- LactMed, National Institutes of Health: http://toxnet.nlm.nih.gov/cgi-bin/sis/htmlgen?
- La Leche League International: www.lalecheleague.org
- Office on Women's Health, U.S. Department of Health and Human Services: www.womenshealth.gov/breastfeeding
- U.S. Department of Health and Human Services. *The Surgeon General's Call to Action to Support* Breastfeeding. Washington, DC: U.S. Department of Health and Human Services, Office of the Surgeon General; 2011. http://www.surgeongeneral.gov/library/calls/breastfeeding/calltoactiontosupportbreastfeeding.pdf. Accessed March 1, 2015.

CODES

ICD10

- P92.5 Neonatal difficulty in feeding at breast
- Q38.1 Ankyloglossia
- P92.6 Failure to thrive in newborn

FAQ

- Q: How do I know if my baby is getting enough milk?
- A: Look for signs of effective feeding as described earlier. Your baby should suck deeply and rhythmically during a feeding, seem satisfied after a feeding, and gain approximately 15–30 g/day. A baby's elimination pattern may be variable, but, in general, most adequately breastfed infants will have 4 or more stools a day by 4 days of life.
- Q: How do I alleviate breast pain with nursing?
- A: Most pain is due to poor latch. Ensure deep latch. Compress the breast and make sure the baby takes as much of the areola as possible. If stinging occurs throughout nursing, consider candidal infection. Seek advice from a lactation expert if pain does not improve.
- Q: How can I increase my milk supply?
- A: Increase frequency and effectiveness of feeding or pumping. Place infant skin to skin. Pump after nursing sessions. If pumping often, use a hospital-grade double pump. Get plenty of sleep and try to reduce stress.
- Q: How long can expressed breast milk be stored safely (applies to term infants only)?
- A: At room temperature (up to 77°F) for 3–6 hours. In the back of a refrigerator for 3 (ideal)–8 days if very clean container. For 6–12 months if in the freezer. Thawed breast milk should be refrigerated and used within 24 hours of thawing.
- Q: How long should breastfeeding be continued?
- A: The AAP recommends breastfeeding at least until 12 months of age, and as long afterward as is mutually desired. The WHO recommends breastfeeding for at least 2 years. Exclusive breastfeeding is nutritionally adequate for the first 6 months.
- Q: Can adoptive mothers breastfeed?
- A: Induced lactation is possible. Lactation experts should be consulted.

BREATH-HOLDING SPELLS

Nailah Coleman

BASICS

DESCRIPTION

- Breath-holding spells are the general term for emotionally provoked attacks that occur in young children. These attacks can progress from a strong emotion to "breath holding" to decreased sensorium and either limpness or stiffness, which can appear as seizure-like activity.
- Disease essentials
  - Provoked by anger, pain, or frustration
  - Association with altered respiratory effort
  - Results in decreased muscle tone
  - Can be classified as simple (brief, no loss of consciousness) or severe (prolonged, associated loss of consciousness)
- Subtypes
  - Cyanotic (80%)
    - Classic breath-holding spells
    - Typically associated with anger
    - Progress from crying to exhalation to apnea and syncope to decreased muscle tone and falling
    - May also note generalized clonic jerks, opisthotonos, and bradycardia
    - Ages: 6 months to a peak at 2 years, with resolution by 5 years
  - Pallid (20%)
    - Typically associated with pain, frustration, or surprise
    - Progress from quieting to apnea (at the end of expiration) to syncope to decreased muscle tone and falling
    - May also note clenched hands and clonic jerks and bradycardia

EPIDEMIOLOGY

- Incidence: not reported
- Prevalence: 4.6% (severe), up to 27% (simple)
- No gender difference
- 20–35% have a positive family history
- Age/frequency
  - Median age of onset 6–12 months of age
  - Typically ages 1–5 years but can occur up to 7 years of age
  - Usually resolve by school age
  - Frequency
    - Can occur several times per day to only once a year
    - Age of peak frequency of spells is from 1–2 years of age.

RISK FACTORS

- Underlying autonomic regulatory dysfunction
- Inheritance
  - 20–35% of patients with breath-holding spells have a positive family history.
  - 11% of patients with epilepsy or other chronic but nonneurologic disorder have a positive family history of breath-holding spells.
  - For 80% of patients with severe spells and a positive family history, the affected family members are mainly on the maternal side.
  - An autosomal dominant trait with reduced penetrance has been noted in some.

GENERAL PREVENTION

- There are no known methods, medications, or treatments for preventing breath-holding spells.
- Although the term breath-holding spells implies volition, these attacks are involuntary and reflexive.
- For a variety of reasons, emotional outbursts are common in this age group; however, appeasing a child to prevent a spell is not recommended as it may lead the child to develop other, similar-appearing behaviors encouraging parental concession.

PATHOPHYSIOLOGY

- Cyanotic breath-holding spells
  - Syncope due to a Valsalva maneuver increasing the intrathoracic pressure, decreasing cardiac blood return and eventually cardiac output, which causes cerebral hypoperfusion and unconsciousness
- Pallid breath-holding spells
  - Abnormal vagal response to emotional stimulation causing bradycardia and/or asystole, leading to decreased cardiac output and cerebral ischemia and unconsciousness

ETIOLOGY

Always provoked by anger, pain, or frustration

COMMONLY ASSOCIATED CONDITIONS

- No definitive associated conditions
- There have been reports of some children with breath-holding spells going on to have syncope and/or seizures.
- Some studies have noted an increased prevalence of anemia in children with breath-holding spells; the anemia and spells improved over time with iron treatment. Although these findings also coincide with the expected timing for resolution of breath-holding spells, anemia might complicate an individual child's picture.

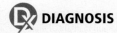

DIAGNOSIS

HISTORY

- Important to elicit history of
  - Provocation by anger, pain, or frustration
  - Altered respiratory effort, decreased responsiveness, and altered muscle tone (either limpness or stiffness)
  - Lack of trauma
  - Not volitional

PHYSICAL EXAM

- Vital signs: normal on exam; perform orthostatic blood pressures
- Focal findings: none, normal cardiac, and neurologic exams

DIFFERENTIAL DIAGNOSIS

- Syncope: not usually preceded by crying; altered muscle tone typically accompanied by efforts to prevent falling
  - Neurocardiogenic (vasovagal syncope, fainting)
    - Associated with bradycardia, vasodepression, and/or hypotension leading to decreased cerebral perfusion
    - More common in adolescents
  - Cardiac
    - Dysrhythmias
      - Prolonged QT syndrome
      - Wolff-Parkinson-White syndrome
      - Complete heart block
    - Structural
      - Hypertrophic cardiomyopathy
      - Severe pulmonary or aortic stenosis
      - Coronary artery aneurysm
      - Anomalous origin of the left coronary artery
      - Pulmonary hypertension
      - Myxoma
  - Orthostatic
  - Neuropsychiatric
    - Panic attacks or hyperventilation syndrome
    - Benign paroxysmal vertigo
    - Cataplexy
    - Hysterical syncope
  - Cough
    - Most common in asthmatics
    - Increased intrapleural pressure from coughing leads to decreased venous return and eventually decreased cardiac output and cerebral perfusion
  - Metabolic: hypoglycemia
- Epilepsy or epilepsy equivalent: altered muscle tone precedes color change; abnormal EEG
- Central or obstructive apnea: not typically associated with crying; abnormal sleep study
- Brainstem pathology such as tumor or malformation: other abnormal findings on history and exam
- Familial dysautonomia: other abnormal findings on history and exam
- Rett syndrome: other abnormal findings on history and exam

DIAGNOSTIC TESTS & INTERPRETATION

Lab

- If anemia is of concern, CBC should be obtained.
- If hypoglycemia is high on differential acutely, plasma glucose should be obtained.

Imaging

- No specific imaging is necessary to diagnosis breath-holding spells. However, if trauma, brain pathology, or abnormal cardiac morphology is suspected, the following imaging could be obtained:
  - Head CT
  - Brain MRI
  - Cardiac echocardiogram (EKG)
  - Cardiac MRI
  - Chest x-ray—evaluate lung hyperinflation in asthmatics (not needed for diagnosis)

Diagnostic Procedures/Other

- For evaluation of potential dysrhythmias, consider the following:
  - EKG
  - Holter monitor
  - Electrophysiology study
  - Stress test
- For evaluation of epilepsy or other neuroelectric disorder, consider an EEG.
- For evaluation of apnea, consider a sleep study.

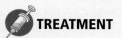

TREATMENT

MEDICATION

- No medication has been found to be definitively useful in preventing or treating breath-holding spells.
- It is important to note that breath-holding spells can occur in the presence of other conditions that can present with syncope and seizure-like activity. Should those conditions be present or suspected, additional treatments may be necessary.
- Multiple studies have evaluated the use of various medications to prevent and/or treat breath-holding spells. However, they are limited by inadequate sample size, power, and/or statistical significance.
  - Iron therapy may be useful in breath-holding spells, particularly in children found to be anemic and/or iron deficient.
  - Atropine and pacemakers have been used for those with severe bradycardia to good effect.
  - Fluoxetine was noted to improve pallid breath-holding spells in another small study.

ADDITIONAL TREATMENT

Reassurance is the primary treatment.

ISSUES FOR REFERRAL

Referral is not necessary unless diagnoses on the differential could not be excluded or if the spells do not conform to the normal pattern and/or the normal age range.

INPATIENT CONSIDERATIONS

- Inpatient hospital admission for breath-holding spells is not necessary as they are a benign condition. However, if other diagnoses are being considered, if the patient required resuscitation, or if the patient requires ongoing support, an inpatient hospital admission and medical evaluation is warranted.
- Should an inpatient admission be warranted, other diagnoses should be considered and evaluated.

ADDITIONAL TREATMENT

- Should loss of consciousness occur with a breath-holding spell, it is important to place the child on his or her side and ensure a clear airway.
- With the potential for altered muscle tone and additional injury, parents should ensure the environment around the child is safe.

ONGOING CARE

PATIENT EDUCATION

The primary goal for ongoing care is parental education as to the natural history of breath-holding spells.

PROGNOSIS

- As they are a benign condition, isolated breath-holding spells have an excellent prognosis without sequelae.
- Breath-holding spells typically resolve by school age.
- Should breath-holding spells not follow the typical course or time frame, additional diagnoses should be considered (could impact the prognosis).

COMPLICATIONS

Although some have postulated the potential for the development of syncope, epilepsy, and neurodevelopmental disorders, no definitive associations have been found.

ADDITIONAL READING

- DiMario FJ Jr. Breath-holding spells in childhood. *Am J Dis Child*.1992;146(1):125–131.
- DiMario FJ Jr. Prospective study in children with cyanotic and pallid breath-holding spells. *Pediatrics*. 2001;107(2):265–269.
- Lombroso CT, Lerman P. Breath-holding spells (cyanotic and pallid infantile syncope). *Pediatrics*. 1967;39(4):563–581.
- Mocan H, Yildiran A, Orhan F, et al. Breath-holding spells in 91 children and response to treatment with iron. *Am J Dis Child*. 1999;81(3):261–261.
- Narchi H. The child who passes out. *Pediatr Rev*. 2000;21(11):384–388.
- Walsh M, Knilans TK, Anderson JB, et al. Successful treatment of pallid breath-holding spells with fluoxetine. *Pediatrics*. 2012;130(3):e685–e689.

CODES

ICD10

R06.89 Other abnormalities of breathing

FAQ

- Q: What is the age range of the typical child with breath-holding spells?
- A: The typical age range of the child with breath-holding spells is 1–5 years of age.
- Q: What is the typical provocation and pathophysiology of the most common type of breath-holding spells?
- A: The most common breath-holding spells are cyanotic (80%). These are typically provoked by anger, which leads to crying, a Valsalva maneuver, decreased cardiac return, decreased cardiac output, decreased cerebral perfusion, and syncope.
- Q: Is there a genetic basis for breath-holding spells?
- A: An autosomal dominant trait has been found in some patients with breath-holding spells.
- Q: What are the common diagnostic tools used to diagnose breath-holding spells?
- A: Breath-holding spells are diagnosed primarily by obtaining a good history and performing a physical exam, the latter of which should be normal. Additional diagnostic tools should only be used if a separate diagnosis is being considered due to unusual history or abnormal physical exam findings.
- Q: How are breath-holding spells managed and prevented?
- A: Breath-holding spells require reassurance provided to the family about acute management and their natural history. At this time, there is no way to prevent breath-holding spells.

BRONCHIOLITIS (SEE ALSO: RESPIRATORY SYNCYTIAL VIRUS)

Alan R. Schroeder

BASICS

DESCRIPTION

Acute infection of the lower respiratory tract in infants and young children leading to mononuclear infiltration of the bronchiolar epithelium, causing edema and mucus plugging of the small airways

EPIDEMIOLOGY

- Peak season is November through April, with some variation by state in the United States (begins earlier in the Southeast).
- Most common cause of infant hospitalization
  - ~150,000 hospitalizations/year in the United States
  - Hospitalization rates tripled from 1980 to 1997 but have decreased over the last decade.
- Most recent estimate ~15 hospitalizations/ 1,000 person-years for children <2 years of age
- Approximately, 1/3 of all children will get bronchiolitis in the first 2 years of life.

ETIOLOGY

- Respiratory syncytial virus (RSV) is the most common causative organism, but other organisms include the following:
  - Human rhinovirus
  - Adenovirus
  - Human metapneumovirus
  - Enterovirus
  - Coronaviruses
  - Influenza viruses
  - Parainfluenza viruses
  - *Mycoplasma pneumoniae*
- Majority of bronchiolitis cases are caused by one virus, but viral coinfections (2 or more viruses) may occur in ~1/4 of cases.

COMMONLY ASSOCIATED CONDITIONS

- Patients at high risk of severe bronchiolitis:
  - Premature infants (<36 weeks' gestation)
  - Young infants (<2–3 months of age)
  - Congenital heart disease
  - Chronic lung disease (including bronchopulmonary dysplasia [BPD])
  - Low birth weight
  - Cystic fibrosis
  - Immunodeficiency
  - Neuromuscular diseases
  - Trisomy 21
- Exposure to cigarette smoke is a risk factor for more severe disease.

DIAGNOSIS

HISTORY

- Generally begins as an upper respiratory infection with rhinorrhea but spreads to lower respiratory tract within 2–3 days
- Often multiple sick contacts in household
- Variable timing of symptoms. The unpredictability of the time course of the disease may be partly explained by viral coinfections.
- Poor feeding and increased insensible water loss may lead to dehydration and decreased urine output.
- Fever in approximately 50% of patients
- Restlessness or lethargy may indicate impending respiratory failure (hypoxemia and/or CO_2 retention).
- Apnea can be sole presenting sign in younger infants.

PHYSICAL EXAM

- General appearance
  - Interactive versus ill-appearing
  - Paroxysmal cough common
- HEENT exam
  - Nasal congestion with copious secretions
  - Otitis media is common.
- Pulmonary exam
  - Pattern of breathing: apnea or periodic breathing
  - Tachypnea: >70/min is associated with severe illness.
  - Grunting, nasal flaring, and accessory muscle use (supracostal, intercostal, subcostal retractions) are signs of more severe disease.
  - Thoracoabdominal asynchrony ("abdominal breathing")
  - Hyperresonance to percussion
  - On auscultation: diffuse, high-pitched heterophonic wheezing; prolonged expiratory phase; inspiratory crackles; diffuse rhonchi
  - Lung exam can change rapidly.
- Other findings:
  - Signs of dehydration
  - Poor peripheral perfusion (delayed capillary refill time, cool extremities, weak peripheral pulses, mottling of skin) is a concerning sign.
  - Liver and spleen often caudally displaced by hyperinflated lungs.

DIAGNOSTIC TESTS & INTERPRETATION

Lab

- The majority of bronchiolitis cases do not warrant any laboratory investigation.
- Blood gas
  - In severe cases, can help determine acid–base status and effectiveness of ventilation; however, decisions to escalate support can generally be based on clinical assessment.
  - Arterial PO_2 generally does not add much information beyond that provided by a pulse oximeter.
- CBC +/− differential: low yield; a bandemia common with RSV
- Serum electrolytes: On occasion, may assist with assessment of hydration (BUN, creatinine), and hyponatremia rarely occurs due to antidiuretic hormone release.
- Viral testing
  - Rarely changes management
  - Some hospitals require it for cohorting, but can be misleading given the broad number of potentially causative viruses and the high frequency of viral coinfections.
  - Best obtained by nasopharyngeal aspirate; can also be obtained by nasal swab
  - Viral cultures are accurate, but may take up to 14 days for results.

Imaging

- Chest radiography is of little value in the majority of bronchiolitis cases, and multiple recent efforts have attempted to limit unnecessary radiographic testing.
- When obtained, findings may include the following:
  - Hyperinflation, flattened diaphragms
  - Peribronchial thickening
  - Patchy or more extensive atelectasis
  - Possible collapse of a segment or a lobe
  - Diffusely increased interstitial markings are common.

DIFFERENTIAL DIAGNOSIS

- Pneumonia (viral or bacterial)
- Foreign body aspiration
- Asthma
- Gastroesophageal reflux (GER)
- Pulmonary edema (e.g., congestive heart failure)
- Cystic fibrosis
- Airway abnormalities (tracheomalacia or bronchomalacia)

TREATMENT

GENERAL MEASURES

- There is substantial variation in the use of diagnostic testing, hospitalization, and treatments, but bronchiolitis is a self-limited condition that generally improves without intervention.
- Most cases are mild and may be managed at home.
  - Ensure adequate fluid intake.
  - Antipyretics may be used for comfort—given concerns of association between acetaminophen use and asthma, consider ibuprofen as first line in infants >6 months of age.
  - For rhinorrhea, nasal suction with bulb syringe may be of use.
- Supplemental oxygen
  - Can be given humidified via nasal cannula, high-flow nasal cannula, face mask cannula, noninvasive positive pressure ventilation, or via endotracheal tube
  - Should be titrated to respiratory distress and/or oxygen saturation
  - Home oxygen use is an alternative and has been shown to successfully and safely reduce hospital admission rates from the emergency department.
- Pulse oximetry
  - Continuous pulse oximetry can be useful as a monitoring device in order to titrate oxygen therapy, but it may also prolong length of stay by contributing to the overdiagnosis of hypoxemia (i.e., transient desaturations in otherwise comfortable infants).
  - Consider intermittent pulse oximetry use in infants who are not requiring oxygen.
- The following medications/therapies are of *no* proven benefit in bronchiolitis and should be avoided:
  - Corticosteroids (systemic or inhaled)
  - Ipratropium bromide
  - Leukotriene modifiers

INPATIENT CONSIDERATIONS

- Common indications for hospitalization include the following:
  - Need for IV hydration
  - Need for frequent suctioning
  - Moderate to severe distress (respiratory rate >60–70 breaths/minute, accessory muscle use, agitation, cyanosis, poor perfusion)
  - Apnea
- Although hypoxemia is often used as an indication for hospitalization, exact oxygen saturation thresholds are uncertain. The American Academy of Pediatrics (AAP) suggests using supplemental oxygen for saturations <90%.
- Hydration
  - Intravenous crystalloid boluses of 10–20 mL/kg should be given to infants with signs of poor perfusion.
  - For infants who are unable to maintain adequate PO intake, hydration can be maintained with nasogastric feeds or maintenance IV fluids. Because of the risk of hyponatremia, hypotonic fluids should be avoided.
- Suctioning
  - Nasal suctioning may improve work of breathing and facilitate feeding. Noninvasive suctioning (i.e., a nasal aspirator placed over the naris) is preferable to deep suctioning, which may cause trauma to the nasopharynx and worsen edema.
- Aerosols
  - β-Adrenergic agonists have no clear benefit in bronchiolitis. While some trials have suggested transient improvements in respiratory scores, none has demonstrated any impact on clinically meaningful outcomes such as hospitalization rates or hospital length of stay.
  - Racemic epinephrine, with its α-adrenergic properties, holds more promise than albuterol given that bronchiolitis is characterized more by airway edema than bronchospasm. Racemic epinephrine has been demonstrated in some studies to reduce hospital admission rates compared to placebo and to shorten length of stay when compared to albuterol.
  - Neither β- or α-adrenergic agonists are recommended by the AAP for routine use.
  - Preliminary studies on nebulized hypertonic saline (HTS) suggest that it might reduce length of stay. Although most studies use HTS in combination with albuterol or racemic epinephrine, at least one large study has suggested that these adjuvants are not necessary.
  - If aerosols are to be used in bronchiolitis, careful attention should be paid to the clinical exam before and after administration (preferably with the use of a respiratory score) in order to support their ongoing use.
- Antimicrobials
  - Antibiotics are overused in bronchiolitis and should be avoided in most cases.
  - Special considerations include the following:
    - Respiratory failure requiring intubation, in which case a substantial portion of patients have bacteria isolated from respiratory cultures
    - Urinary tract infection
    - Otitis media
  - See RSV chapter for discussion of ribavirin and RSV immunoprophylaxis.
- The following inpatient medications/therapies are of *no* proven benefit in bronchiolitis and should be avoided:
  - Corticosteroids (systemic or inhaled)
  - Ipratropium bromide
  - Leukotriene modifiers
  - Methylxanthines (theophylline, aminophylline)
  - Recombinant human DNAse
  - *N*-Acetylcysteine
  - Chest physiotherapy

ONGOING CARE

FOLLOW-UP RECOMMENDATIONS

Patient Monitoring

- Most infants with no underlying disease improve within 1 week.
- A fraction of infants (~20%) will have symptoms for 3 weeks or more.
- Clinical course is prolonged in younger infants (<6 months) and those with comorbid conditions.

PROGNOSIS

- For most previously healthy infants, the prognosis is good.
- A small fraction of infants, especially young or chronically ill ones, need support in the ICU with positive pressure ventilation.
- Mortality rates are very low (<0.1%).
- Infants with chronic underlying disease may have a protracted course and are at risk for repeated hospitalizations.
- Although up to 50% of infants with bronchiolitis develop subsequent episodes of wheezing, the direction of causality between bronchiolitis and asthma is unclear.

COMPLICATIONS

ALERT

Almost all infants with bronchiolitis get better and do not need testing or therapies.

Be aware of viral coinfections—1/4 of hospitalized patients with bronchiolitis have evidence of infection with at least 2 viruses.

ADDITIONAL READING

- Mansbach JM, Piedra PA, Teach SJ, et al. Prospective multicenter study of viral etiology and hospital length-of-stay in children with severe bronchiolitis. *Pediatrics*. 2012;130(3):e492–e500.
- Ralston S, Garber M, Narang S, et al. Decreasing unnecessary utilization in acute bronchiolitis care: results from the value in inpatient pediatrics network. *J Hosp Med*. 2013;8(1):25–30.
- Ralston SL, Lieberthal AS, Meissner HC, et al. Clinical practice guideline: the diagnosis, management, and prevention of bronchiolitis. *Pediatrics*. 2014;134(5):e1474–e1502. doi:10.1542/peds.2014-2742.
- Subcommittee on Diagnosis and Management of Bronchiolitis. Diagnosis and management of bronchiolitis. *Pediatrics*. 2006;118(4):1774–1793.
- Zorc JJ, Hall CB. Bronchiolitis: recent evidence on diagnosis and management. *Pediatrics*. 2010;125(2):342–349.

CODES

ICD10

- J21.9 Acute bronchiolitis, unspecified
- J21.0 Acute bronchiolitis due to respiratory syncytial virus
- J21.8 Acute bronchiolitis due to other specified organisms

FAQ

- Q: How did my child get bronchiolitis?
- A: Viral bronchiolitis is a common, seasonal, respiratory tract infection that is easily transmissible. It is acquired in much the same way as the common cold.
- Q: Can my child become reinfected?
- A: Children can become reinfected with RSV bronchiolitis, and infection can occur more than once during the same respiratory season. Furthermore, some patients can get two viral infections at the same time.
- Q: Do patients with bronchiolitis need to be isolated?
- A: Ideally, all patients with bronchiolitis are kept in isolation from other patients with and without bronchiolitis. If cohorting is necessary, patients with the same virus can be roomed together, although contact precautions should still be taken.
- Q: Will my child develop asthma?
- A: There is an ~50% chance that a patient with bronchiolitis will wheeze again. However, it is not clear whether the virus causes asthma or if infants who are predisposed to asthma are more likely to get bronchiolitis.

BRONCHOPULMONARY DYSPLASIA (BPD)

Vineet Bhandari • Anita Bhandari

BASICS

DESCRIPTION

- A chronic lung disease (CLD) of premature infants defined as the need for supplemental O_2 for 28 days and a need for supplemental oxygen +/−positive pressure at 36 weeks postmenstrual age (PMA).
- It is categorized as mild, moderate, and severe, based on the following at 36 weeks PMA or discharge (whichever comes first).
  - Mild: breathing room air
  - Moderate: need for <30% oxygen
  - Severe: need for >30% oxygen, with or without positive pressure ventilation or continuous positive pressure

EPIDEMIOLOGY

BPD is the most common CLD in infants. Infants with birth weight (BW) <1,250 g account for 97% of all patients with BPD. Prevalence based on BW:

- 501–750 g: 42%
- 751–1,000 g: 25%
- 1,001–1,250 g: 11%
- 1,251–1,500 g: 5%

RISK FACTORS

- Infants with gestational age (GA) <28 weeks and BW <1,000 g
- Invasive ventilation
- Exposure to hyperoxia
- Sepsis (in utero and postnatal; local/systemic)
- Genetic predisposition

GENERAL PREVENTION

- Prevention of premature birth
- Noninvasive ventilation approaches
- Avoidance of hyperoxia
- Decreasing perinatal infections

PATHOPHYSIOLOGY

- Multifactorial with gene–environmental interactions
- Antenatal (AN)—chorioamnionitis
- Postnatal (PN)—ventilator injury, hyperoxia, and sepsis
- AN and PN factors act on a genetically predisposed immature lung, causing release of multiple molecular mediators of inflammation, resulting in activation of cellular death pathways, followed by resolution or repair.
- Repair of the injured developing lung results in decreased alveolarization and dysregulated pulmonary vasculature, the pathologic hallmarks of BPD.

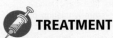

DIAGNOSIS

HISTORY

- Family: premature birth, asthma
- AN: pregnancy-induced hypertension, preterm/prolonged rupture of membranes, chorioamnionitis, steroids
- Perinatal: resuscitation at birth
- PN: GA, BW, small for GA (SGA), respiratory distress syndrome (RDS), surfactant use, duration of invasive/noninvasive ventilation, supplemental O_2

PHYSICAL EXAM

- Early phase (up to 1 PN week): normal to severe RDS (i.e., tachypnea, dyspnea)
- Evolving phase (>1 PN week to 36 weeks PMA): increasing respiratory distress and FiO_2
- Established phase (>36 weeks PMA): tachypnea, dyspnea, crackles, stridor (subglottic stenosis), wheezing, "BPD spells" (tracheobronchomalacia), evidence of pulmonary hypertension (PH), gastroesophageal reflux (GER), poor growth parameters

DIAGNOSTIC TESTS & INTERPRETATION

Labs: Initial Lab Tests

Blood gases: monitoring of acid–base status, hypo/hyperoxia, hypo/hypercapnia

Labs: Follow-Up Tests & Special Considerations

- Echocardiogram: evidence of PH-tricuspid regurgitant jet, flattening of the interventricular septum, accelerated pulmonary regurgitation velocity, right atrial enlargement, right ventricular hypertrophy and dilation
- Cardiac catheterization in selective infants, to confirm PH
- Pulmonary function testing: Majority have abnormal spirometry with decreased forced expiratory flow at 1 second (FEV_1) and decreased small airway expiratory flows (FEF, 25–75%) and impaired diffusion capacity. Majority of studies reveal no decrease in exercise capacity in former premature babies, although response to exercise differs.

Imaging: Initial Approach

Chest radiography: Early— reticular-granular pattern with air bronchograms (RDS); evolving—pulmonary edema, atelectasis; established—hyperinflation, increased interstitial markings, cysts

Imaging: Follow-Up & Special Considerations

CT scan: persistent findings which include linear densities, subpleural triangular densities, and emphysema

Diagnostic Procedures/Other

- Bronchoscopy for subglottic stenosis, trachea/bronchomalacia
- Sleep studies for persistent hypoxia and suspected central or obstructive apnea
- pH probe for GER

DIFFERENTIAL DIAGNOSIS

- Pneumonia
- Aspiration
- Congenital heart disease
- Wilson-Mikity syndrome
- Interstitial lung disease
  - Surfactant protein deficiency
  - Pulmonary lymphangiectasia

TREATMENT

MEDICATION

- O_2 supplementation
  - Prevention of hypoxia and as a pulmonary vasodilator
  - Early/evolving phases: Titrate FiO_2 by pulse oximeter 88–92%, generally, >85–<95%.
  - Established phase: generally ~95%, for prevention of PH
- Methylxanthines
  - Acts as a respiratory stimulant, increases diaphragmatic contractility, weak bronchodilator and diuretic
  - Caffeine use has been associated with decreased BPD and improved neurodevelopmental outcomes.
  - Early/evolving phases: caffeine citrate (IV/PO) 20 mg/kg loading dose, 5 mg/kg/24 h maintenance dose
  - Side effects include feeding intolerance, tachycardia
- Vitamin A
  - Helpful in maintaining epithelial cell integrity of the respiratory tract
  - Early/evolving phases: 5,000 IU IM 3 times per week for 4 weeks
- Steroids
  - Decreases inflammation, pulmonary edema
  - Evolving phase: Dexamethasone (IV/PO, 0.5 mg/kg/24 h × 2 days, then 0.25 mg/kg/24 h × 2 days, then 0.15 mg/kg/24 h × 1 day) may be used to assist with extubation attempts after 3–4 PN weeks.
  - Established phase: Prednisolone (PO, 2 mg/kg/24 h × 5 days, then 1 mg/kg/24 h × 3 days, then 1 mg/kg/24 h every other day for 3 doses) may be helpful in weaning oxygen.
  - Side effects include hyperglycemia and hypertension in the short term.

- Diuretics
  - Evolving/established phases: furosemide (PO/IV, 1–2 mg/kg/24 h or every other day; chlorothiazide (PO/IV, 20–40 mg/kg/24 h) alone or with spironolactone (PO, 2–4 mg/kg/24 h) for transient improvement of lung function
  - Side effects include electrolyte abnormalities, nephrocalcinosis, and osteopenia of prematurity.
- Bronchodilators
  - Evolving/established phases: Inhaled β-agonists (e.g., albuterol 1.25–2.5 mg given via nebulizer or 2 puffs [180 mcg] given via MDI with spacer device, every 3–4 hours as needed) are effective treatment for reversible bronchospasm, although safety and efficacy of long-term use has yet to be established.
  - Muscarinic antagonists (e.g., ipratropium bromide 250–500 mcg via nebulizer or 18 mcg/puff via MDI with spacer device, every 6–8 hours as needed) may be useful adjuncts, especially in patients who are not significantly responsive to albuterol. It may be better tolerated than albuterol in patients with significant tracheomalacia.
  - Cromolyn, although not a bronchodilator, is often used for its anti-inflammatory effects and has a low side-effect profile. It has no role in prevention of BPD.

ALERT

- Many patients have oral aversion and feeding difficulties; close monitoring of growth and nutrition is recommended.
- Patients <2 years of age are candidates for respiratory syncytial virus immune globulin injections (palivizumab; Synagis), and those older than 6 months of age should be offered influenza immunization.
- Childhood immunizations are based on chronologic age rather than corrected age.
- There are no evidence-based guidelines regarding diuretic use or weaning off of supplemental oxygen therapy in established BPD.

ADDITIONAL TREATMENT

- Ventilator strategy
  - Early phase: Avoid intubation; if intubated, give early surfactant (<2 hours of PN life), use short inspiratory times (0.24–0.4 second), rapid rates (40–60/min), low peak inspiratory pressure (14–20 cm H_2O), moderate positive end-expiratory pressure (4–6 cm H_2O), and tidal volumes (3–6 mL/kg), with blood gas targets pH 7.25–7.35, Pao_2 40–60 mm Hg, $Paco_2$ 45–55 mm Hg; "rescue" high-frequency ventilation; attempt extubation to nasal intermittent positive pressure ventilation (NIPPV) or nasal continuous positive airways pressure (NCPAP) in the first PN week.
  - Evolving phase: Use noninvasive ventilation with blood gas targets pH 7.25–7.35, Pao_2 50–70 mm Hg, $Paco_2$ 50–65 mm Hg.
  - Established phase: Use noninvasive ventilation with blood gas targets pH 7.35–7.45, Pao_2 60–80 mm Hg, $Paco_2$ 45–60 mm Hg.

GENERAL MEASURES

Fluids/Nutrition

- Early phase: Restricting fluids to ~140 cc/kg/day may decrease BPD.
- Early/evolving/established phase: Aim to achieve 120–140 kcal/kg/day.

ONGOING CARE

FOLLOW-UP RECOMMENDATIONS

- Multidisciplinary approach with primary care physician, pediatric pulmonologist, pediatric cardiologist, nutritionist, and speech, respiratory, occupational, and physical therapists as well as social worker is recommended.
- Monitor linear growth and nutritional status.
- Immunization: prophylaxis against respiratory syncytial virus (palivizumab injections once a month from October to April) and influenza
- Neurodevelopmental follow-up

PROGNOSIS

- Infants with BPD have high rates of rehospitalization in the first year of life (up to 50%).
- Long-term pulmonary sequelae that may persist into adulthood include airway obstruction, airway hyperreactivity, and concern regarding development of chronic pulmonary obstructive disease (COPD) with aging.
- Long-term neurodevelopmental sequelae associated with BPD is not a specific neuropsychological impairment but more of a global deficit.
- Noninvasive ventilation approaches (NIPPV and NCPAP) hold promise in decreasing BPD.

COMPLICATIONS

- Prolonged intubation may lead to subglottic stenosis, tracheobronchomalacia.
- PH may result in cor pulmonale.

ADDITIONAL READING

- Bhandari A, Bhandari V. The "new" bronchopulmonary dysplasia—a clinical review. *Clin Pulm Med*. 2011;18(3):137–143.
- Bhandari A, Bhandari V. State-of-the-art review article. Pitfalls, problems, and progress in bronchopulmonary dysplasia. *Pediatrics*. 2009;123(6):1562–1573.
- Bhandari A, McGrath-Morrow S. Long-term pulmonary outcomes of patients with bronchopulmonary dysplasia. *Semin Perinatol*. 2013;37(2):132–137.
- Bhandari V. Hyperoxia-derived lung damage in preterm infants. *Semin Fetal Neonatal Med*. 2010;15(4):223–229.
- Bhandari V. The potential of non-invasive ventilation to decrease BPD. *Semin Perinatol*. 2013;37(2):108–114.

CODES

ICD10

P27.1 Bronchopulmonary dysplasia origin in the perinatal period

FAQ

- Q: Can my patient with BPD receive influenza vaccine?
- A: Yes. Influenza vaccination should be considered for babies older than 6 months of age and their contacts.
- Q: The AAP Committee on Infectious Diseases recommends monthly immunoprophylaxis for infants with BPD who are <2 years old and have been on medical therapy for 6 months prior to onset of second respiratory syncytial viral season. What should I do if my patient turns 2 years old, 2 months after the respiratory season started?
- A: Once initiated, immunoprophylaxis should be completed even if the child turns 2 years old before the respiratory season has ended.
- Q: If my patient gets respiratory syncytial virus infection while on immunoprophylaxis (palivizumab; Synagis), should the monthly injections be stopped?
- A: Monthly prophylaxis with palivizumab should be discontinued because of extremely low likelihood of a second RSV hospitalization in the same season based on the revised AAP 2014 policy statement.
- Q: Will my patient with BPD continue to have respiratory problems?
- A: Survivors of BPD are more likely to be rehospitalized with respiratory illnesses in the first 2 years of their life, but the rate of hospitalization decreases after 2 years of age and is rare after 14 years of age. They are more likely to develop asthma, have abnormal pulmonary function tests, and require respiratory medications as compared to their peers. There is also some concern that survivors may develop a COPD phenotype as they age.
- Q: If my patient with BPD has recurrent croup, should I refer the patient to a pediatric pulmonologist for evaluation of asthma?
- A: Survivors of BPD are more likely to develop asthma as compared to peers born full term. However, upper and large airway problems such as subglottic stenosis and tracheomalacia are common in this population. Recurrent croup may result from a narrowing of the upper airway and hence, referral to a pediatric otolaryngologist should be considered to rule out causes such as subglottic stenosis.
- Q: Will my patient with BPD likely to have neurodevelopmental issues as well?
- A: Yes. Children with BPD are more likely to have delayed speech and language development, visual-motor integration impairments, and behavior problems. They may also have low average IQ, memory and learning deficits, and attention problems.

BRUISING

Julie W. Stern

BASICS

DESCRIPTION

- Bruises are the result of extravasation of blood into the skin. Conventional usage often groups petechiae and bruises (or ecchymoses) together as purpura and defines them as follows:
  - Petechiae: flat, red, or reddish purple; 1–3 mm; nonblanching
  - Ecchymoses: larger than petechiae, local extravasation, nonpulsatile, sometimes palpable, color depends on age of lesion

DIAGNOSIS

DIFFERENTIAL DIAGNOSIS

- Congenital/anatomic
  - Coagulation factor abnormality: hemophilia, von Willebrand disease
  - Platelet defect: Bernard-Soulier syndrome, Glanzmann thrombasthenia, and storage pool defects
  - Congenital alloimmune or isoimmune thrombocytopenia
  - Neonatal extramedullary hematopoiesis
  - Hereditary hemorrhagic telangiectasia
- Infectious
  - Meningococcemia
  - Viral infections (coxsackievirus, echovirus)
  - Rocky Mountain spotted fever
  - Syphilis
  - Pertussis—secondary to severe cough
  - Septic or fat emboli
  - Disseminated intravascular coagulation—acquired factor deficiency
- Toxic, environmental, drugs
  - Warfarin—acquired factor deficiency
  - Corticosteroids—striae caused by increased capillary fragility
  - Aspirin and ibuprofen—cause a qualitative platelet abnormality
  - Sulfonamides
  - Bismuth
  - Chloramphenicol
- Trauma
  - Normal activity
  - Child abuse
  - Valsalva, crying, forceful coughing
  - Cupping or coin rubbing
  - Tight garments
- Tumor (quantitative platelet abnormality)
  - Bone marrow replacement—leukemia, myelofibrosis, or (rarely) metastatic solid tumors
- Genetic/metabolic
  - Uremia
  - Vitamin C deficiency
  - Vitamin K deficiency—owing to antibiotics, biliary atresia, malabsorption (acquired factor deficiency)
- Allergic/inflammatory/vasculitic
  - Henoch-Schönlein purpura
  - Bone marrow failure: aplastic anemia (including Fanconi, paroxysmal nocturnal hemoglobinuria)
  - Increased destruction: idiopathic thrombocytopenic purpura, Evans syndrome, lupus
  - Nephrotic syndrome
  - Collagen vascular disease
  - Ehlers-Danlos syndrome, other joint hypermobility syndromes
  - Snake bite (copperhead)
- Miscellaneous (disorders that simulate bruises)
  - Ataxia telangiectasia
  - Cherry angiomas
  - Kaposi sarcoma

DIAGNOSIS

General goal is to determine if the cause of the bruising is thrombocytopenia, a coagulation disorder, or an extrinsic factor (such as trauma, infection).

- **Phase 1:** Determine if the history of bruising and/or petechiae is acute or chronic in onset and if there is known trauma versus spontaneous lesions (see Table 1)

Table 1. How to estimate the age of bruises

1. New	Purple, dark red
2. 1–4 days	Dark blue to brown
3. 5–7 days	Greenish to yellow
4. >7 days	Yellow

  - Acute onset of diffuse subcutaneous bleeding with bruises of different ages may indicate severe thrombocytopenia.
  - Generally, children will not bruise or develop petechiae spontaneously until the platelet count is $<20{,}000/mm^3$.
  - Idiopathic thrombocytopenic purpura, leukemia, aplastic anemia, and so forth, can cause this bleeding.
  - A hematologist should be consulted because of the risk of potentially life-threatening bleeding.
  - Chronic history of recurrent bleeding may indicate an inherited coagulation defect such as von Willebrand disease or hemophilia. Familial history may be positive, although von Willebrand disease often goes undiagnosed into adulthood if there has been no challenge such as surgery.
  - Various bleeding scores available but not fully validated in pediatrics; may be helpful to direct history taking
- **Phase 2:** Perform screening tests for bleeding disorders to categorize the abnormality.
  - Platelet count to assess level of thrombocytopenia
  - PT/PTT: Prolongation of either one or both of these may aid in diagnosis of von Willebrand disease, coagulation factor deficiencies, liver disease, and vitamin K deficiency.
  - Testing for von Willebrand disease and platelet aggregation disorders generally need to be done by a hematologist for accuracy and interpretation.
  - Bleeding time and PFA-100: Both tests are controversial and rarely used in pediatrics.

HISTORY

- **Question:** Significant bruising in the neonatal period?
- *Significance*: May indicate neonatal thrombocytopenia, congenital infections, and sepsis with disseminated intravascular coagulation
- **Question:** Bleeding in the neonatal period?
- *Significance*: Hemophilia. Other inherited disorders of coagulation may not be diagnosed until a child is older; tend to be mild; may be uncovered with preoperative testing or postoperative bleeding complications. Idiopathic thrombocytopenic purpura may occur at any age.
- **Question:** Pattern of bruising?
- *Significance*: In a younger child, may indicate normal toddler activity, child abuse, or religious practices such as coining
- **Question:** Use of aspirin, ibuprofen, cough syrups with guaifenesin, and/or antihistamines?
- *Significance*: Platelet dysfunction; use of these drugs may also unmask an otherwise mild inherited bleeding disorder.
- **Question:** Ecchymosis or petechiae?
- *Significance*: Infections such as meningococcemia or viruses and collagen vascular diseases may present with these.
- **Question:** Familial history?
- *Significance*: Positive familial history of inherited disorders of coagulation factors or platelet aggregation may aid in directing the workup. Negative familial history does not rule out any of these disorders.

PHYSICAL EXAM

- **Finding:** Good appearance, with a history of an antecedent viral illness?
- *Significance*: Those with idiopathic thrombocytopenic purpura often appear well, although often with a history of an antecedent viral illness.
- **Finding:** Ill appearance?
- *Significance*: It should raise concerns about malignancy, infection (especially meningococcemia), or other acquired coagulation factor deficiencies such as those seen with liver failure.
- **Finding:** Bruising in unusual locations (back, genitalia, thorax)?
- *Significance*: Should raise suspicions of child abuse, especially if lesions are in different stages of healing or suggest the pattern of a hand or belt

- **Finding:** Purpura confined mostly to the legs?
- *Significance*: Typical of Henoch-Schönlein purpura

ALERT
- The amount of bruising may not correlate with the amount of internal bleeding that has occurred.
  - Hemophiliacs can significantly drop their hemoglobin during a thigh or psoas bleed without having much in the way of ecchymosis.
  - A child presenting with idiopathic thrombocytopenic purpura may have bruises and petechiae from head to toe without changing the hemoglobin much at all.

- **Finding:** Multiple ecchymoses in the pretibial regions?
- *Significance*: This is typical of normal toddler activity.
- **Finding:** Petechiae entirely above the nipple line?
- *Significance*: Consistent with Valsalva maneuver, severe cough, and viral infections
- **Finding:** Deeper bleeding in muscles and joints?
- *Significance*: Hemophilia
- **Finding:** Bleeding in mucous membranes?
- *Significance*: Severe thrombocytopenia, streptococcal pharyngitis, varicella, measles, and other viral infections can cause this.
- **Finding:** Gingival and/or mucous membrane bleeding?
- *Significance*: Von Willebrand disease can present with this. Severe thrombocytopenia and ITP may also present with oral bleeding.
- **Finding:** Involvement of the reticuloendothelial system?
- *Significance*: Can be found with malignancies such as leukemia or with viral or bacterial infections, indicated by hepatosplenomegaly or lymphadenopathy
- **Finding:** Upper extremity limb malformations and bruising?
- *Significance*: May present with syndromes such as Fanconi anemia and thrombocytopenia absent radii (TAR)

ALERT
Factors that make this an emergency include the following:
- Severe thrombocytopenia below 10,000–20,000/mm^3 carries a higher risk of spontaneous internal bleeding including intracranial bleeding.
- Bleeding or bruising accompanied by evidence of leukemia or other malignancy
- Evidence of sepsis (disseminated intravascular coagulation) or meningococcemia

DIAGNOSTIC TESTS & INTERPRETATION
- **Test:** CBC
- *Significance*: Platelet count is the most important; abnormalities of WBC or Hgb may aid in diagnosis of bone marrow infiltration or failure.
- **Test:** PT
- *Significance*: Elevation may indicate warfarin ingestion or factor VII and/or vitamin K deficiencies.
- **Test:** aPTT
- *Significance*: Prolongation is seen with hemophilia and may be seen in von Willebrand disease.
- **Test:** Both PT and PTT
- *Significance*: Both are prolonged in disseminated intravascular coagulation, liver failure, and severe vitamin K deficiency.
- **Test:** Bleeding time
- *Significance*: Lengthened in platelet aggregation disorders and with drug effects
- **Test:** Fibrinogen
- *Significance*: Decreased in liver failure, disseminated intravascular coagulation
- **Test:** Urinalysis
- *Significance*: Hematuria and/or proteinuria may indicate Henoch-Schönlein purpura, nephrotic syndrome, or other vasculitis.

TREATMENT

GENERAL MEASURES
- Thrombocytopenia precautions for platelets <20,000–50,000—toddlers may need a helmet until platelet count recovers; patients with hemophilia may need restricted activity, generally not needed for patients with von Willebrand disease. Depends on underlying cause.
- Factor replacement for hemophilia
- Platelet transfusion for thrombocytopenia due to decreased production
- IVIG, steroids, Rh immune globulin, thrombopoietin (TPO) mimetics for ITP

ISSUES FOR REFERRAL
- Outpatient evaluation for bruising without significant thrombocytopenia, family history of bleeding disorder
- Suspected child abuse

Admission Criteria
Severe thrombocytopenia, suspected child abuse, significant bleeding, significant head trauma

ONGOING CARE

FOLLOW-UP RECOMMENDATIONS

Patient Monitoring
Recurrent and chronic ITP possible

COMPLICATIONS
Significant bleeding with a bleeding disorder, thrombocytopenia

ADDITIONAL READING

- Berntorp E. Progress in haemophilic care: ethical issues. *Haemophilia*. 2002;8(3):435–438.
- Buchanan GR. Bleeding signs in children with idiopathic thrombocytopenic purpura. *J Pediatr Hematol Oncol*. 2003;25(Suppl 1):S42–S46.
- Geddis AE, Balduini CL. Diagnosis of immune thrombocytopenic purpura in children. *Curr Opin Hematol*. 2007;14(5):520–525.
- Horton TM, Stone JD, Yee D, et al. Case series of thrombotic thrombocytopenic purpura in children and adolescents. *J Pediatr Hematol Oncol*. 2003;25(4):336–339.
- Khair K, Liesner R. Bruising and bleeding in infants and children—a practical approach. *Br J Haematol*. 2006;133(3):221–231.
- Kos L, Shwayder T. Cutaneous manifestations of child abuse. *Pediatr Dermatol*. 2006;23(4):311–320.
- O'Brien SH. An update on pediatric bleeding disorders: bleeding scores, benign joint hypermobility, and platelet function testing in the evaluation of the child with bleeding symptoms. *Am J Hematol*. 2012;87(Suppl 1):S40–S44. doi:10.1002/ajh.23157.
- Wight J, Paisley S. The epidemiology of inhibitors in haemophilia A: a systematic review. *Haemophilia*. 2003;9(4):418–435.

CODES

ICD10
- T14.8 Other injury of unspecified body region
- R23.3 Spontaneous ecchymoses
- D68.9 Coagulation defect, unspecified

FAQ
- Q: Is hemophilia always diagnosed in the newborn period?
- A: No. A familial history may provide clues, but a significant number of patients represent a spontaneous mutation. Additionally, not all boys with hemophilia will bleed with circumcision, and the diagnosis may not be made until the infants become more active.
- Q: What is a common cause of bruising among girls?
- A: Girls may first come to attention at menarche and be diagnosed at that time with von Willebrand disease. Rarely, girls whose fathers have hemophilia may be unfavorably lyonized and, therefore, have decreased factor levels consistent with mild hemophilia.
- Q: Can boys with a family history of von Willebrand disease be circumcised?
- A: Yes, but only within the first few days of life and testing does not need to be completed prior to procedure. If procedure is not completed in the neonatal period, testing may need to be delayed until 6 months of life or later.

BRUXISM

Anupama R. Tate • Karen R. Fratantoni

BASICS

DESCRIPTION
- Bruxism is defined as habitual nonfunctional forceful contact of teeth, which is involuntary. These movements can include excessive grinding, clenching, or rubbing of teeth.
- Other nonfunctional (or "parafunctional") oral habits include movements not involved with normal chewing, swallowing, or speaking, such as chewing pencils, nails, cheek, or lip.
- Sleep bruxism should be distinguished from daytime awake bruxism.
- Awake bruxism is rare with little or no audible sound during clenching, compared to the loud grinding sound commonly occurring in sleep bruxism.

EPIDEMIOLOGY
- May occur throughout life but frequently tends to peak in early childhood, then decreases with age
- Infants have been known to grind their teeth during the eruption of primary teeth.
- May be temporarily or intermittently present, which makes diagnosis difficult
- Recent systematic review of literature reported no gender differences in prevalence. Previous studies suggested girls may be more affected than boys.
- Some studies support higher incidence in children with developmental disabilities, Down syndrome, sleep disorders, and autism.
- No genetic mechanism has been explained. Based on self-reports, 20–50% of children with sleep bruxism have an immediate family member who experienced bruxism as a child.

Prevalence
In children, prevalence in the literature is highly variable with a range of 4–40%. Prevalence decreases with increasing age. Sleep bruxism progressively diminishes around 9–10 years of age.

ETIOLOGY
The exact cause is not known. It is likely to be a multifactorial process including pathophysiologic, psychologic, or morphologic factors.
- Awake bruxism is more commonly associated with psychosocial factors and psychopathologic symptoms.
- Dental factors (current evidence suggests that they play a small role, only ~10% of cases)
  - Occlusal interferences, including malocclusions, in which teeth do not interdigitate smoothly
  - High dental restorations (e.g., fillings or crowns)
  - Intraoral irritation (e.g., sharp tooth cusp)
  - Teething
- Psychological factors
  - Nervous tension (related to stress, anger, and aggression)
  - Personality disorders
  - Posttraumatic stress disorder
- Common systemic factors
  - Moving between levels of sleep
  - Sleep-disordered breathing
  - Snoring and sleep apnea
  - Tonsil/adenoid hypertrophy
  - Neurodevelopmental disorders (e.g., cerebral palsy)
  - Brain injury
  - ADHD
- Other possible factors
  - Asthma
  - Allergies
  - Nasal obstruction
  - Exposure to secondhand smoke
  - Medications (amphetamines, antidepressants—particularly serotonin reuptake inhibitors)

DIAGNOSIS

- Teeth
  - Wearing of facets, abraded areas
  - Extreme wear of primary teeth is occasionally observed; however, pulp or nerve damage is rare.
  - Broken dental restorations
  - Loose teeth
  - Progression of periodontal disease (gingival inflammation, recession, and alveolar bone loss)
  - Pain or sensitivity
- Muscular symptoms of the head and neck muscles, most often seen in the lateral pterygoids followed by the medial pterygoids and masseters
  - Pain
  - Trismus
  - Spasm
- Frequent headache or migraines
- Parasomnias
- Temporomandibular joint (TMJ) disorders
  - Symptoms (pain, clicking, popping when opening or closing)
  - Limited mandibular range of motion

DIFFERENTIAL DIAGNOSIS
- Dental erosion
- Drug reaction
- Gastroesophageal reflux
- Seizures
- Sleep disorder
- Stress

TREATMENT

MEDICATION
- Analgesics or anti-inflammatory medications (e.g., ibuprofen) for management of symptoms
- Rarely used
  - Muscle relaxants for symptoms
  - Mild anxiolytics if anxiety plays an etiologic role

GENERAL MEASURES
- Often, children outgrow bruxism and no treatment is indicated.
- When treatment is needed, it is best managed in a multiprofessional team approach including a dentist.
- Patient and family education: Ensure that the bruxism itself does not become an issue, generating increased stress for the child.
- Plastic or vinyl bite guard (must not interfere with normal dental growth and development)
- Stress counseling
  - Identify and address sources of stress.
  - Meditation
  - Music therapy
  - Biofeedback exercises
  - Acupressure and/or acupuncture
- Counseling/psychotherapy
  - Hypnosis

Additional Therapies

- Rarely used
  - Occlusal adjustment (selective tooth grinding to balance the bite): There is no evidence-based support. Because of inadequate data regarding their usefulness, irreversible therapies should be avoided.
  - Tonsillectomy and adenoidectomy

COMPLEMENTARY & ALTERNATIVE THERAPIES

- Warm compresses for muscle or TMJ symptoms
- Limiting affected muscle activity (e.g., "do not open wide," "take small bites," "avoid chewing gum") may help reduce TMJ symptoms.

INPATIENT CONSIDERATIONS

- Treatment for bruxism is rarely indicated for children in the inpatient setting.
- Therapy is justified if damage to the permanent dentition or periodontal structures is observed.
- For neurologically impaired patients with acute self-injurious issues, bite blocks or mouth props can be protective. Patients who exhibit chronic chewing may require the fabrication of custom-fitted mouth guards, which may require the use of deep sedation or general anesthetic procedures to construct the appliance. The risk of these procedures would need to be weighed against the benefit of the bite guard.

ONGOING CARE

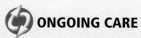

FOLLOW-UP RECOMMENDATIONS

Patient Monitoring

The large majority of bruxism in children stops without any therapy. Monitor for significant associated problems; recommend treatment if damage to permanent dentition and/or periodontal structures occurs.

PROGNOSIS

- There are no data to indicate a cause-and-effect relationship exists for bruxism in childhood continuing into adulthood.
- Preschool- and school-age children
  - Ensure that all children establish a dental home by 1 year of age.
  - Typically ceases without therapeutic intervention
  - Associated problems are rare.
  - Monitor for associated conditions.
- Adolescents
  - More commonly benefit from therapeutic intervention
  - Associated problems (e.g., attrition of teeth; muscular, TMJ symptoms) may also require therapy.
- Special-needs children
  - Long-term prognosis is poor.
  - Children who are comatose or those who have suffered traumatic brain injuries or neurologically impaired may be managed by the use of prefabricated bite blocks or, in rare cases, by the fabrication of custom-fitted mouth guards to minimize risk of damage to lips or tongue. Intraoral botulinum-A injections have relieved the spasticity.

ADDITIONAL READING

- American Academy of Pediatric Dentistry. Guidelines on acquired temporomandibular disorders in infants, children, and adolescents. Reference manual 2012–2013. *Pediatr Dent*. 2012;34:258–263.
- Cheifetz AT, Osganian SK, Allred EN, et al. Prevalence of bruxism and associated correlates in children as reported by parents. *J Dent Child (Chic)*. 2005;72(2):67–73.
- Dahshan A, Patel H, Delaney J, et al. Gastroesophageal reflux disease and dental erosion in children. *J Pediatr*. 2002;140(4):474–478.
- Eftekharian A, Raad N, Gholami-Ghasri N. Bruxism and adenotonsillectomy. *Int J Pediatr Otorhinolaryngol*. 2008;72(4):509–511.
- Lavigne GJ, Khoury S, Abe S, et al. Bruxism physiology and pathology: an overview for clinicians. *J Oral Rehabil*. 2008;35(7):476–494.
- Lindemeyer RG. Bruxism in children. *Dimens Dent Hyg*. 2011;9:60–63.
- Manfredini D, Lobbezoo F. Role of psychosocial factors in the etiology of bruxism. *J Orofac Pain*. 2009;23(2):153–166.
- Manfredini D, Restrepo C, Diaz-Serrano K, et al. Prevalence of sleep bruxism in children: a systematic review of the literature. *J Oral Rehabil*. 2013;40(8):631–642.
- Motta LJ, Martins MD, Fernandes KP, et al. Craniocervical posture and bruxism in children. *Physiother Res Int*. 2011;16(1):57–61.
- Norwood KW Jr, Slayton RL; Council on Children With Disabilities, et al. Oral health care for children with developmental disabilities. *Pediatrics*. 2013;131(3):614–619.
- Ortega AO, Guimarães AS, Ciamponi AL, et al. Frequency of parafunctional oral habits in patients with cerebral palsy. *J Oral Rehabil*. 2007;34(5):323–328.

CODES

ICD10

- F45.8 Other somatoform disorders
- G47.63 Sleep related bruxism

FAQ

- Q: What is the recommendation for nighttime bruxism management in a preschool child?
- A: The majority of bruxism in children stops without any therapy. Considering the controversial nature of treatment modalities, it is prudent to advise no treatment for childhood bruxism and to advise the parents that the condition is common and the child will outgrow the condition.
- Q: Does bruxism in a child result in problems with the permanent teeth or with the TMJ?
- A: There is no evidence that bruxism in children leads to problems during adolescence or later.
- Q: What is the recommendation for bruxism management in a child with snoring or tonsil/adenoid hypertrophy?
- A: Studies have shown a higher incidence of bruxism among children with tonsil hypertrophy and sleep apnea and a decrease in bruxism after adenotonsillectomy. Bruxism alone, without evidence of upper airway obstruction, would not currently be an indication for adenotonsillectomy. Physicians should assess children with bruxism for upper airway obstruction and refer when indicated.

BULIMIA

Sara F. Forman • Melissa B. Freizinger

BASICS

DESCRIPTION

Bulimia nervosa is an eating disorder characterized by the following:

- Recurrent binge eating episodes characterized by rapid consumption of large amounts of food in discrete periods of time, usually <2 hours
- Feeling of lack of control over eating behavior during eating binges
- Compensatory behavior such as self-induced vomiting, laxative or diuretic use, strict dieting, or vigorous exercise to induce weight loss
- Minimum average of one binge eating/compensatory behavior episode per week for at least 3 months
- Associated feelings of guilt, shame, low self-esteem, and depression
- Persistent overconcern with body shape and weight
- Symptoms and psychopathology may overlap with anorexia nervosa but does not occur exclusively during episodes of anorexia nervosa.

EPIDEMIOLOGY

- Onset in adolescence to young adulthood
- Approximately 10:1 female-to-male ratio
- 70% of the adolescents who meet criteria for full and partial syndrome eating disorders also met criteria for an Axis I disorder.

Prevalence

- Adolescents have a 1–1.5% 12-month prevalence of bulimia according to the *Diagnostic and Statistical Manual of Mental Disorders* 5th edition (*DSM-5*).
- 25% of college-aged women use bingeing and purging as a weight management technique.
- Bulimia nervosa prevalence rates in Western countries for females range from 0.3% to 7.3%.

RISK FACTORS

Genetics

Recent studies, including twin studies, suggest that bulimia nervosa and binge eating may have a genetic vulnerability and familial transmission.

GENERAL PREVENTION

- Emphasize healthy self-esteem/body image with preadolescents and adolescents
- Regular family dinners may have some protective effect against eating disorders.

ETIOLOGY

- Personality traits of low self-esteem, self-regulatory difficulties, frustration, intolerance, and impaired ability to recognize and express feelings directly described in bulimia nervosa
- Small positive association between childhood sexual abuse and eating disorders, but size and nature of this association not known
- Neuroendocrine abnormalities may also play a role: Abnormalities in serotonergic and vagal function have been demonstrated in patients with bulimia nervosa.
- Cholecystokinin response to a meal is decreased in bulimia nervosa, which may also indicate abnormal satiety signaling
- May be abnormalities in other hormones or neurotransmitters such as leptin, dopamine, and endorphins. Unclear if cause or effect.

COMMONLY ASSOCIATED CONDITIONS

- Lifetime rates of major depressive disorder in individuals with eating disorders 50–75%
- In adolescents, bulimia is associated with dysthymia more than major depression.
- 63.5% of bulimic patients have lifetime history of an anxiety disorder.

DIAGNOSIS

HISTORY

- Eating disorder specific
  - Eating habits
  - Presence of binge or purge behavior
  - Food rituals
  - Body image
  - Exercise history
  - Actual and desired weights, minimum and maximum weights
  - Use of laxatives, diuretics, diet pills, emetics, ipecac, or weight loss supplements
  - Menstrual history—amenorrhea or oligomenorrhea
  - Unease with others watching them eat
  - Preoccupation with food/eating
  - Preoccupation with body weight/shape
  - Fear of loss of control over one's body
- General
  - Weakness or fatigue or hyperactivity
  - Thirst, frequent urination
  - Headaches
  - Dizziness
  - Abdominal pain, fullness, or bloating; nausea
  - Constipation or diarrhea
  - Dental caries
  - Irregular menses
- Psychiatric
  - Mood disorder
  - Substance abuse
  - Anxiety
  - Personality disorders
  - Suicidal thoughts
  - Low self-esteem
  - Impulsivity
- Family
  - Medical and psychiatric histories
- Specific questions
  - Do you have a weight goal?
  - How do you control your weight?
  - How do you feel about yourself?
  - Do you ever vomit, use diuretics, or laxatives? If so, how often?

PHYSICAL EXAM

- Vital signs: Check for hypotension, orthostasis, and hypothermia.
- Weight: may be normal, overweight, or underweight
- Erosion of dental enamel: exposure to gastric acid secondary to frequent vomiting
- Parotid gland enlargement due to vomiting
- Calluses on knuckle or hands: Russell sign secondary to inducing vomiting
- Muscle weakness or cramps: electrolyte disturbance

DIAGNOSTIC TESTS & INTERPRETATION

Lab

- Part of the diagnostic workup. Most useful for assessing complications; no diagnostic or confirmatory laboratory test for bulimia nervosa. Many patients have normal labs.
- CBC: iron deficiency anemia
- Electrolytes, including calcium, magnesium, and phosphate: Abnormalities may occur as a result of prolonged vomiting or laxative use. Most common pattern for vomiting is hypokalemic-hypochloremic alkalosis.
- BUN and creatinine: Renal function usually normal, but BUN may be elevated secondary to dehydration or altered intake
- Glucose: patient may be hypoglycemic
- Cholesterol, lipids: may be elevated in starvation state
- Amylase: increased secondary to vomiting
- Lipase: increases may indicate severe complications such as pancreatitis
- Total protein, albumin, prealbumin: usually normal, but may be low if with malnutrition
- Liver function tests: Transaminases may be mildly elevated from starvation.
- Erythrocyte sedimentation rate (ESR): almost invariably normal; if elevated, consider occult organic process
- Bicarbonate level: metabolic alkalosis from vomiting or metabolic acidosis if using laxatives or dehydrated
- Urine toxicology screen (optional): may be positive as this disorder often is associated with substance abuse

Imaging

- Electrocardiogram with rhythm strip: may see U waves with hypokalemia, check QTc
- Consider upper GI series with small bowel follow-through if unclear etiology of vomiting
- Consider dual-energy x-ray absorptiometry (DEXA) scan if prolonged amenorrhea to evaluate bone mineral density.

Diagnostic Procedures/Other

Eating disorder questionnaires: Questionnaire assessments may be helpful and augment the diagnostic interview in diagnosing bulimia nervosa.

DIFFERENTIAL DIAGNOSIS

- Psychogenic vomiting
- Drug abuse
- GI obstruction
- Hiatal hernia
- Achalasia, gastroesophageal reflux
- Brain tumor

TREATMENT

MEDICATIONS
- Antidepressants
  - Decrease the binge–purge behavior
  - Improve attitudes about eating
  - Lessen preoccupation with food and weight
  - Fluoxetine (Prozac), sertraline (Zoloft), desipramine, citalopram, and fluvoxamine (Luvox) used with good results
  - Antidepressant effect may diminish over time; may relapse when drug stopped
  - Psychotherapy and cognitive behavioral therapy combined with antidepressant therapy appears to have the best outcome.
  - Low response rate to alternative treatments after cognitive behavioral therapy and 1st-line antidepressant therapy
  - Few studies either of medication or psychotherapy in those <18 years of age; however, cognitive behavioral therapy and family-based therapy appear promising
- Stool softeners: Often of little use for constipation; consider nonstimulating osmotic laxatives if severe
- Ondansetron: Shown in 1 study to decrease vomiting frequency; may help normalize the physiologic mechanism controlling satiation.

ADDITIONAL TREATMENT
- Cognitive behavioral therapy (CBT) with family involvement effective
  - Can be done in group or individual formats
  - More effective than interpersonal psychotherapy or behavioral therapy alone
  - Helps patients determine other ways to cope with the feelings that precipitate purging and to try to correct maladaptive thoughts and beliefs about body image
  - May also be effective in a self-help format, including self-help manual format
  - One study of CBT in adolescents showed considerable promise.
- Family-based treatment (FBT): Therapist empowers parents to disrupt behaviors such as binge eating, purging, restrictive eating, and other compensatory behaviors. The treatment has shown positive research outcomes.
- Individual interpersonal psychotherapy (IPT) is helpful but takes longer to have an effect.
- Dialectical behavioral therapy (DBT): Skill-based treatment shown to be helpful for adult patients with binge eating disorder and less severe symptoms of bulimia nervosa.
- Family therapy
- Group therapy
- Outpatient supportive psychotherapy

ADDITIONAL THERAPIES
Physical activity shown in one study to reduce pursuit of thinness and decrease bingeing/purging behavior. Both physical activity and yoga have shown promise as adjunct treatments.

INPATIENT CONSIDERATIONS
Initial Stabilization
Hospitalize in cases of the following:
- Dehydration
- Severe electrolyte disturbances
- Intractable vomiting
- Acute psychiatric emergencies (e.g., suicidal ideation, acute psychosis)
- Medical complication of malnutrition (e.g., aspiration pneumonia, cardiac failure, pancreatitis, Mallory-Weiss syndrome)
- Comorbid diagnosis that interferes with the treatment of the eating disorder (e.g., severe depression, obsessive-compulsive disorder, severe family dysfunction)
- Failure of outpatient therapy

ONGOING CARE

FOLLOW-UP RECOMMENDATIONS
- Reduction in binge and purge episodes may take time.
- Behavioral and thought disorders associated with bulimia nervosa may be of long duration.

Patient Monitoring
Signs to watch for:
- Weight loss or major weight fluctuations
- Electrolyte abnormalities
- Muscle cramps
- Fatigue
- Depression or mood disturbance
- Mood swings/irritability
- Increasing emotional lability
- Menstrual function/irregular menses

PROGNOSIS
Eating disorders have the highest mortality rate of any mental disorder. Reported mortality rates vary between studies. Part of the variance is because those with an eating disorder may ultimately die of heart failure, organ failure, malnutrition, or suicide. Crude mortality rates reported in 2009 were the following:
- 4% for anorexia nervosa
- 3.9% for bulimia nervosa
- 5.2% for eating disorder not otherwise specified
- Most patients have episodic course with trend toward improvement.
- No studies of long-term prognosis in adolescents
- Adult studies: 5- to 10-year follow-up
  - Up to 85% of patients achieve recovery from bulimia nervosa in various studies.
- Poor prognostic indicators: concomitant depression, personality disorder, substance abuse, frequent vomiting
- Good prognostic indicators
  - High motivation for treatment
  - No concurrent disruptive psychopathology
  - Good self-esteem

COMPLICATIONS
- Pulmonary
  - Aspiration pneumonia
  - Pneumomediastinum
- GI
  - Pancreatitis
  - Parotid or salivary gland enlargement
  - Gastric and esophageal irritation and gastroesophageal reflux
  - Mallory-Weiss tears
  - Paralytic ileus (from laxative abuse/hypokalemia)
  - Severe constipation (due to laxative abuse and subsequent dependence)
- Metabolic
  - Hypokalemia (due to laxative abuse/emesis)
  - Secondary cardiac dysrhythmias, myopathy
  - Electrolyte imbalances, including hypomagnesemia; acid–base disturbances
  - Fluid imbalances
  - Hyperamylasemia
  - Edema (secondary to hypoproteinemia or renal sodium and water retention secondary to hypovolemia and secondary hyperaldosteronism)
  - Bone loss (if amenorrhea; significantly more common in anorexia nervosa)
- Dental
  - Enamel erosion
  - Caries and periodontal disease
- Hormonal
  - Irregular menstrual bleeding

ADDITIONAL READING

- Crow SJ, Peterson CB, Swanson SA, et al. Increased mortality in bulimia nervosa and other eating disorders. *Am J Psychiatry*. 2009;166(12):1342–1346.
- Kreipe RE, Birndorf SA. Eating disorders in adolescent and young adults. *Med Clin North Am*. 2000;84(4):1027–1049.
- LeGrange D, Crosby RD, Rathouz PJ, et al. A randomized controlled comparison of family-based treatment and supportive psychotherapy for adolescent bulimia nervosa. *Arch Gen Psychiatry*. 2007; 64(9):1049–1056.
- Lock J. Treatment of adolescent eating disorders: progress and challenges. *Minerva Psichiatr*. 2010; 51(3):207–216.
- Smink FR, van Hoeken D, Hoek HW. Epidemiology of eating disorders: incidence, prevalence, and mortality rates. *Curr Psychiatry Rep*. 2012; 14(4):406–414.

CODES

ICD10
- F50.2 Bulimia nervosa
- F50.9 Eating disorder, unspecified

FAQ
- Q: How do I determine if a patient has anorexia with vomiting or bulimia?
- A: The key feature of anorexia nervosa that distinguishes it from bulimia nervosa is the degree of malnutrition and presence of bingeing. There is a definite crossover between patients with anorexia nervosa and bulimia nervosa. If bingeing and purging is seen in the setting of significant malnutrition and low weight, the patient is diagnosed with anorexia nervosa.
- Q: What laboratory abnormalities should I look for in my patients with bulimia?
- A: Electrolyte abnormalities, particularly hypokalemia. Patients may develop a hypochloremic metabolic alkalosis. If electrolytes are significantly abnormal, hospitalize until normalized.

C1 ESTERASE INHIBITOR DEFICIENCY

Judith Kelsen

BASICS

DESCRIPTION

- A hereditary and acquired form of recurrent angioedema. The attacks are usually without urticaria.
- Has been classified into a number of types, including
  - Hereditary angioedema (HAE) type I (transmitted as autosomal dominant)
  - HAE type II (transmitted as autosomal dominant)
  - Acquired angioedema (AAE) types I, II, III, and IV
- HAE type I
  - Accounts for ~85% of the C1 esterase deficiencies, insufficient levels of normal C1-esterase inhibitor (C1-INH) protein due to a genetic alteration that leads to impairment of messenger RNA (mRNA) transcription or translation and therefore decreased enzyme synthesis. Often thought of as quantitative deficiency.
- HAE type II
  - Patients have normal levels of less functional C1-INH. May be thought of as a qualitative deficiency.
- HAE type III
  - An estrogen-dependent form; typical clinical features of type I with normal C1-INH level and function and normal C4
  - These cases are all female and have dominant mode of inheritance; poorly understood mechanism.
- In acquired deficiency of C1-INH, there appears to be a normal ability to synthesize the enzyme; however, the enzyme is metabolized at an increased rate. This syndrome may be seen in patients with autoimmune diseases or malignancy and usually occurs after the 4th decade of life.
- AAE type I
  - Very rare syndrome usually associated with lymphoproliferative (usually B-cell) carcinomas, autoimmune diseases, and paraproteinemias. Because of the other disease processes, complement-activating factors and idiotype–anti-idiotype complexes act to increase consumption of C1-INH.
- AAE type II
  - Develops when an autoantibody is produced against the C1-INH protein. When these antibodies adhere to the C1-INH molecule, conformational change occurs, leading to decreased function or enhanced metabolism. This type is often associated with autoimmune disorders.
- AAE type III
  - Associated with sex hormones (specifically in pregnancy)
- AAE type IV
  - Drug-induced AAE, particularly associated with ACE inhibitors or angiotensin receptor blockers
- AAE forms may be differentiated from HAE by genetic studies and serologically by significantly decreased C1q, C1r, and C1s levels and decreased functional activity of the enzyme in AAE.

EPIDEMIOLOGY

Incidence

1:50,000

Genetics

HAE types I and II are transmitted as autosomal dominant.

PATHOPHYSIOLOGY

- C1-INH is a single-chain polypeptide with a molecular weight of 108 kD. The gene has been identified on chromosome 11 (11q12–q13.1). It is involved in the control of vascular permeability.
- C1-INH is a member of the serpin family of serine protease inhibitors produced in the liver.
- This protein inhibits the classic complement pathway by inhibiting activation of C2 and C4. In the fibrinolytic system, C1-INH inhibits formation of plasmin, the activation of C1r and C1s, and the formation of bradykinin from kininogen.
- Deficiency of this enzyme results in activation of the classic complement system along with fibrinolysis and kinin formation, which is felt to participate in the production of angioedema.
- Kinin is known to cause similar histologic lesions to histamine but without pruritus.
- The complement activation leads to production of C2b, a product that also has kinin-like activity, and bradykinin, a vasoactive peptide that may also participate in the formation of angioedema.

DIAGNOSIS

HISTORY

- Presentation: Patients with HAE usually present in the 2nd decade of life with angioedema involving the subcutaneous tissues (mostly involving the extremities).
- Attacks can be precipitated by trauma, infection, or pregnancy.
- Timing
  - Classically, the edema develops gradually over several hours and increases slowly over 12–36 hours.
- GI effects
  - Predominant symptom in 25% of patients
  - Patients may experience abdominal attacks with sudden and very severe onset without visible edema.
  - Angioedema involving the GI tract may lead to severe pain, vomiting, and diarrhea as well as ascites.
  - Secondary to transient edema of small bowel resulting in intestinal obstruction, ascites, and hemoconcentration
- Respiratory complications: 2 of 3 patients will have orofacial or laryngeal swelling.
- Hives: The edema usually occurs without evidence of inflammation; rash resembles urticaria (however, episodes of urticaria have also been documented).
- The variability of clinical manifestations, even among individuals with the same genetic mutation, is striking, implicating nongenetic factors or other genes as possible mediators of clinical presentation.
- Emesis
- Diarrhea
- Hypotension from extravasation of plasma into the skin
- Hemoconcentration
- Azotemia
- CNS complaints, including headache, hemiparesis, and seizures, may be triggered by trauma or stress.
- AAE presents similarly, in the same way but usually in the 4th decade of life; not associated with a familial history.

PHYSICAL EXAM

Depending on the clinical features, angioedema causes pale, well-demarcated, tense, brawny, nonpruritic, and nonpitting single or multiple localized swellings. These may involve the periorbital tissues, genitalia, face, tongue, lips, larynx, extremities, and GI tract.

DIAGNOSTIC TESTS & INTERPRETATION

Lab

- C1-INH concentration
- C1-INH activity
- C4 concentration: low serum level
- C4D: cleavage product of C4, low even when C4 is normal
- C1q concentration (usually lower in patients with AAE)

DIFFERENTIAL DIAGNOSIS

- IgE mediated
  - Episodic angioedema
  - Allergic reactions to food and drugs
  - Physically induced angioedema
- Hypocomplemententemic HAE
- Idiosyncratic
  - NSAIDs
  - Other drugs
- Lupus erythematosus
- Idiopathic

TREATMENT

GENERAL MEASURES

- During an acute episode, management focuses on adequate respiratory and fluid resuscitation and the treatment of pain.
- In HAE, acute attacks are treated with replacement of the C1-INH with IV concentrates. Fresh frozen plasma may also be used.
- Recent studies have shown benefit with recombinant human C1-INH for acute attacks and prophylaxis.
- A recent study has demonstrated that the time to onset of symptom relief is an appropriate end point for assessing the efficacy of C1-INH therapy.
- For prophylaxis, androgens (such as danazol and stanozolol) are used in postpubertal patients with HAE of both types. These androgens stimulate the synthesis of C1-INH, and although the level of activity is not normalized, it is increased sufficiently to be clinically efficacious.
- In prepubertal children, androgens are used only in those with severe attacks; purified C1-INH can be used if available. Antifibrinolytics should be used in prepubertal children over androgens.
- Patients should avoid estrogen oral contraceptive pills (OCPs) or use with caution.
- For patients who do not tolerate androgens, tranexamic acid and ε-aminocaproic acid (antifibrinolytic inhibitors or plasmin activity) may be used, although they carry the risk of significant side effects.
- AAE type I patients may respond to epinephrine for reversal of airway compromise.
- AAE type I requires an intensive search for malignancy, although this form of AAE occasionally appears before the development of clinical signs of the malignancy.
- Androgens are also effective in preventing attacks in individuals with this syndrome.
- AAE type II requires immunosuppression to decrease formation of the autoantibody.
- These patients may respond to C1-INH concentrate.
- Androgen treatment has not led to good clinical response.
- Prophylaxis prior to dental procedures or surgery: high-dose danazol
- Potential treatment: plasma kallikrein antagonists, bradykinin antagonists, serine protease inhibitors
- Genetic counseling: Given the autosomal dominant inheritance, family counseling is important.

INPATIENT CONSIDERATIONS

Initial Stabilization

Therapy is divided into management of the acute attack, maintenance therapy for HAE, and more specific interventions for those with AAE.

ADDITIONAL READING

- Agostoni A, Aygoren-Pursun E, Binkley KE, et al. Hereditary and acquired angioedema: problems and progress: proceedings of the third C1 esterase inhibitor deficiency workshop and beyond. *J Allergy Clin Immunol*. 2004;114(3)(Suppl):S51–S131.
- Bernstein J. Hereditary angioedema: validation of the endpoint time to onset of relief by correlation with symptom intensity. *Asthma Allergy Proc*. 2011;32(1):36–42.
- Csepregi A, Nemesanszky E. Acquired C1 esterase inhibitor deficiency. *Ann Intern Med*. 2000;133(10):838–839.
- Frank MM. Update on preventive therapy (prophylaxis) of hereditary angioedema. *Asthma Allergy Proc*. 2011;32(1):17–21.
- Gompels M, Lock R, Abinun M. C1 inhibitor deficiency: consensus document. *Clin Exp Immunol*. 2005;139(3):379–394.
- Riedl MA. Update on the acute treatment of hereditary angioedema. *Asthma Allergy Proc*. 2011;32(1):11–16.
- Weiler C, van Dellen R. Genetic tests indications and interpretations in patients with hereditary angioedema. *Mayo Clin Proc*. 2006;81(7):958–972.

CODES

ICD10

D84.1 Defects in the complement system

FAQ

- Q: What are other causes of angioedema?
- A:
  - Classic allergic reactions to food and drugs
  - Physically induced angioedema
  - IgE-mediated episodic angioedema
  - Idiosyncratic reactions to nonsteroidal anti-inflammatory and other drugs
  - Lupus erythematosus
  - Idiopathic causes
- Q: What are the usual precipitating factors in causing reactions?
- A: Recurrent episodes of angioedema, abdominal pain, nausea, and vomiting that occur spontaneously or after local trauma, especially to the upper respiratory tract:
  - Vigorous exercise
  - Emotional stress
  - Menstruation

CAMPYLOBACTER INFECTIONS

Matthew P. Kronman

BASICS

DESCRIPTION

- *Campylobacter* species are motile, curved, gram-negative bacilli that are commensal flora of birds, pigs, and cattle and commonly cause bacterial gastroenteritis in humans.

EPIDEMIOLOGY

- *Campylobacter* infections are among the most common causes of enteritis worldwide, with the highest attack rates in children <4 years.
- Asymptomatic infection occurs in 30–100% of chickens, turkeys, and water fowl. Other reservoirs of infection include swine, cattle, sheep, horses, rodents, and household pets (especially young pets).
- Contaminated water and unpasteurized milk are other sources of infection.
- Infections typically occur sporadically, without outbreaks.

Incidence

- Estimated rates of *Campylobacter* infection vary widely worldwide. In the United States, the estimated annual incidence in 2012 was 14.3/100,000 overall, 14% higher than in 2006–2008 (95% CI, 7–21%).
- The highest U.S. incidence is for those <5 years at 24.08/100,000 population.
- Among speciated U.S. infections, 90% were *C. jejuni* and 8% were *C. coli*. Of all U.S. infections, 15% resulted in hospitalization and 0.1% in death.
- The incidence is seasonal and generally peaks in summer worldwide.

Prevalence

- Although surveillance data are limited, the highest prevalence of *Campylobacter* infections occur in resource-poor settings.
- *Campylobacter* is the most common cause of travelers' diarrhea in Southeast Asia, accounting for a third of all infections.

RISK FACTORS

- Approximately 40% of *Campylobacter* enteritis is estimated to be attributable to undercooked chicken consumption, which had an odds ratio (OR) of 3.4 (95% CI, 2.2–4.5) for infection.
- Other risk factors for *Campylobacter* enteritis include international travel (OR 4.9, 95% CI, 2.9–8.2), direct contact with farm animals (OR 2.6, 95% CI, 2.0–3.4), chronic disease, poor food preparation hygiene, consumption of chicken prepared outside the home, and use of acid-suppressive medications.
- Children are at higher risk relative to adults.
- Frequent exposure to *Campylobacter* (e.g., among food handlers and abattoir workers) may protect against disease.
- Person-to-person transmission of *C. jejuni* has been reported when index cases were young children incontinent of feces or as vertical transmission from mother to neonate.
- Asymptomatic hospital personnel or food handlers have not been implicated as sources.

GENERAL PREVENTION

- Hand washing after contact with animals or animal products, cleaning cooking utensils and cutting boards after contact with raw poultry, proper cooling and storage of foods, pasteurization of milk, and chlorination of water supplies decrease the risk for infection.
- Diapered infants with symptomatic infection should be excluded from child care until resolution of diarrhea.
- No licensed vaccines currently exist, but *C. jejuni* strains with decreased risk of secondary Guillain-Barré syndrome (GBS) are being developed as candidates for capsular polysaccharide conjugate vaccines.

PATHOPHYSIOLOGY

- Transmission of disease is by the fecal–oral route from contaminated food and water or by direct contact with fecal material from animals or persons infected with the organism.
- As few as 500 organisms may be required to produce infection.
- *Campylobacter* spp. possess 1 or 2 flagella that provide the organism's motility and facilitate intestinal colonization.
- *C. jejuni* adheres to epithelial cells and mucus, secretes cytotoxins (which play a role in the development of watery diarrhea), can invade intestinal epithelial cells using a microtubule entry system, and induces an inflammatory ileocolitis.
- *Campylobacter* can cause a range of clinical manifestations, including enteritis and rare localized extraintestinal infections.
- Bacteremia, although uncommon, can occur, especially in the neonate and immunocompromised host; *C. fetus* is the species most likely to be isolated. *C. fetus* can also cause neonatal meningitis.
- *C. upsaliensis*, *C. lari*, and *C. hyointestinalis* have been identified in immunocompromised individuals and are usually associated with a self-limiting enteritis but can occasionally cause systemic illness.

ETIOLOGY

- *Campylobacter* is a motile, curved, microaerophilic, non–lactose-fermenting, oxidase-positive, gram-negative rod that requires oxygen and carbon dioxide for optimal growth.
- Three main *Campylobacter* species involved in human infections include *C. jejuni*, *C. coli* (which cause enteritis), and *C. fetus* (implicated in systemic illness in neonates and compromised hosts). Rarer human pathogens include *C. concisus*, *C. curvus*, *C. hyointestinalis*, *C. lari*, *C. rectus*, *C. sputorum*, and *C. upsaliensis*.

COMMONLY ASSOCIATED CONDITIONS

Campylobacteriosis occurs in both healthy and immunocompromised individuals.

DIAGNOSIS

HISTORY

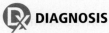

- Enteritis is characterized by fever, abdominal pain, and bloody diarrhea.
- Symptoms can last for 24 hours and be indistinguishable from viral gastroenteritis or appendicitis, or can be relapsing, thus mimicking inflammatory bowel disease.
- In some patients, illness can be severe, resembling dysentery.
- Incubation period is usually 2–5 days and is usually self-limited by 5–7 days.

PHYSICAL EXAM

- Abdominal pain, diarrhea, malaise, and fever are common signs and symptoms of infection.
- Stools can contain occult or visible blood.
- Inflammatory ileocolitis is the most common manifestation in children.
- If the infection establishes a chronic phase (20% of infected patients), symptoms may mimic inflammatory bowel disease and other immunoreactive complications may occur.

ALERT
Not all bacterial colitis presents with blood or mucus in the stool. Therefore, increased suspicion for bacterial colitis should exist if the diarrhea is prolonged or the patient has appropriate exposures.

DIAGNOSTIC TESTS & INTERPRETATION

Lab

- Stool culture requires selective media (Skirrow, Butzler, or campy-BAP), microaerophilic conditions, and an incubation temperature of 42°C to isolate important *Campylobacter* species.
- *C. fetus*, *C. hyointestinalis*, and *C. upsaliensis* may not be detected on *Campylobacter*-selective media due to their sensitivity to antimicrobial agents in the media.

Imaging

Imaging is not often required for diagnosis.

Diagnostic Procedures/Other

- Rapid DNA-based testing to detect and differentiate *Campylobacter* spp. from other enteropathogens is being developed and has moderate sensitivity compared to the current gold standard of stool culture.

Pathologic Findings

- Examination of fecal specimen for darting motility of *C. jejuni* by darkfield or phase-contrast microscopy within 2 hours of passage can permit presumptive diagnosis.

DIFFERENTIAL DIAGNOSIS

- *Campylobacter* infection should be considered in all patients with a diarrheal illness, especially those with blood or mucus in their stool, recurrent gastritis, or in immunocompromised hosts.
- Symptoms can overlap with those of appendicitis or inflammatory bowel disease.
- Additional intestinal bacterial pathogens include *Aeromonas*, *Campylobacter*, *Clostridium difficile*, *Escherichia coli*, *Listeria*, *Plesiomonas*, *Salmonella*, *Shigella*, *Vibrio* species, and *Yersinia*.
- Other viral and parasitic pathogens include amebiasis, adenovirus types 40 and 41, *Cryptosporidium*, *Cyclospora*, *Cystoisospora*, *Giardia*, norovirus, and rotavirus.

TREATMENT

MEDICATION

- Most patients have self-limited infection.
- Select patient populations (HIV and other immunocompromised individuals, pregnant women) may benefit from early therapy.
- If treated in the first 3 days of enteritis, erythromycin (for 5 days) or azithromycin (for 3 days) appear effective in eradicating the organism from the stool within 2–3 days and shortening the course of diarrhea.
- Ciprofloxacin, tetracycline, aminoglycosides, and imipenem are alternatives if resistant or bacteremic strains are present, although fluoroquinolone resistance is increasingly common and thought to be related to human and agricultural antibiotic use.
- Macrolide resistance is approximately 5%.
- Treatment duration for enteritis is 3–5 days.
- Appropriate bacteremia treatment should be based on antimicrobial susceptibility testing.

ADDITIONAL TREATMENT

General Measures

Immunocompetent children with diarrhea usually improve with rehydration alone.

ISSUES FOR REFERRAL

Specific follow-up is unnecessary.

ADDITIONAL THERAPIES

Antimotility agents can prolong symptoms and should be avoided.

INPATIENT CONSIDERATIONS

Initial Stabilization

Correct initial dehydration.

Admission Criteria

Admit those requiring IV fluids.

IV Fluids

Use normal saline to correct dehydration. IV fluids should contain dextrose if being used for maintenance fluid requirements.

Nursing

Contact precautions are recommended for admitted infected infants and children incontinent of stool and should be maintained until they receive 48 hours of antibiotics.

Discharge Criteria

Discharge rehydrated patients able to maintain hydration orally.

ONGOING CARE

FOLLOW-UP RECOMMENDATIONS

Patient Monitoring

In untreated patients, the median organism excretion is 2–3 weeks but can be up to 3 months. Asymptomatic carriage is uncommon.

DIET

Avoid undercooked poultry and unpasteurized milk. Resume a normal diet when tolerated.

PATIENT EDUCATION

Symptoms resolve in 1 week for most people.

PROGNOSIS

For patients with enteritis, the prognosis is very good, regardless of whether antibiotic treatment is given.

COMPLICATIONS

- Postinfectious immunologic complications include reactive arthritis, GBS, Miller-Fisher syndrome (a GBS variant predominantly affecting eye movement), reactive arthritis, and erythema nodosum.
- GBS is estimated to affect 1 in 1,000 patients with *Campylobacter* infection.
- *C. jejuni* (serotypes O:19 and O:41) is the most frequently identified GBS cause and is responsible for up to 40% of U.S. GBS cases.
- HLA-B27 antigen is associated with reactive arthropathy. The estimated incidence of reactive arthritis after *Campylobacter* infection ranges from 0 to 7%.
- Children with high fever may develop seizures.
- Some studies have demonstrated associations between *Campylobacter* infection and both irritable bowel syndrome and inflammatory bowel disease.
- Spontaneous abortion and hemolytic uremic syndrome are described with *C. upsaliensis*.

ADDITIONAL READING

- Centers for Disease Control and Prevention. Incidence and trends of infection with pathogens transmitted commonly through food—foodborne diseases active surveillance network, 10 U.S. sites, 1996–2012. *MMWR Morb Mortal Wkly Rep*. 2013;62(15):283–287.
- Domingues AR, Pires SM, Halasa T, et al. Source attribution of human campylobacteriosis using a meta-analysis of case-control studies of sporadic infections. *Epidemiol Infect*. 2012;140(6):970–981.
- Kirkpatrick BD, Tribble DR. Update on human *Campylobacter jejuni* infections. *Curr Opin Gastroenterol*. 2011;27(1):1–7.
- Lal A, Hales S, French N, et al. Seasonality in human zoonotic enteric diseases: a systematic review. *PLoS One*. 2012;7(4):e31883.
- Liu J, Gratz J, Amour C, et al. A laboratory-developed Taqman Array Card for simultaneous detection of 19 enteropathogens. *J Clin Microbiol*. 2013;51(2):472–480.
- Ross AGP, Olds GR, Cripps AW, et al. Enteropathogens and chronic illness in returning travelers. *N Engl J Med*. 2013;368(19):1817–1825.

CODES

ICD10

A04.5 Campylobacter enteritis

FAQ

- Q: Is treatment necessary for asymptomatic children when *Campylobacter* is isolated as the pathogen causing the enteritis?
- A: No treatment is needed in this situation.
- Q: Can one develop immunity to *Campylobacter* infections?
- A: Immunity to *C. jejuni* is acquired after 1 or more infections. For children living in endemic areas, effective natural immunity is a result of significant repeated early exposure.
- Q: How are *C. jejuni* infection and GBS related?
- A: Many strains of *C. jejuni* have surface glycolipids that are similar to gangliosides, which are abundant in the central and peripheral nervous systems. Anti-*Campylobacter* antibodies bind to the gangliosides through molecular mimicry, causing the demyelinating process characteristic of GBS.

CANCER THERAPY LATE EFFECTS

Kelly L. Neale • Tiffany Chang

BASICS

DESCRIPTION

The majority of children diagnosed with cancer will reach adulthood. Childhood cancer survivors require unique medical follow-up. Risks of late effects depend on the treatments received as well as the type and site of cancer. The Children's Oncology Group's long-term follow-up guidelines serve as the basis for many of the recommendations in this chapter.

EPIDEMIOLOGY

- Long-term survival into adulthood for a child diagnosed with cancer is nearly 80%.
- Among adults treated for childhood cancer:
  - Nearly 2/3 of survivors will develop one or more chronic health condition.
  - Nearly 1/3 of survivors will experience severe or life-threatening complications during adulthood.
- Approximately 270,000 childhood cancer survivors live in the United States.
- These numbers will continue to grow as new cancer therapies become available and more children survive.

RISK FACTORS

Late effects of cancer therapy are influenced by tumor-related treatment and host-related factors.

PATHOPHYSIOLOGY

Risk of organ dysfunction is related to primary cancer location and treatment used. See detailed systems-based evaluations in the following sections.

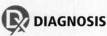

DIAGNOSIS

HISTORY

It is essential for the primary care physician to obtain a thorough cancer treatment summary, including the following:

- Date of diagnosis/age at diagnosis
- Type of cancer, stage, histology
- Site of primary tumor and metastatic sites
- Relapse(s) and date(s)
- Treatment modalities
  - Significant surgical procedures
  - Treatment protocol(s)
  - Chemotherapy
    - Drugs and cumulative dosages
    - Age of first anthracycline therapy
  - Radiation therapy (XRT)
    - Type
    - Site/dose
    - Total/boost doses
  - Hematopoietic stem cell transplant (HSCT)
    - Type and date of transplant
    - Source: bone marrow, cord blood, or peripheral blood stem cells
    - Conditioning regimen
  - Immunotherapy: types/cumulative doses

PHYSICAL EXAM

Annual physical exam of the entire body with particular attention to organ systems as listed in the following sections

SCREENING TESTS & INTERPRETATION (BY AT-RISK ORGAN SYSTEM)

Bladder Toxicity

- Chronic infections
  - Risk factors: cystectomy
- Hemorrhagic cystitis
  - Risk factors: ≥30 Gy XRT to spine, flank, abdomen, pelvis, bladder, or total body irradiation (TBI)
- Bladder fibrosis and hemorrhagic cystitis
  - Risk factors: cyclophosphamide, ifosfamide
- Urinary incontinence or tract obstruction
  - Risk factors: pelvic surgery, hysterectomy
- Screen with annual urinalysis and detailed voiding history.

Bone Toxicity

- Decreased bone mineral density, osteopenia, osteonecrosis, increased risk of fractures
  - Risk factors: corticosteroids, methotrexate, ≥40 Gy XRT to any field, or HSCT
  - Evaluate bone density with DEXA scan.
- Scoliosis or kyphosis
  - Risk factors: spine or thoracic surgery, XRT to spine, chest, lungs, or abdomen
  - Spine exam annually until growth is complete
- Bone growth failure
  - Risk factors: XRT to any field, especially cranium, spine, trunk, or TBI
  - Measure height, weight, sitting height yearly.

Cardiovascular Toxicity

- Cardiomyopathy, left ventricular dysfunction, and arrhythmias
  - Risk factors: anthracyclines (daunorubicin, doxorubicin/Adriamycin, epirubicin, idarubicin, mitoxantrone) and/or XRT to the thorax or abdomen
  - Frequency of echocardiogram (ECHO)/multigated acquisition (MUGA) depends on cumulative dose of anthracyclines, age at first dose, and field of XRT (involving heart).
  - Consider close monitoring during pregnancy.
- Carotid artery or subclavian artery disease
  - Risk factors: ≥40 Gy XRT to head, neck, chest, lungs, or TBI
  - Examine for carotid bruits or diminished carotid/brachial/radial pulses.

ALERT

Anthracycline, antibiotics and XRT to the heart/chest/lungs/neck increases risk of cardiovascular disease; at-risk patients require detailed history, exam, and frequent ECHO/MUGA screening.

- Thrombosis at prior central venous catheter site
  - Inspect site for pain/swelling
- Dyslipidemia
  - Risk factors: TBI
  - Screen with fasting lipid panel every 2 years.
- Vasospastic attacks (Raynaud phenomenon)
  - Risk factors: vincristine or vinblastine

Dermatologic Toxicity

- Skin cancer, dysplastic nevi, fibrosis, alopecia, telangiectasias, nail/pigmentation changes
  - Risk factors: any XRT, HSCT with chronic graft-versus-host disease (cGVHD)
  - Encourage monthly self-skin exams.

Endocrine Toxicity

- Thyroid dysfunction, nodules, and cancer
  - Risk factors: XRT to neck, head, spine, mediastinum, TBI, or therapeutic systemic metaiodobenzylguanidine (MIBG)
  - Thyroid exam and TSH/free T_4 annually
- Growth hormone deficiency
  - Risk factors: XRT to cranium or TBI
  - Height, weight, BMI, Tanner stage every 6 months until mature, then annually
  - If at risk: insulin-like growth factor (IGF)-1, IGF-2, and IGFBP-3
- Central adrenal insufficiency
  - Risk factors: ≥30 Gy XRT to cranium, TBI
  - Screen: annual endocrinology visit
- Hyperprolactinemia
  - Risk factors: ≥40 Gy XRT to cranium, TBI
  - If symptomatic, screen with prolactin level
- Hypopituitarism
  - Risk factors: neurosurgery of brain, ≥30 Gy XRT to cranium, TBI
  - Screening labs: cortisol, prolactin, testosterone/estradiol, IGF-1, TSH, FSH, LH
- Obesity
  - Risk factors: XRT to cranium, brain neurosurgery
  - Height, weight, BMI, BP annually

Gastrointestinal Toxicity

- Esophageal stricture
  - Risk factors: ≥30 Gy XRT to spine, neck, chest, lung, mediastinum, mantle, abdomen, TBI or HSCT with cGVHD
- Cholelithiasis
  - Risk factors: ≥30 Gy XRT to abdomen, flank, liver, kidneys, TBI
- Strictures, fistula, chronic enterocolitis
  - Risk factors: ≥30 Gy XRT to neck, chest, spine, abdomen, liver, kidneys, pelvis, TBI
- Bowel obstruction/adhesions
  - Risk factors: laparotomy or ≥30 Gy XRT to abdomen, pelvis, or spine
- Fecal incontinence
  - Risk factors: pelvic or spinal cord surgery, cystectomy

Hepatic Toxicity

- Chronic hepatitis C
  - Risk factor: blood products prior to 1993
  - Screen with Hep C antibody, PCR if positive
- Hepatic dysfunction
  - Risk factors: methotrexate, mercaptopurine (6-MP), thioguanine (6-TG), HSCT
- Veno-occlusive disease
  - Risk factors: mercaptopurine or thioguanine
- Baseline: ALT/AST/bili; ferritin after HSCT

Neurologic Toxicity

- Peripheral neuropathy
  - Risk factors: cisplatin, carboplatin, vincristine, or vinblastine
- Cerebrovascular complications
  - Risk factors: ≥18 Gy XRT to cranium or TBI
- Neurocognitive difficulties
  - Risk factors: brain neurosurgery, methotrexate, high-dose IV cytarabine, XRT to cranium, TBI
- Seizures, motor/sensory deficits, or hydrocephalus following brain neurosurgery

- Clinical leukoencephalopathy following methotrexate, high-dose IV cytarabine, or XRT to cranium or TBI
- Neuropathic pain risk following amputation
- Neurogenic bowel/bladder, incontinence, sexual dysfunction risk after spinal cord neurosurgery

Ophthalmologic Toxicity
- Cataracts/ocular issues
  - Risk factors: corticosteroids, busulfan, XRT to orbit/eye, cranium, or TBI
  - Annual funduscopic and visual acuity exams
  - Annual ophthalmologist exam as indicated

Ototoxicity
- Hearing loss, vertigo, or tinnitus
  - Risk factors: cisplatin, carboplatin: myeloablative or any does <1 year; XRT ≥30 Gy to ear, cranium, or TBI
  - Baseline audiogram (annually if loss detected)
  - Otoscopic exam annually

Oral Toxicity
- Tooth enamel dysplasia and root/tooth agenesis or root thinning/shortening
  - Risk factors: any chemotherapy (particularly at a young age), XRT to head/neck
- Xerostomia or salivary gland dysfunction
  - Risk factors: head/neck XRT or cGVHD
- Osteoradionecrosis
  - Risk factors: ≥40 Gy XRT to head, neck, TBI
- Oral exam annually; dental cleaning and exam every 6 months

Pulmonary Toxicity
- Fibrosis, dyspnea, decreased lung function
  - Risk factors: bleomycin, busulfan, carmustine, lomustine, XRT to chest or lungs, or TBI
  - If at risk, obtain baseline pulmonary function testing, and as clinically indicated

Psychosocial Disorders
- Neurocognitive, educational, or vocational difficulties
  - Risk factors: any treatment, especially methotrexate, high-dose cytarabine, brain neurosurgery or XRT to head or TBI
  - Educational/vocational assessment annually
  - Formal neuropsychological evaluation as indicated
- Posttraumatic stress, depression, anxiety, risky behaviors, body image disturbance
  - Risk factors: any cancer treatment
  - Assess mental health at each clinic visit.

Renal Toxicity
- Hypertension or renal dysfunction
  - Risk factors: nephrectomy or carboplatin, cisplatin, ifosfamide, methotrexate, or XRT to liver, kidneys, flank, abdomen, TBI, or HSCT
- Hydronephrosis, dysfunctional voiding, vesicoureteral reflux
  - Risk factors: cyclophosphamide, ifosfamide, ≥30 Gy XRT to abdomen, flank, or pelvis
- Urinary incontinence or tract obstruction
  - Risk factor: pelvic surgery
- Baseline: BUN/Cr, Na/K/Cl/CO2, Mg, Phos, Ca
- Annual UA and BP if at risk or after nephrectomy

Reproductive Toxicity
- Gonadal dysfunction: infertility, azoospermia, oligospermia, hypogonadism, delayed or arrested puberty, sexual dysfunction, early menopause
  - Risk factors: spinal neurosurgery, orchiectomy, alkylating agents (busulfan, carmustine, chlorambucil, cyclophosphamide, ifosfamide, lomustine, mechlorethamine, melphalan, procarbazine, thiotepa), carboplatin, cisplatin, dacarbazine, temozolomide, XRT to gonads, pelvis, abdomen, cranium, or TBI
  - Assess Tanner stage yearly until mature.
  - Males: Screen with FSH/LH/testosterone at 14 years or if symptomatic and semen analysis as requested.
  - Females: Screen with FSH/LH/estradiol at 13 years or with delayed puberty/amenorrhea/irregular menses/estrogen deficiency symptoms.

Subsequent Neoplasms
- Increased risk varies by host factors, primary cancer therapy, and environmental exposures.
- The Childhood Cancer Survivor Study reported a 30-year cumulative incidence of 20.5%.
- The risk of subsequent neoplasms (SNs) remains elevated for more than 30 years following primary cancer diagnosis.
- Patients with genetic cancer predisposition syndromes are at increased risk of SNs.
- 80% of SNs are solid tumors and demonstrate a strong relationship with ionizing radiation.
- Blood cancer: acute lymphoblastic leukemia (ALL), acute myeloid leukemia (AML) and therapy-related myelodysplastic syndrome (t-MDS)
  - Risk factors: alkylating agents, anthracyclines, carboplatin, cisplatin, dacarbazine, temozolomide
  - Topoisomerase II inhibitor–associated AML occurs 6 months to 3 years after exposure.
  - Alkylating agent–associated t-MDS/AML occurs 3–5 years after exposure.
  - Screen with annual complete blood count with differential for 10 years following treatment.
  - Perform dermatologic exam for petechiae, purpura, and pallor at each visit.
- Bladder cancer
  - Risk factors: cyclophosphamide, XRT to bladder, prostate, abdomen, pelvis, vagina, flank, inguinal region, or sacral/whole spine
  - Obtain annual detailed voiding history.
- Bone cancer in any XRT field
  - Perform annual inspection/palpation of the bones/soft tissues/skin in XRT field.
- Brain tumors
  - Risk factors: XRT to cranium or TBI
  - Perform annual neurologic exam.
- Breast cancer
  - Risk factors: XRT to chest, lungs, mediastinum, axilla, mantle, or TBI
  - Annual breast exam from puberty to age 25 years; after age 25 years, perform every 6 months
  - ≥20 Gy XRT: annual mammogram and breast MRI beginning at age 25 or 8 years post XRT (whichever is last); 10–19 Gy XRT: consider testing
- Colorectal cancer
  - Risk factors: ≥30 Gy XRT to spine, liver, kidneys, flank, abdomen, pelvis, or TBI
  - Perform colonoscopy at age 35 years or 10 years after XRT (whichever is last), every 5 years.
  - Familial adenomatous polyposis (FAP), start colonoscopy at 21 years; hereditary nonpolysis colorectal cancer (HNPCC), start at puberty
- Skin cancer
  - Risk factors: any XRT
  - Perform annual dermatologic exam in XRT field.
  - Encourage monthly self-skin exams.
- Thyroid cancer
  - Risk factors: XRT to cranium, neck, spine, supraclavicular, mediastinum, mantle, chest, lungs, or TBI
  - Perform annual thyroid exam.

TREATMENT

Treatment depends on long-term effects; see previous discussion for organ system-specific follow-up care.

ONGOING CARE

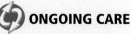

- Regular visits with primary care provider and oncologist or long-term follow-up program
- Dental exams and cleanings every 6 months
- Promptly assess signs or symptoms of SNs.
- Assess psychosocial functioning at each visit.
- Maintain health insurance coverage.
- Immunizations may require updates.

ALERT
- Reimmunize after chemotherapy per oncologist and using Centers for Disease Control and Prevention (CDC) guidelines.
- Psychosocial assessment of the patient should be performed at each clinic visit.

ADDITIONAL READING

- Armstrong GT, Liu Q, Yasui Y, et al. Late mortality among 5-year survivors of childhood cancer: a summary from the Childhood Cancer Survivor Study. *J Clin Oncol*. 2009;27(14):2328–2338.
- Centers for Disease Control and Prevention. Immunization schedules. http://www.cdc.gov/vaccines/schedules/. Accessed February 5, 2015.
- Children's Oncology Group. Long-term follow-up guidelines for survivors of childhood, adolescent, and young adult cancers. http://www.survivorshipguidelines.org/. Accessed February 5, 2015.
- Oeffinger KC, Mertens AC, Sklar CA, et al. Chronic health conditions in adult survivors of childhood cancer. *N Engl J Med*. 2006;355(15):1572–1582. PMID: 17035650.

CODES

ICD10
- T88.7XXS Unspecified adverse effect of drug or medicament, sequela
- Z85 Personal history of malignant neoplasm
- Z92.21 Personal history of antineoplastic chemotherapy

FAQ

- Q: Who is considered a cancer "survivor"?
- A: Anyone from time of cancer diagnosis until end of life. Many long-term follow-up clinics specialize in patients who are 2 years post cancer therapy.
- Q: Where can I find the latest long-term follow-up guidelines for childhood cancer survivors?
- A: http://www.survivorshipguidelines.org/

CANDIDIASIS

Jessica E. Ericson • Daniel K. Benjamin, Jr.

BASICS

DESCRIPTION

Infection caused by species of the yeast, *Candida*; encompasses a spectrum of disease depending on host factors:

- Mucosal infection: oral thrush, esophagitis, vaginitis
- Cutaneous infection: diaper dermatitis, intertriginous dermatitis
- Disseminated candidiasis: candidemia, hepatosplenic candidiasis, meningitis, endocarditis, endophthalmitis

EPIDEMIOLOGY

Incidence

- Mucosal: Thrush occurs in ~5% of normal newborns.
- Disseminated: 3rd most common cause of bloodstream infection in hospitalized patients

RISK FACTORS

Immunocompromise (HIV, malignancy, neutropenia, transplant recipient, corticosteroid use), prematurity, burn injury, central venous catheter, parenteral nutrition, broad-spectrum antibiotic use

GENERAL PREVENTION

- Sterilize bottle nipples and toys to prevent reinfection with oral candidiasis.
- Avoid unnecessary broad-spectrum antibiotic use and limit duration when used.
- Remove indwelling IV catheters as soon as possible and maintain sterility with line care.
- Prophylaxis is indicated for some high-risk populations (preterm infants <750 g in high-incidence nurseries, neutropenic patients).

ETIOLOGY

- 20% of patients have GI or respiratory tract colonization. Neonatal colonization is acquired from infected vaginal mucosa during birth. Incidence of colonization increases with age of the infant especially if exposed to antibiotics or poor hand washing. Colonization increases the risk of invasive infection.
- *Candida albicans* is the most common species isolated in children; non-*albicans* species are increasing in incidence: *Candida parapsilosis* > *Candida glabrata* > *Candida lusitaniae* > *Candida krusei* > other.

COMMONLY ASSOCIATED CONDITIONS

Candida spp. may cause disease at any site.

- Mucosal candidiasis
  - Oropharyngeal candidiasis (thrush) occurs in 5% of normal infants. In older children, it is associated with use of antibiotics, inhaled corticosteroids or immunosuppressive drugs, conditions of endocrine or immune dysfunction, and malignancy.
  - Perlèche (angular cheilosis) is characterized by fissuring, erythema, and pain at the corners of the mouth; more common in children who lick their lips frequently or have vitamin deficiencies
  - Esophageal candidiasis occurs in HIV-infected patients and those on immunosuppressive therapy; 30% have associated thrush.
- Cutaneous candidiasis
  - Diaper dermatitis is most common during infancy because of predisposing factors found with diaper use—warm, moist environment. May co-occur with thrush.
  - Intertriginous candidiasis occurs in skinfolds where there are opposing skin surfaces; generally occurs in healthy patients with the risk factors of chronic moisture, recent antibiotic use, or obesity
- Vaginal candidiasis: Oral contraceptives, antibiotics, pregnancy, corticosteroids, and immunodeficiency are predisposing conditions; classified as uncomplicated or complicated
  - Uncomplicated (90%): mild to moderate; sporadic; organism is *C. albicans*; normal host
  - Complicated (10%): presence of any one of the following factors defines a complicated infection: severe, recurrent (>4 episodes/year) infection by non-*albicans Candida* spp. or predisposing host factor (immunocompromised, diabetes mellitus [DM], etc.)
- Congenital candidiasis: cutaneous infection acquired from infected amniotic fluid. Usually has an excellent prognosis.
- Invasive candidiasis
  - Defined as candidemia and disseminated candidiasis (including hepatosplenic candidiasis). *Candida* from a blood culture should never be considered a contaminant.
  - Risk factors include prematurity, malignancy, immunodeficiency syndromes, DM, broad-spectrum antibiotic therapy, corticosteroids, chemotherapy, hyperalimentation, indwelling catheters, ICU stay, recent complex surgery, and stem cell or organ transplantation.
  - The most frequent sites of involvement are the GI tract, lungs, kidneys (pyelonephritis, mycetoma), liver, spleen, eyes, and brain (meningoencephalitis). Fungal sepsis may occur. Peritoneal, urinary tract, and cardiac valve candidal infections are most often related to instrumentation or catheterization in the immunocompromised host.
- Chronic mucocutaneous candidiasis
  - Noninvasive infection of the skin, hair, mucous membranes, and nails
  - Typically seen in the 1st year of life, and almost all cases occur within the 1st decade
  - Caused by a T-cell defect resulting in decreased production of *Candida*-specific antibody. Patients lack a delayed-type hypersensitivity reaction to intradermal injection of candidal antigens. May be part of polyglandular autoimmune syndrome type 1.

DIAGNOSIS

HISTORY

- Recurrent infection
  - In oral thrush, reinfection may occur from nipples, pacifiers, or toys.
  - In recurrent vaginitis, bacterial or non-*albicans Candida* spp. infections are possible.
- Recent antibiotic use: Thrush often occurs in infants but may occur in normal older children after treatment with systemic antibiotics.
- Predisposing conditions: Systemic dissemination of infection is more likely with impaired immunity.
- Visual changes or discomfort: Features of endophthalmitis include eye pain, blurred vision, scotomata, and photophobia.
- Pain with eating or swallowing: thrush or esophagitis. Esophagitis will often give localized retrosternal pain.

PHYSICAL EXAM

- Oral lesions
  - White cottage cheese–like adherent plaques on tongue, buccal mucosa, pharynx, and gingiva
  - Difficult to scrape away; underlying mucosa may be ulcerated.
- Retinal exam
  - All patients with candidemia should have a dilated retinal exam by an ophthalmologist to assess for endophthalmitis.
  - Chorioretinitis with vitreal haze may be seen.
- Rash
  - Scattered erythema with pustules and papules that become confluent over time. Superficial scale and satellite lesions are classically seen.
  - In neonates with congenital candidiasis, rash is present at birth or develops in 1st week of life. A diffuse macular rash is often accompanied by vesicles and pustules; nails may also be involved.
  - Patients with invasive candidiasis may also present with a diffuse, erythematous rash.
- Vaginitis: white or watery vaginal discharge, erythematous vaginal mucosa with adherent white plaques

DIAGNOSTIC TESTS & INTERPRETATION

Lab

- Direct light microscopic examination of specimen
  - Simple, cost-effective way to confirm clinical diagnosis of mucosal, cutaneous, and vaginal candidiasis; performed using material scraped gently from lesions
  - Potassium hydroxide [KOH] preparation (10% KOH) allows visualization of the long, branching hyphae of *C. albicans*.
- Fungal culture
  - *Candida* spp. can be isolated from culture of mucosal or cutaneous scrapings, blood, urine, CSF, bone marrow, tissue biopsy, abscess aspirate, and bronchoalveolar lavage fluid.

- – However, the sensitivity of blood culture is only 50–60% in patients with invasive candidiasis and may be lower in neonates.
- Adjunctive tests
  - – β-D glucan assay looks for this component of the fungal cell wall in the bloodstream.
  - – Not well studied in children yet but may allow for earlier diagnosis of disseminated disease

Imaging

CT scan, ultrasound, and echocardiogram: Important to identify deep organ lesions (liver, spleen, brain, kidney, or heart) associated with disseminated infection as surgery or more aggressive treatment may be necessary.

DIFFERENTIAL DIAGNOSIS

- Oral lesions: aphthous stomatitis, acute necrotizing gingivitis, herpes gingivostomatitis, coxsackievirus
- Cutaneous: atopy, seborrhea, bacterial skin disease, scabies, irritant dermatitis
- Vaginitis: irritant, bacterial
- Congenital candidiasis: viral infections (especially herpes viruses), bacterial infections, benign neonatal skin conditions
- Invasive candidiasis: bacterial infection

TREATMENT

MEDICATION

- Oral candidiasis: nystatin suspension until 2 days after lesions have cleared. In older patients, nystatin as a swish-swallow suspension or in oral tablet form for >7 days is effective. Clotrimazole lozenges can be used in older patients: 10 mg dissolved in mouth 5 times daily for 7 days.
  - – Fluconazole and ketoconazole are effective for infections that are persistent or occur in immunocompromised hosts. Often, a single dose is effective.
- Esophageal candidiasis
  - – A therapeutic trial with fluconazole for patients with presumed esophageal candidiasis is a cost-effective alternative to endoscopy.
    - ○ Symptoms should resolve within 7 days after the start of therapy.
    - ○ A 14–21-day course is recommended. Itraconazole solution and IV amphotericin B are acceptable alternatives.
- Cutaneous
  - – Keep the area dry. Topical nystatin, clotrimazole 1%, or miconazole 2% 3–4×/day until the rash has cleared. Brief addition of a topical steroid may improve inflammatory changes.
- Uncomplicated vaginal candidiasis
  - – Topical agents are highly effective in uncomplicated infections (cure rates >80%): clotrimazole, miconazole, butoconazole, and terconazole (dose varies with 1-, 3-, or 7-day treatment).
  - – Oral agents are also effective: fluconazole (10 mg/kg up to 150 mg as a single dose)
- Complicated vaginal candidiasis
  - – Extend anti-yeast therapy to 7–14 days.
  - – Non-*albicans* species of *Candida* usually respond to topical boric acid (600 mg/24 h for 14 days). Azole-resistant *C. albicans* infections are extremely rare in the immunocompetent host.
- Recurrent vaginitis (more than 4 episodes of proven infection during a 12-month period, still usually due to azole-susceptible *Candida* sp.)
  - – Induction therapy with 2 weeks of a topical or oral azole is followed by a maintenance regimen for 6 months.
  - – Suitable maintenance regimens include fluconazole (150 mg once weekly), ketoconazole (100 mg daily), itraconazole (100 mg every other day), or daily therapy with a topical azole.
- Systemic or disseminated candidiasis
  - – Begin treatment in hospital because of severity of illness, underlying disease process, and need for the IV route of drug administration.
  - – Address predisposing factors (remove indwelling catheters, reduce immunosuppression if possible).
  - – Antifungal agents commonly used in children include amphotericin B, fluconazole, and, increasingly, echinocandins (micafungin, caspofungin).
- Fluconazole (12 mg/kg/24 h with 25 mg/kg/day loading dose) may be used empirically in those who are less critically ill. Many *C. glabrata* and *C. krusei* are resistant.
- An echinocandin or lipid formulations of amphotericin B should be used for severe illness and in neutropenic hosts. They are also approved for candidal esophagitis.
- Amphotericin B (1 mg/kg/24 h IV) is rarely used due to availability of less toxic agents.
- Lipid-based amphotericin B (3–6 mg/kg/24 h IV)
- Duration of therapy varies based on sites affected: candidemia (3 weeks), candidal meningitis (4 weeks), endophthalmitis (6–12 weeks), endocarditis (>6 weeks following surgical therapy), and osteomyelitis (6–12 months).

ALERT

- Recurrent thrush in a breastfed infant may indicate *C. albicans* colonization of the mother's nipples; this can be eliminated by treatment of the nipples with nystatin cream.
- Candidal diaper dermatitis should prompt an oral exam as thrush is often coexistent.
- Maintain a high index of suspicion for invasive candidiasis in an immunocompromised patient. Persistent fevers despite antibiotic therapy, diffuse rash, and visual complaints are important clues.
- Blood culture growth of *Candida* should never be regarded as a contaminant but should prompt investigation for invasive disease.

C

ADDITIONAL READING

- Benjamin DK Jr, Stoll BJ, Gantz MG, et al. Neonatal candidiasis: epidemiology, risk factors, and clinical judgment. *Pediatrics*. 2010;126(4):e865–e873.
- Hacimustafaoglu M, Celebi S. *Candida* infections in non-neutropenic children after the neonatal period. *Expert Rev Anti Infect Ther*. 2011;9(10):923–940.
- Pappas PG, Kauffman CA, Andes D, et al. Clinical practice guidelines for the management of candidiasis: 2009 update by the Infectious Diseases Society of America. *Clin Infect Dis*. 2009;48(5):503–535.
- Steinbach WJ, Roilides E, Berman D, et al. Results from a prospective, international, epidemiologic study of invasive candidiasis in children and neonates. *Pediatr Infect Dis J*. 2012;31(12):1252–1257.
- Zaoutis T, Walsh TJ. Antifungal therapy for neonatal candidiasis. *Curr Opin Infect Dis*. 2007;20(6):592–597.

CODES

ICD10

- B37.9 Candidiasis, unspecified
- B37.0 Candidal stomatitis
- B37.81 Candidal esophagitis

FAQ

- Q: When should an older child with thrush be evaluated for possible immunodeficiency?
- A: Thrush in the older child is usually caused by recent antibiotic or steroid treatment or diabetes. If no explanatory cause is identified, further evaluation that includes HIV testing should be considered.

CARBON MONOXIDE POISONING

Kevin C. Osterhoudt

BASICS

DESCRIPTION
- Carbon monoxide (CO) is an odorless gas produced via incomplete combustion of carbonaceous fuels.
- CO poisoning occurs when carboxyhemoglobin and CO accumulation leads to impaired physiologic function.

EPIDEMIOLOGY
CO poisoning is a leading cause of death by poisoning within the United States.

Incidence
- More than 13,000 CO exposures were reported to the American Association of Poison Control Centers in 2011, with ~1/3 of such exposures occurring in children.
- Seasonal cold weather and other natural disaster events lead to increases in incidence of exposure.

GENERAL PREVENTION
- Furnaces should receive regular maintenance by skilled technicians.
- Automobiles, gas-powered machinery, and nonelectrical space heaters should only be used with proper ventilation.
- CO detectors should be installed within living spaces.

PATHOPHYSIOLOGY
- On inhalation, some CO binds to hemoglobin to form carboxyhemoglobin.
- Carboxyhemoglobin does not carry oxygen.
- Carboxyhemoglobin produces an allosteric leftward shift of the oxyhemoglobin dissociation curve.
- Carboxyhemoglobin elimination half-life
  - ~4 hours in room air
  - 1–2 hours in 100% oxygen
  - 20 minutes in 100% oxygen at 3 atmospheres
- CO interacts with cellular proteins, leading to impaired mitochondrial function.
- CO is a source of oxidative stress and poisoning may begin a cascade of inflammatory vasculitis within the CNS and heart.

ETIOLOGY
- Common sources of CO exposure include the following:
  - Automobile or boat exhaust
  - Smoke inhalation from house fires
  - Oil, gas, or kerosene space heaters or cooking stoves
  - Portable electricity generators and construction equipment
  - Faulty home furnaces
- The solvent methylene chloride is metabolized to CO by the liver after ingestion, inhalation, or dermal absorption.
- CO is a component of cigarette smoke and environmental air pollution.
- CO is a naturally occurring by-product of the heme biosynthesis pathway.

COMMONLY ASSOCIATED CONDITIONS
Victims of house fires may suffer from thermal injury and/or cyanide poisoning.

DIAGNOSIS

Many emergency medical services crews carry CO detectors.

HISTORY
- Health of family members?
  - CO is an environmental gas that often sickens multiple household members.
- Use of furnace or space heaters?
  - May suggest source of exposure
- Time of exposure?
  - Carboxyhemoglobin levels must be interpreted with consideration to their timing.
- Duration of exposure?
  - Toxicity is related to both magnitude and duration of exposure.
- Loss of consciousness?
  - Syncope appears to be the best clinical predictor of delayed neurologic sequelae.
- Signs and symptoms
  - Mild CO intoxication
    - Malaise
    - Nausea
    - Light-headedness
    - Headache
    - Vomiting
  - Moderate to severe CO intoxication
    - Confusion
    - Syncope
    - Weakness
    - Angina

PHYSICAL EXAM
- Soot on nasal mucosa: suggests possibility of thermal pulmonary injury
- Hypotension: suggests severe CO poisoning
- Cherry red skin: This classic sign is mostly a postmortem finding.

DIAGNOSTIC TESTS & INTERPRETATION

Lab
- CO-oximetry: allows quantitation of carboxyhemoglobin
- Arterial blood gas: allows accurate assessment of oxygenation
- Hemoglobin quantitation: The percentage of carboxyhemoglobin concentration must be considered in relation to the total hemoglobin.
- Serum bicarbonate: A wide anion gap metabolic acidosis suggests the accumulation of lactate, which may result from severe CO poisoning or concomitant cyanide poisoning.
- Creatine kinase: CO poisoning victims are susceptible to rhabdomyolysis.
- Troponin: CO poisoning may lead to myocardial injury.
- ECG: Hypoxemia and metabolic poisoning may lead to cardiac ischemia.
- Transcutaneous carboxyhemoglobin measurement devices are now marketed.

Imaging
- Neuroimaging
  - Not routinely helpful in acute management
- Globus pallidus and subcortical white matter changes may be seen after severe or chronic CO poisoning.

ALERT

Pitfalls

- Pulse oximetry frequently overestimates the percentage of oxyhemoglobin.
- Smokers may have carboxyhemoglobin levels up to 10%.
- Hemolysis, or the presence of fetal hemoglobin, may lead to mild elevation of carboxyhemoglobin.
- In-hospital carboxyhemoglobin levels are not good at predicting risk of delayed neurologic sequelae.

DIFFERENTIAL DIAGNOSIS

- Influenza
- Gastroenteritis
- Vasomotor syncope
- Asphyxia
- Stroke

TREATMENT

GENERAL MEASURES

- Recognize CO exposure.
- Remove patient from source of CO.

Initial Stabilization

Administer 100% oxygen at least until patient is asymptomatic and carboxyhemoglobin level is <5–10%.

ADDITIONAL TREATMENT

- Consider hyperbaric oxygen treatment referral to prevent delayed neurologic sequelae.
- Relative indications
  - Loss of consciousness
  - Seizures
  - Pregnancy
  - Persistent neurologic symptoms
  - CO concentration >25%
- Contraindications
  - Concurrent illness or injury requiring ongoing acute care
  - Unvented pneumothorax
  - Lack of accessible hyperbaric oxygen chamber
- Complications
  - Barotitis media
  - Tympanic membrane rupture
  - Claustrophobic anxiety
  - Seizure
  - Pneumothorax

ALERT

Pitfalls

- Failure to differentiate CO poisoning from winter viral illness
- Syncope may be hard to discern in young infants.
- Undue delay in hyperbaric oxygen therapy, which is most effective in first 6 hours after exposure

ISSUES FOR REFERRAL

- Neuropsychological testing may benefit individuals with perceived neurocognitive deficits.
- Cardiac evaluation for those with myocardial ischemia

INPATIENT CONSIDERATIONS

Admission Criteria

- Perceived merit of hyperbaric oxygen therapy
- Persistent neurologic symptoms
- Evidence of myocardial ischemia
- Associated injuries that merit hospitalization

Discharge Criteria

- Conclusion of hyperbaric therapy
- Stable cardiovascular and neurologic systems after elimination of excess carboxyhemoglobin

ONGOING CARE

FOLLOW-UP RECOMMENDATIONS

Delayed neurologic sequelae may develop 2–40 days after exposure.

PROGNOSIS

- Acute mortality appears to be caused by carboxymyoglobin formation and ischemic ventricular dysrhythmia.
- Patients stable on presentation to medical care have a good prognosis for recovery.
- Delayed neurologic sequelae may manifest in as many as 10–40% of patients after a CO-mediated syncopal episode.

COMPLICATIONS

- Death
- Delayed neurologic sequelae, for example
  - Neurocognitive deficits
  - Personality changes
  - Parkinsonism

ADDITIONAL READING

- Baum CR. What's new in pediatric carbon monoxide poisoning? *Clin Pediatr Emerg Med*. 2008;9:43–46.
- Teksam O, Gumus P, Bayrakci B, et al. Acute cardiac effects of carbon monoxide poisoning in children. *Eur J Emerg Med*. 2010;17(4):192–196.
- Weaver LK. Clinical practice. Carbon monoxide poisoning. *N Engl J Med*. 2009;360(12):1217–1225.

CODES

ICD10

- T58.91XA Toxic effect of carb monx from unsp source, acc, init
- T58.8X1A Toxic effect of carb monx from oth source, accidental, init
- T58.01XA Toxic effect of carb monx from mtr veh exhaust, acc, init

FAQ

- Q: At what carboxyhemoglobin level should hyperbaric oxygen therapy be recommended?
- A: In practice, most dissociation of carboxyhemoglobin occurs with administration of normal-pressure oxygen before hyperbaric therapy can be administered.
- The advocated value of hyperbaric oxygen is to limit cerebral ischemic reperfusion injury in an effort to ameliorate delayed neurologic sequelae.
- Carboxyhemoglobin levels may not directly correlate in this risk stratification, and the occurrence of syncope or seizure may be used as a surrogate marker.
- Currently, patients with CO concentrations >25% may be considered as potential candidates for hyperbaric oxygen.
- Q: In a household, which family member is at greatest risk of CO poisoning?
- A: Smaller and younger children have greater minute ventilation rates and may attain higher carboxyhemoglobin concentrations at a given exposure level.
- It is possible that developing brain tissue is more susceptible to the deleterious effects of CO poisoning.

CARDIOMYOPATHY

Kimberly Molina • Nelangi Pinto

BASICS

DESCRIPTION
Cardiomyopathy (CM) is defined as a disease of the heart muscle, which results in impaired function (systolic, diastolic, or both). It is classified based on structural and functional abnormalities:
- Dilated cardiomyopathy (DCM): The key finding is impairment of ventricular systolic function with cardiac dilation. Predominantly involves the left ventricle (LV) and manifests as congestive heart failure (CHF).
- Hypertrophic cardiomyopathy (HCM): Excessive thickening of the LV that is not secondary to load conditions, such as aortic stenosis or hypertension. Up to 20–25% of patients exhibit LV outflow tract obstruction.
- Restrictive cardiomyopathy (RCM): A myocardial disease in which there is impairment of ventricular diastolic function (or relaxation) from increased stiffness of the ventricle. This results in decreased ventricular filling while systolic function is generally preserved.
- Left ventricular noncompaction (LVNC): A disease where the myocardium of the LV has not completely compacted, resulting in persistence of trabeculations and myocardial dysfunction.

EPIDEMIOLOGY
Incidence
- Overall incidence of CM is 1–2 cases per 100,000 children per year. There is a peak incidence during the 1st year of life and a 2nd peak in adolescence.
  - DCM: 0.3–2.6 cases per 100,000 children per year
  - HCM: 0.3–0.5 cases per 100,000 children per year

Prevalence
- DCM: 36 cases per 100,000 people
- HCM: ~10–20 cases per 100,000 people
- RCM: Least common form of CM (<5%)
- LVNC: ~9% of CM cases

RISK FACTORS
Genetics
- DCM: familial DCM ~20% of cases
  - Autosomal dominant inheritance remains the most common pattern. Although no specific gene has been identified as the cause of familial DCM, 6 genes have been localized in different family cohorts.
  - DCM has also been seen in association with diseases of X-linked inheritance, such as Duchenne and Becker muscular dystrophy and Barth syndrome.
  - May also be inherited via mitochondrial DNA, with differing penetrance
- HCM: ~60% of reported cases are thought to be inherited. Traditionally, HCM is inherited in an autosomal dominant pattern with incomplete penetrance.
- RCM: Idiopathic cases may have a familial occurrence and may be associated with a skeletal myopathy. An autosomal dominant form of the disease with variable penetrance has been associated with Noonan syndrome.
- LVNC: familial in 20–30%. May be X-linked, mitochondrial, autosomal recessive, or dominant

ETIOLOGY
- DCM: There are many etiologies for DCM. Etiology is identified only ~30% of the time.
  - Of known causes, the most common is myocarditis (coxsackievirus B, echovirus, adenovirus). DCM can also occur from toxin exposure (anthracyclines), ischemic coronary artery disease (anomalous left coronary artery from the pulmonary artery, coronary aneurysms), and chronic tachyarrhythmias.
  - Can occur as a finding associated with another disease or syndrome. These include X-linked muscular dystrophies, inborn errors of fatty acid oxidation, disorders of mitochondrial oxidative phosphorylation, nutritional deficiencies, and primary and secondary carnitine deficiency.
  - It may be familial and genetically inherited.
  - DCM is most commonly idiopathic.
- HCM: Etiology is known about 25% of the time. Often genetically inherited. Caused by myocyte hypertrophy with fibrillin disarray.
- RCM: Most commonly idiopathic, although known causes include the following:
  - Systemic disease such as lupus erythematosus, sarcoidosis, amyloidosis, infiltrative diseases (Gaucher disease, Hurler syndrome), storage diseases (Fabry disease), carcinoid syndrome, and radiation-induced fibrosis
  - Familial forms of RCM

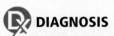

DIAGNOSIS
In the early stages of all 3 forms of CM, the symptoms are nonspecific and can mimic other disease processes. The cardiac examination can be completely normal. Therefore, those patients who raise suspicion for this disease either by family history or clinical presentation should be carefully evaluated.

HISTORY
- DCM: Symptoms usually develop slowly, although they may also be of sudden onset:
  - Irritability
  - Respiratory distress
  - Dyspnea with exertion
  - Anorexia, abdominal pain, nausea
  - Failure to thrive
  - Exercise intolerance
  - Syncope
  - Palpitations
- HCM: Children are often asymptomatic and are first referred for evaluation based on family history or for murmur evaluation. Of those with symptoms, the following may be present:
  - Chest pain with exertion
  - Dizziness
  - Syncope
  - Palpitations
- RCM: Symptoms are usually due to systemic and pulmonary congestion from high atrial pressures. They are usually more evident late in the disease:
  - Dyspnea with exertion
  - Abdominal pain
  - Chest pain
  - Palpitations

PHYSICAL EXAM
- Cardiac
  - DCM: tachycardia, cardiomegaly, hepatomegaly, S_3 or S_4 gallop; evidence of CHF and decreased cardiac output
  - HCM: can be normal or have systolic murmur owing to mitral regurgitation and/or LV outflow tract obstruction. The presence of outflow tract obstruction produces a systolic ejection murmur of variable intensity related to the degree of obstruction; the murmur increases in intensity with Valsalva and decreases in magnitude with squatting. A parasternal or carotid thrill or S_4 gallop may be present.
  - RCM: Jugular venous pulse either fails to fall or rises during inspiration (Kussmaul sign): the presence of S_3 or S_4. Advanced cases may exhibit weak peripheral pulses as evidence of low cardiac output.
- Respiratory (DCM and RCM): tachypnea, rales, wheezing
- Abdominal (DCM and RCM): hepatomegaly, ascites, tenderness to palpation

DIAGNOSTIC TESTS & INTERPRETATION
Lab
Initial lab tests

DCM: In addition to routine inflammatory markers, specific tests should be obtained to establish etiology:
- Metabolic: carnitine level, serum organic acids, and urine organic and amino acids, pyruvate, lactate, thyroid function tests
- Genetic: chromosomal analysis, mutations of the dystrophin gene
- Infectious: enterovirus, coxsackievirus A/B, hepatitis, cytomegalovirus, Epstein-Barr virus, adenovirus, parvovirus, herpes simplex virus, and human immunodeficiency virus
- Brain natriuretic peptide (BNP) is often used to follow heart failure in patients with CM.

Imaging
Echocardiogram
- Allows for assessment of systolic function, ventricular dimensions, outflow tract obstruction, and diastolic filling properties
- DCM: significant dilation of left (and right) ventricle with decreased systolic function
- HCM: gold standard for diagnosis: LV hypertrophy, intraventricular pressure gradient, and systolic anterior motion of the mitral valve
- RCM: disproportionately dilated atria with impaired diastolic filling by Doppler. LV function is normal until late stages.
- LVNC: deep trabeculations and intertrabecular recesses in the LV, ventricular hypertrophy, and systolic dysfunction

Diagnostic Procedures/Other
- Nonspecific tests
  - Chest radiograph: cardiomegaly, pulmonary venous congestion, pulmonary edema, and pleural effusions; segmental atelectasis from bronchiole compression
  - Electrocardiogram: Supraventricular or ventricular arrhythmia may be seen.
    - DCM: sinus tachycardia, nonspecific ST segment, and T-wave changes
    - HCM: hypertrophy, deep Q waves
    - RCM: atrial enlargement, nonspecific ST and T-wave changes
    - LVNC: marked ventricular hypertrophy, T-wave inversion

- Cardiac catheterization
  - DCM: rarely used as the primary diagnostic tool; the procedure is used to delineate coronary anatomy and to perform endomyocardial biopsies.
  - HCM: determination of the presence or absence of LV outflow tract obstruction, evaluation of diastolic dysfunction, classic spike and dome arterial pulse tracing, Brockenbrough phenomenon (a beat following a premature ventricular contraction exhibits an arterial pulse pressure less than that of a control beat)
  - RCM: Atrial pressures are elevated from increased LV and right ventricle (RV) end-diastolic pressures. Ventricular pressures exhibit a rapid and deep early decline at the onset of diastole followed by a rapid rise to a plateau in early diastole (dip and plateau or square root sign).

DIFFERENTIAL DIAGNOSIS

- DCM: Presentation may mimic other diseases:
  - Abdominal distention, right upper quadrant pain, nausea, and anorexia indicate right heart failure but could be mistaken for hepatic or gallbladder disease.
  - Wheezing, tachypnea, and dyspnea on exertion may be diagnosed as asthma.
  - Cardiomegaly on chest radiograph may be mistaken for a large pericardial effusion.
- HCM: This disease must be differentiated from LV hypertrophy seen in a well-trained athlete.
- RCM: should be distinguished from constrictive pericarditis because the latter is usually a remediable process. A history of tuberculosis, trauma, or cardiac surgery may suggest constrictive pericarditis.

TREATMENT

GENERAL MEASURES

- DCM
  - At diagnosis, a trial of IV γ-globulin and/or other immunomodulators (prednisone, azathioprine) to treat possible myocarditis, although impact on outcomes is unclear
  - Diuretics
  - Afterload reduction (enalapril, captopril)
  - Inotropic agents (milrinone, dobutamine, digoxin)
  - Aldactone (improves New York Heart Association [NYHA] functional class)
  - Anticoagulation to avoid embolic complications
  - Antiarrhythmics as needed
  - β-adrenergic blockers (metoprolol, carvedilol)
  - Ventricular assist devices have been used in those with end-stage heart failure either as a bridge to recovery or to transplantation.
- HCM: β-adrenergic blockers remain 1st-line medical therapy. Calcium channel blockers or disopyramide may also be used. Antiarrhythmics may also be part of the medical regimen. There is no evidence that prophylactic medical treatment will reduce the risk of sudden death.
  - If medical therapy is not effective, other options may include septal myectomy (for severe outflow obstruction) and atrioventricular sequential pacing.
  - The placement of an implantable cardioverter-defibrillator (ICD) may be indicated.
- RCM: The mainstay of medical therapy is symptomatic treatment.
  - Diuretics can be used with caution to treat venous congestion without reducing the ventricular filling pressure.
  - Antiarrhythmics are used to treat the high incidence of atrial arrhythmias.
  - ICDs have also been used to treat life-threatening ventricular arrhythmias.
  - Anticoagulation is used owing to the high risk of thrombus formation and embolic complications from hemostasis in the dilated atrium.
  - Due to natural history of disease, most patients eventually require a cardiac transplant.
- Patients with cardiomyopathies are generally restricted from strenuous exercise due to increased risk of sudden cardiac death.

SURGERY/OTHER PROCEDURES

- DCM or RCM: heart or heart–lung (if the pulmonary vascular resistance is elevated) transplantation; transplantation may be necessary if all therapeutic endeavors prove to be futile.
- HCM: septal myectomy if indicated

INPATIENT CONSIDERATIONS

Initial Stabilization

Patients with DCM may present critically ill, requiring intubation and inotropic support.

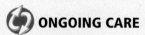

ONGOING CARE

PROGNOSIS

- DCM: The rate of death or transplant is ~30% at 1-year and 40% at 5-year follow-up. Age (<1 month and >6 years), ventricular function, and symptoms of CHF at diagnosis are risk factors for a worse outcome. Biopsy-proven myocarditis is associated with improved outcome.
- HCM: Overall incidence of sudden death is 4–6% in children and adolescents and as low as 1% in adults. Between the ages of 12 and 35 years and in young athletes, HCM is the most common cause of sudden death. Obstruction may slowly develop or progress. Heart failure symptoms usually do not occur until adulthood. Survival is poorer (82%) for those diagnosed at <1 year of age.
- RCM: The reported median survival in RCM is 1.4 years in children with <20% freedom from death or transplant at 5 years.
- LVNC: 5-year survival free of death or transplantation is 75%.

COMPLICATIONS

- CHF can occur in all forms of CM.
- Arrhythmias may be seen and are frequently ventricular in origin.
- Thrombus formation can be seen owing to the stasis of blood in dilated cardiac chambers and the hypocontractile ventricle. Therefore, systemic or pulmonary emboli are possible.

ADDITIONAL READING

- Alexander PM, Daubeney PE, Nugent AW. Long-term outcomes of dilated cardiomyopathy diagnosed during childhood. *Circulation*. 2013;128(18):2039–2046.
- Alvarez JA, Orav J, Wilkinson JD, et al. Competing risks for death and cardiac transplantation in children with dilated cardiomyopathy. *Circ*. 2011;124(7):814–823.
- Ammash NM, Seward JB, Bailey KR, et al. Clinical profile and outcome of idiopathic restrictive cardiomyopathy. *Circ*. 2000;101(21):2490–2496.
- Silva JN, Canter CE. Current management of pediatric dilated cardiomyopathy. *Curr Opin Cardiol*. 2010;25(2):80–87.
- Towbin JA. Hypertrophic cardiomyopathy. *PACE*. 2009;32(Suppl 2):S23–S31.
- Towbin JA, Lowe AM, Colan SD, et al. Incidence, causes, and outcomes of dilated cardiomyopathy in children. *JAMA*. 2006;296(15):1867–1876.
- Wilkinson JD, Landy DC, Colan SD, et al. The pediatric cardiomyopathy registry and heart failure: key results from the first 15 years. *Heart Failure Clin*. 2010;6(4):401–413.

CODES

ICD10

- I42.9 Cardiomyopathy, unspecified
- I42.0 Dilated cardiomyopathy
- I42.5 Other restrictive cardiomyopathy

FAQ

- Q: Should family members be evaluated once CM is diagnosed in a 1st-degree relative?
- A: Yes. In some forms of CM, there is a strong genetic component and family members should be evaluated. If the CM is known to be acquired, evaluation of relatives is not required.
- Q: Does the CM of infants of diabetic mothers carry the same clinical course and outcome as that of patients with HCM?
- A: No. The pathophysiology is initially similar in that asymmetric hypertrophy of the ventricular septum is often seen with or without LV outflow obstruction. However, the clinical course of CM in these infants is usually benign and resolves within the first 6 months of life.
- Q: What are the differentiating features of HCM and the benign physiologic hypertrophy of an athlete's heart?
- A: Several criteria are used to make this distinction. For example, a familial history of HCM raises the suspicion of this entity. Studies have suggested specific echocardiographic LV dimensions to differentiate benign hypertrophy and HCM (i.e., a wall thickness of ≥15 mm or LV cavity dimension <45 mm are more consistent with HCM). Also, evidence of abnormal mitral valve inflow is suggestive of HCM.

CATARACT

M. Edward Wilson • Courtney L. Kraus

BASICS

DESCRIPTION

Cataract is the term used for any opacification of the crystalline lens of the eye.

EPIDEMIOLOGY

- Approximately 4 children per million total population will be born with bilateral congenital cataracts in developed countries.
- Adjusted cumulative incidence is 2.49 per 10,000 in the 1st year of life, increasing to 3.46 by age 15 years.

GENERAL PREVENTION

- There is currently no known way to prevent congenital cataracts. Timely prenatal diagnosis and treatment of intrauterine infections can prevent associated infant morbidities, including secondary cataracts. Correcting an underlying metabolic abnormality and minimizing exposure to inciting agents also reduces risk.
- It is essential that all newborns (and all children) receive screening eye examinations by health care providers. In much of the world, early diagnosis and referral is still the limiting factor for a child's ultimate visual prognosis.

PATHOPHYSIOLOGY

- Derangement of the normal developmental growth of the crystalline fibers of the central lens nucleus or peripheral lens cortex. The location of the opacity often suggests the congenital or early acquired onset.
- Frequently classified according to morphology or etiology
- Dense central opacities of ≥3 mm are visually significant and may produce visual disability.

ETIOLOGY

- Congenital or developmental: About 2/3 are idiopathic, the remainder being inherited or associated with systemic disorders.
- Hereditary: Autosomal dominant transmission is responsible for 75% of bilateral hereditary cataracts. Most affected individuals are otherwise healthy.
  - Phenotypically identical cataracts can occur with mutations at different genetic loci and phenotypically variable cataracts can be found within a single family.
  - Multiple contributing genetic loci have been identified.
  - Rare hereditary syndromes combine cataracts with systemic disease. These are listed in the following discussion.
- Acquired
  - Toxic: may result from chronic steroid use or radiation exposure
  - Traumatic: may result from either blunt or penetrating ocular trauma
  - Inflammatory: from chronic uveitis
- Ocular abnormalities: Cataracts may be associated with primary ocular abnormalities such as aniridia, coloboma, and microcornea.

COMMONLY ASSOCIATED CONDITIONS

- Prenatal factors: intrauterine infection, fetal alcohol syndrome
- Metabolic and endocrine: galactosemia, neonatal hypoglycemia, hypoparathyroidism, diabetes mellitus, homocystinuria, Fabry disease, Wilson disease, mannosidosis
- Chromosomal: trisomy 21 (Down syndrome), 18, 13, or 15; Turner syndrome
- Dermatologic: congenital ichthyosis, hereditary ectodermal dysplasia, infantile poikiloderma, Gorlin syndrome
- Renal: Lowe and Alport syndromes
- Musculoskeletal: Marfan, Conradi, and Albright syndromes; myotonic dystrophy
- Rheumatologic: juvenile idiopathic arthritis, other uveitis (psoriatic, HLA-B27, etc.)
- Other: craniofacial and mandibulofacial syndromes, neurofibromatosis

DIAGNOSIS

HISTORY

- Decreased visual fixation and tracking? Cataracts may decrease vision.
- Sun sensitivity or squinting in bright light? Cataracts may cause glare and light scatter.
- Strabismus (ocular misalignment)? May indicate loss of vision in one eye
- White pupil? Cataracts may appear as a white spot in or under the pupil.
- Asymmetric or abnormal pupillary reflections (red eyes) with flash photography? Cataract may block the normal red reflex.
- Nystagmus (rhythmic oscillations)? May be a sign of severe, usually bilateral, vision loss
- Ocular trauma? Cataract can occur from blunt or penetrating trauma.
- Delayed development? Especially with significant bilateral congenital cataracts
- Careful family and prenatal history? Congenital cataracts can be inherited as an isolated condition. Intrauterine infection or alcohol exposure can cause cataracts.
- Positive family history or known history of an associated systemic condition?

PHYSICAL EXAM

- Decreased visual acuity: In preverbal child, assess and compare ability to fixate and follow with each eye. In verbal child, assess with pictures, HOTV matching, or alphabet (Snellen) eye chart.
- Leukocoria: white pupil
- Red reflex: absent, asymmetric, or irregular. How much of the pupil is obscured? Use direct ophthalmoscope held at an arm's length to illuminate both eyes and compare the red reflex from each eye.
- Strabismus: often an indication; cataract is long-standing and amblyopia likely.
- Nystagmus: will first appear at 2–3 months of age if vision deprivation from cataract is present at birth. Very poor prognostic sign for full vision recovery unless treatment is prompt.
- Laterality of disease: Bilateral cataracts may be due to systemic disease.
- Globe (eyeball) size: Microphthalmia (small eye) suggests congenital cataracts.
- Complete physical exam: to assess for associated conditions

DIAGNOSTIC TESTS & INTERPRETATION

Labs

For cases with a definitive etiology, laboratory evaluation is typically not necessary. For bilateral cataracts without a clear cause, a selective workup to rule out associated conditions may be indicated.

- Serologies: titers to rule out TORCH infections; blood glucose, calcium, and phosphate to exclude metabolic disorders such as diabetes and hypoparathyroidism
- Urine tests: reducing substances to rule out galactosemia; protein, amino acids, and pH to rule out Lowe syndrome
- Red blood cell enzyme levels: galactokinase and gal-1-uridyltransferase as part of galactosemia workup
- Karyotype: in conjunction with genetic consultation and ocular examination of parents and siblings

Imaging

Ophthalmologist may perform ocular ultrasonography if unable to visualize structures posterior to the opacity.

Diagnostic Procedures/Other

- Complete, timely ophthalmic evaluation by a pediatric ophthalmologist, including slit-lamp biomicroscopy and dilated fundus examination
- Examination under anesthesia may be required if office-based exam is inadequate. Coupled with intent to remove cataract when necessary.

DIFFERENTIAL DIAGNOSIS

- Childhood cataracts can be readily identified as such. However, they represent one of the many etiologies on the differential diagnosis for leukocoria.
- Cataracts may also be an expression of an underlying systemic disease, which must be diagnosed for the child's overall benefit.
- Leukocoria or poor red reflex differential diagnosis:
  - Retinoblastoma
  - Retinopathy of prematurity
  - Persistent fetal vasculature
  - Uveitis
  - Retinal detachment
  - Coats disease
  - Toxocariasis

TREATMENT

ADDITIONAL TREATMENT

General Measures

- Importance of timely referral:
  - Congenital cataracts may require surgical removal by 4–6 weeks of age to prevent irreversible deprivation amblyopia, so quick referral is critical.
  - Acquired pediatric cataracts may also cause amblyopia, typically prior to 7 years of age.
- Conservative management:
  - Partial cataracts that do not block the visual axis may be managed with observation, pharmacologic pupillary dilatation, and/or amblyopia treatment as needed (occlusion of the contralateral eye). Glasses may or may not be of additional help.
  - A small or partial cataract may progress, so close follow-up is required.

SURGERY/OTHER PROCEDURES

- Visually significant cataracts must be removed surgically. An intraocular lens (IOL) may be inserted at the time of cataract surgery or later when the child is older.
- Successful intervention must occur very early in life in the case of visually significant congenital cataracts or as soon as possible after progression of later onset or partial cataracts.
- To prevent deprivation amblyopia in bilateral cases, both cataracts are typically removed within 1 or 2 weeks of each other. Rarely the eyes are operated simultaneously, if anesthesia risks are high.
- Postoperative care
  – Overview: Removing the lens leaves the child aphakic (without a lens). Postoperative optical correction with contact lens, glasses, and/or IOL and amblyopia treatment are essential for optimal visual prognosis.
  – Contact lens: In children <1 year of age, optical correction of aphakia is frequently accomplished with contact lenses or spectacles. An IOL is sometimes placed initially but more often is implanted after eye growth as a secondary procedure.
  – IOL: In children >1 year of age, IOLs are frequently placed at the time of cataract surgery. Glasses are needed as well, even when an IOL is placed.
  – Amblyopia therapy: In unilateral cataract cases, successful visual rehabilitation usually requires aggressive occlusion therapy to the normal eye, possibly for years.

ONGOING CARE

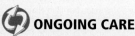

FOLLOW-UP RECOMMENDATIONS

- Without treatment, visually significant cataracts result in progressive visual loss. When an opacity that is present at birth or very early in life is not promptly addressed, the visual loss quickly becomes irreversible.
- Once surgical removal is performed and optical correction is started, the child, the parents, and the ophthalmologist enter into an intensive and long rehabilitation period, lasting until visual maturity is reached (usually 7–10 years of age). Afterward, yearly eye examinations remain a minimum requirement.
- Parental and educational support services as well as special local, state, and federal services for the visually handicapped and blind may be required as not all children with successful surgical results will have good vision.

ALERT

Pitfalls include (i) lack of early diagnosis, referral, and treatment; (ii) lack of understanding of irreversible deprivation amblyopia; (iii) lack of adherence with postoperative optical correction and occlusion therapy; and (iv) lack of continued long-term follow-up to detect and treat late glaucoma or shift in refractive errors with continued eye growth.

PROGNOSIS

- Early surgery and rapid postsurgical optical correction result in best corrected visual acuities of 20/40–20/200 for monocular cataracts and 20/40 or better for bilateral cataracts. 20/20 is obtained in some patients.
- With dense unilateral cataracts, good vision is obtained if the surgery is completed within the first 6 weeks of life. After this time, visual restoration becomes progressively more difficult because of deprivation amblyopia.
- The prognosis for visual rehabilitation in children with bilateral congenital cataracts is better than for unilateral, as long as treatment is before vision deprivation nystagmus develops.
- Later onset and partial, slowly progressing cataracts have the best prognosis.
- Family adherence with both postsurgical optical correction and amblyopia treatment is critical and directly affects the child's ultimate visual outcome later in life.

COMPLICATIONS

- Lack of removal of a visually significant cataract at the appropriate time leads to irreversible deprivation amblyopia.
- Cataract removal in children leaves the eye without the natural crystalline lens—a structure that normally changes to offset the effects of eye growth. Even when an IOL is placed, glasses are often needed and these change frequently as the eyes grow. Unless appropriate optical correction is maintained, irreversible refractive amblyopia may still occur after the cataract is removed, particularly if the cataract is unilateral.
- Congenital cataract eyes often have immature outflow (trabecular meshwork) and 30% or more will eventually develop glaucoma (often years after surgery), requiring drops or surgery to control eye pressure.
- Short- and long-term postoperative complications also include visual axis opacification, retinal detachment, and, very rarely, endophthalmitis (intraocular infection). These complications may lead to vision loss or loss of the eye, and long-term ophthalmology follow-up is required.

ADDITIONAL READING

- Amaya L, Taylor D, Russell-Eggitt I, et al. The morphology and natural history of childhood cataracts. *Surv Ophthalmol*. 2003;48(2):125–144.
- Infant Aphakia Treatment Study Group. A randomized clinical trial comparing contact lens with intraocular lens correction of monocular aphakia during infancy. *Arch Ophthalmol*. 2010;128(7):810–818.
- Lambert SR, Drack AV. Infantile cataracts. *Surv Ophthalmol*. 1996;40(6):427–458.
- Levin AV. Congenital eye anomalies. *Pediatr Clin North Am*. 2003;50(1):55–76.
- Wilson ME Jr, Trivedi RH, Hoxie JP, et al. Treatment outcomes of congenital monocular cataracts: The effects of surgical timing and patching compliance. *J Pediatr Ophthalmol Strabismus*. 2003;40(6): 323–329, quiz 353–354.

CODES

ICD10

- H26.9 Unspecified cataract
- Q12.0 Congenital cataract
- H26.40 Unspecified secondary cataract

FAQ

- Q: Is surgical removal of the cataract a visual cure?
- A: No. Surgery is only the beginning of treatment, which also includes optical correction and amblyopia therapy.
- Q: Once the cataract is removed, will intensive, extensive follow-up be needed?
- A: Yes. The visual prognosis is directly related to postsurgical treatment compliance.
- Q: Is the cataract easier to treat when the child is older?
- A: No. Irreversible deprivation amblyopia develops as the child grows, precluding any chance for normal vision. In newborns, cataracts must typically be removed at 4–6 weeks of age.

CAT-SCRATCH DISEASE

Camille Sabella

BASICS

DESCRIPTION
Cat-scratch disease (CSD) is a zoonotic infection caused by *Bartonella henselae*, which most commonly causes a subacute, regional lymphadenitis syndrome but is also more rarely associated with visceral organ, neurologic, and ocular manifestations.

EPIDEMIOLOGY
- Domestic cat is the primary reservoir for *B. henselae* and the major vector for transmission to humans.
- CSD most commonly results from a cat scratch or bite; flea bites are also implicated in the transmission of CSD.
- Kittens are more likely to transmit the organism than adult cats.
- 90% of patients with CSD have history of recent cat contact.
- Person-to-person transmission is not thought to occur.
- More common in males
- Most cases of CSD occur in the fall and winter.

Incidence
- There are ~22,000 cases each year; annual incidence of CSD is 3.7/100,000 persons.
- Most cases occur in those <21 years of age. Children younger than 10 years of age have highest age-specific annual attack rate (9.3/100,000).
- Most common cause of subacute/chronic regional lymphadenitis in U.S. children

GENERAL PREVENTION
- Avoiding cats is an effective, but unpractical, method of preventing CSD; declawing cats can also be considered.
- Cat bites and scratches should be immediately and thoroughly cleaned.
- Immunocompromised individuals should avoid contact with cats that scratch or bite and avoid kittens as new pets.
- Care of cats should involve effective flea control.

PATHOPHYSIOLOGY
- Infection can result in local invasion, causing lymphadenopathy, or disseminated infection, leading to visceral organ spread.
- Involved nodes initially develop generalized lymphoid hyperplasia, followed by the development of stellate granulomas; the centers are acellular and necrotic and may be surrounded by histiocytes and peripheral lymphocytes.
- Progression leads to microabscesses, which may become confluent and lead to pus-filled pockets within the infected nodes.

ETIOLOGY
The etiologic agent is *B. henselae*, a fastidious, small, curved, pleomorphic gram-negative bacillus.

DIAGNOSIS

HISTORY
- Cat contact
  - 90% of patients have an antecedent cat contact.
- A skin rash
  - A red papule generally appears on the skin at the site of inoculation 7–12 days after the initial cat scratch.
  - This papule persists for 1–4 weeks, often progresses through a vesicular and crusty stage, and then regresses spontaneously.
- Appearance of large lymph nodes
  - Within 1–4 weeks after appearance of a skin lesion, lymphadenopathy in the region of drainage (generally immediately proximal to the skin lesion) is often noted.
- Other symptoms
  - Most persons with CSD do not have fever or other constitutional symptoms; fever and mild systemic symptoms (such as generalized achiness, malaise, and anorexia) are present in up to 30% of patients.

PHYSICAL EXAM
- An erythematous papule at the inoculation site may be detectable.
- Chronic or subacute lymphadenitis involving the 1st or 2nd set of nodes draining the inoculation site is present in approximately 90% of cases:
  - The groups affected, in decreasing order of frequency, are the axillary, cervical, submandibular, periauricular, epitrochlear, femoral, and inguinal lymph nodes.
  - Affected nodes are usually tender, with overlying erythema, warmth, and induration.
  - ~10–30% spontaneously suppurate or form a sinus tract to the skin.
- The finding of conjunctivitis/conjunctival granuloma along with ipsilateral preauricular lymphadenitis is a unique presentation of CSD (Parinaud oculoglandular syndrome), in which the conjunctiva or eyelid is the site of inoculation.

DIAGNOSTIC TESTS & INTERPRETATION

Lab
- Indirect fluorescence antibody (IFA) testing
  - For detection of serum antibodies to *B. henselae*
  - Available at many commercial laboratories and the Centers for Disease Control and Prevention
  - Can be used to confirm CSD
  - A single IgG titer of ≥1:512, a 4-fold rise in titer, or seroconversion is necessary for serologic diagnosis of CSD.
  - IgM titers are less sensitive than IgG titers, even in acute disease.
  - Overall sensitivity and specificity of IFA IgG testing is 88% and 98%, respectively.
- Enzyme immunoassay (EIA) testing
  - Also for detection of serum antibodies to *B. henselae*
  - Similar sensitivity and specificity to IFA
- Blood cultures
  - Using lysed or centrifuged blood may, at times, yield *B. henselae* growth from infected individuals in whom bacteremia is suspected.
  - Growth typically is obtained on blood agar after 12–15 days but may require incubation period of up to 45 days.
- Polymerase chain reaction (PCR)
  - Available in some commercial and research laboratories
  - Sensitive and specific method for diagnosis of *Bartonella* infection in tissue specimens (e.g., needle aspiration of lymph node)
- Histologic findings of lymph nodes are characteristic of CSD but not pathognomonic.
  - Early findings include lymphocytic infiltration with epithelioid granulomas.
  - Later findings include neutrophilic infiltration with necrotic granulomas (stellate microabscesses).
- Warthin-Starry silver stain
  - May demonstrate *B. henselae* bacilli in chains, clumps, or filaments within necrosed areas of lymph node or within primary inoculation site of the skin
  - Not specific for *B. henselae* and not definitively diagnostic of CSD but is strongly suggestive in conjunction with compatible clinical findings

DIFFERENTIAL DIAGNOSIS
- Includes infectious and noninfectious causes of lymphadenopathy
  - Mycobacterial infection (*Mycobacterium tuberculosis* and non-tuberculous mycobacterial infection)
  - Malignancy, especially lymphoma
  - Acute bacterial lymphadenitis caused by *Staphylococcus aureus* and *Streptococcus pyogenes*)
  - Tularemia
  - Viral causes of lymphadenopathy such as EBV, CMV, or HIV
  - Toxoplasmosis

TREATMENT

MEDICATION

- Antimicrobial therapy may hasten recovery in acutely or severely ill patients with systemic symptoms and is recommended for all immunocompromised people.
  - Macrolides, doxycycline, ciprofloxacin, and trimethoprim-sulfamethoxazole appear to be effective.
  - Rifampin may be effective but is often used in combination with a macrolide or doxycycline.
  - Azithromycin or doxycycline is recommended for patients with bacillary angiomatosis and bacillary peliosis.
- The optimal duration of therapy for complicated infections is not clear but may be prolonged for systemic disease.
- Azithromycin (500 mg initially then 250 mg daily for a total of 5 days in patients >45.5 kg and 10 mg/kg on the 1st day and 5 mg/kg for the subsequent 4 days in patients ≤45.5 kg) has been shown to be of modest clinical benefit in children with uncomplicated CSD and is recommended by some experts.

ADDITIONAL TREATMENT

General Measures

- The management of typical CSD is supportive.
- Many experts suggest conservative, symptomatic treatment only, except in severe or systemic disease or in immunocompromised patients.

ISSUES FOR REFERRAL

- Consider infectious disease consult to aid in evaluation, diagnosis, and management, especially in complicated disease or in immunocompromised hosts.
- Consider general surgery consult for needle aspiration if needed.

SURGERY/OTHER PROCEDURES

- Percutaneous needle aspiration of painful, fluctuant nodes can be performed for relief of pain.
- Incision and drainage should be avoided to reduce the risk of sinus tract formation, and surgical excision is generally not necessary.

INPATIENT CONSIDERATIONS

Admission Criteria

- Severe pain refractory to oral analgesics
- Workup to rule out serious other causes of lymphadenopathy or symptomatology
- Severe or unusual complications of CSD

Discharge Criteria

- Pain under adequate control
- No concern for serious or life-threatening complications or other disorders requiring further evaluation or treatment

ONGOING CARE

FOLLOW-UP RECOMMENDATIONS

- Typical CSD is self-limited. Slow resolution of enlarged or painful lymph nodes will occur over 2–4 months.
- ~10–30% of affected lymph nodes will spontaneously suppurate.

PROGNOSIS

- Most immunocompetent patients have a benign course with complete recovery.
- Patients with significant complications, such as encephalopathy, thrombocytopenic purpura, or bone lesions, usually have a more prolonged course but generally have a good long-term prognosis.

COMPLICATIONS

- Systemic CSD
  - Usually characterized by fever, arthralgia, malaise, myalgia, and hepatosplenic involvement
  - Cause of fever of unknown origin (FUO) in children
  - Hepatosplenic involvement may manifest with abdominal pain; microabscesses or granulomas may be visualized on ultrasound or CT of the liver and spleen.
- Encephalopathy/encephalitis
  - May occur 1–3 weeks after the initial symptoms of CSD
  - Seizures, lethargy, combative behavior, and coma may occur.
  - CSF analysis typically normal or slight lymphocytic pleocytosis and elevated protein
  - Recovery is generally complete.
- Optic neuritis or neuroretinitis
  - Acute (usually unilateral) painless vision loss
  - Associated with stellate macular exudates
- Erythema nodosum
  - Likely represents a delayed hypersensitivity reaction to the infection
  - Most often involves the subcutaneous fat of the legs and, at times, dorsum of arms, hands, and feet
- Osteolytic bone lesions
- Endocarditis
- Other, rare complications
  - Thrombotic thrombocytopenic purpura
  - Henoch-Schönlein purpura
  - Mesenteric lymphadenitis
  - Pneumonia
  - Osteomyelitis
  - Hypercalcemia
  - Guillain-Barré syndrome
  - Transverse myelitis
- Endocarditis
- Bacillary angiomatosis and bacillary peliosis can occur in the immunocompromised host.

ADDITIONAL READING

- American Academy of Pediatrics. Cat-scratch disease (*Bartonella henselae*). In: Pickering LK, Baker CJ, Kimberlin DW, et al, eds. *Red Book: 2012 Report of the Committee on Infectious Diseases*. 29th ed. Elk Grove Village, IL: American Academy of Pediatrics; 2012:269–271.
- Bass JW, Freitas BC, Freitas AD, et al. Prospective randomized double blind placebo-controlled evaluation of azithromycin for treatment of cat-scratch disease. *Pediatr Infect Dis J*. 1998;17(6):447–452.
- Biswas S, Rolain JM. *Bartonella* infection: treatment and drug resistance. *Future Microbiol*. 2010;5(11):1719–1731.
- Ciervo A, Mastroianni CM, Ajassa C, et al. Rapid identification of *Bartonella henselae* by real-time polymerase chain reaction in a patient with cat scratch disease. *Diagn Microbiol Infect Dis*. 2005;53(1):75–77.
- English R. Cat-scratch disease. *Pediatr Rev*. 2006;27(4):123–127.
- Forin TA, Zaoutis TE, Zaoutis LB. Beyond cat scratch disease: widening spectrum of *Bartonella henselae* infection. *Pediatrics*. 2008;121(5):e1413–e1425.
- Schutze GE. Diagnosis and treatment of *Bartonella henselae* infections. *Pediatr Infect Dis J*. 2000;19(12):1185–1187.

CODES

ICD10

A28.1 Cat-scratch disease

FAQ

- Q: Can a sibling develop CSD from an infected patient?
- A: No. There is no evidence of person-to-person transmission. However, asymptomatic household contacts of the index case are more likely to be seropositive than the general population, likely related to exposure to the same animal.
- Q: Should the parents of a child with CSD get rid of the cat?
- A: In general, this is not recommended. These animals are not ill; the capacity to transmit disease appears to be transient, and recurrent disease is rare.
- Q: What is the benefit of azithromycin in the treatment of uncomplicated CSD lymphadenitis?
- A: In a prospective, randomized, double-blind study, azithromycin given for 5 days was shown to result in significantly greater decrease in lymph node volume during the 1st month of treatment as compared to placebo. However, there was no difference in outcome between the 2 groups after 30 days.

CAVERNOUS SINUS SYNDROME

Daphne M. Hasbani • Sabrina E. Smith

BASICS

DESCRIPTION

- Cavernous sinus syndrome comprises disease processes that localize to the cavernous sinus—a venous plexus that drains the face, mouth, tonsils, pharynx, nasal cavity, paranasal sinuses, orbit, middle ear, and parts of the cerebral cortex.
- Small lesions in this region may produce dramatic neurologic signs.

EPIDEMIOLOGY

Cavernous sinus syndrome is a rare but serious condition.

PATHOPHYSIOLOGY

- The cavernous sinus is located lateral to the pituitary gland and sella turcica, superior to the sphenoid sinus, and inferior to the optic chiasm.
- Within the cavernous sinus are the carotid artery, the pericarotid sympathetic fibers, and the abducens nerve (VI); within its lateral wall are the oculomotor nerve (III), the trochlear nerve (IV), and the ophthalmic and maxillary divisions of the trigeminal nerve (V1, V2).
- Cavernous sinus syndrome is typically caused by septic or aseptic sinus thrombosis, neoplasm, or trauma. Acute obstruction by mass or thrombosis may progress rapidly if not diagnosed and treated quickly.

ETIOLOGY

- Infectious agents include *Staphylococcus aureus*, *Streptococcus pneumoniae*, Gram-negative rods, and anaerobes; *Mucormycosis* and *Aspergillus* in immunocompromised patients.
- Aseptic venous thrombosis has been associated with sickle cell anemia, trauma, dehydration, vasculitis, pregnancy, oral contraceptive use, congenital heart disease, inflammatory bowel disease, and hypercoagulable states.
- Neoplasms involving the cavernous sinus include pituitary adenomas, meningiomas, trigeminal schwannomas, craniopharyngiomas, lymphomas, neuromas, chordomas, chondrosarcomas, rhabdomyosarcomas, nasopharyngeal carcinomas, and very rarely, teratomas. Neoplasms may present with diplopia, visual field deficits, headache, or isolated cranial nerve deficits.
- The lateral extension of pituitary neoplasms into the cavernous sinus usually affects the 3rd cranial nerve, with the 4th and 6th nerves less commonly involved. Rupture of a cystic craniopharyngioma may present as acute cavernous sinus syndrome.
- Carotid-cavernous fistulas, often with a more chronic course, are direct high-flow shunts between the internal carotid artery and the cavernous sinus. Most often sequelae of trauma, they may present with a history of ocular motility deficits, arterialization of conjunctival vessels, and a bruit usually heard best over the orbit. Less commonly, rupture of a carotid cavernous aneurysm may lead to fistula formation.
- Nonspecific and idiopathic inflammation of the cavernous sinus, also called idiopathic cavernous sinusitis or Tolosa-Hunt syndrome, has been reported in patients as young as 3½ years. This is a diagnosis of exclusion. However, MRI may show enlargement of the affected cavernous sinus with an adjacent soft tissue mass that resolves after treatment with steroids.

DIAGNOSIS

HISTORY

- Recent facial furuncle or cellulitis, sinusitis, dental infection, otitis, or orbital cellulitis may predispose to cavernous sinus syndrome.
- Fever, headache, eye pain, diplopia, and facial paresthesias may be present.

PHYSICAL EXAM

- Conjunctival injection with lid swelling and proptosis indicates cavernous sinus venous congestion.
- Ptosis, anisocoria, ophthalmoparesis, and facial sensory changes are signs of cranial nerve involvement.
- Horner syndrome: Sympathetic nerve fibers traveling with V1 may be affected. Usually occurs in conjunction with an abducens nerve (CN VI) palsy with an inability to abduct the eye.
- Signs and symptoms begin unilaterally but may rapidly spread bilaterally.
- The optic nerve and visual acuity are spared early in cavernous sinus syndrome but can be affected as it progresses.
- Funduscopic findings include venous dilatation and hemorrhages.
- Ocular bruit may be heard in any acute cavernous sinus syndrome but especially in carotid-cavernous fistula.
- Signs of meningitis and systemic toxicity rapidly evolve if infections are untreated.

DIAGNOSTIC TESTS & INTERPRETATION

Lab

- CBC, ESR, PT/PTT, blood culture: Basic studies in any child with suspected acute cavernous sinus syndrome. Blood cultures are positive in 70% of cases of septic venous sinus thrombosis.
  - Lumbar puncture should be performed if there is no contraindication and infection is suspected.
  - ~35% of patients with septic cavernous sinus thrombosis have CSF findings consistent with bacterial meningitis—excess neutrophils, increased protein, and/or decreased glucose.
- Evaluation for a prothrombotic state should be considered in patients with cavernous sinus thrombosis, especially in the absence of infection or trauma. Specific labs include protein C activity, protein S activity, antithrombin III activity, factor V Leiden gene mutation, prothrombin gene mutation, anticardiolipin antibodies, β-2-glycoprotein antibodies, dilute Russell viper venom time, homocysteine, lipoprotein(a), and factor VIII activity.
- Antinuclear antibody panel, angiotensin-converting enzyme level, and HIV test should be obtained before diagnosis of Tolosa-Hunt syndrome (diagnosis of exclusion).

Imaging

Any child with proptosis, cranial nerve findings, or an ocular bruit should have an urgent MRI or CT.

- MRI, with and without gadolinium, with special attention to the cavernous sinus and parasellar region, is the imaging study of choice.
- Magnetic resonance venography may be helpful.
- CT angiography may be the preferred study to evaluate for carotid-cavernous fistula.

Diagnostic Procedures/Other

- Diagnosis of carotid-cavernous fistulas requires angiography.
- Nasopharyngeal biopsy and culture if *Mucormycosis* or *Aspergillus* is suspected.

DIFFERENTIAL DIAGNOSIS

Other disorders that may resemble cavernous sinus syndrome include the following:

- Orbital cellulitis
- Sphenoid sinusitis
- Thyroid eye disease
- Cavernous carotid aneurysm
- Orbital apex tumor
- Orbital pseudotumor
- Ocular migraine
- Ocular trauma
- Burkitt lymphoma

ALERT

- Ophthalmoplegic migraine or cluster headache must be distinguished from cavernous sinus syndrome by neuroimaging studies and history.
  - Proptosis does not occur in migraine or cluster headache.
  - Ophthalmoplegic migraine is a diagnosis of exclusion, especially on first presentation.
- Acute infection and hemorrhage of the pituitary gland—pituitary apoplexy—may present with acute bilateral ophthalmoplegia and signs of acute pituitary insufficiency; most commonly occurs with pituitary neoplasms but may also occur in pregnant women at the time of delivery.
- Chronic granulomatous disorders such as sarcoid and tuberculosis may underlie cavernous sinus syndrome.

TREATMENT

First priority is to rule out septic cavernous sinus thrombosis, life-threatening infections of the face, sinuses, middle ear, teeth, and orbit.

MEDICATION

First Line

- For septic cavernous sinus thrombosis, broad-spectrum antibiotics (including coverage of penicillinase-resistant staphylococci and anaerobes) are begun immediately. Duration of therapy is usually 2–4 weeks beyond the resolution of symptoms.
- Amphotericin B if *Mucormycosis* or *Aspergillus* is suspected
- Idiopathic cavernous sinusitis, a diagnosis of exclusion, responds to corticosteroids. Treatment should not be started until neoplasm and infection have been ruled out.

Second Line

Anticoagulation is controversial, but one study in adults found that heparin reduced morbidity from septic cavernous sinus thrombosis.

SURGERY/OTHER PROCEDURES

- Surgical drainage of the primary infection (i.e., sinusitis) may be indicated (avoiding surgical manipulation of the cavernous sinus itself).
- Posttraumatic carotid-cavernous fistulas rarely close spontaneously and have been treated with endoarterial balloon embolization.

ONGOING CARE

- Septic cavernous sinus thrombosis may relapse or embolic abscesses may develop 2–6 weeks after therapy has been stopped.
- Repeat MRI with gadolinium should be considered, especially if symptoms recur or new symptoms develop.
- Mortality remains 13–30%, and <40% of patients recover fully from cranial nerve deficits.
- Patients with carotid-cavernous fistulas frequently have persistent cranial nerve deficits even after embolization.
- Idiopathic cavernous sinusitis responds to steroids, but relapses can be problematic. Clinical follow-up and serial MRI scans are indicated to rule out a low-grade neoplasm or fungal infection.
- Consultation with a neurooncologist and a neurosurgeon is important for suspected neoplasms or surgical lesions.

PROGNOSIS

- Prognosis depends on the underlying cause.
- Bacterial infections usually respond if diagnosed and treated promptly.

COMPLICATIONS

- Vary with the cause of cavernous sinus syndrome. Septic cavernous sinus syndrome thrombosis and fungal infections may rapidly evolve to bilateral thrombosis, life-threatening sepsis, and meningitis.
- Visual impairment and cranial nerve palsies may persist.
- *Mucormycosis*, usually seen in patients with diabetic ketoacidosis, is especially dangerous.
- Carotid arteritis with resulting stenosis, occlusion, or embolism may occur, resulting in focal neurologic deficits.
- Aseptic cavernous sinus syndrome thrombosis may evolve to more extensive intracranial venous sinus thrombosis.
- Local spread of neoplasms will continue if not treated appropriately.

ADDITIONAL READING

- Chen CC, Chang PC, Shy CG, et al. CT angiography and MR angiography in the evaluation of carotid-cavernous sinus fistula prior to embolization: a comparison of techniques. *Am J Neuroradiol*. 2005;26(9):2349–2356.
- Ebright JR, Pace MT, Niazi AF. Septic thrombosis of the cavernous sinuses. *Arch Intern Med*. 2001;161(22):2671–2676.
- Lee AG, Quick SJ, Liu GT, et al. A childhood cavernous conundrum. *Surv Ophthalmol*. 2004;49(2):231–236.
- Leiba H, Jaqqi GP, Boltshauser E, et al. Prediction of the clinical outcome of cavernous sinus lesions in children. *Neuropediatrics*. 2013;44(4):191–198.

CODES

ICD10

- I67.6 Nonpyogenic thrombosis of intracranial venous system
- G08 Intracranial and intraspinal phlebitis and thrombophlebitis
- H49.889 Other paralytic strabismus, unspecified eye

FAQ

- Q: Will my child's eye movements return to normal?
- A: In most cases, oculomotor nerves regain function as other signs improve, although they may take the longest to recover.
- Q: Can more pain medicine be given?
- A: There is often an attempt to balance side effects of sedation and hypoventilation against the need for pain control, especially when intracranial pressure is a concern.

CAVERNOUS TRANSFORMATION AND PORTAL VEIN OBSTRUCTION

Vani V. Gopalareddy

BASICS

DESCRIPTION

- Cavernous transformation: the collection of collaterals that develop around an obstructed vessel
- Portal vein obstruction
  - Can occur anywhere along the course of the main portal vein or splenic vein, between the hilum of the spleen and the porta hepatis
  - In pediatrics, obstruction is most typically of the portal vein.
- Major cause of prehepatic portal hypertension

EPIDEMIOLOGY

- Most children with portal vein thrombosis present between birth and 15 years of age.
- Acute presentation is rare.
- Chronic cases present with complications of portal hypertension.
- Gastrointestinal (GI) bleeding is more typical in patients presenting <7 years of age.
- Splenomegaly in the absence of symptoms is more typical for patients aged 5–15 years.

RISK FACTORS

Genetics

A genetic basis of this problem has not been identified, although congenital abnormalities of the heart, major blood vessels, biliary tree, and renal system are often found.

PATHOPHYSIOLOGY

- In cirrhosis and hepatic malignancies, the thrombus usually begins intrahepatically and spreads to the extrahepatic portal vein.
- In most other etiologies, the thrombus usually starts at the site of origin of the portal vein.
- Occasionally, thrombosis of the splenic vein propagates to the portal vein, most often resulting from an adjacent inflammatory process (e.g., severe pancreatitis).
- Asymptomatic splenomegaly or upper GI hemorrhage results from extrahepatic portal hypertension.
- Less commonly, ascites or failure to thrive, and portopulmonary hypertension

ETIOLOGY

50% of portal vein obstructions are idiopathic. Identified causes include the following:

- Congenital vascular anomaly
  - Portal vein malformation
  - Webs or diaphragms within the portal vein
- Clot resulting from a hypercoagulable state
- Clot from other causes:
  - Omphalitis
  - Umbilical vein catheterization
  - Portal pyelophlebitis
  - Intra-abdominal sepsis
  - Surgery near the porta hepatis
  - Sepsis
  - Cholangitis
  - Dehydration
  - Trauma
- Other causes for portal vein obstruction in older children:
  - Ascending pyelophlebitis from perforated appendicitis
  - Primary peritonitis, cholangitis, and pancreatitis causing a splenic vein thrombosis
  - Inflammatory bowel disease

DIAGNOSIS

HISTORY

- Splenomegaly (see "Splenomegaly" topic for complete differential)
  - Exposure to infectious mononucleosis
  - Metabolic storage disease (e.g., Gaucher disease)
  - Malignancy (e.g., chronic myelogenous leukemia)
- History of prematurity and admission to NICU should alert the clinician to previous umbilical vein catheterization and increased risk of portal vein thrombosis.

SIGNS AND SYMPTOMS

- Clinical history and examination should concentrate on identifying possible causes predisposing to portal vein obstruction.
- Portal vein obstruction does not affect liver function unless the patient has an underlying liver disease (e.g., cirrhosis). This situation is partially due to a compensatory increased flow of the hepatic artery maintaining the total hepatic blood flow.
- Mild coagulation profile abnormalities

PHYSICAL EXAM

- Splenomegaly
  - Spleen is measured from the left anterior axillary line at the costal margin diagonally toward the umbilicus and inferiorly toward the iliac crest
- Hemorrhoids

DIAGNOSTIC TESTS & INTERPRETATION

Lab

- CBC: Leukopenia and thrombocytopenia will be present if there is hypersplenism.
- Aspartate aminotransferase/alanine aminotransferase/γ-glutamyl transferase: should be normal
- PT/PTT: may be abnormal if malabsorption is present
- Additional testing associated with hypercoagulable states (as clinically indicated)
  - Protein C
  - Protein S
  - Antithrombin III levels
  - Factor V Leiden mutation
  - Activated protein C resistance
  - Lupus anticoagulation evaluation
  - Anticardiolipin antibodies (IgA, IgG, IgM)
  - Antinuclear antibody
  - Blood homocysteine
  - Prothrombin 20-21-0 mutation
  - Methylene tetrahydrofolate reductase mutation evaluation
  - Factor VIII coagulant
  - Reptilase time
  - Heparin cofactor II
  - Tissue plasminogen activator
  - Plasminogen activator inhibitor-1
  - Sticky platelet evaluation
  - Paroxysmal nocturnal hemoglobinuria (genetics or flow cytometry evaluation)

Imaging

- Ultrasound with Doppler
  - To examine portal vein flow and to identify collateral veins if there is cavernous transformation of the portal vein
  - Liver may be slightly small but may be normal in texture.
  - Remains the most useful imaging study
- CT angiography or MRV can give additional information if needed especially prior to planning a surgical portosystemic shunt procedure.

Diagnostic Procedures/Other

- Liver biopsy
  - Not required for diagnosis nor performed routinely
  - Exclude other etiologies
- Upper endoscopy and sigmoidoscopy: to define extent of varices

Pathologic Findings

- Portal hypertension: spider nevi, prominence of abdominal veins, splenomegaly
- Bruising: may be prominent when coexistent consumption of clotting factors
- Normal liver palpation and percussion
- Ascites rarely present

DIFFERENTIAL DIAGNOSIS

The differential diagnosis must exclude other causes of splenomegaly and portal hypertension.

TREATMENT

ADDITIONAL TREATMENT

General Measures

- General goals of therapy are (1) to manage variceal hemorrhage and (2) to identify an underlying cause and/or determine if the patient is at risk for additional venous thrombosis or malignancy.
- Therapy for GI variceal hemorrhage:
  - Octreotide infusion: 1 mcg/kg/h maximum 50 mcg/h
  - Prophylactic variceal banding for large esophageal varices
  - β-Blocker therapy
  - Rex shunt (mesenterico–left intrahepatic portal vein shunt):
    - Can be surgically addressed using the internal jugular vein, internal iliac vein, or dilated coronary vein, which is used to connect the superior mesenteric vein and the umbilical portion of the left portal vein (in the liver)
    - Restores the physiologic intrahepatic portal vein perfusion
    - Avoids the consequences of long-term portosystemic shunting, especially hepatic encephalopathy
- Portosystemic shunts: divert portal blood into the low-pressure systemic venous circulation. Classified into
  - Nonselective shunts: These communicate the entire portal venous system to a systemic venous circulation such as the mesocaval shunt, proximal splenorenal shunt, and portacaval shunts. Nonselective shunts divert more blood into the systemic venous system, and patients are more likely to have encephalopathy.
  - Selective shunts: These divert the gastrosplenic portion of the portal venous flow into the left renal vein or the inferior vena cava. The most common selective shunt is the distal splenorenal shunt (also known as the Warren shunt).

ONGOING CARE

FOLLOW-UP RECOMMENDATIONS

Focus on growth parameters, early detection of malabsorption, presence of GI hemorrhage, and nutritional intervention.

- Aggressive contact sports should be actively discouraged in children with hepatosplenomegaly.
- All patients should be advised to restrict activities that could injure their already enlarged spleen. Spleen guards may be recommended.
- Patients should be told to avoid medicines that interfere with platelet function
- In addition, patients should avoid medications that increase BP, including many over-the-counter cold medications (e.g., phenylephrine), as this can increase splanchnic pressures and may provoke variceal bleeds.

PROGNOSIS

- Long-term prognosis overall is considered good.
- Upper GI hemorrhage becomes less problematic as children become older.
- Rex shunt restores normal physiology and decreases portal pressure. In many centers, Rex shunt is performed as 1st-line therapy.
- Most patients receive β-blockers or undergo prophylactic banding. If the liver function remains normal, as in most cases, it is rare for encephalopathy to develop unless a large portosystemic shunt is created.

COMPLICATIONS

- Variceal hemorrhage from the upper tract or from the perianal varices
- Splenomegaly with hypersplenism
  - Thrombocytopenia
  - Consumption coagulopathy
  - Leukopenia
- Steatorrhea and protein-losing enteropathy occurs secondary to venous congestion of the intestinal mucosa.
- Degree of portal hypertension is variable and depends on the formation of spontaneous shunts that may decompress the portal hypertension. These autoshunts may predispose to the development of complications such as hepatic encephalopathy or hepatopulmonary syndrome.
- Spleen can undergo autoinfarction, resulting in intermittent episodes of pain.
- A large spleen is susceptible to traumatic rupture.
- Spontaneous splenic rupture may also occur (classically associated with infectious mononucleosis).

ADDITIONAL READING

- Fuchs J, Warmann S, Kardorff R, et al. Mesenterico—left portal vein bypass in children with congenital extrahepatic portal vein thrombosis: a unique curative approach. *J Pediatr Gastroenterol Nutr*. 2003;36(2):213–216.
- Mileti E, Rosenthal P. Management of portal hypertension in children. *Curr Gastroenterol Rep*. 2011;13(1):10–16.
- Ryckman FC, Alonso MH. Causes and management of portal hypertension in the pediatric population. *Clin Liver Dis*. 2001;5(3):789–818.
- Superina RA, Alonso EM. Medical and surgical management of portal hypertension in children. *Curr Treat Options Gastroenterol*. 2006;9(5):432–443.
- Superina R, Shneider B, Emre S, et al. Surgical guidelines for the management of extra-hepatic portal vein obstruction. *Pediatr Transplant*. 2006;10(8):908–913.

CODES

ICD10

- I81 Portal vein thrombosis
- K76.6 Portal hypertension
- Q26.9 Congenital malformation of great vein, unspecified

FAQ

- Q: Should I restrict my child's activities and avoid certain medications?
- A: Contact sports should be limited or a spleen guard should be used. NSAIDs, including aspirin, should be avoided because of the risk of hemorrhage. Medications that increase blood pressure, including many nonprescription cold preparations, should also be avoided.

CELIAC DISEASE

Dascha C. Weir

BASICS

DESCRIPTION

- Celiac disease (CD) is a systemic immune-mediated disorder caused by a permanent sensitivity to gluten in genetically susceptible individuals.
- "Gluten" is the collective term for specific alcohol-soluble proteins (called prolamines) that are found in wheat, rye, and barley.
- "Classic CD" refers to children who present predominately with malabsorptive symptoms including diarrhea, abdominal pain, vomiting, and abdominal distention in the setting of suboptimal growth and irritability.
- "Silent CD" defines a minority of people with CD who have no identifiable symptoms but have consistent intestinal mucosal lesions and elevated serum antibodies.
- A rare, but serious, manifestation of CD is termed "celiac crisis" and consists of severe watery diarrhea, electrolyte disturbances, dehydration, hypotension, and lethargy.
- Patients with positive serologic testing but normal intestinal histology are referred to as "potential CD." Some, but not all, of these patients are thought to develop CD overtime on a gluten-containing diet.

PATHOPHYSIOLOGY

- In people with CD, ingestion of gluten leads to an enteropathy of the small intestine characterized by mucosal inflammation and villous atrophy.
- Generation of unique serologic autoantibodies and development of a diverse spectrum of signs and symptoms also occur.
- Elimination of gluten, via implementation of a strict gluten-free diet (GFD), leads to intestinal healing, normalization of elevated antibody levels, and resolution of related symptoms.

EPIDEMIOLOGY

- CD is present in approximately 1% of the U.S. population, but only a small proportion have been diagnosed.
- Average age at diagnosis of pediatric CD in the United States is approximately 9 years old.
- Females are more affected than males.

Genetics

- There is increased prevalence in patients with 1st-degree relatives with CD (10–15%).
- HLA-DQ2 and HLA-DQ8 haplotypes are "necessary but not sufficient" for CD.
  - 90+% of CD patients carry HLA DQ2, 5% carry HLA-DQ8.
  - High negative predictive value for negative DQ2/DQ8 testing
  - Low positive predictive value (30% of general population in North America is HLA-DQ2 positive)
- Numerous other genes have been identified as increasing CD susceptibility.
- A family or personal history of autoimmune disease is also associated with CD.

COMMONLY ASSOCIATED CONDITIONS

- Autoimmune thyroiditis
- Type 1 diabetes mellitus
- Sjögren syndrome
- Selective IgA deficiency
- Williams syndrome
- Down syndrome
- Turner syndrome

DIAGNOSIS

- The range of signs and symptoms secondary to CD is broad. Malabsorptive symptoms such as diarrhea and weight loss are more commonly seen in early childhood. Other more subtle gastrointestinal (GI) symptoms in pediatric CD can be recurrent intermittent abdominal pain, intermittent diarrhea, constipation, and nausea.
- Extraintestinal manifestations of CD may be more prominent, especially in the older child. Atypical" or "nonclassic" symptoms can include the following:
  - Aphthous stomatitis
  - Arthritis/arthralgias
  - Delayed puberty
  - Dental enamel hypoplasia
  - Dermatitis herpetiformis (a pruritic blistering symmetric rash)
  - Elevated transaminases
  - Elevated pancreatic enzymes
  - Fatigue
  - Iron deficiency anemia
  - Neuropsychiatric symptoms (including headaches, cognitive impairment, neuropathy, epilepsy and ataxia)
  - Osteopenia
  - Short stature
  - Thyroiditis
  - Vitamin deficiencies
- Awareness of the wide range of clinical presentation and the high prevalence of CD coupled with a careful history and physical exam is essential to making the diagnosis of CD.
- Obtaining celiac-specific serologic markers is also integral to making the diagnosis.
- Currently, small bowel biopsies remain the gold standard and are required for confirmation of CD.
- Treatment with a GFD should not be initiated before confirmation of disease.

HISTORY

- Review the patient's stooling pattern as well as symptoms of abdominal pain, nausea/ vomiting, low appetite, and bloating/distension.
- Investigate extraintestinal manifestations of CD including fatigue, arthralgias, recurrent oral sores, unusual rashes, and headaches.
- Attention to family history of CD, long-standing undiagnosed GI symptoms, and autoimmune diseases

PHYSICAL EXAM

- Focus on growth patterns:
  - Some patients may have short stature or suboptimal weight gain as the only manifestation of CD.
  - Many children with CD have normal growth or even overweight status.
- Assess pubertal development.
- Although patients with classic CD often have a distended abdomen with wasted buttocks, most patients do not have clear physical signs of CD.
- Observe for dental enamel defects, oral sores, or dermatitis herpetiformis.

DIAGNOSTIC TESTS & INTERPRETATION

All evaluation for CD should be done while a patient is consuming gluten regularly. Testing for the disease while on a GFD can lead to false-negative results. Both serologic testing and histopathologic changes can normalize with gluten removal.

Initial Lab Tests

- Total IgA quantification is essential. IgA deficiency is associated with CD and can contribute to false-negative results.
- Celiac serologic markers with high specificity and sensitivity
  - Tissue transglutaminase antibody IgA (tTG IgA): best general screening test
  - Endomysial antibody IgA (EMA IgA): more subjective and expensive than tTG IgA
- Celiac serologic markers with low specificity and sensitivity
  - Antigliadin IgA and IgG (AGA IgA, AGA IgG) are NOT recommended for screening.
- New serologic markers: Deamidated gliadin peptide antibody IgG is a newer test with high sensitivity and specificity that may be useful to obtain in cases of IgA deficiency.
- Nonspecific testing to screen for associated nutritional deficiencies
  - Vitamin levels
  - CBC
  - Iron panel
  - Bone densitometry
  - Tests of absorption (fecal fat, D-xylose uptake)

Endoscopic Evaluation

- Small bowel biopsies obtained by esophagogastroduodenoscopy (EGD) is required in most cases to confirm CD.
  – It is recommended to obtain multiple small bowel biopsies during endoscopy due to the patchy distribution of lesions.
  – The duodenal bulb, in addition to the duodenum, should be biopsied.
  – The current recommendation is to obtain a small bowel biopsy on a gluten-containing diet.

Pathologic Findings

CD has a number of cardinal histopathologic findings on small bowel biopsy:

- Increased intraepithelial lymphocytosis
- Villous atrophy (partial, subtotal, or total)
- Crypt hyperplasia
- Infiltration of lamina propria with excess lymphocytes (CD4 T cells mainly) and plasma cells

DIFFERENTIAL DIAGNOSIS

- Presumed infectious causes:
  – Giardiasis
  – Rotavirus, parasites
  – Chronic gastroenteritis
  – Postenteritis enteropathy
  – Intractable diarrhea of infancy
  – Tropical sprue
  – Intestinal bacterial overgrowth
  – Immunodeficiency syndromes (HIV)
- Presumed noninfectious:
  – Milk or soy protein intolerance
  – Protein-calorie malnutrition
  – Eosinophilic gastroenteritis
  – Autoimmune enteropathy
  – Graft-versus-host disease
  – Collagenous sprue
  – Peptic duodenitis
  – Immunodeficiency syndromes
  – Crohn disease
  – Congenital enteropathies (microvillus inclusion disease, tufting enteropathy)
  – Bowel ischemia
  – Radiation
  – Chemotherapy

TREATMENT

- Current treatment of CD consists of a strict, lifelong gluten-free diet (GFD).
  – Elimination of all wheat, rye, and barley is essential, with close care to avoid cross-contamination during the preparation and serving of food.
  – Oats, unless specifically certified as gluten free, should also be avoided, as they are standardly contaminated with wheat.
- Consultation with a specialized dietitian with expertise in the GFD is recommended for all cases.

MEDICATION

There are no medications currently available to treat CD. However, people on a gluten-free diet should take a multivitamin. It is imperative to confirm that all medications are also GF.

It may be appropriate to consider recommending the following:

- Calcium and vitamin D
- Iron for iron deficiency anemia
- In patients with symptoms of lactose intolerance, lactase enzyme replacement

ONGOING CARE

FOLLOW-UP RECOMMENDATIONS

Patient Monitoring

- Close clinical monitoring of patients with newly diagnosed CD is important. Patients should be seen several times within the 1st year of diagnosis to monitor symptom response to the GFD, adherence to the GFD, and patient/family coping with the lifestyle changes associated with the GFD. After the 1st year, yearly follow-up is recommended.
- Special attention should be paid to growth at each visit. Catch-up growth is typically noted within the 1st year on the GFD.
- Monitor for other autoimmune disease, especially thyroiditis and diabetes mellitus, with targeted history and exam.
- Assessing for adequate calcium intake and vitamin D deficiency is also recommended to optimize bone health. Bone density in children with CD typically normalizes on a GFD. Bone densitometry can be considered but, in most cases, is recommended after a year on a GFD.
- tTG levels typically normalize within a year on the GFD and, coupled with clinical status, can be helpful in assessing response to the GFD. Obtaining a tTG IgA is recommended after 6 months on a GFD and then on a yearly basis.
- Repeat endoscopic evaluation is not currently recommended in patients who respond clinically to a GFD and who have normalization of tTG IgA. However, repeat endoscopic evaluation in cases of clinical nonresponse to the GFD or persistent serologic elevation should be considered.

PROGNOSIS

In patients with CD, it is strongly recommended to remain on a GFD for life. In patients on a strict GFD, there is lower risk for malignancies and other complications associated with CD. However, increased risk of other autoimmune diseases seems to persist.

COMPLICATIONS

- Adults with CD have increased risk of intestinal lymphoma and other GI malignancies. This risk is magnified in suboptimally treated CD.
- Other complications include the following:
  – Osteopenia/osteoporosis
  – Infertility
  – Development of other autoimmune disorders.
  – Nutritional deficiencies
- Refractory CD is a diagnosis of exclusion that is defined by persistent symptoms and villous atrophy on a strict GFD.
  – Refractory CD is rare in children but affects up to 5% of adults with CD, most of whom harbor an abnormal clonal intraepithelial T-lymphocyte population
  – Complications of refractory sprue: "Cryptogenic enteropathy-associated T-cell lymphoma," ulcerative jejunoileitis, and collagenous sprue.
  – Treatment: immunosuppressives including corticosteroids, azathioprine, cyclosporine, and total parenteral nutrition, in addition to GFD

ADDITIONAL READING

- Fasano A, Catassi C. Clinical practice. Celiac disease. *N Engl J Med*. 2012;367(25):2419–2426.
- Hill ID, Dirks M, Liptak G, et al. Guideline for the diagnosis and treatment of celiac disease in children: recommendations of the North American Society for Pediatric Gastroenterology, Hepatology and Nutrition. *J Pediatr Gastroenterol Nutr*. 2005;40(1):1–19.
- Leffler DA, Schuppan D. Update on serologic testing in celiac disease. *Am J Gastroenterol*. 2010;105(12):2520–2524.
- Olsson C, Hernell O, Hörnell A, et al. Difference in celiac disease risk between Swedish birth cohorts suggests an opportunity for primary prevention. *Pediatrics*. 2008;122(3):528–534.

CODES

ICD10

K90.0 Celiac disease

FAQ

- Q: Is biopsy confirmation necessary if my patient is already doing better on a GFD?
- A: Yes. Referral to a pediatric gastroenterologist who can obtain small bowel biopsy is recommended in almost all cases of suspected pediatric CD.
- Q: Are oats included in the gluten-containing cereal group?
- A: Strictly speaking, wheat, rye, and barley are more closely related in their development from the primitive grains than are oat, rice, corn, sorghum, and millets, which do not activate CD. Gluten-free means a diet devoid of all wheat, rye, and barley. Several studies have shown that ingestion of oats did not cause histologic or clinical deterioration. However, it is important to use a brand of oats that has been tested and demonstrated to not be contaminated with gluten.

CELLULITIS

Nicholas Tsarouhas

BASICS

DESCRIPTION

- Cellulitis is an acute, spreading pyogenic inflammation of the dermis and subcutaneous tissue, often complicating a wound or other skin condition.
- Cellulitis may be further classified by the unique area of the body it affects (e.g., periorbital or orbital cellulitis, peritonsillar cellulitis, etc.).

EPIDEMIOLOGY

- The most common cause of cellulitis in children is *Staphylococcus aureus* or *Streptococcus pyogenes* infection, which develop secondary to local trauma of the integument.
- Community-acquired methicillin-resistant *Staphylococcus aureus* (CA-MRSA) infections continue to increase in incidence, but much more commonly cause purulent abscesses rather than cellulitis.
- The prevalence of CA-MRSA among purulent skin and soft tissue infections is >60% in some communities.
- Clinical failures caused by penicillin-resistant *Streptococcus pneumoniae* have not yet become a significant problem in cases of uncomplicated cellulitis.
- Bacteremic disease is uncommon, owing to the tremendous efficacy of vaccines against both *Haemophilus influenzae* type b (Hib) and *S. pneumoniae*.

GENERAL PREVENTION

- Good wound care is paramount.
- All wounds should be cleaned with soap and water, then covered with a clean, dry cloth.
- Topical antibiotic ointment is optional with minor wounds.

PATHOPHYSIOLOGY

- Cellulitis usually occurs after local trauma that breaches in the integument (abrasions, lacerations, bite wounds, excoriated dermatitis, varicella, etc.).
- Secondary to local invasion or infection (e.g., sinusitis leading to orbital cellulitis)
- Hematogenous dissemination (rarely)

ETIOLOGY

- *S. aureus*: methicillin-susceptible *Staphylococcus aureus* (MSSA) and MRSA
- Group A β-hemolytic streptococci (GABHS, or *S. pyogenes*)
- *S. pneumoniae* (uncommon)
- Group B streptococci (GBS) and gram-negative rods (GNRs): neonates
- Hib (rare)
- *Pseudomonas aeruginosa* and anaerobic bacteria: immunocompromised children
- *Pasteurella* species: from cat and dog bites
- *Eikenella corrodens*: from human bites

COMMONLY ASSOCIATED CONDITIONS

- Periorbital
  - Usually from local trauma (scratch, impetigo, eczema, excoriated varicella)
  - Hematogenous spread is very uncommon.
  - Rarely associated with infectious conjunctivitis
- Orbital
  - Commonly associated with severe sinusitis
  - Less commonly: dental abscess, trauma, hematogenous spread
- Buccal: usually from local trauma; hematogenous seeding also very rare.
- Peritonsillar
  - Commonly due to GABHS pharyngitis
  - Cellulitis may progress to a peritonsillar abscess.
- Extremity: usually secondary to local trauma
- Breast: usually with mastitis (neonates)
- Perianal
  - Seen in infants and young children
  - Etiology: GABHS
  - Perianal pain, pruritus, and erythema; sometimes associated with bloody stools
- Cellulitis–adenitis syndrome
  - Neonates and infants
  - Etiology: GBS, *S. aureus*, GNRs
  - Bacteremia/meningitis commonly associated.

DIAGNOSIS

HISTORY

- An expanding, red, painful area of swelling is the most common presentation.
- Mild constitutional symptoms (with or without fever) are commonly associated with cellulitis.
- A history of local trauma to the integument is the clue to the portal of bacterial entry.
- Visual changes, proptosis, and painful or limited eye movements are classic findings in orbital cellulitis.
- Painful swallowing, pain with opening the mouth (trismus), and muffled ("hot potato") voice are classic presenting symptoms of peritonsillar cellulitis/abscess.

PHYSICAL EXAM

- Erythema, edema, tenderness, and warmth: usual clinical findings of cellulitis
- Distinct demarcation of raised erythema: classic description of erysipelas, a superficial cellulitis usually associated with *S. pyogenes*
- A red streak extending proximally from the extremity: lymphangitis, which usually implies more serious involvement
- Regional adenopathy: commonly associated with minor cellulitis; occasionally complicated by lymphadenitis

DIAGNOSTIC TESTS & INTERPRETATION

Lab

- WBC: normal or elevated
- Blood culture: rarely positive. Ill-appearing children and children with extensive areas of cellulitis may warrant a blood culture.
- Wound culture: As resistance continues to rise (especially MRSA), wound cultures are useful.

Imaging

- Radiographs: sometimes helpful to rule out complications such as osteomyelitis. Also useful in cases of suspected foreign bodies
- Ultrasound: often useful to distinguish cellulitis from abscess, which might need incision and drainage (I&D).
- Head CT scan: important in cases when clinical distinction between periorbital and orbital cellulitis is difficult. Useful in orbital cellulitis to delineate extent of disease

Diagnostic Procedures/Other

In some cases, a cutaneous biopsy, examined by an experienced pathologist, may be needed to identify the correct diagnosis.

DIFFERENTIAL DIAGNOSIS

- Allergic angioedema can be excluded by its lack of tenderness and the absence of fever.
- Allergic reactions to insect stings are usually pruritic and may present with mild to severe local erythema, a bite history confirmatory.
- Red giant urticarial lesions, similarly, may masquerade as cellulitis.
- Contact dermatitis is distinguished by its painlessness, pruritus, and the Koebner phenomenon (appearance of isomorphic lesions in the lines of scratching).
- Nummular eczema is a pruritic dermatitis consisting of one or more circular lesions with papules, scales, and/or crusting, typically distributed on the trunk or extremities.
- The erythema migrans rash of Lyme disease starts as a red macule at the tick bite site, then expands to a large, annular, erythematous lesion; the classic "bulls eye" lesion with central clearing is not always seen.
- A traumatic contusion may be mistaken for cellulitis; the history confirms the diagnosis.
- Severe conjunctivitis presents with conjunctival injection, chemosis, and discharge.
- "Popsicle panniculitis," a cold-induced fat injury to the cheeks of infants; mimics buccal cellulitis; a history of cold weather exposure, eating ice, or popsicle sucking, are classic.

- Erythema nodosum, a panniculitis with raised, tender lesions that are frequently over the shins; may present as a single erythematous lesion. Associated with systemic disorders, including inflammatory bowel disease
- Superficial thrombophlebitis is distinguished by a tender cord palpable along the course of the affected superficial vein.
- An eye malignancy (retinoblastoma), invasive tumor (rhabdomyosarcoma), or metastatic disease (neuroblastoma, leukemia, lymphoma) may simulate periorbital or orbital cellulitis.

TREATMENT

MEDICATION

- Most cases of uncomplicated, superficial "nonpurulent" cellulitis (cellulitis with no purulent drainage or exudate, and no associated abscess) may be treated with β-lactam oral antibiotics active against β-hemolytic streptococci and MSSA (e.g., cephalexin or amoxicillin-clavulanate).
- Coverage for MRSA is indicated in patients who do not respond to initial therapy, patients with signs of systemic illness, patients with recurrent infection in the setting of underlying predisposing conditions, and patients with a previous episode of MRSA infection.
- Additionally, MRSA coverage should be considered in patients with MRSA risk factors, and in areas where the prevalence of MRSA is greater than 30%.
- Patients with purulent cellulitis (cellulitis associated with purulent drainage or exudate, in the absence of a drainable abscess) should be treated with antibiotics active against MRSA.
- Clindamycin is an excellent initial choice due to its activity against β-hemolytic streptococci and both MSSA and MRSA.
- Trimethoprim-sulfamethoxazole covers both MSSA and MRSA, but not β-hemolytic streptococci; consequently, some combine it with amoxicillin.
- Some experts feel that initial coverage against β-hemolytic streptococci is not always mandatory in patients with purulent cellulitis; thus, monotherapy with trimethoprim-sulfamethoxazole is also sometimes used.
- Doxycycline and minocycline are additional alternatives with good MRSA coverage, especially for penicillin-allergic patients.
- Erythromycin is also sometimes used in patients allergic to penicillin; isolates resistant to erythromycin exist, however, and may be cross-resistant to clindamycin as well.
- Ill-appearing children or those with extensive cellulitic lesions require IV antibiotics.
- As MRSA infections continue to rise, most experts now recommend clindamycin as initial parenteral therapy.
- Oxacillin, nafcillin, cefazolin, and ampicillin-sulbactam are reasonable alternatives when MRSA is not strongly suspected.
- Vancomycin is used as empiric therapy in ill-appearing children or with severe or rapidly progressive infections.
- Linezolid, a newer antibiotic that can be given IV or PO, is very effective against MRSA, but it is expensive and should mostly be reserved for multi-resistant organisms.
- If hematogenous dissemination is a strong possibility, an agent active against Hib also should be added (e.g., ceftriaxone, cefotaxime).
- The duration of antibiotics (IV and PO) should generally be 7–10 days.
- Bite wounds should have tetanus and rabies prophylaxis issues addressed.

ALERT

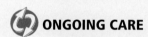

- Remember to consider the possibility of MRSA in all deep, invasive, or persistent infections (i.e., consider clindamycin).
- Penicillin and amoxicillin are never good empiric choices for cellulitis because they have poor *S. aureus* coverage.

ADDITIONAL TREATMENT

General Measures

Local care of cellulitis involves elevation and immobilization of the limb to reduce swelling, and cool sterile saline dressings to remove purulence from open lesions.

SURGERY/OTHER PROCEDURES

Abscesses should always be drained.

ONGOING CARE

FOLLOW-UP RECOMMENDATIONS

- Steady improvement should be expected.
- If daily improvement is not noted, consider the following:
  – Inappropriate antimicrobial coverage
  – A deeper infection or abscess that needs drainage
  – Foreign body

PROGNOSIS

The prognosis for complete recovery is good as long as appropriate antimicrobials are administered in a timely fashion.

COMPLICATIONS

- Local or distant spread of infection is possible.
- Suppuration and abscess formation may occur (e.g., peritonsillar abscess).
- Extremity cellulitis may extend into the deep tissues to produce an arthritis or osteomyelitis, or it may extend proximally as a lymphangitis.
- Orbital cellulitis may be complicated by visual loss and/or cavernous sinus thrombosis.
- Prior to widespread immunization against Hib, the bacteremia associated with facial cellulitis was associated with pneumonia, meningitis, pericarditis, epiglottitis, arthritis, and osteomyelitis.

ADDITIONAL READING

- Elliott DJ, Zaoutis TE, Troxel AB, et al. Empiric antimicrobial therapy for pediatric skin and soft-tissue infections in the era of methicillin-resistant *Staphylococcus aureus*. *Pediatrics*. 2009;123(6):e959–e966.
- Hyun DY, Mason EO, Forbes A, et al. Trimethoprim-sulfamethoxazole or clindamycin for treatment of community-acquired methicillin-resistant *Staphylococcus aureus* skin and soft tissue infections. *Pediatr Infect Dis J*. 2009;28(1):57–59.
- Khawcharoenporn T, Tice A. Empiric outpatient therapy with trimethoprim-sulfamethoxazole, cephalexin, or clindamycin for cellulitis. *Am J Med*. 2010;123(10):942–950.
- Liu C, Bayer A, Cosgrove SE, et al. Clinical practice guidelines by the Infectious Diseases Society of America for the treatment of methicillin-resistant *Staphylococcus aureus* infections in adults and children. *Clin Infect Dis*. 2011;52(3):e18–e55.
- Moran GJ, Krishnadasan A, Gorwitz RJ, et al. Methicillin-resistant *S. aureus* infections among patients in the emergency department. *N Engl J Med*. 2006;355(7):666.
- Odell CA. Community-associated methicillin-resistant *Staphylococcus aureus* (CA-MRSA) skin infections. *Curr Opin Pediatr*. 2010;22(3):273–277.
- Pallin DJ, Binder WD, Allen MB, et al. Comparative effectiveness of cephalexin plus trimethoprim-sulfamethoxazole versus cephalexin alone for treatment of uncomplicated cellulitis: a randomized controlled trial. *Clin Infect Dis*. 2013;56(12):1754–1762.
- Stevens DL, Eron LL. Cellulitis and soft-tissue infections. *Ann Intern Med*. 2009;150(1):ITC11.
- Swartz MN. Clinical practice. Cellulitis. *N Engl J Med*. 2004;350(9):904–912.

CODES

ICD10

- L03.90 Cellulitis, unspecified
- H05.019 Cellulitis of unspecified orbit
- J36 Peritonsillar abscess

FAQ

- Q: Is IV ampicillin-sulbactam adequate initial parenteral therapy for cellulitis with abscess?
- A: No. MRSA should be covered in these patients. IV clindamycin is a better choice.
- Q: When should IV vancomycin be used?
- A: IV vancomycin should be reserved for ill-appearing children or those with severe or rapidly progressive infections. These are cases where any treatment delay waiting for definitive culture and sensitivity results is prohibitive.

CEREBRAL PALSY

Stephen Contompasis

BASICS

DESCRIPTION

Cerebral palsy (CP) describes a group of disorders of movement and posture, limiting activity, attributed to nonprogressive underlying brain pathology. The motor disorders of CP are often accompanied by disturbances of sensation, cognition, communication, perception, and/or behavior or by a seizure disorder:

- Spastic (pyramidal; 75%): increased deep tendon reflexes, sustained clonus, hypertonia, and the clasp-knife response:
  - Spastic diplegia: lower extremity involvement
  - Spastic hemiplegia: 1 side of the body involved
  - Spastic quadriplegia: total body involvement; usually associated with dystonia
- Dyskinetic (10%): fluctuating tone, rigid total body involvement by definition. Persistent primitive reflex patterns (asymmetric tonic neck reflex, labyrinthine)
  - Athetoid: slow writhing movements (or chorea; rapid, random, jerky movements)
  - Dystonic: posturing of the head, trunk, and extremities
- Ataxic (<10%): characterized by cerebellar signs (ataxia, dysmetria, past pointing, tremor, nystagmus) and abnormalities of voluntary movement
- Mixed (10%): 2 or more types codominant, most often spastic and dyskinetic
- Other (10%): Criteria for CP met, but specific subtype cannot be defined.
- Extrapyramidal: sometimes applied to nonspastic types of CP as a group

EPIDEMIOLOGY

- ~50% of cases are associated with prematurity.
- Increased concordance among monozygotic versus dizygotic twins in some studies (not in others)
- Intrauterine growth retardation (IUGR) more common in CP than controls, especially for full-term infants in whom CP develops.
- Male > female (1.3:1)
- Inconsistent relationship to maternal age, socioeconomic status, and parity
- Prenatal factors are more strongly associated with subsequent CP than are perinatal or postnatal factors; however, individual risk factors are poorly predictive of subsequent CP in the individual child.
- Perinatal asphyxia accounts for only ~9% of CP; diagnosis requires evidence of hypoxic-ischemic insult, severe encephalopathy (e.g., neonatal seizures, severe hypotonia), and consistent laboratory/radiologic findings.
- Increased with multiple gestation (10% were twins in 1 study)
- Prevalence ~2–3/1,000

ETIOLOGY

- Not apparent in most cases. A more recently recognized perinatal factor is the presence of chorioamnionitis; mild or even subclinical infection may have increased association with CP.
- Epidemiologic studies indicate 2 types of associated vulnerability to CP:
  - Prematurity: Vulnerability of the periventricular white matter between 28 and 32 weeks of gestation results in periventricular leukomalacia.
  - IUGR: Fetal growth retardation associated with CNS dysgenesis, non-CNS malformation, teratogens, growth retardation, evidence of hypoxic-ischemic encephalopathy.

COMMONLY ASSOCIATED CONDITIONS

- Sensory
  - Sensorineural and conductive hearing loss
  - Impaired visual acuity
  - Oculomotor dysfunction
  - Strabismus
  - Cortical visual impairment
  - Somatosensory impairments
- Cognitive/developmental
  - Intellectual disability in ~50%, especially in spastic quadriparesis
  - Autism, ADHD
  - Language and learning disabilities
  - Dysarthria
  - Sleep and behavioral disturbances
- Neurologic
  - Seizures
  - Hydrocephalus
- Musculoskeletal
  - Contractures
  - Hip subluxation/dislocation
  - Scoliosis
- Cardiorespiratory
  - Upper airway obstruction
  - Aspiration pneumonitis
  - Restrictive lung disease/thoracic deformity
  - Reactive airway disease
- GI/nutritional
  - Poor growth
  - Gastroesophageal reflux
  - Constipation
  - Oral motor dysfunction/dysphagia
- Urinary: neurogenic bladder
- Skin: decubitus ulcers
- Dental
  - Malocclusions
  - Caries
  - Gingival hyperplasia
  - Abnormalities of enamel (congenital)

DIAGNOSIS

HISTORY

- Prenatal
  - Exposure to toxins/drugs
  - Infections or fever
  - HIV/STD risk
  - Vaginal bleeding
  - Abnormal fetal movement
  - Preeclampsia (especially proteinuria)
  - Breech position
  - Poor maternal weight gain
  - Premature labor
  - Fetal distress
  - IUGR
  - Prenatal testing
  - Placental disorders
- Perinatal
  - Premature delivery
  - Neonatal resuscitation
  - Low Apgar scores (<5 at 5 minutes)
  - Birth trauma
  - Evidence of neonatal encephalopathy (seizures, lethargy, hypotonia)
  - Complicated neonatal course (intraventricular hemorrhage, prolonged respiratory support, meningitis, sepsis, hyperbilirubinemia)
- Postnatal
  - Hospitalization for severe infection or trauma
  - Periodic or persistent deterioration in function (suggests neurodegenerative/metabolic disease)
- Development
  - Significant delay in motor milestones/motor quotient (age of typical skill attainment/age of attainment <0.5) (e.g., not rolling at 10 months, not sitting at 12 months, not walking at 24 months)
  - Associated with persistent primitive reflexes (e.g., prominent tonic neck and labyrinthine responses at 1 year of age) and delayed or absent development of protective reactions (e.g., lateral prop at 7 months, parachute at 13 months)
  - Associated delays in language, play, social, and adaptive behavior

PHYSICAL EXAM

- General observation: evidence of dysmorphism/pigmentary skin changes and growth abnormalities
- Head circumference: to evaluate for microcephaly/macrocephaly/hydrocephaly; growth velocity points to timing of brain pathology
- Strabismus/cataracts/iris or retinal abnormalities: eye exam: cranial nerve damage, muscle imbalance, metabolic disease, or congenital infection
- Musculoskeletal
  - Decreased range with contractures
  - Leg length discrepancy: hip dislocation
  - Spinal curvature/scoliosis

- Neurologic
  - Documentation of best level of visual motor/manipulative skills (transfer, hold a cup): to follow course of motor impairment
  - Cranial nerves: strabismus, speech and swallowing, vision and hearing
  - Tone: spasticity versus rigidity versus hypotonia
  - Strength: often decreased
  - Hyperactive deep tendon reflexes and clonus in spasticity; Babinski reflex (extensor response to plantar stimulation)
  - Persistent primitive reflexes
  - Protective reactions: head and trunk righting, prop reactions, parachute; cerebellar signs
  - Balance, stability

ALERT
Pitfalls
- Overdiagnosis of CP in premature infants with spastic hypertonia; normalization of tone/function may take up to 2 years.
- False or premature assumption of cognitive deficit in children with severe dysarthria. May take years of augmentative communication supports to determine true potential
- Slowly progressive neurodegenerative diseases and pediatric neurotransmitter disorders may masquerade as CP.
- Cervical cord lesions may masquerade as quadriparetic spastic CP.
- Determination of ideal body weight/caloric requirements may be complex in CP; skinfold measuring <10th percentile is the best indicator of poor nutrition.
- Pain is a common problem, with more than half of adults and children with CP reporting pain as an ongoing health concern.

DIAGNOSTIC TESTS & INTERPRETATION

Lab
- Genetic and metabolic studies: if history or physical suggests a progressive or hereditary disorder
- Blood chemistries, liver function studies, cell counts: evaluate nutritional/metabolic status, anticonvulsant levels

Imaging
- Brain imaging: perform when hydrocephalus is suspected; can help determine etiology
- Radiography: should be done routinely in spastic diparesis for hip dislocation; consider scoliosis films.
- Radionuclide studies to evaluate gastroesophageal reflux, gastric emptying, aspiration

Diagnostic Procedures/Other
- Hearing and vision: all in 1st year, with regular follow-up exams
- Audiologic evaluation required per guidelines
- Urodynamic studies: spastic bladder in those with recurrent UTIs or voiding dysfunction
- Sleep study: may disclose treatable obstructive sleep apnea in those with somnolence or abnormal sleep–wake cycles
- Pulmonary function studies: document progressive restrictive pulmonary dysfunction (e.g., in severe scoliosis)
- Consider bone density: liability to fracture
- Brain wave (EEG): if seizure suspected

DIFFERENTIAL DIAGNOSIS
- Motor syndromes related to spinal cord, lower motor neuron, peripheral nerve, primary muscular disease, or progressive disorders of the basal ganglia (dopa-responsive dystonia)
- Connective tissue disorders (primary and secondary) resulting in musculoskeletal abnormalities (e.g., arthrogryposis multiplex, skeletal dysplasias)
- Inborn errors of metabolism and CP: protean manifestations, dyskinesia, ataxia, postnatal growth failure, neurologic deterioration, recurrent vomiting

TREATMENT

ADDITIONAL TREATMENT

General Measures
- Family-centered care is directed toward optimizing activity and participation.
- Interdisciplinary clinics: services (medical, surgical, therapy) coordinated with primary physician
- More frequent health maintenance visits and coordination meetings from a medical home practice may assist in managing multiple chronic associated heath conditions.
- Spasticity reduction with IM injections of botulinum toxin is well supported. Oral or intrathecal baclofen used increasingly, although consensus on functional improvement long term is variable.
- Orthopedic management with directed procedures to reduce contractures and improve posture has more evidence on improving functional outcomes long term.
- Education services: recent emphasis on inclusion/mainstreaming; for many, special education services are still required.
- Augmentative communication supports especially for nonverbal/dysarthric children.
- Physical, occupational, speech/language therapy, other allied health professionals: Therapy provided in home, school, and hospital settings; directed primarily at improved mobility, self-care, and communication; orthodontists for braces
- Counseling support for children coping with chronic disability
- Social services: provided in a variety of contexts to aid in the coordination of care
- Vocational counseling and employment options, assistance with transition to adulthood, self-advocacy, self-determination
- Transition to adult health care system

ONGOING CARE

FOLLOW-UP RECOMMENDATIONS
- Requirements for follow-up vary greatly with the degree of disability and impairment. An interdisciplinary clinic setting may be more appropriate for a child with severe CP.
- Early referral to a pediatric orthopedist is indicated, especially for monitoring of the hip.
- Early referral for developmental assessment: need for early intervention to optimize development and promote family coping

DIET
Nutritional assessment and support for those with dysphagia or poor growth (especially calcium, vitamin D intake)

ADDITIONAL READING

- Delgado MR, Hirtz D, Aisen M, et al; Quality Standards Subcommittee of the American Academy of Neurology, Practice Committee of the Child Neurology Society. Practice parameter: pharmacologic treatment of spasticity in children and adolescents with cerebral palsy (an evidence-based review): report of the Quality Standards Subcommittee of the American Academy of Neurology and the Practice Committee of the Child Neurology Society. *Neurology*. 2010;74(4):336–343.
- Liptak GS, Murphy NA. Providing a primary care medical home for children and youth with cerebral palsy. *Pediatrics*. 2011;128(5):e1321–e1329. doi:10.1542/peds. 2011–1468.
- Pakula AT, Van Naarden Braun K, Yeargin-Allsopp M. Cerebral palsy: classification and epidemiology. *Phys Med Rehabil Clin N Am*. 2009;20(3):425–452.
- Rosenbaum P, Paneth N, Leviton A, et al. A report: the definition and classification of cerebral palsy April 2006. *Dev Med Child Neurol Suppl*. 2007;109:8–14. doi:10.1111/j.1469-8749.2007.tb12610.x.
- Strauss D, Brooks J, Rosenbloom L, et al. Life expectancy in cerebral palsy: an update. *Dev Med Child Neurol*. 2008;50(7):487–493.

CODES

ICD10
- G80.9 Cerebral palsy, unspecified
- G80.1 Spastic diplegic cerebral palsy
- G80.2 Spastic hemiplegic cerebral palsy

FAQ
- Q: Is severe clumsiness a form of CP?
- A: Mild spastic diplegia or hemiplegia may present this way, but tone abnormalities and significant functional impairments distinguish CP from milder developmental coordination disorders.
- Q: Do all children with CP also have intellectual disability?
- A: Only ~50% have intellectual disability.

CERVICITIS

Elizabeth M. Wallis • Sarah E. Winters

BASICS

DESCRIPTION

Infection of the endocervix resulting in inflammation, leading to mucopurulent cervical discharge, edema, erythema, bleeding, and friability of the cervix and endocervical canal

EPIDEMIOLOGY

- The true incidence of cervicitis is unknown; however, the primary causes (gonorrhea/chlamydia) are more common in adolescents and young adults than any other age group.
- Because many patients are asymptomatic and the interpretation and presence of the clinical signs is quite variable, many cases go undiagnosed.

RISK FACTORS

- Early age of coitarche
- Multiple sexual partners
- Absent or inconsistent condom use

ETIOLOGY

In most cases of cervicitis, no pathogen is isolated. Common causes include the following:

- *Chlamydia trachomatis*
- *Neisseria gonorrhoeae*
- *Herpesvirus hominis*
- *Trichomonas vaginalis*
- *Mycoplasma genitalium*

COMMONLY ASSOCIATED CONDITIONS

The presence of other sexually transmitted infections (STIs) must be considered, including the following:

- Syphilis
- Hepatitis B
- HIV
- Bacterial vaginosis

DIAGNOSIS

HISTORY

- Often asymptomatic
- If symptomatic: Symptoms consistent with but not diagnostic of cervicitis:
  - Abnormal vaginal bleeding and/or discharge? Inflamed cervix may bleed spontaneously or following sexual intercourse.
  - Dysuria? May indicate urethritis or bladder infection
  - Vulvar itching? May be associated discharge from cervical inflammation or a coexisting vaginal infection
  - Dyspareunia? Common complaint owing to the sensitive cervix
- Past medical history—important to evaluate risk factors related to sexual health but not diagnostic of cervicitis
  - Previous STI? Identifies patients at increased risk for reinfection
  - Last menstrual period? Symptomatic infection often occurs within 7 days of the last menstrual period because of loss of the protective endocervical mucous plug.
  - Birth control method? Condoms are protective.
  - Exposure to infected partner? Identifies patient at increased risk
  - Gravity?
  - Parity?

PHYSICAL EXAM

- Abdominal exam
  - No tenderness on palpation of the abdomen suggests that infection is limited to the cervix.
- Vaginal exam
  - Assess for signs of vaginal/external lesions consistent with herpes simplex virus (HSV).
- Pelvic exam
  - Mucopurulent discharge from the cervical os or yellow exudative discharge present on a cotton-tipped swab from the endocervical canal: clinical evidence of cervical infection
  - No cervical motion or adnexal tenderness or masses: Pathology has not extended beyond the cervix to the upper genital tract.
  - Friability of the exocervix: easily induced bleeding from the cervical canal not to be confused with normal cervical ectopy (area of columnar epithelium around the cervical os presenting as a discrete, nonfriable, reddish circle)

ALERT

Pitfalls:

- Failure to recognize the importance of evaluating the internal pelvic organs by physical examination with the presenting symptoms of dysuria, vaginal discharge, or abnormal menstrual bleeding in the postpubertal female
- Imperative not to confuse normal cervical ectropion in an adolescent with cervicitis

DIAGNOSTIC TESTS & INTERPRETATION

Lab

- Nucleic acid amplification tests done on the patient's urine offers the least invasive method to detect *Chlamydia*, gonococcal, and *Trichomonas* infections. Cervical or vaginal swabs may also be used for nucleic acid amplification tests, provided that there is no bleeding:
  - Cervical swabs, vaginal swabs obtained by the health care provider, and urine have similar sensitivity and specificity.
  - Cervical cultures for chlamydia and gonorrhea will also identify the pathogen but require a speculum examination.
  - Identifies the pathogen, which is important for patient and partner treatment and disease surveillance
- HSV culture if vesicular rash or ulcers are present: important to identify the cause of the ulcers for treatment and patient counseling
- Wet preparation and vaginal pH may be helpful in diagnosing bacterial vaginosis.

DIFFERENTIAL DIAGNOSIS

- It is helpful to consider cervicitis/vaginitis as a single disease in the evaluation process because the symptoms of these 2 entities are the same.
- Inflammation of the vulva, urethra, and/or bladder, and vagina
- In patients presenting with abnormal menstrual bleeding, these infectious causes are common.
- Pregnancy is a frequent cause of abnormal vaginal bleeding.
- Foreign body can be associated with both discharge and bleeding.
- Polycystic ovary syndrome (PCOS), thyroid dysfunction, and hyperprolactinemia can all present with abnormal vaginal bleeding.
- Noninfectious cervicitis occurs and is primarily caused by mechanical or chemical irritation (foreign objects, latex, vaginal douches, contraceptive creams).

C

TREATMENT

MEDICATION
- Gonorrhea
  - Ceftriaxone 250 mg IM or, PLUS azithromycin 1 g PO, single dose or doxycycline 100 mg PO b.i.d. for 7 days. Oral cefixime is no longer recommended as first line due to resistance. If cefixime is used because ceftriaxone is not available, a test of cure is necessary.
  - Recently, noticed patterns of resistance to fluoroquinolones have caused the CDC to no longer recommend this class as first line of treatment of gonococcal cervicitis in the United States.
  - If fluoroquinolones are used, a test of cure is necessary.
- *C. trachomatis*
  - Azithromycin 1 g PO, single dose
  - Doxycycline 100 mg PO b.i.d. for 7 days
  - Erythromycin base 500 mg PO q.i.d. for 7 days
- *T. vaginalis*
  - Metronidazole 2 g PO, single dose
  - Metronidazole 500 mg PO b.i.d. for 7 days
  - Tinidazole 2 g PO in a single dose
- *H. hominis*
  - Acyclovir 400 mg PO t.i.d. for 7–10 days or until resolution
  - Acyclovir 200 mg PO 5 times daily for 7–10 days or until resolution
  - Famciclovir 250 mg PO t.i.d. for 7–10 days or until resolution
  - Valacyclovir 1 g PO b.i.d. for 7–10 days or until resolution

INPATIENT CONSIDERATIONS

Initial Stabilization
Patients meeting the criteria for the clinical diagnosis of cervicitis or those who have a high likelihood of infection should receive presumptive therapy for *N. gonorrhoeae* and *C. trachomatis*. Treat other pathogens if clinically indicated or if documented by laboratory studies.

ONGOING CARE

FOLLOW-UP RECOMMENDATIONS
- The recommended treatment regimens have an excellent cure rate.
- The patient should have resolution of symptoms 3–5 days after starting therapy.
- Patients should abstain from intercourse until 7 days after both partners have been treated to prevent reinfection.
- Routine follow-up cultures are not necessary unless the patient remains symptomatic or in the case of pregnancy.
- Nucleic acid amplification tests done <6 weeks following treatment may yield false-positive results because of persistence of dead organisms.
- Detection of an STI at follow-up is most likely the result of reexposure and reinfection.

Patient Monitoring
- Partners should be referred for evaluation and treatment if laboratory diagnosis of gonorrhea/chlamydia or *Trichomonas* is made.
- Gonorrhea/chlamydia are reportable STIs.

PROGNOSIS
If treated appropriately, patients are cured and have no sequelae from the infection.

COMPLICATIONS
The patient with endocervical infection is at risk for the following:
- Reinfection
- Other STIs
- Pregnancy
- Symptomatic or asymptomatic upper genital tract disease (pelvic inflammatory disease), with all its sequelae:
  - Tubo-ovarian abscess
  - Infertility
  - Ectopic pregnancy
  - Chronic pelvic pain

ADDITIONAL READING

- American Academy of Pediatrics. Sexually transmitted diseases. In: Pickering LK, Baker CJ, Kimberlin DW, et al, eds. *Red Book: 2012 Report of the Committee on Infectious Diseases*. 29th ed. Elk Grove Village, IL: American Academy of Pediatrics; 2012.
- Centers for Disease Control and Prevention. Update to CDC's sexually transmitted diseases treatment guidelines, 2006: fluoroquinolones no longer recommended for treatment of gonococcal infections. *MMWR Morb Mortal Wkly Rep.* 2007;56(14):332–336.
- Centers for Disease Control and Prevention. Update to CDC's sexually transmitted diseases treatment guidelines, 2010: oral cephalosporins no longer a recommended treatment of gonococcal infections. *MMWR Morb Mortal Wkly Rep.* 2012; 61(31):590–594.
- Workowski KA, Berman S; Centers for Disease Control and Prevention. Sexually transmitted diseases treatment guidelines, 2010. *MMWR Recomm Rep.* 2010;59(RR-12):1–110.

CODES

ICD10
- N72 Inflammatory disease of cervix uteri
- A54.03 Gonococcal cervicitis, unspecified
- A56.09 Other chlamydial infection of lower genitourinary tract

FAQ
- Q: How much cervical motion tenderness is present in patients with cervicitis?
- A: None. Patients with cervicitis have inflammation and infection of the cervix only. They do not have any evidence of peritoneal inflammation on physical examination; therefore, patients with tenderness should be treated with the protocols recommended by the CDC for pelvic inflammatory disease. This does not include the use of a single dose of azithromycin.
- Q: Which partners should be referred for treatment?
- A: Sex partners from the preceding 60 days should be referred for evaluation and treatment. Treatment is based on documented or presumptive etiologies.
- Q: What is the appropriate treatment for *M. genitalium*?
- A: *M. genitalium* has clearly been implicated in the development of urethritis in males and is thought to play some role in the development of cervicitis in females (although that role is not entirely clear). Data suggests that azithromycin may be the best treatment for this infection.
- Q: How often should asymptomatic sexually active adolescents be screened for STIs?
- A: Sexually active men and women younger than 25 years of age should be screened annually for STIs.

CHANCROID

Evelyn Porter • Christine S. Cho

BASICS

DESCRIPTION

Sexually transmitted infection caused by *Haemophilus ducreyi* that manifests as painful genital skin ulcerations and inguinal lymphadenopathy

EPIDEMIOLOGY

- Low incidence in the United States with sporadic outbreaks
- In underdeveloped countries, a major cause of genital ulcer syndrome
- Probably underreported due to difficulty with definitive diagnosis via culture in developing areas
- Increases the risk of HIV transmission
- Seen more commonly in males; females are more likely to be asymptomatic.
- Sexual contact is the only known route of transmission.
- If diagnosed in children, sexual abuse should be considered.

Incidence

Cases in the United States steadily declined until 2000; since then, the incidence has fluctuated. In 2012, there were 15 reported cases.

RISK FACTORS

Increased association with sex workers and individuals involved in drug use

GENERAL PREVENTION

Condom use

PATHOPHYSIOLOGY

- Transmission suspected via microabrasions sustained during sexual intercourse, allowing the organism to penetrate the epidermis
- 3–10 days later, an erythematous, tender papule develops and progresses to a pustule.
- The pustule ruptures after 2–3 days, leaving a shallow ulcer with a painful, necrotic base with undermined edges.
- Single or multiple ulcers may be present.

ETIOLOGY

H. ducreyi, a gram-negative coccobacillus

COMMONLY ASSOCIATED CONDITIONS

- Associated with HIV transmission and infection
- Coinfection with syphilis and human herpes virus may occur (10%).

DIAGNOSIS

Diagnosis of chancroid is routinely based on clinical findings after the exclusion of other causes of genital ulcer disease.

HISTORY

- Males usually present with symptoms referable to an acute, painful genital ulcer.
- Females may be asymptomatic or present with nonspecific symptoms (dysuria, vaginal discharge, pain with stooling or sexual intercourse, rectal pain, or bleeding).

PHYSICAL EXAM

Classic findings:

- Extremely painful ulcer with an irregular, undermined border and a gray, necrotic center
  - In males: found on prepuce or coronal sulcus
  - In females: found on the vulva, cervix, or perianal area
- Painful, unilateral, inguinal lymphadenopathy (bubo) in 50% which may spontaneously drain
- Extragenital sites are rare and include the inner thigh area, breasts, fingers, and mouth.

DIAGNOSTIC TESTS & INTERPRETATION

Diagnosis is made by clinical findings and exclusion of other causes of genital ulcers.

Lab

- Gram stain from the base of the ulcer: may show short gram-negative coccobacilli in parallel "school of fish" arrangement. Not reliable as a screening test as ulcers may contain multiple organisms; routine use is not helpful.
- Cultures from the ulcer
  - *H. ducreyi* is a fastidious organism and requires specialized media and technique for successful isolation.
  - Compared with newer amplification techniques, it has been proven to be 75% sensitive.
  - Currently the only method routinely available for the definite diagnosis of chancroid
- DNA amplification
  - A genital ulcer multiplex polymerase chain reaction (GUM) test has been developed for simultaneous amplification of DNA targets from *H. ducreyi*, *Treponema pallidum*, and herpes simplex virus (HSV) types 1 and 2; offers improved sensitivity when compared with culture
  - This technology is not routinely available.
- Monoclonal antibody
  - Monoclonal antibody against the outer membrane protein of *H. ducreyi* using immunofluorescent antibody has also proven to be more sensitive than culture.
  - Could provide easy, rapid, inexpensive, sensitive testing but not available currently

- Additional testing
  - Evaluation for the common causes of genital ulcer syndrome should be done routinely: culture and PCR for HSV 1 and 2, RPR
  - HIV test

DIFFERENTIAL DIAGNOSIS

- Chancroid must be distinguished from the other causes of genital ulcers, including syphilis, HSV, lymphogranuloma venereum, and granuloma inguinale. More than one of these pathogens may be present in individual cases.
- Uncommon etiologies include the following:
  - Trauma
  - Fixed drug eruptions
  - Inflammatory bowel disease
  - Behçet syndrome

TREATMENT

MEDICATION

- Azithromycin 20 mg/kg (max 1 g) PO, once
- Ceftriaxone 50 mg/kg (max 250 mg) IM, once
- Ciprofloxacin 500 mg b.i.d. for 3 days (patients >18 years)
- Erythromycin base (≥18 years) 500 mg PO q.i.d. for 7 days
- One-time directly observed dosing with azithromycin or ceftriaxone is recommended.

SURGERY/OTHER PROCEDURES

Persistent inguinal fluctuant adenitis may be treated with either needle aspiration or incision and drainage.

ONGOING CARE

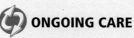

FOLLOW-UP RECOMMENDATIONS

- Symptoms improve within 3–7 days.
- Ulcers heal between 1 and 4 weeks.
- Lymphadenopathy may take longer to regress; may become fluctuant despite adequate therapy
- Patients should be followed weekly until symptoms resolve.
- For patients who do not follow the typical course, consider other causes of genital ulcers; noncompliance; presence of a coexisting sexually transmitted disease, especially HIV; and, rarely, presence of a resistant organism.
- Recent sexual partners (within the preceding 10 days) should be treated.
- If initial HIV and syphilis test results are negative, they should be repeated in 3 months following diagnosis of chancroid.

PATIENT EDUCATION

Prevention: condom use with all sexual activity

COMPLICATIONS

- Draining bubo
- Coinfection with syphilis and HSV
- HIV infection

ADDITIONAL READING

- American Academy of Pediatrics. Chancroid. In: Pickering LK, Baker CJ, Kimberlin DW, et al, eds. *Red Book: 2012 Report of the Committee on Infectious Diseases*. 29th ed. Elk Grove Village, IL: American Academy of Pediatrics; 2012:271–272.
- Centers for Disease Control and Prevention. STD surveillance 2012. http://www.cdc.gov/std/general/other.htm. Accessed February 13, 2014.
- Kaliaperumal K. Recent advances in management of genital ulcer disease and anogenital warts. *Dermatol Ther*. 2008;21(3):196–204.
- Lewis DA. Chancroid: clinical manifestations, diagnosis, and management. *Sex Transm Infect*. 2003;79(1):68–71.
- Mackay IM, Harnett G, Jeoffreys N, et al. Detection and discrimination of herpes simplex viruses, *Haemophilus ducreyi*, *Treponema pallidum*, and *Calymmatobacterium* (*Klebsiella*) *granulomatis* from genital ulcers. *Clin Infect Dis*. 2006;42(10):1431–1438.
- Trager JD. Sexually transmitted diseases causing genital lesions in adolescents. *Adolesc Med Clin*. 2004;15(2):323–352.

CODES

ICD10

A57 Chancroid

CHEST PAIN

Steven M. Selbst

BASICS

DESCRIPTION

Chest pain is a common pain syndrome in childhood. It is less common than abdominal pain and headache. Cardiac disease is an uncommon etiology. Musculoskeletal cause is most common. Boys and girls are equally affected. Etiology is often unclear (idiopathic).

COMMONLY ASSOCIATED CONDITIONS

- Asthma
- Cystic fibrosis
- Diabetes mellitus (long-standing)
- Hypertrophic cardiomyopathy
- Kawasaki disease
- Marfan syndrome
- Sickle cell disease
- Systemic lupus erythematosus

DIAGNOSIS

DIFFERENTIAL DIAGNOSIS

- **Musculoskeletal disorders**
  - Chest wall strain
  - Costochondritis
  - Direct chest trauma
  - Slipping rib syndrome
- **Cardiac pathology**
  - Arrhythmia (supraventricular tachycardia, premature ventricular contractions)
  - Coronary artery anomalies
  - Coronary artery aneurysms (Kawasaki disease)
  - Infections (myocarditis, pericarditis)
  - Myocardial infarction/ischemia
  - Structural abnormalities: hypertrophic cardiomyopathy
- **GI disorders**
  - Caustic ingestions
  - Esophageal foreign bodies
  - Esophagitis (sometimes tetracycline or "pill" induced)
- **Psychogenic causes**
  - Anxiety/stress
  - Hyperventilation
- **Respiratory disorders**
  - Asthma
  - Cough (prolonged)
  - Pleural effusion
  - Pneumonia
  - Pneumothorax: spontaneous, trauma related, drug related (cocaine)
  - Pneumomediastinum
  - Pulmonary embolism
- **Miscellaneous**
  - Breast mass
  - Cigarette smoke
  - Pleurodynia
  - Precordial catch syndrome
  - Shingles
  - Sickle cell crises—acute chest syndrome
  - Thoracic tumor

APPROACH TO PATIENT

Identify the rare child with a serious cause for chest pain (see discussion in "Physical Exam"—[Important Physical Findings on General Examination of Child with Chest Pain])

- **Phase 1:** Is the patient in acute distress? If so, begin emergency management and proceed rapidly to find the cause of pain.
- **Phase 2:** For most stable children with chest pain, determine whether laboratory tests are needed to help identify the cause.
- **Phase 3:** Treat specific conditions as appropriate. Begin analgesics, reassure the family, and arrange for follow-up care.

Hints for Screening Problems

Take a thorough history and perform a careful physical exam. Examine the chest last—do not focus only on this area. Use laboratory tests sparingly, only to confirm clinical suspicions.

HISTORY

- **Question:** How severe, how often is the pain?
- *Significance*: Constant, frequent severe pain is more likely to be distressing and interruptive of daily activity. Serious etiology is not well correlated with frequency and severity of pain.
- **Question:** What is the type of pain? Where is its location?
- *Significance*: Burning pain is associated with esophagitis. Sharp, stabbing pain relieved by sitting up or leaning forward is typical of pericarditis. Young children do not describe or localize chest pain well.
- **Question:** When was the onset of pain?
- *Significance*: Acute pain (<48 hours) is more likely to have an organic cause. Chronic pain (>6 months) is more likely to be psychogenic or idiopathic. In an older child with sudden onset of pain, consider an arrhythmia, pneumothorax, or musculoskeletal injury. In a young child with sudden onset of pain, consider a foreign body (coin) in the esophagus or injury.
- **Question:** Is the pain induced by exercise?
- *Significance*: Exercise-induced chest pain may be related to serious cardiac disease or asthma.
- **Question:** Recent trauma, rough play, or muscle overuse?
- *Significance*: Musculoskeletal (chest wall) pain
- **Question:** Eaten spicy foods? Taken tetracycline or other pills?
- *Significance*: Esophagitis. Teens often take pills with little water and then lie down. The undissolved pill may lodge in the esophagus and cause pain.
- **Question:** Recent use of "street drugs" such as cocaine?
- *Significance*: Hypertension, tachycardia, myocardial ischemia, or pneumothorax
- **Question:** Use of oral contraceptives, clotting disorder, or recent leg trauma?
- *Significance*: Pulmonary embolism. This is rare in the pediatric age group.
- **Question:** Recent significant stress (e.g., move, death of loved one, serious illness)?
- *Significance*: Psychogenic pain. Children may have headaches and abdominal pain related to stress. Chest pain may also relate to unusual stress.
- **Question:** Associated complaints?
- *Significance*: Fever may imply pneumonia (common), myocarditis, and pericarditis (less common but serious). Syncope and palpitations may imply cardiac arrhythmias or severe anemia. Joint pain or rash may relate chest pain to collagen vascular disease. Pain that resolves with parental attention may indicate an emotional cause.
- **Question:** Positive familial history?
- *Significance*: Hypertrophic cardiomyopathy is often familial. Those with this disorder may have familial history positive for sudden death. When there is a positive familial history of heart disease or chest pain, the parents may be unusually concerned about the symptom in a child. The child often has a nonorganic cause.
- **Question:** Past medical history?
- *Significance*: Previous Kawasaki disease, long-standing insulin-dependent diabetes mellitus, and sickle cell disease may have serious cardiac or pulmonary complications leading to chest pain. Marfan syndrome has increased risk for aortic dissection and pneumothorax. Asthma has increased risk for pneumonia and pneumothorax. Collagen vascular disease has increased risk for pleural effusion and pericarditis. Most underlying structural cardiac lesions rarely produce chest pain. Hypertrophic cardiomyopathy is a high-risk situation.

PHYSICAL EXAM

- **Important physical findings on general examination of child with chest pain**
  - Severe distress
  - Chronically ill appearance
  - Fever
  - Skin rash or bruising
  - Abdominal pathology
  - Arthritis present
  - Anxiety apparent
- **Finding:** Child is in significant distress?
- *Significance*: Requires emergency care; stabilization. Consider pneumothorax or arrhythmia.
- **Finding:** Child appears chronically ill?
- *Significance*: Chest pain may be found in serious illnesses such as malignancy (Hodgkin lymphoma) or systemic lupus erythematosus.
- **Finding:** Fever?
- *Significance*: Consider pneumonia, myocarditis, or pericarditis.
- **Finding:** Skin bruising present?
- *Significance*: Chest pain may be related to unrecognized trauma. Osteomyelitis of the rib is a rare cause.
- **Finding:** Abdominal pathology?
- *Significance*: Pain may be referred to the chest.
- **Finding:** Arthritis present?
- *Significance*: Collagen vascular disease may manifest as pleural effusion or chest pain.
- **Finding:** Unusually anxious child?
- *Significance*: Underlying stress may lead to pain.

- **Important physical findings on chest examination of child with chest pain**
  - Breast abnormality
  - Subcutaneous emphysema
  - Heart murmur, rub, arrhythmia
  - Chest wall tenderness
- **Finding:** Breast enlargement, asymmetry, tenderness?
- *Significance*: Physiologic breast changes in young teens may be painful. Consider pregnancy in teenage girls.
- **Finding:** Decreased breath sounds, wheezing?
- *Significance*: May suggest pneumonia, asthma with overuse of chest wall muscles
- **Finding:** Subcutaneous emphysema palpable on chest or neck?
- *Significance*: Pneumothorax, pneumomediastinum
- **Finding:** Heart murmur, rub, arrhythmia?
- *Significance*: Congenital heart disease, hypertrophic cardiomyopathy, cardiac infections such as myocarditis, pericarditis, supraventricular tachycardia, ventricular tachycardia
- **Finding:** Tenderness of chest wall, costochondral junctions?
- *Significance*: Musculoskeletal pain

ALERT

Factors that make this an emergency include the following:

- Pneumothorax: may present with severe sudden chest pain, respiratory distress, cyanosis, hypotension
- Cardiac arrhythmia: Ventricular tachycardia or supraventricular tachycardia in an older child may progress to heart failure or a lethal rhythm.
- Cocaine intoxication: may present with pneumothorax, cardiac arrhythmia, hypertension
- Direct chest trauma: may lead to cardiac contusion and arrhythmia
- Caustic ingestions or esophageal foreign bodies require prompt attention.

DIAGNOSTIC TESTS & INTERPRETATION

- **Test:** EKG
- *Significance*
  - Obtain if history suggests cardiac pathology (e.g., acute onset of pain, pain on exertion, pain associated with syncope, dizziness, palpitations, history of congenital heart disease, serious associated medical problems [Kawasaki disease, diabetes mellitus], use of cocaine)
  - Obtain also if physical exam is abnormal. For instance, respiratory distress, cardiac abnormality, fever, significant trauma
- **Test:** Holter monitor
- *Significance*: Arrange for this study if cardiac arrhythmia is suspected. EKG may fail to detect intermittent arrhythmia.
- **Test:** Exercise stress test
- *Significance*: Obtain if pain is induced by exertion. Usefulness is debated but may identify cardiac disease or asthma.
- **Test:** Drug screen
- *Significance*: Obtain if cocaine use is suspected.

Imaging

Chest radiograph

- Same as for EKG
- Obtain also if history suggests cardiac or pulmonary pathology, tumor, Marfan syndrome, or foreign body (coin ingestion).
- Obtain also if physical exam suggests decreased breath sounds or palpation of subcutaneous air.

TREATMENT

ADDITIONAL TREATMENT

General Measures

Chest pain in children is rarely related to cardiac pathology. However, not all children with chest pain have a benign etiology; pain associated with exertion, syncope, dizziness is concerning for heart disease; if the child is febrile, consider pneumonia or viral myocarditis. Treat specific cause when found. OTC analgesics (acetaminophen 15 mg/kg/dose, ibuprofen 10 mg/kg/dose) suffice for most pain. Antacids may be diagnostic and therapeutic for esophagitis pain. Rest, heat, and relaxation techniques may be useful. Avoid expensive, invasive laboratory studies with chronic pain and normal physical exam or benign history.

ISSUES FOR REFERRAL

- Acute distress
- Significant trauma
- History of heart disease or related serious medical problem
- Pain with exercise, syncope, palpitations, dizziness
- Serious emotional disturbance
- Esophageal foreign body, caustic ingestion
- Pneumothorax, pleural effusion
- Abnormal heart (or sometimes lung) exam
- Abnormal EKG

ONGOING CARE

PROGNOSIS

40% will have continued chest pain for 6–24 months. Follow-up care is important. Serious pathology is unlikely to be found if not diagnosed initially. However, watch for signs of exercise-induced asthma or for emotional problems that were not obvious initially. Encourage return to normal activity if evaluation is negative. Most have an excellent prognosis.

ADDITIONAL READING

- Danduran MJ, Earing MG, Sheridan DC, et al. Chest pain: characteristics of children/adolescents. *Pediatr Cardiol*. 2008;29(4):775–781.
- Drossner DM, Hirsh DA, Sturm JJ, et al. Cardiac disease in pediatric patients presenting to a pediatric ED with chest pain. *Am J Emerg Med*. 2011;29(6):632–638.
- Saleeb SF, Li WY, Warren SZ, et al. Effectiveness of screening for life-threatening chest pain in children. *Pediatrics*. 2011;128(5):e1062–e1068.
- Selbst SM. Approach to the child with chest pain. *Pediatr Clin North Am*. 2010;57(6):1221–1234.
- Selbst SM, Palermo R, Durani Y, et al. Adolescent chest pain—is it the heart? *Clin Ped Emerg Med*. 2011;12:289–300.

CODES

ICD10

- R07.9 Chest pain, unspecified
- R07.89 Other chest pain
- J45.909 Unspecified asthma, uncomplicated

FAQ

- Q: How common is chest pain in children?
- A: Chest pain is a common pain syndrome reported in 6/1,000 children who present to an urban emergency department. The complaint is less common than abdominal pain or headache. Although children of all ages may complain of chest pain, the mean age is about 12 years.
- Q: Which features in the history are worrisome?
- A: Acute onset of pain, it occurs with exercise, associated syncope, dizziness or palpitations, heart disease or chronic conditions that can affect the heart, trauma, fever, drug use (e.g., cocaine)
- Q: Which findings on physical exam are most worrisome?
- A: Respiratory distress, decreased/abnormal breath sounds, cardiac abnormality, fever, trauma, subcutaneous air, Marfan features
- Q: Which children with chest pain do not need extensive evaluation with laboratory studies?
- A: Those with chronic pain (>6 months), and none of the worrisome features mentioned earlier. Individualized management—analgesics, reassurance, and follow-up usually suffice.
- Q: Why should clinicians be concerned about chest pain in children?
- A: Heart disease is an uncommon cause, but serious pathology is found in some cases. Parental fears must be addressed.

CHICKENPOX (VARICELLA, HERPES ZOSTER)

Camille Sabella

BASICS

DESCRIPTION

Varicella-zoster virus (VZV) is a highly contagious herpesvirus. Primary infection with the virus results in varicella (chickenpox), whereas reactivation from latency results in herpes zoster (shingles).

EPIDEMIOLOGY

- Transmission occurs by droplet and airborne transmission of infectious respiratory secretions or direct contact with vesicles and respiratory secretions.
- Incubation 10–21 days (usually 14–16 days) after exposure; cases most contagious 2 days before the rash appears until skin lesions have fully crusted.
  - Immunocompromised patients may have longer or shorter incubation.
  - Post–intravenous immunoglobulin (IVIG), incubation may be up to 28 days.
- The incidence of chickenpox has declined by 90% since the introduction of universal varicella vaccination.
- The attack rate for susceptible household contacts exposed to varicella is 90%.
- Disease is more severe in immunocompromised persons, infants >3 months of age, adolescents, adults, persons with pulmonary disorders (asthma), persons with chronic skin disorders (eczema), and persons on oral and/or intravenous (IV) steroids or long-term aspirin therapy.
- Congenital varicella embryopathy: Risk is 1–2% when maternal primary VZV infection occurs before the 20th week of gestation.
- The rate of complications from varicella has declined dramatically since the licensure of the varicella vaccine.

GENERAL PREVENTION

- Varicella vaccine
  - Live attenuated vaccine (Oka strain)
  - 2-dose series for routine immunization of all healthy, susceptible children; adolescents; and adults
- Immunogenicity: ~85% of immunized children developed protective levels of humoral and cellular immunity after 1 dose, ~100% with 2 doses; 3× less likely to have breakthrough disease when 2 doses of vaccine were administered
- Effectiveness: 70–90% effective against all VZV disease; >97% effective against severe disease (e.g., median number of vesicles was 50 in vaccinated children vs. 250 in unvaccinated children)
- Herpes zoster can occur following varicella vaccination, but clinical severity of the zoster is milder and the risk of acquiring zoster following immunization is lower than following wild-type chickenpox.
- Contraindications
  - Anaphylaxis to vaccine components (e.g., neomycin, gelatin)
  - Pregnant, immunocompromised, or <12 months of age
  - HIV is an exception: It is recommended to vaccinate HIV-positive children if CD4+ T-cell counts are ≥15%. Give doses 3 months apart.
  - High-dose corticosteroid doses of >2 mg/kg/day or >20 mg/day of prednisone, or its equivalent, for ≥14 days are considered immunosuppressive doses: VZV vaccine should not be given until systemic corticosteroid therapy has been discontinued for at least 1 month.
- Postexposure prophylaxis
  - If no contraindication to VZV vaccine: Administer VZV vaccine to susceptible hosts (1st or 2nd dose) within 72 hours (up to 120 hours) of exposure.
  - If with contraindications to VZV vaccine: Consider passive immunization.
- Passive immunization if
  - (i) No evidence of immunity in exposed person, (ii) probability that exposure will result in infection, and (iii) likelihood of complications of VZV in the exposed person due to risk factors
  - Susceptible immunocompromised people, pregnant women, and neonates whose mothers develop varicella infection 5 days prior to 2 days after delivery should be especially considered for passive immunization upon exposure.
  - Administer varicella immunoglobulin (VariZIG) or IVIG as per protocol within 96 hours of exposure.
  - If VariZIG or IVIG is unavailable, or >96 hours have passed, some experts recommend postexposure prophylaxis with oral acyclovir (20 mg/kg q6h for 7 days) beginning 7–10 days after exposure.

PATHOPHYSIOLOGY

- After primary infection, the virus establishes latency in dorsal root ganglia cells.
- Immunity from natural disease is usually lifelong, but symptomatic and asymptomatic reinfections do occur, boosting antibody levels.

DIAGNOSIS

HISTORY

- Chickenpox
  - Fever, malaise; decreased appetite common prior to onset of rash
  - Fever low grade to moderate and persists after rash appears
  - Pruritic rash begins on scalp, face, or trunk.
  - New lesions appear as some begin to crust; all stages (macules, vesicles, crusted lesions) apparent at one time.
  - Vesicles may appear in the mouth, conjunctiva, vagina, and urethra.
- Zoster
  - Prodrome of pain, pruritus, hyperesthesias
  - Vesicular lesions are clustered unilaterally in a dermatomal distribution of one or more adjacent sensory nerves.
  - Mildly painful in children

PHYSICAL EXAM

- Chickenpox
  - Evolution of rash from macules to vesicles, which appear as "dewdrop on a rose petal," then crust
  - Lesions in multiple stages of formation is pathognomonic.
  - Most children have less than 300 lesions; higher numbers are found among children who develop varicella after household contact.
  - New lesions appear for up to 7 days in otherwise healthy children.
  - Assess for complications: interstitial pneumonia, encephalitis, secondary bacterial infection (especially group A *Streptococcus*).
- Zoster
  - Discrete vesicles appear first, then enlarge and coalesce.
  - New lesions cease to form after 3–7 days and crusting occurs within 2 weeks.
  - Severe local dermatomal infection, cutaneous dissemination, and visceral dissemination may occur in immunocompromised children.

DIAGNOSTIC TESTS & INTERPRETATION

Lab

- Not needed for typical cases in healthy children
- VZV is difficult to isolate in cell culture.
- Immunohistochemical staining of epithelial cells from cutaneous lesions may provide a rapid diagnosis.
- PCR testing of clinical specimens must be done by experienced laboratory personnel.
- Serology is used to determine susceptibility to infection.
  - Acute and convalescent sera can determine acute infection: enzyme immunoassay (EIA), immunofluorescence assay (IFA), latex agglutination (LA), fluorescent antibody to membrane antigen (FAMA), and enzyme-linked immunosorbent assay (ELISA).

DIFFERENTIAL DIAGNOSIS

The differential diagnosis includes other causes of vesicular rash:

- Coxsackievirus infection (hand, foot, mouth)
- Eczema herpeticum
- Herpes zoster with dissemination
- Impetigo
- Insect bites
- Monkeypox
- *Mycoplasma* (erythema multiforme)
- *Pseudomonas* (ecthyma gangrenosum)
- Rickettsial pox
- Scabies
- Toxic epidermal necrosis, Stevens-Johnson, and various noninfectious vesicular conditions of the skin

TREATMENT

MEDICATION

- Acyclovir is the drug of choice for varicella or zoster in children.
- IV acyclovir is indicated for infected immunocompromised hosts and neonates and those with associated pneumonia or encephalitis:
  - <1 year old: 10–20 mg/kg q8h
  - ≥1 year old: 500 mg/m^2 q8h or 10–20 mg/kg q8h
  - ≥12 years old: 10 mg/kg q8h
- Treat for 7–10 days or until no new lesions for 48 hours.
- Oral acyclovir may be considered for those with increased risk of severe infection, including those with cutaneous disorders, chronic diseases that

may be exacerbated by acute varicella infection, adolescents, and those who acquire infection after household contact.
  - Acyclovir (PO): 20 mg/kg q6h to max of 800 mg q6h, for 5 days
  - Valacyclovir (PO): (≥2 years old) 20 mg/kg (max 1,000 mg) q8h for 5 days; better bioavailability
- Children with VZV should not receive salicylates because of the risk of Reye syndrome. Use acetaminophen to control fever.

ADDITIONAL TREATMENT

General Measures

- Isolation of hospitalized patients with chickenpox:
  - Contact and airborne precautions of the index case for the duration of vesicular eruption and all vesicles crusted (usually 5 days, longer in immunocompromised patients)
  - Use negative-pressure rooms, if possible.
  - Exposed susceptible persons should be in contact and airborne precautions from day 8 to 21 after the onset of rash in the index patient.
  - Neonates born to mother with VZV: contact and airborne precautions until day 28
  - Embryopathy does not require precautions if there are no active lesions.
  - Persons who received VariZIG or IVIG should be kept in contact and airborne precautions for 28 days after exposure.
- Isolation of hospitalized patients with zoster:
  - Immunocompromised patients who have zoster (localized or generalized) and immunocompetent patients with disseminated zoster should remain in contact and airborne precautions for the duration of the illness, as above.
  - Immunocompetent patients with localized zoster: contact precautions until all lesions crusted.
- Isolation of outpatients with chickenpox:
  - Child should remain at home, away from susceptible and high-risk persons, until no new eruptions and all vesicles have crusted.
- Isolation of outpatients with zoster:
  - For immunocompetent patients with localized zoster, contact precautions are recommended until all lesions are crusted.
  - If lesions can remain completely covered, child may return to school; however, active lesions are infectious.

ONGOING CARE

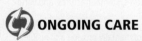

FOLLOW-UP RECOMMENDATIONS

Patient Monitoring

For normal healthy individuals, follow-up is not necessary.

PROGNOSIS

- For most children, this childhood exanthema is a benign disease that lasts 6–8 days.
- Postherpetic neuralgia can cause significant morbidity following zoster in adults but is very rare in children.

COMPLICATIONS

Complications are associated with significant morbidity and may occur regardless of the use of acyclovir:

- Secondary bacterial infection—especially group A streptococcal infections and *Staphylococcus aureus*
- CNS (1 in 4,000): transverse myelitis, myelopathy, encephalitis (60 cases/year prevaccine), meningoencephalitis, acute cerebellar ataxia, necrotizing retinitis
- Varicella interstitial pneumonitis (more common in adults and infants)
- GI: pancreatitis, appendicitis, and hepatitis
- Heme: idiopathic thrombocytopenia, disseminated intravascular coagulation (hemorrhagic VZV)
- Nephritis
- Vasculopathy of small and large cerebral vessels, causing strokes
- Zoster sine herpete: radicular pain without rash but virologic confirmation of reactivation; can be dermatomal or CNS; very rare in the pediatric population
- Individuals with AIDS may have chronic VZV, including progressive myelopathy.
- Congenital varicella syndrome: characterized by limb atrophy and scarring of the extremity (cicatrices), CNS and eye manifestations
- Postherpetic neuralgia: Neuropathic pain is more common in zoster patients >60 years.
- Death: Varicella-related deaths continue to occur despite the recommended vaccine. Secondary bacterial infections and pneumonia are most frequent causes of death.

ADDITIONAL READING

- American Academy of Pediatrics. Varicella- zoster infections. In: Pickering LK, Baker CJ, Kimberlin DW, et al, eds. *Red Book: 2012 Report of the Committee on Infectious Diseases*. 29th ed. Elk Grove Village, IL: American Academy of Pediatrics; 2012:774–789.
- American Academy of Pediatrics, Committee on Infectious Diseases. Prevention of varicella: update of recommendations for use of quadrivalent and monovalent varicella vaccines in children. *Pediatrics*. 2011;128(3):630–632.
- Macartney K, McIntyre P. Vaccines for post-exposure prophylaxis against varicella (chickenpox) in children and adults. *Cochrane Database Syst Rev*. 2008;(3):CD001833.
- Marin M, Güris D, Chaves SS; Advisory Committee on Immunization Practices, Centers for Disease Control and Prevention. Prevention of varicella: recommendations of the Advisory Committee on Immunization Practices (ACIP). *MMWR Recomm Rep*. 2007;56(RR-4):1–40.
- Seward JF, Marin M, Vázquez M. Varicella vaccine effectiveness in the US vaccination program: a review. *J Infect Dis*. 2008;197(Suppl 2):S82–S89.
- Vazquez M, LaRussa PS, Gershon AA, et al. The effectiveness of varicella vaccine in clinical practice. *N Engl J Med*. 2001;344(13):955.

CODES

ICD10

- B01.9 Varicella without complication
- B02.9 Zoster without complications
- B01.89 Other varicella complications

FAQ

- Q: What do you do for a patient on corticosteroids who has not had VZV and is exposed to VZV?
- A: Patients receiving ≥2 mg/kg/day or ≥20 mg/day of prednisone or its equivalent cannot be immunized with VZV vaccine. If the child is susceptible, has had sufficient exposure, and deemed at risk for serious infection, passive immunization with VariZIG or IVIG can be given.
- Q: Can children receiving inhaled steroids for asthma be immunized safely with VZV vaccine?
- A: Yes. Asthmatics on inhaled steroids can be safely immunized because the dose of inhaled steroid is not immunosuppressive.
- Q: For whom is VZV vaccine contraindicated?
- A: Immunosuppressed individuals, pregnant patients, infants <1 year old, and anyone who has a history of an allergic reaction to a vaccine component such as neomycin should not receive the VZV vaccine. Additionally, any child with a moderate to severe acute illness should have his or her VZV vaccination deferred until his or her illness has resolved. Patients with HIV infection can be vaccinated with VZV vaccine if their CD4+ T-cell percentages are ≥15%.
- Q: Can a child get shingles after vaccination with VZV vaccine?
- A: Yes. Zoster can occur following VZV vaccination. However, cases of shingles following vaccination tend to be milder and less frequent than after wild-type varicella.
- Q: What are the most common adverse effects of VZV vaccination?
- A: Mild local reactions are most common, occurring in 20–25% of vaccine recipients. 1–3% of children will develop a localized rash after vaccination, whereas 3–5% will develop a more generalized varicella-like rash. These rashes typically consist of 2–5 maculopapular or vesicular lesions and occur 5–26 days after vaccination.
- Q: What are the characteristics of breakthrough infection in a child who has been immunized with VZV vaccine?
- A: Breakthrough varicella can occur in children who have been appropriately immunized with VZV vaccine. Breakthrough infection is usually milder than that occurring in unimmunized children, often with fewer than 50 lesions, lower fever, and faster recovery. Although these children are less contagious than those with wild virus infection, they can transmit the virus to susceptible individuals.

CHILD ABUSE, PHYSICAL

Allison M. Jackson

BASICS

DESCRIPTION
Physical abuse is an act inflicted on a child or youth by a parent or caregiver resulting in mucocutaneous, musculoskeletal, visceral, or intracranial injury and/or death. Although a medical diagnosis, physical abuse is also defined legally in state statutes.

EPIDEMIOLOGY
Incidence
- Of those cases reported to child protective service agencies in the United States in 2011, 676,569 children were victims of abuse and neglect.
  - Child abuse rate was 9.1 per 1,000 children/year (2011 data).
  - 17.6% of abused children were found to be victims of physical abuse.
  - Over 1,500 child deaths were attributed to maltreatment in 2011, of which nearly 48% resulted from physical abuse.
- Abuse can happen in any family regardless of race, ethnicity, or socioeconomic class.

Prevalence
Not all child maltreatment is reported. In a nationally representative sample of over 4,000 children, more than 18% reported experiencing maltreatment in their lifetime.

GENERAL PREVENTION
- Assessing risk (parental history of mental illness or childhood victimization, parental substance abuse, economic stressors, difficult child temperament, unreasonable developmental expectations, children living with single mothers and an unrelated male)
- Screening for family violence (intimate partner violence)
- Providing anticipatory guidance regarding infant crying/toddler tantrums, toileting, and discipline techniques
- Nurse home visitation for at-risk families
- Parenting classes for all parents, although classes usually only target at-risk parents of young children

ETIOLOGY
- Although child abuse occurs in families regardless of race, ethnicity, or socioeconomic status, there are individual, family, community, and societal factors that place children at increased risk for maltreatment.
- Examples of risk factors include the following:
  - Difficult temperament
  - Parental history of childhood victimization
  - Parental substance abuse
  - Parental mental illness
  - Poverty and unemployment
  - Family violence

COMMONLY ASSOCIATED CONDITIONS
- Emotional abuse
- Neglect
- Sexual abuse
- Domestic violence exposure
- Chronic runaway status
- Domestic sex trafficking
- Posttraumatic stress disorder
- Depression
- Anxiety disorder

ALERT
Pitfalls
- Failing to consider abuse in the differential diagnosis of all pediatric trauma
- Failing to consider abuse in the differential diagnosis of all infants and toddlers with mental status changes (especially apparent life-threatening events [ALTEs]), even without bruising
- Failing to recognize the significance of subconjunctival hemorrhages and bruises in locations on the body atypical for accidental trauma
- Failing to consider trauma as a cause for bloody CSF
- Failing to consider alternative medical diagnoses in children for whom you suspect abuse
- Failing to document the history, physical findings, and assessment clearly

DIAGNOSIS

HISTORY
- As in all of medicine, the history is paramount to diagnosing child physical abuse. The history yields information useful in creating a timeline, determining plausibility of the injury event, and in formulating a differential diagnosis. Tips for gathering history when abuse is suspected:
  - Be curious but nonjudgmental.
  - Use open-ended, nonleading questions.
  - Speak with the verbal child and parent separately when abuse is suspected.
- Eliciting a narrative history about the injury event and the evolution of symptoms helps to establish a timeline and determine plausibility of the explanation. Asking, "Tell me what happened," is the best place to begin. Eliciting achieved developmental milestones also aids in determining plausibility.
- In cases in which no injury event is reported, it is important to gather information of when the child was last well, how signs and symptoms evolved, and what prompted the caregiver(s) to seek medical attention.
- It is also important to elicit who was caring for the child at the time of the injury event or when the child became acutely and persistently ill. When children are verbal, ask them "what happened?" or "how did you get that?" regarding identified injuries.
- Past medical history, review of systems, and family history can also be helpful in formulating a differential diagnosis.

PHYSICAL EXAM
A comprehensive physical exam should be performed on any child for whom maltreatment is suspected. Tips include the following:
- Plot growth parameters.
- Conduct a head-to-toe physical exam, including an anogenital exam.
- Suspicion for physical abuse is raised with injuries in the mouth (such as frenula injuries), subconjunctival hemorrhages, bruises in infants in locations atypical for accidental trauma (ears, neck, abdomen, buttocks, thighs), or cutaneous injuries with a pattern (e.g., loop marks, human bites).
- When head trauma is suspected, a dilated funduscopic exam should be completed by an ophthalmologist. Retinal hemorrhages that are in multiple layers of the retina and that extend to the ora serrata have a high specificity for inflicted head trauma.
- Not all injuries can be detected on physical exam; therefore, it is important to use other modalities to screen for other injuries.

DIAGNOSTIC TESTS & INTERPRETATION
Lab
- In patients with bruising or intracranial hemorrhage and/or a history or exam in which a bleeding disorder should be considered:
  - Urinalysis (UA) for myoglobinuria
  - Creatine kinase for muscle injury
  - Prothrombin (PT)/partial thromboplastin times (PTT) for prolonged bleeding
  - CBC with platelets for anemia and thrombocytopenia
  - Von Willebrand antigen and activity
  - Factors VIII and IX levels for hemophilia
  - Disseminated intravascular coagulation (DIC) panel
- In patients with multiple fractures, screen for metabolic bone disease:
  - Alkaline phosphatase
  - Calcium and phosphorus
  - 25-hydroxy vitamin D
  - Intact parathyroid hormone (PTH)
- To screen for abdominal trauma (bruising not usually present):
  - AST and ALT for liver injury
  - Amylase, lipase for pancreatic injury
  - UA for genitourinary injury
- In patients with altered mental status or concerns for poisoning:
  - Toxicology screen

Imaging
- To evaluate for skeletal trauma:
  - Skeletal survey for all children <2 years old with suspected abuse (occasionally useful in children 2–5 years old)
    - Fractures with high specificity for abuse include posterior rib fractures, classic metaphyseal lesions (i.e., bucket handle or corner fractures), scapular fractures, sternal fractures, and vertebral fractures.
    - A reported injury event that fails to mechanistically or developmentally provide a plausible mechanism should raise suspicions for abuse.
  - Radionuclide bone scans can augment the assessment for skeletal injury.
- To evaluate for head trauma:
  - CT of the brain and MRI of the brain and spine in children <1 year old or with signs or symptoms suggestive of head injury
    - Subdural hemorrhages are associated with abusive head trauma.
    - MRI may be helpful in assessing hemorrhages of different ages and, detecting brain injury and soft tissue neck trauma.
- To evaluate for thoracic, abdominal, and/or pelvic trauma:
  - CT chest, abdomen, and/or pelvis

Pathologic Findings

An autopsy by a qualified medical examiner should be completed when maltreatment is in the differential diagnosis.

DIFFERENTIAL DIAGNOSIS

Should be based on the physical exam, patient history, and family history

- Bruises
  - Trauma: accidental or inflicted
  - Dermatologic: congenital intradermal nevi, hemangiomas, phytophotodermatitis
  - Hematologic: hemophilia, platelet disorders, idiopathic thrombocytopenic purpura, leukemia
  - Infectious: meningococcemia
  - Genetic: Ehlers-Danlos syndrome
  - Congenital indifference to pain
  - Cultural healing practices: coining (*Cao gio*), cupping, spooning (*Quat sha*)
  - Vasculitis: Henoch-Schönlein purpura, hypersensitivity vasculitis
- Burns
  - Trauma: accidental or inflicted
  - Dermatologic: contact dermatitis, fixed drug reaction
  - Infectious: impetigo, staphylococcal scalded skin
  - Genetic: congenital indifference to pain
  - Cultural practices: moxibustion (burning moxa herb at therapeutic points on skin), *Maquas* (small deep burns at therapeutic points), garlic (used topically for infections)
  - Other: brown recluse spider bite
- Fractures
  - Trauma: birth, accidental, or inflicted
  - Metabolic: rickets, scurvy, copper deficiency, osteogenesis imperfecta, hypervitaminosis A, prostaglandin E toxicity
  - Neoplastic: leukemia, Langerhans cell histiocytosis, metastatic
  - Infectious: congenital syphilis, osteomyelitis
  - Other: infantile cortical hyperostosis
- Head injury
  - Trauma: accidental or inflicted
  - Hematologic disorder: late hemorrhagic disease of the newborn (vitamin K), clotting factor deficiencies, thrombocytopenia, platelet function disorder, Von Willebrand disease
  - Infectious: bacterial meningitis
  - Metabolic: glutaric aciduria type I

TREATMENT

GENERAL MEASURES

- Medical treatment according to injuries
- Report suspicions for physical abuse to the Child Protective Services Agency in the jurisdiction of occurrence.
- Incorporate other disciplines into the treatment plan, in particular, social work and trauma-informed mental health care providers.

INPATIENT CONSIDERATIONS

Admission Criteria

- Primarily based on medical needs of patient
- For patient safety to allow for initial investigation to assess for a safe caregiver

Discharge Criteria

When medically prepared for discharge and a safe caregiver has been established by child welfare

ONGOING CARE

FOLLOW-UP RECOMMENDATIONS

Patient Monitoring

- Reports will be investigated by the appropriate child welfare and/or law enforcement agency.
- The child may or may not be placed into foster care. In either case, if a child welfare case is opened, measures to monitor and strengthen the family and parents would be implemented. These measures are not always successful.
- Primary care and ongoing providers should monitor patients for physical and mental health sequelae of the abuse as well as ongoing abuse or neglect.

PROGNOSIS

Depends on nature and extent of injuries, the response of the child welfare and criminal justice system, and the timely implementation of medical and mental health services

COMPLICATIONS

- Death
- Intellectual disability
- Cerebral palsy
- Seizure disorder
- Learning disabilities
- Psychiatric disorders (depression, anxiety, posttraumatic stress disorder)

ADDITIONAL READING

- Anderst JD, Carpenter SL, Abshire TC; American Academy of Pediatrics Section on Hematology/Oncology and Committee on Child Abuse and Neglect. Evaluation for bleeding disorders in suspected child abuse. *Pediatrics*. 2013;131(4):e1314–e1322.
- Finkelhor D, Turner H, Ormrod R, et al. Violence, abuse, and crime exposure in a national sample of children and youth. *Pediatrics*. 2009;124(5):1411–1423.
- Jenny C; Committee on Child Abuse and Neglect. Evaluating infants and young children with multiple fractures. *Pediatrics*. 2006;118(3):1299–1303.
- Kellogg ND; American Academy of Pediatrics Committee on Child Abuse and Neglect. Evaluation of suspected child physical abuse. *Pediatrics*. 2007;119(6):1232–1241.
- U.S. Department of Health and Human Services, Administration for Children and Families, Administration on Children, Youth and Families, Children's Bureau. (2012). *Child Maltreatment 2011*.

CODES

ICD10

- T74.12XA Child physical abuse, confirmed, initial encounter
- T74.4XXA Shaken infant syndrome, initial encounter
- Z69.010 Encounter for mental health services for victim of parental child abuse

FAQ

- Q: When do I need to report child abuse?
- A: Whenever there is suspicion that your patient has experienced maltreatment based on your clinical evaluation. You do not have to prove abuse; you just need to suspect it.
- Q: What happens when a report is taken?
- A: Many jurisdictions proceed with a multidisciplinary investigation. Investigators and attorneys may need to speak with you to clarify your findings and assessment.

CHLAMYDIA TRACHOMATIS INFECTION

Sumit Bhargava

BASICS

DESCRIPTION

Chlamydiae are obligate intracellular bacteria responsible for pulmonary infections, ocular trachoma, sexually transmitted diseases, and infections of the genital tract in the pediatric and adult population.

- The genus *Chlamydophila* has 3 species known to affect humans:
  - *Chlamydia trachomatis*
  - *Chlamydophila psittaci*
  - *Chlamydophila pneumoniae*
- All 3 species can produce the clinical picture of the so-called atypical or interstitial pneumonia.
- *C. trachomatis* can cause afebrile pneumonia in 10–20% of infants born to infected mothers. Infected infants usually present prior to 2 months of age. Up to 50% of patients have a history of inclusion conjunctivitis.
- *C. psittaci* is mainly pathogenic for birds and occasionally affects humans, typically causing interstitial pneumonitis with associated fever, headache, malaise, and nausea.
- *C. pneumoniae* causes pneumonia, pharyngitis, sinusitis, and bronchitis in humans.

ALERT

- *C. trachomatis*
  - Infection can occur in infants delivered by cesarean section, even without rupture of amniotic membranes.
  - Ocular prophylaxis at birth does not reliably prevent conjunctivitis or extraocular infection, even if erythromycin ointment is used. Topical treatment alone is not recommended because it does not eradicate the nasopharyngeal colonization.

GENERAL PREVENTION

- Adequate surveillance and treatment of *C. trachomatis* colonizing the genital tract of pregnant women is the best way of preventing disease in the infant.
- Annual chlamydia screening for all sexually active women younger than age 25 years and for all pregnant women in the 1st trimester of pregnancy is recommended.

EPIDEMIOLOGY

- *C. trachomatis*
  - There are at least 18 serologically distinct variants with different associations:
    - A–K: oculogenital
    - A–C: trachoma
    - B, D–K: genital and perinatal infection
    - L1–L3: lymphogranuloma venereum (LGV)
  - *C. trachomatis* is the most frequent cause of epididymitis in sexually active young men.
  - Incubation period: 5–14 days after delivery for conjunctivitis
  - The possibility of sexual abuse should be considered in older infants and children with vaginal, urethral, or rectal *C. trachomatis*.

Incidence

- This is the most common reportable sexually transmitted infection in the United States. The number of new infections exceeds 4 million annually.
- *C. trachomatis* is responsible for neonatal conjunctivitis, trachoma, pneumonia in young infants, genital tract infection, and LGV.
- Rates of infection in adolescent girls are 15–20%.
- 23–55% of all cases of nongonococcal urethritis in men are caused by *C. trachomatis*. Up to 50% of men with gonorrhea may be coinfected with *C. trachomatis*.
- *C. trachomatis* pneumonia usually develops in infected infants <2 months of age (2 weeks to 5 months). The contagiousness of pulmonary disease is unknown, but is considered low.
- Half of the neonates born to infected mothers via vaginal delivery will acquire *C. trachomatis*. Conjunctivitis may develop in 30–50%.
- Pneumonia may develop in up to 30% of infants with nasopharyngeal infection.
- Ocular trachoma caused by serovars A, B, Ba, and C is the most common cause of preventable blindness in the world, but is rare in the United States.

DIAGNOSIS

HISTORY

- Presents between 4 and 12 weeks of age
- Insidious onset
- Afebrile illness
- Rhinorrhea
- Repetitive cough
  - Staccato type in >50% of infants
  - Sometimes, pertussis-like coughing spells
- Conjunctivitis in up to 50% of infants
- Mild to moderate respiratory distress

PHYSICAL EXAM

- Afebrile
- 50% of patients will have conjunctivitis with discharge (can be seen up to several weeks after birth).
- Rhinitis with mucoid discharge or nasal stuffiness, sometimes causing significant airway obstruction
- Hypoxia is frequently present.
- Apneic episodes may be seen in preterm infants.
- Moderate tachypnea (50–60 breaths/min)
- Staccato cough
- Scattered rales on chest auscultation
- Wheezing is an uncommon finding.

DIAGNOSTIC TESTS & INTERPRETATION

Lab

- Cell culture
  - Definitive diagnosis is by isolation of the organism in tissue culture.
  - Confirmation is by microscopy of the characteristic inclusions by fluorescent antibody staining.
  - Specimens are obtained from the nasopharynx, conjunctiva, vagina, or rectum.
  - Dacron polyester–tipped swabs should be used for collection.

- Nucleic acid amplification methods:
  - FDA-approved nucleic acid amplification methods such as polymerase chain reaction (PCR), strand displacement amplification (SDA), and transcription-mediated amplification (TMA) are more sensitive (98%) than cell culture and more specific and sensitive than DNA probe, direct fluorescent antibody (DFA), or enzyme immunoassay (EIA).
  - In addition, these have been approved for urine studies in both men and women, making them useful noninvasive tests for adolescents.
- Direct antigen tests:
  - DNA probe, DFA, and EIA are the most common nonculture direct antigen-detection tests approved by the FDA.
  - These are most sensitive (90%) and specific (95%) in conjunctival specimens.
  - These methods can have false-positive results when used for vaginal or rectal specimens.
- Serum antibody detection
  - Difficult to perform
  - Tests are not widely available.
- Eosinophilia of 300–400/mm^3, hyperinflation, bilateral diffuse infiltrates on chest radiograph, and elevation of IgM (>110 mg/dL) and IgG (>500 mg/dL) are indirect evidence that indicate *C. trachomatis* pneumonia.
- Only culture should be used for sexual abuse or other forensic purposes.

Imaging

Chest radiography

- Hyperinflation with bilateral diffuse infiltrates

DIFFERENTIAL DIAGNOSIS

- Viral respiratory pathogens:
  - Respiratory syncytial virus (RSV),
  - Adenovirus
  - Influenza A
  - Influenza B
  - Parainfluenza
- Other agents that can cause pneumonitis:
  - Cytomegalovirus
  - *Pneumocystis carinii*
  - *Ureaplasma urealyticum*
  - *Bordetella pertussis*

TREATMENT

MEDICATION

- Erythromycin, 50 mg/kg/day divided q.i.d. for 14 days (therapy is effective in 80–90% of cases). Additional topical therapy is unnecessary. An association between oral erythromycin and infantile hypertrophic pyloric stenosis (IHPS) has been reported in infants <6 weeks of age. Parents should be informed of the possible risk of IHPS and its signs.
- If the patient does not tolerate erythromycin, oral sulfonamides may be used after the immediate neonatal period. Children >8 years can be treated with tetracycline, 25–50 mg/kg/24 h divided q.i.d. for 7 days.
- A single 1-g oral dose of azithromycin may be used in children ≥45 kg or ≥8 years of age.
- In adults and adolescents, a single 1-g dose of azithromycin or doxycycline 100 mg b.i.d. orally for 7 days is 1st-line treatment.

ONGOING CARE

PROGNOSIS

- In general, good
- Infection with *C. trachomatis* has been associated with long-term respiratory sequelae, such as an increased incidence of reactive airway disease and abnormal pulmonary function tests.
- Slow recovery
- Cough and malaise may persist for several weeks.

COMPLICATIONS

- 40% of women whose chlamydial infection is untreated develop pelvic inflammatory disease. 20% of these women may become infertile.
- Role of chlamydia in pathogenesis of asthma and atherosclerosis is under investigation.

ADDITIONAL READING

- Chandran L, Boykan R. Chlamydial infections in children and adolescents. *Pediatr Rev*. 2009;30(7): 243–250.
- Geisler WM. Management of uncomplicated *Chlamydia trachomatis* infections in adolescents and adults: evidence reviewed for the 2006 Centers for Disease Control and Prevention sexually transmitted diseases treatment guidelines. *Clin Infect Dis*. 2007;44(Suppl 3):S77–S83.
- Harris JA, Kolokathis A, Campbell M, et al. Safety and efficacy of azithromycin in the treatment of community-acquired pneumonia in children. *Pediatr Infect Dis J*. 1998;17(10):865–871.
- Sexually transmitted disease guidelines 2002. Centers for Disease Control and Prevention. *MMWR*. 2002;51(RR-6):1–78.
- U.S. Preventative Services Task Force. Screening for chlamydial infection: U.S. Preventative Services Task Force recommendation statement. *Ann Intern Med*. 2007;147(2):128–133.

CODES

ICD10

- A74.9 Chlamydial infection, unspecified
- P23.1 Congenital pneumonia due to Chlamydia
- A71.1 Active stage of trachoma

FAQ

- Q: If the mother has an untreated genital infection, should we treat the asymptomatic newborn?
- A: Yes. The child should receive oral erythromycin for 14 days.
- Q: Do we need to pursue the diagnosis of other sexually transmitted diseases?
- A: Yes. Gonorrhea, syphilis, hepatitis B, and human immunodeficiency virus infection need to be ruled out. If conjunctivitis is present, an ocular swab to exclude *Neisseria gonorrhoeae* infection must be included.
- Q: When do we need to suspect *C. trachomatis* pneumonia?
- A: In any infant <4 months of age who presents with cough, tachypnea, and rales on examination, when the chest radiograph shows bilateral infiltrates with hyperinflation

CHLAMYDOPHILA (FORMERLY CHLAMYDIA) PNEUMONIAE INFECTION

Amanda C. Schondelmeyer • Angela M. Statile

BASICS

DESCRIPTION

Chlamydiae are obligate intracellular organisms classified as bacteria, but which possess qualities of both bacteria and viruses. They cause a variety of infections from the respiratory to the urogenital tract. The genus has been divided into *Chlamydia* (*Chlamydia trachomatis*, others) and *Chlamydophila* (*Chlamydophila pneumoniae*, *Chlamydophila psittaci*, others). Three species are known to affect humans:

- *C. trachomatis*: a leading cause of sexually transmitted infections in the United States, which can be vertically transmitted during childbirth
- *C. pneumoniae*: an important cause of respiratory infections in the school-aged child
- *C. psittaci*: a zoonosis, primarily an avian pathogen, causing the disease psittacosis in exposed humans

EPIDEMIOLOGY

- Spread person to person by respiratory droplets; no specific seasonality
- Asymptomatic carriage and prolonged nasopharyngeal shedding occurs.
- Peak ages of infection are 5–15 years.
- Coinfection with other respiratory pathogens is common.
- Serum antibodies are positive in about 50% of adults by age 20 years.

RISK FACTORS

School-aged children are at highest risk.

GENERAL PREVENTION

Cough etiquette (coughing into elbow or tissue) and proper hand hygiene are important control measures.

PATHOPHYSIOLOGY

- Chlamydiae exist in two forms:
  - Elementary body (EB): infectious form
  - Reticulate body (RB): reproductive form
- Life cycle:
  - EB is taken into cell by endocytosis and reorganizes into a RB to replicate.
  - After replication, RB transformed to EB and are released by exocytosis or cytolysis.
  - Cycle between endocytosis and release is 2–3 days, explaining need for prolonged treatment.

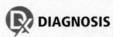

DIAGNOSIS

HISTORY

- *C. pneumoniae* incubation period is approximately 21 days.
- Most commonly presents with prolonged cough (2–6 weeks), developing into atypical pneumonia
- Sore throat may precede onset of cough.
- Patients are mild to moderately ill; infection may be asymptomatic.
- Severe illness occurs in immunocompromised hosts.

PHYSICAL EXAM

- Nasal discharge
- Nonexudative pharyngitis
- Laryngitis, otitis media, and sinusitis may be present.
- Lung exam may be notable for wheezing and rales.

DIAGNOSTIC TESTS & INTERPRETATION

Lab

- No FDA-approved, reliable PCR test available.
- Serologic testing and culture are available, but empiric treatment is recommended.
- Other lab findings are nonspecific including the following:
  - Elevated liver enzymes
  - Left-shifted CBC without neutrophilia

Imaging

Chest radiography

- May have focal or diffuse infiltrates
- Pleural effusion may occur.

DIFFERENTIAL DIAGNOSIS

- Atypical pneumonia due to *Mycoplasma pneumoniae*
- Viral pneumonia
  - Influenza
  - Parainfluenza
  - Adenovirus
  - Respiratory syncytial virus (RSV)
- Less frequently
  - *Coxiella burnetii*
  - *Legionella pneumophila*

TREATMENT

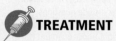

MEDICATION (DRUGS)

First-line therapy is recommended based on national guidelines, as antimicrobial therapy is usually initiated empirically when suspicion is high for atypical pathogens. Alternative therapies are targeted at *C. pneumoniae*.

- First line
  - Azithromycin 10 mg/kg (max 500 mg) for 1 day followed by 5 mg/kg (max 250 mg) for 4 days
  - In hospitalized patients, if clinical picture may also be consistent with typical pathogens, add ampicillin IV 150–200 mg/kg/24 h divided every 6 hours or amoxicillin 90 mg/kg/24 h divided every 12 hours (max 4,000 mg/day) if tolerating oral medications.
- Alternatives:
  - If >8 years, doxycycline
  - Levofloxacin if unable to tolerate macrolides
- Appropriate length of antimicrobial therapy in *C. pneumoniae* infections is unclear.

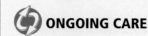

ONGOING CARE

PROGNOSIS

For *C. pneumoniae*, full recovery is expected in general.

COMPLICATIONS

Immunocompromised individuals including those with cystic fibrosis and sickle cell disease can experience a fulminant course.

ADDITIONAL READING

- Bradley JS, Byington CL, Shah SS, et al. The management of community-acquired pneumonia in infants and children older than 3 months of age: clinical practice guidelines. *Clin Infect Dis*. 2011;53(7):e25–e76.
- Burillo A, Bouza E. *Chlamydophila pneumoniae*. *Infect Dis Clin North Am*. 2010;24(1):61–71.
- Centers for Disease Control and Prevention. Sexually transmitted disease guidelines, 2010. *MMWR Recomm Rep*. 2010;59(RR-12):1–114.

CODES

ICD10

A70 Chlamydia psittaci infections

CHOLELITHIASIS

M. Elizabeth Tessier • Eric H. Chiou • Kristin L. Van Buren

BASICS

DESCRIPTION

Cholelithiasis is defined by the presence of cholesterol and/or pigment stones in the gallbladder. Rare in infancy and childhood, it is usually found incidentally on an ultrasound. Risk factors in children include obesity, hemolytic disease, cystic fibrosis (CF), Crohn disease, and long-term total parenteral nutrition (TPN).

EPIDEMIOLOGY

- Cholelithiasis is relatively uncommon in childhood and adolescence; however, the incidence is increasing.
- Gallstones occurring in utero and in infancy have been described.
- Obesity is associated with up to 40% of the gallstones observed in all children and the majority of children with no underlying medical conditions. Obesity is estimated to increase the risk of gallstones in children by over 5-fold.
- Canadian Eskimos and Native Africans have the lowest risk of cholelithiasis.
- Native Americans, Swedes, Scandinavians, and Czechs have the highest risk.
- Pigment stones are more prevalent in prepubertal children, whereas cholesterol stones are predominant in adolescence and adulthood.

Incidence

- Prior to puberty, the incidence of gallstones is equal in males and females. After puberty, the incidence increases in females.

Prevalence

- The prevalence of cholelithiasis in children and adolescents reported in the literature is ~1.9–4.0%.
- In obese children, the prevalence is 2%.
- In children with sickle cell disease, the prevalence is 17–29%.

RISK FACTORS

- Acute renal failure
- Anatomic abnormalities (biliary stricture, duodenal diverticulum)
- CF
- Chronic hemolysis (sickle cell disease, thalassemia, spherocytosis, malaria)
- Chronic overnutrition with carbohydrate and triglyceride-rich, low-fiber diet
- Down syndrome
- Family history
- Female gender (>4 times higher odds than males)
- Hepatobiliary disease/cirrhosis
- Ineffective erythropoiesis (vitamin B_{12} and folate deficiencies)
- Medications (estrogens, octreotide, clofibrate, furosemide, cyclosporine, ceftriaxone, oral contraceptives)
- Necrotizing enterocolitis
- Obesity
- Pregnancy/parity
- Prematurity
- Prolonged fasting/low-calorie diets/rapid weight loss (generally at least ≥10%)
- Severe Crohn disease of the ileum and/or ileal resection
- TPN
- Trauma/abdominal surgery or bariatric surgery
- Hispanic ethnicity

Genetics

- Mutations have been identified in genes encoding the ABC transporters for phosphatidylcholine (adenosine triphosphate–binding cassette, subfamily B), for bile salts (*ABCB11*), or for cholesterol 7a-hydroxylase (*CYP7A1*), the CCK-A receptor (*CCKAR*), and the CF gene (*CFTR*).
- *ABCB4* is also known as *MDR3* (multidrug-resistant 3 glycoprotein). *MDR3* is a phospholipid translocator in the hepatocyte membrane involved in biliary phosphatidylcholine excretion. MDR3 deficiency can cause severe neonatal liver disease, but mutations in MDR3 have also been associated with cholelithiasis, cholestasis of pregnancy, and biliary cirrhosis.
- Variants of ABCG8 and UGT1A1 associated with bile acid metabolism and Gilbert syndrome are risk factors for cholelithiasis.
- Other gene polymorphisms are currently under investigation in humans.

GENERAL PREVENTION

Exercise and dietary modifications can decrease gallstone formation.

PATHOPHYSIOLOGY

- Bile is an aqueous solution of lipids with bile salts, phospholipids, and cholesterol. Changes in the proportion of bile constituents, nucleation (aggregation of cholesterol crystals), changes in gallbladder motility, or infection can lead to stone formation.
- Stone types: pigment, cholesterol, calcium carbonate, and mixed
- Black pigment stones are associated with increased unconjugated bilirubin:
  - Hemolytic diseases
  - Abnormal erythropoiesis
  - Enterohepatic circulation of unconjugated bilirubin
    - Ileal resection, Crohn disease
    - CF
- Brown pigment stones are associated with infection.
- The solubility of cholesterol in bile depends on bile salts and phospholipid concentrations. Cholesterol stones are associated with the following:
  - A decrease in bile salt pool
  - Decreased bile acid synthesis
  - Hypersecretion of cholesterol into the bile
  - Gallbladder stasis (weight loss, pregnancy, long-term TPN)
  - Increased biliary mucus secretion
  - Medications: furosemide, ceftriaxone, cyclosporine

DIAGNOSIS

HISTORY

- Gallstones in children are most commonly incidental findings on abdominal ultrasound.
- Biliary colic, pancreatitis, obstructive jaundice, cholangitis, or other complications should be excluded.
- Intolerance to fatty food rarely exists in children.
- The history should always include questions concerning
  - Previous episodes of right upper quadrant (RUQ) abdominal pain
  - Any risk factors for hemolysis
  - History of prematurity and necrotizing enterocolitis
  - Family history of cholelithiasis
  - Nutritional history
  - Medication use
  - Surgical history
  - Associated medical conditions (e.g., short gut syndrome, ileal disease)

PHYSICAL EXAM

- The physical exam may be completely normal or may uncover the acute abdomen of pancreatitis.
- Murphy sign (tenderness on palpation of the RUQ of the abdomen associated with inspiration) may be elicited in adolescents.
- Silent gallstones present coincidentally in infants and young children.
- Classic symptoms of RUQ pain (Murphy sign) and vomiting are more common in older children and adolescents.
- Younger children present with nonspecific symptoms including obstructive jaundice and mild elevation in transaminases.
- Fever is unusual in all age groups and often indicates the development of rare complications in children:
  - Cholecystitis
  - Choledocholithiasis
  - Cholangitis
  - Gallbladder perforation
    - Pancreatitis develops in 8% of patients with gallstones and is the most common complication.
    - Pancreatitis is more common in obese adolescents who have undergone rapid weight reduction, as reported in the adult population.

DIAGNOSTIC TESTS & INTERPRETATION

Lab

- Laboratory tests should include a complete blood count, urinalysis, amylase, lipase, fractionated bilirubin, alkaline phosphatase, γ-glutamyltransferase (GGT), and transaminase levels.
- Results should typically be within normal ranges.
- Abnormal results may suggest infection, obstruction, or another disease process.

Imaging

- Ultrasound
  - Diagnostic procedure of choice
  - Noninvasive with high sensitivity and specificity
- Plain radiography
  - May not be useful as the majority of gallstones in children are not radiopaque.
- Magnetic resonance cholangiopancreatography (MRCP) is useful to define anatomy in hepatobiliary disease and identify choledocholithiasis.

Diagnostic Procedures/Other

- Endoscopic retrograde cholangiopancreatography (ERCP)
  - Diagnostic for choledocholithiasis
  - Also therapeutic for removal of stones, stenting, or decompression of the biliary tree.
- Surgery should be considered for symptomatic patients.

Pathologic Findings

Black pigment stones are associated with hemolysis and cirrhosis. Brown pigment stones are typically mixed in composition, while cholesterol stones can vary from yellow to green or brown.

DIFFERENTIAL DIAGNOSIS

- Acalculous gallbladder disease
- Biliary dyskinesia
- Cholecystitis
- Common bile duct stones
- Congenital biliary anomalies
- Hydrops of the gallbladder (may be associated with Kawasaki disease)

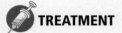

TREATMENT

MEDICATION

- Spontaneous resolution in asymptomatic children is common, without the need for frequent medication use.
- Ursodeoxycholic acid (UDCA) suppresses hepatic cholesterol synthesis and secretion and can improve gallbladder muscle contractility by decreasing muscle cell cholesterol content in the plasma membranes.

ADDITIONAL TREATMENT

General Measures

- Primary prevention
  - High-fiber intake, diet low in saturated fatty acid and nuts, and moderate physical activity
  - Children with asymptomatic gallstones should only be observed.
  - During infancy, there is a chance for spontaneous stone dissolution, especially if cholelithiasis is linked to TPN.
- In children who are dependent on TPN and in patients with short-bowel syndrome, pseudoobstruction, inflammatory bowel disease, or a hemoglobinopathy, gallstones should be removed.
- Prevention of gallstone formation is done by treating underlying risk factors (small enteral feedings in addition to TPN, early pancreatic enzyme supplements in patients with CF, using alternative forms of contraception in high-risk populations, and weight control in obese infants and children with known hemolytic disease).
- Pigment stone formation increases with age.
  - Sickle cell patients should have the gallbladder removed when stones are identified.
  - This strategy will decrease the risk of cholecystitis and other complications and will also help to differentiate between biliary colic and sickle cell crisis.
- Patients with a history of cholecystitis are at increased risk for further episodes (69% will have biliary colic within 2 years and 6% will require cholecystectomy).

SURGERY/OTHER PROCEDURES

- Laparoscopic cholecystectomy is the procedure of choice in symptomatic children.
- Lithotripsy using shock waves has not been approved for use in children.

ONGOING CARE

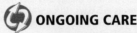

FOLLOW-UP RECOMMENDATIONS

Patient Monitoring

- Asymptomatic patients: Monitor for onset of symptoms; no use for repeat imaging or labs unless symptomatic.
- Symptomatic patients: Consider cholecystectomy.

ADDITIONAL READING

- Buch S, Schafmayer C, Völzke H, et al. Loci from a genome-wide analysis of bilirubin levels are associated with gallstone risk and composition. *Gastroenterology*. 2010;139(6):1942–1951.
- Guarino MP, Cong P, Cicala M, et al. Ursodeoxycholic acid improves muscle contractility and inflammation in symptomatic gallbladders with cholesterol gallstones. *Gut*. 2007;56(6):815–820.
- Lucena JF, Herrero JI, Quiroga J, et al. A multidrug resistance 3 gene mutation causing cholelithiasis, cholestasis of pregnancy, and adulthood biliary cirrhosis. *Gastroenterology*. 2003;124(4):1037–1042.
- Mehta S, Lopez ME, Chumpitazi BP, et al. Clinical characteristics and risk factors for symptomatic pediatric gallbladder disease. *Pediatrics*. 2012;129(1):e82–e88.
- Rosmorduc O, Hermelin B, Boelle PY, et al. ABCB4 gene mutation-associated cholelithiasis in adults. *Gastroenterology*. 2003;125(2):452–459.

CODES

ICD10

- K80.20 Calculus of gallbladder w/o cholecystitis w/o obstruction
- K80.21 Calculus of gallbladder w/o cholecystitis with obstruction
- K80.01 Calculus of gallbladder w acute cholecystitis w obstruction

FAQ

- Q: Does my child with CF have a greater problem with gallstones?
- A: Yes. Children with CF may have more frequent development of gallstones than children without CF. Reports of gallstones while on UDCA therapy have also been noted.
- Q: Why does my child with sickle cell disease have gallstones?
- A: Because the hemolytic process involves breakdown of hemoglobin, which produces bilirubin. This process may accelerate the formation of pigmented gallstones.
- Q: If my child has repeated attacks of RUQ abdominal pain and there are gallstones in the gallbladder, should he have surgery? What kind?
- A: Yes. Laparoscopic cholecystectomy is typically recommended.
- Q: Does obesity increase my child's risk of gallstones?
- A: Yes. Obesity is associated with up to 40% of the gallstones observed in all children.

CHOLERA

Matthew P. Kronman

BASICS

DESCRIPTION

Cholera is an acute-onset infection producing profuse secretory diarrhea with the potential for epidemic spread.

EPIDEMIOLOGY

- Diarrheal disease, including cholera, is the 2nd leading cause of mortality in children <5 years old worldwide.
- The first 6 recorded cholera pandemics occurred prior to 1923, but the current 7th pandemic began in 1961 and has continued through several waves of global transmission.
- Most cholera occurs in Asia and Africa, but *Vibrio cholerae* is now endemic in many countries. Regions previously free of cholera have become susceptible to severe outbreaks, as occurred in Haiti in 2010.
- In the United States, most cases result from travel. Cases have been reported in the Gulf Coast of Louisiana and Texas related to undercooked shellfish consumption.
- Case fatality rates are ~1% with timely treatment but can rise to 35–50% in severe cases in extremely resource-limited settings.

Incidence

- Although underreported, approximately 2.8 million cholera cases occur in endemic countries annually, with an additional 87,000 cases annually in nonendemic countries.
- An estimated 91,000 deaths occur in endemic countries annually.

Prevalence

Given the relatively short duration of illness and lack of chronic carrier state, cholera prevalence generally matches its incidence.

RISK FACTORS

- Inadequate drinking water and sanitation increase transmission; peri-urban slums, refugee camps, disaster areas, etc., are high risk for cholera epidemics.
- Floods and surface water temperature changes lead to increased cholera density.
- Low gastric acidity (which decreases killing of ingested organisms), blood group O, and retinol deficiency are risk factors.
- Young children are at risk for severe cholera.

GENERAL PREVENTION

- Transmission
  - Hand washing after defecation and before food preparation is essential. Boiling or disinfection of water also prevents infection.
  - Thorough cooking of shellfish (which can be naturally contaminated) prevents infection.
  - During travel to endemic areas, avoid swimming or bathing in fresh water.
  - Report confirmed cholera cases to the local department of health.
  - Antibiotic prophylaxis of cholera contacts is debated but was shown in a meta-analysis to prevent disease among the contacts (relative risk, 0.35; 95% CI, 0.18–0.66), although the analysis noted a risk of bias.
- Vaccines
  - No vaccines are available in the United States.
  - Whole cell killed oral cholera vaccines have 52% (95% CI, 35–65%) efficacy in preventing cholera over the subsequent year, but protective efficacy is lower in children <5 years of age at 38% (95% CI, 20–53%).
  - Herd immunity occurs among unvaccinated people living near vaccinees.

PATHOPHYSIOLOGY

- Infection follows ingestion of large numbers of organisms from contaminated water or food (raw or undercooked shellfish and fish, or room temperature damp vegetables).
- The infectious dose for severe cholera is ~10^8 organisms but can be as little as 10^3 organisms in young children or those with decreased gastric acidity (such as those on acid suppression or after certain meals).
- The typical incubation period is usually 2–3 days but ranges from ~12 hours to 5 days.
- 75% are infected asymptomatically; symptomatic illness ranges from moderate to severe.
- Cholera toxin is the key virulence factor responsible for the profuse watery diarrhea.
- Cholera toxin has 1 A and 5 B subunits.
  - The B subunits facilitate toxin attachment to intestinal cells.
  - The A subunit activates adenylate cyclase, increasing intracellular levels of cyclic adenosine monophosphate (cAMP), which causes chloride and sodium to be secreted into the gut lumen.
  - Water follows via osmosis.
- Severely ill patients can progress rapidly to dehydration, circulatory collapse, and death.
- Symptomatic patients may shed as many as 10^{10}–10^{12} organisms per liter of stool and will shed organisms for 2 days to 2 weeks.

ETIOLOGY

- *V. cholerae* is a curved, motile gram-negative rod. Over 200 serogroups exist, but only serogroups O1 and O139 cause epidemics.
- *V. cholerae* serogroup O1 is divided into 2 biotypes: classical and El Tor. The classical biotype was formerly predominant, but the El Tor biotype is causing the 7th pandemic.
- *V. cholerae* serogroup O139 was first identified in 1992 and resembles the O1 El Tor biotype but possesses a distinct lipopolysaccharide and capsule.
- Humans are the only known host, but organisms can also exist freely in water, potentially contaminating fish and shellfish.

COMMONLY ASSOCIATED CONDITIONS

Cholera occurs in healthy individuals.

DIAGNOSIS

HISTORY

- Vomiting and profuse watery diarrhea: Severe illness is characterized by voluminous watery diarrhea (up to 1 L per hour) flecked with mucus ("rice-water stools").
- Sick contacts with similar symptoms: Cholera epidemics can spread rapidly.
- Exposures
  - Return from travel within the last 5 days: Cholera is endemic in much of the world; the incubation period is typically 2–3 days.
  - Patient's water source: Contaminated water serves as a reservoir.
  - History of inadequately cooked shellfish: Shellfish (e.g., oysters, crabs) can harbor the organism.

PHYSICAL EXAM

- Patients with cholera display signs of dehydration (tachycardia, dry mucous membranes, sunken fontanel or eyes, loss of skin turgor, lethargy) varying with severity.
- Arm and leg cramps occur due to secondary hypokalemia and hypocalcemia.
- Fever and obtundation secondary to hypoglycemia are more common in children.

DIAGNOSTIC TESTS & INTERPRETATION

Lab

- Cholera is a generally clinical diagnosis.
- Electrolytes, BUN, creatinine, serum calcium, and glucose can be useful if available. Acidosis can occur from stool bicarbonate losses and lactic acidosis from poor perfusion.

Imaging
No imaging is required for diagnosis.

Diagnostic Procedures/Other
- Use selective media (thiosulfate citrate bile salts sucrose agar) to isolate *V. cholerae*. Alert the microbiology laboratory if culture testing for *V. cholerae* is desired.
- Serologic testing on acute and convalescent sera is also available through the Centers for Disease Control and Prevention (CDC).
- Stool culture may not always be positive in suspected cases of cholera, and rapid dipstick methods to identify cholera toxin and lipopolysaccharide, direct fluorescent antibody assays, and polymerase chain reaction (PCR)–based diagnostic methods also exist and are being studied.

Pathologic Findings
Diagnosis can also be made with the identification of darting, curved bacilli in 400× darkfield microscopy of stool.

DIFFERENTIAL DIAGNOSIS
- Other *Vibrio* species can cause gastroenteritis (commonly caused by *V. parahaemolyticus* but also by *V. fluvialis, V. hollisae*, and *V. mimicus*) or wound infections and sepsis (*V. vulnificus*). Of these, only *V. parahaemolyticus* and *V. vulnificus* cause outbreaks.
- Additional intestinal bacterial pathogens include *Aeromonas*, *Campylobacter*, *Clostridium difficile*, *Escherichia coli*, *Listeria*, *Plesiomonas*, *Salmonella*, *Shigella*, *Vibrio* species, and *Yersinia*.
- Other viral and parasitic pathogens include amebiasis, adenovirus types 40 and 41, *Cryptosporidium*, *Cyclospora*, *Giardia*, norovirus, and rotavirus.

TREATMENT

MEDICATION
First Line
- Give antibiotics as an adjunct to fluid replacement for those with severe cholera.
  – Single-dose doxycycline in those $>$8 years of age
  – Alternately, single-dose azithromycin in children $<$8 years of age and pregnant women
  – Ciprofloxacin is another alternative.
- Single-dose azithromycin can reduce symptom duration by 50% and may reduce excretion of the organism to 1–2 days.
- *V. cholerae* isolates resistant to sulfonamides and tetracyclines are common. Resistance to fluoroquinolones, macrolides, and β-lactams is increasingly reported.
- Administer zinc for 10–14 days: 10 mg/24 h for those $<$6 months of age and 20 mg/24 h for those 6 months to 5 years of age.
- Consider vitamin A supplementation for children in developing countries.
- Avoid antiemetics and antimotility agents.

ADDITIONAL TREATMENT
General Measures
- The mainstay of cholera treatment is rapid rehydration, accounting for both initial and ongoing fluid losses.
- Patients with moderate disease may require only oral rehydration solutions (ORS).
- Administer ORS in frequent small sips to those with vomiting. These solutions should contain at minimum 75 mEq/L of sodium to replete the significant sodium losses associated with cholera.
- ORS with total osmolality $\leq$270 mOsm/L is associated with increased risk of biochemical hyponatremia but not with other symptomatic outcomes compared to ORS $\geq$310 mOsm/L in a meta-analysis of a few existing trials.
- Those with more severe disease (volume loss $>$10%) require intravenous (IV) fluids.

ISSUES FOR REFERRAL
Specific follow-up is unnecessary.

ADDITIONAL THERAPIES
During outbreaks, rapid institution of improved sanitation and safe water availability are critical to decrease the extent of the outbreak.

INPATIENT CONSIDERATIONS
Initial Stabilization
Rapid correction of severe ($>$10%) dehydration is critical.

Admission Criteria
Admit those requiring IV fluids.

IV Fluids
- Dhaka solution is an optimal IV fluid containing dextrose and more bicarbonate and potassium than lactated Ringer (LR).
- LR is an acceptable, more available alternative; D5LR contains 5% dextrose.
- Normal saline lacks potassium and bicarbonate and is second-line.

Nursing
- Measure ongoing fluid losses carefully.
- Use contact precautions for infected infants and children who are incontinent of stool.

Discharge Criteria
Discharge rehydrated patients able to maintain hydration orally.

ONGOING CARE

FOLLOW-UP RECOMMENDATIONS
Patient Monitoring
In the untreated patient, the typical period of *V. cholerae* shedding is 1–2 weeks. Asymptomatic carriage is uncommon.

DIET
Resume a high-energy diet immediately after the initial fluid deficit is replaced. Infants should be encouraged to breastfeed.

PATIENT EDUCATION
- Improved sanitation and safe drinking water can help prevent future episodes.
- Secondary transmission can occur in households with affected members if strict hand washing and hygiene is not followed.

PROGNOSIS
For patients with prompt rehydration, the prognosis is very good regardless of whether antibiotic treatment is given.

COMPLICATIONS
- The main complications are those of severe dehydration: renal failure, thrombosis, stroke, and cardiovascular collapse.
- Cholera itself causes no complications.

C

ADDITIONAL READING

- Ali M, Lopez AL, You YA, et al. The global burden of cholera. *Bull World Health Organ*. 2012;90(3):209–218A.
- Harris JB, LaRocque RC, Qadri F, et al. Cholera. *Lancet*. 2012;379(9835):2466–2476.
- Musekiwa A, Volmink J. Oral rehydration salt solution for treating cholera: $\leq$270 mOsm/L solutions vs $\geq$310 mOsm/L solutions (review). *Cochrane Database Syst Rev*. 2011;(12):CD003754.
- Reveiz L, Chapman E, Ramon-Pardo P, et al. Chemoprophylaxis in contacts of patients with cholera: systematic review and meta-analysis. *PLoS One*. 2011;6(11):e27060.
- Sinclair D, Abba K, Zaman K, et al. Oral vaccines for preventing cholera (review). *Cochrane Database Syst Rev*. 2011;(3):CD008603.

CODES

ICD10
- A00.9 Cholera, unspecified
- A00.0 Cholera due to Vibrio cholerae 01, biovar cholerae
- A00.1 Cholera due to Vibrio cholerae 01, biovar eltor

FAQ
- Q: What foods should I avoid while traveling?
- A: Foods associated with cholera include untreated or unboiled water and ice, undercooked fish and shellfish, raw vegetables, food from street vendors, and cooked food stored at ambient temperature.
- Q: Does cholera pose a risk to pregnant patients?
- A: Given the severe fluid losses, cholera can be life threatening to the fetus; fetal loss occurs in up to 50% of women in their 3rd trimester despite aggressive fluid resuscitation.
- Q: What is the risk of developing cholera among household contacts of those with disease?
- A: Up to 50% of household contacts may develop diarrheal symptoms, typically within 2 days of exposure to the index case.

CHRONIC DIARRHEA

Roberto Gugig

BASICS

DESCRIPTION

- Diarrhea, defined as stool output >200 g/24 h in children and adults or 10 g/kg/24 h in infants, that has occurred for >30 days
- Can be characterized by pattern of stool output with regard to the following:
  - Volume
  - Frequency
  - Consistency
  - Gross appearance
- Should be differentiated from acute diarrhea, which is generally caused by enteric pathogens, is self-limiting, and has a duration of symptoms <14 days; as well as persistent diarrhea, which lasts 14–29 days

EPIDEMIOLOGY

- Gender and genetic factors do not play a significant role in most cases of chronic diarrhea.
- Chronic diarrhea seen in the tropics and developing countries is more likely infectious in nature than in the United States.

PATHOPHYSIOLOGY

The major categories are osmotic and secretory. Inflammatory and motility disorders are important subcategories to consider.

- Osmotic diarrhea occurs when unabsorbable solute accumulates in the lumen of the small intestine and colon, increasing intraluminal osmotic pressure and resulting in excessive fluid and electrolyte losses in stool.
  - Osmotic diarrhea will improve with fasting.
  - Osmotic diarrhea is usually related to malabsorption of dietary products or to the presence of congenital or acquired disaccharidase deficiency or glucose-galactose defects.
- Secretory diarrhea occurs when the net secretion of fluid and electrolyte is in excess of absorption in the intestine:
  - Secretory diarrhea occurs independently of the osmotic load in the intestinal lumen and does not improve with fasting.
  - The mechanisms for secretory diarrhea include the activation of intracellular mediators such as cAMP, cGMP, and calcium-dependent channels.
  - These mediators stimulate active chloride secretion from the crypt cells and inhibit the neutral coupled sodium chloride absorption.
- Inflammation in the intestine can cause an alteration in mucosal integrity resulting in exudative loss of mucus, blood, and/or protein. Increased permeability and altered mucosal surface area may affect absorption and result in diarrhea due to malabsorption.
- Motility disorders affect intestinal transit time. Hypomotility can allow stasis from bacterial overgrowth and can lead to diarrhea.

DIAGNOSIS

HISTORY

- Evaluation of the stool pattern, including consistency, frequency, and appearance
  - The characteristics of the onset of diarrhea should be noted as precisely as possible (e.g., congenital, abrupt, or gradual).
  - Overall duration of the diarrhea and pattern of intermittent versus continuous may also help in determining the underlying process.
  - Stool characteristics should be investigated. Specifically:
    - A history of blood and mucus in stool is strongly suggestive of inflammation.
    - Large-volume stools (>750 mL/24 h) imply small bowel disease and/or a secretory process.
    - Watery stools tend to be more associated with carbohydrate malabsorption, small bowel processes, medications, and functional processes.
    - Steatorrhea (fatty stools) can be greasy, oily, foul-smelling, and bulky and are usually associated with pancreatic disease, bacterial overgrowth, and short bowel syndrome.
- Epidemiologic factors (e.g., travel before onset of illness, antibiotic exposure, and illness in other family members) should be elicited.
- Dietary intake including the types of food and the occurrence of diarrhea in close relationship to specific foods (e.g., dairy products) may be diagnostic. The amount and type of liquid ingested may also be helpful in diagnosis.
- Nutritional status and growth parameters should be assessed. The presence of growth failure or malnutrition has considerable implications compared with a child with normal growth and no history of weight loss.
- Exposure to medications (antibiotics, laxatives, chemotherapeutic agents) or herbal therapies
- Iatrogenic causes of diarrhea should be investigated by obtaining a detailed medication history and history of radiation therapy and surgery.
- Other symptoms associated with the diarrhea are important to assess and include abdominal pain, fever, bloating, tenesmus, soiling, rashes, and joint complaints.
- The presence or absence of abdominal pain should be evaluated. Pain is often present in patients with inflammatory bowel disease, irritable bowel syndrome, and mesenteric ischemia.
- Family history (e.g., celiac disease, inflammatory bowel disease, cystic fibrosis, and other pancreatic processes)
- Previous evaluation should be reviewed whenever possible, objective records should be examined before new studies are ordered.

PHYSICAL EXAM

- Nutritional status: Compare height, weight, and head circumference with normal standards and previous exam measurements.
- Anthropometric measurements are important in assessing loss of body fat and muscle mass.
- Peripheral edema, ascites, rash, dystrophic nails, alopecia, chronic chest findings, and pallor may all be indicative of nutritional deficiencies secondary to chronic diarrhea.
- A rectal exam may reveal stool impaction with overflow diarrhea:
  - Is there blood in the stool?
  - Perianal disease (fistula, skin tags, abscess)
- Evidence of infection should be considered with symptoms such as fever, bloody diarrhea, and vital sign instability.
- Aphthous lesions, arthritis, and clubbing
- The abdominal exam in most patients is generally nonspecific.
- Other features of diagnostic significance include rashes on the skin, mouth ulcers, thyroid masses, wheezing, arthritis, heart murmurs, hepatomegaly or abdominal masses.

DIAGNOSTIC TESTS & INTERPRETATION

Lab

- Stool samples
  - Stool should be cultured for bacteria, ova and parasites, and viral organisms.
  - *Clostridium difficile* toxins A and B are heat-labile, and stool must be kept cool during transport.
  - Collect stool in the correct containers to ensure accurate and reliable analysis.
    - Stool samples can be tested for occult blood and for the presence of fecal leukocytes.
    - Stool pH and reducing substances
      - If stool is positive for reducing substances and/or the pH is <5.5, carbohydrate malabsorption with or without proximal small bowel injury is likely.
      - Note: Sucrose is *not* a reducing substance. If sucrose malabsorption is suspected, stool sample has to be hydrolyzed with hydrochloric acid and heat before analysis.
    - A positive Sudan stain of the stool is indicative of fat malabsorption. However, a 72-hour fecal fat collection remains the gold standard to diagnose fat malabsorption.
    - Stool for fecal elastase can be used to assess fat malabsorption.
    - Stool may be collected for electrolyte and osmolality measurements. Osmotic gap >100 mOsm/kg is indicative of an osmotic diarrhea.
    - Spot or 24-hour collection for fecal α_1-antitrypsin can help assess protein loss.
    - Stool collection for fecal calprotectin to assess for IBD—protein found in neutrophils that enter the bowel during an inflammatory process
- CBC
  - Hemoglobin and RBC may provide evidence and characteristics of anemia (i.e., microcytotic, macrocytotic, normochromic).
  - Leukocytosis suggest the presence of inflammation.
  - Eosinophilia can be seen with neoplasm, allergy, collagen vacular disease, parasitic infection, and eosinophilic gastroenteritis, or colitis.
- Other blood tests:
  - Prealbumin and albumin can provide parameters of protein and overall nutritional status.
  - Erythrocyte sedimentation rate and C-reactive protein (CRP) can serve as markers for inflammatory conditions.
  - Hormonal studies to assess for secretory tumors (vasoactive intestinal peptide [VIP], gastrin, secretin, urine assay for 5-HT)

- In the evaluation for celiac disease, serum antitissue transglutaminase antibody and antiendomysial antibodies (presuming a normal level of total serum IgA)
- Hepatic panel, coagulation profile, and fat-soluble vitamin levels (25-OH vitamin D; vitamins E, A, K) may be helpful to assess fat malabsorption.
- Viral serologies such as HIV and cytomegalovirus need to be considered in the immunocompromised host with diarrhea.
- Thyroid studies in patients with large-volume watery diarrhea

- Specialized studies:
  - A D-xylose absorption test is helpful in screening for small bowel injury. Timed serum D-xylose following oral ingestion is significantly lower in diseases causing diffuse mucosal damage to the small bowel (i.e., postviral enteropathy, celiac disease).
  - A hydrogen breath test may be helpful in evaluating for the possibility of small bowel bacterial overgrowth.
- Sweat chloride if cystic fibrosis is suspected

Imaging
- Plain radiograph studies usually not helpful; may demonstrate presence or absence of formed stool and/or fecal impaction
- Upper GI series with small bowel follow-through may show partial small bowel obstruction, strictures, or evidence of inflammatory bowel disease.
- Abdominal CT scan may help in assessing the pancreas for calcifications and inflammation.

DIAGNOSTIC PROCEDURES/OTHER
- Endoscopy with small bowel biopsy and small bowel aspirate for culture to help diagnose certain congenital, immunologic, or infectious causes of diarrhea
  - Small bowel disaccharidase studies will help detect carbohydrate malabsorption.
- Colonoscopy will diagnose colitis related to inflammatory bowel disease or infection.
- Video capsule endoscopy may also be used to further evaluate the small bowel for evidence of inflammation.

DIFFERENTIAL DIAGNOSIS
- Infants (<1 year of age)
  - Cow's milk and/or soy protein intolerance
  - Intractable diarrhea of infancy is associated with diffuse mucosal injury beginning at <6 months of age, resulting in malabsorption and malnutrition (sucrose and lactase deficiency).
  - Infectious/protracted postinfectious diarrhea
  - Microvillus inclusions disease
  - Tufting enteropathy
  - Autoimmune enteropathy
  - IPEX (immune dysregulation, polyendocrinopathy, enteropathy, X-linked)
  - Congenital glucose-galactose malabsorption
  - Hirschsprung disease with enterocolitis
  - Transport defects (e.g., congenital chloridorrhea)
  - Nutrient malabsorption (e.g., congenital glucose-galactose malabsorption and congenital lactase deficiency, sucrase-isomaltase deficiency)
  - Cystic fibrosis
  - AIDS enteropathy
  - Primary immune defects
  - Munchausen syndrome by proxy (factitious)
  - Drug-, toxin-induced
- Children (1–5 years of age)
  - Chronic nonspecific diarrhea of infancy (toddler's diarrhea)
  - Infectious/postinfectious enteritis
  - Giardiasis
  - Eosinophilic gastroenteritis
  - Sucrase-isomaltase deficiency
  - Tumors (neuroblastoma, VIPoma with secretory diarrhea)
  - Inflammatory bowel disease
  - Celiac disease
  - Cystic fibrosis
  - Small bowel bacterial overgrowth
  - AIDS enteropathy
  - Constipation with (overflow) encopresis
  - Acquired short bowel syndrome
  - Shwachman syndrome
  - Factitious
- Children (>5 years of age)
  - Similar to above
  - Acquired lactose deficiency (early adolescent)
  - Inflammatory bowel disease
  - Celiac disease
  - Constipation with (overflow) encopresis
  - Irritable bowel syndrome (adolescent)
  - Laxative abuse (adolescents)
  - Infection
- Bacterial (*Aeromonas*, *Plesiomonas*, *Campylobacter*, *Salmonella*, *Mycobacterium tuberculosis*, *Yersinia*, recurrent *C. difficile*)
- Viral (rotavirus, adenovirus, Norwalk virus, Norovirus)
- Parasites (*Amoeba*, *Trichuris*, *Cryptosporidium*, *Giardia*, *Schistosoma*, *Cyclospora*)
- Small bowel bacterial overgrowth
- Tumors (neuroblastoma, VIPoma with secretory diarrhea)
- Primary bowel tumors (rare, adolescent)
- Complex congenital heart disease with protein-losing enteropathy
- Pancreatic insufficiency/chronic pancreatitis
- Hyperthyroidism
- Diabetes

TREATMENT

MEDICATION
- Presuming no inflammation or constipation, the use of antimotility agents such as loperamide and Lomotil, and antisecretory agents, such as octreotide, may have a role in noninfectious causes of diarrhea. However, identification and treatment of the underlying cause of diarrhea is always preferable.
- Pancreatic enzymes may be used in specific patients.
- Luminal (nonabsorbed) antibiotics for small bowel bacterial overgrowth

ALERT
- In certain cases in which the diet is altered as a therapeutic intervention, the physician must ensure that the patient is still absorbing adequate calories and micronutrients, so that the nutritional status of the patient is not further compromised.
- Avoid the reinstitution of a regular diet too quickly following a severe and/or protracted insult to the gut because this may further exacerbate the diarrhea.
- The use of antimotility and antisecretory agents should be judicious and as an adjunct to other therapy but not as the mainstay in the treatment regimen.
- In patients with cow's milk and/or soy allergy, rechallenge after 12 months of age in a controlled environment in case anaphylaxis occurs.

- Children with the following symptoms should see a health care provider:
  - Signs of dehydration
  - Failure to thrive
  - Diarrhea for more than 24–48 hours
  - A fever of 102°F or higher
  - Stools containing blood or pus
  - Stools that are black and tarry

ADDITIONAL TREATMENT
- The first goal is to ensure adequate hydration status, nutritional intake, and to permit normal growth and development.
- Antibiotics when infection is suspected
- Many causes of congenital diarrhea do not have specific therapy available, and treatment is supportive.
- Diet: If infection is severe or protracted, an elemental formula may be necessary early in the recovery phase. If oral nutrition appears inadequate, the formula can be given in a slow, continuous fashion via a nasogastric/jejunal tube. Remove offending agent (e.g., cow's milk protein, soy protein, lactose, or gluten).
- In cases in which there is increased motility and thus rapid transit time, such as in chronic nonspecific diarrhea, alterations in the diet can be very helpful.
- Elimination of sorbitol-containing juices, which increases the osmotic load, and low-carbohydrate diet will help to lower the osmotic load delivered to the intestine. Furthermore, a high-fat diet will slow the intestinal transit time and increase the time available to absorb fluid, electrolytes, and nutrients from the intestinal tract.

ADDITIONAL READING

- Bhutta ZA, Nelson EA, Lee WS, et al. Recent advances and evidence gaps in persistent diarrhea. *J Pediatr Gastroenterol Nutr*. 2008;47(2):260–265.
- Lee SD, Surawicz CM. Infectious causes of chronic diarrhea. *Gastroenterol Clin North Am*. 2001;30(3): 679–692.
- Pawlowski SW, Warren CA, Guerrant R. Diagnosis and treatment of acute or persistent diarrhea. *Gastroenterology*. 2009;136(6):1874–1886.
- Salvilahti E. Food-induced malabsorption syndromes. *J Pediatr Gastroenterol Nutr*. 2000;30(Suppl): S61–S66.

CODES

ICD10
K52.9 Noninfective gastroenteritis and colitis, unspecified

FAQ
- Q: If my infant has cow's milk allergy, when can he have cow's milk?
- A: In patients with cow's milk and/or soy allergy, rechallenge should be around 12 months of age and should be in a controlled environment in case anaphylaxis occurs. If the testing is negative, ingestion of cow's milk can be recommended.
- Q: What are the best markers for success in management of chronic diarrhea?
- A: If weight and height normalize, the chances of continued malabsorption are unlikely.

CHRONIC GRANULOMATOUS DISEASE

Benjamin T. Prince • Ramsay L. Fuleihan

BASICS

DEFINITION
Chronic granulomatous disease (CGD) is a rare, primary immunodeficiency caused by a genetic defect that results in an inability of phagocytes to generate superoxide, which is important in microbial killing. Affected individuals are susceptible to recurrent, life-threatening bacterial and fungal infections.

EPIDEMIOLOGY
Incidence
1:200,000 to 1:250,000 live births in the United States and Europe. Rates in other countries vary depending on ethnic practices and degree of intermarriage.

RISK FACTORS
Genetics
- Mutations in any of the 5 genes that code for the 5 subunits of the phagocyte NADPH oxidase complex (phox) can result in CGD.
- Mutations in the gp91phox subunit are responsible for 65% of cases and are inherited in an X-linked manner (1/3 of these cases are the result of a de novo mutation).
- Mutations in p47phox, p22phox, p67phox, and p40phox subunits account for the remaining cases and have an autosomal recessive inheritance.
- Mutations in the p47phox subunit are the most common cause of autosomal recessive CGD (25% of all cases).

PATHOPHYSIOLOGY
- Phagocytes (neutrophils, monocytes, and macrophages) require NADPH oxidase to generate reactive oxygen species (ROS) in a process called the respiratory burst.
- During this process, the NADPH oxidase complex transfers an electron to molecular oxygen forming superoxide, which is eventually converted to hydrogen peroxide.
- Superoxide plays a significant role in killing bacterial and fungal pathogens both directly and through the activation of more important intraphagosomal proteases.
- The clinical phenotype of CGD is related to the level of residual superoxide production; patients who have higher levels of superoxide production have better long-term survival rates.
- Only the X-linked subunit gp91phox is phagocyte specific, and patients with defects in the autosomal subunits may also have other abnormalities such as vascular disease, diabetes, and inflammatory bowel disease.

ETIOLOGY
CGD is the result of a spontaneous or inherited genetic mutation that is present at birth.

DIAGNOSIS

HISTORY
- Patients most commonly present in early childhood with recurrent or severe bacterial or fungal infections of the lung, skin, lymph nodes, liver, bones, and blood.
- Patients may also have a history of failure to thrive, diarrhea, anemia, abnormal wound healing, or granulomatous inflammation.
- Infecting organisms are typically catalase producing; however, catalase alone does not appear to be a significant virulence factor in animal models.
- Most common organisms include *Staphylococcus aureus*, *Burkholderia (Pseudomonas) cepacia*, *Serratia marcescens*, *Nocardia*, *Aspergillus*, *Salmonella*, *Bacillus Calmette-Guérin* (BCG), *Mycobacterium*, *Klebsiella pneumoniae*, and *Candida*.
- Obtain a good maternal family history given that most common inheritance is X-linked. There may also be family history of lupus, especially maternal.

PHYSICAL EXAM
- Skin and mucosa
  - Dermatitis, cellulitis, impetigo, abscesses, stomatitis, gingivitis
- HEENT
  - Conjunctivitis, chorioretinitis, sinusitis
- Lymphatic
  - Lymphadenopathy, suppurative lymphadenitis
- Respiratory
  - Pneumonia, pneumonitis
- Gastrointestinal
  - Gastric outlet obstruction hepatomegaly, splenomegaly, colitis, diarrhea, malabsorption, perirectal abscess, fistulae
- Genitourinary
  - Urethral strictures, urinary tract infections

DIAGNOSTIC TESTS & INTERPRETATION
Lab
- Dihydrorhodamine 123 (DHR) test
  - Uses flow cytometry to directly measure NADPH oxidase function in phagocytes
  - Phagocytes take up nonfluorescent DHR. Oxidation by a normal functioning NADPH oxidase complex causes DHR to fluoresce, which is identified by flow cytometry.
  - More sensitive and quantitative than older nitroblue tetrazolium (NBT) test
  - Can identify NADPH positive and negative subpopulations of phagocytes, easily identifying a carrier of CGD
  - May be falsely positive in patients with myeloperoxidase deficiency and SAPHO (synovitis, acne, pustulosis, hyperostosis, osteitis) syndrome
- NBT test
  - Historical test for CGD that is no longer widely used by immunologists
  - Neutrophils with a normal NADPH complex can reduce the dye, resulting in a color change from yellow to dark blue. Neutrophils from patients with CGD cannot reduce the dye, and it remains colorless.
  - Color change is assessed with microscopy, and results may be inaccurate if not performed by experienced technician.
- Genetic testing
  - A diagnosis of CGD should be confirmed with genetic testing to identify the specific genetic defect.
  - Identification of specific mutation can better predict the patient's clinical course.
  - Identification of specific mutation is necessary for a future prenatal diagnosis.

Imaging
Obtain chest radiograph, ultrasound, CT scan, or MRI as appropriate to aid in the diagnosis and evaluation of acute infections.

DIFFERENTIAL DIAGNOSIS
- Genetic/metabolic
  - Glucose-6-phosphate dehydrogenase (G6PD) deficiency
  - Glutathione synthetase (GS) deficiency
  - Cystic fibrosis
- Immunology
  - Myeloperoxidase deficiency
  - Hyper IgE syndrome
  - Humoral immunodeficiencies
  - IRAK4 deficiency
  - MyD88 deficiency
- Gastrointestinal
  - Inflammatory bowel disease

TREATMENT

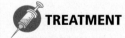

MEDICATION
- Trimethoprim-sulfamethoxazole (TMP-SMX)
  - First line for antibacterial prophylaxis; also can be used for the treatment of acute bacterial infections
  - Prophylaxis dosing: 5 mg/kg/24 h TMP PO divided b.i.d., maximum 320 mg b.i.d.
  - Has been shown to decrease frequency and severity of infections in CGD patients

- Itraconazole
  - First line for antifungal prophylaxis
  - Prophylaxis dosing: 5 mg/kg PO daily, maximum 200 mg daily
- Interferon gamma-1b
  - Effective in reducing the frequency and severity of infections when used prophylactically; however, it is unclear how much additional benefit is gained when used in conjunction with TMP-SMX and itraconazole prophylaxis
  - Prophylaxis dosing: 50 mcg/m^2 subcutaneously 3 times weekly
- Ciprofloxacin
  - Should be started prophylactically before any invasive procedure and continued for at least 24 hours afterward
  - Prophylaxis dosing: 7.5 mg/kg PO q12h, maximum 500 mg q12h
- Acute infections
  - Broad-spectrum IV antimicrobials: Severe infections should be treated empirically until a specific organism is identified. Treatment should cover both gram-negative and gram-positive bacteria along with fungi.
  - First line: TMP-SMX, fluoroquinolones, and voriconazole
  - Carbapenems, vancomycin, and amphotericin B may be considered depending on site or severity of infection.

ISSUES FOR REFERRAL

Factors that may help alert you to make a referral:

- New diagnosis of CGD
  - Immunologists can assist with antibiotic prophylaxis and with parameters for when to seek medical attention.
  - Can help establish the specific molecular diagnosis of the patient and offer genetic counseling for the future
  - Can discuss treatment options, including the possibility of hematopoietic stem cell transplant
- Fever or suspected infection
  - Patients with CGD tend to develop infections in unusual sites with unusual organisms. Both an infectious disease specialist and an immunologist can help with the evaluation and appropriate treatment of infections.
- Gastrointestinal symptoms or malabsorption
  - Gastroenterologists can help identify and treat strictures, obstruction, and colitis.
- The diagnosis of CGD should be considered in patients with
  - Recurrent lymphadenitis
  - Staphylococcal hepatic abscess
  - Infections with *Burkholderia cepacia*, *Serratia marcescens*, *Nocardia*, or *Aspergillus*
  - *Salmonella* sepsis
  - Perirectal or deep tissue abscesses
  - Colitis in infancy
  - Granulomatous lesions of the gastrointestinal or genitourinary systems

COMPLEMENTARY & ALTERNATIVE THERAPIES

- Hematopoietic stem cell transplant (HSCT)
  - HSCT can be a definitive cure for CGD.
  - Younger patients with absence of preexisting overt infection have the best prognosis.
- Gene therapy
  - May be an effective treatment of CGD in the future; however, currently still in research phase

ONGOING CARE

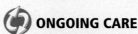

FOLLOW-UP RECOMMENDATIONS

Patient Monitoring

- Regular screening blood tests
  - CBC with differential and LFTs should be performed every 6 months to monitor for any adverse effects of prophylactic medications.
  - CRP and ESR should be performed regularly and at times of acute infection.
- Pulmonary function testing should be followed annually to screen for chronic lung disease.
- Patients should be screened regularly by ophthalmology for chorioretinal lesions.
- Closely monitor CGD patients and carriers for signs of systemic lupus erythematosus and other autoimmune disorders.

PROGNOSIS

- CGD is a lifelong disease.
- Survival beyond the 4th decade is now common with antimicrobial prophylaxis and early and aggressive treatment of infections.
- Successful HSCT is curative.

COMPLICATIONS

CGD patients have an increased susceptibility to bacterial and fungal infections that usually are not pathogenic in normal hosts:

- Recurrent infections (see previous sections)
- Sepsis
- Chronic lung disease (secondary to recurrent infections)
- Chronic liver disease (secondary to recurrent infections)
- Chronic osteomyelitis of large and small bones
- Malabsorption
- Systemic and discoid lupus erythematosus
  - Increased incidence in female carriers

ADDITIONAL READING

- Cole T, Pearce MS, Cant AJ, et al. Clinical outcome in children with chronic granulomatous disease managed conservatively or with hematopoietic stem cell transplantation. *J Allergy Clin Immunol*. 2013;132(5):1150–1155.
- Damen GM, van Krieken JH, Hoppenreijs E, et al. Overlap, common features, and essential differences in pediatric granulomatous inflammatory bowel disease. *J Pediatr Gastroenterol Nutr*. 2010;51(6): 690–697.
- Holland SM. Chronic granulomatous disease. *Hematol Oncol Clin North Am*. 2013;27(1):89–99.
- Kuhns DB, Alvord WG, Meller T, et al. Residual NADPH oxidase and survival in chronic granulomatous disease. *N Engl J Med*. 2010;363(27): 2600–2610.
- Song E, Jaishankar GB, Saleh H, et al. Chronic granulomatous disease: a review of the infectious and inflammatory complications. *Clin Mol Allergy*. 2011;9(1):10.

CODES

ICD10

D71 Functional disorders of polymorphonuclear neutrophils

FAQ

- Q: Should patients with CGD receive dental prophylaxis?
- A: Yes. Antibiotic prophylaxis should be started before and continued for the 24 hours after any dental treatment likely to cause bleeding.
- Q: Can patients with CGD receive live viral vaccines?
- A: Yes. The only routine immunization that adults and children with CGD should NOT receive is BCG as it has been associated with disseminated infection.
- Q: Are all CGD patients with fever automatically admitted to the hospital?
- A: No. Although CGD patients are more prone to invasive and systemic infections, they are not necessarily admitted with every febrile episode. If there is evidence of a minor bacterial or viral infection without any concern for a more serious infection, patients may be treated as an outpatient with close monitoring. Subtle signs of an invasive infection must be taken very seriously.
- Q: Can CGD be diagnosed prenatally?
- A: Yes. Testing involves chorionic villus sampling; however, it can only be done on families with a history of CGD in which the specific mutation is known.

CHRONIC HEPATITIS

Vani V. Gopalareddy

BASICS

DESCRIPTION

- Chronic hepatitis is a continuous inflammation of the liver that can lead to cirrhosis.
- Features include inflammation not caused by acute self-limiting infection or past drug exposure, with raised transaminases and histologic evidence of hepatitis.

EPIDEMIOLOGY

Depends on the cause of the underlying disease

- Nonalcoholic steatohepatitis (NASH) is a leading cause of elevated aspartate aminotransferase (AST)/alanine aminotransferase (ALT).
- Hepatitis B: common in immigrant children from Asia and Eastern Europe
- Hepatitis C: common in those who had blood transfusions and blood products before screening became available, history of IV drug abuse
- Wilson disease presents mainly in older children (>2 years of age) and adults.
- Autoimmune liver disease is more common in females and patients >6 months of age.
- Autoimmune hepatitis (AIH) may be associated with other autoimmune conditions such as diabetes, ulcerative colitis, autoimmune thyroiditis, and celiac disease.
- Cystic fibrosis and α_1 antitrypsin deficiency

PATHOPHYSIOLOGY

Pathology has been traditionally classified by evidence of chronic persistent hepatitis, chronic aggressive hepatitis, and chronic lobular hepatitis. All are associated with damaged hepatocytes as well as inflammatory cellular infiltration accompanied by liver regeneration.

- Chronic persistent hepatitis
  - Minimal portal tract fibrosis
  - Slightly widened portal tracts
  - Limiting plate is intact and inflammation does not extend beyond this.
  - No bridging fibrosis between portal tracts
- Chronic aggressive hepatitis
  - Perilobular hepatitis, with inflammatory cells extending from portal tracts into parenchyma with fibrosis
  - Piecemeal necrosis: necrotic hepatocytes surrounded by lymphocytes and fibroblasts
  - In advanced disease, fibrosis bridges the portal tracts (bridging fibrosis).
  - Cirrhosis occurs when there is loss of architecture owing to fibrosis.
- Chronic lobular hepatitis
  - Liver architecture is preserved with scattered changes of acute hepatitis with hepatocyte necrosis in the lobules (perivenular regions).
  - Associated with hepatitis B and non-A, non-B hepatitis

ETIOLOGY

- Autoimmune liver disease
- Viral hepatitis
- Obesity (NASH)
- Progressive familial intrahepatic cholestasis (PFIC) syndromes
- Congenital hepatic fibrosis
- Cystic fibrosis
- Metabolic disease
  - Mitochondrial disease
  - Lysosomal storage disorders
  - Peroxisomal disease
  - Lipid storage disease
  - Glycogen storage disease
  - Wilson disease and others
- Drug hepatotoxicity
  - Methotrexate
  - Isoniazid
  - Thioguanine
  - 6-Mercaptopurine
  - Valproate
- Liver disease associated with other chronic diseases
  - Cardiac disease
  - Autosomal recessive polycystic kidney disease
  - Diabetes mellitus
  - Langerhans cell histiocytosis
  - Immunodeficiency
  - Total parenteral nutrition cholestasis

DIAGNOSIS

HISTORY

- Preceding clinical signs and symptoms for at least 6 months and complete medical history
  - History of blood transfusions
  - Surgery
  - Medications
  - Foreign travel
  - Social circumstances that predispose to liver diseases
- Symptoms of chronic illness can be nonspecific:
  - Poor growth
  - Intermittent jaundice
  - Abdominal pain
  - Bleeding
  - Malabsorption
  - Fever
  - Amenorrhea
  - Poor school achievement
  - Itching
- Variceal bleeding may be a presenting symptom in patients with portal hypertension.
- A history of jaundice in infancy, family history of liver disease or autoimmune liver disease, blood transfusions, IV drug use, or multiple sexual partners can suggest an etiology of hepatitis.

PHYSICAL EXAM

Stigmata of chronic liver disease are as follows:

- Spider nevi, palmar erythema
- Dilated veins on abdomen/cutaneous shunts
- Palmar erythema
- Cyanosis (hepatopulmonary syndrome)
- Clubbing
- Jaundice
- Pruritus/scratch marks (due to accumulation of bile salts in the epidermis)
- Hypercholesterolemic xanthomas
- Enlarged liver or small, shrunken liver
- Splenomegaly
- Ascites
- Rickets
- Mental changes
- Fetor associated with high ammonia
- Poor weight gain/FTT, weight loss

DIAGNOSTIC TESTS & INTERPRETATION

Lab

- General liver testing: albumin, creatinine, γ-glutamyl transferase, AST, ALT, bilirubin, PT/INR, CBC, ammonia level
- Other testing as indicated by the specific clinical presentation
  - Viral serologies: hepatitis B, hepatitis C, hepatitis D
  - Autoantibodies: type 1: smooth muscle (also called antiactin), antinuclear, antisoluble liver antigen; type 2: liver kidney microsomal, primary sclerosing cholangitis: pericytoplasmic antineutrophil (p-ANCA)
  - Immunoglobulins: IgG elevated in autoimmune liver disease
  - Fasting glucose, insulin levels, CRP, lipid profile (suspected NASH)
  - α_1 Antitrypsin level and phenotype
  - Serum ceruloplasmin, serum copper, 24-hour urine copper (+/− penicillamine challenge), quantitative liver copper (Wilson disease)
  - Cholesterol, triglycerides elevated in cholestatic syndromes, glycogen storage, Alagille syndrome, certain lysosomal disease, steatohepatitis
  - Metabolic workup as indicated
  - CPK level to rule out muscle source of elevated ALT/AST
  - Urinary succinylacetone: tyrosinemia
  - Urinary bile acids: bile acid synthetic defects
  - Sweat test and cystic fibrosis genotyping
  - Alpha fetoprotein (AFP) level
  - Fibrosis markers (FibroSURE; FibroTest; ActiTest) are not validated for children but may be useful in older patients.

Diagnostic Procedures/Other

- Ultrasound with Doppler flow studies: should focus on liver and spleen and may detect steatosis
- Other testing as indicated by specific clinical presentation
  - MRI can demonstrate percentage steatosis.
  - FibroScan can measure liver stiffness/fibrosis.
  - Liver biopsy
  - Endoscopic retrograde cholangiopancreatography (ERCP) or magnetic retrograde cholangiopancreatography (MRCP) may be useful if primary sclerosing cholangitis is suspected.
  - Colonoscopy: sclerosing cholangitis, inflammatory bowel disease
  - Bone marrow aspirate to exclude Niemann-Pick type C or other storage disorders
  - Enzyme analysis to evaluate for lysosomal storage disease, glycogen storage disease
  - Angiography: congenital or acquired venous or arterial malformations, assessment of portosystemic shunt
  - Cardiac catheterization to assess pulmonary hypertension and cardiac status
  - Macroaggregated albumin scan to assess hepatopulmonary syndrome and hepatic encephalopathy
  - Muscle biopsy to assay respiratory chain enzymes in mitochondrial disorders
  - Genotyping: Wilson disease, cystic fibrosis, and others

DIFFERENTIAL DIAGNOSIS

Nonhepatic etiologies of lab or physical exam abnormalities

- Hepatomegaly: elevated right-sided cardiac pressures, such as patients with Fontan operations, right-sided heart failure; respiratory diseases with lung hyperexpansion
- Splenomegaly
  - Blood malignancies
  - Storage diseases
  - Hematologic disease with hemolysis
  - Infection
  - Vascular
- Jaundice: often confused with hypercarotenemia
- Elevated transaminases: consider nonhepatic sources such as skeletal muscles in myopathies; with jaundice, consider hypopituitarism in infancy
- Alkaline phosphatase: may be elevated in growing children and in rickets; may not indicate biliary obstruction
- γ-Glutamyl transferase
  - Produced in renal tubules, pancreatic and biliary ducts
  - Often elevated in patients on antiepileptic drugs and in alcoholics
- Abnormal coagulation: anticoagulant medications, bacterial overgrowth with malabsorption, inherited disorders of coagulation, sepsis

TREATMENT

GENERAL MEASURES

The management of patients is dictated by the underlying diagnosis.

- General management
  - Maintaining growth and development is paramount.
  - Fat-soluble vitamins (A, D, E, K) given orally are poorly absorbed in cholestasis, and levels must be monitored.
  - Anthropometric parameters must be recorded, including skinfold thickness.
  - Body mass index
  - Preference for medium-chain triglyceride (MCT)–rich formulas can reduce fat malabsorption.
  - Branched-chain amino acids may be useful in patients with hepatic encephalopathy.
  - Ursodeoxycholic acid: choleretic
  - Encourage bolus feedings; minimizing continuous feeding and total parenteral nutrition may reduce gallbladder sludge.
  - Proactive involvement of clinical psychologist and play therapist can help alleviate problems such as depression and fear.
  - Aggressive weight management in patients with obesity/hypermetabolic syndrome with steatohepatitis; curbing passive activities such as television, computer games
  - Chronic debilitating pruritus: indication for liver transplantation after failure of medical therapy. Treatment for pruritus includes the following:
    - Actigall (ursodeoxycholic acid)
    - Rifampicin
    - Ondansetron
    - Antihistamines
    - Naltrexone
    - Zoloft
    - Cholestyramine
    - Ultraviolet light
  - Monitoring portal hypertension: Assessment of portal flow on ultrasound and spleen size may provide some indication of disease progression.
  - Treatment of recurrent cholangitis may decelerate the progression of liver disease.
  - Aggressive treatment for spontaneous bacterial peritonitis in patients with ascites
  - Early referral to a liver transplant center
  - Complete immunization schedule including hepatitis A, hepatitis B, and annual flu shots.
- Specific management depends on the underlying liver disease.

ONGOING CARE

FOLLOW-UP RECOMMENDATIONS

Patient Monitoring

- Look for hepatocellular carcinoma developing in patients with chronic liver disease.
- Obtaining an ultrasound scan of liver and AFP every 6 months is considered a reasonable schedule.
- Advise patients with splenomegaly to wear a spleen guard and avoid activities (e.g., contact sports) that can cause splenic rupture.

PROGNOSIS

Some cases of chronic hepatitis are associated with diseases that are treatable. Others are progressive and not amenable to treatment. A subset of patients will progress to end-stage liver disease and require liver transplantation.

ADDITIONAL READING

- Mieli-Vergani G, Vergani D. Autoimmune hepatitis in children: what is different from adult AIH? *Semin Liver Dis*. 2009;29(3):297–306.
- Murray KF, Shah U, Mohan N, et al. Chronic hepatitis. *J Pediatr Gastroenterol Nutr*. 2008;47(2):225–233.
- Nel E, Sokol R, Comparcola D, et al. Viral hepatitis in children. *J Pediatr Gastroenterol Nutr*. 2012;55(5):500–505.

CODES

ICD10

- K73.9 Chronic hepatitis, unspecified
- K73.0 Chronic persistent hepatitis, not elsewhere classified
- B18.9 Chronic viral hepatitis, unspecified

FAQ

- Q: What are the risks of providing very young patients with a liver transplant?
- A: Lifetime risks of immunosuppression and rejection. Although transplant in the very young is more difficult, with the increased use of split liver techniques and improved use of immunosuppressives, outcomes of orthotopic liver transplantation in infants have improved.
- Q: Why should we be aggressive with vitamin supplementation?
- A: Chronic hepatitis is associated with significant malabsorption of vitamins A, D, E, and K. Vitamins D and E deficiencies in particular can cause rickets and neuropathy.
- Q: How can I optimally administer oral supplements of vitamins in the very young?
- A: It is common practice in some centers to give vitamins D and E as an intramuscular injection on a monthly basis, with levels done in between.
- Q: Why do jaundiced children scratch?
- A: The accumulation of bile salts causes pruritus.
- Q: What stigmata of chronic liver disease can be seen in children?
- A: Spider nevi, liver palms (palmar erythema), splenomegaly, cutaneous shunts, and clubbing are very common.

CHRONIC KIDNEY DISEASE

Madhura Pradhan • Susan L. Furth

BASICS

DESCRIPTION

- The Kidney Disease: Improving Global Outcomes (KDIGO) 2012 clinical practice guidelines defines chronic kidney disease (CKD) as abnormalities of kidney structure or function, present for >3 months (except in infants <3 months of age) with implications for health.
- Criteria for CKD include the following:
  - Markers of kidney damage such as albuminuria, urine sediment abnormalities, electrolyte and other abnormalities due to tubular disorders, abnormalities detected by histology, structural abnormalities detected by imaging, and history of kidney transplantation
  - Decreased glomerular filtration rate (GFR) <60 mL/min/1.73 m^2
- CKD is classified based on cause, GFR category, and albuminuria category.
- GFR categories
  - G1: GFR ≥90
  - G2: GFR 60–89
  - G3a: GFR 45–59
  - G3b: GFR 30–44
  - G4: GFR 15–29
  - G5: GFR <15
- Albuminuria categories—albumin to creatinine ratio in mg/g
  - A1 <30
  - A2 30–300
  - A3 >300

EPIDEMIOLOGY

Incidence

~5–12 cases per year per million of age-related population

Prevalence

Prevalence of CKD has been reported to be between 21 and 74 cases per million of age-related population from various studies in Europe and Latin America.

RISK FACTORS

- Risk factors for congenital renal disease include genetic and environmental factors (maternal diabetes, exposure to medications such as ACE inhibitor/NSAIDs)
- Low birth weight, prematurity, and rapid weight gain in early childhood increase risk of CKD.
- Hypertension and proteinuria increase risk of CKD progression.

PATHOPHYSIOLOGY

- Low nephron mass: leads to hyperfiltration injury
- Cardiovascular: Hypertension secondary to activation of renin-angiotensin system, fluid overload, and anemia from erythropoietin deficiency contribute to cardiovascular morbidity.
- Bone and mineral bone disorder of CKD: Decreased synthesis of vitamin D1,25 OHD leads to hyperparathyroidism and bone disease.
- Growth: Metabolic acidosis, anemia, and perturbations in the growth hormone insulin-like growth factor-1 (GH-IGF-1) axis lead to poor growth.

ETIOLOGY

- Congenital anomalies of kidney and urinary tract (CAKUT) constitute ~60% of cases of childhood CKD and include the following:
  - Renal dysplasia/hypoplasia
  - Obstructive uropathy (posterior urethral valves, prune belly syndrome)
- Cystic and hereditary disorders
  - Autosomal recessive and dominant polycystic kidney disease
  - Juvenile nephronophthisis (cystic)
  - Alport syndrome, cystinosis, oxalosis, congenital nephrotic syndrome (hereditary)
- Glomerular diseases
  - Focal segmental glomerulosclerosis (FSGS)
  - Hemolytic uremic syndrome (HUS)
  - Systemic lupus erythematosus (SLE)
  - IgA nephropathy
  - Others—membranoproliferative glomerulonephritis (MPGN), membranous nephropathy, pauci-immune glomerulonephritis

COMMONLY ASSOCIATED CONDITIONS

Several syndromes have associated anomalies of the kidney and urinary tract such as DiGeorge syndrome, Alport syndrome, Alagille syndrome, branchio-oto-renal syndrome, Townes-Brocks syndrome, and Bardet-Biedl syndrome.

DIAGNOSIS

HISTORY

- Past history
  - Birth history for oligohydramnios, perinatal events
  - Recurrent urinary tract infections (UTIs)
  - Enuresis
- Family history
  - Renal disease
  - Hearing impairment

SIGNS AND SYMPTOMS

- Poor growth
- Poor appetite
- Fatigue, malaise
- Headache (if hypertensive)
- Polyuria (in congenital abnormalities)
- Oliguria

PHYSICAL EXAM

- General
  - Short stature
  - Decreased weight for age
  - Pallor
  - Fetid breath
  - Elevated blood pressure (BP)
- Head, ears, eyes, nose, and throat
  - Retinal changes
  - Presence of preauricular tags, branchial cysts
  - Hearing deficit
- Chest
  - Rales
- Heart
  - Flow murmur
  - Gallop
  - Pericardial rub
- Abdomen
  - Palpable kidneys
  - Suprapubic mass
- Extremities
  - Rachitic changes
  - Edema
- Neurologic system
  - Developmental delay
  - Altered mental status
  - Hypotonia
  - Irritability

DIAGNOSTIC TESTS & INTERPRETATION

Lab

- Serum chemistries: azotemia, hyperkalemia, acidemia, hypocalcemia, hyperphosphatemia, elevated alkaline phosphatase
- CBCs: normocytic anemia with low reticulocyte count (CKD stage 3, GFR <60)
- Urinalysis: isosthenuria, proteinuria, hematuria
- Intact parathyroid hormone: elevated
- 25-vitamin D: often low
- GFR measurement
  - Inulin clearance is the gold standard for GFR measurement but is not practical. A simple and commonly used method to estimate GFR in children >1 year of age with CKD is the CKiD bedside equation, an update to the traditional Schwartz formula.
  - The calculation is already corrected for surface area and does not require a urine collection: height (cm) × 0.413 correction factor/Pcreat in mg/dL.

Imaging
- Chest x-ray: pulmonary edema, cardiomegaly
- Bone films: delayed bone age, rickets, osteomalacia, osteitis fibrosa
- Renal ultrasound: small echogenic kidneys, cystic kidneys, hydronephrosis

Diagnostic Procedures/Other
A renal biopsy is indicated for diagnosis of acquired or glomerular kidney diseases such as FSGS. It is not necessary when there is radiologic evidence of structural/congenital cause of CKD such as small or echogenic kidneys.

DIFFERENTIAL DIAGNOSIS
- Differentiate acute kidney injury from CKD
- Usually, CKD is insidious and associated with poor growth, delayed puberty, rickets, polyuria, and anemia. The kidneys may be small on renal ultrasound.

TREATMENT

MEDICATION
- Phosphate binders (e.g., calcium carbonate, calcium acetate, sevelamer; avoid aluminum)
- 1,25-dihydroxy vitamin D and/or 25-hydroxy vitamin D
- Alkali therapy (e.g., sodium bicarbonate/citrate)
- Antihypertensive therapy
- ACE inhibitors (renoprotection)
- Recombinant erythropoietin
- Ferrous sulfate (if iron deficient)
- Recombinant human growth hormone

ADDITIONAL TREATMENT
Renal replacement therapy (dialysis/renal transplantation) is indicated when GFR is <10 mL/min/1.73 m^2 or when medical management fails to control signs/symptoms of CKD.

ISSUES FOR REFERRAL
Pediatric primary care physicians should observe patients with CKD in consultation and with assistance from a pediatric nephrologist.

COMPLEMENTARY & ALTERNATIVE THERAPIES
Treatment of hypertension, proteinuria (with ACE inhibitor/angiotensin receptor blocker [ARB]), and dyslipidemia delays progression of CKD.

ALERT

During episodes of gastroenteritis, infants with CKD may be prone to dehydration because they have obligatory polyuria due to a concentrating defect. Do not use urine output level or specific gravity of urine as indices for hydration. If hospitalized, fluid levels considered "maintenance" may be insufficient due to polyuria.

SURGERY/OTHER PROCEDURES
- Transplantation: In some cases, a preemptive transplant may be offered instead of dialysis.
- Consider arteriovenous fistula or graft placement for patients who will require long-term hemodialysis.

ONGOING CARE

FOLLOW-UP RECOMMENDATIONS

Patient Monitoring
Children with CKD need close outpatient follow-up every 1–3 months, depending on the level of GFR to monitor BP, growth, and lab tests.

DIET
Restrictions mandated by condition
- Phosphate
- Potassium
- Sodium (indicated if patient has edema/hypertension)
- Fluid (indicated in conditions related to oliguria)

PROGNOSIS
Prognosis of CKD depends on the cause of CKD. CKD progression leads to need for renal replacement therapy. Prognosis of children with renal transplantation is excellent with 5-year survival of $>85\%$.

COMPLICATIONS
- Growth retardation is particularly severe when CKD develops in the 1st year of life. Growth failure may be secondary to poor nutrition, bone disease, acidosis, or a direct effect on the GH-IGF-1 axis.
- Mineral and bone disorders may be seen early in association with CKD, manifesting with growth failure, bowing of the lower extremities, and slipped epiphysis. Vitamin D deficiency and secondary hyperparathyroidism are the major factors leading to bone disease.
- Anemia develops secondary to decreased erythropoietin secretion and decreased erythrocyte survival. The anemia is a normocytic variant associated with a low reticulocyte count.
- Cardiovascular disease including left ventricular hypertrophy (LVH) and coronary artery disease often develops in early adulthood. Uncontrolled hypertension, anemia, hyperlipidemia, and hyperparathyroidism all contribute to this leading cause of death in adults with CKD.
- Neurodevelopmental delay increases in children with CKD. This is probably due to uremic effects on the development of the brain.
- Hypertension may be seen in some patients with CKD due either to hyperreninemia or hypervolemia.
- Platelet abnormalities, protein-calorie malnutrition, and immunologic disturbances are also seen in patients with uremia.

ADDITIONAL READING

- Friedman AL. Etiology, pathophysiology, diagnosis, and management of chronic renal failure in children. *Curr Opin Pediatr*. 1996;8(2):148–151.
- Kidney Disease: Improving Global Outcomes (KDIGO) CKD Work Group. KDIGO 2012 Clinical practice guideline for the evaluation and management of chronic kidney disease. *Kidney Inter Suppl*. 2013;3:1–150.
- Schwartz GJ, Muñoz A, Schneider MF, et al. New equations to estimate GFR in children with CKD. *J Am Soc Nephrol*. 2009;20(3):629–637.
- Staples A, Wong C. Risk factors for progression of chronic kidney disease. *Curr Opin Pediatr*. 2010; 22(2):161–169.

CODES

ICD10
- N18.9 Chronic kidney disease, unspecified
- Q63.9 Congenital malformation of kidney, unspecified
- N18.3 Chronic kidney disease, stage 3 (moderate)

FAQ
- Q: Which OTC medications should be avoided in children with CKD?
- A: NSAIDs, pseudoephedrine (if patient hypertensive), enemas containing phosphate, and antacids containing magnesium or aluminum should not be taken.
- Q: Can children with CKD receive immunizations?
- A: Children with CKD should especially receive all necessary immunizations because some vaccines are contraindicated after transplantation. In some cases, booster immunizations are necessary because of an inadequate response to the initial series (e.g., hepatitis B virus, measles, mumps, rubella; varicella). Additionally, children with CKD should receive the polyvalent pneumococcal vaccine after age 2 years.
- Q: When is recombinant human erythropoietin indicated?
- A: Generally, this medication should be considered when the hematocrit level is $<33\%$ (Hgb <11.0 g/dL).

CIRRHOSIS

Rima Fawaz

BASICS

DESCRIPTION

- Cirrhosis is the end stage of progressive hepatic necrosis, fibrosis, and regenerative nodule formation that may occur as a result of many different liver diseases.
- Results in distortion of liver architecture and compression of hepatic vascular and biliary structures
- In its advanced form, cirrhosis is irreversible and often requires liver transplantation for survival of the patient.

EPIDEMIOLOGY

- There are varying causes of cirrhosis; accordingly, no specific epidemiologic pattern can be identified.
- Cirrhosis due to chronic HCV infection, alcoholic liver disease, and nonalcoholic fatty liver disease (NAFLD) are the most common indications for liver transplantation in adults.
- Biliary cirrhosis due to biliary atresia is the most common indication for liver transplantation in children.

Genetics

- Many distinct genetic disorders can cause cirrhosis, such as Wilson disease and hereditary hemochromatosis.
- Human leukocyte antigen (HLA) associations have been identified in several autoimmune disorders, including sclerosing cholangitis and autoimmune hepatitis.

DIAGNOSIS

HISTORY

- Compensated (latent) cirrhosis: asymptomatic, with no signs or symptoms of liver disease. Discovered incidentally either during routine physical examinations with an enlarged liver and/or palpable spleen or as a result of an investigation for an unrelated condition
- Decompensated (active) cirrhosis: As cirrhosis progresses, overt signs and symptoms may occur including failure to thrive, muscle weakness, fatigue, jaundice, pruritus, edema, abdominal pain, ascites, steatorrhea, spontaneous bleeding (i.e., epistaxis) or bruising, and deterioration in school performance or depression.
  - In adults, decompensated cirrhosis is defined by the development of major complications: variceal hemorrhage, ascites, spontaneous bacterial peritonitis, hepatic encephalopathy, hepatorenal syndrome, hepatopulmonary syndrome, and portopulmonary hypertension.
- Based on the varying etiologies, one should elicit pertinent historical features characteristic of specific problems:
  - Exposure to infectious hepatitis, antecedent viral illnesses
  - Exposure to hepatotoxins
  - Family or personal history of genetic, metabolic, or autoimmune diseases
  - Neurologic problems, deteriorating school performance, depression (Wilson disease)

PHYSICAL EXAM

- General: poor growth, malnutrition, fever, cachexia, obesity (NAFLD)
- Skin: jaundice, flushing, pallor, cyanosis, palmar erythema, spider angiomata, fine telangiectasia (face and upper back), easy bruising
- Abdomen: ascites (distention, fluid wave, shifting dullness), caput medusa (prominent periumbilical veins), splenomegaly, rectal varices, hepatomegaly, or a shrunken liver
- Extremities: digital clubbing, hypertrophic osteoarthropathy, muscle wasting, peripheral edema
- Endocrine: gynecomastia, testicular atrophy, delayed puberty
- Central nervous system: asterixis, positive Babinski sign, mental status changes, hyperreflexia, muscle wasting
- Eyes: Kayser-Fleischer rings (Wilson disease)

DIAGNOSTIC TESTS & INTERPRETATION

Lab

Can be useful in determining the etiology and the severity of liver disease prior to a liver biopsy

- Tests of liver cell injury: alanine aminotransferase (ALT), aspartate aminotransferase (AST), lactic dehydrogenase (LDH)
- Tests of synthetic function: albumin and other serum proteins, prothrombin time (PT), international normalized ratio (INR), partial thromboplastin time (prolonged in severe liver disease), ammonia, plasma and urine amino acids, serum lipids and lipoproteins, cholesterol and triglycerides
- Tests of cholestasis: fractionated bilirubin, alkaline phosphatase, γ-glutamyltransferase, cholesterol, serum and urine bile acids
- Tests of fibrosis: Serum markers may be useful to evaluate hepatic fibrosis noninvasively; however, these are still being investigated for clinical use.
- Miscellaneous disease-specific serum tests:
  - Viral serologies: hepatitis B, hepatitis C, other viruses
  - Wilson disease: serum ceruloplasmin, 24-hour urine copper, and slit-lamp exam for Kaiser–Fleischer rings
  - α_1-Antitrypsin deficiency: α_1-Antitrypsin serum level and protease inhibitor (Pi) phenotype
  - Autoimmune hepatitis: autoantibodies (antinuclear, anti–smooth muscle, anti-liver/kidney microsomal, anti–F-actin), serum immunoglobulins
  - Hemochromatosis: serum iron, total iron binding capacity, ferritin
  - Metabolic/genetic: fasting blood sugar, lactate, pyruvate, uric acid, sweat test, carnitine, creatine phosphokinase (CPK), porphyrins, serum amino acids, urine organic acids, urine reducing substances, urine succinylacetone, fatty acid degeneration products, α-fetoprotein

Imaging

- Ultrasound with Doppler images: Evaluate for anatomy of the liver and biliary tree and vessels, presence of ascites, signs of portal hypertension such as splenomegaly, varices, reversal of flow in portal vein.
- Hepatobiliary radioisotope scanning: Assess biliary patency in neonatal cholestasis.
- Cholangiography (magnetic resonance cholangiopancreatography [MRCP]: Assess for intra- and extrahepatic biliary disease (stones, choledochal cyst, sclerosing cholangitis).
- Angiography: CT or magnetic resonance angiography to evaluate for vascular anatomy and portosystemic shunts
- Noninvasive assessment of liver fibrosis: CT, MRI, elastography by ultrasound or MRI

Diagnostic Procedures/Other

- Liver biopsy
  - Percutaneous needle biopsy, intraoperative wedge biopsy, transjugular liver biopsy
  - Confirm the presence (stage), activity (grade), and type of cirrhosis.
  - Various hepatic diseases that progress to cirrhosis have characteristic histologic findings. However, the process of cirrhosis may obscure the nature of the original insult, rendering morphologic and histologic classifications unhelpful.
- Hepatic venous pressure gradient (HPVG): rarely used in children but is the most accurate prognostic indicator of outcome in adults with cirrhosis.
- Cholangiography
  - Intraoperative cholangiography: Assess for extrahepatic biliary atresia in neonates.
  - Endoscopic retrograde cholangiopancreatography (ERCP): Assess for extrahepatic biliary disease in older patients where MRCP is not helpful or therapeutic interventions possible (i.e., stent placement).

DIFFERENTIAL DIAGNOSIS

- Biliary
  - Extrahepatic biliary atresia
  - Choledochal cyst
  - Tumors
  - Common bile duct and biliary lithiasis
  - Alagille syndrome
  - Biliary hypoplasia
  - Sclerosing cholangitis
  - Graft-versus-host disease
  - Vanishing bile duct syndrome due to drugs (e.g., trimethoprim–sulfamethoxazole)
  - Langerhans cell histiocytosis
- Hepatic
  - Infectious hepatitis, including viral hepatitis B, C, D, other viruses
  - Autoimmune hepatitis
  - Nonalcoholic steatohepatitis (NASH)
  - Drugs/toxins and alcohol

- Genetic/metabolic (examples for each category, not a complete list)
  - Cystic fibrosis
  - α_1-Antitrypsin deficiency
  - Congenital hepatic fibrosis
  - Progressive familial intrahepatic cholestasis (PFIC)
  - Wilson disease
  - Hereditary hemochromatosis
  - Carbohydrate defects: galactosemia, hereditary fructose intolerance, glycogen storage III and IV
  - Amino acid defects: tyrosinemia
  - Lipid storage diseases: Gaucher disease, Niemann-Pick type C
  - Mitochondrial disorders: fatty acid oxidation defects, respiratory chain defects
  - Peroxisomal disorders: Zellweger syndrome
  - Porphyrias: erythropoietic protoporphyria
- Vascular
  - Budd-Chiari syndrome
  - Veno-occlusive disease
  - Congestive heart failure

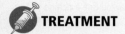

TREATMENT

MEDICATION

First Line

- Fat-soluble vitamin supplementation: vitamins A, D, E, and K
- Diuretic therapy (furosemide, spironolactone) for patients with ascites
- Albumin infusions for patients with refractory ascites
- β-blockers have been shown to decrease portal pressure and reduce the risk of variceal bleeding in adults with portal hypertension.
- Antibiotics, if suspicious for spontaneous bacterial peritonitis (avoid nephrotoxic agents)
- Lactulose and rifaximin (adults) are used for patients with hepatic encephalopathy.

SURGERY/OTHER PROCEDURES

- Endoscopic variceal band ligation or sclerotherapy for variceal GI bleeding
- Paracentesis for refractory ascites or diagnosis of spontaneous bacterial peritonitis
- Portosystemic shunt placement (surgical or radiologic transjugular intrahepatic portosystemic shunting [TIPS] procedure) for complications of uncontrolled portal hypertension
- Liver transplantation

ONGOING CARE

DIET

- Malnutrition is common in chronic liver diseases because of several metabolic derangements, fat malabsorption, anorexia, and increased energy requirements.
- Adequate caloric intake is critical and, often, will require supplemental nasogastric tube feedings.
- Some of the dietary fat should be provided as medium-chain triglycerides, which do not require bile for absorption.
- Fat-soluble vitamin levels should be monitored and supplemented, if necessary.
- Careful attention must also be paid to fluid and electrolyte balance; sodium restriction ($<$2 mEq/kg/day) may be necessary in the presence of ascites.

General Measures

Spleen guard and avoidance of abdominal trauma if significant splenomegaly

PROGNOSIS

- The prognosis for cirrhosis leading to decompensation depends on the underlying cause.
- The underlying condition should be treated when possible (e.g., Wilson disease, autoimmune hepatitis).
- Poor prognostic features in children include prolonged INR unresponsive to vitamin K, ascites, malnutrition, low plasma cholesterol, elevated bilirubin level, and presence of hepatorenal syndrome.

COMPLICATIONS

- Malnutrition and growth failure
- Malabsorption (diarrhea, steatorrhea, fat-soluble vitamin deficiencies)
- Portal hypertension and variceal bleeding
- Chronic gastritis, peptic ulcer disease, gastroesophageal reflux
- Ascites
- Encephalopathy
- Hypersplenism (associated with anemia, thrombocytopenia, and neutropenia)
- Anemia
- Coagulopathy
- Hepatopulmonary syndrome (hypoxemia, cyanosis, dyspnea, digital clubbing)
- Hepatorenal syndrome (rapidly progressive renal failure in patients with cirrhosis)
- Bacterial infections, spontaneous bacterial peritonitis
- Hepatocellular carcinoma

ADDITIONAL READING

- Albilllos A, Garcia-Tsao G. Classification of cirrhosis: the clinical use of HVPG measurements. *Dis Markers*. 2011;31(3):121–128.
- Feldstein AE, Charatcharoenwitthaya P, Treeprasertsuk S, et al. The natural history of non-alcoholic fatty liver disease in children: a follow-up study for up to 20 years. *Gut*. 2009;58(11):1538–1544.
- Kamath BM, Olthoff KM. Liver transplantation in children: update 2010. *Pediatr Clin North Am*. 2010;57(2):401–414.
- Leonis MA, Balistreri WF. Evaluation and management of end-stage liver disease in children. *Gastroenterology*. 2008;134(6):1741–1751.
- Lewindon PJ, Shepherd RW, Walsh MJ, et al. Importance of hepatic fibrosis in cystic fibrosis and the predictive value of liver biopsy. *Hepatology*. 2011;53(1):193–201.
- Mencin AA, Lavine JE. Nonalcoholic fatty liver disease in children. *Curr Opin Clin Nutr Metab Care*. 2011;14(2):151–157.
- Poupon R, Chazouilleres O, Poupon RE. Chronic cholestatic diseases. *J Hepatol*. 2000;32(1)(Suppl):129–140.

CODES

ICD10

- K74.60 Unspecified cirrhosis of liver
- K74.5 Biliary cirrhosis, unspecified
- Q44.2 Atresia of bile ducts

FAQ

- Q: Will my child with cystic fibrosis develop cirrhosis?
- A: The medical literature suggests a 5–10% incidence of cirrhosis in children with cystic fibrosis. Children with cystic fibrosis liver disease who develop cirrhosis are at risk for complications of portal hypertension.
- Q: Will every child with cirrhosis need a liver transplant?
- A: If cause of cirrhosis cannot be treated, most children who develop cirrhosis will ultimately require a liver transplant.

CLEFT LIP AND PALATE

Oksana A. Jackson • Jesse A. Taylor

BASICS

DESCRIPTION

- Cleft lip
  - Deformity of the upper lip that may include a discontinuity of vermilion, skin, muscle, and mucosa as well as the underlying gingiva and bone
  - May be unilateral or bilateral
  - A complete cleft extends into the nose. An incomplete cleft has a bridge of intact tissue between the oral and nasal cavities.
- Cleft palate
  - May involve the gingiva, hard palate, and/or soft palate
  - Represents a visible separation between the 2 halves of the roof of the mouth, involving mucosa, muscle, and often the bones of the hard palate
  - A submucous cleft palate has intact mucosa, but the underlying muscle and bone are at least partially divided.

EPIDEMIOLOGY

Incidence

- Incidence of cleft lip with or without cleft palate is approximately 1 in 700 births.
- Incidence of cleft lip with or without cleft palate increases with parental (especially paternal) age >30 years. Some association with low socioeconomic class may be nutrition related.

Prevalence

- Racial heterogeneity noted in cleft lip and palate (Asians, 2.1 in 1,000 births; whites, 1 in 1,000; blacks, 0.41 in 1,000)
- Isolated cleft palate is present in 1 in 2,000 births across races.
- Gender heterogeneity noted in Caucasians (male-to-female ratio: cleft lip with or without cleft palate, 1.5–2:1; cleft palate only, 0.7:1)

Genetics

- 1/3 of patients with cleft lip and/or cleft palate have a positive family history; positive family history is noted twice as often in cleft lip with or without cleft palate compared to cleft palate alone.
- The recurrence risk for cleft lip with or without cleft palate is 4% if one 1st-degree relative is affected and 9% if two are affected.
- Some recognized patterns of malformation that include cleft lip and/or cleft palate may be caused by exposure to teratogens, but there is little evidence linking isolated clefts to exposure to any single teratogenic agent.
  - Exceptions include phenytoin (use during pregnancy has been associated with a 10-fold increase in the incidence of cleft lip) and isotretinoin (~26 relative risk of congenital malformations including cleft palate).
- Incidence of cleft lip in infants born to mothers who smoke during pregnancy is twice that in those born to nonsmoking mothers.

PATHOPHYSIOLOGY

- Muscle fibers are atrophic and disorganized in the region of the cleft.
- Mitochondrial abnormalities are noted at the cleft margins by histochemical and electromyographic studies.

ETIOLOGY

- Cleft lip may result from failure of the medial nasal and maxillary processes to join in utero or possibly from lack of adequate mesenchymal reinforcement, leading to subsequent breakdown and separation.
- Cleft palate results from failure of the palatal shelves to fuse.
- Prenatal dietary supplementation with folic acid and vitamin B_6 has led to lower-than-expected incidence of cleft lip and cleft palate and to a decreased incidence of neural tube defects.
- Bilateral cleft lip is associated with cleft palate in 86% of cases. Unilateral cleft lip is associated with cleft palate in 68% of cases.
- Cleft lip/cleft palate is more common on the left, particularly in boys.

COMMONLY ASSOCIATED CONDITIONS

- Most clefts are nonsyndromic and may be either multifactorial in origin or the result of changes at a major single-gene locus
- Over 400 genetic syndromes are associated with facial clefts.
- Among patients with clefts of the secondary palate alone, syndromes associated with microdeletions of chromosome 22q11.2 are currently the most common syndromic diagnoses.
  - Collectively known as 22q11.2 deletion syndrome, includes velocardiofacial syndrome, DiGeorge syndrome, and conotruncal anomaly face syndrome
  - Inheritance is autosomal dominant with considerable variability in phenotypic expression, which may include facial dysmorphism, developmental delay, cardiovascular anomalies, immunologic abnormalities, cleft palate, and velopharyngeal dysfunction.
- Next most common syndrome associated with palatal clefts is Stickler syndrome:
  - Characterized by autosomal dominance, cleft palate, epicanthal folds, flat facies, joint hyperflexibility, severe myopia, retinal detachment, and glaucoma
  - Caused by a mutation of the gene for type 2 collagen (chromosome 12q)
- Most common syndrome associated with clefts of the lip and/or palate is Van der Woude syndrome (autosomal dominant, lower lip pits, IRF6 mutations, 1q32)
- Other genetic syndromes associated with cleft lip and/or palate:
  - CHARGE (Coloboma of the eye, Heart defects, Atresia of the choanae, Retardation of growth and/or development, Genital and/or urinary abnormalities, and Ear abnormalities and deafness) syndrome has an autosomal dominant pattern of malformation with majority of patients having *CHD7* microdeletion or mutation.
  - EEC (ectrodactyly–ectodermal dysplasia, cleft) syndrome is associated with p63 gene mutations.
  - Smith-Lemli-Opitz (defect in cholesterol synthesis, DHCR7 gene mutation, 7q34)
  - Pierre Robin sequence is a condition usually associated with a wide U-shaped cleft palate.
    - Characterized by a small mandible, retropositioned tongue, and subsequent upper airway obstruction
    - May occur in infants with or without genetic syndromes (Stickler most common)

DIAGNOSIS

HISTORY

- Prenatal exposure to alcohol, cigarettes, phenytoin, and isotretinoin
- Family history of cleft lip or cleft palate
- Speech problems in 1st-degree relative

PHYSICAL EXAM

- Incomplete or complete cleft of lip, alveolus, hard and soft palate, or uvula. Soft palate and uvula clefts are always midline, whereas lip, alveolar, and hard palatal clefts can be unilateral or bilateral.
- A bifid uvula or a notch in the bone at the posterior hard palate may indicate a submucous cleft.
- A small mandible and retropositioned tongue may indicate a risk for airway obstruction (Pierre Robin sequence).
- Look for associated anomalies of the face, heart, and extremities that may indicate a clefting syndrome.
- Tricks
  - Examine the palate from the top of the patient, with the head in your lap, using a tongue depressor and flashlight.
  - Palpate the posterior hard palate for a possible notch in the bone.
  - Palpate the gums and maxilla for a possible notch in the floor of the nose.

DIAGNOSTIC TESTS & INTERPRETATION

- Hearing evaluation
- Complete ophthalmologic examination to check for myopia, glaucoma, and retinal detachment and rule out Stickler syndrome
- Pulse oximetry to check for desaturation while feeding or while supine
- Polysomnography to distinguish central from obstructive apnea. Increased serum 7-dehydrocholesterol and decreased serum cholesterol to rule out Smith-Lemli-Opitz syndrome
- Karyotype to rule out specific genetic abnormalities
- Fluorescence in situ hybridization to rule out a chromosome 22q11.2 deletion
- Echocardiography, renal ultrasound, and endocrine laboratory studies if indicated

Imaging

- Prenatal diagnosis of cleft lip is reliable by ultrasound; prenatal diagnosis of cleft palate remains unreliable by ultrasound. 3-D ultrasound has improved the reliability of prenatal diagnosis.
- Fetal MRI provides excellent soft tissue definition and can be used when the diagnosis is uncertain on ultrasound or to better delineate the severity of the cleft.
- After birth, no additional radiologic imaging is indicated in patients with isolated cleft lip and/or palate.

C

TREATMENT

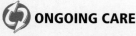

GENERAL MEASURES

Airway management

- Prone positioning if the tongue is causing airway obstruction
- Plastic surgery and ENT consultation if airway obstruction persists

ORTHODONTICS

Preoperative orthodontics may include obturators to facilitate feeding and speech, nasoalveolar molding and lip taping to narrow the cleft and reshape the nose before lip repair, palatal expansion prior to bone grafting, conventional orthodontics including braces, maxillary appliances, prosthetic teeth, bridgework, and maxillary and/or mandibular distraction to advance the mid- or lower face.

SURGERY/OTHER PROCEDURES

- Significant airway obstruction and desaturation in the neonatal period refractory to prone positioning may indicate the need for a tongue–lip adhesion, release of the floor of the mouth musculature, mandibular distraction, or tracheostomy.
- Wide clefts of the lip may benefit from either nasoalveolar molding or preliminary lip adhesion at 2–3 months of age. Timing of definitive lip repair varies from 2 to 6 months of age.
- Palate repair is generally done at <1 year of age to decrease speech and language difficulties.
- Otitis media is more common with cleft palate, and bilateral myringotomy tubes can be inserted at the time of cleft repair.
- Correction of secondary deformities may include the following:
  - Lip scar revision
  - Cleft nasal deformity correction (infancy to adulthood)
  - Alveolar bone grafts (usually when permanent canines are erupting, age 6–10 years)
  - Pharyngoplasty for soft palate–velopharyngeal incompetence (childhood–adolescence)
  - Closure of palatal fistulas
  - Orthognathic surgery for severe jaw deformities (after facial growth is complete)

Admission Criteria

Airway obstruction or severe feeding difficulties in the neonate

Discharge Criteria

- Stable airway
- Tolerating feedings

ONGOING CARE

FOLLOW-UP RECOMMENDATIONS

Multidisciplinary team for routine visits from infancy to adolescence:

- Pediatrician
- Plastic surgeon
- Speech pathologist
- Orthodontist
- Pediatric dentist
- Otolaryngologist
- Oral surgeon
- Psychologist
- Social worker
- Anthropologist (facial growth specialist)
- Geneticist
- Support groups

DIET

- Cleft patients may have significant feeding problems because of an inability to generate negative intraoral pressure necessary to feed efficiently.
- Preemie nipples with enlarged or cross-cut openings, or soft plastic squeezable bottles, can facilitate milk flow.
- Specially designed cleft bottles are commercially available.
- Poor weight gain may necessitate nasogastric tube feedings.

PROGNOSIS

Very good. Most patients undergo normal growth and development. Long-term follow-up by a multidisciplinary team and parental support are critical for optimal outcomes.

COMPLICATIONS

- Airway obstruction and feeding disorders, particularly with Pierre Robin sequence
- Chronic otitis media
- Speech problems, including hypernasality and articulation errors
- Associated malformations
  - ~1/3 of patients with cleft palate has associated anomalies, with isolated cleft palates having the highest. CNS, cardiac, and urinary tract malformations and clubfoot are commonly associated with clefting.
- Potential problems
  - Hypernasal resonance and nasal air emission during speech may indicate velopharyngeal incompetence or palatal fistula. 8–30% of patients may require additional palatal or pharyngeal surgery following initial palate repair.
  - Multiple ear infections may require prolonged use of myringotomy tubes to prevent hearing impairment. Audiograms should be obtained regularly.
  - Delays in speech and language development may require detailed evaluation, early intervention programs, and speech therapy.
  - Poor dentition, occlusal problems (crossbite), gingivitis, and crowding
  - Learning disabilities are increased in children with clefts.
  - Behavior disorders and psychosocial adjustment disorders
  - ~25% of affected individuals will manifest maxillary hypoplasia that requires jaw surgery to correct occlusal abnormalities.

ALERT

- Failure to diagnose airway obstruction in infants with Pierre Robin sequence may lead to failure to thrive or, in severe cases, death.
- Failure to diagnose associated anomalies may lead to missed syndromes and inaccurate genetic counseling.
- A submucous cleft palate can be easily missed until hypernasal speech is noted later in life.

ADDITIONAL READING

- Fisher, DM, Sommerlad BC. Cleft lip, cleft palate, and velopharyngeal insufficiency. *Plast Reconstr Surg*. 2011;128(4):342e–360e.
- Heinrich A, Proff P, Michel T, et al. Prenatal diagnosis of cleft deformities and its significance for parent and infant care. *J Craniomaxillofac Surg*. 2006; 34(Suppl 2):14–16.
- Mulliken JB, Wu JK, Padwa BL. Repair of bilateral cleft lip: review, revisions, and reflections. *J Craniofac Surg*. 2003;14(5):609–620.
- Murray JC. Gene/environment causes of cleft lip and/or palate. *Clin Genet*. 2002;61(4):248–256.
- Nasser M, Fedorowicz Z, Newton JT, et al. Interventions for the management of submucous cleft palate. *Cochrane Database Syst Rev*. 2008:(1):CD006703.
- Redford-Badwal DA, Mabry K, Frassinelli JD. Impact of cleft lip and/or palate on nutritional health and oral-motor development. *Dent Clin North Am*. 2003;47(2):305–317.
- Strong EB, Buckmiller LM. Management of the cleft palate. *Facial Plast Surg Clin North Am*. 2001;9(1): 15–25, vii.

CODES

ICD10

- Q37.9 Unspecified cleft palate with unilateral cleft lip
- Q36.9 Cleft lip, unilateral
- Q35.9 Cleft palate, unspecified

FAQ

- Q: Will there be a scar?
- A: All cleft lip repairs will leave some type of permanent scar, with potential asymmetry that may benefit from later additional lip scar revision or additional nasal surgery.
- Q: What is the goal of surgery?
- A: Goal is to create a lip that does not attract undue attention.
- Q: What is the most difficult part of surgery?
- A: The nose is often the most difficult to correct because of asymmetry in cartilage and skin contour.
- Q: Will my child be able to speak clearly?
- A: Most children will achieve velopharyngeal competence and normal speech but may require additional speech therapy to achieve this goal.
- Q: Is cleft palate inherited?
- A: For nonsyndromic cleft lip with or without cleft palate:
  - Risk of having a second child with a cleft, if neither parent has a cleft: 4%
    - Child's risk of later having a child with a cleft: 4%
    - Risk of having a third child with a cleft, if parents have 2 affected children but neither parent is affected: 9%
    - Risk of having a second child with a cleft, if 1 parent also has a cleft: 17%
  - For nonsyndromic isolated cleft palate:
    - Risk of having a second child with a cleft, if neither parent has a cleft: 2%
    - Child's risk of later having a child with a cleft: 3%
    - Risk of having a third child with a cleft, if parents have 2 affected children but neither parent is affected: 1%
    - Risk of having a second child with a cleft, if 1 parent also has a cleft: 15%

CLUBFOOT

Richard S. Davidson

BASICS

DESCRIPTION

Clubfoot is a congenital or neuromuscular deformity in which the hindfoot is fixed in equinus (plantar flexion) and varus (toward the midline) and the forefoot is fixed in varus, equinus, and often cavus (high midfoot arch with overextension).

EPIDEMIOLOGY

- Risk of deformity increases by 20–30 times when there is an affected 1st-degree relative.
- Male > female (2:1)

Incidence

Incidence is 1–1.4/1,000 live births but can vary among different ethnic groups.

PATHOPHYSIOLOGY

- Many anatomic abnormalities have been postulated as causing clubfoot:
  - Anomalous or deficient muscles, myoblasts, mast cells, abnormal primary bone formation, joint and muscle contractures, vascular anomalies (absent dorsalis pedis artery), and nerve anomalies
  - Abnormalities of the fibrous connective tissue
- Interruption of embryonic foot development has also been suggested.

ETIOLOGY

- Most cases are idiopathic (multifactorial inheritance pattern with significant environmental influence).
- Infrequently, neuromuscular imbalance may underlie the deformity (cerebral palsy, myelomeningocele, lipomas of the cord, caudal or sacral agenesis, polio, arthrogryposis, fetal alcohol syndrome).
- Rapid recurrence should prompt a thorough examination for possible underlying etiologies.

DIAGNOSIS

HISTORY

- Family history of clubfoot (3%)
- Onset of deformity (congenital or developmental)

PHYSICAL EXAM

- Careful examination of
  - The neuromuscular system for neuromuscular etiologies such as lumbosacral sinuses, dimples, and lipomas as well as spasticity, asymmetry, and muscle imbalance
  - The hips for hip dysplasia
  - The neck for torticollis
- Physical exam trick
  - Push the foot into a corrected position. Is the deformity fully correctable? Overcorrectable?
  - About 1 in 15 idiopathic clubfeet have rigid equinus, midfoot (metatarsal) plantarflexion, a deep heel crease at the posterior ankle, a transverse midsole or midfoot crease, and a short hyperextended hallux. This appearance for these feet may not be apparent until after 1–3 casts. They have been called "complex idiopathic clubfoot" and are more difficult to treat.

DIAGNOSTIC TESTS & INTERPRETATION

Lab

- The diagnosis is established clinically.
- Radiographs (after 3 months of age) may confirm bone position but cannot make the diagnosis.
- At 3–6 months of age, anteroposterior and lateral radiograph films in dorsiflexion (maximal correction) may help in defining residual deformity. The beam should be focused on the hindfoot for both the anteroposterior and lateral radiographs as the measured angles will be hindfoot angles.
- Decreased talocalcaneal angle on the anteroposterior and lateral views ($\leq$25 degrees) confirm persistent deformity.
- Medial displacement of the cuboid on the calcaneus and persistent plantar flexion of the forefoot on the hindfoot (talar to 1st metatarsal angle) indicate more complex deformities.

DIFFERENTIAL DIAGNOSIS

Distinguish other deformities of the foot:

- Metatarsus adductus or varus (heel is in neutral position, no fixed equinus)
- Calcaneovalgus (foot is in valgus, no fixed heel equinus)
- Vertical talus (foot is in valgus, heel in equinovalgus)
- Many children with clubfoot also have tibial torsion, which is a normal variant that rarely requires treatment.

TREATMENT

ADDITIONAL TREATMENT

General Measures

- Ponseti method (casting and bracing) and its variations have become the standard of initial treatment.
- Initial treatment:
  - Care can begin in the 1st week after birth, although later treatment is generally successful as well.
- Initial treatment is serial (weekly) manipulation and casting with long leg casts first correcting abduction, then rotation, then dorsiflexion. The talar head is stabilized with the casting physician's thumb while the contralateral hand manipulates the foot.
- Taping may be useful for treatment of the infant requiring ICU care; access to the feet should be maintained for blood tests.
- Surgical intervention should be done if manipulation cannot correct the deformity completely within 8–12 weeks of casting.
- Long leg serial casting by the Ponseti technique improves results so that in most clubfeet, little more than heel cord lengthening and possibly posterior ankle release is required. The operated foot is stabilized for healing for 1 month in a Ponseti-type cast.
- Following surgery, bracing with bars and shoes for 3 months full time and then 3 years nights and naps is an integral part of the Ponseti method.
- With the Ponseti method, 30–45% of patients may have various forms of recurrence requiring repeated casting and/or surgical release through maturity.
- Treatment of complex idiopathic clubfoot require up to 5 additional casts to abduct the forefoot at the midfoot, laterally rotating the anterior tuberosity of the calcaneus under the head of the talus. Recurrence of deformity is more common in this type.

ONGOING CARE

FOLLOW-UP RECOMMENDATIONS

Patient Monitoring

- Realignment of the deformity is the goal and should be achieved with casting and surgery.
- Most surgeons cast the feet for 1 month postoperatively.
- With the Ponseti method, bars and shoes are recommended full time for 3 months and nights for 3 years to maintain the correction.
- Remember, the cause of the deformity is not corrected. Only the alignment of the bones and lengthening of the soft tissues are corrected.
- Depending on the severity of the deformity, all corrected clubfeet can be expected to demonstrate varying amounts of calf narrowing and weakness, ankle and subtalar stiffness, a difference between the feet of 1–2 shoe sizes, and even a leg length discrepancy, usually <2 cm.
- There also will be decreased ankle and subtalar motion as compared to normal.
- Adolescent children with clubfeet often will get leg cramps and tire easily while doing sports.
  - Recurrence of heel cord tightness is common, especially during periods of rapid growth.
  - Additional heel cord stretching and casting and, infrequently, additional surgery may be needed.
- All true recurrences should lead to further evaluation for neuromuscular or syndromic causes that might have been undiagnosed in the infant.

ADDITIONAL READING

- Hamel J, Becker W. Sonographic assessment of clubfoot deformity in young children. *J Pediatr Orthop B*. 1996;5(4):279–286.
- Ponseti IV, Zhivkov M, Davis N, et al. Treatment of the complex idiopathic clubfoot. *Clin Orthop Relat Res*. 2006;451:171–176.
- Roye BD, Hyman J, Roye DP Jr. Congenital idiopathic talipes equinovarus. *Pediatr Rev*. 2004;25(4):124–130.
- Scher DM. The Ponseti method for treatment of congenital club foot. *Curr Opin Pediatr*. 2006;18(1):22–25.
- Scherl SA. Common lower extremity problems in children. *Pediatr Rev*. 2004;25(2):52–62.
- Yamamoto H, Muneta T, Morita S. Nonsurgical treatment of congenital clubfoot with manipulation, cast, and modified Denis Browne splint. *J Pediatr Orthop*. 1998;18(4):538–542.

CODES

ICD10

- Q66.89 Other specified congenital deformities of feet
- Q66.7 Congenital pes cavus
- Q66.0 Congenital talipes equinovarus

FAQ

- Q: How can a rigid clubfoot be distinguished from a positional clubfoot?
- A: During initial evaluation of the child, it is important to assess the amount of flexibility in a clubfoot. This can be most easily done by flexing the hip to 90 degrees, flexing the knee to 90 degrees, and then gently trying to turn the forefoot into a straight position lined up with the thigh. If the foot easily spins around into a normal position, it can be assumed that this is a flexible or positional clubfoot. If deformity persists, this is a rigid deformity. If possible, the examining physician should palpate the heel to see if the os calcis comes out of its equinus position filling the heel pad. In some children, particularly with a rocker-bottom sole, the heel pad looks as if it is in the correct position, but the os calcis remains in equinus with the posterior aspect of the os calcis proximal to the heel pad.
- Q: What percentage of clubfeet are successfully treated by casting?
- A: To some extent, the amount of success depends on how much correction is desired. Occasionally, cast correction will provide a partial correction. Some feet, after casting, can be held in the corrected position, only to spin back to the clubfoot deformity when released. Positional clubfeet are likely to improve with casting in perhaps 98% of cases. Rigid clubfeet are much less likely to be corrected by casting. The success rate with casting alone in the rigid feet is likely to be ~10%. It is important to remember that casting and surgery cannot make the clubfoot normal.
- Q: What will be the permanent disability of a congenital clubfoot deformity?
- A: Although casting and surgical correction of a congenital clubfoot can realign the bones, the surgery does little to correct the underlying neuromuscular problems. As a result, all children with rigid clubfeet are likely to have a leg length inequality (usually <1.5 inches), a smaller foot (usually 1–2 sizes), calf narrowing that cannot be significantly improved with exercise, and joint stiffness (ankle, subtalar, and midfoot). Even children with optimal realignment of the deformity will notice their inability to perform gymnastic activities or running activities requiring normal range of motion of the ankle and foot. Many will complain of the inability to keep up with their peer group during adolescent and young adult sports activities.
- Q: How soon should an infant with congenital clubfoot be referred to an orthopedic surgeon?
- A: Casting begins within the 1st–2nd week of life. Medical and life-threatening conditions should take precedence over the treatment of the clubfoot. Access to the feet for IV or blood studies will interfere with a casting regimen. Casting should begin as soon as is practical. It may even be possible to begin taping of the foot as an alternative to casting, which will still allow IV access to the feet. Referral to an orthopedic surgeon should, therefore, follow as soon as is practical. Studies have shown that excellent results can be obtained from the Ponseti method even when initiated after the 1st year of life.

COARCTATION OF AORTA

Luz Natal-Hernandez

BASICS

DESCRIPTION

- Discrete stenosis of the upper thoracic aorta, usually just opposite the site of insertion of the ductus arteriosus (juxtaductal). A segment of tubular hypoplasia and/or a remnant of ductal tissue give rise to a prominent posterior infolding ("the posterior shelf").
- The hemodynamic lesion is most often discrete but may be a long segment or tortuous in nature. It is usually juxtaductal but may occur in other sites (i.e., the abdominal aorta). The prevalence of other associations (bicuspid aortic valve) and long-term complications (hypertension) indicate that this lesion may be part of a broader spectrum arteriopathy and/or endothelial disorder.

EPIDEMIOLOGY

Prevalence

- ~6–8% of patients with congenital heart disease have coarctation.
- Male > female (1.5–4.0:1)

RISK FACTORS

Genetics

- Multifactorial: occurs in 35% of patients with Turner syndrome (XO)
- Has been described in cases of monozygotic twins
- Many studies document the prevalence of a microdeletion at 22q11 in patients with arch anomalies and ventricular septal defects.

PATHOPHYSIOLOGY

- Decreased systemic blood flow to lower body after ductal closure
- Increased afterload to left ventricle (LV) causes LV hypertrophy. Relative underperfusion of the renal vessels, baroreceptors, and multiple other mechanisms combine to induce compensatory hypertension.
- If the coarctation is severe, LV dysfunction and congestive heart failure (CHF) result, with low cardiac output and increased LV end-diastolic pressure.
- Decreased myocardial perfusion may be present in cases of very low output.

DIAGNOSIS

HISTORY

There are 2 typical patterns for the clinical presentation of coarctation:

- An infant with CHF or shock: Typically precipitated by ductal closure, this presentation is more common in infants with coarctation and other intracardiac malformations (20–30%):
  - Respiratory distress (dyspnea/tachypnea)
  - Poor feeding
  - Pallor
  - Diaphoresis
  - Poor weight gain
  - Oliguria
- An otherwise asymptomatic child or adolescent with systolic hypertension and/or a heart murmur (70–80%)
  - Lower extremity claudication
  - Headaches

PHYSICAL EXAM

- Tachypnea and tachycardia
- Discrepant arterial pulses and systolic blood pressure (BP) in the upper and lower extremities
- Weak, "thready" pulses
- Grade 2–3/6 systolic ejection murmur
- Gallop rhythm in an infant with CHF
- Ejection click of a bicuspid aortic valve
- The most important finding is decreased or absent lower extremity pulses. Are pulses present? Is there a delay between the brachial and femoral pulses?
- Heart murmur: best heard at the upper left sternal border, at the base, and radiating to the left interscapular area posteriorly
- An infant with severe coarctation and a patent ductus arteriosus (PDA) may have "differential cyanosis." The lower part of the body appears cyanotic because the descending aortic flow is provided by the right ventricle (RV) through the PDA (check postductal saturation).

ALERT

- The most reliable clinical findings to diagnose native, residual, or recurrent coarctation are the presence of pressure differences in the upper and lower extremities and decreased or absent femoral pulses. Palpable pulses do not exclude coarctation. What one palpates is pulse pressure, not absolute systolic pressure.
- 4-extremity BP measurement is very important in assessing infants and children with possible congenital heart disease. Proper cuff size must be used.
- Bowel ischemia can be present in the ill patient, and emesis or poor feeding are hallmark signs.

DIAGNOSTIC TESTS & INTERPRETATION

Lab

- Electrocardiogram: RV hypertrophy is usually present in symptomatic infants. The electrocardiogram is often normal in children. LV hypertrophy is apparent with more severe coarctation or longer standing coarctation, particularly in older children.
- Blood tests: In the patient presenting in extremis, management, initial therapy, and timing of surgery can be guided by arterial blood gas analyses and markers of end organ dysfunction.

Imaging

- Chest x-ray: in the infant, moderate to severe cardiomegaly with increased pulmonary vascular markings (PVMs). In an asymptomatic child, the heart size is often normal, with normal PVMs. Rib notching may be seen in older children secondary to dilated intercostal collateral vessels.
- Echocardiography: localization, degree of coarctation, and associated findings (PDA, arch hypoplasia, other defects); assessment of associated left-sided obstruction: mitral valve abnormality, LV outflow obstruction, and aortic stenosis (bicuspid aortic valve)
- Magnetic resonance imaging: clearly defines the location and severity of coarctation; useful for serial postoperative follow-up (especially aortic aneurysms)

Diagnostic Procedures/Other

Cardiac catheterization and angiography: usually not indicated unless there are further questions to be answered and/or a planned intervention

DIFFERENTIAL DIAGNOSIS

- Other left-sided heart obstructive lesions
- Hypoplastic left heart syndrome
- Cardiomyopathy and/or myocarditis
- Critical aortic stenosis (aortic obstruction to a degree that adequate systemic perfusion depends on patency of the ductus arteriosus)
- Sustained tachyarrhythmia
- Shock from sepsis, metabolic disease, or other entities

TREATMENT

GENERAL MEASURES

- For the sick neonate who presents with severe CHF or shock (ductal-dependent systemic blood flow):
  - Alprostadil (PGE1) prostaglandin infusion: 0.05–0.1 mcg/kg/min (anticipating adverse effects, including apnea)
  - Inotropic support: Dopamine 3–5 mcg/kg/min
  - Diuretics for pulmonary venous hypertension or pulmonary edema
  - Surgical intervention should follow as soon as possible.
- For the asymptomatic child, elective repair and assessment for systemic hypertension are appropriate; however, aggressive antihypertensive pharmacotherapy is not indicated prior to surgical intervention.
- Other
  - Interventional cardiology
    - Percutaneous balloon angioplasty of native coarctation in infants and children is pursued in some centers. Others have concern about rates of recurrent stenosis, hypertension, aneurysm formation, and iliofemoral arterial injury.
    - Use of vascular stents to relieve the area of stenosis, particularly in older children and adolescents, has provided an alternative to surgical intervention; may increase the need for reintervention in the future when compared to the surgical approach

SURGERY/OTHER PROCEDURES
- Infancy
  - Surgical repair of severe coarctation and coarctation associated with intracardiac anomalies
  - The surgical mortality rate for infants with coarctation and a large ventricular septal defect ranges from 5 to 15% and is higher for children with more complex intracardiac anomalies.
- Childhood
  - Elective coarctation repair between ages 18 months and 3 years in asymptomatic children without severe upper extremity hypertension. Later repair is associated with an increased risk of sustained hypertension and other late complications.
- Types of surgical repair: end-to-end anastomosis, subclavian flap aortoplasty, prosthetic patch aortoplasty, bypass graft

ONGOING CARE

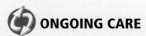

FOLLOW-UP RECOMMENDATIONS
Patient Monitoring
- Reexamine every 12 months with 4-extremity pulse and BP assessment.
- Residual or recurrent coarctation occurs most commonly in those patients requiring repair in early infancy and can depend on the method of intervention (e.g., higher incidence with patch aortoplasty and coarctation ridge resection); most centers delay percutaneous balloon angioplasty of residual or recurrent lesions until 2 months postoperatively.
- Persistent systemic hypertension: most common in patients whose coarctation repair is delayed beyond late childhood
- Aortic aneurysm formation
- Intracranial aneurysms and/or cerebrovascular accidents
- May have hypertension with exercise, even if normotensive at rest
- Exercise-induced hypertension without anatomic stenosis may respond to beta-blocker therapy.

PROGNOSIS
- Untreated coarctation has a poor natural history with the onset of CHF, especially in those patients with other intracardiac malformations. Claudication is common in older children with previously undiscovered coarctation. Generally, the short-term prognosis following successful intervention for isolated coarctation in infancy or childhood is excellent. Procedure-related mortality in every modern series is very near zero.
- Clinical conditions that may affect long-term prognosis after repair of coarctation include the following:
  - Residual or recurrent coarctation
  - Hypertension (rest and exercise)
  - Aortic aneurysm (associated with repair technique)
  - Associated intracardiac lesions
  - Intracranial aneurysms
  - Occurrence or progression of aortic valve disease
  - Premature coronary arterial and cerebrovascular disease
- Associated lesions
  - Bicuspid aortic valve
  - Ventricular septal defect
  - Valvar or subvalvar aortic stenosis
  - Mitral stenosis: often associated with structural mitral valve abnormalities (i.e., supravalvar mitral ring, thickening of mitral leaflet, single papillary muscle with parachute deformity, or short dysplastic chordae tendineae)
  - Shone syndrome: multiple left-sided obstructive lesions, including supravalvar mitral ring, parachute mitral valve, subaortic obstruction, and coarctation
  - Berry aneurysm of the circle of Willis
  - Renal artery stenosis associated with abdominal coarctation
  - Congenital diaphragmatic hernia

COMPLICATIONS
- Shock, if severe untreated obstruction
- CHF, if severe untreated obstruction
- Systemic hypertension, before and after intervention
- Intracranial aneurysms
- Mesenteric ischemia
- Paraplegia
- Postoperative complications
  - Bleeding
  - Postcoarctectomy syndrome/mesenteric ischemia
  - Paradoxical hypertension
  - Spinal cord ischemia (0.4%)
  - Residual coarctation
  - Chylothorax
  - Stridor
  - Diaphragm paralysis
  - Aortic aneurysm or dissection
  - Paralysis

ADDITIONAL READING

- Carr JA. The results of catheter-based therapy compared with surgical repair of adult aortic coarctation. *J Am Coll Cardiol*. 2006;47(6):1101–1107.
- Celermajer DS, Greaves K. Survivors of coarctation repair: fixed but not cured. *Heart*. 2002;88(2): 113–114.
- Cowley CG, Orsmond GS, Feola P, et al. Long-term randomized comparison of balloon angioplasty and surgery for native coarctation of the aorta in childhood. *Circulation*. 2005;111(25):3453–3456.
- Rosenthal E. Coarctation of the aorta from fetus to adult: curable condition or lifelong disease process? *Heart*. 2005;91(11):1495–1502.
- Shah L, Hijazi Z, Sandhu S, et al. Use of endovascular stents for the treatment of coarctation of the aorta in children and adults: immediate and midterm results. *J Invasive Cardiol*. 2005;17(11): 614–618.
- Toro-Salazar OH, Steinberger J, Thomas W, et al. Long-term follow-up of patients after coarctation of the aorta repair. *Am J Cardiol*. 2002;89(5):541–547.

CODES

ICD10
Q25.1 Coarctation of aorta

FAQ
- Q: When is the most appropriate time to perform surgical repair of simple coarctation?
- A: Recommendations vary regarding the age at which asymptomatic children (without severe upper extremity hypertension) should undergo intervention. Advances in technique no longer require patients to be "grown" to a threshold size or weight, and there is increasing evidence that severity and incidence of late complications correlate directly with older age at repair. Although some authors mention 3–5 years of age, others recommend repair as early as 18 months to 2 years of age.
- Q: What is the incidence of systemic hypertension after surgical repair of coarctation?
- A: Greatly depends on age at repair, surgical method or technique, length of follow-up interval, and how one defines or measures hypertension. In no situation is the answer zero, and this important complication is one of several reasons patients require lifelong detailed follow-up. 1 year after a technically perfect repair via resection with end-to-end anastomosis, the patient operated on in early childhood is unlikely to have hypertension at rest. However, 20 years further along, a patient of older age at repair is quite likely to have significant hypertension on exercise stress testing.

COCCIDIOIDOMYCOSIS

Camille Sabella

BASICS

DESCRIPTION

Coccidioidomycosis is an endemic systemic mycosis resulting in both asymptomatic and life-threatening disseminated infections.

EPIDEMIOLOGY

- *Coccidioides* spp. are dimorphic fungi that live in the soil.
- Endemic to the southwestern United States (southern California, Arizona, western and southern Texas, New Mexico), northern Mexico, and parts of South and Central America
- Infection is acquired from exposure to aerosolized spores (arthroconidia) usually during recreational or occupational activities; clusters of cases may involve dust storms and earthquakes.
- The average incubation period is 10–16 days (range 1–4 weeks).
- There is no person-to-person spread.
- 60% of acute infections are subclinical (asymptomatic).

Incidence

- 25,000–150,000 new infections per year in the United States
- Highest rate of infection in the summer and early fall

Prevalence

Seropositivity rates in children living in endemic area for 1 year approach 20%, whereas rates in children living in endemic area for 10 or more years approach 80%.

RISK FACTORS

- The course of illness is highly variable and depend on host immune response and amount of exposure.
- Risk factors for disseminated infection:
  - Immunosuppression (especially organ transplant recipients, those receiving immunosuppressive therapies and immunomodulators, and those with HIV infection)
  - Male gender (adult)
  - Neonates, infants, and the elderly
  - Filipino, African American, Native American, Hispanic ethnicity
  - Pregnancy
- Risk of dissemination is less in children than in adults.

GENERAL PREVENTION

Infection control

- No special isolation or precautions for the hospitalized patient
- Contaminated dressings from skin lesions should be handled and discarded with care.
- Inhalation of aerosolized spores from culture can be hazardous to laboratory personnel.
- Preventive efforts are aimed at dust control and trials to eliminate organisms from soil.
- Immunocompromised people should be counseled to avoid activities that may expose them to aerosolized spores in endemic areas.

PATHOPHYSIOLOGY

- Spores (arthroconidia) are the infectious forms of *Coccidioides* organisms; they are released from the mold and propagate the mold in the soil.
- Inhalation of arthroconidia from disturbed, arid soil is the major route of infection.
- In tissues, arthroconidia enlarge to form spherules. Mature spherules release endospores that propagate in the host and continue the tissue cycle.
- Primary infection occurs in the lungs.
- Most patients have infection limited to a localized area of lung and hilar lymph nodes after mounting an intense inflammatory response with granuloma formation.
- Extrapulmonary dissemination occurs via lymphatic or hematologic spread and usually involves the skin, bones and joints, and central nervous system but can spread to virtually any organ system.

ETIOLOGY

- *Coccidioides immitis* and *Coccidioides posadasii* are the etiologic agents of coccidioidomycosis.
- Asymptomatic infection is the most common outcome, occurring in 60% of infected individuals.
- Primary pulmonary infection accounts for most symptomatic cases; nonspecific illness most common feature (cough, malaise, chest pain, fever); self-limited in most cases; may be accompanied by reactive rashes such as erythema multiforme or erythema nodosum
- Disseminated disease occurs in less than 1% of infected individuals and may manifest with
  - Osteomyelitis: subacute or chronic and frequently involves more than 1 bone (40%). Common sites are the hands, feet, ribs, skull, and vertebrae.
  - Meningitis: develops within 6 months of initial infection. Hydrocephalus is a common complication. Central nervous system vasculitis and intracerebral abscesses are rare.
  - Cutaneous disease: Papules or pustular lesions that ulcerate are most common; most commonly seen on the face but can occur anywhere; regional adenitis is common.

DIAGNOSIS

HISTORY

- Travel or residence in an endemic area is typical. Risk factors for disseminated infection should be sought.
- Acute pneumonia
  - Fever, dry or productive cough, and pleuritic chest pain; hemoptysis is rare in children.
  - Systemic symptoms include headache, malaise, arthralgias, sore throat, and fatigue; rash may be reported.
  - Also known as "valley fever"
- Myalgias, arthralgias, chills, night sweats, and anorexia suggest systemic dissemination.
- Headache, vomiting, and altered mental status suggest meningitis.
- Most infections (60%) are asymptomatic.

PHYSICAL EXAM

- Signs of pneumonia and pleural effusions are often present with symptomatic pulmonary infection.
- Reactive rashes
  - Contain no live organisms
  - Erythematous maculopapular rash and erythema multiforme are seen in 50% of symptomatic children.
  - Erythema nodosum and fever may occur following the onset of symptoms and correlate with the development of cell-mediated immunity (hypersensitivity reactions).
  - Hypersensitivity reactions may occur in the absence of pulmonary symptoms.
- Hematogenous dissemination to the skin
  - Lesions may consist of papules, nodules, abscesses, pustules, sinus tracts, and verrucous ulcers.
  - May be single or multiple
  - Can occur anywhere but are most common on the nasolabial folds
- Stridor is present with infection of the subglottic tissues.
- Signs of increased intracranial pressure are often seen with central nervous system infection. Classic signs of meningeal irritation and fever may be absent.

ALERT

- Clinicians in endemic areas should maintain a high level of clinical suspicion of primary as well as disseminated infection.
- Diagnosis in nonendemic areas may be missed owing to low clinical suspicion or missed travel history.
- False-negative serologic results may occur during the initial weeks of infection or in an immunocompromised host.

DIAGNOSTIC TESTS & INTERPRETATION

Lab

- Direct examination and culture
  - Cytologic examination of bronchoalveolar fluid is diagnostic in only about 1/3 of persons and is less sensitive than culture. Visualization of large spherules is possible in stained specimens of sputum, tracheal aspirates, urine, or tissue biopsy. They are rarely seen in CSF.
  - The organisms can be detected by culture in experienced laboratories. The yield is highest from purulent material. The yield from other sources, such as pleural fluid, blood, and gastric aspirates, is lower.
  - A DNA probe can identify *Coccidioides* species in cultures.
- Coccidioidin or spherulin skin intradermal testing has been used as an epidemiologic tool in the past but is no longer commercially available.
- Serologic studies
  - Serve as valuable diagnostic and prognostic tools but may be hampered by false-negative results early in the course of infection and in immunocompromised hosts; false-positive reactions occur as a result of cross-reactivity with other endemic mycoses.
  - *C. immitis*–specific IgM antibody is detectable in 75% of patients 1–3 weeks after symptom onset and usually is absent after 6 months. False-positive results are seen in 15% of patients with cystic fibrosis.
  - IgG is detected by the complement fixation (CF) assay from serum or CSF. It is positive in 50% of patients at 4 weeks and 83% at 3 months following symptomatic primary infection. In general, higher titers reflect more extensive infection, and rising CF antibody concentrations are associated with worsening disease.
  - Enzyme immunoassay (EIA) for qualitative detection of IgM and IgG is sensitive but can yield false-positive results. It can be useful for screening, but a positive EIA should be confirmed with another test.
  - Hematologic findings include elevated erythrocyte sedimentation rate, leukocytosis, and eosinophilia (in 10%).

- Other studies
  – CSF findings in meningitis include hypoglycorrhachia and pleocytosis with mononuclear cell predominance.

Imaging

Radiologic studies

- Chest radiograph may reveal well-circumscribed nodules, lobar or patchy pulmonary infiltrates, pleural effusions, cavitary lesions, and hilar adenopathy.
- Radiographs of involved bones may reveal lytic lesions. Scintigraphy or MRI of bone is more sensitive for the diagnosis of osteomyelitis.

DIFFERENTIAL DIAGNOSIS

- Other pulmonary mycoses (e.g., *Histoplasma capsulatum*, *Aspergillus fumigatus*, and *Blastomyces dermatitidis*)
- *Mycobacterium tuberculosis* (lung or CSF)
- *Mycoplasma pneumoniae*
- Influenza and other viral infections that present as bronchopneumonia
- Skin lesions may mimic other endemic mycoses, tuberculosis, actinomycetes, or syphilis.

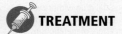

TREATMENT

MEDICATION

- Uncomplicated or minor disease is self-limited and should not be treated with antifungal therapy (>95% of cases).
- Treatment of uncomplicated respiratory infection is recommended for infants, pregnant women, and patients with continuous fever for >1 month, >10% weight loss, extensive or progressive pulmonary disease, or immunodeficiency (either from HIV or as a result of immunosuppressive medications). Use either oral fluconazole or itraconazole for 3–6 months.
- Diffuse pneumonia or immunocompromised host: Start therapy with amphotericin B and replace with oral fluconazole or itraconazole when clinical improvement is demonstrated. The total length of therapy should be at least 1 year, and for patients with severe immunodeficiency, oral azole therapy should be continued as secondary prophylaxis.
- Disseminated infection, nonmeningeal: Treat with oral fluconazole or itraconazole. Amphotericin B may be used initially, especially for patients with severe or rapid progression of disease. The duration of therapy may be longer than for those with pneumonia only.
- Meningitis: Oral fluconazole is preferred (12 mg/kg/24 h once daily or divided b.i.d., max 800–1,000 mg/24 h). Itraconazole (10–20 mg/kg/24 h divided b.i.d.–t.i.d., max 600 mg/24 h) for 3 days, 4–10 mg/kg/24 h divided b.i.d. (max 400 mg/24 h) thereafter, is an alternative agent. Therapy should be continued indefinitely.
- Intrathecal amphotericin B may be useful in central nervous system infections for those who fail to respond to azole therapy.
- Surgical debridement is used for localized and persistent lesions in bone and lung.

ONGOING CARE

FOLLOW-UP RECOMMENDATIONS

Patient Monitoring

- Patients with mild primary respiratory tract infections who are not treated with antifungal therapy should be assessed at 3–6 months intervals for up to 2 years to ensure that their clinical and radiographic findings have resolved.
- Periodic assessment should be done for all patients treated with antifungal therapy throughout their treatment and after cessation of antifungal therapy.
- Patients who are being treated for meningeal infections should undergo CSF assessment every 3 months for life.
- Rising or unchanging CF titers while the patient is receiving treatment may indicate treatment failure, most often due to noncompliance or an occult focus that may require surgical drainage.
- All azoles inhibit P450 enzymes. Consider drug–drug interactions when the patient is taking other medications.

PROGNOSIS

- Most infections are asymptomatic (60%) or mild (35%) and self-limited.
- Primary infection of the lungs is usually self-limited, with a course of illness lasting 1–3 weeks; complications (see below) may prolong the course.
- Fatigue can last for several months.
- Dissemination is infrequent (see earlier section for risk factors). Morbidity and mortality have improved with use of antifungal therapy, but immunocompromised patients still have a poor prognosis after the development of disseminated infection. The mortality rate is 70% in HIV-infected patients with diffuse pulmonary coccidioidomycosis.
- Meningitis, untreated, is nearly always fatal within 2 years of diagnosis.

COMPLICATIONS

- Localized complications of primary pulmonary infection are infrequent and include pleural effusions and pericarditis.
- ~5% of lung infections result in residual pulmonary sequelae, usually nodules or abscess cavities. 1/3 of these cavities spontaneously resolve within 2 years. Hemoptysis and rupture of the abscess, with formation of an empyema, are potential complications in patients with unresolved cavities.
- Extrapulmonary dissemination usually develops within a year after the initial infection but may appear much later if immunity is impaired (e.g., HIV infection, malignancy, immunosuppressive or immunomodulatory therapy).
- Hospital admission seems to be more common in patients with comorbid conditions and frequently necessitates surgical intervention.
- Hydrocephalus may occur with central nervous system involvement.

ADDITIONAL READING

- Ampel NM. New perspectives on coccidioidomycosis. *Proc Am Thorac Soc*. 2010;7(3):181–185.
- Chu JH, Feudtner C, Heydon KH, et al. Hospitalizations for endemic mycoses: a population based national study. *Clin Infect Dis*. 2006;42(6):822–825.
- Deresinski SC. Coccidioidomycosis: efficacy of new agents and future prospects. *Curr Opin Infect Dis*. 2001;14(6):693–696.
- Fisher BT, Chiller TM, Prasad PA, et al. Hospitalizations for coccidioidomycosis at forty-one children's hospitals in the United States. *Pediatr Infect Dis J*. 2010;29(3):243–247.
- Galgiani JN, Ampel NM, Catanzaro A, et al. Practice guidelines for the treatment of coccidioidomycosis. *Clin Infect Dis*. 2000;30(4):658–661.
- Montenegro BL, Arnold JC. North American dimorphic fungal infections in children. *Pediatr Rev*. 2010;31(6):e40–e48.
- Nguyen C, Barker BM, Hoover S, et al. Recent advances in our understanding of the environmental, epidemiological, immunological, and clinical dimensions of coccidioidomycosis. *Clin Microbiol Rev*. 2013;26(3):505–525.
- Shehab ZM. Coccidioidomycosis. *Adv Pediatr*. 2010;57(1):269–286.
- Smith JA, Kauffman CA. Endemic fungal infections in patients receiving tumour necrosis factor-alpha inhibitor therapy. *Drugs*. 2009;69(11):1403–1415.

CODES

ICD10

- B38.9 Coccidioidomycosis, unspecified
- B38.2 Pulmonary coccidioidomycosis, unspecified
- B38.3 Cutaneous coccidioidomycosis

FAQ

- Q: Do all patients with symptomatic primary respiratory infection due to *C. immitis* require treatment?
- A: No. Because >95% of initial pulmonary infections are self-limited, treatment is not always required. Patients with concurrent risk factors (e.g., HIV, organ transplant, or high doses of corticosteroids) or evidence of unusually severe infections should always be treated. Factors suggesting increased severity of infection include weight loss of >10%, symptoms for 3 or more weeks, infiltrates involving more than half of 1 lung or portions of both lungs, and CF antibody to *C. immitis* >1:16.
- Q: What is the best option for treatment of the child with coccidioidal meningitis?
- A: Fluconazole has become the treatment of choice because of its ease of administration, excellent central nervous system penetration, and safety profile. Other azoles such as ketoconazole and itraconazole appear to also be effective in adults. Intravenously and intrathecally administered amphotericin B is considered a 2nd-line agent because of its inconvenience and adverse effect profile.

COLIC

Cori Green

BASICS

DESCRIPTION

Crying is considered a normal part of human behavior and is a baby's most effective form of communication. However, when crying is perceived to be in excess than what is expected, it can cause a family a great deal of distress. Colic is a syndrome of excessive crying for which no organic cause can be identified. It is described as unexplained end of the day crying that begins at age 2–3 weeks, peaks at 8 weeks, and tapers at 12 weeks.

No standard definition of colic exists. The most widely used definition is from 1954 (Wessel) and referred to as the rule of 3's. He defined colic by the amount of crying: >3 hours a day, >3 days a week, and lasting at least 3 weeks. Colic episodes usually begin suddenly, with no clear reason, and at the end of the day or evening. The crying is intense and high pitched. Infants may have a flushed face, furrowed brow, and postural changes such as bending or drawing up of the knees, clenched fists, and tensed abdominal muscles. Episodes may end with a bowel movement or passing of gas.

EPIDEMIOLOGY

- Crying is one of the most common reasons families present to a health care professional during the 1st months of life.
- 1 in 6 families who have children with colic seek care from a health care professional.
- Estimates are difficult to make due to lack of standard definition; literature suggests a prevalence of 3–40%.
- Incidence is similar in male and females and in breast- and bottle-fed infants.

RISK FACTORS

Possible risk factors include maternal smoking, increased maternal age, and being the firstborn child. In addition, colic has been associated with higher levels of maternal stress, anxiety, and depression.

GENERAL PREVENTION

Although no study has shown any certain way to prevent colic, educating parents about infant crying can be helpful. Remind parents that crying is an infant's way to communicate, inform them of the expected average hours a day and infant may cry, and teach them soothing techniques.

ETIOLOGY

- The term colic is now considered a misnomer because it derives from the Greek word for colon. Studies in the early 1900s suggested colic was a result of gastrointestinal (GI) dysfunction, whereas today, there are many theories.
- Typically, colic is considered to result from an interaction between infant factors and the environment at a unique time of biologic vulnerability. No single cause has been identified. Several hypotheses for the etiology exist.
  - GI disturbances are often implicated in colic. Abnormal motility has been hypothesized and is somewhat supported by the fact that anticholinergics may improve symptoms. Other studies have shown infants with colic have decreased amounts of lactobacilli and increased amounts of coliform bacteria. Although another theory is that increased gas production can cause colic, this theory is not supported based on radiographs taken during crying spells. Recent studies have suggested an association with *Helicobacter pylori* and infantile colic. Others theorize that colic is a form of milk protein allergy. However, these studies are limited and no causality has been established.
  - Psychosocial issues have been implicated including family tension, parental anxiety, or inadequate parent–infant interactions. However, in studies where infants are cared for by trained occupational therapists, symptoms did not improve.
  - A neurodevelopmental etiology is supported by the fact that infants with colic have similar patterns of crying to infants without colic and that colic is outgrown. Excessive crying has also been considered a manifestation of normal emotional development where colic is on the end of a spectrum of crying.

DIAGNOSIS

HISTORY

- Obtain details about the infant's behavior around the start of a crying episode and the intensity, time of day, and duration of crying. Documenting this can help both the caregivers and health care providers.
- Prenatal history and history of fever in the infant is important to assess infant's risk of infection.
- History about stooling and vomiting should be elicited to eliminate organic etiologies of crying such as gastroesophageal reflux, malabsorption, or pyloric stenosis.
- History of color changes, apnea, or respiratory distress should help assess for a cardiac or respiratory etiology for crying.

PHYSICAL EXAM

- For the diagnoses of colic, vital signs, growth, and physical exam should be normal.
- Look for signs of trauma or evidence of nonaccidental injuries. Look for bruises and palpate bones to look for fractures. A thorough GI and neurologic exam should also be performed.

DIAGNOSTIC TESTS & INTERPRETATION

No tests are indicated if there are no concerning signs on history or physical.

DIFFERENTIAL DIAGNOSIS

- Normal crying
  - As studied by Brazelton in 1962, at 2 weeks, normal infants cried for a median of 1¾ hour a day, just under 3 hours at 6 weeks, and ~1 hour by 12 weeks. Normal crying, like colic, tends to occur predominantly in the evening and can vary from day to day.
- Organic causes of excessive crying:
  - Cardiac: congenital heart disease, supraventricular tachycardia
  - Respiratory: upper respiratory infection, pneumonia, foreign body aspiration, pneumothorax
  - GI: constipation, cow's milk protein intolerance, gastroesophageal reflux, lactose intolerance, intussusception, rectal fissures, and strangulated inguinal hernias
  - Neurologic: hydrocephalus, subdural hematoma, infantile migraine, neonatal drug withdrawal
  - Metabolic: hypoglycemia, electrolyte abnormalities, ingestions, inborn errors of metabolism
  - Infectious: meningitis, otitis media, urinary tract infections, and viral illnesses
  - Trauma: child abuse, corneal abrasions, foreign bodies in the eye, fractures, and hair tourniquets

ALERT

Although organic causes are found in less than 5% of infants who present with crying, it is important to look for red flags in the history and physical such as the following:

- **Symptoms elicited in history:**
  - Vomiting that is frequent, large quantity (>1 oz), bilious, or projectile
  - Bloody stools
  - Poor weight gain
  - Respiratory difficulties including apneic or cyanotic episodes
  - Fever, lethargy, poor feeding
- **Signs observed on physical exam:**
  - Irritability, tachycardia, pallor, mottling, poor perfusion
  - Abnormal neurologic findings including hypotonia, a full fontanelle, or a head circumference >95%
  - Petechiae, bruising, tachypnea, cyanosis, nasal flaring
  - Weight decreasing

TREATMENT

MEDICATION

The literature does not support the use of pharmacologic interventions in colic. Although some studies have shown certain pharmacologic agents to be effective, these studies lack methodologic rigor or involve medications with serious adverse effects.

- Anticholinergic medications such as dicyclomine hydrochloride and cimetropium have been proven to be effective. However, these medications are contraindicated in infants younger than 6 months in the United States due to side effects such as apnea and drowsiness.
- Simethicone is an over-the-counter drug that decreases intraluminal gas. Studies of its efficacy have been mixed and any reduction of symptoms has been attributed to a placebo effect.
- Probiotics may play a role in reducing symptoms. Studies comparing *Lactobacillus reuteri* DSM 17938 to placebo in breastfed infants have shown a reduction of symptoms. These studies are promising; however, further studies confirming these results are needed.

ADDITIONAL TREATMENT

General Measures

The most important and effective treatment is for health care providers to acknowledge the difficulty of the situation and to provide reassurance. Parents of a colicky infant often feel tired and inadequate and need their concerns to be substantiated by a provider who acknowledges how difficult of a time this must be. Main points to reassure and guide parents include the following:

- The crying of colic can be persistent, but there is no evidence of a physical problem or proof that the infant is in pain. Periods of wellness each day followed by periods of crying is reassuring.
- Colic is benign and self-limited; the majority of infants improve by age 3–4 months.
- During crying spells, the infant is probably overaroused and tired.
- On average, a healthy infant will cry 2–3 hours per day.
- Strategies for soothing their infant such as swaddling, making "Shh" sounds, swinging the baby (no more than 1 inch back and forth), pacifier use, repetitive sounds, and decreasing environmental stimulation
- Anticipatory guidance on child abuse prevention (e.g., encouraging parents to take a break when their infant's crying is causing them excessive distress or to turn to each other or others for support)

Diet Modification

- Breastfeeding mothers are encouraged to continue to breastfeed. There is conflicting evidence about whether mothers should eliminate allergenic foods from their diet.
- Although hydrolyzed formulas have been shown to reduce symptoms of colic, most of these studies lack methodologic rigor. In addition, if symptoms do improve, milk protein allergy must be considered.
- Although soy milk formula has been shown to reduce crying, it is not recommended in the treatment of colic due to the prevalence of allergy to soy.
- High-fiber formulas and lactase drops have not been shown to be effective.

Behavioral Modifications

- Car-ride simulators, crib vibrators, and increased carrying have not been shown to be effective.
- Other interventions such as modified parent and infant interactions involving decreased stimulation, "contingent music," and assisting parents in acquiring effective coping and consoling methods have shown some benefit. However, none of these studies involve randomization and blinding, and most are of small sample size.

COMPLEMENTARY & ALTERNATIVE THERAPIES

- Although teas containing chamomile, vervain, licorice, fennel, and lemon balm have been shown to be effective if used 3 times a day with 150 mL per dose, they are not recommended. Adverse events have been reported. The dose is a large volume. In addition, there is no standard dosing or formulations of these products.
- Sucrose solutions have been found to improve symptoms compared to placebo, yet evidence is limited and there are concerns about nutritional effects and lack of standardization for formulation of preparations.
- Chiropractic care, infant massage, and acupuncture have also been studied, but due to mixed results and lack of methodologic rigor, they are not recommended in treating colic.

ONGOING CARE

FOLLOW-UP RECOMMENDATIONS

Patient Monitoring

- It is important to keep in close touch with parents of an excessively fussy baby. Telephone contact every 2–3 days is essential until improvement.
- Although reexamination may not be needed, consistent follow-up from a supportive physician may help reassure parents.

DIET

Breast milk and formula changes are not recommended unless milk protein allergy is suspected.

PATIENT EDUCATION

Educate parents regarding the average number of hours an infant is expected to cry and provide soothing techniques. Reassure that colic is benign and self-limited.

PROGNOSIS

- Without intervention, this prolonged crying usually diminishes around 3–4 months of age.
- Some studies suggest infants with colic can have difficulties later in life in family communication, dissatisfaction, and sleeping, psychological, or GI disorders; however, other research has shown no long-term consequences.
- There is no association between colic and later diagnosed asthma or allergic disease.

COMPLICATIONS

Most complications are related to the fatigue, anxiety, and distress that colic can cause in families. The most serious outcome is if parental exasperation leads to the physical abuse of the infant.

ADDITIONAL READING

- Brazelton TB. Crying in infancy. *Pediatrics*. 1962;29:579–588.
- Drugs and Therapeutics Bulletin. Management of infantile colic. *BMJ*. 2013;347:f4102.
- Radesky JS, Zuckerman B, Silverstein M, et al. Inconsolable infant crying and maternal postpartum depressive symptoms. *Pediatrics*. 2013;131(6):e1857–e1864.
- Szajewska H, Gryczuk E, Horvath A. *Lactobacillus reuteri* DSM 17938 for the management of infantile colic in breastfed infants: a randomized, double-blind, placebo-controlled trial. *J Pediatr*. 2013;162(2):257–262.
- Wessel MA, Cobb JC, Jackson EB, et al. Paroxysmal fussing in infants, sometimes called "colic." *Pediatrics*. 1954;14(5):421–434.

CODES

ICD10

- R10.83 Colic
- R68.11 Excessive crying of infant (baby)

FAQ

- Q: What is colic?
- A: Excessive crying in an infant for which no organic etiology is identified. Crying usually is for at least 3 hours a day, for 3 days a week, for a minimum of 3 weeks.
- Q: Why do certain infants get colic?
- A: The etiology of colic is poorly understood. Although there is evidence that GI dysfunction can cause colic, most believe colic is a neurodevelopmental syndrome.
- Q: How is colic treated?
- A: Pharmacologic, nutritional, and behavioral interventions are not recommended. The most important treatment a health care provider can provide is to substantiate a parent's concern, provide reassurance, educate, and provide anticipatory guidance about colic.

C

COMA

Jennifer Huffman

BASICS

DESCRIPTION

Coma is defined as a state in which the patient appears to be asleep, shows no awareness of his or her surroundings, and cannot be aroused. Coma frequently is only a transient state, whereby patients recover, die, or progress to a permanent state of impairment. Often a medical emergency, immediate intervention may be required to preserve life and brain function.

- Coma is at the far end of a spectrum of acute impaired consciousness, which also includes the following:
  - Lethargy or stupor: patient arousable but does not stay awake; impaired responses to commands
  - Delirium: a confused, agitated patient with fragmented attention, concentration, and memory
- Coma may progress to
  - Persistent vegetative state: chronic state of unconsciousness with no awareness or cognition, no voluntary responses, and no language abilities; preserved autonomic functions and sleep/wake cycles
  - Brain death: coma, apnea, and lack of cortical and brainstem responses

EPIDEMIOLOGY

Incidence varies by age, season (infection), and ethnicity (inborn errors of metabolism [IEM]).

PATHOPHYSIOLOGY

Dysfunction of the reticular activating system in the brainstem or bilateral cerebral dysfunction causes impaired arousal and consciousness.

ETIOLOGY

Coma etiology can be traumatic or nontraumatic. Infection is a common cause of nontraumatic coma. Traumatic coma is more likely in older children.

DIAGNOSIS

DIFFERENTIAL DIAGNOSIS

- Trauma
  - Epidural/subdural or intracerebral bleeding, cerebral swelling, and/or diffuse axonal injury
- Intoxication
  - Household drug ingestion including barbiturates, opiates, psychotropics, and salicylates; street drugs; alcohol; smoke or carbon monoxide inhalation; ethylene glycol; lead; and others
- Hypoxia/diffuse ischemia
  - Drowning, suffocation/strangulation, cardiac disease, or complications
- Infection
  - Bacterial or viral meningitis, encephalitis, postinfectious encephalomyelitis, toxic or systemic shock, subdural empyema. Pathogens leading to coma include HSV, *Mycoplasma pneumoniae*, influenza, and *Neisseria meningitidis*.
- Postinfectious/autoimmune mediated
  - Anti-NMDA receptor encephalitis, acute disseminated encephalitis (ADEM), acute necrotizing encephalitis (ANE), febrile infection–related epilepsy syndrome (FIRES), CNS lupus
- Metabolic disorders
  - Hypoglycemia (salicylate or ethanol intoxication, insulin overdose/hyperinsulinemia), diabetic ketoacidosis (DKA) (neurologic deterioration on initiation of insulin therapy), hyperglycemic nonketotic coma, Reye syndrome, electrolyte abnormalities (Na, K, Ca, Mg), hepatic/uremic encephalopathy, IEM, endocrine abnormalities (hypothyroidism, Addisonian crisis), hypothermia/hyperthermia
- Tumor
  - Can cause increased intracranial pressure and herniation
- Seizure
  - Nonconvulsive status
- Vascular
  - Infarction, hemorrhage from arteriovenous malformation (AVM), aneurysm, coagulopathy, cerebral venous thrombosis, hypertensive encephalopathy, basilar-type migraine
- Hydrocephalus
  - Ventriculoperitoneal (VP) shunt obstruction, mass/bleed obstructing ventricular outflow

Disorders mimicking coma include the following:

- Psychogenic coma
  - Patient may resist passive eye opening, regard self in a mirror, and avoid passive arm fall over face and other noxious stimuli.
- Catatonia
  - A form of psychogenic coma; patients may hold a posture, sit, or stand.
- Locked-in state/complete paralysis
  - Patient is paralyzed with intact cerebral function; may occur in severe neuromuscular disorders or in ventral pontine lesions

HISTORY

- **Question:** Evidence or history of head trauma, drowning, or other trauma?
- *Significance*: Are there concerns for nonaccidental trauma?
- **Question:** What medications are in the home? Has the patient been depressed or displayed suicidal behaviors? Is there a history of illicit drug use?
- *Significance*: Ingestion/drugs/toxins
- **Question:** Recent fevers, viral or bacterial illnesses, mental status changes, sick contacts, immunosuppression, infectious risk factors?
- *Significance*: Infection
- **Question:** Past medical history risk factors?
- *Significance*: Epilepsy, diabetes, heart disease, neurologic disease including previous episodes of coma, history of failure to thrive (IEM)
- **Question:** Recent nausea, vomiting, mental status change?
- *Significance*: Increased intracranial pressure

PHYSICAL EXAM

- Vital sign changes: Hyperthermia suggests infection, intoxication, and neuroleptic malignant syndrome. Tachycardia suggests fever, pain, hypovolemia, arrhythmia, and heart failure.

ALERT

Hypertension, bradycardia, and irregular respirations (Cushing reflex) herald impending brain herniation.

- Skin changes: Look for rashes suggesting infection, bruising, and other evidence of trauma; neurocutaneous stigmata may be associated with seizures; feel anterior fontanelle in infants for evidence of increased intracranial pressure (ICP).
- Neurologic exam: Focus on general level of awareness, eye movements, and motor responses to accurately define coma versus lethargy or delirium. Findings can be used in various coma scales.
- Eye movements: Persistent eye deviation is associated with contralateral seizure activity or ipsilateral brain lesions. Impaired upward gaze may indicate high ICP. Nystagmus can be seen in intoxications.
- Pupillary reaction: Small reactive or large reactive pupils suggest intoxication. Anisocoria suggests unilateral brainstem compression. Fixed, dilated pupils indicate global herniation/brain death. Perform oculocephalic (doll's eye) and oculovestibular (calorics) to confirm.
- Motor exam: Assess tone, reflexes, and motor responses to stimuli. Flaccid tone and areflexia are serious signs if not related to medications or lower motor neuron disease. Pressure on the supraorbital notch beneath medial eyebrow will avoid reflex pain responses. Localizing pain entails purposeful movements to remove the stimulus. Withdrawal from pain is less purposeful. Decorticate (adduction with elbow and wrist flexion) and decerebrate (extension, internal rotation of arms) may be provoked by stimulation. They can be asymmetric and intermittent and should not be mistaken for seizures.
- Glasgow Coma Scale/Pediatric Glasgow Coma Scale—associated with prognosis in certain situations (see Appendix, Tables 5 and 6)
  - Eye opening (score range 1–4)
  - Verbal response (score range 1–5)
  - Motor response (score range 1–6)

DIAGNOSTIC TESTS & INTERPRETATION

Initial blood studies obtained with placement of an IV line include the following:

- Glucose, electrolytes, blood urea nitrogen/creatinine, calcium, magnesium, phosphorous
- CBC and blood culture
- Arterial blood gas
- Toxicology screen (consider EKG)
- Ammonia, liver transaminases, CK

Other helpful studies based on the clinical picture may include the following:

- Metabolic labs (urine organic acids, serum amino acids, lactate), urinalysis, urine culture, thyroid function tests, cortisol, coagulation studies, carboxyhemoglobin (CO poisoning), ANA, anti-NMDA receptor antibodies

- LP (opening pressure, glucose, cell count, protein, Gram stain, culture) to rule out infection or bleed; defer until after CT if focal exam or signs of increased ICP. If question of traumatic tap, spin out red cells promptly and examine fluid for xanthochromia. Simultaneous fingerstick blood glucose is ideal.
- EEG can be helpful to rule out nonconvulsive status epilepticus, especially in patients with a history of seizures or clinically suspected seizures. Continuous EEG may be needed to make this diagnosis.
- Electrophysiologic studies including somatosensory evoked (SEP), brainstem auditory evoked, and visual evoked potentials may be helpful for diagnosis and prognosis.

Imaging

- Head CT: Quick noncontrast scan can detect hemorrhage, hydrocephalus, herniation, and masses; may be followed by contrast images or MRI; should be done prior to LP to rule out a mass (risk for herniation from LP)
- Cervical spine series (CT or lateral and anterior–posterior radiograph studies): indicated if with evidence of trauma by history or on physical exam. Spine must be stabilized until injury is ruled out.
- Brain MRI: can help with diagnosis and prognosis if prior workup is unrevealing. Consider MRA to evaluate arteries and MRV to rule out venous thrombosis. MRS can help clarify hypoxic and metabolic etiologies.

TREATMENT

SURGERY/OTHER PROCEDURES

Neurosurgical intervention may be required in cases of head trauma, hemorrhage, mass lesion, or hydrocephalus. Neurology consultation is usually indicated.

INPATIENT CONSIDERATIONS

Initial Stabilization

- First priority is airway, breathing, and circulation management.
- If head trauma is suspected, stabilize the cervical spine with a collar while securing the airway.
- Endotracheal intubation: often required for airway protection and adequate oxygenation
- Place large-bore IV lines for isotonic fluids to maintain intravascular volume and blood pressure as needed.
- Evidence of increased ICP
  - Hyperventilate to decrease blood carbon dioxide to 30–35 torr.
  - Consider 3% hypertonic saline (HS) as bolus or continuous infusion, which may be more efficacious than other osmotic agents.
  - Consider mannitol (0.5–1 g/kg IV); can also give dexamethasone 1–2 mg/kg IV
  - Treat fever with antipyretics and environmental cooling methods.
  - Elevate head to 30 degrees above horizontal; avoid head-turned posture to maximize cerebral venous drainage.
  - Hospitalization in the intensive care unit for close monitoring of changes in respiratory status or signs of increased ICP
  - Neurosurgical consultation; consider role for decompression craniectomy.
- If fingerstick glucose is low, give 2–4 mL/kg of 25% dextrose (D25) IV (D10 for infant).
- If opiate ingestion is suspected, administer naloxone (0.1 mg/kg IV for infants <5 years of age or <20 kg; 2 mg for older, larger children).
- Correct electrolyte and acid–base abnormalities.
- Empiric treatment with IV antibiotics and acyclovir should be started if bacterial or viral meningitis is suspected.
- Consider benzodiazepine (lorazepam 0.05–0.1 mg/kg IV) for suspected seizure activity, although this may compromise neurologic examination.

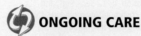

ONGOING CARE

PROGNOSIS

- Prognosis depends on underlying etiology and patient's clinical course. It is not advised to prognosticate too early.
- Serial exams combined with diagnostic tests (electrophysiology, imaging) will provide more complete information.
- The following portend poor prognosis: absent motor responses to painful stimuli on day 3, no spontaneous eye opening after 1 week, bilaterally absent SEP, and isoelectric baseline or burst suppression on EEG at 1 week.
- Conversely, a reactive EEG is associated with improved outcomes. Some of these findings are more firmly established in adults but, in the right clinical context, may be applicable to pediatric patients.

COMPLICATIONS

- Acute coma
  - Brain injury
  - Respiratory failure/aspiration
  - Seizures
  - Infection
- Chronic sequelae
  - Epilepsy
  - New cognitive and/or motor baseline

ADDITIONAL READING

- Abend NS, Licht DJ. Predicting outcome in children with hypoxic-ischemic encephalopathy. *Pediatr Crit Care Med*. 2008;9(1):32–39.
- Gwer S, Gatakaa H, Mwai L, et al. The role for osmotic agents in children with acute encephalopathies: a systematic review. *BMC Pediatr*. 2010;10:23.
- Martin C, Falcone RA Jr. Pediatric traumatic brain injury: an update of research to understand and improve outcomes. *Curr Opin Pediatr*. 2008;20(3):294–299.
- Seshia SS, Bingham WT, Sadanand V. Nontraumatic coma in children and adolescents: diagnosis and management. *Neurol Clin*. 2011;29(4):1007–1043.

CODES

ICD10

- R40.20 Unspecified coma
- R40.1 Stupor
- R40.3 Persistent vegetative state

FAQ

- Q: What is the value of the Pediatric Glasgow Coma Scale (PGCS)?
- A: The PGCS is helpful in predicting prognosis but not for diagnosing the cause of coma. The etiology of coma can impact the usefulness of the scale. For example, PGCS has a better correlation with outcomes following traumatic brain injury than for cold water drowning.
- Q: When a bacterial infection is suspected as a potential etiology of coma, should antibiotic therapy be delayed until CSF has been obtained for testing?
- A: Starting antibiotic therapy prior to obtaining CSF may lead to a false-negative CSF culture. However, if there is any concern for increased ICP or mass effect, a CT should be obtained prior to an LP, and antibiotics should be started in the meantime.

COMMON VARIABLE IMMUNODEFICIENCY

Elena Elizabeth Perez

BASICS

DESCRIPTION

- Common variable immunodeficiency is the most common clinically important primary immunodeficiency syndrome, characterized by
  - Low IgG, IgA, and/or IgM
  - Recurrent infections
  - A wide spectrum of immunologic abnormalities, including autoimmune disease, inflammatory conditions, and the development of lymphomas
- Other terminology for this disease include the following:
  - Acquired hypogammaglobulinemia
  - Adult-onset hypogammaglobulinemia
  - Dysgammaglobulinemia
  - Common variable hypogammaglobulinemia
- Diagnosis of exclusion, requiring low IgG and variable reduction in IgA and/or IgM, impaired specific antibody responses

EPIDEMIOLOGY

- Prevalence is estimated to be 1 in 25,000 to 1 in 66,000 in the general population.
- Can present at any age
  - Most diagnosed between 20 and 40 years old
  - Diagnosis is usually made several years after the onset of recurrent infections (pneumonia, sinusitis, otitis).
- A subgroup of children has been described in which the onset of disease was most often <5 years of age. This group was characterized by a relapsing and remitting course in which autoimmune disease predominated.
- About 20–25% of patients with common variable immunodeficiency have 1 or more autoimmune conditions at time of diagnosis.
- Affects males and females equally

RISK FACTORS

Genetics

- Complex genetics, likely multifactorial
- Rare recessive mutations described in
  - T-cell inducible costimulatory (ICOS) in one kindred, <1% of patients
  - CD19 in a few unrelated families
  - B-cell activating factor (BAFF)
  - CD20 and CD81
  - Transmembrane activator and calcium-modulating cyclophilin ligand interactor (TACI, TNFRSF13B) in 8% of patients, associated with autoimmunity and lymphoid hyperplasia; heterozygous mutation more common than homozygous; significance not clear due to similar mutation found in healthy family members
- IgA deficiency more likely in offspring of parents with common variable immunodeficiency
- Incidence of IgA deficiency, autoimmune disease, and malignancies is increased in family members of patients with common variable immunodeficiency.

PATHOPHYSIOLOGY

- Main characteristic is hypogammaglobulinemia.
- Impaired immunoglobulin and specific antibody production despite normal B cell numbers
- Often increased proportion of immature B cells
- Deficiency of class-switched memory B cells associated with more complex disease (autoimmunity, granulomatous disease, hypersplenism, and lymphoid hyperplasia)
- Functional defects of both B and T lymphocytes are described.

ETIOLOGY

- The primary immunologic defect(s) leading to this syndrome is unknown.
- Multiple defects have been associated with common variable immunodeficiency, including the following:
  - Lack of somatic mutation within variable region genes
  - Lack of memory B cells
  - Impaired maturation, IL-12 secretion, and upregulation of costimulatory molecules by antigen-presenting cells may impair T cells, which are important for providing help to B cells for antibody production.
  - Toll-like receptor 9 (TLR9) response and expression by B cells may also be impaired. TLR signaling pathways are being investigated for their potential role in pathogenesis of common variable immunodeficiency.
- Some genetic defects have been described but do not account for the majority of cases.

DIAGNOSIS

HISTORY

- Recurrent sinopulmonary infections, especially sinusitis and pneumonia, with encapsulated bacteria
- Autoimmune diseases such as autoimmune hemolytic anemia, idiopathic thrombocytopenic purpura, thyroid disease, and chronic active hepatitis
- Localized or systemic granulomatous disease that can be diagnosed years before low IgG is discovered. Lungs, spleen, and lymph nodes are most commonly affected; can be misdiagnosed as sarcoidosis
- Persistent diarrhea of infectious (e.g., *Giardia lamblia*) or noninfectious causes
- Inflammatory bowel disease–like disorder in 6–10% of patients
- Noninfectious, diffuse pulmonary complications described as granulomatous-lymphocytic interstitial lung disease (GLILD) exhibit granulomatous and lymphoproliferative histologic patterns (lymphocytic interstitial pneumonia [LIP], follicular bronchiolitis, and lymphoid hyperplasia).
- Severe or unusual viral infections with herpes simplex, cytomegalovirus, and varicella, such as pneumonitis, hepatitis, or encephalitis. Chronic meningoencephalitis can be seen with enteroviral infection.

PHYSICAL EXAM

- Evaluation should focus on the presence of infection.
- 30% of patients will have lymphadenopathy and/or splenomegaly.

DIAGNOSTIC TESTS & INTERPRETATION

Lab

- IgG, IgA, IgM below age-appropriate norms
- CBC with differential: Examine smear for evidence of hemolysis in autoimmune hemolytic anemia.
- Autoimmune antibody screen: antinuclear antibody, autoantibody panel
- Stool culture for bacteria and ova/parasites to evaluate chronic diarrhea
- Isohemagglutinins as well as functional antibody titers to bacterial antigens such as tetanus, diphtheria, and pneumococcus are usually low to absent.
- Spirometry may be helpful in following chronic lung disease.
- Mitogen/antigen stimulation studies will help assess lymphocyte function.
- T- and B-lymphocyte enumeration by flow cytometry
- B-cell phenotyping becoming more available
- Absent B lymphocytes in males suggests X-linked agammaglobulinemia rather than common variable immunodeficiency.
- Appropriate cultures based on site of infection

Imaging

Chest and sinus x-ray studies/CT scans may be warranted for evaluation of bronchiectasis and chronic disease.

Diagnostic Procedures/Other

- GI endoscopy with biopsies for cases of idiopathic persistent diarrhea
- Lymph node biopsy in suspected malignancy

DIFFERENTIAL DIAGNOSIS

- Other primary antibody deficiency disorders: X-linked agammaglobulinemia, transient hypogammaglobulinemia of infancy, and selective antibody deficiency
- Severe malabsorption with protein-losing enteropathy
- HIV infection
- Chronic lung disease: cystic fibrosis, immotile cilia syndrome, and α_1-antitrypsin deficiency
- Primary autoimmune diseases: immune idiopathic thrombocytopenic purpura, autoimmune hemolytic anemia, systemic lupus erythematosus, thyroiditis

TREATMENT

MEDICATION

First Line

Immunoglobulin replacement therapy

Second Line

Antibiotics as needed for infection may also be used as adjunct to immunoglobulin replacement as prophylaxis.

ADDITIONAL TREATMENT

General Measures

- Monthly IV immunoglobulin replacement
  - Starting dose is usually 400–600 mg/kg/month IV to maintain a trough IgG level of at least 500 mg/dL or FDA-approved formulation(s) for SC administration, given weekly or biweekly following the establishment of intravenous immunoglobulin (IVIG) dosage.
- Appropriate antibiotics for acute infections
- Prophylactic antibiotics may be helpful in chronic/recurrent infections.
- Cautious use of corticosteroids may be necessary in the treatment of GI and autoimmune manifestations.

ISSUES FOR REFERRAL

- Autoimmune manifestations
- GI: chronic abdominal pain or signs of possible lymphoid hyperplasia

INPATIENT CONSIDERATIONS

Nursing

- Supervision during IVIG administration
- Monitor for side effects of therapy.
- Have anaphylaxis medications available.

ONGOING CARE

FOLLOW-UP RECOMMENDATIONS

- Close and frequent follow-up is warranted for patients with severe, recurrent symptoms. It may be as frequent as monthly, depending on symptoms.
- Signs and symptoms suggesting malignancy (e.g., persistent adenopathy in absence of infection, significant weight loss, or abdominal mass) should be evaluated expeditiously.
- Abdominal pain may indicate infection or lymphoid hyperplasia.

Patient Monitoring

CBC with differential, ALT, creatinine, IgG level

PATIENT EDUCATION

Several Web sites available to patients and families:

- Immune Deficiency Foundation: http://primaryimmune.org
- International Patient Organisation for Primary Immunodeficiencies: www.ipopi.org
- The Jeffrey Modell Foundation: www.jmfworld.org
- National Institute of Allergy and Immunology: www.niaid.nih.gov

PROGNOSIS

- Immunoglobulin replacement therapy, prophylactic antibiotics when necessary, and close follow-up by immunology have greatly improved the overall prognosis.
- The newer challenge with this disease is detection and management of autoimmune and other disease-associated complications.
- Phenotypic classifications based on memory B cell numbers divide patients into two major categories: those that do well with IgG replacement alone and others with more likely autoimmune and granulomatous complications.

COMPLICATIONS

- Autoimmune disease in 20% of common variable immunodeficiency patients; most common are autoimmune hemolytic anemia and idiopathic thrombocytopenia purpura.
- GI complications include chronic diarrhea, malabsorption, and weight loss. Inflammatory bowel disease and *Helicobacter pylori* infection have also been observed.
- Granulomatous infiltrations may mimic sarcoidosis.
- Lymphoproliferative disease: Overall risk is 8–10%. The most common are lymphomas, usually non-Hodgkin lymphoma, well differentiated, mostly Epstein-Barr virus negative.
- Chronic sinusitis and lung disease with abnormal pulmonary function tests
- Progressive decline in T-lymphocyte function

ADDITIONAL READING

- Agarwal S, Cunningham-Rundles C. Autoimmunity in common variable immunodeficiency. *Curr Allergy Asthma Rep*. 2009;9(5):347–352.
- Ballow M. Primary immunodeficiency disorders: antibody deficiencies. *J Allergy Clin Immunol*. 2002;109(4):581–591.
- Brant D, Gershwin M. Common variable immune deficiency and autoimmunity. *Autoimmun Rev*. 2006;5(7):465–470.
- Castigli E, Geha R. Molecular basis of common variable immunodeficiency. *J Allergy Clin Immunol*. 2006;117(4):740–746.
- Cunningham-Rundles C. How I treat common variable immunodeficiency. *Blood*. 2010;116(1):7–15.
- Cunningham-Rundles C. Immune deficiency: office evaluation and treatment. *Allergy Asthma Proc*. 2003;24(6):409–415.
- Moratto D, Gulino AV, Fontana S, et al. Combined decrease of defined B and T cell subsets in a group of common variable immunodeficiency patients. *Clin Immunol*. 2006;121(2):203–214.
- Orange JS, Glessner JT, Resnick E, et al. Genome-wide association identifies diverse causes of common variable immunodeficiency. *J Allergy Clin Immunol*. 2011;127(6):1360–1367.e6.
- Park JH, Levinson AI. Granulomatous-lymphocytic interstitial lung disease (GLILD) in CVID. *Clin Immunol*. 2010;134(2):97–103.
- Salzer U, Grimbacher B. Common variable immunodeficiency: the power of costimulation. *Semin Immunol*. 2006;18(6):337–346.
- Simonte S, Cunningham-Rundles C. Update on primary immunodeficiency: defects of lymphocytes. *Clin Immunol*. 2003;109(2):109–118.
- Warantz K, Schlesier M. Flowcytometric phenotyping of common variable immunodeficiency. *Cytometry B Clin Cytom*. 2008;74(5):261–271.

C

CODES

ICD10

- D83.9 Common variable immunodeficiency, unspecified
- D83.0 Com variab immunodef w predom abnlt of B-cell nums & functn
- D83.2 Common variable immunodef w autoantibodies to B- or T-cells

FAQ

- Q: What is the life expectancy of patients with the diagnosis of common variable immunodeficiency?
- A: Because the clinical presentations and symptoms are variable, it is difficult to predict the life expectancy in individual patients. IVIG replacement, in addition to antibiotic therapy, has greatly improved the outlook for these patients. However, despite adequate therapy, a large percentage of patients with common variable immunodeficiency have a progressive decline in immune function. Major morbidity and mortality usually result from the associated complications of malignancy, chronic lung disease, and severe autoimmune disease. In one study, the mortality is estimated at 23–27% over a median follow-up of 7 years (0–25 years). The 20-year survival after diagnosis for males is 64% and for females 67% versus 92% and 94%, respectively, for the general population. Main causes of death include respiratory complications, granulomatous disease of organs, liver disease, malnutrition due to GI pathology, uncontrolled autoimmune manifestations, and lymphoma.
- Q: Should patients with common variable immunodeficiency receive live viral vaccines?
- A: In general, patients receiving IVIG replacement therapy do not require any vaccinations. Live viral vaccines should be avoided in these patients, especially if they have deteriorating immune function.
- Q: Can common variable immunodeficiency be diagnosed prenatally?
- A: Because there are no clear genetic inheritance patterns, prenatal diagnosis is unavailable.

COMPLEMENT DEFICIENCY

Melanie M. Makhija

BASICS

DESCRIPTION

- Complement is a major component of the innate immune system.
  - Consists of plasma and membrane proteins which mediate 3 pathways of cascading enzyme reactions
  - Pathway activation leads to inflammatory and immune responses.
- Deficiencies can arise in any of the proteins, leading to loss of activity of the deficient protein as well as loss of function of proteins that follow in the cascade.
- Inherited deficiencies of the complement components may predispose individuals to infections and autoimmunity.
- Secondary/acquired deficiencies are much more common than inherited deficiencies and are most often caused by increased consumption by immune complexes.

Clinical manifestations of complement deficiencies

Deficiency	Clinical manifestations
C1q,r,s, C2	Systemic lupus erythematosus (SLE), bacterial infections
C4	SLE, autoimmune disorders
C3	Severe infections with encapsulated bacteria (i.e., *Haemophilus influenzae*), glomerulonephritis, immune complex disease
Factor H, I	Secondary C3 deficiency, atypical hemolytic uremic syndrome
Properdin	Males with neisserial and sinopulmonary infections
Factor D	Neisserial infections
MBL, MASP	Infections with encapsulated bacteria, SLE, rheumatoid arthritis
C5, 6, 7, 8, 9	Disseminated neisserial infections
DAF, CD59	Paroxysmal nocturnal hemoglobinuria
C1 inhibitor	Hereditary angioedema (HAE)

EPIDEMIOLOGY

- Complement deficiency accounts for approximately 2% of all primary immune deficiencies.
- Homozygous C2 deficiency 1 in 10,000
- Borderline C4 in 1–3% of Caucasian population
- C9 deficiency almost always found in people of Japanese descent
- C6 deficiency more common in African Americans
- Alternative pathway deficiencies (properdin, factor D) are rare.

RISK FACTORS

Genetics

- Properdin deficiency is X-linked.
- Most other complement deficiencies are autosomal recessive.
- C1 inhibitor deficiency is autosomal dominant.
- Heterozygotes are usually phenotypically normal.

PATHOPHYSIOLOGY

- Classic complement pathway is activated when IgM or IgG antibodies bind to antigen.
- Lectin pathway is activated when a lectin such as mannose-binding lectin (MBL) binds to antigen.
- Alternative pathway does not need antibody or lectins to be activated.
- Main goal of all 3 pathways is to deposit C3b fragments on the target antigen to mark the target for immune response.

ETIOLOGY

- Primary complement deficiencies are hereditary.
- Acquired deficiencies: accelerated consumption by immune complexes (most common), decreased hepatic production (less common), or loss through the urine (rare)

DIAGNOSIS

HISTORY

Indications for evaluating complement system:

- Recurrent pyogenic infections in patients with normal white blood cell count and immunoglobulin levels
- Recurrent neisserial infections (meningitis, sepsis, gonococcal arthritis) at any age
- Multiple family members who have had neisserial infections
- SLE, especially familial lupus: Evaluate for C2 deficiency.
- Recurrent angioedema without urticaria: Evaluate for C1 inhibitor deficiency (HAE).

PHYSICAL EXAM

- Depends on which component is deficient
- Assess for signs and symptoms of autoimmunity (i.e., SLE) and also of bacterial infections and sequelae.
- Failure to thrive
- Recurrent angioedema without urticaria for HAE

DIAGNOSTIC TESTS & INTERPRETATION

Diagnostic Procedures/Other

- Initial lab tests
  - Total hemolytic complement (CH50): Screens for homozygous deficiencies in the classical pathway. All 9 components (C1–C9) required for normal CH50
  - Complement activity is thermolabile and reduced quickly at room temperature. Low levels often due to improper specimen handling
  - Complete deficiency of any component gives undetectable CH50 level.
  - Heterozygotes may have normal CH50.
- AH50
  - To assess integrity of alternate pathway
- Individual component testing
  - Based on clinical history
- C4, C1 esterase inhibitor level and function may be used to evaluate for HAE

DIFFERENTIAL DIAGNOSIS

- Antibody (humoral) deficiency syndromes
- Secondary complement deficiencies

ALERT

- Most common cause of low complement levels is improper specimen handling.
- Secondary deficiency may be caused by consumption of complement components.

TREATMENT

MEDICATION

- There are no specific treatments for most complement deficiencies.
- Aggressive diagnosis and treatment of infections with antibiotics
- HAE prophylaxis and treatment for C1 inhibitor deficiency

ADDITIONAL TREATMENT

General Measures

- Consider prophylactic antibiotics to prevent recurrent infections.
- Vaccination with *Streptococcus pneumoniae* and *Neisseria meningitidis* conjugate vaccines as well as *Haemophilus influenzae* for patients and household contacts
- Can receive other routine vaccines (including live viral vaccines) safely
- Wear medical identification tag identifying condition.
- Plasma infusions impractical over lifetime and risk of development of antibody against missing component

ISSUES FOR REFERRAL

- Should be followed by immunologist
- Monitor for autoimmune disease and refer to rheumatologist for autoimmunity management.
- Genetic counseling for family members

ONGOING CARE

COMPLICATIONS

- Severe infections and sequelae including death
- Immune complex disease
- Autoimmunity

ADDITIONAL READING

- Bonilla FA, Geha RS. Primary immunodeficiency diseases. *J Allergy Clin Immunol*. 2003;111:S571–S581.
- Frank MM. Complement deficiencies. *Pediatr Clin North Am*. 2000;47(6):1339–1354.
- Frank M. Complement disorders and hereditary angioedema. *J Allergy Clin Immunol*. 2010;125(2)(Suppl. 2):S262–S271.
- Walport MJ. Complement. First of two parts. *N Engl J Med*. 2001;344(14):1058–1066.
- Walport MJ. Complement. Second of two parts. *N Engl J Med*. 2001;344(15):1140–1144.

CODES

ICD10

D84.1 Defects in the complement system

FAQ

- Q: When should I evaluate for a complement deficiency?
- A: Any child with recurrent sinopulmonary infections or >1 episode of a neisserial infection.

CONCUSSION

Evelyn Porter • Andrea Marmor

BASICS

DESCRIPTION

- Concussion is a complex pathophysiologic process affecting the brain, induced by traumatic biomechanical forces.
- There is a graded set of clinical symptoms that define concussion, which may or may not involve a loss of consciousness.
- Concussion may be caused either by a direct blow to the head or a blow to the face, neck, or elsewhere on the body with an "impulsive" force transmitted to the head.
- Concussion typically results in the rapid onset of short-lived impairment of neurologic function that resolves spontaneously. In a small percentage of children, postconcussive symptoms may be prolonged.
- Concussion may result in pathologic changes, but the acute clinical symptoms largely reflect a functional rather than structural injury and no abnormality is seen on standard neuroimaging studies.

EPIDEMIOLOGY

- A recent review estimated that up to 3.8 million recreation- and sport-related concussions occur annually in the United States.
- Concussion is underreported.
- Most common sports include football, ice hockey, soccer, wrestling, lacrosse, basketball, baseball, softball, field hockey, and volleyball.
- Although concussion is overall more common in boys, girls have higher rates of concussion than boys in similar sports.
- Risk of injury depends on game, position, prior concussion, and use of helmet.

GENERAL PREVENTION

- Nothing has been shown to prevent concussion.
- Helmet use is essential at reducing the severity of a blow to the head.
- Given that children may have a sense of invulnerability and desire to return to usual activities quickly, preparticipation medical visits should emphasize that reporting concussion immediately is essential and that loss of consciousness is not the only manifestation of concussion.

PATHOPHYSIOLOGY

- The brain is buoyed in the cranium by cerebrospinal fluid that acts as protective insulation. With acceleration–deceleration, the brain continues to experience momentum and strikes against bone. The temporal and frontal lobes are particularly prone to injury because of their location adjacent to irregular parts of the skull.
- Depressed level of consciousness is thought to be the result of rotational stretch injury to the reticular activating system in the dorsal aspect of the brainstem.
- Pathologic changes after concussion include alterations in neuronal depolarization and neurotransmitter release, impaired axonal function, decreased cerebral blood flow, and altered brain autoregulation and glucose metabolism.
- Children may respond to brain trauma differently than adults due to developmental factors such as brain size, brain water content, myelination level, skull and suture geometry and elasticity, and differential skull to body proportions.

DIAGNOSIS

HISTORY

- Detailed history of traumatic event
- Detailed symptom evaluation
- History of prior concussions, including surrounding circumstances
- History of preexisting cognitive or attention problems should be elicited to help guide interpretation of postinjury testing.

SIGNS AND SYMPTOMS

- Standardized, validated instruments for mental status testing are available and can be administered quickly on the sideline (i.e., Sport Concussion Assessment Tool 2 [SCAT-2])
- Postconcussive symptoms may be divided into 4 domains:
  - Somatic: headaches, fatigue, decreased energy, nausea, vision change, tinnitus, dizziness, incoordination, and balance difficulty
  - Emotional/behavioral: irritability, increased emotionality, personality change, depression, or anxiety
  - Cognitive: slowed thinking and response time; impaired concentration, learning, and/or memory; and reduced problem-solving ability
  - Sleep disturbances are common.

PHYSICAL EXAM

- Onsite and acute evaluation should include the usual ABCs and evaluation for potential associated injuries such as cervical spinal injury.
- A detailed neurologic examination should be performed to detect focal signs suggestive of serious neurologic impairment and to allow accurate observation over time.
- Mental status: orientation (person, place, time), concentration (digit span), and memory (anterograde and retrograde)
- Cranial nerves: pupil reactivity, eye movements (particularly smooth pursuit and saccadic movements), visual fields, face movement and sensation, tongue protrusion
- Motor: strength and tone
- Sensory: gross sensory deficits
- Cerebellar: agility, finger-to-nose-to-finger, rapid alternating movements (finger tapping, toe tapping), tandem gait (forward and backward, eyes open and closed)
- Exertion provocative tests: 5 push-ups, 5 sit-ups, 5 knee bends, 40-yard sprint; look for change in symptoms/exam.

DIAGNOSTIC TESTS & INTERPRETATION

Imaging

- Structural lesions are absent on standard CT and MRI in concussion.
- Computed tomography of the head (HCT) is the test of choice in the acute evaluation of suspected intracranial hemorrhage or skull fracture in head trauma.
- Decision rules exist to determine those children at low risk for clinically important brain injury who may not need an HCT.
- There is increased suspicion of intracranial injury in patients with abnormal mental status, non-frontal scalp hematoma, prolonged loss of consciousness, severe injury mechanism, palpable skull fracture, vomiting, and severe headache.
- MRI is the imaging modality of choice in the subacute or chronic evaluation of concussion

Diagnostic Procedures/Other

Neuropsychological testing: Computerized testing is now widely available and baseline testing is being performed by many school athletic departments. Research is still needed regarding the optimum timing of this testing and whether it improves outcome.

TREATMENT

GENERAL MEASURES

- Remove the child from the activity with no return to play if concussion is suspected.
- Monitor the athlete for several hours after the injury to evaluate for any deterioration.
- Consider referral to the emergency department if there is repeated vomiting, severe or worsening headache, seizure, unsteady gait, slurred speech, weakness or numbness in the extremities, unusual behavior, signs of a basilar skull fracture, or a GCS <15.
- There is currently no evidence-based research on the use of any medication in the treatment of the concussed pediatric athlete.

ISSUES FOR REFERRAL

- Neuropsychological evaluation should be considered in children with multiple concussions or when recovery is not progressing as expected. This evaluation can document impairment, identify factors contributing to persisting difficulties, and guide school accommodations or formal intervention.
- If admitted for observation, consults by speech therapy, physical therapy, and psychiatry should be considered to evaluate for subtle sequelae.

SURGERY/OTHER PROCEDURES

Neurosurgical evaluation or transfer to a trauma center should be considered for symptoms of prolonged unconsciousness, persistent mental status alterations, worsening postconcussive symptoms, abnormalities on neurologic examination, or abnormalities on neuroimaging.

INPATIENT CONSIDERATIONS

Admission Criteria

Consider admission if the child continues to have altered level of consciousness, if focal neurologic signs are present, or if patient remains severely symptomatic.

Nursing

If observation is required, nursing staff must be able to perform neurologic assessments at regular intervals.

Discharge Criteria

- Planning must be individualized depending on severity of symptoms, family support, and presence of associated injuries.
- The child and guardian should receive return to play guidelines focused on avoiding repeat concussions as concussions have a cumulative effect and result in increased vulnerability to future injuries.
- No athlete should return to play while still symptomatic from a concussion. This includes physical, cognitive, or behavioral symptoms. There must be no symptoms or signs at rest or during exertion.
- Activities with a high cognitive demand should be limited while symptomatic, including television, computer, videogames, and texting. School accommodations may be needed.
- Before considering return to play, any medication to reduce symptoms must be stopped and the athlete must be symptom-free off medications.
- Return to play should occur in a gradual fashion while monitoring for symptoms because symptoms may be aggravated with exertion. Consider in sequence light aerobic activity, noncontact sport–related activity, full practice, and then game play.
- Retirement should be considered for any athlete who has sustained 3 concussions in an individual season or has had postconcussive symptoms for more than 3 months, when recovery requires an increasing amount of time, or when concussions occur with less forceful injury.

ONGOING CARE

FOLLOW-UP RECOMMENDATIONS

Patient Monitoring

If the patient is discharged home for observation, the guardian should have detailed instruction regarding reasons to return to the ED. These include difficulty awakening or staying awake, worsening headache or dizziness, emesis, seizures, blood or clear fluid from the ears or nose, major changes in behavior, or any focal weakness/sensory/vision changes.

PROGNOSIS

- In general, the prognosis is excellent but depends on the severity of the injury.
- The typical adult patient with a concussion will recover to baseline function in 6–12 weeks.
- Athletes and children usually recover in 48 hours. However, children with previous head injury, learning difficulties, or neurologic, psychiatric, or family problems may continue to show significant ongoing problems at 3 months.
- Chronic headaches, persistent difficulty with short- and long-term memory, and episodic confusion are common sequelae of the cumulative damage that occurs with repeated concussive injuries.

COMPLICATIONS

- Postconcussion symptoms such as confusion; altered concentration, memory, and problem solving; irritability; emotional changes; and headaches may take several months to resolve.
- Serious head injury may occur and requires immediate neurosurgical evaluation and neurocritical care. Serial HCT imaging may be necessary as intracranial lesions, such as contusion or hemorrhages (epidural, subdural, intraparenchymal), can expand. These may occur with or without skull fracture and may occur without an initial loss of consciousness.

ADDITIONAL READING

- Centers for Disease Control and Prevention. Nonfatal traumatic brain injuries related to sports and recreation activities among persons aged ≤19 years—United States, 2001-2009. *MMWR Morb Mortal Wkly Rep*. 2011;60(39):1337–1342.
- Giza CC, Kutcher JS, Ashwal S, et al. Summary of evidence-based guideline update: evaluation and management of concussion in sports: report of the Guideline Development Subcommittee of the American Academy of Neurology. *Neurology*. 2013;80(24):2250–2257.
- Halstead ME, Walter KD; The Council on Sports Medicine and Fitness. Clinical report–sport-related concussion in children and adolescents. *Pediatrics*. 2010;126(3):597–615.
- Kuppermann N, Holmes JF, Dayan PS, et al; Pediatric Emergency Care Applied Research Network. Identification of children at very low risk of clinically-important brain injuries after head trauma: a prospective cohort study. *Lancet*. 2009;374(9696):1160–1170.
- McCrory P, Meeuwisse W, Johnston K, et al. Consensus statement on concussion in Sport 3rd International Conference on Concussion in Sport held in Zurich, November 2008. *Clin J Sports Med*. 2009;19(3):185–200.
- U.S. Department of Health and Human Services. *Centers for Disease Control and Prevention. Heads Up toolkits*. Atlanta, GA: Centers for Disease Control and Prevention; 2005.

CODES

ICD10

- S06.0X0A Concussion without loss of consciousness, initial encounter
- F07.81 Postconcussional syndrome
- R41.3 Other amnesia

CONGENITAL ADRENAL HYPERPLASIA

Erica A. Eugster

BASICS

DESCRIPTION

Congenital adrenal hyperplasia (CAH) refers to a group of autosomal recessive disorders that have in common the deficiency of an enzyme needed for cortisol biosynthesis. The disease exists along a spectrum of severity and is typically subdivided into "classic" (severe) and "nonclassic" (milder) forms.

- There are 5 specific causes of CAH:
  - 21-hydroxylase deficiency
  - 11-hydroxylase deficiency
  - 3β-hydroxysteroid dehydrogenase deficiency
  - 17α-hydroxylase deficiency
  - Congenital lipoid hyperplasia (stAR mutation)
- The vast majority of cases of CAH (~95%) are due to 21-hydroxylase (21OHase) deficiency, which will therefore be the focus of this chapter. The 21OHase enzyme is in the glucocorticoid and mineralocorticoid biosynthetic pathways.

EPIDEMIOLOGY

- The incidence of classic CAH is 1:10,000–1:20,000 live births.
  - More common in certain ethnic groups and in remote areas.
  - ~75% of cases are characterized by overt salt wasting due to mineralocorticoid deficiency, whereas the remaining cases are described as simply virilizing.
- The prevalence of non-classic CAH (also called late-onset) is approximately 1:1,000.
  - More common in some ethnicities such as Ashkenazi, Italian, and Yugoslavian and may be as common as 1:50 individuals in these groups.

RISK FACTORS

Genetics

- CAH is caused by mutations in the *CYP21A2* gene, which is located on chromosome 6p21.3 and encodes for the 21OHase enzyme. This locus is characterized by many overlapping transcripts and a high rate of recombination.
- Most mutations involve large deletions or arise from the transfer of small sequences of the nearby pseudogene *CYP21A1P* during meiosis. More than 100 different *CYP21A2* mutations are known. Most patients are compound heterozygotes, with the phenotype reflecting the milder mutation. Approximately 1% of mutations are estimated to arise de novo and uniparental disomy has been reported in one case.
- Although genotype–phenotype correlations are generally high, the genetic complexity of CAH renders them sometimes problematic.

PATHOPHYSIOLOGY

- The enzymatic block in cortisol biosynthesis results in diminished negative feedback at the level of the hypothalamus and pituitary gland with a subsequent increase in CRH and ACTH. The buildup of precursors proximal to the block results in increased adrenal androgen production. Variable degrees of mineralocorticoid deficiency cause salt wasting and contribute to the risk of adrenal crisis. The clinical consequences of this process vary according to gender and to the severity of the CAH (Appendix, Table 13).
- Classic CAH; genetic females
  - Androgen excess during early prenatal life (1st trimester) results in ambiguous genitalia. Typical features include elongation of the urethra, development of a urogenital sinus, and enlargement of the clitoris.
  - Development of the internal reproductive structures is unaffected.
  - If not diagnosed and treated early, progressive virilization occurs postnatally. Girls with salt-wasting CAH are also at risk for an adrenal crisis.
- Classis CAH; genetic males
  - Prenatal androgen exposure has no clinical consequence in infant boys with CAH. However, infant boys with salt-wasting CAH are at risk for an adrenal crisis.
  - As with girls, if not diagnosed and treated early, progressive virilization occurs postnatally.
- Non-classic CAH; females
  - The far milder degree of androgen excess in non-classic CAH has no effect during embryologic development but can result in symptoms of hyperandrogenism during childhood, adolescence, or adulthood.
- Non-classic CAH; males
  - Symptoms of androgen excess can occur during childhood, adolescence, or adulthood.

DIAGNOSIS

HISTORY

- Any family history of CAH should be sought as well as any history of exposures and/or maternal virilization during pregnancy. In infants, poor feeding, lethargy, and vomiting are important potential clues to an impending adrenal crisis.
- Children with previously undiagnosed CAH typically present with precocious puberty due to androgen excess. Typical symptoms in classic CAH include adult body odor, acne, pubic and axillary hair, penile enlargement in boys, clitoromegaly in girls, and linear growth acceleration. Symptoms of nonclassic CAH during childhood are usually limited to adult body odor and early pubic/axillary hair.
- Symptoms of CAH in adolescent girls include irregular periods, hirsutism, and acne.

PHYSICAL EXAM

- Classic CAH; genetic females
  - Ambiguous genitalia in infant girls with classic CAH exists along a continuum known as the Prader scale. Prader 1 is a typical female, whereas Prader 5 denotes the most extreme degree of masculinization in which the urethral opening is at the tip of the clitoris and complete labial fusion has occurred. Thus, a male sex assignment is sometimes mistakenly made. This scenario is the rationale for the admonition "Never circumcise a male infant with bilaterally nonpalpable testes!"
  - Most girls with classic CAH are Prader 3 or 4. Significant clitoromegaly will be present along with increased rugation and pigmentation of the labioscrotal structures but no palpable gonads. Posterior labial fusion and a single perineal opening is usually found.
  - Physical findings in the setting of salt wasting are nonspecific but would include low weight percentile, poor skin turgor, dry mucous membranes, and vital signs suggesting dehydration.
  - Although the vast majority of infant girls with classic CAH are diagnosed in the newborn period, occasional cases are missed. If this occurs, the external genitalia will exhibit the same features as in infancy. Other signs of hyperandrogenism will be present such as pubic hair and extreme tall stature from linear growth acceleration. The presence of a urogenital sinus and posterior labial fusion indicate 1st-trimester androgen excess, whereas androgen exposure after this critical period results in clitoromegaly only.
- Classic CAH; genetic males
  - Although average penile size in newborn boys with classic CAH is increased, the external genitalia appear normal and thus there is nothing on physical exam to alert providers to the presence of CAH. As is the case in girls, physical exam findings associated with salt wasting include low weight percentile, poor skin turgor, dry mucous membranes, and vital signs indicating dehydration.
  - Boys with classic CAH who are missed in infancy come to medical attention due to early secondary sexual development. On physical exam, tall stature, adult body odor, acne, pubic and axillary hair, and penile enlargement are seen. A hallmark of CAH and other forms of peripheral precocious puberty in boys is a prepubertal testicular volume, indicating a source of sex steroids other than the HPG axis.
- Nonclassic CAH; females
  - Girls with nonclassic CAH have pubic and/or axillary hair, adult body odor, and ± acne. Adolescent girls typically have hirsutism. Mild clitoromegaly may also be seen.

- Nonclassic CAH; males
  - Boys with nonclassic CAH will also have signs of mild androgen excess on physical exam including pubic and axillary hair, adult body odor, and acne.

DIAGNOSTIC TESTS & INTERPRETATION

Lab

- CAH is included on the newborn screen in all 50 states. The biochemical hallmark is an elevated 17-hydroxyprogesterone (17OHP). Depending on the 17OHP concentration, a repeat newborn screen or a serum concentration is obtained. In any presumptive positive case, serum electrolytes need to be monitored closely for early detection of an adrenal crisis. False positives are extremely common in preterm and sick neonates. An elevated plasma renin will confirm overt salt wasting.
- Any report of an abnormal newborn screen for CAH, particularly in a term infant male, should be considered an emergency.
- Serum 17OHP is also the diagnostic test for classic CAH that was missed in the newborn period and for nonclassic CAH. Testosterone, dehydroepiandrosterone-sulfate (DHEAS), and androstenedione should also be measured.

Imaging

- In infants with ambiguous genitalia, a pelvic ultrasound and genitogram are often performed. In girls with CAH, a normal uterus is seen on ultrasound, whereas a urogenital sinus, "male-type" urethra, and cervical impression are typical findings on genitogram. No routine imaging is performed in infant boys with CAH. However, periodic testicular ultrasound to detect adrenal rest tumors is recommended starting in adolescence, particularly in boys whose CAH is poorly controlled as evidenced by chronic elevations in 17OHP concentrations.
- A bone age x-ray is an important part of the evaluation in children with precocious puberty. In the setting of undiagnosed classic CAH, skeletal maturation will be markedly advanced.

Diagnostic Procedures/Other

- In equivocal cases, a full ACTH stimulation test can distinguish between classic and nonclassic CAH, affected individuals and heterozygous carriers, and between 21OHase deficiency and other forms of CAH.
- Genotyping can also confirm the diagnosis and is helpful for genetic counseling. However, complete sequencing (rather than targeted mutation analysis) of the *CYP21A2* gene may be necessary to accurately determine genotype because complex genetic variations are often present.

DIFFERENTIAL DIAGNOSIS

- CAH is the most common 46,XX disorder of sex development. Other causes for ambiguous genitalia are outlined in other chapters.
- The differential diagnosis of classic CAH presenting during childhood includes etiologies of androgen excess such as an androgen-secreting tumor or exogenous exposures. In boys, a β-hCG–producing tumor, McCune-Albright syndrome, and familial male precocious puberty should be considered.
- Nonclassic CAH presenting during childhood is often indistinguishable from premature adrenarche. In adolescent girls, the differential diagnosis includes PCOS, which also shares many clinical features with nonclassic CAH.

TREATMENT

MEDICATION

- Medical treatment of CAH consists of glucocorticoid therapy in doses sufficient to suppress adrenal androgen overproduction, which are generally considered to be 10–15 mg/m^2/24 h hydrocortisone equivalent.
- Regardless of salt-wasting status, current recommendations also endorse mineralocorticoid therapy in all patients with classic CAH in the form of Florinef 0.05–0.2 mg/24 h.
- Salt supplementation (NaCl 3–5 mEq/kg/24 h) is also needed during infancy.

ADDITIONAL TREATMENT

Girls with CAH usually undergo genital surgery in the form of a feminizing genitoplasty. However, whether and when such surgery should be performed is controversial.

General Measures

ALERT

Stress-dose glucocorticoid coverage during illness or injury is essential in patients with CAH.

ONGOING CARE

Ongoing clinic visits and monitoring of growth, puberty, and hormonal studies (including serial measurements of 17OHP) are standard of care. Psychological support and educational materials should be provided on a regular basis.

PROGNOSIS

- Adult height is normal when CAH is well controlled but is compromised in poorly controlled or late-diagnosed cases.
- Girls with classic CAH may exhibit boy-typical behaviors but have normal female gender identity.
- Fertility is decreased in women with classic CAH compared to the general population.
- Fertility may be impaired in men with CAH if testicular adrenal rest tumors are present.
- Transition to adulthood ideally takes place in the context of a multidisciplinary team.

ADDITIONAL READING

- Auchus RJ, Witchel SF, Leight KR, et al. Guidelines for the development of comprehensive care centers for congenital adrenal hyperplasia: guidance from the CARES Foundation initiative. *Int J Pediatr Endocrinol*. 2010;2010:275213.
- Finkielstain GP, Chen W, Mehta SP, et al. Comprehensive genetic analysis of 182 unrelated families with congenital adrenal hyperplasia due to 21- hydroxylase deficiency. *J Clin Endocrinol Metab*. 2011;96(1):E161–E172.
- Nebesio TD, Eugster EA. Growth and reproductive outcomes in congenital adrenal hyperplasia. *Int J Pediatr Endocrinol*. 2010;2010:298937.
- Speiser PW, Azziz R, Baskin LS, et al. Congenital adrenal hyperplasia due to steroid 21-hydroxylase deficiency: an Endocrine Society clinical practice guideline. *J Clin Endocrinol Metab*. 2010;95(9):4133–4160.
- Speiser PW, White PC. Congenital adrenal hyperplasia. *N Engl J Med*. 2003;349(8):776–788.

CODES

ICD10

E25.0 Congenital adrenogenital disorders assoc w enzyme deficiency

FAQ

- Q: When does a salt-wasting crisis usually occur in newborns with CAH?
- A: The most common time is between days 5 and 10 of life. However, it may occur as early as on day 1 of life or not until many weeks or months later.
- Q: When should children with CAH be given a "stress dose" and what does this consist of?
- A: Double or triple the usual glucocorticoid dose is considered a stress dose. This should be given at times of illness or psychological stress. However, if a child is vomiting, an emergency Solu-Cortef injection should be given. Hydrocortisone 100 mg/m^2 IV is given prior to any surgery.
- Q: What is the best form of glucocorticoid treatment in children with CAH?
- A: Hydrocortisone has long been considered the optimal glucocorticoid in CAH. However, this is controversial, and some patients do well on prednisone or dexamethasone.
- Q: Should extremely virilized girls with CAH be sex-assigned male?
- A: Because fertility and gender identity are normal in girls with CAH, the current consensus is to raise these girls female regardless of the extent of virilization.

CONGENITAL HEPATIC FIBROSIS

Mansi D. Amin • Eric H. Chiou • Kristin L. Van Buren

BASICS

DESCRIPTION

- Congenital hepatic fibrosis (CHF) is an inherited, noncirrhotic liver disease.
- Prominent clinical features include the following:
  - Portal hypertension
  - Increased risk of ascending cholangitis
- Liver biopsy shows the classic lesion of ductal plate malformation.
- Majority of patients with CHF have associated autosomal recessive polycystic kidney disease (ARPKD). However, several other genetic diseases also result in CHF.

EPIDEMIOLOGY

- The incidence of ARPKD is 1/20,000–1/40,000 live births.
- Carrier frequency of *PKHD1* mutation in the general population is ~1:70.

RISK FACTORS

Genetics

- Inheritance is autosomal recessive in most families, but X-linked and autosomal dominant patterns are also seen.
- Penetrance is 100% but marked intrafamilial variation in severity is observed.
- *PKHD1*, the ARPKD/CHF disease gene, is located on chromosome 6p12.
  - The gene is large, consisting of at least 86 exons extending over 469 kb of genomic DNA.
  - It is expressed at high levels in fetal and adult kidneys and at lower levels in the liver and pancreas.
- More than 300 mutations of the *PKHD1* gene have been reported with variable rates of progression of hepatic/renal disease, even with the same *PKHD1* mutation, indicating the presence of modifier genes.
  - Mutations of the *PKHD1* gene include frameshift, nonsense, and out-of-frame splicing alterations that are consistent with a loss of function mechanism.
  - The presence of 2 truncating mutations leads to the most severe phenotype, associated with death in the neonatal period.
- The *PKHD1* gene product is a protein called polyductin or fibrocystin.
  - Transmembrane protein
  - Located mostly on the primary cilia and apical surface of renal tubular cells and cholangiocytes
  - It complexes with polycystin 1 and polycystin 2, the mutated proteins in autosomal dominant polycystic kidney disease (ADPKD).
  - Together, the complex is thought to function as mechanotransducer, detecting the shear force from urine and bile flow. Further studies will be needed to identify the biologic function of polyductin and to determine how mutations of the protein cause disease.

PATHOPHYSIOLOGY

- Ductal plate malformation is a characteristic histologic lesion of the liver, implying a disturbance of the normal development of the bile ducts.
- Hallmarks include the following:
  - Irregularly shaped, dilated, proliferating bile ducts, often described as staghorn shaped
  - Noninflammatory periportal fibrosis
  - Normal appearance of hepatocytes and lobular architecture
- The primary defect in ARPKD may be linked to ciliary dysfunction.
  - The ciliary structure is abnormal in ARPKD renal tubule cells and cholangiocytes.
- Developmental abnormalities involve the liver and kidneys and, less commonly, the vasculature and the heart.
- Portal hypertension is thought to result from the fibrosis in the portal tracts as well as, in some patients, from portal vein abnormalities.

COMMONLY ASSOCIATED CONDITIONS

- Portal hypertension leading to varices and hypersplenism
- Hepatomegaly
- Systemic hypertension
- Renal dysfunction
- Cholangitis
- Conditions associated with the finding of ductal plate malformation/CHF:
  - ARPKD; most frequent association
  - ADPKD, rare
  - Caroli syndrome (CHF and intrahepatic bile duct dilation)
  - Juvenile nephronophthisis
  - Congenital disorder of glycosylation type 1b (phosphomannose isomerase deficiency)
  - Congenital malformation syndromes
    - Meckel Gruber syndrome
    - Joubert syndrome
    - Jeune syndrome
    - Bardet-Biedl syndrome

DIAGNOSIS

HISTORY

- Severely affected patients are usually diagnosed in utero or shortly after birth due to massively enlarged cystic kidneys.
  - Prenatal renal dysfunction may result in pulmonary hypoplasia.
- Older patients may present with systemic hypertension or signs of portal hypertension and esophageal variceal bleeding.
- Patients may present with fever and jaundice (cholangitis) or, rarely, with signs of liver failure.

PHYSICAL EXAM

- Firm, enlarged liver with a prominent left lobe
- Splenomegaly
- Kidneys may be palpable on abdominal exam.

DIAGNOSTIC TESTS & INTERPRETATION

Lab

- Thrombocytopenia and leukopenia are associated with hypersplenism.
- Liver enzymes and bilirubin are typically normal; transaminases may be mildly elevated in some patients.
- Usually, hepatic synthetic function (albumin, prothrombin time) is normal.
- May see elevated blood urea nitrogen and creatinine with renal involvement
- Genetic testing is available and consultation is recommended.

Imaging

- Complete abdominal ultrasound with Doppler
  - Increased hepatic echogenicity
  - Splenomegaly
  - Evidence of portal hypertension, portal vein patency, and decreased flow variability
  - Cystic kidneys
- Magnetic resonance cholangiopancreatography (MRCP) can further characterize the biliary system in Caroli syndrome.

Diagnostic Procedures/Other

- Liver biopsy
  - Characteristic histology of ductal plate malformation
  - If cholangitis is suspected clinically, send specimen for bacterial culture.

DIFFERENTIAL DIAGNOSIS

Varies with presentation. Usually, differential diagnosis is that of early cirrhosis or idiopathic portal hypertension.

C

TREATMENT

MEDICATION

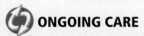

Choleretic agents, including ursodeoxycholic acid, are used in bile stasis.

ADDITIONAL TREATMENT

General Measures

- Monitor growth, weight gain, nutritional status, and for vitamin A, D, E, K malabsorption.
- Suspected cholangitis should be managed with blood culture, antibiotics to cover gram-negative rods, and +/− liver biopsy. Some patients with chronic cholangitis may require antibiotic prophylaxis.
- Endoscopic variceal banding and/or sclerotherapy provide prevention and treatment of esophageal variceal hemorrhage in many cases.
- Activity
  - No contact sports if splenomegaly is present.
  - Spleen guard may be used to protect against injury from abdominal trauma.

SURGERY/OTHER PROCEDURES

- Portosystemic shunting may be needed but should be considered in the context of kidney function given ammonia disposal occurs renally.
- Liver transplant may be indicated for chronic cholangitis, recurrent bleeding, or progressive hepatic disease.
- Children who require transplantation should be considered for combined liver and renal transplantation.

ONGOING CARE

FOLLOW-UP RECOMMENDATIONS

Patient Monitoring

- Acute upper GI tract bleeding or melena requires urgent EGD for bleeding control, frequent Hgb/Hct checks, blood cultures, IV proton pump inhibitor, antibiotics, and possible need for octreotide drip in the ICU setting.
- Platelet count is the best predictor of pulmonary hypertension severity; an acute drop could indicate hepatorenal syndrome.
- Morbidity and mortality occurs mainly from variceal bleeding and cholangitis.
- Systemic hypertension and kidney function must be monitored.
- Early referral to a hepatologist, nephrologist, and transplant center is indicated in neonatal disease.

DIET

No restrictions are needed unless secondary to renal disease.

PROGNOSIS

- Substantial variability in severity and progression of clinical manifestation exists.
- Bleeding from varices is a major cause of morbidity and mortality.
- Ascending cholangitis with resultant sepsis is a major cause of morbidity and mortality.
- Those presenting during childhood have better prognosis compared to those presenting within the neonatal period.
- Need for eventual liver +/− kidney transplantation needs to be considered.

COMPLICATIONS

- Portal hypertension with hypersplenism and variceal bleeding (chronic, common)
- Cholangitis: acute and recurrent, significant cause of morbidity in Caroli syndrome
- Renal and/or hepatic failure
- Associated vascular anomalies in the liver and brain
- Increased risk of hepatocellular or cholangiocarcinoma in adulthood; screening in pediatric population is not warranted.
- Systemic hypertension owing to renal involvement

ADDITIONAL READING

- Badano JL, Mitsuma N, Beales PL, et al. The ciliopathies: an emerging class of human genetic disorders. *Annu Rev Genomics Hum Genet*. 2006;7:125–148.
- Buscher R, Buscher AK, Weber S, et al. Clinical manifestations of autosomal recessive polycystic kidney disease (ARPKD): kidney-related and non-kidney related phenotypes. *Pediatr Nephrol*. 2014;29(10):1915–1925.
- Gunay-Aygun M, Avner ED, Bacallao RL, et al. Autosomal recessive polycystic kidney disease and congenital hepatic fibrosis: summary statement of a first National Institutes of Health/Office of Rare Diseases conference. *J Pediatr*. 2006;149(2):159–164.
- Gunay-Aygun M, Font-Montgomery E, Lukose L, et al. Characteristics of congenital hepatic fibrosis in a large cohort of patients with autosomal recessive polycystic kidney disease. *Gastroenterology*. 2013;144(1):112–121.
- Harris PC, Rossetti S. Molecular genetics of autosomal recessive polycystic kidney disease. *Mol Genet Metab*. 2004;81(2):75–85.
- Rawat D, Kelly DA, Milford DV, et al. Phenotypic variation and long-term outcomes in children with congenital hepatic fibrosis. *J Pediatr Gastroenterol Nutr*. 2013;57(2):161–166.

CODES

ICD10

- P78.89 Other specified perinatal digestive system disorders
- K76.6 Portal hypertension
- K83.0 Cholangitis

FAQ

- Q: Will other children of mine be affected?
- A: Maybe. The inheritance pattern is autosomal recessive, with the possibility of an affected sibling being 1:4.
- Q: Is my child at increased risk if he contracts viral hepatitis?
- A: Yes. The underlying liver disease places these patients at increased risk. They should be immunized against hepatitis A and B.
- Q: If my child has a fever, does she need to be seen by her doctor?
- A: Yes. Patients with CHF who have fever without an obvious source should be evaluated for possible cholangitis, at least by obtaining a blood culture and liver enzymes.

CONGESTIVE HEART FAILURE

Jondavid Menteer

BASICS

DESCRIPTION

Heart failure (HF) is the pathophysiologic state in which the heart is unable to pump sufficient blood to meet the metabolic demands of the body.

RISK FACTORS

- In utero
  - Arrhythmias: supraventricular or ventricular tachycardia, complete heart block (CHB)
  - Volume overload: atrioventricular (AV) valve regurgitation or arteriovenous malformation (AVM)
  - Primary myocardial disease: cardiomyopathy (dilated, hypertrophic), myocarditis
  - Anemia: Rh isoimmune disease, thalassemia, and twin-twin transfusion
  - Premature closure of ductus arteriosus with isolated right ventricular failure
- In neonates
  - Myocardial dysfunction: asphyxia, acidosis, myocarditis, hypoglycemia, cardiomyopathy (dilated, hypertrophic, ventricular noncompaction), ischemia (anomalous left coronary artery from the pulmonary artery), metabolic defects, or pressure overload imposed by aortic stenosis, pulmonary hypertension, or coarctation of the aorta
  - Volume overload: atrial septal defect (ASD) (large), ventricular septal defect (VSD) (large), patent ductus arteriosus (PDA) (moderate to large), truncus arteriosus, aortopulmonary window, anomalous pulmonary venous return, AVM in any location
  - Arrhythmias: supraventricular or ventricular tachycardia, CHB
  - Left heart inlet obstruction: mitral stenosis, cor triatriatum, pulmonary venous obstruction
  - Note: Certain cyanotic heart diseases such as hypoplastic left heart syndrome may present with elevated pulmonary blood flow or depressed systemic blood flow and minimal desaturation. These patients may have HF in the 1st day of life due to increased pulmonary circulation or due to shock from ductal closure.
- In infants
  - Myocardial dysfunction: cardiomyopathy (dilated, hypertrophic, restrictive, ventricular noncompaction), endocardial fibroelastosis, metabolic/mitochondrial diseases, myocarditis, Kawasaki disease, anomalous left coronary artery from pulmonary artery, or chronic pressure overload due to coarctation of the aorta or aortic stenosis
  - Volume overload: ASD (large), VSD, PDA, common AV canal defect, partial anomalous pulmonary venous connections.
  - Secondary causes: renal disease (volume overload, electrolyte disturbance), hypertension, hypothyroidism, sepsis
  - Arrhythmias: supraventricular or ventricular tachycardia, CHB
  - Pericardial effusion due to juvenile rheumatoid arthritis (JRA), systemic lupus erythematosus (SLE), other inflammatory diseases, or following repair of congenital heart disease (CHD)
- In childhood and adolescence:
  - Unrepaired CHD with volume and/or pressure overload
  - Repaired CHD with residual defects that result in volume and/or pressure overload
  - Acquired heart disease: pericarditis, myocarditis, endocarditis, acute rheumatic fever
  - Cor pulmonale (pulmonary hypertension, Eisenmenger syndrome, chronic lung disease)
  - Cardiomyopathy due to primary myocardial disease (dilated, hypertrophic, restrictive, ventricular noncompaction), chemotherapy (anthracyclines), radiation therapy, sickle cell anemia, thalassemia, neuromuscular disease (e.g., Duchenne or Becker muscular dystrophy)

GENERAL PREVENTION

- Limited use of anthracycline drugs in cancer therapy
- Prompt treatment (within 10 days) of streptococcal pharyngitis to prevent rheumatic fever
- SBE prophylaxis to prevent infective endocarditis

ALERT

- In patients with HF due to large left-to-right shunts, long-term spontaneous clinical improvement of HF with decreased murmur may indicate the development of pulmonary vascular disease (Eisenmenger syndrome), eventually leading to cyanosis.
- Care must be used in the administration of oxygen to the undiagnosed infant with heart disease. A patient with single-ventricle physiology (e.g., hypoplastic left heart syndrome) can have manifestations of HF and mild desaturation (92–98%). Providing oxygen in this situation can result in shock due to excessive pulmonary blood flow and inadequate systemic blood flow.

ETIOLOGY

- Low cardiac output HF (e.g., all cardiomyopathy, severe AV valve regurgitation)
- High cardiac output HF
  - Left-to-right shunts (e.g., ASD, VSD, PDA)
  - AVM
  - Severe anemia, beriberi, and hyperthyroidism

DIAGNOSIS

HISTORY

- Infants and neonates
  - Prolonged feedings associated with tachypnea, retractions, or diaphoresis
  - Emesis, inadequate caloric intake, irritability with feeding, and failure to thrive
  - Frequent respiratory infections. Orthopnea: "Spoiled baby" becomes distressed when supine.
  - Family history of HF or sudden unexpected deaths
  - Sweating, especially when supine/sleeping
- Childhood and adolescence
  - Exercise intolerance with exertional dyspnea
  - Palpitations or chest pain, especially during exercise
  - Chronic cough, wheezing, orthopnea, fatigue, weakness, anorexia, nausea, and edema
  - Gradual weight loss (anorexia, nausea, and increased metabolic demands)
  - Sudden weight gain (fluid retention)
  - Family history of HF or unexpected deaths
  - Sweating, especially when supine/sleeping

PHYSICAL EXAM

- Infants and neonates
  - Tachycardia
  - Gallop rhythm
  - Murmur of outflow obstruction, increased flow, AV valve regurgitation, VSD, or semilunar valve incompetence
  - Systolic click (semilunar valve abnormalities)
  - Abnormal second heart sound (fixed split, loud P_2 component)
  - Tachypnea, wheezing, crackles, rales
  - Nasal flaring, grunting, retractions
  - Abdominal or cranial bruit
  - Hepatomegaly, splenomegaly
  - Edema (periorbital)
  - Cool and/or mottled extremities
  - Poor capillary refill or pulses
- Children and adolescents
  - Tachycardia
  - Gallop rhythm
  - Murmur of outflow obstruction, increased flow, AV valve regurgitation, VSD, or semilunar valve incompetence
  - Loud second heart sound (P2 component)
  - Hyperactive precordium, displaced PMI
  - Tachypnea, retractions
  - Wheezing ("cardiac asthma") or rales
  - Jugular venous distension
  - Hepatomegaly, splenomegaly
  - Edema (periorbital, peripheral)
  - Pulsus alternans, pulsus paradoxus
  - Cool extremities, poor pulses, poor capillary refill
  - Manifestations of Kawasaki disease, rheumatic fever, or endocarditis on mucous membranes, skin, and extremities

DIAGNOSTIC TESTS & INTERPRETATION

Diagnostic Procedures/Other

- Chest x-ray
  - Cardiomegaly, increased pulmonary vascular markings, hyperinflation, pleural effusion, Kerley B lines
- Electrocardiography
  - Abnormal P-waves
  - ST–T wave changes (ischemia, strain, inflammation/myocarditis)
  - Heart block (1st-, 2nd-, 3rd-degree) or tachyarrhythmia
  - Disease-specific findings: anomalous left coronary artery from the pulmonary artery (Q waves and inverted T waves in leads I and aVL, left ventricular hypertrophy, right ventricular hypertrophy, ischemic changes), restrictive cardiomyopathy, pericarditis pattern (diffuse ST segment changes, low voltages), hypertrophy (cardiomyopathy, CHD, storage disease)
- Echocardiography
  - Rule out CHD, evaluate coronary origins
  - Assessment of cardiac systolic and diastolic function
- Cardiac catheterization (in select cases)
  - Assessment of cardiac hemodynamics and anatomy
  - Endomyocardial biopsy may be helpful in the diagnosis of myocarditis, storage disease, or cardiomyopathy.
  - Electrophysiologic study to evaluate for the induction of arrhythmia
- Cardiac MRI or CT (in select cases)
  - Delineation of complex anatomic relationships
  - Right ventricular performance
- Other laboratory abnormalities
  - Blood gas: metabolic acidosis with elevated lactate

– Chemistry: hyponatremia (dilutional), prerenal state
– Blood counts: anemia, leukocytosis, or leukopenia (e.g., viral myocarditis)
– Elevated erythrocyte sedimentation rate (e.g., rheumatic fever, Kawasaki disease)
– B-type natriuretic peptide (BNP or NT-BNP) elevation
– Urine: proteinuria, high urine specific gravity, microscopic hematuria
– Evaluation for metabolic causes of cardiomyopathy may include pyruvate, amino acid quantification, urine organic acids, carnitine, selenium, acylcarnitine profile, and liver function tests.
– Viral evaluation (adenovirus, coxsackievirus, Epstein-Barr virus, cytomegalovirus, parvovirus, echovirus)

DIFFERENTIAL DIAGNOSIS

- Tachycardia
  – Fever
  – Dehydration
  – Anemia
  – Supraventricular tachycardia or ventricular tachycardia without HF
  – Hyperthyroidism
  – Pericardial effusion
- Tachypnea
  – Respiratory disease or infection
  – Pulmonary venous obstruction
  – Acidosis (metabolic disease, poisoning)
  – Pneumothorax, pleural effusion
  – Carbon monoxide poisoning
- Edema
  – Hypoalbuminemia
  – Systemic inflammatory conditions/allergies
  – Hypothyroidism
- Sepsis
- Hepatomegaly
  – Liver disease
  – Storage disease
  – Extramedullary hematopoiesis

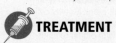

TREATMENT

GENERAL MEASURES

- Treatment of underlying cause
  – Surgical palliation or correction of CHD
  – Interventional cardiac catheterization (e.g., balloon dilation of aortic or pulmonary stenosis, coil embolization of PDA, device closure of ASD, dilation, or stenting of coarctation of the aorta)
  – Carnitine, coenzyme Q10, riboflavin, antioxidant replacement for select cardiomyopathies
  – Targeted medical treatment of endocarditis, myocarditis, anemia, rheumatic fever, Kawasaki disease, or hypertension
  – Radiofrequency ablation of tachyarrhythmia
  – Medical therapy for patients or mothers of fetuses with tachyarrhythmia
  – Pacing for bradyarrhythmias (e.g., heart block)
  – Control of chronic inflammatory conditions, such as SLE or JRA
- Management
  – Assessment of degree of illness:
  – If perfusion is compromised or acidosis is present, ICU care is indicated.
  – Hospitalization may be necessary to initiate treatment or prepare for surgery (e.g., coronary abnormalities, aortic coarctation).
  – Many patients diagnosed as outpatients with CHD or cardiomyopathy may not require inpatient treatment. Immediate consultation with a pediatric cardiologist should be arranged.
- Immediate management
  – General measures: activity restriction as indicated, oxygen as needed (not for patients with pulmonary overcirculation)
  – Tube feedings for severe failure to thrive or parenteral nutrition if there is concern for splanchnic circulation
  – Drainage of pericardial effusion, if needed.
  – Inotropic agents (digoxin, milrinone, dobutamine in refractory cases)
  – Intravenous immunoglobulin (IVIG) for myocarditis or Kawasaki disease
  – Loop diuretics (e.g., furosemide)
  – Nesiritide (synthetic BNP) for refractory fluid overload
  – Mechanical respiratory or circulatory support, if necessary (ventilator, extracorporeal membrane oxygenation, ventricular assist device)
- Chronic therapy
  – Digoxin
  – Loop diuretics (e.g., furosemide) for fluid overload/edema
  – Afterload reduction (e.g., angiotensin-converting enzyme [ACE] inhibitors)
  – Antagonism of activated neurohormonal systems: ACE inhibitor or angiotensin receptor blocker, spironolactone, beta-blocker
  – Anticoagulation or antiplatelet therapy (especially in restrictive and severe dilated cardiomyopathy)
  – Biventricular pacing/resynchronization in some cases
  – Heart and heart/lung transplantation in select cases

ONGOING CARE

FOLLOW-UP RECOMMENDATIONS

- Dependent on the etiology and degree of HF. Generally, initial follow-up of a patient with HF should be intensive, focused on assessing response to therapy. Initial follow-up generally weekly, spreading to monthly or quarterly over time, under the supervision of a pediatric cardiologist.
- Depending on the etiology and degree of HF, echocardiography, ECG, blood chemistry, BNP levels, INR, Holter monitoring, and chest radiography will be evaluated.

ADDITIONAL READING

- Aurbach SR, Richmond ME, Lamour JM, et al. BNP levels predict outcome in pediatric heart failure patients: post-hoc analysis of the Pediatric Carvedilol Trial. *Circ Heart Fail*. 2010;3(5):606–611.
- Kay JD, Colan SD, Graham TP Jr. Congestive heart failure in pediatric patients. *Am Heart J*. 2001;142(5):923–928.
- Kindel SJ, Miller EM, Gupta R, et al. Pediatric cardiomyopathy: importance of genetic and metabolic evaluation. *J Card Fail*. 2012;18(5): 396–403.
- Rosenthal DN. Cardiomyopathy in infants: a brief overview. *Neoreviews*. 2000;1(8):e139–e145.
- Shaddy RE. Optimizing treatment for chronic congestive heart failure in children. *Crit Care Med*. 2001;29(10)(Suppl):S237–S240.
- Towbin JA, Bowles JA. The failing heart. *Nature*. 2002;415(10):227–233.
- Wilkinson JD, Landy DC, Colan SD, et al. The pediatric cardiomyopathy registry and heart failure: key results from the first 15 years. *Heart Fail Clin*. 2010; 6(4):401–413.

CODES

ICD10

- I50.9 Heart failure, unspecified
- P29.0 Neonatal cardiac failure
- Q23.4 Hypoplastic left heart syndrome

FAQ

- Q: My child has a large VSD and is prescribed digoxin and furosemide. Should I take salt out of his diet?
- A: No. Excessive salt restriction is seldom enforceable and is not necessary. A no-added-salt diet is generally sufficient.
- Q: What is the importance of tachycardia and bradycardia in HF?
- A: Tachycardia limits diastolic filling time and may result in decreased cardiac output. However, bradycardia may be poorly tolerated in patients with HF and a relatively fixed stroke volume who are dependent on heart rate to maintain an appropriate output. Either may be problematic for a patient in chronic HF. Most HF patients do not have as much heart rate variation as healthy people.
- Q: What are the major causes of death to HF patients?
- A: Younger children tend to die of progressive HF. Ventricular arrhythmias are the most common cause of sudden death in older children and adults with HF. Other causes of mortality include infection and stroke.
- Q: My patient has a normal blood pressure, but the cardiologist says more ACE inhibition is necessary. Why?
- A: Blood pressure is the weight that the myocardial muscle must "lift" with every beat. By decreasing the blood pressure as much as possible (short of causing dizziness or syncope), the work done by the heart and myocardial oxygen consumption are reduced. Reduction of the systemic blood pressure also potentially reduces the amount of left-to-right shunting through a VSD, PDA, and AP window.

CONJUNCTIVITIS

Shonul A. Jain

BASICS

DESCRIPTION

An inflammatory process of the conjunctiva, the membrane covering the eye and inside of the eyelids, manifested by erythema and edema, frequently with tearing and discharge. There is a wide range in severity and many potential causes. It is critical to rule out gonococcus infection because of the destructive nature of the eye disease and potential for vision loss.

EPIDEMIOLOGY

Incidence

- Children: Viral infection is the most common cause and is highly contagious.
- Neonates: Ophthalmia neonatorum, conjunctivitis in the 1st month of life, is the most common infection in neonates. Remains a significant cause of blindness in children worldwide. *Chlamydia trachomatis* is the most common infectious cause.

PATHOPHYSIOLOGY

- Results from bacterial, viral, allergic, or toxic activation of the inflammatory response that causes dilation and exudation from conjunctival blood vessels
- Pathology involves dilated conjunctival capillaries with leukocytic infiltration and edema of conjunctiva and substantia propria.

ETIOLOGY

- Ophthalmia neonatorum
  - If present in the first 24 hours of life, most likely due to chemical irritation from silver nitrate or povidone-iodine (e.g., Wokadine, Betadine) eyedrops
  - Gonococcal conjunctivitis is treatable if recognized early but devastating if diagnosis is delayed or missed.
  - Chronic *Chlamydia* infection can lead to scarring and corneal opacity. Chlamydial pneumonia develops in 20% of patients with chlamydial conjunctivitis.
- Bacterial
  - Agents include staphylococci, streptococci, *Haemophilus*, *Moraxella*, and *Pseudomonas*.
  - Serious complications of these are rare.
- Viral
  - Adenovirus is the most common agent.
  - Recurrent herpes simplex virus infection can lead to significant visual loss from corneal scarring, even with proper therapy.
  - Other viral etiologies usually follow a benign course but rarely can lead to conjunctival scarring.
- Allergic
  - IgE-mediated hypersensitivity response

DIAGNOSIS

HISTORY

- Ophthalmia neonatorum
  - Gonococcus: typically presents 2–4 days after birth with mucopurulent discharge
  - *Chlamydia*: typically presents 4–14 days after birth with mucopurulent discharge
- Bacterial
  - Eye redness and mucopurulent discharge. Patient may complain of sticky eyelids upon waking. Mild photophobia and discomfort may be present but are typically not painful.
- Viral
  - HSV ocular infection may present as conjunctivitis; often associated with corneal anesthesia, so painless. In neonates, it occurs 1–2 weeks after birth as unilateral serous discharge and conjunctival injection.
  - Other viral causes often present with upper respiratory symptoms, fever, sore throat, eye redness, tearing, serous discharge, eyelid edema, and photophobia. Typically begins in one eye but spreads to the other within a few days. History of similar infection in siblings or contacts is common.
- Allergic
  - Bilateral itching and tearing; classically, a complaint of itching or foreign body sensation in an older child with red eyes

PHYSICAL EXAM

- General
  - Cornea is clear.
  - Vision, pupils, and ocular motility are normal.
  - Refer to an ophthalmologist for vesicular rash on eyelids or corneal changes, as the condition may be caused by herpes simplex virus and can be vision threatening.
- Bacterial
  - Wide range of clinical presentation, from mild hyperemia to significant injection and mucopurulent discharge (opaque and thick)
  - Injected conjunctiva, episcleral vessels, palpebral conjunctival papillae
  - Preauricular lymphadenopathy less common
- Viral
  - HSV ocular infection may involve corneal ulceration or dendritic or disciform keratitis.
  - Serous discharge (clear and watery)
  - May involve pseudomembrane formation, pinpoint subconjunctival hemorrhages, and palpable preauricular lymph nodes
- Allergic
  - Bilateral conjunctival edema and chemosis

ALERT

- Failure to diagnose gonococcal conjunctivitis may lead to corneal perforation or visual loss.
- HSV ocular infection is associated with a significant risk of blindness; have high suspicion for HSV with any recurrent unilateral eye redness, corneal changes, or vesicular rash on eyelids.
- Steroids can activate or accelerate unrecognized herpes simplex virus infection, and chronic use can lead to raised intraocular pressure or cataract formation.
- Chronic use of empiric broad-spectrum antibiotics for self-limited conjunctivitis can promote bacterial resistance, although less so than for systemic antibiotic administration.

DIAGNOSTIC TESTS & INTERPRETATION

Lab

- Gram stain
  - Note: always for ophthalmia neonatorum
  - Gonococcus: gram-negative intracellular diplococcus
  - *Chlamydia*: intracytoplasmic, paranuclear inclusion bodies on Gram stain and conjunctival scraping with Giemsa stain for basophilic intracytoplasmic inclusion bodies
  - Viral or chemical: polymorphonuclear leukocytes without bacteria
- Culture
  - Viral: Cultures for HSV and adenovirus are not clinically useful.
  - Bacterial: blood agar and chocolate agar
  - Gonococcus: Thayer-Martin media
  - *Chlamydia*: Culture techniques are not widely available. However, they remain the gold standard for diagnosis. Specimens should be obtained using an aluminum-shafted Dacron-tipped swab and processed within 24 hours. A positive test is confirmed when the organism is identified using fluorescein-conjugated monoclonal antibody. Other equally effective methods involve polymerase chain reaction or direct fluorescent antibody.
- Conjunctival scrapings
  - Allergic: mast cells and eosinophils
- Serum tests
  - Allergic: IgE may be elevated.
  - *Chlamydia*: The diagnosis of chlamydial pneumonia can be made with a serum test but is not reliable for chlamydial conjunctivitis.

DIFFERENTIAL DIAGNOSIS

- Ophthalmia neonatorum
  - Chemical conjunctivitis: noninfectious, mild, self-limited; result of silver nitrate or povidone-iodine administration
  - Birth trauma: often unilateral subconjunctival hemorrhage, may have associated eyelid contusion, history of forceps use or difficult delivery
  - Congenital glaucoma: mild redness, minimal discharge. Look for enlarged eye, cloudy cornea, tearing, and photophobia.
  - Nasolacrimal duct obstruction: unilateral or bilateral discharge, may be clear to mucopurulent with reflux from nasolacrimal sac. Conjunctiva is usually white and nonerythematous.
- All conjunctivitis
  - Preseptal cellulitis: early eyelid edema/erythema; looks like conjunctivitis, especially in young children with a difficult exam. Motility deficit, proptosis, decreased vision, and afferent pupillary defect are consistent with orbital cellulitis.
  - Foreign body
  - Blepharitis: inflammation of eyelids, history of gritty/burning sensation, excessive tearing, significant eyelid swelling
  - Corneal abrasion: history of pain, associated trauma; significant tearing, photophobia, erythema. Diagnose with fluorescein and blue light.
  - Keratitis: signifies corneal infection; may have associated conjunctivitis. Primary herpes keratitis is associated with vesicular eyelid rash and pain. Consult an ophthalmologist. Bacterial keratitis may be caused by staphylococci, streptococci, and *Pseudomonas*; Lyme spirochete; or vitamin A deficiency.
  - Episcleritis: inflammation of the thick loose connective tissue between the clear conjunctiva and the white-appearing stroma of the sclera; rare disease in childhood; can be associated with rheumatologic disease
  - Scleritis: presents as red eye; severe disease involving inflammation of the sclera; rare in childhood; associated with systemic disease; requires oral or IV steroids
  - Iritis/uveitis: frequently unilateral, with or without a history of trauma; photophobia, decreased vision, and constant pain (except if associated with juvenile rheumatoid arthritis). Contagious history is rare. Consult an ophthalmologist for full evaluation, including pupillary dilation.

- Systemic diseases with red eye
  - Varicella: ocular involvement in rare cases. Treat with antiviral medications.
  - Stevens-Johnson syndrome: secondary to viruses, mycoplasma, or adverse drug reaction. Mucous membrane involvement may lead to conjunctival bullae with risk of rupture and subsequent scarring.
  - Kawasaki disease: acute vasculitis. Classic symptoms include fever × 5 days, plus 4 out of 5 of the following: bilateral, limbic-sparing nonexudative conjunctivitis; oropharyngeal changes (including strawberry tongue); cervical adenopathy; polymorphous rash; and extremity changes/swelling of palms and soles with peeling around nail beds.
  - Measles: presents with fever, rash, cough coryza, and conjunctivitis
  - Cat-scratch disease: Parinaud syndrome includes granulomatous conjunctivitis and adenopathy.

TREATMENT

MEDICATION

- Ophthalmia neonatorum
  - Gonococcus: ceftriaxone, 25–50 mg/kg/dose (max 125 mg) IV or IM as a single dose and ocular irrigation followed by topical 0.5% erythromycin ophthalmic ointment q.i.d. for 14 days. Also treat for *Chlamydia*.
  - *Chlamydia*: oral erythromycin suspension, 12.5 mg/kg/dose q6h for 14 days. Topical 0.5% erythromycin ophthalmic ointment q.i.d. both eyes for 14 days as above. (Povidone-iodine 1.25% ophthalmic drops q.i.d. can be used if other antibiotics are not readily available.)
  - Important to treat both of these conditions systemically as well as topically
- Bacterial
  - Often self-limited; however, studies have shown empiric antibiotic treatment can shorten duration of symptoms and reduce transmission.
  - Treatment includes erythromycin ointment, sulfacetamide 10%, polymyxin-trimethoprim, fluoroquinolone, or azithromycin drops.
- Viral
  - Herpes simplex: topical trifluorothymidine (Viroptic solution), 1 drop q2h while awake (max 9 drops/24 h) until reepithelialization of ulcer; then 1 drop q4h for 7 days (do not exceed 21 days of treatment) with or without systemic acyclovir
  - Topical glucocorticoid therapy is contraindicated.
  - Other viral: over-the-counter antihistamine or decongestant drops for comfort
  - Cidofovir has recently been considered as a potential antiadenoviral therapy, but its clinical use is limited by local toxicity to the skin, eyelids, and conjunctiva.
- Allergic
  - A new class of topical mast cell stabilizers such as olopatadine b.i.d. is effective for more involved cases.

ADDITIONAL TREATMENT

General Measures

- Ophthalmia neonatorum
  - Cases of suspected gonococcal conjunctivitis should be hospitalized for IV antibiotics and workup for sepsis.
  - For suspected chlamydial infection, topical and oral therapy is usually appropriate.
- Bacterial
  - Usually self-limited, but treatment may help shorten course and prevent spread of infection. Contact lens users should remove lenses until infection clears and consider use of fluoroquinolone.
- Viral
  - Suspected HSV warrants hospitalization for IV antiviral therapy.
  - For suspected adenovirus, children should stay home from school until discharge is minimal and discomfort has subsided; cool compresses for comfort
- Allergic
  - Remove offending allergen if possible.
  - Mild symptoms can be treated with preservative-free artificial tears. Consider topical or systemic antiallergy medicine if symptoms persist.
  - Consider treating other atopic conditions which are often present.
- Chemical
  - Close observation only. Remove offending agent; self-limited

ONGOING CARE

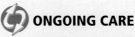

FOLLOW-UP RECOMMENDATIONS

Patient Monitoring

- Daily follow-up is necessary for gonococcus, *Chlamydia*, and herpes simplex virus.
- For epidemic viral conjunctivitis, frequency is dictated by severity (daily to weekly).
- For allergic conjunctivitis, follow-up can be made after a few weeks of treatment.
- No office follow-up is recommended for routine conjunctivitis.
- Follow atypical conjunctivitis closely until a more serious disease can be excluded.
- A nonresponsive or worsening condition needs ophthalmic consultation.

COMPLICATIONS

- Significant complications are extremely rare for common bacterial, viral, or allergic conjunctivitis.
- Blindness may result from untreated neonatal conjunctivitis or from recurrent HSV ocular infection.

ADDITIONAL READING

- American Academy of Ophthalmology. *Conjunctivitis. Preferred Practice Pattern*. San Francisco, CA: American Academy of Ophthalmology; 2013.
- Azari AA, Barney NP. Conjunctivitis: a systematic review of diagnosis and treatment. *JAMA*. 2013; 310(16):1721–1729.
- Bielory L, Mongia A. Current opinion of immunotherapy for ocular allergy. *Curr Opin Allergy Clin Immunol*. 2002;2(5):447–452.
- Brook I. Ocular infections due to anaerobic bacteria in children. *J Pediatr Ophthalmol Strabismus*. 2008; 45(2):78–84.
- Crede CSF. Reports from the obstetrical clinic in Leipzig: prevention of eye inflammation in the newborn. *Am J Dis Child*. 1971;121(1):3–4.
- Greenberg MF, Pollard ZF. The red eye in childhood. *Pediatr Clin North Am*. 2003;50(1):105–124.
- Hillenkamp J, Reinhard T, Ross RS, et al. The effects of cidofovir 1% with and without cyclosporin a 1% as a topical treatment of acute adenoviral keratoconjunctivitis: a controlled clinical pilot study. *Ophthalmology*. 2002;109(5):845–850.
- Isenberg SJ, Apt L, Valenton M, et al. A controlled trial of povidone-iodine to treat infectious conjunctivitis in children. *Am J Ophthalmol*. 2002;134(5):861–868.
- Rietveld RP, van Weert HC, ter Riet G, et al. Diagnostic impact of signs and symptoms in acute infectious conjunctivitis: systematic literature search. *BMJ*. 2003;327(7418):789.
- Sethuraman US, Kamat D. The red eye: evaluation and management. *Clin Pediatr*. 2009;48(6):588–600.
- Sheikh A, Hurwitz B, van Schayck CP, et al. Antibiotics versus placebo for acute bacterial conjunctivitis. *Cochrane Database Syst Rev*. 2012:9:CD001211.
- Strauss EC, Foster CS. Atopic ocular disease. *Ophthalmol Clin North Am*. 2002;15(1):1–5.
- Teoh DL, Reynolds S. Diagnosis and management of pediatric conjunctivitis. *Pediatr Emerg Care*. 2003;19(1):48–55.
- Trocme SD, Sra KK. Spectrum of ocular allergy. *Curr Opin Allergy Clin Immunol*. 2002;2(5):423–427.

CODES

ICD10

- H10.9 Unspecified conjunctivitis
- B30.9 Viral conjunctivitis, unspecified
- P39.1 Neonatal conjunctivitis and dacryocystitis

FAQ

- Q: Is conjunctivitis contagious?
- A: All infectious conjunctivitis is contagious but to varying degrees. Viral or epidemic keratoconjunctivitis (EKC) is the most contagious. Careful handling of secretions, tissues, towels, and bed linens and strict hand washing usually prevent spread. Wipe surfaces with isopropyl alcohol or dilute bleach to prevent recontamination. Gonococcus, *Chlamydia*, and herpes simplex virus can be transmitted through infected discharge or secretions, but this is less common. The most common source is the infected birth canal.
- Q: Should the patient with "pink eye" (non-Gonococcus, non-*Chlamydia*, non–herpes simplex virus conjunctivitis) be treated with empiric antibiotics?
- A: There is some benefit to empiric antibiotic treatment in bacterial conjunctivitis but not in viral or allergic etiologies. Practically, it is often difficult to distinguish viral and bacterial conjunctivitis based on symptoms alone, and return to school is often contingent on initiation of antibiotic therapy. Providers should be aware that empiric treatment with topical antibiotics can cause harm in the case of sulfa-containing compounds. Antibiotic toxicity, including Stevens-Johnson reactions, can occur from sulfa antibiotics, and use of antibiotics long term promotes selection of resistant strains of bacteria. Empiric treatment also increases manipulation of the infected eye and thus increases the risk of spread.
- Q: How long is the patient with pink eye (non-Gonococcus, non-*Chlamydia*, non–herpes simplex virus conjunctivitis) contagious, and when can the patient return to school?
- A: The organism can be recovered from the eye for up 2 weeks after onset of symptoms, demonstrating that patients are infectious during this time. Practically, children should probably be kept out of school at least 24 hours after onset of therapy, if indicated, ideally until discharge is minimal and discomfort has subsided.

CONSTIPATION

Jay Fong

BASICS

DESCRIPTION
Delay or difficulty in defecation; infrequent (<2) stools per week, and resulting in pain, rectal bleeding, as well as fecal soiling. May also refer to a decrease in frequency of bowel movements compared with the patient's usual bowel pattern.

GENERAL PREVENTION
- Dietary measures: high-fiber diet, plenty of fluids, fruits, and vegetables; avoidance of excessive caffeine and milk (calcium) intake
- Regular physical activity

PATHOPHYSIOLOGY
- Delay in colonic passage and/or retention of stool allows fluids mixed in stool to be resorbed across cellular membranes, increasing stool caliber and leading it to be harder in consistency.
- Decreased motility leads to a buildup of desiccated stool causing painful defecation that leads to ongoing stool retention.
- As the rectosigmoid enlarges with retained stool, a child's ability to sense rectal fullness diminishes, and he or she may not appreciate the need to defecate.
- Often there is a family history of motility disturbances or constipation.

ETIOLOGY
- Most patients have idiopathic or functional constipation with no identifiable cause.
- Personal history of constipation may be traceable to an acute event (i.e., passage of large, painful stool) followed by chronicity.
- Intentional or unintentional withholding of stool may result in hard stools, anal pain, and fissures that perpetuate and lead to constipation. Rectal dilatation, decreased sensation of the urge to defecate, shortening of the anal canal, decreased tone of the external anal sphincter, and encopresis can result.
- Precipitating events may include the following:
  - Transition from breast milk to cow's milk
  - Excessive cow's milk intake
  - Insufficient water intake
  - Refusal to use toilets outside the home
  - Premature toilet training
  - Perianal streptococcal infection
  - Food allergies
  - Transient viral illness (diarrhea followed by constipation)
- Constipation also can be caused by anatomic anomalies in the lower GI tract, decreased propulsion, increased rectal sensitivity threshold, a functional outlet obstruction (muscular spastic levator ani or impaired relaxation of the puborectalis).
- Neurologic causes:
  - Abnormalities of the myenteric plexus
  - Intestinal pseudoobstruction
  - Congenital aganglionosis (Hirschsprung disease)
  - Visceral neuropathies
  - Visceral myopathies
  - Familial dysautonomia
- Lesions of the spinal cord can result in loss of rectal tone and sensation and reduced anal closure, affecting the sacral reflex center (e.g., meningocele, myelomeningocele, tethered cord).
- Anatomic disorders of anus and rectum (stricture, stenosis, mass, ectopic anus, imperforate anus, fistula)
- Endocrine abnormalities (hypothyroidism), drugs, electrolyte abnormalities

DIAGNOSIS

HISTORY
- Question: What was the timing after birth of passage of meconium?
  - If it is delayed for >48 hours, consider Hirschsprung disease.
- Is the child able to pass a bowel movement unaided by a suppository or enema?
  - If rectal stimulation is required for passage of a bowel movement, consider Hirschsprung disease or habituation to rectal stimulation.
- What are the size, frequency, and consistency of bowel movements?
  - 1–3 normal (in size and consistency), painless bowel movements may be passed every 1–3 days. The size of bowel movements reflects the caliber of the colon.
- Does the child experience frequent urination, bedwetting, or urinary tract infections?
  - Chronic UTIs are frequently linked to chronic constipation.
- Does fecal soiling occur?
  - Soiling occurs with stool impaction or with nerve damage involving the anus.
- Is there the presence of rectal sensation?
  - Patients with long-standing constipation or stool withholding may develop a dilated rectum and lose the sensation of rectal distention.
- Is there a history of painful bowel movements or rectal fissure?
  - Pain with defecation and/or fissuring can further lead to withholding secondary to fear of painful bowel movements.
- Is the child experiencing any stressful events (i.e., new sibling, family death)?
  - Stress can precipitate stool withholding.
- Is there an unsteady gait?
  - This may suggest neuromuscular problems.
- Did the child experience difficult toilet training?
  - May be associated with encopresis

PHYSICAL EXAM
- General: Look for evidence of systemic illness and alarm signals: weight loss, anorexia, delayed growth, delayed passage of meconium, urinary incontinence, passage of bloody stools (in the absence of anal fissure), fever, vomiting, and diarrhea.
- Abdomen: abdominal distention (indicative of the presence of stool or gas), presence of stool masses (size, location), distended bladder, and bowel sounds (may be decreased in intestinal pseudoobstruction)
- Rectal examination
  - Perianal soiling
  - Size and position of anus (evaluate for signs of imperforate, stenosed, or ectopic anus)
  - Presence of skin tags and fissures
  - Perianal or anal erythema (streptococcal proctitis)
- Evidence of child abuse
- Digital examination is not recommended to diagnose functional constipation. If suspicious for other etiologies, can use to assess anal tone (long and tight anal canal in Hirschsprung); amount and consistency of stool; size of rectum (dilated rectum with chronic constipation; tight and empty anus with Hirschsprung disease); presence of blood
- Absence of anal wink or cremasteric reflex suggests neurologic abnormalities.
- Neurologic examination: decreased reflexes in the lower extremities
- Back: Check for sacral dimple, tuft of hair (underlying sacral abnormality), flat buttocks, and patulous anus.

ALERT
- Grunting baby syndrome: Infants cry, scream, and draw up their legs during a bowel movement. They respond to rectal distention by contracting their pelvic floor. This is not constipation.
- Always rule out an organic cause.
- Always consider medications as a cause.

DIAGNOSTIC TESTS & INTERPRETATION

Lab
Testing for possible underlying thyroid disease and/or celiac disease may be recommended in patients with likely functional constipation. Other lab testing is not routinely recommended.

Imaging
- Abdominal radiography:
  - May demonstrate presence or absence of fecal impaction
  - Should not be used routinely for the evaluation of functional constipation
- Water-soluble contrast enema:
  - An unprepped study is useful to diagnose Hirschsprung disease.
  - A prepped study is useful to diagnose a stricture.
  - Most patients with constipation will not require this test, especially those with functional constipation.

Diagnostic Procedures/Other
- Measurement of abdominal transit time with radio-opaque markers may help discriminate between children with and without clinical constipation, but evidence does not support its routine use in diagnosis.
- Anorectal manometry: analyzes rectal sensation, resting and squeezing pressures, and pelvic floor dyssynergia (anismus)

DIFFERENTIAL DIAGNOSIS

- Celiac disease (more likely in younger children)
- Hypothyroidism, hypercalcemia, hypokalemia
- Diabetes mellitus
- Dietary protein allergy
- Drugs, toxics:
  - Opiates, anticholinergics, antidepressants, chemotherapy, and heavy metal ingestion (lead)
- Vitamin D intoxication
- Botulism
- Cystic fibrosis
- Hirschsprung disease
- Anal achalasia
- Colonic inertia
- Anatomic malformations (imperforate anus, anal stenosis)
- Pelvic mass (sacrococcygeal teratoma)
- Spinal cord anomalies, trauma, tethered cord
- Abnormal abdominal musculature (prune belly, gastroschisis, Down syndrome)
- Pseudoobstruction
- Multiple endocrine neoplasia type 2B

TREATMENT

GENERAL MEASURES

- Treatment of functional constipation:
  - Disimpaction
    - The use of polyethylene glycol (e.g., MiraLAX or other generics) with or without electrolytes orally at 1–1.5 g/kg/24 h for 3–6 days is recommended as first line for children presenting with impaction.
    - If the patient is not tolerating PO, enemas may be required for initial disimpaction.

ALERT

Multiple phosphate enemas can cause severe electrolyte imbalances (hyponatremia, hypokalemia, hypocalcemia, hypomagnesemia).

    - Children >2–3 years of age require adult-size enemas, whereas younger children require pediatric-size enemas. Enemas can be given once per day for 3–6 days.
  - Evacuation
    - Following rectal disimpaction, further evacuation can be achieved by using polyethylene glycol solution (Go-Lytely), orally or via nasogastric tube over 6–8 hours until the effluent is clear.
  - Maintenance stool softeners:
    - Infants ≤6 months of age may be given sorbitol or pectin-containing juices, lactulose, or Karo syrup.
    - Children >6 months of age may be given lactulose (0.7–2 g/kg/24 h [1–3 mL/kg/24 h], max 40 g/24 h [60 mL/24 h]) or MiraLAX (0.5–1 g/kg, max 17 g/24 h).
    - Mineral oil or Kondremul (>15 months of age 1–3 mL/24 h, >6 years 10–25 mL/24 h) is added as an adjunctive lubricant to aid in the passage of stool, but contraindicated in children <15 months as well as in children at risk for aspiration.
- Rescue stimulant laxatives:
  - Bisacodyl or senna may be used as a stimulant laxative for short period of time. Long-term use has been associated with colonic nerve damage in adults.
- Diet: A balanced diet of whole grains, fruits, and vegetables is recommended. A normal-fiber diet is recommended (toddler 14 g/24 h; school-aged 17–25 g/24 h; adolescent 25–31 g/24 h). Fiber should be increased gradually to minimize side effects of flatulence. Caffeine and excessive milk-product intake (>16 oz/24 h of milk) may be constipating.
- Fluid intake: A normal fluid intake is important.
- Toilet sitting: Regular toilet sitting twice a day for 10 minutes, preferably 15–20 minutes after meals, is a key step in retraining the bowel.
- Calendar: It is important to keep a record of stools, accidents, toilet sitting, and medications in order to identify causes of failure.
- Biofeedback has not been shown to be helpful in patients who fail conventional therapy and who have abnormalities on anorectal manometry.
- There may be some benefit in referring a patient with constipation and behavioral abnormalities to a mental health specialist.

ONGOING CARE

FOLLOW-UP RECOMMENDATIONS

- Schedule regular visits to make certain therapy is maintained, decreasing the frequency of visits when patient is doing well.
- Parents should call when problems develop.
- Compliance and good follow-up are key to successful management of constipation.

PROGNOSIS

For functional constipation, the success rate is variable (45–90%). Presence of abdominal pain at the time of presentation, close follow-up, and maintenance use of stool softeners are good prognostic factors. Presence of soiling, use of stimulant laxatives, and lack of follow-up were associated with failure.

COMPLICATIONS

- Anal fissures: Infrequent hard stools can cause a tear of the anal mucosa, causing pain and withholding.
- Encopresis: Chronic constipation leads to progressive rectal dilatation and decreased rectal sensation. Fecal impaction results in secondary soiling or encopresis.
- Intestinal obstruction: manifests as vomiting, abdominal pain, and constipation. Abdominal radiograph films show intestinal obstruction and presence of large amounts of stool.
- Sigmoid volvulus: A chronically constipated child may present with symptoms of acute abdomen, fever, tender abdomen, and palpable mass. Abdominal radiograph shows obstruction in the colon. Barium enema may be both diagnostic and therapeutic by achieving reduction.
- Treatment of complications:
  - Encopresis (soiling or diarrhea): Disimpaction and clean out as necessary, followed by treatment of constipation, is recommended (see previous discussion).
  - Intestinal obstruction from fecal mass: Presents with vomiting, abdominal pain, and constipation. Abdominal radiograph film shows intestinal obstruction. Make nil per os (NPO), provide IV fluids, and rule out an acute abdomen. Then give enemas and clear out stool from below. Avoid oral laxatives or a polyethylene glycol solution in a case of obstruction.
  - Sigmoid volvulus: Chronically constipated child with symptoms of acute abdomen, fever, tender abdomen, and palpable mass. Abdominal radiograph shows obstruction in the colon. Contrast enema may reveal and possibly reduce a volvulus.

ADDITIONAL READING

- Bekkali NLH, van den Berg MM, Dijkgraaf MGW, et al. Rectal fecal impaction treatment in childhood constipation: enemas versus high doses oral PEG. *Pediatrics*. 2009;124(6):e1108–e1115.
- Croffie JM, Fitzgerald J. Idiopathic constipation. In: Walker WA, Kleinman RE, Sherman PM, et al, eds. *Pediatric Gastrointestinal Disease*. 4th ed. Philadelphia: BC Decker; 2004:1000–1055.
- Hyman PE, Milla PJ, Benninga MA, et al. Childhood functional gastrointestinal disorder: neonate/toddler. *Gastroenterology*. 2006;130(5):1519–1526.
- Rasquin A, DiLorenzo C, Forbes D, et al. Childhood functional gastrointestinal disorders: child/adolescent. *Gastroenterology*. 2006;130(5):1527–1537.
- Tabbers MM, Dilorenzo C, Berger MY, et al. Evaluation and treatment of functional constipation in infants and children: evidenced-based recommendations from ESPGHAN and NASPGHAN. *J Pediatr Gastroenterol Nutr*. 2014;58(2):265–281.
- U.S. Department of Health and Human Services. Dietary guidelines for Americans, 2010. http://www.health.gov/dietaryguidelines/2010.asp. Accessed March 1, 2015.

CODES

ICD10

- K59.00 Constipation, unspecified
- K59.09 Other constipation
- K59.02 Outlet dysfunction constipation

FAQ

- Q: When is constipation an emergency?
- A: When intestinal obstruction, sigmoid volvulus, or Hirschsprung enterocolitis occurs.
- Q: Does polyethylene glycol-3350 taste bad?
- A: Advantages of polyethylene glycol-3350 include its lack of taste, smell, or odor and that it can be mixed in any liquid.

CONTACT DERMATITIS

Jocelyn H. Schiller

BASICS

DESCRIPTION

An acute or chronic inflammation of the dermis and epidermis as result of either direct irritation to the skin (irritant contact dermatitis) or delayed-type (type IV) hypersensitivity reaction to a contact allergen (allergic contact dermatitis)

EPIDEMIOLOGY

Incidence

Incidence in children is not known.

Prevalence

- Irritant contact dermatitis: Most cases of contact dermatitis (>80%) are irritant contact dermatitis.
  - Skin reactivity is highest in infants and tends to decrease with age.
- Allergic contact dermatitis
  - Because children have less time to develop sensitivities, it is less common in infants and children than in adults.
  - Prevalence increases with age.
  - Overall prevalence is ~13–23% and has been increasing in children, perhaps due to more frequent exposure to allergens at a younger age or improved diagnosis.

RISK FACTORS

- Irritant contact dermatitis
  - Frequent hand washing or water immersion
  - Atopic dermatitis: Chronically impaired barrier function increases susceptibility to irritants.
  - Genetic factors
  - Environmental factors such as cold/hot temperatures or high/low humidity disrupt the skin barrier.
- Allergic contact dermatitis
  - Atopic dermatitis
  - Genetic factors
  - Increased exposure to allergens

GENERAL PREVENTION

Minimize contact exposure to known or potential irritants and allergens.

PATHOPHYSIOLOGY

- Irritant contact dermatitis does not involve an immune response and thus can occur with the first exposure to the irritant. Multiple mechanisms are involved, including the following:
  - Disruption of the epidermal barrier by chemicals (soaps, detergents) or physical irritants (moisture, friction)
  - Damage to cell membranes and cytotoxic effect on skin cells
  - Chronic exposure may stimulate cell proliferation, resulting in acanthosis and hyperkeratosis. Postinflammatory hypo- or hyperpigmentation may result.
- Allergic contact dermatitis requires initial exposure and sensitization to an allergen and only occurs in susceptible individuals. Repeated exposure leads to the development of a type IV hypersensitivity reaction.
- Both processes result in nonspecific findings of dermal and epidermal edema and inflammation and may be indistinguishable from other forms of inflammatory dermatitis.

ETIOLOGY

- Irritant contact dermatitis
  - Frequent hand washing or water immersion
  - Soaps and detergents
  - Saliva (lip licking or thumb sucking)
  - Urine and feces (see "Diaper Rash")
  - High concentrations of most chemicals can induce irritant contact dermatitis, whereas mild irritants may induce inflammation only in susceptible individuals.
- Allergic contact dermatitis
  - Nickel and other metals (gold, cobalt)
  - Hair products (ammonium, 5-diamine)
  - Solvents (toluene-2)
  - Additives to medications, cosmetics (thimerosal, mercuric chloride)
  - Rubber
  - Fragrances (Balsam of Peru)
  - Clothing dyes
  - Formaldehydes
  - Topical antibiotics (neomycin, bacitracin)
  - Plants (*Toxicodendron* species; e.g., poison ivy, poison oak, and poison sumac, which contain the allergen urushiol)

DIAGNOSIS

HISTORY

- Patients may present with either acute or chronic localized, pruritic dermatitis.
- Patients should be asked about all chemicals and potential irritants or allergens to which they are intermittently or frequently exposed.
- Many patients are unable to associate a specific allergen with symptom development.
- Timing of symptoms
  - Irritant contact dermatitis: immediate inflammation
  - Allergic contact dermatitis: inflammation 48–72 hours but occasionally several days after exposure
- Location of skin changes may provide clues, as reactions are typically localized to the areas that come in contact with the allergen.

PHYSICAL EXAM

- Irritant contact dermatitis
  - Acute: ranges from mild skin dryness and mild erythema to erythematous papules and patches, edema, vesicles, and oozing; in severe cases, may result in a chemical burn (skin necrosis)
  - Chronic: erythema, dryness, lichenification, hyperkeratosis, and cracking
  - A perioral rash often signifies an irritant contact dermatitis from lip licking.
- Allergic contact dermatitis
  - Acute: pruritus, erythema, and edema with vesicles or bullae that often rupture, leaving a crust
  - Chronic: lichenification, erythema, scaling
- Often an unusual pattern or distribution that correlates with pattern of exposure (e.g., a linear pattern as patient brushes against poison ivy, round lesion on abdomen where skin contacts nickel button on jeans)
- Autoeczematization or "id" reaction: A more generalized dermatitis may develop distal to the original site of contact 1 or more weeks after the initial localized dermatitis.

DIAGNOSTIC TESTS & INTERPRETATION

Lab

In general, routine laboratory testing is not helpful in confirming the diagnosis of contact dermatitis.

Diagnostic Procedures/Other

- Formal epicutaneous patch testing distinguishes irritant and allergic contact dermatitis and identifies inciting allergens; may be performed by clinicians experienced in the interpretation of the test
- The patch test involves the controlled exposure of multiple allergens to the skin. Positive reactions manifest with the development of erythema, edema, and vesicles at the site of exposure, usually within 48–96 hours. It may be performed using a standard panel of allergens or by the application of selected allergens at the discretion of the specialist.
- Patch testing for poison ivy or oak is not recommended because reactions may be severe.

Pathologic Findings

- Skin biopsy is rarely necessary but may help differentiate between contact dermatitis and psoriasis or other inflammatory dermatoses.
- Skin biopsy findings may not be specific, and histopathologic features may not differentiate irritant from allergic contact dermatitis.

DIFFERENTIAL DIAGNOSIS

- Infection
  - Impetigo and cellulitis: Bacterial infections of the skin (*Staphylococcus aureus* or group A *Streptococcus*) may manifest as erythematous, edematous, crusted patches and plaques. Pustules and/or deep-seated inflammatory nodules may be present. Infection is usually associated more with pain and tenderness than with pruritus.
  - Fungal infection: KOH examination can clarify the diagnosis.
  - Scabies: intensely pruritic papules and nodules with a predilection for the hands and feet (especially the web spaces), the axillae, and the groin. Close contacts are often affected.
  - Herpes simplex virus may present with vesicles but is less erythematous and pruritic and more painful.
- Metabolic
  - Acrodermatitis enteropathica: a genetic or acquired zinc deficiency with characteristic bullae and erosions involving hands, feet, and periorificial areas (perioral, periocular, and perineal). Associated with failure to thrive, diarrhea, and alopecia
- Immunologic
  - Atopic dermatitis: It may favor the face and extremities or occur more diffusely with truncal involvement; usually spares diaper, perinasal, and periocular areas; usually symmetric; associated with erythematous, excoriated, and crusted papules, patches, and plaques and with chronic pruritus, often worse at night; often accompanied by a personal or family history of atopy
  - Seborrheic dermatitis: usually affects infants <1 year of age or adolescents; erythema and greasy scaling patches that favor scalp, face, ears, and intertriginous areas; usually asymptomatic
  - Nummular eczema: a chronic, often intensely inflammatory and pruritic dermatitis with multiple round, crusted, edematous, erythematous patches and plaques, often on extremities

- Psoriasis vulgaris: a chronic dermatitis with recurrent well-defined erythematous plaques with silvery scale; commonly affects scalp, elbows, and knees; nail changes may be present.
- Other
  - Ichthyoses: diffuse, severely dry, scaly, and hyperkeratotic skin; acquired or inherited
  - Pityriasis rosea: may begin with a single round, sharply demarcated, pink "herald" patch on the torso which becomes scaly and develops central clearing, followed by crops of oval lesions on the trunk and proximal extremities
  - Child abuse: inflicted trauma or burns

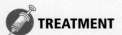

TREATMENT

MEDICATION

First Line

- Topical corticosteroids may help with the pruritus and inflammation associated with both acute and chronic contact dermatitis. Some mild cases may not require treatment and may self-resolve in 1–2 weeks.
- In irritant contact dermatitis, topical corticosteroids are controversial, as efficacy has not been evaluated in randomized controlled studies. Potential benefits must be weighed against the adverse effects.
- Milder forms not involving the face or flexural areas can be treated with class 3–5 topical corticosteroids for a short duration.
- For severe or chronic contact dermatitis with lichenification not involving the face of flexural areas, a medium- to high-potency topical corticosteroid (class 2–4) should be used for a short duration (2 weeks).
- If involving the face or flexural areas, medium- to high-potency topical corticosteroids should be avoided; instead, use a low-potency topical corticosteroid (class 6 or 7).
- Systemic antihistamines (diphenhydramine or hydroxyzine) are generally not necessary but can be considered if pruritus is extreme. There is no evidence that topical antihistamines are useful in treatment of pruritus.
- In severe cases involving a large body surface area or associated with significant facial, genital, or extremity edema, a short course (7–10 days) of systemic corticosteroids (prednisone 1–2 mg/kg/24 h) may be appropriate, with tapering over 1–2 weeks to avoid a rebound of the dermatitis.

Second Line

The intermittent use of a topical calcineurin inhibitor such as tacrolimus or pimecrolimus, which have anti-inflammatory and steroid-sparing properties, may be considered as adjunctive therapy in patients with chronic contact dermatitis. These agents are less effective than mid-potency corticosteroids, and the FDA issued an advisory about the possible link between topical use of calcineurin inhibitors and cancer. They should not be used in children younger than 2 years of age.

ADDITIONAL TREATMENT

General Measures

- The most effective treatment involves identification and avoidance of the offending allergens or exposures. This often requires extensive education of the patient and family regarding potential sources of exposure.
- Emollients restore epidermal barrier function. Petrolatum-based products are preferred to emollients containing lanolin or fragrances to reduce the risk of contact sensitization. Frequent application is recommended.
- Prompt bathing with soap and water immediately after exposure to poison ivy, oak, or sumac may help reduce exposure to the allergen in susceptible individuals.
- Chemical inactivators of urushiol may decrease dermatitis, but oil-removing compounds and soap also decrease dermatitis when used promptly after exposure.
- Acute allergic contact dermatitis: Application of cool compresses and shake lotions with drying properties (e.g., calamine lotion) can be helpful. Products containing colloidal oatmeal may also be helpful in soothing inflamed skin.

ONGOING CARE

FOLLOW-UP RECOMMENDATIONS

Patient Monitoring

Patients who do not improve after 1–2 weeks of therapy should be reevaluated.

PATIENT EDUCATION

Prevention

- Patients should be instructed on allergen avoidance, including the use of protective gloves and clothing where appropriate.
- Barrier creams containing quaternium-18 bentonite (bentoquatam 5%) may prevent exposure to the allergen in poison ivy if applied prior to anticipated exposure. Protective clothing may be helpful but can harbor the allergenic resin for many days.

PROGNOSIS

Complete resolution can be expected after appropriate treatment and elimination of further exposure to the allergen.

COMPLICATIONS

Generally, there are no long-term complications, although secondary bacterial infections may occur.

ADDITIONAL READING

- Bonitsis NG, Tatsioni A, Bassioukas K, et al. Allergens responsible for allergic contact dermatitis among children: a systematic review and meta-analysis. *Contact Dermatitis*. 2011;64(5):245–257.
- De Waard-van der Spek FB, Andersen KE, Darsow U, et al. Allergic contact dermatitis in children: which factors are relevant? (review of the literature) *Pediatr Allergy Immunol*. 2013;24(4):321–329.

CODES

ICD10

- L25.9 Unspecified contact dermatitis, unspecified cause
- L24.9 Irritant contact dermatitis, unspecified cause
- L23.9 Allergic contact dermatitis, unspecified cause

FAQ

- Q: Can the fluid from blisters caused by poison ivy spread the rash to other parts of the body?
- A: The contents of blisters from rhus dermatitis are not contagious. After exposure is eliminated, new lesions may appear because of the variable sensitivity of various areas of the body to the allergen.
- Q: How does saliva cause a perioral rash in some kids?
- A: "Lip-licker dermatitis" is an irritant dermatitis that results from chronic and/or excessive exposure to moisture. It is not caused by any specific substances in the saliva.

CONTRACEPTION

Michelle Forcier

BASICS

DESCRIPTION

- Prevention of conception or pregnancy. Ideal contraceptive is 100% effective, has no side effects, is easily reversed, and is readily used by adolescents.
- Efficacy issues:
  - In practice, contraceptive efficacy is based on two core concepts:
    - Adherence or ability to adequately "do" the method
    - Continuation or length of time over which patient uses method
  - Adherence and continuation improved by superior effectiveness of long-acting reversible contraceptives (LARCs), such as intrauterine devices (IUDs) or subdermal implants. LARCs have failure rates of less than 1% and approximately 80% continuation rates.
  - The most effective methods should be offered as 1st-line contraceptive options for sexually active teens.

Methods of contraception:

- LARCs:
  - Etonogestrel implant
    - Single-rod subdermal implant containing 68 mg of progestin etonogestrel. Implant provides contraception for 3 years.
    - Benefits: easy to insert and remove device, insertion site easy to access (nondominant upper arm)
    - Can be placed in not yet sexually active patients considering future sexual activity or for heavy or painful menses
  - Levonorgestrel-releasing (IUD)
    - T-shaped polyethylene IUDs containing progestin hormones
    - Ovulation may be suppressed in some women but is not the main mechanism of action, with between 45–75% of women ovulating on the 52 mg device, and almost all women ovulating on the lower dose LNG-IUD.
    - Ovulation on the lower dose LNG-IUD may result in less amenorrhea and more regular menses which can be a desired effect for some women.
    - Mirena® contains 52 mg of levonorgestrel and a release rate of 20 mcg/day and is FDA-approved for use for up to 5 years but is effective up to 7 years. Significantly reduces menstrual bleeding and dysmenorrhea
    - Skylar® IUD is slightly smaller, 28 mm × 30 mm, and contains 13.5 mg levonorgestrel with a release rate of 5–14 mcg/day and decline to 5 mcg/day after 3 years.
  - Copper T380 IUD
    - Contraceptive effect related to in utero oxidation with release of copper ions.
    - FDA-approved for use up to 10 years but may be effective for up to 12 years
    - May also be placed as very effective emergency contraceptive and then retained for ongoing pregnancy prevention
- Moderate-duration contraceptives:
  - Depot-medroxyprogesterone acetate (DMPA or Depo-Provera)
    - IM injection administered every 12 weeks. Failure rates in real-world settings estimated as low as 6%, likely much higher for adolescents.
    - 1-year continuation: 56% for users of all ages, likely lower for teens
    - Effective up to 14 weeks, so patients within that dosing window do not need additional pregnancy testing before readministration
- Short-acting estrogen-progestin (EP) contraceptives:
  - General issues:
    - Typically use both estrogen (to minimize break-through bleeding) and progestin (to block ovulation) in variety of delivery systems
    - Typical use failure rates at 9% but higher in adolescent populations. Continuation rates are 67%, likely lower in teens.
    - Some EP agents such as combined oral contraceptive pills (COCs) and vaginal rings may be used almost continuously for extended cycling. Such extended cycling may be useful for patients with dysmenorrhea, heavy periods, anemia, or times (life events) when delaying a period desired.
  - Combined oral contraceptive pills (COCs):
    - Monophasic COCs contain fixed doses of estrogens (ethinyl estradiol [EE]) and progestins. Phasic COCs vary doses of estrogens, progestins, or both. No practical difference between monophasic and phasic COCs.
    - 99.9% effective with perfect use but real-life use, difficulties with adherence, and continuation significantly reduce effectiveness.
    - Benefits: reduce incidence of endometrial and ovarian cancers after as little as 3 months of use, protect against salpingitis (PID) and subsequent ectopic pregnancies, and decrease incidence of benign breast disease and dysmenorrhea
    - Effective treatment for abnormal or heavy uterine bleeding (AUB), perimenstrual mood and physiologic symptoms, hygiene and behavior changes around menses for some developmentally delayed individuals, and sequelae of hyperandrogenism or polycystic ovary syndrome (AUB, hirsutism, acne)
  - Transdermal patch
    - Contains ethinyl estradiol and norelgestromin. Each patch left in place for 7 days, changed weekly, allowing 1 patch-free week per month for menses; convenient due to once-weekly change
    - Typically not recommended for extended cycling, as studies demonstrate 60% more circulating estrogen than with other EP methods
    - Unclear if this increases vascular thrombotic event (VTE) risk
  - Vaginal ring
    - Soft, flexible, polymer ring containing ethinyl estradiol and etonogestrel
    - FDA-approved for vaginal insertion for 3 weeks then removed for 1 week for menses
    - May be effective over a 4-week insertion and for extended cycling
    - Benefits: avoidance of 1st-pass liver effects and lower hormone doses
- Emergency contraceptives (EC): postcoital contraceptives, "morning-after" pills
  - General issues:
    - Safe but less effective (estimated 75%) than other hormonal/inserted contraceptives
    - Not abortifacient but blocks ovulation, as do other hormonal methods of contraceptives
    - Advance provision improves patient use but does not decrease overall pregnancy rates over time.
    - May be offered to all women using short- or moderate-acting contraceptives
  - Ulipristal acetate (UPA) 30 mcg
    - Administered in a single oral dose up to 5 days post unprotected sex with equal effectiveness across time
    - Is more effective in overweight or obese women than progestin methods
    - Not carried by all pharmacies, both community and hospital based as of 2015
    - Often requires insurance preauthorization (unlike progestin only methods) which may delay administration
  - Progesterone-only methods:
    - Most effective when used within 72 hours of intercourse; treatment less likely to be effective up to 5 days
    - Levonorgestrel administered one time at a dose of 1.5 mg available by prescription and over the counter in the United States
    - Male patients should be educated about the use of EC and may purchase this method over the counter as well.

– Yuzpe method of EC with COCs
  ○ Consists of 100 mcg EE + 0.5 mg levonorgestrel given with repeated 2nd dose 12 hours later
  ○ This method has higher rates of nausea and vomiting.
  ○ Generally used as a matter of urgent timing, convenience and expense if a woman has a COC pack of pills at home and prefers to use these for her EC method because the other methods are more effective and have fewer side effects.
- Additional contraceptive methods:
  – General issues:
    ○ Well-known but with significantly lower efficacy
    ○ Include barrier methods to sperm entry (male and female condoms, diaphragms)
  – Male condoms
    ○ 88% effective with typical use; likely higher failure rates in adolescents
    ○ Female condom and diaphragm are 79% and 88% effective, respectively.
    ○ Proper condom use can prevent transmission of sexually transmitted infections such as HIV, HPV, HSV, syphilis, *Neisseria gonorrhoeae*, and *Chlamydia trachomatis*.
    ○ Important to inform teens that condoms are superior for STI prevention but inferior to other methods as a sole agent of contraception.
  – Spermicidal agents
    ○ Include: foam, film, vaginal inserts, as well as nonoxynal-9 as the active agent most widely used
    ○ Only 72% effective in preventing pregnancy with typical use. May reduce transmission of *C. trachomatis* and *N. gonorrhoeae*. When used with condoms, overall efficacy 93% with typical use
    ○ Irritant effect linked in some high-risk populations with increased risk of HIV transmission.
    ○ Spermicides must be inserted with each intercourse, near the time of intercourse; some formulations require 10–15 minutes for activation. Most have an unpleasant taste.
  – Progestin-only pills (POPs) ("mini-pill")
    ○ Much less effective than most other hormonal methods, as effectiveness is highly dependent on perfect use
    ○ May offer some measure of benefit for women who are immediately postpartum (up to 6 months) and breastfeeding on demand
    ○ Typically not a good method for most teens
  – Abstinence
    ○ Abstinence or refraining from vaginal-penile sexual intercourse is the most effective way to prevent unintended or unwanted pregnancy as well as transmission of STIs. However, gaining a mature understanding and experience of one's gender and sexual development is a necessary and desired component of adolescent development.
    ○ Provider counseling and recommendations should promote a 4-pronged approach to sexual decision making: personal maturity and readiness, thoughtful partner selection and communication, family planning and pregnancy prevention, as well as prevention of STIs.

ALERT

- Advising teenagers to abstain from all forms of physical intimacy may be both unrealistic and counterproductive in the context of their psychosocial development.
- Providers should emphasize at every visit that only 100% use of condoms (or abstinence) protects against sexually transmitted diseases but is not the most effective form of birth control available.
- All forms of birth control are not "equal"—long acting reversible contraceptives are significantly more effective contraceptives than all other methods, even sterilization.
- Long acting reversible contraceptive implants are both highly desirable and well tolerated in adolescents and should be offered as first line contraceptives to teens.
- Include male patients in discussions about both condom use as well as contraceptive use.

GENERAL PREVENTION

- Encourage consistent use of latex condoms.
- Patients using oral contraceptive pills may be strongly encouraged to cease tobacco use, but tobacco use does not preclude EP methods in women younger than 35 years.

PATHOPHYSIOLOGY

- Combined EP hormonal therapy suppresses ovulation by directly decreasing release of hypothalamic gonadotropin-releasing hormone (GnRH) and pituitary follicle-stimulating hormone (FSH) and luteinizing hormone (LH).
- Progesterone thickens cervical mucus, thins the endometrium, and decreases tubal motility. Higher dose systemic progestins inhibit the hypothalamic–ovarian axis and halt ovulation.
- Copper: Copper ions inhibit transtubal sperm migration and act in both an ovicidal and spermicidal way to prevent zygote formation.
- EC: Mechanisms of action include ovulation disruption, endometrial impairment to prevent implantation, and possibly sperm or ova transport alteration.
- Spermicides (nonoxynol-9 and octoxynol-9) destroy sperm cell membranes. Most spermicidal preparations contain an inert base (foam, cream, or jelly) to support the spermicidal agent and provide a barrier to sperm entry.

DIAGNOSIS

HISTORY

General considerations in family planning interviews and methods counseling:
- Open queries about family planning intentions should be included in all reproductive age anticipatory guidance or reproductive health visits.
- One Key Question, "Do you want to be pregnant in the next 6 months or year?" opens the conversation to all potential family planning intentions: intention to become pregnant, ambivalence about pregnancy, and desire for contraception and no immediate pregnancy plan.
- Method selection should consider and include the following: past use, failures, and side effects (both real and perceived) of contraceptives, priorities and goals for family planning.
- Does the patient want a pregnancy and parenting? Does his or her partner? Is the teen ambivalent about pregnancy and parenting?
- What is the teen's sexual history? Ask about sexual debut, recent partners, lifetime number of partners, gender and risk behaviors of partners, types of sexual behaviors (may be receptive or giving/insertive, penile-vaginal, penile-anal, oral, digital, dildos and other objects, other)
- Is sexual activity spontaneous or planned? Coerced or desired? Is the teen happy and confident about his or her sexual activity? Does sex give pleasure, feel uncomfortable, any other sexual concerns?
- What methods has the youth tried in the past? What worked, what did not work and why? Does the patient feel that she or he can be compliant with a daily pill or barrier methods? Can the teen demonstrate this ability with other medications or regimens?
- Does the patient require privacy and confidentiality? Does the teen have a parent or guardian's support regarding contraception and safer sex?
- Is the patient comfortable applying a condom or asking their partner to put on a condom?
- Does the patient have open communication with his or her partner? Does the partner respect the patient's decisions? Does the teen feel safe and respected by his or her partner?
- Are there any other barriers to adherence and continuation with the chosen contraceptive method? Is the patient comfortable with the level of efficacy and potential side effects with the current plan?

PHYSICAL EXAM

- Is not essential for some patients who need to start contraception on an urgent or emergency basis. A thorough medical history that excludes current pregnancy, medical conditions that would be a contraindication to particular methods, and a plan for follow-up can allow some providers to begin a method without a physical exam at that time.
- Exams may be helpful in obtaining baseline weight, BP, and other physical stigmata (hirsutism, acne) that may benefit from hormones.
- It is not necessary to perform a pelvic exam on asymptomatic young women initiating hormonal contraception. It is not recommended to perform a pelvic exam (bimanual and speculum) for an adolescent who has never been sexually active but requests contraception.

- A pelvic exam to assess and diagnose an STI or to evaluate for pregnancy in a patient with amenorrhea may be indicated.
  – The Centers for Disease Control and Prevention (CDC) recommends screening for STIs after sexual debut and at least annually until age 25 years.
  – Papanicolaou cancer screening begins after sexual debut and by 21 years of age. Pap guidelines have been evolving and changing over recent years.

DIAGNOSTIC TESTS & INTERPRETATION

- Pregnancy test prior to initiating hormonal contraceptives:
  – Urine pregnancy tests are typically adequate for diagnosing most pregnancies.
  – Serum human choriogonadotropin hormone (B-hCG) is useful when trying to differentiate between normal and abnormal (miscarriage, ectopic) pregnancies.
- It is helpful to ask patients, "when was your last sexual activity without a condom and without birth control?" in order to determine the accuracy of your current pregnancy test, not exclude very early pregnancy, and create a follow-up plan for possible future pregnancy testing in 2–4 weeks.

TREATMENT

GENERAL MEASURES

- Barrier methods: Trained personnel can teach the proper technique for application of condoms and spermicidal agents.
- Fertility (and ovulatory cycles) should return within 6 months of the last DMPA injection.
- Etonogestrel implant is a simple procedure easily done in outpatient settings but requires training and certification by the manufacturer.
- IUDs are also simple outpatient procedures for primary care providers with pelvic and uterine exam skills. Insertion of an IUD should be scheduled when one can be as certain as possible that the adolescent is not pregnant but should not be delayed in a manner that places teen at risk for unintended pregnancy.
- All methods offer contraceptive protection immediately if inserted days 0–5 of their menstrual cycle. Most teens return to ovulation soon after discontinuation of most contraceptives.

ALERT

- Drugs that activate the cytochrome P-450 enzyme will diminish the efficacy of hormonal contraceptives and may include the following: phenobarbital, carbamazepine, primidone, rifampin, griseofulvin, HIV protease inhibitors, and tetracyclines (including doxycycline).
- Hormonal contraceptives can increase concentrations of phenytoin, benzodiazepines, antidepressants, corticosteroids, β-blockers, theophylline, and alcohol.
- Hormonal contraceptives can decrease the efficacy of acetaminophen, oral anticoagulants, hypoglycemics, and methyldopa.

ONGOING CARE

FOLLOW-UP RECOMMENDATIONS

Patient Monitoring

- Patients using hormonal contraceptives should be seen within 6 weeks to 2 months of initiation, to evaluate adherence, continuation and help manage side effects.
- BP, weight, and STIs may continue to be monitored.

PROGNOSIS

- Use of COCs declines over time:
  – 45% in 3 months
  – 33% at 1 year

COMPLICATIONS

Barrier methods

- Latex allergy: Patients may use polyurethane rather than latex condoms. Animal skin condoms are permeable to viral pathogens.
- Breakage or permeability: Oil-based lubricants and most intravaginal medications used with latex condoms will increase the risks of these complications.

Spermicides

- Local irritation or allergic reaction
- May increase the risk of HIV infection in adolescents with high-risk sexual partners

Hormonal EP contraceptives

- Contraindications to COC pills are uncommon in most teens and include the following: pregnancy, history of thromboembolic event, structural heart disease, breast cancer, active liver disease, migraine headaches with an aura, prolonged immobilization, or severe hypertension.
- Caution should be taken with women $<$6 weeks postpartum, with gallbladder disease, and those who use medications that affect liver enzymes.
- Minor, and usually self-limited, side effects of COCs may include intermenstrual spotting, nausea, breast changes, fluid retention, leukorrhea, minor headache, and depression.
- Thromboembolic events and liver disease are extremely rare in nonsmoking adolescents using estrogen-containing oral contraceptive pills. Placing risk in perspective is essential to adequate consent. Estimates of VTE may be communicated as follows:
  – Baseline risk: 10 in 100,000 women-years
  – COC user risk: 15 in 100,000 women-years
  – 3rd generation COC (desogestrel) or patch risk: 30 in 100,000 women-years
  – Pregnancy risk: 60 in 100,000 women-years
- Mortality from estradiol-containing methods is estimated at 1 in 1.5 million per year. Mortality from bike riding, motor vehicle crashes, and other causes is much higher. Death from gynecologic and related causes was 7/100,000 in 15–19-year-old adolescents per year. If no fertility control measures were used, the mortality is 0.3/100,000 per year in nonsmoking oral contraceptive pill users and 2.2/100,000 per year in smoking oral contraceptive pill users.

Progestin-only methods

- POPs' side effects include weight gain, rapid hair turnover, and menstrual irregularities.
- DMPA can reduce bone mineral density (BMD), which typically rebounds to normal after DMPA discontinuation. Because adolescence is the period of peak bone mass accretion, there is concern that DMPA use during adolescence may increase the risk for osteopenia or osteoporosis later in life. This has not been proven or validated at present. For adolescents with anorexia nervosa, chronic steroid use, chronic renal failure, there may be better LARCs available that have no BMD impact.

- Most common side effect reported with etonogestrel implant is abnormal bleeding. A wide range of bleeding patterns may be experienced, and it is not possible to predict the bleeding pattern for any individual.
- Overall, in the 90-day reference periods of clinical trial experience, 33.3% had infrequent bleeding, 21.4% had amenorrhea, 6.1% had frequent bleeding, and 16.9% had prolonged bleeding.
- The lower androgenic effect of etonogestrel may make side effects of acne and weight gain less frequent than with other progestins.

IUDs

- Contraindications to IUD placement are those who are pregnant or suspected to be pregnant, have active PID or puerperal or postabortion sepsis, malignancy of the genital tract, uterine abnormalities that distort the uterine cavity, an allergy to any component of IUDs, or Wilson disease (for the copper T IUD only).
- IUDs have been associated with a slightly higher risk of PID within the first 21 days after insertion, especially if cervical infection is present. IUDs do not increase risk of PID above baseline after this time.
- Younger age may confer an increased risk of IUD failure from expulsion because of smaller uterus and higher incidence of nulliparity.
- The copper T IUD has been associated with increased menstrual bleeding and spotting, especially in first 3–6 months after insertion. In addition, some women may experience menstrual pain and heavy bleeding throughout use.

Emergency contraception

- Nausea and/or vomiting occur in most patients using Yuzpe (EP) EC or "doubling up" on oral contraceptive pills.

ADDITIONAL READING

- Committee on Adolescent Health Care Long-Acting Reversible Contraception Working Group, The American College of Obstetricians and Gynecologists. Committee opinion no. 539: adolescents and long-acting reversible contraception: implants and intrauterine devices. *Obstet Gynecol*. 2012;120(4):983–988.
- Bellanca HK, Hunter MS. ONE KEY QUESTION®: preventive reproductive health is part of high quality primary care. *Contraception*. 2013;88(1):3–6.
- Centers for Disease Control and Prevention. U.S. medical eligibility criteria for contraceptive use, 2010. *MMWR Recomm Rep*. 2010;59(RR-4):1–86.
- Dean G, Schwarz EB. Intrauterine contraceptives (IUCs). In: Hatcher RA, Trussell J, Nelson AL, et al, eds. *Contraceptive Technology*. 20th ed. New York, NY: Ardent Media; 2011:147–191.
- Mestad R, Secura G, Allsworth JE, et al. Acceptance of long-acting reversible contraceptive methods by adolescent participants in the Contraceptive CHOICE Project. *Contraception*. 2011;84(5):493–498.
- Sitruk-Ware R, Nath A, Mishell DR Jr. Contraception technology: past, present and future. *Contraception*. 2013;87(3):319–330.
- Trussell J. Contraceptive efficacy. In: Hatcher RA, Trussell J, Nelson AL, et al, eds. *Contraceptive Technology*. 20th ed. New York, NY: Ardent Media; 2011.
- Winner B, Peipert JF, Zhao Q, et al. Effectiveness of long-acting reversible contraception. *N Engl J Med*. 2012;366(21):1998–2007.

CODES

ICD10

- Z30.9 Encounter for contraceptive management, unspecified
- Z30.09 Encounter for oth general cnsl and advice on contraception
- Z30.8 Encounter for other contraceptive management

FAQ

- Q: My adolescent, minor patient asks for confidentiality regarding contraception. Can I comply?
- A: Yes. Teenagers benefit from private and confidential contraceptive services. Teens should have right to confidentiality regarding contraception and treatment of STIs, even though some states do not have specific laws protecting these rights. The benchmark of care supported by all professional medical societies supports private and confidential contraceptive care for teens. Do not assume, however, that a teen may not have or benefit from parental support in her efforts to prevent pregnancy. It may be in the patient's best interest to have a caring adult involved. Which adult and how he or she is involved should be negotiated with the adolescent.
- Q: My adolescent patient has been on and off short-acting birth control methods? I am worried about her risk of pregnancy? How might I better help her?
- A: There are several parts to managing this issue.
  - First, in an open and supportive manner, ask her whether she wants to become pregnant and parent or would she like to delay pregnancy?
  - Second, if she wishes to delay pregnancy over the next 6–12 months, offer her a LARC. Educate her on the superior efficacy and ease of use. Insert a LARC that day or facilitate an urgent referral to a teen-friendly provider if she continues to express an interest.
  - While she waits for that appointment, offer to help her protect from unintended pregnancy with a single dose of DMPA providing coverage for the next 12 weeks. Offer her EC as well.
  - Applaud efforts to be smart and safely sexually active.
  - Engage her partner, if present and supportive, in contraceptive discussions and discussions about safe, satisfying, and responsible sexuality.
- Q: One of my patients has asked me to prescribe EC in advance for her. Is this something that I should do?
- A: Yes! EC is now over the counter, but if a patient is more likely to access using insurance coverage, this may increase use. Studies done clearly show that use of EC is safe. In fact, there are no absolute contraindications to using progestin-only EC. Because unprotected sexual encounters often take place at a time when adolescents do not have access to their health care providers (e.g., evenings or weekends), advanced prescription may be of benefit for many adolescents.
- Q: What should I tell my patient if she misses a dose of her oral contraceptive?
- A: If she has missed 1 pill, she should take it as soon as she remembers, then take the next pill at the regular time. If she has missed 2 doses, she should take 2 when she remembers, and then 2 the next day. She should use a back-up method during the cycle in which she had to "double up." If she has missed 3 or more pills, she will probably menstruate. After discarding the last pack, she should start a new pack on the 1st Sunday after the start of her next period. She is not protected during the remainder of this cycle.

COR PULMONALE

Brian D. Hanna • Heather L. Meluskey

BASICS

DESCRIPTION

- Cor pulmonale is right ventricular (RV) failure secondary to an altered pulmonary process that results in a loss of functional capillary vascular bed and in excessive pulmonary artery pressure and pulmonary vascular resistance (PVR).
- Cor pulmonale is not the result of a primary congenital heart defect.

ALERT

- In newborns, the RV muscle mass is comparable to that of the left ventricle.
- RV failure from pulmonary hypertension (PH) occurs but is rare in newborns.
- RV failure in newborns is usually a consequence of hypoxemia, ischemia, metabolic acidosis (e.g., persistent fetal circulation), and/or premature restriction/closure of the intrauterine ductus arteriosus.

EPIDEMIOLOGY

- Cor pulmonale may be found at any age but is typically a result of a long-standing pulmonary process. However, severe bronchopulmonary dysplasia is an increasingly common cause of neonatal PH.
- Primary pulmonary hypertension (PPHN) is most often diagnosed in the 2nd or 3rd decade of life with a female predominance, and it is often diagnosed during pregnancy.

Incidence

- PPHN has an annual incidence of 2 per million.

Prevalence

- Upward of 2 per 1,000 neonatal intensive care unit patients will develop significant cor pulmonale.
- 2% of infants undergoing cardiac surgery will have PH, with an associated mortality of 10–20%.

RISK FACTORS

Genetics

- Pediatric patients with trisomy syndromes are at high risk for PH.
- Familial PH has been mapped to chromosome 2q32, but this is less frequently found in patients with secondary etiologies of PH.
- Region 2q32 point mutations encode for a defective bone morphogenic receptor 2, a pulmonary vascular smooth muscle receptor that mediates proliferation.

PATHOPHYSIOLOGY

- Chronic hypoxia is the principal factor, resulting in a cascade of endothelial dysfunction with pulmonary vasoconstriction, followed by the development of PH.
- A variety of vasoactive mediators may be responsible for the effect on vasomotor tone.
- Alveolar hypoventilation, hypoxemia, hypercarbia, and/or acidemia all result in increased RV afterload and decreased RV systolic function.

ETIOLOGY

- Parenchymal lung disease (most common)
- Chronic obstructive pulmonary disease
  - Cystic fibrosis
  - Asthma
- Restrictive lung disease
  - Infectious
  - Pulmonary toxins
  - Pulmonary fibrosis
  - Bronchopulmonary dysplasia (combined)
- Upper airway diseases: tonsillar/adenoidal hypertrophy
- Syndromes (Down, Treacher Collins)
- Neuromuscular disorders: Duchenne muscular dystrophy
- Chest wall deformities

COMMONLY ASSOCIATED CONDITIONS

- Pulmonary vascular abnormalities
- Collagen vascular diseases
- Pulmonary veno-occlusive disease
- Pulmonary thromboembolism
- PPHN

DIAGNOSIS

HISTORY

- Fatigue
- Failure to thrive/weight loss
- Dizziness
- Syncope
- Exercise intolerance
- Chest pain (secondary to RV ischemia)
- Palpitations
- Hemoptysis

ALERT

Hemoptysis is a life-threatening emergency and heralds a poor prognosis for any patient with PH.

PHYSICAL EXAM

- Tachycardia
- Parasternal RV impulse
- Cyanosis may be evident.
- Hepatomegaly, jugular venous distention, peripheral edema
- A loud, narrowly split or single 2nd heart sound (P_2); RV gallop; holosystolic murmur right of the sternum (tricuspid regurgitation); and/or diastolic murmur at the left upper sternal border (pulmonary insufficiency)

ALERT

In the newborn period to puberty, an abnormally increased RV impulse is best felt under the xiphoid sternum.

DIAGNOSTIC TESTS & INTERPRETATION

Lab

- Brain-type natriuretic peptide is an excellent biomarker of RV diastolic dysfunction and is elevated with worsening cor pulmonale.
- Decreased Pao_2, increased $Paco_2$, and a compensatory metabolic alkalosis
- Polycythemia may be consistent with chronic hypoxemia.

Imaging

- Chest radiograph: cardiomegaly from RV dilation and main pulmonary artery enlargement
- Echo: RV dilation, tricuspid annular plane systolic excursion (TAPSE), RV hypertrophy, pulmonic insufficiency, RV pressure estimate from tricuspid regurgitation, and/or intraventricular septal position
- Ventricular/perfusion (V/Q) scan is beneficial to rule out thromboembolic disease.
- Chest CT scan: volumes to assess lung hypoplasia, interstitial lung disease, thromboembolic disease, and large pulmonary vein disease

Diagnostic Procedures/Other

- ECG: may show right atrial enlargement, RV hypertrophy, and T-wave inversion
- 6-minute walk: measures functional capacity and limitations; 2 minute tests are reliable for those younger than 6 years old.
- Cardiac catheterization, although invasive, remains the gold standard.
- Lung biopsy is usually contraindicated in the face of PH and significant lung disease.

Pathologic Findings
- Vascular lesions (plexiform lesions)
- Parenchymal fibrotic lesions
- Concentric and eccentric remodeling

DIFFERENTIAL DIAGNOSIS
- Congenital heart disease with PH and right-to-left shunt (Eisenmenger syndrome)
- Obstruction of pulmonary venous return, both anatomic obstruction and left ventricular failure
- Pulmonary veno-occlusive disease
- Alveolar capillary dysplasia

TREATMENT

MEDICATION
First Line
- Oxygen to keep saturations >90%
- Anticongestive medications (digoxin, diuretics)

Second Line
Vasodilator therapy with care not to worsen the intrapulmonary shunt

ADDITIONAL TREATMENT
General Measures
- The primary goal is reduction of the abnormally elevated pulmonary artery pressure and the RV workload.
- If at all possible, address the primary etiology (i.e., tonsillectomy/adenoidectomy in a patient with obstructive upper airway disease).
- Fluid boluses are poorly tolerated and rarely augment systemic BP.
- Oxygen (nocturnal oxygen)
- Diuretics (if pulmonary congestion)
- Bronchodilators (theophylline)
- Digoxin (may improve RV contractility)
- Anticoagulants
- Pulmonary vasodilators
  - Nitric oxide
  - Calcium channel blockers (only if >1 year of age and cardiac output is not compromised)
  - Phosphodiesterase-5 inhibitors
  - Endothelin receptor antagonists
  - Prostanoid
- Atrial septostomy (in select cases, may improve cardiac output but at the expense of hypoxemia)
- Lung or heart–lung transplantation
- Usually self-limited activity
- No competitive sports
- Arginine, a nitric oxide donor, has been used; however, the increased amino acid concentrations are proliferative and may worsen the long-term prognosis.

SURGERY/OTHER PROCEDURES
Consider tracheostomy, Nissen fundoplication, and gastrostomy tube (G-tube) early

ONGOING CARE

FOLLOW-UP RECOMMENDATIONS
Patient Monitoring
Home oxygen saturation monitoring is indicated when night oxygen is necessary to keep saturations >90%.

PROGNOSIS
- Patients with reversible lung disease usually have a better prognosis.
- Patients with cor pulmonale are at risk for sudden death because of the inability to augment cardiac output with exercise, growth, or febrile illnesses.
- Numerous medical therapies and lung transplantation may improve long-term survival.
- Long-term survival is variable and depends on the age at onset of pulmonary changes and the underlying conditions (e.g., Down syndrome) that may adversely affect survival.
- Death often occurs in the 2nd or 3rd decade of life.

COMPLICATIONS
Aside from the underlying lung process, the chronic hypoxia results in polycythemia, decreased systemic oxygen delivery, and RV failure secondary to the inability of the RV to handle the excessive afterload.

ADDITIONAL READING

- Bandla HP, Davis SH, Hopkins NE. Lipoid pneumonia: a silent complication of mineral oil aspiration. *Pediatrics*. 1999;103(2):E19.
- Brouillette RT, Fernback SK, Hunt CE. Obstructive sleep apnea in infants and children. *J Pediatr*. 1982;100(1):31–40.
- Cerro MJ, Abman S, Diaz G, et al. A consensus approach to the classification of pediatric pulmonary hypertensive vascular disease: report from the PVRI Pediatric Taskforce, Panama 2011. *Pulm Circ*. 2011;1(2):286–298.
- Koestenberger M, Revekes W, Everett AD, et al. Right ventricular function in infants, children and adolescents: reference value of the tricuspid annular plane systolic excursion (TAPSE) in 640 healthy patients and calculation of z score values. *J Am Soc Echocardiogr*. 2009;22(6):715–719.
- Perkin RM, Anas NG. Pulmonary hypertension in pediatric patients. *J Pediatr*. 1984;105(4):511–522.
- Proceedings of the 4th World Symposium on Pulmonary Hypertension, February 2008, Dana Point, California, USA. *J Am Coll Cardiol*. 2009; 54(1)(Suppl):S1–S117.
- Rashid A, Ivy D. Severe paediatric pulmonary hypertension: new management strategies. *Arch Dis Child*. 2005;90(1):92–98.
- Simonneau G, Robbins M, Beghetti M, et al. Updated clinical classification of pulmonary hypertension. *J Am Coll Cardiol*. 2009;54(1)(Suppl):S43–S54.

CODES

ICD10
- I27.81 Cor pulmonale (chronic)
- I26.09 Other pulmonary embolism with acute cor pulmonale

FAQ
- Q: Is cardiac catheterization indicated in all patients with cor pulmonale?
- A: Yes. Although a great deal of information can be learned from echocardiogram, direct pulmonary artery pressure/resistance measurements require an invasive procedure. In addition, assessment of the reactivity of the pulmonary vascular bed to various agents (oxygen, prostacyclin, and calcium channel blockers) is best performed in the catheterization laboratory.
- Q: Is nocturnal oxygen therapy beneficial?
- A: Nocturnal oxygen has been speculated to delay the progression of cor pulmonale in some select patients with obstructive sleep hypoxemia.

COSTOCHONDRITIS

Richard M. Kravitz

BASICS

DESCRIPTION

Costochondritis is chest pain that emanates from a costal cartilage and is reproducible on compression of that cartilage.

EPIDEMIOLOGY

- Frequency of sternal wound infections following median sternotomy is 0.1–1.6%.
- Costochondritis accounts for 10–31% of all pediatric chest pain.
- Peak age for chest pain in children is 12–14 years.

PATHOPHYSIOLOGY

- Inflammation of unknown etiology (histologic examination is usually normal)
- Infection
  - Can present months to years after surgery (the costal cartilage is avascular, making it vulnerable to infection if it has been exposed, injured, or denuded of perichondrium)
  - Complication of median sternotomy
  - Occurs by spread from adjacent osteomyelitis or may arise de novo during surgery

ETIOLOGY

- Infectious
  - Bacterial
    - *Staphylococcus aureus* (especially after thoracic surgery)
    - *Salmonella* (in sickle cell disease)
    - *Escherichia coli*
    - *Pseudomonas* sp.
    - *Klebsiella* sp.
  - Fungal
    - *Aspergillus flavus*
    - *Candida albicans*
- Posttraumatic injury

DIAGNOSIS

HISTORY

- Inflammatory costochondritis
  - Pain usually preceded by exercise or an upper respiratory tract infection
  - Description of pain
    - Usually sharp
    - Affects the anterior chest wall
    - Localized or radiates to the back or abdomen
    - Usually unilateral (left side greater than right side)
  - The 4th–6th costochondral junction is the usual site of pain.
  - Motion of the arm and shoulder on the affected side elicits the pain.
  - Girls are affected more often than are boys.
- Tietze syndrome
  - Onset is usually abrupt but can be gradual.
  - Believed to be caused by a minor trauma, although etiology is unknown
  - Description of pain
    - Radiates to arms or shoulder
    - May last up to several weeks
    - Swelling at the sternochondral junction may persist for several months to years.
  - Usually affects the 2nd or 3rd costochondral joint
  - Pain is aggravated by sneezing, coughing, deep inspiration, or twisting motions of the chest.
  - No differences in frequency between sexes
- Infectious costochondritis
  - Slow, insidious course
  - Usually unimpressive clinical symptomatology

PHYSICAL EXAM

- Usually normal
- Inspect for evidence of trauma, scars, bruising, and swelling.
- Palpation and percussion of the costochondral and costosternal junctions should reproduce and localize the pain.
- In Tietze syndrome, spindle-shaped swelling is visible at the sternochondral junction.

DIAGNOSTIC TESTS & INTERPRETATION

Lab

- WBC count not helpful (even when infection present)
- EKG (may be helpful if cardiac etiology is being considered)

Imaging

- Radiologic studies (chest x-ray, CT) usually not helpful
- Gallium scan
  - May be useful in some cases of infectious origin
  - Not highly specific
  - May show increased radionuclide uptake
  - No evidence of osteomyelitis of the sternum in most cases
- Technetium bone scan
  - Not highly specific

DIFFERENTIAL DIAGNOSIS

- Cardiovascular
  - Myocardial infarction
  - Pericarditis
  - Pericardial effusion
  - Myocarditis
  - Endocarditis
  - Cardiomyopathy
  - Premature ventricular contractions
  - Supraventricular tachycardia
  - Dissecting aneurysm
- Pulmonary
  - Asthma
  - Exercise-induced bronchospasm
  - Pneumonia
  - Pleural effusion
  - Pneumothorax
  - Pulmonary embolism
- GI
  - Gastroesophageal reflux
  - Esophagitis
  - Gastritis
  - Achalasia
- Mechanical
  - Muscle strain
  - Stress fractures
  - Precordial catch syndrome
  - Trauma
- Rheumatologic
  - Rheumatoid arthritis
  - Ankylosing spondylitis
- Oncologic
  - Rhabdomyosarcoma
  - Leukemia
  - Ewing sarcoma
- Miscellaneous
  - Tietze syndrome
  - Psychogenic chest pain
  - Breast tissue pain (both sexes)

TREATMENT

GENERAL MEASURES

- Inflammatory costochondritis
  - Anti-inflammatory and analgesic agents
  - Reassurance
  - If pain disturbs normal activities and sports, infiltration with local anesthetic may prove useful.

ALERT

- Inflammatory costochondritis
  - Important cause of school absence
  - Adolescents tend to limit physical activity unnecessarily for long periods.
  - Restriction of activities is usually not required.
  - Most adolescents still worry about cardiac problems, even after the diagnosis has been made.

- Infectious costochondritis
  - Prolonged course of intravenous (IV) antibiotics
  - Prompt surgical resection of all involved cartilage
  - Reconstructive surgery with muscular flaps should be done.

ALERT

- Infectious costochondritis
  - Long-term IV antibiotics alone do not resolve the problem; surgical resection and repair also are required.
  - There is a tendency for the infection to spread to adjacent costal cartilages and across the sternum to the contralateral chest wall.
  - In general, avoid costochondral junctions when performing surgical procedures in the chest (i.e., chest tube placement).

ONGOING CARE

FOLLOW-UP RECOMMENDATIONS

Patient Monitoring

- Inflammatory costochondritis
  - Long-lasting condition
  - Follow-up once a year is recommended.
- Infectious costochondritis
  - Long-term follow-up after surgery is mandatory.

PROGNOSIS

- Inflammatory costochondritis: excellent
- Infectious costochondritis: prognosis relates to
  - Underlying clinical condition of the patient (i.e., immunocompromised, postradiation therapy for cancer, postcardiac surgery)
  - Extent of surgery required to reconstruct the area damaged by the infection

ADDITIONAL READING

- Brown RT, Jamil K. Costochondritis in adolescents. A follow-up study. *Clin Pediatr*. 1993;32(8):499–500.
- Kocis KC. Chest pain in pediatrics. *Pediatr Clin North Am*. 1999;46(2):189–203.
- Mendelson G, Mendelson H, Horowitz SF, et al. Can (99m)technetium methylene diphosphate bone scans objectively document costochondritis? *Chest*. 1997;111(6):1600–1602.
- Selbst DM. Consultation with the specialist. Chest pain in children. *Pediatr Rev*. 1997;18(5):169–173.
- Son MB, Sundel RP. Musculoskeletal causes of pediatric chest pain. *Pediatr Clin North Am*. 2010;57(6):1385–1395.
- Talner NS, Carboni MP. Chest pain in the adolescent and young adult. *Cardiol Rev*. 2000;8(1):49–56.

CODES

ICD10

M94.0 Chondrocostal junction syndrome [Tietze]

FAQ

- Q: Am I having or will I have a heart attack?
- A: Chest pain does not imply a heart problem. This pain arises from the chest wall; there is no risk of a myocardial infarction. A cardiac etiology to chest pain in an adolescent is usually uncommon.
- Q: Is costochondritis related to arthritis?
- A: There is no relation to any form of arthritis.
- Q: Where does the name Tietze syndrome come from?
- A: The syndrome is named after German surgeon Alexander Tietze (1864–1927), who first described the syndrome in 1921.

C

COUGH

Margaret M. McNamara • Gwynne D. Church

BASICS

DESCRIPTION

A high-velocity expulsion of gas from the airways that serves to clear them of mucus, cellular and microbial debris, or foreign bodies. An absence or inability to cough can lead to recurrent pneumonia. Cough can be acute (<2 weeks), subacute/protracted (2–4 weeks), or chronic (>4 weeks).

EPIDEMIOLOGY

Cough is the most common symptom presenting to primary care physicians in the United States and worldwide. Chronic cough accounts for up to 9% of chief complaints to U.S. pediatricians.

Healthy children can have a nonpathologic cough. School-age children typically experience 10 cough episodes per day.

PATHOPHYSIOLOGY

Cough results from a complex reflex phenomenon initiated by cough receptors that is mediated through the brainstem. The receptors are located in the respiratory tract from the larynx to the segmental bronchi, paranasal sinuses, external auditory canal, and stomach and are triggered by thermal, chemical, mechanical, or inflammatory stimuli. Cough is generally reflexive but may sometimes be voluntarily initiated or suppressed.

DIAGNOSIS

DIFFERENTIAL DIAGNOSIS

Infection and asthma are the most common causes of cough in all pediatric age groups and should always be considered.

Children have an average of 6–8 upper respiratory infections (URIs) per year, with each lasting up to 2–3 weeks. Roughly 1/3 of preschool-aged children cough more than 10 days after a cold, and 10% of preschool children cough more than 25 days after a cold.

- **Causes of acute (<2 weeks) or subacute/ protracted (2–4 weeks) cough**
  - Infection
  - Reactive airway disease (RAD)
  - Sinusitis
  - Irritants
  - Allergy
  - Foreign body
- **Causes of chronic (>4 weeks) cough**
  - Bronchitis
  - Postinfectious
  - Sinusitis
  - Asthma
  - Irritants (cigarette smoke exposure, air pollution)
  - Allergic rhinitis
  - Foreign body
  - Gastroesophageal reflux (GER)
  - Habitual or psychogenic
  - Anatomic abnormalities: tracheoesophageal fistula, tracheobronchomalacia, laryngeal cleft, polyps, adductor vocal cord paralysis, pulmonary sequestration, bronchogenic cyst, cystic hygroma, vascular ring, tumor
  - Cystic fibrosis (CF)
  - Ciliary dyskinesia
  - Immunodeficiency states that result in recurrent respiratory infections: HIV, immunoglobulin deficiencies (IgA, IgG), phagocytic defects, complement deficiency
  - Interstitial lung disease
  - Angiotensin-converting enzyme inhibitors
  - Stimulation of external auditory canal cough receptors (Arnold reflex cough)

APPROACH TO PATIENT

Given the common nature of cough and the large differential diagnosis it generates, an extremely thorough history and physical exam (H&P) should direct a rational, stepwise approach.

HISTORY

- **Question:** How long has the child coughed?
- *Significance*: Most acute and subacute coughs are associated with viral URIs. Pediatric chronic cough is defined as daily cough that lasts for >4 weeks.
- **Question:** Is there a recent history of URI?
- *Significance*: Serial URIs, the most common cause of chronic cough in children, can be diagnosed by a careful history of waxing and waning symptoms and will avoid unnecessary tests. Also consider postinfectious cough (due to heightened cough receptor sensitivity) or sinusitis (which complicates up to 5% of URIs). Overall, 8–12% of children with URIs develop complications.
- **Question:** What are the associated symptoms?
- *Significance*:
  - Fever and nasal discharge suggests infection.
  - Fever with chills or night sweats suggests TB in children with chronic cough.
  - With rhinorrhea, halitosis, headache, or facial edema, consider sinusitis.
  - With respiratory distress, suspect RAD, infection, or foreign body.
- **Question:** What is the quality of the cough?
- *Significance*:
  - Acute wet cough suggests upper or lower airway respiratory infection or asthma.
  - Subacute wet cough suggests sinusitis, bronchitis, or asthma.
  - Chronic wet cough is always abnormal and can be associated with sinusitis, bronchitis, asthma, CF, ciliary dyskinesia, bronchitis, or anatomic lower airway abnormality such as tracheomalacia.
  - Dry cough can suggest asthma.
  - Barking cough is usually associated with croup.
  - Brassy cough is associated with tracheomalacia.
  - A honking or barking chronic cough that increases during times of stress and is absent during sleep is typical for habit cough.
  - Staccato cough suggests chlamydial pneumonia in infants.
  - Paroxysmal cough, with or without whoop, suggests pertussis or parapertussis.
- **Question:** What is the pattern of the cough?
- *Significance*:
  - Chronic nighttime cough suggests RAD, postnasal drip from allergic rhinitis, or GERD.
  - With nighttime/early morning cough, consider sinusitis or allergic rhinitis.
  - Seasonal cough suggests allergy.
- **Question:** Are there any known triggers of cough (e.g., smoke, cold air, dust, URI)?
- *Significance*: Consider irritant, allergy, or RAD.
- **Question:** Is there any personal or familial history of atopy?
- *Significance*: Consider RAD.
- **Question:** Are there recurrent infections?
- *Significance*: Consider immunodeficiency, CF. Consider pulmonary sequestration if patient has recurrent pneumonias in same location.
- **Question:** Is there any relation of cough to feedings?
- *Significance*: Consider aspiration, GER, laryngeal cleft, and tracheoesophageal fistula.
- **Question:** Is there a history of a choking episode?
- *Significance*: Consider retained foreign body.
- **Question:** Is there exercise intolerance?
- *Significance*: Consider asthma, interstitial lung disease
- **Question:** What is the parental level of concern?
- *Significance*: Children's cough generates significant parental stress and concerns, and appreciation of parental worries is valuable when addressing this problem.

PHYSICAL EXAM

Assess patient's general appearance

- **Finding:** Evidence of failure to thrive?
- *Significance*: Consider TB, CF, immunodeficiency, aspiration
- **Finding:** Cyanosis or pallor?
- *Significance*: Consider pneumonia, asthma
- **Finding:** Signs of respiratory distress such as tachypnea, accessory muscle use?
- *Significance*: Consider pneumonia, asthma, congenital anatomic abnormalities
- **Finding:** Barrel chest?
- *Significance*: Suggests air trapping due to chronic disease
- **Finding:** Clubbing?
- *Significance*: Consider CF, ciliary dyskinesia, interstitial lung disease, chronic aspiration
- **Finding:** Nasal polyp?
- *Significance*: Must rule out CF. Also seen with allergic rhinitis.
- **Finding:** Tracheal deviation?
- *Significance*: Suggests mediastinal mass or foreign body aspiration
- **Finding:** Signs of atopic disease such as eczema, allergic shiners, transverse nasal crease, rhinitis, mucosal cobblestoning, injected conjunctivae?
- *Significance*: Allergic rhinitis
- **Finding:** Rhinorrhea/purulent posterior pharyngeal drainage, sniffling, halitosis, periorbital edema, sinus tenderness?
- *Significance*: Suggest sinusitis
- **Finding:** Crackles (rales)?
- *Significance*: Coarse crackles suggest bronchiectasis; fine crackles suggest pneumonia, atelectasis, pulmonary edema, and interstitial lung disease.
- **Finding:** Rhonchi
- *Significance*: Bronchitis, impaired cough (from weakness, tracheostomy)
- **Finding:** Decreased breath sounds
- *Significance*: Suggests pneumonia, pleural effusion, chest mass
- **Finding:** Wheezing?
- *Significance*:
  - Polyphonic inspiratory or expiratory wheezes suggest RAD.
  - Monophonic or fixed wheezes should make one consider foreign body or mass/congenital lesion.

DIAGNOSTIC TESTS & INTERPRETATION

- Laboratory investigation should reflect a rational, stepwise approach based on likely etiologies after a thorough history.
- Evidence-based clinical practice guidelines for evaluating chronic cough in pediatrics were published in 2006. In general, children with chronic cough should have a chest radiograph, and spirometry should be considered for children >4 years of age.
- **Test:** chest x-ray posteroanterior/lateral
- *Significance*: Detect infection, foreign body, chronic aspiration, interstitial lung disease, pulmonary edema, diaphragmatic hernia, signs typical for asthma, CF
- **Test:** Spirometry
- *Significance*: Detect airway obstruction or lung restriction. Pre- and post-bronchodilator response is useful to diagnose asthma.
- **Test:** Microbiology workup as indicated (e.g., polymerase chain reaction [PCR] for pertussis, direct fluorescent antibody [DFA] for viral panel, culture for *Chlamydia*)
- *Significance*: Aids in precise diagnosis and treatment as needed
- **Test:** Paranasal sinus CTscan
- *Significance*: Should be used judiciously to evaluate sinus disease, that is, for complications of sinusitis, recurrent sinusitis
- **Test:** CBC
- *Significance*: Eosinophilia suggests atopic disease or, rarely, parasitic infection; anemia should prompt one to consider chronic disease or, rarely, pulmonary hemosiderosis; leukocytosis suggests infection.
- **Test:** Bronchoscopy
- *Significance*: Diagnose presence of foreign body, and airway anomalies (laryngeal cleft, tracheobronchomalacia, tracheoesophageal fistula [TEF], vascular ring) and perform alveolar lavage for cultures, cytology, hemosiderin-laden macrophages (suggests alveolar bleeding), lipid-laden macrophages (suggest aspiration)
- **Test:** Barium swallow
- *Significance*: Aspiration
- **Test:** Upper GI series
- *Significance*: Vascular ring
- **Test:** Mantoux test: purified protein derivative (PPD) skin test
- *Significance*: To diagnose TB
- **Test:** Serum IgE
- *Significance*: Significant elevation indicates allergy or, rarely, allergic bronchopulmonary aspergillosis
- **Test:** Sweat test
- *Significance*: To diagnose CF, but need to be sure that laboratory has experience with this test
- **Test:** Immune workup
- *Significance*: HIV, immunodeficiency
- **Test:** pH probe
- *Significance*: GER
- **Test:** High-resolution CT scan of the thorax, video fluoroscopy, echocardiogram, or nuclear medicine scans
- *Significance*: May be judiciously used; generally reserved until after referral to a specialist

Imaging

Chest x-ray

- Infiltrates may suggest pneumonia, bronchiolitis, pneumonitis, TB, CF, bronchiectasis, or foreign body.
- Volume loss may be seen with foreign body aspiration; sometimes need to obtain lateral decubitus views in young children who cannot cooperate with inspiratory/expiratory views.
- Hyperinflation suggests RAD or CF.
- Mediastinal nodes may indicate infection (especially TB or fungal) or malignancy.

TREATMENT

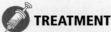

ADDITIONAL TREATMENT

General Measures

- Cough should be treated based on etiology.
- OTC cough medicines are widely prescribed and overused.
- The U.S. Food and Drug administration (FDA) and Consumer Healthcare Products Association recommend avoiding OTC cough and cold medicines in children <4 years of age. An American Academy Pediatrics position statement questions the efficacy and safety of these medications in children <6 years of age.
- To avoid overuse of antibiotics, parents should be informed that viral URI can cause cough that commonly lasts up to 2–3 weeks.
- Educate parents about the beneficial function of cough to remove irritants and about the potential harm of suppressing a productive cough or cough secondary to RAD.
- Honey may be used in children older than age 1 year. Acute cough from URI or chronic nonspecific cough (i.e., dry cough in the absence of asthma or other identifiable disease) may be safely, effectively, and inexpensively treated with honey.
- Specific pharmacologic interventions:
  - RAD: Bronchodilators ± inhaled anti-inflammatory agents, oral or inhaled steroids, removal of irritants
  - Infection: Appropriate antibiotics as indicated. May be considered in cases of chronic productive cough or pneumonia.
  - Antihistamines (nonsedating) should be used only when cough coexists with rhinitis.
- Self-hypnosis is a safe, effective treatment for children with habit cough.
- Children with "nonspecific cough" (i.e., without specific indicators by H&P as noted earlier) generally do not derive much benefit from medications and may undergo a period of "watchful waiting." If medications are used, patients need to be reassessed in 2–3 weeks.

ISSUES FOR REFERRAL

- The vast majority of cases of cough, even when chronic, can be diagnosed and managed by the primary care physician.
- Factors in making a referral:
  - The cough is unresponsive to treatment.
  - The cause is likely to be an anatomic malformation or foreign body aspiration.
  - There appears to be involvement of other organ systems (e.g., failure to thrive, CF, congestive heart failure, immunodeficiency, unusual infection).
- Hemoptysis

Initial Stabilization

- Cough should be considered an emergency if there are associated signs or symptoms of respiratory distress.
- Routine emergency airway assessment should be undertaken on presentation and appropriate supportive measures started in cases in which there is concern.

C

ADDITIONAL READING

- Anbar RD, Hall HR. Childhood habit cough treated with self-hypnosis. *J Pediatr*. 2004;144(2):213–217.
- Carr BC. Efficacy, abuse, and toxicity of over-the-counter cough and cold medicines in the pediatric population. *Curr Opin Pediatr*. 2006;18(2):184–188.
- Chang AB. American College of Chest Physicians cough guidelines for children: can its use improve outcomes? *Chest*. 2008;134(6):1111–1112.
- Chang AB. Cough. *Pediatr Clin North Am*. 2009;56(1):19–31.
- Chang AB, Glomb WB. Guidelines for evaluating chronic cough in pediatrics. *Chest*. 2006; 129(1)(Suppl):260S–283S.
- Goldsobel AB, Chipps BE. Cough in the pediatric population. *J Pediatr*. 2013;156(3):352–358.
- Gupta D, Verma S, Vishwakarma SK. Anatomic basis of Arnold's ear-cough reflex. *Surg Radiol Anat*. 1986;8(4):217–220.
- Marchant JM, Morris PS, Gaffney J, et al. Antibiotics for prolonged moist cough in children (Review). *The Cochrane Library*. 2011;2:1–25.
- Marchant JM, Newcombe PA, Juniper EF, et al. What is the burden of chronic cough for families? *Chest*. 2008;134(2):303–309.
- Mulholland S, Chang AB. Honey and lozenges for children with non-specific cough (Review). *The Cochrane Library*. 2011;(2):1–14.

CODES

ICD10

- R05 Cough
- J00 Acute nasopharyngitis [common cold]
- J45.909 Unspecified asthma, uncomplicated

FAQ

- Q: Is whooping cough still a problem despite routine childhood immunization?
- A: Yes. Pertussis often goes unrecognized as a cause of acute and chronic cough, particularly in infants who have not completed their immunization series and in older children, adolescents, and adults. Immunity from vaccination or natural infection may wane within 5 years, thus providing a reservoir of pertussis in the community. Tdap vaccination is recommended for all 11 years of age and older.
- Q: How can an ear examination help explain the cause of chronic cough?
- A: For some patients, the presence of cerumen, a foreign body, or irritation of the external auditory ear canal can stimulate the auricular branch of the vagus nerve ("Arnold nerve") and trigger a cough. This is also known as the oto-respiratory reflex. One study conducted in India suggests a 4% prevalence of this phenomenon.

CROHN DISEASE

Helen Pappa

BASICS

DESCRIPTION

Crohn disease (CD) is a chronic inflammatory bowel disease (IBD) affecting any part of the gastrointestinal (GI) tract from the mouth to the anus. Crohn disease is generally characterized by transmural skip lesions, as well as periods of exacerbations and quiescence.

EPIDEMIOLOGY

- ~20–25% of patients are diagnosed with CD in childhood or adolescence.
- Family history is present in 30% of patients <30 years old.
- In adulthood, male = female; in childhood, male > female (1.6:1)
- Highest frequency in Caucasian populations; however, CD can be diagnosed in patients of all racial backgrounds.

RISK FACTORS

Genetics

- 1st-degree relatives have a 5–25% higher risk of developing CD than the normal population.
- Children of 1 parent with CD have a 7–16% risk of developing either CD or ulcerative colitis.
- Siblings of patients with IBD are at 30 times higher risk of developing the disease.
- Concordance in monozygotic twins is 50%; in dizygotic twins, 38%
- CD is complex genetic disease:
  - Over 100 gene loci have been associated with CD.
  - Gene mutations in CD involve pathways responsible for microbe recognition and autophagy.
  - The first gene association was with NOD2/CARD15, a protein important in innate immunity.
  - CARD15 mutation is present in ~14–18% of patients. Homozygotes carry 2–4% lifetime risk of developing CD.
  - Additional genetic links found to possibly predict responses to corticosteroids, anti-TNF agents.

PATHOPHYSIOLOGY

- Interaction and combination of environmental factors, genetic susceptibility, host's intestinal microbiota, and a yet, unspecified triggering factor (likely bacterial products) lead to a dysregulated immune response, causing chronic intestinal inflammation.
- CD pathogenesis is now attributed to dysfunction of both innate and adaptive immunity.
  - Innate immunity: Defects have been identified in epithelial barrier, microbial sensing, and autophagy in CD, for example, patients with the CARD15/NOD2 mutation have dysregulated response to bacterial products.
  - Adaptive immunity: abnormal activation of T-helper-1 and Th17 lymphocytes leads to overproduction of inflammatory cytokines such as IL-2, interferon g, IL-6, TNF-α, and IL-17 which cause invasive intestinal inflammation in CD.
- IL-23 is a significant cytokine in CD. Polymorphisms in the IL-23R gene have been associated with aberrant responses of both the innate and adaptive immune systems. In the GI tract, release of inflammatory cytokines causes transmural inflammation with cryptitis, crypt abscesses and distortion of crypt architecture, and pathognomonic formations called granulomas (in 20–40% of biopsies).
- Macroscopically, the following are characteristics of CD:
  - Ulcerations
  - "Creeping fat" (increased mesenteric fat surrounding inflamed small intestinal loops)
  - Sinus tracts (extension of deep ulcerations beyond the intestinal wall)
  - Fistulae (communications between intestine and skin, other intestinal loops or other organs)
  - Strictures
- The most common site to be affected in the GI tract is the terminal ileum. Other sites most often affected, in decreasing frequency, are right colon, isolated colon, proximal small bowel, and upper GI tract (i.e., stomach, duodenum, esophagus).

DIAGNOSIS

HISTORY

- Diarrhea (80%)
- Weight loss (85%)
- Abdominal pain (85%)
- Rectal bleeding (50%)
- Fever (40%)
- Growth failure (35%)
- Perianal disease (25%)
- Nausea and vomiting (25%)
- Delayed puberty
- Menstrual irregularity
- Extraintestinal disease (25%)
  - Arthritis
  - Erythema nodosum
  - Pyoderma gangrenosum
  - Mouth ulcers
  - Episcleritis
  - Uveitis
  - Thromboembolic disease
  - Vasculitis
  - Renal stones
  - Amyloidosis
  - Sclerosing cholangitis
  - Pancreatitis
- Other history could include the following:
  - Enteric infection (including *Clostridium difficile*)

PHYSICAL EXAM

- Growth delay and weight loss, delayed puberty
- Abdominal examination:
  - Hyperactive bowel sounds
  - Right lower quadrant (RLQ) mass and tenderness
  - Palpable thickened loop of intestine
- Rectal and perianal examination: skin tag, fissure, fistula, and abscess

DIAGNOSTIC TESTS & INTERPRETATION

Lab

- CBC; common to see microcytic anemia (due to iron deficiency); can also see a normocytic anemia due to chronic disease or a macrocytosis (suggesting nutrient deficiency, especially iron, B_{12}, folate, zinc)
- Elevated ESR, C-reactive protein, stool calprotectin (disease activity)
- Electrolytes (reflect hydration, renal function)
- Transaminases, alkaline phosphatase, γ-glutamyl transpeptidase (hepatobiliary disease)
- Stool for occult blood and presence of white cells
- Stool cultures, *Clostridium difficile* toxin A and B
- Serologic profiles, including perinuclear antineutrophil cytoplasmic antibody (pANCA) and anti *Saccharomyces cerevisiae* antibody (ASCA), may be helpful in differentiating among types of IBD.
- Genetic screening among healthy, asymptomatic patients is not recommended.

Imaging

- Consider plain abdominal x-ray in acute presentation to rule out obstruction or perforation.
- MRI enterography to assess disease extent and activity is radiation-paring and provides information about small bowel and colonic disease, including abscesses and fistula.
- Barium upper GI and small bowel follow-through may also be used to evaluate extent of disease in small bowel not accessible to endoscopy—involves exposure to radiation.
- CT scan and ultrasound may be necessary to evaluate complications (abscess, phlegmon).
- Colonoscopy and upper endoscopy with multiple biopsies are the gold standard tests for initial evaluation and diagnosis of CD.
- Video capsule endoscopy can be used to access small bowel not visualized at the time of endoscopy.
- Balloon-assisted enteroscopy is useful in the evaluation of small intestinal lesions and has the advantage of providing biopsies for diagnostic purposes.

DIFFERENTIAL DIAGNOSIS

- Ulcerative colitis
- Appendicitis
- Infection:
  - *Mycobacterium tuberculosis*
  - *Salmonella*, *Shigella dysenteriae*
  - *Campylobacter jejuni*, *Aeromonas* spp.
  - *Yersinia enterocolitica*, *Clostridium difficile*
  - *Escherichia coli*, *Giardia lamblia*, *Cryptosporidium*, *Strongyloides*
- Hemolytic uremic syndrome
- Henoch-Schönlein purpura
- Irritable bowel syndrome
- Peptic ulcer disease
- Autoimmune enteropathy, immunodeficiency
- Cow's milk protein allergy
- Small intestinal lymphoma
- Functional disorders

TREATMENT

MEDICATION

- The goal of therapy is resolution of all symptoms in the acute phase (induction), microscopic healing of the intestinal mucosa, steroid-free long-term remission, appropriate growth, and good quality of life. The therapy is used in a stepwise fashion.
- Several 5-aminosalicylic acid (5-ASA) preparations can be trialed according to their intestinal site of activation. These medications can be used for both induction and maintenance of remission of mild to moderate disease but have modest efficacy:
  - Mesalamine (Asacol; terminal ileum, colon): 50–100 mg/kg/24 h (max 4.8 g/24 h for active disease and 3.2 g/24 h to maintain remission)
  - Mesalamine (Pentasa; duodenum, jejunum, ileum, colon): 50–100 mg/kg/24 h (max 4 g/24 h for active disease and 3 g/24 h to maintain remission)

- Sulfasalazine (Azulfidine): 40–60 mg/kg/24 h (max 4 g/24 h) for active disease, and 30 mg/kg/24 h (max 2 g/24 h) for maintenance of remission (liquid preparation available)
- Balsalazide (Colazal; 6.75 g/24 h; 110–170 mg/kg/24 h): can be given to small children as liquid preparation
- Mesalamine (Rowasa): 4-g enemas and 500-mg suppositories daily to b.i.d. PR

- Corticosteroids can control intestinal inflammation in the acute setting; however, they should not be used long-term for maintenance of remission due to their side-effect profile. An effective starting dose to treat CD is 1–2 mg/kg/24 h IV methylprednisolone or oral prednisone (max 60 mg). Initially, patient is treated for 10 days to 2 weeks and tapered off within several weeks. Topical hydrocortisone is useful in localized left-sided colonic disease and is available in liquid and foam enemas. Corticosteroid with controlled ileal release, budesonide (9 mg/24 h) is available.
- Exclusive enteral nutrition (EEN): This approach is frequently used in Europe and Canada as a 1st-line therapy to induce remission in lieu of steroids. With EEN, an exclusive elemental or polymeric diet has been reported to be effective in inducing remission, especially in active small bowel disease. Nutritional supplementation in addition to other treatment is also used to correct growth failure. In this setting, it can be given as overnight nasogastric feeding if not tolerated orally. EEN has the appeal of being drug-free but does involve a large commitment from the patient and may be difficult to maintain long-term.
- Azathioprine, 2–3 mg/kg/24 h PO, and its metabolite 6-mercaptopurine, 1–1.5 mg/kg/24 h, PO are immunomodulators used as maintenance treatment to prevent exacerbations in patients who have been placed in remission with steroids, or biologics and other agents. Adverse events include liver toxicity, leukopenia, and slightly increased risk of malignancy, specifically lymphoma.
- Methotrexate, another immunomodulator is also used for the maintenance of remission, at the dose of 10–25 mg IM or PO once a week. Adverse effects are similar to azathioprine and 6-mercaptopurine, with the addition of nausea and vomiting, and pulmonary fibrosis.
- Frequent laboratory follow-up is necessary when immunomodulators are used. WBC and platelet count should be monitored carefully. In the case of azathioprine and 6-mercaptopurine, thiopurine methyltransferase (TPMT)—an enzyme catabolizing these drugs—activity or genotype should be determined prior to its use. If TPMT activity is absent (homozygous), these immunomodulators should not be used due to severe risk of myelosuppression via reduced drug clearance. If TPMT activity is intermediate (heterozygous), they should be used in adjusted doses with close monitoring of WBC count.
- Other immunomodulatory therapy used infrequently: cyclosporine, tacrolimus (FK-506), thalidomide, etc.
- Antibiotics can be used for induction of remission, fistulizing disease, or postoperative maintenance of remission; however, their efficacy is modest, and side effects frequently preclude their long-term use.
  - Metronidazole: 15 mg/kg/24 h
  - Ciprofloxacin: 20 mg/kg/24 h
  - Rifaximin: 200 mg t.i.d.–800 mg b.i.d.
- Infliximab, a biologic, chimeric anti–tumor necrosis factor-α antibody (5 mg/kg IV infusion, given every 2–3 months, after initial 3-dose induction therapy at 0, 2, and 6 weeks) for severe and fistulizing disease unresponsive to other therapy. Adalimumab, a humanized anti-TNF-α antibody, was recently approved for use in children with moderate to severe CD (80–160 mg SC at week 0, 40–80 mg at week 2, and 20–40 mg at week 4, and bimonthly thereafter). Both agents can be used for both induction and maintenance of remission. Their side effects include serious infections, anaphylactic reactions, and slightly increased risk of malignancy (lymphoma).
- Other biologic therapies including anti-TNF-α antibody certolizumab and the antiadhesion molecule natalizumab are available but not yet approved for use in pediatric CD.
- Complementary therapy (probiotics, prebiotics)

SURGERY/OTHER PROCEDURES

- Surgery is reserved for patients with localized CD that is unresponsive to other therapy and that is causing intractable bleeding.
- Surgery may be necessary in stricturing disease, especially in case of proximal intestinal dilatation, and perforation.
- Several types of procedures are available: stricture-plasty, abscess drainage, and intestinal resection (side-to-side anastomosis is widely accepted).
- Surgery for CD is not curative, and postoperative recurrence at the site of anastomosis is common.

ONGOING CARE

FOLLOW-UP RECOMMENDATIONS

Patient Monitoring

- The morbidity of CD is high. The majority of patients experience recurring disease.
- Most patients have good general health in between episodes and go on to lead productive lives.
- Carcinoma surveillance is necessary on a regular basis.
- After 5 and 20 years of disease, the probability of survival is 98% and 89% of expected survival, respectively.
- Death is a rare complication (2.4% in a large series).

COMPLICATIONS

- Intestinal obstruction due to strictures, or adhesions
- Abscess or phlegmon formation
- Enteroenteric, enterovesical, enterovaginal, and enterocutaneous fistulas
- Perforation
- Gallstones, kidney stones
- Intestinal lymphoma, colon cancer
- Malabsorption resulting in deficiency (e.g., vitamin B_{12} and bile salt deficiency, iron deficiency)
- Short bowel syndrome due to repeated bowel resections
- Massive hemorrhage is rare (1%).
- Growth failure is frequent; final height is reduced, and puberty is delayed in CD affecting prepubertal children.
- Future infertility due to inflammation involving the fallopian tubes and ovaries
- Osteopenia and osteoporosis secondary to inflammation, nutritional deficiency, and therapeutic side effects (corticosteroids)
- Toxic megacolon is a rare but serious complication.

ADDITIONAL READING

- Benchimol EI, Fortinsky KJ, Gozdyra P, et al. Epidemiology of pediatric inflammatory bowel disease: a systematic review of international trends. *Inflamm Bowel Dis*. 2011;17(1):423–439.
- Cabré E, Gassull MA. Nutritional and metabolic issues in inflammatory bowel disease. *Curr Opin Clin Nutr Metab Care*. 2003;6(5):569–576.
- Day AS, Ledder O, Leach ST, et al. Crohn's and colitis in children and adolescents. *World J Gastroenterol*. 2012;18(41):5862–5869.
- Henderson P, van Limbergen JE, Wilson DC, et al. Genetics of childhood-onset disease. *Curr Opin Pediatr*. 2014;26(5):590–596.
- Hildebrand H, Karlberg J, Kristiansson B. Longitudinal growth in children and adolescents with inflammatory bowel disease. *J Pediatr Gastroenterol Nutr*. 1994;18(2):165–173.
- Kugathasan S, Baldassano RN, Bradfield JP, et al. Loci on 20q13 and 21q22 are associated with pediatric-onset inflammatory bowel disease. *Nat Genet*. 2008;40(10):1211–1215.
- Maltz R, Podberesky DJ, Saeed SA. Imaging modalities in pediatric inflammatory bowel disease. *Curr Opin Pediatr*. 2014;26(5):590–596.
- Rufo PA, Denson LA, Sylvester FA, et al. Health supervision in the management of children and adolescents with IBD: NASPGHAN recommendations. *J Pediatr Gastroenterol Nutr*. 2012;55(1):93–108.

CODES

ICD10

- K50.90 Crohn's disease, unspecified, without complications
- K50.913 Crohn's disease, unspecified, with fistula
- K50.911 Crohn's disease, unspecified, with rectal bleeding

FAQ

- Q: Should the diet of patients with CD be restricted?
- A: One approach to inducing remission in active disease can be to use EEN. However, this approach can be difficult to maintain long-term and should be reserved for those patients who are committed to excluding all other foods. In general, a careful, balanced approach to nutrition in children with CD is required to assure appropriate growth and development. The only foods not recommended are "high-residue foods," including poorly digestible vegetables (if eaten raw), nuts, and popcorn, which can cause obstruction in the narrowed, inflamed intestine. Patients with secondary lactose intolerance should use lactase supplements or avoid milk products while ensuring adequate calories and calcium intake.

CROUP (LARYNGOTRACHEOBRONCHITIS)

Daniel Walmsley

BASICS

DESCRIPTION

- Croup (laryngotracheobronchitis) is a common respiratory illness in children that presents with hoarseness, a characteristic barking cough, rhinorrhea, and fever.
- Spasmodic croup (subglottic allergic edema) refers to an illness characterized by sudden inspiratory stridor at night followed by sudden resolution. Mild cold symptoms may be present but are often absent. The child can have frequent attacks on the same night or for multiple, successive nights.

EPIDEMIOLOGY

- Accounts for 15% of the respiratory illnesses seen in children
- Most commonly occurs in children between 6 and 36 months of age
  - Although cases can be seen up to 6 years of age, it is uncommon in children older than 6 years.
  - Mean age at presentation is 18 months.
- Most prevalent in the fall to early winter
  - October is the most common for parainfluenza viruses.
- More common in males (ratio 1.4:1)
- ER visits for croup are most frequent between the hours of 10 p.m. and 4 a.m.

RISK FACTORS

- Anatomic narrowing of the airway such as in subglottic stenosis or Down syndrome
- Prior history of croup
- Hyperactive airway common in atopic children
- Preexisting airway swelling

ETIOLOGY

In children, the cricoid ring of the trachea, located in the immediate subglottic area, is the narrowest part of their upper airway. A small amount of edema in this region can lead to significant airway obstruction, which is what makes children especially susceptible to this illness.

Caused mainly by respiratory viruses including the following:

- Parainfluenza virus types 1–3, most commonly; accounting for 65% of cases
- Adenovirus
- RSV—in some cases, patients may also have wheezing present
- Influenza virus A, B
- Rhinoviruses
- Enteroviruses
- Metapneumovirus
- Enteric cytopathogenic human orphan virus (echovirus)
- Human coronavirus NL63
- Measles—in areas where measles is prevalent
- *Mycoplasma* pneumonia—associated with mild cases of croup
- Bacterial infection may occur secondarily by *Staphylococcus aureus*, *Streptococcus pyogenes*, and *Streptococcus pneumoniae*.

DIAGNOSIS

HISTORY

- Croup typically starts with rhinorrhea, cough, coryza, and congestion.
- After a short period (12–48 hours), upper airway obstruction occurs resulting in hoarseness, "barky cough," and inspiratory stridor.
- Fever is often present.
- Symptoms persist for 3–7 days.
- Usually presents as hoarseness in children older than 6 years of age or adults.

ALERT

The sudden development of inspiratory stridor without other upper respiratory tract infection (URI) symptoms or fever should prompt the consideration of a foreign body aspiration or upper airway mass.

- Recurrent episodes of stridor should lead to the consideration of spasmodic croup, an anatomic abnormality, or an underlying condition such as atopy.
- In a child with truncal or multiple strawberry hemangiomas, a sudden episode of stridor without fever or URI symptoms should raise the concern for a hemangioma in the child's airway.
- Bacterial tracheitis should be suspected in a child who develops marked worsening of symptoms with a high fever after having 5–7 days of mild croup symptoms.

PHYSICAL EXAM

- Examine the child in a comfortable position and make every effort to minimize anxiety, as this can often worsen their symptoms.
- Observe for stridor at rest, irritability, and fatigue. Assess respiratory status and level of consciousness.
- Vital signs:
  - Fever and tachypnea may be present.
  - A child with croup is usually not hypoxic because croup affects the upper airway.
  - Hypoxia is seen only when complete airway obstruction is imminent.
- A child with croup will likely have a hoarse voice, coryza, inflamed pharynx, and varying degrees of respiratory distress.
- The degree of respiratory distress should be observed by assessing for tachypnea, nasal flaring, retractions, grunting, and use of accessory muscles.
- Children with significant upper airway obstruction may sit in a "sniffing" position with their neck mildly flexed and head mildly extended.
  - This position is in contrast to the "tripod" position noted in epiglottitis where the child is in a sitting position with the chin pushed forward and refusing to lie down.
- The presence of inspiratory stridor should be determined.
  - Stridor may be present at rest or only with agitation, and this difference will affect the patient's management.
  - Stridor at rest is a sign of significant upper airway obstruction and needs urgent treatment with racemic epinephrine.
- The hydration status of the child should be assessed.
  - Drooling should not be present with croup.
  - Drooling may indicate a different diagnosis such as epiglottitis or peritonsillar abscess.
- The severity of croup can be determined by a clinical scoring system known as the modified Westley Croup Score (see Table 1).
  - Score <3: mild disease
  - Score of 3–6: moderate disease
  - Score >6: severe disease

DIAGNOSTIC TESTS & INTERPRETATION

Lab

- Croup is a clinical diagnosis, and laboratory tests are not needed.
- The anxiety associated with blood draws may actually worsen the child's condition.
- Rapid antigen tests to determine the viral agent responsible for the illness may be helpful if the child has an atypical presentation or for infection control if the child requires admission.

Imaging

- Radiographs may be helpful to rule out other causes of stridor; they should be considered in children with atypical courses, recurrent episodes, failure to respond to treatment, or if a foreign body is suspected (although of note, most foreign bodies are not radio-opaque).
- Classically, an anteroposterior view demonstrates the "steeple" sign, which is a narrowed air column in the subglottic area.

Table 1. Croup (Laryngotracheobronchitis)—Severity Score for Croup Patients (Westley Croup Score)

Indicator of Severity of Illness	Score
<u>Inspiratory stridor</u>	
None	0
At rest, with stethoscope	1
At rest, w/o stethoscope	2
<u>Retractions</u>	
None	0
Mild	1
Moderate	2
Severe	3
<u>Air entry</u>	
Normal	0
Decreased	1
Severely decreased	2
<u>Cyanosis</u>	
None	0
With agitation	4
At rest	5
<u>Level of consciousness</u>	
Normal	0
Altered mental status	5

Diagnosis Procedures/Surgery

- Pulse oximetry
- Visual inspection of the airway via bronchoscopy and direct or fiberoptic laryngoscopy may be helpful in cases of recurrent croup to rule out an anatomic abnormality. In spasmodic croup, noninflammatory edema may be seen of the airway suggesting atopy.

Pathologic Findings

- Gross pathology: edema and erythema of the subglottic trachea; occasionally, pseudomembranes or exudate are noted.
- Microscopic: edema of airway lining with infiltration of neutrophils, histiocytes, plasma cells, and lymphocytes

DIFFERENTIAL DIAGNOSIS

ALERT
Cases of epiglottitis still occur in unimmunized and underimmunized children; therefore, it is important to check the child's immunization status.

Other important diseases to consider in the differential include the following:

- Infectious
  - Acute epiglottitis
  - Bacterial tracheitis
  - Retropharyngeal abscess
  - Adenotonsillitis
  - Diphtheria
  - Pneumonia
  - Ulcerative laryngitis
- Allergic/inflammatory
  - Asthma
  - Anaphylaxis
  - Angioedema
  - Microaspiration secondary to gastroesophageal reflux or hypotonia
- Environmental
  - Foreign body aspiration
  - Caustic ingestion or burn
  - Smoke inhalation
  - Paraquat poisoning
- Traumatic
  - Subglottic edema/stenosis postintubation
  - Laryngeal or subglottic hematoma
  - Laryngeal fracture
- Obstruction/masses
  - Papillomatosis
  - Hemangioma
  - Cystic hygroma
  - Lymphoma
  - Rhabdomyosarcoma
  - Thymoma
  - Teratoma
  - Thyroglossal duct cyst
  - Branchial cleft cyst
- Congenital anomalies of the upper airway
  - Tracheomalacia/laryngomalacia
  - Vascular ring
  - Laryngeal web
- Genetic/metabolic
  - Hypocalcemia

TREATMENT

INITIAL STABILIZATION

- Racemic epinephrine
- Corticosteroids
- Oxygen (if needed)
- Endotracheal intubation is very rarely required, noted to occur about 1% of the time in studies.

General Measures

- Children with mild symptoms can be treated with humidity, antipyretics, and oral hydration at home. However, randomized controlled trials (RCTs) have not demonstrated a benefit for the use of humidity.
- Short, acute episodes of stridor can be treated with cool mist, a bathroom filled with steam from a shower or cold night air. If the stridor persists, worsens, or occurs at rest, the child should be seen in the emergency room.
- It is important to try to keep the child calm, as agitation or anxiety can worsen symptoms and increase work of breathing.

ALERT
In the child with impending respiratory failure, prompt intubation and direct visualization of the airway in the operating room is imperative. Do not wait for x-rays to confirm a diagnosis.

MEDICATION

- Corticosteroids and nebulized racemic epinephrine, which are the main treatments for croup, have resulted in a dramatic reduction in the number of admissions and length of hospital stays in patients with croup.
- Dexamethasone (PO or IM; half-life 36–54 hours) 0.6 mg/kg single dose (max 10 mg) has been shown to reduce symptoms in patients with moderate to severe croup.
  - Oral dexamethasone is the most cost-effective steroid treatment available.
  - It has been shown to start having an effect within 30 minutes.
- Alternatively, prednisolone 1–2 mg/kg for 1–3 daily doses can be used to treat a patient with croup, although there is no RCT evidence for this method. A recent double-blinded randomized trial demonstrated that a single dose of 1 mg/kg of prednisolone was NOT as effective at keeping children from emergency medical care as 0.15 mg/kg of dexamethasone.
- Budesonide given via nebulizer at a dose of 2 mg administered q12h—shown in recent studies to be as effective as dexamethasone in reducing symptoms; less systemic absorption compared with dexamethasone, with maximum deposition of drug in the upper airway. Although widely accepted, budesonide is not as readily used as dexamethasone because it is not as cost-effective.
- Racemic epinephrine: A nebulized racemic epinephrine treatment offers immediate reduction in swelling of the laryngeal airway in children who present in extreme respiratory distress. Dose: 0.5 mL of 2.25% solution (D- and L-isomers) in 2.5 mL normal saline delivered via nebulizer as needed.
- L-epinephrine: If racemic epinephrine is not available, 5 mL of L-epinephrine 1:1,000 delivered via nebulizer is effective.

INPATIENT CONSIDERATIONS

Admission Criteria

- Severe respiratory distress on presentation (Croup score of >3)
- Persistent hypoxia despite treatment with steroids and racemic epinephrine
- Requirement of treatment of racemic epinephrine more than once over a 3- to 4-hour period
- Dehydration or risk for dehydration
- Admission should be strongly considered for children who present symptomatically to an ER more than once and have significant stridor on day 1 of illness as croup is usually worse on days 2–3.

Discharge Criteria

- Croup score of ≤3 over a 1- to 3-hour period of observation
- Does not require racemic epinephrine in the 3–4 hours prior to discharge
- Able to take adequate PO fluids

ISSUES FOR REFERRAL

- The vast majority of children with croup do well. However, transfer to a facility where trained individuals can address pediatric airway problems should be considered if the patient is inadequately responding to treatment or has increasing respiratory distress.
- A recent study showed heliox during transport for children with severe croup provided added benefit to their prognosis.

PROGNOSIS

- The vast majority of patients do not require hospitalization.
- Almost all patients go on to complete recovery.

COMPLICATIONS

- Poor oral intake/dehydration
- Hypoxia
- Upper airway obstruction
- Respiratory failure (rare)

ONGOING CARE

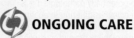

FOLLOW-UP RECOMMENDATIONS

Patient Monitoring

- In most cases, the illness is self-limited, lasting 3–5 days.
- A "rebound phenomenon" with worsening of stridor and respiratory distress after initial relief with the racemic epinephrine treatment may be seen up to 2 hours post treatment in some patients.
- Dexamethasone has a half-life of 36–54 hours so parents should be warned that some children may have worsening in 2 days after treatment with this medication.
- Several studies have shown that children can be safely discharged 3–4 hours after racemic epinephrine treatment.

ALERT
Recurrent croup may signal an underlying anatomic problem and needs evaluation for other causes.

ADDITIONAL READING

- Bjornson C, Russell VF, Vandermeer B, et al. Nebulized epinephrine for croup in children. *Cochrane Database Syst Rev*. 2011;16(2):CD006619.
- Cherry JD. Clinical practice croup. *N Engl J Med*. 2008;358(4):384–391.
- Donaldson D, Poleski D, Knipple E, et al. Intramuscular versus oral dexamethasone for the treatment of moderate-to-severe croup: a randomized, double-blind trial. *Acad Emerg Med*. 2003;10(1):16–21.
- Geelhoed GC, Turner J, Macdonald WB. Efficacy of a small single dose of oral dexamethasone for outpatient croup: a double blind placebo controlled clinical trial. *BMJ*. 1996;313(7050):140–142.
- Kline-Krammes, Reed C, Giuliano JS, et al. Heliox in children with croup: a strategy to hasten improvement. *Air Med J*. 2012;31(3):131–137.
- Miller EK, Gebretsadik, Carroll KN, et al. Viral etiologies of infant bronchiolitis, croup and upper respiratory illness during four consecutive years. *Pediatr Infect Dis J*. 2013;32(9):950–955.
- Scolnik D, Coates AL, Stephens D, et al. Controlled delivery of high vs low humidity vs mist therapy for croup in emergency departments: a randomized controlled trial. *JAMA*. 2006;295(11):1274–1280.
- Sparrow A, Geelhoed G. Prednisolone versus dexamethasone in croup: a randomised equivalence trial. *Arch Dis Child*. 2006;91(7):580–583.
- Westley CR, Cotton EK, Brooks JG. Nebulized racemic epinephrine by IPPB for the treatment of croup: a double-blind study. *Am J Dis Child*. 1978;132(5):484–487.

CODES

ICD10

- J05.0 Acute obstructive laryngitis [croup]
- J40 Bronchitis, not specified as acute or chronic

CRYING

Mark F. Ditmar

BASICS

DESCRIPTION

- Crying is usually a normal physiologic response to stress, discomfort, unfulfilled needs such as hunger, pain, over- or understimulation, or temperature change.
- Crying is felt to be potentially pathologic if it is interpreted by caregivers as differing in quality and duration without apparent explanation and/or persists without consolability beyond a reasonable time (generally 1–2 hours).

EPIDEMIOLOGY

- Excessive crying in the first months of life, per parental reports, occurs in about 1 in 5 infants.

ETIOLOGY

- The most likely cause of inconsolable crying in the first few months of life is infantile colic.
  - However, colic is a diagnosis of exclusion.
  - Practitioners must be familiar with the clinical pattern of infantile colic so that deviations are readily recognized.
- Organic problems are identified in 5% or less of afebrile excessively crying infants.

DIAGNOSIS

HISTORY

- **Question:** Colic?
- *Significance*:
  - Colic less likely as a cause if onset after 1 month of age or persistent in infants >4 months of age
  - Recurrent episodes, particularly with a diurnal or evening pattern, are more likely due to colic.
  - Crying shortly after feeding suggests aerophagia or gastroesophageal reflux; 1 hour after feeding suggests formula intolerance. A rare cause of postprandial crying is anomalous coronary arteries.
  - Overfeeding or underfeeding, excessive air swallowing, inadequate burping, and improper formula preparation may contribute to excessive crying.
- **Question:** Fever?
- *Significance*: Indicates potential need for evaluation of meningitis, other infections
- **Question:** Paradoxically increased crying (attempts at consolation make the crying worse, especially with lifting, rocking)?
- *Significance*: Can be seen in meningitis, peritonitis, long bone fractures, arthritis
- **Question:** Stridor?
- *Significance*: Implies possible upper airway obstruction (mechanical, functional)
- **Question:** Expiratory grunting?
- *Significance*: Indicates higher likelihood of significant pathologic cause of crying (especially cardiac, respiratory, and/or infectious disease)
- **Question:** Cold symptoms and/or day care attendance?
- *Significance*: Increase likelihood of otitis media
- **Question:** Vomiting?
- *Significance*: Increases likelihood of pathologic GI cause (e.g., obstruction, gastroesophageal reflux with possible esophagitis), particularly in infant <3 months of age, or CNS disease
- **Question:** Recent fall or trauma?
- *Significance*: May indicate possible fracture, increased intracranial pressure, abuse
- **Question:** Documented weight loss outside of the 2-week neonatal period?
- *Significance*: Suggests an organic cause

PHYSICAL EXAM

- **Finding:** Infant appears ill (e.g., pallor, grunting, poor arousability, poor response to social overtures)?
- *Significance*: Implies much higher likelihood of an organic cause
- **Finding:** Tenderness on palpation of extremities, clavicle, or scalp or painful or decreased range of motion of joints?
- *Significance*: Suggests fracture, subluxation, osteomyelitis, septic arthritis
- **Finding:** Conjunctival redness, eye tearing, scratches near the eye?
- *Significance*: Suggest corneal abrasion (fluorescein testing of eye warranted) or foreign body in eye (eversion of lid recommended). Cessation of crying with ophthalmic anesthetic drops while doing fluorescein staining suggests corneal injury as a cause.
- **Finding:** Impacted or bloody stool on rectal exam, abdominal mass?
- *Significance*: Suggest constipation or intussusception
- **Finding:** Geographic scars, frenulum tears, retinal hemorrhages, suspicious bruises, burns, decreased weight/height ratio?
- *Significance*: Suggest neglect/abuse (physical, emotional). Bruises are rare in preambulatory children (particularly <6 months of age); if present, consider inflicted injuries.
- **Finding:** Bulging or full fontanel (especially in upright, quiet infant)?
- *Significance*: Indicates possible increased intracranial pressure (meningitis, subdural hematoma, vitamin A toxicity)
- **Finding:** Edema of individual toes, fingers, or penis?
- *Significance*: Suggest hair tourniquet syndrome
- **Finding:** Tender swelling in inguinal or scrotal area?
- *Significance*: May indicate incarcerated hernia, testicular torsion
- **Finding:** Heart rate >200 bpm with minimal variability?
- *Significance*: Indicates possible supraventricular tachycardia
- **Finding:** Hypothermia?
- *Significance*: Suggests infections or hypothyroidism

DIAGNOSTIC TESTS & INTERPRETATION

- **Test:** Stool for occult blood
- *Significance*: Possible intussusception, anal fissure
- **Test:** Fluorescein testing of eye
- *Significance*: Corneal abrasion (may occur without significant conjunctival redness)
- **Test:** Urinalysis/urine culture
- *Significance*: UTI
- **Test:** Urine toxicology screen
- *Significance*: Drug withdrawal (neonatal), ingestions, passive exposures (e.g., cocaine)
- **Test:** Pulse oximetry
- *Significance*: Hypoxia (from cardiac causes) may cause increased irritability.
- **Test:** Electrolyte panel/blood glucose
- *Significance*: Endocrine or metabolic disturbance, especially if abnormal sodium, hypoglycemia, significant acidosis, or elevated anion gap
- **Test:** Skeletal survey
- *Significance*: Suspected abuse; also consider MRI or head CT scan for those <1 year of age with suspicious injuries

DIFFERENTIAL DIAGNOSIS

- Congenital/anatomic
  - Intussusception
  - Gastroesophageal reflux/esophagitis
  - Volvulus
  - Gaseous distention (secondary to improper feeding or burping)
  - Incarcerated inguinal hernia
  - Peritonitis (acute abdomen)
  - Testicular/ovarian torsion
  - Constipation
  - Anal fissure
  - Meatal ulceration
  - Glaucoma
  - Urinary retention (secondary to posterior urethral valves)
  - Cardiac—anomalous coronary artery, hypoxia, congestive heart failure (CHF)
  - Increased intracranial pressure (hydrocephalus, tumor, pseudotumor cerebri)
- Infectious
  - Otitis media/externa
  - UTI/pyelonephritis
  - Stomatitis/gingivitis
  - Meningitis/encephalitis
  - Diskitis
  - Gastroenteritis
  - Mastitis
  - Arthritis, septic
  - Osteomyelitis
  - Perianal cellulitis
  - Balanitis
  - Dermatitis (especially pruritic as in scabies or painful as in staphylococcal scalded skin syndrome)

- Toxic, environmental, drugs
  - Neonatal drug withdrawal
  - Prenatal/perinatal cocaine exposure
  - Immunization reactions (especially DTP)
  - Isolated fructose intolerance
  - Drug reactions (especially antihistamines, pseudoephedrine, phenylpropanolamine), including maternal medications in breast milk
  - Vitamin A toxicity
  - Carbon monoxide exposure
  - Emotional/physical neglect
  - Foreign body ingestion (coin, pin)
  - Ear foreign body (e.g., cockroach)
- Trauma
  - Corneal abrasion
  - Foreign body (hypopharynx, eye, ear, nose)
  - Skull fracture/subdural hematoma
  - Intracranial hemorrhage
  - Retinal hemorrhage (e.g., shaken baby syndrome)
  - Other fractures (especially extremities)
  - Hair tourniquet syndrome (encircling finger, toe, penis, clitoris)
  - Open diaper pin
  - Bite (human, animal, insect)
- Genetic/metabolic
  - Sickle cell crisis
  - Phenylketonuria
  - Hypothyroidism
  - Electrolyte abnormalities (especially sodium)
  - Hypoglycemia
  - Hypocalcemia
  - Hypercalcemia
  - Inborn error of metabolism
- Allergic/inflammatory
  - Cow milk allergy
  - Celiac disease (gluten enteropathy)
  - Hemolytic uremic syndrome
  - Henoch-Schönlein purpura
  - Kawasaki disease
- Functional
  - Parental expectations/responses
- Miscellaneous
  - Overstimulation
  - Persistent night awakening
  - Night terrors
  - Caffey disease (infantile cortical hyperostosis)
  - Dysrhythmia (especially supraventricular tachycardia)
  - IV infiltration
  - Autism
  - Teething
  - Headache/migraine
  - Temperament
  - Colic
  - Discomfort (cold, heat, itching, hunger)

ALERT

Factors that make this an emergency include the following:
- Suspicion of meningitis: stiff neck, bulging fontanel, fever (especially infants <2–3 months of age)
- Suspicion of intestinal obstruction: vomiting (especially bilious or projectile), mass on abdominal palpation, and/or bloody stools
- Suspicion of incarcerated hernia or testicular/ovarian torsion
- Evidence of cardiac compromise (CHF, supraventricular tachycardia): tachycardia, poor perfusion (capillary refill >3 seconds, poor distal pulses), rales
- Evidence of acute dehydration: weight loss, decreased urine output, orthostatic changes, poor perfusion
- Evidence of child abuse or neglect

TREATMENT

APPROACH TO THE PATIENT

General goal is to decide if the crying represents a normal physiologic response, a protracted multifactorial physiologic/developmental response (colic), or a potentially pathologic problem.
- **Phase 1:** How urgent is the need for evaluation? A classic and difficult triage issue. One must identify the periodicity of the problem, associated symptoms, impression of wellness, and parental anxiety/reliability.
- **Phase 2:** When in doubt, particularly if colic seems unlikely, see the patient as soon as possible. Treatment is then based on the most likely diagnosis following evaluation. Be wary of the infant who, despite a period of observation, is not noted at any point to be awake and calm.

ADDITIONAL READING

- Bolte R. The crying child: what are they trying to tell you? Parts I and II. *Contemp Pediatr*. 2007;24:74–81, 90–95.
- Douglas P, Hill P. Managing infants who cry excessively in the first few months of life. *BMJ*. 2011;343:d7772.
- Douglas P, Hill P. The crying baby: what approach? *Curr Opin Pediatr*. 2011;23(5):523–529.
- Freedman SB, Al-Harthy N, Thull-Freedman J. The crying infant: diagnostic testing and frequency of serious underlying disease. *Pediatrics*. 2009;123(3):841–848.
- Herman M, Le A. The crying infant. *Emerg Med Clin North Am*. 2007;25(4):1137–1159.
- McKenzie SA. Fifteen-minute consultation: troublesome crying in infancy. *Arch Dis Child Edu Pract Ed*. 2013;98(6):209–211.
- Poole SR. The infant with acute, unexplained, excessive crying. *Pediatrics*. 1991;88(3):450–455.

CODES

ICD10
- R68.11 Excessive crying of infant (baby)
- R10.83 Colic
- K21.9 Gastro-esophageal reflux disease without esophagitis

FAQ

- Q: How important is lab testing in the evaluation of the crying infant?
- A: History and physical exam, rather than extensive lab testing, are the keys to the diagnosis. In Freedman's emergency department (ED) study of 237 excessively crying infants, less than 1% had testing contribute to the diagnosis in the absence of a suggestive clinical picture.
- Q: How might the quality of cry be helpful in the diagnosis?
- A: Subjective interpretation can be helpful.
  - High-pitched (shrill, piercing) crying in short bursts: associated with CNS pathology, especially with increased intracranial pressure
  - High-pitched crying in longer bursts: seen in small-for-gestational age infants, neonatal drug withdrawal
  - Hoarse crying: seen in hypothyroidism, laryngeal diseases, hypocalcemic tetany
  - Weak crying: may be seen in neuromuscular disorders, infant botulism, and/or the very ill infant
  - Catlike cry: can be associated with cri du chat syndrome (5p- syndrome or absence of short arm of chromosome 5)
- Q: How common is teething as a cause of excessive crying?
- A: Patients' families often suggest teething as a cause of excessive crying (as well as fever, diarrhea, rashes, etc.). Objective data do not support a strong association. Be careful in ascribing symptoms and signs to teething.

CRYPTOCOCCAL INFECTIONS

Eric S. Kirkendall • Samir S. Shah

BASICS

DESCRIPTION

Cryptococcosis is an opportunistic fungal infection caused by *Cryptococcus neoformans* that may involve several organ systems, including the CNS, lungs, bones, visceral organs, and skin. *Cryptococcus gattii* is a less common cause.

EPIDEMIOLOGY

- Most pediatric infections occur in immunocompromised hosts, including those with malignancy, HIV, and solid organ or bone marrow transplantation.
- 20% of infections requiring hospitalization occur in normal hosts.
- There is no person-to-person spread.
- Occurs in 5–15% of HIV-infected adults, usually with CD4+ lymphocyte counts <50 cells/mm^3; occurs in 0.8–2.3% of HIV-infected children. The lower infection rate in children reflects lower exposure to sources of *C. neoformans*. Seroprevalence varies by age: neonates, 0%; school-aged children, 4.1%; and adults, 69%.
- 1–3% of solid organ transplant recipients develop *C. neoformans* infections, typically >1 year after transplantation.

GENERAL PREVENTION

- Use of highly active antiretroviral therapy (HAART) prevents most cases of cryptococcosis in HIV-infected patients.
- Primary prophylaxis with fluconazole prevents new-onset cryptococcal disease in HIV-infected patients but is not routinely recommended except for those with limited access to HAART and with high levels of antiretroviral drug resistance.
- Maintenance (suppressive) therapy after completion of therapy for cryptococcal infection is recommended for HIV-infected patients. In those with low CD4+ lymphocyte counts, relapse is 100% without maintenance antifungal therapy, 18–25% with amphotericin B or itraconazole, and 2–3% with fluconazole.
  - Prophylaxis may be discontinued in patients receiving HAART with CD4+ lymphocytes >100/mm^3 and undetectable viral loads.
- There is no consensus on the duration of fluconazole suppressive therapy after treatment of cryptococcosis in HIV-negative immunocompromised patients. Most experts provide maintenance (suppressive) antifungal therapy with fluconazole PO (6 mg/kg/day) for at least 1 year after the completion of acute treatment and then reassess ongoing use based on the level of immunosuppression.

PATHOPHYSIOLOGY

- Primary infection occurs through the inhalation of aerosolized soil particles containing the yeast forms. The skin and GI tract are also portals of entry.
- Protective immune response requires specific T cell–mediated immunity.
- CNS infection with *C. neoformans* results from hematogenous dissemination.

COMMONLY ASSOCIATED CONDITIONS

- *C. neoformans* is the most common cause of fungal meningitis in the United States.
- Dissemination is rare in immunocompetent patients.
- Concurrent *Pneumocystis jiroveci* pneumonia was detected in 13% of adults with cryptococcal meningitis.
- Pulmonary involvement is asymptomatic in up to 50% of cases, and disease may be either focal or widespread.
- Bone involvement occurs in 10% of cases of disseminated cryptococcal infection.
- Cutaneous involvement mimics acne-type eruptions that ulcerate and results from hematogenous spread of the organism or from direct extension of bone infection.

DIAGNOSIS

HISTORY

- Cryptococcal meningitis may present as either an indolent infection or acute illness.
- Symptoms of cryptococcal meningitis include headache, malaise, and low-grade fever. Nausea, vomiting, altered mentation (including behavioral changes), and photophobia are less common. Stiff neck, focal neurologic symptoms (e.g., decreased hearing, facial nerve palsy, or diplopia), and seizures are rare.
- Primary pulmonary cryptococcal disease is not well described in children because most cases are disseminated at the time of diagnosis. 50% of adults have cough or chest pain, and fewer have sputum production, weight loss, fever, and hemoptysis.
- In immunocompromised hosts, the onset of infection is more rapid and the course more severe. Pulmonary involvement is minimal when dissemination occurs quickly.

PHYSICAL EXAM

- None of the presenting signs of cryptococcal infection are sufficiently characteristic to distinguish it from other infections, particularly in immunocompromised patients.
- CNS involvement: nuchal rigidity, photophobia, and focal neurologic deficits
- Respiratory tract involvement: cough, tachypnea, grunting, and subcostal or intercostal retractions. Decreased breath sounds or dullness to percussion may be present, or the lung exam may be normal.
- Cutaneous manifestations: erythematous or verrucous papules, nodules, pustules, acneiform lesions, ulcers, abscesses, or granulomas. Lesions can occur anywhere but are found most often on the face and neck.
  - Mucocutaneous findings are present in 10–15% of cases of disseminated disease.

DIAGNOSTIC TESTS & INTERPRETATION

Lab

- Lumbar puncture: diagnose cryptococcal meningitis
  - CSF should be sent for cell count and differential; protein; glucose; cultures for bacterial, fungal, and viral pathogens; and cryptococcal antigen. A large quantity of CSF may be needed to recover the organism.
  - Examination of the CSF reveals <500 WBC/mm^3 (usually <100 WBC/mm^3), mostly mononuclear leukocytes, with minimal changes in protein. CSF glucose is <50 mg/dL in ~65% of patients.
  - India ink stain (less commonly performed) shows budding yeast in 50% of cases.
  - CSF cultures are positive in ~90% of cases.
  - The latex agglutination test for cryptococcal polysaccharide antigen is specific, sensitive, and rapid. Titers ≥1:4 suggest the diagnosis of cryptococcal infection if appropriate controls are negative.
  - HIV-infected patients with pneumonia and CD4+ T-lymphocyte counts <200 cells/mm^3 should be evaluated with sputum fungal culture, blood fungal culture, and a serum cryptococcal antigen test. A lumbar puncture to exclude the possibility of occult meningitis should be considered. If any test is positive for *C. neoformans*, then a lumbar puncture should be performed to exclude cryptococcal meningitis.
- Blood culture and serum cryptococcal antigen titers: diagnose disseminated cryptococcal infection. Serum cryptococcal antigen tests are positive in >90% of patients with cryptococcal meningitis.
- Sputum culture: diagnose cryptococcal pneumonia
- Skin or bone biopsy: diagnose cutaneous or osteoarticular cryptococcal infection
- HIV testing: Evaluation for immunodeficiencies, including HIV, is warranted in any patient with cryptococcosis.
- CBC with differential: may reveal hypereosinophilia (absolute eosinophil count >1,500/mm^3)
- Serum electrolytes: detect hyponatremia, a complication of cryptococcal meningitis

Imaging

- Chest x-rays: Focal or solitary nodules, diffuse infiltrates, and pleural effusions may be seen in cryptococcal pneumonia.
- Head CT or MRI: may demonstrate granulomatous lesions (cryptococcomas; ~15% of patients with meningitis) or elevated intracranial pressure. MRI reveals dilation of perivascular spaces in almost half the cases.

DIFFERENTIAL DIAGNOSIS

- Although cryptococcosis occurs most commonly in HIV-infected patients with low CD4+ lymphocyte counts, the diagnosis warrants consideration in all febrile immunocompromised children (e.g., solid organ transplant, leukemia)
- Meningitis: viruses, *Mycobacterium tuberculosis*, and other fungal causes
- Pneumonia: other pulmonary mycoses, including aspergillosis, histoplasmosis, and blastomycosis; also consider *Mycoplasma pneumoniae* and *M. tuberculosis*
- Bone: osteogenic sarcoma
- Cutaneous: molluscum contagiosum, herpes simplex virus infection, pyoderma gangrenosum, and cellulitis

TREATMENT

- Clinical management depends on extent of disease and immune status of the host.
- Pulmonary and extrapulmonary disease (*HIV-negative, nontransplant*)
  - Normal hosts with isolated pulmonary nodules may not need treatment if the serum cryptococcal antigen is negative and the patient is asymptomatic.
  - Patients with symptoms, extensive pulmonary disease, or evidence of extrapulmonary disease require treatment.
  - Fluconazole 6–12 mg/kg/24 h PO (max 400 mg) for 6–12 months for mild/moderate disease. Alternate regimen: itraconazole 5–10 mg/kg/24 h PO (max 400 mg) for 6–12 months (steady-state trough level >1 mcg/mL and ≤10 mcg/mL) or amphotericin B 0.7–1 mg/kg/24 h IV for 3–6 months
  - Severe disease: same as CNS (see below)
  - Maintenance therapy with fluconazole should be considered for immunocompromised patients (see "General Prevention").
- Pulmonary and extrapulmonary disease (*HIV-infected or transplant*)
  - Fluconazole (PO) 6–12 months for mild/moderate disease; same as CNS infection for severe disease
  - Consider surgical debridement for patients with persistent or refractory pulmonary or bone lesions.
- CNS disease (*HIV-negative, nontransplant*)
  - Induction/consolidation: amphotericin B (0.7–1 mg/kg/24 h) plus flucytosine (100–150 mg/kg/24 h PO, divided q6h; therapeutic levels: 25–100 mg/L) for 4 weeks, then fluconazole PO (10–12 mg/kg/day) for a minimum of 8 weeks followed by maintenance therapy with fluconazole PO (6 mg/kg/24 h) for 6–12 months. Alternate induction/consolidation regimen: amphotericin B plus flucytosine for 6–10 weeks
- CNS disease (*HIV-infected or transplant*)
  - Induction/consolidation: amphotericin B (IV) plus flucytosine (PO) for at least 2 weeks, followed by fluconazole PO (10–12 mg/kg/day) for at least 8 weeks; consider subsequent suppressive therapy with fluconazole PO (6 mg/kg/24 h).
  - Intrathecal amphotericin B is very toxic but may be used in refractory cases.
  - HIV-infected patients require continuation of antifungal drugs indefinitely because of the high recurrence rate of cryptococcosis.
  - Liposomal amphotericin (5 mg/kg/24 h) or amphotericin B lipid complex (5 mg/kg/24 h) IV may be substituted for amphotericin B, especially in patients with renal dysfunction and those receiving calcineurin inhibitors.
  - Flucytosine is used only in combination with amphotericin B and not as a single agent because of the rapid emergence of drug resistance.
- Voriconazole, a triazole antifungal agent, demonstrates excellent in vitro activity against *C. neoformans* but requires clinical study. Caspofungin, an echinocandin antifungal agent, is *not active* against *C. neoformans*.

ONGOING CARE

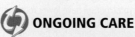

FOLLOW-UP RECOMMENDATIONS

Patient Monitoring

- Because of the risk of relapse, patients should be seen at 3-month intervals for 12–18 months following treatment. Immunocompromised patients should be evaluated every 2–3 months, even while on suppressive therapy, to monitor clinically for relapse.
- Repeat lumbar punctures documenting a decrease in CSF cryptococcal antigen and sterility of culture are useful in evaluating response to treatment. During therapy for acute meningitis, an unchanged or increased titer of CSF antigen correlates with clinical and microbiologic failure to respond to treatment. Serum antigen titers are not helpful for this purpose.
- Evaluate patients with cryptococcal meningitis for neurologic sequelae.
- HIV-infected patients require suppressive antifungal therapy (see "General Prevention").

PROGNOSIS

- Mortality is rare in patients with isolated pulmonary or cutaneous disease.
- In-hospital mortality is ~20% for cryptococcal meningitis and ~8% for non-CNS cryptococcal infections.
  - In normal hosts with meningitis, poor prognostic factors include serum or CSF cryptococcal titers >1:32 or CSF WBC <20/mm^3.
  - In HIV-infected patients with meningitis, poor prognostic factors include hyponatremia, concomitant growth of *C. neoformans* from another site, increased intracranial pressure, and any alteration of mental status.
- Up to 40% of patients with cryptococcal meningitis have residual neurologic deficits.
- Relapse rates are high in HIV-infected patients (see "General Prevention").

COMPLICATIONS

- Elevated intracranial pressure with meningitis
- Pulmonary, cutaneous, and bone involvement may occur (see "Commonly Associated Conditions").
- In solid organ transplant patients, tacrolimus recipients are less likely to have CNS involvement and more likely to have skin, soft tissue, or osteoarticular involvement.
- Cryptococcal immune reconstitution inflammatory syndrome (C-IRIS) may lead to a new presentation of the disease and/or a clinical deterioration after reversal of a host immune deficiency state.

ADDITIONAL READING

- Gonzalez CE, Shetty D, Lewis LL, et al. Cryptococcosis in human immunodeficiency virus-infected children. *Pediatr Infect Dis J*. 1996;15(9):796–800.
- Joshi NS, Fisher BT, Prasad PA, et al. Epidemiology of cryptococcal infection in hospitalized children. *Pediatr Infect Dis J*. 2010;29(12):e91–e95.
- Pappas PG, Perfect JR, Cloud GA, et al. Cryptococcosis in human immunodeficiency virus-negative patients in the era of effective azole therapy. *Clin Infect Dis*. 2001;33(5):690–699.
- Perfect JR, Dismukes WE, Dromer F, et al. Clinical practice guidelines for the management of cryptococcal disease: 2010 update by the Infectious Diseases Society of America. *Clin Infect Dis*. 2010;50(3):291–322.

CODES

ICD10

- B45.9 Cryptococcosis, unspecified
- B45.0 Pulmonary cryptococcosis
- B45.1 Cerebral cryptococcosis

FAQ

- Q: What are the sources of *Cryptococcus* in nature?
- A: Pigeon droppings and soil. Naturally acquired infections occur in lower mammals, especially cats. However, neither animal-to-human nor human-to-human infections have been reported.
- Q: Should all children with *Cryptococcus* infection be evaluated for immunodeficiency?
- A: Yes.

CRYPTORCHIDISM

Hsi-Yang Wu

BASICS

DESCRIPTION

Cryptorchidism is a condition characterized by one or both testes being undescended. An undescended testis does not remain at the bottom of the scrotum after the cremaster muscle has been fatigued by overstretching. Cryptorchidism is commonly confused with a retractile testis. A retractile testis may not always lie in the scrotum but will stay at the bottom of the scrotum after overstretching the cremaster.

EPIDEMIOLOGY

- 3% of full-term newborn boys have cryptorchidism.
- This percentage falls to 1% by 3 months of age.
- There are 2 peaks for detection of undescended testes: at birth and at 5–7 years of age. The latter group probably represents those patients with low undescended testes that become apparent with linear growth.
- Bilateral undescended testes occur in 10% of patients with undescended testicles.
- Unilateral anorchia is found in 5% of patients with cryptorchidism.

Genetics

- Of boys with undescended testes, 4% of their fathers and 6–10% of their brothers also had undescended testes. There is a 23% prevalence of cryptorchidism in family members of cases compared to 7.5% of relatives of controls.
- Androgen receptor gene mutations are not linked to isolated cryptorchidism. Abnormalities in *HOXA10*, *HOXA11*, *HOXD13*, *ESR1*, *INSL3*, and the *LGR8/GREAT* receptor genes are being investigated in patients with cryptorchidism.

PATHOPHYSIOLOGY

- Normal testicular descent occurs during the 7th month of gestation.
- The majority of testes that are undescended at birth but will descend spontaneously do so by 3 months of age, possibly due to the gonadotropin surge that is responsible for germ cell maturation.
- The undescended testis fails to show normal maturation at both 3 months and 5 years of age.
  - At 3 months of age, the fetal gonocytes are transformed into adult dark spermatogonia.
  - At 5 years of age, the adult dark spermatogonia become primary spermatocytes.
  - Both of these steps are abnormal in the undescended testis and, to a lesser extent, the contralateral descended testis.
  - Previous beliefs that the undescended testis was normal between birth and 1 year of age are incorrect because they were derived from counts of all germ cells without taking into account whether maturation was occurring.
  - After 5 years of age, thermal effects on the testis left out of position are seen independent of the endocrinologic effects.

ETIOLOGY

- A multifactorial mechanism involving 2 theories have been postulated:
  - Hypogonadotropic hypogonadism
  - Abnormal mechanical factors (gubernaculum, epididymis, genitofemoral nerve innervation, intra-abdominal pressure)
- Although boys with undescended testes do have abnormal attachment of the gubernaculum, the mechanical theories do not consistently explain the testis histology found in cryptorchidism.
- Many boys with cryptorchidism have lower morning urinary luteinizing hormone and a decreased luteinizing hormone/follicle-stimulating hormone response to gonadotropin-releasing hormone, corresponding to the abnormal germ cell development in both the undescended and contralateral descended testis.
- The normal initial postnatal gonadotropin surge at 60–90 days of age is absent or blunted in some boys with cryptorchidism. Without this surge, Leydig cells do not proliferate, testosterone does not increase, germ cells do not mature, and infertility may develop. This indicates that a mild endocrinopathy is responsible, and cryptorchidism may be a variant of hypogonadotropic hypogonadism.
- Secondary undescended testes can occur after inguinal surgery, either due to scar tissue or difficulty in diagnosing an undescended testis in a young boy with a hernia.

COMMONLY ASSOCIATED CONDITIONS

- Patients with prune belly, Klinefelter, Noonan, and Prader-Willi syndromes have a higher likelihood of undescended testes.
- Cryptorchidism associated with hypospadias should also raise the possibility of a disorder of sex development (DSD), which occurs in 30–40% of patients, mainly consisting of defects in gonadotropin or testosterone synthesis.

DIAGNOSIS

HISTORY

- Exogenous maternal hormones (used in infertility treatments)
- Maternal oral contraceptive use
- Consanguinity
- Family history of urologic abnormalities or neonatal deaths
- Prematurity
- CNS lesions
- Previous inguinal surgery
- Precocious puberty
- Infertility

PHYSICAL EXAM

- The undescended testis may be found at the upper scrotum, in the superficial inguinal pouch, or in the inguinal canal. For treatment purposes, the main distinction that needs to be made is whether or not the testis is palpable.
- The patient should be examined sitting in the frog-leg position.
  - With warmed hands, check the size, location, and texture of the contralateral descended testis.
  - Begin the examination of the undescended testis at the anterior superior iliac spine.
  - Sweep the groin from lateral to medial with the nondominant hand.
  - Once the testis is palpated, grasp it with the dominant hand and continue to sweep the testis toward the scrotum with the other hand.
  - With a combination of sweeping and pulling, it is sometimes possible to bring the testis to the scrotum.
  - Maintain the position of the testis in the scrotum for a minute so that the cremaster muscle is fatigued.
  - Release the testis, and if it remains in place, it is a retractile testis.
  - If it immediately pops back, it is an undescended testis.
- For difficult-to-examine patients (chubby 6-month-olds or obese youth), having them sit with heels together and knees abducted can help relax the cremaster. Wetting the fingers of the nondominant hand with lubricating jelly or soap can increase the sensitivity of the fingers in palpating the small, mobile testis.

DIAGNOSTIC TESTS & INTERPRETATION

Lab

- For the typical patient with a unilateral palpable or nonpalpable undescended testis, no further laboratory evaluation is necessary.
- For the patient with bilateral undescended testis, with 1 testis palpable, no further workup is necessary.
- The patient with bilateral nonpalpable testes should have a chromosomal and endocrinologic evaluation, as should the patient with 1 or 2 undescended testes and hypospadias.
- If the patient has bilateral nonpalpable testes and is <3 months of age, serum luteinizing hormone, follicle-stimulating hormone, testosterone, and anti-müllerian hormone levels will determine whether testes are present.
- After that age, human chorionic gonadotropin stimulation will result in a measurable serum testosterone if testes are present. A failure to respond to human chorionic gonadotropin stimulation in combination with elevated luteinizing hormone/follicle-stimulating hormone levels is consistent with anorchia.

Imaging

Ultrasound, CT, and MRI can detect testes in the inguinal region, but this is also the region where they are most easily palpable. They are only 50% accurate in showing intra-abdominal testes. Imaging is not necessary preoperatively because, for nonpalpable testes, surgical planning is based on the exam performed in the clinic and under anesthesia.

DIFFERENTIAL DIAGNOSIS

- Retractile testes are commonly confused with undescended testes. The key to distinguishing them from undescended testes is the physical exam.
  - All retractile and many undescended testes can be delivered into the scrotum.
  - The retractile testis will stay in the scrotum after the cremaster muscle has been overstretched.
  - The low undescended testis will immediately pop back to its undescended position after being released.
- Atrophic or "vanishing" testes are found anywhere along the normal path to the scrotum.
  - They are believed to be due to neonatal vascular ischemia.
  - The contralateral testis can be hypertrophied in these boys, but this is not a reliable diagnostic sign.
- Anorchia or DSD
  - On evaluation, 80% of nonpalpable testes are present in either the abdomen or in the inguinal canal.
  - A child with bilateral nonpalpable testes should have an endocrine evaluation to rule out anorchia or DSD.

TREATMENT

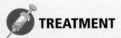

ADDITIONAL TREATMENT

General Measures

- Patients with undescended testes should be referred for surgical evaluation no later than 3 months of age.
- Hormonal therapy
  - Hormonal therapy was widely used in Europe for inducing descent of undescended testes. Both gonadotropin-releasing hormone and human chorionic gonadotropin were used, with long-term success rates of 20%.
    - Treatment is most successful for low undescended testes, but there is a 25% relapse rate.
    - More recent recommendations from European pediatric endocrinologists indicate that surgery is the preferred therapy.
  - For these reasons, as well as that gonadotropin-releasing hormone and human chorionic gonadotropin are not approved for this indication in the United States, most therapy in the United States to bring the testis down to the scrotum is surgical (orchiopexy).
  - The use of hormonal therapy after orchiopexy to improve semen analyses in high-risk patients is in its preliminary stages of investigation in Europe and the United States.

SURGERY/OTHER PROCEDURES

Goals in bringing the testis into the scrotum:

- Prevent ongoing thermal damage to the testis.
- Treat the associated hernia sac.
- Prevent testis torsion/injury against the pubic bone.
- Achieve a good cosmetic result/avoid psychological effects of empty scrotum.
- Allow the older child to perform testicular self-exam for cancer.

ONGOING CARE

FOLLOW-UP RECOMMENDATIONS

Patient Monitoring

After successful orchiopexy, patients are examined at 6–12 months to check on testicular size and position. They are rechecked at puberty to explain the technique and need for monthly testis self-exam concerning early recognition of testis cancer. Patients with retractile testes should be examined annually until age 7 years because ~5% will be found to have a testis out of the scrotum.

PROGNOSIS

- Surgery cannot reverse the maturational failure of the undescended testis, but it can prevent ongoing thermal injury.
- Parents are often concerned about future fertility:
  - In patients who have undergone orchiopexy at an early age, it appears that 90% of boys with unilateral cryptorchidism and 65% with bilateral cryptorchidism will achieve paternity.
  - Patients who are interested in their risk for infertility may have a semen analysis performed at age 18 years.
- Surgery decreases the relative risk of testicular cancer if the surgery is performed before 13 years of age.
  - All patients should be taught proper monthly testicular self-exam at the time of puberty. Some patients with cryptorchidism are at a higher risk of cancer (prune belly syndrome, ambiguous genitalia, karyotypic abnormalities, or the postpubertal boy).

ADDITIONAL READING

- Callaghan P. Undescended testis. *Pediatr Rev*. 2000; 21(11):395.
- Lee PA. Fertility after cryptorchidism: epidemiology and other outcome studies. *Urology*. 2005;66(2): 427–431.
- Pettersson A, Richiardi L, Nordenskjold A, et al. Age at surgery for undescended testis and risk for testicular cancer. *N Engl J Med*. 2007;356(18): 1835–1841.
- Pyorala S, Huttunen NP, Uhari M. A review and meta-analysis of hormonal treatment of cryptorchidism. *J Clin Endocrinol Metab*. 1995;80(9): 2795–2799.
- Ritzen EM. Undescended testes: a consensus on management. *Eur J Endocrinol*. 2008;159(Suppl 1): S87–S90.
- Tasian GE, Yiee JH, Copp HL. Imaging use and cryptorchidism: determinants of practice patterns. *J Urol*. 2011;185(5):1882–1887.
- Virtanen HE, Bjerknes R, Cortes D, et al. Cryptorchidism: classification, prevalence and long-term consequences. *Acta Paediatr*. 2007;96(5): 611–616.
- Virtanen HE, Cortes D, Rajpert-De Meyts E, et al. Development and descent of the testis in relation to cryptorchidism. *Acta Paediatr*. 2007;96(5):622–627.

CODES

ICD10

- Q53.9 Undescended testicle, unspecified
- Q53.10 Unspecified undescended testicle, unilateral
- Q53.20 Undescended testicle, unspecified, bilateral

FAQ

- Q: If there is only 1 testicle in the scrotum, will fertility be affected?
- A: In general, the outlook for paternity is good in a patient with only 1 descended testicle. Paternity is more significantly affected with a history of 2 undescended testicles.
- Q: Why do patients with retractile testes require follow-up?
- A: The ability to distinguish between retractile and undescended testes can be difficult in some patients. Some of the patients will be found to have true undescended testes as they grow. Boys should be taught how to perform a monthly testicular self-exam at puberty.

C

CRYPTOSPORIDIOSIS

Michelle W. Parker

BASICS

DESCRIPTION

Cryptosporidiosis is protozoal infection causing a self-limited acute gastroenteritis characterized by nonbloody watery diarrhea.

- Symptoms, when present, can also include abdominal pain, fever, fatigue, weight loss, vomiting, headache, and joint pain and typically last 1–2 weeks.
- In an immunocompromised patient, gastrointestinal symptoms can be chronic, relapsing, and severe, causing profound and life-threatening wasting and malabsorption.
- Extraintestinal: Pulmonary, biliary tract (sclerosing cholangitis, acalculous cholecystitis, pancreatitis), or disseminated infection rarely occurs among immunocompromised individuals.

EPIDEMIOLOGY

- Oocysts of *Cryptosporidium* are shed in stool of infected hosts (humans, cattle, and other mammals) and are transmitted by fecal–oral contamination.
- Disease is most commonly associated with contamination of water sources, both drinking and recreational, and transmission is also seen in association with child care centers or livestock.
- *Cryptosporidium* has been found in all parts of the world and is a cause of traveler's diarrhea.
- Because of summer recreational water use, the incidence of cryptosporidiosis is highest in children and typically peaks in summer through early fall.

Incidence

In 2010, nearly 9,000 new cases were reported in the United States. The incidence began increasing in 2005, with a peak in 2007 at just over 11,500 cases.

RISK FACTORS

- Those most at risk of infection are children who attend day care centers, people who take care of others with cryptosporidiosis (including child care workers, parents of infected children, and health care workers), those who swim in or drink from contaminated water sources such as streams or unprotected wells, and people who handle livestock including those visiting petting zoos.
- Because *Cryptosporidium* are chlorine tolerant, swimming in chlorinated pools does not decrease the risk of infection.

GENERAL PREVENTION

- Drinking water should be adequately filtered to a particle size of 1 μm or smaller in order to ensure oocyst removal.
- If a recreational water supply becomes contaminated, it should be closed and proper decontamination measures should be implemented.
- Those diagnosed with cryptosporidiosis should not swim for at least 2 weeks after diarrhea stops to help protect others.
- Good hand hygiene, washing with soap and water vigorously for at least 20 seconds, is key after contact with animals or stool.
- Children with diarrhea should not attend day care settings until diarrhea is resolved.
- In day care settings, disinfection of diapering areas after each use and frequent disinfection of toys, tabletops, and highchairs during outbreaks is recommended.
- Oocysts can survive for long periods and are resistant to many disinfectants including chlorine, iodine, and dilute bleach. Boiling water or full-strength bleach disinfectant is most effective.
- Contact precautions are recommended for the length of the hospital stay for hospitalized patients.
- Immunocompromised persons should avoid contact with any person or animal with cryptosporidiosis.

PATHOPHYSIOLOGY

- Transmission occurs via fecal–oral passage of oocysts from food, water, or poor hand hygiene.
- The incubation period is typically 3–14 days with a median of 7 days, and oocyst shedding may occur for weeks to months after symptoms resolve. In the majority of people, shedding stops after 2 weeks. Immunocompromised patients can shed for several months.
- Invasion of intestinal epithelial cells in the small intestine and proximal colon leads to a secretory diarrhea.
- Intestinal destruction occurs with villous atrophy and subsequent malabsorption and increased intestinal permeability.

DIAGNOSIS

HISTORY

- Acute onset of symptoms combined with exposure to any of the transmission sources discussed above should prompt consideration. Fever and vomiting are symptoms more commonly found in children and can lead to the misdiagnosis of viral gastroenteritis.
- Immunocompromised patients such as those with AIDS may have chronic severe symptoms with significant wasting.

PHYSICAL EXAM

- Acute weight loss
- Fever
- Tenderness to palpation of abdomen
- Dehydration

- Immunocompromised patients may rarely exhibit respiratory symptoms (dyspnea) or biliary tract symptoms (colicky right upper quadrant pain).

DIAGNOSTIC TESTS & INTERPRETATION

Lab

- Detection of organisms in stool specimens is diagnostic. Oocysts are small and may be missed on routine light microscopic examination of stool; modified acid-fast staining may aid in diagnosis.
  - Fluorescent stains such as auramine O are rapid but have high false-positive rates.
  - Immunofluorescent assays and enzyme-linked immunosorbent assays for antigen detection are also available.
  - The direct immunofluorescent stain is the diagnostic test of choice.
- Tests for *Cryptosporidium* are not routinely performed and should be specifically requested.

DIFFERENTIAL DIAGNOSIS

- Other infectious etiology of diarrheal illness:
  - Viral gastroenteritis including rotavirus, adenovirus, astrovirus; caliciviruses including norovirus, cytomegalovirus
  - Bacterial gastroenteritis including *Salmonella*, *Shigella*, *Yersinia*, *Campylobacter*, enterotoxigenic *Escherichia coli*, *Vibrio cholerae*
  - *Clostridium difficile* enterocolitis
  - Parasitic gastroenteritis including *Giardia*, *Entamoeba*, *Cyclospora*, *Isospora*, *Microsporidia*
- Noninfectious etiology of diarrheal illness:
  - Allergic colitis, inflammatory bowel disease, irritable bowel syndrome, appendicitis, intussusception, malrotation/volvulus, celiac disease, or other malabsorption

TREATMENT

MEDICATION

- In immunocompetent patients, disease is typically self-limited, and no treatment is necessary.
- For those who are malnourished where treatment is preferred, oral nitazoxanide may be given for 3 days.
- Dosage for children 1–3 years of age is 100 mg b.i.d.; for children 4–11 years of age, 200 mg b.i.d.; and for adults, 500 mg b.i.d.
- For immunosuppressed patients, antiretroviral therapy to improve CD4+ count has been associated with decreasing duration of illness. Nitazoxanide, paromomycin, and bovine immunoglobulin have also been tried without strong data to support efficacy.

ADDITIONAL TREATMENT

General Measures

Fluids and electrolytes should be replaced by oral or intravenous route.

ONGOING CARE

FOLLOW-UP RECOMMENDATIONS

Patient Education

- Because the oocysts can be shed in the stool for weeks after clinical resolution, it is important to realize that asymptomatic patients can still transmit the infection to household and day care contacts.
- Requiring patients whose diarrhea has resolved to have a negative stool test for *Cryptosporidium* before reentry to day care has not been evaluated as an outbreak control measure. Repeated testing is expensive.

PROGNOSIS

- For immunocompetent hosts, gastrointestinal disease is self-limited, usually lasting approximately 10 days. Supportive therapy is usually all that is necessary.
- For immunocompromised patients, diarrhea can be severe, debilitating, and often life threatening. Aggressive supportive therapy is usually required, along with antimicrobial therapy and immune reconstitution.

ADDITIONAL READING

- American Academy of Pediatrics. Cryptosporidiosis. In: Pickering LK, Baker CJ, Kimberlin DW, et al, eds. *Red Book: 2012 Report of the Committee on Infectious Diseases*. 29th ed. Elk Grove Village, IL: American Academy of Pediatrics; 2012:296–298.
- Centers for Disease Control and Prevention. Parasites—*Cryptosporidium* (also known as "Crypto"). http://www.cdc.gov/parasites/crypto/. Accessed November 5, 2013.
- Yoder JS, Wallace RM, Collier SA, et al. Cryptosporidiosis surveillance—United States, 2009–2010. *MMWR Surveill Summ*. 2012;61(5):1–12.

CODES

ICD10

A07.2 Cryptosporidiosis

FAQ

- Q: For whom should cryptosporidiosis be considered as a differential diagnosis?
- A: For anyone with acute onset of watery diarrhea with any of the mentioned risk factors
- Q: When is it safe for a child with cryptosporidiosis to return to day care?
- A: When the diarrhea has resolved
- Q: For how long is an immunocompetent patient with cryptosporidiosis contagious?
- A: A healthy person may continue to shed for weeks to months after diarrhea has resolved.

CUSHING SYNDROME

Maya B. Lodish • Constantine A. Stratakis

BASICS

DESCRIPTION

Cushing syndrome is a multisystem disorder resulting from prolonged exposure to excess glucocorticoids.

- Characterized by growth deceleration, truncal obesity, characteristic skin changes, muscle weakness, and hypertension
- Most common cause in childhood is exogenous administration of glucocorticoids.
- Endogenous Cushing syndrome may be caused by ACTH-secreting tumor of the pituitary gland (Cushing disease), ectopic secretion of ACTH, or ACTH-independent secretion of glucocorticoids by the adrenal glands.
- Accurate diagnosis and classification of Cushing syndrome in children is crucial to guide appropriate therapeutic intervention.
- In endogenous Cushing syndrome, the hypothalamic-pituitary-adrenal axis has lost its ability for self-regulation due to excessive secretion of either ACTH or cortisol and loss of the negative feedback function.
- Diagnostic tests help to distinguish the cause of this disorder.
- Key differences in the diagnosis and management of Cushing syndrome exist between children and adults.

EPIDEMIOLOGY

- The overall incidence of Cushing syndrome is approximately 2–5 new cases per million people per year. Only approximately 10% of the new cases each year occur in children.
- In older children with Cushing syndrome, there is a female-to-male predominance, whereas in younger children there may be a male predominance.
- Exogenous Cushing syndrome caused by chronic administration of glucocorticoids (by any route) or, more rarely, by administration of ACTH (for example, for infantile seizures) is the most common cause of this syndrome in children.
- The pituitary-dependent form (Cushing disease) accounts for more than 80% of all cases of Cushing syndrome in children older than 7 years of age.

ETIOLOGY

- Adrenal sources of Cushing syndrome:
  - In very young children, adrenal sources of Cushing syndrome are the most common causes of the condition.
  - 10–15% of all the cases of Cushing syndrome in childhood are due to ACTH-independent Cushing syndrome from unregulated secretion of cortisol from the adrenal glands.
  - Adrenocortical neoplasms
    - Often malignant in young children.
  - Primary pigmented nodular adrenocortical nodular disease (PPNAD)
    - PPNAD is a genetic disorder often associated with Carney complex and related to mutations of the *PRKAR1A* gene.
    - Cushing syndrome in PPNAD may be cyclical and difficult to diagnose.
  - Isolated micronodular adrenocortical disease (iMAD)
    - If no *PRKAR1A* mutations are found or if the patient does not have Carney complex, and Cushing syndrome is due to bilateral adrenal hyperplasia without massive enlargement of the adrenal glands on imaging, then, the most likely diagnosis is iMAD.
    - Like in PPNAD, Cushing syndrome in iMAD can be difficult to diagnose due to an often atypical and/or cyclical clinical course.
  - Massive macronodular adrenal hyperplasia (MMAD)
    - Another form of ACTH-independent bilateral adrenal disease seen (rarely) in children
    - Easier to diagnose due to massive enlargement of the adrenal glands on imaging studies
  - Adrenal hyperplasia and/or adenomas can also be seen in the McCune Albright and Beckwith-Wiedemann syndromes, usually in the infantile period.
- Ectopic ACTH production accounts for less than 1% of the cases of Cushing syndrome in children and may be due to a variety of neuroendocrine (NE) tumors.
  - NE tumors include carcinoid tumors in the lungs, pancreas (and other locations in the gastrointestinal tract), or thymus; medullary carcinomas of the thyroid; and pheochromocytomas, as well as small cell carcinoma of the lungs that may be seen rarely in adolescents.
  - Other causes of ectopic ACTH secretion include infantile neuroblastomas (and related tumors) and paraneoplastic syndromes in all ages.
- Corticotropin-releasing hormone (CRH) secretion by an ectopic CRH-producing source, typically an NE tumor such as the ones producing ectopically ACTH, is an extremely rare cause of Cushing syndrome in children.
- Exogenous steroids: Iatrogenic Cushing syndrome is the most common cause in pediatrics. Cushing syndrome can be caused by chronic systemic, topical, or intranasal steroid use, or ACTH use.

DIAGNOSIS

HISTORY

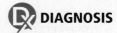

- The most common presenting symptom of the syndrome in childhood is weight gain accompanied by poor linear growth.
- Additional pertinent features in the history of presenting illness often include headaches, hypertension, weakness, hirsutism, irregular menses, and delayed puberty.
- Dermatologic features include facial flushing, striae (in older children and adolescents only), acne, bruising, and acanthosis nigricans.
- Fractures and/or kidney stones related to Cushing syndrome are also relatively frequent manifestations.

PHYSICAL EXAMINATION

- Check growth chart and document height velocity and weight change.
- Note fat distribution (characteristic central obesity, dorsocervical, subclavicular, and bitemporal fat pads).
- Skin examination
  - Document striae (usually wide, violaceous) and acanthosis.
  - Look for characteristic dermatologic features that may be associated with genetic forms of Cushing (café au lait spots for MAS, lentigines for Carney complex).
- Neurologic examination
  - Check for proximal muscular weakness (typically not present in younger children) by having patient rise from a squatting position.
  - Check visual fields and perform funduscopic examination.
- Document Tanner staging and note any discrepancy between pubic hair and gonadal or breast size (which may point to ACTH-dependent or -independent causes of Cushing syndrome).

DIAGNOSTIC TESTS & INTERPRETATION

- Diagnostic tests: The first step in the diagnosis of Cushing syndrome is to document hypercortisolism.
- Screening
  - 24-hour urine free cortisol excretion
  - Low-dose dexamethasone test
    - 1 mg dexamethasone (adjust for pediatric patients 15 mcg × weight [kg]; maximum dose 1 mg) PO at 11 p.m. Measure plasma cortisol at 8 a.m. next day.
  - Circadian cortisol profile
    - Measure serum or salivary cortisol at 8 a.m. and midnight.
- Confirmation: The following results are suspicious for Cushing syndrome:
  - 24-hour urine free cortisol excretion above normal limits for assay (corrected for body surface area)
  - Post low-dose dexamethasone 8 a.m. plasma cortisol >1.8 mcg/dL
  - Blunted circadian rhythm: a single midnight cortisol value of >4.4 mcg/dL highly sensitive and specific for Cushing syndrome

- Differentiate causes:
  - Measure plasma ACTH.
  - If low ACTH (<29 pg/mL) = likely ACTH-independent but need to confirm with dexamethasone testing; only completely undetectable ACTH levels indicate undoubtedly an adrenal source of Cushing syndrome.
  - Proceed with high-dose dexamethasone suppression test (adjust dexamethasone dose for weight 120 mcg × kg; max dose 8 mg).
  - Lack of suppression in response to high-dose dexamethasone indicates that the likely diagnosis is adrenal tumor.
  - If high ACTH (>29 pg/mL) = likely ACTH-independent
    - Proceed with CRH testing (generally done by an endocrine specialist).
    - CRH given at 1 mcg/kg and serial cortisol and ACTH levels are measured. The criterion for the diagnosis of the pituitary-dependent Cushing disease is a mean increase of 20% above baseline for cortisol values at 30–45 minutes and an increase in the mean corticotropin concentrations of at least 35% over basal value at 15–30 minutes after CRH administration.
    - If CRH testing is negative: Likely diagnosis is ectopic ACTH production.
    - If CRH testing is positive: consistent with Cushing disease

Imaging

- When Cushing disease (ACTH-secreting pituitary tumor) is suspected, pituitary magnetic resonance imaging (MRI) should be done in thin sections with high resolution with gadolinium.
- Computed tomography (CT) of the adrenal glands useful in the distinction between pituitary Cushing disease and adrenal causes of Cushing syndrome. MRI of the adrenal glands is less useful for the detection of PPNAD or iMAD, but may be used for the detection of MMAD, single large tumors, and cancer.
- Bilateral inferior petrosal sinus sampling (IPSS) is a catheterization study used to confirm the source of ACTH secretion in ACTH-dependent Cushing syndrome. IPSS needed only when the pituitary MRI is negative or tests are contradictory, but may be performed only if ACTH-dependent disease is confirmed and cortisol levels are consistently high.

TREATMENT

- The treatment of choice for Cushing disease is transsphenoidal surgery (TSS).
- In most specialized centers with experienced neurosurgeons, the success rate of the first TSS is close to, or even higher than, 85%.
- The treatment of choice for adrenal tumors is surgical resection, and if metastatic carcinoma, chemotherapy and radiation may be employed.
- Bilateral total adrenalectomy is usually the treatment of choice in PPNAD, iMAD, and MMAD.
- Adrenalectomy may also be used in patients with refractory Cushing disease or with difficult-to-treat ectopic ACTH-dependent Cushing syndrome.

COMPLICATIONS

- After TSS, patients may have persistent disease or recurrence.
- Postoperative complications may include transient diabetes insipidus and syndrome of inappropriate antidiuretic hormone secretion, central hypothyroidism, growth hormone deficiency, hypogonadism, bleeding, infection (meningitis), and pituitary apoplexy.
- Patients who undergo bilateral adrenalectomy with Cushing disease must be aware of the potential of Nelson syndrome, characterized by increased pigmentation, elevated ACTH levels, and a growing pituitary ACTH-producing pituitary tumor.

ADDITIONAL TREATMENT

- Pituitary irradiation following a failed TSS will lead to remission in approximately 80% of patients, although commonly results in hypopituitarism. Newer forms of stereotactic radiotherapy are now available as options for the treatment of Cushing syndrome, including proton beam and gamma knife.
- A number of medications are available to inhibit corticosteroid biosynthesis, although none of these agents are specifically approved for use in children. These pharmacotherapies include metyrapone and ketoconazole, which may be employed in cases of refractory Cushing or when bridging the patient to definitive therapy. In addition, dopamine receptor agonists such as pasireotide and cortisol receptor antagonists, such as mifepristone, are also under clinical investigation for use in children.

ONGOING CARE

- Following TSS in Cushing disease, patients will be transiently adrenally insufficient while the hypothalamic-pituitary-adrenal axis is recovering.
- Stress doses of cortisol are necessary in the perioperative period.
- These should be weaned relatively rapidly to a physiologic replacement dose.
- The patient should be followed every few months, and the adrenocortical function should be periodically assessed with a 1-hour 250 mcg ACTH test. Most patients recover HPA function within 1 year after TSS.
- Following bilateral adrenalectomy, lifetime replacement glucocorticoids and mineralocorticoids, (fludrocortisone 0.1–0.3 mg daily) is required.
- All patients status post cure of Cushing need to be taught precautions for adrenal insufficiency, including emergency injection of hydrocortisone and medical alert bracelet.

ALERT

- Falsely high urine free cortisol may be obtained because of stress, obesity, pregnancy, chronic exercise, depression, poor diabetes control, alcoholism, anorexia, narcotic withdrawal, anxiety, malnutrition, and high water intake. A combined dexamethasone–CRH test may help to differentiate pseudo-Cushing syndrome from true Cushing syndrome.
- Falsely low urine free cortisol may be present if inadequate collection or intermittent cortisol hypersecretion.

ADDITIONAL READING

- Batista DL, Oldfield EH, Keil MF, et al. Postoperative testing to predict recurrent Cushing disease in children. *J Clin Endocrinol Metab*. 2009; 94(8):2757–2765.
- Batista DL, Riar J, Keil M, et al. Diagnostic tests for children who are referred for the investigation of Cushing syndrome. *Pediatrics*. 2007;120(3): e575–e586.
- Lodish M, Dunn SV, Sinaii N, et al. Recovery of the hypothalamic-pituitary-adrenal axis in children and adolescents after surgical cure of Cushing's disease. *J Clin Endocrinol Metab*. 2012;97(5):1483–1491.
- Stratakis CA. Cushing syndrome in pediatrics. *Endocrinol Metab Clin North Am*. 2012;41(4):793–803.

CODES

ICD10

- E24.9 Cushing's syndrome, unspecified
- E24.0 Pituitary-dependent Cushing's disease
- E24.2 Drug-induced Cushing's syndrome

FAQ

- Q: What clinical clue is most useful to determine which children have obesity alone versus those with Cushing syndrome?
- A: Cushing syndrome is associated with growth failure, whereas obesity is associated with adequate linear growth.
- Q: Are most patients on lifetime glucocorticoid replacement after surgery for Cushing disease?
- A: No. The majority of patients recover their hypothalamic-pituitary-adrenal axis within 1 year of their TSS and can be weaned off glucocorticoids.

CUTANEOUS LARVA MIGRANS

Ross Newman • Jason Newland

BASICS

DESCRIPTION

Infestation of the epidermis by the infectious larvae of certain nematodes, classically manifesting with an intensely pruritic, serpiginous skin lesion

EPIDEMIOLOGY

Worldwide distribution, but most frequent in warmer climates, including the Caribbean, Africa, South America, Southeast Asia, and southeastern United States

RISK FACTORS

- Contracted from soil contaminated with dog and cat feces
- Occupational exposures occur from crawling under buildings, such as among plumbers and pipefitters.

PATHOPHYSIOLOGY

- Route of spread
  - Primary host (dog or cat) passes eggs to ground through feces.
  - Warm, sandy soil acts as an incubator.
  - Eggs mature into *rhabditiform larvae* (noninfectious), which molt in 5 days to *filariform larvae* (infectious).
- Humans are accidental hosts.
- Filariform larvae penetrate the epidermis either through hair follicles or fissures or through intact skin with the use of proteases.
- Larvae are unable to penetrate the basement membrane of the dermis; therefore, the infection remains limited to the epidermis.
- Larvae cannot complete their life cycle in the human host and die within weeks to months.
- Symptoms are due to hypersensitivity to the organism or its excreta.

ETIOLOGY

- Most common organism is the dog or cat hookworm, *Ancylostoma braziliense*.
- Other species include *Ancylostoma caninum*, *Uncinaria stenocephala*, and *Bunostomum phlebotomum*.

DIAGNOSIS

- Diagnosis is usually clinical. Organisms are rarely recovered from biopsy and antibody titers are unreliable.

HISTORY

- Incubation period
  - Usual time from infectious exposure to symptoms is 7–10 days but may last for up to several months.
- Rash
  - Intensely pruritic, raised, serpiginous, and linear
  - Most commonly located on feet, buttocks, and abdomen; also found on face, extremities, and genitalia
- Pruritus
  - Symptoms typically begin with some tingling in the affected area with the development of the typical rash with intense pruritus.
- Speed at which rash spreads
  - Rash typically lengthens by a few millimeters to 2–3 cm daily.
- Source of infection
  - History of contract with beaches in tropical countries where dogs are frequently found
  - In the United States: most frequently contracted from moist soil in southeastern United States contaminated with animal feces

PHYSICAL EXAM

The classic rash is described as an erythematous, raised, serpiginous rash. In addition, it may begin as vesicular and/or form bullae along the track. Tracks under the skin reflect the course of the larvae. The active end is not part of the track.

DIAGNOSTIC TESTS & INTERPRETATION

Lab

- Biopsy: not indicated because it rarely yields organisms
- Serologic testing: not helpful and unreliable, as immunity does not usually develop
- Diagnosis is based on clinical presentation.

DIFFERENTIAL DIAGNOSIS

- Cutaneous larva migrans should be considered in anyone with an intensely pruritic, raised, serpiginous, linear cutaneous eruption.
- Hookworm infections
  - *Strongyloides stercoralis*
  - *U. stenocephala*
  - *B. phlebotomum*
  - *Gnathostoma spinigerum*
- Free-living nematodes (*Pelodera strongyloides*) and insect larvae

- Other cutaneous eruptions that may mimic cutaneous larva migrans include the following:
  - Scabies
  - Tinea pedis
  - Erythema migrans of Lyme disease
  - Jelly fish stings
  - Contact dermatitis
  - Photosensitivity

TREATMENT

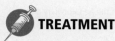

GENERAL MEASURES

- Albendazole
  - First line
  - Administered as 400 mg PO once a day for 3 days
- Ivermectin
  - 200 mcg/kg once a day for 1–2 days
  - Oral ivermectin is contraindicated in children who weigh less than 15 kg or are younger than 5 years old.
- Alternative: topical thiabendazole 10–15% applied three times a day for 5–7 days; not readily available for prescription

ONGOING CARE

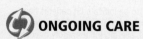

FOLLOW-UP RECOMMENDATIONS

Patient Monitoring

- Symptoms persist for 8 weeks but up to 1 year in untreated patients.
- Those with extensive involvement should be seen after treatment to be certain of improvement in symptoms.

PROGNOSIS

- This is a self-limited disease and will resolve without treatment when the larvae die.
- Cure rates with oral ivermectin range from 77 to 100% after one dose, with a second dose usually providing complete resolution. Oral albendazole for 5–7 days has cure rates of 92–100%.

COMPLICATIONS

- Most common complication is secondary bacterial infection of the involved skin.
- Self-limited disease: If untreated, larvae die within 2–8 weeks but may persist for up to 1 year.
- Rarely, the larvae can invade the dermis and, subsequently, the bloodstream, leading to a peripheral eosinophilia and pulmonary infiltrates (Löffler syndrome).

ADDITIONAL READING

- Blackwell V, Vega-Lopez F. Cutaneous larva migrans: clinical features and management of 44 cases presenting in the returning traveler. *Brit J Dermatol*. 2001;145(3):434–437.
- Bouchaud O, Houze S, Schiemann R, et al. Cutaneous larva migrans in travelers: a prospective study, with assessment of therapy with ivermectin. *Clin Infect Dis*. 2000;31(2):493–498.
- Brenner MA, Patel MB. Cutaneous larva migrans: the creeping eruption. *Cutis*. 2003;72(2):111–115.
- Caumes E. Treatment of cutaneous larva migrans. *Clin Infect Dis*. 2000;30(5):811–814.
- Heukelbach J, Feldmeier H. Epidemiological and clinical characteristics of hookworm related cutaneous larva migrans. *Lancet Infect Dis*. 2008;8(5):302–309.
- Tan SK, Liu TT. Cutaneous larva migrans complicated by Löffler syndrome. *Arch Dermatol*. 2010;146(2):210–212.

CODES

ICD10

- B76.9 Hookworm disease, unspecified
- B76.8 Other hookworm diseases

FAQ

- Q: Can children spread the infection to each other?
- A: The usual spread of infection is from direct contact with the larvae. Person-to-person spread does not occur.
- Q: What is the role of treatment in cutaneous larva migrans?
- A: Although the infestation is self-limited, as the larvae die with time, antiparasitic therapy helps to control the symptoms and prevent complications such as secondary bacterial infection.
- Q: What are preventive strategies for avoiding cutaneous larva migrans when visiting tropical beaches?
- A: When on tropical beaches frequented by dogs, wear shoes, avoid lying directly on dry sand, and only lie in sand that has been washed by the tide.
- Q: What are other names for cutaneous larva migrans?
- A: Creeping eruption, sandworms, and plumber's itch

CYCLIC VOMITING SYNDROME

Desale Yacob

BASICS

DESCRIPTION

- Cyclic vomiting syndrome (CVS) is an idiopathic disorder characterized by recurrent, stereotypical episodes of vomiting with intervening periods of normal health.
- Essential clinical features of CVS are 3 or more discrete episodes of vomiting; intervals of completely normal health between episodes; stereotypical episodes with regard to timing of onset, symptoms, and duration; as well as the absence of an identifiable organic cause for vomiting.

EPIDEMIOLOGY

- CVS commonly starts in early childhood.
- Prevalence of 1.9–2.3% has been reported.
- The syndrome is more common in Caucasians.

COMMONLY ASSOCIATED CONDITIONS

- 2/3 of CVS patients have symptoms of IBS.
- 11% of CVS patients have migraine headaches and a third of patients later develop migraine headaches.

DIAGNOSIS

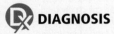

- A consensus statement by the North American Society for Pediatric Gastroenterology, Hepatology and Nutrition (NASPGHAN) expert task force suggests the diagnosis can be made if the following criteria are met:
  - A minimum of 3 attacks during a 6-month period or at least 5 attacks in any interval
  - Episodic attacks of intense nausea and vomiting lasting 1 hour to 10 days and occurring at least 1 week apart
  - Stereotypical pattern and symptoms in the individual patient
  - Vomiting during attacks occurs at least 4 times/h for at least 1 hour.
  - Return to baseline health between episodes
  - Not attributed to another disorder
- If the above criteria is met, the diagnosis should be considered most likely to be CVS and the workup should consist of the following tests only:
  - Electrolytes, glucose, BUN, and creatinine
  - A UGI series to evaluate for malrotation
- Red flags that CVS is not the correct diagnosis include the following:
  - Episode of vomiting is characterized by the presence of the following:
    - Bilious emesis
    - Severe abdominal pain or tenderness
    - Hematemesis
- If episodes are triggered by intercurrent illness, fasting, or high-protein meal, the following labs should be obtained at the beginning of the attack prior to IV fluid:
  - Glucose, electrolytes for anion gap, urine ketones serum lactate, ammonia and amino acids, urine organic acids. Optional metabolic labs include plasma carnitine and acylcarnitine.
- If episodes occur in the context of an abnormal neurologic exam including severe altered mental status, papilledema, abnormal eye movements, motor asymmetry, and gait abnormality, consultation with a neurologist is indicated and a brain MRI should be obtained.
  - Consider at any given time:
    - US of abdomen and pelvis
    - UGI series
    - Amylase and lipase
    - Esophagogastroduodenoscopy
  - During an attack, obtain LFTs, lipase ± amylase.

HISTORY

- Children with CVS experience a stereotypical pattern of vomiting characterized by a consistent time of onset, duration, and associated symptoms.
- Vomiting frequency is high, with median of 6 bouts of emesis per hour, often bilious and associated with severe nausea.
- The intense vomiting results in dehydration and need for IV hydration.
- Accompanying symptoms include nausea, retching, headache, abdominal pain, pallor, listlessness, anorexia, and photophobia.
- Physical and psychological stresses are common triggers.
- CVS episodes are most likely to start in the early morning hours.

PHYSICAL EXAM

Physical exam is often consistent with dehydration, and young children may appear listless.

DIAGNOSTIC TESTS & INTERPRETATION

The consideration of established criteria is important when diagnosing CVS, as is a thorough workup to rule out other etiologies that may explain the symptoms. These tests may include blood, urine, and imaging studies depending on the history and physical exam of the individual child.

Lab

- Basic metabolic panel: Na^+, K^+, Cl^-, HCO_3, glucose, BUN, and creatinine
- Liver and pancreas: ALT, GGT, lipase ± amylase
- Other: urine ketones, lactate, ammonia, serum amino acids, urine organic acids, plasma carnitine, and acylcarnitine

Imaging

- UGI series
  - A UGI should be performed in all patients who present with bilious emesis and who are suspected to have CVS.
- Abdominal US
  - Helpful in evaluation of the hepatobiliary and urinary systems
- Brain MRI
  - Should be obtained when episodes of emesis are associated with progressive or acute, as well as diffuse or focal, neurologic symptoms or signs
  - MRI, rather than CT or skull x-ray is the preferred modality for visualization of the posterior fossa.

DIAGNOSTIC PROCEDURES/SURGERY

Esophagogastroduodenoscopy

- May be indicated if hematemesis occurs following multiple episodes of emesis in a patient with CVS
- Most likely etiologies of hematemesis in a child with CVS are mild esophagitis, Mallory-Weiss tear, or prolapse gastropathy.
- Endoscopy may also be indicated if patients have persistent symptoms between episodes suggestive of peptic/bacterial, allergic, inflammatory or celiac disease, or hematemesis of large quantity that may require endoscopic hemostasis.

DIFFERENTIAL DIAGNOSIS

- Malrotation
- UPJ obstruction
- Rumination syndrome
- Gastroparesis
- Pseudoobstruction
- CNS lesion
- Increased intracranial pressure
- Infectious illness
- Pancreatitis
- Mitochondrial disorder
- Cannabinoid hyperemesis syndrome

TREATMENT

- The treatment strategy should be tailored to an individual taking into account the following:
  - The frequency and severity of attacks as well as how badly it impacts the patient
  - Potential side effects of the treatment have to also be taken into consideration.
- Treatment of children with CVS can be as follows:
  - Prophylactic or preventive measures
  - Abortive and supportive interventions

GENERAL MEASURES

There are a number of lifestyle changes that can be implemented that may prevent recurrence of CVS attacks without resorting to daily medications. Targeted lifestyle changes that can be effective are best found by reviewing a detailed vomiting diary to identify triggers for episodes. Generally speaking, the following are effective measures:

- Reassurance and education of patients and their families about CVS to decrease stress
- Avoidance of triggers and precipitating factors, including prolonged fasting, poor sleep hygiene, chocolate, cheese, monosodium glutamate, antigenic foods, and excessive exercise
- If episodes are induced by fasting, the child should have supplemental carbohydrate by having snacks between meals, before exertion, or at bedtime.
- Considering CVS to be in the migraine spectrum, migraine headache lifestyle interventions by doing regular aerobic exercise, regular meal times, and regulated consumption of caffeine

MEDICATIONS

- Children >5 years of age
  - Amitriptyline, a tricyclic antidepressant (TCA), has been shown to be very effective.
    - It is recommended to initially prescribe a dose of 0.25–0.5 mg/kg PO at bed time.
    - Doses should be increased by 5–10 mg weekly to a maximum dose of 1–1.5 mg/kg if symptoms continue to occur.
    - Patients should be evaluated prior to starting amitriptyline with an EKG for QT_c abnormality and 10 days after achieving peak dose.
    - Side effects of this drug consist of arrhythmia (prolongation of the QT interval), sedation, behavioral changes, and constipation.
    - Nortriptyline is another TCA that can be used as an alternative.
  - Propranolol, a β-blocker, is considered a 2nd-line therapy.
    - This should be dosed at 0.25–1 mg/kg/day PO, with a typical maximum dose of 10 mg b.i.d. or t.i.d.
    - Heart rate should be monitored and maintained ≥60 bpm.
    - Side effects include lethargy and reduced exercise intolerance.
    - Propranolol is contraindicated in children with asthma, diabetes, heart disease, and depression. Propranolol must be tapered for 1–2 weeks when it is discontinued.
- Children 5 years of age or younger can be treated by the following:
  - Cyproheptadine, which is an antihistamine, is first choice.
  - Dosed at 0.25–0.5 mg/kg/day PO divided b.i.d. or t.i.d., the β-blocker propranolol can be used as a second choice as discussed above.
  - Nutritional supplements including the following:
    - L-carnitine 50–100 mg/kg/day PO divided b.i.d. or t.i.d. (Side effects reported include diarrhea and fishy body odor.)
    - Coenzyme Q_{10} 10 mg/kg/day PO divided b.i.d. or t.i.d. (max 100 mg t.i.d.)
  - Other medications and supplements that have been used in treating CVS in a prophylactic measure include the following and are generally only prescribed by neurologists: phenobarbital or alternative anticonvulsants; topiramate, valproic acid, gabapentin, levetiracetam.
- A plan that combines lifestyle changes and medications with careful attention to dosing, side effects, and specialist referrals should be put in place and clearly communicated with the patients and parents.

ADDITIONAL THERAPIES

When children with CVS have an acute episode, they will require both supportive and abortive interventions.

- Decreasing stimulation by situating the patient in a quiet and dark area
- Providing fluid replacements with electrolytes and calories along with antiemetics and analgesics
- Identifying possible metabolic decompensation by paying attention to the following:
  - Anion gap, lactic acidosis, and hyperglycemia
  - Using fluids with higher dextrose concentration such as 10% may also be very helpful.
- Abortive intervention
  - Sumatriptan, an antimigraine drug, can be given at the time of onset at a dose of 20 mg intranasally.
    - Possible side effects: neck pain or burning and coronary vasospasm
    - A contraindication for its use is comorbidity with basilar artery migraines.
- Supportive care
  - Fluids: D10 1/2 NS with or without KCl at 1 1/2 times maintenance
    - Peripheral parenteral nutrition may be necessary if the patient had no enteral intake for 3–5 days.
  - Antiemetic
    - Ondansetron at a dose of 0.15 mg/kg/dose (max dose: 16 mg) IV given every 4–6 hours
  - Sedatives
    - Diphenhydramine 1–1.25 mg/kg/dose (max dose: 50 mg) IV every 6 hours
    - Lorazepam 0.05–0.1 mg/kg/dose (max dose: 2 mg) IV every 6 hours
  - Analgesics
    - Ketorolac 0.4–1 mg/kg IV every 6 hours with a max dose of 30 mg and total daily max of 120 mg. Do not exceed 3–5 days of continuous use.
  - It is also important to treat any abdominal pain, diarrhea, hypertension, and complications that may result from the persistent emesis such as dehydration, weight loss, hematemesis, metabolic acidosis, and syndrome of inappropriate antidiuretic syndrome (SIADH).
  - Once the episode of emesis is over, the child can be fed ad libitum.

FOLLOW-UP RECOMMENDATIONS

Referral to either pediatric gastroenterologists or neurologists with special interest in CVS should be made.

ADDITIONAL READING

- Boles RG. High degree of efficacy in the treatment of cyclic vomiting syndrome with combined co-enzyme Q10, L-carnitine and amitriptyline, a case series. *BMC Neurol*. 2011;11:102.
- Fleisher DR, Matar M. The cyclic vomiting syndrome: a report of 71 cases and literature review. *J Pediatr Gastroenterol Nutr*. 1993;17(4):361–369.
- Li BU, Lefevre F, Chelimsky GG, et al. North American Society for Pediatric Gastroenterology, Hepatology, and Nutrition consensus statement on the diagnosis and management of cyclic vomiting syndrome. *J Pediatr Gastroenterol Nutr*. 2008;47(3):379–393.
- Li BU, Murray RD, Heitlinger LA, et al. Heterogeneity of diagnoses presenting as cyclic vomiting. *Pediatrics*. 1998;102(3, Pt 1):583–587.
- Robinson TL, Cheng FK, Domingo CA, et al. Spicing up the differential for cyclical vomiting. *Am J Gastroenterol*. 2013;108(8):1371.

PATIENT TEACHING

Patients and parents should be directed to visit the following:

- The Cyclic Vomiting Syndrome Association Web site: http://www.cvsaonline.org
- International Foundation for Functional Gastrointestinal Disorders (IFFGD) Web site: http://www.aboutkidsgi.org/site/about-gi-health-in-kids/functional-gi-and-motility-disorders/cyclic-vomiting-syndrome

CODES

ICD10

- G43.A0 Cyclical vomiting, not intractable
- G43.A1 Cyclical vomiting, intractable

FAQ

- Q: How should I evaluate a child with presumed CVS who presents with progressive or focal neurologic findings?
- A: The child should be evaluated for increased intracranial pressure, as well as a metabolic disorder.
- Q: How can one distinguish true encephalopathy from CVS-associated listlessness in child presenting to the ED?
- A: The child with CVS will respond to commands appropriately and is oriented despite the desire to remain low key due to the severe nausea. In contrast, a child with metabolic encephalopathy is most likely to be confused, disoriented, and difficult to arouse.

CYCLOSPORA

Jessica Newman • Jason Newland

BASICS

DESCRIPTION

Cyclospora cayetanensis, a coccidian protozoan, causes a diarrheal illness first described in humans in 1979.

GENERAL PREVENTION

Fresh produce, especially raspberries, cilantro, and salad mixes, should be washed thoroughly before being eaten, although this still may not entirely eliminate the risk of transmission.

EPIDEMIOLOGY

- Worldwide distribution, with areas of endemic infection (Nepal, Peru, Haiti, Guatemala, Indonesia)
- People living in endemic areas have a shorter illness or may be asymptomatic carriers.
- Cyclospora can be an opportunistic infection in human immunodeficiency virus patients.
- In the United States, infection occurs primarily in spring and summer.
- In the United States and Canada, cases are associated with consumption of imported fresh produce.

PATHOPHYSIOLOGY

- Infected patients excrete noninfectious unsporulated oocysts in their stool.
- Sporulation then occurs days to weeks after release into the environment.
- Ingestion of sporulated oocysts occurs and sporozoites are released that invade the intestinal epithelial cells.
- Sporozoites develop into trophozoites, which undergo schizogony and form merozoites.
- Merozoites may develop into macro- or microgametes, which become fertilized, resulting in oocysts.
- Entire life cycle is completed in the host.
- Incubation period is between 2 and 14 days, with an average of 7 days.

ETIOLOGY

- Outbreaks have been associated with the consumption of raspberries, mesclun (young salad greens), salad mixes, cilantro, and basil.
- Infection occurs through the consumption of contaminated food and water.
- Transmission does not occur through person-to-person spread.

DIAGNOSIS

HISTORY

- Fever
  - Low-grade fever is common.
- Clinical prodrome
  - Acute onset of diarrhea is typical, but a flulike prodrome may occur.
- Nature of the diarrhea
  - Profuse, nonbloody, watery diarrhea that may be foul smelling
  - Can alternate with constipation
- Other symptoms experienced:
  - Abdominal cramping
  - Fatigue
  - Anorexia
  - Flatulence
  - Vomiting
- Foods that have been consumed in the past 2 weeks
  - Illness has been attributed to contaminated raspberries, water, mesclun, salad mix, cilantro, and basil.

PHYSICAL EXAM

Dehydration

- Due to profuse diarrhea, signs of dehydration (tachycardia, dry mucous membranes, sunken eyes, poor skin turgor, and weight loss) may be present.

DIAGNOSTIC TESTS & INTERPRETATION

Lab

- Ova and parasites with modified acid-fast staining
  - Identification of *Cyclospora*, *Isospora*, and *Cryptosporidium*
  - Three samples are preferable due to intermittent shedding.
- PCR testing is available from the CDC.
- Ova and parasites: identify common protozoans including *Giardia*
- *Cryptosporidium* and *Giardia* antigen test: immunoassay with high sensitivity and specificity
- Electron microscopy of stool: gold standard for diagnosing microsporidia
- Bacterial stool cultures: identify common bacterial pathogens
- Stool for *Clostridium difficile* PCR: identify a common cause of diarrhea
- Electrolytes, blood urea nitrogen, creatinine: determine extent of dehydration

DIFFERENTIAL DIAGNOSIS

- *Cryptosporidium*
  - Outbreaks are associated with contaminated water sources (municipal pools).
  - Person-to-person transmission may occur.
  - Clinically indistinguishable from *Cyclospora*

- *Isospora belli*
  - Outbreaks are associated with food and water.
  - Clinically indistinguishable from *Cyclospora*, although fever may be more common
- Microsporida
  - Outbreaks are associated with contaminated water sources.
  - Chronic diarrhea occurs in immunocompromised patients, especially HIV patients.
  - Fever is uncommon.
- *Giardia lamblia*
  - Community epidemics are associated primarily with contaminated water sources.
  - Person-to-person transmission may occur and has led to outbreaks in day care centers.
  - Clinical presentation may vary from occasional acute watery diarrhea to a severe, protracted diarrheal illness.
- Viral gastroenteritis
  - Rotavirus
  - Adenovirus
- Bacterial gastroenteritis
  - *C. difficile*
  - *Vibrio cholerae* and non-*cholerae Vibrio* species
  - *Escherichia coli* (especially toxin-producing strains)
  - *Shigella* species
  - *Salmonella* species
  - *Yersinia enterocolitica*
  - *Campylobacter* species

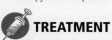

TREATMENT

MEDICATIONS

- Immunocompetent patient: trimethoprim (5 mg/kg)-sulfamethoxazole IV/PO twice a day for 7–10 days
- HIV patient: trimethoprim-sulfamethoxazole 3 times a day for 10 days and then prophylactic dosing 3 times per week to prevent relapse
- Ciprofloxacin or nitazoxanide for 7 days may be alternatives in patients with sulfa allergy.
- Based on severity of dehydration, treatment with IV fluids may be indicated.

INPATIENT CONSIDERATIONS

Admission Criteria

Moderate to severe dehydration

ONGOING CARE

PROGNOSIS

- Most cases are self-limited.
- Diarrhea may last up to 3 months in untreated patients who acquired the parasite in a foreign country where *Cyclospora* is endemic.
- In U.S. outbreaks, the average duration of diarrhea ranged from 10 to 24 days.
- Relapses may occur in untreated patients.
- Patients with HIV have more severe and prolonged diarrhea, which may recur.

COMPLICATIONS

- Dehydration and weight loss are the most common complications.
  - Severe, prolonged diarrhea may lead to dehydration.
  - Malabsorption of D-xylose and excretion of fecal fat occurs, leading to weight loss.
- May cause ascending biliary tract disease in AIDS patients
- Rare associated complications
  - Guillain-Barré syndrome
  - Reactive arthritis

PATIENT MONITORING

- Infected patients need to be observed closely for dehydration.
- Relapse may occur in HIV patients, so close follow-up is essential.

ADDITIONAL READING

- Centers for Disease Control and Prevention. Notes from the field: outbreaks of cyclosporiasis—United States, June–August 2013. *MMWR Morb Mortal Wkly Rep*. 2013;62(43):862.
- Herwaldt BL. Cyclospora cayetanensis: a review, focusing on the outbreaks of cyclosporiasis in the 1990s. *Clin Infect Dis*. 2000;31(4):1040–1057.
- Ortega YE, Sanchez R. Update on *Cyclospora cayetanensis*, a food-borne and waterborne parasite. *Clin Microbiol Rev*. 2010;23(1):218–234.

CODES

ICD10

A07.4 Cyclosporiasis

FAQ

- Q: Does routine ova and parasites testing detect *Cyclospora*?
- A: Rarely. Therefore, modified acid-fast staining must be done to improve the laboratory's ability to detect the oocysts.
- Q: Can person-to-person transmission occur in *Cyclospora* illness?
- A: No. It takes days to weeks for oocysts to sporulate and become infectious.

CYSTIC FIBROSIS

Samuel B. Goldfarb • Bruce A. Ong

BASICS

DESCRIPTION

Cystic fibrosis (CF) is an inherited autosomal recessive disorder, characterized by chronic obstructive lung disease, pancreatic exocrine insufficiency, and elevated sweat chloride concentration.

ALERT

- Most common pitfall is failure to diagnose. Neonatal screening is not performed in all states.
- Not uncommon to delay making the diagnosis in patients with mild symptoms

EPIDEMIOLOGY

- Most common lethal inherited disease in the Caucasian population
- Carrier frequency of mutations in the CF transmembrane conductance regulator (CFTR) gene:
  - 1:29 in Caucasians
  - 1:49 in Hispanics
  - 1:53 in Native Americans
  - 1:62 in African Americans
  - 1:90 in Asians

Prevalence

- 1:3,300 in Caucasians
- 1:9,500 in Hispanics
- 1:11,200 in Native Americans
- 1:15,300 in African Americans
- 1:32,100 in Asians

RISK FACTORS

Genetics

CFTR gene

- Located on the long arm of chromosome 7
- Most common mutation results in deletion of phenylalanine at position 508 in the CFTR glycoprotein.
- The Δ508 mutation occurs in ~70% of CF patients.
- >1,500 mutations have been reported in the CFTR gene.
- Presence of gene modifiers may cause incomplete phenotypic presentations.

GENERAL PREVENTION

Prepregnancy carrier detection

PATHOPHYSIOLOGY

- CFTR
  - Membrane glycoprotein, which functions as a cyclic AMP–activated chloride channel at the apical surface of epithelial cells
  - An abnormality in CFTR results in defective chloride conductance.
  - May have other roles in the regulation of membrane channels and the pH of intracellular organelles; may affect cell apical sodium channel regulation
  - CFTR abnormalities may act as binding sites for *Pseudomonas aeruginosa*, promoting proinflammatory responses in the lung.
- In the respiratory system
  - Increased mucus viscosity
  - Early bacterial colonization despite a robust neutrophilic inflammatory response
  - Mucous plugging and atelectasis
  - Bronchiectasis and emphysema develop.
  - Abnormal nasal sinus development
- In the GI tract
  - Progressive pancreatic damage leads to exocrine pancreatic insufficiency.
  - Endocrine pancreatic dysfunction
  - Focal biliary cirrhosis of the liver
  - Hypoplasia of the gallbladder and impaired bile flow

DIAGNOSIS

HISTORY

- Most common presenting respiratory symptoms: chronic cough, recurrent pneumonia, nasal polyps, chronic pansinusitis
- Most common presenting GI symptoms:
  - Meconium ileus (15–20% of patients present with this symptom); pancreatic insufficiency occurs in 85% of patients. In infants, fat malabsorption may lead to chronic diarrhea and failure to thrive.
  - In older patients, pancreatitis, rectal prolapse (occurs in 2% of the patients; must consider CF until proven otherwise)
  - Distal obstruction of the small intestine (meconium ileus equivalent, seen in older children and adults)
- Evidence of heat intolerance: In summer, increased sweating may lead to dehydration with hyponatremia or hypochloremic metabolic alkalosis.

PHYSICAL EXAM

- Respiratory findings:
  - Frequent cough, often productive of mucopurulent sputum
  - Rhonchi, crackles, wheezing, hyperresonance to percussion
  - Nasal polyposis
- Other common findings:
  - Digital clubbing
  - Hepatosplenomegaly in patients with cirrhosis
  - Growth retardation
  - Delayed puberty
  - Osteoporosis

DIAGNOSTIC TESTS & INTERPRETATION

Lab

- Sweat test: keystone for the diagnosis of CF
  - Sweat chloride >60 mEq/L is abnormal.
    - <40 mmol/L: negative
    - 40–60 mmol/L: borderline
    - >60 mmol/L: consistent with CF
  - In infants up to 6 months of age
    - 30–60 mmol/L: borderline
    - 60 mmol/L: consistent with CF
- Diagnostic criteria include the following:
  - One or more phenotypic features of CF *or* a sibling with CF *or* a positive newborn screening test

    PLUS
  - 2 positive sweat tests *or* 2 CF mutations on genetic screening *or* nasal potential difference (NPD) consistent with CF
- Other causes of elevated sweat chloride:
  - Malnutrition
  - Adrenal insufficiency
  - Nephrogenic diabetes insipidus
  - Ectodermal dysplasia
  - Fucosidosis
  - Hypogammaglobulinemia
  - False negatives seen in CF patients with edema
- Mutation analysis: can detect >90% of CF patients. Failure to identify 2 mutations reduces but does not eliminate CF diagnosis.
- Immunoreactive trypsinogen test (IRT) is used for newborn screening. Blood drawn 2–3 days after birth is analyzed for trypsinogen.
  - Positive IRT tests must be confirmed by sweat test and/or genetic testing.
  - IRT testing may be normal in the presence of meconium ileus
- Frequently recovered organisms in sputum cultures:
  - *Haemophilus influenzae*
  - *Staphylococcus aureus*
  - Methicillin-resistant *Staphylococcus aureus* (MRSA)
  - *P. aeruginosa* (nonmucoid and mucoid)
  - *Burkholderia cepacia*
  - *Stenotrophomonas maltophilia*
  - *Aspergillus* and other fungal species
  - Nontuberculous mycobacterial species
- Pulmonary function test: usually reveals obstructive lung disease, although some patients may have a restrictive pattern
- Analysis of stimulated pancreatic secretions: degree of pancreatic exocrine deficiency
- Fecal elastase measurements can detect pancreatic insufficiency.
- 72-hour fecal fat measurement: fat malabsorption

Imaging

- Chest radiography
  - Typical features include hyperinflation, peribronchial thickening, atelectasis, and bronchiectasis.
- CT scan
  - Bronchiectasis
  - Cystic and interstitial changes
  - Focal consolidation or scarring

DIFFERENTIAL DIAGNOSIS

- Pulmonary
  - Recurrent pneumonia or bronchitis
  - Asthma
  - Aspiration pneumonia
  - Ciliary dyskinesia
  - Airway anomalies
  - Chronic sinusitis
  - Chronic aspiration
  - Non-CF bronchiectasis
  - Allergic bronchopulmonary aspergillosis
  - α_1-Antitrypsin disease
- GI
  - Celiac disease
  - Protein-losing enteropathy
  - GERD
  - Chronic pancreatitis
- Other:
  - Metabolic alkalosis
  - Immune deficiency
  - Shwachman-Diamond syndrome

C

TREATMENT

MEDICATION

First Line

- Antibiotic therapy based on sputum culture results and clinical improvement:
  - Oral antibiotics:
    - Cephalexin
    - Linezolid
    - Trimethoprim-sulfamethoxazole
    - Ciprofloxacin, inhaled tobramycin, colistin, or aztreonam in selected patients
  - IV antibiotics:
    - To treat *S. aureus*, consider oxacillin, ticarcillin with clavulanic acid, linezolid, or vancomycin.
    - To treat *P. aeruginosa* and *B. cepacia*, consider aminoglycoside plus ticarcillin, ceftazidime, or piperacillin.
  - Severe cases with resistant strains may benefit from aztreonam, imipenem, or meropenem.
  - Two or more antibiotics may be used during treatment of pulmonary exacerbations.
  - The use of regular azithromycin is controversial due to emerging mycobacterial resistance.
  - Indwelling catheters may be needed for frequent antibiotic therapy
- Clearance of pulmonary secretions
  - Chest physical therapy or with high-frequency oscillatory vest device. Adjunct therapy such as flutter valve, Acapella, or PEP mask may also be used.
  - Bronchodilator: aerosol or metered-dose inhaler (β_2-agonist)
  - Mucolytics: RhDNase
  - Anti-inflammatory: short-term oral steroid course. Inhaled corticosteroids may benefit patients with asthma and/or those demonstrating an oral steroid response.
  - Hypertonic saline
- GI disease
  - Pancreatic enzyme replacement therapy: used in CF patients who are pancreatic insufficient; dosage adjusted for frequency and character of the stools and for growth pattern; generic substitutes are not bioequivalent to name brands. The maximum recommended dose is 2,500 U of lipase/kg per meal and 10,000 U of lipase/kg/24 h.
  - Vitamin supplements: multivitamin, fat-soluble vitamins A, D, E, and K
  - Salt supplementation
  - Patients with cholestasis may benefit from therapy with ursodeoxycholic acid.

Other Medications

- CFTR potentiators
  - G551D mutations treated with ivacaftor will improve lung function, decrease exacerbations, and, in some cases, normalize sweat test.
  - Ongoing research is underway to determine if other CF genotypes may benefit from this targeted therapy or other therapies.

ONGOING CARE

FOLLOW-UP RECOMMENDATIONS

Patient Monitoring

- Specialized care should be at a CF center.
- Frequency of visits depends on age and severity of illness:
  - Infants should be seen at least monthly for the first 12 months, then every 2–3 months.

DIET

- High-calorie diet with added salt
- Lifelong nutritional support usually required
- Gastrostomy tube placement may be necessary to increase caloric intake and maintain growth.

Respiratory

- Throat and sputum cultures for fungi, acid-fast bacteria, and aerobic organisms are used to direct antimicrobial therapy.
- Duration of antibiotic therapy is controversial; more frequent use is required as pulmonary function deteriorates.

PROGNOSIS

- Current median survival is ~38 years.
- Variable course of the disease
- The median survival has been increasing for the past 4 decades, although the rate of increase in age has slowed in the past decade.

COMPLICATIONS

- Respiratory complications:
  - Recurrent bronchitis and pneumonia
  - Atelectasis
  - Bronchiectasis
  - Pneumothorax
  - Hemoptysis
  - Chronic sinusitis and nasal polyps
- CV complications:
  - Pulmonary hypertension in older patients
- GI complications:
  - Pancreatic insufficiency in 85–90% of CF patients
  - Patients usually have steatorrhea and poor growth and nutritional status.
  - Decreased levels of vitamins A, E, D, and K
  - Rectal prolapse
  - 10–15% of patients have meconium ileus.
  - Distal intestinal obstruction syndrome
  - Clinically significant focal biliary cirrhosis; hepatobiliary disease in 5% of CF patients
  - Esophageal varices
  - Splenomegaly
  - Hypersplenism
  - Cholestasis
- Reproductive complications:
  - Sterility in 98% of males due to absence or atresia of the vas deferens
  - Slight decrease in fertility for females secondary to abnormalities of cervical mucus
- Endocrine complications:
  - Glucose intolerance
  - CF-related diabetes occurs with increasing frequency in adolescent and adult patients.
- Skeletal complications:
  - Osteoporosis

ADDITIONAL READING

- Baumer JH. Evidence based guidelines for the performance of the sweat test for the investigation of cystic fibrosis in the UK. *Arch Dis Child*. 2003;88(12):1126–1127.
- Farrell MH, Farrell PM. Newborn screening for cystic fibrosis: ensuring more good than harm. *J Pediatr*. 2003;143(6):707–712.
- Flume PA, O'Sullivan BP, Robinson KA, et al. Cystic fibrosis pulmonary guidelines: chronic medications for maintenance of lung health. *Am J Respir Crit Care Med*. 2007;176(10):957–969.
- Hammond KB, Abman SH, Sokol RJ, et al. Efficacy of statewide neonatal screening for cystic fibrosis by assay of trypsinogen concentrations. *N Engl J Med*. 1991;325(11):769–774.
- Pier GB. CFTR mutations and host susceptibility to *Pseudomonas aeruginosa* lung infection. *Curr Opin Microbiol*. 2002;5(1):81–86.
- Rowe SM, Verkman AS. Cystic fibrosis transmembrane regulator correctors and potentiators. *Cold Spring Harb Perspect Med*. 2013;3(7):a009761.
- Ryan G, Mukhopadhyay S, Singh M. Nebulised anti-pseudomonal antibiotics for cystic fibrosis. *Cochrane Database Syst Rev*. 2003;(3):CD001021.
- Smyth A, Walters S. Prophylactic antibiotics for cystic fibrosis. *Cochrane Database Syst Rev*. 2000;(2):CD001912.
- Southern KW, Barker PM. Azithromycin for cystic fibrosis. *Eur Respir J*. 2004;24(5):834–838.
- Stallings VA, Stark LJ, Robinson KA, et al. Evidence-based practice recommendations for nutrition-related management of children and adults with cystic fibrosis and pancreatic insufficiency: results of a systematic review. *J Am Diet Assoc*. 2008;108(5):832–839.
- Yankaskas JR, Marshall BC, Sufian B, et al. Cystic fibrosis adult care: consensus conference report. *Chest*. 2004;125(1)(Suppl):1S–39S.

CODES

ICD10

- E84.9 Cystic fibrosis, unspecified
- E84.0 Cystic fibrosis with pulmonary manifestations
- E84.11 Meconium ileus in cystic fibrosis

FAQ

- Q: Should relatives be tested?
- A: All siblings should have a sweat test.
- Q: How well will a child with CF do?
- A: The course of the illness is variable. It is difficult to predict the course of disease in an individual.
- Q: How should a borderline sweat test be interpreted?
- A: Borderline sweat tests should always be correlated with other findings such as physical exam, sputum cultures, pulmonary function, radiographic findings, nutritional evaluation, and/or mutation analysis.

CYTOMEGALOVIRUS INFECTION

Swathi Gowtham • Ravit Arav-Boger

BASICS

DESCRIPTION
Cytomegalovirus (CMV) is a ubiquitous double-stranded DNA virus that is a member of the herpesvirus family. It establishes latency in peripheral blood mononuclear cells and endothelial cells.

EPIDEMIOLOGY
- Primary infection occurs from early childhood into adolescence and childbearing years.
- Transmission occurs by contact with infected body fluids such as saliva, urine, blood, or breast milk through sexual contact or solid organ transplantation. Intrauterine transmission is the most common route of acquiring congenital infection.

Prevalence
Seroprevalence increases with age and varies with socioeconomic status; 50% of middle- and 80% of lower socioeconomic status adults are seropositive.

GENERAL PREVENTION
- Pregnant women should receive education about CMV transmission. Precautions should be instituted for hospitalized patients known to be shedding CMV.
- Seriously ill neonates should receive blood products from CMV-negative donors.
- CMV-seronegative solid organ transplantation recipients should receive organs (and all blood products) from CMV-negative donors whenever possible.
- Hyperimmunoglobulin has been used in high-risk CMV-negative recipients of CMV-positive donors to prevent severe CMV disease.

PATHOPHYSIOLOGY
Infection leads to intranuclear inclusions with massive enlargement of cells. Almost any organ may become infected with CMV in severe disseminated infection.

COMMONLY ASSOCIATED CONDITIONS
- Congenital infection
  - Occurs in about 1% of newborns in United States
  - Intrauterine transmission is more common in pregnant women mothers with primary infection during pregnancy (40–50%) compared to recurrent infection (<1%). Postnatal acquisition of CMV via breast milk: controversy exists over whether this precludes breastfeeding in premature infants (has a lower risk for neurological sequelae than congenital infection).
  - 10% of infected infants are symptomatic at birth, with severe disease characterized by growth retardation, hepatosplenomegaly, thrombocytopenia, and CNS involvement.
  - 10–20% of infants who are asymptomatically infected at birth may develop hearing loss.
  - Of symptomatically infected infants, 90% will have some neurologic sequelae. Degree of impairments may be predicted by CT findings and microcephaly at birth.
- Mononucleosis syndrome
  - CMV can cause a mononucleosis-like syndrome similar to that caused by Epstein-Barr virus (EBV) infection in immunocompetent patients.
  - The most common symptoms are malaise (67%) and fever (50%). ~70% of patients have abnormal liver enzymes.
  - Pharyngitis and splenomegaly less common and severe than observed with EBV-induced mononucleosis.
- Interstitial pneumonitis
  - Seen primarily in severely immunosuppressed children and adults
  - Begins with fever and nonproductive cough but may progress to dyspnea and severe hypoxia over 1–2 weeks
  - Mild, self-limited pneumonitis may occur in immunocompetent patients.
- Retinitis
  - Observed in infants with symptomatic congenital infection and in patients with advanced AIDS
  - Immunosuppressed children should have regular eye exams.
- Hepatitis
  - Occurs in healthy individuals with primary infections and in immunosuppressed patients with either primary or reactivated disease
  - Fever, mild elevation of liver enzymes, and hepatomegaly are typical. Jaundice and severe hepatitis are uncommon.
- GI disease
  - Severely immunosuppressed patients may experience esophagitis, gastritis, colitis, or pancreatitis.
  - Diagnosis requires endoscopy with biopsy.
- CNS disease
  - Commonly seen in infants with symptomatic congenital infection
  - Characterized by microcephaly, periventricular calcifications, seizures, developmental delay, and sensorineural hearing loss
  - Encephalitis or meningoencephalitis may occur in immunocompromised patients and very rarely reported in literature in immunocompetent hosts.
- Hearing loss
  - Congenital CMV is the most common infectious cause of deafness.
  - Onset of deafness often seen after 1st month of life and is progressive. May be missed by newborn hearing screen (if only done in first 2 weeks of life)

DIAGNOSIS

HISTORY
Exposures
- Day care attendance
  - Increased risk of infection
- Recent blood transfusion
  - Transfusion-associated CMV
- Use of immunosuppressive medications
  - Increased cause of serious infection

Symptoms
- Prolonged fever
  - Mononucleosis-like syndrome
- Blurred vision
  - CMV retinitis
- Cough, dyspnea, wheezing
  - CMV pneumonitis
- Vomiting, abdominal pain, diarrhea (watery or bloody)
  - CMV colitis

PHYSICAL EXAM
- Microcephaly
  - Congenital infection
- White, perivascular retinal infiltrates and hemorrhage
  - Retinitis
- Hearing loss (may require audiogram, brainstem evoked auditory responses)
  - Congenital infection
- Photophobia, headache, nuchal rigidity
  - Meningitis/encephalitis
- Tachypnea, rales
  - Pneumonitis
- Hepatomegaly and/or splenomegaly
  - Mononucleosis-like syndrome
- Rash
  - Petechiae, purpura, "blueberry muffin" lesions, rubelliform rash
- Adenopathy
  - Mononucleosis-like syndrome

DIAGNOSTIC TESTS & INTERPRETATION

Lab
- Shell-vial assay: (staining for immediate early antigen production) allows detection of virus 24–48 hours after inoculation
- Viral culture: Virus may be isolated from nasopharyngeal/oropharyngeal secretions, urine, stool, and WBC. Isolation may take up to 4 weeks. Urine or saliva samples are most common way to diagnose congenital disease.
- Highly sensitive CMV quantitative polymerase chain reaction (PCR) assay: Measure viral DNA in plasma, whole blood, urine, and CSF. Real-time PCR has replaced most diagnostic tests in monitoring response to therapy or identifying viral quantitation. Recently standardized to be reported as IU/mL.
- Quantitative antigenemia assay: detection of circulating CMV-infected polymorphonuclear cells by indirect immunofluorescence. In an immunocompromised patient, may monitor response to therapy or identify viral reactivation.
- Serology: Enzyme-linked immunosorbent assay or indirect fluorescent antibody assay to detect the presence of CMV IgM, or IgG has a limited role. IgG avidity test can be used in certain circumstances, particularly in pregnant women, to diagnose a recent infection.

ALERT

- Due to frequency of asymptomatic shedding, mere isolation of virus does not necessarily establish an etiologic association.
- Severely immunocompromised patients who are actively infected with CMV may be seronegative. 4-fold rise in CMV IgG is not diagnostic of primary infection. Increased antibody titers may occur with reactivation. DNA quantification by real-time PCR is useful in these circumstances to make a timely diagnosis.

Imaging

- Noncontrast head CT
  - Periventricular calcifications, cystic abnormalities, ventriculomegaly, periventricular leukomalacia
- Brain MRI
  - Has higher sensitivity than ultrasound for brain abnormalities and greater predictor of symptomatic infection

DIFFERENTIAL DIAGNOSIS

- Congenital infection
  - Congenital rubella syndrome
  - Toxoplasmosis
  - Syphilis
  - Neonatal herpes simplex virus
  - Human immunodeficiency virus
  - Enteroviral infection
- Mononucleosis syndrome
  - EBV infection
  - Toxoplasmosis
  - Hepatitis A or B infection
- Interstitial pneumonitis
  - Respiratory syncytial virus
  - Adenovirus
  - Measles
  - Varicella
  - *Pneumocystis jiroveci* (previously *carinii*)
  - *Chlamydia*
  - *Mycoplasma*
  - Fungal
  - Drug/toxin-induced pneumonitis
- Retinitis
  - Ocular toxoplasmosis
  - Candidal retinitis
  - Syphilis
  - Herpes simplex virus
- Hepatitis
  - EBV infection
  - Hepatitis A, B, or C infection
  - Enterovirus
  - Adenovirus
  - Herpes simplex virus
  - Drug/toxin-induced
- GI disease
  - Herpes simplex virus
  - Adenovirus
  - *Salmonella*
  - *Shigella*
  - *Campylobacter*
  - *Yersinia*
  - *Clostridium difficile*
  - *Giardia*
  - *Cryptosporidium*
- CNS disease
  - Congenital disease (see congenital infection earlier)
  - Meningoencephalitis in immunocompetent host: herpes simplex virus, EBV, varicella-zoster virus, enterovirus, arbovirus
- Meningoencephalitis in immunocompromised host: in addition to organisms listed previously, should include HIV encephalitis, fungal meningitis, toxoplasmosis

TREATMENT

Majority of transplant experts prefer prophylaxis over preemptive therapy in high-risk patients (donor CMV positive, recipient negative).

MEDICATION

First Line

- Ganciclovir: suppresses viral replication by inhibiting the viral DNA polymerase
  - Indications: symptomatic congenital CMV in a neonate meeting clinical criteria; CMV chorioretinitis in immunocompromised patients; tissue diagnosis (hepatitis, enteritis, pneumonitis) of CMV infection; and in immunocompromised patients with CMV disease (viremia + symptoms)
  - Side effects: neutropenia (60%), thrombocytopenia (~5%)
- Foscarnet: suppresses viral replication by inhibiting viral DNA polymerase
  - Indications: same as earlier, but in patients who have failed to improve on ganciclovir therapy or who has experienced significant bone marrow toxicity related to ganciclovir use or with resistance to ganciclovir
  - Side effects: renal impairment (12–33%), headache (26%), seizures (10%)

ONGOING CARE

PROGNOSIS

Varies with nature of infection (see "Commonly Associated Conditions")

COMPLICATIONS

Varies with nature of infection (see "Commonly Associated Conditions")

ADDITIONAL READING

- Alexander BT, Hladnik LM, Augustin KM, et al. Use of cytomegalovirus intravenous immune globulin for the adjunctive treatment of CMV in hematopoietic stem cell transplant patients. *Pharmacotherapy*. 2010;30(6):554–561.
- Boeckh M, Ljungman P. How we treat cytomegalovirus in hematopoetic cell transplant recipients. *Blood*. 2009;113(23):5711–5719.
- Cannon MJ, Schmid DS, Hyde TB. Review of cytomegalovirus seroprevalence and demographic characteristics associated with infection. *Rev Med Virol*. 2010;20(4):202–213.
- Dollard SC, Schleiss MR, Grosse SD. Public health and laboratory considerations regarding newborn screening for congenital cytomegalovirus. *J Inherit Metab Dis*. 2010;33(Suppl 2):S249–S254.
- Foulon I, Naessens A, Foulon W, et al. Hearing loss in children with congenital cytomegalovirus infection in relation to the maternal trimester in which the maternal primary infection occurred. *Pediatrics*. 2008;122(6):e1123–e1127.
- Grangeot-Keros L, Mayaux MJ, Lebon P, et al. Value of cytomegalovirus (CMV) IgG avidity index for the diagnosis of primary CMV infection in pregnant women. *J Infect Dis*. 1997;175(4):944–946.
- Istas AS, Demmler GJ, Dobbins JG, et al. Surveillance for congenital cytomegalovirus disease: a report from the National Congenital Cytomegalovirus Disease Registry. *Clin Infect Dis*. 1995;20(3):665–670.
- Kimberlin DW, Lin CY, Sanchez PJ, et al. Effect of ganciclovir therapy on hearing in symptomatic congenital cytomegalovirus disease involving the central nervous system: a randomized, controlled trial. *J Pediatr*. 2003;143(1):16–25.
- Noyola DE, Demmler GJ, Nelson CT, et al. Early predictors of neurodevelopmental outcome in symptomatic congenital cytomegalovirus infection. *J Pediatr*. 2001;138(3):325–331.
- Revello MG, Zavattoni M, Sarasini A, et al. Human cytomegalovirus in blood of immunocompetent persons during primary infection: prognostic implications for pregnancy. *J Infect Dis*. 1998;177(5):1170–1175.
- Wreghitt TG, Teare EL, Sule O, et al. Cytomegalovirus infection in immunocompetent patients. *Clin Infect Dis*. 2003;37(12):1603–1606.

CODES

ICD10

- B25.9 Cytomegaloviral disease, unspecified
- P35.1 Congenital cytomegalovirus infection
- B25.0 Cytomegaloviral pneumonitis

FAQ

- Q: Should children with congenital CMV infection be excluded from day care settings?
- A: No. Due to the high frequency of shedding of CMV in the urine and saliva of asymptomatic children, especially those younger than 2 years of age, exclusion from out-of-home care is not justified for any child known to be infected with CMV. Careful attention to hygienic practices, especially hand washing, is important.

DAYTIME INCONTINENCE

Amanda K. Berry • Michael C. Carr

BASICS

DESCRIPTION
- Daytime wetting in a child ≥5 years of age warrants evaluation.
- Causes of functional incontinence include an array of bladder storage and voiding disorders.
- Voiding dysfunction is abnormal behavior of the lower urinary tract without a recognized organic cause, generally in the form of pelvic floor hyperactivity or bladder–sphincter discoordination.
- Dysfunctional elimination syndrome describes the association between abnormal bladder and bowel behavior.

Prevalence
- Studies in children 6–7 years of age have shown that 3.1% of girls and 2.1% of boys had an episode of wetting at least once per week.
- Spontaneous cure rate of 14% per year without treatment
- Of all children who wet, 10% have only daytime wetting, 75% wet only at night, and 15% wet during the day and at night.

RISK FACTORS
- Constipation
- Recurrent urinary tract infections (UTIs)
- Diabetes mellitus/diabetes insipidus
- Attention-deficit disorder/attention-deficit/hyperactivity disorder (ADD/ADHD)
- Developmental delay

Genetics
- Only anecdotal relationships have been seen in functional daytime incontinence, unlike studies showing genetic tendencies in nocturnal enuresis.
- Increased rates of daytime wetting have been reported in urofacial (Ochoa) syndrome, an autosomal recessive condition, and Williams syndrome, which is the result of a deletion involving the elastin gene in chromosome 7.

ETIOLOGY
- Neurogenic bladder (e.g., myelomeningocele)
- Anatomic anomalies (e.g., ectopic ureter)
- Obstructive uropathy (e.g., posterior urethral valves)
- Bladder irritability caused by UTI
- Constipation
- Increased urinary output—polyuria
- Infrequent or deferred voiding
- Overactive bladder
- Low functional bladder capacity, with detrusor instability during filling
- Vaginal reflux
- Giggle incontinence
- Temperamental factors (e.g., short attention span, inattentiveness to body signals) in children who ignore the urge to void
- Developmental differences in age at which toilet training is achieved

COMMONLY ASSOCIATED CONDITIONS
- Constipation (common)
- Nocturnal enuresis (common)
- UTIs (common)
- Vesicoureteral reflux is more common in children with voiding dysfunction due to elevated detrusor pressures that overcome a marginal vesicoureteral junction.

DIAGNOSIS

SIGNS AND SYMPTOMS
- Urgency
  - Posturing, Vincent curtsy
- Frequent urination
- Deferred voiding
- Weak or intermittent stream
- Large, hard, or infrequently passed bowel movements
- Recurrent UTIs

HISTORY
- Onset (primary vs. secondary)
- Frequency of voiding
- Frequency and degree of wetting
- Presence or absence of any dry interval
- Signs of urgency, use of hold maneuvers, waiting until the last minute to void
- Description of stream (i.e., strong/weak, continuous/interrupted)
- Straining or pushing during voiding
- Frequency and description of bowel movements
- Presence or history of fecal soiling
- Quality and quantity of fluid intake
- History of UTIs, vesicoureteral reflux
- ADD/ADHD, learning disabilities, or developmental delays
- Level of concern on part of child/family
- Medications

PHYSICAL EXAM
- Abdomen: signs of constipation, distended bladder
- Rectal: if constipation is suspected
- Spine: sacral abnormalities
- Genitalia: labial adhesions, labial erythema, phimosis, urethral stenosis, evidence of leakage
- Neurologic: sensation, reflexes, and gait

DIAGNOSTIC TESTS & INTERPRETATION

Lab
- 1st morning urinalysis to check concentrating ability, rule out occult renal disease
- Urine culture to rule out infection

Imaging
- Renal and bladder ultrasound in children who wet with a history of UTIs and in children with persistent wetting despite regular voiding
- Kidneys, ureter, and bladder (KUB) x-ray to assess for constipation
- MRI of lumbosacral spine if sacral abnormality or refractory to treatment

Diagnostic Procedures/Other
- Uroflowmetry and assessment of postvoid residual urine
- Invasive urodynamic testing is not indicated in neurologically normal children unless refractory to treatment.

DIFFERENTIAL DIAGNOSIS
- UTI
- Constipation
- Developmental variations in toilet training
- Neurogenic bladder
- Spinal cord abnormality
- Giggle incontinence
- Stress incontinence
- Genitourinary tract abnormality (posterior urethral valve, ectopic ureter)

- Vaginal reflux
- Benign increased urinary frequency (pollakiuria)
- Sexual abuse

TREATMENT

GENERAL MEASURES

- Aggressive management of bowels so that child is passing at least 1 soft bowel movement daily (see "Constipation")
- Elimination schedule, with voids every 2–3 hours and time to defecate at least once a day. A reminder watch may be helpful.
- Voiding diary provides concrete data and focus for child.
- Positive reinforcement for regular voiding
- Avoid acidic/diuretic beverages (caffeine, carbonation, chocolate, citrus).
- Adequate hydration
- Local management of perineal irritation/vulvovaginitis to ensure comfort during voiding
- Girls with postvoid dribbling due to vaginal reflux should void with their legs wide apart, sitting backward on the toilet when possible, to minimize backflow of urine into the vagina. Wipe after standing up.

ALERT

- Failure to recognize and manage constipation before attempting to manage wetting
- Use of anticholinergic medications in children with benign frequency of childhood is generally ineffective.
- Increased risk of UTIs when child is placed on anticholinergic medication due to infrequent voiding/incomplete emptying

MEDICATION

- A trial of an anticholinergic may be indicated if the child wets despite conservative medical/behavioral management.
- Extended-release formulations are available.
- Common side effects include dry mouth, decreased diaphoresis with flushing, and constipation. Blurred vision and dizziness are less common.

First Line (≥5 years old)

- Oxybutynin (Ditropan/Ditropan XL): 5–15 mg/24 h
- Tolterodine (Detrol/Detrol LA): 2–4 mg/24 h (adult dose; pediatric dose not established)
- Solifenacin (Vesicare): 5–10 mg/24 h (adult dose; pediatric dose not established)

ADDITIONAL TREATMENT

Pelvic floor muscle retraining through biofeedback can help children learn to identify and relax the pelvic floor muscles to empty the bladder smoothly and completely.

ISSUES FOR REFERRAL

Referral to pediatric urologist

- When wetting is accompanied by recurrent UTIs
- When wetting is refractory to behavioral management, child may benefit from a noninvasive urodynamic evaluation to assess flow pattern, voiding mechanics, and ability to empty the bladder.

ONGOING CARE

PROGNOSIS

- Spontaneous cure rate of 14% per year without treatment
- 72% of patients sustained improvement 1 year after simple behavioral therapy.

COMPLICATIONS

- Local irritation and inflammation of the perineum
- Functional daytime incontinence is primarily a social problem that affects children's self-esteem and interactions with peers.

ADDITIONAL READING

- Deshpande AV, Craig JC, Smith GH, et al. Management of daytime urinary incontinence and lower urinary tract symptoms in children. *J Paediatr Child Health*. 2012;48(2):E44–E52.
- Herndon CDA, Joseph DB. Urinary incontinence. *Pediatr Clin North Am*. 2006;53(3):363–377.
- Loening-Baucke V. Urinary incontinence and urinary tract infection and their resolution with treatment of chronic constipation of childhood. *Pediatrics*. 1997;100(2, Pt 1):228–232.
- Thibodeau BA, Metcalfe P, Koop P, et al. Urinary incontinence and quality of life in children. *J Pediatr Urol*. 2013;9(1):78–83.
- Wiener JS, Scales MT, Hampton J, et al. Long-term efficacy of simple behavioral therapy for daytime wetting in children. *J Urol*. 2000;164(3, Pt 1): 786–790.

CODES

ICD10

- R32 Unspecified urinary incontinence
- N39.498 Other specified urinary incontinence

FAQ

- Q: What findings can distinguish functional incontinence from an ectopic ureter?
- A: An ectopic ureter in girls usually empties below the sphincter or elsewhere, such as in the vagina. Therefore, these girls wet all the time, with no dry period. They do not have symptoms such as urgency. Because in most cases the ureter draining the kidney is duplicated, an ultrasound may be obtained but is not always diagnostic. MR urography provides superior imaging of the urinary tract and is useful in diagnosing ectopic ureter.
- Q: What is a normal bladder capacity for a child?
- A: Normal bladder capacity (in ounces) can be estimated as the child's age plus 1 oz. A child's bladder capacity can be determined by measuring voided volumes for 2 consecutive days when the child is well hydrated. The largest voided volume (not including the first morning void) is considered the child's functional capacity.
- Q: How much water should a child drink each day to cycle the bladder well?
- Adequate water drinking is important to keep the urine more dilute and less irritating to the bladder and to help cycle the bladder. In addition to other fluids, children 5–7 years old should drink at least 20–28 oz of water/day, children 8–12 years old should drink 28–32 oz of water/day, and teens should drink 36–48 oz of water/day.

D

DEHYDRATION

Marc H. Gorelick

BASICS

DESCRIPTION

- Dehydration is a negative balance of body fluid, usually expressed as a percentage of body weight. Mild, moderate, and severe dehydration correspond to deficits of <5%, 5–10%, and >10%, respectively.
- Dehydration is classified into 3 types on the basis of serum sodium concentration: isotonic (Na 130–150 mmol/L), hypotonic (Na <130 mmol/L), and hypertonic (Na >150 mmol/L).

GENERAL PREVENTION

Many cases of frank dehydration may be prevented by early institution of adequate oral maintenance fluid therapy in children with gastroenteritis, with particular attention to replacement of ongoing stool losses and slow administration of fluids to children with vomiting. Use of appropriate solutions is essential to prevent electrolyte disturbance and worsening of diarrhea.

EPIDEMIOLOGY

- ~10% of children in the United States with acute gastroenteritis develop at least mild dehydration.
- Although it accounts for 10% of all nonsurgical hospital admissions for children younger than 5 years of age, up to 90% of cases can be managed on an outpatient basis.
- Incidence of moderate to severe dehydration has declined since the introduction of routine rotavirus immunization

PATHOPHYSIOLOGY

- Dehydration is caused by either excessive fluid losses or inadequate intake of fluids.
- Some conditions leading to dehydration include the following:
  - GI losses: vomiting, diarrhea (most common cause of dehydration in pediatric patients)
  - Renal losses: diabetes mellitus, diabetes insipidus, diuretic agents
  - Insensible losses: sweating, fever, tachypnea, increased ambient temperature, large burns
  - Poor oral intake: stomatitis, pharyngitis, anorexia, oral trauma, altered mental status
  - Note that infants and debilitated patients are at particular risk due to lack of ability to satisfy their thirst freely.

DIAGNOSIS

HISTORY

- Frequency and duration of emesis and/or diarrhea gives an estimate of risk of dehydration.
- If there were large quantities of water taken, be alert for hypotonic dehydration. If inadequate free water is used for hydration, patient may have hypertonic dehydration.
- Frequency and quantity of urination may be difficult to estimate in infants with diarrhea.
- Decreased urination indicates possibility of dehydration but is nonspecific.
- Fever increases insensible water loss.
- Exertion or heat exposure increases insensible water loss.

PHYSICAL EXAM

- Acute change in weight is the best indicator of fluid deficit. If the child's recent preillness weight is not available for comparison, a reasonable estimate of the degree of dehydration may be made from physical findings (see Appendix, Table 2).
- General appearance: lethargy, irritability, thirst
- Vital signs: tachycardia, orthostatic increase in heart rate or hypotension, hyperpnea
- Skin: Prolonged capillary refill at fingertip (<2 seconds is normal in warm environment), mottling, poor turgor
- Eyes: decreased or absent tears, sunken eyes
- Mucous membranes: dry or parched
- Anterior fontanelle: sunken

ALERT

Diagnostic pitfalls

- Physical signs generally appear when the deficit is as small as 2%.
- No single finding is pathognomonic of dehydration. A reasonable guideline is that the presence of 3 or more findings indicates at least mild dehydration. The number and severity of physical signs increase with the degree of dehydration.
- Urine output decreases early in the course of dehydration, and a history of decreased urination is a sensitive but nonspecific finding.
- Capillary refill time is a specific but insensitive indicator. It may be falsely prolonged by cool ambient temperature (<20°C [<68°F]). It is not affected by fever.
- Children with a deficit >15% will show signs of cardiovascular instability such as severe tachycardia and hypotension.
- Physical findings may be more significant for a given degree of dehydration in children with hyponatremia, leading to overestimation of the deficit. Conversely, the clinical picture is reported to be somewhat moderated in hypernatremia.

DIAGNOSTIC TESTS & INTERPRETATION

Lab

- Diagnosis of dehydration is best made on clinical grounds. The following laboratory tests are sometimes helpful adjuncts.
- Serum sodium
  - Classifies type of dehydration
  - Hyponatremia and hypernatremia are uncommon in dehydration due to gastroenteritis (<5% of cases).
  - Measure sodium levels in cases of clinically severe disease or if risk factors are present (e.g., infant <2 months of age, history of excessive free water intake, children with significant neurologic impairment limiting their ability to regulate their own intake).
- Rapid glucose test or serum glucose: to detect hypoglycemia due to prolonged fasting
- Urine specific gravity: This is elevated early in dehydration but may not become elevated at all in young infants or in children with sickle cell disease.
- Serum bicarbonate: This is frequently low with diarrheal illness, even in the absence of dehydration. Useful to detect significant acidosis when dehydration is clinically severe
- Blood urea nitrogen (BUN): may rise late in dehydration in children

TREATMENT

ADDITIONAL TREATMENT

General Measures

Oral rehydration therapy (ORT):

- Most children can be managed successfully with ORT, either at home or in a health care setting.
- Use rehydration solution containing 2.0–2.5% glucose and 75 mmol/L Na (e.g., WHO solution) or 45–50 mmol/L Na (e.g., Pedialyte [Ross Laboratories, Columbus, OH], Infalyte [Mead Johnson, Evansville, IN]).
- Replace entire deficit in 4–6 hours: For mild dehydration, 50 mL/kg; for moderate to severe dehydration, 80–100 mL/kg. Include ongoing losses, ~5 mL/kg for each diarrheal stool.
- Begin with slow administration, with strict limits when vomiting is present: 5 mL q1–2 min. For infants, use a syringe or spoon rather than a bottle. After 30–60 minutes, if the oral liquids have been tolerated, increase the volume and rate.
- Have the child's caregiver participate in giving the fluids and provide education with regard to fluid replacement and signs of dehydration.
- Monitor weight, intake and output, and clinical signs. Failure of ORT includes intractable vomiting, clinical deterioration, or lack of improvement after 4 hours.

IV Fluids

- IV fluids are required when ORT fails or is contraindicated, such as in severe dehydration or shock, poor gag or suck, depressed mental status, severe hypernatremia (Na >160 mmol/L), severe hyponatremia (Na <125 mmol/L), and suspected surgical abdomen.
- Administer IV bolus of normal saline or Ringer lactate, 20 mL/kg, over 10–30 minutes. Repeat as needed to restore cardiovascular stability. Avoid dextrose-containing solutions for boluses except to correct documented hypoglycemia.
- Calculate maintenance fluid requirements: 100 mL/kg/day for the first 10 kg, plus 50 mL/kg/day for the next 10 kg, plus 20 mL/kg/day over 20 kg.
- Calculate fluid deficit based on clinical estimate or known weight loss. For isotonic or hypotonic dehydration, give 1/3–1/2 normal saline with 5% dextrose at a rate adequate to provide maintenance and replace deficit over 24 hours. For hypertonic dehydration, replace deficit over 48 hours using 1/5–1/4 normal saline with 5% dextrose.
- Monitor weight, intake and output, and clinical signs. With hypernatremia, measure serum sodium q4–6h; do not exceed rate of fall of 1 mmol/L/h.
- For mild to moderate isonatremic dehydration, rapid replacement of deficit over 2–6 hours may be possible. Give normal saline at a rate to replace the estimated deficit at a rate of 25–50 mL/kg/h.

Alternative routes of fluid administration

- Enteral fluids may be given via nasogastric (NG) tube when oral fluids are refused.
- Recent studies suggest subcutaneous administration of fluids, facilitated by use of recombinant human hyaluronidase, may be an alternative to the IV route.

MEDICATION

First Line

Most children with dehydration do not require specific medication therapy. For children with significant vomiting, several studies indicate that ondansetron 0.15 mg/kg PO decreases vomiting and facilitates oral rehydration.

INPATIENT CONSIDERATIONS

Admission Criteria

- Failure of oral or IV rehydration within 4 hours
- Severe hypernatremia or hyponatremia
- Substantial ongoing losses indicating a high likelihood of recurrence of dehydration

Discharge Criteria

After initiating ORT, children who are tolerating oral fluids at an acceptable rate to replace their deficit over 4–6 hours may be discharged with a willing and reliable caregiver and complete the ORT at home.

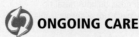

ONGOING CARE

PROGNOSIS

Excellent with appropriate rehydration therapy

COMPLICATIONS

- Severe dehydration may lead to hypovolemic shock and acute renal failure.
- Hyponatremia is associated with hypotonia, hypothermia, and seizures.
- Overly rapid correction of chronic (>36–48 hours) severe hypernatremia or hyponatremia can produce cerebral edema.

PATIENT MONITORING

- After rehydration, children with ongoing losses, as in gastroenteritis, should receive a maintenance solution in addition to regular feedings to maintain a positive fluid balance.
- Recommend 5–10 mL/kg for each diarrheal stool.
- Avoid clear liquids with excessive glucose, such as fruit juices, punches, and soft drinks, as these can promote osmotic fluid losses in the stool.
- In infants <6 months old, do not give large amounts of plain water, which can lead to hyponatremia.

ADDITIONAL READING

- Allen CH, Etzwiler LS, Miller MK, et al. Recombinant human hyaluronidase-enabled subcutaneous pediatric rehydration. *Pediatrics*. 2009;124(5):e858–e867.
- DeCamp LR, Byerley JS, Doshi N, et al. Use of antiemetic agents in acute gastroenteritis: a systematic review and meta-analysis. *Arch Pediatr Adolesc Med*. 2008;162(9):858–865.
- Hartling L, Bellemare S, Wiebe N, et al. Oral versus intravenous rehydration for treating dehydration due to gastroenteritis in children. *Cochrane Database Syst Rev*. 2009;(3):CD004390.
- Holliday MA, Ray PE, Friedman AL. Fluid therapy for children: facts, fashions and questions. *Arch Dis Child*. 2007;92(6):546–550.
- King CK, Glass R, Bresee JS; Centers for Disease Control and Prevention. Managing acute gastroenteritis among children: oral rehydration, maintenance, and nutritional therapy. *MMWR Recomm Rep*. 2003;52(RR-16):1–16.
- Steiner MJ, DeWalt DA, Byerley JS. Is this child dehydrated? *JAMA*. 2004;291(22):2746–2754.

CODES

ICD10

- E86.0 Dehydration
- E87.1 Hypo-osmolality and hyponatremia

D

22Q11.2 DELETION SYNDROME (DIGEORGE SYNDROME, VELOCARDIOFACIAL SYNDROME)

Anne S. Bassett • Donna M. McDonald-McGinn

BASICS

DESCRIPTION

22q11.2 deletion syndrome, formerly known as DiGeorge or velocardiofacial syndrome, is a multisystem disorder with variable severity and number of associated features classically including developmental delay, learning difficulties, congenital cardiac anomalies, palatal abnormalities, especially velopharyngeal insufficiency, hypocalcemia, and subtle facial dysmorphism.

- Rarely (≤1%), neonates have a severe T-cell immunodeficiency.
- Learning disabilities are usually borderline; rarely severe
- Treatable psychiatric illness is common.

EPIDEMIOLOGY

Prevalence is estimated at up to 1 in 2,000 live births.

RISK FACTORS

Genetics

- Associated hemizygous microdeletion of 22q11.2
- Up to 10% of newly diagnosed cases are inherited.
- 50% recurrence risk at each pregnancy for affected individuals

PATHOPHYSIOLOGY

A developmental defect of the 3rd and 4th pharyngeal arches may be part of the mechanism.

DIAGNOSIS

HISTORY

- The syndrome is underrecognized at all ages; thus, an index of suspicion is needed for any child with multisystem features.
- Neonatal and late-onset hypocalcemia may be present secondary to hypoparathyroidism in up to 60% of cases.
- Congenital anomalies of any organ system, classically cardiac defects, particularly interrupted aortic arch type B, septal defects, tetralogy of Fallot ± pulmonary atresia, truncus arteriosus, and vascular ring
- Failure to thrive/dysphagia/gastroesophageal reflux disease (GERD), occasional growth hormone deficiency
- Recurrent infections/autoimmune disease
- Developmental delays, especially speech
- Seizures
- Anxiety, OCD and attention-deficit disorder, schizophrenia

PHYSICAL EXAM

Subtle facial dysmorphism (e.g., malar flatness, hooded eyelids, auricular anomalies, small mouth, micrognathia; tubular nose, bulbous nasal tip with hypoplastic alae nasi), not as recognizable in non-Caucasians

- Cognitive/behavioral disorders
- Hypernasal speech
- Heart murmur
- Hypothyroidism; hyperthyroidism
- Renal/urogenital abnormalities
- Scoliosis; other skeletal abnormalities, for example, polydactyly and butterfly vertebrae
- Recurrent otitis media; hearing deficits
- Thrombocytopenia; splenomegaly
- Juvenile rheumatoid arthritis
- Enamel hypoplasia; chronic caries

DIAGNOSTIC TESTS & INTERPRETATION

Lab

- Genome-wide microarray, MLPA, or fluorescence in situ hybridization (FISH) using specific probe (may miss smaller deletions)
  - Most common microdeletion in humans
  - Parents also require testing for the deletion.
- CBC with differential
- Calcium and parathyroid hormone (PTH)
- TSH
- Newborns
  - Flow cytometry
- Age 9–12 months (before live vaccines)
  - Flow cytometry
  - Immunoglobulins
  - T-cell function

Imaging

- Echocardiogram
- Renal ultrasound
- Cervical spine radiographs
- Other, as indicated by history and signs

Other

- Audiology assessment
- Opthalmology assesment

TREATMENT

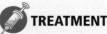

ADDITIONAL TREATMENT

General Measures

- Cardiac monitoring for aortic root dilation
- Vitamin D supplements (those with hypocalcemia will likely need 1,25-D supplementation and calcium supplements)
- Standard treatments are generally effective for each associated feature.
- Depending on the features, the child manifests, issues may need consultation and/or follow-up:
  - Neurology
  - Cardiology to define aortic arch anatomy (side and branching pattern)
  - Palate team, otolaryngology
  - Gastroenterology/feeding team
  - Endocrinology
  - Infant stimulation; educational consultant
  - Speech and cognitive intervention for speech and language delays
  - Child psychiatry
  - Dentistry
  - Immunology to monitor T-cell disorder, recurrent infections, allergy, autoimmune disease
  - Severe immunodeficiency may require matched sibling bone marrow transplant or thymic transplant.
- Special consideration with surgery/obstetrics/acute injury
  - Risk of hypocalcemia with biologic stress
- Special consideration for infants:
  - Initially withhold live vaccines.
  - Cytomegalovirus-negative irradiated blood products
  - Influenza vaccinations
  - Respiratory syncytial virus prophylaxis.
  - Avoid live viral vaccines in cases of severe T-cell dysfunction. These patients may need immunoglobulin replacement therapy to protect from infections.
  - Most patients with CD4+ cell counts >500 cells/mm^3 can be safely and effectively vaccinated with live viral vaccines.
  - Consider varicella immune globulin in a patient with either unknown humoral immunity status or definitive humoral abnormalities and a history of exposure. IV acyclovir may be necessary if varicella develops and patient has severe T-cell defect.

ONGOING CARE

FOLLOW-UP RECOMMENDATIONS

Patient Monitoring

- Cardiac monitoring for aortic root dilation
- Monitor growth and development.
- Monitor hearing.
- Monitor for emerging endocrine, psychiatric, autoimmune, skeletal, and other disorders.
- Genetic and reproductive counseling for adolescents and at transition to adult care

PROGNOSIS

- Most patients survive childhood. Exceptions include those with severe congenital cardiac anomalies or severe immunodeficiency.
- Associated conditions that arise through development and into adulthood include an increased risk for treatable psychiatric illness (e.g., about 1 in 4 develop schizophrenia), autoimmune phenomena, and neurologic sequelae.
- Functioning in adults is correlated most highly with the degree of intellectual deficit and to a lesser degree with severe psychiatric illness. Mortality in adults is elevated compared to unaffected siblings.

COMPLICATIONS

- In the newborn period, patients may present with hypocalcemic tetany/seizures, manifestation of cardiac abnormality, nasal regurgitation, GERD, dysphagia, and recurrent infections.
- Later on, patients present more commonly with speech, neurologic, developmental, and/or behavioral issues.
- Patients are at increased risk for developing multiple later onset conditions, including autoimmune disease, obesity, and psychiatric illness.

ADDITIONAL READING

- Al-Sukaiti N, Reid B, Lavi S, et al. Safety and efficacy of measles, mumps, and rubella vaccine in patients with DiGeorge syndrome. *J Allergy Clin Immunol*. 2010;126(4):868–869.
- Bassett AS, Chow EW, Husted J, et al. Premature death in adults with 22q11.2 deletion syndrome. *J Med Genet*. 2009;46(5):324–330.
- Bassett AS, McDonald-McGinn DM, Devriendt K, et al; International 22q11.2 Deletion Syndrome Consortium. Practical guidelines for managing patients with 22q11.2 deletion syndrome. *J Pediatr*. 2011;159(2):332.e1–339.e1.
- Butcher NJ, Chow EW, Costain G, et al. Functional outcomes of adults with 22q11.2 deletion syndrome. *Genet Med*. 2012;14(10):836–843.
- Carotti A, Digilio MC, Piacentini G, et al. Cardiac defects and results of cardiac surgery in 22q11.2 deletion syndrome. *Dev Disabil Res Rev*. 2008;14(1):35–42.
- Fung W, Butcher N, Costain G, et al. Practical guidelines for managing adults with 22q11.2 deletion syndrome [published online ahead of print January 8, 2015]. *Genet Med*.
- Habel A, McGinn MJ II, Zackai EH, et al. Syndrome-specific growth charts for 22q11.2 deletion syndrome in Caucasian children. *Am J Med Genet A*. 2012;158A(11):2665–2671.
- McDonald R, Dodgen A, Goyal S, et al. Impact of 22q11.2 deletion on the postoperative course of children after cardiac surgery. *Pediatr Cardiol*. 2013;34(2):341–347.
- McDonald-McGinn DM, Sullivan KE. Chromosome 22q11.2 deletion syndrome (DiGeorge syndrome/velocardiofacial syndrome). *Medicine*. 2011;90(1):1–18.
- McLean-Tooke A, Barge D, Spickett GP, et al. Immunologic defects in 22q11.2 deletion syndrome. *J Allergy Clin Immunol*. 2008;122(2):362–367.
- Repetto GM, Guzmán ML, Puga A, et al. Clinical features of chromosome 22q11.2 microdeletion syndrome in 208 Chilean patients. *Clin Genet*. 2009;76(5):465–470.
- Adult Guidelines Paper Practical guidelines for managing adults with 22q11.2 deletion syndrome. FungW, Butcher, Costain, Andrade, Boot E, Chow E, Chung B, Cytrynbaum, Faghfoury, Fishman L, García-Miñaúr, George S, Lang A, Repetto G, Shugar, Silversides, Swillen, van Amelsvoort, McDonald-McGinnD, Bassett. (2015). Genetics in Medicine.

D

CODES

ICD10

- Q93.81 Velo-cardio-facial syndrome
- D82.1 Di George's syndrome

FAQ

- Q: Can patients have severe intellectual impairments?
- A: Most patients with 22q11.2 deletion syndrome have IQs in the borderline range, about 30% fall in the mild intellectual deficit range; a minority are in the average range, and a small minority fall in the moderate to severe intellectual deficit range. Many children have a >10 point split between their verbal and performance IQ; and thus, the full-scale IQ may not reflect the true functional potential; cognitive remediation should be tailored to the individual's relative strengths and weaknesses.

DENTAL CARIES

Ray J. Jurado

BASICS

DESCRIPTION

Dental caries is the process of tooth structure demineralization, ultimately leading to cavitation (cavities). Bacterial metabolism of carbohydrates produces acid, leading to tooth demineralization over time. The presence of 1 or more decayed, missing, or filled primary tooth surfaces in children younger than 6 years old constitutes "early childhood caries" (ECC).

EPIDEMIOLOGY

- 28% of 2–5-year-olds suffer from ECC, which is most prevalent in disadvantaged populations, with those younger than 3 years old largely untreated.
- ECC may lead to increased emergency room visits and admissions, delayed growth and development, and diminished ability to learn.

RISK FACTORS

Dental caries is multifactorial:

- Factors increasing duration of sugar on teeth: frequent consumption of sugars (including prolonged bottlefeeding), sugary beverages, sticky sugars, medications sweetened with sucrose, inconsistent brushing/flossing after meals, pouching of food, tightly spaced teeth that are difficult to clean
- Factors leading to dry mouth (less saliva, less acid buffering): mouth breathing, albuterol inhalers, psychiatric medications
- Factors leading to weaker tooth enamel: lack of systemic or topical fluoride, developmental enamel defects
- Epidemiologic factors (e.g., low socioeconomic status, previous caries experience)

PATHOPHYSIOLOGY

Dental caries develops when oral bacteria, primarily mutans streptococci (MS), ferment carbohydrates into organic acids, over time demineralizing tooth enamel. Continuous demineralization of tooth enamel leads to enamel cavitation.

ALERT

MS has been shown to be vertically transmitted from caregiver to child, leading to the concept of ECC as an infectious disease.

DIAGNOSIS

HISTORY

- Reactive tooth pain to cold or hot foods, sweets, or biting. Spontaneous pain may be a sign of advanced caries and infection.
- Frequent carbohydrate challenge (bottle, juice, snacks, sweets, meds, etc.)
- Inconsistent brushing and flossing after meals

ALERT

Spontaneous or nocturnal pain (waking up at night) may be a sign of advanced caries and dental infection. See chapter on "Dental Infections."

PHYSICAL EXAM

- Tooth discoloration: chalky white (initial caries demineralization), yellow, or brown (advanced cavitation)
- Locations on teeth: in-between (interproximal) front incisors, biting surfaces (occlusal) of molars, at gum line (cervical)
- Soft tissue swelling (advanced caries with infection)
- Dental instrument exploration necessary to help confirm diagnosis
- To document and communicate the location of the lesion, a Universal Numbering System is used to identify the specific tooth/teeth involved (Appendix; Figure 2). Each tooth has a unique letter or number.
- Primary teeth are identified by uppercase letters (A–T).
- Permanent teeth are identified by numbers (1–32).

DIAGNOSTIC TESTS & INTERPRETATION

Lab

None

Imaging

Intraoral radiographs (bitewing and periapical views) help to identify radiolucent/carious tooth structure.

Other

Tooth percussion testing and hot and cold testing (inconsistent diagnostic potential) help to identify extent of caries and/or infection.

Diagnostic Procedures/Other

None

DIFFERENTIAL DIAGNOSIS

Developmental tooth hard tissue defects such as

- Hypoplastic or hypomineralized enamel
- Dental fluorosis

TREATMENT

MEDICATION

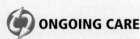

Acetaminophen or ibuprofen for symptomatic pain management. See antibiotic therapy in the chapter "Dental Infections."

ADDITIONAL TREATMENT

- Timely restorative care (fillings, crowns) by a pediatric dentist
- Supplemental topical fluoride (high concentration, prescription only, dentifrice, mouthwash, gel, varnish) with the goal of temporarily arresting caries
- Tooth extraction or root canal of infected teeth

ONGOING CARE

FOLLOW-UP RECOMMENDATIONS

- Dental caries essentially results from sugar in addition to time. Prevention of dental caries should focus on minimizing frequency of sugary beverages/snacks and brushing (with fluoridated toothpaste) and flossing after as many meals/medication administrations as possible.
- Children should have their first dental visit 6 months after the eruption of their first tooth, or around 1 year of age. This first visit is to assess for dental caries risk factors and give appropriate anticipatory guidance to the parent with the goal of preventing ECC.
- Dental caries can advance quickly, therefore periodic preventive visits (at least every 6 months) are recommended throughout childhood.

PROGNOSIS

- Timely caries risk assessment as well as restoration of tooth structure and function will minimize the child's caries experience and its consequences.
- Initial signs of caries (chalky white demineralization) may be remineralized with excellent oral hygiene and fluoride supplementation. Untreated advanced dental caries leads to irreversible pulpitis, dental infection, and tooth extraction.

ADDITIONAL READING

- American Academy of Pediatric Dentistry. 2014-15 Definitions, oral health policies, and clinical guidelines. http://www.aapd.org/policies/. Accessed March 16, 2015.
- Kawashita Y, Kitamura M, Saito T. Early childhood caries. *Int J Dent*. 2011;2011:725320.
- Meyer-Leuckel H, Paris S, Elkstrand KR. *Caries Management—Science and Clinical Practice*. New York, NY: Thieme Medical Publishers; 2013.
- U.S. Department of Health and Human Services, U.S. Public Health Service. Oral health in America: a report of the surgeon general (Executive Summary). http://www.nidcr.nih.gov/datastatistics/surgeongeneral/report/executivesummary.htm. Accessed March 16, 2015

CODES

ICD10

- K02.9 Dental caries, unspecified
- K04.0 Pulpitis
- K04.7 Periapical abscess without sinus

FAQ

- Q: When should I refer my patient for his/her first dental visit?
- A: Children should have their first dental visit 6 months after the eruption of their first tooth, or around 1 year of age. This first visit is to assess for dental caries risk factors and give appropriate anticipatory guidance to the parent, with the goal of preventing ECC.
- Q: Why do baby teeth need to be treated if they are just going to fall out?
- A: Dental pain can affect a child's daily activities, leading to delayed growth and development and diminished ability to learn. Premature primary tooth loss due to infection and extraction can lead to eruption and crowding issues in the permanent dentition.

D

DENTAL HEALTH AND PREVENTION

Johnny I. Kuttab

BASICS

DESCRIPTION

- Dental health and prevention is the practice of maintaining proper oral health to prevent the initiation or progression of oral disease. It is composed of effective oral hygiene, appropriate dietary practices, fluoride exposure, and the establishment of a dental home.
- Dental caries is a disease that generally is preventable. Early risk assessment allows for identification of parent–infant groups who are at risk for early childhood caries (ECC) and would benefit from early preventive intervention. The ultimate goal of early assessment is the timely delivery of educational information to populations at high risk for developing caries in order to prevent the need for later surgical intervention.

EPIDEMIOLOGY

- 42% of children 2–11 years old have had dental caries in their primary teeth.
- 23% of children 2–11 years old have untreated dental caries.
- Children 2–11 years old have an average of 1.6 decayed primary teeth and 3.6 decayed primary surfaces.
- 21% of children 6–11 years old have had dental caries in their permanent teeth.
- Tooth decay is five times more common than asthma and seven times more common than hay fever.
- More than 51 million school hours are lost due to dental-related illness each year.

RISK FACTORS

- Poor oral hygiene
- Poor dietary practices
  - Frequent nighttime bottlefeeding with milk or juice
  - Breastfeeding >7 times daily after 12 months of age
  - Ad libitum breastfeeding after introduction of other dietary carbohydrates
  - A diet high in natural or added sugars
  - Frequent sugar-containing snacking between meals
- Delayed establishment of dental home
- Previous caries
- Lack of exposure to fluoride
- Low socioeconomic status
- Immigrant status
- Poor salivary flow
- Special health care needs or chronic conditions

GENERAL PREVENTION

Establishment of a dental home no later than the child's 1st birthday allows the dental practitioner to educate and promote the use of caries-preventing strategies such as dietary recommendations and appropriate oral hygiene.

- The American Academy of Pediatrics (AAP) recommends children 1–6 years of age consume no more than 4–6 oz of fruit juice per day from a cup (i.e., not a bottle or covered cup) and as part of a meal or snack.
- Dietary guidelines include the following:
  - Eating a variety of nutrient-dense foods and beverages
  - Balancing foods eaten with physical activity to maintain a healthy body mass index
  - Maintaining a caloric intake adequate to support normal growth and development
  - Choosing a diet with plenty of vegetables, fruits, and whole grains and low in fat
  - Using sugars and salt (sodium) in moderation

ALERT

- 54% of U.S. preschool children were given some form of over-the-counter medications, most commonly as analgesics, antipyretics, and cough and cold medications. Numerous oral liquid medications contain a high sugar content to increase palatability and acceptance by children. Frequent ingestion of sugar-sweetened medications has demonstrated a higher incidence of caries in chronically ill children.
- To motivate children to consume vitamins, numerous companies have made "gummy" vitamin supplements. Cases of vitamin A toxicity have been reported as a result of excessive consumption. The AAP recommends that the optimal way to obtain adequate amounts of vitamins is to consume a healthy and well-balanced diet.

- Oral hygiene measures should be implemented no later than the time of eruption of the first primary tooth.
  - Brushing the infant's teeth after eruption with a toothbrush will help reduce bacterial concentrations. Brushing should be performed for children by a parent twice daily.
  - Flossing should be initiated when adjacent tooth surfaces touch. Parents and caregivers should help or watch over their kids' tooth brushing abilities until they're at least 8 years old.
- Optimal exposure to fluoride is an important preventive measure for children. The use of fluoride for the prevention and control of caries is documented to be both safe and effective.
  - When determining the risk–benefit of fluoride, the key issue is mild fluorosis versus preventing devastating dental disease. In children considered at moderate or high caries risk younger than the age of 2 years, a "smear" of fluoridated toothpaste should be used. In all children ages 2–5 years, a "pea-size" amount should be used.
  - Professionally applied topical fluoride, such as fluoride varnish, should be considered for children at risk for caries. Systemically administered fluoride should be considered for all children at caries risk who drink fluoride-deficient water (<0.6 ppm) after determining all other dietary sources of fluoride exposure.

ALERT

Dental caries is a common chronic infectious and transmissible disease resulting from primarily mutans streptococci (MS) that metabolize sugars to produce acid which, over time, demineralizes and cavitates tooth structure (enamel). MS colonization of an infant may occur from the time of birth by "vertical transmission" from mother to infant. The higher the levels of maternal salivary MS, the greater the risk of the infant being colonized, the greater risk for caries. Along with salivary levels of MS, mother's oral hygiene, periodontal disease, snack frequency, and socioeconomic status also are associated with infant colonization. The initial acquisition of MS occurs at the median age of 26 months during the "window of infectivity." Mothers are recommended to minimize or eliminate saliva-sharing habits such as sharing spoons.

PATHOPHYSIOLOGY

The oral cavity contains a diverse microbiota that is essential for maintaining normal physiology in the oral cavity. Oral bacteria metabolize sugar and produce lactic acid. Lactic acid is responsible for the demineralization of tooth structure and may lead to cavitation and the advancement of caries through the various dental structures. Furthermore, lactic acid alters the oral environment to a more acidic one and thus disrupts the balance of the oral microbiota, causing the appearance of more pathogenic organisms, thereby enhancing the process.

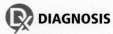

DIAGNOSIS

HISTORY

- Poor oral hygiene
- Poor dietary practices
  - Frequent nighttime bottlefeeding with milk or juice
  - Breastfeeding >7 times daily after 12 months of age
  - Ad libitum breastfeeding after introduction of other dietary carbohydrates
  - A diet high in natural or added sugars
  - Frequent sugar-containing snacking between meals
- Delayed establishment of dental home
- Previous caries
- Lack of exposure to fluoride
- Low socioeconomic status
- Immigrant status
- Poor salivary flow
- Special health care needs or chronic conditions
- Maternal caries
- Dental pain

PHYSICAL EXAM
- Visible plaque buildup
- "Chalky" teeth
- Cavitated teeth
- Gingivitis
  - Red, swollen gingival
  - Spontaneous bleeding
- Abscessed teeth
- Lymphadenopathy
- Pain

ALERT
- Caries risk assessment is a key element of preventive care. Its goal is to prevent disease by identifying and minimizing causative factors and optimizing protective factors.
- Causative factors include maternal caries, low socioeconomic status, frequent sugar snacking, nighttime bottle use, special health care needs.
- Protective factors include brushing twice daily with fluoride toothpaste, proper diet, and having a regular dental home. However, the best predictor of future caries is previous caries.

DIAGNOSTIC TESTS & INTERPRETATION
- Oral swabbing to assess MS bacterial load
- Plaque index
  - Use of disclosing tablets to highlight plaque and score teeth
- Caries risk assessment

Imaging
- Dental x-rays
  - As needed at discretion of the pediatric dentist

DIFFERENTIAL DIAGNOSIS
- Viral infections such as primary herpetic gingivostomatitis, hand-foot-and-mouth disease, herpangina
- Gingivitis
- Periodontal disease

TREATMENT

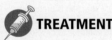

MEDICATION
Treatment of dental caries does not involve medication but rather the restoration of decayed teeth along with the establishment of a dental home. Proper oral hygiene and dietary measures need to be introduced to the patient and the parent.

ADDITIONAL THERAPIES
- Probiotics
  - Probiotics are living microbes that beneficially influence the health of the host when used in adequate numbers. Dental probiotics have been shown to act as antagonists toward pathogenic bacteria by a variety of different mechanism. Restoring the oral health to a more balanced one creates a more suitable environment for the prevention of dental caries and proper oral health.
- Increased fluoride exposure
  - When used appropriately, fluoride is both safe and effective in preventing and controlling dental caries.
  - Topically, low levels of fluoride in plaque and saliva inhibit the demineralization of sound enamel and enhance the remineralization of demineralized enamel.
- Sealant application
  - Sealants reduce the risk of pit and fissure caries in susceptible teeth and are cost-effective when maintained. They are indicated for primary and permanent teeth with pits and fissures that are predisposed to plaque retention. At-risk pits and fissures should be sealed as soon as possible.
- Xylitol chewing gum
  - Xylitol is a five-carbon sugar alcohol derived primarily from forest and agricultural materials. Xylitol reduces plaque formation and bacterial adherence (i.e., is antimicrobial), inhibits enamel demineralization (i.e., reduces acid production), and has a direct inhibitory effect on MS.

ONGOING CARE

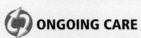

FOLLOW-UP RECOMMENDATIONS
The most common interval of examination is 6 months; however, some patients may require examination and preventive services at more or less frequent intervals based on historical, clinical, and radiographic findings.

PROGNOSIS
The practice of pediatric dentistry is based on prevention. If a dental home is established early, a pediatric dentist can guide the parent and the child on proper oral hygiene and diet, minimizing the risk for the development of caries.

ADDITIONAL READING

- American Academy of Pediatric Dentistry. 2014-15 Definitions, oral health policies, and clinical guidelines. http://www.aapd.org/policies/. Accessed September 2013.
- American Academy of Pediatric Dentistry. Symposium on the prevention of oral disease in children and adolescents. Chicago, Ill; November 11–12, 2005: Conference papers. *Pediatr Dent*. 2006;28(2): 96–198.
- Dye BA, Shenkin JD, Ogden CL, et al. The relationship between healthful eating practices and dental caries in children aged 2-5 years in the United States, 1988-1994. *J Am Dent Assoc*. 2004;135(1): 55–66.
- Dye BA, Shenkin JD, Ogden CL, et al. The relationship between healthful eating practices and dental caries in children aged 2-5 years in the United States, 1988-1994. *J Am Dent Assoc*. 2004;135(1):55–66.
- U.S. Department of Health and Human Services, Office of the Surgeon General. *A National Call to Action to Promote Oral Health*. Rockville, MD: U.S. Department of Health and Human Services, Public Health Service, National Institutes of Health, National Institute of Dental and Craniofacial Research; 2003.

CODES

ICD10
- K02.9 Dental caries, unspecified
- K05.10 Chronic gingivitis, plaque induced
- K05.6 Periodontal disease, unspecified

FAQ
- Q: It's just a baby tooth. Isn't it going to fall out?
- A: Untreated dental caries in children can lead to pain and infection and affect speech and communication, eating and dietary nutrition, sleeping, learning, playing, and quality of life, even into adulthood.
- Q: My child cannot spit yet and swallows the toothpaste. Can I use a fluoride-free "safe-to-swallow" toothpaste?
- A: Latest research has strongly and unequivocally supported the safety and efficacy of fluoride toothpaste in children. The benefit of fluoride far outweighs any potential risks of toxicity. However, use of fluoride should be based on individual risk factors. In children considered at moderate or high caries risk younger than the age of 2 years, a smear of fluoridated toothpaste should be used. In all children ages 2–5 years, a pea-size amount should be used.

DENTAL INFECTIONS

Johnny I. Kuttab

BASICS

DESCRIPTION

A dental infection is an acute or chronic inflammatory response of the dental pulp (pulpitis) tissue caused by the invasion of bacteria secondary to caries or trauma. Pulpal infection can lead to necrosis of the pulp tissue and cause an abscess (localized collection of pus) to form.

- Reversible pulpitis is a condition when pulpitis can be reversed such as the placement of a filling in a tooth.
- Irreversible pulpitis is a condition that cannot be reversed and rather leads to necrosis of the nerve and eventual abscess deposition.

EPIDEMIOLOGY

- Periapical abscesses account for 47% of all dental-related attendances at pediatric emergency rooms in the United States.

RISK FACTORS

- Poor diet (high in sugar)
- Poor hygiene (visible plaque on teeth)
- Dental caries
- Low socioeconomic status
- Lack of dental home due to access to care

PATHOPHYSIOLOGY

- Most dental infections are a result of the advancement of dental caries from the enamel, into the dentin, and finally, into the pulp tissue of the tooth.
  - Advancement occurs due to the production of acid by a group of bacteria that metabolize sugar from diet.
  - As more acid is created, the pH of the oral cavity is lowered, which further enhances the cycle.
  - Demineralization of the tooth layers occurs. As the caries process progresses, the bacteria then invade the pulp where an inflammatory response is initiated.
  - Necrosis of the pulp tissue occurs and forms an abscess at the apex of the root, resulting in bone destruction.
- Depending on host factors, infection may remain localized and drain through a sinus tract or may spread into the marrow, perforate the cortical plate, and invade surrounding tissues and facial planes.
- Typically, once full necrosis of the nerve has occurred, the pain subsides, and abscess formation is present.
  - This is particularly dangerous because the abscess can remain localized at the apex of the tooth or proceed between muscles, arteries, and veins into fascial spaces and cause significant and potentially life-threatening problems.
  - However, most are self-limiting and establish intraoral localized drainage.

DIAGNOSIS

HISTORY

- Nocturnal pain
  - Waking up due to pain
- Inability to eat due to pain
- Sensitivity to cold
- Fever
- Swelling
- Typically, symptoms of reversible pulpitis include sensitivity to hot/cold/sugary foods or sensitivity to air/brushing. Pain is acute in nature. When the stimulus is removed, the spontaneous pain subsides. When the tooth is restored, the pain disappears.
- Irreversible pulpitis symptoms include a dull achy pain that is constant, whether a stimulus is present or not. Most patients present to the dentist or the emergency room with irreversible pulpitis or abscess/infection.

PHYSICAL EXAM

- Lymphadenopathy
- Extraoral asymmetry due to swelling
- Intraoral swelling
  - Sublingual, submandibular, vestibular, palatal swelling adjacent to tooth
- Sinus tract or fistula adjacent tooth
- Limited oral opening
- Tenderness to palpation
- Low-grade fever
- Dehydration

DIAGNOSTIC TESTS & INTERPRETATION

Imaging

- Periapical or panoramic radiograph
  - Localized bone destruction or widened periodontal ligament (PDL) space
- CT scan in cases of serious extraoral swelling

Diagnostic Procedures/Other

Dentists perform pulp vitality tests to assess the health of the nerve, which can dictate treatment. Depending on the response of the nerve to cold, electricity, or percussion, a proper diagnosis can be reached.

- Percussion test (tapping on tooth elicits pain)
- Vitality test
  - Cold test
  - Electric pulp test (EPT)
- Mobility of tooth

DIFFERENTIAL DIAGNOSIS

- Reversible pulpitis
- Gingival abscess due to foreign body
- Ulceration (herpetic or aphthous)
- Eruption of permanent tooth

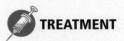

TREATMENT

MEDICATION

Antibiotic use should be considered when symptoms include nocturnal pain, fever, lymphadenopathy, and extraoral swelling.

First Line

- Amoxicillin 20–40 mg/kg/day in divided doses
- Augmentin 25–45 mg/kg/day in divided doses
- Tylenol 10–15 mg/kg/dose every 4–6 hours
- Ibuprofen 4–10 mg/kg/dose every 6–8 hours

Second Line

- Clindamycin 8–20 mg/kg/day in divided doses
- Azithromycin 5–12 mg/kg/day in one dose

ADDITIONAL THERAPIES

- Treatment of irreversible pulpitis or dental infection in primary teeth includes extraction of offending primary tooth or pulpectomy (primary tooth root canal). Extraction is preferred, as the goal is to create the most ideal environment for the permanent tooth to continue to develop. It is not uncommon for the permanent tooth to undergo damage in the presence of a long-term chronic infection.
- Treatment of irreversible pulpitis in permanent teeth includes root canal therapy (removal of the nerve and replacing the nerve with a synthetic filling material) followed by crown.

GENERAL MEASURES
- Space maintenance
  - Space maintenance is important to allow proper growth and development of the permanent teeth.
  - The primary tooth is the best space maintainer.
  - Without opposing or adjacent primary teeth, others may drift or tip into the space left by the extracted tooth, causing the development of malocclusions.
  - Spacers are used for space maintenance.

INPATIENT CONSIDERATIONS
Admission Criteria/Initial Stabilization
- Significant extra- or intraoral swelling due to abscess
- Unusual drowsiness, headache, or a stiff neck; weakness or fainting
- Difficulty swallowing or breathing
- Significant eyelid swelling (e.g., eye swollen shut)
- A rising fever, dehydration, and inability to eat
- Although rare, a dental infection or abscess may spread to fascial planes and cause facial cellulitis.
  - An infection in the buccal space can cause extraoral swelling in the infraorbital, zygomatic, and buccal regions. This most often involves maxillary molars.
  - An infection in the submental space can cause extraoral swelling secondary to infection the mandibular incisors.
  - An infection in the submandibular space can cause extraoral swelling unilaterally in the submandibular region secondary to infection in the mandibular molars.
  - The spread of dental infection through the fascial planes can end at the parapharyngeal or retropharyngeal spaces.
- Dental infections can also spread via lymphatics, veins, and arteries. The cavernous sinus is involved in most fatal spread of dental infection due to the lack of retrograde valves in the veins leading into the sinus. The result may be a cavernous sinus thrombosis.

ALERT

An infection in the submental, sublingual, and bilateral submandibular spaces is referred to as Ludwig angina. Infection may spread down the anterior cervical triangle to the clavicles. Speaking, swallowing, and breathing are severely compromised. This is a medical emergency and requires establishment of a safe airway (intubation).

ONGOING CARE

FOLLOW-UP RECOMMENDATIONS
- Referral to pediatric dentist for treatment
  - Extraction, root canal therapy, restorative treatment
- Thorough dental workup for other caries
- Resolution of abscess/swelling
- Management of space issues caused by extraction
- Establish proper dental home with proper dietary and hygiene intervention and guidance.

PROGNOSIS
The prognosis for a dental infection or abscess is good with proper medical and dental treatment.

ADDITIONAL READING

- American Academy of Pediatric Dentistry. 2014-15 Definitions, oral health policies, and clinical guidelines. http://www.aapd.org/policies/. Accessed September 2013.
- American Academy of Pediatrics, American Society for Microbiology. *Your Child and Antibiotics: Unnecessary Antibiotics Can Be Harmful*. Atlanta, GA: Centers for Disease Control and Prevention; 1997.
- American Association of Oral and Maxillofacial Surgeons. Parameters of care: clinical practice guidelines for oral and maxillofacial surgery (AAOMS ParCare 07 Ver 4.0). *J Oral Maxillofac Surg*. 2007;32(Suppl):238–245.
- Centers for Disease Control and Prevention, Food and Drug Administration, National Institutes of Health. A public health action plan to combat antimicrobial resistance. 1999. http://www.cdc.gov/drugresistance/actionplan/aractionplan.pdf. Accessed September 2013.
- Dodson T, Perrott D, Kaban L. Pediatric maxillofacial infections: a retrospective study of 113 patients. *J Oral Maxillofac Surg*. 1989;47(4):327–330.
- Graham DB, Webb MD, Seale NS. Pediatric emergency room visits for nontraumatic dental disease. *Pediatr Dent*. 2000;22(2):134–140.
- Kaban L, Troulis M. Infections of the maxillofacial region. In: Kaban L, Troulis M, eds. *Pediatric Oral and Maxillofacial Surgery*. Philadelphia, PA: Saunders; 2004:171–186.
- Seow W. Diagnosis and management of unusual dental abscesses in children. *Aust Dent J*. 2003;43(3):156–168.

CODES

ICD10
- K04.0 Pulpitis
- K04.1 Necrosis of pulp
- K04.7 Periapical abscess without sinus

FAQ
- Q: It's just a baby tooth. Isn't it going to fall out?
- A: Dental pain can affect a child's daily activities, leading to delayed growth and development and diminished ability to learn. Delayed treatment for a dental infection may cause damage to the permanent teeth or may proceed to a facial cellulitis. Premature primary tooth loss due to infection and extraction can lead to eruption and crowding issues in the permanent dentition.
- Q: I had horrible teeth growing up. Is this genetic?
- A: Genetic variation of the host factors may contribute to increased risks for dental caries; however, research suggests that other risk factors contribute greater such as diet and hygiene.
- Q: I see a pimple on my child's gums, but he does not complain of pain and is sleeping fine. Does this require treatment?
- A: All dental infections involving primary or permanent teeth require some form of treatment. If the body's host factors have localized the infection, drainage may occur with the absence of pain; however, the source of the infection remains. This may lead to damage to succedaneous (permanent) teeth or spread of the infection into a cellulitis.
- Q: I started the course of antibiotics and my child is feeling better. Is it necessary to complete the antibiotic?
- A: It is necessary to complete the entire course of the antibiotic unless an allergic reaction is occurring. Resolution of pain or swelling does not ensure the infection has fully responded to the antibiotic. Follow-up studies suggest that antibiotic use should continue at least 5 days beyond the point of improvement of symptoms.

DENTAL TRAUMA

Ray J. Jurado

BASICS

DESCRIPTION

Dental trauma is defined as fractured, displaced, or lost primary or permanent teeth.

EPIDEMIOLOGY

- 30% of children suffer from traumatic dental injuries to the primary dentition, with the highest incidence at 2–3 years of age.
- 22% of children suffer from traumatic dental injuries to the permanent dentition occurring secondary to falls, traffic accidents or bicycles, violence, sports, and physical abuse.
- 70% of cases involve maxillary incisors, with displacement injuries being the most common.

RISK FACTORS

- Sex: In the primary dentition, the prevalence of injuries ranges from 31 to 40% in boys and from 16 to 30% in girls. In the permanent dentition, the prevalence of dental trauma in boys ranges from 12 to 33% as opposed to 4–19% in girls.
- Age: The most common age for trauma in the primary dentition is from 1.5 to 2.5 years of age when the child is learning to walk. In the permanent dentition, the peak age ranges from 8 to 10 years of age.
- Season: Injuries occur more in summer months than in winter, depending on the population and demographics being studied.
- Occlusion: Increased "overjet" (protrusion of upper incisors) and insufficient lip closure are predisposing factors to traumatic injuries.

PATHOPHYSIOLOGY

- Basic tooth structures: enamel (white outer layer), dentin (yellow inner layer), pulp (nerves, blood vessels, connective tissue), cementum (layer covering roots), periodontal ligament (PDL; supports tooth in socket)
- Types of injuries (Figure 3)
  – Infraction: fracture of the enamel without loss of tooth structure. A "crack" in the enamel
  – Uncomplicated crown fracture: fracture with loss of tooth substance confined to enamel or dentin and not involving the pulp
  – Complicated crown fracture: fracture involving enamel and dentin with a pulp exposure
  – Crown/root fracture: fracture involving enamel, dentin, and cementum
  – Root fracture: dentin and cementum fracture involving the pulp
  – Concussion: injury to tooth-supporting structures, no abnormal loosening or displacement
  – Subluxation: injury to tooth-supporting structures with abnormal loosening, no displacement
  – Lateral luxation: lateral displacement of the tooth in its socket with fracture of alveolar bone plate
  – Intrusion: tooth forced into the socket and locked into position in the bone
  – Extrusion: tooth displacement partially out of the socket
  – Avulsion: complete displacement totally out of the socket
  – Alveolar process fracture: fracture of alveolar bone containing tooth

DIAGNOSIS

HISTORY

- Medical history: allergies, bleeding disorders
- Where did the injury occur: possible contamination, tetanus prophylaxis
- How did the injury occur: Mechanism of impact should be consistent with injury.
- When did the injury occur: affects treatment and prognosis (e.g., avulsions)
- Loss of consciousness: may indicate need to assess for other injuries
- Bite discrepancy: may indicate luxation injury or jaw fracture
- Sensitivity to cold or hot: may indicate crown fracture

ALERT

- Missing teeth should be located. If not, consider aspiration, swallowing, or even displacement to a sinus.
- The history of injury should correlate with the trauma to rule out physical abuse.

PHYSICAL EXAM

- Pediatric advanced life support if life-threatening emergency (ABCD, cervical assessment, etc.)
- Clean face and oral cavity with water or saline.
- Extraoral exam: Assess face and lips for soft tissue injuries and palpate mandible and maxilla for possible fractures.
- Intraoral exam: Assess for intraoral soft tissue injuries, tooth fractures, abnormal tooth position, and tooth mobility.

ALERT

To help determine whether the tooth is primary or permanent, classify the dentition according to age: primary dentition (younger than 6 years of age), mixed dentition (6–12 years of age), permanent dentition (12 years of age and older). Upper primary incisors begin to loosen and exfoliate around 6 years of age.

DIAGNOSTIC TESTS & INTERPRETATION

Lab

None

Imaging

- A soft tissue radiograph helps to identify foreign bodies. A dental film is placed in the vestibule between the lips and a radiograph is taken at 25% normal exposure time.
- Intraoral radiographs (periapical and occlusal views) help to identify root fractures and/or extent of displacements.
- Panoramic radiograph helps to identify jaw fractures.
- CT helps to identify tooth fractures in relation to surrounding bone as well as accurately determine alveolar fracture location and morphology.

Other

- Tooth percussion testing helps to identify severity of tooth concussions.
- Hot and cold testing assess tooth vitality.

Diagnostic Procedures/Other

None

DIFFERENTIAL DIAGNOSIS

Soft tissue lesions must correlate with history and mechanism of trauma to rule out physical abuse.

TREATMENT

MEDICATION

- Acetaminophen for pain management
- Consider antibiotic therapy for severe injuries in cases of infection risk (subacute bacterial endocarditis [SBE] risk, immunosuppression, etc.).

ADDITIONAL TREATMENT

General Measures

- Primary dentition
  - Infraction: no treatment necessary
  - Crown fracture: restoration of tooth structure (tooth colored filling); pulp therapy if indicated
  - Root fracture: extraction of crown and root
  - Luxation: soft diet × 1 week if minor; if severe or interfering with bite, extraction is recommended
  - Intrusion: allow to reerupt if not impinging on permanent tooth bud (determined by intraoral radiograph); extract if impinging
  - Extrusion: if minor: allow for spontaneous realignment; if severe: extraction
  - Avulsion: leave out, do not reimplant, to protect permanent tooth bud
  - Alveolar fracture: reposition alveolar segment and tooth-bonded splint
- Permanent dentition
  - Infraction: tooth sealant
  - Crown fracture: restoration of tooth structure (tooth colored filling); pulp therapy if indicated
  - Root fracture: reposition, tooth-bonded splint
  - Luxation: reposition, tooth-bonded splint
  - Intrusion: immediate repositioning or spontaneous reeruption
  - Extrusion: reposition, tooth-bonded splint
  - Alveolar fracture: reposition alveolar segment and tooth-bonded splint
- Permanent avulsion
  - Rinse tooth in cold water if dirty and reimplant into socket immediately and stabilize with finger. Refer to dentist immediately for assessment and splint stabilization.
  - If reimplantation is not possible, place tooth in physiologic media—milk, saline, or Hanks balanced storage medium (avoid touching root).
  - Refer to dentist *immediately* for reimplantation, tooth-bonded splint, and root canal therapy.
  - Treatment options and prognosis depend on stage of tooth development, time out of socket, and storage medium.
- Mandibular fracture
  - Immediate referral to an oral surgeon who will be able to determine management options

ALERT

- Every minute counts! Permanent tooth avulsions require immediate reimplantation. Prognosis worsens the longer the tooth is out of the socket.

ONGOING CARE

FOLLOW-UP RECOMMENDATIONS

- For most dental traumas, the child should be seen by a pediatric dentist as soon as possible for immediate assessment and treatment to optimize prognosis. Regular follow-up is necessary to reassess site of trauma.
- It is very difficult to prevent the majority of trauma. It is recommended that mouth/tongue piercings be avoided.
- Most sports injuries can be prevented with appropriate use of mouth guards. The American Academy for Sports Dentistry lists 40 sports for which it recommends the use of mouth guards, including acrobatics, baseball, basketball, cycling, discus, shot put, horseback riding, gymnastics, handball, racquetball, squash, judo, karate, rollerblading, rugby, motor cross, parachuting, skiing, soccer, surfing, skateboarding, ice skating, trampoline, tennis, volleyball, wrestling, weight lifting, and water polo.
- The social impact of dental trauma can be emotional (e.g., school, pictures, social) and financial. The total costs for replacing a single knocked-out tooth can be more than 20 times the preventive cost of a professionally, custom-made mouth guard.

PROGNOSIS

- Prognosis depends on severity of trauma. Minor traumas have relatively good outcomes with timely treatment. Severe traumas highly depend on timely, skilled management and the child's healing abilities.
- In the case of any primary tooth trauma, informing parents about possible pulpal complications, appearance of a vestibular sinus tract, or color change of the crown associated with a sinus tract can help assure timely management.
- Primary tooth displacement may also result in complications involving the developing permanent tooth, including enamel hypoplasia, hypocalcification, crown/root dilacerations, or disruptions in eruption patterns or sequence.

ADDITIONAL READING

- American Academy of Pediatric Dentistry. Guideline of management of acute dental trauma. http://www.aapd.org/media/Policies_Guidelines/G_Trauma.pdf.
- The Dental Trauma Guide. http://www.dentaltraumaguide.org/. Accessed November 25, 2014.

CODES

ICD10

- S02.5XXA Fracture of tooth (traumatic), init for clos fx
- S02.5XXB Fracture of tooth (traumatic), init encntr for open fracture
- K08.119 Complete loss of teeth due to trauma, unspecified class

FAQ

- Q: Why not reposition or reimplant primary teeth?
- A: The treatment strategy in primary teeth trauma is dictated by the concern for the safety of the permanent tooth bud. If the displaced primary tooth has invaded the developing permanent tooth bud, extraction is indicated to minimize damage. Reimplantation may encroach on the permanent tooth bud as well.

DEPRESSION

John I. Takayama • Renée Marquardt

BASICS

DESCRIPTION

- General term that includes major depressive disorder (MDD), dysthymic disorder, depression associated with bipolar disorder, and adjustment disorder with depressed mood
- Syndrome of persistent sadness or irritability associated with a variety of symptoms, resulting in functional impairment in the following:
  - Interpersonal (family, friends) relationships
  - Health (somatic complaints, unhealthy habits)
  - Work or school (task completion, grades)
  - Safety (high-risk behaviors including suicide)

EPIDEMIOLOGY

- Point prevalence: 6–11% of adolescents (age 13–18 years), 3–4% in younger children
- Lifetime prevalence: up to 20% will have diagnosable depression by adolescence
- Ratio of females to males: 1:1 in school-aged children, 2–3:1 in adolescents
- Often chronic with high rate of recurrence
- Often unrecognized; up to 80% of affected adolescents do not receive appropriate care.

RISK FACTORS

- Family history of depression, bipolar disorder, suicidal behavior in 1st-degree relative
- Prior depressive episodes
- Personal history of anxiety disorders, ADHD, learning disabilities, and early losses
- Family dysfunction or caregiver–child conflict
- Negative style of interpreting events and coping with stress
- Substance abuse
- Trauma history (e.g., victim of abuse, bullying)
- Chronic illness (including obesity)

COMMONLY ASSOCIATED CONDITIONS

- 40–70% of children and adolescents with depression have comorbid psychiatric disorders:
  - Anxiety disorders
  - Somatization disorders
  - Disruptive behavioral disorders (e.g., ADHD, oppositional defiant and conduct disorders)
  - Eating disorders
  - Substance abuse
  - Physical or sexual abuse

DIAGNOSIS

SCREENING

- U.S. Preventive Services Task Force recommends routine screening of adolescents for depression in clinical settings that can ensure accurate diagnosis and appropriate management and follow-up; and universal surveillance for younger children.
- If screening identifies depression, diagnosis should be established through formal assessment, and risk for suicidal behavior assessed.
- Screening tools include Patient Health Questionnaire for Adolescents (PHQ-A; sensitivity 73%, specificity 94%), Beck Depression Inventory Primary Care (BDI-PC, sensitivity 91%, and specificity 91%), and Strengths and Difficulties Questionnaire (SDQ, sensitivity 33–63%) for identifying depression in adolescents.
- Additional tools: Kutcher Adolescent Depression Scale, Reynolds Adolescent Depression Screen, Mood and Feeling Questionnaire

HISTORY

- Obtain detailed history of child's mood and functioning at home, at school, and with parents, siblings, teachers, and peers.
- Determine onset and duration of depressive symptoms, associated stressors, and personal impact (distress or impairment).
- Diagnosis of MDD has not changed between *DSM-IV-TR* (*Diagnostic and Statistical Manual of Mental Disorders*) and the recently published *DSM-5*; requires at least 2 weeks of symptoms 1 or 2; and 4 or more of the remaining symptoms:
  1. Depressed or irritable mood: feeling down, sad, or blue most of the time or being "annoyed" or "bothered" by everything and everyone
  2. Diminished interest or pleasure in previously enjoyable activities (events, hobbies, interests)
  3. Change in appetite or weight
  4. Sleep disturbance: not feeling well rested, difficulty in waking up in the morning or in falling asleep at night, waking up in the middle of the night or too early in the morning, daytime napping or sleeping, and nighttime arousal
  5. Psychomotor retardation or agitation: talk or move more slowly than typical, exhibit less speech, and longer response latencies; difficulty sitting still, pacing, hand wringing, tantrums, yelling, shouting, and nonstop talking
  6. Fatigue or loss of energy: feeling chronically tired, exhausted, listless, and without energy or motivation (parents may interpret as laziness)
  7. Feelings of worthlessness or guilt leading to reluctance to do things, excessive self-criticism, difficulty identifying positive self-attributes, "I don't care" attitude, envy or preoccupation with success of others, marked self-reproach or guilt for events that are not their fault
  8. Impaired concentration or indecisiveness: problems with attention and concentration, slowed thinking and processing of information, indecisiveness and procrastination, helplessness or paralysis in taking action
  9. Running or recurrent thoughts of death or suicide or attempts suicide
- Diagnosis should also include assessment of distress and impairment of functioning.
- Patient should not have manic or hypomanic behavior, and symptoms should not be attributable to substance use or another medical condition.
- If symptoms do not fulfill criteria of MDD, consider dysthymic disorder or depressive disorder not otherwise specified (*DSM IV-TR*).
- Dysthymic disorder: symptoms less intense but more persistent; depressed or irritable for at least 1 year with two of the following: appetite disturbance, sleep disturbance, fatigue, low self-esteem, poor concentration, difficulty making decisions, or feelings of hopelessness
- Depressive disorder not otherwise specified: clinically significant depressive symptoms that do not meet criteria for MDD or dysthymic disorder
- In *DSM-5*, dysthymic disorder and chronic MDD are combined in a new category, persistent depressive disorder.
- Adjustment disorder with depressed mood is diagnosed when depressive symptoms occur only in the context of a specific stressor. Important to assess for the following symptoms:
  - Manic symptoms
    - Ask about episodes of elevated or irritated mood associated with increased energy and activity, decreased need for sleep, grandiose thinking, and impulsive behavior.
    - History of manic symptoms suggests bipolar disorder.
  - Premenstrual timing of symptoms
    - If depressed mood is primarily in the days prior to menses, diagnosis may be premenstrual dysphoric disorder.
  - Psychotic symptoms
    - Ask about auditory or visual hallucination, paranoid ideation, and odd beliefs, which suggest either a more serious depression, or a separate psychotic diagnosis.
    - If family reports patient as withdrawn and less motivated, with no clear evidence for sad or irritable mood, this may also suggest a psychotic disorder.

PHYSICAL EXAM

Weight loss or gain may be associated with depression. Somatic complaints (i.e., headaches, abdominal pain) are common in depression. Physical exam should focus on identifying medical conditions that cause depressive symptoms (hypothyroidism, neurologic conditions, and underlying chronic illness) and evaluating for signs of comorbid conditions such as eating disorders.

- Vital signs: weight loss or weight gain
- Goiter (hypothyrodism)
- Lymphadenopathy (chronic illness, infection)
- Sexual development (delayed puberty may be related to hypothyroidism, anorexia nervosa)
- Extremities: arthritis (rheumatologic disease)
- Neurologic exam (postconcussive symptoms)
- Skin: pale, cool, dry (hypothyroidism); evidence of self-injurious behavior (i.e., scars from repetitive wrist cutting)
- Mental status exam
  - Appearance, alertness, speech, behavior
  - Awareness of environment (orientation)
  - Assessment of mood and affect
  - Memory, judgment, reasoning
  - Motoric slowing indicates severe depression.
  - Abnormal thought content, such as current suicidal ideation or psychotic thoughts, should prompt immediate referral.

DIAGNOSTIC TESTS & INTERPRETATION

Lab

- Vitamin B_{12}, free T4, TSH, or other labs based on history and exam to identify contributing or associated medical condition
- Screening for substance abuse as indicated

DIFFERENTIAL DIAGNOSIS

- Medical
  - Mood disorder related to a medical condition
  - Endocrine: hypothyroidism, Addison disease
  - Neurologic: postconcussive syndrome
  - Metabolic: vitamin B_{12} deficiency
  - Autoimmune: systemic lupus erythematosus
  - Infectious: mononucleosis, HIV/AIDS
- Behavioral
  - Substance-induced mood disorder
- Psychiatric
  - Adjustment disorder with depressed mood
  - Bipolar disorder

TREATMENT

- Assessment of severity of depression
  - Determine severity by considering number of symptoms, thought content and process, risk for suicidal behavior, and impact on functioning.
  - Mild depression: 5 or 6 symptoms with mild impairment in functioning
  - Moderate depression: 6–8 symptoms with mild to moderate impairment in functioning
  - Severe depression: all 9 symptoms or 5 or more symptoms and reports specific suicide plan, clear intent, or recent attempt; psychotic symptoms; severe impairment in functioning (i.e., inability to leave home)
- Safety assessment and planning
  - Instruct family to remove lethal means and monitor risk factors for suicidal behavior.
  - Provide patient and family with emergency contacts if risks for suicidal behavior increase.
  - Establish clear follow-up plan.
- Initial management of mild depression
  - Supportive management including education of patient and family about depression and stress reduction, clinical and community support, and management of identified stressors
  - Schedule visits with primary care clinician weekly or biweekly for 6–8 weeks for monitoring.
  - If depression worsens or does not improve in 4–6 weeks, additional intervention is needed.
- Management of moderate or persistent (lasting more than 6–8 weeks) depression
  - Education, support, stress reduction
  - Psychosocial interventions (counseling, therapy), antidepressant medication, or combination of both
  - Among adolescents, psychosocial and medical interventions are equally effective, with slightly increased benefit with combination. Choice of intervention depends on resources, patient/family preference, and individual clinical factors (i.e., age, severity of depression, family history of treatment response).
  - Among adolescents, 1st-line antidepressant medication is selective serotonin reuptake inhibitors (SSRIs).
  - Among preadolescent children, little evidence for effectiveness of antidepressant medication with elevated risk of serious side effects; refer to child psychiatrist if antidepressants needed
  - Antidepressant use in adolescents and young adults are associated with a slight increase in risk of suicidal thoughts and behaviors. These medications, however, have a favorable risk benefit ratio and can be used safely with appropriate patient education and monitoring.
  - Omega-3 fatty acids (1,000 mg/day) may be effective in both children and adolescents.
  - If patient is referred for therapy, continue frequent monitoring until depression is resolved.
  - Several types of therapy can be used for depression. For adolescents, evidence for effectiveness of cognitive behavioral therapy (CBT) and interpersonal psychotherapy (IPT)
- Special diagnostic considerations
  - Premenstrual dysphoric disorder: SSRIs can be used as the 1st-line treatment.
  - Adjustment disorder: When depressed mood is only in context of a specific stressor, psychosocial interventions, rather than medications, are recommended.

ISSUES FOR REFERRAL

Patients with depression can be successfully managed by primary care clinicians. Referral to a mental health provider is recommended for the following:

- Risk for acute suicidal behavior: Refer to emergency services (child crisis).
- History of suicide attempts
- Presence of substance abuse
- Presence of manic or psychotic symptoms
- No improvement after 6–8 weeks of treatment
- Recurrent or chronic depression
- Severe functional impairment
- Psychiatric comorbidities
- Complicated psychosocial factors, such as dysfunctional family dynamics
- After initiating referral to a mental health provider, primary care clinician should continue to follow patient while he or she waits for an appointment and throughout treatment course.

ONGOING CARE

FOLLOW-UP RECOMMENDATIONS

- In the initial phase (6–9 months or longer), the primary care clinician must identify medical conditions associated with depression, provide support and resources, assess patient safety and review safety plan, and monitor response to psychosocial and medical treatments.
- In the continuation phase (6–12 months), patients continue psychosocial or pharmacologic treatments used to achieve remission in the acute phase for at least 6 months, 12 months if difficulties in achieving remission, history of recurrent depression, or presence of ongoing risk factors; patients are typically seen biweekly or monthly by mental health providers depending on clinical status, functioning, support systems, stressors, motivation for treatment, and comorbid psychiatric or medical disorders.
- When asymptomatic for 6–12 months, patients may be recommended for either maintenance phase or discontinuation of treatment.

PROGNOSIS

- Up to 30–40% of patients with MDD can be expected to recover by 6 months and 70–80% by 12 months; 5–10% have protracted episodes lasting longer than 2 years.
- Time to recovery is influenced by age at onset of illness, severity, presence of comorbid disorders, and parental history of depression.
- Shorter duration of symptoms at the time of diagnosis is associated with better outcomes; thus, early identification is recommended.
- Probability of recurrence following recovery of a major depressive episode is approximately 40% by 2 years and 70% by 5 years.

ADDITIONAL READING

- Cheung AH, Zuckerbrot RA, Jensen PS, et al. Guidelines for adolescent depression in primary care (GLAD-PC): II. Treatment and ongoing management. *Pediatrics*. 2007;120(5):e1313–e1326.
- Greydanus DE, Calles JL, Patel DR. *Pediatric and Adolescent Psychopharmacology: A Practical Manual for Pediatricians*. Cambridge, United Kingdom: University Press; 2008.
- Lewandowski RE, Acri MC, Hoagwood KE, et al. Evidence for the management of adolescent depression. *Pediatrics*. 2013;132(4):e996–e1009.
- March J, Silva S, Petrycki S, et al; Treatment for Adolescents with Depression Study (TADS) Team. Fluoxetine, cognitive behavioral therapy, and their combination for adolescents with depression: treatment for adolescents with depression study (TADS) randomized controlled trial. *JAMA*. 2004;292(7):807–820.
- Rao U, Chen LA. Characteristics, correlates, and outcomes of childhood and adolescent depressive disorders. *Dialogues Clin Neurosci*. 2009;11(1):45–62.
- Williams SB, O'Connor EA, Eder M, et al. Screening for child and adolescent depression in primary care settings: a systematic evidence review for the US Preventive Services Task Force. *Pediatrics*. 2009;123(4):e716–e735.
- Zuckerbrot RA, Cheung AH, Jensen PS, et al; GLAD-PC Steering Group. Guidelines for adolescent depression in primary care (GLAD-PC): I. Identification, assessment, and initial management. *Pediatrics*. 2007;120(5):e1299–e1312.

D

CODES

ICD10

- F32.9 Major depressive disorder, single episode, unspecified
- F33.9 Major depressive disorder, recurrent, unspecified
- F34.1 Dysthymic disorder

FAQ

- Q: What is the PHQ-9?
- A: The PHQ-9 is a self-completed screening survey composed of 9 questions that ask about the frequency of symptoms of depression. If a patient reports 5 or more symptoms more than half the days during the past 2 weeks, the clinician must consider MDD as a diagnosis.
- Q: How should clinicians interpret the "Black Box Warning" about SSRIs?
- In 2004, the Food and Drug Administration issued the Black Box Warning, the most serious type of warning in prescription drug labeling, to inform the public about increased risk of suicidal thoughts or behavior in children and adolescents treated with SSRI. Given evidence for improvement of depression with SSRIs, clinicians should weigh the risks and benefits with the patient and family in deciding treatment; adolescents treated with SSRIs must be closely monitored for any worsening in depression, emergence of suicidal thinking or behavior, or unusual changes in behavior, such as sleeplessness, agitation, or withdrawal from normal social situations.
- Q: What is CBT?
- A: In CBT, the therapist guides and helps a patient to understand and modify dysfunctional thoughts, feelings, and behaviors. If a patient believes that he is worthless, the therapist may encourage him to challenge the negative and irrational belief by understanding patterns in his thinking that relate to such a belief.

DERMATOMYOSITIS/POLYMYOSITIS

Megan L. Curran

BASICS

DESCRIPTION

Juvenile dermatomyositis (JDM) and juvenile polymyositis (JPM) are inflammatory myopathies in which inflammation of capillary endothelium of muscle, skin, and other tissues causes vascular and tissue damage. JDM patients present with characteristic rashes and muscle weakness. JPM patients have inflammatory myopathy but lack skin findings. Both disorders have a wide range of severity and presenting findings.

EPIDEMIOLOGY

- The average age of onset is 7 years, but 25% of cases are diagnosed by 4 years of age.
- Male-to-female ratio in the United States is 1:2.3.
- JDM incidence is 3.2 new cases per 1 million children per year; JPM is extremely rare.

RISK FACTORS

- Underlying genetic susceptibility
- Environmental triggers
  - Ultraviolet light exposure
  - Infectious triggers are inconsistently reported, including group A β-hemolytic streptococci, coxsackievirus B, toxoplasma, enterovirus, and parvovirus.
  - Reports of drug exposure, vaccination, and psychological stress prior to diagnosis, but no causation has been found

Genetics

- Genetic factors, including the following:
  - HLA alleles: B8, DRB1*0301, DQA1*0501, DQA1*0301
  - Cytokine polymorphisms: TNFα-308A promoter, various IL1 genes, interferon regulatory factor 5, and others, all resulting in upregulated inflammation
  - Polymorphisms of immunoglobulin constant regions
- Epigenetic factors likely exist: Monozygotic twin studies show low concordance.

PATHOPHYSIOLOGY

- Vasculopathy in patients with underlying inflammatory genetic susceptibility, triggered by environmental factors
- JDM: immune attack on muscle capillary endothelium with infiltration of plasmacytoid dendritic cells causing a type I interferon response and upregulation of myofiber MHC class I expression
  - Immune complex deposition and complement activation drive vasculopathy
  - Upregulation of ICAM-1 and von Willebrand factor antigen indicates endothelial injury.
  - After vasculopathy and MHC class I upregulation, plasmacytoid dendritic and other immune cells infiltrate perivascular and perimysial tissue, resulting in upregulated type I interferon response which perpetuates inflammatory processes including increased production of proinflammatory cytokines
- JPM: CD8 T cell and myeloid dendritic cell-mediated attack on myofibers causing myonecrosis; no increased interferon response
- Myositis-specific and associated autoantibodies directed against vascular and muscle antigens implicated in pathogenesis of JDM and JPM
- Maternal cell chimerism reported in peripheral blood T cells and muscle tissue of JDM patients may be autoreactive toward host cells.

COMMONLY ASSOCIATED CONDITIONS

- Dermatomyositis in children is not associated with presence of malignancy as seen in adults.
- Celiac disease is rarely associated with JDM.

DIAGNOSIS

Bohan and Peter criteria (1975): not validated in children but nonetheless used. Definite JDM requires rash plus three other criteria; probable JDM requires rash plus two other criteria:

- Characteristic rashes: heliotrope discoloration of eyelids and/or erythematous papules over extensor surfaces of joints (Gottron papules)
- Symmetric proximal muscle weakness
- Elevated serum skeletal muscle enzymes
- Electromyographic (EMG) findings of myopathy and denervation; characteristic MRI findings are often substituted to fulfill EMG criteria in children, although are not specific.
- Muscle biopsy with characteristic abnormalities

HISTORY

- Onset is often insidious but can be rapid.
- Constitutional
  - Fever and adenopathy in some children
  - Anorexia, weight loss
  - Fatigue is a sign of muscle weakness and immune activation.
- Skin: characteristic rashes, ulceration, mouth sores, sun sensitivity, limb edema, calcinosis cutis; Raynaud phenomenon and erythema around fingernails due to vasculopathy
- Weakness (e.g, difficulty rising, climbing stairs, getting out of bed or chair, combing hair)
- Gastrointestinal (GI)
  - Dysphonia, dysphagia, choking, and regurgitation of liquids through nose indicate pharyngeal muscle weakness.
  - Constipation, early satiety from muscle weakness, and gut vasculopathy
  - Abdominal pain and hematochezia from gut vasculopathy
- Musculoskeletal: myalgia, arthralgia, arthritis, joint contractures
- Often strong family history of various autoimmune diseases

PHYSICAL EXAM

- Classic rashes in JDM:
  - Heliotrope rash: violaceous discoloration of upper eyelids; can be accompanied by lid swelling, capillary telangiectasia, discoloration below eyes
  - Gottron papules: scaly, erythematous, symmetric, usually hypertrophic but sometimes atrophic papules over extensor surfaces of joints, especially fingers, elbows, knees, and ankles

ALERT

- Findings requiring immediate evaluation: tachycardia, dyspnea, dysphagia, hematochezia, severe abdominal pain, and inability to stand up from the floor or walk

- Other cutaneous findings in JDM:
  - Malar rash
  - V-sign: erythema of upper chest; shawl-sign includes erythema of shoulders
  - Nailfold capillary telangiectasia
  - Overgrown, ragged cuticles
  - Edema of skin overlying inflamed muscles
  - Erythema, dilated vessels, ulcerations of hard palate and buccal mucosa
  - Dermatitis of scalp
  - Ulcerations of skin especially of inner canthi, elbows, or at sites of calcinosis
  - Calcinosis cutis is a late finding:
    - Tumorlike calcium deposits at pressure points: elbows, scapulae, ischia
    - Sheetlike or nodular calcification around joints, axillae
- Musculoskeletal
  - Core weakness: neck, abdominal muscles
  - Proximal weakness: symmetric weakness of shoulder abductors, hip flexors
  - Distal muscle weakness in severe cases
  - Muscle tenderness
  - Waddling (Trendelenburg), wide-based or marching gait due to weak hip flexors
  - Arthritis and joint contractures

ALERT

- Some JDM patients have little to no muscle weakness (amyopathic/hypomyopathic JDM). Patients seemingly without weakness with facial, hand, and/or other vasculopathic rashes can be misdiagnosed with eczema or psoriasis.
- Rarely, patients may have myositis and vasculopathic skin findings but lack heliotrope changes and Gottron papules.

- GI: diffuse abdominal tenderness, distension, palpable stool
- CV: tachycardia, murmurs, tachypnea
- Physical exam tips
  - Gower sign: inability to rise from floor without using hands
  - Lying supine on flat exam table without a pillow, patients with neck and abdominal weakness will have difficulty lifting head (chin to chest) or shoulders off bed.
  - Objective measure of strength: duration of straight-leg raise (normal = 20 seconds)
  - Use ophthalmoscope or otoscope to examine nailfolds for telangiectasia.
  - Evaluate for dysphonia by asking child to say "Nancy" or "jug"—listen for a nasal quality to voice.

DIAGNOSTIC TESTS & INTERPRETATION

Lab

- Muscle enzymes: creatine kinase, aldolase, lactate dehydrogenase, aspartate aminotransferase, alanine aminotransferase
  - One or more is elevated in most cases

ALERT

Creatine kinase and/or other muscle enzymes can be normal or low in patients with hypomyopathic JDM or long duration of untreated disease.

- Markers of immune activation
  - ESR and C-reactive protein often normal
  - Inflammatory findings in complete blood count often not present
  - Elevated neopterin: secreted by activated macrophages and dendritic cells
  - Elevated von Willebrand factor antigen: marker of endothelial activation
  - Complement generally normal; if low, consider overlap syndrome
- Autoantibodies
  - Antinuclear antibodies with various antigen specificities may be present.

- – ~63% of JDM/JPM patients have a myositis-specific antibody (MSA). Anti-p-155 and MJ antibodies most common; anti-synthetase antibodies (i.e., Jo-1), anti-Mi-2, and anti–signal recognition particle are rare in childhood-onset disease.
  - – Myositis-associated antibodies (MAAs) are seen in ~16% of JDM/JPM patients, including anti-Ro, anti-U1RNP, and anti-PM-Scl.
  - – MSAs and MAAs should be tested by immunoprecipitation using validated assays.
  - – Rheumatoid factor and double-stranded DNA antibodies are usually negative; if positive, consider overlap syndrome.
  - – Consider celiac disease testing if with GI symptoms, anemia, and weight loss.
- Occult blood in stool; anemia if blood loss

Imaging

- MRI: Inflamed muscles are identified by signal enhancement on short T1 inversion recovery (STIR) or fat-suppressed T2 sequences; useful to locate site for biopsy
- Video swallow study to identify palatal or proximal esophageal weakness, aspiration
- PFTs to evaluate for respiratory musculature weakness and interstitial lung disease
- EKG and possibly ECHO to evaluate for myocarditis, myocardial dysfunction

Diagnostic Procedures

- Muscle biopsy
- Skin biopsy
- EMG is rarely used in children but can help support diagnosis.

Pathologic Findings

- Skeletal muscle: perifascicular atrophy; variation in fiber size due to degeneration and regeneration; focal necrosis; lymphocytic and mononuclear infiltrates in the perimysium and perivascular spaces (perifascicular), overexpression of MHC class I
- Skin: epidermal atrophy, dermal and perivascular lymphocytic infiltrates

DIFFERENTIAL DIAGNOSIS

- Infectious/postinfectious: influenza A and B, coxsackievirus B, schistosomiasis, trypanosomiasis; bacterial/pyomyositis if focal
- Trauma (physical, toxic, or drug-induced)
- Myositis with other connective tissue diseases
  - – Systemic lupus erythematosus
  - – Systemic sclerosis
  - – Overlap syndromes including mixed or undifferentiated connective tissue disease
  - – Other forms of idiopathic inflammatory myopathy (extremely rare in children): inclusion body myositis, cancer-associated myositis, eosinophilic myositis/fasciitis
- Childhood neuromuscular diseases
  - – Muscular dystrophies
  - – Congenital myopathies (nemaline rod)
  - – Myotonic disorders
  - – Metabolic myopathies (glycogen metabolism disorders, mitochondrial myopathies, familial periodic paralysis, lipid myopathies [carnitine deficiencies], myoadenylate deaminase deficiency, myopathy secondary to endocrinopathy)
  - – Neurogenic atrophies (spinal muscular atrophy and anterior horn cell dysfunction, peripheral nerve dysfunction, neuromuscular transmission disorders)
- The differential diagnosis for JPM is broader than JDM due to lack of skin findings.

TREATMENT

MEDICATION

- Early aggressive therapy improves overall outcome and reduces frequency of calcinosis.
- Prednisone 1–2 mg/kg/24 h PO (maximum 60 mg) for 1 month, taper over months to years
- IV methylprednisolone 30 mg/kg/24 h (maximum 1,000 mg) for 3 infusions at treatment onset; may also be given weekly
- Methotrexate, usually 15 mg/m^2 (maximum generally 25 mg) weekly; SC or IV preferred—PO absorption is poor due to gut vasculopathy
- IV gammaglobulin, especially helpful for rash
- Hydroxychloroquine, especially useful for rash
- 2nd-line immunosuppressants: cyclosporine, mycophenolate mofetil
- Biologic agents for refractory disease including rituximab and abatacept under investigation
- Topical calcineurin inhibitors for rash
- Aggressive broad-spectrum photoprotection with physical blockers (i.e., titanium dioxide) and chemical blockers (i.e., avobenzone)
- Calcium and vitamin D supplementation
- Treatment of calcinosis may include sodium thiosulfate, diltiazem, and bisphosphonates.

ISSUES FOR REFERRAL

- Pediatric rheumatologist for diagnosis and management
- Speech therapist for dysphagia
- Gastroenterology, cardiology, or pulmonary referral depending on involved organ system
- Plastic surgery referral may be indicated for excision of severe calcifications, but there is risk of recurrence and infection.

ADDITIONAL THERAPIES

- Physical and occupational therapy
  - – Initially to maintain range of movement
  - – Strengthening after acute inflammation resolves
  - – Depending on disease severity, patients may require extensive, long-term therapy.

INPATIENT CONSIDERATIONS

Respiratory compromise occasionally requires mechanical ventilation.

ONGOING CARE

FOLLOW-UP RECOMMENDATIONS

Patient Monitoring

- Serial evaluation of muscle strength and function using validated measures such as the Childhood Myositis Assessment Scale or Manual Muscle Testing
- Muscle enzyme levels to monitor treatment efficacy and flare of inflammation
- Joint range of motion
- Skin exams to check for ulceration, calcinosis
- Steroid-induced myopathy is possible; consider if weakness worsens or does not improve during treatment

PATIENT EDUCATION

- Lifelong sun avoidance and sun protection
- Steroid side effects and warnings about physiologic dependence

PROGNOSIS

- Presence of myositis-specific or associated antibodies can predict disease course.
- Normal to good functional outcome: 65–80%
- Minimal atrophy or joint contractures: 24%
- Calcinosis cutis: 12–40%
- Wheelchair dependent: 5%
- Death: 1–3% (sepsis, GI bleeding or perforation, respiratory failure, myocarditis)

COMPLICATIONS

- Infections, sepsis due to immunosuppression
- Ulcerative rash and scarring
- Calcinosis cutis
- Skin infections at sites of ulceration, calcinosis
- Lipoatrophy, lipodystrophy
- Muscle fibrosis or arthritis causing joint contractures
- Restrictive, interstitial lung disease
- Aspiration pneumonia due to respiratory weakness and swallowing dysfunction
- Myocarditis (rare)
- GI tract vasculitis causing ulcerations, perforation
- Osteoporosis due to inflammation and glucocorticoids

ADDITIONAL READING

- Feldman BM, Rider LG, Reed AM, et al. Juvenile dermatomyositis and other idiopathic inflammatory myopathies of childhood. *Lancet*. 2008;371(9631): 2201–2212.
- Khanna S, Reed AM. Immunopathogenesis of juvenile dermatomyositis. *Muscle Nerve*. 2010;41(5): 581–592.
- Ravelli A, Trail L, Ferrari C, et al. Long-term outcome and prognostic factors of juvenile dermatomyositis: a multinational, multicenter study of 490 patients. *Arthritis Care Res*. 2010;62(1):63–72.
- Rider LG, Lindsley CB, Cassidy JT. Juvenile dermatomyositis. In: Cassidy JT, Petty RE, Laxer RM, et al, eds. *Textbook of Pediatric Rheumatology*. 6th ed. Philadelphia, PA: Elsevier; 2011:375–413.
- Rider LG, Pachman LM, Miller FW, et al, eds. *Myositis and You: A Guide to Juvenile Dermatomyositis for Patients, Families, and Healthcare Providers*. Washington, DC: The Myositis Association; 2007.
- Rider LG, Shah M, Mamyrova G, et al. The myositis autoantibody phenotypes of the juvenile idiopathic inflammatory myopathies. *Medicine*. 2013;92(4): 223–243.
- Wedderburn LR, Rider LG. Juvenile dermatomyositis: new developments in pathogenesis, assessment and treatment. *Best Pract Res Clin Rheumatol*. 2009; 23(5):665–678.

CODES

ICD10

- M33.00 Juvenile dermatopolymyositis, organ involvement unspecified
- M33.02 Juvenile dermatopolymyositis with myopathy

FAQ

- Q: Is it mandatory to perform a muscle biopsy to confirm the diagnosis?
- A: Biopsy is indicated if diagnosis is in any way uncertain. In patients with classic rash, weakness, and elevated muscle enzymes, MRI may suffice. However, biopsy results potentially provide prognostic information.

DEVELOPMENTAL DELAY

Rita Panoscha

BASICS

DESCRIPTION

- Developmental delay is a descriptive term, not a specific diagnosis, comprising many disorders and encompassing a broad category of etiologies.
- The term describes any situation where a child is not meeting age-appropriate milestones as expected in 1 or more streams of development. These streams of development include gross motor, fine motor, receptive and expressive language, adaptive, and social (Appendix, Table 1).
- The key feature is that the rate of progress has been slow over time in the area(s) of delay.

ALERT

- Children with behavioral problems may also be masking developmental delays.
- Children with delays in 1 stream of development may also have delays in other areas of development. For example, language delay may be an indication of general cognitive delays.
- Hearing impairment may present as a delay in development.

EPIDEMIOLOGY

Found in both sexes and all racial and socioeconomic groups

Prevalence

This is a heterogeneous group of disorders with different prevalence rates.

GENERAL PREVENTION

There is no known prevention of developmental delays, although prevention of some of the underlying causes is possible.

PATHOPHYSIOLOGY

- This is highly variable depending on etiology, which can include genetic, familial, metabolic, infectious, endocrinologic, traumatic, anatomic brain malformations, environmental toxins, and degenerative disorders as causes. These disorders often result in some neurologic or neuromuscular injury causing the delay. In many cases, the etiology is never determined.
- Prevalence of this group of disorders may vary depending on the inclusiveness of the definition. The milder delays are quite common and can be found in any pediatric practice. Some disorders in this grouping are more prevalent in boys. The long-term outcome depends on the severity and type of delay, with the more involved children usually having lifelong disability.

ETIOLOGY

Specific etiologies are too numerous to list completely, but a partial list of the more common causes includes the following:

- Genetic/familial
  - Fragile X syndrome
  - Trisomy 21 (Down syndrome)
  - Other chromosomal abnormalities
  - Tuberous sclerosis
  - Neurofibromatosis
  - Phenylketonuria
  - Muscular dystrophy
- Nervous system anomalies
  - Hydrocephalus
  - Lissencephaly
  - Spina bifida
  - Seizures
- Infections
  - Prenatal cytomegalovirus
  - Rubella
  - Toxoplasmosis
  - HIV
  - Postnatal bacterial meningitis
  - Neonatal herpes simplex
- Endocrinologic
  - Congenital hypothyroidism
- Environment
  - Heavy metal poisoning such as lead
  - In utero drug or alcohol exposure
- Trauma/injury
  - Closed head trauma
  - Asphyxia
  - Stroke
  - Perinatal cerebral hemorrhages

COMMONLY ASSOCIATED CONDITIONS

- There are numerous associated findings including seizures, sensory impairments, feeding disorders, psychiatric disorders (especially depression), and behavioral disorders.
- Having a child with significant developmental delays can also add stress to the family in terms of time, finances, and emotions.

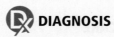

DIAGNOSIS

HISTORY

A complete and detailed history is needed, including the following:

- Pregnancy history
  - Maternal age and parity
  - Maternal complications (including infections and exposures)
  - Medications/drugs used
  - Tobacco or alcohol used, along with quantities
  - Fetal activity
- Birth history
  - Gestational age
  - Birth weight
  - Route of delivery
  - Maternal or fetal complications/distress
  - Apgar scores
- General health
  - Significant illnesses, hospitalizations, or surgeries
  - Accidents or injuries
  - Hearing and vision status
  - Medications used
  - Known exposures to toxins
  - Any new or unusual symptoms
- Developmental history
  - Current developmental achievement in each stream of development
  - Age when developmental milestones were achieved
  - Any loss of skills
  - Where parents think their child is functioning developmentally
- Educational history
  - Type of schooling and services received, if any
  - Any previous educational/developmental testing
- Behavioral history
  - Any perseverative or stereotypical behaviors
  - Interaction skills
  - Attention and activity level
- Family history
  - Anyone with developmental delays, neurologic disorders, syndromes, consanguinity

PHYSICAL EXAM

- A complete physical exam including growth parameters is needed looking for etiology.
- Key features to include:
  - Observation of interactions and behavior: any atypical behaviors and general impression
  - Head circumference: Assess for macrocephaly or microcephaly.
  - Skin: Examine for neurocutaneous lesions
  - Major or minor dysmorphic features: any indication of a syndrome or anatomic malformation
  - Neurologic examination: Assess for cranial nerve deficits, neuromuscular status, reflexes, balance and coordination, and any soft signs.
  - Developmental testing: Although considerable information will already be available on history and observation, a more formal developmental screening or testing should be done. Possible office tests include the Ages & Stages Questionnaires, the Parents' Evaluation of Developmental Status, or the Cognitive Adaptive Test/Clinical Linguistic and Auditory Milestone Scale (CAT/CLAMS). Referral to a specialist or a multidisciplinary team for more detailed testing is indicated when delay is suspected.

DIAGNOSTIC TESTS & INTERPRETATION

Lab

Initial lab tests

- There is no specific laboratory test battery for general developmental delays. The testing needs to be tailored to the individual situation based on the history and physical exam. A high index of suspicion should be maintained for any associated findings and delays in the other streams of development.
- Some of the more common studies ordered for developmental delay workup:
  - Genetic testing: warranted for any dysmorphic features, a family history of delays, or genetic disorder. A karyotype and fragile X DNA testing should be considered, particularly for significant cognitive delays. The comparative genomic hybridization (CGH) microarray is now increasingly recommended as a 1st-line test for developmental delays.
  - Metabolic tests: Tests such as quantitative plasma amino acids, quantitative urine organic acids, lactate, pyruvate, or ammonia should be considered if there is any loss of skills or indication of a metabolic disorder.
  - Thyroid function tests: Most infants will have had screening for hypothyroidism shortly after birth. This should be rechecked if symptoms indicate.

Imaging

Head MRI: Consider a head MRI for head abnormalities, significant neurologic findings, loss of skills, or for workup of a specific disorder such as trauma or leukodystrophy.

Diagnostic Procedures/Other

- Audiologic: Hearing should be checked in any child with speech and language and/or cognitive delays.
- EEG: An EEG should be considered if there is any concern about seizures.
- Subspecialists: Referral to other medical specialists may also be indicated. These specialists may include developmental pediatrics, neurology, genetics, orthopedics, or ophthalmology.

DIFFERENTIAL DIAGNOSIS

- The differential can be extensive and may become more evident with further workup.
- Broad diagnoses include the following:
  - Intellectual disability
  - Developmental language disorder
  - Autism
  - Learning disability
  - Cerebral palsy
  - Attention-deficit/hyperactivity disorder
  - Significant visual or hearing impairment
  - Degenerative disorders

TREATMENT

ADDITIONAL TREATMENT

General Measures

- Therapy should include appropriately treating any medical conditions and associated findings, for example, anticonvulsants for seizures or hearing aids when appropriate for hearing impairment. In addition, traditional therapy has included early intervention or special education services specifically addressing the areas of delay.
- Therapy could include physical therapists, occupational therapists, speech/language therapists, special educators, psychologists, and audiologists, depending on the needs of the child.

ONGOING CARE

FOLLOW-UP RECOMMENDATIONS

Patient Monitoring

- General pediatric care for well-child visits and to monitor any underlying medical conditions is indicated.
- These children need ongoing monitoring of their therapy and educational programs to ensure that it is still meeting their individual needs as these needs change over time.
- The families will also need ongoing counseling and support in dealing with a child having special needs.

PROGNOSIS

Variable depending on the type and severity of delay and the etiology

ADDITIONAL READING

- Battaglia A, Carey JC. Diagnostic evaluation of developmental delay/mental retardation: an overview. *Am J Med Genet C Semin Med Genet*. 2003;117C(1):3–14.
- Council on Children With Disabilities. Identifying infants and young children with developmental disorders in the medical home: an algorithm for developmental surveillance and screening. *Pediatrics*. 2006;118(1):405–420.
- Gerber RJ, Wilks T, Erdie-Lalena C. Developmental milestones: motor development. *Pediatr Rev*. 2010;31(7):267–276.
- Gropman AL, Batshaw ML. Epigenetics, copy number variation, and other molecular mechanisms underlying neurodevelopmental disabilities: new insights and diagnostic approaches. *J Dev Behav Pediatr*. 2010;31(7):582–591.
- Liptak GS. The pediatrician's role in caring for the developmentally disabled child. *Pediatr Rev*. 1996;17(6):203–210.
- Marks KP, LaRosa AC. Understanding developmental-behavioral screening measures. *Pediatr Rev*. 2012;33(10):448–457.
- McQuiston S, Kloczko N. Speech and language development: monitoring process and problems. *Pediatr Rev*. 2011;32(6):230–238.
- Moeschler JB, Shevell M; American Academy of Pediatrics Committee on Genetics. Clinical genetic evaluation of the child with mental retardation or developmental delays. *Pediatrics*. 2006;117(6):2304–2316.
- Shevell M. Global developmental delay and mental retardation or intellectual disability: conceptualization, evaluation, and etiology. *Pediatr Clin North Am*. 2008;55(5):1071–1084.

CODES

ICD10

- F89 Unspecified disorder of psychological development
- F82 Specific developmental disorder of motor function
- F80.9 Developmental disorder of speech and language, unspecified

FAQ

- Q: When do you test a child for delays?
- A: A child can have developmental assessments at any age, including infancy. Making a specific diagnosis, for example, for level of intellectual disability, may need to wait until the child is older.
- Q: When can a child start receiving services?
- A: Children who qualify can receive therapy services starting at birth and in some cases extending up to age 21 years.
- Q: The parents are raising a concern about delays, but the general impression in the office is that the child is doing okay. What should be done next?
- A: Parents or grandparents may be the first to express concerns, especially in a child with milder delays. A more detailed developmental history and more formal developmental screening or testing may be indicated as an initial step.

DEVELOPMENTAL DYSPLASIA OF THE HIP

Syed I. Ahmed • John E. Tis

BASICS

DESCRIPTION

Developmental dysplasia of the hip (DDH) is a range of hip pathology including dysplasia (shallow acetabulum), subluxation (partial femoral head–acetabulum contact), and dislocation (no hip joint contact). Abnormalities can be present at birth or develop over time. A teratologic dislocation is a different condition that occurs during fetal development usually from genetic/syndromic causes. Discussion of teratologic dislocation is beyond the scope of this chapter.

EPIDEMIOLOGY

- Female-to-male ratio is 4:1.
- Incidence varies from 1.5 to 25 in 1,000 births.
- Dislocation incidence is about 1 in 1,000 births.

RISK FACTORS

- Compressive factors:
  - Breech position (newborn DDH risk: male 2.6%, female 12%)
  - Oligohydramnios
  - Firstborn child
  - High birth weight
- Demographic factors:
  - Female gender (newborn DDH risk 1.9%)
  - Family history (newborn DDH risk: male 0.9%, female 4.4%)
  - Ethnicity: Native American, Laplander

Genetics

No defined mode of inheritance; family history, gender, and ethnicity association

GENERAL PREVENTION

Although DDH cannot be prevented, treatment is directed at preventing early arthritis. Screening programs have reduced the newborn dislocation rate to 1 in 5,000 children by the age of 18 months.

PATHOPHYSIOLOGY

The acetabular depth (growth) is determined by healthy cartilage and development around a concentrically reduced/stable femoral head. Cartilage damage occurs from continued instability. Untreated subluxation/dislocation can result in an everted labrum, hypertrophic cartilage/labrum complex (neolimbus), and false acetabulum (pseudoacetabulum). In early adulthood, this can lead to abnormal wear of the joint, limb length differences, and arthritic pain. Compensatory problems may include spinal malalignment (scoliosis/lordosis) and gait abnormalities.

ETIOLOGY

- Mechanical factors: attributed to a smaller in utero environment from oligohydramnios, breech position, increased birth weight, or an unstretched uterus (first pregnancy)
- Female predominance: attributed to estrogen-induced ligamentous laxity
- Left side predominance: attributed to fetal positioning of left hip adduction against the mother's lumbosacral spine
- Native American predominance: attributed to the hip extension/adduction position of swaddling

COMMONLY ASSOCIATED CONDITIONS

- Neurologic conditions (e.g., myelomeningocele)
- Connective tissue disorders (e.g., Ehlers-Danlos)
- Syndromic conditions (e.g., Larsen syndrome)
- Myopathic disorders (e.g., arthrogryposis)

DIAGNOSIS

HISTORY

Gestational age, gender, birth weight/order, delivery method/position (breech), and family history (DDH or associated conditions [see earlier]) should be asked.

PHYSICAL EXAM

- Ensure that the child is relaxed and calm.
- Screening should be done at all well-child visits until normal ambulatory development.
- Newborn exam
  - Hard signs (<3 months old):
    - Ortolani test: The contralateral hip is flexed, abducted, and held with one hand to stabilize the pelvis. The other hip is held with the thumb in the groin crease and the index/middle finger over the trochanter. With the hip flexed (90 degrees), the trochanter is lifted (anteriorly) as the hip is abducted. An unstable hip will "clunk" as it reduces.
    - Barlow test: similar hand position as the Ortolani test. The hip is flexed (90 degrees), and as the hip is adducted, a posterior stress is applied. An unstable hip will palpably slip out of socket.
    - Galeazzi sign: With bilateral hip and knee flexion, an asymmetry in knee height occurs from apparent femoral shortening on the dislocated side.
  - Soft signs:
    - "Packaging" abnormalities: torticollis, limb deformity (metatarsus adductus), joint contractures, or dislocation of other joints
    - Asymmetric skinfolds (low sensitivity)
    - Sacral dimple
- Ambulatory child exam:
  - Stiffness: limited abduction (normally abduction >75 degrees, adduction >30 degrees)
  - Limb length difference: unilateral toe walking, abnormal Galeazzi sign, scoliosis
  - Gait: lurching to one side (Trendelenburg gait)
  - Bilateral dislocation: may have waddling gait and hyperlordosis. Galeazzi sign will be normal. May be difficult to recognize.

ALERT

- Early diagnosis and referral are paramount.
- Main instability indicators are the Barlow and Ortolani exams. Perform these gently.
- Soft tissue clicks superficial in sound and most asymmetric thigh folds are normal.
- An unreducible hip may have a falsely normal Ortolani/Barlow exam but will be Galeazzi positive.
- Exam and risk factors guide future screening and referral.

DIAGNOSTIC TESTS & INTERPRETATION

Imaging

- If the clinical exam findings are clearly abnormal, then refer the patient. No further imaging is needed for referral.
- Imaging is used to clarify an equivocal examination and to monitor treatment progress.
- Ultrasound
  - Optimal age: 3 weeks to 5 months
  - Static examination: Superior acetabular coverage (α-angle) and femoral head position (β-angle) can be assessed.
  - Dynamic examination: assesses stability
- Plain radiographs (AP pelvis ± frog lateral)
  - Optimal age: after 3–6 months
- CT scan/MRI
  - Used to assess concentric hip reduction after orthopedic surgical intervention

DIFFERENTIAL DIAGNOSIS

- Septic hip
- Congenital coxa vara
- Proximal femoral focal deficiency

TREATMENT

ADDITIONAL TREATMENT

General Measures

- Treatment principle: Acetabular remodeling potential rarely exists after 4 years of age. When remodeling potential exists, treatment goals are to redirect the femoral head into the acetabulum with minimal force while avoiding complications of avascular necrosis and cartilage damage.

ISSUES FOR REFERRAL

Primary care providers (PCPs) algorithm of care:

- Initial (newborn) exam
  - Abnormal (hard exam findings): orthopedic referral
  - Inconclusive (soft exam findings only): send for ultrasound after 2–3 weeks of age. If abnormal, refer.
  - Normal exam
    - If no risk factors: Reexamine at every well-child visit until normal ambulatory development.
    - If lower risk (female, male with family history):
      - Reexamine during well-child visits until normal ambulatory development.
    - If intermediate risk (female with family history, male born breech):
      - Consider future imaging: ultrasound (~4–6 weeks), radiographs (~6, 12 months)
    - If intermediate risk (female with breech position)
      - Obtain future imaging: ultrasound (~4–6 weeks) and radiographs (~6, 12 months)
- Follow-up (postnewborn) exam: if abnormalities exist after the initial newborn period, then referral with ultrasound (if <5 months of age) or radiographs (if >4–6 months of age)

ADDITIONAL THERAPIES

Pavlik Harness

- Indications: if earlier criteria is met for referral but referral is not possible and child is <6 months of age or the PCP is trained in Pavlik harness use
- NOTE: Abduction brace (more rigid) can be used if treatment extends past 6 months of age when the child becomes more ambulatory.
- For a hip that reduces:
  - Place harness full time with joint reduced (may confirm with ultrasound).
  - Reexamine hips and readjust harness every 3 weeks.
  - Repeat ultrasound ~6–12 weeks.
  - Once hip exam is normal, continue full-time Pavlik use for additional 6–12 weeks.
  - Radiograph at 6, 12 months
- For hip dislocation (nonteratologic):
  - Follow the earlier protocol except
    - Initial ultrasound and radiographs for documentation of dislocation
    - Clinically reassess every 7–10 days until hip reduces.
    - If hip reduces, document with ultrasound.
    - Radiographs at 3 months
    - Refer patient and abandon harness treatment if not reduced by 3 weeks.
- Pavlik harness application:
  - Chest strap: nipple level, snug
  - Shoulder strap: should cross posteriorly, snug
  - Stirrup: should start distal to the popliteal fossa
  - Anterior strap: midaxillary line strap adjusted so hip is flexed at 90–100 degrees
  - Posterior strap: attaches over the scapula, adjusted so hips do not adduct (do not force abduction)

ALERT

- Pavlik harness use is safe when properly placed.
- Never force the hip into position.
- Improper use can lead to cartilage damage, femoral nerve palsy, and avascular necrosis.

SURGERY/OTHER PROCEDURES

- Closed reduction: used when Pavlik harness treatment fails. Spica cast is applied for 2–6 months.
- Open reduction: used when closed reduction fails usually due to soft tissue interposition and/or muscle contracture. Common after 6 months of age. Adductor tenotomy is usually done. Spica cast is applied after.
- Osteotomy: After about age 2 years, excessive force is needed for a closed/open reduction. Femoral osteotomy reduces this risk along with an open reduction. For residual dysplasia, acetabular osteotomies are performed.

ONGOING CARE

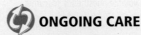

FOLLOW-UP RECOMMENDATIONS

Patient Monitoring

See "Issues for Referral" section.

PROGNOSIS

- 95% successful resolution of an abnormal Ortolani exam when Pavlik harness treatment is initiated in a newborn
- 85% success when the same treatment is started after 1 month of age

COMPLICATIONS

- Pavlik harness
  - Tight shoulder strap: brachial plexopathy
  - Hip hyperflexion: femoral nerve palsy, inferior dislocation
  - Forced abduction: femoral head damage resulting in growth arrest or avascular necrosis. Growth arrest can cause trochanteric overgrowth and abductor lurch.
  - Poor hygiene: skin breakdown (groin crease and popliteal fossa)
- Failure or lack of treatment: residual dysplasia/instability/growth arrest resulting in limb length difference, scoliosis/lordosis, arthritis, gait disturbance, and toe walking

ADDITIONAL READING

- American Academy of Pediatrics. Clinical practice guideline: early detection of developmental dysplasia of the hip. *Pediatrics*. 2000;105(4, Pt 1):896–905.
- American Institute of Ultrasound in Medicine. AIUM practice guideline for the performance of an ultrasound examination for detection and assessment of developmental dysplasia of the hip. *J Ultrasound Med*. 2013;32(7):1307–1317.
- Guille JT, Pizzutillo PD, MacEwen GD. Developmental dysplasia of the hip from birth to six months. *J Am Acad Orthop Surg*. 2000;8(4):232–242.
- Mahan ST, Katz JN, Kim YJ. To screen or not to screen? A decision analysis of the utility of screening for developmental dysplasia of the hip. *J Bone Joint Surg Am*. 2009;91(7):1705–1719.
- Nemeth BA, Narotam V. Developmental dysplasia of the hip. *Pediatr Rev*. 2012;33(12):553–561.
- Storer SK, Skaggs DL. Developmental dysplasia of the hip. *Am Fam Physician*. 2006;74(8):1310–1316.
- Vitale MG, Skaggs DL. Developmental dysplasia of the hip from six months to four years of age. *J Am Acad Orthop Surg*. 2001;9(6):401–411.
- Weinstein SL, Mubarak SJ, Wenger DR. Developmental hip dysplasia and dislocation: part I. *Instr Course Lect*. 2004;53:523–530.
- Weinstein SL, Mubarak SJ, Wenger DR. Developmental hip dysplasia and dislocation: part II. *Instr Course Lect*. 2004;53:531–542.
- Westacott D, Pattison G, Cooke S. Developmental dysplasia of the hip. *Community Pract*. 2012;85(11):42–44.

CODES

ICD10

Q65.89 Other specified congenital deformities of hip

FAQ

- Q: Are screening protocols unified?
- A: Screening and treatment protocols can vary, but the principles are the same. The earlier screening protocol is adopted from the American Academy of Pediatrics Clinical Practice Guideline and Johns Hopkins Pediatric Orthopaedics.
- Q: Why are ultrasound and radiographs used at different age ranges?
- A: After about 3 months of age, radiographs become easier to assess, as radiographs require ossification and ultrasound waves cannot penetrate ossified bone. The hip is not fully ossified at birth, rendering early radiographic examination difficult.
- Q: Why are the Barlow/Ortolani exams used before 3 months of age but not as useful later?
- A: These exams become less useful as the hip naturally stiffens after 3 months, as stiffness results in asymmetric motion but not instability.

DIABETES INSIPIDUS

Todd D. Nebesio • Sheela N. Magge

BASICS

DESCRIPTION

Polyuria and polydipsia caused by the inability to produce or respond to antidiuretic hormone; also called arginine vasopressin

EPIDEMIOLOGY

Incidence

Because most cases are secondary to another disease, the incidence depends on the primary cause.

RISK FACTORS

Genetics

- Rare genetic causes of central diabetes insipidus (DI) are usually autosomal dominant mutations (neuronal degeneration) and rarely recessive (biologically inactive hormone).
- Nephrogenic DI is usually familial (autosomal recessive or dominant and X-linked).

PATHOPHYSIOLOGY

- Antidiuretic hormone stimulates the formation of cyclic adenosine monophosphate (cAMP) in the renal collecting ducts, thereby increasing water permeability and increasing reabsorption of free water.
- Lack of antidiuretic hormone effect results in urinary loss of free water.
- Patients with an intact thirst mechanism drink copiously (polydipsia) to compensate for free water loss.
- If the thirst mechanism is not present or if access to free water is limited (e.g., infants, developmentally delayed child, or vomiting), severe dehydration can occur.

ETIOLOGY

- Insufficient antidiuretic hormone secretion
  - Traumatic or postsurgical
  - Nonaccidental injury
  - Related to tumor invasion of posterior pituitary
  - Extension from anterior pituitary/suprasellar: optic glioma, rarely adenomas
  - Hypothalamic: germinoma, craniopharyngioma, meningioma
  - Lymphoma
  - Granulomas: histiocytosis, sarcoidosis
  - Metastatic carcinoma
  - Post–severe ischemic or hypoxic injury to the brain
  - Familial (autosomal dominant)
  - Congenital malformation of CNS
  - Infection: viral encephalitis, meningitis, tuberculosis
  - Increased metabolic clearance of antidiuretic hormone (gestational DI)
  - Drug or toxin related: snake venom, tetrodotoxin
  - Autoimmune disorders: hypophysitis (inflammation of the pituitary gland)
  - Psychogenic: excessive water drinking
  - Idiopathic: must observe for many years to exclude slow-growing tumors
- Unresponsive to antidiuretic hormone
  - Familial or nephrogenic (X-linked dominant and autosomal recessive forms)
  - Tumor related
  - Urinary tract obstruction, especially in utero
  - Renal medullary cystic disease
  - Electrolyte disturbances: hypokalemia, hypercalcemia (hypercalciuria)
  - Drugs: usually reversible (diuretics, diphenylhydantoin, reserpine, cisplatin, rifampin, lithium [may become permanent], demeclocycline, ethanol, chlorpromazine, volatile anesthetics, foscarnet, amphotericin B)
  - Loss of the medullary concentrating gradient due to excessive free water intake relative to solute intake

ALERT

Pitfalls

- Management of patients without an intact thirst mechanism and of newborns is difficult.
- Patients with psychogenic polydipsia may fail a water deprivation test because prolonged excessive water intake can wash out the renal medullary gradient required for concentrating the urine.
- Surreptitious water intake during water deprivation test
- Idiopathic, acquired DI can be caused by slowly growing brain tumors not visible on the initial magnetic resonance image.

DIAGNOSIS

HISTORY

- Abnormal growth can be a sign of DI.
- Waking up during the night to drink or void:
  - True DI is associated with polyuria throughout the day and night. Enuresis may be the first sign in a child who previously acquired bladder control. Patients, including infants, prefer ice-cold water to other liquids.
- Number of hours the patient goes without drinking:
  - Patients with complete DI do not voluntarily stop drinking for >1–2 hours unless the thirst mechanism is also abnormal.
  - Patients with DI have such overwhelming thirst that they will drink anything, including bath and toilet water.
- Volume of urine output in a day (not just frequency of urination):
  - The daily volume of urine can be as high as 4–10 L. Younger or dehydrated children with DI tend to make less urine daily than older or hydrated children with DI.
- Familial history of DI:
  - Nephrogenic DI will typically affect maternal uncles during infancy, and mothers may have a mild form.
- Frequent episodes of dehydration requiring medical attention:
  - Families may disregard the polydipsia as normal behavior. Repeated episodes of severe dehydration can damage the brain.
- Treatment of adrenal insufficiency in a patient with panhypopituitarism can unmask DI (i.e., one needs cortisol in order to excrete free water).

PHYSICAL EXAM

- Signs of dehydration:
  - DI is typically associated with dry, pale skin and mucous membranes. Because this is hyperosmolar dehydration, the patient may not look as severely dehydrated as she or he is.
- Complete neurologic exam:
  - Check for impaired visual fields, which can be the first sign of brain tumor.

DIAGNOSTIC TESTS & INTERPRETATION

Lab

- Morning urinary osmolality with simultaneous serum sodium and serum osmolality
  - If urine osmolality is at least 2 times higher than serum osmolality, patient does not have complete DI but may still have partial DI.
- Water deprivation test
  - Although definitive, it requires admission to the hospital for controlled testing under the close supervision of a pediatric endocrinologist. Patient fails test if urinary osmolality cannot concentrate more than twice serum osmolality at the same time that serum osmolality exceeds 305 mOsm/kg; serum osmolality exceeds 305 mOsm/kg at any time; or patient loses >5% of body weight and becomes symptomatic from hypovolemia.
  - Once patient fails the water deprivation test, a dose of aqueous vasopressin should be given followed by close monitoring of urinary osmolality to document responsiveness to antidiuretic hormone.
  - Never attempt a water deprivation trial at home. Tell parents to allow free access to water at home in any suspected cases.
- Urinary specific gravity (nonspecific)
  - Insufficient by itself and nondiagnostic during a water deprivation test
- 24-hour urine collection (home testing)
  - To obtain accurate urinary volume while patient has free access to water

Imaging

MRI of the brain with and without contrast, with special cuts of the pituitary and hypothalamus: to confirm the bright spot normally seen in the posterior pituitary and to search for tumors. Its absence is not pathognomonic of central DI.

ALERT

Do not restrict water intake unless the patient is in the hospital under close surveillance.

DIFFERENTIAL DIAGNOSIS

- Psychogenic polydipsia
- Abnormal thirst mechanism (dipsogenic DI)
- Hypernatremic dehydration
- Diabetes mellitus
- Polyuric renal failure (e.g., renal tubulopathy)
- Hypercalcemia
- Cerebral salt wasting
- Hyperthyroidism
- Hypokalemia

TREATMENT

MEDICATION

- DDAVP: intranasal spray or oral tablets
- Aqueous vasopressin: subcutaneous (SC):
  - Comes as 4 mcg/mL solution and doses range from 0.05 mcg up to 1 mcg SC b.i.d. daily. Titrate dose as you would with DDAVP.
- Duration of action of DDAVP is variable from patient to patient. Titration and frequency of dosing should be made under supervision of a pediatric endocrinologist.
- Control of DI in infants is more difficult. These patients may increase fluid intake because of hunger or increase caloric intake because of thirst, thereby causing an imbalance between free water intake and output. Infants can be treated with diluted formula—the volume and frequency of feedings will be increased, but intake of free water will better match urine output. DDAVP should not be used in infants. In some cases, low renal solute load formula (e.g., Similac PM 60/40) and/or thiazide diuretics have been used in infancy. Strict record keeping of intake/output and accurate daily weighing are usually necessary for infants or patients without an intact thirst mechanism. All infants with DI must be treated by experienced providers.
- Nephrogenic DI may be treated with diuretics and solute restriction as these patients are resistant to DDAVP.
- Side effects:
  - Facial flushing
  - Increased blood pressure
  - Headache
  - Nasal congestion
  - Hyponatremia: caused by water overdose (intoxication), not by overdose of drug. Taking a higher dose of DDAVP will generally extend the period of antidiuresis but will not cause hyponatremia. Drinking too much water in the setting of antidiuresis causes hyponatremia. Water intoxication most often occurs in antidiuresed patients who also are on intravenous fluids, lack an intact thirst mechanism, or have psychogenic polydipsia.
- Treatment duration is generally lifelong; some tumors regress with radiation, allowing recovery of antidiuretic hormone secretion.
- Possible conflicts with other treatments:
  - Nasal congestion or gastrointestinal illness can affect the absorption of DDAVP administered.

ONGOING CARE

FOLLOW-UP RECOMMENDATIONS

Patient Monitoring

- Depends on the patient and underlying disease causing the DI
- When to expect improvement:
  - Effects of DDAVP are immediate.
  - Most cases of DI are lifelong; one exception is DI that occurs during the 7–10 days immediately after neurosurgery because this postsurgical DI may resolve spontaneously within 1–2 weeks after surgery (part of the triple-phase response).
- Signs to watch for:
  - Lethargy
  - Somnolence
  - Irritability
  - Hyperpyrexia
  - Any sign of dehydration
  - Seizures

DIET

- Patients with an intact thirst mechanism should drink only when thirsty.
- Patients without an intact thirst mechanism should drink only a carefully calculated fluid volume.

PROGNOSIS

- Generally good but depends on the primary cause
- May cause developmental delay if the hypernatremia is prolonged

COMPLICATIONS

- Without treatment and without access to water:
  - Hypernatremia
  - Dehydration
  - Coma
- When overdosed with water:
  - Hyponatremia
  - Seizures
  - Cerebral edema

ADDITIONAL READING

- Di Iorgi N, Napoli F, Allegri AE, et al. Diabetes insipidus—diagnosis and management. *Horm Res Paediatr*. 2012;77(2):69–84.
- Ghirardello S, Garrè ML, Rossi A, et al. The diagnosis of children with central diabetes insipidus. *J Pediatr Endocrinol Metab*. 2007;20(3):359–375.
- Linshaw MA. Back to basics: congenital nephrogenic diabetes insipidus. *Pediatr Rev*. 2007;28(10):372–380.
- Maghnie M, Cosi G, Genovese E, et al. Central diabetes insipidus in children and young adults. *N Engl J Med*. 2000;343(14):998–1007.
- Rivkees SA, Dunbar N, Wilson TA. The management of central diabetes insipidus in infancy: desmopressin, low renal solute load formula, thiazide diuretics. *J Pediatr Endocrinol Metab*. 2007;20(4):459–469.

CODES

ICD10

- E23.2 Diabetes insipidus
- N25.1 Nephrogenic diabetes insipidus

FAQ

- Q: In a patient with an intact thirst mechanism and partial DI, is the use of DDAVP necessary?
- A: No, as long as the patient has constant access to free water.
- Q: How does therapy of DI affect daily life? Is it easily integrated into normal activity and eating patterns?
- A: DDAVP is used in a patient with an intact thirst mechanism to facilitate the daily routine as well as to allow patients to sleep without the need to void frequently during the night.
- Q: Is there a longer acting preparation or an implantable pump for dosing?
- A: The longest acting form of antidiuretic hormone is an injected medication and can have effects for 3 days, increasing the risks of hyponatremia. Home use of the nasal spray or tablets, therefore, is easier and safer than the use of injections.
- Q: In cases of central DI, is it necessary to screen for anterior pituitary hormone deficiencies?
- A: Yes—at diagnosis of DI and during follow-up as other pituitary hormone deficiencies can occur over time.

DIABETES MELLITUS, TYPE I

R. Paul Wadwa

BASICS

DESCRIPTION

Type 1 diabetes is an autoimmune disorder that causes pancreatic B-cell destruction. This destruction leads to insulin deficiency that results in hyperglycemia and disrupts energy storage and metabolism. Severe insulin deficiency can lead to ketosis, acidosis, dehydration, shock, and death.

EPIDEMIOLOGY

- Most common endocrine disorder of childhood
- More common in whites of Northern European descent

Incidence

- Annual U.S. incidence is ~19/100,000 in children 10–19 years old.
- Incidence of type 1 diabetes is rising by 3% per year but faster in young children.

Prevalence

- Prevalence of type 1 diabetes in youth 0–19 years in United States is ~2/1,000.
- Note: At least 2% of diabetes in children may be due to maturity onset diabetes of youth (MODY) or other genetic forms.

RISK FACTORS

Genetics

- Increased susceptibility to type 1 diabetes associated with HLA region of chromosome 6, 5-fold greater risk with MHC antigen types DR3 and DR4
- MODY is a group of autosomal dominant syndromes of partial insulin deficiency due to monogenic defects of pancreatic development or insulin secretion; they comprise a small fraction of childhood diabetes.

PATHOPHYSIOLOGY

- Loss of pancreatic B cells results in insulin deficiency, leading to hyperglycemia, and predominance of catabolic processes.
- Hyperglycemia causes hyperosmolality, polyuria, and damage to small blood vessels.
- Catabolic processes produce ketosis, weight loss, and metabolic acidosis.

ETIOLOGY

- Type 1 diabetes
  - An environmental trigger (likely viral) induces expression of antigens on B-cell surface.
  - Recruitment of cytotoxic lymphocytes
  - Production of anti-insulin and anti-islet cell antibodies (including GAD65, ICA512, ZnT8)
  - Progressive inflammatory, autoimmune loss of B-cell mass results in insulin deficiency.
  - The autoimmune destruction of B cells is more likely in genetically susceptible persons.

COMMONLY ASSOCIATED CONDITIONS

- Autoimmune thyroid disease
  - Hashimoto (hypothyroidism) more common than Graves (hyperthyroidism)
- Celiac disease
- More rarely other autoimmune diseases, such as alopecia areata, rheumatoid arthritis
- Depression
- After prolonged hyperglycemia: vascular complications:
  - Microvascular
    - Nephropathy
    - Retinopathy
    - Neuropathy
    - (See "Patient Monitoring" for screening recommendations)
  - Macrovascular
    - Peripheral vascular disease
    - Cardiovascular disease

DIAGNOSIS

HISTORY

- Duration of symptoms prior to diagnosis varies by age: may be days in toddlers, months in adolescents.
- Polyuria, nocturia, and enuresis are related to hyperglycemia >180 mg/dL.
- Polydipsia: due to polyuria, hyperosmolality
- Polyphagia: appetite amplified by loss of calories from glycosuria; this is often absent.
- Weight loss: dehydration, loss of calories
- Malaise, nausea, vomiting, abdominal pain, hyperventilation, lethargy due to ketosis, acidosis, electrolyte depletion, hyperosmolality
- MODY is usually asymptomatic.

PHYSICAL EXAM

- Weight loss common at presentation of type 1 diabetes.
- Candidal vaginitis and balanitis common in young children with type 1 diabetes
- In ketoacidosis: dehydration, hyperventilation

DIAGNOSTIC TESTS & INTERPRETATION

Lab

- Diagnosis based on BG level:
  - Fasting BG ≥126 mg/dL, random BG ≥200 mg/dL, or 2-hour BG ≥200 mg/dL on oral glucose tolerance test (OGTT), and exclusion of stress hyperglycemia
  - Asymptomatic hyperglycemia requires repeat confirmation.
- Glycosuria may be intermittent.
- Ketonuria may occur with both types 1 and 2.
- With presence of ketonuria or ketosis, DKA should be ruled out by checking serum bicarbonate.
- HgbA1c reflects BG levels of previous 2–3 months and is nearly always elevated at diagnosis of both types.
- GAD, islet cell, ZnT8, and/or insulin autoantibodies are positive in most persons with type 1 diabetes at onset (85–90%)
- In some patients presenting with hyperglycemia and ketosis, not possible to distinguish type 1 from type 2 until the course over several months has been followed

DIFFERENTIAL DIAGNOSIS

- MODY
- Type 2 diabetes (in obese pubertal youth)
- UTI (polyuria)
- Renal glycosuria
- Stress-related hyperglycemia
- Drug-induced hyperglycemia (steroids)
- Psychogenic polydipsia
- Pneumonia (in DKA)
- Sepsis (in DKA)
- Acute surgical abdomen (in ketoacidosis)

TREATMENT

MEDICATION

(See insulin regimens under "General Measures.")
Insulin is required to treat type 1 diabetes.

- Insulins:
  - Rapid-acting analogs:
    - Aspart (Novolog), lispro (Humalog), glulisine (Apidra)
    - Onset of action 5–15 minutes, peak action 60–90 minutes, and duration 2–5 hours
  - Short-acting
    - Regular insulin—used for IV delivery, can be used for SC injection
    - Onset of action when given SC—30–60 minutes, peak action—2–3 hours, duration—6–9 hours
  - Intermediate-acting
    - NPH (Humulin N, Novolin N)
      - Onset 1–2 hours, peak action 3–8 hours, duration 12–15 hours
      - Use is less common when long-acting analogs available.
  - Long-acting analogs
    - Detemir (Levemir), glargine (Lantus)
    - Onset—3–4 hour, no significant peak, duration 20–24 hours
    - Other long-acting analogs under investigation but are not FDA-approved in 2014 including insulin degludec, which is approved for use in the European Union

ADDITIONAL TREATMENT

General Measures

- Insulin is given as a fixed or flexible regimen.
- TDD—calculated by adding up all short- and long-acting insulin given over 24 hours—usually ~0.7–1.2 U/kg/24 h; choose higher range for ketoacidosis presentation, obesity, and puberty.
- Doses may decline during "honeymoon period."
- Fixed insulin regimens require fewer shots but consistent schedule and eating.
- Historically, common fixed regimen is split-mixed: 2/3 of TDD in morning (1/3 as short-acting and 2/3 long-acting), and 1/3 of TDD in evening (with 1/2 as short-acting and 1/2 as long-acting), either at dinner or split between dinner and bedtime.
- Flexible insulin regimens consist of basal insulin plus a short-acting bolus for every carbohydrate meal and for high blood sugar.
- Basal dosing
  - 40–50% of TDD is given as 1 injection of a long-acting insulin such as glargine (Lantus) or detemir (Levemir).
  - Sometimes, these long-acting insulins are split into twice daily doses given ~12 hours apart.

- Boluses of short-acting insulin (lispro or aspart) are given for meals and snacks based on carbohydrate content and BGs.
  - Carbohydrate coverage (grams of carbohydrate covered by 1 unit) can be estimated by dividing the TDD to 500.
  - Hyperglycemia coverage ("corrective dose") can be estimated by dividing the TDD to 1,800 to find how much 1 unit of insulin may lower blood sugar.
- Another flexible method uses SC insulin infusion by pump that administers a continuous basal infusion.
  - Patient gives manually administered bolus doses of rapid-acting analog insulin at mealtimes and corrective doses.
  - Dosing guidelines are similar.

ONGOING CARE

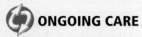

PATIENT MONITORING

- Regular appointments with diabetes specialist every 3 months to assess management:
  - HgbA1c assessment at each visit (with generally recommended goal of <7.5% for children)
  - Is diabetes interfering with emotional health, family relationships, school attendance, athletic activities, or social development?
  - Is family minimizing hospitalization risks from hypoglycemia or DKA with appropriate adjustment of insulin, recognition of lows, glucagon availability, ketone testing, and telephone contact?
  - Is family reducing long-term complication risk by keeping HgbA1c lower and by avoiding or treating other risk factors?
  - Exam: growth, weight, blood pressure, thyromegaly, liver size, pubertal status, injection/infusion sites, feet, skin lesions
- Meet with nutritionist periodically/as needed to reassess meal plan.
- Meet with psychologist or social worker as needed to address psychosocial issues.
- Regular screening for long-term complications:
  - Annual urine for microalbumin after 12 years of age, 3–5 years diabetes duration
  - Periodic lipid profile, thyroid screening (T_4, TSH or TSH and thyroid antibodies), celiac screen
  - Annual eye exam to detect early retinopathy after 10 years of age, 3–5 years diabetes duration

DIET

- Dietary education for type 1 diabetes is directed toward healthy distribution and matching of carbohydrate intake with insulin action:
  - Recommended distribution of calories: 55% from carbohydrates (mostly complex); 30% from fats; 15% from protein
  - Fixed insulin regimens require snacks spaced between meals and before bedtime.
  - Carbohydrate counting is essential for flexible insulin regimens and helpful for maintaining consistency for fixed regimens.
- Reduction of saturated and trans fats, rapidly digested carbohydrates, and salt may be beneficial in both types of diabetes.

PATIENT EDUCATION

- Home BG monitoring at least 6 times per day. Many patients will need to test more frequently: before meals, when feeling hypoglycemic or ill.
- Insulin injection and site rotation
- Oral carbohydrate for mild hypoglycemia; glucagon 0.5–1 mg IM for severe hypoglycemia (lower dose given in children <20 kg)
- Activity:
  - Frequent exercise reduces BG and insulin requirements in both types of diabetes.
  - Exercise may require extra carbohydrate intake or reduced insulin doses to prevent hypoglycemia in type 1 diabetes.
  - Detecting or preventing hypoglycemia during or after physical exercise
- Diet: carbohydrate counting
- Prevention: checking urine for ketones when blood sugar is high or child feels ill; extra insulin for ketones

COMPLICATIONS

- DKA: most common cause of hospitalization and death in type 1 diabetes in childhood. See "Diabetic Ketoacidosis."

ALERT

DKA should be treated in the emergency department or inpatient setting. The risk for morbidity and mortality due to cerebral edema or other complications of DKA is high.

- Hypoglycemia
  - This most common acute complication. Limits achievable glycemic control
  - If severe, may cause seizure, unconsciousness
- Long-term harm may be reduced by better glycemic control:
  - Nephropathy: Microalbuminuria and hypertension are 1st manifestations before adulthood.
  - Retinopathy: Blood vessel changes may occur in childhood but not vision loss.
  - Neuropathy: diminished nerve conduction velocity common; paresthesias are earliest symptoms.
  - Vasculopathy: Large vessel disease begins in childhood, but clinical effects occur in adults.
  - Prenatal harm to infants of diabetic mothers: Birth defects occur early, large size late.
  - Growth failure (Mauriac syndrome) and delayed sexual maturation
- Depression, family stress, higher divorce rate

ADDITIONAL READING

- American Diabetes Association. Clinical practice recommendations: 2013. *Diabetes Care*. 2013; 36(Suppl 1):S1.
- Atkinson MA, Eisenbarth GS, Michels AW. Type 1 diabetes. *Lancet*. 2014;383(9911):69–82.
- Chiang JL, Kirkman MS, Laffel LM, et al; Type 1 Diabetes Sourcebook Authors. Type 1 diabetes through the lifespan: a position statement of the American Diabetes Association. *Diabetes Care*. 2014;37(7):2034–2054.
- Juvenile Diabetes Research Foundation Continuous Glucose Monitoring Study Group, Tamborlane WV, Beck RW, Bode BW, et al. Continuous glucose monitoring and intensive treatment of type 1 diabetes. *N Engl J Med*. 2008;359(14):1464–1476.
- Nguyen TM, Mason KJ, Sanders CG, et al. Targeting blood glucose management in school improves glycemic control in children with poorly controlled type 1 diabetes mellitus. *J Pediatr*. 2008;153(4):575–578.
- Steinke JM, Mauer M; International Diabetic Nephropathy Study Group. Lessons learned from studies of the natural history of diabetic nephropathy in young type 1 diabetic patients. *Pediatr Endocrinol Rev*. 2008;5(Suppl 4):958–963.

CODES

ICD10

- E10.9 Type 1 diabetes mellitus without complications
- E10.8 Type 1 diabetes mellitus with unspecified complications
- E10.21 Type 1 diabetes mellitus with diabetic nephropathy

FAQ

- Q: What is the risk of diabetes in a sibling or child of a person with type 1 diabetes?
- A: It is 5–10% in 1st-degree relatives (siblings, offspring) and 40–50% in identical twins.
- Q: What are the newest management tools?
- A: Continuous glucose sensors allow patients to avoid symptomatic high and low glucoses by detecting trends, to see the outcome of management decisions, and to reduce the risk of severe nocturnal hypoglycemia. Insulin pumps using data from sensors are in development ("artificial pancreas" systems). A pump with a feature to suspend insulin delivery for low glucose detected by sensor is now available.

DIABETES MELLITUS, TYPE 2

Wendy J. Brickman

BASICS

DESCRIPTION

Hyperglycemia, fitting criteria for diabetes, in a setting of insulin resistance with insufficient insulin secretion for given insulin resistance

EPIDEMIOLOGY

- Increased prevalence over past three decades
- Type 2 diabetes mellitus (T2DM) accounts for 15–86% of newly diagnosed cases of diabetes in youth (10–19 years). Wide variation depending on population affected.
- Incidence (per 100,000 person-years, 0–19 years)
  - Pima Indians = 330
  - African American = 10
  - Non-Hispanic whites = 2.8
- Prevalence (per 100,000 youth 10–19 years)
  - Pima Indians = 5,100
  - African American = 106
  - Hispanic = 46
  - Non-Hispanic whites = 18

RISK FACTORS

- Female gender
- Ethnic minorities
- Adolescence (10–19 years)
- Pubertal
- Offspring of mothers with gestational diabetes
- Family history of type 2 diabetes
- History of the following:
  - Large for gestational age at birth
  - Intrauterine growth retardation
- Impaired fasting glucose
  - Fasting glucose 100 mg/dL (5.6 mmol/L)–125 mg/dL (6.9 mmol/L)
- Impaired glucose tolerance
  - Based on 2-hour glucose from oral glucose tolerance test (OGTT; see the following) of 140 mg/dL (7.8 mmol/L)–199 mg/dL (11 mmol/L)

PATHOPHYSIOLOGY

- Characterized by insulin resistance and beta cell dysfunction
- Insulin resistance
  - Major abnormality in youth with T2DM
  - A disorder in which tissues (muscle, hepatic, adipose) have a decreased response to insulin, mediated by abnormal phosphorylation of insulin receptor
- Ideally, a compensatory hyperinsulinemia develops to maintain euglycemia.
- In the presence of beta cell dysfunction, inadequate amounts of insulin are secreted to meet demands from insulin resistance.
- This relative deficiency in beta cell function leads to hyperglycemia and diabetes.

DIAGNOSIS

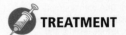

- T2DM usually presents in setting of the following:
  - Family history of type 2 diabetes
  - Overweight or obesity (BMI ≥85th percentile for age, gender)
  - Other abnormalities associated with insulin resistance (i.e., acanthosis nigricans)
  - Residual (yet abnormal) beta cell function
  - No diabetes autoimmunity

HISTORY

- Asymptomatic (most common)
- Polyuria
- Polydipsia
- Weight loss
- Blurry vision
- Increase in nocturia
- Improvement in acanthosis nigricans
- Family history of type 2 diabetes
- Maternal gestational diabetes
- Medications associated with hyperglycemia:
  - For example: glucocorticoid, growth hormone, atypical psychotics, tacrolimus

PHYSICAL EXAM

- Overweight (BMI ≥85th percentile but <95th percentile) or obesity (BMI ≥95th percentile)
- Hypertension
- Acanthosis nigricans
- Vaginal candidiasis

DIAGNOSTIC TESTS & INTERPRETATION

Lab

- Diagnosis of diabetes mellitus:
  - HgbA1c ≥6.5%
    - Using NGSP-certified method
    - False negatives when increased blood cell turnover is present
  - Fasting glucose ≥126 mg/dL (7 mmol/L)
  - 2-hour OGTT glucose ≥200 mg/dL (11.1 mmol/L)
    - At time 0, give oral glucose 1.75 g/kg (maximum dose 75 g) over 5 minutes.
    - At time 120 minutes, measure glucose.
    - If asymptomatic, do 2nd OGTT on a subsequent day to confirm.
  - Random glucose >200 mg/dL with symptoms of hyperglycemia
- Distinguish type 1 from type 2 diabetes.
  - C-peptide or insulin in setting of hyperglycemia
    - Normal or elevated in type 2 diabetes
    - Low C-peptide or insulin does not rule out type 2 diabetes.
  - Diabetes autoimmune panel
    - Negative usually in type 2 diabetes
    - Pancreatic autoantibodies; insulin, islet cell, IA-2, GAD, ZnT8
- Evaluate for acute complications of diabetic ketoacidosis (DKA) and/or hyperglycemic hyperosmolar state (HHS).
  - Check urine for ketones.
  - If urine ketones present (in setting of hyperglycemia), check for DKA.
    - Venous gas: pH <7.30
    - Metabolic panel: HCO_3^- <15 mEq/L
  - If urine ketones negative or low and patient appears ill, check for HHS.
    - Serum glucose: >600 mg/dL (33 mmol/L)
    - Serum osmolality: >330 mOsm/kg
    - Metabolic panel: HCO_3^- >15 mEq/L

DIFFERENTIAL DIAGNOSIS

- Type 1 diabetes
- Atypical diabetes
- Medication-induced diabetes
- Maturity onset diabetes of youth (MODY)
  - Monogenic disorders of glucose regulation
  - Abnormalities of beta cell function common
  - However, youth can be overweight or obese.
  - Genetic testing for MODY is available.
- Renal glycosuria
- Stress-induced hyperglycemia

ALERT

Treat youth with possible type 2 diabetes with insulin, as if they have type 1 diabetes, until clinical course and laboratory findings prove otherwise.

TREATMENT

- Treatment will focus on youth presenting with type 2 diabetes who don't have DKA or HHS.
- Goal of treatment is glucose regulation in order to 1) limit hypoglycemia and hyperglycemia and 2) minimize and delay onset of microvascular and macrovascular disease.

MEDICATION

Insulin

- Initiate treatment with insulin unless clinical picture and laboratory studies support type 2 diabetes and not type 1 diabetes.
- If diagnosis is type 2 diabetes, but initial glucose is >250 mg/dL or HgbA1c ≥9%, insulin therapy is still recommended.
- Initiate basal-bolus insulin regimen (may need to individualize)
  - Total daily dose 0.5–1.0 unit/kg/day (TDD)
  - 40% in long-acting (detemir, glargine) usually given at bedtime
  - For meals and snacks, calculate number of carbohydrates to be eaten and cover with short-acting insulin (lispro, aspart, glulisine).
    - Calculate carbohydrate coverage: 1 unit of insulin for every X grams of carbohydrates, often start with X = 500/TDD.
  - For hyperglycemia prior to mealtimes, give correction doses of short-acting insulin by using the sensitivity factor.
    - Insulin sensitivity factor: 1 unit of insulin will drop glucose by X, often start with X = 1800/TDD.
    - Correct until goal blood glucose is reached: begin with goal 120–150 mg/dL.
- Insulin regimen outlined above gives increased flexibility and decreased risk of hypoglycemia with at least 4 injections a day.

- When hyperglycemia is improved and diagnostic tests supportive of type 2 diabetes, introduce metformin and attempt insulin wean.
- Insulin regimen needs to be tailored to the patient and family, and often alternative regimens with fewer injections but more rigid eating schedules and higher risk of hypoglycemia are preferred.
  - Two injections per day: premixed insulin
    - 2/3 of TDD with breakfast
    - 1/3 of TDD with dinner
  - Three injections per day: split-mixed
    - 2/3 of TDD with breakfast (2/3 NPH, 1/3 short-acting)
    - 1/9 of TDD with dinner (short-acting)
    - 2/9 of TDD at bedtime (NPH)
- Side effect of all insulin regimens is hypoglycemia, especially with increased activity, decreased oral intake, addition of oral antihyperglycemic. Adjust dose to prevent.

Metformin

- Only FDA-approved medication for type 2 diabetes in youth
- First line of therapy for youth with type 2 diabetes with random glucose <250 mg/dL and HgbA1c <9%
- Begin at 500 mg once a day. Increase by 500 mg every 1–2 weeks as tolerated to reach goal of 2,000 mg daily.
- Side effects:
  - Short-term: anorexia, flatus, abdominal pain
  - Long-term: lactic acidosis (avoid with renal failure, hypoxia, liver disease) and vitamin B_{12} deficiency
  - Stop 48 hours prior to elective surgery or contrast study with dye.

ADDITIONAL TREATMENT

Weight management

- Physical activity
  - 60 minutes moderate to vigorous activity a day
  - Can be split throughout the day
  - Start with shorter periods of daily activity and gradually increase to 60-minute goal.
  - Treat orthopedic, respiratory issues.
  - Individualize plan: walking to formal sports.
- Sedentary activity
  - Decrease sedentary activity.
  - Limit screen time (handheld devices, computers, television) to <2 hours a day.
  - Remove televisions/screens from bedrooms.
- Nutrition
  - Healthy eating choices
  - Guidelines from *Pediatric Weight Management Evidence-based Nutrition Practice Guidelines*, Academy of Nutrition and Dietetics
- Surgical intervention (i.e., gastric bypass)
  - Rarely, as part of weight loss program

ONGOING CARE

FOLLOW-UP RECOMMENDATIONS

- Blood glucose monitoring
  - Insulin Rx: preprandial, bedtime
  - Oral medication: Consider fasting, bedtime.
    - Increase when ill, changing dose, concern for low or high glucose.
    - Decrease when stable, in good control.
- Clinic visit with HgbA1c every 3 months
- Goal HgbA1c <7% (may need to individualize); modify treatment as needed.
- Recent study suggests adolescents fail metformin monotherapy rapidly. May need to add additional therapy to reach goals
- Address postprandial glucose excursions to possibly limit risk of macrovascular disease.
- Suggestions for modifying treatment regimen:
  - Introduce long-acting insulin at night.
  - Introduce short-acting insulin at meals.
  - Introduce additional oral antihyperglycemic (not FDA-approved, many with concerns for longer term complications; i.e., rosiglitazone).
- Prevention of DKA and HHS by increasing adherence to treatment plan
- Monitor for hypoglycemia and modify regimens to decrease episodes.
- Little is known regarding disease course in adolescents with T2DM. The SEARCH and TODAY studies have increased our knowledge of prevalence of abnormalities and raised concern for progression of microvascular and risks for macrovascular disease early in course of T2DM.
- Microvascular disease has been noted at presentation or early in course of T2DM.
- Recommendations based on adults (in addition to improving glucose control)
  - Retinopathy
    - Examination at diagnosis, then annually
    - Tx includes laser photocoagulation
  - Microalbuminuria
    - Measure at diagnosis, then annually.
    - Abnormal: random: 30–200 mg/kg
    - Perform timed overnight collection. Need 2/3 abnormal samples: 20–199 mcg/min.
    - Treat with ACE inhibitor until microalbumin excretion is normalized.
  - Peripheral neuropathy
    - Examination at diagnosis, then annually
    - Changes in sensation in feet, leg
  - Autonomic neuropathy
    - Assess at diagnosis, then annually.
    - May present as tachycardia, orthostasis, gastroparesis
  - Cardiovascular disease
    - Optimize therapy for hypertension, dyslipidemia, smoking cessation.

ISSUES FOR REFERRAL

- Other disorders are commonly associated with type 2 diabetes and may contribute to development of complications.
- If present, referral/treatment should occur:
  - Hypertension
  - Dyslipidemia
  - Depression
  - Obstructive sleep apnea
  - Nonalcoholic fatty liver disease
  - Orthopedic abnormalities (i.e., SCFE)
  - Polycystic ovary syndrome
  - Dental abnormalities

ADDITIONAL READING

- American Diabetes Association. Standards of medical care in diabetes—2014. *Diabetes Care*. 2014;37(Suppl 1):S14–S80. doi:10.2337/dc14-S014.
- Copeland KC, Silverstein J, Moore KR, et al. Management of newly diagnosed type 2 diabetes mellitus (T2DM) in children and adolescents. *Pediatrics*. 2013;131(5):364–382. doi:10.1542/peds.2012-3494.
- Fazeli Farsani S, van der Aa MP, van der Vorst MM, et al. Global trends in the incidence and prevalence of type 2 diabetes in children and adolescents: a systematic review and evaluation of methodological approaches. *Diabetologia*. 2013;56(7):1471–1488. doi:10.1007/s00125-013-2915-z.
- Springer SC, Silverstein J, Copeland K, et al. Management of type 2 diabetes mellitus in children and adolescents. *Pediatrics*. 2013;131(2):e648–e663. doi:10.1542/peds.2012-3496.
- TODAY Study Group, Zeitler P, Hirst K, et al. A clinical trial to maintain glycemic control in youth with type 2 diabetes. *N Engl J Med*. 2012;366(24):2247–2256.
- Writing Group for the SEARCH for Diabetes in Youth Study Group, Dabelea D, Bell RA, et al. Incidence of diabetes in youth in the United States. *JAMA*. 2007;297(24):2716–2724.

CODES

ICD10

- E11.9 Type 2 diabetes mellitus without complications
- Z83.3 Family history of diabetes mellitus
- E11.51 Type 2 diabetes w diabetic peripheral angiopath w/o gangrene

FAQ

- Q: What are some of the challenges of follow-up care in youth with type 2 diabetes?
- A: Possible challenges include the following:
  - Competing financial/time constraints
  - Adolescent age
  - Lack of symptoms from hyperglycemia and early complications of hyperglycemia
  - Lack of social support networks
  - Pervasiveness of type 2 diabetes in families

DIABETIC KETOACIDOSIS

Nicole S. Glaser

BASICS

DESCRIPTION
- Severe metabolic derangement in patients with diabetes mellitus (DM) secondary to insulin deficiency and/or stress hormone excess
- Clinical features include hyperglycemia, ketosis, metabolic acidosis, dehydration, and electrolyte deficits.

EPIDEMIOLOGY
Incidence
- Diabetes ketoacidosis (DKA) occurs more commonly in type 1 DM but can also occur in type 2 DM.
- 20–40% of children with new-onset type 1 DM present in DKA.
- Risk of DKA in established type 1 DM is 1–10% per patient per year (most episodes caused by insulin omission/diabetes mismanagement).
- DKA accounts for majority of diabetes-related deaths in childhood (most secondary to cerebral edema/brain injury).

RISK FACTORS
- For type 1 DM presenting as DKA:
  - Very young children (<5 years)
  - Ethnic minority
  - Inadequate health insurance
  - A missed diagnosis of DM in preceding clinic visits is frequent in DKA patients (~35%).
- For DKA in established diabetes:
  - Adolescence
  - Lack of health insurance
  - Poor glycemic control
  - Ethnic minority
  - Low socioeconomic status (SES).

GENERAL PREVENTION
- Prompt diagnosis of new-onset diabetes (e.g., urinalysis in patients with poor weight gain, polyuria, flulike symptoms/vomiting)
- Patient/parental education regarding ketone testing (with any symptoms of illness or unexplained high blood glucose level)
- Strict supervision of long-acting (glargine, detemir) insulin injections by parents
- Detection and avoidance of insulin pump interruptions by frequent blood glucose testing and strict protocols for changing infusion sets

PATHOPHYSIOLOGY
- Excess of counterregulatory "stress" hormone concentrations (glucagon, cortisol, and epinephrine) in relation to insulin concentrations occurs, either as a result of insulin absence (new-onset diabetes or insulin omission) or illness (raising stress hormone levels)
- Imbalance between counterregulatory hormones and insulin results in increased glycogenolysis and gluconeogenesis and decreased peripheral glucose uptake (causing hyperglycemia) as well as lipolysis and ketogenesis (causing ketosis).
- Hyperglycemia causes osmotic diuresis resulting in dehydration and electrolyte losses.
- Ketogenesis results in metabolic acidosis, causing vomiting and tachypnea.
- Dehydration causes poor tissue perfusion, raising lactate levels and is contributing to metabolic acidosis.

ETIOLOGY
- Insulin deficiency
  - New diagnosis of diabetes
  - Insulin omission (diabetes mismanagement or insulin pump malfunction)
- Acute illness (leading to rise in counterregulatory hormone levels)

COMMONLY ASSOCIATED CONDITIONS
- Acute illness as a precipitating factor
- Autoimmune disorders (especially hypothyroidism) for persons with type 1 DM

DIAGNOSIS

HISTORY
- Symptoms of new-onset diabetes (polyuria, polydipsia, weight loss)
- Nausea, vomiting, abdominal pain, weakness, lethargy

PHYSICAL EXAM
- Vital signs: tachycardia, tachypnea (deep, "Kussmaul" respirations), occasional hypothermia
- Dehydration: dry mucous membranes, sunken eyes, poor distal perfusion
- Fruity breath odor
- Abdominal tenderness and decreased bowel sounds (intestinal ileus)
- Altered mental status, lethargy, obtundation

DIAGNOSTIC TESTS & INTERPRETATION
Lab
- Glucose: >200 mg/dL (usual range 200–1,200 mg/dL)
- Urinalysis: glucosuria and ketonuria
- Electrolytes: total body depletion of sodium, chloride, potassium, phosphate, calcium, magnesium (*depletion generally not reflected in serum electrolyte concentrations which may be low, normal, or high at presentation*)
- Sodium: initial Na usually normal or low
  - Hyperglycemia depresses serum Na by about 1.6 mEq/L for every 100 mg/dL–elevation in glucose greater than 100 mg/dL.
  - Elevated Na at presentation implies extreme dehydration.
- Potassium: Initial serum levels typically normal or elevated, may fall rapidly with therapy.
- Serum bicarbonate (total CO_2) is low, consistent with metabolic acidosis.
  - Bicarbonate <18 mEq/L suggests pH <7.3.
  - Bicarbonate <10 mEq/L suggests pH <7.1.
- Phosphate: typically normal or slightly elevated at presentation
- Blood pH low (<7.3) due to metabolic acidosis. Low P_{CO_2} secondary to respiratory compensation for metabolic acidosis
- CBC: White blood cell counts frequently elevated and may be left shifted (even in the absence of infection). Hematocrit may be elevated due to hemoconcentration.
- Serum ketones (β-hydroxybutyrate) are elevated (typically >5 mmol/L).
- Liver enzymes (ALT, AST) may be mildly elevated.
- Amylase and lipase are often mildly elevated.

DIFFERENTIAL DIAGNOSIS
- Gastroenteritis
- Acute abdomen (pancreatitis, appendicitis, bowel ischemia)
- UTI
- Pneumonia, bronchiolitis
- Stress hyperglycemia (particularly during gastroenteritis in young children—ketosis may also be present due to lack of oral intake and may be difficult to differentiate from DKA)
- Salicylate ingestion
- Rare inborn errors of ketolysis (succinyl-CoA: 3-ketoacid CoA transferase deficiency)

TREATMENT

GENERAL MEASURES

Initial emergency treatment consists of fluid resuscitation to insure hemodynamic stability. Most DKA patients require admission to a pediatric critical care unit or other unit with similar capabilities.

ISSUES FOR REFERRAL

The pediatric endocrinology service should be advised of all DKA admissions. New-onset diabetes patients will require diabetes education. Patients with recurrent DKA may require reeducation or other counseling.

INPATIENT CONSIDERATIONS

IV Fluids

- Initial isotonic IV fluid bolus (0.9% saline) of 10–20 cc/kg—may be repeated as necessary to restore perfusion and hemodynamic stability.
- IV fluid rate after initial bolus(es)
  - Average fluid deficit is ~7% of body weight.
  - Replace deficit evenly over 24–48 hours.
  - Add maintenance fluids to deficit replacement (minus initial boluses) to calculate total rate.
  - Replacement of ongoing urinary fluid losses is generally unnecessary, but urine output should be monitored.
  - Urine output and specific gravity do not reflect state of hydration.
  - Adjust fluid infusion rate based on fluid intake and output balance, clinical measures of perfusion, and laboratory indicators of hydration.
- Composition of IV fluids:
  - After initial isotonic fluid bolus(es), IV fluids should consist of 0.45–0.9% saline.
  - Potassium replacement is essential and should be added to IV fluids as soon as renal failure or extreme hyperkalemia is ruled out.
  - Typical initial K replacement is 40 mEq/L, using 1/2 KCl and 1/2 K phosphate.
  - Dextrose should be added to IV fluids when serum glucose level is below ~250 mg/dL. The "2 bag method" (see reference) is ideal.
  - Dextrose concentrations in IV fluids should be adjusted to maintain serum glucose in the range of 100–200 mg/dL. Rates of insulin infusion generally should not be decreased until acidosis resolves.

Insulin

- Insulin treatment should begin after initial isotonic fluid bolus(es).
- Insulin should be administered via continuous IV infusion at a rate of 0.1 units/kg/h.
- An initial insulin "bolus" or "loading dose" is not necessary.

Other

Treatment with bicarbonate is generally unnecessary and has been associated with increased risk of cerebral edema.

ONGOING CARE

PATIENT MONITORING

- Recommended monitoring:
  - Frequent (at least hourly) assessment of mental status and perfusion
  - Hourly vital signs
  - Cardiac monitor and pulse oximeter
  - Hourly intake and output
  - Hourly fingerstick or serum glucose
  - Electrolytes and venous blood gas every 2–4 hours
  - Ca, Mg, phosphate every 4–6 hours

PROGNOSIS

Mortality of DKA in children is ~0.2–0.3%, (most frequently caused by cerebral edema/ cerebral injury).

COMPLICATIONS

- Cerebral injury is the most frequent DKA-related cause of death (57–87% of DKA deaths).
  - Patients at highest risk for cerebral injury are those with the most severe dehydration and acidosis (often younger children).
  - The cause of brain injury in DKA is unclear but may be related to reduced cerebral perfusion during untreated DKA, followed by injury related to reperfusion.
  - Commonly occurs 2–12 hours after starting treatment with insulin and saline
    - Symptoms may include mental status changes in association with severe headache, recurrence of vomiting, inappropriate slowing of heart rate or hypertension.
    - Loss of consciousness, seizures, apnea, or signs of increased intracranial pressure may also occur.
  - Treatment of suspected cerebral edema includes mannitol (0.5–1 g/kg by IV infusion over 15 minutes) or hypertonic saline.
  - Cerebral imaging studies should be done to evaluate edema or other signs of cerebral injury, but treatment should not be delayed to obtain imaging studies.
- Cardiovascular collapse from shock is rare and usually due to delayed or inadequate IV fluids.
- Other complications:
  - Hypokalemia is frequent and can be avoided with frequent serum K reassessments and adjustment of potassium content of IV fluids.
  - Hypoglycemia may occur but can be avoided with frequent glucose checks and adjustment of dextrose concentration of IV fluids.
  - Mild hypophosphatemia is common, but severe hypophosphatemia is rare. Severe hypophosphatemia has been associated with rhabdomyolysis and hemolytic anemia.
  - Hyperchloremic acidosis may occur, particularly with higher NaCl concentrations in IV fluids.
  - Other rare complications include the following:
    - Pulmonary edema or acute respiratory distress syndrome (ARDS)
    - Pneumomediastinum from hyperventilation
    - Arrhythmias due to electrolyte disturbances
    - Thrombosis, especially at central line site
    - Disseminated intravascular coagulation (DIC)
    - Rhinocerebral mucormycosis
    - Pancreatitis

ADDITIONAL READING

- Glaser N. Cerebral injury and cerebral edema in children with diabetic ketoacidosis: could cerebral ischemia and reperfusion injury be involved? *Pediatric Diabetes*. 2009;10(8):534–541.
- Glaser N, Barnett P, McCaslin I, et al. Risk factors for cerebral edema in children with diabetic ketoacidosis. *N Engl J Med*. 2001;344(4):264–269.
- Orlowski JP, Cramer CL, Fiallos MR. Diabetic ketoacidosis in the pediatric ICU. *Pediatr Clin North Am*. 2008;55(3):577–587.
- Wolfsdorf JI, Allgrove J, Craig ME, et al. Diabetic ketoacidosis and hyperglycemic hyperosmolar state. *Pediatr Diabetes*. 2014;(15)(Suppl 20):154–179. doi:10.1111/pedi.12165

D

CODES

ICD10

- E10.10 Type 1 diabetes mellitus with ketoacidosis without coma
- E13.10 Oth diabetes mellitus with ketoacidosis without coma

FAQ

- Q: Is DKA in children with known diabetes usually caused by infection or other illness?
- A: Diabetes mismanagement resulting in inappropriate insulin omission is a far more frequent cause of DKA in children than infection. It is generally unnecessary to evaluate children with DKA for infection unless fever or other symptoms of infection are present.
- Q: Does rapid infusion of intravenous fluids or excessive administration of insulin cause cerebral edema in DKA?
- A: At present, neither the IV fluid administration rate nor the rate of insulin administration has been convincingly shown to increase the risk of DKA-related cerebral edema. Recent data suggest that cerebral edema is more likely related to alterations in cerebral perfusion during DKA, and that rates of fluid and insulin administration (within a reasonable range) do not play a primary role.
- Q: How can DKA episodes in children with diabetes be prevented?
- A: Greater supervision of diabetes care by parents or guardians can decrease the likelihood of insulin omission. Parents should also be instructed to test for ketones at the first sign of any illness or with unexplained high glucose levels and to contact the diabetes care team immediately if ketones are positive.

DIAPER RASH

Jocelyn H. Schiller

BASICS

DESCRIPTION

Diaper dermatitis is a general term used to describe any inflammatory skin rash that develops in the perineal region. Also known as diaper or napkin rash, there are several causes of diaper dermatitis. Most often, diaper rash is caused by an acute irritant contact dermatitis, which is the focus of this chapter.

ALERT

- Severe cases of diaper dermatitis may be complicated by bacterial or fungal infection which may require treatment with topical or systemic antibiotics and/or antifungals.
- If severe cases fail to respond to conventional therapies, consider other diagnoses such as Langerhans cell histiocytosis, acrodermatitis enteropathica, or seborrheic dermatitis.

EPIDEMIOLOGY

Incidence

- The reported incidence varies worldwide due to differences in diaper use, toilet training, hygiene, and child-rearing practices.
- Can develop in the 1st week of life, but unlikely once the child is no longer in diapers

Prevalence

- Estimated prevalence ranges from 7 to 35%.

RISK FACTORS

- Diarrhea increases the risk of irritant diaper rash.
- The presence of oral thrush or recent antibiotic use increases the risk of secondary *Candida albicans* infection.
- Formula-fed infants may have higher risk of diaper dermatitis due to higher stool pH.

GENERAL PREVENTION

- Frequent diaper changes and proper skin care help prevent diaper rash.
- Diapers should be changed as often as every 2 hours or sooner if diaper is wet and/or soiled.
- Super absorbent diapers (disposable diapers containing gelling materials) keep moisture away from skin and may prevent diaper dermatitis compared to cloth diapers.
- Some experts recommend soft cloths and water for cleansing due to preservatives in baby wipes. As manufacturers have decreased the number of additives, contact dermatitis due to wipes has become less common.
- Petrolatum and/or zinc oxide provide effective barriers against potential perineal skin irritants and moisture. Several authors advise caregivers to refrain from rubbing barrier products off completely during diaper changes to prevent further skin damage.

ETIOLOGY

The pathophysiology is multifactorial, including moisture, friction, warmth, urine and feces.

- Friction: Rubbing of wet diapers against exposed skin can result in chafing, maceration, and irritation.
- Moisture trapped against skin causes increased permeability and susceptibility to damage from friction.
- Irritation: Urine raises the pH which activates fecal enzymes resulting in skin damage.
- As the skin barrier breaks down, microbes are more likely to cause a secondary infection.
  - Common causes of secondary infections include *C. albicans*, group A β-hemolytic *Streptococcus*, and *Staphylococcus aureus*.

DIAGNOSIS

HISTORY

- Associated symptoms: Acute or chronic diarrhea suggests a primary irritant dermatitis.
- The presence of oral thrush or recent antibiotic use increases the risk of secondary *C. albicans* infection. Presence of the rash for >3 days also increases likelihood of candidal infection.
- Treatment with topical corticosteroid, antifungal, or antibacterial products can change the appearance of the rash.
- Chemicals, dyes, and fragrances in lotions, wipes, diapers, and detergents can cause irritant or allergic contact dermatitis.
- Infrequent or poor hygiene can result in diaper rash, whereas excessive bathing may result in increased friction on the skin and worsening of a preexisting rash.
- Moderate to severe rashes and rashes infected with group A β-hemolytic *Streptococcus* or *Staphylococcus aureus* cause discomfort for the child.

PHYSICAL EXAM

- Ranges from asymptomatic, generalized erythema to skin breakdown leading to an open wound
- Irritant and allergic dermatitis occurs on skin surfaces in direct contact with the diaper, urine, and feces. Skinfolds are typically spared.
  - Affected intertriginous areas suggest seborrheic dermatitis, candidal infection, or group A β-hemolytic *Streptococcus* infection.
  - Perianal rashes suggest group A β-hemolytic *Streptococcus* (more common) or *S. aureus* (less common) infection.
- The morphology of the dermatitis is important:
  - Well-demarcated, shiny, erosive, erythematous perianal patches suggest group A β-hemolytic *Streptococcus*.
  - Scattered inflammatory papules or pustules suggest *S. aureus*.
  - Erythematous patches with peripheral erythematous papules (satellite lesions) suggest candidal infection.
  - Greasy erythema and scaling suggests seborrheic dermatitis.
- A complete physical exam may reveal other features of the underlying diagnosis:
  - Scalp seborrhea (cradle cap) suggests seborrheic dermatitis.
  - Thrush (oral candidiasis) raises the possibility of a candidal infection.
  - Hepatosplenomegaly suggests Langerhans cell histiocytosis.

DIAGNOSTIC TESTS & INTERPRETATION

Lab

- Rarely helpful
- Candidal infections can be verified by a potassium hydroxide preparation or fungal culture of skin scraping if diagnosis is unclear.
- Group A β-hemolytic *Streptococcus* and *S. aureus* infection can be confirmed by swabbing affected area for bacterial culture.

Pathologic Findings

- Skin biopsy is rarely required unless the rash is atypical and unresponsive to therapy.
- Helpful in diagnosing psoriasis, Langerhans cell histiocytosis, or granuloma gluteale infantum

DIFFERENTIAL DIAGNOSIS

- Candidal dermatitis: Irritant dermatitis may become secondarily infected with *C. albicans*, which results in beefy red plaques with satellite lesions and superficial pustules. Common during or after antibiotic use.
- Allergic contact dermatitis: can result from allergens in the diaper, wipes, or topical creams including dyes, detergents, fragrances, or elastic
- Impetigo: due to group A β-hemolytic *Streptococcus* (common) or *S. aureus* (less common): 1–2 mm pustules and honey-colored, crusted erosions. Bullous impetigo appears as large, fluid-filled bullae.
- Perianal group A β-hemolytic *Streptococcus* presents as bright red, sharply demarcated perianal rash with pain or pruritus. May also have streptococcal pharyngitis.
- Seborrheic dermatitis: associated with scalp, face, and skinfold involvement. In the diaper region, it is characterized by well-circumscribed erythematous papules and plagues.
- Atopic dermatitis: usually spares the diaper region due to the moist environment. If affected, characterized by increased skin lines and excoriations due to scratching.
- Psoriasis: may involve the diaper area either exclusively or may occur in the setting of more diffuse presentation, including other intertriginous areas and the face and scalp. Presents with sharply demarcated erythematous and silvery scaly papules and plaques.
- Scabies: Pruritic, erythematous papules and nodules may involve the genitalia, abdomen, web spaces of extremities, and axilla; often there is a history of multiple affected family members and more widespread involvement.

- Herpes simplex virus may manifest as grouped vesicular, papular, or pustular lesions. May be transmitted through sexual contact or herpetic whitlow.
- Child abuse: An unusual history or morphology suggests the possibility of abuse, especially if the lesions appear geometric or resemble scalds, burns, or bruises or if sexually transmitted disease diagnosed.
- Langerhans cell histiocytosis: usually presents with multiple reddish-brown crusted papules and/or vesicles and petechiae in conjunction with hepatosplenomegaly and anemia
- Acrodermatitis enteropathica, which is caused by impaired zinc metabolism (either inherited or acquired), leads to an erosive acrodermatitis involving the face in a perioral and periocular distribution, the diaper area, and the hands and feet.
- Jacquet erosive diaper dermatitis is rare and likely represents severe irritant diaper dermatitis. Characterized by well-demarcated papules, nodules, and punched out ulcerations.
- Granuloma gluteale infantum is a rare, benign inflammatory dermatosis associated with use of high-potency topical corticosteroids. Characterized by reddish-purple nodules.

TREATMENT

ADDITIONAL TREATMENT

General Measures

- Similar to primary prevention, frequent diaper changes and proper skin care are the primary treatments for diaper dermatitis.
- Skin should be gently washed with a mild cleanser and/or infant wipe and patted dry or air-dried. Vigorous rubbing of the skin or use of washcloths may cause further irritation and skin breakdown.
- Frequent diaper changes are helpful in minimizing exposure to irritants.
- If feasible, remove diaper and expose skin to air to avoid friction and trapped moisture.
- Routine use of a barrier ointment and pastes such as zinc oxide with each diaper change is recommended. Barriers should be applied thickly and can be covered with petroleum jelly to prevent sticking to the diaper.
- Candidal infections should be treated with topical antifungal cream such as nystatin, miconazole, ketoconazole, or clotrimazole cream.
- If secondary bacterial infection is present, topical antibiotics such as mupirocin or oral antibiotics are necessary. Neomycin and bacitracin can incite an allergic contact dermatitis, so they should be avoided.
- Low-potency topical steroids, such as hydrocortisone and hydrocortisone acetate, may be used sparingly in moderate to severe cases.
- Topical application of sucralfate suspension can be useful in recalcitrant cases. It acts as a physical barrier and has antibacterial activity.

ALERT

- Mid- to high-potency topical corticosteroids should not be used because absorption is increased in areas of thin skin and under occlusion. Skin atrophy or systemic effects may result.
- Similarly, prolonged use of any potency topical steroids (>7 days) in the diaper area should be avoided.
- Combination topical corticosteroids and antifungal creams should not be used because these contain mid- to high-potency corticosteroids. Separate corticosteroid and antifungal creams allow the discontinuation of corticosteroid earlier (when the rash starts to improve) while continuing antifungal until rash resolves.
- Products containing boric acid, camphor, phenol, benzocaine, and salicylates should be avoided because of the potential for systemic toxicity.
- Use of powders such as talcum is controversial. Powders can reduce moisture and friction but pose the risk of accidental aspiration.

ONGOING CARE

FOLLOW-UP RECOMMENDATIONS

Patient Monitoring

With proper care, the rash should improve within 4–7 days. If it does not resolve with appropriate treatment, other causes must be sought.

PROGNOSIS

- Diaper dermatitis usually resolves with the institution of appropriate skin care and the treatment of any underlying cause.
- Irritant diaper dermatitis resolves once the child is potty trained.

COMPLICATIONS

- Generally no longer term complications, although secondary bacterial or fungal infections may lead to ulceration.
- Chronic topical corticosteroid use in diaper area may lead to skin atrophy or systemic effects.
- Some experience postinflammatory hypo- or hyperpigmentation that is typically self-limited.

ADDITIONAL READING

- Adam R. Skin care of the diaper area. *Pediatr Dermatol*. 2008;25(4):427–433.
- Kazaks EL, Lane AT. Diaper dermatitis. *Pediatr Clin North Am*. 2000;47(4):909–919.
- Ravanfar P, Wallace JS, Pace NC. Diaper dermatitis: a review and update. *Curr Opin Pediatr*. 2012;24(4):472–479.
- Scheinfeld N. Diaper dermatitis: a review and brief survey of eruptions of the diaper area. *Am J Clin Dermatol*. 2005;6(5):273–281.

CODES

ICD10

- L22 Diaper dermatitis
- B37.2 Candidiasis of skin and nail

FAQ

- Q: Should I switch from cloth to disposable diapers?
- A: This is controversial, although there are some studies that indicate that the superabsorbent disposable diapers may be better for preventing diaper rashes. Cloth diapers used with plastic outer layer probably irritate the skin more because they trap moisture against the skin. Frequent changing of diapers and the use of a barrier paste are very helpful in preventing diaper rash.
- Q: Is the diaper rash due to not keeping the skin clean enough?
- A: Although stool and urine may release enzymes that help break down skin integrity, vigorous and frequent scrubbing with relatively abrasive materials on the damaged skin can be more harmful. This rough cleaning allows introduction of bacteria and yeast into the skin and results in a diaper rash. Gentle cleaning materials should be used. It is not usually necessary to clean the skin of barrier ointments every time; rather, patting the infant dry with a soft cloth or baby wipe, gently reapplying barrier products, and then replacing the diaper is all that is generally required.

DIAPHRAGMATIC HERNIA (CONGENITAL)

Ngoc P. Ly • Fiona Marion

BASICS

DESCRIPTION

- Defect in the diaphragm allowing herniation of abdominal contents into the thoracic cavity, causing varying degrees of pulmonary hypoplasia
- There are 4 types of congenital diaphragmatic hernia (CDH):
  - Bochdalek hernia (posterolateral location)
  - Morgagni hernia (lateral retrosternal location)
  - Pars sternalis (medial retrosternal)
  - Anterolateral

EPIDEMIOLOGY

- 1:2,000–5,000 live births
- Left sided in 85–90%
- Right-sided and bilateral defects less common
- Familial recurrence 2%

PATHOPHYSIOLOGY

- Diaphragm arises from 4 elements and is complete by 8 weeks' gestation.
  - Septum transversum, which becomes the central tendon of the diaphragm
  - Pleuroperiotoneal membranes, which extend from the lateral body wall and fuse with the septum transversum and esophageal mesentery
  - Mesentery of the esophagus, which becomes the crura of the diaphragm
  - Lateral body wall from which myocytes migrate to muscularize the diaphragm
- Posterolateral (Bochdalek defect) in 70%, anterior (Morgagni) in 25–30%, central in 2–5%
- Main problem concerns pulmonary hypoplasia, which results in pulmonary hypertension.
  - Smaller lungs with fewer airway branches, fewer alveoli per terminal lung unit, and decreased surfactant production
  - Decreased pulmonary vascular surface area and smaller muscular arterioles with abnormal vasoreactivity results in pulmonary hypertension.
- Both ipsilateral and contralateral lungs are hypoplastic, worse on ipsilateral side.
- Degree of pulmonary hypoplasia and pulmonary hypertension determines illness severity both in acute and chronic settings.

ETIOLOGY

- Unknown
- Experimental rat models suggest role of vitamin A deficiency in pathogenesis.

COMMONLY ASSOCIATED CONDITIONS

- 40–50% of cases associated with another type of congenital malformation
  - Cardiac: 10–35%
  - Genitourinary: 23%
  - Gastrointestinal malformations: 14%
  - Central nervous system abnormalities: 10%
- Estimated that 10% of patients with associated congenital anomalies have a syndrome
- Associated syndromes include Beckwith-Wiedemann and trisomies 13, 18, and 21.

DIAGNOSIS

HISTORY

- Prenatal imaging and follow-up testing:
  - CDH detected by prenatal ultrasound in >70% cases
  - Larger defects easier to detect by ultrasound. Thus, prognosis is poorer in those CDH cases detected antenatally.
  - Magnetic resonance imaging (MRI) can be used to confirm the diagnosis and may predict degree of pulmonary hypoplasia by estimation of lung volume.
  - Amniocentesis and genetic consultation to screen for chromosomal anomalies advised
  - Important to evaluate for associated congenital abnormalities to guide management
- During the prenatal period, the degree of pulmonary hypoplasia and thus prognosis may be determined by the following:
  - Observed/expected lung-to-head ratio as determined by ultrasound
  - Observed/expected fetal lung volume ratio by fetal MRI
  - Presence of liver in thorax implies worse prognosis.
- Fetal surgery is a possibility for large lesions; however, results have been disappointing.
- Postnatal history
  - Large defects present at birth with respiratory distress.
  - May be easily identified on chest radiograph; however, CT scan may be required to confirm the diagnosis.
  - Smaller defects may be undetected until late childhood/adolescence or even adulthood.
  - Symptoms may include the following:
    - Recurrent cough
    - Recurrent chest infections
    - Intestinal obstruction
    - Feeding intolerance

PHYSICAL EXAM

- Scaphoid abdomen (abdominal contents in thoracic cavity) and asymmetry of chest wall
- Decreased breath sounds with dullness to percussion on the affected side
- Bowel sounds heard in the chest
- Heart sounds shifted to the contralateral chest

DIAGNOSTIC TESTS & INTERPRETATION

Imaging

- Chest radiograph (CXR)
  - Opacified hemithorax with contralateral shift of mediastinum
  - Decreased lung volumes
  - Esophageal portion of nasogastric tube deviated toward opposite side
  - May see loops of bowel in the thoracic cavity
  - Bowel remaining in the abdomen usually gasless

ALERT

- CXR findings in the newborn period may be subtle. In addition, small CDH defects may present outside of newborn period.

- Echocardiogram
  - Right ventricular function is an important determinant of illness severity.
  - Can estimate degree of pulmonary hypertension
  - Determine presence of associated congenital cardiac defects

Lab

- Arterial blood gas
  - Po_2 low: reflects significant hypoxemia
  - Po_2 high: reflects inadequate ventilation
  - pH, bicarbonate, lactate: acid–base balance
- Karyotype: to assess for associated syndromes and chromosomal abnormalities

DIFFERENTIAL DIAGNOSIS

- Pulmonary
  - Pulmonary sequestration
  - Congenital pulmonary airway malformation (CCAM)
  - Pneumatocele
  - Pulmonary cyst
  - Diaphragmatic eventration
  - Hiatal hernia
  - Congenital lobar emphysema
  - Pulmonary agenesis
  - Anterior mediastinal mass
  - Pneumonia
  - Atelectasis
  - Pleural effusion
  - Pneumothorax
- Cardiac
  - Dextrocardia
  - Congenital heart disease

TREATMENT

ACUTE

General Measures

- Aim for delivery of infant in the hospital where defect is to be repaired as this situation is associated with better outcomes.
- Insertion of a nasogastric tube to decompress herniated contents and allow venting
- Mechanical ventilation
  - Avoid bag and mask ventilation.
  - Goal is to limit barotrauma, maintain peak pressures ≤25 mm Hg and positive end-expiratory pressure (PEEP) of at least 5 mm Hg
  - Permissive hypercapnia: tolerate Pa_{CO_2} up to 60 mm Hg
  - Aim for preductal oxygen saturation >85%
  - Consider high-frequency oscillatory ventilation and extracorporeal membrane oxygenation (ECMO) when earlier measures are not effective (e.g., pH <7.25, Pa_{CO_2} >60 mm Hg, preductal saturation <85% on FiO_2 0.6)
- Cardiovascular support
  - In setting of pulmonary hypertension, aim for higher mean arterial blood pressure.
- Pulmonary hypertension
  - Severity predicts outcome.
  - 50% of patients are responsive to inspired nitric oxide (iNO), but the effect may be temporary. iNO has no influence on overall outcome.
  - Sildenafil: Phosphodiesterase 5 inhibitor may be used as an adjunct to iNO to prevent rebound hypertension when weaning iNO or in management of chronic pulmonary hypertension.
  - In setting of left ventricular dysfunction with a right ventricle–dependent systemic circulation, milrinone and prostaglandin may be used to decrease afterload and maintain ductal patency.

ALERT

- It is important to assess and treat pulmonary hypertension.
- Avoid aggressive ventilation. It is important to minimize barotrauma.

Surgical Correction

- Delaying surgery until infant is stabilized has been associated with better outcome.
- Primary repair versus prosthetic patch
- Minimally invasive thoracoscopic approach now possible, although is associated with an increased recurrence rate compared with the open approach
- Up to 50% will require patch repair of diaphragmatic defect.
- Recurrence of hernia occurs in up to 50% of patch closures.
- Patch closure of abdomen or creation of surgical silo may be required with very large defects.

ONGOING CARE

FOLLOW-UP RECOMMENDATIONS

- Long-term multidisciplinary follow-up required to monitor for complications and recurrence of hernia
- Pulmonary
  - Chronic lung disease: Up to 50% require supplemental oxygen at 28 days and 16% at the time of discharge from hospital.
  - Prevalence of long-term pulmonary morbidity unclear—some series report chronic pulmonary symptoms in up to 50% of survivors.
  - Spirometry shows obstructive pattern of lung disease.
  - Scoliosis and chest wall defects may cause restrictive lung disease.
- Gastrointestinal/nutrition
  - Growth failure secondary to chronic lung disease, increased work of breathing, gastroesophageal reflux, and oral aversion
  - Failure to thrive is common—up to 1/3 require gastrostomy tube
  - Gastroesophageal reflux (45–90%): may lead to recurrent bronchitis, worsening bronchopulmonary dysplasia, aspiration pneumonia. Persists into adulthood. Consider an H_2 blocker in all patients
- Cardiac
  - Pulmonary hypertension may persist in up to 30%.
- Neurodevelopmental
  - Behavioral, cognitive, and motor problems common
  - Greater risk in those with large defects or those requiring ECMO
- Sensorineural hearing loss
  - Incidence varies: up to 40% described by some
  - Underlying cause unknown
  - Deficit is progressive, so regular long-term follow-up is recommended.
- Surgical
  - Orthopedic: pectus deformity and scoliosis
  - Recurrence of hernia (in up to 50%): risk greater in those who required patch closure
    - May present with vomiting, bowel obstruction, pulmonary symptoms, or may be asymptomatic
    - Serial CXR recommended for screening

ALERT

- Recurrence of CDH is common and typically presents with vague gastrointestinal symptoms (in contrast to a dramatic presentation of the newborn period).
- Hearing impairment may be progressive. Therefore, serial screening through childhood is essential.

PROGNOSIS

- Depends on the degree of pulmonary hypoplasia and pulmonary hypertension
- 70% postnatal survival, with up to 90% survival described by some centers
- 50% survival in those requiring ECMO
- Prematurity associated with worse prognosis

ADDITIONAL READING

- American Academy of Pediatrics Section on Surgery; American Academy of Pediatrics Committee on Fetus and Newborn, Lally KP, Engle W. Post discharge of infants with congenital diaphragmatic hernia. *Pediatrics*. 2008;121(3):627–632.
- Bohn D. Congenital diaphragmatic hernia. *Am J Respir Crit Care Med*. 2002;166(7):911–915.
- Danzer E, Gerdes M, D'Agostino JA, et al. Longitudinal neurodevelopmental and neuromotor outcome in congenital diaphragmatic hernia patients in the first 3 years of life. *J Perinatol*. 2013;33(11): 893–898.
- Kotecha S, Barbato A, Bush A, et al. Congenital diaphragmatic hernia. *Eur Respir J*. 2012;39(4): 820–829.
- Van Den L, Sluiter I, Gischler S, et al. Can we improve outcome of congenital diaphragmatic hernia? *Pediatr Surg Int*. 2009;25(9):733–743.

CODES

ICD10

- Q79.0 Congenital diaphragmatic hernia
- Q33.6 Congenital hypoplasia and dysplasia of lung

FAQ

- Q: What is the recurrence rate?
- A: Reported rates of recurrence vary from 10 to 50%. Serial screening with CXR and a high index of suspicion is necessary. The typical presentation includes emesis, gastrointestinal obstruction, or respiratory symptoms.
- Q: Is pulmonary impairment lifelong?
- A: Although pulmonary function improves with growth, studies (spirometry, plethysmography, ventilation–perfusion [V/Q] scanning) show persisting deficits. Most patients report decreased pulmonary morbidity/symptoms with increasing age.
- Q: What follow-up is necessary?
- A: Long-term multidisciplinary follow-up is essential. Complications involving multiple organ systems are common.
- Q: Why is long-term gastrointestinal follow-up necessary?
- A: Although complications such as failure to thrive and oral aversion are less common with increasing age, the risk of reflux is lifelong. Treatment into adulthood may be required to control reflux and prevent Barrett esophagus.

DIARRHEA

Roberto Gugig

BASICS

DESCRIPTION

- Diarrhea is an increase in frequency, volume, or fluidity of a patient's stool as compared to the normal bowel movement pattern.
- On the basis of its duration, diarrhea can be classified as acute (<14 days), persistent (14–29 days), or chronic (> 30 days).
- Acute diarrhea typically presents abruptly with increased fluid content of the stool >10 mL/kg/day and lasts <14 days. Usually involves the passage of >250 g/day of unformed stool
- Persistent diarrhea can also begin acutely, but last for ≥14 days.
- Diarrhea is caused whenever there is disruption of the normal absorptive and secretory functions of intestinal mucosa resulting in water and electrolyte imbalance.
- Malabsorption, maldigestion, cellular electrolyte pump dysfunction, and intestinal colonization or invasion by microorganisms can cause diarrhea.
- Tenesmus, perianal discomfort, and incontinence may occur with all diarrhea.

DIAGNOSIS

DIFFERENTIAL DIAGNOSIS

Acute diarrhea

- Dietary causes
  - Sorbitol, fructose, lactose, and intolerance to specific foods (beans, fruit, peppers, etc.)
- Infectious causes:
  - Bacterial (e.g., *Escherichia coli*, *Clostridium difficile*) and viral (e.g., rotavirus, Norwalk agent, adenovirus)
  - Parasites (*Giardia*, *Cryptosporidium*, *Entamoeba*)
- Medications
  - Antibiotics, laxatives
- Vitamin deficiency
  - Zinc, niacin

Chronic diarrhea

- Allergic/autoimmune
  - Milk/soy protein allergy, eosinophilic enteritis, Henoch-Schönlein purpura (HSP), celiac disease, or autoimmune enteropathy
- Immunodeficiency
  - HIV/AIDS, chronic granulomatous disease, hyper IgM, severe combined immunodeficiency
- Anatomic abnormalities
  - Short intestinal tract (e.g., h/o necrotizing enterocolitis, Hirschsprung, malrotation, inflammatory bowel disease)
- Bile acid malabsorption
- Congenital
  - Cystic fibrosis, microvillus inclusion disease, tufting enteropathy, or IPEX syndrome
- Encopresis
- Endocrine disorders
  - Hyperthyroidism, diabetes, congenital adrenal hyperplasia
- Bacterial overgrowth (e.g., blind loop, ostomy)
- Inflammatory bowel disease
  - Ulcerative colitis, Crohn disease
- Intestinal lymphangiectasia
  - Primary and secondary
- Irritable bowel syndrome
- Lactose intolerance
  - Primary, secondary, and congenital
- Pancreatic exocrine dysfunction
  - Shwachman-Diamond syndrome, cationic trypsinogen deficiency, Jeune syndrome, Pearson syndrome, and Johanson-Blizzard syndrome
- Postinfectious enteropathy
- Secretory tumors
  - VIPoma, somatostatinoma, gastrinoma, carcinoid, glucagonoma

APPROACH TO PATIENT

- The first step in the clinical appraisal of the patient with diarrhea is to identify what the patient "means" by diarrhea; exclude the possibility of fecal incontinence; rule out drug-induced diarrhea; distinguish acute from chronic; categorize as inflammatory, fatty, or watery; and consider the possibility of factitious diarrhea.
- It is important to determine the type of diarrhea (osmotic vs. secretory), as this will alter your diagnostic and therapeutic plan.
  - Secretory diarrhea
    - Absorption of intestinal fluid and electrolytes is accomplished through multiple cellular pumps transporting sodium, glucose, and amino acids.
    - Factors that interrupt these pumps (e.g., cholera toxin, prostaglandin E, vasoactive intestinal peptide, secretin, acetylcholine) can cause a severe active isotonic secretory state manifested by profuse diarrhea, dehydration, and acidosis. Other causes include bile acid malabsorption, inflammatory bowel disease, disordered regulation (postvagotomy, diabetic neuropathy), peptide-secreting endocrine tumors, and neoplasia (colon carcinoma, lymphoma, villous adenoma).
  - Osmotic diarrhea
    - In general, the solute composition of intestinal fluid is similar to that of plasma.
    - Osmotic diarrhea occurs when poorly absorbed or nonabsorbable solute is present in the intestinal lumen (this may result in low stool pH <6).
    - This can occur with the ingestion of nonabsorbable sugars (e.g., sorbitol), cathartics (e.g., magnesium citrate), carbohydrate malabsorption secondary to mucosal damage (e.g., lactose), maldigestion (e.g., pancreatic dysfunction), rapid transit of intestinal fluid, or with a rare congenital transport defect.

HISTORY

- **Question:** Duration? (<14 days, >30 days)
  Significance: A distinction should be made between acute and chronic diarrhea. The cause of acute diarrhea is almost always related to an infection, a medication, or the addition of a new food.
- **Question:** Travel history?
  Significance: Questions should be asked regarding travel to areas where drinking water is contaminated (e.g., *Entamoeba* in Mexico) or food handling/preparation is prolonged or unsanitary (e.g., *Campylobacter*, *Bacillus cereus*, or *E. coli*). Exposure to freshwater streams or ponds (e.g., *Cryptosporidium*, *Giardia*) may also be important to address.
- **Question:** Recent use of antibiotics?
  Significance: A variety of antibiotics can be associated with *C. difficile* colitis or antibiotic-related diarrhea.
- **Question:** Adolescents?
  Significance: Questions should be asked regarding body image and weight. Laxative abuse causing an osmotic diarrhea is common among adolescents who have an eating disorder or athletes attempting to lose weight rapidly.
- **Question:** Family history?
  Significance: conditions with genetic susceptibility (e.g., inflammatory bowel disease, celiac disease)
- **Question:** Systemic symptoms?
  Significance: It is important to ask about concomitant fever, GI bleeding, rashes, or vomiting. Certain GI infections and inflammatory bowel disease have specific associated systemic symptoms.
- **Question:** Hematochezia?
  Significance: The occurrence of acute, bloody stools and fever generally indicates a bacterial infection. However, these same symptoms coupled with fatigue, poor urine output, and history of easy bruising may suggest hemolytic uremic syndrome. Bloody stools in combination with a history of crampy abdominal pain, arthritis, and purpuric rash can indicate HSP, a completely different entity. Chronic bloody diarrhea, abdominal pain, and weight loss are characteristic of inflammatory bowel disease.
- **Question:** Steatorrhea? (greasy or bulky stools)
  Significance: indicates fat malabsorption (e.g., cystic fibrosis)
- **Question:** Age? (congenital vs. acquired)
  Significance: The age of the child is important because a number of diseases present between birth and 3 months of life including cystic fibrosis, milk or soy protein allergy, and congenital enteropathies.
- **Question:** Previously well infant with recent viral illness and subsequent protracted diarrhea?
  Significance: Postviral enteritis should be suspected. This disorder is characterized by severe mucosal injury resulting in transient disaccharidase deficiency and potentially prolonged malabsorption.
- **Question:** Normal preschool-aged children who have 2–10 watery stools per day without other symptoms and/or cause who have increased juice intake?
  Significance: Chronic nonspecific diarrhea of childhood or "toddler's diarrhea" should be considered.
- **Question:** Lactose intolerance?
  Significance: commonly occurs in many older children and adults, with >95% occurrence rate in some ethnic groups
- **Question:** Chronic diarrhea with weight loss?
  Significance: Inflammatory or immunologic disorders such as ulcerative colitis, Crohn disease, and celiac disease must be ruled out. Celiac disease is an immune-mediated enteropathy caused by a permanent sensitivity to gluten and related prolamine in genetically susceptible individuals. Occurs in ~1:130 of the U.S. population with a genetic predisposition and should be considered in any child with chronic diarrhea and poor weight gain

PHYSICAL EXAM

- **Finding:** Child's growth parameters?
  Significance: Previous measurements and growth curves are necessary to make an accurate evaluation. Findings of a chronically malnourished child with years of weight loss or poor growth velocity would indicate a divergent differential diagnosis from that of a healthy-appearing child with a history of normal growth.

- **Finding:** Arthritis and rash?
  Significance: Diarrhea accompanied by these signs can occur in diseases such as inflammatory bowel disease, celiac disease, HSP, and specific bacterial infections.
- **Finding:** Oral ulcers?
  Significance: occur in inflammatory bowel disease and celiac disease
- **Finding:** Hydration?
  Significance: Capillary refill >3 seconds, tachycardia without pain or fever, and dry mucous membranes provide clues to dehydration.
- **Finding:** Nail bed clubbing?
  Significance: This finding may direct questioning to rule out cystic fibrosis or chronic inflammatory bowel disease.
- **Finding:** Masses?
  Significance: A right lower quadrant mass could suggest an abscess (e.g., terminal ileitis in Crohn disease or appendiceal abscess) or intussusception (e.g., irritable child with currant jelly-like stools).

DIAGNOSTIC TESTS & INTERPRETATION

- **Test:** stool culture
  Significance: Stool examination for blood, mucus, inflammatory cells, and microorganisms is an important first step in determining the cause of the diarrhea. Stool cultures for parasites (e.g., *Giardia*, *Cryptosporidium*, *Entamoeba*), bacterial pathogens (e.g., *Salmonella*, *Campylobacter*, *Shigella*, *Yersinia*, *Aeromonas*, *Plesiomonas*), viral particles, and *C. difficile* toxin should be appropriately obtained in all children with unexplained diarrhea.
- **Test:** stool pH and reducing substances
  Significance: These tests are useful in identifying carbohydrate malabsorption. A stool pH <5–6 and stool-reducing substances >0.5–1% is suggestive of malabsorption.
- **Test:** stool osmolality and electrolytes
  Significance: Stool osmolality, stool Na, and stool K can be used to calculate an ion gap and differentiate between secretory and osmotic diarrhea.
  – Stool osmotic gap = measured stool osmolality − estimated stool osmolality
  – Estimated stool osmolality = 2 (Na stool + K stool)
  – An increased stool osmotic gap is >50 mOsm/kg.
- **Test:** Hemoccult
  Significance: Sensitive and specific test is helpful in distinguishing truly heme-positive stools from ingested foods/drinks with artificial or natural red coloring. Stool positive for blood is suggestive of infectious (*C. difficile*) and organic etiologies (inflammatory bowel disease).
- **Test:** 72-hour quantitative fecal fat evaluation
  Significance: This is a sensitive test for steatorrhea. Patients need to be placed on a high-fat diet (2–4 g/kg) for a minimum of 1 day prior to testing.
  – Over 3 days, all stool is collected, refrigerated, and tested. A diet record needs to be performed for the 3 days that correspond to the stool collection period.
  – The coefficient of fat absorption is calculated: grams of fat ingested − grams of fat excreted/grams of fat ingested × 100.
  – Normal values are as follows:
    ○ Premature infants: 60–75%
    ○ Newborns: 80–85%
    ○ Children 10 months to 3 years: 85–95%
    ○ Children >3 years: 93%.
  – When fat malabsorption is present, disorders of pancreatic function (e.g., cystic fibrosis, Shwachman-Diamond syndrome) or severe intestinal disease should be suspected.
- **Test:** lactose breath test
  Significance: This noninvasive test measures hydrogen levels and or methane. It is based on the principle that hydrogen gas is produced by colonic bacterial fermentation of malabsorbed carbohydrates. When abnormal in older healthy-appearing children, primary lactase deficiency is likely. However, in young children, a secondary lactase deficiency should be considered and small-bowel disease should be ruled out.
- **Test:** D-xylose test
  Significance: This serum test is an indirect measure of functional small bowel surface area. D-xylose absorption in the blood occurs independent of bile salts, pancreatic enzymes, and intestinal disaccharidases. A specific dose of D-xylose (1 g/kg, maximum 25 g) is given orally after an 8-hour fast, and the serum level of D-xylose is determined after 1 hour. Levels <15–20 mg/dL in children is abnormal and suggestive of disorders that alter or disrupt intestinal mucosa absorption.
- **Test:** fecal calprotectin
  Significance: Calprotectin is a neutrophilic protein detected in stools in inflammatory conditions.
- **Test:** endoscopy and colonoscopy
  Significance: Direct visualization of the intestinal mucosa as well as intestinal culture, disaccharidase collection, and biopsies can provide clues to diagnosis.
- **Test:** celiac panel
  Significance: This includes a tissue transglutaminase, IgA level, and endomysial antibody.

TREATMENT

GENERAL MEASURES

- The key elements in treatment of diarrhea are as follows: (a) correction of hydration, (b) correction of electrolytes, and (c) specific treatment of underlying cause when indicated.
- Rehydration is the cornerstone of treatment.
- Oral rehydration therapy with glucose concentrations of 111 mmol/L and 90 mmol/L sodium is recommended.
- IV rehydration is indicated for patients who are severely dehydrated and unable to tolerate oral feedings.

ISSUES FOR REFERRAL

Children who present with growth failure, noninfectious heme-positive diarrhea, or unexplained chronic diarrhea should be considered for referral to a pediatric gastroenterologist.

INPATIENT CONSIDERATIONS

Initial Stabilization

Diarrhea can lead to significant dehydration and electrolyte imbalance. Any child suspected of clinical dehydration should be closely observed. Only if oral rehydration is ineffective is IV therapy indicated. Culture-negative GI bleeding associated with severe abdominal pain and diarrhea should always be treated urgently.

- Antibiotics
  – *Vibrio cholerae*, *Shigella*, and *Giardia lamblia* require antimicrobial therapy (i.e., trimethoprim/sulfasoxazole, azithromycin, tetracycline, ciprofloxacin, metronidazole).
  – Prolonged courses of enteropathogenic *E. coli*, *Yersinia* in sickle cell patients, and *Salmonella* species infections in the very young febrile or bacteremic infant require antimicrobial therapy.

ONGOING CARE

DIET

- Breastfeeding should continue during episodes of gastroenteritis, as it promotes mucosal healing and recovery.
  – It was traditionally believed that bowel rest was beneficial for formula-fed infants.
  – Many studies have now shown that return feeding after 4–6 hours promotes a faster recovery.
- Micronutrient supplementation
  – Zinc supplementation at a dose of 20 mg/day for children older than 6 months and 10 mg/day in those younger than 6 months for 10–14 days during episodes of acute diarrhea has been shown to decrease severity and duration as well as preventing future episodes in malnourished children.
- Probiotics and Prebiotics
  – Have been used for both prevention and treatment of diarrhea
  – *Lactobacillus rhamnosus GG* has been shown to shorten the duration of diarrheal illness and viral shedding (e.g., rotavirus).
  – May help patients with Crohn disease, ulcerative colitis, irritable bowel syndrome, and pouchitis

ADDITIONAL READING

- Ali SA, Hill DR. *Giardia intestinalis*. *Curr Opin Infect Dis*. 2003;16(5):453–460.
- Aomatsu T, Yoden A, Matsumoto K, et al. Fecal calprotectin is a useful marker for disease activity in pediatric patients with inflammatory bowel disease. *Dig Dis Sci*. 2011;56(8):2372–2377.
- Castelli F, Saleri N, Tomasoni LR, et al. Prevention and treatment of traveler's diarrhea: focus on antimicrobial agents. *Digestion*. 2006;73(Suppl 1):109–118.
- Gore JI, Surawicz C. Severe acute diarrhea. *Gastroenterol Clin North Am*. 2003;32(4):1249–1267.
- Hartling L, Bellemare S, Wiebe N, et al. Oral versus intravenous rehydration for treating dehydration due to gastroenteritis in children. *Cochrane Database Syst Rev*. 2006;(3):CD004390.
- Patel K, Thillainayagam AV. Diarrhea. *Medicine*. 2009;37(1):23–27.
- Surawicz CM. Mechanisms of diarrhea. *Curr Gastroenterol Rep*. 2010;12(4):236–241.
- Thielman NM, Guerrant RL. Clinical practice. Acute infectious diarrhea. *N Engl J Med*. 2004;350(1):38–47.

CODES

ICD10

- R19.7 Diarrhea, unspecified
- K52.9 Noninfective gastroenteritis and colitis, unspecified
- A09 Infectious gastroenteritis and colitis, unspecified

DIPHTHERIA

Michael J. Smith

BASICS

DESCRIPTION

Acute infectious disease caused by *Corynebacterium diphtheriae*; affects primarily the membranes of the upper respiratory tract with the formation of a gray-white pseudomembrane

EPIDEMIOLOGY

- The only known reservoir for *C. diphtheriae* is humans; disease is acquired by contact with either a carrier or a diseased person.
- Most cases occur during the cooler autumn and winter months in individuals <15 years of age who are unimmunized.
- Recent outbreaks have occurred, most notably in the countries of the former Soviet Union, and supply additional evidence that disease occurs among the socioeconomically disadvantaged living in crowded conditions.

Incidence

- Although the disease is distributed throughout the world, it is endemic primarily in developing regions of Africa, Asia, and South America.
- In the Western world, the incidence of diphtheria has changed dramatically in the past 50–75 years as a result of the widespread use of diphtheria toxoid after World War II.
- The incidence has declined steadily and is now a rare occurrence.

GENERAL PREVENTION

Active immunization with diphtheria toxoid is the cornerstone of population-based diphtheria prevention. Current recommendations from the Advisory Committee on Immunization Practices (ACIP) of the Centers for Disease Control and Prevention (CDC) are as follows:

- Ages 2 months–7 years: 5 doses of diphtheria vaccine (with tetanus toxoid and acellular pertussis)
  - First 3 given as DTaP vaccine 0.5 mL IM at 2-month intervals beginning at 2 months of age
  - 4th dose of DTaP should be given at 15–18 months of age.
  - 5th dose of DTaP at 4–6 years of age
- In 2005, 2 tetanus toxoid, reduced diphtheria toxoid, and acellular pertussis (Tdap) vaccines were licensed for use in adolescents 11–18 years of age.
- 1 booster dose of Tdap should be given to all adolescents at the 11–12-year-old visit, provided they have completed the childhood series. Subsequent tetanus and diphtheria (Td) boosters should be administered every 10 years.
- Tdap should replace the 1st dose of Td in children 7–10 years of age who are undergoing primary immunization.
- Isolation of patients with diphtheria is required until culture from the site of infection is negative on 2 consecutive specimens.

PATHOPHYSIOLOGY

- The initial entry site for *C. diphtheriae* is via airborne respiratory droplets, typically the nose or mouth but occasionally the ocular surface, genital mucous membranes, or preexisting skin lesions.
- Following 2–4 days of incubation at one of these sites, the bacterium elaborates toxin.
- Locally, the toxin induces formation of a necrotic coagulation of the mucous membranes (pseudomembrane) with underlying tissue edema; respiratory compromise may ensue.
- Elaborated exotoxin may also have profound effects on the heart, nerves, and kidneys in the form of myocarditis, demyelination, and tubular necrosis, respectively.

ETIOLOGY

C. diphtheriae, a gram-positive pleomorphic bacillus

DIAGNOSIS

- Respiratory tract diphtheria
  - Nasal diphtheria starts with mild rhinorrhea that gradually becomes serosanguineous, then mucopurulent, and often malodorous; it occurs most often in infants.
  - Tonsillar and pharyngeal diphtheria begin with anorexia, malaise, low-grade fever, and pharyngitis.
    - A membrane appears within 1–2 days.
    - Cervical lymphadenitis and edema of the cervical soft tissues may be severe.
    - Disease course varies with extent of toxin elaboration and membrane production.
    - Respiratory and cardiovascular collapse may occur.
  - Laryngeal diphtheria most often represents extension of a pharyngeal infection.
    - Clinically presents as typical croup
    - Acute airway obstruction may occur.
    - In severe cases, the membrane may invade the entire tracheobronchial tree.
  - Cutaneous diphtheria occurs in warmer tropical regions.
    - It is characterized by chronic nonhealing ulcers with gray membrane.
    - May serve as a reservoir in endemic and epidemic areas of respiratory diphtheria
- Other sites: Rarely, vulvovaginal, conjunctival, or aural forms occur.

HISTORY

- Exposure to an individual with diphtheria is not necessarily elicited because contact with an asymptomatic carrier may be the only source of infection.
- Incubation period
  - Incubation period is 1–6 days.
  - Respiratory diphtheria, depending on the site of infection, may begin with nasal discharge alone or with pharyngitis accompanied by mild systemic symptoms.
  - Progression of symptoms thereafter occurs as outlined earlier (see "Diagnosis").
- Previous diphtheria immunization history, diphtheria exposure

PHYSICAL EXAM

- Classic findings
  - Nasal discharge
  - Nasal or pharyngeal membrane
  - Heart rate out of proportion to body temperature
  - Respiratory distress
  - Stridor
  - Cough
  - Hoarseness
  - Palatal paralysis
  - Neck swelling
  - Cervical lymphadenitis
  - Attempt to remove any membrane present results in bleeding.
- Conjunctival diphtheria: palpebral conjunctival involvement with a red, edematous, membranous appearance
- Aural diphtheria: otitis externa with a purulent, malodorous discharge
- Cutaneous diphtheria: See "Diagnosis."

DIAGNOSTIC TESTS & INTERPRETATION

Diagnosis should be on clinical grounds: Delay in treatment increases morbidity and mortality.

Lab

- Culture of material from the membrane or beneath the membrane. Because special growth media are required, the lab should be notified of suspicion of diphtheria.
- If a strain of *C. diphtheriae* is isolated, additional testing for presence or absence of toxin production should be done by a laboratory prepared to conduct an animal neutralization test or, alternatively, neutralization (with antitoxin) in tissue culture.

DIFFERENTIAL DIAGNOSIS

- Nasal diphtheria
  - Common cold
  - Nasal foreign body
  - Sinusitis
  - Adenoiditis
  - Snuffles (congenital syphilis)

- Tonsillar or pharyngeal diphtheria
  - Streptococcal pharyngitis
  - Infectious mononucleosis
  - Primary herpetic tonsillitis
  - Thrush
  - Vincent angina
  - Posttonsillectomy faucial membranes
  - Oropharyngeal involvement caused by toxoplasmosis, cytomegalovirus, tularemia, and salmonellosis
- Laryngeal diphtheria
  - Croup
  - Acute epiglottitis
  - Aspirated foreign body
  - Peripharyngeal and retropharyngeal abscess
  - Laryngeal papillomas
  - Other masses

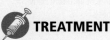

TREATMENT

MEDICATION

Antibiotic therapy: Use in addition to, not in place of, diphtheria antitoxin (DAT).

- Respiratory diphtheria
  - Penicillin G
    - Aqueous crystalline 100,000–150,000 U/kg/24 h in 4 divided doses for 14 days or
    - Procaine 25,000–50,000 U/kg/24 h in 2 divided doses for 14 days or
  - Erythromycin 40–50 mg/kg (maximum 2 g/24 h) PO or parenterally for 14 days
- Cutaneous diphtheria: requires local care of the lesion with soap and water and administration of antimicrobials for 10 days

INPATIENT CONSIDERATIONS

Initial Stabilization

- DAT antiserum, produced in horses, must be administered as soon as possible. DAT is available from the CDC. (Note: For patients with known horse serum sensitivity, a test dose should be administered first; if positive, the patient should be desensitized.)
- Pharyngeal or laryngeal disease of <48 hours duration: 20,000–40,000 U IV
- Nasopharyngeal lesions: 40,000–60,000 U IV
- Extensive disease of ≥3 days' duration or diffuse neck swelling: 80,000–120,000 U IV

ONGOING CARE

FOLLOW-UP RECOMMENDATIONS

- Mild cases: After membrane sloughs off in 7–10 days, recovery is usually uneventful.
- More severe cases: Recovery may be slower; serious complications may occur.

PROGNOSIS

- Most strongly dependent on the immunization status of the host. Those without prior adequate immunization have significantly higher morbidity and mortality.
- Delay in onset of treatment also increases mortality.
  - When appropriate treatment has been administered on day 1 of illness, mortality may be as low as 1%.
  - When treatment has been delayed until day 4, the mortality rate is ≤20-fold higher.
- Organism virulence: Toxigenic strains are associated with more severe disease and a poorer prognosis.
- Location of membrane: Laryngeal diphtheria has a higher mortality due to airway obstruction.
- A megakaryocytic thrombocytopenia and WBC count <25,000 are associated with poor outcome.

COMPLICATIONS

- Cardiac toxicity: Myocarditis may develop secondary to elaborated toxin anytime between the 1st and 6th week of illness. Although cardiac failure may occur, most cases are transient.
- Neurologic toxicity occurs secondary to toxin elaboration and mainly reflects bilateral motor involvement.
- Paralysis of the soft palate is most common, but ocular paralysis, diaphragm paralysis, peripheral neuropathy of the extremities, and loss of deep tendon reflexes also occur.
- The frequency of all complications, including those listed above, increases with increasing time between symptom onset and antitoxin administration and also with extent of membrane formation.

ADDITIONAL READING

- American Academy of Pediatrics. Diphtheria. In: Pickering LK, Baker CJ, Kimberlin DW, et al, eds. *Red Book: 2012 Report of the Committee on Infectious Diseases*. 29th ed. Elk Grove Village, IL: American Academy of Pediatrics; 2012:307–311.
- Broder KR, Cortese MM, Iskander JK, et al. Preventing tetanus, diphtheria, and pertussis among adolescents: use of tetanus toxoid, reduced diphtheria toxoid and acellular pertussis vaccines recommendations of the Advisory Committee on Immunization Practices (ACIP). *MMWR Recomm Rep*. 2006;55(RR-3):1–34.
- Centers for Disease Control and Prevention. Updated recommendations for use of tetanus toxoid, reduced diphtheria toxoid and acellular pertussis (Tdap) vaccine from the Advisory Committee on Immunization Practices, 2010. *MMWR Morb Mortal Wkly Rep*. 2011;60(1):13–15.
- Enhanced surveillance of non-toxigenic *Corynebacterium diphtheriae* infections. *Commun Dis Rep CDR Wkly*. 1996;6(4):29–32.
- Galazka A. The changing epidemiology of diphtheria in the vaccine era. *J Infect Dis*. 2000;181(Suppl 1): 52–59.

CODES

ICD10

- A36.9 Diphtheria, unspecified
- A36.1 Nasopharyngeal diphtheria
- A36.3 Cutaneous diphtheria

FAQ

- Q: What is the incidence of diphtheria in the United States?
- A: No locally acquired case of respiratory diphtheria has been reported in the United States since 2003. Cutaneous diphtheria still occurs but is not a reportable disease.
- Q: Are there currently places in the world where diphtheria is a problem?
- A: Yes. An epidemic began in 1990 in Russia, spread in 1991 to Ukraine, and during 1993 and 1994 spread to the remaining countries of the former Soviet Union. Other endemic regions include the Middle East and Asia and some countries in Africa and Central and South America. Travelers to these regions should check the CDC Web site for the latest information.
- Q: What precautions should be taken by travelers to areas of the world with diphtheria outbreaks?
- A: The ACIP recommends that travelers to such areas be up-to-date with diphtheria immunization. Infants traveling to areas where diphtheria is endemic or epidemic should ideally receive 3 doses of DTaP before travel.

DISKITIS

Melissa L. Mannion • Randy Q. Cron

BASICS

DESCRIPTION
Often benign, self-limited inflammatory process of an intervertebral disk

EPIDEMIOLOGY
>50% of the cases occur in children <4 years of age.

Incidence
- Peak incidence is between 0 and 2 years of age.
- Second peak: >10 years

Prevalence
Rare

PATHOPHYSIOLOGY
- Probably of infectious etiology by an indolent organism
- Usually none identified; occasionally, *Staphylococcus aureus*, *Moraxella*, or the Enterobacteriaceae are cultured.

ETIOLOGY
Idiopathic, infectious, or traumatic

DIAGNOSIS

HISTORY
- Uncomfortable, irritable child
- Refusal to walk
- Fever
- Back or abdominal pain
- Symptoms of short duration prior to presentation

PHYSICAL EXAM
- Usually, rigid posture and pain elicited on movement (sits in tripod position)
- Loss of lumbar lordosis
- Focal tenderness to palpation
- Most common locations: L4–L5 and L3–L4

DIAGNOSTIC TESTS & INTERPRETATION

Lab
Initial lab tests
- Purified protein derivative (PPD)
- WBC count
- Erythrocyte sedimentation rate (ESR)
- C-reactive protein (CRP)
- Blood cultures

Imaging
- Plain radiographic studies
  - Usually normal, although may demonstrate disk narrowing as illness progresses
- MRI
  - Useful to confirm diagnosis and location of pathology
  - Demonstrates disk edema
- Bone scan
  - Demonstrates increased uptake at affected area
  - May be used to screen for other sites of infection

DIFFERENTIAL DIAGNOSIS
- Infection
  - Vertebral osteomyelitis (e.g., *Staphylococcus*, *Salmonella*)
  - Pott disease (tuberculous spondylitis)
  - Pyelonephritis
  - Retrocecal appendicitis
  - Psoas or epidural abscess
- Trauma
  - Fracture
  - Disk herniation
- Tumors
  - Osteoid osteoma
  - Langerhans cell granulomatosis of the spine
- Vascular: avascular necrosis of vertebral body
- Congenital: spondylolisthesis
- Immunologic
  - Ankylosing spondylitis
  - Nonbacterial osteitis
- Miscellaneous: Scheuermann disease (osteochondritis of the vertebral bodies)

ALERT
There is difficulty distinguishing early vertebral body osteomyelitis from diskitis.

TREATMENT

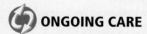

MEDICATION
- Usually quite responsive to NSAIDs
- Toddlers are usually treated with anti-staphylococcal antibiotics.

COMPLEMENTARY & ALTERNATIVE THERAPIES
- Physical therapy
  - Patient should be immobilized during acute period.
  - Casting may be required.

INPATIENT CONSIDERATIONS
Initial Stabilization

Duration
- Follow CBC, CRP, and ESR.
- Continue treatment until child is asymptomatic.

ONGOING CARE

FOLLOW-UP RECOMMENDATIONS
Patient Monitoring
- When to expect improvement: Most patients are asymptomatic in 6–8 weeks.
- Signs to watch for:
  - Recurrence of symptoms due to reactivation of the disease
  - Progressive loss of disk height
  - Destruction of adjacent vertebral bodies

PROGNOSIS
- Usually excellent
- Scoliosis may occur.
- Radiologic disk space narrowing almost always occurs.

COMPLICATIONS
- Occasionally, scoliosis or kyphosis
- Ankylosis of adjacent vertebrae may occur.

ADDITIONAL READING

- Arthurs OJ, Gomez AC, Heinz P, et al. The toddler refusing to weight-bear: a revised imaging guide from a case series. *Emerg Med J*. 2009;26(11):797–801.
- Chandrasenan J, Klezl Z, Bommireddy R, et al. Spondylodiscitis in children. *J Bone Joint Surg Br*. 2011;93(8):1122–1125.
- Early SD, Kay RM, Tolo VT. Childhood diskitis. *J Am Acad Orthop Surg*. 2003;11(6):413–420.
- Fernandez M, Carrol CL, Baker CJ. Discitis and vertebral osteomyelitis in children: an 18-year review. *Pediatrics*. 2000;105(6):1299–1304.
- Garron E, Viehweger E, Launay F, et al. Nontuberculous spondylodiscitis in children. *J Pediatr Orthop*. 2002;22(3):321–328.
- Karabouta Z, Bisbinas I, Davidson A, et al. Discitis in toddlers: a case series and review. *Acta Paeditr*. 2005;94(10):1516–1518.
- Kayser R, Mahlfeld K, Greulich M, et al. Spondylodiscitis in childhood: results of a long-term study. *Spine*. 2005;30(3):318–323.
- Marin C, Sanchez-Alegre ML, Gallego C, et al. Magnetic resonance imaging of osteoarticular infections in children. *Curr Probl Diagn Radiol*. 2004;33(2):43–59.
- McCarthy JJ, Dormans JP, Kozin SH, et al. Musculoskeletal infections in children: basic treatment principles and recent advancements. *Instr Course Lect*. 2005;54:515–528.

CODES

ICD10
- M46.40 Discitis, unspecified, site unspecified
- M46.46 Discitis, unspecified, lumbar region
- M46.42 Discitis, unspecified, cervical region

FAQ
- Q: When are a biopsy and tissue culture indicated?
- A: If there is bony destruction of adjacent vertebral bodies or if clinical course is prolonged or recurrent
- Q: When are antibiotics indicated?
- A: Obviously, in situations with positive cultures or clear infective focus, or if course is atypical or prolonged

D

DISSEMINATED INTRAVASCULAR COAGULATION

Char Witmer

BASICS

DESCRIPTION

- Disseminated intravascular coagulation (DIC) is an acquired syndrome that is always secondary to an underlying etiology.
- It is a systemic life-threatening process characterized by an uncontrolled activation of the coagulation and fibrinolytic systems with excessive thrombin generation and the consumption of coagulation factors and platelets.
- Widespread deposition of microthrombi can compromise perfusion and lead to organ failure.
- Ongoing activation and consumption of coagulant factors and platelets can result in diffuse and profuse bleeding.

EPIDEMIOLOGY

- Most commonly secondary to infections
- Overall incidence is difficult to determine secondary to the many conditions that cause DIC.

PATHOPHYSIOLOGY

- Not a disorder in itself; occurs as a result of various initiating events
- Characterized by microvascular thrombosis and hemorrhage
- May be acute (e.g., meningococcemia) or chronic (e.g., malignancy/leukemia)
- There is a systemic intravascular deposition of fibrin as a result of increased thrombin generation, suppression of anticoagulant pathways, impaired fibrinolysis, and activation of inflammatory pathways.
- The initiation of coagulation activation leading to thrombin formation in DIC is mediated via the tissue factor/factor VIIa pathway.
- The tissue factor/factor VIIa pathway is activated via tissue factor expression from damaged endothelial cells.
- Anticoagulant pathways are diminished because of a decrease in the plasma levels of antithrombin and the protein C system through impaired production and increased destruction.
- The increase in fibrinolytic activity is likely secondary to the release of plasminogen activators from damaged endothelial cells.

ETIOLOGY

Most common causes are sepsis (particularly gram-negative), hypotensive shock, and trauma.

- Sepsis/severe infection
  - Bacterial: gram-negative and gram-positive
  - Malaria: *Plasmodium falciparum*
  - Fungal: Aspergillus
  - Rickettsial: Rocky Mountain spotted fever
  - Viral
- Trauma
  - Multiple fractures with fat emboli
  - Massive soft tissue injury
  - Severe head trauma
  - Multiple gunshot wounds
- Malignancies
  - Acute promyelocytic leukemia
  - Widespread solid tumors (e.g., neuroblastoma, adenocarcinoma)
- Obstetric
  - Retained intrauterine fetal demise
  - Preeclampsia/eclampsia
  - Amniotic fluid embolism
  - Abruptio placentae
  - Posthemorrhagic shock
- Neonatal
  - Necrotizing enterocolitis
  - Perinatal asphyxia
  - Amniotic fluid aspiration
  - Obstetric complications (see above)
  - Sepsis (bacterial and viral)
  - Erythroblastosis fetalis
  - Respiratory distress syndrome
- Vascular malformations
  - Kasabach-Merritt syndrome
  - Large vascular aneurysms
- Miscellaneous
  - Acute hemolytic transfusion reaction
  - Snake bite
  - Homozygous protein C/S deficiency (purpura fulminans)
  - Transplant rejection
  - Severe collagen vascular disease
  - Recreational drugs
  - Profound shock or asphyxia
  - Hypothermia or hyperthermia
  - Extensive burn injuries
  - Fulminant hepatitis/hepatic failure
  - Severe pancreatitis

DIAGNOSIS

HISTORY

- Presence of one of the underlying conditions (see "Etiology")
- Abrupt onset of bleeding
- Prolonged bleeding from venipuncture sites
- Bleeding from multiple sites, especially venipunctures, cutdown sites, mucous membranes, skin, GI tract, and genitourinary tract
- Pulmonary or intracranial hemorrhage
- Major organ dysfunction: pulmonary, renal, hepatic

PHYSICAL EXAM

- Signs of underlying disease
- Generally, a very toxic-appearing patient
- Ecchymosis and petechiae
- Bleeding from previously intact venipuncture sites or surgical wounds
- Skin infarctions (purpura fulminans) secondary to thrombosis of dermal vessels

DIAGNOSTIC TESTS & INTERPRETATION

Lab

- There is no single test that can reliably diagnose DIC.
- Laboratory testing for DIC should be followed closely because results can change rapidly.
- CBC: Decreased platelet count is often the earliest abnormality, but this finding is nonspecific.
- Peripheral smear: schistocytes, microspherocytes (50% of cases)
- Prothrombin time (PT) and activated partial thromboplastin time (aPTT): normal to prolonged
  - Prolonged PT in 50–75% of cases
  - Prolonged aPTT in 50–60% of cases
- Fibrinogen: in the initial phase is increased as an acute-phase reactant and then decrease with consumption
  - Sensitivity is only 28%
- Fibrin degradation products or fibrin split products: increased
  - Sensitivity 90–100% but low specificity

- Soluble fibrin monomer complexes (D-dimers): increased
  - Elevated D-dimer in 93–100% of patients with DIC but low specificity
  - A normal D-dimer rules out DIC
- Antithrombin, protein C or S levels: decreased
  - Not routinely sent to assess for DIC
- Factor VIII: in the initial phase could be increased as an acute-phase reactant and then decrease with consumption
  - Factor VIII is normal in coagulopathy associated with liver disease.
- Multiple scoring systems using common laboratory results have been developed to help determine if a patient is in DIC. These scoring systems have not been validated in pediatric patients.

DIFFERENTIAL DIAGNOSIS

- Coagulopathy of liver disease
- Vitamin K deficiency
- Pathologic fibrinolysis
- Other microangiopathic diseases, for example, thrombotic thrombocytopenic purpura or hemolytic uremic syndrome

TREATMENT

ADDITIONAL TREATMENT

General Measures

- The most important therapy for DIC is to treat the underlying disorder.
- Supportive therapy may be required to treat symptomatic coagulation abnormalities.
- Hemostatic therapy should not be used to treat isolated laboratory abnormalities.
- Correction of the coagulopathy should only occur to treat bleeding or prior to an invasive procedure.
- Replacement therapy
  - Cryoprecipitate: for fibrinogen replacement
  - Platelets
  - Fresh frozen plasma: contains all pro and anticoagulant proteins
- The role of heparin for DIC is controversial. It has been used in chronic DIC, arterial thromboses, or large vessel venous thromboses.
- Antithrombin at supraphysiologic dosing has been studied with mixed results.
  - Antithrombin is currently not recommended for the treatment of DIC in pediatric patients.
- In pediatric DIC, recombinant activated protein C has not been shown to be beneficial and was associated with an increased risk of bleeding.
- Off-label use of recombinant activated factor VII has been reported for patients with severe bleeding that is refractory to replacement therapy. There are significant concerns about the prothrombotic potential of this medication.
- Antifibrinolytic agents (aminocaproic acid or tranexamic acid) have been used for patients with intense fibrinolysis (e.g., Kasabach-Merritt, acute promyelocytic leukemia, or trauma). These medications are not routinely recommended for the treatment of DIC.
- Supportive care: Manage other organ system failure.

ONGOING CARE

PROGNOSIS

- Poor unless underlying disease is treated
- The intensity and duration of DIC depend on the degree of activation of the coagulation system, liver function, blood flow, and ability to reverse underlying etiology that has led to DIC.

COMPLICATIONS

- Hemorrhage
  - Pulmonary
  - Intracranial
- Thrombosis
- Multiorgan system failure

ADDITIONAL READING

- Levi M. Disseminated intravascular coagulation. *Crit Care Med*. 2007;35(9):2191–2195.
- Levi M, Meijers JC. DIC: which laboratory tests are most useful? *Blood Rev*. 2011;25(1):33–37.
- Montagnana M, Franchi M, Danese E, et al. Disseminated intravascular coagulation in obstetric and gynecologic disorders. *Semin Thromb Hemost*. 2010;36(4):404–418.
- Veldman A, Fischer D, Nold MF, et al. Disseminated intravascular coagulation in neonates and preterm neonates. *Semin Thromb Hemost*. 2010;36(4):419–428.

CODES

ICD10

- D65 Disseminated intravascular coagulation
- P60 Disseminated intravascular coagulation of newborn

DOWN SYNDROME (TRISOMY 21)

Esther K. Chung • Julia Belkowitz

BASICS

DESCRIPTION

Syndrome first described by John Langdon Down in 1866 consisting of multiple abnormalities, including hypotonia, flat facies, upslanting palpebral fissures, and small ears; also called "trisomy 21"

Other abnormalities include the following:

- Congenital heart disease (40–50%; most not symptomatic as a newborn)
  - Atrioventricular (AV) canal (60% of those with congenital heart disease)
  - Ventriculoseptal defect (VSD)
  - Patent ductus arteriosus (PDA)
  - Atrioseptal defect (ASD)
  - Aberrant subclavian artery
  - Tetralogy of Fallot
- Hearing loss (66–75%): sensorineural and conductive
- Strabismus (33–45%)
- Nystagmus (15–35%)
- Fine lens opacities (by slit-lamp examination 59%), cataracts (1–15%)
- Refractive errors (50%)
- Nasolacrimal duct stenosis
- Delayed tooth eruption
- Tracheoesophageal fistula
- Gastrointestinal atresia (12%)
- Celiac disease
- Meckel diverticulum
- Hirschsprung disease (<1%)
- Imperforate anus
- Renal malformations
- Hypospadias (5%)
- Cryptorchidism (5–50%)
- Testicular microlithiasis
- Thyroid disease (15%): hypothyroidism, hyperthyroidism
- Transient myeloproliferative disorder (3–10%), neonatal (leukemoid reaction)
- Transient neonatal polycythemia, neutrophilia, thrombocytopenia
- Leukemia (<1%; 10–20 times greater risk than in general population, acute lymphoblastic and myeloid leukemias)
- Decreased T and B lymphocytes
- Testicular germ cell tumors
- Airway anomalies, including tracheo- and laryngomalacia
- Infertility, especially in males
- Obesity
- Alopecia areata (10–15%)
- Seizures (5–10%), usually myoclonic
- Alzheimer disease (nearly all older than age 40 years show neuropathologic signs)
- Mild to moderate mental retardation (IQ range 25–70)
- Dry, hyperkeratotic skin (75%)

EPIDEMIOLOGY

- Male > female (1.3:1)
- Best recognized and most frequent chromosomal syndrome of humans
- 1 of the 3 most common autosomal trisomies in humans (others are trisomies 18 and 13)
- Most common autosomal chromosomal abnormality causing mental retardation
- >50% of trisomy 21 fetuses are spontaneously aborted in early pregnancy.

Incidence

1/600–1/800 live births, although incidence varies with maternal age:

- 1/1,500 for maternal ages 15–29 years
- 1/800 for maternal ages 30–34 years
- 1/270 for maternal ages 35–39 years
- 1/100 for maternal ages 40–49 years

Genetics

- Approximately 90% of cases are the result of chromosomal nondisjunction (failure to segregate during meiosis) in the maternal DNA.
- <5% of cases are the result of paternal nondisjunction.
- 3–4% of cases are the result of translocations; mostly chromosomes 21 and 14 [t(14q21q)]; rarely between 21 and 13 or 15; 75% of translocations are sporadic de novo events; the others result from balanced translocations in one parent.
- Of live births, 1–2% are mosaic (nondisjunction occurs after conception; 2 cell lines are present); generally less severely affected

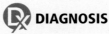

DIAGNOSIS

HISTORY

- Check for previous history of infant with Down syndrome in the family.
- Growth and developmental status
- Feeding problems
- Snoring, signs of sleep apnea (e.g., restless sleep)
- Stool habits
- Hearing concerns

PHYSICAL EXAM

The phenotype is variable from person to person.

- General
  - Short stature
  - Hypotonia (80–100%), with an open mouth and a protruding tongue
  - Midface hypoplasia
- Head
  - Brachycephaly with a flattened occiput
  - Microcephaly
  - False fontanelle (95%)
  - Late closure of fontanelles
- Eyes
  - Upslanting palpebral fissures (98%)
  - Inner epicanthal folds
  - Brushfield spots (speckling of the iris)
  - Fine lens opacities on slit-lamp examination
  - Cataracts, refractive error, strabismus, and nystagmus
- Ears
  - Small, prominent, low set; overfolding of upper helix and small canals
- Nose: small (85%); flat nasal bridge
- Tongue
  - Relative but not true macroglossia (tongue mass is normal)
  - Fissuring of tongue
- Mouth: high-arched or abnormal palate
- Teeth
  - Missing (50%), small, hypoplastic
  - Irregular placement
- Neck
  - In infancy, excess skin at the nape
  - Short appearance
  - Occasionally webbed
- Heart: murmur, arrhythmia, cyanosis
- Abdomen
  - In neonate, distention may be present owing to obstruction or atresia.
  - Diastasis recti
- Genitals
  - In adolescents, straight pubic hair
  - In males, small penis, cryptorchidism
- Extremities
  - Broad hands, with short metacarpals and phalanges
  - 5th finger with hypoplasia of the midphalanx (60%) and clinodactyly (50%)
  - Simian crease (single transverse palmar crease) in ~50%. A newborn with a simian crease has a 1 in 60 chance of having Down syndrome.
  - Wide gap between the 1st and 2nd toes (96%)
  - Syndactyly of 2nd and 3rd toes
  - Hyperflexibility of joints
- Skin
  - Cutis marmorata (43%)
  - In older children, hyperkeratotic dry skin (75%)
  - Fine, soft, sparse hair

DIAGNOSTIC TESTS & INTERPRETATION

Prenatal

- 2nd-trimester prenatal quad screen test (alpha-fetoprotein [AFP], unconjugated estriol, human chorionic gonadotropin [hCG], and inhibin A):
  - Performed at 15–18 weeks
  - These serum markers together can detect 67–76% of pregnancies affected by trisomy 21, with a false-positive rate of ~5%.
  - A positive test is an indication for karyotyping with amniocentesis.
- 1st-trimester maternal serum screening (pregnancy-associated plasma protein A and free β-hCG)
- When 1st- and 2nd-trimester tests are combined, there is a detection rate of 95%.
- New 2nd-trimester noninvasive prenatal screening (NIPS) tests are available to assess fetal DNA in the maternal circulation as a supplement to other tests.

Postnatal

- Chromosomal karyotype on cultured lymphocytes from peripheral blood: may be performed postnatally for confirmation if there is a clinical suspicion of Down syndrome
- Complete blood count (CBC)
  - In the newborn period to check for polycythemia and transient myeloproliferative disorder; repeat test in adolescence.
- Down syndrome patients may have an increased mean corpuscular volume (MCV), making the diagnosis of iron deficiency anemia difficult.
- Thyroid function tests: to rule out hypothyroidism or hyperthyroidism

Imaging

- 1st-trimester ultrasound measurement of nuchal translucency: performed in the 1st trimester along with maternal serum screening
- Fetal ultrasound
  - May show polyhydramnios if bowel obstruction is present
  - A thickened nuchal fold, an absent nasal bone in the 1st trimester, and echogenic intracardiac foci have been associated with an increased risk for Down syndrome.
- Echocardiography and chest radiography: done in the 1st month of life to rule out cardiac disease

- When symptoms suggestive of atlantoaxial instability (e.g., neck and/or radicular pain, weakness, change in tone, difficulties walking, or changes in bowel and bladder function) are present, lateral cervical spine radiographs in flexion, neutral, and extension: to rule out atlantoaxial instability, defined as >5-mm space between atlas and odontoid process of the axis. Important measures include the following:
  - Atlantodens interval (ADI; normal <4.5 mm): the distance between the posterior surface of the anterior arch of C1 and the anterior surface of the dens
  - Neural canal width (NCW; normal ≥14 mm): the distance between the posterior surface of the dens and the anterior surface of the posterior arch of C1
  - Distance of subluxation at the occipitoatlantal joint: normally ≥7 mm

Diagnostic Procedures/Other

- Prenatal karyotyping via amniocentesis (16–18 weeks' gestation) or chorionic villus sampling (9–11 weeks' gestation)
  - Performed for any woman who presents with a positive triple or quad screen
  - May be offered if prenatal ultrasound reveals a finding associated with Down syndrome
  - Because this test fails to detect 10–15% of Down syndrome in older women, amniocentesis is typically offered to all women >35 years of age.
- Tissue sample other than blood (usually skin): to check for mosaicism

Follow-up Recommendations

- Genetic counseling and evaluation is recommended.
- Referral to organizations (e.g., Down Syndrome International), parent-to-parent support groups, and other community supports available to families of children with Down syndrome

Prognosis

- Life expectancy is mildly decreased, with many living into the 6th decade; median age of death is 49 years.
- Clinical signs of Alzheimer disease occur later in life, with reports as high as 51% in the 4th decade.
- As adults, most patients with Down syndrome can work in supported positions.

Complications

- Otitis media with effusion (50–70%)
- Sinusitis
- Tonsillar and adenoidal hypertrophy
- Obstructive airway disease with associated sleep apnea (50–79%), cor pulmonale
- Obstructive bowel disease (12%, newborn period)
- Constipation (owing to low tone and decreased gross motor mobility)
- Subluxation of the hips (secondary to ligamentous laxity)
- Atlantoaxial instability (10–30%; secondary to ligamentous laxity, which is most severe prior to age 10 years)

Patient Monitoring

- Annually: growth and development:
  - Current recommendations by the American Academy of Pediatrics (AAP) are to use standard growth charts for all children including those with Down syndrome because the previously used Down syndrome growth charts are no longer felt to represent the current body proportion.
  - Average age for acquiring developmental milestones differs from normal population.
  - Early intervention program for hypotonia and developmental delay is recommended.
  - Review need for physical, occupational, and speech therapy at each health maintenance visit.
  - Discuss psychosocial and behavioral progress and concerns and screen for mental health disorders (e.g., autism, ADHD).
- Assessment of nutrition and activity for obesity prevention/counseling
- Evaluation/referrals for available family support including medical, financial, and social services and school transitions
- Injury and abuse prevention
- Cardiac: Early evaluation in newborn period, with follow-up until the presence or absence of disease is evident. Subacute bacterial endocarditis prophylaxis for patients with certain types of cardiac disease.
- Ophthalmologic
  - Early evaluation for cataracts and glaucoma
  - Visit to ophthalmologist by 6 months, annually until age 5 years, then every 2–3 years
- Ear, nose, and throat (ENT)/audiologic
  - Audiologic evaluation; if newborn evaluation was normal, repeat at 6 months of age in the first 3 years of life, then every other year.
- Obstructive sleep apnea
  - Review symptoms with family in first 6 months and screen for symptoms at each well child visit.
  - Refer all children for sleep study or polysomnography by 4 years of age and at any age if symptomatic.
- Orthopedic: Routine screening by x-ray for atlantoaxial instability in asymptomatic children is no longer routinely recommended by the AAP, although it is still required for participation in the following Special Olympics activities: butterfly stroke and diving starts in swimming, diving, pentathlon, high jump, equestrian sports, artistic gymnastics, soccer, alpine skiing, and any warm-up exercise placing undue stress on the head and neck.
- Endocrine: thyroid function tests in newborn period, ages 6 months and 12 months, then yearly
- Gastrointestinal: Screen for symptoms of celiac disease (i.e., diarrhea, poor growth, failure to thrive, etc.), and if symptomatic, obtain tissue transglutaminase immunoglobulin A (IgA) level and quantitative IgA.
- For adolescents, discuss personal hygiene and issues related to reproductive health.

ALERT

- Use caution with endotracheal intubation if absence or presence of atlantoaxial instability is unknown in order to avoid spinal cord injury, which may be seen in rare cases.
- Hearing loss may be misinterpreted as a behavioral problem.
- Use care with atropine and pilocarpine for ophthalmologic evaluation because of possible cholinergic hypersensitivity.

ADDITIONAL READING

1. Bull MJ and the Committee on Genetics. Health supervision for children with Down syndrome. *Pediatrics*. 2011;128(2):393–406.
2. Bruwier A, Chantrain DF. Hematological disorders and leukemia in children with Down Syndrome. *Eur J Pediatr*. 2012;171(9):1301–1307.
3. Crissman BG, Worley G, Roizen N, et al. Current perspectives on Down syndrome: selected medical and social issues. *Am J Med Genet C Semin Med Genet*. 2006;142C(3):127–130.
4. Dykens EM. Psychiatric and behavioral disorders in person with Down syndrome. *Ment Retard Dev Disabil Res Rev*. 2007;13(3):272–278.
5. Hickey F, Hickey E, Summar KL. Medical update for children with Down syndrome for the pediatrician and family practitioner. *Adv Pediatr*. 2012;59(1):137–157.
6. Mik G, Gholve PA, Scher DM, et al. Down syndrome: orthopedic issues. *Curr Opin Pediatr*. 2008;20(1):30–36.
7. Pandit C, Fitzgerald DA. Respiratory problems in children with Down syndrome. *J Paediatr Child Health*. 2012;48(3):E147–E152.
8. Gregg AR, Gross SJ, Best RG, et al. ACMG statement on noninvasive prenatal screening for fetal aneuploidy. *Genet Med*. 2013;15(5):395–398.

CODES

ICD10

- Q90.9 Down syndrome, unspecified
- Q90.2 Trisomy 21, translocation
- Q90.1 Trisomy 21, mosaicism (mitotic nondisjunction)

PATIENT TEACHING

- Participation by individuals with Down syndrome who have atlantoaxial instability. See: http://sports.specialolympics.org/specialo.org/special_/English/coach/coaching/basics_o/Down_syn.htm
- Down syndrome. See: http://kidshealth.org/parent/medical/genetic/down_syndrome.html

FAQ

- Q: Why was Down syndrome referred to as mongolism in the past?
- A: There was a mistaken notion about a racial cause for this syndrome because of the facial appearance, which was thought to be similar to that of those of Mongoloid origin.
- Q: Do all children with Down syndrome have mental retardation?
- A: No. Although all persons with nonmosaic Down syndrome have some degree of cognitive disability, some have IQs >70 and are not considered to have mental retardation.
- Q: Can a normal cardiac examination rule out the presence of a cardiac anomaly?
- A: No. The AAP recommends that all patients with Down syndrome have a cardiology consultation within the 1st month of life. Timely surgery may be necessary to prevent serious complications.
- Q: Are patients with atlantoaxial instability symptomatic?
- A: No. Most are asymptomatic, but symptoms of cord compression may be seen in 1–2% of patients. Patients with neck and/or radicular pain, weakness, change in tone, difficulties walking, or changes in bowel and bladder function should undergo radiologic evaluation for atlantoaxial instability.

DROWNING

Mercedes M. Blackstone

BASICS

DESCRIPTION

- Drowning is defined as respiratory impairment from submersion in a liquid medium.
- The term "drowning" does not imply outcome; drowning can be fatal or nonfatal.
- Historically "near drowning," or submersion injury, was defined as survival, at least temporarily, after suffocation by submersion in water.
  - The World Congress on Drowning and the World Health Organization advocate abandoning confusing terms such as "near drowning," "wet drowning," and "dry drowning"; they suggest that the literature should only use the term "drowning."

EPIDEMIOLOGY

- Drowning is second only to motor vehicle collisions as the most common cause of death from unintentional injury in childhood.
- For every drowning death, another 5 children present to emergency departments for nonfatal submersion events.
- Bimodal age distribution, with peak in children <5 years of age and again among adolescents 15–19 years of age
- Bathtub drowning is common in babies; child neglect or abuse should be considered.
- Adolescent submersion injuries usually involve substance abuse or risk-taking behavior.

RISK FACTORS

- Males, children <5 years of age, African Americans, and children of low socioeconomic status are at greatest risk.
- Other significant risk factors include the following:
  - Direct access to swimming pools
  - Poor swimming ability or overestimation of ability
  - Use of alcohol and illicit drugs
  - Inadequate adult supervision
  - Children with seizure disorders or primary cardiac arrhythmias such as long QT syndrome

GENERAL PREVENTION

- Most drowning are preventable.
- Legislation to require adequate 4-sided isolation fencing and rescue equipment for public and residential pools
- Restriction of sale and consumption of alcohol in boating areas, pools, and beaches
- Life vests for children of all ages near bodies of water
- Parental education regarding adequate supervision during bathing and around swimming pools
- Cardiopulmonary resuscitation (CPR) courses for pool owners, parents, and older children

PATHOPHYSIOLOGY

- Drowning begins with a loss of the normal breathing pattern as panic ensues and subsequent apnea, laryngospasm, or aspiration occurs.
- Water aspirated into the trachea and lungs washes out surfactant and leads to atelectasis, intrapulmonary shunting, poor lung compliance, increased capillary permeability, and hypoxemia, ultimately resulting in acute respiratory distress syndrome (ARDS).
- Severe hypoxemia is the final common pathway and results in multisystem organ failure.
- Cerebral hypoxia results in cerebral edema and increased intracranial pressure and causes the majority of morbidity and mortality associated with drowning.

COMMONLY ASSOCIATED CONDITIONS

- Cervical spine injuries should be considered in older children who have experienced diving accidents but are otherwise relatively rare in drowning events.
- Signs of child abuse or neglect should be sought in young children.
- Adolescents may have associated toxic ingestions.

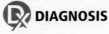

DIAGNOSIS

HISTORY

- Mechanism
  - History of diving or other high-impact injury
  - Intoxication
  - Seizure disorder
  - Cardiac arrhythmia
  - Child abuse
- Prognostic indicators; the following have been correlated with a poor prognosis and may be helpful to ask about:
  - Age <3 years
  - Length of submersion >5 minutes
  - Time to effective CPR >10 minutes
  - Lack of vital signs at the scene
  - Length of resuscitation >25 minutes
  - Warmer water: Submersion in cold water (<5°C [41°F]) may have a good prognosis despite submersion time >5 minutes.

PHYSICAL EXAM

- Vital signs with core temperature
- Drowning victims with unclear histories must be treated as trauma victims.
- Neurologic
  - Pupillary response, cranial nerve findings, Glasgow Coma Scale (GCS) score, gag reflex
  - Serial neurologic exams should be performed to assess neurologic outcome. Children with a GCS score <5 after resuscitation usually have a poor neurologic outcome.
- Respiratory
  - Lower airway findings (rales, tachypnea, wheezing, retractions, nasal flaring)
  - Drowning victims may have deteriorating pulmonary involvement despite an initially normal exam. Watch closely for signs of lower airway involvement.
- Circulation
  - Perfusion, strength of distal pulses, capillary refill, urine output, cardiac rhythm
- GI tract
  - Abdominal distention from swallowed water or ventilation
- Musculoskeletal
  - Neck injuries in high-impact drownings

DIAGNOSTIC TESTS & INTERPRETATION

Lab

- Arterial blood gases
  - To detect and facilitate treatment of metabolic acidosis in the child with respiratory distress or apnea
- Electrolytes
  - Not indicated in the seemingly well child; aspiration of huge amounts of water is required to generate electrolyte shifts.
- Blood glucose
  - An elevated level correlates with poor outcome for comatose submersion victims.
- Anticonvulsant levels for victims with seizure disorders
- Toxicology screening when ingestion suspected
- Children with severe submersion injuries are at risk of multiorgan system failure, and in these patients, end organ labs should be checked including coagulation studies.

Imaging

- A chest radiograph is indicated for children with signs of pulmonary involvement and after intubation.
  - Caution: Initial chest radiographs may be normal in the drowning victim.
- Cervical spine films are indicated for victims of high-impact events.
- Neuroimaging for cerebral anoxic injury

Diagnostic Procedures/Other

- ECG to document normal rhythm and evaluate for prolonged QT_C if indicated by history
- Serial pulse oximetry to detect early signs of pulmonary involvement

TREATMENT

MEDICATION

- Patients may experience bronchospasm and typically respond to conventional management with inhaled beta-agonists.
- Prophylactic antibiotics or steroids are not indicated.
- For patients who develop pneumonia, antimicrobial therapy should cover waterborne pathogens (e.g., *Pseudomonas*, *Aeromonas*).
- Seizures should be aggressively controlled with antiepileptics because they increase oxygen consumption.

ADDITIONAL TREATMENT

General Measures

- Good prehospital care and effective bystander CPR dramatically improve chances of neurologically intact survival.
- Attempts to remove water from the lungs such as abdominal thrusts or Heimlich maneuver delay care and are not recommended.
- Cervical spine immobilization can interfere with airway management and should only be performed when injury is suspected.
- Patients who are breathing spontaneously should be placed in the right lateral decubitus position to prevent aspiration.
- CPR in drowning victims should follow the traditional ABC approach rather than compression-only CPR because prompt rescue breathing increases the chance of survival.
- Even patients who respond well to bystander resuscitation need to be transported to an emergency department for further monitoring.

- Pulses may be difficult to appreciate as they can be weak and slow due to hypothermia; some common arrhythmias such as sinus bradycardia and atrial fibrillation need no immediate treatment.
- The hypothermic patient who is a warm water (>20°C [86°F]) drowning victim does not have a good prognosis or need vigorous rewarming.

INPATIENT CONSIDERATIONS

Initial Stabilization

- Airway
  - Protect the cervical spine if indicated by history.
  - Ensure a patent airway in the comatose victim or patient in cardiac arrest.
- Breathing
  - Supplemental oxygen via facemask with any compromise or desaturation following their submersion event
  - Intubate for apnea, airway protection, or inadequate oxygenation or ventilation
  - Treatment of bronchospasm
- Circulation
  - For the victim with cardiopulmonary arrest, the asystole protocol should be followed.
  - Because capillary leak may occur after an ischemic/anoxic episode, isotonic fluids (e.g., normal saline solution or Ringer lactate, 10-mL/kg aliquots) should be given for signs of intravascular volume depletion until normalized.
  - ECG monitoring should be provided with appropriate response to dysrhythmias, especially for the hypothermic, cold water drowning victim.
  - For severely hypothermic patients with a core temperature <28°C (82.4°F), aggressive rewarming is indicated. Electrical defibrillation and pharmacotherapy may not be successful.
- Disability
  - Maintenance of eucapnia and adequate oxygenation to prevent further hypoxemia
  - Elevate the head of the bed once cervical spine is cleared and consider mild hyperventilation for elevated intracranial pressure (ICP).
  - Other measures for reducing ICP have not proven effective, likely because the brain injury and swelling is secondary to hypoxic cell injury as opposed to a traumatic lesion.
- Exposure
  - The drowning victim should be dried and warmed.
  - Most thermometers do not register temperatures below 34°C (93.2°F) so a hypothermia thermometer may be necessary:
    - For core temperatures 32°C (89.6°F) to 35°C (90.5°F), active external rewarming with heating blankets or radiant warmers
    - For <32°C (89.6°F), active internal rewarming added (heated aerosolized oxygen and IV fluids, gastric and bladder lavage with warm saline)
    - For severe hypothermia (<28°C [82.4°F]) and where available, peritoneal dialysis or hemodialysis, mediastinal irrigation, and cardiac bypass
    - The cold water drowning victim with hypothermia must be rewarmed to a temperature >34°C (89.6°F) before CPR is terminated.
- Remember: The saying, "The patient is not dead until he or she is warm and dead" only applies to drownings in very cold water.

Admission Criteria

- Severely ill children require admission to the intensive care unit.
- Children who were apneic, cyanotic, or pulseless at the scene should be admitted for close observation even if they appear well.
- Patients who are at all symptomatic should be admitted to a monitored setting.
- A subset of asymptomatic children may be discharged from the emergency department after being monitored for 6–8 hours.

ONGOING CARE

FOLLOW-UP RECOMMENDATIONS

- Long-term follow-up of apparently neurologically intact survivors has shown mild coordination or gross motor deficiencies.
- Potential increased risk for chronic lung disease, depending on pulmonary involvement

Patient Monitoring

- Victims who appear well and had relatively minor event:
  - Monitor with pulse oximetry for progressive respiratory distress.
  - If asymptomatic at 6–8 hours postimmersion, can be discharged
- Victims with significant neurologic injury: Key is to prevent secondary injury.
  - Maintain euvolemia and euglycemia.

PROGNOSIS

- Most children (about 75%) recover with intact neurologic survival.
- Duration and severity of initial hypoxic insult are most important determinants of brain injury and death.
- See prognostic factors in "History" section. Additional indicators of poor prognosis:
  - Coma on arrival
  - Needing CPR in the emergency department
  - Initial arterial blood pH <7.1
- Children with warm water submersion time >4 minutes who do not receive CPR at the scene and who have absent vital signs or a GCS score <5 in the emergency department usually have a poor prognosis.
- Victims who have prolonged submersions in very cold water (<5°C [41°F]) may have a good prognosis because of core cooling with a concomitant decrease in metabolic rate while the brain is still being perfused.
- A good prognostic indicator is continuing improvement in the neurologic examination over the first several hours.

COMPLICATIONS

- Pneumonia
- Pneumomediastinum or pneumothorax in the patient undergoing ventilation therapy
- Brain injury secondary to hypoxia
- Pulmonary injury with intrapulmonary shunting secondary to damage of the alveoli
- ARDS
- Metabolic acidosis secondary to hypoxemia
- Ischemic injury to organs such as liver, kidneys, and intestines
- Disseminated intravascular coagulation
- Hypothermia in cold water drowning

ADDITIONAL READING

- American Academy of Pediatrics Committee on Injury, Violence, and Poison Prevention. Prevention of drowning. *Pediatrics*. 2010;126(1):178–185.
- Brenner RA. Prevention of drowning in infants, children, and adolescents. *Pediatrics*. 2003; 112(2):440–445.
- Centers for Disease Control and Prevention. Web-based injury statistics query and reporting system (WISQARS) [online]. http://www.cdc.gov/injury/wisqars. Accessed November 30, 2014.
- Hwang V, Shofer FS, Durbin DR, et al. Prevalence of traumatic injuries in drowning and near drowning in children and adolescents. *Arch Pediatr Adolesc Med*. 2003;157(1):50–53.
- Noonan L, Howrey R, Ginsburg CM. Freshwater submersion injuries in children: a retrospective review of seventy-five hospitalized patients. *Pediatrics*. 1996;98(3, Pt 1):368–371.
- Papa L, Hoelle R, Idris A. Systematic review of definitions for drowning incidents. *Resuscitation*. 2005;65(3):255–264.
- Szpilman D, Bierens JJ, Handley AJ, et al. Drowning. *N Engl J Med*. 2012;366(22):2102–2110.
- Thompson DC, Rivara F. Pool fencing for preventing drowning of children. *Cochrane Database Syst Rev*. 2000;(2):CD001047.
- Vanden Hoek TL, Morrison LJ, Shuster M, et al. Part 12: cardiac arrest in special situations: 2010 American Heart Association Guidelines for Cardiopulmonary Resuscitation and Emergency Cardiovascular Care. *Circulation*. 2010;122(18)(Suppl 3):S829–S861.

CODES

ICD10

T75.1XXA Unsp effects of drowning and nonfatal submersion, init

FAQ

- Q: Should the drowning victim who arrives at the hospital with cardiopulmonary arrest be resuscitated?
- A: Yes. A brief (10–15 minutes) attempt at resuscitation is indicated until circumstances of the drowning and core temperature are known. Warm water drowning victims who require CPR in the emergency department may rarely (0–25%) have good neurologic recovery, but these patients usually respond quickly (<15 minutes) to therapy.
- Q: Is artificial surfactant useful in drowning victims?
- A: Surfactant has not been found to be beneficial for acute lung injury secondary to drowning. Further investigation is needed before it can be recommended for clinical use.

DYSFUNCTIONAL ELIMINATION SYNDROME

Kara N. Saperston • Laurence Baskin

BASICS

DESCRIPTION

- Dysfunctional elimination syndrome (DES) is seen in children with bladder and bowel dysfunction in the setting of normal neurologic findings.
- We define dysfunctional voiding as tightening the pelvic floor muscles before completely emptying the bladder, which may leave a large amount of urine in the bladder.
  - DES also encompasses the underactive ("flaccid") bladder, which is seen in children who postpone voiding and only empty a few times a day.
  - Constipation has a major role to play in affecting the bladder's ability to store urine and also affects the bladder's ability to empty completely and in a timely fashion.
- Patients with DES may also experience daytime and/or nighttime incontinence.

EPIDEMIOLOGY

- 15% of 6-year-olds have abnormal voiding patterns. Children with DES often have
  - Abnormal renal ultrasounds
  - Higher rates of urinary tract infections (UTIs)
  - A decreased ability to resolve vesicoureteral reflux (VUR)
- 89% of children who are treated for their constipation completely resolve their daytime urinary incontinence, and 63% resolve their nighttime incontinence.

RISK FACTORS

- Recurrent UTIs
- Constipation

PATHOPHYSIOLOGY

- A child who is holding his or her stool and not having regular daily bowel movements has increased stool in the rectal vault.
- As stool builds up in the rectal vault (constipation), it begins to push on the bladder. This process causes decreased bladder filling.
- In addition, the rectal vault shares sensory input in the sacral spinal cord with the bladder, and the full rectal vault can be sensed as a full bladder, triggering bladder spasms and leakage and/or incomplete emptying of the bladder.
- As a child struggles to stay dry in the face of bladder spasms, he or she overcontracts the external sphincter of the bladder, has a hard time relaxing the external sphincter during voiding, and develops increased pressure during voiding. This increased pressure can be transmitted to the kidneys.

DIAGNOSIS

HISTORY

- A child will present after toilet training with symptoms of daytime and/or nighttime incontinence.
- In addition, he or she may have a history of recurrent UTIs or VUR.
- Bowel dysfunction may present as encopresis, constipation, or as fecal impaction.

PHYSICAL EXAM

- Most commonly, the exam will be normal.
- Abdomen: palpable bladder or stool in the colon
- Evaluate the spine for skin discoloration, dimples, or hair patches to rule out occult spinal dysraphism.
- Evaluate female genitalia and rule out labial adhesions that can trap urine and cause incontinence.
- Consider possible ectopic ureter if there is vaginal pooling of urine.
- Evaluate male genitalia and rule out prior hypospadias repair or severe phimosis in which urine trapping can occur.
- Rectal exam can reveal fecal impaction.

DIAGNOSTIC TESTS & INTERPRETATION

Lab

- Urinalysis to rule out bacteriuria or glucosuria
- First morning urine osmolality to assess renal concentrating ability in nocturnal enuresis

Imaging

- Radiograph of kidneys, ureters, and bladder (KUB): constipation, normal spine
- Renal ultrasound: pre- and postvoid images to evaluate the bladder and kidneys

Diagnostic Procedures/Other

- Voiding/drinking
  - Diary is a tool used to define the nature of the incontinence.
- Voiding cystourethrogram (VCUG)
  - Used to evaluate for VUR and to look at the urethra and bladder neck during voiding
- Urodynamic studies
  - Tools used to define bladder function if there is a poor response to initial management
  - Uroflow is used to evaluate bladder outflow.
  - Cystometry and perineal EMG studies give information about bladder function during filling and voiding.

DIFFERENTIAL DIAGNOSIS

- Ectopic ureter to the vagina
- Spinal cord abnormalities (tethered cord)
- Brain tumors

TREATMENT

BEHAVIOR MODIFICATION

- Educate proper voiding mechanics.
- Timed voiding every 2 hours; may use a watch with a repeating alarm
- Correct sitting and standing positions during voiding

- Modify drinking and voiding habits based on diaries to attain frequent voiding and regular stooling.
- Encourage plenty of water intake; fiber for management of constipation
- Time set aside to attempt regular morning bowel movements

MEDICATION

- Bowel management
  - Goal: full clean out
    - Clean out usually lasts 3 days.
    - Use polyethylene glycol 3350 (MiraLax)/ lactulose and enemas and/or mineral oil.
  - If severe, can use KUB to confirm clean out is complete
- Daily management
  - Goal: 1–2 soft bowel movements daily
  - Polyethylene glycol 3350 (MiraLax)/lactulose daily dosing and/or mineral oil help for daily maintenance.
- Antimuscarinics
  - Are used for overactive bladders
  - Work by reducing the frequency and intensity of the bladder contraction
  - Can be supplied in short-acting and long-acting formulas or transdermally

ALERT
Make sure the patient has truly had a good bowel clean out and is focusing first on 1–2 daily soft bowel movements before adding medications to treat the bladder symptoms.

ADDITIONAL THERAPIES

- Biofeedback
- Acupuncture
- Neuromodulation

GENERAL MEASURES

- When a provider is treating a child with bladder and bowel dysfunction, it is imperative that the focus begins with daytime management first, specifically focusing on soft daily bowel movements and timed voiding.
- The nighttime wetting will not improve until the daytime wetting and the constipation have been properly managed.

ONGOING CARE

FOLLOW-UP RECOMMENDATIONS

- Children with recurrent febrile UTIs should be referred to pediatric urology.
- Children with abnormal renal ultrasound should be referred to pediatric urology.
- Children who don't resolve their incontinence after initial management of the bowel dysfunction should be referred to pediatric urology.

PROGNOSIS

- 80% of children are able to resolve their symptoms, with attention given to their bowel function and timed voiding.
- Because this treatment predominantly involves making behavioral changes, this process does not occur quickly. Time and patience are required by both the parents and the children.

ADDITIONAL READING

- Dohil R, Roberts E, Jones KV, et al. Constipation and reversible urinary tract abnormalities. *Arch Dis Child*. 1994;70(1):56–57.
- Issenman RM, Filmer RB, Gorski PA. A review of bowel and bladder control development in children: how gastrointestinal and urologic conditions relate to problems in toilet training. *Pediatrics*. 1999;103(6, Pt 2):1346–1352.
- Koff SA, Wagner TT, Jayanthi VR. The relationship among dysfunctional elimination syndromes, primary vesicoureteral reflux and urinary tract infections in children. *J Urol*. 1998;160(3, Pt 2):1019–1022.
- Loening-Bauke V. Urinary incontinence and urinary tract infection and their resolution with treatment of chronic constipation of childhood. *Pediatrics*. 1997;100(2, Pt 1):228–232.

CODES

ICD10

- R32 Unspecified urinary incontinence
- K59.00 Constipation, unspecified
- R15.9 Full incontinence of feces

FAQ

- Q: Should children with DES have urodynamic evaluation?
- A: Rarely. A patient should undergo standard therapy with timed voiding and treatment of constipation as the 1st-line therapy. If that fails, then a referral to pediatric urology is appropriate, and the need for further testing will be assessed.

DYSFUNCTIONAL UTERINE BLEEDING

Leonard J. Levine • Jonathan R. Pletcher

BASICS

DESCRIPTION

- Bleeding beyond the range of normal menses, with "normal" defined as duration of 2–8 days, occurring every 21–40 days, with blood loss of 20–80 mL/cycle
- May vary in presentation from heavy, long menses followed by long periods of amenorrhea to short, heavy menses occurring every 1–2 weeks
- In teens, dysfunctional uterine bleeding (DUB) most commonly results from anovulatory cycles, which are secondary to an immature hypothalamic–pituitary–ovarian axis.

EPIDEMIOLOGY

- DUB commonly occurs within the first 2 years of menarche when >50% of cycles are anovulatory.
- Later age at menarche associated with longer duration of anovulation
- Most females who experience anovulatory cycles do not develop DUB.

RISK FACTORS

Genetics

Patients with disorders, such as blood dyscrasias and polycystic ovary syndrome (PCOS), usually have familial histories of similar disorders.

PATHOPHYSIOLOGY

- Anovulation (failure to ovulate) results in corpus luteum absence.
- Without the secretory effect of progesterone from the corpus luteum, endometrial proliferation continues because of unopposed estrogen.
- The thickened endometrium eventually outgrows support from the basal endometrium, resulting in sloughing of the highest endometrial levels. Alternatively, cyclic estrogen withdrawal may occur, which will lead to sloughing of the endometrium in the absence of progesterone.
- As subsequent levels of endometrium are shed, bleeding increases. Profuse bleeding may result when the basal endometrium is exposed.

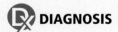

DIAGNOSIS

HISTORY

- Abnormal bleeding
  - Assess the amount of bleeding, and confirm if it is vaginal bleeding.
  - Important to know when bleeding began and some estimate of blood loss to know if the patient is at risk for anemia or hemodynamic instability
- The pattern of DUB in relation to the menstrual cycle can help guide the diagnostic workup.
  - Normal cyclic intervals with increased bleeding during each cycle may suggest a bleeding disorder.
  - Normal intervals with bleeding between cycles may suggest infection or foreign body.
- Abnormal intervals with no cycle regularity may suggest anovulatory cycles or endocrinopathy or be a side effect of hormonal contraception.
  - Increased time lapse between menarche and onset of DUB lessens the likelihood of anovulatory cycles.
  - Teens with chronic diseases and active health problems may have prolonged anovulatory cycles.
- Easy bruisability, epistaxis, and/or bleeding gums may be suggestive of a bleeding disorder.
- A family history of thyroid disease, bleeding disorder, PCOS, or DUB will help guide the laboratory workup.
- Personal and immediate family history of thromboembolism or known familial risk factors
- Ask about sexual activity and abuse in a safe, confidential setting.

PHYSICAL EXAM

- Often normal in patients with DUB
- Assess vital signs, including orthostatic BPs, for signs of cardiac instability resulting from severe blood loss.
- Skin or mucosal pallor, elevated heart rate, or flow murmur may be indicative of anemic state.
- Assess sexual maturity rating (SMR, or Tanner stage). Menarche usually does not occur before SMR 3, so bleeding before this stage suggests a nonmenstrual source of bleeding.
- Look for signs of androgen excess (e.g., hirsutism, acne), which may be reflective of disrupted ovulatory function.
- Bitemporal hemianopsia is suggestive of a pituitary adenoma leading to hyperprolactinemia.
  - Hyperprolactinemia can result in anovulation.
  - Only 1/3 of adolescents with hyperprolactinemia will experience galactorrhea.
- Assess for evidence of thyroid disease, hematologic disorder (e.g., bruising, petechiae), or systemic disease (e.g., poor nutritional status).
- Speculum-assisted pelvic examination may help determine source of bleeding. Bimanual examination is helpful in assessing ovarian or uterine masses, cervical motion or adnexal tenderness, and uterine sizing.

DIAGNOSTIC TESTS & INTERPRETATION

Lab

- Obtain urine or serum human chorionic gonadotropin (β-hCG), regardless of sexual history. Urine hCG testing can reliably detect pregnancy as early as 2 weeks postconception; however, it may be positive for up to 2 weeks following a miscarriage or abortion.
- CBC: Degree of anemia guides treatment plan. Assess for thrombocytopenia. In the setting of acute blood loss, a normal hemoglobin may be falsely reassuring. It is wise to recheck hemoglobin after IV hydration, as decreases may be dramatic.
- For *Chlamydia trachomatis* and *Neisseria gonorrhoeae*, obtain cervical cultures or use nucleic acid amplification tests (NAATs) (e.g., PCR or LCR) on urine, vaginal, or cervical swabs. Be careful to check with laboratory or NAAT manufacturers' information regarding reliability with blood in sample and based on collection site.
- Wet mount or vaginal swab may be unreliable but should be attempted for presence of WBCs and *Trichomonas*. In some labs, *Trichomonas vaginalis* antigen tests may be available.
- Consider prolactin level and thyroid function tests (TSH, T_4): Hyperprolactinemia may have several causes, including pituitary microadenoma, and result in amenorrhea or DUB.
- Prothrombin and partial thromboplastin time, von Willebrand factor: to assess for hematologic causes of bleeding
- Androgen levels, including testosterone (total and free), dehydroepiandrosterone sulfate (DHEAS), androstenedione: Abnormal levels are supportive of PCOS or other hyperandrogenic state.

Imaging

- Pelvic ultrasound
  - Indicated when pregnancy is suspected (ectopic or intrauterine)
  - Consider when a pelvic mass is felt, uterine anomaly is being considered, or bimanual examination cannot be completed
- MRI of the pelvis: Indicated for patients with a suspected pelvic mass when ultrasonography does not clearly define the anatomy

ALERT

Pitfalls

- Neglecting to perform pregnancy testing in an adolescent who denies sexual activity
- Neglecting to reassess hemoglobin concentration after volume expansion

DIFFERENTIAL DIAGNOSIS

Although most cases of abnormal uterine bleeding in adolescents can be attributed to anovulatory cycles, it is important to rule out underlying and alternate causes of irregular or heavy bleeding.

- Pregnancy: should be considered and ruled out in every patient, regardless of patient's reported sexual history
  - Ectopic pregnancy
  - Threatened abortion, incomplete abortion
  - Placenta previa
  - Hydatidiform mole
- Infection
  - Vaginitis (e.g., trichomoniasis)
  - Cervicitis or endometritis (e.g., gonorrhea or chlamydia)
  - Pelvic inflammatory disease

- Hematologic conditions
  - Thrombocytopenia (e.g., immune thrombocytopenic purpura [ITP], leukemia)
  - Platelet dysfunction
  - Coagulation defect (e.g., von Willebrand disease)
- Endocrinologic disorders
  - Hyper- or hypothyroidism
  - Hyperprolactinemia
  - PCOS
  - Adrenal disorders
- Trauma: laceration to vagina or cervix
- Foreign body: usually associated with strong, foul odor
- Medications
  - Direct effect on hemostasis (e.g., Coumadin, chemotherapeutic agents)
  - Hormonal effects (e.g., oral contraceptives, Depo-Provera, other exogenous steroid hormones)
- Systemic disease
  - Disruption of hypothalamic–pituitary–ovarian axis
  - Other examples include systemic lupus erythematosus and chronic renal failure.
- Primary gynecologic disorders
  - Endometriosis
  - Uterine polyps, submucosal myomas
  - Hemangioma, arteriovenous malformation

TREATMENT

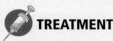

GENERAL MEASURES

- For mild DUB (inconvenient, unpredictable bleeding, and the patient has a normal hemoglobin in setting of hemodynamic stability)
  - Reassurance until ovulatory cycles resume. Encourage maintenance of a menstrual calendar, with follow-up in 3–6 months.
  - Iron supplementation
  - If anxiety is unresponsive to reassurance, hormonal therapy with a daily combined oral contraceptive pill (OCP), 1 tablet daily, should be considered to regulate menstrual cycle; if estrogen is contraindicated, may use progesterone-only pill, medroxyprogesterone acetate 5–10 mg/24 h PO for 10–14 days every month
  - For mild to moderate DUB, a progestin-containing intrauterine device may be indicated.
- For moderate DUB (irregular, prolonged, heavy bleeding with a hemoglobin >10 g/dL)
  - Hormonal therapy, as described previously; may start OCP containing 35 mcg of ethinyl estradiol twice a day until bleeding stops, then taper to once a day
  - Menstrual calendar with follow-up every 1–3 months
- For severe DUB (i.e., heavy, prolonged bleeding with a hemoglobin <10 g/dL), treatment depends on the presence of active bleeding.
  - If no active bleeding, hemodynamically stable patients can be started on daily OCPs and iron supplementation, with follow-up in 1–2 months.
  - In the presence of active bleeding: Hormonal therapy using combined OCP containing higher dose of estrogen (50 mcg ethinyl estradiol)—1 pill q.i.d. until bleeding stops, followed by pill taper (q.i.d. for 4 days, t.i.d. for 3 days, b.i.d. for 2 weeks, then 1 pill daily); switch to lower dose pill (30–35 mcg) after taper is complete.
  - Hospitalization of patient during treatment if with severe anemia (hemoglobin <7 g/dL), if hemodynamically unstable, or with compliance concerns; blood transfusion as necessary
  - If patient is unstable or unable to tolerate oral pill regimen, can give IV conjugated estrogen q4h for 24 hours to stop bleeding. Add PO or IM progesterone as soon as possible.
  - Iron replacement
  - Dilation and curettage rarely necessary; may be needed if hormonal therapy fails
- Possible side effects
  - Estrogen, given in high doses, will cause nausea and/or vomiting. An appropriate antiemetic should be used for prophylaxis against these symptoms.
  - High-dose estrogen may have vascular side effects and should be used with caution in patients particularly at risk for vascular events (e.g., patients with a history of lupus, stroke, or thrombotic phenomena and those who smoke cigarettes). In these cases, consult a gynecologist or adolescent medicine specialist for an alternative progesterone-only therapy.

ALERT

Pitfalls

- Neglecting to provide both estrogen and progesterone in a timely fashion
- Neglecting to adequately assess or mediate risk for thromboembolic event related to estrogen therapy
- Neglecting to consider a retained foreign body (e.g., tampon)

INPATIENT CONSIDERATIONS

Initial Stabilization

If DUB is attributed to anovulatory cycles, or if a complete workup fails to yield a diagnosis, treatment is guided by the severity of DUB and the presence of active bleeding.

ONGOING CARE

FOLLOW-UP RECOMMENDATIONS

Patient Monitoring

When to expect improvement

- Bleeding usually tapers after the first few doses of hormone therapy.
- After 6–12 months, if patient does not wish to remain on OCPs, a trial off medication might reveal normal ovulatory cycles.
- Ongoing follow-up with an adolescent medicine or adolescent gynecologist may be warranted.

PROGNOSIS

DUB persists for 2 years in 60% of patients, 4 years in 50%, and up to 10 years in 30%.

COMPLICATIONS

Mild to severe anemia resulting from blood loss

ADDITIONAL READING

- Hickey M, Higham JM, Fraser I. Progestogens with or without oestrogen for irregular uterine bleeding associated with anovulation. *Cochrane Database Syst Rev*. 2012;9:CD001895.
- LaCour DE, Long DN, Perlman SE. Dysfunctional uterine bleeding in adolescent females associated with endocrine causes and medical conditions. *J Pediatr Adolesc Gynecol*. 2010;23(2):62–70.
- Levine LJ, Catallozzi M, Schwarz DF. An adolescent with vaginal bleeding. *Pediatr Case Rev*. 2003;3(2):83–90.

CODES

ICD10

- N93.8 Other specified abnormal uterine and vaginal bleeding
- N92.3 Ovulation bleeding
- N93.9 Abnormal uterine and vaginal bleeding, unspecified

FAQ

- Q: If most girls have anovulatory cycles, why do only some present with DUB?
- A: Most girls do have irregular menstrual cycles during the first 2 years after menarche. However, in most, the negative-feedback system of estrogen leads to cyclic endometrial shedding in an anovulatory pattern.
- Q: If DUB from anovulatory cycles is caused by lack of progesterone, why does the initial treatment of severe DUB with active bleeding involve large doses of estrogen?
- A: Estrogen has procoagulation effects that promote hemostasis (e.g., effects on platelet aggregation and levels of fibrinogen and clotting factors). In addition, severe DUB may lead to an exposed endometrial base that bleeds profusely; for progesterone to exhibit its secretory effects, the endometrium in that area must be restored by estrogen.
- Q: When hormonal therapy fails, and the basal endometrium continues to bleed, how does a dilation and curettage act as the final treatment?
- A: The curettage removes any remaining bleeding vessels and stimulates local prostaglandins to create a uterine contracture that inhibits bleeding. This procedure is rarely needed in adolescent patients, as they usually respond to hormonal therapy.

DYSMENORRHEA

Zeev Harel

BASICS

DESCRIPTION

Bothersome menses, usually presenting as cramping pain in lower abdomen or back

- Primary dysmenorrhea—in absence of any pelvic abnormalities
- Secondary dysmenorrhea—due to pelvic abnormalities, most commonly endometriosis or reproductive tract anomalies

EPIDEMIOLOGY

- Primary dysmenorrhea
  - Typically begins in adolescence; prevalent in mid- to late adolescence when menstrual cycles become ovulatory
  - Less common in the first 2–3 years following menarche when cycles are anovulatory
- Secondary dysmenorrhea is more common later in adolescence and in young adults; it has been estimated that 15% of young adult women suffer from chronic pelvic pain, with up to 97% of these women having endometriosis.

Prevalence

- Very common gynecologic complaint that affects up to 90% of adolescents
- 15% of adolescents report that the pain is "severe," limiting their daily activities.
- Many adolescents with dysmenorrhea either do not seek medical attention or are undertreated.

RISK FACTORS

- Early menarche
- Increased duration and amount of menstrual flow
- Nulliparity
- Cigarette smoking
- Low fish consumption
- Family history of dysmenorrhea

Genetics

- Dysmenorrhea is more common in patients with a positive family history.
- Particularly, there is a hereditary predisposition to endometriosis; mode of inheritance is polygenic, multifactorial, with expression related to interaction with environmental factors.

PATHOPHYSIOLOGY

- Ovulation leads to increased progesterone release in the second half of the menstrual cycle. With the drop in progesterone late in the menstrual cycle, arachidonic acid and other omega-6 fatty acids are released, triggering an inflammatory response cascade involving prostaglandins (PGs) and leukotrienes (LTs).
- Uterine PGs and LTs cause myometrial contractions and endometrial artery vasoconstriction, resulting in uterine ischemia and in ensuing pain.
  - PGF_{2alpha} is thought to stimulate the myometrium and cause vasoconstriction.
  - Severity of dysmenorrhea is directly proportional to endometrial PGF_{2alpha} concentrations.
- Vasopressin, also elevated among women with dysmenorrhea, may play a secondary role by potentiating uterine contractions and ischemic pain.
- PGs and LTs can affect other body systems/organs, leading to dysmenorrhea-associated symptoms such as nausea/vomiting, diarrhea, and headaches.
- In endometriosis lesions, there is an inappropriate local aromatase activity, leading to a local rise in estrogen, which induces transcription of cyclooxygenase (COX)-2 and synthesis of PGE2. Aberrant expression of cytokines also mediates inflammation/pain.
- The distinct possibility of a müllerian anomaly must also be considered as a cause for secondary dysmenorrhea.

DIAGNOSIS

- Primary dysmenorrhea
  - Painful, often spasmodic cramps of varying severity in the lower abdomen or back, starting hours to a few days prior to menses and lasting up to 2–3 days after the start of menses
  - Pain is strongest in intensity initially, waning by the end of menses. Referred pain to lower back or thighs may occur.
- Secondary dysmenorrhea
  - More likely to present with both cyclic and acyclic pain (chronic pelvic pain), metrorrhagia, and dyspareunia

HISTORY

- Given the high prevalence, screen all adolescent females for dysmenorrhea.
- Pain
  - Ask about quality and intensity of pain (use pain scales); constant or intermittent occurrence; location; onset, timing, and duration; aggravating or alleviating factors; extent to which the pain limits activities (work, school, sports, social).
- Menstrual history
  - Age at menarche: Dysmenorrhea is more common in girls with earlier menarche.
  - Menstrual flow: Dysmenorrhea is more common in women with heavy/long menstrual flow.
  - Last menstrual period (and previous one, if known)
  - Cycle regularity
- Sexual history
  - Parity, current sexual activity, contraception, and history of sexually transmitted infections (STIs) or pelvic inflammatory disease (PID). Adhesions may cause painful menses.
- Menstruation-associated symptoms: nausea, vomiting, diarrhea, headache, irritability, fatigue, breast tenderness, dizziness, bloating, and acne exacerbation
- History of sexual, physical, or emotional abuse
- Family history of gynecologic (GYN) diseases, including endometriosis, GYN or breast cancer, and complications with oral contraceptive pills (OCPs) including deep vein thrombosis (DVT), stroke, or myocardial infarction
- Medications: response to analgesic medications including name, dose, and perceived effectiveness
- Diet: Higher intake of omega-6 polyunsaturated fatty acids correlates with increased dysmenorrhea symptoms.

ALERT

- The adolescent health care provider should screen for menstrual symptoms at every encounter with the adolescent female.
- Menstrual pain that started at menarche or immediately after menarche is unlikely to be primary dysmenorrhea, as most girls are still having anovulatory cycles.
- Cigarette smoking may increase duration of dysmenorrhea.
- Consider a workup of endometriosis for hard to manage dysmenorrhea.

PHYSICAL EXAM

- Abdominal exam
  - Lower abdomen/suprapubic tenderness
  - Enlarged uterus can be palpated in vaginal outlet obstruction.
- Inspection of external genitalia: A cotton-tipped swab can be inserted into the vagina to evaluate for the presence of a transverse vaginal septum or vaginal agenesis.
- Pelvic exam
  - Defer in younger girls with mild, classic symptoms and normal external genitalia who have never been sexually active.
  - Perform in girls with history suggesting secondary dysmenorrhea, particularly if the patient failed treatment with nonsteroidal anti-inflammatory drugs (NSAIDs).

DIAGNOSTIC TESTS & INTERPRETATION

- Lab studies are generally not warranted.
- Consider testing for pregnancy, STIs, and PID as indicated by history and physical exam.

Imaging

- Consider pelvic ultrasound (US) for patients who fail a trial of NSAIDs.
  - US can rule out genital tract abnormalities and ovarian pathologies.
  - Pelvic US or pelvic magnetic resonance imaging (MRI) may be indicated, particularly to exclude obstructive anomalies.
- Although US and MRI can detect ovarian, vaginal, and bladder endometriosis and deeply infiltrative lesions, there are no good imaging modalities to detect intraperitoneal endometriosis lesions.

Diagnostic Procedures/Other

Consider a diagnostic laparoscopy with resection/ablation of lesions if indicated in patients with dysmenorrhea refractory to treatments with NSAIDs and OCPs, particularly if they have a 1st-degree relative with endometriosis.

DIFFERENTIAL DIAGNOSIS
Primary dysmenorrhea is a diagnosis of exclusion; secondary dysmenorrhea should be ruled out based on history, physical exam, response to initial treatment, and imaging if warranted.
- Causes of secondary dysmenorrhea
  - Endometriosis, congenital vaginal or uterine anomalies, adenomyosis, ectopic pregnancy, ovarian cysts or tumors, pelvic adhesions, PID, uterine adhesions, fibroids, or polyps
- Other diagnoses to rule out:
  - Gastrointestinal: constipation, diverticulitis, inflammatory bowel disease, irritable bowel syndrome
  - Urologic: interstitial cystitis, kidney stones, urinary tract infection
  - Neurologic: fibromyalgia, herniated disk, lower back pain

TREATMENT

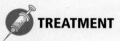

MEDICATION
First Line
- NSAIDs
  - Conventional PG synthetase (COX) inhibitors
  - If a patient fails to respond to the first choice at a therapeutic level, try a different NSAID.
- A COX-2 inhibitor should be considered in patients with prior history of peptic ulcer or gastrointestinal bleeding.
- 90% of patients have relief with proper dosing.
- Most effective when used on a regular basis for the first 2–3 days of menses
- If possible, start 1 day prior or at the onset of menses.
- Choices
  - Ibuprofen: 800 mg initially, followed by 400–800 mg PO q8h as needed
  - Naproxen sodium: 440–550 mg initially, followed by 220–550 mg PO q12h as needed
  - Mefenamic acid: 500 mg PO initially, followed by 250 mg PO q6h as needed
  - Celecoxib: 400 mg initially, followed by 200 mg q12h as needed (COX-2 inhibitor approved for girls ≥18 years)
- Side effects of conventional NSAIDs
  - Black box warnings: increased risk of adverse cardiovascular events, including myocardial infarction, stroke, and new-onset or worsening of preexisting hypertension; increased risk of gastrointestinal irritation, ulceration, bleeding, and perforation

Second Line
- OCPs
  - OCPs suppress ovulation and decrease uterine PG secretion following reduction in progesterone levels.
  - Good choice for patients who fail NSAIDs as monotherapy, desire pregnancy prevention, or who have acne
  - Patients may need 3 months to see improvement.
  - Extended cycling OCPs: can prescribe formulation for a 91-day cycle (e.g., Seasonale, Seasonique) or use multiple OCP packs to achieve same effect
  - Side effects: nausea, vomiting, breast tenderness, breakthrough menstrual bleeding, headaches from the estrogen; rare: DVT, stroke, myocardial infarction
- Long-acting hormonal contraceptives
  - Long-acting combined estrogen and progestin hormonal contraceptives such as the transdermal patch and the vaginal ring as well as long-acting progestin-only hormonal contraceptives such as the injectable depot-medroxyprogesterone acetate, etonorgestrel subdermal implant, and the levonorgestrel-releasing intrauterine system can also alleviate dysmenorrhea symptoms.
- Secondary dysmenorrhea is treated by addressing the underlying cause. Extended OCP regimen is the first line of treatment for endometriosis. Medical management in patients refractory to noncyclic OCP may proceed to treatment with a gonadotropin-releasing hormone (GnRH) agonist.

ISSUES FOR REFERRAL
Consider referral to adolescent gynecologist for possible laparoscopy or management of endometriosis.

COMPLEMENTARY & ALTERNATIVE THERAPIES
- Supplementation with vitamin B_1, magnesium, or omega-3 fatty acids have been shown to alleviate dysmenorrhea symptoms.
- Transcutaneous electrical nerve stimulation (TENS): Electrodes on the skin stimulate nerves at different current frequencies and intensities. Better results are reported with high frequency than with low frequency.
- Exercise may help to reduce symptoms of dysmenorrhea (due to release of endorphins).
- Acupuncture, yoga, and heat therapy may also reduce dysmenorrhea symptoms.

SURGERY/OTHER PROCEDURES
Laparoscopic techniques for interruption of the uterosacral nerves may be used as treatment for primary dysmenorrhea when other modalities have failed.
- Laparoscopic uterine nerve ablation (LUNA) is effective for long-term (≥12 months) pain relief in primary dysmenorrhea.
- Laparoscopic presacral neurectomy is more effective than LUNA for pain relief at ≥6 months follow-up but has significant side effects especially constipation; it should only be performed by pelvic laparoscopic surgeons with special training.

ALERT
- There are a number of over-the-counter medicines that are marketed for treating cramps in women. Only those formulations that contain NSAIDs are effective in treating dysmenorrhea.
- Start an adequate dose of pain medication at first awareness of approaching menses.
- Estrogen and progestin hormones are also used for treatment of dysmenorrhea and do not lead to adolescent sexual activity.

ONGOING CARE

DIET
Encourage patients to increase consumption of fish rich in omega-3 fatty acids.

PATIENT EDUCATION
- Stress to patients the importance of keeping a pain diary indicating days of menses, days of pain, pain ratings (0–10 scale), days of limited activities (school or work) due to pain, and associated symptoms.
- Web site for patient education materials
  - American College of Obstetricians and Gynecologists. Dysmenorrhea. http://www.acog.org/~/media/For%20Patients/faq046.pdf?dmc=1&ts=20121119T1244369567

PROGNOSIS
Improvement in dysmenorrhea symptoms may occur after childbirth.

COMPLICATIONS
Missed school or work, decreased academic performance, sports participation, and peer socialization

ADDITIONAL READING

- Falcone T, Lebovic DI. Clinical management of endometriosis. *Obstet Gynecol*. 2011;118(3):691–705.
- Harel Z. Dysmenorrhea in adolescents and young adults: an update on pharmacological treatments and management strategies. *Expert Opin Pharmacother*. 2012;13(15):2157–2170.
- Harel Z. Dysmenorrhea in adolescents and young adults: from pathophysiology to pharmacological treatments and management strategies. *Expert Opin Pharmacother*. 2008;9(15):1–12.

CODES

ICD10
- N94.6 Dysmenorrhea, unspecified
- N94.4 Primary dysmenorrhea
- N94.5 Secondary dysmenorrhea

FAQ
- Q: What percentage of patients report dysmenorrhea?
- A: Although dysmenorrhea affects up to 90% of adolescents, fewer than 15% will seek medical care. It is important to screen all adolescent women for dysmenorrhea. Barriers to seeking physician advice include fears of pelvic exam and lack of knowledge of effective treatments.
- Q: When to refer a patient with dysmenorrhea to laparoscopy?
- A: Although pelvic US and MRI can detect some endometriosis lesions, there are no good imaging modalities to detect intraperitoneal endometriosis lesions. Therefore, a diagnostic laparoscopy with resection/ablation of lesions is indicated in patients with dysmenorrhea refractory to treatments with NSAIDs and hormones.

DYSPNEA

Thomas G. Saba • Amy G. Filbrun

BASICS

DESCRIPTION

A subjective experience of breathing discomfort that consists of qualitatively distinct sensations that vary in intensity

PATHOPHYSIOLOGY

Abnormality in one of the following elements:

- Respiratory controller (breathing rate, depth)
- Ventilatory pump (chest wall, pleura, airways)
- Gas exchanger (alveoli, capillaries)
- Cardiovascular derangements (cardiac output)

ETIOLOGY

- Respiratory
  - Upper airway
    - Infection (croup, tracheitis, peritonsillar abscess, epiglottitis)
    - Foreign body
    - Anaphylaxis
    - Anatomic abnormalities
    - Vocal cord dysfunction (VCD)
  - Lower airway
    - Asthma
    - Aspiration
    - Airway malacia
    - Hemorrhage
    - Internal/external fixed compression (tumor, cyst, vascular)
  - Parenchymal lung disease
    - Infection (viral, bacterial, fungal)
    - Interstitial lung disease (ILD)
    - Atelectasis
    - Chronic lung disease (chronic obstructive pulmonary disease [COPD], cystic fibrosis)
  - Chest wall disorder
    - Neuromuscular weakness (Duchenne muscular dystrophy [DMD], spinal muscular atrophy [SMA])
    - Scoliosis
    - Pectus excavatum
  - Pleural
    - Pleural effusion
    - Pneumothorax
- Cardiovascular
  - Cardiac
    - Elevated pulmonary venous pressure
    - Congestive heart failure (CHF)
  - Vascular
    - Pulmonary hypertension (PHTN)
    - Pulmonary embolism (PE)
- Toxic/metabolic
  - Metabolic acidosis (diabetic ketoacidosis, salicylate intoxication, renal tubular acidosis [RTA])
  - Renal failure causing fluid overload
- Other
  - Anemia
  - Deconditioning
  - Obesity
  - Panic attack
  - Pregnancy
  - Trauma
  - Gastroesophageal reflux disease (GERD)

DIAGNOSIS

APPROACH TO PATIENT

- Secure the airway and address life-threatening emergencies.
- Identify those who will need intensive/emergency care and those who can be worked up in the office.
- Distinguish new-onset dyspnea from deterioration of chronic disease.
- Detailed history is key to diagnosis.

HISTORY

- Onset
  - Recurrent, discrete episodes associated with anxiety
    - Panic attacks
  - Sudden
    - Foreign body, pneumothorax
- Associated signs and symptoms
  - "Tightness"
    - Bronchoconstriction (asthma)
  - Stridor
    - Upper airway obstruction
  - Wheezing
    - Lower airway obstruction
  - Chest pain
    - Pneumothorax, PE, pleural effusion
  - Hemoptysis
    - Hemorrhage
  - Worse when supine
    - Pulmonary edema
- Temporal association
  - Exercise-induced
    - VCD, asthma, deconditioning, GERD
  - Nocturnal
    - Asthma, GERD
  - Persistent and progressive
    - Neuromuscular disease, ILD
- Infectious signs and symptoms
  - Fever, cough, rhinorrhea
    - Pneumonia, bronchiolitis
  - Stridor, cough, rapid onset
    - Croup, tracheitis, abscess, epiglottitis
- Gastrointestinal signs and symptoms
  - Choking, gagging with feeds
    - Aspiration
  - Epigastric pain, discomfort
    - GERD
- Exposures
  - Salicylates, allergens
- PE risk factors include immobilization, surgery, smoking, pregnancy, central catheter, history of deep vein thrombosis
- History of cardiac disease
  - PHTN, CHF
- Diabetes history
  - Polyuria, polydipsia, polyphagia

PHYSICAL EXAM

- Vital signs, oxygen saturation, temperature
  - Fever
    - Infection
  - Hypoxia suggestive of pulmonary and cardiac causes
- Weight, BMI
  - Chronic disease, obesity
- Breath sounds
  - Generalized decreased air entry
    - Bronchoconstriction, atelectasis
  - Localized decreased intensity
    - Pneumothorax, pleural effusion, local obstruction, elevated hemidiaphragm, foreign body, pneumonia
  - Egophony, bronchial breath sounds
    - Consolidation/pneumonia
  - Wheezing
    - Bronchoconstriction, foreign body, bronchiolitis
  - Crackles
    - Infection, ILD (especially if crackles don't clear with coughing)
  - Barking quality of cough
    - Croup
  - Stridor
    - Upper airway obstruction
- Cardiac exam
  - Crackles, peripheral edema, hepatomegaly, gallop
    - CHF
  - Loud P_2
    - PHTN
- Extremities
  - Clubbing
    - Chronic pulmonary/cardiac disease
  - Cyanosis
    - Shunting
  - Calf tenderness
    - DVT
- Musculoskeletal
  - Generalized muscle weakness
    - DMD, SMA, other neuromuscular diseases
- Head and neck
  - Pharyngeal cobblestoning
    - GERD, allergic rhinitis
  - Allergic shiners, nasal crease, swollen nasal turbinates
    - Allergic rhinitis
  - Rhinorrhea
    - Allergic rhinitis, infection
  - Pharyngeal erythema, uvular deviation
    - Peritonsillar abscess

DIAGNOSTIC TESTS & INTERPRETATION

Lab

First line
- Arterial blood gas
  - Hypercarbia suggests impending respiratory failure; distinguishes metabolic from respiratory acidosis
- Complete blood count with differential
  - Anemia; leukocytosis with left shift is a sign of infection.
- Glucose
  - Hyperglycemia can lead to diabetic ketoacidosis (DKA).
- Viral testing (polymerase chain reaction [PCR], direct fluorescent antibody [DFA], culture)
  - Diagnose viral infection; consider influenza in winter months.

Special considerations
- B-type natriuretic peptide (BNP)
  - Diagnostic marker to help recognize heart disease when access to echocardiography not readily available

Imaging

First line
- Chest radiograph
  - Identify pleural effusion, pneumothorax, consolidation, cardiomegaly, hyperinflation

Special considerations
- CT
  - High-resolution CT to diagnose ILD; spiral CT angiography to diagnose PE
- Echocardiography
  - Signs of PHTN; heart failure; structural abnormalities

Diagnostic Procedures/Other
- Pulmonary function tests
  - Spirometry
    - Obstructive lung disease (asthma); distinguish upper from lower airways obstruction
  - Lung volumes
    - Restrictive lung disease (ILD, neuromuscular and chest wall diseases)
  - Diffusion capacity
    - ILD
  - Mean inspiratory and expiratory pressure
    - Neuromuscular disease/weakness
- Bronchoscopy with bronchoalveolar lavage (BAL)
  - Dynamic visualization of airways to diagnose fixed (vascular) or dynamic (bronchomalacia) airway compression; bacterial, viral, and fungal cultures; lipid-laden macrophages (aspiration); hemosiderin-laden macrophages (hemorrhage)
- Electrocardiogram
  - Readily available test to rapidly diagnose heart disease
- Cardiopulmonary exercise testing
  - Indicated when initial evaluation fails to yield diagnosis; distinguish cardiac and respiratory causes and deconditioning

TREATMENT

- Secure airway and stabilize the patient.
- Treatment should be directed at the underlying cause of dyspnea.
- Consider palliative/symptomatic treatment once underlying or reversible cause has been addressed.

MEDICATIONS
- Opioids (parenteral/oral/inhaled)
- Anxiolytics

ADDITIONAL TREATMENT

General Measures
- Oxygen
- Pulmonary rehabilitation
- Movement of cool air (face fan)

ALERT
In patients with hypercapnic chronic respiratory failure, hypoxemia might be the primary drive to breathe; supplemental oxygen will remove the hypoxic respiratory drive and cause apnea.

ISSUES FOR REFERRAL
- Unstable vital signs, unsecure airway, inability to oxygenate, and need for critical care services
- Surgical consultation for foreign body removal with rigid bronchoscopy
- Pulmonary referral for severe asthma, hemorrhage, ILD, CF, DMD, SMA, flexible bronchoscopy, chronic mechanical ventilation
- Cardiac referral for cardiac disease, PHTN
- Endocrinology referral for diabetes
- Nephrology referral for RTA and renal failure

SURGERY/OTHER PROCEDURES
- Evacuation of tension pneumothorax with chest tube
- Pleural drainage/video-assisted thoracic surgery for loculated empyema
- Rigid bronchoscopy for foreign body retrieval
- Flexible bronchoscopy and laryngoscopy for visual diagnosis and BAL

ADDITIONAL READING

- Birnkrant DJ, Bushby KMD, Amin RS, et al. The respiratory management of patients with Duchenne muscular dystrophy: a DMD care considerations working group specialty article. *Pediatr Pulmonol*. 2010;45(8):739–748.
- Deutch GH, Young LR, Deterding RR, et al. Diffuse lung disease in young children: application of a novel classification scheme. *Am J Respir Crit Care Med*. 2007;176(11):1120–1128.
- Maher KO, Reed H, Cuadrado A, et al. B-type natriuretic peptide in the emergency diagnosis of critical heart disease in children. *Pediatrics*. 2008;121(6):e1484–e1488.
- Morris MJ, Christopher KL. Diagnostic criteria for the classification of vocal cord dysfunction. *Chest*. 2010;138(5):1213–1223.
- National Asthma Education and Prevention Program. *Expert Panel Report 3: Guidelines for the Diagnosis and Management of Asthma*. Bethesda, MD: National Asthma Education and Prevention Program; 2007. NIH Publication No. 07-4051.
- Parshall MD, Schwartzstein RM, Adams L, et al. An official American Thoracic Society Statement: update on the mechanisms, assessment, and management of dyspnea. *Am J Respir Crit Care Med*. 2012;185(4):435–452.
- Ullrich CK, Mayer OH. Assessment and management of fatigue and dyspnea in pediatric palliative care. *Pediatr Clin North Am*. 2007;54(5):735–756, xi.

CODES

ICD10
- R06.00 Dyspnea, unspecified
- R06.1 Stridor
- R06.2 Wheezing

FAQ
- Q: In most pediatric cases, is dyspnea pulmonary in nature?
- A: In most cases, yes. Nonetheless, a systematic approach looking at all organ systems should be employed when addressing a patient with dyspnea.
- Q: How does the etiology of dyspnea differ in adults?
- A: In adults, the most common causes of dyspnea are asthma, COPD, ILD, myocardial dysfunction, and obesity/deconditioning. Whereas asthma and obesity are common in children, COPD, ILD, and myocardial disease are much more common in adults.

DYSURIA

Stephanie Clark • Rebecca Ruebner

BASICS

DESCRIPTION

Painful urination

DIAGNOSIS

DIFFERENTIAL DIAGNOSIS

- Infectious
  - Cystitis
  - Viral infection
  - Gonorrhea
  - Chlamydia
  - Herpes simplex
  - Varicella
  - Tuberculosis
  - Candidiasis
  - Urethritis
  - Pinworms
  - Prostatitis
  - Balanitis
- Congenital/anatomic
  - Meatal stenosis
  - Urethral stricture
  - Posterior urethral diverticula
  - Urethral stones
  - Vesicovaginal fistula
  - Labial adhesions
- Toxic/environmental/drugs
  - Bubble bath urethritis
  - Spermicides, douches
  - Cytoxan
- Trauma
  - Diaper dermatitis
  - Foreign body
  - Bicycle injury
  - Masturbation
  - Sexual abuse
  - Irritation (e.g., from sand, tight pants)
- Tumor
  - Sarcoma botryoides
- Genetic/metabolic
  - Cystinuria
- Allergic/inflammatory
  - Food allergy
  - Stevens-Johnson syndrome
  - Contact dermatitis (e.g., poison ivy)
- Functional
  - Attention mechanism
  - Dysfunctional voiding
- Miscellaneous
  - Appendicitis
  - Hypercalciuria

APPROACH TO PATIENT

- General goal: Determine the cause and begin treatment.
  - Phase 1: Rule out common causes such as trauma, infection, chemical irritant, constipation, and masturbation.
  - Phase 2: Continue investigation—look for congenital or acquired problems that cause infection, strictures, or calculi.
  - Phase 3: Begin treatment.
- Hints for screening problems:
  - Ask about medications and food allergies.
  - Ask about special situations (e.g., travel, sand in bathing suit causing irritation).

HISTORY

- **Question:** Do the symptoms occur any special time of day?
- *Significance*: May indicate an attention mechanism if occurs before school
- **Question:** What kinds of medication do you take?
- *Significance*: Some medications (e.g., Cytoxan) may cause irritation of the urethra.
- **Question:** Have there been any new foods or known food allergens?
- *Significance*: Milk is a possible food allergen that may cause dysuria. Citrus fruits may increase the acidity of the urine and cause dysuria in some patients. Best to determine whether symptoms regress on elimination of possible offending food.
- **Question:** Do you use bubble bath?
- *Significance*: Bubble bath may deplete the protective lipids in the urethra.
- **Question:** Any signs of bleeding?
- *Significance*: May indicate trauma, infection, or congenital anomalies. Calcium excretion may cause dysuria as well as hematuria.
- **Question:** Fever?
- *Significance*: Fever is a common sign of urinary tract infection (UTI).
- **Question:** Frequency?
- *Significance*: Both frequency and dysuria are common findings in UTIs.
- **Question:** Past history of urologic operations?
- *Significance*: Antireflux surgery may have a side effect of dysuria.
- **Question:** What have you taken for discomfort?
- *Significance*: Although cranberry juice is used for many urinary problems, the volume needed is usually more than what can be easily ingested.
- **Question:** Quality and strength of the urinary stream?
- *Significance*: Patients with posterior urethral valves may have urinary dribbling, poor urinary stream, difficulty potty training, or diurnal enuresis.
- **Question:** Sexual activity?
- *Significance*: Urethritis from gonorrhea or chlamydia
- **Question:** Frequency?
- *Significance*: It can sometimes be difficult to differentiate dysuria from frequency, which may cause an uncomfortable feeling or pressure that is described by the child as pain with urination.
- **Question:** Vaginal discharge?
- *Significance:* Vaginal discharge with dysuria suggests gonococcal or chlamydial infection.

PHYSICAL EXAM

- **Finding:** Any signs of redness or ecchymoses?
- *Significance*: May indicate trauma from masturbation or abuse
- **Finding:** Any bleeding?
- *Significance*: Seen in trauma, tumors, and infection
- **Finding:** Any change in behavior?
- *Significance*: May be an attention-seeking device
- **Finding:** Abnormal swelling?
- *Significance*: May occur in trauma or rare tumors

- **Finding:** Abnormal urethra?
- *Significance*: Prolapsed urethra or diverticula
- **Finding:** Grapelike structures in vagina?
- *Significance*: Sarcoma botryoides
- **Finding:** Abdominal pain?
- *Significance*: Intra-abdominal abscess or low-lying inflamed appendix may cause dysuria. A low-lying inflamed appendix may also cause bladder irritation and dysuria.

DIAGNOSTIC TESTS & INTERPRETATION

Lab

- Test: Urinalysis
- *Significance*: In most UTIs, there are WBCs in the urine.
- Test: Urine culture
- *Significance*: Check for infection.
- Test: Metabolic screens
- *Significance*: If sediment shows crystals or if familial history of metabolic disease
- Test: Urinary screen for gonorrhea and chlamydia
- *Significance*: DNA amplification by polymerase or ligase chain reaction on freshly voided urine has 95% sensitivity and 100% specificity.

Imaging

Ultrasound: not routinely requested unless a congenital anomaly is suspected

TREATMENT

ADDITIONAL TREATMENT

General Measures

- See treatment of UTI, vaginitis, urethritis
- Phenazopyridine (Pyridium) may be used for symptomatic relief while documenting cause of dysuria.
- Warm water sitz baths may be helpful for symptomatic treatment.

ISSUES FOR REFERRAL

- Evidence of congenital anomaly
- Increasing severity of symptoms
- Failure to respond to symptomatic or specific treatment

ADDITIONAL READING

- Claudius H. Dysuria in adolescents. *West J Med*. 2000;172(3):201–205.
- Hellerstein S, Linebarger JS. Voiding dysfunction in pediatric patients. *Clin Pediatr (Phila)*. 2003;42(1):43–49.
- Lee HJ, Pyo JW, Choi EH, et al. Isolation of adenovirus type from the urine of children with acute hemorrhagic cystitis. *Pediatr Infect Dis J*. 1996;15(7):633–634.
- Rushton HG. Urinary tract infections in children: epidemiology, evaluation, and management. *Pediatr Clin North Am*. 1997;44(5):1133–1169.

CODES

ICD10

- R30.0 Dysuria
- N39.0 Urinary tract infection, site not specified
- N34.2 Other urethritis

FAQ

- Q: How does bubble bath cause dysuria?
- A: The bubble bath depletes lipids that protect the urethra, causing the tissue to swell and become inflamed.
- Q: Can allergies cause dysuria?
- A: It is difficult to directly prove allergies as a cause of dysuria; however, in some cases, elimination of certain foods such as spices, citrus fruits, or known skin allergens has improved symptoms.
- Q: How do children get infected with gonorrhea?
- A: This is a red flag for sexual abuse, which must be investigated.
- Q: Which viruses cause dysuria?
- A: Adenovirus has been associated with dysuria.

D

EARACHE

Vanessa S. Carlo

BASICS

DESCRIPTION

- *Otalgia*, classified as primary or secondary, means ear pain or an earache.
- Primary (or otogenic) otalgia is ear pain that originates inside the ear, either from the external auditory canal or from the middle ear structures.
- Secondary (or referred) otalgia is ear pain that originates from outside of the ear. Any anatomic area that shares innervation with the ear can be the primary source of perceived ear pain.

DIAGNOSIS

DIFFERENTIAL DIAGNOSIS

Primary otalgia

- Infectious
  - Acute otitis media (AOM)—most common cause of otalgia in children
  - Otitis externa—inflammation of external auditory canal, usually associated with swimming and/or localized trauma; second most common cause of otalgia in children
  - Cellulitis of the auricle—usually caused by *Streptococcus pyogenes*; typically involves the earlobe
  - Perichondritis—inflammation of the auricle without earlobe involvement
  - Furunculosis—infection of the cartilaginous portion of the external auditory canal. Most commonly caused by *Staphylococcus aureus*. Pain is usually made worse by chewing.
  - Mastoiditis—now a rare complication of AOM, characterized by the auricle being pushed out and forward, away from the head
  - Myringitis (bullous myringitis)—inflammation of the tympanic membrane, usually with painful blisters on the eardrum
  - Varicella and herpes zoster infection within the ear
  - Herpes simplex virus infection within the ear
- Trauma
  - Blunt trauma
  - Laceration or abrasion—if inside the ear canal, usually due to cleaning with cotton swabs
  - Thermal injury—frostbite of the ear or burn from a heat source
  - Barotrauma—associated with pressure changes on airplanes and scuba diving
  - Traumatic perforation of the tympanic membrane—frequently presents with tinnitus
- Tumors—rare; usually associated with weight loss, voice changes, dysphagia, and persistent cervical lymphadenopathy
- Allergic/inflammatory
  - Otitis media with effusion
  - Eczema
  - Psoriasis
  - Allergic reaction to topical antibiotics and cerumenolytic agents
- Functional
  - Eustachian tube dysfunction—symptoms are due to pressure differences between the middle ear and the Eustachian tube.
- Miscellaneous
  - Foreign body—can lead to pain, fullness, and minor hearing loss
  - Impacted cerumen—may cause pain if the cerumen presses against the tympanic membrane

Note: Serous otitis media or otitis media with effusion (OME) is common in pediatrics but is usually painless. Children usually complain of fullness or hearing loss.

Secondary otalgia

- Infectious
  - Dental infections—cavities, abscesses, gingivitis
  - Pharyngitis
  - Parotitis
  - Tonsillitis
  - Peritonsillar abscess
  - Retropharyngeal abscess
  - Sinusitis
  - Cervical lymphadenitis
  - Neck abscess
  - Stomatitis
  - Sialadenitis
  - Ramsay Hunt syndrome—viral neuritis of the facial nerve secondary to herpes zoster infection
- Trauma
  - Dental trauma
  - Postsurgical—tonsillectomy, adenoidectomy
  - Oropharyngeal trauma—penetrating injuries, burns
  - Neck and cervical spine injuries
- Allergic/inflammatory
  - Allergic rhinitis
  - Cervical spine arthritis
  - Subacute thyroiditis
  - Esophagitis—secondary to gastroesophageal reflux
  - Bell palsy
- Functional
  - Temporomandibular joint (TMJ) dysfunction—less common in children. Pain is usually unilateral and aggravated by chewing and biting.
- Miscellaneous
  - Foreign body—in oropharynx or esophagus
  - Aphthous ulcers
  - Esophagitis
  - TMJ disease
  - Migraine
  - Aural neuralgia
  - Pillow otalgia (otalgia from sleep position)
  - Psychogenic pain

APPROACH TO THE PATIENT

The first decision that must be made is whether the patient's symptoms require emergent, urgent, or nonurgent intervention. Emergency treatment is rarely required for pediatric patients with otalgia.

- **Phase 1:** Thorough history—must include a full assessment of ear symptoms, followed by questions to determine possible involvement of other head and neck structures
- **Phase 2:** Physical exam—thorough examination of external and internal ear, followed by inspection of the head, neck, and inside of the mouth
- **Phase 3:** Treatment of identifiable conditions
- **Phase 4:** Referral to otolaryngologist (ENT physician), dentist, or other specialist as needed

HISTORY

- **Question:** Duration of symptoms?
- *Significance*: acute (more likely infection or trauma) versus chronic
- **Question:** Quality of the pain?
- *Significance*:
  - Constant (more likely otogenic) versus intermittent (more likely referred)
  - Dull (more likely due to inflammation) versus sharp (more likely due to trauma or neuralgia)
- **Question:** Severity of pain?
- *Significance*:
  - Severe—usually otogenic
  - Mild to moderate—more likely to be referred

Worsening factors

- **Question:** Movement of auricle or pressure on tragus?
- *Significance*: Characteristic of otitis externa; can also be associated with furunculosis.
- **Question:** Movement of the jaw (biting, chewing)?
- *Significance*: TMJ dysfunction; furunculosis

Associated symptoms

- **Question:** Fever?
- *Significance*: Infection
- **Question:** Upper respiratory infection (URI) symptoms?
- *Significance*: AOM or OME
- **Question:** Sore throat?
- *Significance*: Referred otalgia
- **Question:** Ear discharge, tinnitus, or vertigo?
- *Significance*: Otogenic causes
- **Question:** Mouth pain?
- *Significance*: Dental issues or stomatitis
- **Question:** Hoarseness?
- *Significance*: Gastroesophageal reflux
- **Question:** Multiple somatic complaints?
- *Significance*: Psychogenic
- **Question:** Recent swimming?
- *Significance*: Otitis externa

- **Question:** Recent travel? Hobbies?
- *Significance*:
  – Barotrauma from scuba diving or air travel
  – Wrestling—auricular trauma
- **Question:** History of recurrent AOM or OME?
- *Significance*: Cholesteatoma

PHYSICAL EXAM

- **Finding:** Erythematous, dull, bulging tympanic membrane, with decreased mobility?
- *Significance*: Suggestive of AOM
- **Finding:** Retracted, immobile tympanic membrane?
- *Significance*: Suggestive of OME or eustachian tube dysfunction
- **Finding:** Pain with pressure on the tragus or traction on the pinna?
- *Significance*: Suggestive of otitis externa or furunculosis
- **Finding:** Erythema and edema of the external auditory canal?
- *Significance*: Suggestive of otitis externa
- **Finding:** Purulent discharge in external auditory canal?
- *Significance*: Suggestive of otitis externa or AOM with a ruptured tympanic membrane
- **Finding:** Redness, swelling, and/or tenderness of the auricle?
- *Significance*:
  – With earlobe involvement—cellulitis
  – Without earlobe involvement—perichondritis
- **Finding:** Swelling behind the pinna with its lateral displacement?
- *Significance:* Suggestive of mastoiditis
- **Finding:** Normal ear exam?
- *Significance*: Suggestive of secondary otalgia, thus other possible sources must be carefully examined
- **Finding:** Multiple dental caries?
- *Significance*: May be the source of pain; can indicate the presence of a dental abscess
- **Finding:** Foreign body within the ear or in the oropharynx?
- *Significance*: May be the source of pain from direct pressure or secondary to inflammation
- **Finding:** Enlarged, asymmetric tonsils or uvular deviation from midline?
- *Significance*: Suggestive of tonsillitis or peritonsillar abscess

Look for signs of trauma inside or outside of the ear.

DIAGNOSTIC TESTS & INTERPRETATION

Labs, imaging studies, and other diagnostic tests are usually unnecessary as a thorough history and physical exam can lead to a diagnosis in the majority of cases.

- **Test:** Culture of ear discharge
- *Significance*: Indicated when otitis externa or AOM with perforation of the tympanic membrane does not resolve as expected with routine antibiotic treatment
- **Test:** Audiometry
- *Significance*: Evaluate for hearing loss, which would suggest primary otalgia
- **Test:** Tympanometry
- *Significance*: Evaluate for OME, eustachian tube dysfunction, or tympanostomy tube obstruction

Imaging

- CT scan: rarely needed
  – CT of neck—evaluate for retropharyngeal abscess, mass, or hematoma
  – CT of sinuses—evaluate for sinusitis
  – CT of temporal bone—evaluate for AOM, mastoiditis, and other bony pathology
- MRI: rarely needed unless intracranial lesion is suspected

TREATMENT

ADDITIONAL TREATMENT

General Measures

- Therapy is directed at the identified underlying cause.
- Pain medications such as acetaminophen, ibuprofen, or topical benzocaine are important because many of the infectious causes are exquisitely painful.
- Observation without antibiotic therapy ("watchful waiting") is indicated in certain groups of children with AOM.

EMERGENCY CARE

- Rarely needed with most causes of otalgia but may be required if
  – Potential airway compromise from foreign body, mass, or abscess
  – Significant trauma—possible basilar skull fracture
  – Infection with a toxic-appearing child
- For all of the above situations, first establish "ABCs" as needed, hospitalize, and consult ENT promptly.

ISSUES FOR REFERRAL

Referral to ENT when otalgia is primary in origin and any of the following:

- Pain with unexplained hearing loss, vertigo, or tinnitus
- Unexplained or persistent otorrhea
- Suspected neoplasm
- History suggestive of severe barotrauma
- AOM with complications
- Foreign bodies that cannot be removed easily from the ear
- Potential for auricle destruction (e.g., perichondritis may lead to permanent deformation, cauliflower ear)
- Persistent ear pain without an identifiable source should prompt a referral.

ADDITIONAL READING

- American Academy of Pediatrics Subcommittee on Management of Acute Otitis Media. Diagnosis and management of acute otitis media. *Pediatrics*. 2004;113(5):1451–1465.
- Conover K. Earache. *Emerg Med Clin North Am*. 2013;31(2):413–442.
- Leung AK, Fong JH, Leong AG. Otalgia in children. *J Natl Med Assoc*. 2000;92(5):254–260.
- Licameli GR. Diagnosis and management of otalgia in the pediatric patient. *Pediatr Ann*. 1999;28(6):364–368.
- Majumdar S, Wu K, Bateman N, et al. Diagnosis and management of otalgia in children. *Arch Dis Child Educ Pract Ed*. 2009;94(2):33–36.
- Shah RK, Blevins NH. Otalgia. *Otolaryngol Clin North Am*. 2003;36(6):1137–1151.

CODES

ICD10

- H92.09 Otalgia, unspecified ear
- H66.90 Otitis media, unspecified, unspecified ear
- H60.90 Unspecified otitis externa, unspecified ear

FAQ

- Q: What are the most common organisms that cause AOM?
- A:
  – *Streptococcus pneumoniae*
  – *Haemophilus influenzae*
  – *Moraxella catarrhalis*
  – Viruses
- Q: What are the most common organisms that cause otitis externa?
- A:
  – *Pseudomonas aeruginosa*
  – *Staphylococcus aureus*
  – *Staphylococcus epidermidis*
  – Gram-negative rods
  – Fungal (*Aspergillus*) or yeast (*Candida*)—rare
- Q: What is the most common cause of referred ear pain?
- A: Dental disease

E

EDEMA

Stephanie Clark • Rebecca Ruebner

BASICS

DESCRIPTION

Presence of abnormal amount of fluid in the interstitial spaces of the body; usually secondary to low albumin, obstruction of venous or lymphatic channels, or trauma

DIAGNOSIS

DIFFERENTIAL DIAGNOSIS

- Localized
  - Trauma: pressure or sun damage
  - Infection
  - Allergy
  - Lymphatic obstruction (less common)
    - Filariasis
    - Radiation therapy
  - Bee stings or insect bites
  - Sickle cell dactylitis
- Generalized
  - Congenital: lymphatic obstruction of legs or thoracic duct
  - Infection: hepatitis and liver failure; pericarditis
  - Toxic, environmental, drugs
    - Sodium poisoning
    - Toxic effect on liver and/or heart (chemotherapy)
    - Cirrhosis
    - Drug reaction
  - Tumor
    - Obstruction of venous return from enlarged abdominal lymph nodes or tumor
  - Allergic/inflammatory: protein-losing enteropathy
  - Renal
    - Nephrotic syndrome
    - Renal failure
    - Acute glomerulonephritis
  - Cardiac
    - Congestive heart failure (CHF)
    - Pericarditis
  - GI
    - Intestinal protein loss
    - Postpericardiotomy or congenital heart surgery
    - Hepatobiliary disease
  - Endocrine: hypothyroidism

ETIOLOGY

- Excessive losses of protein
  - Renal losses
  - GI losses
- Inadequate production of protein
  - Liver disease
  - Malnutrition
- Local trauma
- Increased hydrostatic pressure
  - CHF
  - Cirrhosis
  - Pericardial effusion
  - Post–cardiac surgery
  - Venous obstruction
    - Superior vena cava syndrome
    - Deep vein thrombosis
- Lymphatic obstruction

APPROACH TO THE PATIENT

Determine the cause of swelling: Is it localized? Are there any sources of protein loss? Is there underproduction of protein?

- **Phase 1:** Is the swelling localized as seen in trauma, lymphatic, or venous obstruction?
- **Phase 2:** Are there urinary or GI losses?
  - Associated with decreased serum albumin
  - Most likely source of loss is renal disease, less frequently GI losses
- **Phase 3:** Search for other causes of edema, such as CHF, cirrhosis, lymphatic obstruction

HISTORY

- **Question:** Is the edema localized or generalized?
- *Significance*: See "Differential Diagnosis"
- **Question:** Is the patient asymptomatic or in some distress specifically because of the edema?
- *Significance*: Determine treatment urgency
- **Question:** Evidence of cardiac, renal, or GI disease?
- *Significance*: Major causes of edema
- **Question:** Waist size has become larger, difficulty putting shoes on, clothes too tight?
- *Significance*: Evidence of edema in body
- **Question:** Excess salt intake in diet?
- *Significance*: In some patients, contributes to edema
- **Question:** Shortness of breath?
- *Significance*: There may be ascites, which compresses the diaphragm, or pleural effusions.
- **Question:** Chronic diarrhea?
- *Significance*: Seen in protein-losing enteropathy or lymphatic obstruction
- **Question:** Has a urinalysis been performed in the past?
- *Significance*: May help date the onset of the problem
- **Question:** Swelling around the eyes or face?
- *Significance*: May suggest allergies but should also consider other causes of edema such as nephrotic syndrome
- **Question:** Anemia?
- *Significance*: Seen in protein-losing enteropathy

PHYSICAL EXAM
- **Finding:** Lumbosacral area, pretibial, scrotum/labia?
- *Significance*: Dependent edema
- **Finding:** Percussion of chest?
- *Significance*: Pleural effusion
- **Finding:** Shifting dullness?
- *Significance*: Early sign of ascites
- **Finding:** Soft ear cartilage?
- *Significance*: Common finding in nephrotic syndrome
- **Finding:** Pitting edema?
- *Significance*: Seen in cases of protein loss
- **Finding:** Nonpitting edema?
- *Significance*: May be caused by venous/lymphatic obstruction or salt poisoning.

DIAGNOSTIC TESTS & INTERPRETATION
- **Test:** Dipstick urinalysis
- *Significance*: If there is generalized edema with heavy proteinuria, this is suggestive of nephrotic syndrome.
- **Test:** Serum albumin
- *Significance*:
  - Hypoalbuminemia in the setting of edema and proteinuria supports diagnosis of nephrotic syndrome.
  - If there is generalized edema with no proteinuria but hypoalbuminemia, consider cardiac, GI, or hepatobiliary disease and direct additional studies to evaluate these 3 organ systems specifically.
  - If there is either localized edema or generalized edema but a normal urinalysis and a normal serum albumin, consider other unusual causes for edema, such as mechanical or lymphatic obstruction, certain endocrine disorders, or the effects of drugs or toxins.
- **Test:** Alpha-1-antitrypsin in stool
  - *Significance*: Seen in protein-losing enteropathy
- **Test:** Cholesterol
  - *Significance*: Only high in hypoalbuminemia associated with nephrotic syndrome

TREATMENT

ADDITIONAL TREATMENT
General Measures
- Moisturize skin.
- Avoid pressure sores.
- Decrease sodium intake.
- Active or passive leg exercise to avoid venous thromboses.
- If edema is massive, the patient may awaken with swollen eyelids. Place blocks under the head of the bed to keep the patient's head elevated.
- If there is scrotal edema, jockey shorts will help support the scrotum and protect the skin from breaking down.
- For severe edema with respiratory distress, severe abdominal discomfort, or severe scrotal edema, consider treatment with albumin and/or furosemide infusion.

ISSUES FOR REFERRAL
- Nephrotic syndrome—pediatric nephrologist
- Protein-losing enteropathy or hepatobiliary disease—pediatric gastroenterologist
- CHF—pediatric cardiologist
- Endocrine-mediated edema—pediatric endocrinologist
- Lymphatic or other mechanical obstructions—vascular surgeon or pediatric surgeon

INITIAL STABILIZATION
Any child or adolescent with an edema-forming state that compromises either cardiorespiratory function or the vascular integrity of a peripheral organ or limb should be referred immediately to an appropriate specialist for emergency care.

ADDITIONAL READING

- Braamskamp MJAM, Dolman KM, Tabbers MM. Clinical practice. Protein-losing enteropathy in children. *Eur J Pediatr*. 2010;169(10):1179–1185.
- Holliday MA, Segar WE. Reducing errors in fluid therapy management. *Pediatrics*. 2003;111(2):424–425.
- Jacobs ML, Rychik J, Byrum CJ, et al. Protein-losing enteropathy after Fontan operation: resolution after baffle fenestration. *Ann Thorac Surg*. 1996;61(1):206–208.
- Molina JF, Brown RF, Gedalia A, et al. Protein losing enteropathy as the initial manifestation of childhood systemic lupus erythematosus. *J Rheumatol*. 1996;23(7):1269–1271.
- Moritz ML, Ayus JC. Prevention of hospital acquired hyponatremia: a case for using isotonic saline. *Pediatrics*. 2003;111(2):227–230.
- Rosen FS. Urticaria, angioedema, and anaphylaxis. *Pediatr Rev*. 1992;13(10):387–390.
- Vande Walle JG, Donckerwolcke RA. Pathogenesis of edema formation in the nephrotic syndrome. *Pediatr Nephrol*. 2001;16(3):283–293.

CODES

ICD10
- R60.9 Edema, unspecified
- R60.0 Localized edema
- R60.1 Generalized edema

FAQ
- Q: At what level of serum albumin does edema occur?
- A: Edema is generally associated with serum albumin <2.5 g/dL.
- Q: Why does pericardial effusion cause edema?
- A: Pericardial effusion is associated with decreased lymphatic flow and increased venous pressure.

E

EHRLICHIOSIS AND ANAPLASMOSIS

Gordon E. Schutze

BASICS

DESCRIPTION

Two common clinically described infections are human monocytic ehrlichiosis (HME), caused by *Ehrlichia chaffeensis*, and human granulocytic anaplasmosis (HGA), caused by *Anaplasma phagocytophilum*. Human ehrlichiosis can be caused by 2 other *Ehrlichia* species in the United States: *ewingii* and *muris*-like agent.

EPIDEMIOLOGY

- HME typically occurs in the midwest, south central, and southeastern United States, mirroring the pattern of Rocky Mountain spotted fever (RMSF). In addition, it has been found in Europe, South America, Asia, and Africa.
- HGA typically occurs in the north central, northeastern United States, and northern California, similar to Lyme disease. Most patients are infected during April through September, the months of greatest tick and human outdoor activity.
- A second peak of HGA occurs from late October to December.

GENERAL PREVENTION

- Avoid tick-infested areas.
- Clothes should cover arms and legs.
- Use tick repellents, but with caution in young children.
- A thorough body search should always be done after returning from a tick-infested area:
  - If a tick is found, the area should be cleaned with a disinfectant, and the tick should be removed immediately.
  - To remove the tick, grasp the tick at the point of origin with forceps, staying as close to the skin as possible.
  - Applying steady, even pressure, slowly pull the tick off the skin. After the tick has been removed, clean the skin with a disinfectant.
- Instruct parents to seek medical attention only if symptoms develop.
- No vaccine is available.

PATHOPHYSIOLOGY

- Obligate intracellular, pleomorphic, gram-negative bacteria.
- Transmission to humans by a tick vector
- Incubation period from 2 to 21 days
- HME infects monocytes and macrophages, whereas HGA infects neutrophils.
- The bacteria reside and divide within cytoplasmic vacuoles of circulating leukocytes, called morulae.
- There is overinduction of the inflammatory and immune response, resulting in clinical manifestations of disease, including multiorgan system involvement.

ETIOLOGY

- HME is transmitted by *Amblyomma americanum*, the Lone Star tick. The white-tailed deer is the major reservoir.
- HGA is transmitted by *Ixodes scapularis*, the black-legged or deer tick, or the Western black-legged tick (*Ixodes pacificus*). Small mammals such as the white-footed mouse are the major reservoirs.
- Congenital infection is very rare but has been described in case reports.

DIAGNOSIS

Classic presentation: fever, headache, and myalgias, followed by the development of a progressive leukopenia, thrombocytopenia, and anemia

HISTORY

- History of tick bite or exposure to wooded areas that are endemic for tick-borne diseases is helpful but is not always present.
- Fever, severe headache, chills, and myalgias
- Complaints of abdominal pain, vomiting, anorexia, and diarrhea may be present.
- Cough and sore throat are often described.

PHYSICAL EXAM

- Fever is described in all children.
- A pleomorphic rash occurs in ~66% of pediatric patients with HME:
  - Rash is described as macular, maculopapular, petechial, erythematous, vesicular, or a combination of these.
  - Usually distributed on the trunk and extremities; spares palms, soles, and face
- Mental status change due to meningoencephalitis
- Cardiac murmur (II/VI systolic ejection murmur at the left lower sternal border)
- Hepatosplenomegaly
- Conjunctival or throat injection

DIAGNOSTIC TESTS & INTERPRETATION

Lab

- CBC with differential (with smear)
  - Thrombocytopenia, $<$150,000/mm^3 (77–92% incidence)
  - Lymphopenia, $<$1,500/mm^3 (75%) with HME
  - Neutropenia, $<$4,000/mm^3 (58–68%) with HGA
  - Anemia, hematocrit $<$30% (38–42%)
  - Intracytoplasmic morulae within leukocytes (20–60%), more common with HGA
- Electrolytes with BUN and creatinine: hyponatremia (33–65%)
- Liver function tests: elevated alanine aminotransferase, $>$55 U/L (90%)
- Coagulation labs, type and cross, as indicated
- CSF
  - Leukocytosis, with an average cell count of 100/mm^3
  - Lymphocytic predominance
  - Elevated protein and borderline low glucose (less common in children, more common in adults)
  - Microbiology cultures are negative.
  - Intraleukocytoplasmic *Ehrlichia* microorganisms (morulae) have been described on CSF smears.
- Serum studies
  - Acute and convalescent antibody titers of *Ehrlichia* (a 4-fold rise or fall is considered positive) obtained 2–4 weeks apart
  - An acute antibody titer of $\geq$1:128 is considered diagnostic.
  - Polymerase chain reaction is also available for both HME and HGA.
  - The detection of intraleukocytoplasmic *Ehrlichia* microcolonies (morulae) on blood or bone marrow monocytes or granulocytes is diagnostic but is not present in all patients.

Diagnostic Procedures/Other

- Bone marrow biopsy is not necessary to diagnose the ehrlichiosis but may be carried out amid concern for other hematologic diseases.
- Bone marrow is usually hypercellular, but normocellularity and hypocellularity have also been found.

ALERT

- Failing to consider the diagnosis of ehrlichiosis or a delay in treatment pending confirmatory serum titers increases morbidity and mortality.
- Thus, treatment should be started if infection is suspected based on history, physical, and initial laboratory data.
- Alternative diagnoses should be considered in children who do not rapidly improve with doxycycline.
- Simultaneous infections have been documented with HGA and Lyme disease.

DIFFERENTIAL DIAGNOSIS
- Tick-borne infection
  - RMSF
  - Tularemia
  - Relapsing fever
  - Lyme disease
  - Colorado tick fever
  - Babesiosis
- Other infections
  - Toxic shock syndrome
  - Kawasaki disease
  - Meningococcemia
  - Pyelonephritis
  - Gastroenteritis
  - Hepatitis
  - Leptospirosis
  - Epstein-Barr virus
  - Influenza
  - Cytomegalovirus
  - Enterovirus
  - Streptococcus pharyngitis
- Miscellaneous
  - Leukemia
  - Idiopathic thrombocytopenia purpura
  - Hemolytic uremic syndrome

TREATMENT

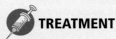

MEDICATION
First Line
- Doxycycline, either PO or IV
- Drug of choice regardless of age of child who is severely ill
- Dose: 4.4 mg/kg/day divided q12h (max dose 200 mg q12h)
- Treatment duration: minimum 5–10 days. Continue for 3–5 days after defervescence, longer if there is CNS involvement.

Second Line
- Rifampin has been reported to be an effective antibiotic for children <8 years of age who are less toxic and are experiencing an HGA infection.
- Dose: 20 mg/kg/day divided q12h for 5–10 days
- This is also the drug of choice for pregnant mothers.
- Unlike Lyme disease, neither amoxicillin nor ceftriaxone has been shown to be effective for the treatment of ehrlichiosis.

ADDITIONAL TREATMENT
General Measures
- Volume and BP medications as needed
- Intubation for respiratory failure
- Dialysis for renal failure
- Platelets for thrombocytopenia
- Packed red blood cells for anemia
- Fresh frozen plasma, cryoprecipitate, and vitamin K for DIC
- Antifungal or antibiotics for secondary infections

ONGOING CARE

PROGNOSIS
- >60% of patients are hospitalized.
- Case fatality rate for HME is 2–5%; for HGA, 7–10%.
- Elevated BUN and creatinine have been associated with a more severe course.
- Children appear to have an excellent outcome: Blood, renal, and liver abnormalities resolve in 1–2 weeks after initiating antibiotics.
- Cognitive and behavioral problems have been reported.
- Neuropathy has been described.

COMPLICATIONS
- Neurologic
  - Headache, described as severe
  - Mental status changes
  - Seizures
  - Coma
  - Focal neurologic findings
  - Cognitive learning deficits
- Hematologic
  - Disseminated intravascular coagulation (DIC)
  - Thrombocytopenia
  - Leukopenia
  - Lymphopenia
  - Anemia
- GI
  - Hemorrhage
  - Elevated liver enzymes
  - Hepatosplenomegaly
- Respiratory
  - Pulmonary hemorrhage
  - Interstitial pneumonia
  - Pleural effusions
  - Noncardiogenic pulmonary edema
- Infectious
  - Fungal superinfection
  - Nosocomial infections
  - Opportunistic infections
- Renal
  - Renal failure
  - Proteinuria
  - Hematuria
- Cardiac
  - Cardiomegaly
  - Murmurs

ADDITIONAL READING

- Dhand A, Nadelman RB, Aguero-Rosenfeld M, et al. Human granulocytic anaplasmosis during pregnancy: case series and literature review. *Clin Infect Dis*. 2007;45:589–593.
- Havens NS, Kinnear BR, Mató S. Fatal ehrlichial myocarditis in a healthy adolescent: a case report and review of the literature. *Clin Infect Dis*. 2012;54:e113–e114.
- Schutze GE, Buckingham SC, Marshall GS, et al. Human monocytic ehrlichiosis in children. *Pediatr Infect Dis J*. 2007;26:475–479.
- Dumler JS, Madigan JE, Pusterla N, et al. Ehrlichioses in humans: epidemiology, clinical presentation, diagnosis, and treatment. *Clin Infect Dis*. 2007;15:S45–S51.

CODES

ICD10
- A77.40 Ehrlichiosis, unspecified
- A77.41 Ehrlichiosis chafeensis [E. chafeensis]
- A77.49 Other ehrlichiosis

FAQ
- Q: If a tick is removed from my child, should antibiotics be started?
- A: No. Antibiotics should be started if a child becomes symptomatic because prophylactic use of antimicrobial agents will not prevent the development of disease.
- Q: What is the most common chief complaint in children with ehrlichiosis?
- A: Intense, unremitting headache and fever are the most common features.

E

ENCEPHALITIS

Lily C. Wong-Kisiel • Elaine C. Wirrell

BASICS

DESCRIPTION
Encephalitis is inflammation of the brain parenchyma, which results in alterations in mental status, motor or sensory symptoms, speech problems, or seizures. This inflammation may be due to direct brain invasion by an infectious pathogen or immune-mediated from an inflammatory processes due to acute or chronic illnesses.

EPIDEMIOLOGY
- Exact incidence is unknown, but infants and children are predominantly affected.
- Encephalitis due to enterovirus or arbovirus has a peak incidence between summer and early autumn. Many cases of viral encephalitis occur in epidemics.

GENERAL PREVENTION
- Routine immunization for measles, mumps, rubella, and influenza and, if travelling to endemic area (e.g., Southeast Asia), consideration of immunization for Japanese encephalitis
- Careful hand washing, avoid tick and mosquito exposure (DEET [*N*,*N*-diethyl-meta-toluamide] repellant, mosquito netting, appropriate dress), and insect control (drainage of stagnant water, insecticides)

PATHOPHYSIOLOGY
- Transmission of infectious pathogens can be by the blood-borne route, by retrograde spread through peripheral nerves (such as HSV or rabies), or rarely by direct inoculation of the brain.
- Encephalitis may also result indirectly, by immune-mediated injury due to parainfectious (i.e., acute disseminated encephalomyelitis or mycoplasma) or inflammatory/paraneoplastic causes (i.e., anti-NMDA receptor encephalitis). Such immune-mediated mechanisms involve cytokine effects and cytotoxic antibodies on neurons.

ETIOLOGY
- In most cases, the underlying cause remains unknown. Of those with known etiology, the majority are due to viral agents, followed by bacterial, autoimmune, parasitic, and fungal causes.
- The most common viral causes include HSV 1 and 2, enteroviruses, arboviruses (West Nile virus [WNV]), and other herpesviruses (CMV, EBV, HHV-6, VZV). HSV-1 typically presents with focal seizures, often of temporal lobe origin and encephalopathy. HSV-2 is the predominant cause of neonatal HSV infection. Enteroviruses and arboviruses typically cause disease in the summer and fall. WNV presents as an acute flaccid paralysis, extrapyramidal symptoms, and cranial nerve palsies. Other viruses may be considered given specific historical features (rabies with animal bite or bat exposure or with prominent hydrophobia) or history of travel (Japanese encephalitis virus).
- Bacterial causes include *Listeria, Francisella tularensis, Bartonella, Mycobacterium, Rickettsia, Mycoplasma, Borrelia, and Chlamydia.*
- Fungal and parasitic causes include *Cryptococcus, Blastomyces, Histoplasma, Paracoccidioides, Naegleria, Toxoplasma, Plasmodium*, and *Toxocara*.
- Parainfectious etiologies include acute disseminated encephalomyelitis (ADEM), acute hemorrhagic leukoencephalitis, postinfectious cerebellitis, and *Mycoplasma* encephalopathy. ADEM typically presents with encephalopathy and focal neurologic symptoms, with an MRI showing multifocal white matter lesions.
- Other inflammatory or paraneoplastic etiologies include anti-NMDA receptor encephalitis, voltage-gated potassium channel complex antibody, aquaporin-4 autoimmunity, SREAT (steroid-responsive encephalopathy associated with thyroid disease), systemic lupus erythematosus, and other vasculitis. Anti-NMDA receptor encephalitis typically presents subacutely with encephalopathy, sleep disturbance, seizures, perioral dyskinesias, and autonomic disturbances.

DIAGNOSIS

HISTORY
- Symptoms include fever, headache, photophobia, altered mental status, irritability, gait disturbance, and seizures.
- Ask for focal neurologic symptoms. A recent viral illness, recent travel, animal exposures, tick or mosquito bites, immunizations, and immune status may provide clues to etiology.
- A history of maternal herpes infection or prolonged rupture of membranes should be queried in neonates.

PHYSICAL EXAM
- Hypertension, bradycardia, or apnea may suggest impending herniation due to brain swelling.
- Altered mental status is the hallmark of encephalitis and ranges from mild confusion to stupor and coma. Distinguishing infectious from postinfectious encephalitis usually cannot be done reliably on clinical grounds.
- Specific neurologic findings suggestive of a specific etiology include focal seizures and focal neurologic findings (HSV); hydrophobia, pharyngeal spasms, and mood disturbance (rabies); facial nerve palsy (Lyme disease); flaccid paralysis or polio-like syndrome (WNV); and ataxia (VZV).
- Nonneurologic findings suggesting a specific etiology include respiratory symptoms (*Mycoplasma*), adenopathy and splenomegaly (EBV), petechial skin rash (*Rickettsia*), morbilliform rash (measles), erythematous maculopapular rash (enterovirus), and parotitis (mumps).

DIAGNOSTIC TESTS & INTERPRETATION

Lab
- Routine labs such as electrolytes, glucose, renal and liver function, and CBC are usually nonspecific.
- Selected serologic testing depending on the suspected agent (e.g., WNV and *Mycoplasma*) can provide confirmatory diagnosis of underlying etiology.
- Toxicology screen should be done to rule out overdose or toxin exposure as the cause for altered mental status.
- Lumbar puncture is performed urgently, once the patient is stabilized and signs and symptoms of intracranial pressure are excluded (broad-spectrum treatment should commence if these conditions are not met).
- In addition to measuring opening pressure (frequently elevated), other studies should include CSF cell count and differential (lymphocytic predominance suggests a viral process, whereas neutrophilic predominance suggests bacterial or early viral processes), red blood cells (in the absence of a traumatic tap, red blood cells are suggestive of necrotizing encephalitis associated with HSV), protein (often elevated), glucose (usually normal), Gram stain and bacterial culture (20% of patients with suspected encephalitis are diagnosed with bacterial meningitis), and HSV polymerase chain reaction (PCR). Initial studies may be normal, which does not rule out the diagnosis of encephalitis if clinical suspicion is high.
- Other PCR-based tests on CSF including enterovirus, *Borrelia burgdorferi*, and WNV may be considered depending on the situation.
- In immunocompromised hosts, CSF should be sent for fungal stains and culture (and serum for cryptococcal serum antigen).
- In those patients suspected of paraneoplastic etiology, an extended panel of autoimmune antibodies should be investigated in the serum and CSF.

Imaging
Imaging is performed urgently to rule out surgically remediable conditions (e.g., abscess or hematoma). MRI (or if not available, CT) of the brain with and without contrast medium is preferred. Neuroimaging can be normal or demonstrate focal or diffuse parenchymal enhancement (HSV-2 has a preference for the medial temporal lobe).

Diagnostic Procedures/Other
- An EEG usually shows diffuse generalized slowing. Findings of periodic lateralized discharges are suggestive but not diagnostic of HSV.
- Brain biopsy: rarely performed

DIFFERENTIAL DIAGNOSIS
Several conditions can resemble encephalitis including metabolic (acute electrolyte disturbance, inborn errors of metabolism), toxic (ingestions), structural (acute obstructive hydrocephalus or shunt obstruction),

vascular (cerebral vasculitis, ischemic or hemorrhagic stroke, septic embolization, sinus thrombosis), endocrine (hypothyroid crisis, pituitary infarction), infectious (bacterial meningitis, brain abscess, subdural empyema, viral meningitis), or epileptic disorders (status epilepticus).

TREATMENT

MEDICATION

Initial treatment should target bacterial and viral agents until culture results are confirmed or negative.

- Bacterial meningitis: vancomycin (15–20 mg/kg IV q6–8h, monitor levels) plus either cefotaxime (225–300 mg/kg/24 h IV q6–8h) or ceftriaxone (100 mg/kg/24 h IV divided q12–24h; use for ≥1 month old). Treat until cultures are negative at 48 hours.
- HSV encephalitis: acyclovir (>28 days–<12 years: 20 mg/kg/dose IV q8h; ≥12 years: 10 mg/kg/dose IV q8h). Acyclovir is continued for a minimum of 21 days if HSV is confirmed. PCR may be falsely negative in 5–10% of cases—contact an infectious diseases consultant if there is a high clinical suspicion. Monitor renal function while on acyclovir.
- Rickettsial infection (characteristic rash with exposure to ticks in an endemic region) or ehrlichiosis (headache, rash, leukopenia, thrombocytopenia, typical blood smear, transaminase elevation, with exposure to ticks in an endemic region): Consider empiric doxycycline.
- There is no evidence from controlled clinical trials that corticosteroids, IVIG, and therapeutic hypothermia are useful in cases of infectious encephalitis.
- *Mycoplasma* encephalopathy: erythromycin (benefit sustained from this medication is controversial given probable parainfectious mechanism)
- ADEM: high-dose IV corticosteroids 20–30 mg/kg/day × 3 days followed by prednisolone taper. In refractory cases, either IVIG or plasmapheresis can be considered.
- Anti-NMDA receptor encephalitis: high-dose IV corticosteroids, IVIG, or plasmapheresis. Rituximab has been used in combination with 1st-line agents.
- Immunotherapy is also recommended for other inflammatory or paraneoplastic causes of encephalitis.

INPATIENT CONSIDERATIONS

Initial Stabilization

- Careful attention to cardiorespiratory status is essential as is ruling out potential cerebral herniation. Children with severe encephalitis require intensive care with careful cardiorespiratory monitoring. Isolation precautions are based on type of suspected organism.
- Seizures: IV benzodiazepines (lorazepam, midazolam, or diazepam) are used acutely. Status epilepticus should be aggressively managed with a loading dose of fosphenytoin or levetiracetam. Barbiturate coma or midazolam infusion may be needed in refractory cases. In children with reduced level of consciousness, or those treated for refractory status epilepticus, EEG monitoring should be considered.
- Cerebral edema: Cerebral perfusion pressure should be kept at 70 mm Hg or higher for children older than 2 years of age. Conservative measures including fluid restriction, elevation of the head of the bed, and hyperventilation are most commonly used. With impending herniation, mannitol should be considered. Rarely, in malignant cases of cerebral edema, craniectomy can be considered for decompression.
- Investigation for occult tumors should be done with anti-NMDA receptor or other autoantibody-mediated encephalitis. Among girls with anti-NMDA receptor encephalitis, 9% younger than age 14 years and 30% younger than age 18 years were found to have an ovarian teratoma. Tumor resection is required to improve symptoms. Testicular teratoma has been rarely reported

IV Fluids

Closely monitor electrolytes, anticipating possible syndrome of inappropriate antidiuretic hormone or diabetes insipidus.

ONGOING CARE

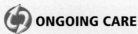

FOLLOW-UP RECOMMENDATIONS

- Physical and occupational therapists should be consulted early in the course and will be helpful during the convalescence.
- Neuropsychologic testing is helpful to identify cognitive deficits and direct appropriate services.
- Follow-up with speech pathologists and developmental pediatricians may be indicated.

PROGNOSIS

- Outcome varies greatly and depends on age, etiologic agent, and disease severity at the time of presentation (e.g., patients presenting in coma do worse).
- Outcomes range from complete recovery to focal neurologic deficits, persistent vegetative state, and death.
- Potential complications include aphasia, ataxia, developmental delay, learning disabilities, quadriparesis/hemiparesis, and epilepsy.

ADDITIONAL READING

- DuBray K, Anglemyer A, LaBeaud AD, et al. Epidemiology, outcomes and predictors of recovery in childhood encephalitis: a hospital based study. *Pediatr Infect Dis J*. 2013;32(8):839–844.
- Gable MS, Sheriff H, Dalmau J, et al. The frequency of autoimmune N-methyl-D-aspartate receptor encephalitis surpasses that of individual viral etiologies in young individuals enrolled in the California Encephalitis Project. *Clin Infect Dis*. 2012;54(7):899–904.
- Rosenfeld MR, Dalmau J. Anti-NMDA-receptor encephalitis and other synaptic autoimmune disorders. *Curr Treat Options Neurol*. 2011;13(3):324–332.
- Sonneville R, Klein IF, Wolff M. Update on investigation and management of postinfectious encephalitis. *Curr Opin Neurol*. 2010;23(3):300–304.
- Tunkel AR, Glaser CA, Bloch KC, et al. The management of encephalitis: clinical practice guidelines by the Infectious Diseases Society of America. *Clin Infect Dis*. 2008;47(3):303–327.

CODES

ICD10

- G04.90 Encephalitis and encephalomyelitis, unspecified
- A85.8 Other specified viral encephalitis
- B00.4 Herpesviral encephalitis

FAQ

- Q: Will the child suffer permanent brain injury from encephalitis?
- A: The complications following encephalitis vary greatly from severe mental retardation and cerebral palsy to full recovery. There is a correlation between degree of brain destruction and outcome; however, children frequently recover better than adults with a similar degree of illness.
- A: Outcomes depend on the neurologic status of the patient at presentation and the causative organism. Although many children will make a full recovery, some have persisting neurologic problems including cognitive or motor difficulties, vision or hearing deficits, epilepsy, or personality change. Children with focal deficits or markedly impaired level of consciousness in the acute stage or those with HSV encephalitis are at highest risk of sequelae.
- Q: Is encephalitis highly contagious?
- A: Most cases of encephalitis are not highly contagious, although precautions should be followed with blood or body fluid exposure.

E

ENCOPRESIS

Jay Fong

BASICS

DESCRIPTION

- Repeated unintentional soiling of underwear
- Most commonly associated with functional constipation with severe stool retention and subsequent overflow incontinence:
  - 90% of cases of encopresis fall into this category.
- Another less common type of encopresis refers to the entity of repeated passage of feces into inappropriate places (usually clothing or floor) after the age of 4 years in the absence of constipation and structural or inflammatory diseases, also known as functional nonretentive fecal incontinence (FNRFI).

EPIDEMIOLOGY

- The reported ratio of boys to girls with encopresis ranges from 2:1 to 6:1.
- Boys are more likely to experience nonretentive fecal incontinence than girls at a ratio of 9:1.
- There is no association with family size, ordinal position in the family, age of parents, or socioeconomic status.
- Encopresis is reported in 1.5–2.8% of children >4 years of age.
- Between 10 and 30% of children with encopresis have nonretentive fecal incontinence.

RISK FACTORS

Genetics

Monozygotic twins have a 4-fold higher incidence than do dizygotic twins.

ALERT

- Constipation with a rectal fecal mass is most common risk for encopresis.
- Children with FNRFI have more behavioral problems, poor self-esteem, and higher prevalence of attention deficit disorder.

PATHOPHYSIOLOGY

Chronic constipation with fecal impaction results in overflow incontinence and reduced sensation secondary to rectal distention. The pattern of holding fecal matter, leading to chronic constipation and overflow incontinence, may result from a variety of causes, such as a painful experience from a fissure, difficult toilet training, or refusal to use school bathrooms. However, eliciting a medical history often does not reveal a triggering event.

ETIOLOGY

- Chronic constipation leads to a dilated rectum, decreased rectal sensation, shortening of the anal canal, and decreased anal sphincter tone in some patients.
- Findings on anorectal manometry include increased rectal sensory threshold and paradoxic contraction of the external anal sphincter during attempts at defecation (known as anismus).
- FNRFI occurs in children without constipation. The soiling may be a manifestation of an emotional disturbance, and it may be associated with specific triggers (person or place) or may represent an impulsive action triggered by unconscious anger. All studies in these patients are normal, including normal anorectal manometry and normal colonic transit times.

COMMONLY ASSOCIATED CONDITIONS

Enuresis is more frequently seen in patients with FNRFI (45% have daytime and 40% have nighttime enuresis) compared to constipated children.

DIAGNOSIS

HISTORY

- Toileting habits:
  - Constipation: frequency and size of bowel movements (large-diameter bowel movements are common in children with encopresis associated with functional constipation)
  - Bowel movements that obstruct the toilet and/or chronic abdominal pain relieved by enemas or laxatives
  - Retentive posturing: avoiding defecation by contraction of pelvic floor, squeezing the buttocks together (leg scissoring, crossing the legs, standing on tiptoes)
- Irritability, abdominal cramps, decreased appetite (symptoms improve after passage of large stool)
- Onset: Elicit history of triggering events (perianal infection, diet changes, toilet training, avoidance of school bathrooms, sexual abuse, or other stressful events).
- Enuresis (secondary daytime enuresis may occur in patients with megarectum compressing the bladder)
- Timing in the neonatal period of meconium passage, as well as past surgeries, medical history, and medications, are relevant.
- Unsteady or clumsy gait may suggest a neuromuscular disorder.
- Children with FNRFI do not have any history of constipation and have daily bowel movements. The incontinence is diurnal, usually in the afternoon.

PHYSICAL EXAM

- Encopresis with functional constipation
  - Fecal mass palpable in 40% of patients; fecal soiling in the perianal region
  - Dilated rectum with a normally positioned anus
- Digital rectal exam is not recommended to routinely diagnose fecal impaction or FNRFI.
  - Anal sphincter tone may be normal or slightly decreased; the anal canal is usually shorter than normal.
  - Hard stool or a large amount of "mushy" stool present in rectal vault
- FNRFI
  - No palpable fecal mass
  - Normal-size rectum
  - Normal sphincter length
- Examine deep tendon reflexes, anal wink, rectal exam, lumbosacral spine exam to look for sacral dimpling, and documentation of normal growth.
- In patients with extreme fear of anal exam, attempt a perianal inspection and obtain a plain radiograph of the abdomen to establish a fecal impaction.

DIAGNOSTIC TESTS & INTERPRETATION

Referral to a pediatric gastroenterologist for further evaluation, including anorectal manometry, may be useful for patients who are not responding to standard management.

Lab

No tests are needed if both the history and physical exam are consistent with functional constipation and associated encopresis. If the patient's history or physical exam is atypical and a systemic disorder is suspected, appropriate diagnostic tests should be done.

Imaging

- Abdominal radiography is often necessary for patients who refuse a rectal exam, or when a rectal impaction is not palpable on abdominal exam (e.g., in obese patients).
- Enema with water-soluble contrast material can be both helpful diagnostically to look for areas of narrowing and therapeutically as a clean out procedure.
- MRI of the spine can be done for children with suspected spinal abnormalities. This is rarely necessary if the neurologic exam is normal.
- Colonic transit study with radio-opaque markers to confirm the patients' complaints or assess for slow transit constipation

Diagnostic Procedures/Other

- Rectal suction biopsy can be performed to evaluate for ganglion cells within the colonic mucosa and definitively evaluate for Hirschsprung disease.
- Anorectal manometry can be done in selected cases to evaluate anorectal function. The main indication is to demonstrate the rectoanal inhibitory reflex to exclude Hirschsprung disease and ultra-short-segment Hirschsprung disease. It may also show an increased threshold to rectal sensation, providing important information to the patient and the parents.

DIFFERENTIAL DIAGNOSIS

Determine whether stool leakage is caused by functional constipation or an underlying anatomic, metabolic, or neurologic abnormality. Fecal incontinence may be secondary to diarrheal diseases or defective neuromuscular control, such as in children with spinal defects.

- Neuromuscular
  - Spinal cord tumor
  - Tethered spinal cord
  - Meningomyelocele
- Anal abnormalities:
  - Anteriorly displaced anus
  - Ectopic anus
- Inflammatory
  - Proctitis (infectious or ulcerative)
  - Fistula secondary to Crohn disease
  - Celiac disease
- Stricture (after necrotizing enterocolitis or inflammatory bowel disease)
- Abdominal pelvic mass (sacral teratoma, meningomyelocele)
- Hypotonia (cerebral palsy, amyotonia congenita, familial visceral myopathy)
- Hirschsprung disease (constipation common, fecal incontinence rarely seen) or ultra-short-segment Hirschsprung disease
- Postsurgical repair of imperforate anus or Hirschsprung disease
- Endocrine
  - Hypothyroidism
  - Panhypopituitarism
  - Diabetes mellitus
- Constipating drugs:
  - Opiates
  - Calcium supplements
  - Psychotropics

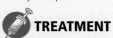

TREATMENT

MEDICATION

- Evidence suggests fecal disimpaction can be equally achieved with either oral PEG (with or without electrolytes at 1–1.5 g/kg/24 h) for 3–6 days of enemas or enema therapies. Sedated manual disimpaction is rarely required.
  - Severe cases may require PEG ingestion by NG tube after disimpaction in a hospital setting.
- Stimulant laxatives:
  - Magnesium citrate
  - Bisacodyl
  - Senna
- Oral stool softeners:
  - PEG-3350 (0.75 mg/kg/24 h) is the preferred agent because of its palatability and ease of administration.
  - Lactulose (2.5–10 mL/24 h for infants and 40–90 mL/day in older children) is recommended as the 1st-line treatment if PEG-3350 is not available.
  - Milk of magnesia (0.5–1 mL/kg/24 h) is a good option.
  - Mineral oil (5–20 mL in divided doses) may also be used in older children who have no risk of aspiration.

ISSUES FOR REFERRAL

Patients with nonretentive fecal incontinence usually require referral to a mental health professional for more intensive behavioral intervention.

COMPLEMENTARY & ALTERNATIVE THERAPIES

- Behavior modification therapy: decrease family stress. Have the child sit on toilet for defined amount of time (1 min/year of age to a maximum of 10 minutes) 1–2 times per day (ideally after a meal, tailored to the age of the child) and try to perform a Valsalva maneuver. Have young children blow into a pinwheel or a balloon to try to make them bear down.
- Use a sticker incentive chart if age-appropriate.
- Delay toilet training if the child is in diapers (to reduce stress).
- Motivate using positive reinforcement strategies. Biofeedback can be successful in some cases.

INPATIENT CONSIDERATIONS

Initial Stabilization

Management combines pharmacology, behavioral modification, and dietary alterations.

ONGOING CARE

FOLLOW-UP RECOMMENDATIONS

Patient Monitoring

- First follow-up visit is at 2 weeks to ensure compliance and success with the initial management.
- If the fecal impaction has been successfully removed, a reward system is started.
- The patient is followed at monthly intervals to ensure motivation and to be supportive.
- Treatment with stool softeners is needed until behavior and diet have improved and until rectal dilation has resolved.
- Medication is often needed for 6 months or longer.

ALERT

- Parents may misconstrue stool-withholding behavior as an attempt to defecate.
- Parents may think that the soiling represents diarrheal illness, causing a delay in diagnosis and treatment.
- Parents may think their child's soiling is deliberate. They may not understand that the child can neither feel the passage of stool nor prevent it. The usual urge to defecate, which comes from stretching of the ampulla and internal anal sphincter, is not felt because the rectal ampulla is massively distended.
- Patients or their parents often stop stool softeners as soon as a normal stool pattern starts. If therapy has been ended prematurely, the patient's constipation and encopresis returns immediately because rectal tone is still poor and no other behavior or dietary modifications have been made.

DIET

- Normal fiber intake
- Adequate fluid intake

COMPLICATIONS

- Social problems
- UTIs, especially in girls
- Abdominal discomfort
- Decreased appetite and weight loss

ADDITIONAL READING

- Burgers RB, Benninga MA. Functional nonretentive fecal incontinence in children: a frustrating and long-lasting clinical entity. *J Pediatr Gastroenterol Nutr*. 2009;48(Suppl 2):S98–S100.
- Desantis DJ, Leonard MP, Preston MA, et al. Effectiveness of biofeedback for dysfunctional elimination syndrome in pediatrics: a systematic review. *J Pediatr Urol*. 2011;7(3):342–348.
- Di Lorenzo C, Benninga MA. Pathophysiology of pediatric fecal incontinence. *Gastroenterology*. 2004;126(Suppl 1):S33–S40.
- Griffiths DM. The physiology of continence: idiopathic fecal constipation and soiling. *Semin Pediatr Surg*. 2002;11(2):67–74.
- Har AF, Croffie JM. Encopresis. *Pediatr Rev*. 2010; 31(9):368–374.
- Tabbers MM, Dilorenzo C, Berger MY, et al. Evaluation and treatment of functional constipation in infants and children: evidence-based recommendations from ESPGHAN and NASPGHAN. *J Pediatr Gastroenterol Nutr*. 2014;58(2):265–281.

CODES

ICD10

- R15.9 Full incontinence of feces
- F98.1 Encopresis not due to a substance or known physiol condition

FAQ

- Q: Is it possible to become "addicted" to laxative medicines?
- A: Stool softeners, rather than cathartic laxatives or per rectal therapies are chosen for long-term therapy because the colon does not become dependent.
- Q: Will my child become sick if this problem is not resolved?
- A: Most children with chronic constipation and encopresis grow well and do not develop other health problems. The major problems are social and should be taken seriously. Social continence is crucial for the school-aged child.

ENDOCARDITIS

Jenifer A. Glatz

BASICS

DESCRIPTION

Infective endocarditis (IE) is a microbial infection of the endocardium of the heart.

EPIDEMIOLOGY

Incidence

- IE is relatively uncommon. The estimated incidence is 0.3 per 100,000 children per year.
- The overall incidence of endocarditis decreased with the advent of antibiotics. However, a recent increase in frequency has been associated with improved survival of patients with congenital heart disease and the more widespread and often prolonged use of central vascular catheters, especially in premature infants.

RISK FACTORS

- Preexisting heart disease (congenital or acquired)
- Prior history of endocarditis
- Cardiac surgery
- Intracardiac pacemakers and implantable cardioverter-defibrillators
- Prosthetic valves or conduits
- Indwelling catheters/IV drug use

GENERAL PREVENTION

- Dental hygiene
- Minimal use of central lines
- Correction of the cardiovascular anomaly by surgery or interventional catheterization techniques
- Subacute bacterial endocarditis (SBE) prophylaxis regimes as per the 2007 American Heart Association (AHA) recommendations. Give as a single dose 30–60 minutes prior to procedure:
  - Oral: amoxicillin (50 mg/kg, max 2.0 g)
  - IV or IM: ampicillin (50 mg/kg, max 2.0 g) or ceftriaxone/cefazolin (50 mg/kg, max 1.0 g)
  - Oral for penicillin-allergic patients: cephalexin, if no history of urticaria, angioedema, or anaphylaxis (50 mg/kg, max 2.0 g); clindamycin (20 mg/kg PO/IV, max 600 mg); or azithromycin/clarithromycin (15 mg/kg PO, max 500 mg)
  - IV or IM for penicillin-allergic patients: cefazolin, ceftriaxone, or clindamycin (doses as above)
- SBE prophylaxis is recommended by the AHA only for the following cardiac conditions:
  - Prosthetic cardiac valve or prosthetic material used for cardiac valve repair
  - Prior history of IE
  - Unrepaired cyanotic congenital heart disease, including palliative shunts and conduits
  - Congenital heart defect repaired with prosthetic material or device for the first 6 months after the procedure
  - Repaired congenital heart disease with residual defect near the site of prosthetic patch or device
  - Cardiac transplantation recipients with cardiac valvulopathy
- SBE prophylaxis is recommended only for the following procedures:
  - Dental procedures involving manipulation of the gingival or periapical region of teeth or perforation of the oral mucosa
  - Invasive respiratory tract procedures involving incision or biopsy, such as tonsillectomy/adenoidectomy or abscess drainage
  - Surgery involving prosthetic intravascular or intracardiac material, including heart valves
- Procedures that do not require SBE prophylaxis:
  - Placement of removable prosthodontic or orthodontic appliances
  - Bleeding from trauma to the lips or oral mucosa or shedding of deciduous teeth
  - Routine anesthetic injections through noninfected oral mucosa tissues
  - Bronchoscopy without a biopsy
  - Gastrointestinal (GI) or genitourinary procedures: Prophylaxis solely to prevent IE is not recommended.

PATHOPHYSIOLOGY

- IE is primarily seen in patients with preexisting heart disease (congenital or acquired) who develop bacteremia with organisms that are likely to cause infection.
- IV drug abusers and patients with indwelling central venous catheters may develop endocarditis even in the absence of prior heart disease.
- Local turbulence secondary to the cardiovascular abnormality is thought to result in damage of the endocardial surface. The development of a fibrin and platelet network occurs in which bacteria may then become entrapped, causing infection.
- Bacteremia may be a complication of focal infection (e.g., pneumonia, cellulitis, or urinary tract infection) or may be associated with various dental and surgical procedures. Bacteremia, however, also occurs spontaneously with usual activities, such as chewing, flossing, and brushing teeth.
- Peripheral manifestations in chronic endocarditis are mediated by immune complex reactions.

ETIOLOGY

- Gram-positive cocci account for 90% of culture-positive endocarditis. There has been a recent shift in the microbial etiology, corresponding with a more acute presentation:
  - *Streptococcus viridans and Staphylococcus aureus* are the most common agents.
  - Other organisms that can cause endocarditis are coagulase-negative staphylococci, β-hemolytic streptococci, enterococci, the HACEK group (*Haemophilus aphrophilus*, *Haemophilus paraphrophilus*, *Haemophilus parainfluenzae*, *Actinobacillus actinomycetemcomitans*, *Cardiobacterium hominis*, *Eikenella corrodens*, *Kingella* species), *Candida* species, *Aspergillus* species, *Pseudomonas* species, pneumococci, and *Neisseria* species.
- <20% of endocarditis cases are reported as culture negative.

DIAGNOSIS

- The Modified Duke criteria define diagnostic categories (definite endocarditis, possible endocarditis, and rejected cases) based on combinations of major and minor criteria.
- Criteria:
  - Major: organism specific for IE demonstrated by positive blood culture or histologic specimen and definitive echocardiographic data
  - Minor: predisposing heart disease, fever, vascular/immunologic phenomena, or microbiologic evidence not within major criteria
- Definitive endocarditis requires 2 major, or 1 major plus 3 minor, or 5 minor criteria.
- Several studies have confirmed the high sensitivity and specificity of these criteria.

HISTORY

- Fever
- Malaise
- Anorexia
- Weight loss
- Heart failure symptoms
- Arthralgia/myalgia
- Neurologic symptoms
- GI symptoms
- Chest pain
- Occasionally, a recent infection, dental visit, or surgical procedure can be identified.
- Acute endocarditis is associated with a more rapidly progressive, fulminant course.

PHYSICAL EXAM

- General
  - Fever (usually low grade with α-hemolytic streptococci and high grade with *S. aureus*)
  - Petechiae (occurring in 1/3 of cases)
- Embolic or immunologic phenomena
  - Renal: glomerulonephritis, infarct
  - Splinter hemorrhages
  - Retinal hemorrhages (Roth spots)
  - Osler nodes (painful)
  - Janeway lesions (painless)
  - Splenomegaly (occurring in about 50% of cases)
  - Arthralgia/arthritis
  - Neurologic: cerebral infarction, embolism, or hemorrhage. Mycotic aneurysms may also occur.
- Cardiac/valvulitis
  - New or change in heart murmur
  - Signs of congestive heart failure (CHF)
- Newborns with IE may present with feeding difficulty, respiratory distress, tachycardia, hypotension, seizures, apnea, and septic emboli.

DIAGNOSTIC TESTS & INTERPRETATION

Lab

- Blood cultures
  - Most important diagnostic test for endocarditis
  - Positive in 85–90% of reported cases
  - Obtain 3–5 sets from different sites during the first 24 hours of suspected endocarditis.
  - Collect the largest volume that is clinically reasonable.
  - The bacteremia of endocarditis is continuous; therefore, it is not necessary to wait to obtain the blood cultures during a fever spike.
- Nonspecific data
  - Elevated erythrocyte sedimentation rate (ESR) (80%) and C-reactive protein
  - Anemia (44%)
  - Positive rheumatoid factor (38%)
  - Hematuria (35%) and red cell casts
  - Leukocytosis
  - Decreased complement

Imaging

- Echocardiography, transthoracic
  - Valuable noninvasive technique in the identification of vegetations
  - Specificity is 98%, but sensitivity is <60%, so a negative echocardiogram does not rule out endocarditis.
  - Also invaluable for follow-up, including evaluation for potential cardiac complications
- Echocardiography, transesophageal
  - Especially in older or obese patients, provides better visualization of smaller vegetations, with sensitivity of 76–100%
  - Recommended in patients with an inconclusive transthoracic study but a high index of suspicion for endocarditis

ALERT

- The absence of vegetation(s) by echocardiography does not rule out endocarditis.
- In patients with a prosthetic valve, echocardiography is not always helpful as there is frequently artifact from the prosthetic valve. Abnormal movements of the valve leaflets may suggest a vegetation.
- The ESR may remain elevated for some time, even after cessation of bacteremia.

Diagnostic Procedures/Other

Electrocardiogram: New-onset abnormalities such as atrioventricular block (even 1st-degree) may represent conduction system and myocardial involvement from invasive disease.

DIFFERENTIAL DIAGNOSIS

- Other infections
- Acute rheumatic fever
- Malignancy
- Connective tissue disorders

TREATMENT

MEDICATION

Antibiotics

- Prolonged IV therapy (at least 4 weeks) is needed.
- Choice of antibiotic(s) and duration of treatment depend on the infecting organism, sensitivity pattern, and patient risk factors.
- For staphylococcal or fungal endocarditis, IV therapy is given for at least 6–8 weeks.

SURGERY/OTHER PROCEDURES

- Severe/worsening CHF
- Valvular disease with unstable hemodynamics
- Failing medical therapy
- Large (>10 mm), mobile vegetations
- ≥2 major embolic events
- Fungal endocarditis
- Abscess formation/periannular extension
- Prosthetic valve endocarditis

INPATIENT CONSIDERATIONS

Initial Stabilization

- Rest
- Antipyretics
- Optimal nutrition and hydration
- Careful dental hygiene

ONGOING CARE

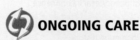

FOLLOW-UP RECOMMENDATIONS

Patient Monitoring

- Obtain repeat blood cultures after a few days of antibiotic or antifungal therapy to ensure the eradication of bacteria.
- Obtain blood cultures again 2 months after completion of a full course of antibiotic therapy.

PROGNOSIS

If diagnosed in a timely fashion and appropriate therapy is instituted, prognosis is relatively good for bacterial endocarditis. *S. aureus* and fungal endocarditis are associated with higher morbidity and mortality.

COMPLICATIONS

Despite improvements in diagnosis and treatment, IE continues to be a disease with significant morbidity and mortality (~10–20%):

- Cardiac: valve destruction and perforation leading to incompetence, abscess and fistula formation, heart failure, or conduction abnormalities
- Embolic events (22–50%) may occur to multiple organ systems (central nervous system, bowel, coronary arteries, kidneys, spleen, skin, lungs).

ADDITIONAL READING

- Ferrieri P, Gewitz MH, Gerber MA, et al. Unique features of infective endocarditis in childhood. *Circulation*. 2002;105(17):2115–2126.
- Knirsch W, Nadal D. Infective endocarditis in congenital heart disease. *Eur J Pediatr*. 2011;170(9):1111–1127.
- McDonald JR. Acute infective endocarditis. *Infect Dis Clin North Am*. 2009;23(3):643–664.
- Wilson W, Taubert KA, Gewitz M, et al. Prevention of infective endocarditis: guidelines from the American Heart Association. *Circulation*. 2007;116(15):1736–1754.

CODES

ICD10

- I38 Endocarditis, valve unspecified
- I33.0 Acute and subacute infective endocarditis

FAQ

- Q: I forgot to give my child antibiotics prior to the procedure. Should I give him a dose afterward?
- A: The dosage may be administered up to 2 hours after the procedure.
- Q: SBE prophylaxis is recommended for my child, but she already is on long-term antibiotic therapy with that recommended antibiotic. Should she use an additional antibiotic or increase her current dose for the procedure?
- A: An antibiotic from a different class should be selected.
- Q: My child has a congenital heart defect. Does he/she require SBE prophylaxis?
- A: The answer depends on the type of the congenital heart defect and the status of any needed intervention. The child's physician should be contacted regarding the need for prophylaxis.

ENURESIS

Eugene R. Hershorin • Marissa Janel DeFreitas

BASICS

DESCRIPTION

- Involuntary, urinary incontinence after age of expected bladder control; term generally reserved for children ≥5 years of age. May be
  - Primary: has never been dry for 6 months (80%)
  - Secondary: patient previously dry for 6 months or longer
- Classified as
  - Monosymptomatic nocturnal enuresis (MNE)
  - Nonmonosymptomatic nocturnal enuresis (NMNE) if there is evidence of lower urinary tract malfunction (e.g., delayed voiding, frequency, urgency, holding maneuvers)

EPIDEMIOLOGY

- Male > female (3:1)
- Prevalence of 10–15% in children at age 5 years, 7–15% at 7 years, 5% at 10 years, and 0.5–1% in teenagers and adults.

Genetics

- 60–70% have a positive family history of enuresis.
- Risk of severe enuresis is greater with maternal enuresis history compared with paternal history (odds ratio 3.6 vs. 1.8).
- Risk is twice as high in monozygotic compared with dizygotic twins.
- Autosomal dominant pattern seen in 50%, whereas 30% of cases are sporadic.
- Several loci on chromosomes 13q, 12q, and 22q associated with a nocturnal enuresis phenotype, but no candidate genes have been identified.

RISK FACTORS

- Constipation
- Lower urinary tract dysfunction
- Sleep disorders
- Neuropsychiatric disorders

ETIOLOGY

- Primary nocturnal enuresis: the interplay of one or more of the following:
  - Nocturnal polyuria
  - Decreased functional bladder volume
  - Increased arousal threshold when asleep
- Daytime incontinence and enuresis, day and night
  - As above. More concerning for underlying urologic and neurologic disorder
  - Urinary reflux into vagina with seepage after conclusion of voiding
  - Insertion of ureter into urethra or vagina
  - Stress incontinence with increased abdominal pressure (laughing, coughing, increased intravesicular pressure)
- Secondary enuresis
  - Any condition causing polyuria
  - Urinary tract infection (UTI)
  - Encopresis
  - Emotional stress or trauma including physical and sexual abuse, parental divorce, depression, new sibling, household moving, new school

COMMONLY ASSOCIATED CONDITIONS

Neuropsychiatric comorbidities: ADHD, anxiety, and oppositional behavior are more commonly associated with secondary nocturnal enuresis.

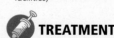

DIAGNOSIS

HISTORY

- Onset
  - Nocturnal versus diurnal
  - Dry period (even if only weeks)
    - Concomitant recent onset of polydipsia (sometimes accompanied by candidal infection) suggests new-onset diabetes.
  - Frequency
    - A frequency–volume chart provides information on daily fluid intake and volumes and timing of voids; identifies subtle lower urinary tract symptoms and can aid in treatment approach
  - Pattern of urination
    - Constantly wet pants (dribbling)
    - Frequent small amounts of urine
    - Presence of weak urinary stream
    - Dysuria
    - Frequency
    - Hesitancy
    - Urine holding maneuvers (e.g., pressing the heel into perineum)
    - Nocturia
- Past medical history
  - Obstipation/constipation/fecal incontinence (encopresis)
  - History of UTI
  - Behavioral/developmental history
  - Toilet training history
  - Medications
  - Neurologic symptoms
  - Other medical problems
- Family history
  - 1 parent or both parents
- Social history
  - For whom does this pose problem—parent or child?
  - Effect on child
    - Ability to sleep away from home without embarrassment
    - Teasing at school
    - Emotional effects
- Social changes
  - Divorce
  - New significant other for parent
  - New sibling
  - Household move
  - New school

PHYSICAL EXAM

- Vital signs
- Growth parameters and pattern
- Neurologic exam
  - Gait, tone, sensory, motor, deep tendon reflexes, cremasteric reflex
- Funduscopy: to rule out raised intracranial pressure
- Abdominal exam: to rule out masses, especially renal mass, fecal impaction, bladder distention
- Genitalia: rule out adhesions, vulvovaginitis, balanitis, stenosis, foreign bodies
- Urinary stream
- Rectal exam: tone, perianal sensation, anal wink
- Spine: bony defects, cutaneous signs of underlying spinal defects

DIAGNOSTIC TESTS & INTERPRETATION

Lab

- Urinalysis
  - Specific gravity (first morning void)
  - Glucose
  - Protein
  - Blood
- Urine culture: usually not necessary if no symptoms are present

Imaging

- Rarely necessary in primary enuresis
- Perform if suggestion of anatomic or functional abnormality of genitourinary tract
- Ultrasound least invasive modality
- Renal/bladder ultrasound with pre/post void bladder images to assess residual urine volume and look at bladder contour
- Noninvasive uroflow with pelvic floor electromyography—done by pediatric urologists

ALERT

Laboratory evaluation rarely yields a specific diagnosis. Balance risks and costs with unlikelihood of yield. Evaluation should generally not involve more than urinalysis.

DIFFERENTIAL DIAGNOSIS

- UTI/urethritis
- Obstipation/constipation
- Water intoxication
- Type 1 or type 2 diabetes
- Diabetes insipidus
- Sickle cell disease or trait
- Nephritis/nephrosis
- Anatomic abnormalities of the urinary tract
- Sleep disorders
- Depression
- Anxiety
- Behavioral disorders
- Medications (sedatives, soporifics, antihistamines, diuretics, caffeine, methylxanthines)
- Spinal cord disease
  - Cognitive disorders
  - Seizure disorders
- Legitimate safety issues in going to bathroom alone
- Substandard living conditions (cold bathrooms, poor facilities)

TREATMENT

GENERAL MEASURES

- If the problem is affecting only the parents and child is not affected, the treatment should be education and support for the parents.
- Avoid all negative interventions.

- Minimize fluid intake during evening.
  - Success rate: low
- Encourage child to void regularly during the day and immediately prior to retiring to bed.
- Alarm therapy
  - Most effective in motivated patient and family
  - Improves arousal and nocturnal bladder function as a reservoir through conditioning
  - Use nightly for at least 2–3 months until 14 consecutive dry nights are achieved.
  - "Overlearning" (after dryness is achieved, have child drink modest amount of water 1 hour before bedtime) reduces risk of relapse if dryness is maintained for 1 month on this regimen.
  - High relapse rate; 2nd remission very frequent with reintroduction of alarm system; 2nd relapse rare

MEDICATION

- Avoid medication use before age 6–8 years.
- Desmopressin (DDAVP)
  - Dose not based on age or weight.
    - Standard dose 0.2–0.4 mg PO given 1 hour before bedtime
    - Use oral formulation only (nasal formulation is associated with increased risk of hyponatremia and seizures).
  - Caution against excessive fluid intake
  - Can be used intermittently or continuously
  - Drug holidays are advised to assess for resolution of symptoms.
- Anticholinergics (e.g., oxybutynin)
  - Often used in combination with DDAVP
  - Usual dose: 5 mg given at bedtime
  - Exclude postvoid residual bladder volume.
  - Adverse effects: constipation, decreases saliva (hence, stress proper dental hygiene), hallucinations/agitation
- Imipramine
  - Tricyclic antidepressant
  - 80% effective
  - No longer 1st- or 2nd-line choice for benign condition because of risk of QTc prolongation and controversial risk of sudden cardiac death and risk of ingestion by siblings.

ADDITIONAL TREATMENT

- Urotherapy: aims towards normalizing bladder emptying and storage by teaching relaxed voiding techniques (e.g., biofeedback programs)
- Cognitive behavioral interventions
  - Formal programs developed and used by pediatric psychologists: high rate of success; involve "overcorrection techniques"—frequent practice and rewards for voiding procedures along with enuresis alarm
  - Positive reinforcement for dry nights
  - Use of praise, stickers, token economies
- Hypnotism
  - Appears to work by increasing subconscious awareness of bladder pressure during sleep, allowing increased awareness during sleep of intravesicular pressure

INPATIENT CONSIDERATIONS

Initial Stabilization

- Specific therapy to address specific anatomic, infectious, or functional genitourinary problems
- Address constipation and lower urinary tract dysfunction, as both may lead to treatment failure, whereas addressing these problems may result in spontaneous enuresis resolution.

ALERT

Decision to treat is a balance of the effect on the child of nontreatment (social, emotional) with the potential side effects of medication.

ONGOING CARE

PROGNOSIS

- 99% of cases resolve without treatment.
- Spontaneous resolution is ~15% per year after age 5 years.

COMPLICATIONS

- Physical
  - Vulvovaginitis
  - Diaper dermatitis
- Emotional
  - Embarrassment
  - Poor self-esteem
  - Reluctance to sleep out with peers or nonimmediate family
  - Depression

ADDITIONAL READING

- Franco I, von Gontard A, De Gennaro M; International Children's Continence Society. Evaluation and treatment of nonmonosymptomatic nocturnal enuresis: a standardization document from the International Children's Continence Society. *J Pediatr Urol*. 2013;9(2):234–243.
- Maternik M, Krzeminska K, Zurowska A. The management of childhood urinary incontinence. *Pediatr Nephrol*. 2015;30(1):41–50.
- Neveus T, Eggert P, Evans J, et al; International Children's Continence Society. Evaluation of and treatment for monosymptomatic enuresis: a standardization document from the International Children's Continence Society. *J Urol*. 2010;183(2):441–447.
- von Gontard A, Heron J, Joinson C. Family history of nocturnal enuresis and urinary incontinence: results from a large epidemiological study. *J Urol*. 2011;185(6):2303–2306.
- International Children's Continence Society: www.i-c-c-s.org

CODES

ICD10

- R32 Unspecified urinary incontinence
- N39.44 Nocturnal enuresis

FAQ

- Q: Do the medications cure the enuresis?
- A: None of the medications cure the problem. DDAVP increases reabsorption of water in the kidney, resulting in decreased bladder volumes. Tricyclic antidepressants cause urinary retention by the noradrenergic effects on bladder contraction and detrusor relaxation. Oxybutynin decreases detrusor irritability, resulting in larger bladder capacity before emptying. The medications result in nonemptying of the bladder during sleep but do not affect the underlying cause. Any resolution that occurs after cessation of medication treatment is probably from the natural resolution of the problem with age.
- Q: Isn't it important to treat the enuresis when the parents bring it up as a problem?
- A: Developmental resolution of nocturnal enuresis occurs at a range of ages, and in almost all cases, the enuresis resolves spontaneously. It is important to elicit for whom the enuresis is a problem. If the child is not affected by the enuresis, and it is only the parents who desire a cure, the important intervention is to educate them on the natural history of the problem and to let them know about the available interventions and their success rates for when the child desires a cure.
- Q: Are there any other interventions available for use only on sleep-out nights?
- A: One helpful tip is to allow the child to take a sleeping bag with him or her on sleep-outs. Place a pull-up inside the sleeping bag. When the child gets into the sleeping bag, he or she can change into the pull-up without anyone knowing. In the morning, the child puts his or her underwear back on, leaving the damp pull-up in the sleeping bag; the parent can take it out when the child gets home.

EOSINOPHILIC ESOPHAGITIS

Elizabeth H. Yen • Hemant P. Sharma

BASICS

DESCRIPTION

- Eosinophilic esophagitis (EoE) is a chronic immune-mediated esophageal disease characterized clinically by variable symptoms of esophageal dysfunction and pathologically by localized eosinophilic inflammation.
- The diagnosis is established in symptomatic patients who have the following:
  - At least 15 eosinophils/HPF isolated to the esophagus on endoscopic biopsies
  - Persistent eosinophilic infiltrate in esophageal biopsies after a trial of proton pump inhibitor (PPI) therapy

EPIDEMIOLOGY

- Incidence rates range from 0.7 to 10 per 100,000 person-years, and prevalence from 0.2 to 43 per 100,000.
- 3:1 male-to-female ratio
- Peaks of onset in childhood and 3rd–4th decade

PATHOPHYSIOLOGY

- The exact pathophysiology of EoE is unknown but likely involves an immune response to environmental antigens in genetically predisposed individuals.
- Environmental factors (food and possibly aeroallergens) trigger inflammatory response mediated by type 2 T-helper (Th2) cells.
- Genetic polymorphisms which predispose to EoE include eotaxin-3, thymic stromal lymphopoietin, and filaggrin.

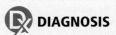

DIAGNOSIS

ALERT

Any patient who presents with esophageal food impaction should be evaluated for EoE. More than half of patients with food impaction are ultimately diagnosed with EoE.

HISTORY

Symptoms of EoE vary with age:

- In younger children, symptoms may include feeding difficulty or refusal (median age 2 years), vomiting (median age 8 years), and abdominal pain (median age 12 years).
  - Assess for:
    - Failure to thrive (poor weight gain, weight loss)
    - Feeding difficulties (not advancing past liquids, refusal of previously tolerated solids)
    - Gastroesophageal reflux (arching, irritability/fussiness)
    - Vomiting
- In adolescents and adults, symptoms include dysphagia, food impaction, refractory heartburn, epigastric abdominal pain, chest pain.
- Questions to assess dysphagia:
  - Sensation of difficulty swallowing or food getting stuck?
  - Is the child a slow eater? Does the child overchew or overcut food? Does the child avoid specific foods?
  - Personal history of esophageal food impaction?
- EoE is often associated with atopic disease (asthma, allergic rhinitis, atopic dermatitis, food allergy). Ask about the following:
  - Personal or family history of atopic disease?
  - Family history of EoE, dysphagia, refractory GERD, esophageal food impactions or dilations?
- No relief of symptoms after acid-blocking medication (minimum 8 weeks)

PHYSICAL EXAM

- Typically normal
- Growth failure (rare but may occur if feeding dysfunction or significantly decreased appetite)
- Signs of comorbid atopic disease: allergic shiners, wheezing, eczematous skin lesions

DIAGNOSTIC TESTS & INTERPRETATION

Labs

- Blood tests:
  - No diagnostic serum markers for EoE
  - Peripheral eosinophilia observed in <50% of patients
  - Elevated serum IgE present in 50–60%.
- Food allergy testing
  - Performed after biopsies confirm EoE
  - In vitro–specific IgE testing: serum testing for food-specific IgE antibodies; no studies of predictive value, limited or no role
  - Skin prick testing (SPT): assesses for IgE-mediated reactions; good specificity (>82%) for identifying EoE triggers, but poor sensitivity
  - Atopy patch testing (APT): assesses for non–IgE-mediated reactions; application of fresh or rehydrated food in occlusive chambers for 48 hours on back; similar specificity as SPT but better sensitivity
  - Combination of SPT and APT identified causative food antigens in 70% of patients at one center. More studies, especially prospective randomized controlled studies, are needed.
- Aeroallergen testing
  - SPT may identify aeroallergen triggers of EoE and inform timing of follow-up endoscopies relative to pollen seasons.

Imaging

- Upper GI series fluoroscopy
  - Provides complementary information to an upper endoscopy
  - Evaluates esophageal anatomy for strictures, hiatal hernia, Schatzki ring (lower esophageal ring), and achalasia
  - Is not sufficient to make a diagnosis of EoE
- Use upper GI series to evaluate worsening dysphagia for development of stricture that may require dilation.

Diagnostic Procedures/Other

- Esophagogastroduodenoscopy (EGD)
  - Required for diagnosis of EoE
  - Used to evaluate appearance of esophagus and obtain biopsies for pathology
  - As some forms of EoE are responsive to high doses of PPI, the diagnostic endoscopy is usually performed after an 8-week trial of a twice daily PPI.
  - 4–6 esophageal biopsies are obtained by cold forceps. The distal and proximal esophagus should be sampled separately. A pathologist experienced with the diagnosis of EoE should examine the biopsies for the presence of ≥15 eosinophils/HPF. Corroborating features include surface layering of eosinophils, eosinophilic microabscesses, extracellular eosinophilic granules, basal zone hyperplasia, dilated intercellular spaces, and lamina propria fibrosis.
  - Gastric and duodenal biopsies should also be obtained to rule out other causes of esophageal eosinophilia. In EoE, there is no associated gastric or duodenal eosinophilic infiltrate.
- pH/impedance probe
  - Use in diagnosis and management of EoE is unclear.
  - Some patients clearly suffer from both pathologic reflux and EoE. pH/impedance monitoring may clarify who should be treated with PPI.
- Endoscopic ultrasound
  - Findings include thickened mucosal and muscular layer.

DIFFERENTIAL DIAGNOSIS

- GERD
- Crohn disease
- Eosinophilic gastroenteritis
- Parasitic infection
- Connective tissue disease
- Drug allergy
- Hypereosinophilic syndrome
- Autoimmune enteropathy
- *Candida* esophagitis
- Viral esophagitis (HSV, CMV)
- Achalasia
- Peptic stricture

TREATMENT

MEDICATION

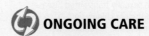

- Proton pump inhibitors (PPIs)
  - Part of the diagnostic criteria for EoE is that the esophageal eosinophilia persists after treatment with high-dose PPI (e.g., omeprazole, pantoprazole, esomeprazole, lansoprazole, dexlansoprazole, or rabeprazole). If the eosinophilia persists after an 8-week course of PPI, then the diagnosis of EoE is applied.
  - Useful as adjunctive therapy to treat associated reflux symptoms
  - Insufficient to treat EoE
- Non-systematic corticosteroids
  - Description
    - Swallowed topical steroids (fluticasone propionate and budesonide) are an alternative to dietary therapy.
    - Discontinuation is associated with recurrence of disease. They are safe for short-term administration.
    - Local fungal infections are known complications.
    - Data on long-term safety are lacking.
  - Fluticasone propionate
    - Use metered-dose inhaler.
    - Dose is sprayed into mouth and swallowed.
    - Initial doses:
      - Adults: 440–880 mcg twice daily
      - Children: 88–440 mcg 2–4 times daily
    - Avoid eating or drinking for 30 minutes after each dose.
  - Budesonide (viscous suspension)
    - Liquid budesonide inhaled solution ampules are mixed with sucralose/maltodextrin (e.g., Splenda, 5 packets per ampule) or other sweetener to form thick slurry that coats the esophagus when ingested (see Liacouras CA, Furuta GT, Hirano I, et al, 2011 in "Additional Reading").
    - Initial doses:
      - Adults: 2 mg daily
      - Children (<10 years): 1 mg daily
    - Avoid eating or drinking for a minimum of 30 minutes after dose.
    - Bedtime dosing is optimal.
- Systemic corticosteroids
  - Are effective but should only be used in cases of severe dysphagia and weight loss affecting growth
  - Long-term use should be avoided.
  - Prednisone or methylprednisolone:1–2 mg/kg/24 h (max 60 mg daily)

Dietary Therapy

- Elemental diet
  - Use amino acid–based formula for 100% of caloric requirements.
  - Highest efficacy for clearing eosinophilic inflammation
  - Reintroduction of foods into diet should be stepwise and guided by allergist.
- Six food elimination diet (SFED)
  - Avoid most common food allergens: (1) milk, (2) soy, (3) wheat, (4) egg, (5) peanuts and tree nuts, (6) fish and shellfish.
  - Efficacy not as high as with elemental diet but comparable to topical swallowed steroids
- Targeted elimination diet
  - Use results from multimodal allergy testing to guide food eliminations from diet.
  - Efficacy comparable to SFED

When reintroducing foods into the diet following one of the above dietary therapies, caution should be taken to do so stepwise with reevaluation of esophageal biopsies after each food reintroduction to determine the actual dietary trigger that should continue to be avoided.

ONGOING CARE

COMPLICATIONS

- Failure to thrive
- Esophageal strictures
- Small-caliber esophagus
- Esophageal perforation
- Esophageal fungal or viral superinfection

ENDOSCOPIC THERAPY

- Dilation of esophageal strictures
  - Useful in alleviating dysphagia
  - Does not address underlying problem
  - A trial of medical or dietary therapy is advisable prior to dilation unless a high-grade stricture is present.
  - Complications include chest pain (5%) and esophageal rupture (<1–5%).
- Removal of esophageal food impaction
  - Should be performed within 24 hours of food impaction to decrease risk of esophageal rupture

ADDITIONAL READING

- Greenhawt M, Aceves SS, Spergel JM, et al. The management of eosinophilic esophagitis. *J Allergy Clin Immunol Pract*. 2013;1(4):332–340.
- Kagalwalla AF, Shah A, Li BU, et al. Identification of specific foods responsible for inflammation in children with eosinophilic esophagitis successfully treated with empiric elimination diet. *J Pediatr Gastroenterol Nutr*. 2011;53(2):145–149.
- Liacouras CA, Furuta GT, Hirano I, et al. Eosinophilic esophagitis: updated consensus recommendations for children and adults. *J Allergy Clin Immunol*. 2011;128(1):3–20.
- Soon IS, Butzner JD, Kaplan GG, et al. Incidence and prevalence of eosinophilic esophagitis in children. *J Pediatr Gastroenterol Nutr*. 2013;57(1):72–80.
- Spergel JM, Brown-Whitehorn TF, Beausoleil JL, et al. 14 years of eosinophilic esophagitis: clinical features and prognosis. *J Pediatr Gastroenterol Nutr*. 2009;48(1):30–36.

CODES

ICD10

K20.0 Eosinophilic esophagitis

FAQ

- Q: What are the goals of EoE treatment?
- A: There is no agreed upon definition of EoE remission. Treatment goals include symptom reduction, decrease in esophageal eosinophilia to <15 eosinophils/HPF, and improvement in histologic and visual endoscopic changes. However, several studies show discordance between symptoms and histologic findings.
- Q: Do patients who have symptom response but persistent esophageal eosinophilia require further treatment?
- A: There is insufficient natural history data to answer this question. The concern is that untreated esophageal eosinophilia may progress to dysphagia, strictures, and esophageal fibrosis, but predictors of this progression are not well-defined.
- Q: Why might the SFED and targeted elimination diet have similar efficacy?
- A: The targeted elimination diet is guided by allergy testing (SPT and APT) results, but data on their diagnostic use are poorly reproducible. For certain foods (milk, wheat), they have poor reliability. Also, the APT process is not standardized and interpretation may be subjective and variable. More prospective controlled trials are needed to evaluate the diagnostic use of these tests.
- Q: What is the best 1st-line therapy for EoE?
- A: The approach to each patient is individualized, as there is no agreement on the single best 1st-line therapy for EoE. Younger children may be more amenable to dietary restrictions. Children with failure to thrive benefit from elemental formula either as monotherapy, or as a nutritional supplement in conjunction with either an elimination diet or topical corticosteroids. Dietary compliance in teenagers makes topical corticosteroids a popular option.

EPIDIDYMITIS

Melissa T. Sanford • Hillary L. Copp

BASICS

DESCRIPTION

Epididymitis is an acute inflammation of the epididymis that can cause severe scrotal pain. It is important to differentiate epididymitis from testicular torsion or testicular appendage torsion.

EPIDEMIOLOGY

- Epididymitis is the most common cause of acute scrotum, approximately 37–65% of cases. The incidence ranges between 0.8 and 1.2 cases/1,000 persons per year.
- There is a bimodal distribution with a peak in incidence in infants younger than 1 year of age and peripubertal boys.

RISK FACTORS

Urologic manipulation (cystoscopy, intermittent self-catheterization, surgery of the urethra)

PATHOPHYSIOLOGY

- The majority of epididymitis is idiopathic (73%).
- Viral epididymitis: 2nd most common cause
  - Urinalysis and culture are negative.
  - Often elevated titers of enterovirus, *Mycoplasma pneumoniae*, and adenoviruses
  - New research shows that some epididymitis might be due to postinfectious inflammation, as 50% of patients had respiratory symptoms within 1 month of presentation and presentations appear to peak in concert with rotavirus and enterovirus.
- Bacterial epididymitis: 2–6% of cases and is related to age
  - Due to ascending infection from the urethra or bladder, reflux of infected urine into the vas deferens, or hematogenous dissemination
  - Infants <1 year of age
    - Typically due to genitourinary anomalies (73% vs. 21% in children >1 year of age)
    - Abnormalities include meatal stenosis, neurogenic voiding dysfunction, urethral stenosis, posterior urethral valves, ectopic ureter.
    - Typical bacteria include *Escherichia coli*, *Klebsiella*, and *Enterococcus*.
    - Postpubertal sexually active boys may have infection with sexually transmitted diseases such as gonorrhea or chlamydia.
- Chemical epididymitis: due to reflux of sterile urine into the vas deferens or drugs (amiodarone)
- Posttraumatic

COMMONLY ASSOCIATED CONDITIONS

- Systemic serositis (familial Mediterranean fever, sarcoidosis, Kawasaki disease)
- Systemic vasculitis (Henoch-Schönlein purpura, polyarteritis nodosa)

DIAGNOSIS

HISTORY

- It is not always possible to distinguish between testicular torsion, testicular appendage torsion, and epididymitis based on history and physical exam.
- Duration of symptoms is longer than in testicular torsion, typically >12 hours.
- The majority of patients complain of scrotal pain (91–98%), scrotal swelling (83%), and scrotal erythema (74%).
- Patients who have bacterial epididymitis are more likely to have prior urologic history than patients without bacterial epididymitis (73% vs. 0%).
- 16–33% of patients have a fever, almost always in bacterial epididymitis

PHYSICAL EXAM

Inflamed, swollen scrotum with localized epididymal pain early in the course that can spread to generalized testicular inflammation late in the course.

DIAGNOSTIC TESTS & INTERPRETATION

Lab

- Urinalysis and urine culture are only positive in a minority of presentations (7% and 1–6% respectively), but they should be sent for all patients to help guide therapy if they are positive for bacterial epididymitis.
- WBC, CRP, and ESR are most elevated in systemic serositis or vasculitis.
- Any sexually active boy or boy with an unclear sexual history should have gonorrhea and chlamydial testing performed.

Imaging

ALERT
For acute scrotum, perform scrotal ultrasound with Doppler to differentiate between testicular torsion, testicular appendicular torsion, or epididymitis.

- Epididymitis typically appears as an enlarged epididymis with hypervascular flow and mixed echogenicity with reactive fluid.

DIFFERENTIAL DIAGNOSIS

- Testicular torsion
- Testicular appendage torsion
- Incarcerated inguinal hernia
- Hydrocele
- Systemic vasculitis
- Recent urologic surgery
- Idiopathic scrotal edema
- Testicular tumor
- Appendicitis
- Mumps orchitis

TREATMENT

GENERAL MEASURES

Given that the majority of acute epididymitis is nonbacterial, initial treatment should be supportive with analgesics, nonsteroidal anti-inflammatory drugs, bed rest, scrotal ice packs, and scrotal elevation.

MEDICATION

- Any children younger than 1 year of age or with pyuria should be empirically begun on antibiotics based on a local antibiogram.
- If a child has culture-proven bacterial epididymitis, they should be started on culture-sensitive antibiotics for a 2-week course.

ONGOING CARE

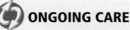

FOLLOW-UP RECOMMENDATIONS

- Schedule for follow-up appointment in 2–4 weeks to ensure resolution of epididymitis.
- Recommend referral to pediatric urology.
- Children <1 year of age and any child with a positive urine culture should be evaluated with a renal bladder ultrasound to rule out genitourinary anomalies.

ADDITIONAL READING

- Cappele O, Liard A, Barret E, et al. Epididymitis in children: is further investigation necessary after the first episode? *Eur Urol*. 2000;38(5):627–630.
- Halachmi S. Inflammation of the gonad in prepubertal healthy children. Epidemiology, etiology, and management. *ScientificWorldJournal*. 2006;6: 1081–1085.
- Makela E, Lahdes-Vasama T, Rajakorpi H, et al. A 19-year review of paediatric patients with acute scrotum. *Scand J Surg*. 2007;96(1):62–66.
- Somekh E, Gorenstein A, Serour F. Acute epididymitis in boys: evidence of post-infectious etiology. *J Urol*. 2004;171(1):391–394; discussion 394.
- Tekgul S, Riedmiller E, Gerharz P. Guidelines on Paediatric Urology. European Society for Paediatric Urology. 2008. http://www.uroweb.org/fileadmin/user_upload/Guidelines/19%20Paediatric%20Urology.pdf. Accessed June 23, 2014.

CODES

ICD10

- N45.1 Epididymitis
- N45.3 Epididymo-orchitis
- N45.4 Abscess of epididymis or testis

FAQ

- Q: What is the best empiric antibiotic?
- A: Empiric antibiotic choice should be based on local antibiogram. Typically reasonable choices include cephalexin, sulfamethoxazole and trimethoprim (Bactrim, Septra), or fluoroquinolone.
- Q: What should be done if the epididymitis has not resolved after 2 weeks?
- A: The child should have repeat urinalysis and urine culture to ensure he or she has not developed a resistant bacterial infection and repeat scrotal ultrasound to ensure he or she has not developed an abscess.
- Q: What is a Prehn sign?
- A: A Prehn sign (named after Douglas T. Prehn, MD) is a historical diagnostic maneuver that was previously used to help diagnose epididymitis. This maneuver is inferior to Doppler ultrasound. To conduct the Phren maneuver, elevate the testicles from below. The elevation of the testes should decrease pain if it is due to epididymitis; however, it does not theoretically relieve pain due to testicular torsion.

E

EPIGLOTTITIS

Laura H. Brower • Erin E. Shaughnessy

BASICS

DESCRIPTION

Acute life-threatening bacterial infection consisting of cellulitis and edema of the epiglottis, aryepiglottic folds, arytenoids, and hypopharynx, resulting in narrowing of the glottic opening and airway obstruction; also known as supraglottitis

EPIDEMIOLOGY

- Disease due to *Haemophilus influenzae* type B occurs most often between the ages of 1 and 7 years (overall range: infancy to adulthood).
- Epiglottitis and other invasive disease secondary to *H. influenzae* have been reduced by 99% since the introduction of the conjugate vaccines in 1987 (approved for use at 15 months) and 1990 (approved for use at 2, 4, and 6 months).
- Nontypeable *H. influenzae* now appears to be a more common cause of invasive disease than type B.
- Year-round occurrence
- All geographic areas
- Can have secondary cases in households or child care centers
- May be more frequent in children with sickle cell anemia, asplenia, immunoglobulin defects, or hematologic malignancies (e.g., leukemia)
- Increasing ratio of adult to pediatric cases

Incidence

- Incidence of pediatric epiglottitis due to any organism has declined in the postvaccine era (0.3–0.7/100,000 per year from 3.47 to 6.0/100,000 per year).
- Incidence in adults has remained steady (1–4/100,000 per year).

GENERAL PREVENTION

- Universal immunization with *H. influenzae* type B capsular polysaccharide conjugate vaccines at 2 and 4 months (potential dose at 6 months, depending on the vaccine), with booster at 12–15 months.
- Isolation of hospitalized patient: Droplet precautions should be continued for at least 24 hours from the initiation of effective antimicrobial therapy.
- Control measures: prophylaxis for *H. influenzae* type B index case and susceptible children in household and child care setting and intimate contacts with the assistance of infection control
  - Rifampin: 20 mg/kg/day in single dose for 4 days

PATHOPHYSIOLOGY

Edema of the supraglottic structures (uvula, aryepiglottic folds, arytenoids, epiglottis, and vocal cords) that reduces the airway aperture. Respiratory arrest can be caused by airway obstruction, aspiration of oropharyngeal secretions, or mucous plugging.

ETIOLOGY

- *H. influenzae*, nontypeable and type B (type B accounted for up to 90% of cases prior to the introduction of Hib vaccine)
- *Streptococcus pneumoniae*
- *Streptococcus pyogenes* (group A β-hemolytic *Streptococcus*)
- *Staphylococcus aureus*
- Groups C and G β-hemolytic *Streptococcus*
- *Candida albicans* may be an etiologic agent in immunocompromised patients and those receiving prolonged corticosteroid treatment.
- *Pasteurella multocida* has been implicated in a few cases after exposure to nasopharyngeal secretions from a cat.
- Other rare isolates: *Moraxella catarrhalis*, *Klebsiella pneumoniae*, *Neisseria meningitidis*, *Pseudomonas* species
- Bacterial superinfection of viral infections including herpes simplex, parainfluenza, varicella, Epstein-Barr
- Varicella can cause primary infection or lead to a secondary infection, often with *S. pyogenes*.
- Noninfectious etiologies include thermal injuries, trauma, and caustic ingestions.

DIAGNOSIS

HISTORY

- Abrupt onset of high fever (39–40°C), sore throat, and dysphagia
- Drooling or difficulty handling secretions
- Very limited or no prodrome of mild upper respiratory tract infection (URI)
- "Hot potato" voice (muffled)
- Rapid onset of toxicity and respiratory distress
- Cough and hoarseness are late symptoms, if they occur at all.
- Time from onset of symptoms to presentation with progressive respiratory distress is generally <12 hours.
- Immunization against *H. influenzae* type B
- Child's preferred position or way of sitting (i.e., sitting upright, leaning forward with chin hyperextended)

PHYSICAL EXAM

- Extremely anxious appearance
- Child prefers to remain sitting up.
- Child often leaning forward with chin hyperextended to maintain airway in a "tripod" position
- Slow and labored respiratory effort
- Drooling is seen as a manifestation of dysphagia.
- Inspiratory stridor, retractions, and late cyanosis
- Diagnosis can be suspected on history and observation of child's appearance alone.
- Do *not* attempt to examine the throat if epiglottitis is a serious consideration.

DIAGNOSTIC TESTS & INTERPRETATION

Lab

- Complete blood count: increased white blood cell count with left shift
- Cultures of blood and epiglottis (performed only in the operating room)

Imaging

Lateral neck radiography (should not be performed until airway team is in place): characteristic "thumb sign" of edematous epiglottis, with narrowing of the posterior airway and ballooning of the hypopharynx

Diagnostic Procedures/Other

Definitive diagnosis requires direct visualization of erythematous and edematous epiglottis.

ALERT

- Ensure appropriate airway management prior to any other interventions, including intrusive examination components, radiographs, and blood collection.
- A radiograph is indicated only when the diagnosis is in doubt and should not delay airway management.

DIFFERENTIAL DIAGNOSIS

- Viral laryngotracheobronchitis (croup) with or without secondary bacterial tracheitis
- Severe parainfluenza or influenza infection
- Uvulitis
- Peritonsillar, retropharyngeal, or lingual abscess
- Foreign body aspiration in a child with URI
- URI, including croup, in a child with a congenital or acquired airway problem (e.g., premature infant with subglottic stenosis, laryngeal web, vascular ring, tracheal stenosis)
- Hereditary angioedema (deficiency of complement C1 esterase inhibitor) can present with edema of the airway including the epiglottis.
- Diphtheria: rare in the United States
- Laryngeal infections

TREATMENT

MEDICATION

First Line

- Empiric parenteral antibiotic coverage to include gram-positive cocci and *H. influenzae* (type B and nontypeable)
  - Cephalosporins
    - Cefotaxime: 200–225 mg/kg/24 h (max 12 g/24 h) divided q4–6h
    - Ceftriaxone: 100 mg/kg/24 h (max 2 g/24 h) divided q12–24h
    - Cefuroxime: 100–200 mg/kg/24 h (max 9 g/24 h) divided q6–8h
  - Ampicillin/sulbactam: ampicillin 200 mg/kg/24 h (max 8 g/24 h) IV divided q6h
  - Serious penicillin/cephalosporin allergies
    - Levofloxacin (IV or PO): <5 years: 10 mg/kg/dose twice daily; >5 years: 10 mg/kg/dose once daily; max dose: 750 mg/24 h
- Duration of therapy: 7–10 days for all but staphylococcal disease (14–21 days).
- Switch may be made to oral medication after extubation and resumption of oral intake.
- Steroids are used commonly but without convincing evidence for their efficacy.

Second Line
- Discuss with infectious disease consultant.
- Chloramphenicol: 50–75 mg/kg/24 h (max 4 g/24 h) IV divided q6h; monitor levels
- Ampicillin: 200–400 mg/kg/24 h (max 12 g/24 h) IV divided q6h
- Penicillin: 200,000–300,000 U/kg/24 h (max 24 million U/24 h) IV divided q6h for streptococcal disease
- Oxacillin: 150–200 mg/kg/24 h (max 4 g/24 h) IV divided q4–6h for susceptible staphylococcal disease

ISSUES FOR REFERRAL
Airway should be secured by clinician skilled in airway management (e.g., otolaryngologist, anesthesiologist) prior to any attempt to transport a child with suspected epiglottitis.

INPATIENT CONSIDERATIONS
Initial Stabilization
- Airway management: Maintain child upright, never supine. Personnel experienced in airway management should accompany the child at all times, including during transport and in radiology.
- Rapid assembly of a team, which should include an anesthesiologist, an otolaryngologist, and a pediatrician, if possible
- Allow the child to assume his or her most comfortable position (usually in the parent's arms/lap).
- Oxygen by mask or blown by face
- Transport to operating room as soon as possible for anesthesia.
- Secure airway via direct laryngoscopy and bronchoscopy with intubation.
- Institute intravenous catheterization and blood collection and culturing of epiglottis only after the airway is secured.
- Perform emergent cricothyrotomy if obstruction occurs prior to controlled airway management.
- Use fluid resuscitation in cases of septic shock.

Admission Criteria
Admit all children with suspicion of epiglottitis for airway management.

ONGOING CARE

FOLLOW-UP RECOMMENDATIONS
Patient Monitoring
- Extubation is usually possible within 24–48 hours. Criteria include decreased erythema and edema of the epiglottis on direct inspection and development of an air leak around the endotracheal tube.
- Defervescence is usually prompt after initiation of appropriate antimicrobial therapy.

PROGNOSIS
Mortality is estimated to be 5–10%.

COMPLICATIONS
- Without prompt medical intervention: complete airway obstruction leading to respiratory arrest, hypoxia, and death
- Necrotizing cervical fasciitis (rarely)
- Therapeutic complications
  - Aspiration
  - Endotracheal tube dislodgment and extubation
  - Tracheal erosion or irritation
  - Pneumomediastinum
  - Pneumothorax
  - Pulmonary edema
- Complications of *H. influenzae* type B bacteremia:
  - Septic shock
  - Pneumonia
  - Cervical lymphadenopathy
  - Rarely, arthritis, meningitis, and pericarditis

ADDITIONAL READING

- Guardiani E, Bliss M, Harley E. Supraglottitis in the era following widespread immunization against *Haemophilus influenzae* type B: evolving principles in diagnosis and management. *Laryngoscope*. 2010;120(11):2183–2188.
- Rafei K, Lichenstein R. Airway infectious disease emergencies. *Pediatr Clin North Am*. 2006;53(2): 215–242.
- Shah RK, Roberson DW, Jones DT. Epiglottitis in the *Hemophilus influenzae* type B vaccine era: changing trends. *Laryngoscope*. 2004;114(3):557–560.
- Shah RK, Stocks C. Epiglottitis in the United States: national trends, variances, prognosis, and management. *Laryngoscope*. 2010;120(6):1256–1262.
- Stroud RH, Friedman NR. An update on inflammatory disorders of the pediatric airway: epiglottitis, croup, and tracheitis. *Am J Otolaryngol*. 2001;22(4): 268–275.

CODES

ICD10
- J05.10 Acute epiglottitis without obstruction
- J05.11 Acute epiglottitis with obstruction

FAQ
- Q: What is the incidence of epiglottitis since the introduction of conjugate vaccines against *H. influenzae* type B?
- A: Because *H. influenzae* type B caused 90% of epiglottitis and the incidence of all invasive disease due to *H. influenzae* type B has decreased by 99% in children <5 years of age, it is estimated that the incidence of epiglottitis has been reduced by more than 90%.
- Q: Have there been reports of epiglottitis caused by *H. influenzae* type B after complete vaccination?
- A: Yes. Several cases due to *H. influenzae* type B have been reported in the United States and abroad after partial and complete vaccination. Therefore, even a history of having received a full vaccination series does not eliminate the possibility of Hib-associated epiglottitis. In one case series from 2004, 5/6 patients with Hib epiglottitis had completed the Hib vaccination series.
- Q: Should a fully vaccinated child who develops invasive disease due to *H. influenzae* type B be tested for an underlying immunodeficiency?
- A: Probably. In one study, about 1/3 of children diagnosed with invasive disease due to *H. influenzae* type B were found to have a previously undiagnosed immunoglobulin deficiency.
- Q: Can epiglottitis recur?
- A: Yes, but rarely.
- Q: Are corticosteroids of any value in the management of epiglottitis?
- A: They are used commonly, but there is no evidence to support their benefit.

E

EPSTEIN-BARR VIRUS (INFECTIOUS MONONUCLEOSIS)

Jessica Newman • Jason Newland

BASICS

DESCRIPTION
A double-stranded DNA virus implicated as a causative agent for infectious mononucleosis by an infected laboratory worker in 1968

GENERAL PREVENTION
- No vaccine is clinically available.
- Standard precautions should be used in the hospitalized patient.
- Restriction of intimate contact with immunosuppressed individuals may be advisable.
- Patients with recent Epstein-Barr virus (EBV) infection, either proven or suspected, should not donate blood or solid organs.

EPIDEMIOLOGY
- Worldwide distribution
- Humans are the only known reservoir.
- Transmission occurs through saliva and, occasionally, via blood transfusions and solid organ transplant (SOT).
- Incubation period is 4–7 weeks.
- Antibodies to EBV are almost universally present in adult populations.
- Areas with a high population density or low socioeconomic status usually become primarily infected within the first 3 years of life.

Incidence
In developed countries, acquisition of EBV is biphasic.
- Initial peak in incidence occurs before the age of 5 years.
- Second peak occurs during adolescence, coinciding with an increased frequency of intimate oral contacts.

Prevalence
90–95% of adults have demonstrable EBV titers.

PATHOPHYSIOLOGY
- Replicates initially in the oropharyngeal epithelium
- Selective infection of B lymphocytes occurs.
- The clinical syndrome of infectious mononucleosis results from proliferation of cells in the tonsils, lymph nodes, and spleen.
- Nonspecific humoral immune responses include the formation of heterophile antibodies and autoantibodies.
- Specific antibodies to EBV antigens are produced.
- Despite humoral responses, cellular immunity is responsible for controlling EBV infection.
- Latent, lifelong infection of B lymphocytes occurs.
- Latent virus may be reactivated during periods of immunosuppression.

COMMONLY ASSOCIATED CONDITIONS
- Subclinical infection
  - Most EBV infections in children, and even in adolescents, are clinically inapparent.
  - Mild, nonspecific symptoms may include coryza, diarrhea, and/or fever.
  - Immunologic seroconversion does occur.
- Infectious mononucleosis ("glandular fever"): most commonly observed with late primary acquisition of EBV. The classically defined illness is characterized by the following:
  - Fatigue
  - Malaise
  - Fever
  - Tonsillopharyngitis (often exudative)
  - Lymphadenopathy
  - Splenomegaly
  - Usually associated with increased atypical lymphocytes in the peripheral blood
- Rare illnesses of the nervous system have been reported, including the following:
  - Guillain-Barré syndrome
  - Bell palsy
  - Aseptic meningitis
  - Meningoencephalitis
  - Peripheral and/or optic neuritis
- Hematologic complications have been reported in association with EBV.
  - Aplastic anemia
  - Hemolytic anemia
  - Agranulocytosis
  - Hemophagocytic syndrome
- Other illnesses associated with EBV in case reports include the following:
  - Hemolytic uremic syndrome
  - Hepatitis
  - Pancreatitis
  - Myocarditis
  - Mesenteric adenitis
  - Orchitis
  - Genital ulcerative disease
- Lymphoproliferative disorders
  - Burkitt lymphoma
  - Nasopharyngeal carcinoma
  - Lymphoma and non-Hodgkin lymphoma (in immunocompromised children)
  - Lymphomatoid granulomatosis
  - Posttransplant lymphoproliferative disorders (PTLD)
  - X-linked lymphoproliferative disease (Duncan disease)

DIAGNOSIS

HISTORY
- A prodrome may occur.
  - Most often, lasts 3–5 days
  - Malaise, fatigue, with or without fever
- In the acute phase, the following features are common:
  - Fever: begins abruptly, lasts 1–2 weeks
  - Fatigue
  - Malaise
  - Anorexia
  - Sore throat
  - "Swollen glands"
  - Rash; more common with ampicillin administration
- Young children are more likely to have rash or abdominal pain.

PHYSICAL EXAM
- Tonsillopharyngitis
  - May be exudative and mimic streptococcal pharyngitis
  - Often accompanied by palatal petechiae
- Lymphadenopathy
  - Occurs in 90%
  - Most prominent in cervical chains
  - May be diffuse
  - Usually nontender, nonerythematous, and discrete
- Hepatosplenomegaly
  - Splenomegaly occurs in more than half the cases.
  - Even if not palpable, splenomegaly may be demonstrated on ultrasound.
  - Most prominent in 2nd–4th week of illness
  - Hepatomegaly is less common.

DIAGNOSTIC TESTS & INTERPRETATION

Lab
- Complete blood count with differential
  - Leukocyte count up to 20,000/mm^3
  - Lymphocytosis
  - Atypical lymphocytes often constitute >10% of total leukocyte count.
  - Thrombocytopenia may occur.
  - False positives: Atypical lymphocyte counts >10% of the total leukocyte count also occur with cytomegalovirus and toxoplasmosis infections.
- Liver enzymes
  - Mild hepatitis is often found.
  - Jaundice is rare.
- "Monospot" (mononucleosis rapid slide agglutination test for heterophile antibodies)
  - Detects heterophile antibodies (nonspecific IgM antibodies to unrelated antigens)
  - Appears in first 2 weeks of illness, usually slow decline over 6 months
  - Detects 85% of cases in adolescents/adults
  - False positives: infrequent; heterophile antibodies are also produced in serum sickness and neoplastic processes; heterophile antibodies may persist for months after acute infection and be indicative of past illness.
- EBV serology
  - Usually reserved for heterophile-negative patients or children <4 years of age when strong clinical suspicion persists
  - Antibodies are detected by indirect immunofluorescence or enzyme-linked immunosorbent assay techniques.
  - Acute or past infection can usually be detected and differentiated.
  - EBV IgM is consistent with acute infection, whereas EBV nuclear antibody (EBNA) is indicative of past infection.
- Other technology
  - Tissue culture of EBV is difficult and, therefore, not clinically useful.
  - Polymerase chain reaction (PCR) may detect EBV genetic material.
  - Real-time PCR may quantify the amount of EBV genome present, which is useful in patients with PTLD.

ALERT
- Heterophile antibodies may not appear early in the illness.
- Up to 10% of patients with acute EBV infection may have no heterophile response 3 weeks into the illness.
- The heterophile response is less common in infants and children and should not be used in children <4 years of age.

DIFFERENTIAL DIAGNOSIS
- Infectious
  - Group A *Streptococcus*
  - Adenovirus
  - Cytomegalovirus
  - *Toxoplasma gondii*
  - Human herpesvirus-6
  - *Mycoplasma pneumoniae*
  - Human immunodeficiency virus
  - Rubella
  - Diphtheria
  - Viral hepatitis (A, B, C)
- Noninfectious
  - Leukemia/lymphoma

TREATMENT

MEDICATION
- Acetaminophen or ibuprofen reduces fever and provides analgesia.
- Corticosteroids (prednisone 1 mg/kg/24 h PO, maximum of 20 mg/24 h) may reduce swelling of lymphoid tissues (see "FAQ")
  - Indicated for patients with impending airway obstruction
  - May be considered for patients with severe tonsillopharyngitis requiring IV hydration
  - May be considered for patients with rare, life-threatening manifestations of EBV infection, such as hepatitis, aplastic anemia, and central nervous system dysfunction
  - 7-day treatment followed by tapering
- Acyclovir has not been shown to provide clinical benefit; sometimes, used in cases of active replicating EBV in posttransplant situations
- Patients with PTLD should have immunosuppression reduced.
- Advise avoidance of contact sports until resolution of symptoms and no further splenomegaly.

INPATIENT CONSIDERATIONS
Admission Criteria
- Respiratory distress secondary to airway obstruction
- Dehydration secondary to severe pharyngitis and poor oral intake

Discharge Criteria
- Resolved airway obstruction
- Good oral intake

ISSUES FOR REFERRAL
- PTLD
- EBV in immunocompromised host
- EBV-associated lymphoproliferative disorders
- Considering steroid use as treatment

ONGOING CARE

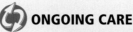

FOLLOW-UP RECOMMENDATIONS
Patient Monitoring
- Immunocompetent individuals usually recover uneventfully in 1–4 weeks.
- Recovery is often biphasic, with a worsening of symptoms after a period of improvement.
- Splenomegaly may persist for weeks after primary infection (see "FAQ").
- Fatigue may persist months after recovery.

PROGNOSIS
- Most patients with primary EBV infection will recover uneventfully in 1–4 weeks.
- Long-lasting immunity generally ensues.
- Prognosis of patients with unusual manifestations of EBV infection depends on the severity of the illness and the organ system involved.
- Patients with inherited or acquired immunodeficiency are at higher risk of complications and neoplasms.

COMPLICATIONS
- Dehydration
  - Severe pharyngitis often limits fluid intake.
  - Most common problem requiring hospitalization
- Antibiotic-induced rash
  - Morbilliform in appearance
  - Most common after administration of ampicillin or amoxicillin
  - Rare association with penicillin
  - Usually benign; resolves with discontinuation of the aminopenicillin
- Splenic rupture
  - Incidence of ~1 in 1,000 patients
  - More common in males
  - 50% of the cases of splenic rupture are spontaneous; 50% follow blunt trauma.
- Airway obstruction: may result from massive lymphoid hyperplasia and mucosal edema

ADDITIONAL READING

- Bravender T. Epstein-Barr virus, cytomegalovirus, and infectious mononucleosis. *Adolesc Med State Art Rev*. 2010;21(2):251–264.
- Hurt C, Tammaro D. Diagnostic evaluation of mononucleosis-like illness. *Am J Med*. 2007;20(10): 911.e1–911.e8.
- Macsween KF, Crawford DH. Epstein-Barr virus—recent advances. *Lancet Infect Dis*. 2003;3(3):131–140.
- Okano M. Overview and problematic standpoints of severe chronic active Epstein-Barr virus infection syndrome. *Crit Rev Oncol Hematol*. 2002;44(3): 273–282.
- Putukian M, O'Connor FG, Stricker P, et al. Mononucleosis and athletic participation: an evidence-based subject review. *Clin J Sport Med*. 2008;18(4):309–315.

CODES

ICD10
- B27.90 Infectious mononucleosis, unspecified without complication
- B27.99 Infectious mononucleosis, unsp with other complication
- B27.91 Infectious mononucleosis, unspecified with polyneuropathy

FAQ
- Q: Should all patients with infectious mononucleosis be given corticosteroids?
- A: No. Symptomatic EBV infection is most often self-limited. EBV has been linked to certain lymphoproliferative disorders, and theoretic risks to modulating the host immune response with corticosteroids have been proposed.
- Q: How long after infectious mononucleosis may a patient return to athletic activity?
- A: More than half of patients with "mono" will have a boggy, enlarged spleen, which is prone to rupture even if it is not palpable. Athletic activity should be restricted until no evidence exists for a clinically enlarged spleen. Return to contact sports is not advised until 4–6 weeks after resolution of illness. Some experts recommend ultrasound of the spleen before a return to heavy contact sports such as rugby, football, lacrosse, and hockey.

ERYTHEMA MULTIFORME

Minnelly Luu • Kelly M. Cordoro

BASICS

DESCRIPTION

- Erythema multiforme (EM) is an acute, self-limited mucocutaneous eruption characterized by distinct targetoid lesions on the skin.
- Although classically defined by the presence of target lesions, at various stages of evolution, EM may appear as erythematous macules, papules, vesicles, or bullae.
- EM is considered an immune-mediated reaction, usually to infectious triggers; numerous additional triggers have been reported in the literature.
- Ranges from relatively mild cutaneous disease (EM minor) to severe forms with significant mucosal involvement (EM major)
- Historically viewed as a spectrum of diseases, most authors now regard EM to be a separate entity from Stevens-Johnson syndrome (SJS) and toxic epidermal necrolysis (TEN). SJS and TEN are distinguished from EM by differing patterns of cutaneous involvement, precipitating factors, and prognosis.

EPIDEMIOLOGY

- Predominantly affects healthy young adults but can also affect younger children
- Possible seasonal variation with increased frequency in spring and summer. The more severe form (EM major) has been reported to occur more frequently in winter.
- Recurrences are common.

ETIOLOGY

- ~90% of cases are caused by an infectious agent, most commonly herpes simplex virus (HSV) or *Mycoplasma pneumoniae*.
- <10% of cases are secondary to drug exposure. Common culprits include NSAIDs, sulfonamides, antiepileptics, and antibiotics.
- Reported causes are numerous. Rare precipitants include the following:
  - Chemical and physical exposures
  - Immunizations
  - Autoimmune disease
- Often, the causative factor is not identified.
- HSV is the major cause of recurrent EM.
- *M. pneumoniae* is associated with more severe bullous skin disease and significant mucosal involvement.

DIAGNOSIS

HISTORY

- Prodrome of fever and malaise may precede skin eruption. The prodrome is generally uncommon except in cases of EM major, where symptoms are usually indistinguishable from those of the underlying illness.
- Onset is abrupt with rapid evolution of lesions over the course of 3–5 days.
- Although usually appearing at the same time, mucosal lesions occasionally precede or follow cutaneous lesions by a few days.
- Lesions may be associated with pruritus or burning.
- Elicit careful drug (prescription and OTC) and exposure history, including personal and family history of herpetic lesions.
- Symptoms of HSV, mycoplasma, or other infections may be present.
- Assess for symptoms of mucosal involvement, including dysphagia, dysuria, and ocular symptoms.

PHYSICAL EXAM

- Early lesions are usually round, well-defined erythematous, edematous papules.
- Classically, some of these will evolve to the characteristic target lesion defined by three zones of concentric color change:
  - Dark, dusky center
  - Pale, edematous middle zone
  - Well-defined erythematous outer border
- The center of well-formed lesions will have signs of necrosis: duskiness, blistering, or erosion.
- Atypical target lesions may also be present, defined by only two zones of color change and/or a poorly defined border.
- Lesions may have multiple morphologies including macules, papules, and vesicles/bullae.
- Distribution is typically symmetric and favors acral sites.
- Oral mucosal involvement (labial and buccal mucosa, vermillion lip) is most common, although any mucosal site may be affected.
- Mucosal involvement usually starts with erythema and edema and progresses to painful erosions with crusting.

DIAGNOSTIC TESTS & INTERPRETATION

Lab

- Laboratory tests do not establish diagnosis, although they may provide supporting evidence and reveal the underlying cause.
- Eosinophilia may suggest drug as etiology.
- Any lesions suspicious for herpes should be evaluated with culture, direct fluorescent antibody testing (DFA), or polymerase chain reaction (PCR).
- Consider evaluation for *Mycoplasma* with chest radiograph and cold agglutinins, serology, or PCR.
- Erythrocyte sedimentation rate, white blood cell count, and liver function tests may be elevated in severe EM.

Diagnostic Procedures/Other

Diagnosis of EM can usually be made on clinical grounds. Biopsy is often not required, although it can help confirm diagnosis and exclude other possibilities. Of importance, pathology does not reliably distinguish EM from SJS/TEN and thus differentiation between these entities requires clinical correlation.

Pathologic Findings

- Necrotic keratinocytes
- Vacuolar basal layer degeneration (liquefactive or hydropic degeneration)
- Subepidermal blistering may be seen in cases of extensive basal layer degeneration.
- Perivascular inflammation in the upper and mid dermis composed mainly of mononuclear cells
- Spongiosis, papillary dermal edema, and exocytosis of lymphocytes may also be seen.

DIFFERENTIAL DIAGNOSIS

- SJS/TEN should be considered when a drug is suspected or morphology consists of predominantly macular atypical targets or dusky, ill-defined macules/patches with or without epidermal detachment.
- Urticaria
- Urticaria multiforme
- Vasculitis/urticarial vasculitis
- Fixed drug eruption
- Atypical hand foot and mouth disease
- Pemphigus vulgaris
- Paraneoplastic pemphigus
- Bullous pemphigoid
- Polymorphous light eruption
- Serum sickness reaction
- Systemic lupus erythematosus (Rowell syndrome)
- Sweet syndrome
- Kawasaki disease
- Varicella (chickenpox)

TREATMENT

GENERAL MEASURES

- Treat the underlying cause (e.g., acyclovir for HSV-related cases) or withdraw the offending agent.
- EM minor
  - Care is supportive and symptom-based.
  - White petrolatum +/− topical corticosteroids
  - Oral antihistamines for pruritus
- EM major
  - Skin-directed therapy as above
  - White petrolatum and nonstick dressings for bullous lesions
  - Pain control
  - "Swish and spit" oral preparations composed of diphenhydramine or viscous lidocaine for painful oral lesions.
  - Ophthalmology consultation; consider ENT and urology based on signs and symptoms.
  - Avoid aggressive debridement of crust, which can lead to further scarring.
  - Monitoring of fluid and electrolyte balance and observation for secondary infection
  - The role of systemic steroids is controversial and randomized controlled trials are lacking. Generally thought to be most beneficial when given early in the course of disease. The risks and benefits of corticosteroid therapy must be weighed carefully in the setting of potential infection.

INPATIENT CONSIDERATIONS

Admission Criteria

- Severe mucositis with inability to adequately hydrate
- Atypical progression with suspicion for SJS/TEN or other potentially life-threatening process

ONGOING CARE

PROGNOSIS

- The course of EM is self-limited. Lesions resolve in 2–4 weeks with postinflammatory pigment alteration. Severe cases of EM may take longer to heal.
- Recurrences may occur and are often associated with HSV. Prophylactic therapy with acyclovir may be considered with frequent episodes.

COMPLICATIONS

- Complications of the triggering/underlying infection may occur in individual cases.
- EM minor generally heals without significant sequelae.
- In EM major, mucosal involvement may lead to sequelae at individual sites: stricture formation of the oral cavity, trachea, esophagus, and urethra. Ophthalmologic consequences include conjunctivitis, corneal erosions, scarring, and rarely, blindness.
- Skin scarring in severe, ulcerated, or secondarily infected sites

ADDITIONAL READING

- Auquier-Dunant A, Mockenhaupt M, Naldi L, et al. Correlations between clinical patterns and causes of erythema multiforme major, Stevens-Johnson syndrome, and toxic epidermal necrolysis: results of an international prospective study. *Arch Dermatol*. 2002;138(8):1019–1024.
- Huff JC, Weston WL, Tonnessen MG. Erythema multiforme: a critical review of characteristics, diagnostic criteria, and causes. *J Am Acad Dermatol*. 1983;8(6):763–775.
- Riley M, Jenner R. Towards evidence based emergency medicine: best BETs from the Manchester Royal Infirmary. Bet 2. Steroids in children with erythema multiforme. *Emerg Med J*. 2008;25(9):594–595.
- Sokumbi O, Wetter DA. Clinical features, diagnosis, and treatment of erythema multiforme: a review for the practicing dermatologist. *Int J Dermatol*. 2012;51(8):889–902.

CODES

ICD10

- L51.9 Erythema multiforme, unspecified
- L51.8 Other erythema multiforme
- L51.0 Nonbullous erythema multiforme

ERYTHEMA NODOSUM

Vikash S. Oza • Erin Mathes

BASICS

DESCRIPTION
Delayed, cell-mediated hypersensitivity panniculitis characterized by red, tender, nodular lesions most often seen on the pretibial surface of the legs

EPIDEMIOLOGY
- Girls are affected more often than boys.
- Incidence peaks in adolescence and is rare under 2 years of age.

Incidence
Greatest seasonal incidence in spring and fall

PATHOPHYSIOLOGY
- Most likely a host hypersensitivity immune response to circulating immune complexes secondary to infectious and/or inflammatory stimuli
- The response results in chronic injury to the blood vessels of the reticular dermis and subcutaneous fat.

ETIOLOGY
- Most cases are idiopathic (~50% of cases).
- Infectious associations
  - Bacterial: β-hemolytic streptococcal infection is the most common cause in children.
  - Other bacteria: *Mycoplasma*, *Yersinia*, *Shigella*, *Brucella*, *Neisseria meningococcus* and *gonococcus*, chlamydia, cat-scratch disease, rickettsial diseases including syphilis
  - Viral: Epstein-Barr virus (EBV), HIV, hepatitis B virus (HBV)
  - Mycobacterial: tuberculosis and atypical mycobacteria, leprosy
  - Fungal: histoplasmosis, coccidioidomycosis
- Systemic associations
  - Sarcoidosis
  - Inflammatory bowel disease
  - Behçet disease
  - Malignancy (lymphoma, leukemia)
- Pregnancy
- Medications
  - Oral contraceptives
  - Sulfonamides
  - Phenytoin
  - Halides

DIAGNOSIS

HISTORY
- Arthralgia is commonly noted 2–8 weeks prior.
- Prodromal symptoms of fatigue/malaise or upper respiratory infection often occur by 1–3 weeks.
- Pain and tenderness of the extremities is common, sometimes causing difficulty in ambulation.
- Important questions to ask:
  - Recent streptococcal infection
  - Medication history (oral contraceptives, sulfonamides, iodides/bromides)
  - Last menses (erythema nodosum is seen in pregnancy)
  - History of diarrhea (inflammatory bowel disease or infectious diarrhea)
  - Tuberculosis exposure

PHYSICAL EXAM
- Red, often tender nodules on anterior lower legs, 2–6 cm in diameter
- Lesions can also be present in other areas with subcutaneous fat such as the thighs, arms, trunk, and face.
- Overlying skin is normal except for erythema.
- Initially, lesions are slightly elevated, bright to deep red nodules with palpable warmth.
- Later, lesions develop a brownish red or violaceous, bruise-like appearance.
- Exam pearls
  - Symmetric distribution
  - Erythema nodosum never ulcerates or suppurates.
  - Usually, there are no more than 6 lesions at a time.

DIAGNOSTIC TESTS & INTERPRETATION

Lab
- Throat culture
- Antistreptolysin-O titer
- Tuberculin skin test
- CBC
- Erythrocyte sedimentation rate (ESR)
- Stool culture, if history of diarrhea
- Serologic testing, if yersiniosis, rickettsial disease, histoplasmosis, or coccidioidomycosis suspected

Imaging
Chest radiograph can help screen for possible underlying tuberculosis or sarcoidosis.

Diagnostic Procedures/Other
- Erythema nodosum is a clinical diagnosis.
- Biopsy for histopathology and culture (bacterial, fungal, mycobacterial) is used if diagnosis is in doubt.

Pathologic Findings
- Septal panniculitis: lymphocytic perivascular infiltrate in the dermis; lymphocytes and neutrophils in the fibrous septa in the subcutaneous fat
- Older lesions: Histiocytes, giant cells, and occasionally plasma cells can be seen.
- No fat cell destruction or vasculitis is present.

DIFFERENTIAL DIAGNOSIS
- Infection
  - Erysipelas/cellulitis
  - Erythema induratum (nodular vasculitis)
  - Deep fungal infection or Majocchi granuloma
- Superficial or deep thrombophlebitis
- Trauma: accidental or from child abuse
- Palmoplantar hidradenitis
- Metabolic
  - Panniculitis secondary to pancreatic disease
  - Pretibial myxedema
- Major insect bite reaction
- Psychosocial (self-injection with foreign material)
- Cutaneous sarcoidosis
- Polyarteritis nodosa
- Granuloma annulare

TREATMENT

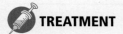

FIRST LINE
- Bed rest
- Leg elevation
- Salicylates or other NSAIDs, such as ibuprofen, naproxen, or indomethacin

ADDITIONAL THERAPIES
- Potassium iodide 300 mg PO t.i.d. for 3–4 weeks, especially for cases diagnosed early in course
- Colchicine
- Corticosteroids (rarely used) for severe cases; courses generally last 2–4 weeks

ONGOING CARE

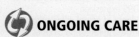

FOLLOW-UP RECOMMENDATIONS
Patient Monitoring
- Can expect improvement within 1 week
- If lesions recur after cessation of treatment, an underlying infection/inflammatory trigger may still be present.
- If atypical locations or exuberant or suppurative nodules are present, a biopsy is warranted to rule out a disseminated infection.

PROGNOSIS
- Most individual lesions will completely resolve in 10–14 days.
- In general, erythema nodosum resolves in 3–6 weeks with or without treatment unless the underlying cause is a chronic infection or systemic disorder.
- Aching of legs and swelling of ankles may persist for weeks; rarely, symptoms may persist for up to 2 years.
- In children, the recurrence rate is 4–10% and is often associated with repeated streptococcal infection.

ADDITIONAL READING

- Chachkin S, Cheng JW, Yan AC. Erythema nodosum. In: Burg FD, Ingelfinger JR, Polin RA, et al, eds. *Current Pediatric Therapy*. 18th ed. Philadelphia, PA: WB Saunders; 2006.
- Garty BZ, Poznanski O. Erythema nodosum in Israeli children. *Isr Med Assoc J*. 2000;2(2):145–146.
- Gonzalez-Gay MA, Garcia-Porrua C, Pujol RM, et al. Erythema nodosum: a clinical approach. *Clin Exp Rheumatol*. 2001;19(4):365–368.
- Kakourou T, Drosatou P, Psychou F, et al. Erythema nodosum in children: a prospective study. *J Am Acad Dermatol*. 2001;44(1):17–21.
- Paller A, Mancini A. The hypersensitivity syndromes. In: Paller AS, Mancini AJ, eds. *Hurwitz Clinical Pediatric Dermatology: A Textbook of Skin Disorders of Childhood and Adolescence*. 4th ed. Philadelphia, PA: Elsevier Health Sciences; 2011.
- Pettersson T. Sarcoid and erythema nodosum arthropathies. *Best Pract Res Clin Rheumatol*. 2000;14(3):461–476.

CODES

ICD10CM
- L52 Erythema nodosum
- A18.4 Tuberculosis of skin and subcutaneous tissue

FAQ
- Q: Will the lesions leave a scar?
- A: In the vast majority of cases, erythema nodosum heals without scarring.

E

EWING SARCOMA

Erin E. Karski • Steven G. DuBois

BASICS

DESCRIPTION

- Family of cancers with common biology and treatment:
  - Ewing sarcoma of bone
  - Extraskeletal Ewing sarcoma (arises in soft tissue adjacent to bone)
  - Peripheral neuroectodermal tumor (PNET) of bone or soft tissue
  - Askin tumor (Ewing sarcoma of the chest wall)
- Most common primary tumor sites are as follows:
  - Pelvic bones (26%)
  - Femur (20%)
  - Chest wall (16%)

EPIDEMIOLOGY

- 2nd most common primary bone cancer of children and young adults after osteosarcoma
- Median age of diagnosis is 15 years, although can occur in any age group
- Slight male predominance

Incidence

- ~200–250 new cases are diagnosed in the United States each year.
- Annual incidence in the United States of 2.7 cases per million children younger than 15 years of age
- Most (~65%) occur in the 2nd decade of life.
- Strikingly lower incidence in sub-Saharan Africa and in African American population

RISK FACTORS

- Most cases occur sporadically.
- Not associated with familial cancer syndromes
- Only rarely reported as a second malignancy
- One genome-wide association study identified several single nucleotide polymorphisms (SNPs) associated with higher risk.
- Epidemiologic studies suggest higher risk in patients with history of inguinal or umbilical hernia.

GENERAL PREVENTION

There are no known preventive measures.

PATHOPHYSIOLOGY

- Rearrangement of the *EWSR1* gene on chromosome 22 is detected in >95% of cases.
  - 85% of cases have a t(11;22) translocation resulting in a fusion EWS-FLI1 protein.
  - 10% of cases have a t(21;22) translocation between EWS and ERG.
  - Other translocation partners occur in <1% of cases and include other members of the ETS transcription factor family, such as ETV1.
- Fusion proteins thought to play a role as aberrant transcription factor

DIAGNOSIS

HISTORY

- Pain is most common symptom.
- Pain is often attributed to minor injuries that are common in this age group.
- Other presenting symptoms are as follows:
  - Palpable mass
  - Fever
  - Limp
- Systemic symptoms (fever, weight loss) are more common among patients with metastatic disease and more common compared to patients with osteosarcoma.

PHYSICAL EXAM

- Palpable mass (35%)
- Local tenderness (70%)
- Painful movement of joint (35%)
- Fever (30%)
- Regional node involvement uncommon, although more likely with a soft tissue primary tumor

DIAGNOSTIC TESTS & INTERPRETATION

Lab

- CBC as a screen for bone marrow involvement
- Serum lactate dehydrogenase (LDH) is often elevated at diagnosis and may be prognostic.
- Prechemotherapy labs include liver function tests and tests of renal function.

Imaging

- To evaluate primary site:
  - Plain radiographic findings may include the following:
    - Destructive lesion with "moth-eaten" appearance
    - Periosteal reaction with layers of reactive bone can give an "onionskin" appearance.
    - Raised periosteum may result in a Codman triangle.
    - When arising in long bones, tends to arise from diaphysis rather than metaphysis
- CT or preferably MRI scan in addition to radiograph is essential to fully characterize the extent of the primary tumor.
- 25% have detectable metastases at diagnosis.
  - Lung
  - Bone
  - Bone marrow
- To evaluate for distant metastases:
  - Chest CT scan
  - Fluorine-18-fluorodeoxyglucose positron emission tomography (FDG PET) or 99m-Tc-diphosphonate bone scan

Diagnostic Procedures/Other

- Biopsy
  - Consultation with a pediatric oncologist and orthopedic oncologist is essential before biopsy.
  - Should be performed by an experienced orthopedic surgeon
  - Avoid contamination of surrounding tissues.
  - Include testing for *EWSR1* translocation, either by fluorescence in situ hybridization (FISH), cytogenetics, or reverse transcription-polymerase reaction (RT-PCR).
  - Small round blue cell tumor with nearly universal membranous CD99 expression
  - PNET shows evidence of neural differentiation.
- Bilateral bone marrow aspirates and biopsies to complete metastatic staging
- Echocardiogram in anticipation of starting chemotherapy

DIFFERENTIAL DIAGNOSIS

- Malignant
  - Osteosarcoma
  - Neuroblastoma
  - Non-Hodgkin lymphoma
  - Rhabdomyosarcoma
  - Other soft tissue sarcoma
  - Bone metastasis from other malignancy
- Benign
  - Osteomyelitis
  - Tendonitis
  - Trauma
  - Langerhans cell histiocytosis
  - Other benign bone tumor

TREATMENT

CHEMOTHERAPY

- Chemotherapy is essential for cure.
  - Prior to the use of chemotherapy, only 10% of patients survived.
  - Patients with nonmetastatic disease now have an overall survival rate approaching 70% with the use of chemotherapy and appropriate local control.
  - Suggests that patients have small amounts of occult micrometastatic tumor cells that cannot be detected by current technology
- In North America, standard chemotherapy traditionally includes vincristine, doxorubicin, and cyclophosphamide alternating every 2 weeks with etoposide and ifosfamide.
- Other agents under investigation include camptothecins (irinotecan and topotecan) as well as IGF-1R inhibitors.

ADDITIONAL TREATMENT

General Measures

- In addition to systemic treatment with chemotherapy, patients need local control treatment to the site of the primary tumor and metastases (if present) with surgery, radiation, or both.
- The type of local control used depends on the location and extent of the tumor, the morbidity associated with resection, and the presence of tumor cells at the resection margin in those who have surgery.
- The usual sequence of treatment is
  - Neoadjuvant chemotherapy
  - Local control
  - Adjuvant chemotherapy
- Most children are treated on or according to large cooperative group clinical trials.
- Myeloid growth factor (e.g., granulocyte colony-stimulating factor [G-CSF]) is usually given following chemotherapy to shorten the duration of neutropenia.

SURGERY/OTHER PROCEDURES

- If surgical local control is pursued, goal is to remove the entire tumor with negative tissue margins.
- Limb salvage surgery is often possible but may not be best in some cases.
- Amputation is less commonly performed given the radiosensitive nature of Ewing sarcoma.

RADIATION

- Definitive radiation provides reasonable local control in cases not amenable to surgical resection.
- Radiation also used for
  - Attempted surgical resection, but margins positive
  - Treatment of cytology-proven malignant pleural effusions in patients with chest wall tumors
  - Treatment of metastatic disease, including whole lung radiotherapy for patients with lung metastasis
- Carries risk of second malignancy

ADDITIONAL THERAPIES

- Physical therapy
  - All patients who receive surgery should be referred to physical therapy following surgery.
  - Patients regardless of surgery may need physical therapy for deconditioning associated with treatment.
- Reproductive endocrinology
  - Given the role of alkylating chemotherapy in the treatment of Ewing sarcoma, all patients should be encouraged to meet with reproductive endocrinology to discuss fertility preservation strategies prior to initiating therapy.

ISSUES FOR REFERRAL

Consultation with a pediatric oncologist is essential before any attempt is made at a diagnostic biopsy.

ONGOING CARE

PROGNOSIS

- 5-year overall survival rate for all patients is ~60%.
- Presence of metastases is the most important prognostic factor.
  - Estimated overall survival in those with metastatic disease at diagnosis is less than 30% at 5 years.
- Other unfavorable prognostic features:
  - Older age (age >18 years)
  - Pelvic primary tumor
  - Large primary tumor
- Other prognostic factors under investigation:
  - LDH
  - Race
  - Aberrations in p53/p16
- Subtype of *EWSR1/FLI1* translocation not prognostic

COMPLICATIONS

- Acute toxicity
  - Alopecia
  - Bone marrow suppression
    - Platelet and packed red blood cell transfusions are usually necessary.
    - Neutropenia: increased risk of bacterial and fungal infections
  - Gastrointestinal side effects
    - Nausea and vomiting
    - Mucositis
  - Kidney and bladder side effects
    - Electrolyte wasting
    - Hemorrhagic cystitis
  - Complications from radiation
    - Skin breakdown and erythema
    - Bone marrow suppression
  - Complications from surgery
    - Wound dehiscence
    - Infection

Late Effects

- Cardiotoxicity (See "Cancer Therapy Late Effects.")
  - Anthracyclines (doxorubicin) can lead to cardiomyopathy and heart failure.
  - Risk depends on cumulative dose of doxorubicin.
  - Radiation to the heart can increase the risk of cardiotoxicity.
  - Patients should have yearly echocardiogram for evaluation.
  - Reduced fertility
- Second malignancy
  - Sarcomas may occur within the radiation field.
  - Myelodysplastic syndromes and acute myeloid leukemia may occur secondary to chemotherapy.

ADDITIONAL READING

- Grier HE, Krailo MD, Tarbell NJ, et al. Addition of ifosfamide and etoposide to standard chemotherapy for Ewing's sarcoma and primitive neuroectodermal tumor of bone. *N Engl J Med*. 2003;348(8):694–701.
- Postel-Vinay S, Veron AS, Tirode F, et al. Common variants near TARDBP and EGR2 are associated with susceptibility to Ewing sarcoma. *Nat Genet*. 2012;12(3):323–327.
- Rodriguez-Galindo C, Liu T, Krasin MJ, et al. Analysis of prognostic factors in Ewing sarcoma family of tumors: review of the St. Jude Children's Research Hospital studies. *Cancer*. 2007;110(2):375–384.
- Rodriguez-Galindo C, Spunt SL, Pappo AS. Treatment of Ewing sarcoma family of tumors: current status and outlook for the future. *Med Pediatr Oncol*. 2003;40(5):276–287.
- Valery PC, Holly EA, Sleigh AC, et al. Hernias and Ewing's sarcoma family of tumours: a pooled analysis and meta-analysis. *Lancet Oncol*. 2005;6(7):485–490.
- Womer RB, West DC, Krailo MD, et al. Randomized controlled trial of interval-compressed chemotherapy for the treatment of localized Ewing sarcoma: a report from the Children's Oncology Group. *J Clin Oncol*. 2012;30(33):4148–4154.

CODES

ICD10

- C41.9 Malignant neoplasm of bone and articular cartilage, unsp
- C41.4 Malignant neoplasm of pelvic bones, sacrum and coccyx
- C40.20 Malignant neoplasm of long bones of unspecified lower limb

FAQ

- Q: At what time point is a child with Ewing sarcoma considered cured?
- A: Most cases of recurrence in Ewing sarcoma occur within 2 years of initial diagnosis. However, late relapses beyond 5 years from initial diagnosis have been seen with Ewing sarcoma.
- Q: Should an Ewing sarcoma be completely resected at the time of diagnosis?
- A: Ewing sarcoma tumors are typically large at initial diagnosis. The standard approach is to treat with chemotherapy first, both to reduce the size of the tumor and to treat any distant tumor cells.
- Q: Is surgery or radiation better for local control of the primary tumor in Ewing sarcoma?
- A: This is an area of controversy. Most specialists favor surgical resection when feasible without significantly jeopardizing function, reserving radiation for cases that are less amenable to surgical resection with negative margins.
- Q: Why do Africans and African Americans have such low rates of Ewing sarcoma?
- A: It is not known why these populations are at lower risk for developing Ewing sarcoma, although it suggests a genetic component that influences the risk of developing this disease. Studies are ongoing to investigate this consistent finding.

EXSTROPHY–EPISPADIAS COMPLEX

Brian M. Inouye • John P. Gearhart

BASICS

DESCRIPTION

The exstrophy–epispadias complex is a rare spectrum of multisystem birth defects involving the genitourinary and gastrointestinal tracts, musculoskeletal system, pelvic floor, and bony pelvis. It is composed of epispadias, bladder exstrophy, and cloacal exstrophy. The latter two conditions present with an open bladder through the anterior abdominal wall.

- The least common variant of the complex, complete epispadias presents with a closed bladder and dorsally open urethral meatus.
- Cloacal exstrophy is the most severe variant, presenting with a large omphalocele, imperforate anus, shortened colon, bladder halves with cecum interposed between, associated cord defects, and multiple upper urinary tract and limb anomalies. All three forms are associated with a pubic diastasis.

EPIDEMIOLOGY

Incidence

- Bladder exstrophy
  - Male-to-female ratio is between 2:1 and 4:1.
  - Between 1:10,000 and 1:50,000 live births
  - Risk in offspring of individuals with bladder exstrophy and epispadias is 1:70 (500-fold greater than general population).
  - Risk of recurrence in family is approximately 1:100.
- Epispadias
  - Risk of male epispadias: 1:117,000 live births
  - Risk of female epispadias: 1:484,000 live births
- Cloacal exstrophy
  - Male-to-female ratio is between 1:1 and 2:1.
  - Cloacal exstrophy is exceedingly rare, with an incidence between 1:200,000 and 1:400,000 births (decreasing incidence with prenatal diagnosis and termination).

RISK FACTORS

Bladder exstrophy: only known association is related to offspring of in vitro fertilization pregnancies

PATHOPHYSIOLOGY

Embryology

- Normal development
  - By week 2 of gestation, the cloacal membrane is located at the caudal end of the infraumbilical abdominal wall.
  - At week 4 of gestation, mesenchyme from the primitive streak migrates between the layers of the cloacal membrane to reinforce the abdominal wall while the cloacal membrane regresses.
- Bladder exstrophy
  - Unclear pathogenesis, but there is an error in embryogenesis
  - The cloacal membrane may overdevelop and prevent mesenchymal migration, which inhibits formation of normal lower abdominal wall.
  - Without reinforcement, the cloacal membrane ruptures. The timing of this rupture determines the variant of the exstrophy–epispadias complex. In bladder exstrophy, rupture of the membrane occurs after the urorectal septum has descended, dividing the genitourinary and gastrointestinal tracts.
- Cloacal exstrophy
  - Abnormally large cloacal membrane ruptures prior to division of the cloaca by the urorectal septum.

DIAGNOSIS

PHYSICAL EXAM

- Bladder exstrophy
  - All cases have pubic diastasis (mean of 4.8 cm) caused by outward rotation of the innominate bones and iliac wings.
  - The exstrophied bladder and posterior urethra are exposed through a triangular defect in the anterior abdominal wall and are bound by the umbilicus superiorly, the two separated pubic bones laterally, and the anus inferiorly.
  - The anus is anteriorly displaced, shortening the distance between it and the umbilicus.
  - Boys commonly have indirect inguinal hernias that are prone to incarceration because the perineum is short and broad due to the compromised pelvic floor. Less common when osteotomy is used.
  - Male genital anomalies
    - Penis is 50% shorter and 30% wider than nonexstrophy boys.
    - Corpora cavernosa are short and widely separated secondary to the pubic diastasis.
    - There is a short urethral plate and a marked dorsal chordee causing the penis to curve upward.
    - Epispadias always presents with the lower tract open from the tip of the penis to the dome of the bladder.
  - Female genital anomalies
    - Mons pubis is laterally displaced, with a bifid clitoris secondary to the diastasis.
    - Vagina is short and wide.
    - Vagina and introitus are displaced anteriorly, with the cervix in the anterior vaginal wall.
    - All female patients are at an increased risk for uterine prolapse in adolescent and adult life.
  - Urinary defects
    - Bladder mucosa at birth usually appears normal but may be ectopic or contain polyps.
    - Exstrophic bladder may develop slowly prior to closure.
    - Upper urinary tract usually normal but may observe horseshoe, pelvic, hypoplastic, solitary, or dysplastic kidney.
    - Most children have vesicoureteral reflux requiring correction at the time of their continence procedure.
- Cloacal exstrophy
  - Two halves of the exstrophied bladder are separated by an exstrophied ileocecal bowel segment with various amount of hindgut present.
  - Omphalocele usually present; varies in size.
  - Imperforate anus is usually present.
  - Vertebral and neurologic abnormalities (lumbar myelodysplasia, hemivertebrae) are present in >50% of children.
  - Upper urinary tract anomalies (duplicated systems, horseshoe kidney, pelvic kidney) are seen in up to 70% of children.
  - Penis may be duplicate or diminutive.
  - Bifid vagina and uterine abnormalities

DIAGNOSTIC TESTS & INTERPRETATION

Imaging

- Prenatal sonographic findings between 15th and 32nd weeks of pregnancy demonstrating absence of normal fluid-filled bladder, an anterior abdominal mass increasing in size, low-set umbilicus, and wide pubic ramus are suggestive of bladder exstrophy.
- A baseline renal ultrasound and KUB after birth will demonstrate renal abnormalities and the pubic diastasis, respectively.

TREATMENT

SURGERY/OTHER PROCEDURES

Goals: Provide urinary continence with a compliant bladder, preserve renal function, and surgically reconstruct the phallus for cosmesis.

- Modern staged repair of bladder exstrophy (MSRE)
  - In the early neonatal period, bladder, posterior urethra, and abdominal wall closure is performed with or without osteotomy.
  - Closure of the urethra occurs at 6–12 months of age.
    - Bladder capacity is annually measured with gravity cystogram.
  - If bladder has adequate capacity and patient desires continence (between 5 and 9 years), a continence procedure is performed with ureteral reimplantation.
    - Noncandidates or those who fail continence may require bladder neck transection, augmentation cystoplasty, and continent urinary diversion.
  - Results and complications: Daytime continence in 60–80% following bladder neck surgery may require clean intermittent catheterization (long-term follow-up). Minimal risk for upper urinary tract changes or hydronephrosis.
    - Small bladder capacity and failed primary closure are predictors of postsurgical incontinence.
- Complete primary repair of exstrophy (CPRE)
  - Bladder and abdominal wall closure, bladder neck reconstruction, and epispadias repair completed in single procedure. May be performed with or without osteotomy.
  - Total penile disassembly dissects the urethral plate from corporal bodies to posteriorly position the bladder neck into the pelvis.
  - Results and complications: Daytime continence and volitional voiding in selected patients in up to 20% over 5 years of age; additional bladder neck surgery to gain continence is usually required; >50% require subsequent hypospadias repair and bladder neck fistula rate is up to 40%. Penile disassembly may cause penile soft tissue loss.
- Role of osteotomy and immobilization in all closures
  - Recommended in patients with a diastasis >4 cm who no longer have a malleable pelvis, which usually occurs after 72 hours of age
  - Bilateral transverse anterior innominate and vertical posterior iliac osteotomies performed by pediatric orthopedic surgeon.
  - Fixator pins and external fixation devices can be placed and left postoperatively for 4–6 weeks.
  - Pelvis immobilized and patient is placed in modified Buck or Bryant traction to increase chance of success.
  - Complications: increased risk of transient nerve and muscle palsies (which typically resolve), delayed ileal union, and superficial infection at pin sites
- Complications for both types of closure:
  - Dehiscence, bladder prolapse, bladder outlet obstruction, stone formation, hydronephrosis, and vesicocutaneous fistula formation may occur. Patients must be followed carefully.
  - Chance of long-term continence decreases with each additional closure attempt.
  - Failed bladder neck repair in 20–50% may require further reconstruction.
  - 60–95% cosmetic and functional success of epispadias repair with a straight penis with erections
    - Urethral strictures and urethrocutaneous fistula are the most common complications of epispadias repair seen in ≤25% of patients.
  - Adenocarcinoma of the bladder is 400 times more likely than in the normal population. This disease is not reported in adults who have had bladder closure after infancy.
- Fertility and pregnancy
  - Following successful repair, sexual function and libido are normal.
  - Following epispadias repair, up to 87% of boys have erections.
  - Expect retrograde and small-volume ejaculation.
  - Males can have successful impregnation with assisted reproductive techniques.
  - Females can achieve pregnancy, but uterine and cervical prolapse are common following pregnancy. Cesarean section is recommended.

INPATIENT CONSIDERATIONS

Initial Stabilization

Postnatal and nursery care:

- Instead of umbilical clamp, tie umbilical cord with 2-0 silk to avoid trauma
- Cover bladder and other exstrophied bowel/omphalocele with a hydrated gel dressing or plastic wrap to prevent mucosa from sticking to clothing or diapers.
- Transfer immediately to an appropriate center for evaluation and management by a pediatric urologist and an experienced team.

Discharge Criteria

- Prophylactic antibiotics should be continued in all children until antireflux procedure or resolution of vesicoureteral reflux.
- Maintain close follow-up with surgeon.

ONGOING CARE

PROGNOSIS

Current treatments preserve the bladder in nearly every patient and allow for continence through the urethra, providing an excellent overall prognosis. There can be favorable long-term outcome with early intervention by a pediatric urologist.

ADDITIONAL READING

- Baird AD, Nelson CP, Gearhart JP. Modern staged repair of bladder exstrophy: a contemporary series. *J Pediatr Urol*. 2007;3(4):311–315.
- Ebert AK, Reutter H, Ludwig M, et al. The exstrophy-epispadias complex. *Orphanet J Rare Dis*. 2009;4:23.
- Gargollo PC, Borer JG, Diamond DA, et al. Prospective followup in patients after complete primary repair of bladder exstrophy. *J Urol*. 2008;180 (Suppl 4):1665–1670.
- Gearhart JP, Baird AD. The failed complete repair of bladder exstrophy: Insights and outcomes. *J Urol*. 2005;174(4):1669–1672.
- Grady RW, Mitchell ME. Complete primary repair of exstrophy. *J Urol*. 1999;162(4):1415–1420.
- Inouye BM, Massanyi EZ, Di Carlo H, et al. Modern management of bladder exstrophy repair. *Curr Urol Rep*. 2013;14(4):359–365.
- Schaeffer, AJ, Stec AA, Purves JT, et al. Complete primary repair of bladder exstrophy: a single institution referral experience. *J Urol*. 2011;186(3):1041–1046.
- Stec AA, Tekes A, Ertan G, et al. Evaluation of the pelvic floor muscular redistribution after primary closure of classic bladder exstrophy by 3-dimensional magnetic resonance imaging. *J Urol*. 2012;188(4)(Suppl):1535–1542.

CODES

ICD10

- Q64.10 Exstrophy of urinary bladder, unspecified
- Q64.0 Epispadias
- Q64.12 Cloacal extrophy of urinary bladder

FAQ

- Q: Will the child have normal sexual function?
- A: Yes. Following a completed, successful repair, the sexual function will be normal.
- Q: Will the child be fertile?
- A: Females commonly achieve pregnancy without the need for in vitro fertilization. Males require in vitro fertilization to impregnate.
- Q: Can an exstrophy patient play sports?
- A: After successfully exstrophy closure, patients are able to play sports.
- Q: Is there risk of recurrence of bladder exstrophy in a family?
- A: Yes. There is a 1:100 chance for bladder exstrophy to recur in a family.

FAILURE TO THRIVE (WEIGHT FALTERING)

Tanya Hinds • Allison M. Jackson

BASICS

DESCRIPTION

Failure to thrive (FTT) or weight faltering describes *a pattern of growth* that is below established standards for age and gender. Anthropometric FTT is defined as any one of the following:

- Weight (or weight for length/height) <2 standard deviations below mean
- Weight deceleration of more than 2 major percentile lines after a previously established pattern
- Weight <75% of median weight for chronologic age
- Weight <80% of median weight for length
- Weight for chronologic age <5th percentile
- Body mass index for chronologic age <5th percentile
- Length for chronologic age <5th percentile

EPIDEMIOLOGY

- FTT often begins in the first 6 months of life but may not be diagnosed until after 1 year of age.
- It is difficult to accurately determine FTT incidence or prevalence as there is neither consensus on the best definition of FTT nor concordance between definitions. Depending on definition selected, prevalence can range from 1% to 22% based on an analysis of infants from a Danish Birth Registry.

RISK FACTORS

No single risk factor uniformly predicts FTT.

- Substantiated child abuse or neglect is 4 times more likely in FTT children compared to non-FTT children. However, maltreatment is a primary concern in only 4–5% of FTT cases.
- Family poverty was traditionally believed to be an important risk for FTT. However, recent prospective studies of large populations seen in general pediatric clinics have either been equivocal or failed to show poverty to be an important risk factor.
- Maternal mental health vulnerabilities, maternal education, and infant characteristics have also been equivocal.
- Currently, there is consensus that FTT involves a multiplicity of overlapping dietary, developmental, social, and medical concerns.

GENERAL PREVENTION

Advice should be straightforward, practical, and tailored to specific needs.

- Primary prevention
  - Addresses proper formula and food preparation, feeding quantities and frequencies, community-based nutrition support programs, and mental health resources
- Secondary prevention
  - Involves early identification by regular growth monitoring
- Tertiary prevention
  - Requires creation of an individualized treatment plan that addresses specific factors (dietary, developmental, social, and medical) adversely affecting a child's ability to meet caloric needs
  - Long-term, coordinated multidisciplinary efforts involving home visiting nurses, dietitians, social workers, primary care providers, and medical subspecialists are critical to success.

PATHOPHYSIOLOGY

Inadequate Caloric Intake

- Dietary
  - Breastfeeding difficulties
  - Diluted or inappropriately prepared formula
  - Food fads or restrictions
- Developmental/neurologic
  - Oral motor difficulties
  - Central nervous system abnormalities
- Social
  - Unavailability of food
  - Parent–child interaction disorders
  - Mental health or behavioral disorders affecting child's appetite
  - Mental health disorders affecting caregiver's parenting abilities
  - Disorganized meal times
  - Neglect (omitting feeds or creating environment not conducive to feeding)
- Medical
  - Adenotonsillar hypertrophy
  - Cleft lip and/or palate
  - Dental pain and decay
  - Congenital cardiac disease
  - Gastroesophageal reflux disease
  - Dysphagia

Inadequate Absorption or Utilization

- Food allergies or intolerances
- Inflammatory bowel disease
- Gastrointestinal malformations
- Pyloric stenosis
- Hepatitis
- Cystic fibrosis
- Parasitic infections
- Inborn errors of metabolism

Increased Caloric Expenditure

- Hyperthyroidism
- Chronic infections
- Chronic immunodeficiencies
- Malignancy
- Pulmonary disease
- Cardiac disease
- Renal disease

ETIOLOGY

- Historically, FTT was classified as organic (secondary to medical illness) or inorganic (secondary to psychosocial concerns). This categorization is obsolete. It places inordinate emphasis on organic conditions. In outpatient primary care settings, an identifiable organic disease likely contributes to FTT in <18% of children age 2 years or younger.
- Children with FTT may eat less. An undemanding child temperament, low appetite, and disinterest in food may either cause or result in FTT.
- FTT children also have significantly fewer positive mealtime interactions with caregivers. Family dysfunction, caregiver incompetence, lack of knowledge about child development, and caregiver mental health vulnerabilities can affect a caregiver–child feeding relationship.

COMMONLY ASSOCIATED CONDITIONS

Severe, chronic FTT may have significant adverse effects on cognition, attention, and behavior.

DIAGNOSIS

HISTORY

Responses to questions about the following can help guide evaluation:

- Prenatal
  - Multiple miscarriages (suggesting a genetic disorder)
  - Maternal health and/or medical diagnoses
  - Tobacco, alcohol, or illicit substances
  - Other teratogens or toxins (prescribed medication, radiation exposure)
- Birth
  - Gestational age at delivery
  - Weight, length, and head circumference
  - Asphyxia, infection, other perinatal complications
- Medical
  - Newborn metabolic screening results
  - Medical diagnoses: reflux, cardiac disease, obstructive sleep apnea, respiratory infections, urinary tract infections, other chronic or recurrent conditions
  - Hospitalizations, surgeries, immunizations
  - Event(s) at time of significant loss or gain of weight
- Developmental
  - Personal–social, language, fine and gross motor milestones
  - Loss of previously acquired milestones
- Family
  - Weight, height of biologic parents and siblings
  - Parental history of childhood growth delay
  - Medical, mental, and developmental diagnoses of parents and siblings
  - Maternal postpartum depression
  - Caregiver(s) use of illicit substances
- Review of systems
  - Activity level compared to peers
  - Chronic rhinorrhea, congestion, cough
  - Mouth breathing, snoring, frequent awakenings from sleep
  - Difficulty or pain with sucking, chewing, or swallowing
  - Vomiting or excessive spitting up
  - Breathlessness, sweating, or tiring during feeds
  - Frequent, large, bloody, or oily stools
  - Constipation
  - Urinary frequency or dysuria
  - Polyuria, polydipsia, polyphagia
  - Eczema or urticaria exacerbated by select foods

- Psychosocial
  - Difficulty purchasing or preparing food
  - Distractions during feeds/meals
  - Perception of child's behavior during meals
  - Eating habits of siblings when at a similar age as infant/child with FTT
  - Individual and family stressors and strengths
  - Supplemental food and community resources
  - Travel to less developed countries
- Dietary
  - Frequency, duration of active suck
  - Frequency, type, preparation, quantity of typical formula feed
  - Feeding changes at night or on weekends
  - Age of weaning/shift in feeding practices
  - Foods consumed over typical 24 hours
  - Water, juices, sodas over typical 24 hours
  - Food allergies or intolerances
  - Feeding habits and techniques (bottle propping, grazing)
  - Eating habits outside the home (day care, school)
  - Vitamin, herbal, other supplements

PHYSICAL EXAM

Helps identify chronic illness, syndromes

- Weight, length/height, head circumference
- Vital signs, pain
- General: activity level (lethargic, hyperactive), caregiver–child interactions (eye contact, physical approximation, checking), hygiene, dysmorphic features, lymphadenopathy
- Head: dry, dull, or absent hair; fontanelle size
- Eyes: palpebral fissures, conjunctival pallor, strabismus, cataracts, retinal hemorrhages
- Ears: malposition, otitis
- Mouth, throat: anatomic abnormalities of palate or tongue, glossitis, cheilosis, gum bleeding, thrush, dental abnormalities, enlarged tonsils
- Cardiac: murmur; abnormal femoral pulses
- Chest, lungs: retractions, wheezes, crackles
- GI: distention, masses, hepatomegaly
- Anogenital: malformations; severe rashes; anal fissures, hemorrhoids
- Musculoskeletal: frontal bossing, rachitic rosary, extremity bowing, wrist widening, edema, decreased muscle mass
- Skin: eczema; hives; scaling; spoon-shaped nails; patterned bruises, scars, burns
- Neurologic: cranial nerve palsies, hyper- or hypotonia, retention of primitive reflexes

DIAGNOSTIC TESTS & INTERPRETATION

Initial Lab Tests

- CBC: anemia; leukemia
- Comprehensive metabolic panel (CMP), phosphorus: malnutrition; metabolic abnormalities; chronic endocrine, liver, and renal disease
- Thyroid function tests
- UA and culture: renal tubular acidosis, infection

Follow Up Tests & Special Considerations

- Ferritin
- Lead
- Vitamin D
- Purified protein derivative (PPD)
- HIV, hepatitis B and C
- Stool pathogens, *Giardia* antigen
- Stool fat
- Sweat test
- Serum IgA, antitransglutaminase antibodies: celiac disease
- Karyotype: Turner syndrome

Diagnostic Procedures/Other

- Wrist x-rays: bone age
- Chest x-ray: cardiac anomalies, cystic fibrosis
- Lateral neck x-ray: adenotonsillar hypertrophy
- Skeletal survey: suspected maltreatment
- Upper GI series, pH probe: anatomic abnormalities, reflux
- ECG

TREATMENT

MEDICATION

Medications that stimulate appetite and growth hormone therapy have not been extensively studied in FTT. Nutritional supplements and calorie-dense foods help promote catch-up growth.

ADDITIONAL THERAPIES

- Community-based nutritional and psychosocial counseling program when no underlying illness. Multidisciplinary interventions including home nursing visits improve weight gain, parent–child relationships, and cognitive development.
- Goal is catch-up growth (growth faster than normal rate for age). Normal growth rates for age average about 30 g/day until 3 months, 20 g/day from 3 to 6 months, 10 g/day from 6 to 12 months, and 8 g/day from 1 to 3 years.
- Daily multivitamins, zinc, and iron

ISSUES FOR REFERRAL

- **Subspecialty consultation**
  - Minimize risk of refeeding syndrome
  - Genetic syndrome or disease suspected

INPATIENT CONSIDERATIONS

Hospitalize when

- FTT persists despite community-based dietary interventions
- Severe malnutrition. Weight for age <60% of median or weight for height <70% of median increases morbidity.
- Suspicion of abuse or neglect; note, this necessitates mandatory CPS report.

ONGOING CARE

Monitoring should continue until weight for height deficit is repaired and child no longer needs a specialized diet to maintain normal growth. The Centers for Disease Control and Prevention (CDC) suggests World Health Organization growth charts for all children up to age 2 years and CDC growth charts for older children. Specialty growth charts for patients with genetic conditions can supplement these charts.

ADDITIONAL READING

- Mash C, Frazier T, Nowacki A, et al. Development of a risk-stratification tool for medical child abuse in failure to thrive. *Pediatrics*. 2011;128(6):e1467–e1473.
- Olsen EM, Petersen J, Skovgaard AM, et al. Failure to thrive: the prevalence and concurrence of anthropometric criteria in a general infant population. *Arch Dis Child*. 2007;92(2):109–114.
- Rudolf MCJ, Logan S. What is the long term outcome for children who fail to thrive? A systematic review. *Arch Dis Child*. 2005;90(9):925–931.
- Shields B, Wacogne I, Wright CM. Weight faltering and failure to thrive in infancy and early childhood. *BMJ*. 2012;345:e5931.
- Wright C, Birks E. Risk factors for failure to thrive: a population-based survey. *Child Care Health Dev*. 2000;26(1):5–16.

CODES

ICD10

- P92.6 Failure to thrive in newborn
- R63.4 Abnormal weight loss
- R63.3 Feeding difficulties

FAQ

- Q: How should weight gain while hospitalized be interpreted?
- A: Children with and without medical illnesses will grow with sufficient caloric intake. Growth during hospitalization is not diagnostic of inorganic FTT.
- Q: How often is organic disease the cause of FTT?
- A: Organic disease is rare in children with FTT who are otherwise asymptomatic.

FEEDING DISORDERS

Elizabeth J. Hait

BASICS

DESCRIPTION

- Feeding disorder: inability to consume by mouth in quantity or quality the nutrition that is developmentally appropriate for that child
- Dysphagia: disorder of swallowing characterized by difficulty in oral preparation for the swallow or in moving food or liquid from the mouth to the stomach
- Aspiration: Food or fluid enters the trachea and passes through the vocal cords to lungs.
- Penetration: Food or fluid enters the trachea but remains above vocal cords and can be cleared by patient through coughing to prevent aspiration.
- Oral motor disorder: inability to manipulate age-appropriate diet; often related to incoordination of facial muscles and/or tongue
- Pharyngeal dysphagia: inability to protect airway during swallow; may be due to anatomic abnormality or neurologic dysfunction
- Voluntary food or fluid refusal associated with maladaptive interactions at mealtimes; associated with learned fear when foods or textures are advanced before a child is developmentally or medically ready to swallow without dysfunction

RISK FACTORS

- Congenital heart disease
- Cystic fibrosis
- Metabolic disorders
- Autism spectrum disorder
- Developmental delay/cerebral palsy
- Prolonged tube feeders (>4 weeks)
- Prematurity
- Neuromotor dysfunction
- Anatomic deformities (i.e., Pierre Robin sequence, laryngomalacia, tracheotomy, cleft palate)
- GI disorders: gastroesophageal reflux, eosinophilic esophagitis, celiac disease
- Tachypnea (respiratory rate >40 breaths per minute)

GENERAL PREVENTION

- Monitor weight, height, head circumference, weight for height, and BMI percentiles at regular interval office visits to identify changes in nutritional status early, especially in high-risk populations.
- Selective eater: Educate parents on age-appropriate portion sizes and foods.
- Provide vitamin and mineral supplementation or refer to nutritionist for complete assessment if patient is at risk for deficiencies.
- Developmental delay: Evaluate diet and feeding skills to manipulate nutrition provided.
- Ensure foods offered match developmental readiness rather than chronologic age.

DIAGNOSIS

HISTORY

- Past and present medical diagnoses
- Therapeutic management or procedures in past or at present, especially those aversive to face and upper body (e.g., suctioning, tracheostomy, intubation)
- 24-hour diet: Recall food and fluid consumed over a 24-hour period.
- Previous hospitalizations, especially those involving respiratory illnesses
- Allergies or food intolerances
- Growth history
- Developmental history
- History of snoring or sleep apnea (may indicate adenoidal or tonsillar hypertrophy)
- GI history: stool pattern, vomiting, gagging, spitting up, pain
- Family history: GI disease, allergies, developmental delays, genetic abnormalities
- Failure to thrive
  - Poor linear growth
  - Sucking and swallowing incoordination: Infant should demonstrate 1:1:1 suck, swallow, breathe pattern when sucking from breast or bottle.
  - Recurrent pneumonia
  - Coughing during or after feeding
  - Refractory asthma
  - Drooling
  - Refusal to drink or eat
  - Feeding selectivity
  - Difficulty with texture progression

PHYSICAL EXAM

- HEENT: dysmorphic facial features, shape of head and sutures, facial tone, intact soft and hard palate, shape of mandible, tonsillar size, patency of nares, movement of lips and tongue, presence of stridor, mouth closure, dentition, drooling
- Pulmonary: rate of breathing, use of accessory muscles for respiration, rales
- Cardiac: murmur, rate, and rhythm
- GI: bowel sounds, masses, stool palpable, tenderness, distension
- Neurologic: tone, positioning, cranial nerves, gait, affect, head control
- Extremities: subcutaneous stores, muscle development, adipose tissue
- Skin: rashes, alopecia

DIAGNOSTIC TESTS & INTERPRETATION

Perform feeding observation: Watch caregiver feed child, preferably thru 1-way observation mirror. Monitor child's behavioral response to placement in the feeding chair and presentation of bottle, breast, or cup and a variety of food types and textures; observe parental reaction to child's behaviors and child's ability to manipulate foods and fluids.

Lab

- Tailor labs obtained based on nutritional and/or developmental concerns, including the following:
  - Failure to thrive: celiac panel, CBC, comprehensive metabolic panel, lead, urine analysis, thyroid function; other tests if suspect vitamin or mineral deficiency (i.e., zinc, iron)
  - Developmental and/or genetic concerns: chromosomes, FISH test for 22q11 deletion, FISH test for Prader-Willi syndrome, fragile X (males), serum and urine organic acids, lactate, pyruvate, CPK
  - Sweat test if suspected cystic fibrosis: failure to thrive, diarrhea, and/or recurrent pulmonary infections

Imaging

- Tests indicated based on history and physical
- Suspected pharyngeal dysphagia: modified barium swallow study (MBSS) (videofluoroscopic swallow study) evaluates swallow function and can visualize aspiration during swallow; usually performed by radiologist and speech therapist. Study visualizes function of pharyngeal muscles and structures. See below:
  - Upper GI series (including esophagram) ensures normal anatomy of esophagus, stomach, and duodenum (evaluate for TEF, malrotation).
  - Chest x-ray: determine if infiltrates or atelectasis is present; right upper and/or middle lobe changes indicative of potential aspiration.
  - Gastric emptying scan: Assess gastric emptying and assess if gastroparesis is present
  - Salivagram: radionucleotide study to evaluate if patient is aspirating oral secretions
  - Chest CT scan: allows detection of subtle changes from silent aspiration not detectable by pulmonary exam or chest x-ray

Diagnostic Procedures/Other

- MBSS
  - Speech therapist feeds a variety of textures: thin and thickened liquid of honey and nectar consistency, thin and thick purees, and chewable foods to determine safety of oral feeding.
  - Allows visualization of oral and pharyngeal phases of swallowing
  - Can determine appropriate positioning and type of infant bottles and cups to minimize the risk for aspiration
  - Timing of aspiration is evaluated to determine if volume and fatigue result in aspiration; the patient may be safe to drink or eat for short periods of time before the swallow becomes uncoordinated and leads to aspiration.
- Fiberoptic endoscopic evaluation of swallowing (FEES)
  - Usually performed by ENT specialist; direct visualization of airway structures and swallowing mechanism
  - Provides information on pharyngeal phase of swallowing but not oral phase. Best used if pharyngeal or laryngeal abnormality is suspected, tracheostomy in place, and there is difficulty managing secretions.
  - Can observe food or fluid falling below vocal cords (aspiration)

- Bronchoscopy
  - Visualizes tracheobronchial tree and lungs, sample for lipid-laden macrophages in lungs indicative of aspiration
- Endoscopy
  - To perform esophageal, gastric, and small bowel biopsies to determine presence of eosinophilic esophagitis, celiac disease (positive or inconclusive celiac panel), or presence of gastroesophageal reflux disease (GERD)

DIFFERENTIAL DIAGNOSIS
- Cardiorespiratory
  - Congenital heart disease
    - Infectious pneumonia
    - Bronchopulmonary dysplasia
- Neurologic
  - Diencephalic syndrome
    - Congenital myopathy
    - Arnold-Chiari malformation
    - Hypoxic-ischemic encephalopathy
- GI/nutritional
  - GERD
  - Gastroparesis
  - Eosinophilic esophagitis
  - Failure to thrive
  - Celiac disease
- Metabolic syndromes
- Psychological disorders
  - Behavioral refusal
  - Psychosocial deprivation
  - Anxiety disorder
- Food allergies
- Anatomic
  - Laryngeal cleft
  - Tracheoesophageal fistula
- Genetic disorders
- Developmental disorders:
  - Autistic spectrum disorder
  - Sensory integration disorder

TREATMENT
- Pharyngeal dysphagia: Pulmonary referral, oral stimulation program, NPO as indicated by clinical exam and studies, initiate tube feeds; monitoring by speech therapist
- Feeding disorders are complex and should be evaluated and managed by multidisciplinary team involving medical, nutrition, psychology, occupational therapy, and speech therapy.

MEDICATION
Medications are administered to treat underlying medical condition (e.g., GERD); refer to specific sections for treatment of identified medical issues resulting in feeding disorder.

ADDITIONAL TREATMENT
General Measures
- Calorie counts
- Ensure adequate hydration

ADDITIONAL THERAPIES
- Obtain a list of all supplemental vitamins, minerals, herbs, etc., that the parent may be providing to the patient.
- Investigate if parent is following any special diets (e.g., casein/gluten-free diet in autistic spectrum disorder).

COMPLEMENTARY & ALTERNATIVE THERAPIES
- Speech therapy: Evaluate oral motor skill and safety of swallowing mechanism; perform MBSS when indicated.
- Occupational therapy: Evaluate fine motor skills, sensory processing, and posture to support feeding.
- Psychology: may identify behaviors interfering with food acceptance and recommend strategies to improve oral acceptance
- Nutrition: Perform complete nutritional assessment, including evaluation of growth parameters, identifying patient's nutrition requirements, and adequacy of current diet. The nutritionist can develop a care plan to meet patient's nutritional requirements and monitor intake and weight gain during hospitalizations.

SURGERY/OTHER PROCEDURES
- Consider gastrostomy tube placement if tube feedings for >3 months are anticipated.
- For GERD not responding to medications, consider bypassing stomach and feeding into intestine with jejunostomy tube or placement of gastrostomy tube in conjunction with Nissen fundoplication.

INPATIENT CONSIDERATIONS
Initial Stabilization
- Prior to initiation of behavioral program, ensure weight gain and growth are adequate.
- Evaluate and treat vitamin and mineral deficiencies.
- If weight-for-height ratio or BMI is <5%, inappropriate weight gain crossing down 2 percentiles on growth chart occurs, or weight loss occurs, consider initiating supplemental nasogastric tube feeds.
- If aspiration pneumonia is suspected, obtain blood cultures, chest x-ray; keep NPO and start IV fluids and antibiotics. Measure oxygen saturation and initiate supplemental oxygen if <95%.

ONGOING CARE

FOLLOW-UP RECOMMENDATIONS
Appointment with multidisciplinary feeding team, if available within reasonable geographic radius

Patient Monitoring
- Patient's weight should be checked within 2 weeks of discharge.
- Pediatrician should monitor patients with respiratory difficulties related to aspiration every 2 weeks until stable.

DIET
- Keep patient NPO if aspiration is suspected until further evaluation (MBSS) can be performed.
- Order diet appropriate for child's current level of feeding skills (i.e., accepts baby food; may trial pureed diet).
- If nutritional intake is inadequate, offer nutritional supplements, monitor calorie counts, and initiate supplemental nasogastric tube feeds if unable to meet nutritional requirements.
- Caregiver education regarding administration of supplemental tube feeds

PROGNOSIS
- Nutritional rehabilitation can be achieved with tube feedings if patient is monitored closely.
- Patients with pharyngeal dysphagia resulting in aspiration may improve over time.
- Static or degenerative neurologic conditions resulting in aspiration generally do not resolve.
- Patient demonstrating dysphagia during illness may improve when healthy.

ADDITIONAL READING

- Kral TV, Souders MC, Tompkins VH, et al. Child eating behaviors and caregiver feeding practices in children with autism spectrum disorders [published ahead of print August 11, 2014]. *Public Health Nurs*.
- Rudolph CD, Thompson LD. Feeding disorders in infants and children. *Pediatr Clin North Am*. 2002;49(1):97–112.
- Williams KE, Field DG, Seiverling L. Food refusal in children: a review of the literature. *Res Develop Disabil*. 2010;31(3):625–633.

CODES

ICD10
- R63.3 Feeding difficulties
- R13.10 Dysphagia, unspecified
- T17.928A Food in resp tract, part unsp causing oth injury, init

FAQ
- Q: What is the difference between aspiration and penetration in a swallowing disorder?
- A: Penetration occurs when food or fluid enter the trachea but remains above the vocal cords and is cleared by the patient. Aspiration occurs when the food or fluid falls below the vocal cords, thus entering the lungs.
- Q: How is a modified barium swallow study used to evaluate dysphagia?
- A: A speech therapist in conjunction with the radiologist feeds the patient a variety of textures, including thin and thickened liquids, thin honey and nectar, thick purees, and chopped food if indicated, visualizing the pathway during swallowing to determine if it moves safely into the esophagus without entering the airway. The speech therapist also will engage in therapeutic endeavors, such as repositioning the patient, to determine if they can eliminate aspiration.

FETAL ALCOHOL SYNDROME

Tracey A. McLean • Seth J. Bokser

BASICS

DESCRIPTION

- The four major features of classic fetal alcohol syndrome (FAS) are as follows:
  - CNS neurodevelopmental abnormalities
  - Facial dysmorphisms
  - Growth retardation
  - Maternal alcohol use during pregnancy.
- First described in 1973; classic FAS has since been recognized as one of the fetal alcohol spectrum disorders (FASDs), which include the following:
  - FAS, partial FAS (pFAS), alcohol-related neurodevelopmental disorder (ARND), and alcohol-related birth defects (ARBD)
  - Taken together, FASDs are three times more common than classic FAS, and the effects range from very mild symptoms to very severe.

EPIDEMIOLOGY

Incidence

- Classic FAS: 3.1 per 1,000 live births
- FASDs: 9.1 per 1,000 live births

RISK FACTORS

- Binge drinking seems to be the primary risk factor.
- The highest prevalence of reported alcohol use during pregnancy are among those who are aged 35–44 years, white, college graduates, or employed.
- Poor maternal nutrition appears to increase risk in the presence of maternal binge drinking.
- Maternal polymorphisms of the alcohol dehydrogenase gene (*ADH*): The presence of the *ADH1B*3* allele appears to protect the fetus.
- Concordance of FAS is higher in monozygotic than in dizygotic twins.

GENERAL PREVENTION

- Women who are pregnant or may become pregnant should avoid alcohol. No "safe" level of alcohol consumption has been determined during pregnancy.
- Women with alcohol addiction who are or may become pregnant should enter a treatment program.
- According to the Centers for Disease Control and Prevention (CDC), 7.6% of pregnant women reported alcohol use during the month prior to being surveyed and 1.4% reported binge drinking.
- The highest risk for FAS occurs in children whose mothers consume ≥4 drinks per occasion per week (peak blood alcohol level is more important than a lower sustained blood alcohol level).
- In the United States, Alcoholic Beverage Labeling Act passed in 1998 requires heath warning labels, including risk of alcohol consumption during pregnancy.

PATHOPHYSIOLOGY

- Malformation of the developing brain is the primary pathophysiologic event resulting in secondary neurodevelopmental pathology and facial dysmorphisms in classic FAS.
- May involve increased susceptibility to cell damage by free radicals in the developing fetus, especially in the first trimester
- Alcohol and its metabolite acetaldehyde are teratogens.

DIAGNOSIS

HISTORY

- Neurodevelopmental and behavioral symptoms. No specific neurobehavioral pattern has been defined. See below for examples of age-specific presentations.
- Fine motor function abnormalities may be present.
- Birth and subsequent growth deficit (weight, height, head circumference)
- Maternal history of alcohol use (binge drinking, average number of drinks per day, timing in pregnancy) and other drug use
- Family history
  - Neurobehavioral abnormalities may not be typical of other family members who were not exposed to alcohol prenatally.
- Neurobehavioral problems in infancy:
  - May or may not have alcohol withdrawal as newborn
  - Irritability, irregular sleep, poor feeding, hypotonia, delayed motor function
- Neurobehavioral problems in preschool and school age:
  - Hyperactivity
  - Slow verbal learning
  - Slow visual–spatial learning
  - Poor abstract thinking (planning and organizing)
  - Perseveration (inability to abandon ineffective strategies)
  - Attention problems
  - Difficulty with peer interactions
- Neurobehavioral problems in adolescence and adulthood:
  - Substance abuse
  - Criminal behavior
  - Inability to work
  - Inability to live independently

PHYSICAL EXAM

- Birth weight (≤10th percentile)
- Birth length (≤10th percentile)
- Microcephaly at birth (≤10th percentile)
- Postnatal growth deficiency persists throughout life.
- Facial manifestations include the following:
  - Short palpebral fissures (measurement from inner to outer canthus of eyes)
  - Long and smooth philtrum (area from nasal septum to vermillion border of lip)
  - Thin vermillion border (upper lip)
- Ptosis, epicanthal folds, and flat face are also common in FAS.

DIAGNOSTIC TESTS & INTERPRETATION

Neuropsychological testing

- Simple IQ tests cannot distinguish children with FAS from those with other developmental disabilities.
- No specific neurobehavioral phenotype yet defined

Lab

No laboratory marker exists for FAS.

Diagnostic Procedures/Other

Classic FAS diagnosis requires all four of the following markers.

- Facial features:
  - Short palpebral fissures (≤10th percentile)
  - Thin vermilion border upper lip (score of 4 or 5 on the lip/philtrum guide [see Astley reference])
  - Smooth philtrum (4 or 5 on lip/philtrum guide)
  - Other findings such as ptosis; maxillary hypoplasia; and short, upturned nose are not diagnostic but are commonly seen in children with FAS.
- Documentation of growth deficits
  - Height or weight ≤10th percentile at any time in patient's history
- Documentation of CNS abnormality (any 1 below)
  - Structural
    - Structural brain abnormalities (e.g., agenesis of corpus callosum, cerebellar hypoplasia)
  - Neurologic
    - Seizures, poor coordination, impaired memory, or other soft neurologic signs not attributable to postnatal insult or fever
  - Functional: performance substantially below that expected for an individual's age and circumstances, as evidenced by either
    - Global cognitive deficits (IQ or developmental delays in multiple domains) >2 standard deviations (*SD*) below the mean *OR*
    - Functional deficits 1 *SD* below the mean in at least 3 specific domains (e.g., attention, executive functioning, motor functioning, social skills, language, or specific learning disabilities)

- Maternal alcohol exposure
  - Confirmed maternal exposure to alcohol is defined as substantial regular intake or heavy episodic drinking.
  - Evidence may include self-report or that of a reliable informant, medical records showing an elevated blood alcohol level or alcohol-related medical problems (e.g., hepatic disease), and legal problems related to drinking.
  - If there is no available history, or conflicting reports, then diagnosis can be "FAS without confirmed maternal alcohol exposure."

DIFFERENTIAL DIAGNOSIS

- By physical features
  - Normal variant
  - Aarskog syndrome
  - Williams syndrome
  - Noonan syndrome
  - Brachmann-De Lange syndrome
  - Dubowitz syndrome
  - Fetal valproate syndrome
  - Fetal hydantoin syndrome
  - Maternal phenylketonuria fetal effects
  - Toluene embryopathy
- By neurobehavioral features
  - Fragile X syndrome
  - 22q11 deletion syndromes
  - Turner syndrome
  - Opitz syndrome

TREATMENT

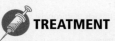

GENERAL MEASURES

- The role of the pediatrician is early identification, appropriate referrals, and development of a multidisciplinary case plan, including the pediatrician, specialists, early intervention providers, psychologists, and social and educational resources in the community to support family and child.
- Specific medical referrals should include
  - Comprehensive neuropsychological evaluation (IQ, achievement, executive function, memory, adaptive function, language, reasoning and judgment, behavior)
  - Ophthalmologic exam (consider routine screening prior to school, then every 2 years)
  - Hearing test (consider brainstem auditory evoked response [BAER] at 6–12 months)

ONGOING CARE

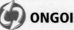

FOLLOW-UP RECOMMENDATIONS

Patient Monitoring

- Growth and nutrition in infancy: Failure to thrive is a common problem.
- Regular evaluations of vision and hearing: Problems occur at a high rate.
- As indicated by other medical/psychological problems

PROGNOSIS

- 50% have intellectual disability (IQ <70). Average IQ in individuals with FAS is in the 60s (mild mental retardation); however, a wide range of IQ exists, from 16 to 115.
- 62% have severe behavioral problems, even if a normal IQ exists.
- The major disabilities of FAS caused by the neurocognitive/neurobehavioral effects can lead to poor academic performance, legal problems, employment difficulties, and secondary mental health problems.
- Many are unable to live independently as adults.

ADDITIONAL READING

- American Academy of Pediatrics. Fetal alcohol syndrome and alcohol-related neurodevelopmental disorders. *Pediatrics*. 2000;106(2, Pt 1):358–361.
- Astley SJ, Clarren SK. Diagnosing the full spectrum of fetal-alcohol exposed individuals: introducing the 4-digit code. *Alcohol Alcohol*. 2000;35(4):400–410.
- Bertrand J, Floyd RL, Weber MK, et al; National Task Force on Fetal Alcohol Syndrome and Fetal Alcohol Effect. *Fetal Alcohol Syndrome: Guidelines for Referral and Diagnosis*. Atlanta, GA: Centers for Disease Control and Prevention; 2004. http://www.cdc.gov/ncbddd/fasd/documents/FAS_guidelines_accessible.pdf. Accessed February 14, 2015.
- Bertrand J, Floyd RL, Weber MK, et al; National Task Force on Fetal Alcohol Syndrome and Fetal Alcohol Effect. *Fetal Alcohol Syndrome: Guidelines for Referral and Diagnosis*. 3rd rev ed. Atlanta, GA: Centers for Disease Control and Prevention; 2005.
- Hoyme HE, May PA, Kalberg WO, et al. A practical clinical approach to diagnosis of fetal alcohol spectrum disorders: clarification of the 1996 Institute of Medicine criteria. *Pediatrics*. 2005;115(1):39–47.
- National Institute on Alcohol Abuse and Alcoholism. *Fetal Alcohol Exposure and the Brain*. Alcohol Alert no. 50. Bethesda, MD: National Institutes of Health; 2000.
- Riley EP, Infante MA, Warren KR. Fetal alcohol spectrum disorders: an overview. *Neuropsychol Rev*. 2011;21(2):73.
- Sampson PD, Streissguth AP, Bookstein FL, et al. Incidence of fetal alcohol syndrome and prevalence of alcohol-related neurodevelopmental disorder. *Teratology*. 1997;56(5):317–326.

CODES

ICD10

- Q86.0 Fetal alcohol syndrome (dysmorphic)
- P04.3 Newborn affected by maternal use of alcohol

FAQ

- Q: What is partial FAS?
- A: No diagnostic consensus; however, criteria include two of the key facial features, growth retardation OR CNS involvement, and confirmed prenatal alcohol exposure.
- Q: What is ARND?
- A: No diagnostic consensus; however, criteria include CNS involvement with functional impairment and onset in childhood, facial features and growth retardation not necessary (but may be present), not better explained by other conditions (teratogens, genetic, neglect), and confirmed prenatal alcohol exposure.
- Q: How much alcohol does it take to produce damage?
- A: The highest risk for FAS occurs in children whose mothers consume ≥4 drinks per occasion at least once per week. However, NO minimum safe level of alcohol consumption has been determined
- Q: Do most children with FAS have ADHD?
- A: Although hyperactivity appears to be common in FAS, many of these children are misdiagnosed as having ADHD. Instead of difficulty focusing and sustaining attention, children with FAS often have difficulty shifting attention from one task to another. Use of stimulant medication is not routinely supported, although a small proportion may respond to stimulant medication in educational settings.

FEVER AND PETECHIAE

Angela M. Statile • Craig H. Gosdin

BASICS

DESCRIPTION

- Petechiae
  - Small hemorrhages (<3 mm in size) into the superficial layers of the skin
  - Manifest as a reddish purple, macular, nonblanching skin rash
- Purpura
  - Larger skin hemorrhages (>3 mm in size)
  - Often macular like petechiae but may be raised or tender

EPIDEMIOLOGY

- Most patients (70–80%) presenting with fever and petechiae have defined or presumed viral infections, which are often caused by enteroviruses or adenovirus.
  - Parvovirus B19 may also be responsible for many cases of fever and generalized petechiae in children.
- Approximately 0.5–11% of children presenting with fever and petechiae will have an invasive bacterial disease, most commonly *Neisseria meningitidis*.
  - Infants and toddlers are at greatest risk of having an invasive bacterial infection with fever and petechiae.
  - Teenagers and young adults are most commonly affected by outbreaks of meningococcemia, presenting with fever and petechiae.
- Streptococcal pharyngitis may cause fever and petechiae in the well-appearing child.
- Other etiologies, such as acute leukemia, idiopathic thrombocytopenic purpura (ITP), and Henoch-Schönlein purpura (HSP), are responsible for a minority of cases of fever and petechiae.

GENERAL PREVENTION

- Vaccine recommendations
  - All children should complete the *Streptococcus pneumoniae* and *Haemophilus influenzae* type B immunization series that begins at 2 months of age.
  - Routine childhood immunization with meningococcal vaccine is recommended for all children at 11–12 years of age and a booster dose at 16–18 years of age.
  - Infants and children at high risk for meningococcal disease such as those with asplenia or terminal complement deficiencies should receive meningococcal vaccine as early as 2 months of age.
  - Annual immunization against influenza viruses is recommended for all children >6 months of age.
- Chemoprophylaxis is recommended for close contacts of patients with meningococcal disease. Ideally, treatment should begin within 24 hours; rifampin is the drug of choice in most children (dosing <1 month of age: 5 mg/kg PO every 12 hours × 2 days, ≥1 month of age: 10 mg/kg PO every 12 hours × 2 days). Alternatives include ceftriaxone, ciprofloxacin, and azithromycin.

PATHOPHYSIOLOGY

Petechiae may result from several different mechanisms:

- Disruption of vascular integrity—due to infections, vasculitis, or trauma
- Platelet deficiency or dysfunction—typically thrombocytopenia due to sepsis, disseminated intravascular coagulation (DIC), ITP, or leukemia
- Factor deficiencies, although these are more likely to manifest as ecchymoses or deep bleeding

DIAGNOSIS

DIFFERENTIAL DIAGNOSIS

- Viral infections (see "Etiology")
- Invasive bacterial infections
  - Most commonly *N. meningitidis*
  - Less often *Staphylococcus aureus* or other bacteria (see "Etiology")
- Streptococcal pharyngitis—due to *Streptococcus pyogenes*
- Rickettsial infections: diagnosis aided by season, history of tick bite accompanied by fever, petechiae, headache, and myalgias
- Petechiae above the nipple line may be noted after significant coughing or vomiting.
- Coining or other traumatic causes
- Acute leukemias: diagnosis aided by clinical findings of pallor, adenopathy, hepatosplenomegaly, and laboratory findings
- ITP: diagnosis aided by findings of mucous membrane bleeding and isolated thrombocytopenia on laboratory testing
- HSP: diagnosis aided by clinical findings consistent with HSP, including palpable purpura on dependent areas such as the buttocks and lower extremities, often without fever
- Endocarditis: diagnosis aided by bacteremia and a history of congenital heart disease, cardiac surgery, or rheumatic fever

ETIOLOGY

Petechiae, when accompanied by fever, most often have an infectious cause. Multiple organisms are associated with fever and petechiae. Less commonly, fever and petechiae may be caused by other entities such as acute leukemia, ITP, HSP, and bacterial endocarditis.

- Bacterial
  - *N. meningitidis*
  - *S. pneumoniae*
  - *H. influenzae* type B
  - *S. aureus*
  - *S. pyogenes*
  - *Escherichia coli*
- Viral
  - Enterovirus
  - Adenovirus
  - Influenza
  - Parainfluenza
  - Parvovirus B19
  - Epstein-Barr virus (EBV)
  - Rubella
  - Respiratory syncytial virus
  - Hepatitis viruses
- Rickettsial diseases
  - *Rickettsia rickettsii*
  - Ehrlichiosis

ALERT

Unsuspected invasive bacterial disease is the most common pitfall in the differential diagnosis of fever and petechiae. A thorough history and physical exam accompanied by laboratory testing, a period of close observation, and empiric antimicrobial therapy may minimize missed serious diagnoses.

HISTORY

Important historical factors to obtain include the following:

- Age of the child
- Any underlying immunodeficiency
- Immunizations received
- Exposure to infectious contacts, particularly *N. meningitidis*
- Duration and height of fever
- Duration and progression of rash
- Excessive coughing or vomiting
- Pallor or other bleeding
- Level of activity, excess fatigue
- Travel or history of tick bites
- History of trauma in location of rash

PHYSICAL EXAM

- Important components of exam:
  - Vital signs, noting tachycardia, hypotension, or delayed capillary refill
  - Mental status
  - Meningismus/nuchal rigidity
  - Character of rash: petechiae or purpura, body distribution, number of lesions, progression during exam
- Important findings suggesting specific diagnoses:
  - **Finding:** Pallor, adenopathy, organomegaly
  - *Significance*: May suggest leukemia, EBV infection
  - **Finding:** Mucous membrane bleeding
  - *Significance*: May suggest thrombocytopenia, such as with ITP
  - **Finding:** Headache, myalgias, centripetal rash distribution
  - *Significance*: May suggest Rocky Mountain spotted fever

DIAGNOSTIC TESTS & INTERPRETATION

Most children with fever and petechiae require laboratory testing. Consider obtaining a CBC with differential, C-reactive protein (CRP), and a blood culture even in non–toxic-appearing children.

- Consider rapid antigen testing for group A *Streptococcus* and throat culture if with signs of pharyngitis.
- Children who are ill-appearing may warrant lumbar puncture for cerebrospinal fluid (CSF) studies and coagulation studies including prothrombin time (PT), partial thromboplastin time (PTT), and DIC screen.
- Viral testing, including cultures, serology, and antibody immunofluorescence, is not routinely required and may be ordered at the discretion of the managing practitioner based on exposures, need for specific therapeutic interventions, admission to the hospital, and severity of illness.
- Although no one factor is 100% sensitive in identifying children with invasive bacterial disease, a constellation of factors is useful in identifying children with fever and petechiae in whom invasive bacterial disease is unlikely:
  – Multiple studies have demonstrated that well-appearing children with a normal WBC count (between 5,000 and 15,000 cells/microliter), a normal absolute neutrophil count (between 1,500 and 9,000 cells/microliter), an absolute band count <500 cells/microliter, and petechiae limited to above the nipple line are exceedingly unlikely to have an invasive bacterial infection. A CRP <6 mg/L has also been shown to have a high negative predictive value for ruling out invasive bacterial infection.

TREATMENT

MEDICATION

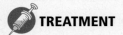

- Empiric antibiotic use should be decided on a case-by-case basis. Due to the high morbidity and mortality of *N. meningitidis*, the most likely bacterial pathogen in this circumstance, empiric ceftriaxone should be strongly considered in children with fever and petechiae who are not at low risk for bacterial infection.
- 3rd-generation cephalosporins such as ceftriaxone and cefotaxime are effective against most bacterial pathogens causing fever and petechiae.
- Doxycycline should be administered if rickettsial disease is considered.
- Vancomycin should be added to the regimen for children with suspected bacterial meningitis to cover penicillin and cephalosporin-resistant strains of *S. pneumoniae*.

INPATIENT CONSIDERATIONS

Initial Stabilization

- The management of children who are ill-appearing and have meningismus or purpura consists of a full sepsis evaluation, admission to the hospital with parenteral antibiotics, and fluids and vasoactive infusions to maintain normal hemodynamics.
- Because sporadic as opposed to epidemic cases of meningococcemia appear to occur in children in the first 2 years of life, and these children have less competent immune systems in fighting encapsulated organisms, full sepsis evaluation and admission for all children in this young age group are recommended.
- The well-appearing child with fever and petechiae and a positive streptococcal antigen test and an illness compatible with streptococcal pharyngitis may be treated as an outpatient with antistreptococcal antibiotics.
- After a several-hour period of observation, children who remain well-appearing, are not tachycardic, have no progression of petechiae, and have normal lab studies may be considered for management as outpatients.

ONGOING CARE

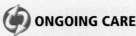

FOLLOW-UP RECOMMENDATIONS

Patient Monitoring

- Children managed as outpatients:
  – Give instructions to return immediately for progression of rash or worsening illness.
  – Follow-up in 12–18 hours.
  – Monitor cultures closely.
- Most children with viral causes have little progression of their petechiae and are clinically better within several days with the resolution of fever.

PROGNOSIS

- Depends on the underlying cause
- Because most cases of fever and petechiae are caused by viral infections, particularly enteroviruses and adenovirus, the prognosis is excellent.
- Case fatality rate of meningococcemia is 10–14%.

COMPLICATIONS

- Related to the underlying cause
- Most common complications of invasive bacterial disease causing fever and petechiae include sepsis and meningitis.
- Serious sequelae from *N. meningitidis* occur in 11–19% of patients and include neurologic deficits such as hearing loss, digit or limb loss, and skin scarring.

ADDITIONAL READING

- Brayer AF, Humiston SG. Invasive meningococcal disease in childhood. *Pediatr Rev*. 2011;32(4):152–161.
- Klinkhammer MD, Colletti JE. Pediatric myth: fever and petechiae. *CJEM*. 2008;10(5):479–482.
- Wells LC, Smith JC, Weston VC, et al. The child with a non-blanching rash: how likely is meningococcal disease? *Arch Dis Child*. 2001;85(3):218–222.

CODES

ICD10

- R50.9 Fever, unspecified
- R23.3 Spontaneous ecchymoses
- D69.2 Other nonthrombocytopenic purpura

FAQ

- Q: What are the most common causes of fever and petechiae in children?
- A: Viruses are the most common overall cause of fever and petechiae in children. The most common invasive bacterial disease causing fever and petechiae in children is *N. meningitidis*.
- Q: Is there ever a role for outpatient management of children with fever and petechiae?
- A: Practitioners may consider outpatient management in well-appearing children >2 years of age with the following criteria after a period of close observation in which they have normal vital signs and no progression of petechiae:
  – A normal WBC count (between 5,000 and 15,000 cells/microliter)
  – A normal absolute neutrophil count (between 1,500 and 9,000 cells/microliter)
  – An absolute band count <500 cells/microliter
  – A CRP <6 mg/L

FEVER OF UNKNOWN ORIGIN

Samir S. Shah

BASICS

DESCRIPTION

Fever of unknown origin (FUO) implies

- A febrile illness (38.3°C on multiple occasions)
- Present for >14 days
- No apparent source despite careful history taking, physical exam, and preliminary lab studies

DIAGNOSIS

DIFFERENTIAL DIAGNOSIS

FUO is more often an unusual presentation of a common disease than a common presentation of an unusual disease. Possible causes include the following:

- **Common infectious causes**
  - Respiratory infections (otitis media, mastoiditis, sinusitis, pneumonia, pharyngitis, peritonsillar/retropharyngeal abscess)
  - Systemic viral syndrome
  - Infectious mononucleosis (Epstein-Barr virus [EBV], cytomegalovirus [CMV])
  - Urinary tract infection (UTI)
  - Bone or joint infection
  - Enteric infection (*Salmonella*, *Yersinia enterocolitica*, *Yersinia pseudotuberculosis*, *Campylobacter jejuni*)
  - Cat-scratch disease
- **Less common infectious causes**
  - Tuberculosis (TB)
  - Lyme disease
  - Rickettsial disease (Rocky Mountain spotted fever, ehrlichiosis, anaplasmosis)
  - Malaria
  - CNS infection (bacterial or viral meningoencephalitis, intracranial abscess)
  - Dental or periodontal abscess
  - Subacute bacterial endocarditis (SBE)
  - HIV infection
  - Acute rheumatic fever
- **Other infectious causes**
  - Q fever
  - Brucellosis
  - Toxoplasmosis
  - Syphilis
  - Parvovirus B19
  - Endemic fungi (histoplasmosis, blastomycosis, coccidioidomycosis)
  - Psittacosis
  - Typhoid (*Salmonella* spp.)
  - Chronic meningococcemia
- **Possible noninfectious causes**
  - Collagen vascular disease (systemic juvenile idiopathic arthritis [JIA], systemic lupus erythematosus, dermatomyositis, sarcoidosis, vasculitis syndrome)
  - Malignancy
  - Kawasaki syndrome
  - Inflammatory bowel disease (IBD)
  - Drug fever
  - Hyperthyroidism
  - Factitious fever or Munchausen syndrome by proxy
  - Centrally mediated fever
  - Periodic fever syndrome
  - Kikuchi-Fujimoto disease (histiocytic necrotizing lymphadenitis)

ETIOLOGY

Etiology has changed as the use of more sensitive tests (e.g., MRI, polymerase chain reaction [PCR] tests) permits earlier detection of many conditions that caused FUO in the past. Fever resolves in 40–60% of children without identification of a specific cause.

APPROACH TO THE PATIENT

Find the cause of the fever and begin treatment of the underlying illness.

- **Phase 1**
  - Document fever.
  - Thorough history and physical exam
  - Determine whether constitutional symptoms (e.g., growth failure, developmental arrest) suggest a serious underlying disease.
  - Create broad differential diagnosis.
  - Begin initial laboratory evaluation while tailoring the cadence of evaluation to patient's severity of illness.
- **Phase 2**
  - Begin invasive studies to seek rarer forms of fever, such as lymphoma, brucellosis, and SBE, only if clinically indicated.
- **Phase 3**
  - Reexamine patient, consider additional testing, and reconsider causes such as systemic JIA, sarcoidosis, and factitious fever.

Repeat history and physical exam combined with the results of previous testing should guide the subsequent evaluation.

HISTORY

Initial studies should include a CBC, liver function tests, blood culture, urinalysis, urine culture, stool culture, and stool ova and parasite testing.

- **Question:** Temperatures and how they were measured (tympanic, oral, axillary, rectal)?
- *Significance*:
  - As many as 50% of children referred for evaluation of FUO have multiple unrelated infections, parental misinterpretation of normal temperature variation, or complete absence of fever at time of evaluation.
  - Parents are sometimes told to add a 1–2°F "correction" onto a temperature measured in the axilla to better approximate the core temperature. Such practices may further cloud the evaluation of the febrile child.
- **Question:** Ethnicity?
- *Significance*: Some hereditary periodic fever syndromes have ethnic predilection. Consider familial Mediterranean fever (Armenian, Arab, Turkish, Sephardic Jew), hyper-IgD syndrome (Dutch, French), and tumor necrosis factor receptor–associated periodic fever syndrome (TRAPS) (Irish, Scottish)
- **Question:** Exposure to animals?
- *Significance*
  - Household exposures including pets and rodents
  - Recreational activities (e.g., hunting)
  - Household contacts with occupational exposure to animals
  - Consider cat-scratch disease, brucellosis, tularemia, leptospirosis, and lymphocytic choriomeningitis virus (from mice)
- **Question:** Ingestion of raw meat, fish, or unpasteurized milk?
- *Significance*: Trichinosis, brucellosis
- **Question:** Travel history, including past residence?
- *Significance*: Malaria, endemic fungi (e.g., coccidioidomycosis in Southwest, blastomycosis in Southeast, histoplasmosis in Midwest), typhoid (Indian subcontinent), TB
- **Question:** Pica or dirt ingestion?
- *Significance*: *Toxocara canis* or *Toxoplasma gondii* infection
- **Question:** Change in behavior or activity?
- *Significance*: Brain tumor, TB, EBV, Rocky Mountain spotted fever
- **Question:** Pattern of fever?
- *Significance*: May correlate with underlying cause. A fever diary kept by the parent or caretaker may provide more objective documentation of the fever pattern than simple recall.
- **Question:** Medications (including OTC medications and eyedrops)?
- *Significance*: Drug fever, atropine-induced fever, methylphenidate, and antibiotics (especially penicillin, cephalosporins, and sulfonamides)
- **Question:** Well-water ingestion?
- *Significance*: Giardiasis

PHYSICAL EXAM

- **Finding:** Impaired weight gain or linear growth?
- *Significance*: Collagen vascular disease, malignancy, IBD
- **Finding:** Toxic appearance?
- *Significance*: Kawasaki syndrome
- **Finding:** Conjunctivitis?
- *Significance*: Kawasaki syndrome (limbic sparing), adenovirus, measles
- **Finding:** Ophthalmologic exam?
- *Significance*: Papilledema—consider CNS mass lesion; uveitis—consider TB, systemic lupus erythematosus, Kawasaki syndrome, and sarcoidosis
- **Finding:** Sinus tenderness, nasal discharge, or halitosis?
- *Significance*: Sinusitis
- **Finding:** Pharyngitis?
- *Significance*: Kawasaki syndrome, EBV, CMV
- **Finding:** Tachypnea?
- *Significance*: SBE, pneumonia
- **Finding:** Rales?
- *Significance*: Histoplasmosis, sarcoidosis, coccidioidomycosis
- **Finding:** Cardiac murmur, gallop, or friction rub?
- *Significance*: SBE, acute rheumatic fever, pericarditis
- **Finding:** Hepatosplenomegaly?
- *Significance*: Hepatitis, EBV, CMV, ehrlichiosis, anaplasmosis
- **Finding:** Rectal abnormalities?
- *Significance*: Pelvic abscess, IBD
- **Finding:** Arthritis?
- *Significance*: JIA, IBD, acute rheumatic fever
- **Finding:** Bony tenderness?
- *Significance*: JIA, leukemia, osteomyelitis

DIAGNOSTIC TESTS & INTERPRETATION

The laboratory evaluation for a child with FUO should be directed toward the most likely diagnostic possibilities. Consider the following initial studies:

- **Test:** CBC with differential and careful examination of WBC morphology
- *Significance*: Kawasaki syndrome, cyclic neutropenia, malignancy, ehrlichiosis, anaplasmosis (morulae in WBC cytoplasm), and babesiosis
- **Test:** ESR, C-reactive protein, or procalcitonin
- *Significance*: Collagen vascular disease, IBD, occult infection. ESR is generally normal in drug fever and central fever.
- **Test:** Blood cultures
- *Significance*: Endocarditis, salmonellosis, other bloodstream infections
- **Test:** Urinalysis and urine culture
- *Significance*: UTI, Kawasaki syndrome (sterile pyuria)
- **Test:** Tuberculin skin test (by purified protein derivative)
- *Significance*: TB
- **Test:** Stool bacterial culture and examination for ova and parasites
- *Significance*: *Salmonella*, *Giardia*
- **Test:** Specific antibody testing
- *Significance*: Depending on clinical suspicion, consider the following:
  - First line: Streptococcal enzyme titers (antistreptolysin O, anti-DNase B); EBV; CMV; cat-scratch disease; Lyme disease; hepatitis A, B, or C; or HIV (by PCR)
  - Second line: Rocky Mountain spotted fever; ehrlichiosis/anaplasmosis, toxoplasmosis, brucellosis, Q fever, leptospirosis, tularemia, dengue fever
- **Test:** Viral testing of nasopharyngeal aspirates
- *Significance:* systemic viral syndrome (adenovirus)
- **Test:** Evaluation for immune deficiency
- *Significance*: underlying predisposition
- **Test:** Bone marrow examination and culture
- *Significance: Salmonella* infection, *Mycobacterium avium* complex, histoplasmosis, brucellosis, malignancy
- **Test:** Lumbar puncture
- *Significance:* CNS infection

Imaging

- Guided by history, physical examination, and epidemiologic factors; indiscriminate use of imaging not likely to be helpful.
- Sinus CT: sinusitis
- Chest radiograph: TB, endemic fungi, pneumonia
- Chest and/or abdominal CT scan: TB, liver abscess, hepatosplenic cat-scratch disease
- Pelvic or extremity MRI: osteomyelitis, pyomyositis
- Gallium or bone scan: osteomyelitis, malignancy

ADDITIONAL READING

- Chow A, Robinson JL. Fever of unknown origin in children: a systematic review. *World J Pediatr*. 2011;7(1):5–10.
- Drenth JPH, van der Meer JWM. Hereditary periodic fever. *N Engl J Med*. 2001;345(24):1748–1757.
- Gattorno M, Caorsi R, Meini A, et al. Differentiating PFAPA syndrome from monogenic periodic fevers. *Pediatrics*. 2009;124(4):e721–e728.
- Jacobs RF, Schutze GE. *Bartonella henselae* as a cause of prolonged fever and fever of unknown origin in children. *Clin Infect Dis*. 1998;26(1):80–84.
- Talano JM, Katz BZ. Long-term follow-up of children with fever of unknown origin. *Clin Pediatr*. 2000;39(12):715–717.

CODES

ICD10

R50.9 Fever, unspecified

FAQ

- Q: Do all of the mentioned tests need to be performed?
- A: A "shotgun" approach to testing is rarely useful in making the diagnosis, and unanticipated abnormalities (e.g., false-positives) may lead to additional invasive tests with potential for harm.
- Q: Is hospitalization required for the diagnosis of FUO?
- A: Many tests, including MRI, can now be performed in the outpatient setting. Hospitalization is not routinely required for diagnosis but should be considered in patients who appear ill, have progression of symptoms, or when fever needs to be documented.
- Q: How is cat-scratch disease acquired?
- A: Cat-scratch disease, caused by *Bartonella henselae*, can be acquired through cat (usually kittens or young cats) scratches or licks. Rarely, dogs may transmit the organism. If the family does not own a kitten or young cat, remember to ask about other sources of exposure (e.g., friends, family, school trips).

FLOPPY INFANT SYNDROME

Mayada A. Helal • Ronald D. Cohn

BASICS

DESCRIPTION

- "Floppy infant" refers to the newborn/infant presenting at birth or early in life with hypotonia, a symptom of diminished tone of skeletal muscles associated with decreased resistance of muscles to passive stretching.
- Hypotonia can be caused by abnormalities of the CNS (central hypotonia), peripheral neuromuscular system (peripheral hypotonia), or combined abnormality involving both (combined hypotonia).
- Nonspecific transient hypotonia occurs in nonneurologic conditions and may suggest gastrointestinal (GI), cardiac, pulmonary, infectious, renal, or endocrine disease.

EPIDEMIOLOGY

No comprehensive prevalence known owing to presence of hypotonia as a feature of many distinct disorders; overall, central hypotonia is more common than peripheral hypotonia.

RISK FACTORS

Genetics

Substantial proportion (>50%) of infantile hypotonia cases accounted for by genetic-metabolic disorders.

ETIOLOGY

Causes may be divided into two major categories:

- Central: hypotonia with decreased alertness, developmental delay, and lack of or minimal weakness; caused by upper motor neuron defect
- Peripheral: hypotonia with profound weakness, paucity of antigravity movements, decreased or absent deep tendon reflexes (DTRs), and visual alertness; caused by lower motor neuron defect (i.e., disorders of anterior horn cell, peripheral nerve, neuromuscular junction, or skeletal muscle)

COMMONLY ASSOCIATED CONDITIONS

- Respiratory problems (apnea/hypoventilation)
- Feeding/swallowing difficulties
- Hip dislocation/contractures/joint laxity
- Seizure disorder
- Cognitive/developmental delay
- Hypersomnolence

DIAGNOSIS

History and physical exam findings used to categorize patients as having central, peripheral, or combined hypotonia.

HISTORY

- Pregnancy and delivery
  - Pregnancy
    - Maternal illness
    - Drug or teratogen exposure
    - Abnormalities on prenatal ultrasound
    - Polyhydramnios (poor prenatal swallow)
    - Reduced fetal movements (neuromuscular disorders)
  - Delivery
    - Gestational age and presentation
    - Birth trauma, anoxia, or complications
    - Shortened umbilical cord
    - Low Apgar scores
    - Maternal perinatal infection
- Medical history
  - Seizures
  - Apnea
  - Feeding difficulties
  - Review of systems for associated malformations or health conditions
  - Delayed motor milestones
  - Delayed social, fine motor, or language milestones point to CNS defect.
- Course of hypotonia
  - Age at onset
  - Improved or worsened
- Family history
  - Parental consanguinity
  - Three-generation pedigree specifically inquiring about history of neuromuscular disease, birth defects, intellectual disability, and recurrent infantile deaths

PHYSICAL EXAM

Exam findings will help determine if hypotonia is suggestive of an upper motor neuron versus a lower motor neuron problem or both. Perform the following:

- General physical exam
  - Dysmorphic features (may lead to particular syndromic diagnosis)
  - Alertness: Infants with neuromuscular disease are typically alert.
  - Poor spontaneous movements
  - Abnormal head size and/or shape
  - High-arched palate (neuromuscular disorders)
  - Tongue fasciculations (anterior horn cell)
  - Large tongue (storage disorders)
  - Ophthalmologic exam: cataracts (peroxisomal disorders), pigmentary retinopathy (peroxisomal disorders), cherry red spot (storage disorders), lens dislocation (sulfite oxidase/molybdenum cofactor deficiency)
  - Abnormal fat pads, inverted nipples (congenital disorders of glycosylation)
  - Cardiac enlargement and signs of cardiac failure (Pompe disease)
  - Visceral enlargement (storage disorders)
  - Arthrogryposis (central, neuromuscular, or connective tissue disorders)
  - Hip dislocation (intrauterine hypotonia)
  - Joint laxity (connective tissue disorders)
- Neurologic exam
  - Strength
    - Low-pitched or progressively weaker cry
    - Poor suck
    - Paucity of facial expression ("myopathic" facies) indicates facial weakness (myotonic dystrophy, congenital muscular dystrophy, congenital myopathies).
    - Ptosis and external ophthalmoplegia (congenital myasthenic syndromes, congenital myopathies, and congenital muscular dystrophies)
    - Regional strength differences: Spinal muscular atrophy (SMA) spares diaphragm, face muscles, and pelvic sphincters. Neuropathies present with distal limb weakness and proximal sparing. Myasthenic syndromes affect bulbar and oculomotor muscles.
  - Muscle tone
    - Abnormal resting posture (abducted, externally rotated legs, flaccid arms) and prominent head lag with pull-to-sit
    - Fisting indicates spasticity.
    - Abnormal posture and tone in supine position, ventral and horizontal suspension, and traction
    - Elbow may easily extend beyond midsternum (scarf sign).
    - Generalized hypotonia with increased tone in thumb adductors, wrist pronators, and hip adductors: early cerebral palsy
    - Fatigability: cardinal feature of myasthenic syndromes but may occur in other neuromuscular diseases
  - DTRs
    - Hyperreflexia implies central dysfunction.
    - Diminished DTRs in proportion to degree of weakness in myopathic diseases
    - Absent DTRs in setting of minimal weakness typical of neuropathic disease
- Examination of the mother
  - Signs of myotonia (myotonic dystrophy)
    - Handgrip myotonia (inability to release handgrip quickly)
    - Percussion myotonia (inability to release muscle tapped with reflex hammer), including tongue myotonia, a more reproducible feature than handgrip myotonia
    - Action myotonia (delayed muscle relaxation after voluntary contraction)

DIAGNOSTIC TESTS & INTERPRETATION

Lab

- Initial tests may include the following:
  - Electrolytes (including Ca and Mg)
  - Thyroid function tests
  - Creatine kinase (normal in central, may be high in peripheral or combined cases)
  - Arterial blood gas
- Toxoplasmosis, other viruses, rubella, cytomegalovirus, or herpes (TORCH) screen; blood, urine, and CSF cultures (infection)
- Screen for inborn error of metabolism:
  - Ammonia (high in urea cycle defects, organic acidemias, fatty acid oxidation disorders)
  - Lactate in blood, urine, CSF (high in carbohydrate metabolism and mitochondrial disorders)
  - Quantitative amino acid analysis in blood and urine (aminoacidopathies)
  - Plasma acylcarnitine profiles and urine organic acid analysis (organic acidemias, fatty acid oxidation defects)
  - Plasma very-long-chain fatty acids (peroxisomal disorders)
  - Uric acid (low in molybdenum cofactor deficiency)
  - Transferrin isoelectric focusing (abnormal pattern seen in congenital disorders of glycosylation)
  - 7-dehydrocholesterol (high in Smith-Lemli-Opitz syndrome)
  - WBC lysosomal enzyme assays
  - Urine GAA/GMT(creatine deficiency disorders)
  - Urine purine/pyrimidine (purine/pyrimidine metabolism disorders)
  - CSF neurotransmitters
  - Stools for *Clostridium* toxin when botulism suspected (endemic in Pennsylvania, some Northwestern states)
- Molecular studies
  - Karyotype (Down syndrome)
  - Microarray/SNP array (microdeletion/microduplication syndromes)
  - DNA methylation/MS-MLPA (Prader-Willi/Angelman syndrome)
  - DNA-based molecular testing
  - Exome sequencing

Imaging

- MRI for structural brain abnormalities; CT for intracranial calcifications
- Magnetic resonance spectroscopy (MRS): assesses neuronal integrity (*N*-acetylaspartate [NAA] peaks), intracerebral accumulation of unusual metabolites (lactate, glycine), or deficiency of a key metabolite (creatine)
- Muscle imaging: used in some centers to delineate a neuromuscular problem
- Abdominal/pelvic ultrasound: Assess other organ involvement.

Diagnostic Procedures/Other

- Evaluation of vision and hearing
- Echocardiography
- Anticholinesterase administration in suspected myasthenia may be diagnostic.
- Electromyography (EMG) and nerve conduction velocity: useful tools to assess the lower motor unit and localize involved site
- EEG: if seizures are suspected
- Skin biopsy: for lysosomal enzyme assay in fibroblasts and electron microscopy for abnormal organelles, inclusions, or storage material (Pompe disease)
- Muscle biopsy: for histopathology, electron microscopy and respiratory chain studies (congenital myopathies, storage myopathies [Pompe disease], or muscular dystrophies)

DIFFERENTIAL DIAGNOSIS

Generalized nonneurologic conditions including the following:

- Acute systemic disorders
  - Sepsis
  - Trauma
  - Malnutrition
  - GI obstruction or bleed
  - Toxic (hyperbilirubinemia, maternal sedative, analgesic, and/or anesthetic exposure)
- Chronic systemic disorders
  - Congenital heart disease
  - Endocrinopathies (hypothyroidism, rickets, hypercalcemia)
  - Renal tubular acidosis
  - Cystic fibrosis
  - Malabsorption
  - Connective tissue disorders
    - Ehlers-Danlos syndrome
    - Marfan syndrome
    - Loeys-Dietz syndrome
    - Osteogenesis imperfecta
    - Chondrodysplasia
    - Benign joint laxity

Neurologic diagnoses including the following:

- Central hypotonia
  - Disorders involving cerebral cortex, cerebellum, and brainstem
    - Structural brain abnormalities (lissencephaly, holoprosencephaly)
    - Hypoxic-ischemic encephalopathy
    - Intracranial hemorrhage
    - Infections (meningitis, encephalitis)
  - Chromosomal disorders
    - Down syndrome
    - Williams syndrome
    - Prader-Willi syndrome
    - Angelman syndrome
  - Single-gene disorders
    - Fragile X syndrome
    - Rett/Rett-like syndrome
    - PTEN-related disorders
    - Smith-Lemli-Opitz syndrome
    - Peroxisomal disorders (Zellweger syndrome, infantile Refsum, neonatal adrenoleukodystrophy)
    - Congenital disorders of glycosylation
    - Creatine deficiency disorders
    - Purine/pyrimidine metabolism disorders
  - Disorders of spinal cord
    - Myelodysplasias (meningomyeloceles, diplomyelia, diastematomyelia)
  - Benign congenital hypotonia: mild transient hypotonia without dysmorphology; weakness; or other neurologic, physical, or laboratory abnormalities
- Peripheral hypotonia
  - Disorders of anterior horn cell including the following:
    - Spinal muscular atrophy (SMA)
    - SMA with respiratory distress (SMARD)
    - Arthrogryposis multiplex congenita
    - Pompe disease (glycogen storage type II)
    - Neonatal poliomyelitis
  - Disorders of peripheral nerve
    - Dejerine-Sottas disease
    - Guillain-Barré syndrome
    - Charcot-Marie-Tooth disease
    - Familial dysautonomia
  - Disorders of neuromuscular junction
    - Myasthenia gravis (congenital, transient)
    - Infantile botulism
    - Toxic (hypermagnesemia, antibiotics [especially aminoglycosides], nondepolarizing neuromuscular blockers)
  - Disorders of muscle
    - Congenital myotonic dystrophy
    - Congenital muscular dystrophies
    - Congenital structural myopathies: central core, nemaline, centronuclear myopathy
    - Metabolic myopathies (mitochondrial and storage disorders)
    - Organic aciduria (Barth syndrome)
    - Fatty acid oxidation disorders
- Combined hypotonia
  - Dystroglycanopathies
  - Leukodystrophies (Canavan disease, Pelizaeus-Merzbacher disease)
  - Marinesco-Sjögren syndrome
  - Mitochondrial encephalomyopathies

TREATMENT

MEDICATION

- Anticholinesterase inhibitors and 3,4-diaminopyridine in congenital myasthenic syndromes
- IV immunoglobulin and plasmapheresis have been used in treatment of infants with Guillain-Barré syndrome.

ADDITIONAL TREATMENT

General Measures

- Address apnea, hypoventilation, hypoxia:
  - Intubation or positive pressure devices may be required.
  - Chest physiotherapy, antibiotics, bronchodilators, and oxygen may be needed.
  - Hypermagnesemia can cause apnea.
  - Weak infants in car seats may be at risk for acute respiratory problems.
- Underlying toxic or metabolic causes should be addressed and treated appropriately.

COMPLEMENTARY & ALTERNATIVE THERAPIES

- Physical therapy
  - May help maintain maximum muscle function and reduce secondary deformities
  - Orthopedic consultation to evaluate hips and contractures
- Occupational therapy
- Speech therapy

SURGERY/OTHER PROCEDURES

Surgical intervention in later childhood to correct primary as well as secondary deformities

INPATIENT CONSIDERATIONS

Admission Criteria

Respiratory insufficiency, feeding intolerance, failure to thrive, metabolic abnormality

ONGOING CARE

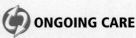

FOLLOW-UP RECOMMENDATIONS

Individualized multidisciplinary care including specialists in neurology, pulmonology, orthopedics, development, physiotherapy, and nutrition; attention to vision and hearing; as well as psychosocial support to caregivers/families

DIET

Feeding and swallowing difficulties may necessitate nutritional supplementation and/or feeding tube placement.

PROGNOSIS

Many of the paralytic hypotonias are quite variable in their clinical course. Severity of disease depends on underlying cause and associated respiratory and nutritional factors.

COMPLICATIONS

- Respiratory insufficiency/recurrent pneumonia
- Orthopedic deformities
- Poor nutritional status

ADDITIONAL READING

- Bodensteiner JB. The evaluation of the hypotonic infant. *Semin Pediatr Neurol*. 2008;15(1):10–20.
- Harris SR. Congenital hypotonia: clinical and developmental assessment. *Dev Med Child Neurol*. 2008;50(12):889–892.
- Lisi E, Cohn R. Genetic evaluation of the pediatric patient with hypotonia: perspective from a hypotonia specialty clinic and review of the literature. *Dev Med Child Neurol*. 2011;53(7):586–599.
- Peredo DE, Hannibal MC. The floppy infant: evaluation of hypotonia. *Pediatr Rev*. 2009;30(9):e66–e76. 19726697.
- Prasad A, Prasad C. Genetic evaluation of the floppy infant. *Semin Fetal Neonatal Med*. 2011;16(2):99–108.

CODES

ICD10

P94.2 Congenital hypotonia

FAQ

- Q: By what age should one expect resolution of benign congenital hypotonia?
- A: Hypotonia typically resolves by the time the infant is walking, up to 18 months of age.
- Q: What clinical sign can help distinguish between SMA and infantile botulism?
- A: Tongue fasciculations are seen in SMA. Also, decreased pupillary light reflex is seen in botulism.

F

FOOD ALLERGY

Jackie P-D. Garrett • Terri Brown-Whitehorn

BASICS

DESCRIPTION

Food allergy has recently been defined as "an adverse health effect arising from a specific immune response that occurs reproducibly on exposure to a given food." Most commonly, the protein component of the food is responsible for the adverse immunologic response.

- Classifications of food allergies:
  - IgE mediated, including
    - Anaphylaxis
    - Acute urticaria
    - Oral allergy syndrome
  - Non–IgE mediated (cell mediated), including
    - Food protein–induced enterocolitis syndrome (FPIES)
    - Food protein–induced allergic proctocolitis
    - Celiac disease
  - Mixed IgE and non–IgE mediated, including
    - Atopic dermatitis
    - Eosinophilic gastroenteropathies (eosinophilic esophagitis, eosinophilic gastroenteritis)
- Most common IgE-mediated food allergies:
  - Children
    - Milk
    - Egg
    - Soy
    - Peanut
    - Wheat
    - Fish
  - Adults
    - Peanuts
    - Tree nuts
    - Fish
    - Shellfish
- Most common non–IgE-mediated food allergies associated with food protein enterocolitis and proctocolitis:
  - Milk
  - Soy
  - Rice
  - Oat
  - Barley
  - Chicken

EPIDEMIOLOGY

Food-induced anaphylaxis is the most common cause of anaphylactic reactions treated in emergency departments in the United States. The prevalence of food allergy has increased over the past 10–20 years.

Prevalence

- 5% of children <5 years of age, 4% of teens and adults
- Nearly 2.5% of infants have hypersensitivity reactions to cow's milk during 1st year (½ of these cases are thought to actually represent GI diseases); outgrown by most (80%) by 5 years of age.
- 1.6% have egg allergy by 2.5 years (based on population-based studies); 66% of children outgrow egg allergy by 7 years of age.
- 0.6% of U.S. population have peanut allergy.
- 37% of children <5 years of age with moderate to severe atopic dermatitis have a food allergy.
- 34–49% of children with food allergy have asthma.
- 33–40% of children with food allergy have allergic rhinitis.
- Fatal and near-fatal reactions are associated with uncontrolled asthma.

RISK FACTORS

- Genetic
- Family history
- Presence of atopic dermatitis
- Other unknown factors suspected

ETIOLOGY

- Oral tolerance to food proteins believed to develop through T-cell anergy or induction of regulatory T cells. Food hypersensitivity develops when oral tolerance fails to develop or breaks down.
- IgE mediated: T cells induce B cells to produce IgE antibodies that initially bind on the surface of mast cells and basophils; when reexposed, the food protein binds to IgE antibodies, leading to degranulation of those cells and release of histamine and other chemical mediators.
- Non–IgE mediated (cell mediated): T cells react to protein-inducing proinflammatory cytokines, leading to inflammatory cell infiltrates and increased vascular permeability. These factors lead to subacute and chronic responses primarily affecting the GI tract.
- Mixed IgE and non–IgE mediated: Eosinophilic esophagitis and eosinophilic gastroenteropathy are characterized by eosinophilic infiltration of intestinal wall, occasionally reaching to serosa.

COMMONLY ASSOCIATED CONDITIONS

- Asthma (4-fold more likely)
- Allergic rhinitis (2.4-fold more likely)
- Other atopic diseases
- Dermatitis herpetiformis (celiac)

DIAGNOSIS

Varies depending on the individual and the type of food hypersensitivity (see Table for symptoms of specific illnesses)

- IgE mediated
  - Urticaria
  - Angioedema
  - Immediate GI reactions (emesis, cramping, etc.)
  - Oral allergy syndrome
  - Rhinitis
  - Anaphylaxis (hypotension, dyspnea, dysphonia, wheezing, coughing, angioedema)
  - Nausea, abdominal pain, colic, and vomiting develop within 2 hours of ingesting offending foods.
  - Diarrhea: develops within 2–6 hours
- Mixed IgE and non–IgE (cell mediated)
  - Eosinophilic gastroenteropathy
    - Weight loss (key feature), pain, emesis, failure to thrive (FTT), anorexia
    - Some infants have a large protein-losing enteropathy component causing low serum albumin and hypogammaglobulinemia.
  - Eosinophilic esophagitis
    - Dysphagia
    - Food impaction
    - Intermittent vomiting
    - Food refusal
    - Abdominal pain
    - Irritability
    - Failure to respond to reflux medication
    - FTT
    - Gastroesophageal reflux
- Non–IgE mediated
  - Food protein enterocolitis
    - Severe vomiting 2 hours after ingestion; profuse diarrhea
    - Shock due to fluid/electrolyte loss
    - Very ill appearing
  - Food protein proctocolitis
    - Blood in stool
  - Food protein–induced enteropathy
    - Diarrhea, bloating, FTT, anemia

PHYSICAL EXAM

- IgE mediated
  - Hives/angioedema (however, in 12% of patients with anaphylaxis, there are no skin findings and often these are most severe cases)
  - Wheezing/dyspnea
  - Hypotension/tachycardia
  - Vomiting, abdominal tenderness
  - Ill-appearing
- Mixed IgE mediated, non–IgE mediated:
  - Eosinophilic esophagitis: abdominal tenderness (variable), growth concerns (in some)
  - Eosinophilic gastroenteropathy
    - Abdominal tenderness
    - Weight loss
- Cell mediated
  - Food protein–induced enterocolitis
    - Abdominal distention
    - FTT
    - Severe dehydration (may present in shock)
  - Celiac disease
    - Abdominal distention
    - FTT

DIAGNOSTIC TESTS & INTERPRETATION

Lab

Initial lab tests

Depends on clinical presentation and patient symptoms, may include

- CBC with differential
  - Anemia in patients with enteropathy
  - Eosinophilia may be seen in patients with eosinophilic gastroenteritis, enteropathy, and, on occasion, eosinophilic esophagitis (but cannot be used to monitor therapy).
- Serum IgE: may be elevated in
  - IgE-mediated hypersensitivities
  - Eosinophilic esophagitis, eosinophilic gastroenteritis
- Albumin: low in
  - Protein-losing enteropathies
  - Non–IgE-mediated protein enterocolitis (chronic version)
  - Eosinophilic gastroenteritis
- Serologic tests: may aid in diagnosis of celiac disease
- Tryptase: may be elevated in anaphylaxis; obtain within 4 hours of initial reaction.
- ImmunoCAP assay may be helpful in IgE-mediated illness.
  - ImmunoCAP has many false positives (do not send food allergy panels).

Diagnostic Procedures/Other

- Skin prick testing
  - Used in conjunction with clinical history for IgE-mediated food allergies
  - 50% positive predictive value; 95% negative predictive value
  - Performed upon evaluation of patients with eosinophilic esophagitis
- Food challenges
  - Gold standard for diagnosis of food allergy is double-blind placebo-controlled challenge but impractical in many clinical settings.
  - Most sites use single-blind or open food challenge.
  - Used to confirm food allergy in patients when unsure of diagnosis or to assess whether someone has outgrown food allergy (either IgE-mediated or food protein–induced enterocolitis)
  - Challenge must be performed in setting equipped to treat severe allergic reactions.

Food Allergy/Hypersensitivity

Classification	Illness	Symptoms	Diagnosis
IgE mediated	Anaphylaxis	Rapid onset; nausea, vomiting; abdominal pain; hives, coughing, wheezing; involvement of other organ systems—skin, respiratory system	History + skin prick or ImmunoCAP test; oral challenge only in monitored setting with emergency access and anaphylaxis therapy
IgE mediated	Oral allergy syndrome (children and adults); due to cross-reactivity between food protein and pollen	Mild pruritus, angioedema of lips and oropharynx, sense of tightness in throat, rare systemic symptoms	History + skin prick tests; oral challenge positive with fresh foods and negative with cooked foods
IgE and cell mediated	Allergic eosinophilic gastroenteritis	Failure to thrive, weight loss, abdominal pain, irritability, early satiety, vomiting, protein-losing enteropathy, edema, ascites	History + skin prick, endoscopy and colonoscopy with biopsy, elimination diet; monitor closely, may need immunosuppressants
IgE and cell mediated	Eosinophilic esophagitis	GERD with failure to respond to proton pump inhibitor, vomiting, FTT, dysphagia, intermittent abdominal pain, irritability	History, endoscopy with biopsy, elimination diet based on testing or history, elemental diet, or "swallowed" steroids
Cell mediated	Allergic proctocolitis "breast milk colitis" (infants)	Bloody stool, melena in first few months of life; no diarrhea or failure to thrive	Elimination of food (cow's milk or soy most commonly) clears bleeding in 72 hours, reexposure causes recurrence; RAST/skin prick not helpful; typically outgrown by 12–18 months of age
Cell mediated	Food protein–induced enterocolitis syndrome (FPIES)	Severe symptoms; vomiting 2 hours after meal; severe vomiting; 6–8 hours later, diarrhea ± blood, abdominal distention, failure to thrive, dehydration, hypotension	Elimination of protein clears symptoms in 1–3 days. ImmunoCAP/skin prick *not* helpful; patch testing may be helpful
Cell mediated	Food protein enteropathy (infants)	Diarrhea, steatorrhea, abdominal distention, flatulence, failure to thrive or weight loss, nausea/vomiting, oral ulcers	Endoscopy with biopsy; elimination diet resolves symptoms. Similar symptoms to celiac but resolves by 2 years of age.
Cell mediated	Celiac disease (infants to adults)	Diarrhea, steatorrhea, failure to thrive, abdominal distention, flatulence, weight loss, nausea/vomiting, oral ulcers	Endoscopic biopsy when patient is on gluten; gluten-free diet resolves symptoms. Anti-gliadin and TTG antibodies; HLA-DQ2 and DQ8 are often found.

- Endoscopy with biopsies of esophagus, stomach, and small bowel
  - Patients should be on proton pump inhibitor prior to endoscopy if there are concerns for eosinophilic esophagitis, as GERD may also lead to eosinophils in esophagus.
- Colonoscopy
  - If lower GI symptoms are present
- Patch skin testing
  - May be used to evaluate for mixed (IgE/non–IgE mediated) or cell-mediated sensitivities
  - Standards for interpretation and methods for reliability are under development.
- Elimination diets
  - Should be conducted with care
  - May lack critical nutrients
  - Oral rechallenge should be carefully planned because a more severe reaction may ensue after a food has been temporarily removed.

Pathologic Findings

- Increased eosinophils in eosinophilic gastroenteropathy
- Presence of intraepithelial lymphocytes and variable villous damage in celiac disease

TREATMENT

MEDICATION

First Line

- Anaphylaxis
  - Epinephrine for severe allergic reaction or anaphylaxis
  - H_1 antihistamines (diphenhydramine) may be given for milder symptoms.
  - H_2 antihistamines may be given in conjunction with H_1 antihistamines.
  - Systemic steroids
- Eosinophilic gastroenteritis
  - Systemic steroids (briefly)
  - "Swallowed" steroids
    - Refers to having the patient use a corticosteroid inhaler
    - However, the patient swallows after spraying rather than inhaling.
  - Elemental formulas
  - Dietary restrictions

ADDITIONAL TREATMENT

General Measures

- Avoidance of food allergen
- Anaphylaxis
  - Full monitoring of vital signs
  - Epinephrine for severe allergic reaction or anaphylaxis given intramuscularly: may be repeated
  - IV fluid bolus
  - Antihistamines may be given for hives or mild skin swelling.
  - Antihistamines (H_1 and H_2 blockers) and bronchodilators may be used as adjunct to epinephrine for severe reactions.
  - Glucocorticoids may prevent biphasic reaction.
  - Trendelenburg positioning: helps decrease risk of empty ventricle syndrome
- Nonanaphylactic food allergies: eosinophilic esophagitis
  - Systemic steroids for a brief course
  - Swallowed steroids (NPO for 30 minutes after use)
  - Hydrolyzed or elemental formulas: Patients may respond to hypoallergenic formulas.

ISSUES FOR REFERRAL

Allergy/immunology and/or gastroenterology and/or nutrition follow-up needed for most patients for diagnosis and long-term management.

ONGOING CARE

DIET

Nonanaphylactic and anaphylactic food allergies: removal of the offending food agent from diet

PATIENT EDUCATION

- Epinephrine self-administration, if anaphylaxis
- Anaphylaxis plan for families to know which medication to use and when, along with education regarding when to go to the emergency department
- Education regarding specific food avoidance and label reading

PROGNOSIS

- Generally good after offending food antigens are removed from diet and adequate nutrients are ensured
- Tolerance to food allergens may develop over time. Current research trials to help induce tolerance are underway.
- IgE-mediated disease may persist longer than non–IgE mediated.
- Eosinophilic esophagitis and eosinophilic gastroenteritis are considered chronic illnesses.

COMPLICATIONS

- Food protein allergy can be associated with
  - Poor growth
  - Feeding disorder
  - Protein-losing enteropathy
  - Anemia
- Eosinophilic esophagitis
  - Strictures
  - Hiatal hernia concerns
  - Poor growth
  - Feeding disorder
- Respiratory food-hypersensitivity reactions
  - Heiner syndrome: rare food-induced pulmonary hemosiderosis

ADDITIONAL READING

- Bock SA. Diagnostic evaluation. *Pediatrics*. 2003;111(6, Pt 3):1638–1644.
- Burks W. Skin manifestations of food allergy. *Pediatrics*. 2003;111(6, Pt 3):1617–1624.
- Cianferoni A, Spergel JM. Food allergy: review, classification and diagnosis. *Allergol Int*. 2009;58(4):457–466.
- James JM. Respiratory manifestations of food allergy. *Pediatrics*. 2003;111(6, Pt 3):1625–1630.
- Järvinen KM, Nowak-Węgrzyn A. Food protein induced enterocolitis syndrome (FPIES): current management strategies and review of the literature. *J Allergy Clin Immunol Prac*. 2013;1(4):317–322.
- NIAID-Sponsored Expert Panel. Guidelines for the diagnosis and management of food allergy in the United States: report of the NIAID-sponsored expert panel. *J Allergy Clin Immunol*. 2010;126(6)(Suppl):S1–S58.
- Sampson HA. Update on food allergy. *J Allergy Clin Immunol*. 2004;113(5):805–819.
- Sicherer SH, Sampson HA. Food allergy: recent advances in pathophysiology and treatment. *Annu Rev Med*. 2009;60:261–277.

CODES

ICD10

- T78.1XXA Oth adverse food reactions, not elsewhere classified, init
- T78.00XA Anaphylactic reaction due to unspecified food, init encntr
- L27.2 Dermatitis due to ingested food

FAQ

- Q: What are the most common food allergens leading to IgE-mediated allergic reactions in childhood?
- A: The most common allergens to which children are sensitive are milk, egg, soy, wheat, fish, peanuts, and nuts.
- Q: Do you recommend elimination diets?
- A: Elimination diets are recommended when necessary to treat underlying disease. Nutrition evaluation is often necessary to avoid nutrient-deficient diets and malnutrition. Elimination diets are used only in extreme circumstances because they can result in nutrient deficiency and malnutrition without identifying the offending allergen. Double-blinded food challenges are a better method for identifying the offending agent.

F

FOOD HYPERSENSITIVITY (NON–IgE-MEDIATED, GASTROINTESTINAL)

Kirsten Kloepfer

BASICS

DESCRIPTION

- A non–IgE-mediated reaction to a food protein that involves the gastrointestinal (GI) tract
- Previously referred to as milk protein intolerance
- Includes the following:
  - Food protein–induced proctocolitis
  - Food protein–induced enteropathy
  - Food protein–induced enterocolitis syndrome (FPIES)

EPIDEMIOLOGY

- Proctocolitis: Over 60% of infants with rectal bleeding have proctocolitis.
- Enteropathy: may occur after infectious gastritis
- FPIES
  - Slight male predominance (60%)
  - 30% of infants with FPIES have atopic disease(s).
  - Family history of atopy present in 40–80%.

RISK FACTORS

- Proctocolitis
  - 40% react to both milk and soy.
  - 50–60% of infants are breastfed and react to milk and/or soy in mom's diet.
- Enteropathy: usually formula-fed and given intact cow's milk prior to 9 months of age
- FPIES: Exclusive breastfeeding appears to protect against FPIES, but a few cases have been reported.
- Currently, no reports that non–IgE-mediated GI food hypersensitivities are inherited.

PATHOPHYSIOLOGY

- Unclear
- Assumed to be a cell-mediated reaction due to delayed onset

ETIOLOGY

- Cow's milk is number 1 cause of proctocolitis, enteropathy, and FPIES, followed by soy, egg and wheat.
- FPIES: can also react to solid foods thought to be hypoallergenic (rice, oat, barley, chicken, turkey, peanut, potato, corn, fruit protein, fish, and mollusks)

DIAGNOSIS

HISTORY

- Proctocolitis
  - Occurs between 1 and 6 months of age (usually between 2 and 8 weeks)
  - Specks or streaks of blood (± mucus) in the stool of an otherwise healthy infant
  - Absence of vomiting and diarrhea
  - Blood-tinged stools resolve with elimination of offending food protein.
  - Rare in older children
- Enteropathy
  - Persistent diarrhea (rarely bloody)
  - Vomiting
  - Abdominal pain
  - FTT with hypoproteinemia and anemia
  - Usually formula-fed
  - Do not experience an acute reaction with reexposure
- FPIES
  - Can begin anytime from within a few days of life through 12 months of age
  - FPIES due to solid food usually begins when solids are first introduced (rice cereal).
  - Profuse protracted emesis 1–3 hours after exposure to offending food protein
  - Profuse diarrhea 4–8 hours after food ingestion in 25% of cases
  - May appear acutely ill with 15% of cases presenting with dehydration and shock
- All non–IgE-mediated GI food hypersensitivities resolve when offending food protein removed from diet.

PHYSICAL EXAM

- Proctocolitis: usually healthy-appearing child with normal physical exam
- Enteropathy
  - Diffuse abdominal pain with distention
  - Weight loss
- FPIES
  - Profuse vomiting and watery diarrhea with signs of dehydration
  - Lethargy, may appear septic

DIAGNOSTIC TESTS & INTERPRETATION

Diagnostic Procedures/Other

- All non–IgE-mediated GI food hypersensitivities are as follows:
  - Diagnosed clinically
  - No laboratory test available to diagnose hypersensitivity
  - Serum-specific IgE testing and skin testing often negative
- Proctocolitis
  - No endoscopy unless prolonged rectal bleeding, anemia, and/or FTT
  - Eosinophils and lymphoid nodular hyperplasia may be present in the colon.
- Enteropathy
  - Endoscopy shows villous injury with increase in crypt length and villous atrophy.
- FPIES
  - Labs may also show anemia, leukocytosis, eosinophilia, neutrophilia, thrombocytosis, and hypoalbuminemia.
  - If reaction to food is severe, patient may have metabolic acidosis.
  - May see methemoglobinemia in up to 35% of cases that require hospitalization
  - Stool may contain blood, mucus, leukocytes, eosinophils, and/or increased carbohydrate content due to malabsorption.
  - Abdominal x-ray may show intramural gas (may be confused with necrotizing enterocolitis [NEC] or ileus).
- With FPIES, if the offending food is discontinued and restarted, the patient will experience vomiting and diarrhea within a few hours (not recommended to be performed at home).

DIFFERENTIAL DIAGNOSIS

- Proctocolitis
  - Anal fissures
  - Vascular malformations
  - Intussusception
  - Meckel diverticulum
- Enteropathy
  - Lactose intolerance
  - Celiac disease
  - Inflammatory bowel disease (IBD)

- FPIES
  - Anaphylaxis
  - Sepsis
  - NEC
  - GI infection
  - Reflux
  - Metabolic disorder
  - Surgical abdomen

TREATMENT

ADDITIONAL TREATMENT

General Measures

- Proctocolitis
  - Exclusively breastfed infant: Continue breastfeeding with mom eliminating all forms of dairy including casein and whey in packaged food.
  - Symptoms should improve within 72 hours, but it may take up to 2 weeks to completely resolve.
  - If no improvement, eliminate soy in mom's diet, followed by egg.
  - If the infant is formula-fed, consider changing formula to a hydrolysate formula (e.g., Pregestimil, Nutramigen, Alimentum) because many patients are sensitive to both milk and soy protein.
  - If bleeding continues, consider changing formula to an amino acid–based formula (e.g., Neocate, PurAmino, EleCare).
- Enteropathy
  - Eliminate milk from diet.
  - Symptoms should improve in 1–3 weeks.
- FPIES
  - Acute episodes should be treated with IV fluids, methylprednisolone (1 mg/kg) to decrease possible cell-mediated intestinal inflammation, plus vasopressors, epinephrine, and/or bicarbonate for shock and possible metabolic acidosis.
  - Long-term management involves strict avoidance of trigger food(s).
  - Stop cow's milk or soy formula and start hydrolysate formula due to possible intolerance to both milk and soy protein.
  - For solid food FPIES:
    - Eliminate trigger food and allow the patient to continue eating foods previously tolerated.
    - Consult allergist for future solid food introduction.

ALERT

If suspect FPIES (patient with vomiting, acute dehydration, lethargy and acidosis), fluid resuscitation and refeeding should be performed in the hospital.

ONGOING CARE

FOLLOW-UP RECOMMENDATIONS

- Proctocolitis
  - 95% tolerate reintroduction of food(s) at 9 months of age. Patient can reintroduce offending food at home 4–6 months after beginning protein elimination diet.
  - Prognosis: excellent. Nearly all infants tolerate cow's milk and soy products by 12 months of age.
  - Proctocolitis is not inherited; therefore, subsequent children should not be started on hydrolysate or amino acid formula.
- Enteropathy
  - Most cases resolve spontaneously by 2 years of age.
  - Food can be reintroduced at home 1–2 years after beginning protein elimination diet.
- FPIES
  - The trigger food may be reintroduced 12–18 months after the last reaction, preferably under the supervision of a physician.
  - Cow's milk and soy FPIES resolve in most patients by 3 years of age.
  - Patients with solid food FPIES may experience protracted courses.
  - Nutritional counseling may be helpful for children with multiple non–IgE-mediated reactions to food.
  - Because close follow-up is needed to determine if tolerance has developed and if an oral food challenge can be performed, an allergy consult is warranted when FPIES is suspected.

ADDITIONAL READING

- Boyce JA, Assa'ad AH, Burks AW, et al. Guidelines for the diagnosis and management of food allergy in the United States: summary of the NIAID-sponsored expert panel report. *J Allergy Clin Immunol*. 2010;126(6):1105–1118.
- Elizur A, Cohen M, Goldberg MR, et al. Cow's milk associated rectal bleeding: a population based prospective study. *Pediatr Allergy Immunol*. 2012;23(8):766–770.
- Järvinen KM, Nowak-Węgrzyn A. Food protein-induced enterocolitis syndrome (FPIES): current management strategies and review of the literature. *J Allergy Clin Immunol Pract*. 2013;1(4):317–322.
- Lake AM. Food-induced eosinophilic proctocolitis. *J Pediatr Gastroenterol Nutr*. 2000;30(Suppl):S58–S60.
- Mehr S, Kakakios A, Frith K, et al. Food protein-induced enterocolitis syndrome: 16-year experience. *Pediatrics*. 2009;123(3):e459–e464.
- Sampson HA, Anderson JA. Summary and recommendations: classification of gastrointestinal manifestations due to immunologic reactions to foods in infants and young children. *J Pediatr Gastroenterol Nutr*. 2000;30(Suppl):S87–S94.
- Sicherer SH, Eigenmann PA, Sampson HA. Clinical features of food protein-induced enterocolitis syndrome. *J Pediatr*. 1998;133(2):214–219.
- Walker-Smith JA. Cow's milk-sensitive enteropathy: predisposing factors and treatment. *J Pediatr*. 1992;121(5, Pt 2):S111–S115.
- Xanthakos SA, Schwimmer JB, Melin-Aldana H, et al. Prevalence and outcome of allergic colitis in healthy infants with rectal bleeding: a prospective cohort study. *J Pediatr Gastroenterol Nutr*. 2005;41(1):16–22.

CODES

ICD10

- Z91.011 Allergy to milk products
- E73.9 Lactose intolerance, unspecified
- K90.4 Malabsorption due to intolerance, not elsewhere classified

FAQ

- Q: Will my child outgrow this?
- A: For proctocolitis, most children outgrow milk and/or soy intolerance by 12 months of age. For enterocolitis, symptoms resolve within 1–2 years. For FPIES, symptoms may resolve within 1–2 years, however, they may persist which is why food challenges are important to determine if symptoms have improved and the food can be safely reintroduced into the diet.
- Q: Should I refer the patient to an allergist?
- A: Infants with suspected FPIES should be referred to an allergist for both evaluation and future food challenges. A patient with proctocolitis or enteropathy that resolves with formula change does not need to be seen by a specialist unless symptoms persist despite a strict elimination diet.
- Q: Can my child have FPIES and an IgE-mediated food allergy?
- A: Although not as common as FPIES alone, there are reports of children with FPIES and elevated food-specific IgE levels. These children tend to have a more protracted course of FPIES and are at increased risk of developing IgE-mediated immediate-type symptoms when challenged. This supports the recommendation to refer children with suspected FPIES to an allergist for further evaluation.

F

FOOD POISONING OR FOODBORNE ILLNESS

Kacy A. Ramirez

BASICS

DESCRIPTION

Any illness resulting from the ingestion of food or drink contaminated with an infectious organism or associated toxin

EPIDEMIOLOGY

Incidence (U.S. Annual Estimates)

- 31 major pathogens caused
  - 9.4 million episodes of foodborne illness
  - 56,000 hospitalizations
  - 1,350 deaths
- Highest incidence in children <5 years
- Hospitalizations and death more common in persons >64 years
- See Appendix, Table 8 regarding epidemiologic aspects by organism.

GENERAL PREVENTION

- Vaccination
  - Oral rotavirus vaccine
  - Hepatitis A vaccine
- Preventive strategies
  - Hand washing (soap and water)
  - Proper food handling (adequate cooking and refrigeration)
  - Avoidance of unpasteurized dairy products and juices
  - Avoidance of raw or undercooked eggs, meat, and shellfish
  - Avoidance of honey in children <1 year old
  - Avoidance of well water, which may contain nitrates, in preparing infant formulas

PATHOPHYSIOLOGY

- Gastroenteritis
  - Viral epithelial invasion/replication or ingestion of preformed elaborated toxin
- Noninflammatory diarrhea
  - Selective destruction of absorptive cells in mucosa, leaving secretory cells intact
  - Toxin elaboration (secretory diarrhea)
  - Impairment of brush border enzymes and lactose intolerance (osmotic diarrhea)
- Inflammatory diarrhea/dysentery
  - Direct mucosal invasion of intestinal epithelial cells (colon)
  - Toxin elaboration
  - Inflammatory infiltration destroys villous cells and transporters and leads to exudation of mucus/protein/blood into gut.
- Local/remote invasion (bacteremia, meningitis, dissemination, hepatitis, osteomyelitis)
- Immune-mediated extraintestinal manifestations (hemolytic uremic syndrome, reactive arthritis, Guillain-Barré)

ETIOLOGY

- Viruses
  - Most common cause of foodborne illness
  - Caliciviruses (norovirus)
  - Rotavirus (infant/child)
  - Astrovirus
  - Enteric adenovirus
  - Hepatitis A
- Bacteria
  - *Salmonella* (*typhi*, *paraptyphi*, non-typhoidal)
  - *Clostridium perfringens*
  - *Campylobacter*
- Other bacteria
  - *Salmonella typhi/Salmonella paratyphi*
  - *Shigella*
  - *Escherichia coli*
    - *Enterohemorrhagic E. coli* [EHEC] including Shiga toxin–producing *E. coli* [STEC]
    - Enteropathogenic *E. coli* [EPEC]
    - Enterotoxigenic *E. coli* [ETEC]
    - Enteroinvasive *E. coli* [EIEC]
    - Enteroaggregative *E. coli* [EAEC]
  - *Vibrio* (*cholerae*, *parahaemolyticus*, *vulnificus*)
  - *Staphylococcus aureus* (preformed toxin)
  - *Bacillus cereus* (preformed and diarrheal toxin)
  - *Clostridium botulinum* (toxin)
  - *Listeria monocytogenes*
  - *Brucella*
- Parasites
  - *Entamoeba histolytica*
  - *Giardia intestinalis*
  - *Cryptosporidium*
  - *Cyclospora cayetanensis*
  - *Toxoplasma gondii*

DIAGNOSIS

SIGNS AND SYMPTOMS

- Gastroenteritis
  - Sudden onset vomiting
  - Fever and diarrhea may also be present
  - Associated with viral etiology, preformed toxin ingestion
- Noninflammatory diarrhea
  - Acute watery diarrhea, abdominal pain, without fever/dysentery
  - Some may present with fever
  - Consider: ETEC, viral or parasitic etiology
- Inflammatory diarrhea:
  - Bloody stool, abdominal pain and fever
  - Consider: *Shigella*, *Campylobacter*, *Salmonella*, EIEC, EHEC, STEC O157H7, EAEC, *Vibrio parahaemolyticus*, *Yersinia enterocolitica*, *Entamoeba*
- Chronic diarrhea >14 days
  - 3 or more unformed stools/day
  - Consider: parasitic etiology
- Neurologic manifestations
  - Paresthesias, respiratory depression, bronchospasm, cranial nerve palsies
  - Consider: *Clostridium botulinum* toxin, organophosphate, fish toxin poisons, Guillain-Barré [*Campylobacter jejuni*]
- Systemic illness
  - Fever, weakness, arthritis, jaundice
  - Consider: *Listeria*, *Brucella*, *Trichinella*, *Toxoplasma*, *Vibrio vulnificus*, *Hep A*, *S. typhi*, *S. paratyphi*

HISTORY

- Incubation period
- Duration of illness
- Predominant symptoms
- Population involved in outbreak
- Similarly exposed persons with related symptoms
- Suspected similarly ill contacts
- Type of food ingested and type of exposure (location of exposure, pet contact, travel, occupation, institutional/daycare)
- See Appendix, Table 9 regarding clinical symptoms by organism.

PHYSICAL EXAM

- Detailed neurologic examination
- Assessment of dehydration status (examination of mucous membranes, skin turgor)
- Assessment of potential liver involvement (hepatomegaly, jaundice, icterus)
- Assessment of disseminated disease (MS exam for septic arthritis and osteomyelitis)
- Careful abdominal examination

DIAGNOSTIC TESTS & INTERPRETATION

Lab

- Routine bacterial stool culture
  - Cultures for *Vibrio* and *Yersinia*, EC0157H7, and *Campylobacter* require additional media or incubation conditions and may require communication with laboratory if suspected.
  - Toxin testing, serotyping, and molecular techniques may only be available from large commercial or public health labs.
- Blood/CSF cultures as clinically indicated
- Serology (hepatitis A, *Brucella*, *Toxo*)
- Ova/parasite examination
- Direct antigen testing/DFA (*Giardia*, *Cryptosporidium*)
- Polymerase chain reaction (PCR) identification of multiple pathogens in stool (viral, bacterial, parasitic) are most sensitive.
- Careful monitoring of patients with hemorrhagic colitis during illness and 3 days after resolution of diarrhea to detect changes of HUS (CBC with smear, BUN/Cr)

DIFFERENTIAL DIAGNOSIS

- Systemic viral illness (myalgias/arthralgias) or infection (e.g., pharyngitis)
- Appendicitis, peritonitis, pelvic inflammatory disease
- Irritable bowel syndrome
- Inflammatory bowel disease
- Malignancy
- Medication use
- *Clostridium difficile* enterocolitis
- Malabsorption syndromes (celiac disease, cystic fibrosis, malnutrition)
- Food intolerance or allergy
  - Cow's milk (protein allergy)
  - Carbohydrate intolerance (e.g., lactose)
- Dietary manipulations
  - Hyperosmolar formulas
  - Food additives (dyes, processing materials, coloring)
  - Caffeine
  - Overfeeding
  - Low fat intakes
  - Excessive fluids
  - Munchausen by proxy
- Ingestion of noninfectious foodborne illness (contaminated seafood, mushroom poisoning, chemical poisoning)

TREATMENT

ADDITIONAL TREATMENT

General Measures

- Gastroenteritis
  - Treat dehydration with oral rehydration solution (ORS):
    - Standard ORS contains 75–90 mEq of sodium and 74–111 mmol/L of glucose
    - Alternative ORS, including rice-based carbohydrate or amylase-based solutions, may be more effective for *Vibrio cholerae* infections.
  - Transition rapidly (after 3–4 hours of ORS tolerance) to regular diet (see below).
  - Continue breastfeeding infants if possible.
- Botulism
  - Continuous cardiac and respiratory monitoring, may need assisted ventilation

DIET

Balanced, varied diet; providing easily digestible, complex carbohydrates will promote improved stool consistency.

SPECIAL THERAPY

Botulism: For suspected infant botulism cases, human-derived antitoxin, BabyBIG (Human Botulism Immune Globulin, BIG-IV), may be obtained from the Infant Botulism Treatment and Prevention Program, California Department of Public Health (24-hour line: 510-231-7600).

IV Fluids

If patient is unable to be rehydrated via oral route (because of ileus, circulatory failure, CNS complications) or if >10% dehydration

COMPLEMENTARY & ALTERNATIVE THERAPIES

Supplements with specific probiotic strains (e.g., *Lactobacillus GG*) have been shown to reduce duration of less severe, non-rotaviral diarrhea and hospital stays.

MEDICATION

Use of antibiotics is

- Always indicated
  - *Shigella*
  - *Brucella*
  - *L. monocytogenes* (invasive disease)
  - Invasive *Salmonella* (*typhi, paratyphi,* non-tyhoidal)
  - Typhoid fever (*Salmonella typhi, paratyphi*)
  - *Salmonella typhi*
  - *Salmonella paratyphi*
  - *Vibrio* spp.
  - *Cyclospora cayetanensis*
  - *Cryptosporidium* (severe or children <12 years old)
  - *Trichinella*
  - *E. histolytica*
  - *Campylobacter* (in severe cases, early treatment limits duration, prevents relapse, and shortens duration of shedding)
  - *G. intestinalis*
- Sometimes indicated
  - *E. coli* (severe ETEC in a traveler in resource limited country)
  - Non-*typhi Salmonella*
    - Treatment indicated to reduce risks of bacterial translocation only in a few select populations: patients <3 months old as well as those who are immunocompromised, have a hemoglobinopathy, or have chronic GI condition (IBD)
    - Other patients should not be treated, as antibiotics prolong organism shedding in the stool and promote disease spread.
  - *Y. enterocolitica* (sepsis)
  - *T. gondii* (pregnant and immunocompromised patients)
  - *Cryptosporidium* (severe, <12 years of age)
- Contraindicated
  - *Clostridium botulinum* (aminoglycosides potentiate paralytic effects)
  - No antimotility agents for children with inflammatory or bloody diarrhea

ONGOING CARE

PROGNOSIS

- Most gastroenteritis is mild and self-limited.
- Recovery is complete in 2–5 days in most individuals.
- In the very young, prognosis is more guarded because these patients can become dehydrated quickly.
- After the patient has survived the paralytic phase of botulism, the outlook for complete recovery is excellent.

REPORTING REQUIREMENTS

- Foodborne diseases and conditions generally notifiable at the national level include the following:
  - Botulism, brucellosis, STEC O157H7, hemolytic uremic syndrome, listerosis, salmonellosis (other than *S. typhi*), shigellosis, typhoid fever (*S. typhi and S. paratyphi* infections), *Vibrio*, hepatitis A
- Additional reporting requirements may be mandated by state and territorial laws and regulations: Full reporting instructions are available:
  - 1-800-CDC-INFO (1-800-232-4636)
  - http://www.cdc.gov/foodsafety/fdoss/reporting/how-to-report.html

ADDITIONAL READING

- Centers for Disease Control and Prevention. Diagnosis and management of foodborne illnesses. *MMWR Recomm Rep*. 2004;53(RR-4):1–33.
- Centers for Disease Control and Prevention. Incidence and trends of infection with pathogens transmitted commonly through food —Foodborne Disease Active Surveillance Network, 10 U.S. sites, 1996-2012. *MMWR Morb Mortal Wkly Rep*. 2013;62(15):283–287.
- Davidson G, Barnes G, Bass D, et al. Infectious diarrhea in children: Working group report of the first World Congress of Pediatric Gastroenterology, Hepatology, and Nutrition. *J Pediatr Gastroenterol Nutr*. 2002;25(Suppl 2):143–150.
- Greer FR, Shannon M. Infant methemoglobinemia: the role of dietary nitrate in food and water. *Pediatrics*. 2005;116(3):784–786.
- NASPGHAN Nutrition Report Committee. Clinical efficacy of probiotics: review of the evidence with a focus on children. *J Gastroenterol Hepatol Nutr*. 2006;43(4):550–557.
- Scallan E, Hoekstra RM, Angelo FJ, et al. Foodborne illness acquired in the United States—major pathogens. *Emerging Infect Dis*. 2011;17(1):7–15.

CODES

ICD10

- T62.91XA Toxic effect of unsp noxious sub eaten as food, acc, init
- A05.9 Bacterial foodborne intoxication, unspecified
- A02.0 Salmonella enteritis

FAQ

- Q: What are the most common causes of food poisoning?
- A: Viruses, particularly norovirus, are the leading cause of foodborne illnesses. The most common bacterial infections include *Salmonella*, *Clostridium perfringens*, and *Campylobacter jejuni*.
- Q: How are the signs and symptoms of food poisoning different from those of a viral gastroenteritis?
- A: The signs and symptoms of food poisoning and gastroenteritis are similar in that the patient displays diarrhea, vomiting, and fever. Historically, food poisoning is distinguished by its association with a common food that affects multiple individuals who consumed it.
- Q: Which foods are most likely to be contaminated?
- A: Poorly cooked foods (e.g., eggs, meats, fish, shellfish), unpasteurized milk and juices, inadequately washed fresh produce, home canned goods, soft unpasteurized cheeses. Use of well water, which may be contaminated with nitrates, to prepare infant formula can result in infant methemoglobinemia.

FRAGILE X SYNDROME

Chad R. Haldeman-Englert • Marni J. Falk

BASICS

DESCRIPTION

- Most common cause of inherited intellectual disability (ID)
- Caused by mutations in the *FMR1* gene on chromosome Xq27.3

EPIDEMIOLOGY

- Affects ~1 in 4,000–6,000 in males; prevalence in females is ~1/2 that in males
- Carrier prevalence in females for *FMR1* premutation is 1:382 and for intermediate allele(s) is 1:143

RISK FACTORS

Genetics

- Caused by loss-of-function mutations in the *FMR1* gene on chromosome Xq27.3
- >99% of affected individuals have a trinucleotide (CGG) repeat expansion (>200 repeats) within the 5′ untranslated region of the *FMR1* gene.
- Repeat size categories (based on guidelines from the American College of Medical Genetics):
  - Normal number of repeats: 5–44
  - Intermediate ("gray zone"): 45–54
  - Premutation: 55–200
  - Full mutation: >200
- Other *FMR1* gene mutations may rarely occur (<1% cases).
- Fragile X syndrome is inherited in an X-linked manner.
- Fragile X is a CGG trinucleotide repeat disorder that shows anticipation, in which the phenotype can be more severe in subsequent generations due to an expansion in the number of CGG repeats.
- Expansion only may occur in the germline of mothers who carry a premutation range repeat allele of *FMR1*.
  - Expansion does not always occur in offspring of female premutation carriers. In general, the larger the number of CGG repeats (>50), the higher the probability that expansion to a full mutation will occur.
- A male with a premutation will pass on the premutation to 100% of his daughters and none of his sons.
- Females with a full mutation are typically less severely affected than males because their 2nd *FMR1* allele is typically normal and, assuming random X-inactivation occurs, produces variable amounts of fragile X mental retardation protein (FMRP).
- Males with mosaicism for the *FMR1* full mutation (some cells with the full mutation and other cells with the premutation) are generally less severely affected (average IQ 60) relative to males with the full mutation in all the cells
- Patients with larger chromosomal deletions involving *FMR1* and other nearby genes typically have a more severe phenotype

GENERAL PREVENTION

- Prenatal diagnosis by chorionic villous sampling (~10–12 weeks' gestation) or amniocentesis (~16–20 weeks' gestation) is possible for at-risk pregnancies.
- Preimplantation genetic diagnosis in the setting of in vitro fertilization is possible for at-risk couples when a familial *FMR1* mutation is known.

PATHOPHYSIOLOGY

Residual FMRP protein levels directly correlate with the severity of fragile X syndrome manifestations:

- Absence of FMRP results in characteristic craniofacial, neurologic, and connective tissue abnormalities.
- Decreased FMRP levels may cause long-term depression of hippocampal synaptic transmission via specific glutamate receptors, with resulting behavioral and neuronal phenotypes.

COMMONLY ASSOCIATED CONDITIONS

Other *FMR1*-related disorders include fragile X–associated tremor/ataxia syndrome (FXTAS) and premature ovarian insufficiency (POI):

- FXTAS can be seen in older (age >50 years) male and female premutation carriers. Clinical features include intention tremors, abnormal gait with frequent falling, cerebral atrophy, and memory deficits.
- POI can be seen in 20–25% of female premutation carriers, with menopause occurring prior to age 40 years.

DIAGNOSIS

HISTORY

- Birth/neonatal history
  - Normal to increased birth weight
  - May have large head circumference at birth
  - Feeding problems and frequent emesis due to gastroesophageal reflux may occur but improves with growth.
  - Irritability may result from sensory integration difficulties and tactile defensiveness.
- Past medical history
  - Strabismus and hyperopia occur in 40%
  - Frequent ear infections in 60%: Conductive hearing loss is possible.
  - Mitral valve prolapse (MVP) and aortic root dilation can occur, typically in adults.
  - Seizures occur in ~20% of children and may resolve by adolescence.
  - Periventricular heterotopia seen on magnetic resonance imaging (MRI)
  - Pes planus
  - Scoliosis
- Developmental/behavioral history
  - Motor delay due to hypotonia
  - Speech may be absent to minimally affected.
  - Autism (60% of males with full mutation)
  - Severe intellectual disability in males (average IQ of males with the full mutation is 41, with range of 30–55)
  - Borderline or mild intellectual disability in 50% of females with the full mutation (IQ range 70–85)
  - Tantrums occur around age 2 years.
  - Hyperactivity can be severe.
  - Obsessive and compulsive behaviors
  - Often requires routine for daily activities
  - Social anxiety: Patients are shy and easily overwhelmed by noisy environments.
- Family history
  - Fragile X syndrome
  - Intellectual disability or autism, especially in males related through the maternal side
  - Tremors or ataxia developing >50 years
  - Premature ovarian insufficiency in females <40 years
  - No male–male transmission

PHYSICAL EXAM

- Growth parameters
  - Height, weight, and head circumference
- Characteristic facial features
  - Large head, prominent forehead
  - Long face
  - Large and protruding ears
  - High palate
  - Prominent chin (after puberty)
- Murmur or midsystolic click (MVP)
- Large testicles (after puberty)
- Joint hypermobility, pes planus, scoliosis
- Skin often feels soft and smooth

DIAGNOSTIC TESTS & INTERPRETATION

Lab

Initial lab tests

- Consider *FMR1* mutation testing in the following:
  - Males or females with features of autism, developmental delays, or intellectual disability
  - Males or females with clinical findings consistent with fragile X syndrome
  - Family history of fragile X syndrome, recurrent intellectual disability or autism, especially through the maternal side
  - Males or females with tremor and/or ataxia developing age >50 years
  - Females with premature ovarian insufficiency age <40 years
- Southern blot or polymerase chain reaction (PCR)–based analyses are the 1st-line genetic tests to determine if there is a repeat expansion and define the number of CGG repeats within the *FMR1* gene.

Follow-Up Tests & Special Considerations

- Methylation status can be determined by using a restriction enzyme that selectively cuts nonmethylated DNA or by methylation-sensitive PCR techniques. This may be considered for higher functioning males with a full mutation to establish their degree of *FMR1* methylation.
- Standard karyotype analysis will typically not be able to detect the repeat expansion.
- If the patient has many clinical features of fragile X syndrome and Southern blot analysis is normal, consider further molecular techniques to detect point mutations or whole/partial *FMR1* gene deletions.

Diagnostic Procedures/Other

- Echocardiogram if cardiac exam is consistent with MVP (usually in adults)
- Aortic root dilation may be seen but typically does not progress or require specific treatment
- Evaluate for hypertension.
- Assess for seizure activity.
- Developmental evaluations
  - Feeding assessment in infants
  - Education planning
    - Speech and language
    - Hearing assessment
    - Occupational and physical therapy
    - Behavioral/neuropsychological testing

DIFFERENTIAL DIAGNOSIS

- In early childhood, the symptoms of fragile X syndrome are often nonspecific.
- Other genetic syndromes with overlapping features include the following:
  - Fragile XE syndrome (FRAXE): Patients have a milder degree of intellectual disability as well as less specific physical characteristics compared to patients with typical fragile X syndrome (FRAXA). Mutations of *FMR2* on Xq28 are associated with FRAXE.
  - Sotos syndrome: Patients have overgrowth (macrocephaly), intellectual disability, behavioral abnormalities, and cardiac and renal defects. Mutations or deletions of *NSD1* are causative of this syndrome.
  - Abnormal parent-specific imprinting of chromosome 15q11-q13:
    - Paternal chromosome affected: Prader-Willi syndrome—infantile hypotonia, obesity, hyperphagia, developmental delay, cognitive deficits, and behavioral abnormalities
    - Maternal chromosome affected: Angelman syndrome—severe developmental delay or intellectual disability, minimal to no speech development, gait ataxia and/or tremulousness of the limbs, and inappropriate happy demeanor that includes frequent laughing, smiling, and excitability
  - A range of other genes is now recognized to cause syndromic autism and X-linked intellectual disability. *PTEN* mutations can be associated with macrocephaly and autism. Clinical diagnostic testing either individually or through gene panels is available (www.genetests.org).

TREATMENT

MEDICATION

- No specific medications are available.
- Some medications are used to treat specific symptoms in individual patients:
  - Medications for hyperactivity (e.g., methylphenidate, clonidine, others)
  - Selective serotonin reuptake inhibitors (e.g., fluoxetine) for obsessive and compulsive behaviors, social phobia, anxiety, and depression
  - Atypical antipsychotic medications (e.g., risperidone) for psychosis or paranoia
  - Valproic acid or carbamazepine for seizures and/or mood stabilization

ADDITIONAL TREATMENT

General Measures

- Treatment is aimed at supportive measures.
- Per American Academy of Pediatrics (AAP) guidelines, routine evaluation for ocular, ENT, skeletal, and neurologic abnormalities. Refer to appropriate specialists as needed.
- Early developmental services
  - Physical therapy for joint laxity/hypotonia
  - Occupational therapy
  - Speech and language therapy
  - Social integration therapy
- Some patients do well in a mainstream school with appropriate support, whereas others require a school for children with special needs.
- Behavioral therapies involve avoidance of overstimulation and providing positive reinforcement.

ADDITIONAL THERAPIES

- Experimental therapies
  - Glutamate receptor antagonists, gamma-aminobutyric acid (GABA) receptor agonists, minocycline, carnitine, valproic acid, and lovastatin have shown some improvement in the neurologic and behavioral symptoms.
- Surgery/other procedures
  - Myringotomy tubes if with frequent ear infections and/or conductive hearing loss
  - Inguinal hernia repair, if present
  - Strabismus repair, if necessary
  - Corrective lenses for refractive errors

ONGOING CARE

FOLLOW-UP RECOMMENDATIONS

Patient Monitoring

- Regular follow-up with a behavioral and developmental pediatrician as well as a psychiatrist/psychologist is recommended for patients with behavioral problems.
- Hypertension can occur in adults with fragile X syndrome. Therefore, annual blood pressure and cardiac exam should be performed. Hypertension can be treated with typical medications used in the general population. If hypertension is refractory to treatment, evaluate for other causes of high blood pressure (e.g., renal).

DIET

No specific dietary requirements.

PROGNOSIS

Most patients generally have a normal lifespan.

ADDITIONAL READING

- American Academy of Pediatrics. Health supervision for children with fragile x syndrome. *Pediatrics*. 2011;127(5):994–1006.
- Bagni C, Oostra BA. Fragile X syndrome: from protein function to therapy. *Am J Med Genet A*. 2013;161A(11):2809–2821.
- Fragile X mental retardation syndrome. Online Mendelian Inheritance in Man. http://www.omim.org/entry/300624. Accessed December 3, 2014.
- Monaghan KG, Lyon E, Spector EB; American College of Medical Genetics. ACMG Standards and Guidelines for fragile X testing: a revision to the disease-specific supplements to the Standards and Guidelines for Clinical Genetics Laboratories of the American College of Medical Genetics and Genomics. *Genet Med*. 2013;15(7):575–586.
- Saul RA, Tarleton JC. FMR1- related disorders. In: Pagon RA, Adam MP, Bird TD, et al, eds. *GeneReviews*™ [Internet]. Seattle, WA: University of Washington, Seattle; 1993–2013.

See Also: National Fragile X Foundation: www.fragilex.org

CODES

ICD10

Q99.2 Fragile X chromosome

FAQ

- Q. Why is it called "fragile X syndrome"?
- A. Early cytogenetic studies of male patients with intellectual disability identified a site on the X chromosome that would appear constricted when the patient's cells were grown with special culture techniques to induce "fragile" sites.
- Q. How many repeats are necessary to cause the full mutation resulting in fragile X syndrome?
- A. More than 200 repeats.
- Q. What are typical facial features seen in patients with fragile X syndrome?
- A. Prominent forehead, long face, protruding ears, and a prominent chin.
- Q. When does the macroorchidism associated with fragile X syndrome typically develop?
- A. After puberty.

FROSTBITE

Denise A. Salerno

BASICS

DESCRIPTION

- Localized injury of epidermis and underlying tissue resulting from exposure to extreme cold or contact with extremely cold objects
- Distal extremities and unprotected areas (i.e., fingers, toes, ears, nose, and chin) most commonly affected
- Feet and hands account for 90% of frostbite injuries.
- Classified according to severity:
  - Superficial, 1st degree: partial skin freezing
  - Superficial, 2nd degree: full-thickness skin freezing
  - Deep, 3rd degree: full-thickness skin and subcutaneous tissue freezing
  - Deep, 4th degree: full-thickness skin, subcutaneous tissue, muscle, tendon, and bone freezing
- New classification of severity at day 0 has been proposed based on findings that correlate extent of frostbite with outcome of involved body part along with results of bone scans:
  - 1st degree: leads to recovery
  - 2nd degree: leads to soft tissue amputation
  - 3rd degree: leads to bone amputation
  - 4th degree: leads to large amputation with systemic effects

RISK FACTORS

- Alcohol use
- Arthritis
- Atherosclerosis
- Constricting clothing
- Diabetes mellitus
- High altitude
- Hypothermia
- Immobilization
- Improper use of aerosol sprays
- Previous cold injury
- Smoking tobacco
- Trauma
- Vasoconstrictive drugs
- Body parts most affected:
  - Fingers
  - Toes
  - Nose
  - Cheeks
  - Ears
  - Male genitalia
- Groups at risk:
  - Mentally ill patients
  - Patients with impaired circulation
  - Winter sports enthusiasts and fans
  - Homeless persons
  - Very thin individuals
  - Malnourished people
  - Outdoor laborers
  - Military personnel, especially those of African American and Afro-Caribbean descent, exposed to cold, wet climates
  - Elderly people
  - Very young people

GENERAL PREVENTION

- Avoid prolonged cold exposure whenever possible.
- Maintain adequate nutrition and hydration when spending time in cold weather.
- Dress appropriately for cold weather:
  - Dress in layers: Clothing should be made of material that absorbs perspiration and prevents heat loss, and outerwear should be windproof and water repellent.
  - Cover head, ears, and neck.
  - Mittens help to conserve heat better than gloves do.
  - Footwear should be water-repellent and insulated.

PATHOPHYSIOLOGY

- Tissue damage and cell death result from initial freeze injury and inflammatory response that occurs with rewarming.
- Direct cellular damage can occur from frostbite. As temperature of freezing tissue approaches −2°C, extracellular ice crystals form and cause increased osmotic pressure in the interstitium, leading to cellular dehydration. As freezing continues, these shrinking, hyperosmolar cells die due to abnormal intracellular electrolyte concentrations. With rapid freezing, intracellular ice crystal formation occurs, resulting in immediate cell death.
- Indirect cellular damage results from progressive microvascular insult. Initial tissue response to extreme cold exposure is vasoconstriction. Blood flow to extremities is reduced as freezing continues. Ice crystals form in plasma, blood viscosity increases, and decreased circulation and formation of microthrombi occur in distal extremities, resulting in hypoxia, tissue damage, and ischemia.
- Oxygen free radicals and inflammatory mediators, especially prostaglandin F2 and thromboxane A2, contribute to tissue injury following rewarming and reperfusion of damaged tissue.
- Most severe injuries are seen in tissues that freeze, thaw, and freeze again.

DIAGNOSIS

- Depends on severity
- Superficial, 1st degree: transient tingling, stinging, and burning followed by throbbing and aching with possible hyperhidrosis (excess sweating)
- Superficial, 2nd degree: numbness, with vasomotor disturbances in more severe cases
- Deep, 3rd degree: no sensation initially, followed by shooting pains, burning, throbbing, and aching
- Deep, 4th degree: absence of sensation, presence of muscle function, pain, and joint discomfort

HISTORY

- Was there prolonged exposure to cold environment? In frostbite, history of prolonged cold exposure is typical.
- Was there contact with a cold object, especially metal? Metal will drain heat from skin through conduction and increase the risk of frostbite.
- What was the timing and duration of exposure?
- Was there any treatment prior to presentation?
- Does the patient have any underlying conditions or behaviors that put him or her at risk?
  - Peripheral vascular disease, medications, smoking, etc.

PHYSICAL EXAM

- Superficial, 1st degree: waxy appearance, erythema, and edema of involved area without blister formation
- Superficial, 2nd degree
  - Erythema, significant edema, blisters with clear fluid within 6–24 hours
  - Desquamation may occur with eschar formation 7–14 days after initial injury.
- Deep, 3rd degree: hemorrhagic blisters, necrosis of skin and subcutaneous tissues, skin discoloration in 5–10 days
- Deep, 4th degree: initially, little edema with cyanosis or mottling; eventually, complete necrosis, then becomes black, dry, and mummifies; occasionally results in self-amputation

DIAGNOSTIC TESTS & INTERPRETATION

Lab

Usually not necessary but may be indicated when infection is suspected

Imaging

- No diagnostic studies done immediately after rewarming can accurately predict amount of nonviable tissue.
- Radionucleotide angiography with 99m-Tc-pertechnetate or triple-phase bone scanning with 99m-Tc-methylene diphosphonate 1–2 weeks after initial injury is advocated by some to assess tissue viability in cases of 3rd- and 4th-degree frostbite.
- MRI and MRA are being advocated by some as superior techniques for severe frostbite. They allow for direct visualization of occluded vessels and tissue, giving a more clear-cut demarcation of ischemic tissue injury, which may allow for earlier surgical intervention.

DIFFERENTIAL DIAGNOSIS

- Frostnip: mild form of cold injury with pallor and painful, tingling sensation. Warming of cold tissue results in no tissue damage.
- Hypothermia
- Thermal injury: easily excluded based on history but can result from warming techniques

TREATMENT

MEDICATION

- Tetanus prophylaxis: dT, dTap, or DT/DTaP, depending on age, and tetanus immunoglobulin if patient not fully immunized
- Anti-thromboxane agents (NSAIDs, prostaglandin E_1 [PGE1]) to prevent intravascular thrombosis
- Pentoxifylline (a phosphodiesterase inhibitor) should be considered with severe frostbite. It has been shown to enhance tissue viability by increasing blood flow and reducing platelet activity.
- Analgesics: as indicated
- Antibiotics: given prophylactically by some; others recommend waiting for signs of infection or necrotic tissue.
- Tissue plasminogen activator (tPA) is being used by frostbite specialists within 24 hours of acute, severe frostbite. It is useful when microvascular thrombosis has already developed. Studies show it can significantly reduce digital amputation rates

ADDITIONAL TREATMENT

General Measures

- Check core temperature to rule out hypothermia, which would need to be addressed first.
- Remove constrictive clothing and jewelry.
- Rapid rewarming in warm water (40–42°C) for 15–45 minutes
  - Do not rewarm slowly.
  - Rewarming is complete when skin is soft and sensation returns.
  - Usually all that is needed for superficial, 1st-degree frostbite
- Apply dry, sterile dressings to affected areas and between frostbitten toes and fingers.
- Intact nontense clear blisters should be left in place and wrapped with loosely applied dry gauze dressings. Rupturing may increase the risk of infection.

- Tense or hemorrhagic blister may be carefully aspirated, but this increases the risk for infection.
- Ruptured blisters should be debrided and covered with antibiotic ointment and nonadhesive dressings.
- Elevate affected parts to minimize edema.
- Daily hydrotherapy with hexachlorophene or povidone-iodine added to water
- Topical application of aloe vera (for its antiprostaglandin effect) to debrided blisters and intact hemorrhagic blisters to minimize further thromboxane synthesis

ALERT
- Prohibit nicotine use because of its vasoconstrictive properties.
- Full extent of injury may not be apparent at presentation. Close observation is important.

SURGERY/OTHER PROCEDURES
- Conservative surgical intervention: recommended because it usually takes 6–8 weeks for injured tissue to declare viability
- Escharotomy: performed on digits with impaired circulation or movement
- Fasciotomy: performed if significant edema causes compartment syndrome
- Early amputation and debridement with closure of wound site: necessary for uncontrolled infection
- Debridement of mummified tissue: performed after 1–3 months

INPATIENT CONSIDERATIONS
Initial Stabilization
- Do not rub the area; it may cause mechanical injury.
- Do not expose the area to direct heat; it may cause burn injury.
- Refreezing after thawing leads to increased injury.
- Remove wet clothing and constricting jewelry.

ONGOING CARE

PROGNOSIS
- Depends on degree of cold injury
- Superficial, 1st-degree frostbite heals in a few weeks.
- Favorable indicators: sensation in affected area, healthy-looking skin color, blisters filled with clear fluid
- Unfavorable indicators: cyanosis, blood-filled blisters, unhealthy-looking skin color
- Early rehabilitation often needed for functional recovery.
- Long-term follow-up for 6–12 months to monitor for sequelae
- Education to avoid reexposure and reinjury

COMPLICATIONS
- Arthritis
- Changes in skin color
- Chronic numbness
- Chronic pain
- Cold hypersensitivity
- Digital deformities
- Gangrene
- Growth plate abnormalities (only in children)
- Hyperesthesias
- Neuropathy
- Premature closure of the physis (in children)
- Reduced sensitivity to touch
- Rhabdomyolysis
- Squamous cell carcinoma (rare)
- Tetanus
- Tissue loss
- Wound infection

ADDITIONAL READING

- Biem J, Koehncke N, Classen D, et al. Out of the cold: management of hypothermia and frostbite. *CMAJ*. 2003;168(3):305–311.
- Hallam MJ, Cubison T, Dheansa B, et al. Managing frostbite. *BMJ*. 2010;341:c5864.
- Murphy JV, Banwell PE, Roberts AH, et al. Frostbite: pathogenesis and treatment. *J Trauma*. 2000;48(1):171–178.
- Noonan B, Bancroft RW, Dines JS, et al. Heat- and cold-induced injuries in athletes: evaluation and management. *J Am Acad Orthop Surg*. 2012;20(12):744–754.
- Twomey JA, Peltier GL, Zera RT. An open-label study to evaluate the safety and efficacy of tissue plasminogen activator in treatment of frostbite. *J Trauma*. 2005;59(6):1350–1354.
- Woo EK, Lee JW, Hur GY, et al. Proposed treatment protocol for frostbite: a retrospective analysis of 17 case based on a 3-year single-institution experience. *Arch Plast Surg*. 2013:40(5):510–516.

CODES

ICD10
- T33.90XA Superficial frostbite of unspecified sites, init encntr
- T34.90XA Frostbite with tissue necrosis of unsp sites, init encntr
- T33.829A Superficial frostbite of unspecified foot, initial encounter

FAQ
- Q: Why did I need to get a tetanus shot when I had frostbite?
- A: Injuries, such as frostbite, that cause dead skin are at risk for causing tetanus. The absence of oxygen in dead tissues allows tetanus spore to reproduce and produce the toxin that leads to tetanus.
- Q: I've heard that your eyes can get frostbite. Is that true?
- A: Frozen corneas (the surface layer of the eye) have been reported in persons partaking in high windchill activities such as snowmobiling and skiing. Prevention is possible with the use of protective goggles/sunglasses.
- Q: My children's doctor recommended that we use sunscreen when we go skiing. Will the sunscreen help prevent frostbite?
- A: Although sunscreen is necessary to prevent getting sunburn that can occur from the sunlight's reflection off the snow, it will not decrease the risk for frostbite from the cold exposure.
- Q: I live in Buffalo, New York, where the winters are very cold and the windchill factor is often below zero. My children like playing outside, especially in the snow. How can I prevent them from getting frostbite?
- A: Because there is a risk of frostbite with a windchill factor of −25°C, try to encourage indoor play when the temperature dips this low. It is important to have the children come inside frequently to warm up and for you to check for signs of cold injury.
- Q: My family members are avid skiers. While traveling in Europe last winter, I purchased a protective emollient that was sold there. Can protective emollients prevent frostbite if used on the face and exposed areas while skiing?
- A: No. Research has shown that the use of "protective" emollients and creams leads to a false sense of safety and leads to an increased risk of frostbite. This is thought to be due mostly to the failure to use more efficient protective measures when the emollients and creams are used.
- Q: If my child has had frostbite in the past, can she get it again?
- A: Yes. Children who have had a previous frostbite injury are at increased risk for repeat injury, especially in the location of previous damage. Appropriate clothing and limitation of cold exposure should be strictly enforced.
- Q: To prevent frostbite, is there a temperature below which I should not let my child go out to play?
- A: Although body tissue freezes more quickly at lower temperatures, the degree of damage from frostbite is related to the length of time tissue remains frozen. Therefore, the amount of time spent outside during cold weather should never be prolonged.
- Q: How can I tell if my child has frostbite or just cold fingers?
- A: Cold fingers are red and may be painful but do not become numb or white. Frostbitten fingers are painful, white, and waxy prior to rewarming and turn red with rewarming. The sequential development of digital blanching, occasional cyanosis, and erythema of the fingers or toes following cold exposure and subsequent rewarming is known as Raynaud phenomenon.
- Q: If I suspect frostbite in my child and we are outdoors without access to warm water, are there any options for treatment?
- A: If there is a delay in reaching shelter, you can start to thaw your child's body part by using your body as a warmer by placing the exposed body part under your armpit and keeping it there until further care can be initiated. Before starting the rewarming process, you must be sure refreezing will not recur.
- Q: When should I call the doctor?
- A: The doctor should be called if, after rewarming, the skin is not soft and/or sensation does not return to normal. Call the doctor immediately if the skin is discolored and cold, blisters develop during rewarming, or there are signs of infection, such as the appearance of red streaks leading from the affected area, pus accumulation, or fever.
- Q: We are going on a winter vacation this year and expect to spend a lot of time outside skiing and sledding. What types of clothing should I pack for my 6-year-old son?
- A: It would be a good idea to pack a few pairs of waterproof mittens, a ski suit or ski pants, waterproof boots, thick cotton socks, and cotton thermal under garments. Try to make sure your son stays dry and warm. Take frequent breaks indoors to warm up and check your child for any early signs of cold injury.
- Q: Is frostnip the same thing as frostbite?
- A: No. Frostnip is the mildest form of cold injury, which commonly occurs on exposed parts of the body, such as the fingers, nose, and ears. The symptoms of frostnip are numbness and pallor of the involved body parts. Warming of these areas is the only treatment that is needed, and there is no associated tissue damage.

FUNCTIONAL DIARRHEA OF INFANCY (TODDLER'S DIARRHEA)

Roberto Gugig

BASICS

DESCRIPTION

- Benign chronic diarrhea in a toddler or a preschool child who appears healthy and is normally active and who is growing, without evidence of systemic illness, infection, malabsorption, or malnutrition
- Also known as chronic nonspecific diarrhea of childhood, toddler's diarrhea, and irritable bowel of childhood

RISK FACTORS

Genetics

Family members often report nonspecific GI complaints or functional bowel disorders.

GENERAL PREVENTION

- Limit the consumption and delay the introduction of sorbitol or fructose-rich fruit juices to the infant diet.
- In the treatment of acute gastroenteritis, parents should be instructed to give an oral rehydration solution (ORS) and resume normal feeding early, avoiding diet restrictions.
- Avoid restrictive diets that may cause caloric deprivation.

PATHOPHYSIOLOGY

- Carbohydrate malabsorption
  - Diarrhea is often preceded by acute gastroenteritis or other viral infection that results in dietary restrictions. Increased oral fluids, including juices, are used to compensate for stool losses and to prevent dehydration.
  - Capacity of the small intestine to absorb fructose is limited. Foods that contain equivalent amounts of fructose and glucose are more readily absorbed because of the additive effect of a glucose-dependent fructose cotransport mechanism.
  - Excessive consumption of juices high in sorbitol (which inhibits fructose absorption) and those with a high fructose-to-glucose ratio (e.g., apple juice) result in fructose malabsorption and increased intraluminal gas caused by fermentation. The end result is abdominal distension, excessive flatulence, and diarrhea.
  - Colonic function: possibly, disruption of colonic ability to ferment unabsorbed carbohydrates into short-chain fatty acids (SCFA), which maintain colonic function and prevent colon-based diarrhea
- Disturbed motility: short mouth-to-anus transit time
  - Persistence of immature bowel motility pattern. Failure of initiation of normal postprandial delayed gastric emptying
  - Low-fat meals. Meals with high dietary fat delay gastric emptying.
  - Excess fluid intake. Infant's colon already operates in high efficiency (in children, higher volume of fluids reach the cecum). Excessive fluids can lead to diarrhea.
  - Low-fiber diet. Dietary fiber serves as a bulking agent.
  - Excessive fecal bile acids. Rapid transit resulting in excess conjugated bile salt entering the colon. Bacterial degradation produces unconjugated bile salts, which decrease net water absorption in the colon.

ETIOLOGY

- Nutritional factors: excessive consumption of fruit juice; high-carbohydrate, low-fat, and low-fiber diet
- Disordered intestinal motility (i.e., variant of irritable bowel syndrome of infancy) with rapid transit

DIAGNOSIS

- The typical age is 12–36 months, but range is 6 months to 5 years.
- Diagnostic criteria (Rome III):
  - Daily, painless, recurrent passage of ≥3 large unformed stools
  - Symptoms that last >4 weeks
  - Onset of symptoms that begins between 6 and 36 months of age
  - Passage of stools that occurs during waking hours
  - There is no failure to thrive (FTT) if caloric intake is adequate:
    - There is no definite diagnostic test. The diagnosis is primarily clinical based on age of onset, the history, symptoms, clinical course, and limited number of laboratory tests. Usually, it is an evident condition and not a diagnosis of exclusion.

HISTORY

- Nutritional history is essential, with attention to the 4 Fs (fiber, fluid, fat, and fruit juices) and dietary changes.
- Diarrhea
  - For a toddler, it may not be abnormal to have >3 soft and occasionally loose stools a day with visible food remnants.
  - Children, typically, have intermittent symptoms, and are often diagnosed with recurrent viral gastroenteritis.
- Stool characteristics
  - Stools that smell foul and contain undigested food particles. Presence of blood or mucus suggests another diagnosis.
- Timing of diarrhea
  - No stools passed at night, and typically, the first stool of the day is large and has firmer consistency than those occurring later on in the day.
- Recent enteric infection
  - Presence of other affected family members, history of travel, day care, and infectious contacts suggests infectious cause.
- Signs and symptoms:
  - Thorough history is required because all illnesses in the differential diagnosis are associated with morbidity if diagnosis is delayed.

PHYSICAL EXAM

- Normal: Children look healthy, eat well, and are growing normally according to serial plots on the growth chart.
- There are no signs of malnutrition or malabsorption. Weight might be influenced by the dietary measures.
- Fecal mass(es) found on abdominal palpation may signal constipation.

DIAGNOSTIC TESTS & INTERPRETATION

- The following tests would be helpful only if indicated by history and physical exam:
  - Cystic fibrosis: sweat test, stool for pancreatic enzymes, and genetic testing
  - Celiac disease is common and warrants a serologic testing (antiendomysial antibodies, tissue transglutaminase antibodies with IgA serum levels).
  - CBC, iron studies, vitamin levels, serum albumin
  - Allergy testing for suspected food proteins (commonly milk, soy, egg, and wheat)
  - Inflammatory markers
- Diarrhea as the sole symptom of malabsorption in a normally thriving child is rare.

Lab

- Stool tests and culture: negative for white blood cells, blood, fat, and pathogens including ova, parasites, and *Giardia* antigen
- Serum electrolytes normal: no dehydration
- Celiac serology: negative
- CBC normal: no anemia
- Food allergen testing: negative

Imaging

Usually unnecessary: Plain abdominal radiograph may demonstrate colonic fecal retention.

Diagnostic Procedures/Other
- A trial of lactose and fruit juice–free diet done separately is practical and diagnostic.
- Breath hydrogen test has limited benefit and is inferior to a trial of milk avoidance.
- Small bowel biopsy is rarely indicated unless strong evidence suggests another cause (e.g., positive celiac serology).

DIFFERENTIAL DIAGNOSIS
- All causes of chronic diarrhea should be considered.
- Infection: bacterial, viral, and parasite (giardiasis, cryptosporidiosis)
- Celiac disease
- Malabsorption: carbohydrate: postinfectious secondary lactose intolerance, sucrase-isomaltase deficiency
- Pancreatic: cystic fibrosis, Shwachman-Diamond syndrome, Johannson-Blizzard syndrome, chronic pancreatitis
- Bile acid disorders: chronic cholestasis, terminal ileum disease, bacterial overgrowth
- Immunologic: cow's milk and soy protein intolerance, food allergy, immunodeficiency
- Food allergies
- Miscellaneous: antibiotic-associated diarrhea, laxatives, fecal retention constipation, UTI, abetalipoproteinemia, inflammatory bowel disease, short-bowel syndrome, hormone-secreting tumors, Munchausen by proxy
- Common conditions that may cause diarrhea without FTT: constipation, lactose intolerance, and persistent infective diarrhea
- Constipation-related diarrhea is frequently overlooked. Consider it if diarrhea alternates with hard stools.

TREATMENT

MEDICATION
- Medications are unwarranted for a condition primarily caused by food that does not hamper growth.
- Metronidazole may be beneficial for patients with undetected giardiasis.
- Loperamide is effective in normalizing bowel patterns, but only for duration of therapy.
- Studies have shown that certain probiotic preparations such as *Lactobacillus rhamnosus* and *Saccharomyces boulardii* may be effective at reducing symptoms.

ADDITIONAL TREATMENT
General Measures
Daily diet and defecation diary may document a specific food responsible for loose stools.

ADDITIONAL THERAPIES
Reassure parents that there is no underlying GI disease, infection, or inflammation.

ISSUES FOR REFERRAL
- Failure of response to diet
- Weight loss despite adequate intake
- Presence of other symptoms (e.g., anorexia, irritability, fever, vomiting)
- Fat, blood, and mucus in the stool

ONGOING CARE

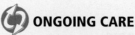

FOLLOW-UP RECOMMENDATIONS
- Improvement with dietary changes confirms the diagnosis and reassures the parents.
- Follow up phone call to parents within a few days of instituting diet. If no improvement within 2 weeks despite good compliance with dietary recommendations, then reconsider diagnosis; consider more diagnostic tests and referral to a specialist.

Patient Monitoring
- Follow growth parameters.
- Monitor symptoms indicating nonfunctional illness.

DIET
- The child's feeding pattern should be normalized according to the 4 Fs:
  - Overconsumption of *fruit juices* should be discouraged, especially those that contain sorbitol and a high fructose-to-glucose ratio (e.g., apple juice, pear nectar).
    - Cloudy apple juice or white grape juice may be safe as alternatives.
  - *Fiber intake* should be normalized by introduction of whole-grain bread and fruits.
  - Increase *dietary fat* to at least 35–40% of total energy intake. Substitution of low-fat milk with whole milk may be sufficient.
  - Restrict *fluid intake* to $<$90 mL/kg/24 h if history is significant for fluid consumption $>$150 mL/kg/24 h.
- Improvement occurs within a few days to a couple of weeks after initiating the earlier discussed therapy.

PROGNOSIS
- Good
- Symptoms resolve by school age.
- Long-term benefit of low-carbohydrate diet: contributes to balanced nutrition and the prevention of obesity

COMPLICATIONS
Although children tend not to suffer from the symptoms, parents are often worried and frustrated and require frequent reassurance.

ADDITIONAL READING

- Hoekstra JH. Toddler diarrhoea: more a nutritional disorder than a disease. *Arch Dis Child*. 1998;79(1):2–5.
- Huffman S. Toddler's diarrhea. *J Pediatr Health Care*. 1999;13(1):32–33.
- Hyman PE, Milla PJ, Benninga MA, et al. Childhood functional GI disorders: neonate/toddler. *Gastroenterology*. 2006;130(5):1519–1526.
- Judd RH. Chronic nonspecific diarrhea. *Pediatr Rev*. 1996;17(11):379–384.
- Kneepkens CM, Hoekstra JH. Chronic nonspecific diarrhea of childhood: pathophysiology and management. *Pediatr Clin North Am*. 1996;43(2):375–390.
- Moukarzel AA, Lesicka H, Ament ME. Irritable bowel syndrome and nonspecific diarrhea in infancy and childhood: relationship with juice carbohydrate malabsorption. *Clin Pediatr*. 2002;41(3):145–150.
- Vernacchio L, Vezina RM, Mitchell AA, et al. Characteristics of persistent diarrhea in a community-based cohort of young US children. *J Pediatr Gastroenterol Nutr*. 2006;43(1):52–58.

CODES

ICD10
- K59.1 Functional diarrhea
- K90.4 Malabsorption due to intolerance, not elsewhere classified

FAQ
- Q: How do I know that my toddler's diarrhea is not serious?
- A: Growth is usually normal and your child looks and feels well. His or her activity and development seem unaffected by the diarrhea. The change of diet results in improvement.
- Q: What are the components of a successful treatment plan?
- A: Attention to the 4 Fs in the diet: decreased fruit juice intake, increased fat intake, decreased fluid, and increased fiber intake
- Q: Are probiotics useful in the treatment of toddler's diarrhea?
- A: There is no adequate data to support such a recommendation, but evidence is emerging that probiotics may be effective in treating "irritable bowel syndrome like diarrhea and bloating."
- Q: When should care by a pediatric gastroenterologist be sought?
- A: If no response after 2 weeks of compliance with dietary therapy, if growth is delayed, or if other GI or systemic complaints are present, seek a pediatric gastroenterologist's care.
- Q: Did my child get diarrhea because he goes to child care or because he is not clean?
- A. No. Functional diarrhea is not caused by infection.

FUNGAL SKIN INFECTIONS (DERMATOPHYTE INFECTIONS, CANDIDIASIS, AND TINEA VERSICOLOR)

Sonal Shah • Renee Howard

BASICS

DESCRIPTION

Superficial fungal infections of the skin, hair, and nails are characterized by erythema, scaling, changes in color, and pruritus.

EPIDEMIOLOGY

- Dermatophyte infections
  - Tinea capitis
    - Most common fungal infection in pediatric population
    - Occurs mainly in prepubescent children (between ages 3 and 7 years)
    - Asymptomatic carriers are common and contribute to spread.
  - Tinea corporis is usually seen in younger children or in young adolescents with close physical contact to others (i.e., wrestlers).
  - Onychomycosis: Overall prevalence is 0–2.6% in children; often occurs with concomitant tinea pedis or in 1st-degree relatives with infection
- Candidiasis: majority of infants colonized with *Candida albicans*
- Tinea versicolor: seen in adolescents and young adults

GENERAL PREVENTION

- Measures should be taken to avoid transmission between hosts, including not sharing combs, brushes, hats, etc.
- Hair utensils and hats should be washed in hot, soapy water at onset of therapy.
- Pets should be watched and treated early for any suspicious lesions.
- In patients in whom appropriate therapy has not led to improvement in symptoms, siblings and close contacts should be examined and fungal cultures performed.
- Isolation of hospitalized patient is unnecessary.

PATHOPHYSIOLOGY

- Fungal elements (arthroconidia) adhere to stratum corneum or hair shaft. Proteases work to degrade keratin, which allows for invasion of dermatophytes.
- Predisposing factors may include moisture, macerated skin, and immunocompromise.
- Host immune response is usually able to contain infection.
- Inflammatory response is variable; highly inflammatory forms may lead to pustules and kerion (large inflammatory mass) formation.

ETIOLOGY

- Varies by geographic region
- Dermatophyte infections
  - Tinea capitis: >90% caused by *Trichophyton tonsurans* in North America; spread from human to human (anthropophilic); increasing incidence of *Microsporum canis* infection spread from animals such as cats and dogs to humans (zoophilic).
  - Tinea corporis: preadolescent children: *M. canis, Microsporum audouinii*; older children: *Trichophyton rubrum, Trichophyton mentagrophytes, T. tonsurans*
  - Onychomycosis: *T. rubrum, T. mentagrophytes*
- Candidiasis: usually *C. albicans*
- Tinea versicolor: *Malassezia furfur*

DIAGNOSIS

HISTORY

- Determine onset and duration.
- Elicit signs and symptoms such as expanding areas of erythema, scaling, or color change with associated pruritus.
- Determine contacts, including exposure to pets.
- Determine if patient is immunocompromised.
- List of medications previously prescribed or used

PHYSICAL EXAM

- Dermatophyte infections
  - Tinea capitis: Presentation varies.
    - Round patches of alopecia with erythema or black dots (broken hair shafts at surface of skin)
    - Diffusely dry scalp with scaling
    - Follicular pustules resembling bacterial folliculitis
    - Boggy, tender plaque with follicular pustules or purulent discharge (kerion): represents exaggerated immune response
    - Cervical or occipital lymphadenopathy
  - Tinea corporis
    - One or more, asymmetrically distributed, annular, well-demarcated erythematous scaling plaques with central clearing
    - Inflammatory forms may be frankly pustular or vesicular at the borders.
    - Lesions may occur anywhere on the body.
  - Onychomycosis
    - *Distal subungual* type: invasion of the underlying nail bed and inferior portion of the nail plate, which leads to detachment of the nail plate from the nail bed and subungual thickening and debris with yellowing of the plate
    - *Proximal subungual* type: invasion of the nail unit at the proximal nailfold (most common in HIV patients)
    - *White superficial* type: Superficial infection presents with white plaques on the dorsal nail plate.
- Candidiasis
  - Diffuse erythema (often "beefy" red) with sharp, marginated border
  - Pinpoint satellite pustules at edge of erythema
  - Prefers warm, moist environments
  - Favors skinfolds/creases (axillae, groin, below breasts, and, in infants, diaper area)
- Tinea versicolor
  - Scaling, oval patches that are either hypo- or hyperpigmented
  - Distributed on upper trunk, neck, and proximal arms and in areas where there is high amount of sebum and free fatty acids, which the organism requires; occasionally on face

DIAGNOSTIC TESTS & INTERPRETATION

Lab

- KOH preparation
  - Clean area with alcohol.
  - Using a no. 15 scalpel blade, gently scrape the outer edge of the active border, broken off hairs, or subungual debris.
  - Place material flat on a glass side in a single layer. Apply coverslip on top.
  - Place a few drops of 10–20% KOH to edge of coverslip until space between slide and coverslip is filled, and apply mild pressure.
  - Warm slide gently or let sit for 30 minutes.
  - Examine slide under microscope at low power under low light.
    - Dermatophytes: arthrospores around or within hair shaft; long, branching fungal hyphae with septations
    - Candidiasis: budding yeast, pseudohyphae
    - Tinea versicolor: short hyphae and clusters of spores ("spaghetti and meatballs")
- Fungal culture
  - Obtain specimen with scalpel blade from outer active edge of scaling.
  - For scalp, gently rub a wet sterile toothbrush, cytobrush, or cotton-tipped swab over the area of scaling, then plate on fungal medium.
  - Results can take up to 4 weeks.
  - Some laboratories provide drug susceptibility testing as well as identification of fungus.

Diagnostic Procedures/Other

- Wood's lamp examination (~360-nm wavelength of ultraviolet light): Infected hairs may fluoresce (not useful in skin or nail infections).
  - Examine in completely darkened room.
  - Ectothrix infections (organisms outside of hair shaft): bright green fluorescence (*M. canis* and *M. audouinii*); endothrix infections (organisms inside hair shaft): do not fluoresce (*T. tonsurans*)
  - Tinea versicolor: yellow, copper, or bronze fluorescence

DIFFERENTIAL DIAGNOSIS

- Dermatophyte infections
  - Dermatologic conditions
    - Tinea capitis: seborrheic dermatitis, psoriasis, alopecia areata, trichotillomania, folliculitis, impetigo, atopic dermatitis
    - Tinea corporis: herald patch of pityriasis rosea, nummular dermatitis, psoriasis, contact or atopic dermatitis, granuloma annulare
    - Onychomycosis: psoriasis, nondermatophyte infection
  - Systemic diseases: cutaneous T-cell lymphoma, histiocytosis, sarcoidosis

- Candidiasis
  - Dermatologic conditions: contact dermatitis, seborrheic dermatitis, atopic dermatitis, bacterial infection
- Tinea versicolor
  - Dermatologic conditions: pityriasis alba, postinflammatory hypopigmentation, vitiligo, seborrheic dermatitis, pityriasis rosea

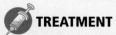

TREATMENT

MEDICATION

First Line

- Dermatophyte infections
  - Tinea capitis: systemic therapy warranted to penetrate hair shaft
    - Oral griseofulvin: 20–25 mg/kg/24 h (max 1 g/24 h) once daily or divided b.i.d. of microsize griseofulvin for 6–8 weeks (10–15 mg/kg/24 h [max 750 mg/24 h] once daily or divided b.i.d. if ultramicrosize form is used), taken with high-fat food (e.g., milk or ice cream) for 6–12 weeks. In addition, topical therapy of 2.5% selenium sulfide or ketoconazole shampoo twice weekly suppresses viable spores. Laboratory monitoring is not needed.
  - Tinea capitis with kerion
    - Treat for tinea capitis.
    - Systemic steroids may be needed to treat significant inflammation.
  - Tinea corporis
    - Topical azole antifungals (1% clotrimazole, 2% ketoconazole) or 1% terbinafine cream applied twice daily for 2–4 weeks
  - Onychomycosis
    - Oral terbinafine 3–6 mg/kg/dose (max 250 mg) once daily for 6–12 weeks; can be associated with hepatic failure; avoid use in patients with liver disease. Check liver enzymes before and during treatment.
    - Oral itraconazole (adolescent and adult) in weekly pulses for 3–4 months; 200 mg twice daily for 7 days, then off for 3 weeks
- Candidiasis: topical nystatin cream or ointment 3–4 times daily for 7–10 days
- Tinea versicolor: selenium sulfide 2.5% applied to affected skin for 10 minutes. Wash off thoroughly. Apply daily for 7–10 days. Monthly applications may help prevent recurrences.

Second Line

- Dermatophyte infections
  - Tinea capitis
    - Oral itraconazole: 3–5 mg/kg once daily for 4–6 weeks. May also use oral terbinafine 3–6 mg/kg once daily for 4 weeks or oral fluconazole 5 mg/kg once daily for 4–6 weeks. All of these may be associated with hepatic failure and should be avoided in patients with liver disease. Liver enzymes should be checked before and during treatment.
  - Tinea corporis
    - Oral griseofulvin 15–25 mg/kg once daily or divided b.i.d. for 4 weeks for persistent or extensive involvement
- Candidiasis
  - Oral fluconazole
    - 6 mg/kg on day 1, then 3 mg/kg once daily for 2 weeks if poor response to topical therapy
- Tinea versicolor
  - Topical azole antifungals (ketoconazole 2% shampoo applied daily for 3 days)
  - Oral ketoconazole (adolescent and adult) 200–400 mg once daily for 5–10 days or itraconazole (adolescent and adult) 200 mg once daily for 5–7 days if severe, recurrent, or persistent

ONGOING CARE

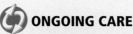

FOLLOW-UP RECOMMENDATIONS

Patient Monitoring

- Monitor for secondary bacterial infection.
- Highly inflammatory lesions (kerion) may require concomitant systemic steroids.
- Repeated infection may indicate a source that needs to be diagnosed and treated (e.g., family member or pet).

DIET

Griseofulvin is better absorbed with a fatty meal and should be taken with foods such as milk, eggs, or ice cream.

PROGNOSIS

- Dermatophyte: Inflammation improves within several days but may take several weeks to completely resolve; nail infections take 6–12 months to show improvement and are prone to recurrence.
- Areas with significant inflammatory component may become scarred and permanently alopecic.
- Candidal skin lesions improve within 24–48 hours and resolve by 1 week.
- Tinea versicolor: Resolution of dyspigmentation may take months to occur.
- Relapses and recurrences are common.

COMPLICATIONS

- Dermatophyte infections
  - Secondary bacterial infection
  - Kerion formation can lead to permanent alopecia and scarring.
- Candidiasis
  - Scarring in severe disease
  - Fungemia in immunocompromised host

ADDITIONAL READING

- Ameen M. Epidemiology of superficial fungal infections. *Clin Dermatol*. 2010;28(2):197–201.
- Andrews MD, Burns M. Common tinea infections in children. *Am Fam Physician*. 2008;77(10): 1415–1420.
- Baldo A. Mechanisms of skin adherence and invasion by dermatophytes. *Mycoses*. 2012;55(3):218–223.
- Elewski BE. Terbinafine hydrochloride oral granules versus oral griseofulvin suspension in children with tinea capitis: results of two randomized, investigator-blinded, multicenter, international, controlled trials. *J Am Acad Dermatol*. 2008;59(1): 41–54.
- Gupta AK. Superficial fungal infections: an update on pityriasis versicolor, seborrheic dermatitis, tinea capitis, and onychomycosis. *Clin Dermatol*. 2003;21(5):417–425.
- Shemer A. Update: medical treatment of onychomycosis. *Dermatol Ther*. 2012;25(6):582–593.

CODES

ICD10

- B35.9 Dermatophytosis, unspecified
- B35.4 Tinea corporis
- B37.2 Candidiasis of skin and nail

FAQ

- Q: What is the role of combination topical antifungals and corticosteroids in the treatment of superficial fungal infections of the skin?
- A: Combination products containing high-potency topical steroid antifungals should be avoided. High-potency topical steroids may lead to a decrease in inflammation; however, they can mask the clinical features of tinea infection (so-called tinea incognito) and can allow for rapid expansion of infection. In addition, prolonged use of high-potency topical steroids used particularly in intertriginous areas can lead to side effects such as striae formation and atrophy of the skin.
- Q: What can be done to prevent recurrent tinea versicolor infection?
- A: *M. furfur* is a normal part of skin flora and lives in lipid-rich areas of skin. Tropical climates, humid environments, and excessive sweating result in infection in adolescents and young adults. Recurrences are common and can be prevented by regular application of selenium sulfide 2.5%. In addition, itraconazole has been shown to be effective in prevention of tinea versicolor. In one study, the recurrence of tinea versicolor was prevented in 88% of patients over a 6-month period using itraconazole 200 mg b.i.d. 1 day per month.
- Q: How can a clinician adequately assess for complete clearance when treating tinea capitis?
- A: At the end of treatment course, a repeat fungal culture should be performed to ensure complete clearance of spores.

GASTRITIS

Richard Lirio

BASICS

DESCRIPTION

Microscopic inflammation of mucosa of stomach

EPIDEMIOLOGY

- Most common cause of upper GI tract hemorrhage in older children
- 8 out of every 1,000 people are estimated to have gastritis.
- >2% of ICU patients have heavy bleeding secondary to gastritis.

ETIOLOGY

- Physiologic stress (e.g., chronic disease, CNS disease, overwhelming sepsis, ICU patients)
- Peptic disease
- Drug-induced (e.g., NSAIDs, steroids, valproate; more rarely, iron, calcium salts, potassium chloride, antibiotics)
- Infection (e.g., tuberculosis, *Helicobacter pylori*, cytomegalovirus, parasites)
- *H. pylori* (children more likely to have more severe gastritis, specifically located in antrum of stomach)
- Celiac disease: lymphocytic gastritis
- Major surgery; severe burns; renal, liver, respiratory failure; severe trauma
- Caustic ingestions (e.g., lye, strong acids, pine oil)
- Protein sensitivity (e.g., cow's milk-protein allergy), allergic enteropathy
- Eosinophilic gastroenteritis
- Crohn disease: Up to 40% of Crohn patients have gastroduodenal involvement.
- Gastric Crohn disease may manifest itself as highly focal, non–*H. pylori*, nongranulomatous gastritis.
- Direct trauma (nasogastric tubes)
- Ethanol
- Idiopathic
- Less common causes:
  - Radiation
  - Hypertrophic gastritis (Ménétrier disease)
  - Autoimmune gastritis
  - Collagenous gastritis
  - Zollinger-Ellison syndrome
  - Vascular injury

DIAGNOSIS

HISTORY

- Epigastric pain
- Abdominal indigestion
- Nausea
- Vomiting postprandially
- Vomiting blood or coffee ground–like material
- Diarrhea
- Dark or black stools (or bright red blood from rectum, if bleeding is brisk and intestinal transit time is short)
- Irritability
- Poor feeding and weight loss
- Less often: chest pain, hematemesis, melena

PHYSICAL EXAM

- Epigastric tenderness is physical finding that most closely correlates with gastritis on endoscopy.
- Normal bowel sounds

DIAGNOSTIC TESTS & INTERPRETATION

Lab

- CBC
  - Evaluate for anemia with other signs of chronic blood loss (e.g., microcytosis, low reticulocyte count).
- Heme testing stool may be helpful.
- *H. pylori* identification
  - Noninvasive *H. pylori* tests, including antibody (from serum, whole blood, saliva, or urine), antigen (from stool), or urea breath testing (UBT)
  - UBT (using C_{13}) and stool antigen tests are more reliable and sensitive than antibody testing; serologic testing is not recommended. However, UBT is not widely available and is used primarily in adults.
  - Rapid urease test from gastric biopsy specimen for *H. pylori*

Imaging

- Upper GI radiography when endoscopy not available
- Chest radiograph may detect free abdominal air secondary to perforation.

Endoscopy

Upper endoscopy with biopsies

- Greatest sensitivity for gastritis
- Possible gross findings:
  - Erythema, granularity, edema, small ulcerations
  - Thickened hyperemic mucosa
  - Atrophic mucosa
  - Antral micronodules (represent lymphoid follicles) commonly seen in children with *H. pylori* infection
  - Antral and prepyloric edema with retained gastric secretions
- Biopsies will show chronic and/or active inflammation.
  - Can order special staining (Silver Warthin-Starry stain, Genta stain, modified Giemsa stain, or cresyl violet stain) of gastric biopsy for *H. pylori*
  - Culture and sensitivities of homogenized gastric biopsy for *H. pylori* (difficult to perform outside of research setting)

DIFFERENTIAL DIAGNOSIS

- Gastroesophageal reflux with esophagitis
- Peptic ulcer disease
- Biliary tract disorders
- Pancreatitis
- Inflammatory bowel disease
- Genitourinary pathology (renal stones, infection)
- Nonulcer dyspepsia
- Functional pain
- Allergic enteropathy

TREATMENT

MEDICATION

- Proton pump inhibitors: drug of choice as 1st-line therapy. Can also use antacids or H_2 blockers to maintain gastric pH >4–5
  - Ranitidine: 2–3 mg/kg/dose b.i.d.–t.i.d. in children
  - Famotidine: 0.5–2 mg/kg/24 h divided b.i.d.
  - Omeprazole, lansoprazole, rabeprazole, or esomeprazole: 1–2 mg/kg/24 h divided b.i.d.
  - Interactions: Cimetidine is less effective and can increase toxicity when given to patients receiving other medicines metabolized by cytochrome P450 system (e.g., theophylline). Proton pump inhibitors can also interfere with the absorption of other medicines and may interact with other medicines metabolized by specific cytochrome P450 isoenzymes.

- Misoprostol
  - Synthetic prostaglandin E1 (PGE1)
  - May reduce risk of progression of gastritis to ulcers in patients taking NSAIDs
  - Concerns exist for increased cardiovascular events in adults when using misoprostol.
- Discontinue NSAIDs.
- Treatment of *H. pylori*:
  - Triple therapy with proton pump inhibitor and antibiotics (e.g., omeprazole, amoxicillin, and clarithromycin)
  - If eradication unsuccessful, quadruple therapy is recommended for 7–14 days, including the following:
    - Bismuth (of note, may need to avoid bismuth subsalicylate and choose instead bismuth subcitrate)
    - Metronidazole
    - A proton pump inhibitor
    - Another antibiotic (either amoxicillin, clarithromycin, or tetracycline)
  - Drug regimens change frequently; clarithromycin resistance becoming increasingly problematic

ALERT

- Antacids are not palatable to children and can lead to diarrhea or constipation. Prolonged use of large doses of aluminum hydroxide–containing antacids may lead to phosphate depletion and aluminum-related CNS toxicity (particularly in patients with renal disease).
- If *H. pylori* eradication is attempted, important to use a tested regimen. Untested substitutions in the triple or quadruple regimens should be avoided.

ONGOING CARE

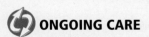

FOLLOW-UP-RECOMMENDATIONS

Patient Monitoring

- For stress gastritis with hemorrhage, provide vigilant supportive care with close monitoring of hemodynamics, fluids, and electrolytes.
- Monitor for Hemoccult-positive stools.
- Follow CBCs.
- May elect to repeat endoscopy in severe cases

DIET

- Benefit of changes in diet is inconclusive.
- Eliminate alcohol, tobacco, and caffeine, as well as NSAIDs.

PROGNOSIS

Significant gastritis relapse rates for children who remain infected with *H. pylori*

COMPLICATIONS

- Bleeding (from mild to hemorrhagic)
- When gastritis caused by acid/alkali ingestions, outlet obstruction may result from prepyloric strictures (4–8 weeks after ingestion).

ADDITIONAL READING

- Aanpreung P. Hematemesis in infants induced by cow milk allergy. *Asian Pac J Allergy Immunol*. 2003;21(4):211–216.
- Drumm B, Koletzko S, Oderda G. *Helicobacter pylori* infection in children: a consensus statement. European Paediatric Task Force on *Helicobacter pylori*. *J Pediatr Gastroenterol Nutr*. 2000;30(2):207–213.
- Hino B, Eliakim R, Levine A, et al. Comparison of invasive and non-invasive tests diagnosis and monitoring of *Helicobacter pylori* infection in children. *J Pediatr Gastroenterol Nutr*. 2004;39(5):519–523.
- Pashankar DS, Bishop WP, Mitros FA. Chemical gastropathy: a distinct histopathologic entity in children. *J Pediatr Gastroenterol Nutr*. 2002;35(5):653–657.
- Vesoulis Z, Lozanski G, Ravichandran P, et al. Collagenous gastritis: a case report, morphologic evaluation, and review. *Mod Pathol*. 2000;13(5):591–596.
- Weinstein WM. Emerging gastritides. *Curr Gastroenterol Rep*. 2001;3(6):523–527.
- Zheng PY, Jones NL. Recent advances in *Helicobacter pylori* infection in children: from the petri dish to the playground. *Can J Gastroenterol*. 2003;17(7):448–454.
- Zimmermann AE, Walters JK, Katona BG, et al. A review of omeprazole use in the treatment of acid-related disorders in children. *Clin Ther*. 2001;23(5):660–679.

CODES

ICD10

- K29.70 Gastritis, unspecified, without bleeding
- K29.71 Gastritis, unspecified, with bleeding
- K29.60 Other gastritis without bleeding

FAQ

- Q: Will a bland diet help to resolve gastritis?
- A: Dietary changes have not been shown to affect the natural course of gastritis.
- Q: What is *H. pylori*?
- A: *H. pylori* is a bacterium frequently found in the gastric mucosa of patients with gastritis and peptic ulcer disease. It can be diagnosed by a variety of means, often including a combination of upper endoscopy and urea breath tests. Relapse rates for gastritis secondary to *H. pylori* are high when the infection is left untreated.
- Q: Is it appropriate to treat cases of gastritis with antibiotics not proven to be *H. pylori*?
- A: No. It is important to treat only confirmed *H. pylori* infections, not to treat on suspicion of infection, especially with increasing issues with antibiotic resistance.
- Q: If a patient is treated for *H. pylori* and they still have symptoms and a positive stool *H. pylori* Ag, what would be the next course of action?
- A: Consider retreating with a proton pump inhibitor, amoxicillin, and Flagyl, as clarithromycin resistance in *H. pylori* infection is an increasingly frequent cause for treatment failure.
- Q: What are newly recognized complications of treating patients with proton pump inhibitors?
- A: Some adult studies show hypomagnesemia, increased risk of pneumonia, hip fracture, and *Clostridium difficile* infection are associated with proton pump inhibitor use.

GASTROESOPHAGEAL REFLUX

Peter D. Ngo

BASICS

DESCRIPTION

- Effortless regurgitation of gastric contents. Occurs physiologically at all ages, and most episodes are brief and asymptomatic
- Divided into physiologic and pathologic processes:
  - Some degree of physiologic gastroesophageal reflux (GER) is normal at all ages.
  - Physiologic infant reflux (normal GER of infancy) is very common. Symptoms peak around 4 months of age and generally have resolved by 1 year of age.
  - Pathologic reflux or gastroesophageal reflux disease (GERD) is defined by troublesome symptoms or complications of GER.
  - Complications may include reflux esophagitis, bleeding, esophageal stricture, failure to thrive, chronic/recurrent respiratory tract disease, or vomiting.

EPIDEMIOLOGY

Pathologic GERD: 10% of adults, 2–8% of children

RISK FACTORS

- Neurologic disorders (cerebral palsy/quadriplegia)
- Esophageal atresia
- Tracheoesophageal fistula
- Cystic fibrosis
- Asthma
- Gastroparesis
- Hiatal hernia

PATHOPHYSIOLOGY

Transient relaxation of the lower esophageal sphincter during episodes of increased abdominal and gastric pressure. GERD is a multifactorial process involving number of reflux events, acidity, esophageal clearance, gastric emptying, mucosal barriers, visceral hypersensitivity, and airway responsiveness.

DIAGNOSIS

HISTORY

- General symptoms of GERD:
  - Vomiting
  - Irritability
  - Chest/abdominal pain
  - Heartburn
  - Hematemesis, melena
  - Blood loss
  - Dysphagia
  - Food refusal
  - Cough, wheezing
  - Obstructive apnea
  - Dysphonia
  - Aspiration pneumonia
  - Posturing (Sandifer syndrome)
- GERD may be asymptomatic and still carry risk of complications.
- Infant
  - Many common conditions in infancy such as physiologic GER, infant colic, milk protein allergy, or multifactorial feeding difficulties/aversion can present with symptoms that can be difficult to distinguish from GERD and history should also assess for these conditions.
  - Pay attention to feeding volume and frequency in addition to weight gain, failure to thrive, and irritability in association with regurgitation events.
  - Identify episodes of pneumonia, obstructive apnea, chronic cough, stridor, wheezing.
  - Identify additional signs/symptoms that suggest food protein allergy (hematochezia, rash, diarrhea, irritability, failure to thrive).
  - Evaluate for evidence of bowel obstruction (forceful emesis, polyhydramnios during pregnancy).
  - If vomiting is atypical or associated with other signs/symptoms, rule out infection, metabolic disease, anatomic abnormality, or neurologic disease.
  - Special questions:
    - Presence of polyhydramnios or bilious emesis?
    - Family history of metabolic disease?
    - Family history of allergies/atopy?
    - Perinatal asphyxia (and other neurologic disorders)?
    - History of prematurity?
- Older child
  - Identify typical adult GERD complaints (chest pain, heartburn, regurgitation, dysphagia), but recognize that children describe discomfort poorly (often isolated abdominal pain).
  - Identify episodes of pneumonia, choking, chronic cough, laryngitis, stridor, and wheezing (may need to assess swallowing function).
  - Assess for solid food dysphagia (more common with eosinophilic esophagitis).
  - Evaluate for presence of nocturnal GERD symptoms.
  - Special questions:
    - Family history of GERD?
    - Family history of allergies/atopy?
    - Family history of eosinophilic esophagitis or other chronic GI disease such as celiac disease or inflammatory bowel disease.

PHYSICAL EXAM

- May be normal
- Growth failure
- Reactive airway disease and other manifestations of pulmonary complications
- Anemia or blood in stool (uncommon)
- Erosive dental disease (possibly linked to GERD, but common unrelated finding)

DIAGNOSTIC TESTS & INTERPRETATION

- Diagnosis of GERD is frequently made clinically.
- Testing is typically only needed to evaluate for other conditions, evaluate questionable cases, potential causes, complications, or symptom-reflux correlations. Evaluation may include the following:
  - Common screening laboratories (CBC, routine chemistries, transaminases)
  - Allergen testing (i.e., milk, soy, egg, etc.)
  - Celiac serology
  - Stool occult blood
  - Stool *Helicobacter pylori* antigen

Imaging

- Upper GI contrast study: Evaluate anatomy.
- Chest x-ray: Evaluate for recurrent pneumonia (if warranted by respiratory symptoms).
- Modified barium swallow: Evaluate swallowing function and for aspiration.
- Gastric-emptying study (gastric scintigraphy): Evaluate gastric motility and/or pulmonary aspiration.

Diagnostic Procedures/Other

- Empiric trial of medication (recommended for 4 weeks)
- pH probe study
  - To quantify and correlate esophageal acid exposure with symptoms over a 24-hour period (commonly performed off of acid blockade therapy)
- Combined pH/multichannel intraluminal impedance (MII):
  - Allows detection of both acid and nonacid GER events. May detect more pathologic reflux than pH probe alone (can be performed on or off of acid blockade)
  - Wireless pH monitoring (disposable probe placed endoscopically and clipped to esophageal mucosa)
- Esophagogastroduodenoscopy with biopsies
- Laryngoscopy
- Bronchoscopy
- Esophageal manometry
- Antroduodenal manometry

Pathologic Findings

Evidence of reflux esophagitis, allergic esophagitis, Barrett esophagus, adenocarcinoma, stricture

DIFFERENTIAL DIAGNOSIS

- Toxin
  - Lead
  - Fe
  - Medications
- Renal
  - Obstructive uropathy
  - Uremia
- Infection
  - Gastroenteritis
  - *H. pylori*
  - Urinary tract infection
  - Sepsis
  - Pneumonia
  - Hepatitis
  - Otitis media
  - Pancreatitis
  - Cholecystitis
- Neurologic
  - Meningitis/encephalitis: intracranial injury
  - Brain tumor
  - Hydrocephalus
  - Subdural hematoma
- Metabolic
  - Urea cycle defects
  - Aminoacidopathies (phenylketonuria, maple syrup urine disease)
  - Adrenal hyperplasia
  - Galactosemia, fructosemia
- Allergy/food intolerance
  - Milk/soy protein allergy
  - Eosinophilic esophagitis
  - Celiac disease
  - Hereditary fructose intolerance
- Anatomic malformation
  - Diaphragmatic hernia
  - Gastric outlet obstruction
  - Esophageal atresia
  - Pyloric stenosis
  - Antral/duodenal web
  - Volvulus/malrotation
  - Meconium ileus
  - Enteral duplications
  - Intussusception
  - Trichobezoar
  - Foreign body
  - Incarcerated hernia

- Drugs that affect lower esophageal sphincter pressure:
  - Nitrates
  - Nicotine
  - Narcotics
  - Caffeine
  - Theophylline
  - Anticholinergic agents
  - Estrogen
  - Somatostatin
  - Prostaglandins
- Other:
  - Pregnancy
  - Cyclic vomiting syndrome

TREATMENT

Treatment should be individualized, and cost effectiveness should be considered.

MEDICATION

First Line

H_2 blockers: Good for intermittent or PRN dosing. Can be used for maintenance of chronic GERD in some patients and/or promote mucosal healing.

- Ranitidine (PO)
  - < 1 month: 6 mg/kg/24 h divided t.i.d.
  - ≥ 1 month to 16 years of age: 5–10 mg/kg/24 h divided b.i.d.–t.i.d. (max 300 mg/24 h)
  - Adults 150 mg b.i.d. or 300 mg nightly
- Famotidine (PO)
  - <3 months: 0.5 mg/kg daily
  - 3 months to 1 year: 0.5 mg/kg b.i.d.
  - 1–12 years: 1 mg/kg/24 h divided b.i.d. (max 80 mg/24 h)
  - 12 years–adults: 20 mg b.i.d.

Second Line

Proton pump inhibitors (PPI):

- Demonstrated to be more effective at blocking gastric acid as compared to H_2 blockers. Can be used for symptoms as well as mucosal injury, refractory to H_2 blockers. May be appropriate for short-term empiric trial of medication
  - Omeprazole (PO)
    - <1 year: 1–2 mg/kg/24 h (daily or divided b.i.d.); multiple studies demonstrate no improvement of clinical symptoms (crying, irritability).
    - >1 year: 1–2 mg/kg/24 h (daily or divided b.i.d.) to adult dose range
    - >20 kg: 20 mg once or twice daily
    - Up to 3.5 mg/kg/24 h have been used.
  - Lansoprazole (PO)
    - <1 year: 0.4–1.8 mg/kg/24 h (daily or divided b.i.d.); multiple studies demonstrate no improvement of clinical symptoms (crying, irritability).
    - 1–11 years: <10 kg 7.5 mg/24 h
    - 10–30 kg: 15 mg/dose daily up to b.i.d.
    - >30 kg: 30 mg/dose daily up to b.i.d.
  - Several other PPIs are available.
  - Side effects of PPIs may include headache, abdominal pain, and diarrhea.
  - Recent reports of increased risk for acute gastroenteritis, *Clostridium difficile* infection, and pneumonia in children. Adult studies report increased risk of osteopenia and bone fracture associated with higher dose and long-term use. Benefits should outweigh risks, especially for long-term use.
- Prokinetics: as adjunctive therapy for more severe GERD complications and hypomotility
  - No single drug has optimal prokinetic effect without significant side effects.
  - Not recommended as routine therapy
  - Erythromycin (PO)
    - 3–4 mg/kg/dose b.i.d.–t.i.d. (used in lower dose than for antibiotic purposes for gastric prokinetic effect)
    - Can prolong QT interval
    - Can develop tachyphylaxis
    - Short-term use can be considered for treatment of GERD symptoms seen in postinfectious gastroparesis which typically resolves spontaneously.
  - Metoclopramide (Reglan)
    - Dosage is significantly less for GERD indication as compared to the antiemetic indication.
    - Side effects: may cause dystonia or oculogyric crisis, black box warning regarding risk of tardive dyskinesia
- Calcium and aluminum/magnesium-containing antacids
  - Offers short-term symptom relief, requires multiple dosing
  - Side effects: carry risk of diarrhea and aluminum toxicity
  - Interactions: may lead to malabsorption of other medications
- Mucosal protective agents: sucralfate (Carafate) for erosive esophagitis; maximally effective at pH 4 and on mucosal lesions

ADDITIONAL TREATMENT

General Measures

- Parental reassurance and education, especially in infants with physiologic GER
- Small, frequent infant feedings
- Encourage burping in infants.
- Reassure parents that infant GER/GERD is not associated with sudden infant death syndrome.
- Thickening of infant feedings (~2–3 teaspoons cereal/ounce of formula): may help with volume of regurgitation, does not stop GER
- Positioning: keeping infant upright after feeds, head elevation in bed of older children only; prone positioning not recommended

SURGERY/OTHER PROCEDURES

- Fundoplication (open or laparoscopic)
  - To increase lower esophageal sphincter tone by wrapping portion of gastric fundus around lower esophagus
  - Variations may include addition of a gastric emptying procedure (i.e., pyloroplasty).
  - Indications: failure of aggressive medical management and/or persistent, life-threatening complications (i.e., esophageal stricture; intestinal metaplastic changes as in Barrett esophagus), presence of large hiatal hernia, poor airway protection leading to aspiration of gastric contents (i.e., severe neurodevelopmental delay)
- Fundoplication complications include the following:
  - Gas bloating syndrome
  - Intractable retching
  - Bowel obstruction
  - Dumping syndrome
  - Dysphagia
  - Paraesophageal hernia
  - Wrap failure with recurrent GERD (up to 6% failure at 48 months)
  - Limited long-term clinical effectiveness
- Greater morbidity may be associated with fundoplication in children with severe physical and mental disabilities.

ONGOING CARE

FOLLOW-UP RECOMMENDATIONS

May be appropriate to recommend repeat endoscopy for evidence of pathologic changes of esophagus

DIET

Dietary modifications in older child: Avoid large high-fat meals, especially before bedtime. Avoid caffeine, chocolate, acidic/spicy food, peppermint, but recent adult studies show this is on an individual basis only.

ADDITIONAL READING

- Colletti RB, Di Lorenzo C. Overview of pediatric gastroesophageal reflux disease and proton pump inhibitor therapy. *J Pediatr Gastroenterol Nutr*. 2003;37(Suppl 1):S7–S11.
- Craig WR, Hanlon-Dearman A, Sinclair C, et al. Metoclopramide, thickened feedings, and positioning for gastro-oesophageal reflux in children under two years. *Cochrane Database Syst Rev*. 2004;(4):CD003502.
- El-Serag HB, Gilger M, Carter J, et al. Childhood GERD is a risk factor for GERD in adolescents and young adults. *Am J Gastroenterol*. 2004;99(5): 806–812.
- Lightdale JR, Gremse DA. Gastroesophageal reflux: management guidance for the pediatrician. *Pediatrics*. 2013;131(5):e1684–e1695.
- Lobe TE. The current role of laparoscopic surgery for gastroesophageal reflux disease in infants and children. *Surg Endosc*. 2007;27(2):167–174.
- Thakkar K, Boatright RO, Gilger MA, et al. Gastroesophageal reflux and asthma in children: a systematic review. *Pediatrics*. 2010;125(4):e925–e930.
- Vandenplas Y, Rudolph CD, Di Lorenzo C, et al. Pediatric gastroesophageal reflux clinical practice guidelines. *J Pediatr Gastroenterol Nutr*. 2009;49(4):498–547.

CODES

ICD10

- K21.9 Gastro-esophageal reflux disease without esophagitis
- K21.0 Gastro-esophageal reflux disease with esophagitis
- P78.83 Newborn esophageal reflux

FAQ

- Q: How long will my baby suffer with GERD?
- A: Most infant reflux resolves by 9–12 months of age, but symptoms may persist up to 24 months. If GERD continues after 2–3 years, it is more likely to behave clinically like adult GERD and require chronic management.
- Q: Should all babies with reflux be treated with medication?
- A: No. Often infant reflux is physiologic and education is all that is needed. Conservative treatments such as thickened feedings, frequent small feedings, and postprandial upright positioning can be tried first, especially as data do not support acid blockade therapy in children younger than 12 months. It is often helpful to explain to parents that physiologic infant reflux tends to worsen from 1 to 3 months of age then typically starts to improve when children can sit upright at 6–7 months of age.

G

GERM CELL TUMORS

Esteban I. Gomez • James Feusner

BASICS

DESCRIPTION

Germ cell tumors (GCTs) are a heterogeneous group with a suspected common cell of origin, the primordial germ cell.

- Their location can be gonadal or extragonadal.
- The numerous histologic subtypes are broadly classified as mature or immature teratomas and malignant GCTs.
- See "Brain Tumor" chapter for primary CNS GCT.

EPIDEMIOLOGY

The incidence has a bimodal distribution with a smaller peak in early infancy and a larger peak in adolescence.

- In children younger than 15 years of age, GCTs occur at a rate of 2.4 cases per million children, and they account for 2–3% of all malignancies.
- Between 15 and 19 years of age, extracranial GCTs account for approximately 14% of cancer diagnoses.
- Teratomas and germinomas are the predominant histologic subtypes of early infancy and adolescence respectively.
- Sacrococcygeal teratomas account for 50% of childhood teratomas. They are most prevalent in infants (1:40,000 live births); with a female predominance (4:1)

RISK FACTORS

- Sex chromosome abnormalities are associated with an increased risk for GCTs.
- Klinefelter syndrome is associated with an increased risk of mediastinal GCTs.
  - Approximately 50% of adolescent mediastinal GCTs are associated with a cytogenetic diagnosis of Klinefelter syndrome.
- Turner syndrome with any portion of Y chromosome material, Swyer syndrome, nonscrotal partial androgen insensitivity, Frasier syndrome, and males with Denys-Drash syndrome are all associated with streak gonads at increased risk for developing GCTs.
- History of cryptorchidism is associated with an increased risk of testicular GCT.

Genetics

Familial GCT has been described in 1.5–2% of adult GCTs and a similar contribution to adolescent GCTs is presumed.

GENERAL PREVENTION

- Prophylactic gonadectomy is recommended for streak gonads in the specific syndromes mentioned above because of the increased risk of developing GCTs.
- Guidelines on the management of cryptorchidism recommend the following to decrease the future risk of testicular GCT:
  - Orchidopexy by 18 months of age
  - Consideration of orchiectomy of an undescended testis in all boys with a normal contralateral testis when orchidopexy is not feasible
  - Consider orchiectomy or biopsy in a post pubertal boy with cryptorchidism.
  - Counsel all men with a history of cryptorchidism and/or their parents regarding the long-term risk of testicular cancer.

ETIOLOGY

- GCTs are hypothesized to originate from primordial germ cells containing neoplastic genetic aberrations.
- Arrested migration of primordial germ cells is presumed to explain the midline location of extragonadal GCTs.
- The postpubertal peak in the incidence of GCTs suggests hormonal factors are involved in their growth.
- Isochromosome 12p or i(12)p is present in more than 80% of postpubertal GCTs. GCTs without the i(12)p typically have gain of 12p chromosomal material.
  - Mature and immature ovarian tumors are biologically distinct in their lack of association with the i(12)p.
  - A number of other genetic mutations have been observed in testicular GCTs.
- Malignant GCTs in children younger than age 4 years typically contain cytogenetic abnormalities of chromosomes 1, 3, 6, and others.
  - The i(12)p is rarely seen in this group.
  - Deletion of 1q36 is present in 80–100% of infantile malignant GCTs in testicular and extragonadal sites.
  - Recurrent genetic changes of infantile yolk sac tumors include loss of 6q24-qter, gain of 20q and 1q, loss of 1p, and c-myc or n-myc amplification.

DIAGNOSIS

HISTORY

- Acute or chronic abdominal pain is the presenting symptom in up to 80% of ovarian GCTs.
  - Vaginal bleeding, amenorrhea, and constipation may also be present.
- Pediatric testicular tumors typically present as nontender scrotal masses.
- GCTs can present with severe, acute abdominal or testicular pain secondary to gonadal torsion.
- A history of abnormal sexual development may be an indication of an underlying sex chromosome abnormality associated with an increased risk of a GCT.
- Sacrococcygeal teratomas typically present with swelling.
  - Pregnancies may be associated with polyhydramnios or high-output cardiac failure.
  - Other congenital anomalies are seen in up to 18% of patients.
- Mediastinal tumors can present with respiratory compromise in younger children, whereas adolescents may have a more insidious presentation.

PHYSICAL EXAM

- A palpable abdominal mass may be present with an ovarian GCT.
- A palpable nontender testicular mass is typical of testicular GCT.
- Sacrococcygeal GCTs can present with a palpable mass or signs of spinal cord compression.
- Especially in younger children, a mediastinal GCT may present with potentially critical respiratory compromise or superior vena cava syndrome.
- Inappropriate absence or presence of sexual development may be seen with hormonally active GCTs.

DIAGNOSTIC TESTS & INTERPRETATION

Lab

- Serum tumor markers include AFP and beta-hCG help to diagnose, monitor, and stage GCTs.
  - An acute rise can be seen after initiating chemotherapy.
- Workup should include a CBC and differential, chemistry panel, liver function tests, uric acid, and LDH to evaluate for other malignancies or organ dysfunction.

Imaging

- Plain radiograph: may reveal mature calcified tissues, such as bone or teeth, within tumor
- Chest radiograph: shows mediastinal mass
- CT scan: necessary to evaluate the primary site and regional disease
- Transscrotal ultrasound: initial imaging of testicular mass, can reveal calcifications or heterogenous features.
- Prenatal MRI: helpful for prenatal counseling and preoperative planning of fetal sacrococcygeal teratomas
- Chest CT and bone scan: indicated to evaluate for metastatic disease when malignancy is suspected

Diagnostic Procedures

Tissue is mandatory, since histology is essential to the classification of GCTs.

Pathologic Findings

- GCTs are broadly classified as teratomas or malignant GCTs.
- Teratomas contain elements of all three germ cell layers (ectoderm, mesoderm, and endoderm).
  - They can be mature, immature, or immature with malignant elements.
- Major malignant histologic subtypes include yolk sac tumor, embryonal carcinoma, gonadoblastoma, choriocarcinoma, and mixed malignant GCT.
  - Histologic subtype does not necessarily correlate with tumor biology, patient age, site of origin, or patient prognosis.

DIFFERENTIAL DIAGNOSIS

- Sacrococcygeal: pilonidal cyst, meningocele, lipomeningocele, hemangioma, abscess, bone tumor, epidermal cyst, chondroma, lymphoma, ependymoma, neuroblastoma, glioma
- Abdominal: Wilms tumor, neuroblastoma, lymphoma, rhabdomyosarcoma, hepatoblastoma, retained twin fetus
- Vaginal: rhabdomyosarcoma (sarcoma botryoides), clear cell carcinoma
- Ovarian: cyst, appendicitis, pregnancy, pelvic infection, hematocolpos, sarcoma, lymphoma, other ovarian tumors
- Testicular: epididymitis, testicular torsion, infarct, orchitis, hernia, hydrocele, hematocele, rhabdomyosarcoma, lymphoma, leukemia, other testicular tumors
- Mediastinal: Hodgkin and non-Hodgkin lymphoma, leukemia, thymoma

TREATMENT

MEDICATION

- The administration of chemotherapy is based on malignant potential, local tumor extent, surgical outcomes, and the patient's medical history.
- The typical 1st-line chemotherapy regimen for malignant GCTs includes cisplatin, etoposide, and bleomycin or PEB.
  - Cyclophosphamide in addition to PEB is being investigated in the treatment of high-risk GCTs.
  - Cisplatin is associated with a risks of ototoxicity and nephrotoxicity.
  - PEB therapy is associated with a risk of secondary myelodysplasia or acute myeloid leukemia.
  - Bleomycin is associated with a risk of pulmonary toxicity.

SURGERY/OTHER PROCEDURES

- Every effort should be made to preserve fertility in gonadal teratomas. An experienced pediatric–gynecology oncologic surgeon is critical.
- Sacrococcygeal teratoma
  - A complete surgical resection including the coccyx is curative.
  - Close postoperative follow-up should include monitoring of tumor markers.
  - Fetal surgery should be considered if signs of hydrops are seen.
- Mature teratoma
  - Full surgical excision, irrespective of site, is curative in prepubescent patients.
  - Postpubescent patient with testicular teratoma (mature or immature) is at risk for retroperitoneal metastatic recurrence, so adjuvant chemotherapy and retroperitoneal lymph node resection are additional treatment considerations.
- Immature teratoma
  - Complete surgical resection is therapy of choice; close observation and tumor marker evaluation for normalization
  - In cases of elevated AFP and incomplete surgical resection, chemotherapy should be offered given risk of microscopic foci of endodermal sinus tumor.
- Teratoma with malignant components
  - Surgery plus chemotherapy with etoposide, cisplatin or carboplatin, and bleomycin
  - Patients with residual disease should have additional surgery and additional chemotherapy if total resection is not possible.
  - High-dose chemotherapy with autologous stem cell support and radiation are reserved for salvage therapy in recurrent disease.

ONGOING CARE

- Serial physical exams and imaging studies of primary site
- Tumor markers (AFP or β-hCG) if elevated at diagnosis
- If chemotherapy or radiation therapy used, need to monitor for secondary malignancies, long term (See "Cancer Therapy Late Effects" chapter); short term, need to monitor blood counts, chemistries, renal function, and audiology

ADDITIONAL READING

- Barksdale EM, Obokhare I. Teratomas in infants and children. *Curr Opin Pediatr*. 2009;21(3):344–349.
- Hedrick HL, Flake AW, Crombleholme TW, et al. Sacrococcygeal teratoma: prenatal assessment, fetal intervention, and outcome. *J Pediar Surg*. 2004;39(3):430–438.
- Koulouris CR, Penson RT. Ovarian stromal and germ cell tumors. *Semin Oncol*. 2009;36(2):126–136.
- Lakhoo K. Neonatal teratomas. *Early Hum Dev*. 2010;86(10):643–647.
- Mannuel HD, Hussain A. Update on testicular germ cell tumors. *Curr Opin Oncol*. 2010;22(3):236–241.

CODES

ICD10

- C80.1 Malignant (primary) neoplasm, unspecified
- D48.0 Neoplasm of uncertain behavior of bone/artic cartl
- C38.3 Malignant neoplasm of mediastinum, part unspecified

FAQ

- Q: What is the chance of cure for immature/malignant teratomas?
- A: With current chemotherapy as outlined earlier, overall survival is 85–97% (dependent on disease stage).
- Q: Can a benign tumor recur? If so, can it then be malignant?
- A: Yes. If there is residual tissue left behind, the tumor can recur. If there were unrecognized areas of malignancy, the recurrence can be a malignant teratoma. The greatest risk for the latter is with the immature teratomas.

GERMAN MEASLES (THIRD DISEASE, RUBELLA)

Michael J. Smith

BASICS

DESCRIPTION

- *Rubella* derived from Latin, meaning "little red."
- Disease initially considered variant of measles
- Viral infection characterized by mild symptoms (often subclinical), with an erythematous rash progressing from head to toes
- Congenital rubella syndrome can be devastating.

EPIDEMIOLOGY

- Spread person to person via airborne transmission; worldwide infection
- Infection most contagious when rash is erupting. However, virus may be shed beginning 7 days before rash to 14 days after.
- Infants with congenital rubella syndrome may shed virus for up to 1 year.
- In temperate regions, peaks in late winter and early spring
- Infection occurs equally in following age groups: <5 years, 5–19 years, and 20–39 years.
  - In prevaccine era, annual incidence of infection in the United States was ~58 per 100,000 population.
  - 2004: No longer endemic in the United States.
  - 2004–2011: 77 reported cases, mostly in unvaccinated individuals born overseas
- Congenital rubella syndrome
  - 1964: 20,000 newborns
  - 1980s: reported rarely, with <5 cases annually
  - 1990–1991: ~30 cases reported annually
  - 2004–2011: Total of 4 cases reported to CDC, only 1 with mother born in the United States.

GENERAL PREVENTION

- Prevention of congenital rubella syndrome is main objective of vaccination programs.
- Rubella vaccine
  - Current strain of vaccine (RA 27/3, developed at the Wistar Institute in Philadelphia) was licensed in 1979 and has replaced all other strains.
  - Given as part of MMR vaccine at 12–15 months and again at 4–6 years
  - Immunity occurs in 95% of those vaccinated and is thought to be lifelong.
  - Important to ensure full vaccination for preschool-aged children
  - Vaccine virus is not communicable: Pregnant women and persons who are immunodeficient (except asymptomatic HIV infection) should not receive vaccine, but household contacts should.
- Isolation
  - Pregnant women should avoid contact with source patient.
  - Postnatal: Droplet precautions and/or school exclusion is indicated for 7 days after onset of rash.
  - Congenital: Contact isolation until 1st birthday, or until 2 nasopharyngeal and urine cultures consecutively negative

PATHOPHYSIOLOGY

- Respiratory transmission
- Replication in nasopharynx and regional lymph nodes
- Viremia 5–7 days after exposure, with spread of virus throughout body
- In congenital rubella syndrome, transplacental infection of fetus occurs during viremia.

ETIOLOGY

- Rubella virus
  - Classified as a *Rubivirus* in the Togaviridae family
  - RNA virus with single antigenic type
  - First isolated in 1962 by Parkman and Weller

DIAGNOSIS

If rubella is suspected, case should be reported to local public health authorities.

HISTORY

- In children, prodrome is not often recognized.
- In adults, a 1–5-day prodrome of low-grade fever, malaise, and cervical adenopathy may precede rash.
- Inquire about immunizations and exposures.

PHYSICAL EXAM

- Rash
  - Begins on face, then progresses to trunk and extremities
  - Does not usually coalesce
  - Lasts for 3 days
- Adenopathies, especially postauricular, posterior cervical, and suboccipital, are commonly noted along with conjunctivitis.
- Arthralgia/arthritis may be seen in adolescents and adults.

DIAGNOSTIC TESTS & INTERPRETATION

Lab

- Congenital infection
  - Serologic testing should be performed on both mother and infant.
  - Rubella-specific IgM in infant is highly suggestive.
  - Viral isolation from throat or nasal specimen can confirm diagnosis. Blood, urine, and CSF samples may also be diagnostic.
  - Diagnosis is difficult to verify after neonatal period.
- Postnatally acquired
  - Rubella-specific IgM or a ≥4-fold rise in rubella-specific IgG antibodies between acute and convalescent titers is diagnostic.

DIFFERENTIAL DIAGNOSIS

Infections that are sometimes confused with rubella include the following:

- Modified measles
- Scarlet fever
- Roseola
- Erythema infectiosum (fifth disease, parvovirus B19 infection)
- Enteroviral infections
- Infectious mononucleosis
- Drug eruptions

TREATMENT

Supportive care

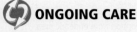

ONGOING CARE

PROGNOSIS

- Quite good; as many as 50% of infections are asymptomatic.
- Rubella infection in pregnant woman can be devastating for infant (see "Complications").

COMPLICATIONS

- Tend to occur in adults; most are uncommon.
- Arthritis or arthralgia
  - Occur in 70% of adult women, lasting up to 1 month
  - Usually affects small joints
- Encephalitis
  - 1 in 5,000 cases
  - May be associated with mortality
- Bleeding
  - 1 in 3,000 cases
  - Occurs in children more than in adults
- Thrombocytopenia: commonly noted
- Orchitis and neuritis: rare
- Congenital rubella syndrome
  - Rubella infection in early gestation can lead to fetal death, premature delivery, and congenital defects.
  - Severity of defects is worse the earlier in gestation the infection occurs.
  - 85% of infants are affected if infection occurs in 1st trimester.
  - Defects are rare if infection occurs after 20th week.
  - Common defects of congenital rubella syndrome:
    - Deafness: most common defect
    - Ophthalmologic defects: cataracts, glaucoma, microphthalmia
    - Cardiac defects: patent ductus arteriosus, ventricular septal defect, pulmonic stenosis, coarctation of aorta
    - Neurologic defects: mental retardation, microcephaly
  - Some manifestations of congenital rubella syndrome (diabetes mellitus, progressive encephalopathy) may be delayed for years.

ADDITIONAL READING

- American Academy of Pediatrics. Rubella. In: Pickering LK, Baker CJ, Kimberlin DW, et al, eds. *2012 Red Book: Report of the Committee on Infectious Diseases*, 29th ed. Elk Grove Village, IL: American Academy of Pediatrics; 2012:629–634.
- Atkinson W, et al. *Epidemiology and prevention of vaccine-preventable diseases*. 2nd ed. Bethesda, MD: Centers for Disease Control and Prevention; 1995.
- Centers for Disease Control and Prevention. Elimination of rubella and congenital rubella syndrome—United States, 1969–2004. *MMWR Morb Mortal Wkly Rep*. 2005;54(11):279–282.
- Papania MJ, Wallace GS, Rota PA, et al. Elimination of endemic measles, rubella, and congenital rubella syndrome from the Western Hemisphere: the U.S. experience. *JAMA Pediatr*. 2014;168(2):148–155.
- Retraction—Ileal-lymphoid-nodular hyperplasia, non-specific colitis, and pervasive developmental disorder in children. *Lancet*. 2010;375(9713):445.

CODES

ICD10

- B06.9 Rubella without complication
- P35.0 Congenital rubella syndrome
- B06.89 Other rubella complications

FAQ

- Q: Although pregnancy is a contraindication to rubella vaccination, if a pregnant woman is inadvertently vaccinated, will there be harm to the fetus?
- A: Data collected since 1979 by the CDC show no evidence of congenital rubella syndrome in 321 susceptible women who were vaccinated while pregnant. Therefore, inadvertent vaccination is not an indication for termination of pregnancy.
- Q: Is there any evidence that the MMR vaccine causes autism spectrum disorder?
- A: No. Multiple epidemiologic studies have shown no difference in the rates of autism spectrum disorder in children who received the MMR vaccine versus those who did not. The original paper that suggested a link between vaccines and autism was retracted in 2010.

GIARDIASIS

Kacy A. Ramirez

BASICS

DESCRIPTION

Infection of small intestine (duodenum and jejunum) and biliary tract with flagellated protozoan *Giardia intestinalis* (formerly *Giardia lamblia* and *Giardia duodenalis*)

EPIDEMIOLOGY

Giardia is the most common parasitic enteric pathogen diagnosed across the world, including in the United States.

Incidence

- U.S. average is 7.3–7.6 cases per 100,000 and approximately 20,000 cases are reported each year.
- Affects all age groups, but peaks at 1–9 years and less so at 35–49 years of age
- Highest in early summer through early fall and among residents of northern United States

Prevalence

- In the United States, nondysenteric diarrheal stool specimens ranges from 5 to 7%, with higher rates in children (up to 15–30% in United States and developing countries, respectively).
- Acquired by ingestion of cysts directly from infected person (rarely animals) or ingestion of fecally contaminated water or food
- Cysts infectious for as long as person excretes them (weeks to months), and infectious dose is low (10 cysts can produce infection).
- Incubation period usually 1–3 weeks
- Direct person-to-person transmission accounts for the very high prevalence rates in institutions, day care centers, and family contacts.
- Waterborne transmission is an important source of endemic or epidemic spread, especially when water is supplied by surface source such as streams and reservoirs (outdoor recreation and international travel).
- Foodborne infection is less common and generally from food (lettuce) washed by contaminated water source.

RISK FACTORS

- Day care attendance (poor fecal–oral hygiene)
- Travel to endemic areas
- International adoption
- Contact with recreational fresh water, backpacking, camping, swimming (swallowing water)
- Contact with some animal species
- Certain sexual practices
- Hypochlorhydria (previous gastric surgery)
- Hypogammaglobulinemia, immunodeficiency

GENERAL PREVENTION

- Practice good hygiene (hand washing after toileting, changing diapers, handling animal waste, gardening, tending to a person with diarrheal illness, and when preparing food).
- Exclusion from child care and pool/recreational water during diarrheal illnesses
- Avoiding potentially contaminated water (recreational/drinking) and food
- Examine water source in endemic areas.
- Boiling (1 minute) or filter (National Sanitation Foundation [NSF] Standard 53 or 58) water treatments
- Prevent contact with feces during sex.
- Vitamin A given in children of developing countries may improve host defenses against *Giardia* infection.

ETIOLOGY

- *G. intestinalis*
  - 2-form life cycle: cyst (transmission) and trophozoite (infection)
    - Gastric acid and pancreatic enzymes initiate excystation of ingested cysts.
    - Trophozoites divide asexually and adhere to brush border of proximal small bowel enterocytes.
    - Cyst formation (encystation) occurs in the colon and is passed into the environment.

PATHOPHYSIOLOGY

- Trophozoite causes direct damage to intestinal brush border and mucosa (but does not invade mucosa) leading to the following:
  - Disruption of tight junctional zonula occludens
  - Increased permeability via myosin light chain kinase dependent phosphorylation of F-actin
  - Induction of epithelial apoptosis
  - Induction of host immune response that results in secretion of fluid and damage to the gut
  - Secondary lactase deficiency

DIAGNOSIS

- Most (50–75%) infected individuals are asymptomatic, or have acute self-limiting diarrhea (25–50%) lasting 7–10 days.
- Clinical presentation (acute):
  - Sudden-onset watery, foul-smelling diarrhea without blood/pus/mucus
  - Malaise
  - Bloating/flatulence
  - Steatorrhea
  - Abdominal cramps
  - Anorexia/nausea
  - Dyspepsia
- Clinical presentation (chronic):
  - Loose, semiformed stool >14 days
  - Steatorrhea
  - Profound malaise
  - Abdominal distention
  - Weight loss
  - Anorexia
  - Flatulence
  - Depression
  - Alternation of diarrhea/constipation until spontaneous resolution or treatment begun
- Malabsorption syndrome may include the following:
  - Steatorrhea
  - Deficiencies of iron, D-xylose, vitamins A, B_{12}, and E
  - Protein-losing enteropathy

HISTORY

- Exposures:
  - Habitation or adoption from endemic area
  - Attendants of child care centers or inhabitants of institutions
  - Camping or hiking near fresh water/recreational water exposure
  - Exposure to infected individual
- Underlying immunodeficiency or irritable bowel syndrome (IBS)
- Previous gastric surgery
- Asymptomatic infection can occur.

PHYSICAL EXAM

- Abdominal distention
- Aphthous ulcers in oral mucosa
- Urticaria
- Arthralgia/arthritis

DIAGNOSTIC TESTS & INTERPRETATION

Lab

Initial lab tests

- Identification of trophozoites or cysts in stool specimens (multiple [3] ova/parasite [O/P] samples collected every other day can be sent to microscopy to increase sensitivity) AND
- Direct fluorescent antibody staining (DFA)
- Real-time PCR is most sensitive and preferred test for diagnosis, as available.
- Other immunodiagnostic kits that do not require microscopy (enzyme immunoassay [EIA]) should not replace O/P and DFA.
- If immunodeficiency is suspected, evaluate humoral immunodeficiency (total immunoglobulins includes IgA).
- WBC usually normal and eosinophilia absent

Diagnostic Procedures/Other

- Consider duodenal aspiration or string test (Enterotest) and rarely biopsy.

PATHOLOGIC FINDINGS

Mucosal lesions vary from normal to subtotal villous atrophy, with crypt hyperplasia and proliferation of intraepithelial and lamina propria lymphocytes. Trophozoites may be seen on biopsies.

DIFFERENTIAL DIAGNOSIS

- Celiac disease
- Cystic fibrosis
- Lactose intolerance
- Irritable bowel syndrome
- Inflammatory bowel disease
- Nonulcer dyspepsia

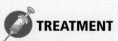

TREATMENT

MEDICATION

- Metronidazole (not approved by FDA)
  - Most effective and best tolerated
  - Dose: 15 mg/kg/24 h divided t.i.d. PO for 5–10 days
- Tinidazole (approved for children ≥3 years)
  - 50 mg/kg, max 2 g; single oral dose
  - Available in tablet form only
  - Fewer adverse effects than metronidazole
- Nitazoxanide (approved for ages 1–11 years)
- Furazolidone: lower efficacy but better tolerated than metronidazole
- Paromomycin (for symptomatic infection in pregnant women in the 2nd and 3rd trimesters)
- Asymptomatic giardiasis, in absence of risk factors, should not be treated.
- Treatment failures:
  - High dose courses of original agent
  - Combination of nitroimidazole plus quinacrine for at least 2 weeks
- Treatment of asymptomatic carriers in patients with IBS or in households of patients with cystic fibrosis or hypogammaglobulinemia may be considered.

ONGOING CARE

FOLLOW-UP RECOMMENDATIONS

Patient Monitoring

- Symptom recurrence can be attributable to reinfection, secondary lactose intolerance, insufficient treatment, or drug resistance.
- Detailed exposure history and O/P and antigen detection with recurrence of symptoms
- If reinfection suspected, a course can be repeated with similar drug, otherwise alternative agent if resistance suspected.
- If symptoms persist, with negative diagnostic studies, consider alternative etiology or enteropathogen.

DIET

Consider lactose avoidance to prevent bloating and diarrhea for 1 month after treatment.

PROGNOSIS

- Remains good for symptomatic patients
- Combination therapy with 2 medications has been successful when repeated courses of single drug have failed.

COMPLICATIONS

- Malabsorption syndrome
- Steatorrhea
- Lactose deficiency
- Deficiencies of iron, folic acid, and vitamins A, B_{12}, and E
- Protein-losing enteropathy
- Urticaria
- Arthralgia
- In pediatric patients:
  - Growth retardation
  - Failure to thrive
  - Lower IQ
  - Urticaria

ADDITIONAL READING

- Ali SA, Hill DR. *Giardia intestinalis*. *Curr Opin Infect Dis*. 2003;16(5):453–460.
- American Academy of Pediatrics. *Giardia intestinalis* (formerly *Giardia lamblia* and *Giardia duodenalis*) infections. In: Pickering LK, Baker CJ, Kimberlin DW, et al, eds. *Red Book: 2012 Report of the Committee on Infectious Diseases*. 29th ed. Elk Grove Village, IL: American Academy of Pediatrics; 2012:333–335.
- Huang DB, White AC. An updated review on *Cryptosporidium* and *Giardia*. *Gastroenterol Clin North Am*. 2006;35(2):291–314.
- Katz DE, Taylor DN. Parasitic infections of the gastrointestinal tract. *Gastroenterol Clin North Am*. 2001;30(3):797–815.
- Lima AA, Soares AM, Lima NL, et al. Effects of vitamin A supplementation on intestinal barrier function, growth, total parasitic, and specific *Giardia* spp infections in Brazilian children: a prospective randomized, double-blind, placebo-controlled trial. *J Pediatr Gastroenterol Nutr*. 2010;50(3):309–315.
- Yoder JS, Gargano JW, Wallace RM, et al. Giardiasis surveillance—United States, 2009–2010. *MMWR Surveill Summ*. 2012;61(5):13–23.

CODES

ICD10

A07.1 Giardiasis [lambliasis]

FAQ

- Q: How is *G. intestinalis* likely contracted?
- A: Most community-wide epidemics occur from a contaminated water supply (drinking water), as well as person-to-person transmission in child care and institutional settings. Food and food handler–associated outbreaks are less reported.
- Q: What do I do if I suspect *Giardia*, but the stool sample is negative?
- A: 3 O/P samples are needed and should optimally be done every other day on a diarrheal stool specimen with a DFA to increase diagnostic sensitivity. Stool samples should be examined as soon as possible or placed immediately in a preservative, such as neutral buffered 10% formalin or polyvinyl alcohol. If endemic areas, it may be appropriate to treat empirically. If stool testing is negative and the diagnosis is strongly suspected, you can consider ordering a commercially available string test (designed to obtain bile-stained mucus from duodenum to reveal trophozoites on wet mount) or refer to a pediatric gastroenterologist, who can perform endoscopy with duodenal aspiration and biopsy.

GINGIVITIS

Daniel Walmsley

BASICS

DESCRIPTION

Gingivitis is a reversible dental plaque–induced inflammation of the gingival tissues. Symptoms may include bleeding, swelling, ulceration, and pain, although gingivitis is usually mild and asymptomatic.

EPIDEMIOLOGY

- Affects >90% of children between the ages of 4 and 13 years. Most of these children have low-grade gingivitis.
- 13–40% of children aged 6–36 months have eruption gingivitis, which commonly resolves after teeth eruption.
- The prevalence of gingivitis increases with age; by puberty, nearly 100% of all children are affected. This pubertal peak is likely due to hormonal influences and inconsistent dental hygiene.
- After puberty, the prevalence remains relatively constant at 50% of all adults.

RISK FACTORS

- Behavioral factors: smoking, stress, alcohol consumption
- Medications: antiepileptic, cyclosporine, calcium channel blockers
- Hormonal changes: puberty, pregnancy
- Chronic illnesses: diabetes mellitus, chronic renal failure, histiocytosis X, scleroderma, secondary hyperparathyroidism
- Immunologic deficiencies: HIV, Chédiak-Higashi, cyclic neutropenia
- Neurologic problems: cerebral palsy, mental retardation, seizures, and other conditions where routine dental care is difficult
- Miscellaneous: chronic mouth breathing, malnutrition, viral illnesses

GENERAL PREVENTION

- Consistent daily oral hygiene described as the following by age:
  - Infants: gum massage, washcloth to remove plaque; toothbrush using baby toothpaste (i.e., enzyme-based; no fluoride)
  - Young children: assistance with brushing with a small amount of fluoridated toothpaste
  - School-aged children: Supervise brushing and assist if necessary.
  - Older children and adolescents: Brush teeth twice a day with fluoridated toothpaste in addition to daily flossing. Some dentists recommended flossing as early as age 4 years.
  - Children with fixed orthodontics: Careful brushing and flossing is critical.
- Fluoride: Supplements are appropriate if the water supply is not fluoridated. It is important to be careful to treat with the appropriate amount of fluoride in order to prevent fluorosis.
- Sealants: Adherent plastic coating may be applied to the pits and fissures of the permanent teeth to provide a mechanical barrier.
- The American Academy of Pediatrics (AAP) recommends that children at high risk for dental caries should establish routine dental care by their first birthday. Children should then continue routine dental checkups at a minimum of every 6 months.

ETIOLOGY

- Poor dental hygiene
- Bacterial plaque, calcified and noncalcified
- Caries
- Orthodontic appliances
- Malocclusion
- Crowded teeth
- Mouth breathing
- Erupting teeth margins
- Poor nutrition
  - Vitamin deficiencies (e.g., vitamin C deficiency)
  - Diet low in coarse detergent like foods (e.g., raw carrots, celery, apples)
  - High prevalence of anaerobic microflora
- Infections
  - Herpes simplex virus (HSV) type I
  - *Candida albicans*
  - HIV
  - Bacterial pathogens
- Drugs
  - Phenytoin
  - Cyclosporine
  - Nifedipine
  - Oral contraceptive pills
- Trauma

DIAGNOSIS

HISTORY

- Review the frequency of dental care visits and the home dental hygiene regimen.
- Review significant medical history, asking about chronic illnesses, bleeding disorders, and immunodeficiency.
- Review the diet of the child to assess for nutritional deficiencies.
- Dental appliances worn by patient:
  - Orthodontic equipment makes gingiva more difficult to clean, and reactive tissue growth is more common.
- Regular medications taken by patient:
  - Phenytoin may result in gingival hyperplasia, and chemotherapeutic agents, exogenous hormone therapy, and calcium channel blockers may result in gingivitis.
- Signs and symptoms:
  - Edema and erythema of the gingiva
  - Bleeding at gum line
  - Pain near the gingival margin

PHYSICAL EXAM

- Evaluate the gingival tissue for erythema, swelling, ulceration, fluctuance, or drainage. Erythema and edema are the most common findings in gingivitis.
- In severe cases, the gingival tissues may bleed spontaneously from ulcerations in the sulcus and there may be significant gingival hypertrophy.
- In herpetic gingivostomatitis, there is often significant ulceration and swelling of the gingiva associated with systemic symptoms such as fever and malaise.
- Evaluate the teeth for caries, fractures, looseness, malocclusion, pain, and plaque.
- Examine the face and neck for signs of swelling, erythema, warmth, or enlarged maxillary lymph nodes which may be signs of more extensive bacterial infection.
- Tanner staging: Normal pubertal changes seem to aggravate gingival inflammation, so paying special attention to the gingiva of patients entering puberty is important.
- Assess the patient's oral hygiene technique in the office. This is the single largest contributor to gingivitis.

DIAGNOSTIC TESTS & INTERPRETATION

Lab

- Most patients will not need laboratory evaluation.
- If there is a concern for excessive bleeding, a CBC with differential, PT, and PTT may be helpful to rule out thrombocytopenia, pancytopenia, or a clotting disorder.
- Blood culture: if there is concern for sepsis
- Direct fluorescent antibody testing for HSV-1: If herpes is suspected (stomatitis is usually present), swab the base of a stoma/vesicle and smear on a slide. HSV culture is the gold standard.
- Biopsy is rarely necessary.

Imaging

Panoramic or individual tooth radiographic imaging is important to assess the bones for evidence of periodontal extension of the gingivitis in the more severe cases.

DIFFERENTIAL DIAGNOSIS

- Infectious
  - Abscess
  - Herpetic gingivostomatitis—ulcerative lesions of the gingiva and mucous membranes of the mouth
- Traumatic
  - Food impaction
  - Orthodontic appliances
  - Self-inflicted minor injury
- Hematologic
  - Gingival bleeding due to hemophilia (factor VIII or IX deficiency)
  - Thrombocytopenia

- Immunologic
  - Neutrophil disorders
  - Leukemia
  - HIV
  - Graft-versus-host disease (infiltrative gingivitis)
- Miscellaneous
  - Gingival hyperplasia due to medications (i.e., phenytoin and nifedipine)
  - Periodontitis
  - Aphthous stomatitis
  - Vitamin C deficiency
  - Behçet disease
  - Acute necrotizing ulcerative gingivitis (ANUG)—painful gingivitis associated with rapid onset and tissue ulceration and necrosis
    - Peaks in adolescence and young adulthood
    - Related to high oral concentrations of spirochetes and/or *Prevotella intermedia*

TREATMENT

MEDICATION

Mouth rinses for plaque inhibition can be used to augment daily oral care routine. The most commonly used rinses include 0.12% chlorhexidine and 0.075% or 0.1% cetylpyridinium chloride.

ADDITIONAL TREATMENT

General Measures

A daily oral care routine, including brushing and flossing, is essential to prevent gingivitis.

- Mild gingivitis
  - Careful daily dental hygiene, including meticulous brushing and flossing
  - Mechanical plaque and calculus removal by scaling or root planing. This is then followed by frequent dental cleanings every 3–6 months to prevent recurrence.
- Moderate to severe gingivitis
  - Care as outlined for mild gingivitis
  - Should be evaluated by a pedodontist in addition to a general dentist
  - Mouth rinses for plaque inhibition using either 0.12% chlorhexidine or 0.075% or 0.1% cetylpyridinium chloride
  - Irrigation devices
  - Sonic toothbrushes
  - Gingivectomies in cases of overgrowth to permit better cleaning
  - Antibiotics to cover mouth flora in more severe cases when bacterial superinfection is suspected

ISSUES FOR REFERRAL

- It is important for providers to evaluate the oral health of all children. When gingival inflammation is noted, the patient should be referred to a dentist.
- Routine dental care with professional cleaning and plaque removal is recommended for all children and adults.
- If the extent of involvement is great or the underlying disease of the patient requires more aggressive care, a periodontist should be consulted.
- The inability to resolve gingivitis by oral hygiene measures necessitates the consideration of other causes such as leukemia, vitamin C deficiency, or other chronic disease.

SURGERY/OTHER PROCEDURES

Only the most severe cases require gingivectomy.

ONGOING CARE

FOLLOW-UP RECOMMENDATIONS

- Routine dental care with professional cleaning and plaque removal is recommended for all children and adults.
- Children with gingivitis should have frequent dental visits; most dentists recommend every 3 months.

Patient Monitoring

Routine dental exam and cleaning should be performed every 6 months to monitor for signs of inflammation.

DIET

- Avoid high sugar content food and beverages.
- Xylitol-containing chewing gum can improve oral hygiene by reducing plaque adherence to the gum line.

PATIENT EDUCATION

- Establish a daily mouth care routine.
- Brushing and flossing each morning and at bedtime will reduce plaque formation.
- Mouth rinses, if recommended by your dentist, can also reduce plaque formation.
- See the dental health professional every 6 months beginning at your child's first birthday for examination and cleaning.

PROGNOSIS

- Good oral hygiene may reverse mild to moderate gingivitis within several months.
- Periodontal disease is not reversible; therefore, prevention is essential.

COMPLICATIONS

- Periodontal disease
- Osteomyelitis
- Tooth decay

ADDITIONAL READING

- American Academy of Pediatric Dentistry. Guideline on periodicity of examination, preventive dental services, anticipatory guidance, and oral treatment for children. http://www.aapd.org/media/Policies_Guidelines/G_Periodicity.pdf. Accessed February 14, 2015.
- Bacci C, Sivolella S, Pellegrini J, et al. A rare case of scurvy in an otherwise healthy child: diagnosis through oral signs. *Pediatr Dent*. 2010;32(7):536–538.
- Califano JV, American Academy of Periodontology—Research, Science and Therapy Committee. Periodontal diseases of children and adolescents. *J Periodontol*. 2003;74(11):1696–1704.
- Kallio PJ. Health promotion and behavioral approaches in the prevention of periodontal disease in children and adolescents. *Periodontology*. 2001;26:135–145.
- Mankodi S, Bauroth K, Witt JJ, et al. A 6-month clinical trial to study the effects of a cetylpyridinium chloride mouth rinse on gingivitis and plaque. *Am J Dent*. 2005;18:9A–14A.

CODES

ICD10

- K05.10 Chronic gingivitis, plaque induced
- K05.00 Acute gingivitis, plaque induced
- A69.1 Other Vincent's infections

FAQ

- Q: Are there differences among toothpastes and prevention of gingivitis?
- A: Yes. A study demonstrated that stabilized stannous fluoride toothpaste is effective in preventing gingivitis. When essential oil mouthwashes (e.g., Listerine) are added, there is additional reduction in the amount of gingivitis noted.
- Q: What dietary changes may improve gingival health?
- A: Avoiding frequent carbohydrate intake may reduce gingivitis. Carbonated beverages, sugared chewing gum, and candy often adhere to teeth. When daily dental care is inconsistent, plaque formation is increased and gingivitis is much more likely.
- Q: Why do children generally not have the significant periodontal disease that adults get?
- A: No one knows for sure; however, it is known that the gingiva of the primary dentition is rounder and thicker and contains more blood vessels and less connective tissue than the gingival seen later in life. Whether these differences mask disease or are helpful is unclear.
- Q: How do intraoral piercings impact gum health?
- A: In addition to fractured teeth, gingival recession and gingivitis are complications of the trauma inflicted by a foreign body in the oral cavity.
- Q: Why is smoking associated with gingival disease?
- A: Nicotine inhibits phagocyte and neutrophil function, reduces bone mineralization, impairs vascularization, and reduces antibody production. Smokers do not respond as well as nonsmokers to surgical and nonsurgical treatments.

GLAUCOMA–CONGENITAL

Hee-Jung Park

BASICS

DESCRIPTION

- Elevation of intraocular pressure (IOP) due to congenital anomalies that prevent outflow of aqueous humor, leading to damage to the optic nerve
- Neonatal primary congenital glaucoma (PCG), presents at birth
- Depending on the degree of the malformation, presentation can occur even later in life.
- About 80% of childhood glaucoma presents in the 1st year of life. Secondary congenital glaucoma is associated with systemic conditions.

EPIDEMIOLOGY

- PCG accounts for ~1/2 of all cases of childhood glaucoma.
- 1:10,000 births (ranging from 1:2,500 in Saudi Arabia to 1:38,000 in Spain)
- Male > female (3:2)
- ~70% bilaterally affected

PATHOPHYSIOLOGY

- PCG is caused by immature anatomic relationship between the iris, trabecular meshwork, and cornea.
- Secondary glaucoma is mostly due to damage or alteration of the trabecular meshwork.

GENETICS

- Most are sporadic, but 10–40% are familial.
- Autosomal recessive is most common.
- PCG is associated with mutations in cytogenic locations 2p22.2 (GLC3A), 1p36.2-p36.1 (GLC3B), 14q24.3 (GLC3C), and 14q24.2-q24.3 (GLC3D).

ETIOLOGY

- Aqueous humor, a clear fluid produced by the ciliary body at the posterior base of the iris, passes through the pupil and exits through the trabecular meshwork and Schlemm canal, which are located at the junction of the cornea and iris.
- Outflow blockage of aqueous humor causes pressure to build in eye.
- The blockage may be microscopic (open-angle glaucoma) or due to obstruction of the outflow by the iris (angle-closure glaucoma).
- High IOP in young children leads to enlargement of eye and destruction of fibers of the optic nerve.

COMMONLY ASSOCIATED CONDITIONS

- Sturge-Weber syndrome
- Neurofibromatosis type 1
- Oculocerebrorenal (Lowe) syndrome
- Marfan syndrome
- Rubinstein-Taybi syndrome
- Stickler syndrome
- Walker-Warburg syndrome
- Hepatocerebrorenal syndrome (Zellweger)
- Pierre Robin syndrome
- Homocystinuria
- Rubella
- Trisomy 13
- Trisomy 21 (Down syndrome)
- Axenfeld-Rieger syndrome
- Ocular Anomalies
  - Aniridia
  - Peters anomaly
  - Sclerocornea
  - Congenital iris ectropion syndrome
  - Congenital cataract

ALERT
Intraocular neoplasms such as retinoblastoma can cause glaucoma. Other causes of secondary glaucoma include trauma and chronic uveitis.

DIAGNOSIS

HISTORY

- Classic triad of symptoms that develop from corneal edema caused by increased IOP
  - Epiphora (excessive tearing)
  - Blepharospasm (squeezing of eyelids)
  - Photophobia (light sensitivity)
- Cloudy corneas
- Red eyes (can be mistaken for conjunctivitis)
- Fussiness
- Large eyes

PHYSICAL EXAM

- Unlike adult glaucoma, PCG presents with physical changes due to high pressure.
- Buphthalmos (ocular enlargement) due to stretching of immature collagen in infants
- Corneal asymmetry or enlargement (diameter >11 mm at birth or >12 mm in the 1st year of life)
- Corneal haze from edema and/or scarring
- Myopic shift in refractive error
- Rapid changes in IOP present with redness and pain but usually painless without redness from gradual change in pressure.
- Optic nerve cupping develops rapidly in infants but may be reversible with control of glaucoma in very young children.
- Nystagmus may be present if there is early sensory deficit.
- Common to develop amblyopia and strabismus from insult on developing visual system
- General signs of many systemic syndromes associated with glaucoma (neurofibromatosis, Sturge-Weber syndrome)

Imaging

Ultrasound: axial length using A-scan

- Eye is usually abnormally long for age.
- Longitudinal data are very useful in determining progression of glaucoma.

Diagnosis Procedures/Other

- IOP measurement
  - An awake child is ideal; use bottle or breast to quiet, along with low lighting.
  - If examination under anesthesia is needed, check IOP as soon as possible after induction, as IOP decreases with anesthetic agents.
- Corneal inspection
  - Diameter measured with calipers
  - Normal newborn: 10–10.5 mm
  - >11.0 mm suspicious
  - Watch for asymmetry.
  - Clarity: Haze may be due to edema or breaks in the Descemet membrane (Haab striae).
- Optic disc evaluation
  - Increase in cupping of the optic nerve head is early sign.
  - May reverse with good IOP control in the very young
- Refractive error
  - Myopic shift from enlargement of the eye
  - Anisometropia (difference in refractive error between the two eyes)
  - Astigmatism from change in ocular shape or corneal scar
  - Early signs of glaucoma and useful office test for monitoring control of glaucoma
- Gonioscopy: evaluation of anterior chamber angle (between iris and cornea)
  - In trabeculodysgenesis, insertion of iris into corneoscleral angle often flat or concave
  - Iris defects may suggest type of abnormality causing glaucoma.
  - Abnormal iris vessels may influence surgical plan.
  - In angle-closure glaucoma: diagnostic apposition of iris on cornea
- Pachymetry: measurement of corneal thickness to assess corneal edema as an indicator of pressure control

DIFFERENTIAL DIAGNOSIS

- Excessive tearing: commonly due to nasolacrimal duct obstruction in neonates
- Megalocornea
  - May be associated with high myopia
  - Contralateral microphthalmia
- Corneal haze
  - Birth trauma, forceps
  - Congenital corneal dystrophies
  - Mucopolysaccharidoses
  - Cystinosis
  - Intrauterine inflammation (rubella, syphilis)
- Photophobia
  - Uveitis
  - Retinal cone dystrophy
- Enlarged optic nerve cupping
  - Physiologic cupping
  - Optic atrophy from hydrocephalus can look similar to glaucomatous damage.

TREATMENT

GENERAL MEASURES

- Surgery is considered definitive therapy.
- Medical treatment for glaucoma in children is usually a temporizing measure or adjunctive therapy.
  - In other types of pediatric glaucoma, medical treatment involves use of the same medications as those used in adults such as β-blockers, adrenergic agents, and carbonic anhydrase inhibitors. In general, miotics are not used because they may cause a paradoxical rise in IOP in children.

MEDICATION

ALERT

Topical α-adrenergic agonists are contraindicated in infants and young children, as they can cause CNS suppression leading to apnea, sedation, and fatigue.

First Line

- Carbonic anhydrase inhibitors: Side effects include metabolic acidosis, growth retardation, loss of appetite, paresthesias, polyuria, diarrhea, and nausea.
  - Systemic
    - Acetazolamide (10 mg/kg/24 h PO divided t.i.d.)
    - Methazolamide
  - Topical
    - Brinzolamide
    - Dorzolamide
- β-Blockers, topical: Side effects include bronchospasm, apnea, and bradycardia.
  - Timolol
  - Betaxolol
  - Levobunolol
  - Metipranolol
  - Carteolol
- Prostaglandins, topical: Side effects include iris and eyelid pigmentation and growth of lashes.
  - Latanoprost
  - Bimatoprost
  - Travoprost

SURGERY/OTHER PROCEDURES

- Goniotomy/trabeculotomy: Both procedures open portions of Schlemm canal into anterior chamber, allowing easier outflow of aqueous humor (goniotomy approaches the Schlemm canal from inside the eye and trabeculotomy from the outside).
- Trabeculectomy: creates a sclerotomy covered with a partial-thickness scleral flap to create a controlled outflow that bypasses the Schlemm canal and trabecular meshwork. Fluid drains in the sub-Tenon space.
- Seton procedures: various drainage devices placed in subconjunctival space with tube inserted into the anterior chamber, allowing free flow of aqueous humor from eye
- Cyclodestructive procedures: procedures involving destruction of the ciliary body, which produces aqueous humor
- Iridectomy: If the mechanism of glaucoma is angle closure (limited outflow of aqueous humor due to anatomic blockage with iris), then creating a window in the iris allows bypass for aqueous humor to access the anterior chamber.

ONGOING CARE

FOLLOW-UP RECOMMENDATIONS

Early postoperative

- Postoperative steroids and cycloplegic drops to decrease pain and prevent adhesions due to inflammation
- Corneal edema clears slowly, but IOP falls quickly if surgery is successful.
- Adjusting pressure-lowering medications based on the success of the surgery

Longer term

- Follow-up is needed throughout life.
- Examination under anesthesia may be required frequently during the first 3–4 years of life to ensure adequate control of IOP.
- Contact social services for children suspected of having visual impairment.

PATIENT EDUCATION

Children and parents must understand that glaucoma may recur at any point and that continued, long-term surveillance is essential.

PROGNOSIS

Guarded; even if pressure is well controlled and amblyopia treatment undertaken rigorously, child is still at high risk for visual impairment. Must be carefully followed for the following:

- Amblyopia
- Abnormal refractive errors
- Recurrence of glaucoma

COMPLICATIONS

- Severe visual impairment or blindness due to optic nerve damage, amblyopia, and corneal scarring likely if glaucoma is undetected or uncontrollable
- Corneal edema and decompensation requiring corneal transplant especially from Seton procedures
- Development of cataract
- If glaucoma is controlled, the following are relatively common:
  - Unrecognized and untreated amblyopia (most serious threat to child's vision)
  - High degrees of myopia
  - Anisometropia (difference in refractive error between fellow eyes)
  - Buphthalmos and corneal scarring

ADDITIONAL READING

- Beck AD. Diagnosis and management of pediatric glaucoma. *Ophthalmol Clin North Am*. 2001;14(3):501–512.
- Bejjani B, Edward D. Primary congenital glaucoma. In: Pagon RA, Adam MP, Ardinger HH, et al, eds. *Gene Reviews* [Internet]. Seattle, WA: University of Washington, Seattle; 2007.
- De Silva DJ, Khaw PT, Brookes JL. Long-term outcome of primary congenital glaucoma. *J AAPOS*. 2011;15(2):148–152.
- Kipp MA. Childhood glaucoma. *Pediatr Clin North Am*. 2003;50(1):89–104.
- Mandal AK, Gothwal VK, Bagga H, et al. Outcome of surgery on infants younger than 1 month with congenital glaucoma. *Ophthalmology*. 2003;110(10):1909–1915.
- Papadopoulos M, Khaw PT. Advances in the management of paediatric glaucoma. *Eye*. 2007;21(10):1319–1325.
- Yeung HH, Walton DS. Clinical classification of childhood glaucomas. *Arch Ophthalmol*. 2010;128(6):680–684.

CODES

ICD10

Q15.0 Congenital glaucoma

FAQ

- Q: Can glaucoma be painful?
- A: If the ocular pressure rises quickly (hours), pain occurs frequently. Very high IOPs may be present without pain if they occur slowly (months to years). However, most patients with glaucoma are asymptomatic until they have advanced vision loss.
- Q: Can glaucoma occur after eye trauma?
- A: Yes. This is a very common cause of glaucoma and may be asymptomatic, thus requiring periodic follow-up ophthalmic examinations for early detection and treatment.
- Q: Can infantile glaucoma be inherited?
- A: Yes. Both primary infantile glaucoma and glaucoma related to systemic or ocular syndromes may be inherited. Siblings and children of affected individuals should be examined for glaucoma.

GLOMERULONEPHRITIS

Kevin V. Lemley

BASICS

DESCRIPTION

- Glomerulonephritis presents with the nephritic syndrome: hematuria with RBC casts, hypertension, azotemia, and edema. Proteinuria and oliguria may also be present.
- Acute glomerulonephritis is associated with inflammation and cell proliferation in the glomerular tuft. It may be rapidly progressive.
- Chronic glomerulonephritis indicates permanent damage has occurred.

EPIDEMIOLOGY

- Acute poststreptococcal glomerulonephritis (APSGN) can occur in anyone >2 years but is most frequently found in boys 5–15 years old. It can be sporadic or epidemic.
- Incidence of APSGN has declined over the last 2 decades.
- Chronic glomerulonephritis occurs more often at the end of the 1st decade of life and in adults.

Genetics

Genetic predisposition: hereditary nephritis (e.g., X-linked Alport syndrome)

ETIOLOGY

Can be categorized based on serum complement levels and presence of renal versus systemic disease

- Low serum complement level: systemic diseases
  - Vasculitis and autoimmune disease (e.g., systemic lupus erythematosus [SLE])
  - Subacute bacterial endocarditis (SBE)
  - Shunt nephritis
  - Cryoglobulinemia
- Low serum complement level: renal diseases
  - APSGN
  - Membranoproliferative glomerulonephritis, C3 glomerulopathy
- Normal serum complement level: systemic diseases
  - Microscopic polyangiitis
  - Granulomatosis with polyangiitis (Wegener)
  - Henoch-Schönlein purpura (HSP)
  - Hypersensitivity vasculitis
  - Anti-GBM disease (Goodpasture syndrome)
- Normal serum complement level: renal diseases
  - IgA nephropathy
  - Idiopathic rapidly progressive glomerulonephritis
  - Pauci-immune glomerulonephritis (renal-limited ANCA vasculitis)
  - Immune-complex disease

DIAGNOSIS

HISTORY

- Macroscopic hematuria (tea-colored urine) in many
- Reduced urine output, edema
- Dyspnea, fatigue, lethargy
- Headache
- Seizures (hypertensive encephalopathy)
- Symptoms of a systemic disease such as fever, rash (especially on the buttocks and legs, posteriorly), arthralgia, and weight loss
- Preceding sore throat, upper respiratory infection (7–14 days), *or* preceding impetigo (14–28 days) suggests APSGN.
- An upper respiratory infection in the few days prior to macroscopic hematuria may suggest IgA nephropathy.

PHYSICAL EXAM

- Hypertension
- Signs of volume overload (e.g., edema, jugular venous distention, hepatomegaly, basal pulmonary crepitation, a gallop rhythm)
- Impetigo or pyoderma
- Signs of vasculitis such as rash, Raynaud phenomenon, and vascular thrombosis
- Signs of other systemic disorder (SLE)
- Signs of chronic kidney disease, such as short stature, pallor, sallow skin, edema, pericardial friction rub, pulmonary rales, breath that smells of urine, clonus

DIAGNOSTIC TESTS & INTERPRETATION

Lab

Initial lab tests

- Urine
  - Microscopy of the urine for dysmorphic erythrocytes and erythrocyte casts: hallmark of nephritis
  - Proteinuria
- Evidence of prior strep infection
  - Throat culture for β-hemolytic *Streptococcus* (result is positive in only 15–20% with sporadic APSGN)
  - Antistreptolysin O and anti-DNAse B titers: positive result in patients with preceding acute poststreptococcal infection
  - Streptozyme test: A mixed antigen test for β-hemolytic *Streptococcus* (ASO, anti-DNAse, anti-streptokinase, anti-hyaluronidase, etc.) has 85–90% sensitivity and specificity; sensitivity is increased by serial testing.
- Complement C3 serum level will be low in APSGN and in several other causes of acute glomerulonephritis.
- Blood chemistry
  - Can be normal in acute glomerulonephritis
  - Serum creatinine generally <1.5× normal in uncomplicated APSGN
  - In chronic glomerulonephritis, serum chemistries will reflect the degree of chronic kidney disease (i.e., raised serum urea and creatinine). The serum potassium and phosphate levels may be elevated and the calcium level decreased.
  - In chronic kidney disease: normocytic, normochromic, or hypochromic microcytic anemia

Imaging

- Chest radiograph to look for pulmonary edema and determine cardiac size if severe edema or respiratory symptoms are present
- Renal ultrasound if presentation or course not typical of APSGN. The ultrasound is to assess the size and parenchymal texture.

Diagnostic Procedures/Other

Electrocardiogram to assess ventricular size and for T-wave changes in cases of hyperkalemia

Pathologic Findings

In APSGN, light microscopy reveals enlarged, swollen glomerular tufts and mesangial and endothelial cell proliferation, with polymorphonuclear leukocyte infiltration. There is granular deposition of C3 and IgG on immunofluorescence, and electron-dense subepithelial deposits or humps are seen on electron microscopy. The histology varies in chronic glomerulonephritis and depends on the cause. Rapidly progressive glomerulonephritis is associated with crescent formation.

DIFFERENTIAL DIAGNOSIS

- Acute postinfectious glomerulonephritis (nephritogenic strains of group A β-hemolytic streptococci, *Pneumococcus*, *Staphylococcus*, *Mycoplasma*, Epstein-Barr virus)
- Infection-related (hepatitis B and C, syphilis)
- IgA nephropathy
- Membranoproliferative glomerulonephritis
- Autoimmune glomerulonephritis (e.g., SLE)
- Immune-complex glomerulonephritis
- Hereditary glomerulonephritis
- Tubulointerstitial nephritis
- Hemolytic uremic syndrome
- Pyelonephritis

TREATMENT

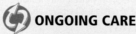

Aimed toward treating hypertension, renal failure, and the underlying cause of glomerulonephritis

MEDICATION

- The following may be required:
  - Loop diuretics (furosemide) for volume, BP, and potassium control
  - Antihypertensive agents; vasodilators such as calcium channel blockers (e.g., nifedipine, isradipine, amlodipine) as 1st-line agents; IV hydralazine, labetalol, nicardipine, or nitroprusside may be required to treat severe refractory hypertension or posterior reversible encephalopathy syndrome (PRES). Avoid ACE inhibitors or angiotensin receptor blockers (ARBs) in case of hyperkalemia or acute kidney injury (AKI).
  - Serum potassium-lowering agents (sodium polystyrene sulfonate [Kayexalate], furosemide, bicarbonate, insulin/glucose, β-agonists). IV calcium is used to stabilize the myocardium in severe hyperkalemia (with T-wave changes); dialysis in severe renal failure with significant hyperkalemia
  - Phosphate binders (calcium carbonate)
  - Immunosuppressive agents such as prednisone, cyclophosphamide, mycophenolate mofetil, and rarely rituximab or eculizumab are used in the treatment of vasculitis-associated glomerulonephritis, membranoproliferative glomerulonephritis, rapidly progressing glomerulonephritis, or disorders of complement regulation. Plasmapheresis may be used to treat rapidly progressing glomerulonephritis, especially with multisystem (pulmonary, CNS) involvement or severe acute renal failure requiring dialysis.
  - Penicillin is used in active poststreptococcal glomerulonephritis to prevent rheumatic fever and the spread of nephritogenic strains but generally does not affect the course of the renal disease. It may be indicated in exposed individuals in epidemic APSGN and household contacts of sporadic cases.

ADDITIONAL TREATMENT

General Measures

- APSGN is typically a self-limited disease. Acute supportive therapy is usually sufficient.
- Dietary salt restriction
- The therapy of chronic glomerulonephritis depends on the underlying disease process; it may include immunosuppressive medications and, ultimately, the management of chronic kidney disease.

INPATIENT CONSIDERATIONS

Initial stabilization

Treat hypertensive encephalopathy and life-threatening electrolyte disturbances immediately.

Admission Criteria

- Hypertension
- Severe edema, pulmonary edema
- Acute kidney injury

ONGOING CARE

FOLLOW-UP-RECOMMENDATIONS

In APSGN, improvement usually occurs within 3–7 days, hypertension is not sustained, and macroscopic hematuria is transient. Watch for ongoing oliguria, unresolved hypertension, increasing proteinuria, or progressive azotemia. Complement levels return to normal within 6–8 weeks of the initial presentation.

ALERT

- Microscopic hematuria may be present up to 2 years after an episode of poststreptococcal glomerulonephritis.
- Recurrent gross hematuria calls the diagnosis of APSGN into question.
- If complement levels do not return to normal after presumed APSGN, consider SLE and MPGN.

PATIENT MONITORING

- To control seizures, treat the hypertension; anticonvulsants play a secondary role.
- Look for and treat hyperkalemia.
- Monitor the degree of acute kidney injury.
- Home testing: BP monitoring may be required.
- Be certain to recognize fluid overload.
- Be certain to recognize the type of renal failure: acute versus chronic.
- Long-term monitoring for hypertension and/or progressive proteinuria may be indicated in some populations (5–10% may develop progressive proteinuria within 20 years).

DIET

Restrictions of intake of fluid, sodium, potassium, and phosphate are initially required.

PROGNOSIS

- Prognosis is excellent in APSGN and variable for other causes of glomerulonephritis in childhood.
- APSGN rarely recurs.

COMPLICATIONS

- Hypertension
- Acute renal failure
- Hyperkalemia
- Volume overload (e.g., congestive cardiac failure, pulmonary edema, hypertension)
- Chronic kidney disease

ADDITIONAL READING

- Ahn SY, Ingulli E. Acute poststreptococcal glomerulonephritis: an update. *Curr Opin Pediatr*. 2008;20(2):157–162.
- Lau KK, Wyatt RJ. Glomerulonephritis. *Adolesc Med*. 2005;16(1):67–85.
- Ornstein BW, Atkinson JP, Densen P. The complement system in pediatric systemic lupus erythematosus, atypical hemolytic uremic syndrome, and complocentric membranoglomerulopathies. *Curr Opin Rheumatol*. 2012;24(5):522–529.
- Pan CG. Evaluation of gross hematuria. *Pediatr Clin North Am*. 2006;53(3):401–412.
- Wong W, Morris MC, Zwi J. Outcome of severe acute post-streptococcal glomerulonephritis in New Zealand children. *Pediatr Nephrol*. 2009;24(5): 1021–1026.

CODES

ICD10

- N05.9 Unsp nephritic syndrome with unspecified morphologic changes
- N00.9 Acute nephritic syndrome with unsp morphologic changes
- N03.9 Chronic nephritic syndrome with unsp morphologic changes

FAQ

- Q: When do serum complement levels return to normal?
- A: Serum complement levels (C3) return to normal within a 6–8-week period in APSGN. Persistently low C3 levels suggest a cause other than APSGN and renal biopsy should be considered with persistent urinary abnormalities (hematuria and/or proteinuria).
- Q: What are the indications for renal biopsy in acute glomerulonephritis?
- A: Patients in whom there is sustained hypertension, ongoing or progressive azotemia, or persistent proteinuria of >1.5 mg/mg should be biopsied.

GLUCOSE-6-PHOSPHATE DEHYDROGENASE DEFICIENCY

Michele P. Lambert

BASICS

DESCRIPTION

Deficiency of the enzyme glucose-6-phosphate dehydrogenase (G6PD) in the RBC, which may result in hemolytic anemia. Several types of genetic mutations result either in deficient enzyme production or in production of an enzyme with diminished activity.

- Although most patients with this deficiency are never anemic and have mild to no hemolysis, the classic manifestation is acute hemolytic anemia in response to oxidative stress.
- World Health Organization classification of G6PD:
  - Class 1: congenital nonspherocytic hemolytic anemia: rare. Chronic hemolysis without exposure to oxidative stressors—splenomegaly in 40%. Affected individuals tend to be white males of Northern European background.
  - Class 2: severe deficiency (1–10% enzymatic activity): oxidative stress–induced hemolysis. Prototype is G6PD-Mediterranean.
  - Class 3: mild deficiency (10–60% enzymatic activity): most common type. Acute hemolytic anemia uncommon, occurs only with stressors
  - Class 4: nondeficient variant (60–100% enzymatic activity): no symptoms, even during oxidant stressors (e.g., G6PD A+ [variant with normal activity]); 20–40% allelic frequency in Africans
  - Class 5: >150% of normal activity
- Deficient neonates may have hyperbilirubinemia out of proportion to their anemia.
  - May, in part, account for increased prevalence of African Americans among patients with bilirubin encephalopathy
  - Should be considered as cause of hyperbilirubinemia in neonates of appropriate racial background and may contribute to kernicterus

GENERAL PREVENTION

Avoid drugs and toxins known to cause hemolysis. Prompt follow-up with febrile illness and signs of hemolysis.

EPIDEMIOLOGY

Prevalence

- Most common of all clinically significant enzyme defects, affecting ~400 million people worldwide
- X linked (Xq28): primarily affects males
- Almost 400 allelic variants
- Frequency of different mutations varies by population:
  - Africans: 20–40% of X chromosomes are G6PD A+ (mutant enzyme with normal activity).
  - Sardinians (some regions): 30% have G6PD-Mediterranean.
  - Saudi Arabians: 13% have G6PD deficiency.
  - African Americans: 10–15% have G6PD A− (mutant enzyme with decreased activity).
- High incidence of mutant genes in some regions may relate to survival advantage against malarial infection (*Plasmodium falciparum*).

Genetics

Gene is on the X chromosome (Xq28).

- Males express the enzyme (mutant or normal) from their single X chromosome (hemizygotes).
- Female homozygotes (rare) are more severely affected than female heterozygotes.
- Heterozygote females show variable intermediate expression because of random X inactivation.

PATHOPHYSIOLOGY

- RBCs lose G6PD activity throughout their lifespan; therefore, older cells are more prone to oxidative hemolysis.
- Normal RBC lifespan of ~120 days is unaffected in unstressed states, even with severe enzyme deficiency, but may be shortened during oxidant stress.
- Enzyme-deficient RBCs are destroyed by intravascular hemolysis on exposure to the oxidative stressor and acute hemolytic anemia results.
- Oxidant stressors include infections and chemicals (mothballs, antimalarials, some sulfonamides, methylene blue).
- Hemolysis usually follows stressor by 1–3 days, and nadir occurs 8–10 days postexposure. Obtain hemoglobins for >1 week after the initial exposure.
- Favism: severe hemolytic anemia in patients with more severe forms of G6PD deficiency after fava bean ingestion
- Normal G6PD activity is 7–10 IU/g hemoglobin.

DIAGNOSIS

HISTORY

- Symptoms of anemia include fatigue, irritability, and malaise.
- Dark urine (cola or tea colored) may follow moderate to severe hemolysis. May develop jaundice (particularly scleral icterus).
- Patient may have required phototherapy in newborn period for hyperbilirubinemia.
- Recent drug, chemical, or food (fava bean) exposures may precipitate moderate to severe hemolysis.
- Family history of intermittent jaundice, splenectomy, cholecystectomy, or blood transfusion may indicate an inherited condition.
- Ethnicity may help determine type/severity of disease.

PHYSICAL EXAM

- Tachycardia, a flow murmur, or pallor: signs of anemia
- Jaundice or scleral icterus: signs of hemolysis

DIAGNOSTIC TESTS & INTERPRETATION

Lab

- CBC
  - Usually reveals a normochromic normocytic anemia with appropriate reticulocytosis
  - Hemoglobin can drop precipitously; should be monitored closely until stable or trending upward; checking a single hemoglobin the day of exposure to the stressor is not sufficient.
- Peripheral blood smear
  - Often shows bizarre RBC morphology with marked anisocytosis and poikilocytosis
  - Can see schistocytes, hemighost cells (uneven distribution of hemoglobin), bite cells, blister cells, and occasional Heinz bodies (on supravital staining)
- Hemoglobinemia: seen as plasma (pinkish red supernatant) or measured as free serum hemoglobin
- Hemoglobinuria: occurs when hemoglobin-binding sites in the plasma (haptoglobin and hemopexin) are saturated; may be visible as dark urine—heme positive on dipstick and no RBC on microscopy
- Free haptoglobin levels decrease.
- Direct and indirect Coombs tests
  - Must be done to exclude autoimmune hemolytic anemia
  - Should be negative in G6PD deficiency
- Other: Plasma indirect bilirubin, lactate dehydrogenase, and aspartate aminotransferase may be elevated; hemosiderin may be found in the urine several days after hemolysis. Liver function tests should be normal. Renal functions to rule out thrombotic thrombocytopenic purpura and hemolytic uremic syndrome:
  - Rapid screening tests for G6PD activity in RBCs are qualitative; will miss some female heterozygotes with measurable but low enzyme levels
  - Necessary to confirm a deficiency or to diagnose a suspected heterozygote with a test to quantify G6PD activity
  - Normal activity: 7–10 IU/g hemoglobin
    - Accurately detects deficiency in males and homozygous females with no recent hemolysis
    - Helpful with heterozygous women/
- Newborn screening for G6PD deficiency
  - Included in some panels of genetic screening tests performed on newborns
  - Typically performed by DNA-based methods that detect a few of the most common variants in U.S. populations. Does not screen for all G6PD variants and can miss severe but rare variants.
  - Results may be reported in terms of predicted enzyme levels but not a true measurement of enzymatic activity.

ALERT

- Screening tests may be falsely negative during rapid red cell turnover (reticulocytosis).
- Most cost-effective approach: Defer screening until 1–2 weeks after resolution of hemolysis. Smear may be normal during steady state.
- Heterozygote female detection:
  - 2 RBC populations exist because of mosaicism from random X inactivation.
  - On average, 50% are normal and 50% are deficient, but there may be variability.

DIFFERENTIAL DIAGNOSIS

Intravascular hemolysis is very rare in children, but other causes include the following:

- Acute hemolytic transfusion reactions (Coombs test is positive)
- Microangiopathic hemolytic disease, such as hemolytic uremic syndrome, thrombotic thrombocytopenic purpura, and prosthetic cardiac valves
- Physical trauma (e.g., March hemoglobinuria); severe burns (uncommon)
- Other inherited RBC enzyme deficiencies
- Paroxysmal nocturnal hemoglobinuria
- Extravascular hemolysis can also be confused with G6PD deficiency and includes the following:
  - Hereditary spherocytosis (spherocytes on smear)
  - Autoimmune hemolysis and delayed hemolytic transfusion reactions (both Coombs positive)
  - Hemoglobinopathies
  - Hypersplenism
  - Severe liver disease
  - Gilbert disease

TREATMENT

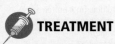

GENERAL MEASURES

- Removal of the oxidant stressor is of primary importance:
  - Discontinue the suspected drug and/or treat the infection.
    - In class 3 and 4 patients, essential drug therapy may be continued while monitoring for signs of severe hemolysis.
    - Transfusion may be necessary (especially in some class 1 and 2 deficiencies), but any patient who is symptomatic with anemia or has a low hemoglobin and signs of ongoing brisk hemolysis should be transfused immediately with packed RBCs.
  - Supportive care, evaluation of renal function (risk of acute tubular necrosis with brisk hemolysis), and monitoring degree of anemia and ongoing hemolysis are important.
- For the affected neonate:
  - Monitor the bilirubin closely and start phototherapy early.
    - If necessary, exchange transfusion should be carried out.
    - Phenobarbital may decrease bilirubin level.
    - Early discharge is not recommended in newborn infants with jaundice and known risk for G6PD deficiency.

ONGOING CARE

FOLLOW-UP RECOMMENDATIONS

- Most deficient individuals remain asymptomatic.
- When hemolysis does occur, it tends to be self-limited and resolves spontaneously, with a return to normal hemoglobin levels in 2–6 weeks.
- Development of renal failure is extremely rare in children, even with massive hemolysis and hemoglobinuria.

DIET

- Avoid fava beans (*Vicia faba*). Fava beans have a variety of names in different cultures (e.g., faba bean, broad bean, tick bean, field bean, bell bean, bakela [Ethiopia], faviera [Portugal], ful masri [Sudan], winter field bean [United Kingdom]).

PROGNOSIS

- For those with the milder forms, the prognosis is excellent.
- Can cause significant morbidity, but rarely mortality, in those with the more severe forms

COMPLICATIONS

Neonates can be at risk for hyperbilirubinemia, requiring treatment. Kernicterus has been reported in infants with G6PD deficiency.

ADDITIONAL READING

- Cappellini MD, Fiorelli G. Glucose-6-phosphate dehydrogenase deficiency. *Lancet*. 2008; 371(9606):64–74.
- Frank JE. Diagnosis and management of G6PD deficiency. *Am Fam Physician*. 2005;72(2):1277–1282.
- Nkhoma ET, Poole C, Vannappagari V, et al. The global prevalence of glucose-6 phosphate dehydrogenase deficiency: a systematic review and meta-analysis. *Blood Cells Mol Dis*. 2009;42(3):267–278.
- Youngster I, Arcavi L, Schechmaster R, et al. Medications and glucose-6-phosphate dehydrogenase deficiency: an evidence-based review. *Surg Saf*. 2010;33(9):713–726.
- Watchko JF. Hyperbilirubinemia in African American neonates. *Semin Fetal Neonatal Med*. 2010;15(3):176–182.

CODES

ICD10

D55.0 Anemia due to glucose-6-phosphate dehydrogenase deficiency

FAQ

- Q: Do I need to follow a special diet or avoid medications if I have G6PD deficiency?
- A: Although most patients will have no symptoms of their disease, certain medications may cause transient hemolytic anemia, and these should be avoided. When prescribing medications, your physician and pharmacist should know about your G6PD, but most necessary medications are safe and well tolerated. People with severe variants of the deficiency should also avoid fava beans, but otherwise no dietary restrictions are necessary.
- Q: Do I need to know which variant of G6PD I have?
- A: It may be clear which variant you are likely to have based on your clinical symptoms and ethnic background.
- Q: Should my family be screened if someone has G6PD deficiency?
- A: In families of patients with G6PD, screening members may help provide meaningful genetic counseling to female carriers and affected but asymptomatic males.
- Q: How does G6PD affect sickle cell anemia and vice versa?
- A: Having sickle cell disease is somewhat protective in patients with G6PD A deficiency because their RBC population is young and, therefore, has higher enzymatic activity. On the other hand, G6PD has no effect on the clinical characteristics of sickle cell disease.

G

GOITER

Adda Grimberg

BASICS

DESCRIPTION
Goiter is enlargement of the thyroid gland.

EPIDEMIOLOGY
- The most common cause of pediatric goiter in the United States is chronic lymphocytic thyroiditis.
- The prevalence of goiter in the United States is 3–7%, although the incidence is much higher in regions of iodine deficiency.
- Thyroid cancers make up 0.5–1.5% of all malignancies in children and adolescents.
- Both thyroid tumors and autoimmune thyroid disease are more common in females than males.

Prevalence
World Health Organization (WHO) Global Database on Iodine Deficiency (1993–2003)
- Goiter prevalence globally is 15.8% of the general population.
- Insufficient iodine intake among school-aged children ranges from 10.1% in the Americas to 59.9% in Europe.
- 54 countries had iodine deficiency, 29 countries had excessive iodine intake, and 43 countries achieved optimal iodine intake.

ETIOLOGY
- Multinodular goiter (MNG) loci have been identified on chromosome 14q and on chromosome Xp22 and 3q26.
- Germline mutations in *DICER1* (chromosome 14q31) have been found in familial MNG-1, with and without ovarian Sertoli-Leydig cell tumors.
- Germline mutation in thyroid transcription factor-1 (TITF-1/NKX2.1) has been found in patients with papillary thyroid carcinoma and a history of multinodular goiter.
- Other genes implicated in simple goiter formation: thyroglobulin, thyroid-stimulating hormone (TSH) receptor, and Na^+/I^- symporter
- Thyroid peroxidase mutations lead to iodide organification defects and goitrous congenital hypothyroidism.
- Twin and family studies show a modest to major effect of environmental factors, especially iodine deficiency and cigarette smoking.
- Excessive maternal ingestion of iodine during pregnancy can lead to congenital goiter with increased iodine uptake on scan and in some babies, a transient hypothyroidism.
- Autoimmune goiters, such as chronic lymphocytic thyroiditis, occur in children with a genetic predisposition.
- Thyroid cancers are usually sporadic. Medullary carcinoma can be familial (autosomal dominant), as part of multiple endocrine neoplasia (MEN) type 2A and 2B, or as isolated malignancy.
- Pendred syndrome (autosomal recessive) causes congenital sensorineural deafness and an iodine organification defect that leads to goiter.

DIAGNOSIS

HISTORY
- Symptoms of hypothyroidism:
  - Increase in sedentary behavior
  - Lethargy
  - Weight gain
  - Constipation
  - Cold intolerance
  - Dry skin and/or hair
  - Hair loss
- Symptoms of hyperthyroidism:
  - Hyperactivity
  - Irritability
  - Difficulty concentrating or focusing in school
  - Hyperphagia
  - Weight loss
  - Diarrhea
  - Heat intolerance
- Careful dietary and medication history
- History of head, neck, or chest irradiation is associated with increased risk of carcinoma.
- Family history of thyroid carcinoma or MEN syndrome

PHYSICAL EXAM
Inspect, palpate, and auscultate the neck:
- Neck extension aids inspection.
- Palpation is best performed standing behind the child:
  - Determine if the thyroid is diffusely enlarged or asymmetric, evaluate gland firmness, and assess for any nodularity.
  - Check for cervical lymphadenopathy.
  - Pain on palpation suggests acute inflammation.
- Auscultate with the stethoscope diaphragm (while patient holds his or her breath) for a bruit, which indicates hyperthyroidism-associated hypervascularity.
- Careful examination for signs of hypothyroidism or hyperthyroidism
  - Linear growth and weight pattern
  - Pulse
  - Sexual development
  - Deep tendon reflexes
  - Skin
- Have patient drink water during inspection of gland.

DIAGNOSTIC TESTS & INTERPRETATION
- Thyroid function tests: Total T_4 and TSH are best screens for hypothyroidism or hyperthyroidism.
- T_3 radioimmunoassay in cases of suspected hyperthyroidism (note: radioimmunoassay, which measures total T_3, and not resin uptake, which indirectly assesses thyroid hormone–binding capacity)
- In cases of suspected chronic lymphocytic thyroiditis: antithyroglobulin and antimicrosomal (antiperoxidase) antibodies
- In cases of suspected Graves disease: thyroid-stimulating immunoglobulins (or TSH-receptor antibodies)
- Fine-needle aspiration biopsy in children should be considered only for evaluation of low-risk or purely cystic thyroid nodules. (A higher percentage of solitary thyroid nodules are malignant in children compared with adults.)
- Calcitonin levels: elevated in 75% of patients with medullary thyroid carcinoma

Lab
Urinary iodine (UI) concentration is the best measure of the adequacy of iodine intake.

Imaging
- Ultrasound to determine the number, size, and nature (cystic, solid, or mixed) of nodules
- ^{123}I thyroid scans in cases of solitary nodules to establish whether the nodule concentrates iodide
  - "Cold" nodules (no I uptake) suggest neoplasia and require immediate evaluation by a pediatric endocrinologist and surgeon.
- Barium swallow studies can reveal a fistulous tract between the left piriform sinus and the left thyroid lobe in children with recurrent acute suppurative thyroiditis. Such fistulas are amenable to surgical resection.

DIFFERENTIAL DIAGNOSIS
- Fat neck
  - Adipose tissue
  - Large sternocleidomastoid muscles
- Thyroglossal duct cysts
- Nonthyroidal neoplasms: lymphoma, teratoma, hygroma, ganglioneuroma
- Immunologic
  - Chronic lymphocytic thyroiditis (often referred to as Hashimoto thyroiditis)
  - Graves disease
  - Amyloid deposition (familial Mediterranean fever, juvenile rheumatoid arthritis)
- Infectious
  - Acute suppurative thyroiditis (most often *Streptococcus pyogenes*, *Staphylococcus aureus*, and *Streptococcus pneumoniae*)
  - Subacute thyroiditis (often viral)
- Environmental
  - Goitrogens: iodide, lithium, amiodarone, oral contraceptives, perchlorate, cabbage, soybeans, cassava, thiocyanate in tobacco smoke (smoking is especially goitrogenic in iodine-deficient areas)
  - Iodine deficiency (exacerbated by pregnancy)
- Neoplastic
  - Thyroid adenoma/carcinoma
  - Follicular adenoma: benign
  - Follicular, papillary, or mixed carcinoma: well-differentiated; follicular 90%
  - Medullary carcinoma: 4–10% as part of the MEN type 2 syndrome
  - TSH-secreting adenoma
  - Lymphoma
- Congenital
  - Ectopic gland
  - Unilateral agenesis of gland
  - Dyshormonogenesis
  - T_4 resistance
- Miscellaneous:
  - Simple colloid goiter
  - Multinodular goiter

TREATMENT

ALERT

Possible conflicts: In manic depressive patients on lithium and cardiac patients on amiodarone, medication-induced thyroid abnormalities can be a significant problem that should be addressed by the endocrinologist and appropriate subspecialist.

MEDICATION

- Goiters with hypothyroidism: L-thyroxine
- Goiter with hyperthyroidism: Treatment consists of antithyroid drugs (methimazole); if remission is not achieved after 1 or 2 years, radioactive iodine ablation (^{131}I) or surgery (near-total or total thyroidectomy) may be considered.
- Duration depends on the cause of the goiter.

ALERT

FDA issued a black box warning (6/4/2009) against propylthiouracil (PTU) use in treating Graves disease owing to risk of severe liver injury including life-threatening acute liver failure.

ADDITIONAL TREATMENT

Additional Therapies

Intraamniotic injections of L-thyroxine may treat fetal goitrous hypothyroidism. Large fetal goiters pose a risk of airway compromise at birth.

SURGERY/OTHER PROCEDURES

- Surgery solely to decrease size of goiter indicated only if adjacent structures are compressed.
- Rates of complications after pediatric total thyroidectomy are similar for benign and malignant thyroid diseases; most common is transient hypocalcemia.
- Cancer
  - Surgery is recommended for a nonfunctioning nodule if there is:
    - A history of radiation
    - Rapid growth of a firm nodule
    - Evidence of satellite lymph nodes
    - Evidence of impingement on other neck structures
    - Evidence of distant metastases
- Following surgery, radioiodide therapy is administered if a follow-up iodine scan reveals any residual tissue or metastases.
- Suppressive doses of exogenous thyroid hormone are then given to maintain TSH levels <0.2 mIU/L.
- Thyroglobulin levels are useful as markers of thyroid tissue; calcitonin level serves as tumor marker for medullary carcinoma.

ONGOING CARE

FOLLOW-UP RECOMMENDATIONS

- Potential for goiter regression depends on its cause. Goiters associated with chronic lymphocytic thyroiditis and Graves disease may or may not decrease in size with treatment.
- A goiter patient who is clinically and biochemically euthyroid still requires careful follow-up for the detection of the early signs of developing thyroid dysfunction.
- Potential complications of thyroid surgery include laryngeal nerve damage and hypoparathyroidism. Complication rates are lower in high-volume centers.
- Long-term follow-up of patients with thyroid cancer is recommended, as disease can recur decades after initial diagnosis and therapy.

ALERT

- Work up solitary thyroid nodules aggressively. Remember: Incidence of malignancy in these nodules in children is 15–40% (less in adults).
- Malignancy is more likely in euthyroid pediatric patients with nodules that have palpable lymph nodes, compressive signs, microcalcifications, intranodular vascularization, and lymph node alterations.
- Differentiated thyroid carcinoma in prepubertal children, compared to pubertal adolescents, has a more aggressive presentation and more frequently a family history of thyroid carcinoma.

DIET

- Depends on the cause of the goiter
- Incidence of iodine deficiency (endemic) goiter has greatly declined since the addition of potassium iodide to table salt.
- Iodide can also be added to communal drinking water or administered as iodized oil in isolated rural areas.

PROGNOSIS

- Depends on the cause of the goiter
- Thyroid cancers usually follow an indolent course with excellent prognosis, especially the well-differentiated follicular cell carcinoma. Mortality is most common in medullary and undifferentiated carcinomas, which are relatively rare in children.

COMPLICATIONS

- Depending on gland size, goiters can produce a mass effect on midline neck structures. If the goiter is intrathoracic, it may cause pleural effusions or chylothorax.
- Typically, the child is euthyroid, but clinical hypothyroidism or hyperthyroidism may result from certain types of goiters.
- Therapy for thyroid cancer may induce permanent hypothyroidism.

ADDITIONAL READING

- Aghini Lombardi F, Fiore E, Tonacchera M, et al. The effect of voluntary iodine prophylaxis in a small rural community: the Pescopagano survey 15 years later. *J Clin Endocrinol Metab*. 2013;98(3):1031–1039.
- Corrias A, Mussa A, Baronio F, et al. Diagnostic features of thyroid nodules in pediatrics. *Arch Pediatr Adolesc Med*. 2010;164(8):714–719.
- Hashimoto H, Hashimoto K, Suehara N. Successful in utero treatment of fetal goitrous hypothyroidism: case report and review of the literature. *Fetal Diagn Ther*. 2006;21(4):360–365.
- Lazar L, Lebenthal Y, Steinmetz A, et al. Differentiated thyroid carcinoma in pediatric patients: comparison of presentation and course between pre-pubertal children and adolescents. *J Pediatr*. 2009;154(5):708–714.
- Raval MV, Browne M, Chin AC, et al. Total thyroidectomy for benign disease in the pediatric patient—feasible and safe. *J Pediatr Surg*. 2009;44(8):1529–1533.
- Rivkees SA. Pediatric Graves' disease: controversies in management. *Horm Res Paediatr*. 2010;74(5):305–311.
- Rivkees SA, Mazzaferri EL, Verburg FA, et al. The treatment of differentiated thyroid cancer in children: emphasis on surgical approach and radioactive iodine therapy. *Endocr Rev*. 2011;32(6):798–826.
- Stevens C, Lee JK, Sadatsafavi M, et al. Pediatric thyroid fine-needle aspiration cytology: a meta-analysis. *J Pediatr Surg*. 2009;44(11):2184–2191.
- Zimmermann MB, Hess SY, Molinari L, et al. New reference values for thyroid volume by ultrasound in iodine-sufficient schoolchildren: a World Health Organization/Nutrition for Health and Development Iodine Deficiency Study Group report. *Am J Clin Nutr*. 2004;79(2):231–237.

CODES

ICD10

- E04.9 Nontoxic goiter, unspecified
- E04.2 Nontoxic multinodular goiter
- E06.3 Autoimmune thyroiditis

FAQ

- Q: Does a bigger thyroid gland mean increased thyroid functioning?
- A: Goiters can be euthyroid, hypothyroid, or hyperthyroid, depending on cause.
- Q: Will the goiter decrease in size with treatment?
- A: This depends on the cause of the goiter.
- Q: Does a bigger thyroid gland mean cancer?
- A: Most pediatric goiters are benign, and thyroid cancers often are detected as solitary nodules within an otherwise normal gland (in children with solitary nodules, up to 40% are carcinomas). Patients with a history of goiter or benign nodules/adenomas have an increased risk of developing thyroid cancer.
- Q: Does thyroid cancer usually present with hyperthyroidism?
- A: No. The usual chief complaint is a solitary, hard, painless nodule in an euthyroid patient.
- Q: Is there an increased risk of thyroid cancer from diagnostic radiographs (chest radiographs, lateral neck films)?
- A: Routine diagnostic radiographs should fall well below the levels of radiation thought to increase risk of thyroid neoplasia. During more prolonged radiologic procedures that might expose the thyroid to higher doses of radiation, a lead neck shield is used.
- Q: Should prophylactic thyroidectomy be performed in children identified genetically as having familial medullary carcinoma?
- A: Yes. Because of the poorer prognosis associated with development of this cancer

GONOCOCCAL INFECTIONS

Angela M. Statile • Samir S. Shah

BASICS

DESCRIPTION

Neisseria gonorrhoeae, an aerobic gram-negative diplococcus, is the etiologic agent of gonorrhea.

EPIDEMIOLOGY

- Gonorrhea is the second most common sexually transmitted infection (STI) in the United States.
- Coinfection with *Chlamydia trachomatis* commonly occurs in sexually active patients.

Incidence

- In the United States, there are >800,000 new cases of gonorrhea each year. Rates of infection are highest among adolescents and young adults.
- Racial disparities are present, with a disproportionately high incidence in ethnic minorities.

Prevalence

- Less than half of all infections are estimated to be detected or reported.

RISK FACTORS

- Vaginal delivery to an infected mother is a risk factor for neonatal disease.
- Sexual abuse should be considered in all prepubertal children presenting with gonorrhea.
- Risk factors for sexually active adolescents include multiple sexual partners, lack of condom use, and inconsistent screening by health care providers.
- The risk of male-to-female transmission is 50% per episode of vaginal intercourse; the risk of female-to-male transmission is ~20% per episode. Rectal intercourse is also a mode of transmission.

GENERAL PREVENTION

- Ophthalmia neonatorum: Prophylactic ophthalmic ointment is mandatory in the United States regardless of method of delivery. Instillation of 0.5% erythromycin ophthalmic ointment in both eyes occurs immediately after birth.
- Maternal infection: Routine screening cervical cultures should be performed at the 1st prenatal visit; repeat at term if high risk.

PATHOPHYSIOLOGY

- Incubation period is 2–7 days.
- Transmission results from contact with infected mucosa and secretions, usually through vaginal delivery, sexual activity, and (rarely) household contact in prepubertal children.
- In prepubertal children, genital infection is mild; ascending or disseminated infection rarely occurs. In adolescents, estrogenization protects the vagina from infection and instead serves as a conduit for cervical exudate.
- Immunity is not induced by infection.

COMMONLY ASSOCIATED CONDITIONS

Pediatric gonococcal infections can be categorized by age group: neonates, prepubertal children, and sexually active adolescents.

- Neonatal gonococcal diseases include ophthalmia neonatorum, scalp abscess (complication of fetal scalp monitoring), and, rarely, disseminated disease.
- Prepubertal gonococcal disease usually occurs in the genital tract. Vaginitis is the most common manifestation. Pelvic inflammatory disease (PID), perihepatitis (Fitz-Hugh–Curtis syndrome), urethritis, proctitis, and pharyngitis rarely occur. Consider sexual abuse.
- Gonococcal diseases in sexually active adolescents resemble those found in adults and may be asymptomatic.
  - Both sexes: pharyngitis, anorectal infection, tenosynovitis-dermatitis syndrome, or arthritis
  - Females: Genital tract infection may cause urethritis, vaginitis, and endocervicitis. Ascending genital tract infection may lead to PID and perihepatitis.
  - Males: Acute urethritis is the predominant manifestation. Epididymitis also occurs.

DIAGNOSIS

HISTORY

- In neonates, assess for risk factors such as premature or prolonged membrane rupture, presence of fetal scalp monitoring, and maternal history of infection.
- Onset of eye findings in ophthalmia neonatorum is usually between 2 and 5 days of age but ranges from 1 day to several weeks.
- Sexual history should be thoroughly reviewed with all adolescents.
- Vaginal itching and discharge may indicate vaginitis.
- Urethritis: purulent urethral discharge and dysuria without urgency or frequency
- Abdominal pain
  - Ascending infection is characterized by diffuse lower quadrant abdominal pain, including discomfort with ambulation. Low back pain, dyspareunia, and abnormal vaginal bleeding occasionally occur. Fever, chills, nausea, and vomiting may be present. Acute perihepatitis causes right upper quadrant pain and results from direct extension of infection from the fallopian tube to the liver capsule.
- Symptoms of extragenitourinary disease including sore throat, joint pain, or rash

PHYSICAL EXAM

- Ophthalmia neonatorum
  - Bilateral eyelid edema, chemosis, and copious purulent discharge
- Neonatal scalp abscess
- PID
  - Signs include cervical motion tenderness, pelvic adnexal tenderness (usually bilateral), and lower or right upper quadrant abdominal pain (with perihepatitis). Many females with PID also have mucopurulent cervical discharge.
- Cervicitis or urethritis: purulent vaginal or penile discharge
- Rash: classically discrete, tender, necrotic pustules on distal extremities, although macules, papules, and bullae occasionally occur
- Joint findings: tenosynovitis, migratory arthritis

DIAGNOSTIC TESTS & INTERPRETATION

Lab

Initial lab tests

- Gram stain (low sensitivity) and culture of infected exudate or body fluid
  - Intracellular gram-negative diplococci on gram stain. Confirmation depends on isolation of *N. gonorrhoeae* from culture. Specimens are immediately inoculated onto Thayer-Martin or chocolate–blood agar–based media at room temperature and incubated in an enriched CO_2 environment. In cases of suspected sexual abuse, collect genital, rectal, and pharyngeal cultures.
- Nonculture gonococcal tests
  - Nucleic acid amplification tests (NAATs) for urine specimens (freshly voided specimens), male urethral, female endocervical or vaginal (self-administered introital) swabs are highly sensitive and specific but should not be used in investigations of possible sexual abuse (possibility of false-positive results). NAATs also cannot provide antimicrobial susceptibility test results.
- STI panel
  - Test for other STIs including *C. trachomatis*, *Treponema pallidum* (syphilis), *Trichomonas vaginalis*, and HIV in children in whom sexual abuse is suspected or when evaluating sexually active adolescents.
- CBC, ESR, C-reactive protein, and blood culture may be obtained to evaluate for inflammation and disseminated disease.
- Synovial fluid cell count and culture in patients with joint swelling (cell count often >50,000 WBC/μL with differential of >90% PMNs)
- Synovial fluid cultures are positive in 50% with gonococcal arthritis; blood cultures are positive in less than 1/3, although cultures from other sites (e.g., cervix, urethra) are frequently positive.

Imaging

Pelvic ultrasound may detect ectopic pregnancy and, in PID, may reveal thick, dilated fallopian tubes or tuboovarian abscess.

DIFFERENTIAL DIAGNOSIS

- Ophthalmia neonatorum: Other causes of neonatal conjunctivitis include infection with *C. trachomatis*, *Staphylococcus aureus*, *Streptococcus pneumoniae*, *Haemophilus* species, chemical conjunctivitis, and herpes simplex virus (HSV).
- Scalp infection: Gonococcal scalp abscesses may be difficult to distinguish from abscesses caused by staphylococcal species, group B *Streptococcus*, *H. influenzae*, Enterobacteriaceae, and HSV.
- Vaginitis: In the prepubertal child, other causes include chemical or environmental irritants, pinworms, foreign body, and infections (i.e., streptococci, *T. vaginalis*). In cases of sexual abuse, *C. trachomatis* and syphilis may occur.

- Genitourinary tract infection: In adolescents, other causes include *C. trachomatis*, syphilis, and *T. vaginalis*.
- Arthritis: other bacterial causes of septic arthritis, Reiter syndrome, and reactive arthritis
- Abdominal pain: ectopic pregnancy, appendicitis, cholecystitis, UTI/pyelonephritis, and ovarian torsion

TREATMENT

MEDICATION

First Line

- Changing resistance patterns in the United States led to extended-spectrum cephalosporin as initial therapy.
- Neonates
  - Ophthalmia neonatorum: ceftriaxone 25–50 mg/kg IV or IM (single dose; maximum, 125 mg); alternate agent for infants with hyperbilirubinemia is cefotaxime 100 mg/kg IV or IM (single dose).
  - Neonates with gonococcal ophthalmia also require eye irrigation with sterile saline at presentation and at frequent intervals until mucopurulent drainage has ceased.
  - Disseminated infection: cefotaxime for 7 days for bacteremia, 10–14 days for meningitis
- Older children and adolescents
  - Uncomplicated gonococcal infection (including cervicitis, epididymitis, or pharyngeal infection): Cefixime is no longer recommended as 1st-line treatment. Give a single IM dose of ceftriaxone 250 mg. Follow with a treatment regimen for *C. trachomatis*.
  - If ceftriaxone is not available, give single-dose cefixime 400 mg orally, along with *C. trachomatis* treatment. In cases of severe cephalosporin allergy, give single dose azithromycin 2 g. Alternative regimens to ceftriaxone require tests of cure in 1 week.
  - PID: See Pediatric *Red Book* or 2010 CDC guidelines for treatment regimens.
  - Complicated gonococcal infection: ceftriaxone or cefotaxime for 7 days (arthritis and septicemia), 10–14 days (meningitis), or ≥28 days (endocarditis). Include concomitant *C. trachomatis* therapy.
  - Pursue empiric treatment of sexual partners.

INPATIENT CONSIDERATIONS

Admission Criteria

- Neonates: Hospitalize and obtain appropriate cultures (conjunctivae, blood, CSF, or those from any other site of infection).
- Prepubertal children: safety concerns present or complicated disease
- Sexually active adolescents: PID with inability to tolerate oral antibiotics, complicated disease requiring further monitoring

ONGOING CARE

FOLLOW-UP RECOMMENDATIONS

- Provide risk reduction education.
- Sexual contacts (including mother and her partner[s]) of patients with gonorrhea should be counseled and treated.
- Evaluate for concurrent infection with other sexually transmitted diseases, including syphilis, *C. trachomatis*, *T. vaginalis*, hepatitis B, and HIV. Patients whose age has progressed beyond the neonatal period should be treated presumptively for *C. trachomatis* infection.
- All cases of gonorrhea must be reported to public health officials.
- Contact isolation precautions are recommended for all hospitalized patients with gonococcal disease in the neonatal and prepubertal age groups; no special policies are recommended for other patients.
- Evaluate prepubertal children for abuse.

ALERT

Pitfalls

- Failure to consider the diagnosis of sexual abuse in a prepubertal child with a gonococcal infection. Cases of transmission via nonsexual contact have been reported (i.e., from freshly infected towels/fomites, childhood sexual play, or by digital transmission from an infected caregiver), but such mode cannot be assumed without first excluding sexual abuse.
- Failure to use culture to diagnose infection in cases of suspected abuse
- Failure to differentiate *N. gonorrhoeae* by culture from other *Neisseria* species, especially in prepubertal children, given concern for sexual abuse
- Failure to consider acute gonococcal perihepatitis/Fitz-Hugh–Curtis syndrome in females with right upper quadrant pain

PROGNOSIS

Prognosis has been improved by treating all forms of infection with a 3rd-generation cephalosporin.

COMPLICATIONS

- Gonococcal infection during pregnancy is associated with spontaneous abortion, preterm labor, and perinatal infant mortality.
- Ophthalmia neonatorum may rapidly progress to corneal ulceration and perforation, with subsequent scarring and blindness.
- PID
  - Endometritis, salpingitis, tuboovarian abscess, and pelvic peritonitis occur as a consequence of untreated vaginal disease.
  - Scarring secondary to salpingitis causes sterility in ≤20% of women with a single infection and ≤50% of women after 3 episodes of infection.
  - Risk of ectopic pregnancy increases 7-fold after 1 episode of PID.
- In males, rare complications include periurethral abscess, acute prostatitis, seminal vesiculitis, and urethral strictures.
- Disseminated disease
  - Consider evaluation for complement deficiency in those with multiple episodes.
  - In neonates, arthritis is the most frequent systemic manifestation; symptoms develop 1–4 weeks after delivery. Involvement of multiple joints is typical, and most infants do not have ophthalmia neonatorum.
  - In older children and adolescents, septic arthritis (1 joint) and a characteristic poly–arthritis-dermatitis syndrome are possible manifestations.
  - Gonococcal meningitis, endocarditis, and osteomyelitis are rare in children.
- Gonococcal infection can serve as a cofactor in increasing HIV infection and transmission.

ADDITIONAL READING

- American Academy of Pediatrics. Gonococcal infections. In: Pickering LK, Baker CJ, Kimberlin DW, et al, eds. *Red Book: 2012 Report of the Committee on Infectious Diseases*. 29th ed. Elk Grove Village, IL: American Academy of Pediatrics; 2012:336–344.
- Centers for Disease Control and Prevention. Update to CDC's sexually transmitted diseases treatment guidelines, 2010: oral cephalosporins no longer a recommended treatment for gonococcal infections. *MMWR Morb Mortal Wkly Rep*. 2012;61(31):590–594.
- Comkornruecha M. Gonococcal infections. *Pediatr Rev*. 2013;34(5):228–234.
- Kellogg N; American Academy of Pediatrics Committee on Child Abuse and Neglect. The evaluation of sexual abuse in children. *Pediatrics*. 2005;116(2):506–512.

CODES

ICD10

- A54.9 Gonococcal infection, unspecified
- P39.8 Other specified infections specific to the perinatal period
- P39.1 Neonatal conjunctivitis and dacryocystitis

FAQ

- Q: What are the advantages of the NAATs for making a diagnosis?
- A: The transcription-mediated amplification (TMA) test of urine samples, approved by the FDA for women, can be used to simultaneously test for *C. trachomatis* and *N. gonorrhoeae*.
- Q: When is this test not approved?
- A: For rectal and pharyngeal swabs and for cases of suspected abuse

GRAFT-VERSUS-HOST DISEASE

Valerie I. Brown

BASICS

DESCRIPTION

Graft-versus-host disease (GVHD) is a multiorgan inflammatory process that develops when immunologically competent T lymphocytes from a histoincompatible donor are infused into an immunocompromised host unable to reject them. Divided into acute and chronic, historically based on time of presentation but best delineated by clinicopathologic findings.

- Acute: develops within 100 days after allogeneic hematopoietic stem cell transplant (HSCT); affects skin, GI tract, and/or liver
- Chronic: develops 100 days after allogeneic HSCT; presents with diverse features resembling autoimmune syndromes
- Chronic subtypes
  - Progressive: extension of acute GVHD
  - Quiescent: after resolution of acute GVHD
  - De novo: no prior acute GVHD

EPIDEMIOLOGY

- Acute GVHD (grades II–IV): 10–80% of patients receiving T-cell–replete HSCT
  - 35–45% for human leukocyte antigen (HLA)–identical related donor bone marrow
  - 60–80% if 1-antigen HLA-mismatched unrelated donor bone marrow or peripheral stem cells
  - 35–65% if 2-antigen HLA-mismatched unrelated umbilical cord blood
- Chronic GVHD: most common cause of late morbidity and mortality of allogeneic HSCT
  - 15–25% if HLA-identical related marrow
  - 40–60% if HLA-matched unrelated marrow
  - 54–70% if HLA-matched unrelated peripheral stem cells
  - 20% if unrelated umbilical cord blood
- Flare-ups triggered by infection (usually viral)

RISK FACTORS

- HLA disparity (both major and minor antigens)
- Older donor or recipient age
- Stem cell source and dose
  - Highest risk: with peripheral stem cells
  - Lowest risk: with umbilical cord blood
- Donor leukocyte infusions
- Reactivation of viruses (e.g., HHV-6, CMV)
- T-cell depletion decreases incidence.
- Acute GVHD-specific
  - Higher intensity conditioning regimen
  - Prior pregnancies in female donors
  - Gender mismatch
- Chronic GVHD specific
  - Severity of acute GVHD
  - Malignancy as indication for transplantation
  - Use of total-body irradiation
  - Type of immunosuppressive prophylaxis

Genetics

- HLA gene complex on chromosome 6; inherited as haplotype
- Full siblings: 25% chance HLA identical
- Minor histocompatibility antigen differences likely account for GVHD in HLA-identical sibling stem cell transplants.

GENERAL PREVENTION

- Transfusion: irradiation of all cellular blood products for patients at risk
- Stem cell transplantation
  - Selection of a histocompatible donor
  - Immunosuppression (gold standard): cyclosporine or tacrolimus with a short course of methotrexate
  - Other options: corticosteroids, sirolimus, mycophenolate mofetil, and low-dose cyclophosphamide
  - Donor T-cell depletion with anti–T-cell antibodies ex vivo in graft or in vivo in recipient

PATHOPHYSIOLOGY

- Acute GVHD: interaction of donor and host innate and adaptive immune responses
  - Severity related to degree of HLA mismatch
  - 3 phases ending in "cytokine storm"
    - Tissue damage by conditioning regimen
    - Priming and activation of donor T cells
    - Infiltration of activated T cells into skin, GI tract, and liver resulting in apoptosis
- Chronic GVHD: findings similar to autoimmune disorders: donor T cells directed against host antigens, donor T-cell autoreactivity, B-cell dysregulation, regulatory T-cell deficiency; marked collagen deposition in target organs and lack of T-cell infiltration

ETIOLOGY

- Hematopoietic stem cell transplantation
- Transfusion of nonirradiated blood products to immunodeficient hosts: caused by viable donor lymphocytes engrafting in the recipient
- Transfusion of nonirradiated blood from a donor homozygous for 1 of the recipient's HLA haplotypes (1st- or 2nd-degree relative)
- Intrauterine maternal–fetal transfusions and exchange transfusions in neonates
- Solid organ grafts: contain immunocompetent T cells, into immunosuppressed recipient

DIAGNOSIS

HISTORY

- Acute GVHD
  - Rash: usually 1st manifestation; pruritus or burning sensation can precede rash.
  - Diarrhea, abdominal pain, and intestinal bleeding: unusual to precede skin disease
  - Anorexia, nausea, vomiting, and dyspepsia
  - Jaundice (liver involvement)
- Chronic GVHD
  - Dry eyes and/or dry mouth, blurry vision, eye irritation, photophobia, eye pain
  - Difficulty swallowing or retrosternal pain
  - Sensitivity to mint, spicy foods, or tomatoes
  - Weight loss, failure to thrive, anorexia, nausea, vomiting, diarrhea
  - Dyspnea, wheezing, cough
  - Poor wound healing, especially post trauma
  - Joint stiffness, muscle cramps
- Infections: pneumococcal sepsis, *Pneumocystis jiroveci*, fungal infections

PHYSICAL EXAM

- Acute/transfusion-associated GVHD
  - Skin (most common site)
    - Maculopapular rash of palms, soles; can become confluent erythroderma
    - Severe form: bullae formation, to even full-thickness necrosis
  - GI tract: weight loss; profuse, watery, often green, and often bloody diarrhea
  - Liver: jaundice; atypical findings: painful hepatomegaly, ascites, rapid weight gain
- Chronic GVHD
  - Skin (involved in almost every patient)
    - Hyper- or hypopigmentation, xerosis (skin dryness), pruritus, scaling, patchy erythema, poikiloderma, skin atrophy; lichenoid, eczematous, and/or sclerodermatous changes
    - Advanced scleroderma: thickened, tight, and fragile skin
  - Hair: thin, fragile; premature graying
  - Scalp: dry or seborrheic
  - Nails: dystrophic, fragile; entire nail loss
  - Mouth: xerostomia, mucositis, ulcers; whitish, lacy plaques on tongue and buccal surfaces, may be painful; tight oral aperture
  - Esophageal strictures, stenosis, webs
  - Blood: thrombocytopenia, anemia, eosinophilia, autoantibodies, hypo- or hypergammaglobulinemia
  - Joints: stiffness, contractures, swelling
  - Muscles: eosinophilic fasciitis, myositis
  - Lung: bronchiolitis obliterans (obstructive), bronchiolitis obliterans organizing pneumonia (restrictive), pleural effusions
  - Other: pericardial effusions, pericarditis, cardiomyopathy, nephrotic syndrome, peripheral neuropathy, genital ulceration

DIAGNOSTIC TESTS & INTERPRETATION

Diagnosis is often made on clinical grounds.

Lab

- Complete blood count with differential and Coombs test: autoimmune thrombocytopenia (most common), hemolytic anemia, and neutropenia; eosinophilia, resolves with treatment
- Blood smear: Howell-Jolly bodies due to functional asplenia of chronic GVHD

- Elevated ALT/AST without hyperbilirubinemia
- Vitamin D: often low; risk for osteoporosis
- Urinalysis: may show protein, glucose, blood
- Schirmer test: decreased tear production
- Pulmonary function tests
- Echocardiogram/electrocardiogram
- Fluorescein microscopy: punctate keratopathy

Imaging

- High-resolution chest CT: bronchiolitis obliterans
- Barium swallow: strictures, webs

Diagnostic Procedures/Other

- Endoscopy or colonoscopy with biopsy: apoptosis and loss of villi; GI tract GVHD
- Skin biopsy: localized epidermal atrophy
- Liver biopsy: bile duct damage reminiscent of primary biliary cirrhosis
- Rule out viral/fungal infections
- Analysis of pleural, pericardial fluid

DIFFERENTIAL DIAGNOSIS

- Acute GVHD
  – Skin: drug reaction, chemoradiotherapy, viral exanthema, engraftment syndrome; TEN for grade IV skin GVHD
  – Liver: hepatic veno-occlusive disease, total parenteral nutrition, drug toxicity, bacterial sepsis, or viral infection
  – GI: diarrhea secondary to transplant conditioning regimen, infectious causes (e.g., *Clostridium difficile*, CMV, adenovirus), or opiate withdrawal
- Chronic GVHD
  – Skin: keratosis pilaris, eczema, psoriasis

ALERT

- In chronic GVHD, do not give live vaccines; may lead to symptomatic infection
- Sudden high fevers may indicate bacterial sepsis, may be overwhelming. Chronic GVHD patients often functionally asplenic; have profoundly impaired immune function

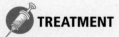

TREATMENT

MEDICATION

- Acute GVHD (grades II–IV)
  – 1st line: systemic steroids at 2 mg/kg/24 h for 7–14 days then quick taper; cyclosporine or tacrolimus if not taking as prophylaxis
  – 2nd line: mycophenolate mofetil, sirolimus (rapamycin), antithymocyte globulin, and etanercept (experimental)
  – Infliximab: steroid-refractory GI disease
  – Visceral organ involvement requires urgent start of 2nd-line therapy.
  – For isolated, mild skin GVHD, topical tacrolimus ointment and triamcinolone
- Chronic GVHD
  – Steroids alone or with cyclosporine, sirolimus, tacrolimus, or mycophenolate mofetil
  – Goal: steroids <0.5 mg/kg alternating days; with cyclosporine or tacrolimus
- Steroid-refractory GVHD
  – Mycophenolate mofetil, sirolimus, pentostatin (investigational)
  – Other options many off-label: antithymocyte globulin; rituximab; low-dose methotrexate in liver GVHD; thalidomide; hydroxychloroquine; imatinib; low-dose cyclophosphamide; etanercept; alefacept; alemtuzumab: high infection risk
- Oral rinses with dexamethasone: oral GVHD
- Ursodeoxycholic acid: hepatic GVHD

ADDITIONAL TREATMENT

General Measures

- Prophylaxis for *P. jiroveci* pneumonia and pneumococcal infection
- Antifungal coverage if on multiple immunosuppressive agents
- Hypogammaglobulinemia: IVIG
- Monitor closely for viral reactivation.
- Skin care: Lubricate dry skin with petroleum jelly. Protect skin from injury. Avoid sunburn.
- Correct electrolyte imbalances for muscular aches and cramps.
- Nutrition consults for malnutrition and wasting.
- If chronic GVHD persists past 2–3 months or prednisone is needed at 1 mg/kg/day, alternative therapy should be used.
- Hospitalization may be required for hydration, nutritional support, IV medications, monitoring, treatment of infections, and other supportive care.

ADDITIONAL THERAPIES

- Extracorporeal photophoresis: very effective for chronic skin GVHD; lower response rate if visceral organs involved
- Psoralen plus ultraviolet A is of some benefit in skin GVHD (lichenoid, not sclerotic).
- Mesenchymal stem cells (experimental)
- Artificial tears for sicca syndrome
- Physical therapy/range-of-motion exercises to prevent contractures
- Inhaled corticosteroids and azithromycin (experimental) for bronchiolitis obliterans

ONGOING CARE

FOLLOW-UP RECOMMENDATIONS

Patient Monitoring

- Steroids: osteoporosis, diabetes
- Calcineurin inhibitors: hypertension, renal dysfunction, hypomagnesemia
- Sirolimus: hyperlipidemia, leukopenia, microangiopathic hemolytic anemia
- Mycophenolate mofetil: GI discomfort, diarrhea, leukopenia

PROGNOSIS

Prognosis of GVHD is based on severity.

- Acute GVHD: graded from I to IV based on organ involvement, percent of body surface area involved (skin), volume of diarrhea (gut), and/or elevation of serum bilirubin (liver). The higher the grade, the lower the long-term survival. Grade I survival is the same as for patients without GVHD; grade II, 60%; grade III, 25%; grade IV, 5–15%
- Acute GVHD: 50–60% of patients respond to corticosteroids plus cyclosporine or tacrolimus.
- Poor prognosis for survival: extensive skin involvement, progressive onset, GI involvement, thrombocytopenia, weight loss, and low Karnofsky performance status (40–60% survival)
- 50% of patients still require therapy 5 years after diagnosis of chronic GVHD.

COMPLICATIONS

- Mortality from GVHD after HSCT is usually related to infection.
- Rarely, patients die of hepatic failure or abdominal catastrophe.
- In transfusion-associated GVHD, death is usually from bone marrow aplasia with destruction of the host's marrow by donor lymphocytes.

ADDITIONAL READING

- Carpenter PA, MacMillan ML. Management of acute graft versus host disease in children. *Pediatr Clin North Am*. 2010;57(1):273–295.
- Jacobsohn DA. Optimal management of chronic graft-versus-host disease in children. *Br J Haematol*. 2010;150(3):278–292.
- Schlomchik WD. Graft-versus-host disease. *Nat Rev Immunol*. 2007;7(5):340–357.
- Wolff D, Schleuning M, von Harsdorf S, et al. Consensus conference on clinical practice in chronic GVHD: second-line treatment of chronic graft-versus-host disease. *Biol Blood Marrow Transplant*. 2011;17(1):1–17.

G

CODES

ICD10

- D89.813 Graft-versus-host disease, unspecified
- D89.810 Acute graft-versus-host disease
- D89.811 Chronic graft-versus-host disease

FAQ

- Q: Do all patients with acute GVHD get chronic GVHD?
- A: No. ~30% of patients <10 years of age who receive HLA-identical sibling HSCT will get acute GVHD, whereas only 13% will develop chronic GVHD. Chronic GVHD can develop in a patient who did not have acute GVHD; the prognosis is much more favorable than for the progressive form.
- Q: Do all severe chronic GVHD patients die?
- A: No. Occasionally, the GVHD will "burn out." This is rare, and the process by which it happens is not understood.

GRAVES DISEASE

Adda Grimberg

BASICS

DESCRIPTION

Multisystem autoimmune disorder that presents with the classic triad of hyperthyroidism (goiter), exophthalmos, and dermopathy (rare in children)

EPIDEMIOLOGY

- Female > male (4–5:1)
- 10–15% of all childhood thyroid disorders
- Incidence increases with age, peaking in adolescence and in the 3rd–4th decades.

Genetics

- No simple hereditary pattern (i.e., genetic susceptibility plus environmental factors)
  - Up to 60% of patients have a family history of autoimmune thyroid disease (hyperthyroidism or hypothyroidism).
  - Concordance rates of Graves disease: 17% in monozygotic twins (of note, another 17% had chronic lymphocytic thyroiditis and 10% had other nonthyroid autoimmune conditions), 2% in dizygotic twins, 4% of 1st-degree relatives
- Often associated with HLA-DR3
- Increased incidence in genetic syndromes
  - Down syndrome: presents at a younger age, no female predominance unlike the general population; usually milder course
  - Turner syndrome

PATHOPHYSIOLOGY

- Autoimmune process that includes production of immunoglobulins against antigens in the thyroid, orbital tissue, and dermis
- IgG1 anti-TSH (thyroid-stimulating hormone receptor autoantibody, thyroid-stimulating immunoglobulin [TSI]) activates the TSH receptor, causing constitutive stimulation, leading to increased thyroid follicular cell production and release of thyroid hormone.

DIAGNOSIS

ALERT

Thyroid storm can constitute an endocrinologic medical emergency.

HISTORY

- Growth acceleration that can be associated with precocious puberty (hyperthyroidism can accelerate the bone age)
- Declining school performance, mind racing, difficulty concentrating; may be mistaken for ADHD
- Symptoms of hyperthyroidism and their duration (if child complains of these symptoms, evaluate for possible hyperthyroidism):
  - Restlessness, emotional lability, nervousness
  - Fine tremor
  - Disturbed sleep pattern and insomnia; may result in daytime fatigue
  - Weight loss despite increased appetite
  - Palpitations or chest pain with minimal exertion or at rest; low exercise tolerance
  - Heat intolerance
  - Increased urination and diarrhea
  - Muscle weakness (proximal)
  - Plummer nails (separation of nail from bed)
  - Menstrual irregularities
- Thyroid gland enlargement: Graves disease can present with goiter. Tenderness suggests infectious cause.
- Exophthalmos (bulging of the eyes), increased staring, change in vision or in facial appearance: Exophthalmos due to retro-orbital immune depositions is a hallmark of Graves disease.
- Familial history: increased incidence of Graves disease in families with thyroid disease

PHYSICAL EXAM

- Accelerated growth or height above expected genetic potential due to bone age advancement
- Symmetrically enlarged, smooth, nontender goiter in >95% of cases
- Auscultate the thyroid gland for bruit while patient holds his or her breath (glandular hyperperfusion is associated with hyperthyroidism).
- Resting tachycardia with widened pulse pressure; hyperdynamic precordium: cardiac effects of excessive thyroid hormone
- Slightly elevated temperature: Thyroid hormone controls basal metabolic rate and upregulates catecholamine-induced thermogenesis.
- Lid lag/stare; exophthalmos and proptosis: Severe ophthalmopathy is rare.
- Fine tremor, especially visible in hands and tongue in ~60% of children with Graves disease
- Proximal muscle weakness is common but seldom severe.
- Exaggerated deep tendon reflexes are variable.
- Skin warmth and moisture: heat intolerance and excessive sweating in >30% of children

DIAGNOSTIC TESTS & INTERPRETATION

Lab

- Total or free thyroxine: elevated
- Triiodothyronine assessment by radioimmunoassay: elevated (triiodothyronine radioimmunoassay, as direct measurement of triiodothyronine, and not triiodothyronine resin uptake, which indirectly evaluates thyroid hormone–binding capacity)
- TSH: significantly suppressed or undetectable
- TSI titer: positive in 90% of children
- False-positive test results: Elevated total thyroxine levels can also be caused by increased protein binding and so are not necessarily diagnostic for hyperthyroidism: Increased estrogen states (e.g., pregnancy and oral contraceptive use) lead to augmented hepatic thyroid-binding globulin (TBG) production. Familial dysalbuminemic hyperthyroxinemia: Mutation affecting thyroxine binding affinity leads to increased protein-bound pool.

Imaging

I^{123} scan: not needed to diagnose Graves disease. If done, shows diffuse increased uptake at 6 and 24 hours. If palpation suggests nodule, scan may reveal a hot nodule within a suppressed gland.

DIFFERENTIAL DIAGNOSIS

- Infectious
  - Acute suppurative thyroiditis (i.e., transient thyroxine elevations)
  - Subacute thyroiditis after viral illness (also transient)
- Environmental
  - Thyroid hormone ingestion
  - Ingestion of excess iodine (escape from Wolff-Chaikoff block due to impaired autoregulation)
- Tumors (all rare in childhood)
  - TSH-producing pituitary adenoma
  - Thyroid adenoma/hyperfunctioning autonomous thyroid nodule (most pediatric patients are euthyroid; incidence of nodule hyperfunctioning rises with patient age)
  - Thyroid carcinoma (rarely presents with hyperthyroidism)
- Congenital
  - Neonatal Graves disease (transplacental antibody transfer from mothers with Graves disease or chronic thyroiditis)
- Genetic and developmental
  - Pituitary resistance to thyroid hormones (dominant negative thyroid-receptor gene mutations causing loss of pituitary negative feedback loop and inappropriately elevated levels of TSH; can be isolated, with clinical hyperthyroidism, or associated with peripheral thyroid resistance and clinical euthyroidism or hypothyroidism)
  - TSH-receptor gene mutations (rare; germline activating TSH-receptor mutations cause autosomal dominant nonautoimmune hereditary hyperthyroidism)
  - McCune-Albright syndrome: Activating G-protein mutation can lead to indolent hyperthyroidism in addition to the classic features of this syndrome.
  - Ectopic thyroid tissue
- Other causes of hyperthyroidism: See "Goiter."

TREATMENT

MEDICATION

ALERT

- Antihistamines and cold medications may worsen sympathetic nervous system symptoms.
- Stopping antithyroid drugs because of low thyroxine values when TSH is still suppressed, reflecting continued TSI activity, will likely result in relapse. Antithyroid medication dosage should be decreased, or L-thyroxine should be added.
- FDA issued a black box warning (June 4, 2009) against propylthiouracil (PTU) use in treating Graves disease owing to risk of severe liver injury including life-threatening acute liver failure.

First Line

- Drug therapy is the 1st-line choice in children. Antithyroid medications (thiourea derivatives): 65–95% effective: Medications block thyroid hormone synthesis but not the release of existing hormone.
  - Methimazole
  - PTU: Note black box warning. Limited, short-term use of PTU may be considered for patients requiring antithyroid medication (neither I^{131} ablation nor prompt surgery are options) or after a toxic reaction to methimazole. PTU is preferred during 1st trimester of pregnancy (teratogenic effects of methimazole).
- Propranolol and atenolol block adrenergic symptoms; should be used with antithyroid medications at start of treatment and whenever cardiac symptoms are prominent.

- Duration of treatment:
  - Antithyroid medications can be tapered and potentially discontinued after 2–3 years of therapy, depending on the patient's course.
  - β-Blockers: Continue until thyroxine and triiodothyronine are under control (~6 weeks).
  - If remission not achieved in 1–2 years, ablation with I^{131} or total or subtotal thyroidectomy may be considered.

SURGERY/OTHER PROCEDURES

Radiotherapy: I^{131} ablation therapy

- 90–100% effective; safe and definitive, with predictable outcome
- Results in permanent hypothyroidism requiring lifelong thyroxine replacement
- Adequate dose should be used (>150 μCi/g of thyroid tissue) to prevent residual tissue that would be at risk of developing thyroid cancer.
- Current recommendations advise avoiding I^{131} ablation in children <5 years of age owing to theoretical concerns relating radiation exposure and cancer risks.
- Radioiodine ablation may exacerbate ophthalmopathy, but this effect can be prevented with concomitant glucocorticoid administration.

Total or near-total thyroidectomy

- Effective, rapid, and definitive (vs. 30% recurrence rate for subtotal thyroidectomy)
- Lifelong thyroxine replacement needed
- Surgical complication rates higher for children age 0–6 years and for children treated in lower volume centers

ISSUES FOR REFERRAL

Treatment for severe ophthalmopathy: must refer patient to an ophthalmologist:

- 3 options: high-dose glucocorticoids, orbital radiotherapy, or surgical orbital decompression
- Rehabilitative surgery for eye muscles or eyelids is often needed after the ophthalmopathy has been treated.

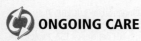

ONGOING CARE

PROGNOSIS

- Good, if adherent with treatment
- Mortality in severe thyrotoxicosis is possible from cardiac arrhythmias or cardiac failure.
- Spontaneous remission occurs in 20–30% of children after 1–2 years but can relapse in 30%. Large thyroid gland size (by ultrasound) and high titers of TSH-receptor antibody (TRAb) predict lower chance of remission.
- Neonatal hyperthyroidism remits by 48 weeks and more commonly by 20 weeks.
- Propranolol or atenolol should result in rapid relief of symptoms of sympathetic hyperactivity.
- 4–6 weeks of medical treatment should result in normalization of levels of thyroxine and triiodothyronine, although TSH levels may remain suppressed owing to persistent underlying activity of the thyroid-stimulating Ig.
- Persistent suppression of TSH is associated with pretreatment presence of thyrotropin-binding inhibitory Ig, severity of thyrotoxicosis, and time to recovery of thyroid hormone levels.
- Duration and type of treatment depend on patient age and remission and relapse pattern.

COMPLICATIONS

- Endocrine disturbances: delayed/early puberty, menstrual irregularity, hypercalcemia
- Ophthalmologic: 3–5% of patients develop severe ophthalmopathy, including eye muscle dysfunction and optic neuropathy, requiring specific treatment by an ophthalmologist. Pediatric ophthalmologic findings (lid lag, soft tissue involvement, and proptosis) are more common but usually less severe than in adults.
- Bone: low bone mineral density for age/sex common at diagnosis due to high bone turnover. Corrects with Graves disease therapy and return to euthyroid status.
- Fetal/neonatal: intrauterine growth retardation (IUGR), nonimmune hydrops fetalis, craniosynostosis, intrauterine death, goiter that complicates labor and can cause life-threatening airway obstruction at delivery, hyperkinesis, failure to thrive, diarrhea, vomiting, cardiac failure and arrhythmias, systemic and pulmonary hypertension, hepatosplenomegaly, jaundice, hyperviscosity syndrome, thrombocytopenia
- Medication side effects: agranulocytosis (in 0.2–0.5% of patients), rash (most common side effect), gastrointestinal upset, headache, transient transaminitis/hepatitis and life-threatening liver failure with PTU, vasculitis with PTU (frequently associated with perinuclear antineutrophil cytoplasmic antibody [p-ANCA] titers)

ADDITIONAL READING

- Bahn RS, Burch HB, Cooper DS, et al; American Thyroid Association; American Association of Clinical Endocrinologists. Hyperthyroidism and other causes of thyrotoxicosis: management guidelines of the American Thyroid Association and American Association of Clinical Endocrinologists. *Endocr Pract*. 2011;17(3):456–520.
- Bauer AJ. Approach to the pediatric patient with Graves' disease: when is definitive therapy warranted? *J Clin Endocrinol Metab*. 2011;96(3):580–588.
- De Luca F, Corrias A, Salerno M, et al. Peculiarities of Graves' disease in children and adolescents with Down's syndrome. *Eur J Endocrinol*. 2010;162(3):591–595.
- Hemminki K, Li X, Sundquist J, et al. The epidemiology of Graves' disease: evidence of a genetic and an environmental contribution. *J Autoimmun*. 2010;34(3):J307–J313.
- Langley RW, Burch HB. Perioperative management of the thyrotoxic patient. *Endocrinol Metab Clin North Am*. 2003;32(2):519–534.
- Marcocci C, Marinò M. Treatment of mild, moderate-to-severe and very severe Graves' orbitopathy. *Best Pract Res Clin Endocrinol Metab*. 2012;26(3):325–337.
- Papendieck P, Chiesa A, Prieto L, et al. Thyroid disorders of neonates born to mothers with Graves' disease. *J Pediatr Endocrinol Metab*. 2009;22(6):547–553.
- Rahhal SN, Eugster EA. Thyroid stimulating immunoglobulin is often negative in children with Graves' disease. *J Pediatr Endocrinol Metab*. 2008;21(11):1085–1088.
- Rivkees SA. Pediatric Graves' disease: controversies in management. *Horm Res Paediatr*. 2010;74(5):305–311.
- Wilhelm SM, McHenry CR. Total thyroidectomy is superior to subtotal thyroidectomy for management of Graves' disease in the United States. *World J Surg*. 2010;34(6):1261–1264.

CODES

ICD10

- E05.00 Thyrotoxicosis w diffuse goiter w/o thyrotoxic crisis
- E05.01 Thyrotoxicosis w diffuse goiter w thyrotoxic crisis or storm
- P72.1 Transitory neonatal hyperthyroidism

FAQ

- Q: Does Graves disease lead to thyroid cancer?
- A: No, although controversy surrounds the role of TSH and the closely related TSH-receptor antibodies of Graves disease in thyroid cancer's incidence and aggressiveness. There is an increased incidence of benign thyroid adenoma from 0.6–1.9% after therapy involving I^{131} ablation.
- Q: Does hyperthyroidism affect long-term growth or final adult height?
- A: No. Hyperthyroidism can cause tall stature and acceleration of skeletal maturity but does not typically affect final adult height.
- Q: Should WBC counts be monitored routinely while patients are on antithyroid medications?
- A: No. Routine monitoring is not cost-effective because agranulocytosis is rare and sudden in onset. WBC counts should be checked when a patient on antithyroid medication develops fever.
- Q: Will the ophthalmopathy correct with antithyroid treatment?
- A: Not necessarily. It may require specific intervention by an ophthalmologist.
- Q: Can mothers breastfeed while they are being treated for Graves disease?
- A: Yes. PTU has a lower milk/serum concentration ratio than methimazole (0:1 and 1:0, respectively). In 1 study, 3 of 11 infants exclusively breastfed by women on 300–750 mg daily PTU had high levels of TSH; of these 3, 1 was just above the normal range and the other 2 completely corrected while the mother was still being medicated.

GROWTH HORMONE DEFICIENCY

Paul Hofman

BASICS

DESCRIPTION

- Growth hormone deficiency (GHD) is a rare cause of growth failure due to a lack of growth hormone action caused by a defect in GH synthesis (insufficient hormone), release, or signaling (decreased responsiveness to normal or high levels of hormone).
- GHD can be associated with other pituitary hormone deficiencies.

EPIDEMIOLOGY

- Prevalence in the United States is approximately 1:4,000.
- Males are more commonly diagnosed than females.
- 2 peak ages of diagnosis:
  - Infancy (<1 year of age) usually because of associated hypoglycemia
  - Childhood at >4 years of age, usually because of poor linear growth

Genetics

- Spontaneous
- Autosomal recessive (AR)
- Autosomal dominant (AD)
- X-linked forms

PATHOPHYSIOLOGY

GH has a number of anabolic actions, but its principal one is increasing linear growth. This occurs predominantly due to direct GH action on the growth plate, although there are also some indirect GH actions on growth via stimulation of secretion of hepatic and growth plate insulin-like growth factor 1 (IGF-1).

ETIOLOGY

- Idiopathic: Although idiopathic GH deficiency is a relatively common diagnosis, it is a diagnosis of exclusion. Sometimes misdiagnosed in normally growing children
- Congenital
  - Congenital malformation of the pituitary can be associated with the following:
    - Holoprosencephaly
    - Septo-optic dysplasia
    - Midline defects: cleft lip, cleft palate, central maxillary incisor
    - Ectopic posterior pituitary, small anterior pituitary, and/or hypoplastic infundibulum
  - Genetic mutations
    - Familial multiple anterior pituitary hormone deficiency (Pit-1, Prop-1)
    - GH gene mutations (Type Ia, Ib, II, III)
  - GH insensitivity
    - Laron dwarfism, AR disorder classically caused by GH receptor mutations, presents with the phenotype of severe GH deficiency (severe short stature, hypoplastic nasal bridge, sparse hair, high-pitched voice, and delayed bone age).
    - Postreceptor and second messenger defects such as IGF-1 gene deletion, IGF-1 receptor mutation, STAT5b mutation
- Acquired idiopathic
  - CNS tumors: craniopharyngioma, germinoma, medulloblastoma, glioma, pinealoma
  - Pituitary or hypothalamic irradiation
  - Trauma: child abuse or closed head injury
  - Surgical resection/damage of the pituitary gland/stalk
  - Birth injury/perinatal insult
  - Infection: viral encephalitis, bacterial or fungal infection, tuberculosis
  - Vascular: pituitary infarction or aneurysm
  - Infiltration affecting pituitary gland or sella turcica: histiocytosis, sarcoidosis
  - Hypophysitis
  - Psychosocial deprivation

DIAGNOSIS

HISTORY

- Family history
  - Parental heights
  - Family history of short stature (women <4 feet 11 inches [150 cm] or men <5 feet 4 inches [163 cm]) indicates genetic shortness.
  - Family history of delayed puberty "late bloomer" (growth after high school, menarche at ≥14 years): Constitutional delay of growth and development tends to occur in family members.
- Birth history
  - Babies born small for gestational age. 10–15% will not show "catch-up growth," but are not typically GHD.
  - Babies with congenital GHD may not be short at birth but will grow poorly over the next few years.
- Medication history: Look for overuse of corticosteroids, either systemic or inhaled. Ask about nonprescription drugs and health food store supplements.
- Past history of chronic illness (e.g., cyanotic cardiac disease, renal tubular acidosis, asthma, celiac disease, chronic anemia, etc.)
- Psychosocial history: Poor growth occurring at the time of a major stressful event may be due to psychosocial deprivation.

PHYSICAL EXAM

- Measure accurate weight and height with wall-mounted stadiometer. Perform a sitting height and arm span if possible.
- Neurologic examination, including visual fields and funduscopic examination for evaluation of brain tumors
- Assess for signs of Turner syndrome:
  - Cubitus valgus, low posterior hair line, abnormal dentition, abnormal ears, and/or shortened 4th metacarpals in girls suggest Turner syndrome.
  - Turner syndrome is the most common pathologic cause of short stature in girls, and short stature may be the only manifestation.
- Midline facial defects such as submucous cleft, cleft lip, and palate are associated with hypopituitarism.
- Tanner stage
  - Micropenis is associated with congenital hypopituitarism.
  - Delayed puberty suggests constitutional delay but may also be indicative of panhypopituitarism.
- Cherubic facies with frontal bossing, thin hair, high-pitched voice, and relative truncal obesity with adiposity are seen in GHD.

DIAGNOSTIC TESTS & INTERPRETATION

Lab

- CBC with differential: anemia, malignancy, cell-based immunodeficiency, and inflammatory processes
- Sedimentation rate and CRP: inflammatory processes such as Crohn disease
- Hepatic and renal function tests: hepatic or renal disease
- Celiac screen
- Urinalysis including pH
- Thyroid function tests (thyroid-stimulating hormone [TSH] and either a T_4 or a free T_4)
- Chromosomes in females (to exclude Turner syndrome)
- IGF-1 and IGF-binding protein-3 (IGFBP-3) production is regulated directly by GH. However, there is a poor correlation with GH deficiency. IGF-1 values are low early in life and in conditions such as hypothyroidism, diabetes, renal failure, and undernutrition.
- GH-provocative testing (performed by an endocrinologist)
  - A random GH level is of little value to diagnose GHD beyond the neonatal period.
  - After neonatal period, GH is mostly secreted only in brief pulses during deep sleep (at night). However, false-positive results are common.
  - NOTE: Using two GH provocation tests and strict GH cutoffs (<5.0 ng/mL), approximately 5% of normally growing children would be diagnosed as GH-deficient, whereas fully 20% of healthy GH-replete children can fail any one provocative test.

Imaging

- Bone age: radiography of left hand and wrist to assess skeletal maturation
- If provocative testing shows GH deficiency, obtain MRI with contrast of the pituitary and hypothalamus to look for central nervous system tumor or anomaly of the hypothalamus/pituitary.

DIFFERENTIAL DIAGNOSIS

- Abnormal body proportions:
  - Skeletal dysplasia (e.g., hypochondroplasia, achondroplasia)
- Normal skeletal proportions with prenatal growth failure (birth weight <10th percentile):
  - Small for gestational age
  - Congenital infection
  - Maternal drug use (tobacco, alcohol etc.)
  - Chromosomal short stature (Turner, Down syndrome, etc.)
  - Syndromes (Noonan, Prader Willi, Russell Silver syndrome, etc.)
- Normal skeletal proportions with postnatal growth failure (birth weight >10th percentile):
  - Constitutional delay of growth and adolescence
  - Familial short stature
  - Malnutrition
  - Renal failure
  - Inflammatory bowel disease
  - Celiac disease
  - Congenital heart disease
  - Hypothyroidism
  - Hypercortisolism
  - Metabolic disorders
  - Rickets
  - Psychosocial deprivation

ALERT

- Children with constitutional growth delay or pubertal delay show poor growth when peers are going through their pubertal growth spurts, and have a delayed bone age, mimicking GH deficiency.
- GH-provocative testing may yield false-positive or false-negative results:
  - 20% of normal children will fail at least 1 GH-provocative test.
  - Obese but otherwise normal children are more likely to fail GH-provocative testing.
  - When GH testing is done in a child at high risk for GHD or if the growth pattern is concerning, the predictive value of GH testing is markedly improved. Assessing growth velocity over a 6–12-month period is very useful.
- Malnutrition can cause low IGF-1.
- Psychosocial deprivation mimics GHD. Such deprived patients may have low growth factors and respond poorly to GH-provocative testing.

TREATMENT

MEDICATION

- Recombinant human growth hormone (rhGH) was approved by FDA for use in 1985 by SQ injection daily.
- Duration of therapy (in children and adolescents)
  - Until growth velocity drops to 2.5 cm/year
  - When puberty is complete
  - GH-deficient adults may benefit from lifelong rhGH therapy due to its effects on body composition, lipids, bone density, and general sense of well-being.
  - Before adult GH is initiated, adult patients should undergo repeat GH-provocative testing in all instances, as GH testing can normalize even with known central structural lesions.

ALERT

- rhGH is associated with idiopathic intracranial hypertension (pseudotumor cerebri). This side effect is usually transient and often reverses without cessation of therapy.
- rhGH is usually not given in cancer patients until 1 year has elapsed without recurrence.
- Carefully evaluate any limp or hip or knee pain in patients on rhGH therapy because these symptoms may be associated with slipped capital femoral epiphysis (SCFE); SCFE necessitates orthopedic consultation.

ONGOING CARE

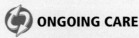

FOLLOW-UP-RECOMMENDATIONS

Every 3 months by an endocrinologist

- When to expect improvement:
  - Immediate effect on hypoglycemia
  - Growth velocity improves within 3–6 months
- Signs to watch for:
  - Pseudotumor cerebri (headache, vision problems)
  - SCFE
  - Scoliosis
  - In adults, edema and carpal tunnel syndrome, but uncommon in children
  - The risk of malignancy is generally NOT increased in children receiving GH therapy, although there may be a small increased risk of a secondary malignancy in those already who have previously survived a malignancy.

PROGNOSIS

Response to GH therapy is excellent in truly GH-deficient patients. Those who are not GH-deficient have a variable but generally positive growth response. The main cause of poor growth in all children receiving GH therapy, however, is noncompliance. In one national study, 66% of patients missed at least one injection per week, and this affected growth.

COMPLICATIONS

- Short stature
- Lack of self-esteem because of short stature
- Delay in pubertal changes (sexual characteristics and growth spurt) due to delayed bone age
- Hypoglycemia (in the newborn period)
- Osteopenia

ADDITIONAL READING

- Clayton PE, Cohen P, Tanaka T, et al. Diagnosis of growth hormone deficiency in childhood. On behalf of the Growth Hormone Research Society. *Horm Res*. 2000;53(Suppl 3):30.
- Cutfield WS, Derraik JGB, Gunn AJ, et al. Non-compliance with growth hormone treatment in children is common and impairs linear growth. *PLoS One*. 2011;6(1): e16223.
- Pitukcheewanont P, Desrosiers P, Steelman J, et al. Issues and trends in pediatric growth hormone therapy—an update from the GH Monitor observational registry. *Pediatr Endocrinol Rev*. 2008;5(Suppl 2):702–707.
- Richmond E, Rogol AD. Current indications for growth hormone therapy for children and adolescents. *Endocr Dev*. 2010;18:92–108.
- Wit JM, Kiess W, Mullis P. Genetic evaluation of short stature. *Best Pract Res Clin Endocrinol Metab*. 2011;25(1):1–17.

CODES

ICD10

- E23.0 Hypopituitarism
- Q89.2 Congenital malformations of other endocrine glands

FAQ

- Q: Does GH improve the body composition in patients with GH deficiency?
- A: Not only is growth impressive in these patients, but there is a normalization of body composition with a loss of fat and increased muscle mass due to the lipolytic and anabolic effects of growth hormone therapy.
- Q: Will GH use cause long-term safety issues?
- A: Although a study from France suggested increased long-term mortality, several similar studies have refuted this observation. Currently, there is no credible evidence suggesting there are long-term safety issues with GH treatment.

GUILLAIN-BARRÉ SYNDROME

Jennifer A. Markowitz

BASICS

DESCRIPTION

Guillain-Barré syndrome (GBS) is an acute monophasic inflammatory disorder of the peripheral nervous system. It causes progressive weakness in the limbs, face, and respiratory muscles. Autonomic and sensory disturbances, including pain, are present. Neurologic deficits peak by 4 weeks or sooner. Various forms include the most common acquired inflammatory demyelinating polyradiculoneuropathy (AIDP), followed by acute motor axonal neuropathy (AMAN), Miller Fisher syndrome, and others.

EPIDEMIOLOGY

Incidence

Overall yearly incidence rate of 0.6–1.9 cases per 100,000. Of 95 reported pediatric GBS patients in one study, 45 were aged 1–5 years, 36 were aged 6–10 years, and 14 were aged 11–15 years. Another found that 67% of pediatric patients had AIDP; 7%, AMAN; and 7%, Miller Fisher syndrome.

RISK FACTORS

Genetics

Particular subtypes of GBS are more common among certain human leukocyte antigen (HLA) types. No data indicate an increase in GBS among 1st-order relatives.

PATHOPHYSIOLOGY

Inflammatory cell–mediated and humoral-mediated immune mechanisms play a role in segmental demyelination on nerve biopsy; lymphocytes and macrophages participate in myelin destruction. Axonal variants of GBS feature axonal degeneration without demyelination. Circulating antiganglioside antibodies (e.g., GM1, GM2, GQ1B) found in particular subtypes suggest a molecular mimicry mechanism stimulated by infection. Some variants (e.g., Bickerstaff encephalitis) involve central and peripheral demyelination.

ETIOLOGY

- Follows viral infection in >50% of cases; cytomegalovirus, Epstein-Barr virus, varicella-zoster virus, acute HIV infection, H1N1, others
- Also associated with bacterial infection (especially *Campylobacter jejuni*), surgery, and vaccination
- Tetanus toxoid is the only vaccination in common use with a clear link to GBS. Often, no precipitating event can be identified.

COMMONLY ASSOCIATED CONDITIONS

- GBS is seen in a higher than expected rate in patients with sarcoidosis, systemic lupus erythematosus, lymphoma, HIV infection, Lyme disease, and solid tumors.
- Muscle atrophy, joint contractures, pressure ulcers, chronic pain, hypertension, voiding difficulty

DIAGNOSIS

HISTORY

- GBS has a variety of clinical presentations so that index of suspicion is critical. Typical features are progressive motor weakness and areflexia, often following distal sensory changes. Common presentations include decreased ambulation (or crawling in toddlers), unsteady gait (which may be due to sensory ataxia), facial weakness, leg or back pain, or sensory changes in the extremities.
- After respiratory status has been stabilized, address autonomic dysfunction and pain. Close monitoring is required for dysautonomic symptoms: arrhythmias, BP lability/orthostasis, ileus, urinary retention.
- Most patients first note leg weakness or gait instability that progresses over days to weeks. 60% are unable to walk at peak of symptoms.
- Paresthesias and pain typically occur in a stocking/glove distribution frequently early in the course.
- 2/3 of patients will report symptoms of an infection 2–3 weeks earlier. Consider direct infection (e.g., polio, West Nile virus) if fever is present at symptom onset.
- Weakness may lead to respiratory paralysis in up to 20% of children with GBS.

PHYSICAL EXAM

- Weakness and sensory changes, classically symmetric with distal greater than proximal involvement
- A proximal predominance of symptoms does not preclude the diagnosis (radicular involvement).
  - Deep tendon reflexes are usually lost within 1 week, although retention of reflexes has been reported.
- Respiratory difficulty: impaired upper airway or restrictive/neurogenic, with decreased vital capacity and maximum inspiratory (PiMax) and expiratory (PeMax) pressures
  - Respiratory failure leads to intubation in up to 20% of patients. Bulbar weakness and poor airway protection can also necessitate intubation. Impending respiratory failure can often be unpredictable, and blood gas determination is not a useful indicator of neuromuscular respiratory failure until intubation is imminent. If close monitoring of vital capacity, inspiratory, or expiratory pressures suggests >30% decline in 24 hours, monitor patient in ICU.
- Bilateral facial weakness occurs in ≤50% of cases.
- Ophthalmoplegia, ataxia, and areflexia in Miller Fisher variant
- Neonates and infants may (rarely) present as floppy infants.

DIAGNOSTIC TESTS & INTERPRETATION

Lab

- In atypical cases, consider heavy metal screen, HIV titer, Lyme titer, porphyria screen, acetylcholine receptor antibodies (myasthenia), tick paralysis, and conversion disorder.
  - See "Differential Diagnosis."
- IgA level should be considered if the child has a history of frequent pulmonary infections: IgA deficiency could contraindicate intravenous immunoglobulin (IVIG) therapy (risk of anaphylaxis depending on how IVIG is prepared).

Imaging

MRI of the spine (with gadolinium enhancement). Consider MRI for spinal cord compression syndrome in a child presenting with paraparesis. Spinal nerve root enhancement on MRI can support the diagnosis of GBS.

Diagnostic Procedures/Other

- Electrodiagnosis
  - Nerve conduction studies (NCS) and electromyography (EMG) can confirm diagnosis of GBS and are helpful when clinical or CSF findings are ambiguous. NCS and EMG are abnormal in 50% of patients in the first 2 weeks and in 85% of patients afterward.
  - Initially, needle EMG may be normal; consider serial studies if initially nondiagnostic, high clinical suspicion.
- Lumbar puncture: elevated levels of CSF protein after the 1st week of symptoms; classically an albuminocytologic dissociation with normal cell count. Minimal pleocytosis (<20 leukocytes/mm^3), largely mononuclear leukocytes, may occur.

DIFFERENTIAL DIAGNOSIS

- Myasthenia gravis
- Botulism
- Intoxication (e.g., heavy metals, organophosphates)
- Myopathy/myositis
- Poliomyelitis and other acute (i.e., viral) motor neuron diseases
- Acute cerebellar ataxia (sometimes associated with neuroblastoma)
- Transverse myelitis
- Chronic inflammatory demyelinating polyneuropathy (CIDP)
- Vasculitic neuropathy
- Diphtheritic neuropathy (rare)
- Porphyric neuropathy
- Tick paralysis
- Locked-in state
- Conversion, psychogenic weakness, astasia/abasia

ALERT
- Initially, gait instability may mistakenly be interpreted as having a psychogenic source.
- Reflexes may be preserved in early stages of illness.
- Proximal symptoms may predominate early on.
- Check for reflexes in patients with bilateral Bell palsy. Close observation for further development of symptoms or signs of GBS.

TREATMENT

ALERT
- Respiratory failure may occur quickly and is of a neuromuscular, rather than obstructive, nature (i.e., work of breathing may not be increased).
- Treat hypertension cautiously; catastrophic refractory hypotension may ensue.

A combination of supportive therapy and immunotherapy is the mainstay of treatment for patients with GBS.
- Regular monitoring of vital capacity; strongly consider intubation if vital capacity reaches <50% of normal.
- IVIG and plasmapheresis have equivalent efficacy as 1st-line immunotherapy. Combination of the 2 therapies has not proven more effective than monotherapy alone. Complications and discontinuation of therapy are less common with IVIG.
- Pediatric studies have shown IVIG and plasmapheresis to be well tolerated and efficacious.
- IVIG at 0.4 g/kg (body weight) for 5 consecutive days and initiated in ambulatory patients within 2–4 weeks of symptom onset. Alternatively, dosages of 1 g/kg for 2 consecutive days or 2 g/kg as a single dose may be used.
- Plasmapheresis may be performed peripherally in children big enough for large-bore IVs but requires placement of a central catheter in others. Total plasma exchange volume of 200–250 mL/kg divided in 3–5 treatments over 7–14 days. Therapy initiation is recommended within 4 weeks of symptom onset for patients who cannot walk and 2 weeks for patients who can.
- Corticosteroids have not been shown to be helpful and are not recommended.
- Pain from nerve root inflammation is common in GBS and should be treated aggressively. Agents such as gabapentin can be useful.

ADDITIONAL THERAPIES
Physical therapy: Avoid contractures with lower extremity splinting and early passive range of motion. Aggressive physical and occupational therapy are essential for good outcomes.

INPATIENT CONSIDERATIONS
Initial stabilization
Key elements center around respiratory management and deciding on hospitalization to monitor/treat progressive symptoms including heart block, hypotension, urinary retention, and neuropathic pain.

Admission Criteria
Admit patients with symptoms progressing over hours to days, with any respiratory or bulbar complaints, or who are nonambulatory.

Nursing
Particular attention to preventing skin breakdown, contractures, venous thrombosis, and secondary compressive neuropathies

Discharge Criteria
- Completion of immunotherapy
- Stabilization of symptoms
- Severity of bulbar, respiratory, and autonomic involvement dictates duration of hospital stay. Consider intensive inpatient rehabilitation.

ONGOING CARE

FOLLOW-UP RECOMMENDATIONS
- Improvement typically begins 2–3 weeks after onset of symptoms up to 2 months in some patients.
- Improvement continues for up to 2 years.

PATIENT EDUCATION
Parent Internet information: Guillain–Barré Syndrome GBS/CIDP Foundation International: http://www.gbs-cidp.org/

PROGNOSIS
- Most children recover, although 25% may have some residual symptoms; ultimate functional recovery depends on the degree of axonal injury. Follow-up electrodiagnostic studies can be helpful in some cases.
- Early prognosticators include the severity of weakness at the disease nadir and fulminant onset.
- Overall prognosis in children is better than in adults.

COMPLICATIONS
- Complications include respiratory failure, BP dysregulation (hypotension and/or hypertension), urinary retention, aspiration, pain syndromes, deep venous thrombosis, and infection.
- Death from early respiratory failure, autonomic instability, or other complications occurs in 3–6%.

ADDITIONAL READING

- Devos D, Magot A, Perrier-Boeswillwald J, et al. Guillain-Barré syndrome during childhood: particular clinical and electrophysiological features. *Muscle Nerve*. 2013;48(2):247–251.
- Hughes RA, Raphaël JC, Swan AV, et al. Intravenous immunoglobulin for Guillain-Barré syndrome. *Cochrane Database Syst Rev*. 2006;(1):CD002063.
- Hughes RA, Swan AV, van Koningsveld R, et al. Corticosteroids for Guillain-Barré syndrome. *Cochrane Database Syst Rev*. 2006;(2):CD001446.
- Hughes RA, Wijdicks EF, Barohn R, et al. Practice parameter: immunotherapy for Guillain–Barré syndrome: report of the Quality Standards Subcommittee of the American Academy of Neurology. *Neurology*. 2003;61(6):736–740.
- Korinthenberg R. Acute polyradiculoneuritis: Guillain-Barré syndrome. *Handb Clin Neurol*. 2013;112:1157–1162.
- Lawn ND, Fletcher DD, Henderson RD. Anticipating mechanical ventilation in Guillain-Barré syndrome. *Arch Neurol*. 2001;58(6):893–898.
- Lin JJ, Hsia SH, Wang HS, et al. Clinical variants of Guillain-Barré syndrome in children. *Pediatr Neurol*. 2012;47(2):91–96.
- Tekgul H, Serdaroglu G, Tutuncuoglu S. Outcome of axonal and demyelinating forms of Guillain-Barré syndrome in children. *Pediatr Neurol*. 2003;28(4):295–299.

CODES

ICD10
G61.0 Guillain-Barre syndrome

FAQ
- Q: Is GBS contagious?
- A: No.
- Q: Will I get GBS again?
- A: Acute relapses occur in 1–5% of patients in large series. Treatment-related fluctuations (worsening after completion of immunotherapy) can also occur in CIDP and can be indistinguishable from GBS initially.
- Q: Do all cases require hospitalization and immunomodulatory treatment?
- A: Some youngsters with mild, nondisabling symptoms may be observed as outpatients (≤10%).

GYNECOMASTIA

Chirag R. Kapadia • Zoe M. Gonzalez-Garcia

BASICS

DESCRIPTION
Visible or palpable proliferation of unilateral or bilateral breast glandular tissue in a male

EPIDEMIOLOGY
- 2 age distribution peaks: neonatal, pubertal
- Neonatal gynecomastia occurs in 60–90% of all newborns.
- Peak incidence for pubertal gynecomastia in males is 14 years of age (range: 10–16 years). Onset usually at 5–10-mL testicular size and pubic hair Tanner III or IV.
- ~40% of pubertal boys develop transient gynecomastia (measuring ≥0.5 cm). This percentage varies greatly in studies, perhaps due to examination technique.

RISK FACTORS
Any state that leads to an increase in the net effect of estrogen relative to androgens on breast glandular tissue, such as the following:
- Increased endogenous estrogen
- Increased exogenous estrogen or estrogen-like compounds in commercial products
- Increased sensitivity of breast tissue to estrogen action
- Decreased androgen concentrations
- Androgen receptor defects
- Pharmacologic or commercial product interference with androgen receptors
- Increased aromatase action. Aromatase converts androgens to estrogens. This can be intrinsic as in aromatase excess syndrome or as a result of tumors or hyperthyroidism.
- Elevated leptin concentrations, which may increase aromatase enzyme activity, stimulate growth of mammary cells or increase breast receptor sensitivity to estrogens.
- High serum gonadotropin concentrations altering sex steroid production ratios
- Increased sex hormone–binding globulin, which reduces free testosterone levels
- Hyperthyroidism, which increases aromatization of androgens to estrogens
- Hyperprolactinemia interfering with gonadotropin production, thus altering sex steroid production
- Obesity: may increase leptin levels and may increase aromatization. Obesity correlates with true gynecomastia in some studies only. Other studies find obesity correlates with pseudogynecomastia but not true ductal breast tissue development.

ETIOLOGY
- Physiologic
  - Neonatal: Transient palpable breast tissue develops in newborns, owing to elevated estrogen levels in the fetoplacental unit. Resolves as estrogen levels decline
  - Pubertal: benign transient gynecomastia occurring in otherwise healthy males. In this setting, breast tissue measuring <5 cm in diameter has high likelihood of spontaneous regression.
  - Involutional: Breast enlargement occurs in elderly men.
  - Physiologic gynecomastia usually bilateral
- Pathologic
  - Drug-induced
    - Hormones: estrogen, androgens, gonadotropins, growth hormone, antiandrogens, commercial products containing estrogenic or antiandrogenic compounds
    - Anti-infective agents: Can cause gynecomastia through antiandrogenic properties. Ethionamide, isoniazid, ketoconazole, metronidazole, antiretrovirals
    - Antiulcer drugs: usually cause gynecomastia through antiandrogenic properties. Cimetidine, ranitidine, omeprazole
    - Chemotherapeutic agents: usually cause gynecomastia by causing hypogonadism. Alkylating agents, methotrexate, vinca alkaloids
    - Cardiovascular agents: spironolactone—androgen receptor blocker; unknown mechanism of action: amiodarone, captopril, digitoxin, diltiazem, enalapril, methyldopa, nifedipine, reserpine, verapamil
    - Psychotropic agents: may act by increasing prolactin levels or decreasing androgen levels: diazepam, risperidone, haloperidol, phenothiazines, antidepressants
    - Drugs of abuse: alcohol, heroin, amphetamines, marijuana, methadone
    - Miscellaneous: metoclopramide, phenytoin, penicillamine, theophylline, gabapentin, clonidine, pregabalin
- Hypogonadism
- Infectious: breast abscess
- Tumors: testicular (including Sertoli cell and germ cell), adrenal, ectopic tumors that produce human chorionic gonadotropin
- Chronic disease: renal failure, liver cirrhosis, malnutrition with refeeding, HIV infection
- Congenital disorders causing gonadal hypofunction, androgen receptor issues, or increased aromatization: Klinefelter syndrome, vanishing testes syndrome, androgen resistance syndromes, true hermaphroditism, excessive peripheral tissue aromatase
- Acquired testicular failure (viral, torsion, other)
- Late-onset congenital adrenal hyperplasia–elevated androgens converted to estrogen
- Spinal cord injury leading to testicular failure over the long term
- Neoplasms: breast carcinoma, neurofibroma, lymphangioma, lipoma, neuroblastoma metastasis
- Trauma: hematoma
- Miscellaneous masses: dermoid cyst

DIAGNOSIS

ALERT
- Do not mistake pseudogynecomastia (i.e., fatty enlargement of the breasts) for true gynecomastia.
- Do not overlook drug-related causes. Drug-related gynecomastia is usually reversible if diagnosed during year of onset.

HISTORY
- Family history: 1/2 of adolescents with gynecomastia have positive family history.
- Time of onset relative to puberty: Onset usually at testicular size 5–10 mL and Tanner stage III or IV pubic hair.
- Prepubertal more concerning than pubertal.
- Unilateral more concerning than bilateral.
- Rate of progression
  - Rapidly enlarging, painful gynecomastia with acute onset is of more concern than long-standing enlargement.
- Drug exposures, including alcohol, marijuana, and heroin, along with exposure to exogenous estrogen and commercial products containing estrogens, lavender, tea tree oil, phthalates, ginseng, and others
- Symptoms suggestive of hyperthyroidism
- Symptoms suggestive of liver disease, such as cirrhosis
- Symptoms suggestive of renal failure
- Symptoms suggestive of neoplastic disease
- Symptoms suggestive of hypogonadism, such as decreased libido, erectile dysfunction, or infertility, may indicate an abnormal estrogen-to-androgen ratio.

PHYSICAL EXAM
- Assess for malnourishment: may result in hepatic dysfunction causing higher estrogen-to-androgen ratio
- Perform a complete breast exam:
  - With patient supine, grasp breast between thumb and forefinger and move digits toward the nipple: Look for a firm, rubbery, mobile, discoid mound of glandular tissue arising concentrically below the nipple and areola. Measure diameter of the disc. Asymmetry and tenderness are common.
  - Check for galactorrhea, which is a sign of drug ingestion or hyperprolactinemia.
  - Masses not concentric around the areola, that are hard, firm, fixed, that are unilateral, or have any skin dimpling, nipple retraction, nipple bleeding, or discharge, are concerning for carcinoma. This is very rare in male adolescents.
  - Check for pseudogynecomastia: (fatty enlargement): If present, no glandular disc will be palpable under areola.
  - If disc diameter is >5 cm, regression is very unlikely.

- Thyroid exam: Goiter may indicate hypothyroidism.
- Testicular exam: Consider testicular tumors with masses or significant asymmetry of testes. Consider gonadal failure for small, firm testes. Gynecomastia more likely to be pathologic if testes <5 mL (in this case, not defined as pubertal gynecomastia).

DIAGNOSTIC TESTS & INTERPRETATION

Lab

- Benign presentations do not need extensive workup. Neonatal gynecomastia can be monitored without workup for regression by 1 year of age. Bilateral pubertal gynecomastia arising after pubertal onset, <5 cm in diameter can be monitored as well for further growth.
- In other cases, direct workup to suspected causes based on history and exam:
  - LH for pituitary function
  - FSH to rule out testicular failure
  - Prolactin for hyperprolactinemia
  - TSH for hyperthyroidism
  - Testosterone for gonadal function
  - Estrogen for aromatization excess, estrogen excess, or estrogen-secreting tumors (Although in some cases, local aromatase activity can cause gynecomastia without high circulating estrogen.)
  - DHEA-S for adrenal tumors
  - hCG for germ cell tumors (Note that this specific lab is to be ordered, not a qualitative pregnancy test.)
  - Karyotype to rule out Klinefelter syndrome (only indicated in suspicious cases via history or exam, or those with proven testicular failure via high FSH)
  - Most of these labs are best done in the morning if possible.

Imaging

- None indicated for benign presentations.
- Testicular ultrasound in cases with concerns of testicular tumor via asymmetric exam, elevated estradiol or hCG, or pubertal level testosterone with suppressed LH
- Abdominal/adrenal CT or MRI
  - To rule out adrenal neoplasm, if estradiol elevated, DHEA-S elevated, or in cases concerning for testicular tumor that turn out to have negative testicular ultrasound
  - Consider chest CT in such cases as well.
- Brain MRI or CT, with and without contrast: if pituitary tumor is suspected
- Bone age can be an adjunct evaluation in cases with concerns for estrogen excess; estrogen results in bone age advance.

DIFFERENTIAL DIAGNOSIS

See "Etiology."

TREATMENT

MEDICATION

- Generally, drug therapy should proceed under the guidance of an endocrinologist.
- Tamoxifen and aromatase inhibitors in off-label use have shown some benefit in benign pubertal gynecomastia if started within 1 year of onset.
- If hypogonadal, replace testosterone.
- If gynecomastia has been present for >1 year, pharmacologic therapy is of little benefit because of an increase in fibrosis.

ADDITIONAL TREATMENT

Additional Therapies

- Reassurance for patients with pubertal gynecomastia measuring <5 cm
- Discontinue drugs or commercial products known or suspected to induce gynecomastia, and follow up in 1–2 months.
- Reexamine at 3–6-month intervals for size change.
- For gynecomastia >5 cm, consider surgical consultation once history, exam, and lab evaluation for pathology (along with imaging in indicated cases) have been conducted.

ISSUES FOR REFERRAL

Consider surgical consultation in patients with >5-cm diameter glandular tissue near the end of puberty. Surgery prior to completion of puberty may increase risk of recurrence.

SURGERY/OTHER PROCEDURES

- Surgery is therapy of choice for macrogynecomastia or persistent gynecomastia refractory to medical therapy, although obtaining insurance coverage may be difficult.
- Obesity should not preclude surgical intervention.
- Surgical options include periareolar incision with adjunctive liposuction or glandular tissue removal through 2 incisions in the anterior axillary regions.
- Ultrasound-assisted liposuction has emerged as a new alternative surgical option.

ONGOING CARE

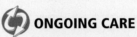

FOLLOW-UP RECOMMENDATIONS

- Reexamine every 3–6 months for size and characteristics.
- Watch for signs of psychological stress.
  - Significant issue in some male adolescents and should not be dismissed
  - Reassure that eventually, they shall be referred for treatment.
  - In those with significant psychological stress, referral before completion of puberty may result in repeat surgery later, but this can be considered after discussion with patient and family.

PROGNOSIS

- In benign cases, prognosis is good.
- Neonatal gynecomastia usually resolves within the 1st year of life.
- Pubertal gynecomastia <5 cm: 50–75% disappear spontaneously within 2 years, 90% within 3 years. If size >5 cm, regression unlikely
- Medical therapy effective only if treatment initiated within a year of onset.

COMPLICATIONS

- In benign cases
  - Pain (may interfere with sports)
  - Psychological stress
  - Embarrassment
  - Skin erosion of the nipple owing to rubbing against clothing

ADDITIONAL READING

- Braunstein GD. Clinical practice. Gynecomastia. *N Eng J Med*. 2007;357(12):1229–1237.
- Goldman RD. Drug-induced gynecomastia in children and adolescents. *Can Fam Physician*. 2010;56(4);344–345.
- Ma NS, Geffner ME. Gynecomastia in prepubertal and pubertal men. *Curr Opin Pediatr*. 2008;20(4): 465–470.
- Mauras N, Bishop K, Merinbaum D, et al. Pharmacokinetics and pharmacodynamics of anastrazole in pubertal boys with recent onset gynecomastia. *J Clin Endocrinol Metab*. 2009;94(8):2975–2978.
- Nordt CA, DiVasta AD. Gynecomastia in adolescents. *Curr Opin Pediatr*. 2008;20(4):375–382.
- Rosen H, Webb ML, DiVasta AD, et al. Adolescent gynecomastia: not only an obesity issue. *Ann Plast Surg*. 2010;64(5):688–690.

CODES

ICD10

- N62 Hypertrophy of breast
- P83.4 Breast engorgement of newborn

FAQ

- Q: When should a neonate with gynecomastia be referred to a specialist?
- A: For male neonates, if galactorrhea persists at 3 months of age, or the gynecomastia not resolved by 1 year of age.
- Q: When should a nonneonatal, but prepubertal, male with gynecomastia be referred to a specialist?
- A: Gynecomastia in a prepubertal boy is rare and concerning. Urgent referral should be made to a pediatric endocrinologist.
- Q: When should a pubertal adolescent with gynecomastia be referred to a specialist?
- A: If gynecomastia is unilateral; if size is >5 cm; if size is <5 cm but with visible enlargement ongoing within 1 year of onset of problem; if started before onset of puberty; if nipple bleeding, discharge or retraction. Also, if testes are <5 mL or testicular mass present; if abnormal hormonal workup or imaging study.
- Q: How can gynecomastia be distinguished from breast cancer?
- A: Breast cancer usually presents as a unilateral, eccentric hard or firm mass fixed to underlying tissues. Location usually outside the nipple–areolar complex. Associated findings can include dimpling of the skin, retraction of the nipple, nipple discharge, and/or axillary lymphadenopathy. Breast cancer in the pediatric population is extremely rare: <0.1% of all breast cancers occur in patients <20 years of age. Benign tumors, such as fibroadenomas, much more common than malignant tumors. If differentiation between gynecomastia and breast carcinoma cannot be made by physical exam alone, patient should undergo diagnostic mammography.
- Q: Has the incidence of gynecomastia increased?
- A: As the prevalence of childhood and adolescent obesity has increased, the presence of *pseudo* gynecomastia has also increased. Pseudogynecomastia is best treated with diet and exercise.

HAND, FOOT, AND MOUTH DISEASE

Ross Newman • Jason Newland

BASICS

DESCRIPTION

Hand, foot, and mouth disease is a viral illness with the characteristic clinical features of the following:

- Vesiculoulcerative stomatitis
- Papular or vesicular exanthem on the hands and/or the feet
- Mild constitutional symptoms such as fever and malaise

GENERAL PREVENTION

- Frequent hand washing, especially after changing diapers, and good personal hygiene are the most useful means to prevent spread of enteroviral illnesses.
- Contact precautions should be maintained with all hospitalized patients.
- The prodromal and enanthem periods appear to be the most contagious; however, some may shed virus in the stool 3 months after infection.

EPIDEMIOLOGY

- In temperate climates, hand, foot, and mouth disease is most common in the summer and fall (a pattern common to many of the enterovirus infections).
- In tropical climates, disease is present year-round.
- Transmitted by oral–fecal route. Respiratory secretions may also transmit the virus.
- Incubation period is 3–6 days.
- Highly contagious, afflicting up to 50% of those exposed
- Close household contacts are particularly susceptible.
- Most common in children younger than 5 years but may affect adults
- May occur as an isolated case or in an epidemic distribution

PATHOPHYSIOLOGY

- Enteroviruses are acquired primarily from oral–fecal contamination.
- Lymphatic invasion leads to viremia and spread to secondary sites.
- Viremia ceases with antibody production.
- Direct inoculation of the extremities from oral lesions has been hypothesized with regard to hand, foot, and mouth disease.

ETIOLOGY

Coxsackie A16 virus is the most common causative agent. Other serotypes include the following:

- Coxsackieviruses A5, A7, A9, A10, A16, B1, and B3
- Enterovirus 71
- Echoviruses
- Other enteroviruses

DIAGNOSIS

HISTORY

- History of ill contacts
  - Family members or close contacts are often similarly affected.
  - Incubation period 3–6 days
- Any fever, pain, or other symptoms
  - A mild prodrome occasionally precedes the characteristic enanthem and exanthem by 1 or 2 days
  - Low-grade fever (usually near 101°F [38.3°C])
  - Malaise, sore mouth, anorexia, coryza, diarrhea, abdominal pain
- Lesions in mouth
  - Oral lesions typically occur shortly before the hand and foot manifestations.
- Hydration status
  - Determine quality and amount of oral intake, quality and amount of urine output, recent weight loss, duration of symptoms.

PHYSICAL EXAM

- Enanthem
  - Oral lesions begin as small, red papules.
  - Papules quickly evolve to small vesicles on an erythematous base.
  - Lesions progress to ulcerations.
  - Tongue, buccal mucosa, palate, gingiva, uvula, and/or tonsillar pillars may be involved.
  - Typically 2–10 lesions that may persist up to 1 week
- Exanthem
  - Less consistently present than oral lesions occurring in 1/4–2/3 of patients
  - Maculopapular eruptions progress to vesicles.
  - Rarely tender or pruritic
  - Most frequent on the dorsal aspects of fingers and toes
  - May also occur on the palms, soles, arms, legs, buttocks, and face
- Adenopathy
  - Enlarged anterior cervical or submandibular nodes are present in 1/4 of cases.
- Other
  - Attention should be given to the patient's vital signs; general appearance; and respiratory, cardiac, and neurologic functioning to help identify the rare patient with a threatening complication of hand, foot, and mouth disease.

DIAGNOSTIC TESTS & INTERPRETATION

Lab

- Hand, foot, and mouth disease has unique clinical features and a relatively benign course. Laboratory confirmation of the diagnosis is seldom needed or indicated.
- Culture
  - Causative viruses may be cultured from many sites:
    - Oral ulcers
    - Cutaneous vesicles
    - Nasopharyngeal swabs
    - Stool (Isolation of an enterovirus from the stool does not confirm it to be the cause of disease because the virus can be shed for many weeks after infection.)
    - Cerebrospinal fluid (CSF) (in cases where meningoencephalitis is suspected). Reverse transcription-polymerase chain reaction (RT-PCR) can be used and is more sensitive than culture in the CSF.

DIFFERENTIAL DIAGNOSIS

Few infectious diseases have such characteristic clinical findings. Oral ulcerations followed by lesions on the distal extremities are virtually pathognomonic. The most difficult diagnostic dilemmas may occur early in the disease course when isolated oral lesions predominate:

- Herpangina
  - Also caused by coxsackie A viruses
  - Associated with higher fever
  - Usually limited to the posterior oropharynx
- Herpetic gingivostomatitis
  - Most common cause of stomatitis in children
  - Associated with higher fever
  - More frequently associated with lymphadenopathy
  - Gingival involvement severe
  - Aphthous ulcers
  - Can occur without fever or upper respiratory symptoms
  - Does not occur in outbreaks
  - No seasonal predilection
- Stevens-Johnson syndrome
  - Ulcerations frequently coalesce.
  - Usually affects other mucous membranes
  - Often appears with separate cutaneous manifestations
- The Boston exanthem
  - Caused by echovirus 16
  - Mild febrile illness with a macular rash on the palms and soles occurring at time of or after defervescence
  - Oral lesions absent

TREATMENT

SUPPORTIVE CARE

No specific therapy is indicated or usually necessary. Most cases are mild and self-limiting and only require parental reassurance.

SPECIAL THERAPY

- Symptomatic relief from particularly painful oral ulcers may be accomplished by application of a topical antihistamine or anesthetic directly to the sores.
- Dehydration should be treated when present. IV fluids may be required in the more severe cases, especially in infants and young children.
- Good supportive care is generally sufficient to treat most complications.

MEDICATION

Acetaminophen may relieve malaise and minor discomfort associated with the oral ulcers. It also may be used as an antipyretic in those children with fever.

INPATIENT CONSIDERATIONS

Admission Criteria

Dehydration and inability to maintain adequate oral hydration

Discharge Criteria

Rehydration and good oral intake

ONGOING CARE

FOLLOW-UP RECOMMENDATIONS

Small children must be followed closely for signs of dehydration.

DIET

Dietary adjustments often improve oral intake from painful oral lesions and prevent or relieve dehydration:

- Avoid spicy or acidic foods.
- Provide cool or iced liquids in small quantities frequently.

PROGNOSIS

- In nearly all instances, hand, foot, and mouth disease will resolve quickly, usually within 1 week after diagnosis, requiring only supportive care.
- Careful history and examination should distinguish those patients with the rare aforementioned complications.
- Rare cases may recur at intervals for up to 1 year.

COMPLICATIONS

- Hand, foot, and mouth disease is usually self-limited and uncomplicated, resolving within 7–10 days.
- Dehydration is the most frequent morbid complication:
  - Oral ulcerations are painful and interfere with feeding.
  - Infants and children are at highest risk.
- Rare complications include the following:
  - Neurologic complications such as aseptic meningitis, encephalitis, and acute flaccid paralysis
  - Pneumonia
  - Myocarditis
  - A possible association with 1st-trimester spontaneous abortions in previously infected women

ADDITIONAL READING

- American Academy of Pediatrics. Herpes simplex. In: Pickering LK, Baker CJ, Kimberlin DW, et al, eds. *Red Book: 2012 Report of the Committee on Infectious Diseases*. 29th ed. Elk Grove Village, IL: American Academy of Pediatrics; 2012.
- Robinson CR, Doane FW, Rhodes AJ. Report of an outbreak of febrile illness with pharyngeal lesions and exanthem: Toronto, summer 1957; isolation of group A coxsackie virus. *Can Med Assoc J*. 1958;79(8):615–621.
- Ruan F, Yang T, Ma H, et al. Risk factors for hand, foot, and mouth disease and herpangina and the preventive effect of hand-washing. *Pediatrics*. 2011;127(4):e898–e904.
- Scott LA, Stone MS. Viral exanthems. *Dermatol Online J*. 2003;9(3):4.
- Slavin KA, Frieden IJ. Picture of the month: hand-foot-and-mouth disease. *Arch Pediatr Adolesc Med*. 1998;152(5):505–506.

CODES

ICD10

- B08.4 Enteroviral vesicular stomatitis with exanthem
- B34.1 Enterovirus infection, unspecified

FAQ

- Q: What is in the "magic mouthwash" often used to relieve the pain of stomatitis?
- A: Many health care providers will prescribe a magic mouthwash for symptomatic relief of oral ulcers, pharyngitis, and teething pain. The most common such treatment consists of an aluminum hydroxide/magnesium hydroxide gel suspension and diphenhydramine elixir (12.5 mg/5 mL) in a 1:1 formulation. It can be applied directly to the sores with a cotton swab or a small syringe before meals. Note: Some people will have a reaction to topical diphenhydramine.
- Q: Should lidocaine be used topically or in suspension with magic mouthwash for symptomatic relief of oral ulcers?
- A: The routine use of lidocaine in this situation is not recommended. Lidocaine is an effective topical anesthetic and comes in a 2% viscous suspension. In practice, the pain relief is short lived, which encourages frequent administration. Lidocaine is absorbed from the mucous membranes (bypassing 1st-pass liver metabolism) and has been frequently reported to cause poisoning of the cardiovascular and central nervous systems. Both pediatric and adult fatalities have occurred. Topical viscous lidocaine should be reserved for use by physicians knowledgeable about its proper dosage and potential side effects and by educated, compliant parents or caregivers.
- Q: When may children with hand, foot, and mouth disease return to school?
- A: Good hygiene will greatly reduce viral transmission. Isolation from school or day care contacts should occur while fever remains and/or while the enanthem persists. As mentioned, some patients may shed the virus in their stool for weeks after symptoms have resolved (again stressing the need for good personal hygiene).

HEAD BANGING

Ana Catarina Garnecho • Yvette E. Yatchmink

BASICS

DESCRIPTION

- Head banging (HB) is defined as the hitting of head on solid object such as a wall, side of crib, mattress, or floor.
- Tend to hit the front or side of the head
- Usually last for 15 minutes but can go on for >1 hour
- Regular rhythm of 60–80 bpm
- Can be seen along with body rocking or head rolling

EPIDEMIOLOGY

- Average age of onset is 9 months; usually extinguished by 3 years of age. Older patients with head banging are more likely to have a developmental delay or other medical problems
- More common in boys than girls (3:1)
- Occurs in 3–15% of typically developing children
- Estimated that 2–3% of kids with intellectual disability have stereotypic movement disorder (SMD) (HB) and 5% of kids with Tourette syndrome have SMD (HB)

ETIOLOGY

- Can be comforting and be a part of other self-soothing activities such as body rocking or head rolling
- Can be seen during a temper tantrum secondary to frustration or anger
- Can be seen with typically developing children as an expression of happiness or as a method of self-stimulation (sometimes secondary to sensory deprivation)
- Need to rule out medical causes specifically if head banging occurs suddenly and is associated with other symptoms
- Can be part of a sleep rhythmic disorder called *Jactatio capitis nocturna* (partial arousal during light, non-REM sleep); head banging occurs when drowsy or falling asleep.
- Can be described as SMD, which is a repeated, rhythmic, purposeless movement or activity; these usually cause self-injury or severely interfere with normal activities. These are most prevalent in adolescence and tend to occur in clusters of symptoms. Diagnosis requires 4 weeks of duration.

COMMONLY ASSOCIATED CONDITIONS

- Medical causes: teething (pain), ear infection, seizures, meningitis, headaches, drug use (cocaine, amphetamines)
- SMD associated with cerebral palsy, intellectual disability, schizophrenia, autism spectrum disorders, Down syndrome, Lesch-Nyhan syndrome, blindness, deafness
- Tic disorder or Tourette syndrome
- Rule out child abuse if significant scalp laceration, skull fracture, or intracerebral or subdural hemorrhage

DIAGNOSIS

- Dependent on multiple factors
- Determine factors associated with behavior, including age of child, degree of parental concern, location of behavior, associated behaviors, motivations of the child, benefits to the child, etc.
- Determine if a medical cause exists, particularly if sudden onset.
- Determine if psychological factors are involved.

DIAGNOSTIC TESTS & INTERPRETATION

- Usually, no laboratory testing is needed for diagnosis.
- Physical examination to look for bruising, swelling, scratches, or minor lacerations.
- If swelling or blood loss is involved, brain imaging may be necessary to rule out damage.
- If severe and persistent head banging is reported, an ophthalmology exam is warranted to rule out complications.
- Developmental screening to rule out possible developmental delay
- If developmental delay is suspected, formal psychoeducational testing can be recommended.

TREATMENT

- Typically, developing children will outgrow the habit by age 3 years.
- Older children may need psychological/developmental follow-up to determine delay/cognition status and to determine if behavioral modification therapy could be beneficial in decreasing symptomatology.
- If severe, head banging can lead to ophthalmologic complications, including cataracts, glaucoma, or retinal detachment. Referral to ophthalmologist is recommended.
- For patients with particularly violent movements of *Jactatio capitis nocturna*, trials with clonazepam and citalopram have shown some success.
- For patients with stereotypic movement disorder, medications may help, including antipsychotics, tricyclic antidepressants, SSRIs, and benzodiazepines. These should be closely monitored.

ONGOING CARE

PROGNOSIS

- Normally disappears by age 3–4 years
- *Jactatio capitis nocturna* is usually benign and resolves by age 5 years.
- Stereotypic movement disorder usually peaks in adolescence and then declines.

ADDITIONAL READING

- Harris KM, Mahone EM, Singer HS. Nonautistic motor stereotypes: clinical features and longitudinal follow-up. *Pediatr Neurol*. 2008;38(4):267–272.
- Leekam S, Tandos J, McConachie H, et al. Repetitive behaviours in typically developing 2-year-olds. *J Child Psychol Psychiatry*. 2007;48(11):1131–1138.
- Miller JM, Singer HS, Bridges DD, et al. Behavioral therapy for treatment of stereotypic movements in nonautistic children. *J Child Neurol*. 2006;21(2):119–125.
- Sallustro F, Atwell CW. Body rocking, head banging, and head rolling in normal children. *J Pediatr*. 1978;93(4):704–708.
- Vinston R, Gelinas-Sorrell D. Head banging in young children. *Am Fam Phys*. 1991;43(5):1625–1628.

CODES

ICD10

- F98.4 Stereotyped movement disorders
- G47.69 Other sleep related movement disorders

FAQ

- Q: Can head banging lead to serious head injury or neurologic damage?
- A: Typically, developing children rarely bang their heads hard enough to cause bleeding or fracture.
- Q: What can a parent do to prevent injury or diminish head banging behavior?
- A: Remove sharp or breakable objects from child's environment to avoid accidental injury.
  - Place a rubber pad on the floor or a thick rug.
  - Secure the crib to the wall to decrease noise and vestibular input to the child.
  - Pad crib with bumpers.
  - If behavior occurs during temper tantrums, ignore the behavior once safety is established. Reward the child for appropriate behaviors.

H

HEADACHE AND MIGRAINE

Christopher B. Oakley

BASICS

DESCRIPTION

- Primary headache: headache without an identifiable underlying etiology; includes but not limited to migraine, tension headache, cluster headache, and other trigeminal autonomic cephalgias; may be episodic or chronic in nature
- Secondary headache: headache attributed to an identifiable underlying etiology
- Other: unusual headaches, especially in children, that include various cranial neuralgias and central and primary facial pain

EPIDEMIOLOGY

- Headache prevalence can approach 30–50% by school age, 60–80% by early adolescence, and as high as 85% by adulthood.
- Tension-type headache is most common type of headache, with migraine second.
- Mean age of onset for migraine is 7 years for boys and 11 years for girls. Migraine precursors such as abdominal migraine, cyclic vomiting syndrome, and benign paroxysmal vertigo of childhood can be seen even younger. These may transform into migraines by puberty.
- Overall migraine reported prevalence ranges between 8 and 23%. Suspicion is that migraine prevalence may be as high as 30–35% due to underreporting. Prevalence of chronic daily headache in younger children is 2–4% and 4–5% in adolescence/adulthood.
- Until puberty, migraines more common in males (55–60%), post puberty in females (75%)
- Genetics plays a role with some reports of 90% family history noted. Genes have been identified for some migraine subtypes including familial hemiplegic migraine.
- Ethnicity plays a role, with majority of reported chronic migraine sufferers being Caucasian.

DIAGNOSIS

Migraine in children is classified into the following groups:

- Migraine without aura: "Common" migraine represents most cases
- Migraine with aura: "Classic" migraine must include aura, a reversible focal neurologic symptom that gradually develop over 5–20 minutes and typically resolve within 1 hour.
- Basilar-type migraine (up to 20% of childhood migraines): often seen migraine with aura with occipital pain often and must include two of the following: dysarthria, vertigo, tinnitus, hyperacusis, diplopia, ataxia, visual symptoms, bilateral paresthesias, and decreased consciousness
- Childhood periodic syndromes that are precursors to migraine: benign paroxysmal vertigo of childhood, cyclic vomiting, abdominal migraine, benign paroxysmal torticollis
- Hemiplegic migraine: type of migraine with aura, with symptoms that must include motor weakness along with one of the following: sensory symptoms, visual symptoms, dysphasic speech
- Others: "Alice in Wonderland syndrome" has distortions of vision, space, and/or time; confusional migraine has impaired sensorium, agitation, and lethargy.

General migraine diagnostic criteria set by the *International Classification of Headache Disorders* 3rd edition, beta (*ICHD III*, beta) in children/adolescents

- 5 attacks not attributed to another condition
  - Lasting 2–72 hours
  - 2 of the following:
    - unilateral or bilateral pain
    - moderate to severe pain
    - pulsating quality
    - aggravated by routine activity
  - 1 of the following:
    - photophobia and phonophobia (may be inferred)
    - nausea or vomiting
- Aura has separate criteria.

Tension-type headache differs from migraine as follows: more episodes typically seen, lasts 30 minutes to 7 days, typically describes as bilateral pain, pressing/tightening quality, mild to moderate intensity, not worse with activity, not associated with sensitivity to light or sound, nausea, or vomiting

HISTORY

The history should help clarify the diagnosis of which type of headache is present and help guide workup and treatment.

- The following questions should be asked:
  - Is there more than 1 type of headache?
  - Have headaches gotten worse?
  - How often do they occur?
  - Where is the pain located?
  - What is the quality of the pain?
  - Do the headaches occur at any special time of day?
  - What associated symptoms are present?
  - Is there a warning sign or aura noted?
  - What triggers a headache?
  - What helps the headache feel better?
  - Any symptoms present between episodes?
  - What treatments have been tried? (include dose, duration, and outcome)
  - Any migraine precursors noted or other common comorbidities such as motion sickness or psychiatric concerns?
- "Red flags": age of onset younger than 3 years of age; first or worst headache; occipital location; recent headache onset; increasing severity or frequency; headache in the morning associated with vomiting; headache causing awakening from sleep; worse with straining; change in mood, mental status, or school performance; or underlying neurocutaneous syndrome or other neurologic concern
- Lifestyle considerations that affect headaches: amount and quality of sleep, hydration status, consistent diet/meals, caffeine consumption, level of fitness and amount of cardiovascular exercise, stress, and anxiety

PHYSICAL EXAM

- Vital signs: blood pressure, heart rate, and weight. Consider orthostatic blood pressure and pulse for dizziness or syncope; if obese, consider pseudotumor or sleep apnea syndrome.
- Skin changes consistent with neurocutaneous syndrome
- Sinus tenderness, limitation of jaw excursion, or occipital trigger points
- Complete neurologic exam including vision screen and funduscopic exam: should be normal in primary headaches. Exception is during aura: Exam may show temporary deficit.
- Basic depression and psychiatric screen
- Any abnormality on exam warrants further investigation, as it may suggest secondary headache with possible underlying etiology.

DIAGNOSTIC TESTS & INTERPRETATION

Practice parameters are established in 2002 for the evaluation of children and adolescents with recurrent headaches. The guidelines address laboratory evaluation, ancillary testing, and imaging.

Imaging

- Neuroimaging studies (CT or MRI): generally not recommended if neurologic exam is normal and no red flags. If exam is abnormal or red flags are present, imaging should be obtained with determining which study to obtain based on clinical concern and situation.
  - CT if there is any suspicion for any acute process such as hemorrhage, but otherwise MRI is preferred.
  - Consider risk of imaging (e.g., younger children require anesthesia for MRI; radiation exposure with CT).
  - Consider MRA/MRV if vascular cause/etiology in differential diagnosis.
- Neuroimaging guidelines are based on multiple studies with more than 600 images reviewed. Only 3% of those images obtained led to specific treatments geared toward imaging findings, and in all those who had abnormal imaging that required treatment, their neurologic exams were found to be abnormal.

Diagnostic Procedures/Other

- EEG: no role for EEG in routine testing of patients with headache
- Laboratory investigation: generally not recommended in primary headaches
- Lumbar puncture (LP): not recommended unless concern for secondary headache or underlying etiology such as infection, hemorrhage, sinus thrombosis, pseudotumor cerebri, and low-pressure headache. Imaging should be done first to ensure it is safe to perform LP.

DIFFERENTIAL DIAGNOSIS

The pattern of headache can help clarify the differential. There are 5 patterns.

- Acute, 1st severe headache
  - CNS infection, cocaine or other substance abuse, medication (methylphenidate, steroids, psychotropic drugs, analgesics, cardiovascular agents), hypertension (usually secondary), hydrocephalus, pseudotumor cerebri (idiopathic intracranial hypertension), post-LP, CNS hemorrhage, ventriculoperitoneal shunt malfunction, sinus thrombosis, migraine, other infection including upper respiratory, somatization
- Acute recurrent headache
  - Much of what is listed above in acute, 1st severe headache can be recurrent as well. Additional consideration would include migraine and variants, cluster, and tension.
- Chronic progressive headache
  - Brain tumor, chronic CNS infection including abscess, hydrocephalus, vascular malformation, hematoma, sinus thrombosis, idiopathic intracranial hypertension, depression or other psychiatric condition, anemia, rheumatologic diseases
- Chronic nonprogressive or daily headache
  - Much of what is listed above in chronic progressive headache can be nonprogressive as well. Additional consideration would include medication overuse, substance abuse including caffeine, chronic infection such as sinusitis, occipital neuralgia, temporomandibular joint syndrome, orthostatic headache, post-LP, other systemic disease, posttraumatic, sleep disorder, tension headache, fibromyalgia.
- Mixed headache: migraine-superimposed tension headache with broad differential including much of what is listed above

TREATMENT

MEDICATION

Practice parameters are established in 2004 for the pharmacologic treatment of migraine in children and adolescents. The guidelines addressed acute and prophylactic medical management.

- Acute treatment: generally most effective if given early in the acute headache/migraine
  - 1st line is ibuprofen (10 mg/kg PO) – level A.
  - Acetaminophen (10–15 mg/kg PO) – level B
  - Naproxen sodium 5.5–7.7 mg/kg PO per dose: longer acting NSAID than ibuprofen
  - Sumatriptan nasal spray can be 1st line in adolescent migraine – level A.
  - Many options noted to be level U (not enough data).
- Additional acute treatments often used especially in refractory patients
  - Antiemetics (prochlorperazine, metoclopramide, ondansetron) also enhance effectiveness of analgesics and may abort migraines. Prochlorperazine has best evidence of this class, with up to 95% improvement noted in some studies.
  - Triptans: generally safe, but only almotriptan is currently FDA approved for use in children or adolescents. Rizatriptan and zolmitriptan have been shown effective in children and adolescents. Seven triptans are available in various forms, including tablet, nasal spray, dissolvable, and injection.
  - Any agent that may lead to vasoconstriction such as triptans and ergotamines are not recommended in basilar, hemiplegic, or any migraine with vascular risk factors.
  - Most over-the-counter or prescription pain/headache/migraine medications may cause rebound headaches.
- Status migrainosus
  - Migraine lasting >72 hours
  - General treatment involved a combination of medications/treatments.
  - Not well studied, but some evidence that the following combinations are successful:
    - Fluids, triptan if used successfully prior, NSAID (ibuprofen/naproxen/ketorolac), antidopaminergic (prochlorperazine [Compazine] with best evidence), and Benadryl
    - Valproic acid can be used as second tier.
    - No definitive evidence for steroids or magnesium despite often being used
  - Dihydroergotamine (DHE-45) noted to be highly effective in small studies; can be IV, IM, or intranasal; given with combination of treatments including antiemetic
  - Narcotics are not recommended.
- Prophylaxis
  - When to start is controversial, but generally if there is more than 1 day per week with disability or dysfunction, daily medication is recommended.
  - Goal is reduction in headache frequency or severity by ≥50%. There is no cure for headaches/migraines. Keeping realistic expectations is key to treatment.
  - Start at a low dose and titrate as needed while being mindful of adverse effects.
  - Can take 4–6 months for effects to be seen
  - Choose a drug that may address comorbidities as well. Be careful to avoid drug classes that may exacerbate other medical conditions (e.g., beta-blockers in asthma patients).
  - Practice parameters from 2004 very limited: Flunarizine (not available in United States) only prophylactic medication with any recommendation other than level U
  - Amitriptyline (TCA) and topiramate (anticonvulsant) most commonly used and studied options in children
  - Cyproheptadine (antihistamine) frequently used 1st line in younger children as well as for migraine precursors and GI symptoms
  - Other options would include the following:
    - Calcium channel blockers: verapamil
    - Beta-blockers: propranolol, nadolol
    - Tricyclic agents: nortriptyline, imipramine
    - SNRI: venlafaxine, duloxetine
    - Anticonvulsants: valproic acid, gabapentin, carbamazepine (neuralgias), and oxcarbazepine (neuralgias)

COMPLEMENTARY & ALTERNATIVE THERAPIES

- Physical therapy, exercise (aerobic, yoga, Pilates), massage therapy, relaxation techniques (meditation, progressive muscle relaxation, self-hypnosis), stress management, cognitive behavioral therapy, biofeedback
- Some evidence for vitamins, supplements, and herbs such as butterbur (50–75 mg b.i.d.), riboflavin (50–400 mg daily), magnesium oxide (50–200 mg b.i.d.). Of note, supplements and vitamins are not regulated by the FDA. Melatonin as low as 3 mg nightly is reported to be as effective as low-dose amitriptyline.

ADDITIONAL READING

- Abu-Arafeh I, Razak S, Silvaraman B, et al. Prevalence of headache and migraine in children and adolescents: a systematic review of population-based studies. *Dev Med Child Neurol*. 2010;52(12):1088–1097.
- Lewis D. Pediatric migraine. *Pediatr Rev*. 2007;28(2):43–53.
- Lewis DW, Ashwal S, Dahl G, et al. Practice parameter: evaluation of children and adolescents with recurrent headaches: report of the Quality Standards Subcommittee of the American Academy of Neurology and the Practice Committee of the Child Neurology Society. *Neurology*. 2002;59(4):490–498.
- Lewis D, Ashwal S, Hershey A, et al. Practice parameter: pharmacological treatment of migraine headache in children and adolescents: report of the American Academy of Neurology Quality Standards Subcommittee and the Practice Committee of the Child Neurology Society. *Neurology*. 2004;63(12):2215–2224.
- Papetti L, Spalice A, Nicita F, et al. Migraine treatment in developmental age: guidelines update. *J Headache Pain*. 2010;11(3):267–276.
- Termine C, Ozge A, Antonaci F, et al. Overview of diagnosis and management of paediatric headache. Part II: therapeutic management. *J Headache Pain*. 2011;12(1):25–34.

CODES

ICD10

- R51 Headache
- G43.909 Migraine, unsp, not intractable, without status migrainosus
- G44.209 Tension-type headache, unspecified, not intractable

H

HEAT STROKE AND RELATED ILLNESS

Patrick B. Solari • George Anthony Woodward

BASICS

DESCRIPTION

- Heat stroke occurs during imbalance in heat production, absorption, and dissipation. It can result from excessive body heat generation and storage without appropriate dissipation, high ambient temperature, low radiation or convective heat loss, decreased evaporation, or inadequate fluid/electrolyte replacement in response to losses through sweat or GI disturbance.
- 2 forms of heat stroke exist.
  - Exertional heat stroke, which occurs during periods of intense exertion
  - Nonexertional heat stroke, in which the body is unable to compensate for an increase in ambient temperature; more common in very young and elderly and during heat waves

RISK FACTORS

- Environmental predisposition
  - Hot and humid without wind, heat wave, overheated indoor environment, lack of air conditioning; social isolation, inability to care for self, or entrapment in closed space (e.g., car, trunk; internal automobile temperature in sunlight with poor ventilation can reach 131–172°F; the sharpest temperature increase occurs within the first 15 minutes)
- Medical
  - Obesity, low fitness level, cardiac disease, diabetes mellitus and insipidus, diarrhea, hyperthyroidism, dehydration, vascular disease, sweat gland dysfunction, sunburn, viral illness
- Drugs/medications
  - Anticholinergics
  - Antihistamines
  - Stimulants
  - Beta-blockers
  - Diuretics
  - Psychiatric medications
  - Recreational drugs and alcohol
- Behaviors
  - Lack of recognition of risk factors or warning signs
  - Overexertion or inadequate fluid intake
  - Inappropriate clothing; heavy, dark, tight-fitting, overbundling
  - Lack of acclimatization and conditioning
  - Children in enclosed space within vehicle

GENERAL PREVENTION

- Avoid enclosed spaces (e.g., children in closed cars).
- Reduce activity levels, keep cool, and use shaded areas. Adaptation to warmer climates may take 8–10 exposures of 30–45 minutes each daily or every other day.
- Air conditioning or fans during hot weather
- Cool or tepid baths
- Fluid intake
  - Increase fluid intake before, during, and after scheduled exercise or strenuous activity.
  - Up to 200–300 mL q10–20 min
  - Do not wait until there is a sensation of thirst.
- Precooling using external (cold water immersion, cooling vests) or internal (drinking cold liquid/ice slurry) methods may improve performance before endurance events in heat.
- Appropriate clothing
  - Loose, light-colored clothing
  - Protective hat
- Acclimatization via gradual conditioning over 10–14 days in hotter environment
- Liberal dietary sodium
  - Avoid NaCl tablets (possible hypernatremia, potassium depletion, gastric irritation, delayed gastric emptying).
- Frequently flex leg muscles when standing.
- Avoid prolonged standing in hot environments.
- Avoid caffeine and alcohol.

PATHOPHYSIOLOGY

- Heat production increases 10–20 times by strenuous exercise.
- When environmental temperature is greater than body temperature, body gains heat by conduction and radiation and can lose heat by evaporation and convection.
- Children have greater body surface-to-mass ratio, higher metabolic rate, inability to increase cardiac output, decreased sweat production, and inability to independently change environments compared to adults.
  - Dehydration results in loss of sweating, hence decreased evaporation.
  - Above 40°C, cell volume, membrane integrity, metabolism, and acid–base balance is affected.
  - Extreme core temperatures >42°C can uncouple oxidative phosphorylation and allow enzyme systems to cease functioning.

COMMONLY ASSOCIATED CONDITIONS

- Miliaria rubra (prickly heat)
  - Heat rash, usually caused by obstruction of sweat glands by clothes or lotions
  - Erythematous papular rash; usually self-limited
- Heat cramps/spasms
  - Related to physical exercise in people who have not trained or are poorly acclimatized with mild dehydration
  - Related to water and sodium depletion
- Heat tetany
  - Paresthesias and carpopedal spasm help distinguish tetany from heat cramps.
- Heat syncope
  - Alteration of consciousness (i.e., dizziness, syncope) at end of strenuous or upright event
- Heat edema
  - Swollen feet and ankles (i.e., vascular leak, orthostatic pooling)
- Heat exhaustion
  - Relatively slow onset
  - Water and/or salt depletion
  - Copious perspiration with headache, nausea, vomiting, malaise, myalgias, pallor, lightheadedness, visual disturbances, syncope, temperature 38–40°C, dehydration, electrolyte imbalance, hemoconcentration
  - Can evolve into heat stroke
- Heat stroke
  - Core body temperature exceeding 40°C with altered mental status ranging from confusion, disorientation, and incoherent speech to delirium, decerebrate posturing, seizure, and coma
  - May have acute, sudden onset (80%) or slower onset (minutes to hours, 20%)
  - Classic heat stroke is associated with dry skin and prolonged exposure to elevated temperatures at rest.
  - Exertional heat stroke may present with anhidrosis or profuse sweating.

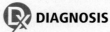

DIAGNOSIS

HISTORY

- Heat exhaustion
  - Weakness, lethargy, thirst, malaise, diminished ability to work or play, headache, nausea, vomiting, myalgias, pale skin, dizziness
- Heat stroke
  - History of CNS dysfunction in environment consistent with, or predisposing conditions conducive to, development of heat-related illness should suggest heat stroke.

PHYSICAL EXAM

- Heat exhaustion
  - Visual disturbances, syncope, mild CNS dysfunction, impaired judgment, cramps, vertigo, hypotension, tachycardia, hyperventilation, paresthesias, agitation, ataxia, psychosis, temperature <40°C, sweating, environmental exposure, and activity; no coma or seizures
- Heat stroke
  - Temperature >40°C (may be cooler after prehospital interventions and maneuvers)
  - Altered level of consciousness (confusion, drowsiness, irritability, neurologic deficits, euphoria, combativeness, obtundation), ataxia, posturing, incontinence, seizures, coma, purpura, or petechiae
  - 2/3 with constricted pupils
  - May have muscle rigidity with tonic contractions and dystonia that mimic seizures
  - Shock: tachycardia, hypotension, widened pulse pressure, tachypnea
  - Hot, dry (classic), or clammy (exercise-induced) skin; pink or ashen color
  - Weakness, nausea, vomiting, anorexia, headache, dizziness

- Temperature measurement (continuous best)
  - Esophageal thermometry is probably the best.
  - Deep rectal thermometry is a good approximation of core temperature.
  - Tympanic, oral, axillary, and temporal artery temperatures are less accurate measures of core temperature.

DIAGNOSTIC TESTS & INTERPRETATION

Lab

Initial lab tests

Tests are only to confirm diagnosis, evaluate extent of injury, or rule out other processes because treatment should be empiric.

- Heat cramps: decreased levels of serum and urine sodium and chloride; BUN level normal or slightly increased
- Heat exhaustion: may see hyponatremia or hypernatremia (free water loss), hypochloremia, low urine sodium, and chloride hemoconcentration; normal LFTs
- Heat stroke
  - Electrolyte abnormalities: sodium, chloride level normal or high, hypokalemia, elevated BUN/creatinine; hypoglycemia
  - Hematologic: hemoconcentration, leukocytosis, thrombocytopenia
  - Prerenal azotemia
  - Elevated AST/ALT
  - Metabolic acidosis: lactate high, especially with exertional heat stroke
  - Coagulopathy
- Arterial blood gases (classic heat stroke: respiratory alkalosis and hypokalemia early; lactic acidosis later; exertional heat stroke; lactic acidosis)
- Others: creatine phosphokinase (rhabdomyolysis), urinalysis (casts, brownish color proteinuria, microscopic hematuria, myoglobinuria), CSF, EKG, chest radiograph

DIFFERENTIAL DIAGNOSIS

- Heat cramps: rhabdomyolysis, tetany
- Heat edema: thrombophlebitis, lymphedema, congestive heart failure
- Heat stroke: CNS process with fever (cerebrovascular stroke, meningitis, encephalitis), other infections, anticholinergic poisoning (dilated pupils), drug/medication induced, temperature rise, severe dehydration. Chills suggest febrile illness, not heat stroke.
- Neuroleptic malignant syndrome
- Serotonin syndrome
- Malignant hyperthermia

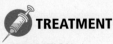

TREATMENT

MEDICATION

- Antipyretics are not useful because an intact hypothalamus is required for action.
- Avoid anticholinergic drugs, which inhibit sweating.
- May require inotropic support
- Chlorpromazine may improve peripheral vasodilatation and prevent shivering.
- Benzodiazepine for sedation and/or seizures
- Dantrolene not shown to be effective

ADDITIONAL TREATMENT

General Measures

- Heat stroke: Treat empirically, and then rule out other causes of presentation. Maintain airway, breathing, and circulation including securing airway as indicated and supplemental oxygen delivery.
  - Cooling is mainstay of treatment, external, internal, or both.
  - Fluid replacement: IV 0.9% NS or LR solution. Rule out hypoglycemia.
  - Miscellaneous therapies
    - Foley catheter to monitor urine output
    - Nasogastric tube
    - Myoglobinuria therapy (mannitol, bicarbonate, dialysis if necessary)
    - Electrolyte replacement if symptomatic from hypokalemia or hypocalcemia
    - Fresh frozen plasma for disseminated intravascular coagulation (DIC)

INPATIENT CONSIDERATIONS

Initial Stabilization

- Rapid recognition and cooling imperative
- Specific therapy
  - Heat cramps: rest, salt and water replacement
  - Heat syncope: self-limited, as return to horizontal position is treatment; rest and fluids, salted liquids
  - Heat exhaustion: Clinical findings (heart rate, BP, orthostatic changes, urine output) should direct therapy. Most treated as outpatient with rapid rehydration, cooling; mild case: oral electrolyte solution; if with nausea, vomiting, inability to drink: IV (0.45 [similar to sweat losses]–0.9% NS); avoid rapid overcorrection of hypernatremia (treat as with hypernatremic dehydration); if with hyponatremic seizures, treat with 3% saline at ~5 mL/kg.
  - Heat stroke: immediate cooling and support of cardiovascular system. Remove clothing, remove patient from hot environment; use air conditioning, open vehicle for transport if possible; esophageal or rectal temperature probe (continuous temperature measurements); cooling should exceed 0.1°–0.2°C/min; slow cooling down at 38.5°–39°C to avoid overshoot.
  - Cooling options: Cold water immersion (15°–16°C) has lowest morbidity and mortality for exertional heat stroke and is as effective as ice bath without discomfort, shivering, or vasoconstriction.
    - Also: ice packs to neck, groin, axillae; wet sheet over patient; moisten skin with water spray, convection increase (fan) to increase evaporative cooling; cooling blankets; cool/ice water lavage (peritoneum, rectum, gastric); cold to room temperature IV fluids; massage with ice (decreases shivering response).

Admission Criteria

- Patients with symptoms suggestive of heat stroke require immediate cooling and should be closely observed.
- Patients with evidence of multisystem disease (altered mental status, electrolyte imbalances, hematologic abnormalities) should be admitted until such issues are resolved.
- Patients with respiratory or hemodynamic instability may require intensive care.

ONGOING CARE

PROGNOSIS

- Heat-related illness (e.g., heat rash, edema, cramps, tetany, syncope, exhaustion): rapid recovery with supportive care
- Heat stroke: poor prognosis if not recognized and aggressively managed; morbidity and mortality directly proportional to how rapidly core temperature is reduced

ADDITIONAL READING

- Bouchama A, Knochel JP. Heat stroke. *N Engl J Med*. 2002;346(25):1978–1988.
- Grubenhoff JA, du Ford K, Roosevelt GE. Heat-related illness. *Clin Pediatr Emerg Med*. 2007:8:59–64.
- Jardine DS. Heat illness and heat stroke. *Pediatr Rev*. 2007;28(7):249–258.
- Nelson NG, Collins CL, Comstock RD, et al. Exertional heat-related injuries treated in emergency departments in the U.S., 1997-2006. *Am J Prev Med*. 2011;40(1):54–60.

CODES

ICD10

- T67.0XXA Heatstroke and sunstroke, initial encounter
- T67.1XXA Heat syncope, initial encounter
- L74.0 Miliaria rubra

FAQ

- Q: How can one distinguish between heat exhaustion and heat stroke?
- A: Heat stroke involves temperature >40°C with CNS and LFT abnormalities, whereas heat exhaustion refers to inability to continue exercise.
- Q: When should heat stroke be suspected?
- A: Suspect heat stroke in a patient with or without sweating and who demonstrates alterations of CNS function.
- Q: Does the presence or absence of sweating help with the diagnosis of heat exhaustion versus heat stroke?
- A: No. Sweating will be present with heat exhaustion and may or may not be present with heat stroke.
- Q: Are children at increased risk of heat illness?
- A: Yes. They have a number of predisposing factors: greater surface area–to–body mass ratio than adults, higher metabolic rate, slower rate of sweating than adults, temperature when sweating starts is higher, lower cardiac output at a given metabolic rate than adults, rate of acclimatization is slower, thirst response is blunted, and access to fluids may be limited.

H

HEMANGIOMAS AND OTHER VASCULAR LESIONS

Katherine B. Püttgen

BASICS

DESCRIPTION

- Vascular tumors: neoplasms of the vasculature
  - Infantile hemangioma (IH)
  - Congenital hemangiomas: noninvoluting congenital hemangioma (NICH) and rapidly involuting congenital hemangioma (RICH)
  - Tufted angioma (TA)
  - Kaposiform hemangioendothelioma (KHE)
  - Pyogenic granuloma
  - Hemangiopericytoma
- Vascular malformations (VaM): anomalous blood vessels without endothelial proliferation
  - Capillary malformations (CM) (e.g., salmon patch, port-wine stain, nevus flammeus)
  - Venous malformations (VM)
  - Arterial malformations: arteriovenous malformations (AVM) or arteriovenous fistula (AVF)
- Lymphatic malformations (LM) (macrocystic and microcystic)
- Combined malformations (e.g., capillary-venous-lymphatic)
- Other types of VaM may occur in any part of the body and may be associated with soft tissue overgrowth of the involved part.

EPIDEMIOLOGY

Incidence

Infantile hemangiomas

- 4–5% of infants
- ~10% of Caucasian infants by age 12 months
- Increased incidence in low-birth-weight and premature infants
- Other demographic risk factors include white non-Hispanic race, female sex, multiple gestation pregnancy, advanced maternal age, chorionic villus sampling during pregnancy, and positive family history.

COMMONLY ASSOCIATED CONDITIONS

- Infantile hemangiomas
  - PHACES
    - Segmental hemangioma (usually facial) associated with other developmental anomalies (Posterior fossa malformations; hemangiomas; arterial anomalies; cardiac anomalies, including aortic coarctation; eye abnormalities; sternal defects/supraumbilical raphe)
    - Cerebral malformations occur in >50% and cerebrovascular anomalies in 33%.
  - Lumbosacral
    - An underlying spinal dysraphism may be present.
    - PHACE-like syndromes of the lower body with associated GI and GU anomalies have been described.
  - Segmental
    - Commonly located on the face and involving a developmental unit (segment) and frequently associated with complications, even without meeting full PHACES criteria
    - Segmental IHs are much more likely to have complications and to receive treatment than focal IHs.
- Kaposiform hemangioendothelioma
  - Kasabach-Merritt phenomenon (consumptive coagulopathy, severe thrombocytopenia)
- VaM
  - CM may be present as part of syndromes (e.g., Sturge-Weber, *RASA-1* mutations associated with fast-flow VaM, von Hippel-Lindau, Rubinstein-Taybi, Beckwith-Wiedemann, Cobb syndrome).
  - VM can be inherited autosomal dominantly due to *TIE2/TEK* gene mutations.
  - CM-AVM: due to *RASA-1* gene mutation and associated with fast-flow VaM
  - Generalized LM and lymphedema have been associated with *VEGFR3* mutations.

DIAGNOSIS

HISTORY

- Onset of lesions and timing of changes
- IHs are often inapparent at birth or present with nascent telangiectatic patches followed by a rapid growth phase.
  - Proliferative phase: During the first 2 months of life, nearly all IHs double in size.
  - Most rapid period of growth occurs between 5.5 and 7.5 weeks of age; majority of rapid growth phase is in the first 8 weeks of life.
  - Most IHs reach 80% of their maximum size by 3–5 months of age.
- Segmental and deep IH grow longer.
- Congenital hemangiomas (RICH and NICH) are present fully formed at birth.
- VaM are present (although may not be noticed) at birth. Most slowly enlarge over time.
- Past medical history for IH
  - Low birth weight, twin or other multiple gestation, prematurity
- Family history
  - Present in up to 15% of IH
  - CM-AVM is autosomal dominantly inherited.

PHYSICAL EXAM

- Infantile hemangiomas
  - Neonate: flat pale patch, superficial telangiectasia with halo border
  - Superficial IH: raised red, partially compressible, nontender plaque or nodule with well-demarcated borders. Overlying skin is usually intact, although sometimes ulceration may be present.
  - Deep IH: raised soft mass with bluish-purplish discoloration with smooth, intact, overlying skin
  - Mixed IH: Lesions will have both superficial and deep components.
  - Morphology may be localized (most common), segmental, indeterminate (looks "sub"-segmental), or multifocal (>5 IH).
  - Ulceration occurs in up to 25% in a referral setting; risk of ulceration peaks by age 4 months.
  - Involuting lesion: flat, atrophic pale or gray center with surrounding raised reddish border with stippled texture
  - The presence of large numbers of small- to moderate-sized IH may indicate a rare condition called diffuse neonatal hemangiomatosis. Internal organ involvement (liver, lungs, GI tract, CNS) may be present.
- VaM
  - Salmon patches (nevus simplex)
    - Most notable at birth as pinkish-red macules that often blanch and are most commonly found at the nape of the neck, glabella, and upper eyelids
    - Frequently, all three locations are involved in an individual newborn.
  - Port-wine stains (nevus flammeus)
    - Easily seen at birth and are deep pink to red-purplish, nonblanching macules with well-demarcated borders
    - Most commonly located on the face and often cover a large area
    - Matured port-wine stains are deeper in color and frequently develop raised nodules and vascular blebs.
    - If an extremity is heavily involved, there may be underlying bony and soft tissue overgrowth with limb hypertrophy.
  - AVMs
    - Raised pulsating lesions with bruits audible by stethoscope if large in size
    - Smaller lesions may vary in appearance from macular erythema to thin vascular plaques.
    - Signs of cardiac compromise (i.e., tachycardia, gallop rhythm, shortness of breath, hepatomegaly) may be associated with very large AVMs.
  - VMs
    - Deep blue to purplish, soft, fleshy compressible nodules in the skin; may be surrounded by superficial venules
    - The drainage pattern is generally obvious upon inspection.
    - Mature lesions may include small calcifications (phleboliths).
  - LM
    - Present differently depending on size
    - Large lesions are rubbery, skin-colored, massive nodules with ill-defined borders, most often located in the head, neck, axilla, or chest (cystic hygromas in older, less preferred nomenclature).
    - Lesions in the neck area may be associated with respiratory compromise if the airway is constricted.
    - Microcystic LM present as nodules or plaques, sometimes in clusters, with overlying skin changes such as discoloration. Complicated lesions may be hemorrhagic or leak translucent lymph fluid.

DIAGNOSTIC TESTS & INTERPRETATION

Diagnosis is usually made by recognition of the typical physical exam findings.

Imaging

- Occasionally helpful in distinguishing vascular tumors like IH from VaM but primarily useful in determining subtype and extent of VaM for treatment planning

- For multifocal IH, abdominal ultrasound to rule out hepatic involvement should be ordered.
- Preoperative MRI/MRA, CT angiography, or venography aids in treatment planning of VaM.

Diagnostic Procedures/Other

- Biopsy: rarely required but may be helpful to differentiate lesions suspicious for malignancy; should be avoided if lesion is highly suspected to be vascular, as significant bleeding may ensue
- Other diagnostic tests should be considered if concerns for syndromes or other complications (e.g., cardiac or respiratory compromise) exist.

TREATMENT

GENERAL MEASURES

- Infantile hemangiomas
  - Most patients will not need treatment, as lesions will spontaneously involute without complications.
  - Consider treatment of lesions interfering with critical organ functions, such as vision or breathing, or lesions significantly affecting appearance, such as on the face.
  - Timing of surgical treatment of IH should be carefully determined to minimize the risk of undesirable cosmetic outcome. Surgery during the proliferative phase in infancy is rare. Most surgery is performed between 3 and 6 years of age.
  - Propranolol, given orally at 2 mg/kg/24 h in divided doses (range 1–3 mg/kg/24 h) is now accepted as 1st-line therapy for IH.
  - Oral corticosteroids (generally given as prednisolone at 2–3 mg/kg/24 h) are now 2nd-line treatment.
  - Topical timolol maleate 0.5% gel-forming solution or solution (ophthalmic dosage forms used topically) may be used for small, superficial IH.
  - Interferon may be useful in refractory or severe lesions. The development of spastic diplegia in up to 20% of treated infants (highest risk group is <12 months of age) is a known complication and has drastically limited modern use of this therapy.
  - Vincristine is another 3rd-line therapy and is rarely used.
  - For ulcerated IH, petrolatum, zinc oxide paste, and topical dressings are used; pulsed dye laser may be used. Propranolol has been shown to speed ulcer healing.
- VaM
  - Pulsed dye laser
    - The treatment of choice for port-wine stains and other superficial VaM
    - Serial treatments over several years may be necessary. Large lesions may not completely respond.
    - Better outcomes are noted in children treated in infancy and early childhood.
  - Sclerotherapy or surgery may be appropriate for complicated, symptomatic VaM.

ISSUES FOR REFERRAL

Consider referral to specialty services if the following conditions are present:

- Lesions in locations where function may be impacted such as periorbital, ear canal, tip of nose, lips, or anogenital areas
- Lesions distributed in a "beard-like" distribution, which may be associated with airway IH
- Presence of numerous cutaneous lesions increasing the likelihood of visceral involvement (including the GI tract, liver, CNS, lungs)
- Lesions causing or likely to cause significant disfigurement
- Lesions located over the lumbosacral spine, which may be associated with spinal dysraphism
- Lesions located in a segmental distribution about the head and face
- Large AVMs impacting circulation and cardiac function (e.g., resulting in high-output heart failure)
- Presence of dysmorphic features along with vascular lesions
- Lesions that are ulcerating or bleeding
- Suspected VaM of unknown type or extent

ONGOING CARE

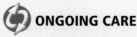

PATIENT EDUCATION

Vascular Birthmarks Foundation (www.birthmark.org)

PROGNOSIS

- Infantile hemangiomas
  - All IHs undergo spontaneous involution. By 9–10 years of age, 90% will have completed involution. Greater than 85% will resolve without need for treatment.
  - Residual areas of skin atrophy and/or discoloration occur in up to 50%.
  - Complicated lesions marked by ulceration result in scarring.
- VaM
  - VaM do not generally involute or resolve.
  - Salmon patches fade over time and generally are not a cosmetic problem.
  - Port-wine stains may darken and become nodular with age; bleeding can occur.
  - Larger lesions can be associated with excessive growth of the involved body area resulting in hypertrophy.
  - Malignant transformation is rare.

COMPLICATIONS

- Infantile hemangiomas
  - Bleeding, ulceration, superinfection
  - Interference with function of important organs (including vision, airway, GI tract, CNS)
  - Disfigurement
  - Hypothyroidism may occur with large hemangiomas that stimulate increased breakdown of thyroid hormone.
  - KHE and TA may be associated with Kasabach-Merritt phenomenon with severe thrombocytopenia (due to platelet trapping, consumptive coagulopathy, and microangiopathic hemolytic anemia).
- VaM
  - High-output cardiac failure due to circulatory "steal" associated with AVMs
  - Skeletal overgrowth of the involved limb can occur with disfigurement and orthopedic complications.
  - Limitation of movement and pain from localized ischemia
  - Problems associated with lymphedema
  - Airway compromise from constriction by large neck lesions

ADDITIONAL READING

- Chang LC, Haggstrom AN, Drolet BA, et al. Growth characteristics of infantile hemangiomas: implications for management. *Pediatrics*. 2008;122(2):360–367.
- Drolet BA, Frommelt PC, Chamlin SL, et al. Initiation and use of propranolol for infantile hemangiomas: report of a consensus conference. *Pediatrics*. 2013;131(1):128–140.
- Greene AK. Current concepts of vascular anomalies. *J Craniofac Surg*. 2012;23(1):220–224.
- Haggstrom AN, Drolet BA, Baselga E, et al. Prospective study of infantile hemangiomas: clinical characteristics predicting complications and treatment. *Pediatrics*. 2006;118(3):882–887.

CODES

ICD10

- D18.00 Hemangioma unspecified site
- Q27.9 Congenital malformation of peripheral vascular system, unsp
- Q27.30 Arteriovenous malformation, site unspecified

FAQ

- Q. When will the IH go away?
- A. Growth in nearly all IH stops by 12 months of age. Regression occurs over a period of years, with most involution occurring in the first 3 years of life; further regression will occur until about age 10 years.
- Q. Is the risk of bleeding in IH significant?
- A. No. Risk of significant bleeding is less than 1%. Even with ulceration, bleeding is more of an "ooze."

HEMATURIA

Stephanie Nguyen • Jennifer Yang

BASICS

DESCRIPTION

- Hematuria is defined as $\geq$3–5 RBCs per high-power field (hpf) using a standard urinalysis technique on a centrifuged sample.
- Persistent hematuria: hematuria on >2 separate examinations
- Macroscopic or gross hematuria: hematuria visible to the naked eye
- Microscopic hematuria: hematuria detected by urinalysis or microscopy only

EPIDEMIOLOGY

- Asymptomatic microscopic hematuria (on >1 sample): 0.5–2% of school-aged children
- Gross hematuria: 0.13% children in walk-in clinic
- Gross hematuria is more common in boys.

RISK FACTORS

Hematuria, hypercalciuria, nephrolithiasis, and nephritis can be inherited.

PATHOPHYSIOLOGY

Bleeding can occur from anywhere along the urinary tract or kidney. In glomerular hematuria, RBCs cross the glomerular basement membrane (GBM) into the urinary space.

DIAGNOSIS

No identifiable cause is found in the majority (up to 80%) of children with asymptomatic microscopic hematuria and in up to 30% of children with a single episode of gross hematuria.

DIFFERENTIAL DIAGNOSIS

Hematuria may originate at any site along the urinary tract. Nonglomerular causes are more common than glomerular causes.

- Factitious causes: Urine appears bloody, but no RBCs are present.
  - Endogenous pigments
    - Myoglobin (rhabdomyolysis)
    - Hemoglobin (hemolysis)
    - Porphyria
    - Bile pigments
    - Urate crystals (pink diaper syndrome)
    - Beets, blackberries
  - Exogenous pigments
    - Food and beverage dyes
    - Drugs that cause urinary discoloration:
      - Phenazopyridine (Pyridium)
      - Senna (Ex-Lax)
      - Rifampin
      - Sulfa
      - Others
  - *Serratia marcescens*
- Glomerular causes
  - Common:
    - Strenuous exercise
    - Acute postinfectious glomerulonephritis (GN)
    - IgA nephropathy
    - Thin basement membrane disease (benign familial hematuria)
  - Uncommon:
    - Alport syndrome, hereditary nephritis
    - Membranoproliferative GN
    - Nephritis of systemic disease (Henoch-Schönlein purpura [HSP], systemic lupus, or other vasculitis)
- Nonglomerular causes
- Upper urinary tract
  - Common:
    - Pyelonephritis
    - Hypercalciuria/nephrolithiasis/nephrocalcinosis
    - Renal trauma (contusion), particularly in hydronephrotic or cystic kidneys
    - Ureteropelvic junction obstruction
    - Hemoglobinopathies (sickle cell disease, sickle cell trait)
  - Uncommon:
    - Drug-induced interstitial nephritis (penicillins, cephalosporins, NSAIDs, phenytoin, cimetidine, omeprazole)
    - Cystic disease (simple cyst, polycystic kidney disease)
    - Neoplasm: Wilms tumor
    - Coagulopathy
    - Renal venous thrombosis, renal arterial thrombosis
    - "Nutcracker" phenomenon
- Lower urinary tract
  - Common:
    - Bladder catheterization, Foley catheter
    - Cystitis (bacterial, viral, occasionally chemical)
    - Perineal trauma or irritation
    - Urethrorrhagia
    - Meatal stenosis
    - Urethritis
    - "Terminal hematuria" syndrome (trigonitis)
    - Epididymitis
  - Uncommon:
    - Bladder tumor
    - Arteriovenous malformation
    - Polyp
    - Urethral or bladder trauma
    - Foreign body or calculus in bladder or urethra
    - Schistosomiasis
- External causes of "hematuria"
  - Menstrual contamination
  - Diaper rash, perineal irritation

APPROACH TO THE PATIENT

Evaluate all children with gross hematuria and those children with microscopic hematuria confirmed on 2 of 3 consecutive samples over several weeks:

- Phase 1: Determine if the pigment in urine is from blood or another source. Are RBCs present on microscopy?
- Phase 2: Determine the source of bleeding: glomerular or nonglomerular, kidney or urinary tract?
- Phase 3: Select those who will require referral versus those who will simply require follow-up.

HISTORY

- **Question:** Blood on voiding?
- *Significance*: Glomerular or renal source will be constantly bloody; urethral bleeding is more likely at initiation or end of stream.
- **Question:** Prior episodes of gross hematuria or abnormal urinalyses?
- *Significance*: Chronic versus acute process
- **Question:** Antecedent infection, streptococcal pharyngitis, or impetigo?
- *Significance*: Suggests postinfectious GN
- **Question:** Concurrent upper respiratory infection (URI) or gastroenteritis?
- *Significance*: Suggests IgA nephropathy
- **Question:** Any precipitating factors (trauma, exercise)?
- *Significance*: Renal contusion, exercise hematuria, or myoglobinuria
- **Question:** Voiding symptoms, dysuria, urgency, frequency?
- *Significance*: Suggests bacterial or viral (adenovirus) hemorrhagic cystitis
- **Question:** Renal colic or other pain?
- *Significance*: Suggests stones or other obstructive process
- **Question:** Drops of blood or spotting in underwear after or between voiding in prepubertal boys?
- *Significance*: Suggests urethrorrhagia
- **Question:** Fever, rash, arthritis?
- *Significance*: Signs or symptoms of systemic illness or immune-mediated process
- **Question:** Bleeding from any other source (i.e., gums, GI tract)?
- *Significance*: Suggests coagulopathy
- **Question:** Symptom-less "terminal" hematuria?
- *Significance*: Suggests trigonitis, hemorrhagic cystitis
- **Question:** Medications and diet?
- *Significance*: Food or drug pigment, drug nephrotoxicity
- **Question:** Sexually active? STD?
- *Significance*: Urethritis, epididymitis
- **Question:** Family history?
- *Significance*:
  - Hematuria in family members: Familial hematuria, kidney failure, or premature deafness suggests Alport syndrome.
  - Sickle cell disease or trait in child or family members: Suggests sickle nephropathy, papillary necrosis, or hemoglobinuria
  - Renal stone disease in family members: Suggests renal stones, hypercalciuria, or metabolic disease
  - Cystic kidney disease in family members: Autosomal recessive or autosomal dominant polycystic kidney disease

PHYSICAL EXAM

- **Finding:** Head, ears, eyes, nose, throat (HEENT) exam (periorbital edema)?
- *Significance*: GN, renal failure, volume overload
- **Finding:** Cardiovascular exam (hypertension, tachycardia, murmur, gallop)?
- *Significance*: GN, renal failure, volume overload
- **Finding:** Abdominal exam (ascites, organomegaly, tenderness, or masses)?
- *Significance*: Volume overload, tumor, polycystic or hydronephrotic kidneys, venous thrombosis
- **Finding:** Back exam (flank tenderness)?
- *Significance*: Pyelonephritis, renal calculi, large cysts
- **Finding:** Genital exam (blood at urethral meatus, normal urethral opening)?
- *Significance*: Urethral trauma, meatal stenosis
- **Finding:** Perineal exam (skin breakdown, irritation)?
- *Significance*: External source of bleeding or infection
- **Finding:** Extremities (pretibial edema, arthritis)?
- *Significance*: GN, volume overload, systemic illness
- **Finding:** Skin and mucosal exam (petechial, vasculitic rash, ulcerations)?
- *Significance*: Systemic illness (lupus, HSP)

DIAGNOSTIC TESTS & INTERPRETATION

Positive test for blood on urine dipstick may be myoglobin or hemoglobin. If the urinary sediment does not show RBCs, investigate for problems such as rhabdomyolysis (elevated creatinine phosphokinase [CPK]) or hemolysis.

- **Test:** Repeated urinalysis to confirm persistent microscopic hematuria
- *Significance*:
  - Patient should be told not to exercise before the urine collection.
  - 2 of 3 positive specimens over several weeks should be documented in an otherwise well child before diagnostic testing is initiated.
- **Test:** Gross and microscopic analyses of fresh urine specimen
- *Significance*:
  - Absence of RBCs suggests factitious hematuria.
  - Dysmorphic RBCs suggest glomerular source.
  - Eumorphic RBCs suggest nonglomerular source/collecting system etiology.
  - RBC casts: Diagnostic for GN
  - WBCs suggest cystitis.
  - WBC casts suggest pyelonephritis.
- **Test:** Screening of the family members for occult hematuria
- *Significance*: Familial benign hematuria or Alport syndrome
- **Test:** Testing for hypercalciuria (random urine calcium/creatinine ratio >0.2 mg/mg in children >6 years; >0.6 in children 6–12 months; >0.8 in children <6 months)
- *Significance*: If elevated, 24-hour urine calcium collection >4 mg/kg/day in children >2 years of age: Hypercalciuria
- **Test:** Culture
- *Significance*: Bacterial, viral—cystitis, *S. marcescens*, adenovirus
- **Test:** Serum electrolytes, BUN, and creatinine levels
- *Significance*: Impaired renal function suggests inflammation, infection, or obstruction.
- **Test:** Evaluation for GN
- *Significance*:
  - Hematuria with RBC casts in combination with proteinuria, edema, hypertension, and/or impaired renal function
  - Streptococcal serology (ASO titer, streptozyme): Acute postinfectious GN
  - Complement studies (C3,C4): Hypocomplementemic GN—immune complex–mediated (lupus nephritis, postinfectious GN, membranoproliferative GN)
  - Antinuclear antibody (ANA) titer or anti–double-stranded DNA if hypocomplementemic or signs of systemic vasculitis: Vasculitis (lupus)
  - Quantitation of proteinuria and serum albumin concentration
    - 3–4+ proteinuria, urine protein/creatinine ratio >2 mg/mg, and hypoalbuminemia suggest glomerular disease/nephrosis.
    - 24-hour urine protein ≥1 g/day
- **Test:** CBC with platelets, coagulation times
- *Significance*: May suggest hemolysis, clotting disorder, or systemic illness
- **Test:** Hemoglobin electrophoresis should be considered in black patients.
- *Significance*: Sickle cell disease or sickle trait may cause hematuria.
- Rarely, additional studies, such as voiding cystourethrogram, renal angiography, cystoscopy, and renal biopsy, will be required with an appropriate referral to urology or nephrology.
- Audiometry and ophthalmologic exam may be indicated if hereditary (Alport) nephritis is suspected; should be performed on boys with familial hematuria

Imaging

Every child with gross hematuria should have imaging of the kidneys and urinary tract. It may or may not be indicated in children with microscopic hematuria.

- Ultrasound of kidneys and bladder: urinary tract obstruction, congenital malformation, cysts, stones, nephrocalcinosis, malignancy
- Abdominal CT scan: after trauma if there are >50 RBCs/hpf; if mechanism (deceleration injury, multiple organ injury) or signs or symptoms (flank pain or ecchymosis) are significant, even if <50 RBC/hpf
- Helical CT without contrast: study of choice for the visualization of stones; however, must consider radiation exposure risk. Ultrasound is reasonable first test for stones.

TREATMENT

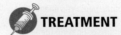

ADDITIONAL TREATMENT

General Measures

- For children with microscopic hematuria, in the absence of other clinical, laboratory, or imaging findings, no specific treatment is indicated besides routine follow-up.
- For children with glomerular hematuria, treatment depends on the histopathologic diagnosis, clinical features, renal function, and degree of proteinuria.
- For children with an anatomic/structural etiology, treatment is specific to abnormality.

ISSUES FOR REFERRAL

- Nephrology: recurrent gross hematuria, proteinuria, RBC casts, nephrosis, edema, hypocomplementemia, hypertension, azotemia, cysts, hypercalciuria, family history of renal failure, hereditary nephritis, deafness, or cystic kidney disease
- Urology: congenital anomaly of urinary tract, uncontrollable bleeding after trauma, recurrent, painful or large stones, recurrent urinary infections
- Hematology: bleeding secondary to coagulopathy or sickle cell disease papillary necrosis

ONGOING CARE

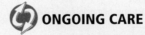

FOLLOW-UP RECOMMENDATIONS

Patient Monitoring

A healthy child with asymptomatic isolated hematuria and a negative workup should be reassessed annually with a complete physical exam, measurement of BP, and urinalysis. If hematuria is persistent, periodic assessment of renal function should also be performed. The development of significant proteinuria, hypertension, elevated creatinine, family history of renal failure, or other concerns should prompt evaluation by a pediatric nephrologist.

PROGNOSIS

- Most children with asymptomatic isolated microscopic hematuria detected on a well-child examination, without proteinuria, hypertension, or azotemia, will NOT be found to have serious underlying pathology and will simply require longitudinal follow-up.
- Many children with hematuria will not have an identifiable cause; however, long-term prognosis is still generally good.
- Children with asymptomatic microscopic or gross hematuria combined with proteinuria have a higher likelihood of glomerular disease.
- Children with a history of stones or hypercalciuria are at increased risk of developing renal stones in the future.
- Familial hematuria secondary to thin GBM disease is a diagnosis of exclusion. Although it often has a benign prognosis, in some families, it can progress to chronic kidney disease. Children should be examined yearly for the development of proteinuria or hypertension.

ADDITIONAL READING

- Bergstein JB, Leiser J, Andreoli S. The clinical significance of asymptomatic gross hematuria and microscopic hematuria in children. *Arch Pediatr Adolesc Med*. 2005;159(4):353–355.
- Cohen RA, Brown RS. Clinical practice. Microscopic hematuria. *N Engl J Med*. 2003;348(23):2330–2338.
- Diven SC, Travis LB. A practical primary care approach to hematuria in children. *Pediatr Nephrol*. 2000;14(1):65–72.
- Feld LG, Meyers KE, Kaplan BS, et al. Limited evaluation of microscopic hematuria in pediatrics. *Pediatrics*. 1998;102(4):E42.
- Patel HP, Bissler JJ. Hematuria in children. *Pediatr Clin North Am*. 2001;48(6):1519–1537.
- Vivante A, Afek A, Frenkel-Nir Y, et al. Persistent asymptomatic isolated microscopic hematuria in Israeli adolescents and young adults and risk for end-stage renal disease. *JAMA*. 2011:306(7):729–736.
- Youn T, Trachtman H, Gauthier B. Clinical spectrum of gross hematuria in pediatric patients. *Clin Pediatr*. 2006;45(2):135–141.

CODES

ICD10

- R31.9 Hematuria, unspecified
- R31.1 Benign essential microscopic hematuria
- R31.0 Gross hematuria

HEMOLYSIS

Julie W. Stern

BASICS

DESCRIPTION
Premature destruction of RBCs, either intravascularly or extravascularly, leading to a shortened red cell survival time. The premature destruction can be caused by intrinsic factors (defects within the RBC itself) or extrinsic factors (factors outside the RBC leads to premature destruction).

EPIDEMIOLOGY
Incidence depends on the cause of hemolysis.

ETIOLOGY

Table 1. Common mechanisms of hemolysis

Acquired (extrinsic) disorders	Hereditary (intrinsic) disorders
Infectious	Hemoglobinopathies
Drug induced	RBC membrane defects
Immune mediated	RBC enzyme defects
Microangiopathic	

RISK FACTORS
- Acquired (extrinsic): ABO and/or Rh incapability is a risk factor in the newborn period.
- Hereditary (intrinsic): Although many hereditary disorders are autosomal dominant, 20% of these patients represent new spontaneous mutations and have no affected family members.

GENERAL PREVENTION
- Acquired (extrinsic): Most causes of acquired, non–transfusion-related hemolytic disease are not preventable.
- Hereditary (intrinsic): Although there is no way to prevent hereditary forms of hemolysis, newborn screening can help identify and allow proper management of some of these conditions. Patients with glucose-6-phosphate dehydrogenase (G6PD) deficiency should be counseled to avoid triggers such as fava beans, broad beans, and mothballs.

DIAGNOSIS

DIFFERENTIAL DIAGNOSIS

Acquired (Extrinsic)
- Allergic/inflammatory/immune
  - Autoimmune hemolytic anemia
    - Warm antibody mediated
    - Cold antibody mediated
    - Hemolytic transfusion reaction
- Congenital/anatomic
  - ABO blood type incompatibility and Rh incompatibility between infant and mother
  - Cardiac lesions with turbulent flow; left-sided more common than right-sided
  - Prosthetic heart valve (especially aortic)
  - Kasabach-Merritt syndrome
  - Hypersplenism
- Infectious
  - Congenital infections with syphilis, rubella, cytomegalovirus, and toxoplasmosis
  - Malaria
  - Bartonellosis
  - *Clostridium perfringens* (via a toxin)
  - *Mycoplasma pneumoniae*
  - HIV
  - Hemolytic uremic syndrome
- Toxic, environmental, drugs
  - Immune complex "innocent bystander" mechanism
    - Quinidine
    - Acetaminophen
    - Amoxicillin
    - Cephalosporins
    - Isoniazid
    - Rifampin
  - Immune complex drug adsorption mechanism
    - Penicillin
    - Cephalosporins
    - Erythromycin
    - Tetracycline
    - Isoniazid
  - Drug-induced autoimmune hemolytic anemia: alpha-methyldopa
  - Toxic drug-induced hemolysis: ribavirin (generally mild and not clinically significant)
  - Snake and spider venoms
  - Extensive burns
- Mechanical hemolysis
  - Cardiac hemolysis
  - Abnormal microcirculation
    - Thrombotic thrombocytopenic purpura (TTP)
    - Disseminated intravascular coagulation (DIC)
    - Malignant hypertension
    - Eclampsia
    - Hemangiomas
    - Renal graft rejection
  - March hemoglobinuria (prolonged physical activity)
- Tumor
  - Lymphomas
  - Thymoma
  - Lymphoproliferative disorders

Hereditary (Intrinsic)
- Genetic/metabolic
  - RBC membrane defects
    - Hereditary spherocytosis (HS)
    - Hereditary elliptocytosis
    - Pyropoikilocytosis
    - Paroxysmal nocturnal hemoglobinuria (can be acquired)
  - Enzyme defects
    - PK deficiency
    - G6PD deficiency
  - Thalassemias (β-thalassemia major is the most severe)
  - Hemoglobinopathies
    - Sickle cell anemia (Hgb SS and SC variants)
    - Unstable hemoglobins

> **ALERT**
> Factors that constitute an emergency:
> - Hemoglobin <5 g/dL, especially with signs of cardiovascular compromise
>   - Attempts to stabilize cardiovascular compromise with volume should be undertaken with care because hemodilution may occur.
>   - Transfusion may be riskier in autoimmune hemolysis because of potential problems with cross-matching.
> - Renal failure may accompany severe hemolysis in TTP or hemolytic uremic syndrome.
> - Hemolysis in the neonatal period secondary to ABO or Rh incompatibility may require exchange transfusion either for anemia or for hyperbilirubinemia.

APPROACH TO THE PATIENT
General goal is to establish existence of hemolysis rather than other causes of anemia, such as blood loss and hypoproduction.
- **Phase 1:** Determine acuity and severity of the anemia and hemolysis:
  - With acute onset, there will be evidence of unstable vital signs and possibly heart failure.
  - Parents may give a history of a rapid deterioration of the child's physical and/or mental state.
  - Patients with chronic anemia that has progressed slowly may have a low hemoglobin yet be well compensated with fairly normal vital signs (except for tachycardia).
  - CBC with a corrected reticulocyte count will help determine if there is an appropriate bone marrow response to the level of anemia and, therefore, whether the process is hypoproductive or hemolytic.
- **Phase 2:** Determine the cause of hemolysis. Treatment approaches will vary depending on the underlying etiology.

HISTORY
- Hemoglobinuria is a sign of intravascular hemolysis, whereas pallor, fatigue, and jaundice may occur with either intravascular or extravascular hemolysis.
- **Question:** History of anemia, splenectomy, or early cholecystectomy in multiple family members?
  - While many hereditary membrane defects and enzyme deficiencies are autosomal dominant, some are autosomal recessive or X-linked. Thus, a negative familial history does not always rule out these diagnoses.
  - In some cases, the diagnosis of HS has not been made, yet multiple family members have had their gallbladders removed at an early age, which may indicate the presence of this defect.
  - Thalassemia (especially β-thalassemia) and sickle cell anemia may present in early childhood with chronic hemolysis with or without a familial history.
- **Question:** History of travel?
  - Malaria is endemic to Africa, India, and parts of Central America.

- **Question:** Drugs and diet history?
  - Specifically ask about exposure to fava beans, mothballs, and antibiotics. Drugs can themselves cause hemolysis or can induce hemolysis if there is an underlying disorder such as G6PD deficiency.
- **Question:** Age at first signs and symptoms of hemolysis (pallor or jaundice)?
  - Hereditary causes of hemolysis are most often chronic or recurrent, although the diagnosis may be delayed until the child is older if the process is mild.
  - Acute, acquired hemolytic disorders may also recur.

PHYSICAL EXAM

Hemolysis that is a secondary problem (e.g., related to infection, tumors) may be found incidentally during evaluation of the primary process.

- **Finding:** Acute processes such as autoimmune hemolytic anemia (both warm and cold antibody mediated) may present with a child in extremis.
  - Tachycardia is a common finding in nearly all cases of acute hemolysis.
  - BP instability is a late finding.
- **Finding:** More chronic processes, such as HS, G6PD, PK deficiencies, thalassemia intermedia, and sickle cell disease, may be picked up at well visits or by laboratory examination.
  - These children often appear well (except for jaundice) but may become more anemic with an acute illness.
- **Finding:** Splenomegaly (often impressive) and hepatomegaly are common findings in extravascular hemolysis.
  - Hepatomegaly may be more pronounced if the child is in heart failure due to acute, severe anemia.
  - Splenomegaly may be either the cause of or, more frequently, a result of a hemolytic process.
  - If significant lymphadenopathy is present, look for an underlying cause such as lymphoproliferative disorders or malignancy.
- **Finding:** Skin changes
  - Pallor is nearly a universal finding in acute hemolysis and in exacerbations of chronic hemolysis.
  - Jaundice is more common in intravascular hemolysis.
  - Presence of ecchymoses or petechiae suggests DIC or thrombocytopenia.

DIAGNOSTIC TESTS & INTERPRETATION

- CBC with differential and reticulocyte count
  - Interpret level of anemia and the reticulocyte count together. Chronic hemolysis in HS, for example, may have a nearly normal hemoglobin count but usually has an increased reticulocyte count.
  - With a rapid fall in hemoglobin, as in acute autoimmune hemolytic anemia, the reticulocyte count may be low at the start, rise in response to anemia, and fall during recovery.
  - Thrombocytopenia should raise suspicions about TTP or hemolytic uremic syndrome.
- Peripheral blood smear
  - Fragmented RBCs, schistocytes, and helmet cells are seen in DIC, TTP, hemolytic uremic syndrome, and cardiac valve hemolysis.
  - Helmet or bite cells are nearly pathognomonic for G6PD deficiency.
  - Other findings on the smear that may be helpful are spherocytes (HS and warm autoimmune hemolytic anemia), target cells (hemoglobin C and thalassemias), and acanthocytes (anorexia nervosa).
- Bilirubin
  - Total and unconjugated bilirubins are elevated in most cases.
- Urinalysis
  - Hemoglobinuria is present in intravascular hemolysis; established by a urine dipstick positive for heme with no intact red cells microscopically
  - Myoglobinuria can also give this picture.
- Coombs test
  - Direct Coombs test (direct antiglobulin test) detects antibodies or complement fragments present on the patient's RBCs.
  - Indirect antiglobulin test detects antibodies in the patient's serum that can bind normal RBCs.
  - Direct antiglobulin test provides direct evidence of immune-mediated hemolysis.
  - Warm antibody autoimmune hemolytic anemia is caused by an IgG antibody that coats RBCs, which are subsequently removed by the spleen.
  - Cold antibody autoimmune hemolytic anemia is caused by an IgM antibody that binds RBCs, fixes complement, and can cause both extravascular and intravascular hemolysis.
- Haptoglobin, hemopexin, and lactate dehydrogenase (LDH)
  - In intravascular hemolysis, haptoglobin levels may be undetectable, hemopexin is reduced, and LDH increased.
  - In extravascular hemolysis, haptoglobin is decreased (but detectable) and LDH may be increased but not to the level seen in intravascular hemolysis.
- Bone marrow aspiration
  - Rarely indicated, but if done, erythroid hyperplasia may be seen.
- Blood for diagnostic RBC enzyme or hemoglobinopathy studies must be drawn prior to transfusion.

TREATMENT

ADDITIONAL TREATMENT

General Measures

- Red cell transfusion may be indicated for symptomatic anemia regardless of cause: Rate and volume of blood to be transfused will depend on severity of anemia and speed of onset (generally slower transfusion rate needed in chronic anemia).
- Plasmapheresis for TTP
- Withdrawal of inducing drug/agent (G6PD)

ISSUES FOR REFERRAL

- Most patients with severe, acute hemolysis or an underlying chronic hemolytic disorder will need to be evaluated by a hematologist.
- Suspected RBC membrane and enzyme defects, as well as hemoglobinopathies, should be referred for initial evaluation.

Admission Criteria

Unstable vital signs with acute hemolysis, significant exacerbation of chronic hemolysis

ADDITIONAL READING

- Gallagher PG. Update on the clinical spectrum and genetics of red blood cell membrane disorders. *Curr Hematol Rep*. 2004;3(2):85–91.
- Lo L, Singer ST. Thalassemia: current approach to an old disease. *Pediatr Clin North Am*. 2002;49(6):1165–1191.
- Maisels MJ, Kring E. The contribution of hemolysis to early jaundice in normal newborns. *Pediatrics*. 2006;118(1):276–279.
- Old JM. Screening and genetic diagnosis of haemoglobin disorders. *Blood Rev*. 2003;17(1):43–53.
- Perkins SL. Pediatric red cell disorders and pure red cell aplasia. *Am J Clin Pathol*. 2004;122:S70–S86.
- Shah S, Vega R. Hereditary spherocytosis. *Pediatr Rev*. 2004;25(5):168–172.

CODES

ICD10

- D58.2 Other hemoglobinopathies
- D59.1 Other autoimmune hemolytic anemias
- P58.9 Neonatal jaundice due to excessive hemolysis, unspecified

FAQ

- Q: When are blood transfusions indicated in patients with active hemolysis?
- A: Patients with severe, acute hemolysis that is causing cardiovascular compromise may require a transfusion if the process cannot be stopped with standard therapy (e.g., steroids for warm autoimmune hemolytic anemia, plasmapheresis for TTP). Transfusions must be given slowly if the hemolytic process has been chronic and the patient's blood volume is expanded.
- Q: Can hemolysis always be identified on a peripheral blood smear?
- A: No. Schistocytes, fragments, spherocytes, targets, and other morphology may provide clues to specific diagnoses but are not always present. The presence of a hemolytic process is inferred from a fall in hemoglobin, rise in the reticulocyte count, and elevation of the bilirubin and LDH levels.

HEMOLYTIC DISEASE OF THE NEWBORN

Janice E. Hobbs • Maureen M. Gilmore

BASICS

DESCRIPTION

A hemolytic anemia in newborns due to the destruction of fetal and newborn RBCs by maternal antibodies passively transferred across the placenta; primarily related to ABO blood group or RhD incompatibility

EPIDEMIOLOGY

- ABO incompatibility
  - Occurs in 12% of first pregnancies
  - Only 10–20% become significantly jaundiced, requiring phototherapy.
- Rh incompatibility
  - Incidence of Rh hemolytic disease: 6–7/1,000 live births
  - Prevalence of RhD positive (RhD+) fetus in RhD negative (Rh−) mother: 15%
  - RhD(−) status in 15% of white, 7–8% of black and Hispanic, and 2% of Asian persons
  - 48–55% are heterozygous (Dd)
  - 35–45% are homozygous (DD)
  - Of all Rh-sensitized pregnancies:
    - 9% require intrauterine transfusion.
    - 10% are delivered early and require newborn exchange transfusion.
    - 31% require treatment after a full-term delivery.
    - 50% require no treatment.

RISK FACTORS

- Type O mother pregnant with either type A, B, or AB fetus
- RhD(−) mother becomes pregnant with an RhD(+) fetus; D-antigen is inherited from the father.
- Omitted or failed RhIG (anti-D) prophylaxis
- Only a fraction of women at risk develop antibodies.

GENERAL PREVENTION

- Rh incompatibility: RhIG is given to an RhD(−) woman after any exposure to RhD(+) blood.
  - RhIG is also known by trade names RhoGAM and HyperRHO.
  - Given at 28 weeks, 34 weeks (prophylaxis), and within 72 hours of birth, or following, for example, amniocentesis, abortion, antepartum bleeds
- No prophylaxis for HDN caused by other blood group incompatibilities.

PATHOPHYSIOLOGY

- Isoimmunization—general principles:
  - Passage of fetal RBCs into maternal circulation occurs as a result of asymptomatic transplacental hemorrhage.
  - Initial sensitization of mother from fetomaternal hemorrhage can occur with placental abruption, abortion, ectopic pregnancy, or procedures (CVS, amniocentesis, or cordocentesis).
  - Exposure triggers maternal immune response (anti-D antibodies).
  - Maternal IgG antibodies (Ab) cross the placenta and bind to fetal RBCs. Coated RBCs are then destroyed in the reticuloendothelial system, primarily the spleen.
  - Isoimmunization may lead to hyperbilirubinemia, severe anemia, and potentially hydrops.
  - Extramedullary hematopoiesis in the fetal liver and spleen is a response to severe fetal anemia, leading to hepatosplenomegaly.
- ABO isoimmunization
  - Occurs in type O mothers with a type A or B fetus; clinically a milder hemolysis compared to Rh incompatibility and rarely requires intervention
  - 1% of type O mothers have high titers of IgG Ab against both A and B that cross the placenta and cause HDN.
  - Hemolysis due to anti-A is more common.
  - Hemolysis due to anti-B can be more severe and may require exchange transfusion in the newborn.
- Rh isoimmunization
  - Passage of RhD(+) fetal RBCs which cross the placenta into the circulation of an Rh(−) mother
  - RhD(−) state is the absence of D antigens on RBCs.
  - Decreased risk of RhD sensitization of mother if fetus is also ABO incompatible
  - Rh isoimmunization rarely occurs in first pregnancy.

ETIOLOGY

- Fetomaternal hemorrhage, usually asymptomatic, with maternal immune response to foreign fetal RBC antigens
- Most common systems involved: ABO blood group antigens, with mild HDN, and RhD antigens, with more severe HDN
- 1% of cases involve other RBC antigens, such as Kell, Kidd, Duffy, or MNS blood groups.

DIAGNOSIS

HISTORY

- Maternal exposure to incompatible blood products
- Previous stillbirths and/or abortions
- Neonatal hyperbilirubinemia requiring exchange transfusion in previous pregnancy
- RhIG not given after previous pregnancy or abortion

PHYSICAL EXAM

- Milder cases—hyperbilirubinemia only
- Minimal jaundice at birth but rapidly develops within 24 hours
- Pallor, tachycardia, tachypnea due to CHF secondary to severe anemia
- Generalized edema and massive hepatosplenomegaly in cases with severe anemia and hydrops

DIAGNOSTIC TESTS & INTERPRETATION

Lab

- Antenatal
  - ABO and Rh blood typing of all mothers at first prenatal visit
  - Indirect Coombs test: detects anti-D Ab in maternal serum
  - Father's ABO and Rh type and zygosity (D/D or D/d)
  - Fetal blood group typing from amniotic fluid or fetal cord blood
  - Fetal blood sample to assess degree of anemia in severe cases
- Neonatal
  - Cord blood or neonate red blood cells for ABO and Rh types
  - Hemoglobin (Hgb), hematocrit (Hct), bilirubin (direct and indirect), reticulocyte count
  - Direct Coombs test: detects maternal anti-D Ab already bound to fetal/newborn RBCs
  - Kleihauer-Betke test or flow cytometry: estimates proportion of fetal RBCs in maternal circulation
  - Peripheral smear: nucleated RBCs (spherocytes in ABO disease)

Imaging

- Fetal ultrasound (estimate fetal size, weight, and organomegaly)
- Doppler ultrasonography of fetal middle cerebral artery: peak systolic velocity

Diagnostic Procedures/Other

- Fetal cordocentesis (for fetal anemia)
- Amniocentesis

Pathologic Findings
- Kernicterus
- Extramedullary hematopoiesis
- Hepatosplenomegaly

DIFFERENTIAL DIAGNOSIS
- Hydrops fetalis
  - Hematologic: α-thalassemia, severe G6PD deficiency, twin-to-twin transfusion
  - Cardiac: hypoplastic left heart syndrome, myocarditis, endocardial fibroelastosis, heart block
  - Congenital infections: parvovirus, syphilis, cytomegalovirus (CMV), rubella
  - Renal: renal vein thrombosis, urinary tract obstruction, nephrosis
  - Placental: umbilical vein thrombosis, true knot of umbilical cord
  - Genetic: trisomy 13, 18, 21; triploidy; aneuploidy
  - Other: diaphragmatic hernia

TREATMENT

ADDITIONAL TREATMENT
General Measures
- Antenatal
  - Serial fetal monitoring
  - Intrauterine RBC transfusion: for severely affected fetuses (fetal Hct <25–30%) where early delivery is not possible; usually performed after 20 weeks gestation
  - Early delivery and neonatal resuscitation may be required if with severe HDN.
    - For high-risk fetus after amniocentesis or history of a prior stillbirth or hydrops
- Neonatal
  - Phototherapy, IV hydration, and serial bilirubin monitoring begins immediately.
  - Exchange transfusion: removes sensitized fetal RBCs and circulating bilirubin and also
    - Corrects anemia in severely anemic infants
    - Removes circulating antibodies
- Indications for early exchange transfusion:
  - Cord blood bilirubin >3 mg/dL and Hgb <13 g/dL
  - Bilirubin rising at rate >1 mg/dL/h despite optimal phototherapy
  - Indirect bilirubin ≥20–25 mg/dL or rising to reach that level
  - Hgb of 11–13 g/dL and bilirubin rising at rate >0.5 mg/dL/h despite optimal phototherapy
  - Lower indirect bilirubin triggers are used in preterm or high-risk infants.
- In hydropic infants, immediate partial exchange may be needed to correct anemia and CHF.
- Double-volume exchanges may be needed for hyperbilirubinemia.
- Selection of blood for exchange transfusion:
  - Fresh, washed, CMV-safe, and irradiated, hemoglobin S negative
  - For Rh disease: type O, Rh(−) cross-matched against mother's blood
  - For ABO disease: type O, Rh(−) or Rh compatible cross-matched against mother or infant's serum
  - For other antibodies: antigen-negative RBCs selected to avoid the clinically significant antibody. ABO type-specific blood can be used if baby's type confirmed.
- Risks of exchange transfusion include prolonged neutropenia, thrombocytopenia, late anemia, metabolic abnormalities, arrhythmias, thrombosis, and death.
- Most infants with ABO incompatibility require no treatment or phototherapy only.
- Some infants with milder Rh isoimmunization may have only exaggerated physiologic anemia at 8–12 weeks.
- Avoid drugs that interfere with bilirubin metabolism or its binding to albumin (e.g., sulfonamides, caffeine, and sodium benzoate).

ISSUES FOR REFERRAL
Late anemia: Infants who had HDN are at risk due to reticulocytopenia related to persistent high titers of circulating maternal antibody. Small-volume RBC transfusion may be required.

ADDITIONAL THERAPIES
- Intravenous immunoglobulin (IVIG): in some studies shown to diminish hemolysis and may prevent the need for exchange transfusion
- Oral iron supplementation
- Erythropoietin, with iron, may be used to support infants at high risk for late anemia.

ONGOING CARE

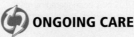

FOLLOW-UP RECOMMENDATIONS
Patient Monitoring
- Hct and reticulocyte count every 1–2 weeks for first 2–3 months, especially for infants who had exchange transfusion, due to risk of late anemia at 8–12 weeks
- Assess for neurodevelopmental delays or neurologic injury.

PROGNOSIS
- ~50% of affected infants have minimal anemia and hyperbilirubinemia and require either no treatment or phototherapy only.
- ~25% with severe HDN will require exchange transfusions.
- Hydropic infants have an ~30% mortality rate.

COMPLICATIONS
- Hydrops fetalis
- Stillbirths
- Kernicterus

ADDITIONAL READING

- Alcock GS, Liley H. Immunoglobulin infusion for isoimmune haemolytic jaundice in neonates. *Cochrane Database of Syst Rev*. 2009;(3):CD003313.
- Chen WX, Wong VC, Wong KY. Neurodevelopmental outcome of severe neonatal hemolytic hyperbilirubinemia. *J Child Neurol*. 2006;21(6):474–479.
- Moise KJ Jr. Management of rhesus alloimmunization in pregnancy. *Obstet Gynecol*. 2008;112(1):164–176.
- Ross MB, Alearcon P. Hemolytic disease of fetus and newborn. *NeoReviews*. 2013;(14):e83–e88.

CODES

ICD-10
- P55.1 ABO isoimmunization of newborn
- P55.0 Rh isoimmunization of newborn
- P55.8 Other hemolytic diseases of newborn

FAQ
- Q: Why does the Rh isoimmunization become worse with each pregnancy?
- A: Most sensitizing fetomaternal hemorrhages occur at delivery. In the first exposure, mother produces IgM Ab, which does not cross the placenta; IgG Ab slowly develops. In second or subsequent pregnancies, repeat exposure to even small amounts of fetal RhD causes rapid production of IgG anti-D, which crosses the placenta and attacks fetal RBCs. Other antibodies, such as Kell, may result in severe HDN even in a first pregnancy.
- Q: Can maternal blood be used to transfuse the affected baby?
- A: Washed maternal blood may be used, but donor infectious disease testing protocols would need to be followed so it would not be routinely available in an emergency situation.
- Q: How does IVIG work, and does it decrease the need of an exchange transfusion?
- A: HDN occurs by destruction of RBCs via an antibody-dependent cytotoxic mechanism mediated by Fc receptors of the neonatal reticuloendothelial system. IVIG nonspecifically blocks these Fc receptors, decreasing hemolysis. In a 2009 Cochrane analysis of IVIG in HDN, results showed a significant decrease in the need for exchange transfusion in those treated with IVIG.

HEMOLYTIC UREMIC SYNDROME

Erica Winnicki • Marsha Lee

BASICS

DESCRIPTION

- HUS is characterized by the triad of acute kidney injury, thrombocytopenia, and hemolytic anemia with fragmentation of erythrocytes (schistocytes noted on peripheral smear).
- Kidney dysfunction may manifest as hematuria and/or proteinuria and/or azotemia.
- HUS is one of the leading causes of acute kidney injury in infants and young children.
- ~90% of childhood cases are associated with Shiga toxin, primarily Shiga toxin–producing *Escherichia coli* (STEC-HUS, or typical HUS), and follow a diarrheal prodrome. *Shigella dysenteriae* is also a well-recognized infectious cause.
- The term "atypical HUS" is used for non-STEC HUS and primarily refers to familial, complement-mediated HUS but encompasses a variety of sporadic causes of HUS including malignancies, *Streptococcus pneumoniae* infection, organ transplantation, pregnancy, collagen vascular disorder, or drugs such as calcineurin inhibitors and antiplatelet agents.
- Atypical forms of HUS have a worse outcome than STEC-HUS.

EPIDEMIOLOGY

- STEC-HUS
  - Tends to occur in the summer months and may be sporadic or occur in epidemic outbreaks
  - Occurs mainly in older infants and young children, between 6 months and 5 years of age
- Atypical HUS
  - Has no seasonal variation and can occur at any age (including early infancy); may be sporadic or familial

GENERAL PREVENTION

- STEC is primarily found in the intestine of ruminants, particularly cattle, and can be transmitted by undercooked beef, unpasteurized milk, or by contamination of water and produce.
- For adequate prevention, practice good hand hygiene, wash food well, and cook food, especially meat, thoroughly.

PATHOPHYSIOLOGY

- Vascular endothelial cell injury is central to the pathogenesis of all forms of HUS.
- STEC colonize colonic mucosa, adhere to mucosal villi, and release Shiga toxin (Stx).
- Stx enters the systemic circulation, where it causes endothelial cell injury via inflammation, upregulation of chemokine and cytokine production, and by binding to endothelial cell surface receptors (Gb_3) and interrupting protein synthesis.
- Endothelial cell injury exposes the thrombogenic basement membrane, causing platelet activation and local intravascular thrombosis.
- In vitro studies show that glomerular endothelial cells and proximal tubular epithelial cells have receptors with very high affinity for the Stx.
- Atypical HUS is caused by dysregulation of the alternate complement pathway.

ETIOLOGY

- STEC-HUS: Most cases are caused by the O157:H7 strain of *E. coli*.
  - STEC most commonly infects children from 6 months to 5 years of age in the summer and the fall. The primary reservoir is cattle.
  - A negative stool culture in a patient who has HUS does not rule out STEC.
- Atypical HUS: Mutations of complement regulatory proteins are identifiable in ~60% of cases, with either an autosomal dominant or recessive inheritance. Reported mutations include complement factor H (most frequent), I, and B; membrane cofactor protein; and C3. Autoantibodies to complement factor H have also been reported.
- One of the common causes of sporadic non–STEC-HUS is *Streptococcus pneumoniae* infection.

DIAGNOSIS

HISTORY

- GI prodrome: STEC-HUS typically develops 5–13 days after the onset of diarrhea (usually bloody). There can be associated vomiting and fever.
- Symptoms of pneumonia or meningitis: *S. pneumoniae*–associated HUS is associated with severe disease.
- Consumption of undercooked meat, particularly hamburger; consumption of unpasteurized milk, cheese, or juice; consumption of raw seed sprouts
- Direct animal contact (petting zoos)
- Family history of HUS (reported in up to 20% of patients with atypical HUS)
- Note that atypical HUS may be triggered by mild infections; presence of diarrhea does not exclude the diagnosis of atypical HUS.

PHYSICAL EXAM

- Pallor and petechiae
- Dehydration secondary to the gastroenteritis
- Edema
- Pulmonary edema (volume overload)
- Hypertension
- Irritability
- Behavioral changes

DIAGNOSTIC TESTS & INTERPRETATION

Lab

- CBC
  - Anemia (Coombs negative), thrombocytopenia ($<150{,}000/mm^3$), leukocytosis (often seen in typical HUS)
- Blood smear: schistocytes
- Markers of hemolysis:
  - Elevated LDH, circulating free hemoglobin, decreased haptoglobin, elevated unconjugated bilirubin, increased reticulocyte count
- Renal function: elevated BUN and serum creatinine
- Serum electrolytes
  - Hyperkalemia (hypokalemia can be observed with severe GI involvement), metabolic acidosis, hyponatremia, hypocalcemia, hyperphosphatemia
- Serum albumin: usually low due to enteral losses and/or hypercatabolic state
- Amylase/lipase: elevated with pancreatic involvement
- Stool culture
  - Should be screened for *E. coli* O157:H7
  - Preferably <6 days after the onset of diarrhea
  - The local health department should be notified of any isolates.
- Identification of Stx from stool

Imaging

- Plain film of the abdomen often demonstrates colonic distension and may show evidence of bowel perforation.
- Barium enema may show "thumb-printing" secondary to bowel wall edema and submucosal bleeding.

Pathologic Findings

Renal biopsy shows thrombotic microangiopathy: hyaline thrombi involving the glomerular capillaries and afferent arterioles with swelling of endothelial cells.

DIFFERENTIAL DIAGNOSIS

- Sepsis
- Diffuse intravascular coagulation
- Vasculitis
- Thrombotic thrombocytopenic purpura (TTP)
- Severe hemolytic anemia
- Malaria

TREATMENT

GENERAL MEASURES

- Treatment of HUS is generally supportive. The mainstay of therapy involves the following:
  - Strict fluid balance
  - Nutritional support
  - Control of hypertension
  - Treatment of seizures

MEDICATION

- Antihypertensives
  - Vasodilators, such as calcium-channel blockers or hydralazine, are useful in the acute phase.
  - After recovery, if a patient persists with hypertension and/or proteinuria, then ACE inhibitors are indicated.
- In patients with seizures, diazepam or lorazepam is preferred. In patients with recurrent seizures or cerebral infarcts, long-term anticonvulsant therapy is indicated.
- Treatment with insulin may be needed in patients with pancreatic necrosis.
- Antibiotics are not indicated for treatment of STEC but would be indicated for patients with invasive bacterial infections or abscesses.
- Avoid antiperistaltic agents for treatment of colitis.

ADDITIONAL TREATMENT

- Renal replacement therapy
  - Intermittent or continuous hemodialysis or peritoneal dialysis
  - For severe acidosis, fluid overload, electrolyte imbalance, or uremia (required in ~2/3 of patients with STEC-HUS).
- Treatment of severe anemia
  - Packed RBCs are transfused slowly if the hemoglobin decreases below 6 g/dL (BP can increase during transfusion).
- Platelet transfusion
  - Indicated only if there is active bleeding and severe thrombocytopenia or the patient needs surgery or invasive procedure (as platelet transfusion can contribute to microthrombi formation).

ADDITIONAL THERAPIES

- Plasma exchange should be initiated in atypical (complement mediated) forms of HUS.
- Eculizumab, a humanized anti-C5 monoclonal antibody that inhibits complement activation, is approved for treatment of atypical HUS. Patients on this medication are at increased risk of serious bacterial infections, including meningococcal infection.
- Patients with typical or atypical forms of HUS who progress to end-stage renal disease should be considered for kidney transplant. Depending on the genotype, patients with atypical HUS should also be considered for liver transplant.

SURGERY/OTHER PROCEDURES

Some patients can have extensive bowel necrosis requiring resection.

INPATIENT CONSIDERATIONS

IV Fluids

Any fluid deficit should be corrected, and additional fluids should be limited to ongoing losses (insensible water loss plus urine and/or GI losses).

Monitoring

Patients generally require ICU-level care. Along with frequent laboratory monitoring and assessment of fluid balance, frequent neurologic assessments should be performed.

ONGOING CARE

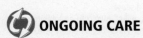

FOLLOW-UP RECOMMENDATIONS

- Resolution is usually heralded by a rise in platelet count and a gradual decrease in the frequency of blood transfusions.
- Pancreatic insufficiency may persist, requiring long-term insulin therapy beyond resolution of acute illness.

DIET

- Adequate nutritional support is important due to the hypercatabolic state of these patients.
- Enteral feeding should be trialed if GI symptoms are not severe, and total parenteral nutrition is used in patients with severe GI involvement.
- Close attention should be paid to fluid, sodium, potassium, and phosphorus intake.
- Some patients can have pancreatic involvement with subsequent exocrine or endocrine pancreatic insufficiency.

PROGNOSIS

- Patients with STEC-HUS can be mildly or severely affected. ~25% of survivors demonstrate long-term renal sequelae such as proteinuria, hypertension, and chronic kidney disease.
  - Mildly affected patients do not develop anuria, almost never have seizures, are rarely hypertensive, do not require dialysis, and have an excellent outcome.
  - Severely affected patients develop anuria and require dialysis, develop hypertension, and may have seizures.
  - They can also progress to end-stage renal disease.
  - Recurrence after kidney transplantation is very uncommon.
- Atypical HUS is associated with a poor prognosis, with mortality in up to 25% of patients and end-stage renal disease in 50% of patients.

COMPLICATIONS

- GI
  - Acute colitis is usually transient.
  - Rectal prolapse, toxic megacolon, bowel wall necrosis, intussusception, perforation, and stricture
  - Pancreatic involvement may result in pancreatitis or insulin-dependent diabetes mellitus.
- CNS
  - CNS involvement occurs in 20–25% of patients and may be acutely life threatening.
  - Most patients have mild CNS symptoms that include irritability, lethargy, and behavioral changes.
  - Major symptoms such as stupor, coma, seizures, cortical blindness, posturing, and hallucinations may also occur. Thrombotic or hemorrhagic stroke may occur.
- Cardiac: Cardiomyopathy may occur.
- Musculoskeletal: rarely, rhabdomyolysis

ADDITIONAL READING

- Joseph C, Gattineni J. Complement disorders and hemolytic uremic syndrome. *Curr Opin Pediatr*. 2013;25(2):209–215.
- Noris M, Remuzzi G. Atypical hemolytic-uremic syndrome. *N Engl J Med*. 2009;361(17):1676–1687.
- Pennington H. *Escherichia coli* O157. *Lancet*. 2010;376(9750):1428–1435.
- Scheiring J, Andreoli S, Zimmerhackl LB. Treatment and outcome of Shiga-toxin-associated hemolytic uremic syndrome (HUS). *Pediatr Nephrol*. 2008;23(10): 1749–1760.
- Trachtman H, Austin C, Lewinski M, et al. Renal and neurological involvement in typical Shiga toxin-associated HUS. *Nat Rev Nephrol*. 2012;8(11): 658–669.

CODES

ICD10

D59.3 Hemolytic-uremic syndrome

FAQ

- Q: What factors should raise concern for atypical HUS?
- A: Age <6 months at presentation, insidious onset, relapsing disease, or failure to identify STEC or Stx in the stool
- Q: How many patients with gastroenteritis from *E. coli* O157:H7 will develop HUS?
- A: 10–15%
- Q: What should the family tell the day care staff and neighbors?
- A: If the patient has enteropathic HUS, contacts should be informed that any episodes of gastroenteritis merit close follow-up for evidence of anemia, thrombocytopenia, and kidney injury. No prophylaxis is indicated. Exclusion of infected children from day care centers until 2 consecutive stool cultures are negative for *E. coli* O157:H7 has been shown to prevent additional transmission.

HEMOPHILIA

Char Witmer

BASICS

DESCRIPTION

- Hemophilia A is factor VIII deficiency, and hemophilia B is factor IX deficiency.
- Deficiency or absence of factor VIII or factor IX leads to a delay and disruption of blood clotting that results in prolonged bleeding.
- The severity of bleeding depends on the baseline percentage of clotting activity.

EPIDEMIOLOGY

- Most common severe inherited bleeding disorder
- Distribution
  - Hemophilia A: 80–85%
  - Hemophilia B: 10–15%
- No geographic or ethnic associations

Incidence

- Hemophilia A: 1 per 5,000 male births
- Hemophilia B: 1 per 30,000 male births

RISK FACTORS

Genetics

- X-linked recessive disorder
- Daughters of fathers with hemophilia are obligate carriers for the hemophilia gene mutation. An obligate carrier has a 50% chance of passing the hemophilia gene mutations to her offspring.
- Carrier status and prenatal testing available
- Hemophilia A
  - The intron 22 inversion mutation in the factor VIII gene is found in ~40–50% of patients with severe hemophilia A.
- Hemophilia B
  - Most factor IX gene defects are single base pair changes that result in missense, frameshift, or nonsense mutations. Mutations have been detected in all regions of the factor IX gene.

GENERAL PREVENTION

- Prophylaxis: the regularly scheduled infusion of clotting factor concentrate with the goal of preventing bleeding episodes; primarily used in patients with severe disease
- Anticipatory guidance and prevention
  - Good dental hygiene
  - Immunizations: no intramuscular injections; give subcutaneously with a small-gauge needle and apply direct pressure.
  - Rapid treatment of hemarthrosis to avoid chronic joint damage
  - Avoidance of contact sports (e.g., football, hockey, rugby)
  - Encourage physical fitness to ensure strong muscles to maintain joint health and prevent joint bleeding.
  - Head trauma precautions

PATHOPHYSIOLOGY

- Both factors VIII and IX are crucial for normal thrombin generation via the intrinsic pathway. The absence or decrease in activity of either protein severely impairs the ability to generate thrombin and fibrin.
- Hemophilia patients do not bleed more rapidly; rather, there is delayed formation of an abnormal clot resulting in prolonged bleeding.

DIAGNOSIS

HISTORY

- Family history
  - Familial history of hemophilia in male offspring of female blood relatives is present in only 70% of cases.
- Excessive bleeding in a male neonate
  - Excessive bleeding with circumcision may be an initial presentation of hemophilia, although only 50% of patients with hemophilia will bleed with circumcision.
  - Muscle bleeding from intramuscular injections (e.g., vitamin K or immunizations); presents as increasing swelling at the site of injection
  - Prolonged bleeding from a torn frenulum, venipuncture, or heel puncture can be seen.
  - 3.5–4% of neonates with hemophilia may present with an intracranial hemorrhage.
- Pattern of bleeding in severe hemophilia
  - Characterized by easy, excessive, and palpable bruising with normal activity, spontaneous joint and muscle hemorrhages, and prolonged hemorrhage after trauma or surgery
- Age of onset of bleeding
  - Bleeding events occur frequently when the child begins to crawl and walk or with the eruption of teeth.
  - Patients with mild hemophilia may not present until they are older.
- Location of hemarthroses
  - Large weight-bearing joints are most often involved: knees, ankles, and hips.
  - Other non–weight-bearing joints can be involved including elbows and shoulders.
- Early symptoms of a hemarthroses:
  - Aura of tingling or warmth, visible swelling
  - Followed by increasing pain and decreasing range of motion (ROM) and inability to bear weight

PHYSICAL EXAM

Joint exam

- Acute hemarthrosis: limitation and pain with ROM, warmth, swelling, tenderness
- Chronic joint changes: crepitus, decreased ROM, synovial hypertrophy, bony abnormalities, and proximal muscle weakness
- Intramuscular hemorrhage: may not have external bruising; pain with motion and swelling; discrepancy in limb circumference
- Distal extremity neurovascular compromise can be a sign of compartment syndrome from bleeding into the forearm.

DIAGNOSTIC TESTS & INTERPRETATION

ALERT

- Neonates have a normal physiologic reduction in the vitamin K–dependent factors, including factor IX, making a determination of the degree of factor IX deficiency difficult in the neonatal period. The factor IX level must be confirmed after 6 months of age.
- When interpreting coagulation testing in a neonate, neonatal normal values for the PT and aPTT are different from those in adults.

Lab

Patients with hemophilia either A or B will have a normal PT and a prolonged aPTT. Assay for factor VIII and factor IX levels:

- <1%: severe hemophilia, characterized by spontaneous bleeding, hemarthroses, and deep tissue hemorrhages
- 1–5%: moderate hemophilia; bleeding following mild to moderate trauma; seldom spontaneous hemorrhage
- 5–30%: mild hemophilia; bleeding only from trauma

DIFFERENTIAL DIAGNOSIS

- Isolated prolonged aPTT associated with increased bleeding tendency:
  - von Willebrand disease
  - "Acquired hemophilia" owing to an inhibitory antibody to factor VIII or IX (extremely rare in children)
  - Hereditary factor deficiency of either VIII, IX, or XI
- Prolonged aPTT without increased bleeding tendency:
  - Factor XII deficiency
  - High-molecular-weight kininogen deficiency
  - Prekallikrein deficiency
  - Antiphospholipid antibody
  - Heparin artifact
  - Underfilling of the specimen tube

TREATMENT

MEDICATION

Acute bleeding episodes:

- Factor replacement
  - Factor VIII replacement products
    - Recombinant, non–plasma-derived factor VIII
    - Plasma-derived, monoclonal antibody–purified factor VIII concentrate; heat or solvent detergent treated for viral inactivation
    - Cryoprecipitate (rarely used)
  - Factor IX replacement products
    - Recombinant, non–plasma-derived factor IX
    - Plasma-derived, immunoaffinity-purified factor IX concentrate; heat or solvent detergent treated for viral inactivation
    - Fresh frozen plasma (rarely used)
- Calculation of dose for pediatrics:
  - Recombinant factor VIII dosing (units) = % desired rise in plasma factor VIII × body weight (kg) × 0.5
  - Recombinant factor IX dosing (units) = % desired rise in plasma factor IX level × body weight (kg) × 1.4
- Target factor levels:
  - Joint bleed: 30–50% for 24–48 hours
  - Large muscle bleed: 70–100% for 24–48 hours
- CNS bleeding: 80–100% maintained for 10–14 days
- Desmopressin (DDAVP)
  - Synthetic vasopressin analog that stimulates release of endogenous factor VIII and von Willebrand factor
  - Only suitable for patients with mild or moderate factor VIII deficiency who have shown a response to DDAVP in a trial
  - Tachyphylaxis (unresponsiveness) may occur with repeated dosing.
  - Hyponatremia may also occur. Fluid restriction is recommended after each dose. Should not be used in neonates.
- Antifibrinolytic therapy (aminocaproic acid or tranexamic acid)
  - Antifibrinolytic therapy is used to stabilize a clot by inhibiting the normal process of clot lysis by the fibrinolytic system.
  - Used for the treatment of oral hemorrhages and to minimize bleeding from dental and some surgical procedures

ADDITIONAL TREATMENT

General Measures

- Joint hemorrhage
  - Factor replacement
  - Immobilization: splints, casts, crutches, and/or bed rest (24–48 hours)
  - Prolonged immobilization may reduce recovery of joint ROM.
  - Initiation of physical therapy with factor coverage may be recommended, particularly after joint surgery.
- Special bleeding situations
  - Intracranial hemorrhage
    - Significant bleeding can occur despite a minor mechanism of head injury and the absence of external bruising.
    - In severe hemophilia, spontaneous intracranial bleeding can occur.
    - Factor replacement to 100% should be administered immediately followed by the diagnostic evaluation.
  - Major surgery
    - Factor replacement to 100% preoperatively and postoperatively
    - Regular dosing of factor for a minimum of 1 week postoperatively, even in mild hemophilia
  - Compartment syndrome
    - Bleeding within the fascial compartments of muscles
    - Most often occurs in the forearm
    - Neurovascular compromise can lead to shortening of the forearm muscles and clawlike deformity of the hand (Volkmann contracture).
  - Iliopsoas bleed
    - Lower abdominal or upper thigh pain may be the first symptom.
    - Exam is notable for inability to extend hip with preservation of internal and external rotation (allows distinction from hemarthrosis of hip joint).
    - Diagnosis confirmed by ultrasound or CT scan
    - Treat with factor replacement and bed rest.
  - Oral bleeding/epistaxis
    - Constant pressure for 15–20 minutes
    - Aminocaproic acid or tranexamic acid
    - Topical thrombin directly to the site of bleeding
    - Factor replacement if these measures don't work.
  - Dental care
    - Factor replacement is required for significant dental procedures like tooth extraction or procedures that require a mandibular block.
    - Factor replacement is not required for routine teeth cleaning.
  - Lacerations
    - Factor replacement is necessary at time of placement and removal of the sutures.
  - Hematuria
    - Increased fluid intake and bed rest as initial treatment
    - If hematuria persists 24–48 hours, 30–40% factor replacement
    - Antifibrinolytics are contraindicated in the setting of hematuria because of the concern of obstructive uropathy from excessive clot formation.
- Patients should be followed regularly at a comprehensive hemophilia treatment center.

INPATIENT CONSIDERATIONS

Initial Stabilization

Life-threatening hemorrhages

- Prompt therapy with clotting factor concentrate should start immediately and prior to any diagnostic procedures.
  - CNS bleeding
  - Bleeding into and around the airway
  - Exsanguinating hemorrhage

ONGOING CARE

COMPLICATIONS

- Complications of disease:
  - Hemophilic arthropathy: Repeated joint hemorrhages lead to synovial thickening and joint cartilage erosion. Joint space becomes narrowed and eventually fuses. Patients can develop joint contractures, limited ROM, and chronic pain.
- Complications of therapy:
  - Inhibitors: antibodies against factor VIII or IX, which can inactivate infused factor. This is currently the most significant complication in hemophilia and is associated with significant morbidity and decreased quality of life. Bleeding episodes are treated with less effective bypassing agents (activated prothrombin complex concentrates or activated recombinant factor VIIa).
  - Anaphylaxis: seen primarily with infusions of factor IX

ADDITIONAL READING

- Ljung R. Intracranial haemorrhage in haemophilia A and B. *Br J Haematol*. 2007;140(4):378–384.
- Pruthi RK. Hemophilia: a practical approach to genetic testing. *Mayo Clin Proc*. 2005;80(11):1485–1499.
- Raffini L, Manno C. Modern management of haemophilic arthropathy. *Br J Haematol*. 2007;136(6):777–787.
- Witmer C, Young G. Factor VIII Inhibitors in hemophilia A: rationale and latest evidence. *Ther Adv Hematol*. 2013;4(1):59–72.
- Zimmerman B. Hemophilia: in review. *Pediatr Rev*. 2013;34(7):289–295.

CODES

ICD10

- D66 Hereditary factor VIII deficiency
- D67 Hereditary factor IX deficiency
- D68.1 Hereditary factor XI deficiency

FAQ

- Q: Are there any medications contraindicated in a child with hemophilia?
- A: Aspirin should not be given as it interferes with platelet function. NSAIDs cause a milder effect on platelets and should also be avoided when possible. Patients with hemophilia should use acetaminophen for fever or pain.
- Q: Can immunizations be given to a child with hemophilia?
- A: To prevent bleeding from immunizations, they can be given SQ (instead of IM) with the smallest gauge needle available. Ice or cold packs should be applied to the area to minimize hematoma formation.

HEMOPTYSIS

Stamatia Alexiou • Suzanne E. Beck

BASICS

DESCRIPTION

- Hemoptysis is the expectoration of blood from the respiratory tract. The term comes from the Greek words *haima*, meaning blood, and *ptysis*, meaning spitting.
- Bleeding from the respiratory tract can range from blood-streaked sputum to massive hemoptysis from the lung. The amount and nature of bleeding should be characterized by taking a careful history.
- The source of bleeding can be anywhere in the respiratory tract, from the nose to the alveolus.
- Consequences of hemoptysis may include exsanguination, hypoxemia, and anemia, or there may be none.

EPIDEMIOLOGY

Large series of pediatric patients with massive hemoptysis have not been described. Most instances of massive hemoptysis take place in older children, usually with an underlying cardiac abnormality.

PATHOPHYSIOLOGY

- Related to the underlying pulmonary or cardiac disease
- Vascular origin of hemoptysis is from 2 locations:
  - Pulmonary arteries: higher volume, lower pressure
  - Bronchial arteries: lower volume, higher pressure

ETIOLOGY

- More common causes:
  - Infection (pneumonia, bronchitis, viral illnesses)
  - Bronchiectasis
  - Cavitary infections (e.g., tuberculosis, abscess, histoplasmosis)
  - Cystic fibrosis
  - Congenital heart disease with collateral vessels or pulmonary hypertension
  - Foreign body aspiration
  - Tracheostomy-related complications
  - Trauma (pulmonary contusion, bronchoscopy, airway manipulation)
  - Aspiration
- Less common causes:
  - Factitious hemoptysis
  - Congenital vascular or airway lesions (pulmonary arteriovenous malformation, hemangioma, bronchogenic cyst, pulmonary sequestration)
  - Hemorrhagic diathesis, including anticoagulant therapy
  - H-type tracheoesophageal fistula
  - Pulmonary embolism
  - Pulmonary hemosiderosis
  - Tumors (teratomas, lymphomas)
  - Immune mediated: Henoch-Schönlein purpura, Goodpasture syndrome, Wegener granulomatosis, polyarteritis nodosa, systemic lupus erythematosus, Heiner syndrome
  - Sarcoidosis

DIAGNOSIS

HISTORY

- Associated symptoms vary and may include cough, chest pain, rhinorrhea, or dyspnea, or there may be none.
- Distinguish the source of bleeding: nose, mouth, gastrointestinal (GI) tract versus lungs:
  - Bleeding from the nose and mouth may be associated with recurrent episodes, recent trauma, or pain at the site and is usually self-limited.
  - Bleeding from the GI tract may be associated with vomiting, history of gastritis, or abdominal pain.
  - Bleeding from the lungs may be associated with chest discomfort or sensations, shortness of breath, or coughing.
  - Blood from the GI tract is often darker and acidic, whereas blood from the airway tends to be bright red and alkaline or pink and frothy.
- Determine amount of bleeding:
  - *Massive*: >240 cc in 24 hours or >100 cc per day for several days
  - *Minor*: smaller volumes
  - Life-threatening hemoptysis is typically defined as greater than 8 cc/kg/day
- Determine associated symptoms/conditions:
  - Familial history of pulmonary disease or bleeding disorder
  - Systemic symptoms (weight loss, may indicate tumor)
  - Exposure to environmental toxins (mold or flood-damaged homes)
  - Exposure to tuberculosis
  - Medication/drug use: cocaine, marijuana, propylthiouracil
  - Recurrent episodes of cough associated with blood-tinged sputum or hemoptysis suggests underlying bronchiectasis or chronic pulmonary infection.
  - Acute pleuritic chest pain raises the possibility of pulmonary embolism with infarction or other pleural lesion.

PHYSICAL EXAM

- Respiratory distress or hypoxemia: indicates significant ventilation–perfusion mismatch due to airspace disease, shunt due to pulmonary embolism, or acidosis due to hypovolemia from blood loss
- Pallor: indicates anemia or poor perfusion
- Pleural friction rub: may be associated with pulmonary embolism
- Loud 2nd heart sound: suggests primary pulmonary hypertension, mitral stenosis, or Eisenmenger syndrome
- Localized wheeze over a major lobar airway: suggests an intramural lesion such as hemangioma, foreign body, or carcinoma
- Presence of a murmur over the lung fields: may suggest pulmonary arteriovenous malformation
- Clubbing: indicates the presence of underlying pulmonary disease such as cystic fibrosis, congenital cardiovascular disease, bronchiectasis, or liver disease

DIAGNOSTIC TESTS & INTERPRETATION

Lab

- Complete blood count, reticulocyte count, and coagulation profile: may indicate the degree of blood loss or evidence of a bleeding diathesis
- Comprehensive metabolic panel: to determine hepatic and renal function, acid–base status
- Sputum for bacterial culture, Gram stain, and acid-fast bacilli
- Purified protein derivative (PPD) testing
- Drug screen: if appropriate
- Electrocardiogram: to determine presence of right ventricular hypertrophy
- Erythrocyte sedimentation rate and C-reactive protein can help identify the chronicity of the bleed.
- Antinuclear antibodies (ANA), antineutrophil cytoplasmic antibody (ANCA), and antibodies to double-stranded DNA (anti-dsDNA) can help identify an immune-mediated etiology.

Imaging

- Chest radiograph, both anteroposterior and lateral
  - May reveal pleural effusion, bronchiectasis, foreign bodies, or consolidation
  - Fleeting alveolar infiltrates suggest pulmonary hemorrhage.
- Computed tomography (CT)
  - Useful when chest radiographs and fiberoptic bronchoscopy are normal
  - High-resolution CT may identify an area of bleeding, especially if bronchiectasis and arteriovenous malformation are suspected.
  - A CT angiography is helpful to directly visualize the vessel during interventional treatment.
- Ventilation–perfusion scans: helpful if a pulmonary embolism or infarct is suspected

Diagnostic Procedures/Other

- Flexible fiberoptic bronchoscopy
  - Usually performed to localize the site of bleeding; preferred over rigid bronchoscopy to identify a distal or alveolar bleed
  - If a bronchoalveolar lavage is performed, the presence of hemosiderin-laden macrophages can help identify the time of onset because they usually appear 48 hours after the onset of bleeding and can remain present for up to several weeks following the event.
- Rigid bronchoscopy is preferred for removal of foreign objects or masses in the proximal airway. The wide lumen provides airway stabilization and a means to ventilate the patient during the procedure.

DIFFERENTIAL DIAGNOSIS

- Infections
  - Pneumonia
  - Pulmonary abscess
  - Tuberculosis
  - Bronchitis
- Pulmonary disease
  - Cystic fibrosis
  - Bronchiectasis
  - Foreign body aspiration
  - Arteriovenous malformation
  - Congenital lung malformation
  - Pulmonary emboli
  - Pulmonary hemosiderosis
  - Alveolar capillaritis
  - Aspiration
  - Isolated unilateral pulmonary agenesis
  - Bronchogenic cysts
- Cardiovascular disease
  - Congenital heart malformations
  - Pulmonary hypertension
- Collagen vascular disease
  - Systemic lupus erythematosus
  - Vasculitis
  - Goodpasture disease
  - Wegener granulomatosis
  - Heiner syndrome
- Trauma
- Coagulation disorder
- Other
  - Munchausen syndrome
  - Pseudohemoptysis (red-colored sputum secondary to *Serratia marcescens* production of red pigment)
  - Neoplasms
  - Hemangiomas

TREATMENT

GENERAL MEASURES

- Initial management is supportive and should be aimed at identifying the underlying cause.
- Blood loss should be replaced using colloidal solutions (i.e., normal saline, Ringer lactate) until red blood cells become available.
- Methods used to stop localized bleeding:
  - Tamponade with balloon-tipped catheter
  - Ice water lavage
  - Local instillation of epinephrine
  - Catheter-directed umbilication
  - IV vasopressin
  - Bronchial artery embolization
  - Surgical resection is usually reserved for the most difficult cases such as extensive collateralization of bronchial arteries or arteriovenous malformations unresponsive to embolization.
  - Other techniques include endoscopic instillation of fibrinogen/thrombin and endobronchial argon plasma coagulation.

ONGOING CARE

PROGNOSIS

- Depends on the etiology and severity of hemoptysis
- Immediate airway management reduces morbidity and mortality.

COMPLICATIONS

- Respiratory insufficiency
- Acute airway obstruction
- Hypovolemic shock
- Anemia
- Pneumonia
- Death

ADDITIONAL READING

- Gaude GS. Hemoptysis in children. *Indian Pediatr*. 2010;47(3):245–254.
- Hurt K, Bilton D. Haemoptysis: diagnosis and treatment. *Acute Med*. 2012;11(1):39–45.
- Salih ZN, Akhter A, Akhter J. Specificity and sensitivity of hemosiderin-laden macrophages in routine bronchoalveolar lavage in children. *Arch Pathol Lab Med*. 2006;130(11):1684–1686.
- Susarla SC, Fan LL. Diffuse alveolar hemorrhage syndromes in children. *Curr Opin Pediatr*. 2007;19(3):314–320.

CODES

ICD10

- R04.2 Hemoptysis
- P26.9 Unsp pulmonary hemorrhage origin in the perinatal period

H

HENOCH-SCHÖNLEIN PURPURA

Blaze Robert Gusic

BASICS

DESCRIPTION

- Henoch-Schönlein purpura (HSP) is an immunologically mediated, purpuric, nonthrombocytopenic, and systemic vasculitis involving the small blood vessels of the skin, gastrointestinal (GI) tract, joints, and kidneys.
- Defined by the presence of 2 of the following:
  - Palpable purpura (without thrombocytopenia)
  - Age of onset <20 years
  - Abdominal pain
  - Granulocytic infiltration of vessel walls
    - In children, only palpable purpura with normal platelet count needs be documented.
    - Although most children do have purpura, colicky abdominal pain, and arthritis, up to 1/2 may present with symptoms other than purpura.

EPIDEMIOLOGY

Incidence

- Incidence of 13.5 cases per 100,000 school-aged children per year (90% of patients are <10 years)
- Most common acute vasculitis in childhood
- Slight male predominance

RISK FACTORS

Genetics

Familial history of IgA-related disorders or inherited defects in complement (C2, C4 deficiency) may predispose to HSP.

PATHOPHYSIOLOGY

- Considered to be an immune-mediated vasculitic disorder involving primarily IgA, specifically subclass IgA1
- IgA from mucosal B cells interacts with IgG to form immune complexes that activate the alternate pathway of the complement system.
- Circulating IgA is deposited in the affected organs, causing the inflammatory process.
- Capillaries, arterioles, and venules are affected in HSP as opposed to polyarteritis nodosa, granulomatosis with polyangiitis (Wegener granulomatosis), and systemic lupus erythematosus (SLE), where small arteries are affected.
- Biopsy of the involved kidneys shows endocapillary proliferative glomerulonephritis involving endothelial and mesangial cells. Crescent formation may also be present. IgA, IgG, C3, and fibrin are commonly found in the mesangial regions.

ETIOLOGY

- No single etiologic agent has been identified.
- Most cases are associated with preceding upper respiratory tract infections (URIs), usually group A β-hemolytic streptococci. A recent study shows a significant association with *Bartonella henselae*. Also reported following infections with parvovirus, adenovirus, hepatitis A virus, *Helicobacter pylori*, and *Mycoplasma pneumoniae*; parvovirus B19 previously proposed, but evidence is inconclusive
- Also reported after drug ingestion (e.g., thiazides) and insect bites

DIAGNOSIS

HISTORY

- Previous illness: especially infections such as hepatitis, URI, and streptococcal infections
- Abdominal pain
  - Pain is the most common GI tract symptom and may precede the rash by up to 2 weeks.
  - 2/3 of children have GI tract symptoms. Emesis and melena are also reported.
- Transient, nondeforming, nonmigratory arthritis of knees, ankles, wrists, elbows, and digits is a frequent problem and most common in knees and ankles.
- Presence of testicular pain or scrotal swelling, headache, cough, and hematuria suggests vasculitic lesions in the associated system.

PHYSICAL EXAM

- Pay particular attention to blood pressure: Hypertension is common.
- Low-grade fever is present in 50% of the cases.
- Rash that is petechial or purpuric in a pressure-dependent symmetric distribution, usually around the lateral malleoli of the ankles, on the ventral surfaces of the feet, and on the buttocks
- Purpura may be briefly preceded by maculopapular or urticarial lesions.
- Lesions may ulcerate or present as hemorrhagic bullae.
- Joints should be examined for swelling and limitation of motion: Redness and warmth are not common. Symptoms precede the rash by up to 2 weeks in 25% of patients.
- Nonpitting subcutaneous edema of the scalp, periorbital region, hands, and feet is often noted.
- Generalized edema is more common in children <3 years of age. The edema may lead to acute hemorrhagic edema, now considered to be a variant of HSP.
- Abdomen is often tender to palpation but without rebound tenderness. Hepatosplenomegaly may be found. Because intussusception and appendicitis are possible complications, serial examinations may be necessary to determine if radiographic studies are indicated.
- Symptoms of pancreatitis may appear after the onset of the rash but may be a rare presenting symptom.
- Orchitis, where affected testicle may be tender and swollen
  - Swelling and bruising may be noted on the scrotum.
  - Testicular torsion has also been reported in HSP and may mimic orchitis.
- Neurologic changes
  - CNS involvement may present with headaches, seizures, or behavioral changes.
  - Guillain-Barré syndrome has been reported.

DIAGNOSTIC TESTS & INTERPRETATION

There are no definitive diagnostic tests.

Lab

- CBC
  - Normal platelet count differentiates from thrombocytopenic purpura.
  - Hemoglobin is usually normal.
  - Leukocytosis (especially eosinophilia), may be present.
- ESR: elevated in about 60% of cases
- Prothrombin (PT) and partial thromboplastin time (PTT): normal
- IgA: often elevated in the acute phase of illness, with normal or increased IgG and IgM
- C3: normal (decreased in poststreptococcal glomerulonephritis and SLE)
- Antinuclear antibody: negative (elevated in SLE)
- Von Willebrand factor antigen elevated with active HSP due to endothelial damage
- Throat swab for group A β-hemolytic streptococci: positive in up to 75% of cases
- Serum chemistries: Elevated BUN and creatinine levels and decreased protein and albumin are seen with renal involvement.
- Urinalysis
  - Gross hematuria and proteinuria are present in many patients.
  - Proteinuria alone is rare.
  - Microscopic blood, RBCs, WBCs, and casts suggest glomerulonephritis.
- Stool guaiac: GI tract involvement may present as guaiac-positive stools, bloody stools, or melena.

Imaging

- Chest radiograph: may show interstitial lung disease
- Abdominal ultrasound: may be helpful if intussusception or appendicitis suspected
- Barium enemas are *not* indicated for suspected intussusception.
  - They will not reduce the ileoileal intussusception common to HSP (idiopathic intussusception is usually ileocolic in location).
  - Barium enema may damage or perforate the inflamed bowel.
- Testicular ultrasound if torsion of the testes or appendix testes, known complications of HSP, suspected on clinical exam

Diagnostic Procedures/Other

- Renal biopsy: With severe renal failure, a biopsy should be performed to determine the extent of disease.
- Skin biopsy: Direct immunofluorescence for IgA can be helpful in confirming the diagnosis.

DIFFERENTIAL DIAGNOSIS

- Petechial and purpuric rashes seen in thrombocytopenia from the following:
  - Idiopathic thrombocytopenic purpura (ITP)
  - Meningococcemia
  - Rocky Mountain spotted fever
  - Leukemia
  - Hemolytic uremic syndrome (HUS)
  - Coagulopathies

- Vasculitic rashes may result from primary and secondary vasculitides.
  - Polyarteritis nodosa
  - Granulomatosis with polyangiitis (Wegener granulomatosis)
  - Infection related
  - Connective tissue diseases (e.g., SLE), Berger disease (IgA nephropathy)
  - Glomerulonephritis similar to HSP both clinically and immunologically but not associated with the skin, GI tract, or joint manifestations of HSP streptococcal glomerulonephritis
  - Infantile acute hemorrhagic edema
  - Vasculitis that presents with urticarial or maculopapular rash, which then becomes purpuric
  - It is differentiated from HSP in that it usually affects children from 4 months to 2 years of age and is not associated with systemic symptoms.
  - On biopsy, IgA deposits are not as consistent a finding as with HSP.
  - Juvenile idiopathic arthritis
  - Rheumatic fever

TREATMENT

MEDICATIONS

- HSP usually resolves spontaneously without specific therapy.
- Analgesics and NSAIDs may be used for control of joint pain and inflammation, but salicylates and other agents that affect platelet function should be avoided if GI tract bleeding is present.
- Steroids are used for painful cutaneous edema, arthritis, and abdominal pain (2 mg/kg/24 h of prednisone until clinical resolution); however, steroids have not been shown to affect purpura or to decrease duration of disease or frequency of recurrences.
  - No consensus on management of GI and renal involvement. Oral prednisone at 2 mg/kg/24 h has shown faster resolution of abdominal pain, whereas other studies indicate that the symptoms will resolve similarly without intervention.
  - Steroids may mask associated problems such as intussusception and bowel perforation.
  - In nephritis, immediate treatment with steroids may prevent more serious renal disease; however, most will improve spontaneously. Treatment should be considered for children at high risk for chronic renal insufficiency or failure (those presenting with nephrotic syndrome or renal insufficiency).
- >50% crescentic glomerulonephritis on renal biopsy has a greater risk of future renal failure. Such cases should be considered for aggressive therapy with pulse or oral steroids and/or immunosuppressants (azathioprine, cyclophosphamide, cyclosporine) or plasmapheresis and intravenous immunoglobulin (IVIG). There are rare reports of treatment with danazol and fish oil.
- Treatment of hypertension may delay or prevent progression of renal disease in patients with glomerulonephritis.

ONGOING CARE

FOLLOW-UP RECOMMENDATIONS

Patient Monitoring

- Patients should be seen weekly during the acute illness. Visits should include history and physical exam, along with BP measurement and urinalysis. Urine spot protein-to-creatinine ratio should be followed when proteinuria is present.
- All patients, even those who did not present with renal involvement, should have urine monitored for 6 months; however, there is no consensus on frequency. Previous evidence recommended weekly for 6 months. Recent studies recommend weekly studies only for the first 2 months. This recommendation is based on findings that the risk for developing nephritis is less than 2% after 2 months. Others suggest less frequent urinalysis (day 7; day 14; then 1,3, and 6 months) may be sufficient, with more intense follow-up if renal involvement is noted.
- Women with a history of HSP should be monitored during pregnancy.

PROGNOSIS

- Generally excellent: Most (>60%) children are better within 4 weeks of the onset.
- Better prognosis associated with younger age
- Recurrence within the first 6 weeks in up to 40%, usually as rash and abdominal pain
- No laboratory or clinical findings have been found to be predictive of recurrence.
- Most have only 1–3 episodes of purpura; however, a few will continue to experience symptoms for months or years. These patients have a poor prognosis and are more likely to develop severe nephritis.
- GI tract disease accounts for the most significant morbidity in the short term.
- Renal involvement is the cause of the most serious long-term morbidity. Microscopic hematuria alone or with mild proteinuria generally has a good outcome. A nephritic and nephrotic combination is more guarded, and those patients with a high percentage of crescent formation have worse outcomes.

COMPLICATIONS

- Persistent hypertension
- End-stage kidney disease (acute or as a late sequela)
- Intussusception (most common GI tract complication; affecting 1–5% of patients)
- Protein-losing enteropathy
- Hemorrhagic pancreatitis
- Hydrops of the gallbladder
- Strictures of the esophagus and ileus
- Bowel perforations, ischemia, and infarctions
- Pseudomembranous colitis
- Appendicitis
- Skin necrosis
- Subarachnoid, subdural, and cortical hemorrhage and infarction
- Peripheral mononeuropathies and polyneuropathies (Guillain-Barré syndrome)
- Pulmonary hemorrhage (uncommon, but may result in death)
- Torsion of the testis and appendix testes and priapism, scrotal swelling, and pain

ADDITIONAL READING

- Gedalia A, Cuchacovich R. Systemic vasculitis in childhood. *Curr Rheumatol Rep*. 2009;11(6):402–409.
- Jauhola O, Ronkainen J, Koskimies O, et al. Renal manifestations of Henoch-Schonlein purpura in a 6-month prospective study of 223 children. *Arch Dis Child*. 2010;95(11):877–882.
- Peru H, Soylemezoglu O, Bakkaloglu SA, et al. Henoch Schönlein purpura in childhood: clinical analysis of 254 cases over a 3-year period. *Clin Rheumatol*. 2008;27(9):1087–1092.
- Piram M, Mahr A. Epidemiology of immunoglobulin A vasculitis (Henoch-Schonlein): current state of knowledge. *Curr Opin Rheumatol*. 2013;25(2):171–178.
- Prais D, Amir J, Nussinovitch M. Recurrent Henoch-Schonlein purpura in children. *J Clin Rheumatol*. 2007;13(1):25–28.
- Sinclair P. Henoch-Schönlein purpura—a review. *Curr Allergy Clin Immunol*. 2010;23(3):116–120.
- Watson L, Richardson AR, Holt RC, et al. Henoch Schonlein purpura—a 5-year review and proposed pathway. *PLoS ONE*. 2012;7(1):e29512.
- Zaffanello M, Fanos V. Treatment-based literature of Henoch-Schönlein purpura nephritis in childhood. *Pediatr Nephrol*. 2009;24(10):1901–1911.

CODES

ICD10

D69.0 Allergic purpura

FAQ

- Q: When should I consider hospitalization for HSP?
- A: Often it is not necessary. Severe complications require admission. These include GI hemorrhage, orchitis, protein-losing enteropathy requiring total parenteral nutrition (TPN), decreased glomerular filtration rate (GFR) or hypertension, and pulmonary hemorrhage.
- Q: Is there a role for prophylactic penicillin?
- A: In patients with frequent relapses in whom group A β-hemolytic streptococci is often the inciting agent, administration of penicillin may be helpful.
- Q: Who are Henoch and Schönlein?
- A: The clinical finding of joint pain associated with purpura was named "purpura rheumatica" in 1837 by Schönlein. Henoch, a student of Schönlein's, later described the association of GI tract and renal involvement. However, the 1st report was by Heberden in 1801. Of note, it has been speculated that Mozart—whose symptoms included fever, vomiting, exanthem, arthritis, anasarca, and coma—died of HSP.

HEPATOMEGALY

Sivan Kinberg • Sarah S. Lusman

BASICS

DESCRIPTION

Hepatomegaly is enlargement of the liver beyond age-adjusted normal values. It can be due to intrinsic liver disease or associated with systemic diseases seen in infants and children.

- Normal liver size
  - Depends on age, gender, and body size
  - Average liver span is 4.5–5 cm (neonates), 6–6.5 cm (12-year-old girls), 7–8 cm (12-year-old boys), and up to 16 cm (adults).

PATHOPHYSIOLOGY

- Inflammation (hepatitis)
- Excessive storage
- Infiltration
- Vascular congestion
- Biliary obstruction

DIAGNOSIS

HISTORY

Obtain a detailed history to identify potential risk factors for liver disease and to evaluate for underlying systemic disease.

- **Question:** Prenatal history suggesting possible TORCH infection or HIV infection?
  - Infections may cause hepatomegaly.
- **Question:** Prolonged hyperbilirubinemia after 2 weeks of age?
  - Could suggest biliary atresia, cystic fibrosis, alpha-1 antitrypsin deficiency
- **Question:** Developmental delay or poor growth?
  - Could suggest a metabolic disorder
- **Question:** Family history of early infant death or hepatic, neurodegenerative, or psychiatric disease?
  - Could suggest a metabolic disorder
- **Question:** Sexual activity, intravenous (IV) drug use, tattoo?
  - Risk factors for hepatitis B and C infections and HIV; also consider gonococcal perihepatitis (Fitz-Hugh–Curtis syndrome) and syphilis
- **Question:** Foreign travel?
  - Parasitic infection or liver abscess
- **Question:** Pruritus?
  - Can be a subtle sign of cholestasis
- **Question:** Contaminated shellfish?
  - Source of large outbreaks of hepatitis A
- **Question:** Previous total parenteral nutrition (TPN)?
  - Can lead to cholestasis, bile duct proliferation, fatty infiltration, and early cirrhosis
- **Question:** Medications, supplements, and recreational drug use?
  - Many commonly used medications can be hepatotoxic; ask about vitamin A, alcohol, and certain mushroom species.
- **Question:** Other chronic illnesses?
  - Heart disease: liver enlargement from CHF
  - Cystic fibrosis: related liver disease
  - Diabetes mellitus: increased glycogen secretion
  - Severe anemia: extramedullary hematopoiesis
  - Inflammatory bowel disease: increased likelihood of primary sclerosing cholangitis
  - Obesity: nonalcoholic fatty liver disease

PHYSICAL EXAM

Perform a careful physical exam to look for clues to etiology and for signs of chronic liver disease.

- **Finding:** Liver edge?
  - Children <2 years: can be normal up to 3.5 cm below costal margin; however, if >2 cm, further workup or referral may be indicated.
  - Children >2 years: normal up to 2 cm
  - Verify all suspected cases of hepatomegaly by checking the liver span.
- **Finding:** Signs of chronic liver disease?
  - Liver is usually firm and enlarged; can decrease in size with advanced disease
  - Splenomegaly, ascites, caput medusae, spider angiomas, esophageal varices, and hemorrhoids suggest portal hypertension.
  - Also look for signs of occult bleeding or bruising due to vitamin K deficiency.
- **Finding:** Tender liver?
  - May indicate hepatitis or acutely congested liver secondary to right-sided heart failure or Budd-Chiari syndrome
- **Finding:** Splenomegaly?
  - In the context of chronic liver disease, implies portal hypertension
  - In the context of other signs of viral illness, suggests acute viral hepatitis
  - In the absence of these signs, suggests storage disease or malignancy
- **Finding:** Coarse facial features?
  - Suggests mucopolysaccharidoses
- **Finding:** Kayser-Fleischer rings or cataracts?
  - Suspect Wilson disease

DIAGNOSTIC TESTS & INTERPRETATION

All patients with hepatomegaly should have a laboratory evaluation. History and physical exam should direct laboratory and further testing.

Lab

- CBC with differential
  - Thrombocytopenia may suggest portal hypertension.
- Comprehensive metabolic panel
  - Elevated aspartate aminotransferase (AST) and alanine aminotransferase (ALT) can reflect the amount of damage to hepatocytes. Elevations >1,000 IU/L indicate severe damage. ALT is more liver-specific.
  - Albumin assesses synthetic function.
  - Hyperbilirubinemia suggests cholestasis (direct hyperbilirubinemia) or hemolytic disease (indirect hyperbilirubinemia).
- Prothrombin time (PT)
  - Assesses synthetic function
  - Prolongation can occur with an acute injury or illness.
  - Can also be prolonged due to vitamin K deficiency
- Gamma-glutamyl transferase (GGT) and alkaline phosphatase
  - Elevation of GGT out of proportion to elevation in aminotransferases can indicate an obstructive or infiltrative process.
  - If an elevated GGT is associated with elevations in bilirubin, cholesterol, and alkaline phosphatase, an obstructive process is more likely.
- Ammonia level
  - Important to send on ice
  - Increasing ammonia levels, with prolonged PT, can suggest liver failure.
- Viral hepatitis serology
  - Hepatitis A IgM, hepatitis B surface antigen, hepatitis B surface antibody, hepatitis B core antibody, hepatitis C antibody
  - Should be obtained in patients with suggestive prodromal illness
- EBV and CMV IgM/IgG
- Monospot
  - Nonspecific heterophile antibody test for Epstein-Barr virus infection; can be predictive in association with an elevation of atypical lymphocytes
  - High false-negative rate in children <4
- α-Fetoprotein and carcinoembryonic antigen
  - Tumor markers for hepatoblastoma and hepatocellular carcinoma, respectively
- TORCH titers
  - Consider in newborns with hepatomegaly
- Autoimmune markers
  - Serum immunoglobulins, antinuclear antibody, anti–smooth muscle antibody, anti-liver/kidney microsomal antibody, soluble liver antigen
- Ceruloplasmin and urinary copper excretion
  - Wilson disease: decreased ceruloplasmin and increased urinary copper excretion
  - Consider for patients with unexplained liver disease and neurologic symptoms
- Iron, total-iron binding capacity (TIBC), ferritin
  - To assess for hemochromatosis
- Alpha-1 antitrypsin phenotype
  - To look for alpha-1 antitrypsin deficiency
  - Only send if no blood transfusion in last month

Imaging

- Abdominal ultrasound with Doppler
  - Most helpful initial study
  - Perform in all patients with acholic stools, asymmetric liver enlargement or mass
  - Can measure liver size and consistency, masses, cysts, abscesses, biliary tree abnormalities, and venous blood flow
- CT or MRI can be done for further evaluation.
- Echocardiogram to assess heart function

Pathologic Findings

Liver biopsy is often needed for definitive diagnosis.

ALERT

Refer to gastroenterologist or hepatologist if

- Unexplained or persistent elevation of liver enzymes
- Decreased synthetic function or signs of portal hypertension

DIFFERENTIAL DIAGNOSIS

Inflammation (hepatitis)

- Infections
  - Viral infections
    - Hepatitis types A–E
    - Epstein-Barr virus
    - Cytomegalovirus
    - Coxsackievirus
  - Congenital infections
    - TORCH
    - HIV
  - Bacterial infections
    - Hepatic abscess
    - Tuberculosis
    - Sepsis

- Parasitic infections
  - Amebiasis
  - Flukes
  - Schistosomiasis
  - Malaria
- Fungal diseases
  - Candidiasis
  - Histoplasmosis
- STDs
  - Gonococcal perihepatitis
  - Syphilis
  - HIV
- Zoonotic diseases
  - Brucellosis
  - Leptospirosis
  - *Bartonella henselae*
  - *Pasteurella multocida*

- Toxic, metabolic, drugs
  - Acetaminophen
  - Alcohol
  - Corticosteroids
  - Erythromycin
  - Hypervitaminosis A
  - Iron
  - Isoniazid
  - Nitrofurantoin
  - Oral contraceptives
  - Phenobarbital
  - Valproate
- Autoimmune
  - Autoimmune hepatitis
  - Sarcoidosis
  - Systemic lupus erythematosus

Storage disorders

- Glycogen
  - Glycogen storage disease
  - Diabetes mellitus
  - TPN
- Lipids
  - Wolman disease
  - Niemann-Pick disease
  - Gaucher disease
- Fat
  - Nonalcoholic fatty liver disease
  - Cystic fibrosis
  - Fatty acid oxidation defect
  - Mucopolysaccharidoses
  - Reye syndrome
- Iron
  - Hemochromatosis
- Copper
  - Wilson disease
- Abnormal proteins
  - Alpha-1 antitrypsin deficiency

Infiltration

- Tumors
  - Benign tumors
    - Hemangioma
    - Hemangioendothelioma
    - Mesenchymal hamartoma
    - Focal nodular hyperplasia
    - Adenoma
  - Malignant tumors
    - Hepatoblastoma
    - Hepatocellular carcinoma
  - Metastatic tumors
    - Leukemia
    - Lymphoma
    - Neuroblastoma
    - Wilms tumor
    - Histiocytosis
- Cysts
  - Choledochal cysts
  - Parasitic cysts
  - Polycystic liver disease
- Amyloidosis
- Granulomatous disease
- Hemophagocytic syndromes
- Extramedullary hematopoiesis

Vascular congestion

- Intrahepatic
  - Veno-occlusive disease
  - Budd-Chiari syndrome (hepatic vein thrombosis)
- Suprahepatic
  - Congestive heart failure
  - Pericardial disease
  - Suprahepatic web

Biliary obstruction

- Biliary atresia
- Alagille syndrome
- Choledochal cyst
- Cholelithiasis
- Tumors
- Primary sclerosing cholangitis

ALERT

Indications for immediate hospitalization:

- Persistent anorexia and vomiting
- Mental status changes
- Worsening jaundice
- Relapse of symptoms after initial improvement
- Known exposure to a liver toxin
- Rising PT/INR
- Rising ammonia level
- Bilirubin >20 mg/dL
- AST $>2{,}000$
- Development of new ascites
- Hypoglycemia
- Leukocytosis and thrombocytopenia
- Hematemesis

TREATMENT

Depends on underlying etiology of hepatomegaly.

ADDITIONAL READING

- Clayton PT. Diagnosis of inherited disorders of liver metabolism. *J Inherit Metab Dis*. 2003;26(2–3): 135–146.
- Diehl-Jones WL, Askin DF. The neonatal liver part II: assessment and diagnosis of liver dysfunction. *Neonatal Netw*. 2003;22(2):7–15.
- Wolf AD, Lavine JE. Hepatomegaly in neonates and children. *Pediatr Rev*. 2000;21(9):303–310.

CODES

ICD10

- R16.0 Hepatomegaly, not elsewhere classified
- B19.9 Unspecified viral hepatitis without hepatic coma
- K76.1 Chronic passive congestion of liver

FAQ

- Q: Why does cholestasis cause pruritus?
- A: This phenomenon probably reflects an abnormal accumulation of bile acids in the skin.
- Q: Do patients with chronic liver disease have any different nutritional needs?
- A: Yes. Patients may have impaired fat absorption and therefore may have deficiencies of fat-soluble vitamins A, D, E, and K, which can lead to visual disturbances, rickets, pathologic fractures, neuropathy, hemolytic anemia, or bleeding. Consider supplementing the diet with medium-chain triglycerides, which are more easily absorbed.
- Q: What causes TPN-associated cholestasis?
- A: It is likely multifactorial. TPN components act as toxins; bacterial endotoxins and lack of enteral feeding also play significant roles.
- Q: What conditions can mimic hepatomegaly?
- A: Riedel lobe is an extended, tongue-like, right lobe of the liver and is a normal variant. A normal liver can be displaced by pulmonary hyperinflation, subdiaphragmatic abscesses, retroperitoneal mass lesions, or rib cage anomalies.

HEREDITARY ANGIOEDEMA

Barry Pelz • Anna B. Fishbein

BASICS

DESCRIPTION

Hereditary angioedema (HAE) is an autosomal dominant condition characterized by recurrent, unpredictable, and potentially life-threatening swelling. Deficiency or dysfunction of C1 esterase inhibitor (C1-INH) leads to unregulated activation of complement and plasma kinin–forming pathways, leading to angioedema. There are 3 main classifications of HAE:

- Type I HAE: deficiency of C1-INH (~85% of patients)
- Type II HAE: dysfunction of C1-INH (~15%)
- HAE with normal C1-INH (previously called type III HAE): unclear mechanism (very rare)
- Acquired or ACE inhibitor–induced angioedema (are not HAE and will be minimally discussed here)

EPIDEMIOLOGY

- HAE type I or II
  - Prevalence between 1 in 10,000 and 150,000
  - All genders and races affected equally
  - Onset before puberty in ~50% of patients
  - Symptoms tend to worsen during puberty and persist into adulthood.
- HAE with normal C1-INH
  - Only a few families described, mostly women of childbearing age

ETIOLOGY

Genetics

- HAE type I or II
  - Autosomal dominant, high penetrance
  - 25% spontaneous mutations
  - Mutations on chromosome 11 in SERPING1 gene which codes for C1-INH
- HAE with normal C1-INH
  - Autosomal dominant, low penetrance
  - Some patients with mutation in coagulation factor XII gene

PATHOPHYSIOLOGY

- Deficiency/dysfunction of C1-INH leads to unopposed activation of the classical complement pathway, and conversion of prekallikrein to kallikrein.
- Kallikrein increases formation of bradykinin which produces angioedema.
- Histamine and other mast cell mediators are NOT involved.

COMMONLY ASSOCIATED CONDITIONS

Mildly increased risk of autoimmunity

DIAGNOSIS

Decide if symptoms consistent with HAE; if so, laboratory testing should be used to confirm the diagnosis (C4 + C1-INH antigen and function are confirmatory tests.).

SIGNS AND SYMPTOMS

Any of the following symptoms may be present:

- Recurrent "attacks" of angioedema worsening in first 24 hours, lasting 2–5 days
- Tingling sensation as prodrome to symptoms
- Abdominal pain (with possible nausea, vomiting, diarrhea) even without angioedema
- Laryngeal edema (tightness in throat, dyspnea is a late sign)

HISTORY

- Ask about potential triggers of attacks: minor trauma, emotional distress, surgery, infections, stress, menstruation, and/or pregnancy.
- Explore recurrent nature of symptoms can be intermittent or more chronic.
- Family history of angioedema

PHYSICAL EXAM

- Angioedema, nonpruritic, nonpitting
- 30% with transient serpiginous rash, erythema marginatum, on trunk/medial extremities
- Swelling of face, lips, larynx, gastrointestinal tract, genitals, and/or extremities
- Abdominal tenderness

ALERT

Be aware of laryngeal swelling in absence of facial swelling; can be severe enough to lead to asphyxiation

DIAGNOSTIC TESTS & INTERPRETATION

HAE type I or II

- C4 (natural substrate for C1-INH) and CH50 (general screen of complement) can be used as screening tests.
  - Will be very low or absent
  - CH50 needs to be sent on ice, as it will otherwise degrade, causing falsely low levels.
- C1-INH antigen (protein) level
  - Type 1 = <50% of normal value
  - Type 2 = normal
- C1-INH function
  - Type 1 = <50% of normal value
  - Type 2 = <50% of normal value
- Genetic testing available, not required to confirm diagnosis, helpful in children <1 year of age
- Lab testing should be repeated (ideally at least 1 month later) to confirm results.
- Labs preferably drawn during attacks but usually abnormal in-between episodes as well.

HAE with normal C1-INH

- Positive family history of angioedema
- Normal C4, C1-INH level and function (when drawn during an attack)
- Consider factor XII gene mutation analysis.

Acquired angioedema

- No family history of angioedema
- Low C4, C1-INH level and function usually low
- Low C1q (<50% normal)

Imaging

- Imaging rarely necessary
- Abdominal CT scan or ultrasound might demonstrate bowel wall edema in abdominal attacks.

DIFFERENTIAL DIAGNOSIS

- Allergic reactions and anaphylaxis:
  - IgE-mediated allergic reactions: drug, food, and insect allergies
  - Transfusion reactions
  - Idiopathic anaphylaxis
  - Exercise-induced anaphylaxis
- Drug-induced angioedema (particularly to ACE inhibitors or NSAIDs)
- Idiopathic angioedema—typically involves urticaria and not posterior oropharynx
- Allergic contact dermatitis
- Rheumatologic diseases (low C3 + low C4)
- Superior vena cava syndrome
- Oncologic diseases such as head and neck tumors or lymphomas
- Physical urticarias such as cold-induced urticaria, cholinergic urticaria, aquagenic urticaria, solar urticaria, pressure urticaria (or angioedema), or vibratory angioedema
- Psychological
  - Panic attacks
  - Globus sensation
  - Vocal cord dysfunction
- Presence of C4 null alleles can cause low C4 levels.

TREATMENT

MEDICATION

First Line

- C1-INH replacement protein (C1INHRP) from pooled human plasma, rare risk of thrombosis
  - Berinert
    - FDA-approved for acute attacks
    - IV dose for ≥6 years: 20 mg/kg or ≤50 kg = 1,000 U, >50–100 kg = 1,500 U, >100 kg = 2,000 U up to 3 doses per attack
  - Cinryze for prophylaxis
    - ≥6 years: 1,000 U IV q3–4d
- Bradykinin receptor antagonist
  - Icatibant (Firazyr)
    - ≥18 years: 30 mg SQ q6h up to 3 doses per 24 hours
- Recombinant plasma kallikrein inhibitor
  - Ecallantide (Kalbitor)
    - Rare risk of anaphylaxis
    - ≥16 years (new study used in children as young as 9 years): 30 mg SQ × 1; if attack persists, an additional dose may be administered within a 24-hour period.

Second Line

- Plasma: Solvent/detergent-treated plasma or fresh frozen plasma (FFP) may be used in the setting of an acute attack if the above medications are not available.
- Attenuated androgens (danazol or stanozolol)
  - Increase production of C1-INH significantly
  - Androgenic side effects
  - No longer preferred in pediatric patients
- Plasmin inhibitors (β-aminocaproic acid or tranexamic acid)
- Recombinant C1-INH: Ruconest (Rhucin)
  - A rabbit-derived protein currently approved in Europe only
  - It may become approved for use in the United States in the near future.
- HAE symptoms do not respond to epinephrine, corticosteroids, or antihistamines.

Short-term prophylaxis

- Medications may be given prior to dental procedures, intubations, or other anticipated traumas or stressors.
- None of the therapies confer complete protection from HAE attacks, so procedures should be performed in a setting where emergency intubation can be performed.

Long-term prophylaxis

- May be indicated for patients who have
  - Frequent and severe attacks
  - Rapid progression of attacks
  - Poor access or response to on-demand therapy for acute attacks
  - History of intubation(s) due to HAE
  - Excessive absences from work or school
  - Significant decrease in quality of life due to HAE

ISSUES FOR REFERRAL

- Any patient with angioedema should be referred to a physician with experience managing HAE.
- An allergist/immunologist can help with the evaluation, treatment, and management of these patients.

ONGOING CARE

FOLLOW-UP

- Patients should be seen at least annually.
- Education should be provided to the patient and patient's family regarding the disease.
- Testing family members should be considered.
- Care should include identification and avoidance of triggers when possible and plan in the event of an acute attack.
  - Medical identification band or wallet card
  - A written emergency action plan should outline treatment during an acute attack.
- Follow-up should include the following:
  - Review of triggers
  - Prospective genetic counseling
  - Review of attacks during the previous year
  - Reconsideration of the need for prophylaxis
  - Review of an emergency plan
- Regular follow-up with an endocrinologist is indicated for patients requiring androgen therapy.

PATIENT EDUCATION

- General education provided by physician
- Support groups, handouts, ID bands
- www.haea.org
- www.haei.org

PROGNOSIS

Variable. Once attacks begin, they generally persist throughout the patient's life, although the frequency and severity can be dramatically improved with available therapies.

COMPLICATIONS

- Upper airway obstruction may be life threatening or lead to asphyxiation.
- Severe abdominal pain may be mistaken for a surgical abdomen.
- Diagnosis may be delayed.
- Patients may be frustrated by the nature of the recurrent attacks and the significant impact on quality of life.

ADDITIONAL READING

- Bowen T, Cicardi M, Farkas H, et al. 2010 International consensus algorithm for the diagnosis, therapy and management of hereditary angioedema. *Allergy Asthma Clin Immunol*. 2010;6(1):24.
- Longhurst H, Cicardi M. Hereditary angio-oedema. *Lancet*. 2012;379(9814):474–481.
- Morgan BP. Hereditary angioedema—therapies old and new. *N Engl J Med*. 2010;363(6):581–583.
- Sardana N, Craig TJ. Recent advances in management and treatment of hereditary angioedema. *Pediatrics*. 2011;128(6):1173–1180.

CODES

ICD10

D84.1 Defects in the complement system

FAQ

- Q: What is a good screening test for HAE?
- A: C4 is a good screening test. C1 inhibitor functional and quantitative assays are readily available from commercial labs and are the definitive tests of choice for HAE.
- Q: What is the mode of inheritance in HAE?
- A: Autosomal dominant
- Q: What are the side effects of prophylactic androgen therapy?
- A: Side effects include virilization, menstrual irregularities, enhanced epiphyseal growth plate closure, weight gain, water retention, hypertension, cholestatic hepatitis, hepatic carcinoma, decreased spermatogenesis, and gynecomastia.

HEREDITARY SPHEROCYTOSIS

Michele P. Lambert

BASICS

DESCRIPTION

- Hemolytic anemia with shortened RBC survival due to selective destruction of RBCs in the spleen secondary to an inherent defect of the RBC membrane.
- Pathophysiologically related to hereditary elliptocytosis and hereditary ovalocytosis
- Membrane loss is gradual; it results in spherocytosis, which results in increased osmotic fragility.
- Severity related to degree of membrane loss
  - Mild (20% of patients)
    - Hemoglobin near normal
    - Slight reticulocytosis (<6%)
    - Compensated hemolysis, mild splenomegaly
    - Often not diagnosed until adulthood due to gallstones
  - Moderate (60% of patients)
    - Hemoglobin 8–10 mg/dL
    - Reticulocytes generally >8%
    - >50% patients have splenomegaly.
  - Moderately severe (10%)
    - Hemoglobin 6–8 mg/dL
    - Reticulocytes >15%
    - Intermittent transfusions
  - Severe (3–5%)
    - Life-threatening anemia requiring regular transfusions
    - Almost always recessive

EPIDEMIOLOGY

Most common in people of Northern European extraction (~1:3,000)

RISK FACTORS

Genetics

- ~75% of cases are inherited in an autosomal dominant pattern.
- The other 25% are autosomal recessive forms, dominant disease with reduced penetrance, or new mutations.

PATHOPHYSIOLOGY

- The most common abnormality is a deficiency of ankyrin and subsequent decrease in spectrin, 2 major proteins of the erythrocyte membrane skeleton (50–60% Northern European decent; 5–10% Japan).
  - Spectrin deficiency alone accounts for 20% of HS.
  - Mutations in other erythrocyte surface proteins also occur, including the following:
    - Beta-spectrin (typically mild to moderately severe), alpha-spectrin (severe HS)
    - Band 3 (15–20% generally mild to moderately severe)
    - Protein 4.2 (<5% HS, recessive and results in almost complete absence)
    - Rh antigen (<10% mild to moderate hemolytic anemia)
- The membrane skeletal defect causes RBC membrane fragility, resulting in membrane loss.
- The sequelae are as follows:
  - Loss of cell surface area relative to volume (spherocytosis) causes a decrease in cellular deformability.
  - The spleen detains and "conditions" the nondeformable spherocytic RBC.
  - Conditioning of cells involves depletion of adenosine 5′-triphosphate (ATP), increased glycolysis, increased influx and efflux of sodium, and loss of membrane lipid.
- Ultimately, these events lead to premature RBC destruction.

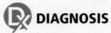

DIAGNOSIS

HISTORY

- Fatigue (a sign of anemia)
- Jaundice, scleral icterus, dark urine (signs of hemolysis)
- Phototherapy required in newborn period (50% of cases): hyperbilirubinemia due to hemolysis
- Positive familial history (for disease, gallstones, or splenectomy) is significant because of autosomal dominant inheritance.

PHYSICAL EXAM

- Splenomegaly is present in most older patients and may worsen with intercurrent illness.
- Icterus/jaundice and pallor are present with increased hemolysis.
- Linear growth, weight gain, and sexual development may be delayed. Delayed growth is indication for splenectomy.

DIAGNOSTIC TESTS & INTERPRETATION

Lab

- CBC
  - Mild to moderate anemia
  - Mean corpuscular volume (MCV) usually normal
  - Mean corpuscular hemoglobin concentration (MCHC) elevated (useful screening test with high specificity)
  - Reticulocyte count: may be only slightly elevated
  - Often accompanied by elevated RBC distribution width (RDW)
  - Indirect hyperbilirubinemia: present in 50–60% of cases
  - Peripheral smear: microspherocytes, polychromasia
- Coombs test: negative
  - Important differential test in a patient with hemolytic anemia and spherocytes
- Urinalysis
  - Hemoglobinuria
  - Increased urobilinogen
- Special tests:
  - Osmotic fragility (most useful test in diagnosis but can be normal in 10–20% of patients)
    - Spherocytes are more fragile, less resistant to osmotic stress, and therefore lyse in higher concentrations of saline than normal RBCs.
    - Test can result in a false-negative, especially in newborns whose RBCs may be more dehydrated and with high fetal hemoglobin.
    - Important to use an age-matched control if possible
    - Any anemia that results in spherocytes will give increased osmotic fragility (especially autoimmune hemolytic anemia) and must be excluded.
  - Eosin-5-maleimide (EMA) binding
    - Flow cytometric analysis of RBCs with much higher sensitivity and specificity for HS
    - Is now the test of choice for diagnosis but not available at all centers

DIFFERENTIAL DIAGNOSIS

- Hemolysis secondary to intrinsic RBC defects
  - Membrane defects secondary to inherited disorders of membrane skeleton (HS and elliptocytosis) and RBC cation permeability and volume (stomatocytosis and xerocytosis)
  - Enzyme defects: Embden-Meyerhof pathway (i.e., pyruvate kinase deficiency) and hexose monophosphate pathway (i.e., glucose-6-phosphate dehydrogenase deficiency)
  - Hemoglobin defects
    - Congenital erythropoietic porphyria;
    - Qualitative hemoglobin S (sickle cell), Hgb C, Hgb H, Hgb M
    - Quantitative: thalassemias
  - Congenital dyserythropoietic anemias
- Hemolysis secondary to extracorpuscular RBC defects
  - Immune-mediated (important in differential because spherocytes are present on smear and can give increased osmotic fragility if sent): isoimmune (e.g., hemolytic disease of the newborn, blood group incompatibility) and autoimmune (e.g., cold agglutinin disease, warm autoimmune hemolytic anemia)
  - Non–immune-mediated: idiopathic and secondary to underlying disorder (e.g., hemolytic uremic syndrome, thrombotic thrombocytopenic purpura)

ALERT

- A patient with HS may become extremely anemic during an aplastic crisis, hyperhemolysis episode, or folic acid deficiency, requiring transfusion.
- False-negative osmotic fragility tests can occur in several situations; therefore, index of suspicion must be high to follow the clinical course and repeat test (e.g., in neonatal period, during megaloblastic crisis, and recovery from aplastic crisis after transfusion when cells are youngest and least spherocytic).
- 20–25% of HS patients have normal unincubated osmotic fragility (incubated test almost always positive; therefore, it may be necessary to conduct both tests).
- Spherocytes are often present in immune-mediated hemolysis.

TREATMENT

GENERAL MEASURES

- Folic acid supplement
- Penicillin prophylaxis (if splenectomized)
- Pneumococcal, meningococcal, and *Haemophilus influenza* B vaccines (prior to splenectomy)

SURGERY/OTHER PROCEDURES

Splenectomy: high response rate (most patients normalize their blood counts):

- Indications: moderate to severe anemia with significant hemolysis resulting in transfusion dependence, decreased exercise tolerance, skeletal deformities, or delayed growth
- Complications: risk of postsplenectomy sepsis, emerging data on increased risk of later pulmonary hypertension, and increased risk of thrombosis

Cholecystectomy

- Indications: symptomatic gallbladder disease; sometimes done simultaneous with splenectomy if gallstones evident by ultrasound
- Complications: morbidity of surgical procedure and postoperative period

ONGOING CARE

- Physical exam
  - Check for splenomegaly.
  - Follow growth curves closely.
- CBC with reticulocyte count as needed: If patient develops fatigue, pallor, or increased jaundice especially in setting of viral illness
- Penicillin prophylaxis after splenectomy

PROGNOSIS

Severity of disease is extremely variable, ranging from an incidental diagnosis in adulthood to severe anemia requiring transfusions.

COMPLICATIONS

- Gallstones
  - Most common complication of HS
  - Pigment stones can lead to cholecystitis and/or biliary obstruction.
- Cholelithiasis in HS manifests in 2nd and 3rd decades of life.
- Aplastic crises
  - Can result in severe life-threatening anemia; often caused by parvovirus B19 infection
  - Epstein-Barr virus (EBV), influenza, and cytomegalovirus (CMV) can also cause worsening anemia and reticulocytopenia.
- Hyperhemolysis
  - Increased RBC destruction
  - Often precipitated by infection
- Postsplenectomy sepsis
  - Lower risk of infection if postponed until 4–5 years of age and immunized with pneumococcal vaccine
  - 50–70% of sepsis caused by *Streptococcus pneumoniae*
- Folate deficiency
  - Caused by insufficient dietary intake of folic acid for increased bone marrow requirement
  - Can result in megaloblastic crisis
- Pulmonary hypertension
  - Long-term complication of splenectomy due to recurrent small vessel thrombosis in the lungs (either local clot or thromboembolic events)
  - Long-term risk that weighs against splenectomy in patients with mild or well-compensated disease
- Other rare complications
  - Gout
  - Indolent leg ulcers
  - Chronic erythematous dermatitis on legs

ADDITIONAL READING

- An X, Mohandas N. Disorders of red cell membrane. *Br J Haematol*. 2008;141(3):367–376.
- Barcellini W, Bianchi P, Fermo E, et al. Hereditary red cell membrane defects: diagnostic and clinical aspects. *Blood Transfus*. 2011;9(3):274–277.
- Bolton-Maggs PHB, Stevens RF, Dodd NJ, et al. Guidelines for the diagnosis and management of hereditary spherocytosis. *Br J Haematol*. 2004;126(4):455–474.
- Delhommeau F, Cynober T, Schischmanoff P, et al. Natural history of hereditary spherocytosis during the first year of life. *Blood*. 2000;95(2):393–397.
- Gallagher P. Red cell membrane disorders. *Hematology Am Soc Hematol Educ Program*. 2005;13–18.
- Shah S, Vega R. Hereditary spherocytosis. *Pediatr Rev*. 2004;25(5):168–172.

CODES

ICD10

D58.0 Hereditary spherocytosis

FAQ

- Q: Will my child require blood transfusions?
- A: It depends on the clinical severity of your child's disease.
- Q: If a parent has HS, how should the newborn be followed?
- A: The infant has a 50% chance of having HS. In infants with HS, the CBC is usually normal in the first 72 hours of life but then drops because of an inability to mount an appropriate erythropoietic response to increased destruction. Therefore, infants at risk should have a CBC with reticulocyte count after 72 hours. These infants also need to be monitored closely for hyperbilirubinemia.
- Q: What are the risks and benefits of splenectomy?
- A: Splenectomy is almost always successful in ameliorating anemia but adds the risk of postsplenectomy infections and later risks for pulmonary hypertension and maybe increased risk of thrombosis and/or cardiovascular disease. The risks and benefits need to be carefully weighed and, in patients with mild, well-compensated hemolysis, splenectomy is not indicated.

HEROIN INTOXICATION

Jeannine Del Pizzo • Fran Balamuth

BASICS

DESCRIPTION

Heroin is a semisynthetic derivative of opium. The opioid family includes the following:

- Drugs that occur naturally in opium (from the poppy plant)
- Codeine
- Morphine
- Semisynthetic derivatives (e.g., hydromorphone, oxycodone)
- Synthetic compounds (e.g., meperidine, fentanyl, methadone)

EPIDEMIOLOGY

- General
  - 23 years of age: mean age of 1st use (2012)
  - ~50% of those who have used an opioid pain reliever for nonmedical uses state they obtained it for free from a friend or relative.
  - Nonmedical use of opioid pain relievers can lead to eventual injection heroin use.
- Neonatal
  - Fetal exposure commonly involves polysubstance abuse.
  - 60–80% of heroin-exposed infants develop withdrawal—dependent on maternal dosing and length of use.
- Adolescents
  - Most use experimentally or intermittently; few become addicted and use daily.
  - Use of opioid analgesics has increased dramatically over the last 10 years and has become more common than heroin use.
  - Most common substances were oxycodone, hydrocodone, and methadone
- Overdose
  - Up to 1/3 of heroin users experience nonfatal overdose.
  - Most occur in the home and with other people present.
  - Risk factors include length of injecting history, concurrent use of CNS depressants, recent completion of substance abuse program, and recent release from prison.
- Deaths
  - Most heroin deaths occur when drug is administered IV.
  - Most deaths in patients in their late 20s or 30s, with significant drug dependence
  - Males are 4 times more likely to die than females from heroin-related causes.
  - Multiple drug use common in heroin-related death
  - As of 2011, opioid pain relievers are responsible for more overdose fatalities than heroin and cocaine combined.

Prevalence

- Precise estimates of prevalence of use difficult
- ~2.9 million people used at least once.
- ~467,000 used in 2012 (double since 2001).
- Prevalence of fetal exposure <1–3.7%

PATHOPHYSIOLOGY

- Well-absorbed from gastrointestinal (GI) tract, nasal mucosa, pulmonary capillaries, and SC and IM injection sites
- Oral dose less potent than parenteral because of 1st-pass hepatic metabolism
- IV heroin peaks in <1 minute; intranasal and IM heroin peak in 3–5 minutes.
- Very lipid soluble; crosses blood–brain barrier within 15–20 seconds
- Extensive distribution into skeletal muscle, kidneys, liver, intestine, lungs, spleen, brain, and placenta
- Rapidly crosses the placenta, entering fetal tissues within 1 hour
- Crosses into breast milk in quantities sufficient to cause addiction
- Excreted in urine as morphine
- Receptor types
  - Mu (or OP3)
    - Located in CNS, GI tract, and sensory nerve endings
    - Effect: analgesia, euphoria, respiratory depression, physical dependence, GI dysmotility, miosis, pruritus, bradycardia
  - Kappa (or OP2)
    - Located in CNS
    - Effect: analgesia, miosis, diuresis, dysphoria
  - Delta (or OP1)
    - Located in CNS
    - Effect: spinal analgesia, modulation of mu receptors/dopaminergic neurons

DIAGNOSIS

HISTORY

- Neonate
  - Maternal history of heroin or other drug use
  - Extent of prenatal care
  - Time from most recent use to delivery
  - Breastfeeding
- Older child/adolescent
  - History of heroin use
  - Observed overdose
  - Found in setting consistent with possible drug use

PHYSICAL EXAM

- Neonate with in utero exposure
  - Prematurity
  - Low birth weight
  - Perinatal depression with 5-minute Apgar <5
  - Hypotonia
- Intoxication/overdose
  - Classic toxidrome: depressed level of consciousness, very decreased respiratory effort, miotic pupils, with or without diminished bowel sounds
  - More severe overdose: bradycardia, hypotension, noncardiogenic pulmonary edema
- Withdrawal
  - Early signs (8–24 hours): anxiety, restlessness, insomnia, yawning, rhinorrhea, lacrimation, diaphoresis, stomach cramps, mydriasis
  - Late signs (up to 3 days): tremor, muscle spasms, vomiting, diarrhea, hypertension, tachycardia, fever, chills, piloerection, seizures
- Additional neonatal withdrawal signs and symptoms
  - Hyperirritability
  - Hypertonicity
  - Posturing
  - Exaggerated startle reflex
  - Tachypnea
  - Hyperpyrexia
  - Poor suck/swallow coordination
  - High-pitched cry
  - Poor weight gain
  - Timing of neonatal symptoms depends on maternal substance used: See withdrawal from heroin within 48 hours, can be longer for methadone; can see delayed withdrawal up to 4 weeks with both drugs

DIAGNOSTIC TESTS & INTERPRETATION

Diagnostic Procedures/Other

- Therapy should not be withheld pending laboratory results.
- Urine toxicology screen (heroin easily detected; synthetic opioids are not)
- Serum toxicology screen for acetaminophen level, etc., if suspect polydrug use
- Serum tests to rule out other causes, if needed (e.g., glucose)
- Urine testing in neonates and mothers. Meconium testing is also helpful but not readily available, and results can take days to weeks.

DIFFERENTIAL DIAGNOSIS

- Neonatal exposure
  - Sepsis
  - Hypoglycemia
  - Hypocalcemia
  - Hyperthyroidism
  - CNS abnormality
  - Metabolic disorder
  - Withdrawal from other maternal drug use
- Intoxication/overdose
- Other pharmacologic agents
  - Clonidine, sedative hypnotics, barbiturates, antipsychotics, gamma hydroxy butyrate
- Hypoglycemia
- Hypothermia
- Hypoxia
- Heat stroke
- Pontine or subarachnoid hemorrhage

TREATMENT

ADDITIONAL TREATMENT

General Measures

- Intoxication/overdose
  - ABCs (airway, breathing, circulation)
  - Antidote is naloxone (Narcan).
  - Assessment of respiratory status/adequacy of ventilation
  - If adequate respiratory effort, observe until normal level of consciousness.
    - Consider naloxone as diagnostic challenge.
  - If inadequate respiratory effort
    - Bag-valve-mask ventilation
    - Naloxone (IV preferred route, SC, IM)
    - If <20 kg, 0.1 mg/kg; 2 mg if ≥20 kg. Dose may be repeated.
    - ET route: optimal dose unknown but some recommend using 2–3 times the above IV dosage
    - Intranasal route: 2 mg (1 mg per nostril) has been used in adolescents ≥13 years and a slightly delayed onset of action compared to IV/IM route has been reported.
  - If suspect dependence, start with lower dose (0.4-mg ampule)
  - If no response to large dose, question diagnosis of heroin toxicity—heroin exquisitely sensitive to naloxone.

– Naloxone loses efficacy in 20–40 minutes.
  ○ May need repeat dosing
  ○ Can give as continuous infusion if necessary; dosing recommendations vary.
  ○ One method: 2/3 of effective bolus dose given on an hourly basis with gradual wean
– Consider low-dose naloxone (0.01 mg/kg) in apneic infants exposed to opiates in utero but caution, as naloxone can precipitate seizures in opioid-dependent neonates.
– Endotracheal intubation if no response to naloxone in 5–10 minutes, or other reason for invasive airway management
– Observe in emergency department for a minimum of 2–3 hours for respiratory status stabilization.
– Consider chest radiograph to evaluate for pulmonary edema.
– Consider glucose testing to evaluate for hypoglycemia.
– Consider whole bowel irrigation with GoLYTELY for symptomatic body packers and consult local poison control center.

- Withdrawal
  – Standard treatment methadone maintenance (adolescents/adults)
    ○ Blocks euphoria and prevents withdrawal symptoms
    ○ Patients generally treated in established methadone maintenance programs
    ○ Stabilize with 20–40 mg/24 h; wean by 2–5 mg/week over several months.
    ○ Adjust wean if signs of withdrawal appear.
    ○ Some programs use heroin maintenance when methadone fails; research ongoing
  – Buprenorphine is also an option.
  – Clonidine (0.2 mg q4–6h PRN for 5–7 days) can control acute withdrawal symptoms. Monitor blood pressure.
  – Rapid and ultrarapid detoxification (using opioid antagonist with or without general anesthesia) a possibility in selected patients; recent review suggests high-rate adverse events.
    ○ Should be used only by experienced team with appropriate resources
- Children receiving prescription opioids for pain likely will exhibit symptoms of withdrawal after 14 days of daily use and will need a weaning schedule. Use of daily opioids for less than 7 days usually does not result in withdrawal symptoms.
- In neonates
  – Nonmedical management of neonatal opioid withdrawal includes minimizing environmental stimulation (light, noise, cold), swaddling, and comfort measures.
  – Treatment
    ○ Paregoric (0.4 mg/mL) not recommended owing to high alcohol content (45%) and toxic compounds such as camphor, anise oil, benzoic acid, and glycerin
    ○ Oral tincture of opium (10 mg/mL) best diluted 25-fold to a concentration equal to paregoric (0.4 mg/mL)
      ▪ 0.1 mL/kg q4h; increase 0.1 mL/kg q4h as needed to control symptoms.
      ▪ After 3–5 days, wean dose by 0.1 ml/kg/24 h. Observe infant for 3–5 days after stopping therapy.
  – May need IV morphine in severe cases
  – Methadone and buprenorphine have also been shown to be effective.
  – Clonidine gaining favor for use in infants; pharmacokinetic data not available, although use is currently recommended only in the context of a randomized clinical trial.
  – Phenobarbital is not a 1st-choice agent owing to long half-life, CNS depression, induction of drug metabolism, and rapid tolerance to sedative effect; however, it has been shown to be effective in conjunction with diluted tincture of opium.
  – Infants with opioid withdrawal have elevated metabolic demands: Consider higher calorie (24 kcal/oz) feeds.
- Breastfeeding is not recommended in mothers using heroin but can be considered for mothers on methadone treatment.

FOLLOW-UP

DISPOSITION

Most patients with overdose warrant hospitalization.

ONGOING CARE

FOLLOW-UP RECOMMENDATIONS

Developmental follow-up for exposed neonates

ISSUES FOR REFERRAL

- Social services and referral to substance abuse program
- Consider referral for testing for HIV and hepatitis B and C.

PROGNOSIS

- Neonatal
  – Long-term morbidity from neonatal heroin dependence unclear owing to confounding variables (e.g., developmental environment)
- Intoxication/overdose
  – With adequate early treatment, patients with uncomplicated overdoses do well—key is to prevent respiratory arrest.
- Addiction
  – Dependent on involvement in other risky behaviors (polydrug use, high-risk sexual practices, school failure, delinquency, etc.)
  – Longer treatment likely produces a better outcome.
  – Most relapses require lifetime of therapy.

COMPLICATIONS

- Intoxication/overdose
  – Respiratory arrest
  – Noncardiogenic pulmonary edema
  – CNS depression/coma
  – Hypotension
  – Aspiration pneumonia
- Pregnancy
  – Poor prenatal care
  – Preterm labor
  – Premature rupture of membranes
  – Breech presentation
  – Antepartum hemorrhage
  – Toxemia
  – Anemia
  – Uterine irritability
  – Infection (e.g., HIV, hepatitis B)
  – Infantile dependence
- Naloxone use
  – May precipitate withdrawal syndrome in opioid-dependent patients
  – Symptoms: agitation, hypertension, tachycardia, emesis
  – May cause acute severe withdrawal in infants born to addicted mothers

ADDITIONAL READING

- Centers for Disease Control and Prevention. Vital signs: overdoses of prescription opioid pain relievers—United States, 1999–2008. *MMWR Morb Mortal Wkly Rep*. 2011;60(43):1487–1492.
- Coyle MG, Ferguson A, La Grasse L, et al. Neurobehavioral effects of treatment for opiate withdrawal. *Arch Dis Child Fetal Neonatal Ed*. 2005;90(1):F73–F74.
- Ferri M, Davoli M, Perucci CA. Heroin maintenance for chronic heroin dependents. *Cochrane Database Syst Rev*. 2005;(2):CD003410.
- Galinkin J, Koh JL. Recognition and management of iatrogenically induced opioid dependence and withdrawal in children. *Pediatrics*. 2014;133(1):152.
- Gonzalez G, Oliveto A, Kosten TR. Treatment of heroin (diamorphine) addiction: current approaches and future prospects. *Drugs*. 2002;62(9):1331–1343.
- Gowing L, Ali R, White J. Opioid antagonists under heavy sedation or anaesthesia for opioid withdrawal. *Cochrane Database Syst Rev*. 2006;(2):CD002022.
- Hudak ML, Tan RC. Neonatal drug withdrawal. *Pediatrics*. 2012;129(2):e540.
- Johnson K, Gerada C, Greenough A. Treatment of neonatal abstinence syndrome. *Arch Dis Child*. 2003;88(1):F2–F5.
- Jones HE, Kaltenbach K, Heil S, et al. Neonatal abstinence syndrome after methadone or buprenorphine exposure. *New Engl J Med*. 2010;363(24): 2320–2331.
- Osborn DA, Jeffery HE, Cole M. Opiate treatment for opiate withdrawal in newborn infants. *Cochrane Database Syst Rev*. 2010;(10):CD002059.
- Osborn DA, Jeffery HE, Cole M. Sedatives for opiate withdrawal in newborn infants. *Cochrane Database Syst Rev*. 2010;(10):CD002053.
- Perron BE, Bohnert AS, Monsell SE. Patterns and correlates of drug-related ED visits: results from a national survey. *Am J Emerg Med*. 2011;29(7): 704–710.
- Substance Abuse and Mental Health Services Administration. Results from the 2012 national survey on drug use and health: summary of national findings and detailed tables. http://archive.samhsa.gov/data/NSDUH/2012SummNatFindDetTables/Index.aspx. Accessed February 7, 2015.

CODES

ICD10

- F11.929 Opioid use, unspecified with intoxication, unspecified
- F11.23 Opioid dependence with withdrawal
- P96.1 Neonatal w/drawal symp from matern use of drugs of addiction

FAQ

- Q: Is nalmefene an appropriate substitute for naloxone in a heroin overdose?
- A: Nalmefene, a long-acting specific narcotic antagonist, has not proved to be as effective as naloxone in a randomized, double-blind trial. It also may result in prolonged, dangerous withdrawal. It therefore has limited usefulness in this setting.

HERPES SIMPLEX VIRUS

Paul K. Sue • W. Christopher Golden

BASICS

DESCRIPTION

Herpes simplex virus (HSV) is an enveloped double-stranded DNA virus. It exists as two distinct subtypes, HSV-1 and HSV-2, and is responsible for a wide spectrum of illness ranging from fever blisters to genital ulcers and fatal encephalitis. It establishes lifelong latency and can lead to interval episodes of asymptomatic shedding and disease recurrence.

EPIDEMIOLOGY

- HSV-1 infects 40–80% of the U.S population by young adulthood, and 60–85% by age 60.
- HSV-2 incidence increases during adolescence and adulthood, and infects 20–35% of U.S. adults by age 40.
- In the United States, approximately 1,500 cases of neonatal HSV (1:3,200 live births) occur every year, primarily due to HSV-2.
- Following the neonatal period, HSV-1 infections predominate among children.
- Risk factors for HSV-1 and HSV-2 infection include older age and lower socioeconomic status. Additional risk factors for HSV-2 include number of lifetime sexual partners and female gender.

GENERAL PREVENTION

- Perinatal infection
  - The majority of neonatal HSV infections (85%) occur through contact with maternal HSV shed within the birth canal. A smaller proportion (5%) of infections occur in utero.
  - The majority (60–80%) of mothers of infected infants have no symptoms of HSV infection at the time of delivery.
  - Children born to mothers with primary genital HSV infection at time of delivery are at highest risk (~60%). In contrast, the risk of neonatal infection with recurrent maternal genital herpes is significantly lower (2–5%).
  - In the setting of active genital herpes (lesions or pain), cesarean delivery is recommended, preferably within 4 hours of rupture of membranes. However, infections may still occur despite cesarean delivery and intact amniotic membranes.
  - Cesarean delivery is not recommended for mothers with a history of genital HSV in the absence of lesions or symptoms.
  - Fetal scalp monitors should be avoided in women with suspected genital HSV.
  - The use of antiviral therapy (acyclovir or valacyclovir) after 36 weeks' gestation decreases viral shedding and reactivation of genital lesions in mothers with a history of genital HSV, although breakthrough infections may still occur.
- Postnatal infection (neonates and children)
  - Secretions of active HSV lesions are highly infectious, and asymptomatic viral shedding is common. 10% of neonatal HSV infections are contracted postpartum through direct contact with infectious fluids.
  - Standard universal precautions are appropriate in caring for recurrent/localized lesions in immunocompetent persons.
  - Contact precautions should be considered in neonates, immunocompromised persons with active lesions, and in severe primary mucocutaneous HSV.
  - Contact with genital/cutaneous HSV lesions (e.g., sexual intercourse, wrestling) should be avoided until lesions resolve.

PATHOPHYSIOLOGY

- Spread occurs typically via contact with abraded skin or mucous membranes.
- The incubation period for primary infection is approximately 2–12 days.
- Viral replication begins at the portal of entry (epithelia) and commences within sensory ganglia. Migration occurs back to the site of inoculation, with subsequent destruction of epithelial cells.
- Following initial infection, the virus remains latent in sensory neural ganglia and can be reactivated by UV exposure, trauma, stress, hormonal changes, or immunosuppression.
- Viral dissemination occurs most often in neonates, pregnant women, or immunosuppressed patients.
- HSV antibodies provide a degree of cross protection across serotypes; previous infection with one HSV serotype (e.g., HSV-1) can decrease the severity of infection with the alternate serotype (e.g., HSV-2).

COMMONLY ASSOCIATED CONDITIONS

- Gingivostomatitis
- Encephalitis
- Herpes gladiatorum
- Herpetic whitlow
- Eczema herpeticum
- Erythema multiforme

DIAGNOSIS

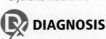

SIGNS AND SYMPTOMS

- The majority of primary HSV infections are asymptomatic in healthy individuals.
- Infections "above the waist" are classically due to HSV-1, whereas HSV-2 most commonly causes genital infection. However, both serotypes can cause genital and/or mucocutaneous infection.
- Recurrent infections occur due to reactivation of latent virus and are usually less severe than primary infections.
- Neonatal infection
  - Neonates may present with classic skin lesions or with nonspecific findings of irritability, fever, temperature instability, and poor feeding with or without a rash.
  - Skin, eye, and/or mouth (SEM) disease (40–45% of neonatal HSV) presents in the 1st–2nd week of life with rash, chorioretinitis, or keratitis. Approximately 85% of patients have visible skin lesions.
  - Disseminated neonatal HSV disease (25% of neonatal HSV) presents with a sepsis-like syndrome in the 1st–2nd week of life, commonly involving the lungs, liver, adrenals, and the central nervous system (CNS). Approximately 60% have visible skin lesions.
  - HSV CNS disease (30–35% of neonatal HSV) usually presents in the 2nd–3rd week of life with seizures, fever, and/or temperature instability.
- Oropharyngeal infection
  - Primary infection is characterized by fever, irritability, and severe pain/burning of the oral mucosa, with vesicular and ulcerative lesions on the lips, gingiva, and tongue.
  - Pharyngitis is also common in older children and adolescents.
  - Illness lasts for 2–3 weeks, with viral shedding continuing for several weeks.
- Genital infection
  - Infection is characterized by genital pain and itching, associated with tender inguinal adenopathy, fever, malaise, and rash.
  - Lesions begin as vesicles and progress to ulcers before crusting over by 2–3 weeks.
- Keratoconjunctivitis (ocular infection)
  - Presents as unilateral or bilateral conjunctivitis with preauricular adenopathy, associated eyelid edema, photophobia, tearing, and/or chemosis
- Encephalitis (CNS infection)
  - Infection is characterized by fever, headache, altered mental status, focal neurologic symptoms, and seizures.
- Disseminated HSV infection
  - Infection presents with fever or temperature instability and a sepsis-like syndrome with end-organ involvement (e.g., lungs, liver).
  - Neonates, pregnant women, transplant recipients, and other immunocompromised hosts are at increased risk for disseminated infection.

PHYSICAL EXAM

- The "classic" HSV rash consists of vesicles on an erythematous base, which subsequently ulcerate, become friable, and bleed easily.
- Lesions may not be readily apparent, particularly in cases of disseminated disease and CNS infection.

DIAGNOSTIC TESTS & INTERPRETATION

- Neonatal infection
  - Newborn conjunctival, oropharyngeal, nasal, and rectal samples should be sent for viral culture approximately 24 hours after birth (sooner if suspicious lesions are present).
  - Suspicious vesicles should be unroofed and the vesicle base thoroughly swabbed for viral culture.
  - Cerebrospinal fluid (CSF) should be sent for cell count, differential, chemistries, and HSV-polymerase chain reaction (PCR), in addition to evaluation (blood, urine, CSF) for bacterial and other viral infections.
  - Repeat HSV CSF PCR testing may be required, as false negatives of the CSF can occur early in the disease course.
  - Serum HSV PCR and liver function tests (specifically alanine aminotransferase [ALT]) should be sent in cases of suspected disseminated HSV.
  - Additional testing (ophthalmoscopy, electroencephalogram [EEG], CNS imaging [MRI], chest x-ray) is recommended in cases of disseminated, CNS, or ophthalmologic disease.
  - In asymptomatic neonates of women with genital lesions, maternal serologic status should be used to assess the risk of neonatal herpes and should, along with clinical findings, guide subsequent testing and therapy. See the 2013 clinical report from the AAP Committee on Infectious Diseases and Committee on Fetus and Newborn (reference in the "Additional Reading" section).
- Oropharyngeal HSV infection is typically diagnosed based on history and clinical exam. Viral culture and DFA are recommended for testing of questionable lesions.
- Genital herpes lesions should be diagnosed using both viral culture and HSV PCR, as the sensitivity of viral culture alone may be as low as 27% in genital ulcers and recurrent lesions.
- Encephalitis
  - CSF PCR is the diagnostic test of choice. Samples should be sent to a reliable laboratory with a low rate of false-positive results.
  - In HSV encephalitis, CSF analysis reveals a lymphocytic, progressive pleocytosis (average 100 WBCs/mm^3) and rising protein (median 80 mg/dL), although these may be normal in 5–10% of early disease.

- EEG can reveal a characteristic pattern of periodic unilateral or bilateral focal spikes.
- MRI of the brain may show temporal lobe enhancement, deep gray matter involvement, and ischemic changes in watershed distribution areas.

• HSV keratoconjunctivitis
  - Ophthalmology referral is recommended.
  - Characteristic dendritic corneal ulcerations with linear branching pattern are observed on slit-lamp examination.
  - Viral culture and HSV PCR are highly sensitive but often unnecessary.

• Disseminated HSV
  - HSV serum PCR is useful in detecting viremia in disseminated infection.
  - CNS involvement is noted in up to 70% of cases.

DIFFERENTIAL DIAGNOSIS

- Neonatal HSV disease should be distinguished from severe enteroviral and bacterial sepsis, especially in the first 4–6 weeks of life.
- Intrauterine HSV should be considered in newborns born with microcephaly, intracranial calcifications, chorioretinitis, hepatosplenomegaly, and/or skin lesions and must be distinguished from other congenital viral infections (such as cytomegalovirus [CMV] and rubella).
- Oropharyngeal HSV should be distinguished from enteroviral (e.g., coxsackie) herpangina.
- Genital HSV should be distinguished from chancroid and syphilis. Syphilis lesions are usually nonpainful, indurated ulcers. Chancroid lesions are painful, purulent ulcers due to *Haemophilus ducreyi* infection.
- Ocular HSV should be distinguished from other infectious causes of conjunctivitis (adenovirus, *Haemophilus influenzae*, *Staphylococcus aureus*, *Streptococcus pneumoniae*) and rheumatologic or traumatic etiologies.

TREATMENT

MEDICATION

• Neonatal disease
  - Intravenous (IV) acyclovir (20 mg/kg/dose every 8 hours). The recommended minimum duration of therapy is 14 days (if the disease is limited to the skin, eye, and mouth) or 21 days (for encephalitis or disseminated disease).
  - Infants with ocular HSV should also receive topical antiviral therapy (trifluridine 1%, vidarabine 3%, or iododeoxyuridine 0.1%) in addition to parenteral therapy.
  - In cases of neonatal HSV infection (without proven disease), preemptive therapy with IV acyclovir (20 mg/kg/dose every 8 hours) should be given for 10 days (see 2013 AAP clinical guidance report).
  - Acyclovir prophylaxis (300 mg/m^2/dose orally three times per day) for 6 months following initial treatment improves infant neurodevelopmental outcomes and prevents recurrent skin outbreaks.

• Oropharyngeal herpes
  - Symptomatic treatment with antipyretics and analgesia is recommended. IV hydration is sometimes needed in cases of decreased oral intake.
  - Oral acyclovir (15 mg/kg/dose five times per day for 7–10 days; max 200 mg per dose) may decrease the duration of illness if started within 72 hours at the onset of symptoms.

• Genital herpes
  - Patients ≥12 years old with primary genital HSV infection should receive oral acyclovir (400 mg/dose three times per day), valacyclovir (1 g/dose twice per day), or famciclovir (250 mg/dose three times per day) for 7–10 days or until resolution of lesions, whichever is longer. Topical therapy is not recommended.
  - Early treatment of recurrent herpes lesions (within 24 hours) with short-course acyclovir, valacyclovir, or famciclovir can reduce severity and duration of symptoms.
  - Suppressive oral therapy with acyclovir (400 mg/dose twice per day) or valacyclovir (500–1,000 mg once daily) has been shown to reduce recurrence of genital HSV. Patients should be reassessed after 1 year of therapy to determine if ongoing suppression is needed.
  - Suppressive therapy (valacyclovir [500 mg/dose twice per day] or acyclovir [400 mg/dose three times per day]) should be offered to pregnant women with a history of genital herpes from 36 weeks' gestation to delivery.

• Encephalitis
  - IV acyclovir (15–20 mg/kg/dose every 8 hours if <12 years old, otherwise 10 mg/kg/dose every 8 hours) for 14–21 days is recommended for treatment of HSV encephalitis.

• HSV keratoconjunctivitis
  - Topical antiviral therapy: trifluridine 1% (every 2 hours while awake), ganciclovir ophthalmic gel 0.15% (every 3 hours while awake), or vidarabine 3% ointment (every 3 hours while awake) for 7–14 days until resolution of lesions
  - Oral acyclovir (100–400 mg/dose, three times per day; max child dose: 80 mg/kg/24 h) may be considered if topical therapy is not feasible. Oral suppression may be necessary to prevent recurrences.

• Immunocompromised patients and severe cutaneous disease (e.g., eczema herpeticum)
  - HSV lesions should be treated with oral acyclovir 200 mg/dose five times per day (patients >2 years old; max child dose: 80 mg/kg/24 h) OR IV acyclovir (750–1,500 mg/m^2/24 h divided every 8 hours) for 7–14 days
  - IV acyclovir should be considered initially in patients who are immunocompromised, have severe disease (e.g., eczema herpeticum), or cannot tolerate oral therapy.

ALERT

- Use of acyclovir in therapeutic and suppressive doses has been associated with neutropenia in infants. Monitoring of the patient's absolute neutrophil count (ANC) is recommended.
- Common side effects of acyclovir therapy in children include diarrhea, nausea, and headache. Rare, but serious side effects of acyclovir therapy may include acute renal failure, hemolytic uremic syndrome, and thrombotic thrombocytopenic purpura.

ONGOING CARE

PROGNOSIS

- Despite antiviral therapy, mortality is approximately 30% among infants with disseminated HSV disease.
- Among neonates with encephalitis, mortality is around 5% with treatment, although 70% will have neurodevelopmental sequelae.
- HSV encephalitis mortality outside the neonatal period is 70% without therapy. With treatment, mortality declines to 19%, with 38% return to normal neurologic function.
- Herpes simplex keratoconjunctivitis frequently recurs and can lead to corneal ulceration and permanent scarring.

COMPLICATIONS

The major morbidities in survivors are brain damage, seizures, and blindness.

ADDITIONAL READING

- American Academy of Pediatrics. Herpes simplex. In: Pickering LK, Baker CJ, Kimberlin DW, et al, eds. *Red Book: 2012 Report of the Committee on Infectious Diseases*. 29th ed. Elk Grove Village, IL: American Academy of Pediatrics; 2012:398–408.
- Corey L, Wald A. Maternal and neonatal herpes simplex virus infections. *N Engl J Med*. 2009;361(14):1376–1385.
- Kimberlin D, Baley J; Committee on Infectious Diseases, Committee on Fetus and Newborn. Guidance on management of asymptomatic neonates born to women with active genital herpes lesions. *Pediatrics*. 2013;131(2):e635–e646.
- Kimberlin DW, Whitley RJ, Wan W, et al. Oral acyclovir suppression and neurodevelopmental outcomes after neonatal herpes. *N Engl J Med*. 2011;365(14):1284–1292.
- Liu S, Pavan-Langston D, Colby KA. Pediatric herpes simplex of the anterior segment: characteristics, treatment, and outcomes. *Ophthalmology*. 2012;119(10):2003–2008.
- Pinninti S, Kimberlin D. Maternal and neonatal herpes simplex virus infections. *Am J Perinatol*. 2013;30(2):113–120.
- Vossough A, Zimmerman RA, Bilaniuk LT, et al. Imaging findings of neonatal herpes simplex virus type 2 encephalitis. *Neuroradiology*. 2008;50(4):355–366.
- Waggoner-Fountain LA, Grossman LB. Herpes simplex virus. *Pediatr Rev*. 2004;25(3):86–93.
- Workowski KA, Berman S; Centers for Disease Control and Prevention. Sexually transmitted diseases treatment guidelines, 2010. *MMWR Recomm Rep*. 2010;59(RR-12):1–110.

CODES

ICD10

- B00.9 Herpesviral infection, unspecified
- A60.00 Herpesviral infection of urogenital system, unspecified
- B00.1 Herpesviral vesicular dermatitis

FAQ

- Q: What is the role of suppressive therapy in immunocompromised HIV and solid organ and stem cell transplant recipients?
- A: Suppressive therapy with oral acyclovir is recommended in immunosuppressed transplant patients with a history of HSV infection or positive HSV antibody titers, and may be considered in HIV positive persons with clinical or serologic evidence of HSV-2 infection.
- Q: Is a repeat lumbar puncture necessary at the end of therapy for neonates or for children with HSV encephalitis?
- A: Repeat HSV PCR should be performed on the CSF of all children with HSV encephalitis prior to stopping therapy. If virus is detected, therapy should be prolonged until repeat CSF PCR testing is negative.

HICCUPS (SINGULTUS)

Bradley J. Monash

BASICS

DESCRIPTION
- The hiccup (or hiccough) is an onomatopoeic name stemming from the sound made by the abrupt glottic closure following involuntary contraction of the diaphragm and intercostal muscles.
- The medical term for hiccup is singultus, which stems from the Latin *singult*, originally used to describe the sharp intake of breath associated with prolonged sobbing.
- Usually a benign, yet recurrent nuisance
- Prolonged bouts of hiccups can be indicative of an underlying or serious condition.

EPIDEMIOLOGY
- Fetal hiccups are common in the 3rd trimester of pregnancy, and mothers often feel the rhythmic movement.
- Newborns may spend as much as 2.5% of their time hiccupping, which decreases in infancy.
- There is no seasonal, geographic, racial, or socioeconomic predilection.
- Persistent (>48 hours) and intractable (>1 month) hiccups more commonly occur in men and adults.

GENERAL PREVENTION
Avoid precipitating factors (e.g., eating rapidly, carbonated beverages, alcohol, tobacco).

PATHOPHYSIOLOGY
- A hiccup reflex arc has been elucidated through the study of pathologic hiccups.
  - Afferent limb: receptors in the distal esophagus, stomach, and abdominal side of the diaphragm; signals travel through the phrenic nerve, vagus, and sympathetic (T6–T12) chain branches.
  - Central component: the middle and dorsolateral medulla; independent from the respiratory center, the hypothalamus, and the phrenic nerve nuclei
  - Efferent limb: phrenic nerve to the diaphragm; accessory nerves to the intercostal and scalene muscles, glottis structures, and the esophagus
- Hiccups are often unilateral, involving the left hemidiaphragm.

ETIOLOGY
- Hiccups have many causes, which can be characterized as environmental, peripheral or central nervous system (CNS), toxic-metabolic, psychogenic, or unknown:
  - Environmental
    - Changes in the ambient or gastrointestinal (GI) temperature, cold showers, ingestion of hot or cold beverages
  - Peripheral nervous system (any process that irritates or stimulates the phrenic or vagus nerves or other afferent receptors)
    - GI: aerophagia, ingestion of excessive food or carbonated beverages, gastric insufflation during endoscopy, gastroesophageal reflux, esophagitis, gastritis, peptic ulcer disease, GI malignancies, pancreatitis, gallbladder disease, hepatic or renal disorders, ascites, inflammatory bowel disease, appendicitis, intra-abdominal abscess
    - Thoracic: goiter, cysts, hiatal hernia, pneumonia, bronchitis, asthma, mediastinal lymphadenopathy, lung cancer
    - Cardiovascular: pericarditis, pericardial effusion, myocardial infarction, central catheter migration
  - CNS (any process that may impact the "hiccup center")
    - Neuromyelitis optica, hydrocephalus ventriculoperitoneal shunt, stroke, arteriovenous malformation, CNS trauma, encephalitis, meningitis, brain abscess
  - Toxic-metabolic
    - Alcohol or tobacco use
    - Meds: anesthetic agents, epidural injections, corticosteroids, barbiturates, benzodiazepines, antibiotics, opioids, chemotherapy
    - Metabolic: uremia, hypocalcemia, hyponatremia, hypokalemia, hyperglycemia
    - Infectious: thrush, sepsis, influenza, herpes zoster, malaria, tuberculosis
  - Psychogenic
    - Excitement or stress
    - Conversion disorder
    - Anorexia nervosa
    - Personality disorders
    - Malingering

DIAGNOSIS

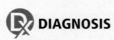

HISTORY
- Hiccups are typically discernible by their classic appearance.
- Ascertain the onset, duration, and any adverse sequelae of hiccups.
- Obtain a complete medical and surgical history, including a thorough review of systems.
- Inquire about prescription and nonprescription medications, tobacco, alcohol, and illicit drug use.
- Screen for anxiety, depression, and other psychiatric disorders.
- Hiccups persisting during sleep suggest an organic cause.

PHYSICAL EXAM
- Head and neck exam may reveal evidence of trauma, foreign body in the ear canal, nuchal rigidity, lymphadenopathy, or goiter.
- Assess the chest for evidence of pneumonia, bronchitis, or pericarditis.
- Examine the abdomen for evidence of an inflammatory process or masses.
- Neurologic examination should be detailed, including cranial nerve assessment.

DIAGNOSTIC TESTS & INTERPRETATION
Hiccup bouts are common and do not routinely require extensive investigations. The history and physical examination will often identify the etiology.

ALERT
Persistent or intractable hiccups require a thorough evaluation.

Lab
- CBC
- Electrolytes (e.g., Na, K, Ca)
- Glucose
- Renal function (BUN and Cr)
- Liver function tests, amylase/lipase
- Toxicology screen

Imaging
Additional testing should be guided by the patient's history, physical examination, and laboratory findings:
- Chest radiograph to look for pulmonary, cardiac, and mediastinal abnormalities
- Chest or abdominal ultrasound or other advanced imaging (e.g., CT, MRI) to assess for occult tumor, infection, or other pathology
- EKG to assess for pericarditis or ischemia
- EGD or esophageal manometry if patient has dysphagia or other esophageal symptoms
- Brain MRI +/− LP to assess for tumor, CNS lesions, stroke, or infection

DIFFERENTIAL DIAGNOSIS
Hiccups present uniquely and are not often mistaken for another entity.

TREATMENT

MEDICATION
- Pharmaceutical intervention is rarely recommended for children and should be reserved for severe or refractory cases.
- There are limited high-quality data supporting any particular medication or intervention for hiccups. Most treatments stem from case series and case reports, primarily involving adult patients. A recent Cochrane review found insufficient evidence to recommend any particular treatment for hiccups.
- When trialed, medications should target the underlying cause if possible.
- Chlorpromazine is the only FDA-approved intervention for hiccups in adults and can be given in low doses PO or IV if no response.
- A variety of other medications have been used to treat hiccups. Careful attention should be paid to risk/benefit ratio prior to initiating pharmacotherapy:
  - Promotility: metoclopramide
  - Anticonvulsants: gabapentin, phenytoin, valproic acid, carbamazepine
  - Muscle relaxants: baclofen, cyclobenzaprine
  - Antipsychotics: chlorpromazine, haloperidol, olanzapine
  - CNS stimulants: methylphenidate
  - Antiarrhythmics: quinidine sulfate
  - Antidepressants: sertraline, amitriptyline
  - Anesthetics: nebulized, oral, and IV lidocaine
  - Antihypertensives: nifedipine, nimodipine, carvedilol
  - Other: amantadine
- For refractory cases, combination therapy has been used.

ADDITIONAL TREATMENT

General Measures

- Treat the underlying cause if identified (e.g., correct electrolyte disturbances, discontinue potential culprit medications).
- Physical maneuvers often serve as the 1st-line treatment for hiccups. Consider harmful effects prior to trying any intervention:
  - Interruption of normal respiratory function: sneezing, coughing, breath-holding
  - Disruption of phrenic nerve transmission: tapping over the 5th cervical vertebra, ice applied to the skin over the area of the phrenic nerve
  - Nasopharyngeal or uvula stimulation: traction on the tongue, stimulating the pharynx with a cotton swab, lifting the uvula with a spoon, sipping ice water, gargling, swallowing a teaspoon of granulated sugar
  - Increased vagal stimulation: applying a bag of ice to the face, Valsalva maneuver
  - Combining physical maneuvers has also been championed (e.g., plugging both ears tightly, pushing both right and left tragus, and drinking a glass of water through a straw without pause and without releasing the pressure over the ears).

COMPLEMENTARY & ALTERNATIVE THERAPIES

- Acupuncture
- Behavioral modification
- Hypnosis
- Suboccipital release

SURGERY/OTHER PROCEDURES

- Surgical treatment is rarely performed.
- Success has been reported with phrenic nerve blockade, percutaneous phrenic nerve pacing, vagus nerve stimulation, and short-term positive pressure ventilation but mostly in adults and in those with underlying chronic illnesses.

ONGOING CARE

FOLLOW-UP RECOMMENDATIONS

- Frequency of follow-up depends on the underlying etiology of the hiccups.
- Patients should be monitored for adverse effects of any medications trialed.
- Successful interventions can usually be stopped the day after hiccups subside.
- If a medication is ineffective after 7–10 days, an alternative treatment should be considered.

PROGNOSIS

- Usually self-limited and resolve within hours.
- Persistent (>48 hours) and intractable (>1 month) hiccups may indicate underlying disease and may lead to complications.

COMPLICATIONS

- Adverse effects that have been associated with intractable hiccups:
  - Vomiting
  - Malnutrition and dehydration
  - Insomnia
  - Fatigue
  - Psychological distress
- Rare complications:
  - Reflux esophagitis
  - Wound dehiscence
  - Pulmonary edema
  - Cardiac dysrhythmia
  - Death

ADDITIONAL READING

- Becker D. Nausea, vomiting, and hiccups: a review of mechanisms and treatment. *Anesth Prog*. 2010;57(4):150–157.
- Buyukhatipoglu H, Sezen Y, Yildiz A, et al. Hiccups as a sign of chronic myocardial ischemia. *South Med J*. 2010;103(11):1184–1185.
- Chang FY, Lu CL. Hiccup: mystery, nature and treatment. *J Neurogastroenterol Motil*. 2012;18(2):123–130.
- Howes D. Hiccups: a new explanation for the mysterious reflex. *BioEssays*. 2012;34(6):451–453.
- Lierz P, Felleiter P. Anesthesia as therapy for persistent hiccups. *Anesth Analg*. 2002;95(2):494–495.
- Moretto EN, Wee B, Wiffen PJ, et al. Interventions for treating persistent and intractable hiccups in adults. *Cochrane Database Syst Rev*. 2013;1:CD008768.
- Pearce JMS. A note on hiccups. *J Neurol Neurosurg Psychiatry*. 2003;74(8):1070.
- Petroianu G, Hein G, Stegmeier-Petroianu A, et al. Gabapentin "add-on therapy" for idiopathic chronic hiccup. *J Clin Gastroenterol*. 2000;30(3):321–324.
- Rizzo C, Vitale C, Montagnini M. Management of intractable hiccups: an illustrative case and review. *Am J Hosp Palliat Care*. 2014;31(2):220–224.
- Roberts H. Bloodletting and miraculous cures. *BMJ*. 2006;333:1127.
- Takahashi T, Miyazawa I, Misu T, et al. Intractable hiccup and nausea in neuromyelitis optica with anti-aquaporin-4 antibody: a herald of acute exacerbations. *J Neurol Neurosurg Psychiatry*. 2008;79(9):1075–1078.
- Viera AJ, Sullivan SA. Remedies for prolonged hiccups. *Am Fam Physician*. 2001;63(9):1664, 1668.
- Wilcox SK, Garry A, Johnson MJ. Novel use of amantadine: to treat hiccups. *J Pain Symptom Manage*. 2009;38(3):460–465.
- Woelk CJ. Managing hiccups. *Can Fam Physician*. 2011;57(6):672–675.

CODES

ICD10

- R06.6 Hiccough
- F45.8 Other somatoform disorders

FAQ

- Q: Why do we hiccup?
- A: The true physiologic function is unknown, although hiccups have recently been postulated as a mechanism to remove air from the stomachs of young suckling mammals. Despite extensive activation of the muscles of respiration, hiccups serve no known respiratory function.
- Q: How good is the evidence supporting the treatment of hiccups?
- A: Most treatments are based on observational studies, case reports, and small case series involving adults. A recent Cochrane review found insufficient evidence to recommend any particular treatment for hiccups.
- Q: Does rebreathing into a paper bag work?
- A: As a fall in P_{CO_2} may increase the frequency of hiccups, rebreathing air may increase P_{CO_2} and thus terminate hiccups. However, this runs the risk of causing hypoxia.
- Q: Will hiccups harm my baby?
- A: Hiccups are usually harmless and are very common in babies. They can be caused by a variety of stimuli, including the swallowing of air or exposure to cold. If they are truly persistent, intractable, or disrupt sleep, they may lead to adverse effects as listed.

HIRSCHSPRUNG DISEASE

Lusine Ambartsumyan

BASICS

DESCRIPTION

- Congenital motor disorder of the gut characterized by lack of ganglion cells in the distal bowel beginning at the anal verge and extending proximally to varying lengths
- Lack of internal anal sphincter (IAS) relaxation and failure of relaxation of the aganglionic segment during peristalsis, producing a functional obstruction.

EPIDEMIOLOGY

Incidence

- Most common cause of lower intestinal obstruction in neonates: 1 in 5,000 births
- Involves the rectum and sigmoid in 75%, descending colon in 14%, whole colon in 8%, and, rarely, small bowel in 3%
- There is familial incidence in total colonic (15–21%) and total intestinal aganglionosis (50%).

Prevalence

- Male predominance with short segment disease ranging from 3:1 to 4:1
- Gender predominance <1:1 in long segment disease.
- Syndromic and nonsyndromic Hirschsprung disease (HD): In the former, there are other congenital anomalies (30% of cases), whereas in the latter, it occurs as an isolated trait.

RISK FACTORS

Genetics

- Loci implicated include those at chromosomes 3p21, 10q11, 5p13, 22q13, 1p36, and19q12.
- *RET* proto-oncogene is the major susceptibility gene; mutations of *RET* account for 50% of familial and 20% of sporadic cases.
- ~5% of patients with HD have mutations in endothelin signaling pathways

PATHOPHYSIOLOGY

- Defects in and failure of caudal migration of the neural crest cells result in congenital absence of distal enteric nervous system (ENS).
- Basic histologic findings are the absence of ganglion cells in the Meissner and Auerbach plexuses as well as hypertrophied nerve bundles between the circular and the longitudinal muscles and in the submucosa.

COMMONLY ASSOCIATED CONDITIONS

- Isolated trait in 70% (nonsyndromic HD)
- Associated malformations in 30% (syndromic HD)
  - Chromosomal abnormalities (12%): the most common is trisomy 21 (2–10% of trisomy 21 have HD)
  - Congenital birth anomalies (18%): cardiac, limb, sensorineural deafness, central nervous system, genitourinary, and gastrointestinal malformations (anal stenosis, imperforate anus, and small/large bowel atresias)
- Other syndromes associated with HD: Waardenburg syndrome type 4, congenital central hypoventilation syndrome, MEN2, and Smith-Lemli Opitz; dysautonomias

DIAGNOSIS

HISTORY

- 80% of patients present in the neonatal period.
- 15% diagnosed in 1st month, 40–50% within 3 months, 60% within 1 year, and 85% within 4 years.
- Adult diagnosis of HD reported in 2% of population.
- Presentation varies with age:
  - Neonatal period: delay in passage of meconium (>48 hours of life); bilious emesis, abdominal distention, complete intestinal obstruction, perforation of cecum or appendix
  - Infancy: constipation associated with fecal impactions and/or episodes of enterocolitis
  - Infancy to adulthood: mild to severe constipation, recurrent fecal impactions, intractable constipation
- Neonates usually have normal weight, but growth retardation may occur when the disease is severe.
- Children with HD may have small-volume and small-diameter stools. Some may have overflow diarrhea as well.
- Enterocolitis (chronic infectious colitis of the colon) is primary presentation in up to 16.6% of patients

PHYSICAL EXAM

- On rectal exam, the sphincter tone is usually normal or increased. Removal of the finger may be followed by explosive diarrhea. In most instances, especially in older children, the rectum is empty.
- Patients may be anemic owing to chronic blood loss from the large bowel secondary to enterocolitis

DIAGNOSTIC TESTS & INTERPRETATION

Lab

CBC: anemia, leukocytosis in the presence of enterocolitis

Imaging

- Plain film of abdomen
  - May show distended intestinal loops
  - Diffuse intestinal pneumatosis has been reported as a rare presentation.
- Barium enema
  - May be suggestive or supportive but not diagnostic
  - Normal barium enema does not exclude HD.
  - Transition zone is a funnel-shaped area of intestine with normal distal area and dilated proximal area.
  - Reveals large intestinal mucosal pattern, prominently thickened folds, and irregular margins secondary to ulceration
  - Significant delay in excretion of barium should also raise one's suspicion for HD.
  - Normal barium enema is commonly seen in the neonate (<30 days old).

Diagnostic Procedures/Other

- Anorectal manometry
  - Safe and noninvasive way to exclude HD in patients older than 3 months of age
  - Lack of IAS relaxation with rectal balloon distention is suggestive of HD.
  - Abnormal study must be confirmed with rectal biopsies.
- Rectal suction biopsy
  - Should be done ~2–4 cm from the anal verge depending on the age of the patient
  - Biopsies must have adequate submucosa.
  - The presence of ganglion cells on histology excludes HD.
  - If the suction biopsies are not conclusive, a full-thickness rectal biopsy (gold standard) is mandatory.

Histologic Findings

- Absence of ganglion cells
- Hypertrophy of preganglionic cells
- Increased acetylcholinesterase staining in the lamina propria

Pathologic Findings

- Aganglionic segment
- Zone of hypoganglionosis proximal to the aganglionic segment
- Incomplete maturation of enteric nerve plexus
- Hypertrophy of nonmyelinated nerve fibers within bowel wall

DIFFERENTIAL DIAGNOSIS

- Mechanical obstruction
- Meconium ileus
- Meconium plug syndrome
- Neonatal small left colon syndrome
- Malrotation with volvulus
- Intestinal atresia
- Intussusception
- Necrotizing enterocolitis
- Functional obstruction
- Intestinal neuronal dysplasia
- Sepsis
- Metabolic disorders (e.g., uremia, hypothyroidism)
- Disorders of intrinsic enteric nerves (diabetes or dysautonomia)
- Disorders of smooth muscle function
- Electrolyte disturbances
- Chronic constipation

ALERT

Early recognition is of utmost importance in reducing the morbidity and mortality of HD.

TREATMENT

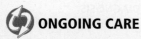

Surgical resection of the aganglionic segment and subsequent pull-through of the ganglionic segment to the anus

GENERAL MEASURES

Stabilizing treatment if child presents with suspected enterocolitis or obstruction:

- Fluid and electrolyte resuscitation
- Nasogastric decompression
- Broad-spectrum antibiotics
- Rectal decompression via rectal tubes and irrigations with saline enemas

SURGERY/OTHER PROCEDURES

- Initial operation
  - Defunctionalizing colostomy or ileostomy for total colonic aganglionosis or if child presents with obstruction not relieved by rectal irrigations
  - Performed to avoid the hazards of enterocolitis
- Definitive surgery
  - Performed 6 months to 1 year after the initial colostomy
  - May be performed as initial procedure in stable, nonobstructed child
- A multitude of surgical techniques have been described.
- Most common surgical procedures are Swenson (rectosigmoidectomy), Duhamel (retrorectal transanal pull-through), and Soave (endorectal pull-through).
- Recent advances include the following:
  - The introduction of entirely transanal techniques
  - Increasing use of laparoscopic assistance with various procedures
  - Transition away from multistaged procedures to a variety of definitive single-stage operations

ALERT
Clinicians must have *high* suspicion for enterocolitis both *before* and *after* definitive pull-through.

ONGOING CARE

FOLLOW-UP RECOMMENDATIONS

Most children are followed on a regular basis for the 1st decade after surgery.

COMPLICATIONS

- Enterocolitis (chronic infectious colitis of the colon) with initial presentation
  - Mortality rates between 20% and 50%
  - Develops in 15–50% of patients
- Early (<4 weeks postoperation, usually related to technical issues)
  - Anastomotic leak
  - Cuff abscess and retraction of pull-through segment
  - Disturbance of micturition
  - Wound infection, intra-abdominal adhesions
- Late
  - Voiding dysfunction: urinary incontinence
  - Sexual dysfunction due to dissection around pelvic nerve plexus
  - Defecation disorders present in >50%
  - Normal bowel function reported in ~68.7%
  - Obstructive symptoms (~11–42%): constipation, abdominal distention, difficulty passing stool
    - Anatomic (anal stenosis, anastomotic strictures, residual aganglionosis
    - Functional (IAS dysfunction, colonic dysmotility)
  - Fecal incontinence (3–53%)
  - Enterocolitis (preop: 15–32%, postsurgically in 2–42%)
- Enterocolitis is major cause of morbidity and mortality:
  - Secondary to obstruction causing an increase in intraluminal pressure and decreased intramural capillary blood flow
  - Affects the protective mucosal barrier, enabling fecal breakdown products, bacteria, and toxins to enter the bloodstream
  - Usually presents with abdominal distention, explosive diarrhea, fever, vomiting
  - Can occur both before and after definitive pull-through
  - Clinicians must have *high* suspicion; can be rapidly progressive and FATAL

ADDITIONAL READING

- Dasgupta R, Langer JC. Evaluation and management of persistent problems after surgery for Hirschsprung disease in a child. *J Pediatr Gastroenterol Nutr*. 2008;46(1):13–19.
- de Lorijn F, Boeckxstaens GE, Benninga MA. Symptomatology, pathophysiology, diagnostic work-up, and treatment of Hirschsprung disease in infancy and childhood. *Curr Gastroenterol Rep*. 2007;9(3):245–253.
- Kenny SE, Tam PK, Garcia-Barcelo M. Hirschsprung's disease. *Semin Pediatr Surg*. 2010;19(3):194–200.
- Menezes M, Corbally M, Puri P. Long-term results of bowel function after treatment for Hirschsprung's disease: a 29 year review. *Pediatr Surg Int*. 2006;22(12):987–990.
- Rangel S, de Blaauw I. Advances in pediatric colorectal surgical techniques. *Semin Pediatr Surg*. 2010;19(2):86–95.
- Rintala RJ, Pakarinen MP. Long-term-outcomes of Hirschsprung's disease. *Semin Pediatr Surg*. 2012;21(4):336–343.
- Swenson O. Hirschsprung's disease: a review. *Pediatrics*. 2002;109(5):914–918.
- Teitelbaum DH, Coran AG. Primary pull-through for Hirschsprung's disease. *Semin Neonatol*. 2003;8(3):233–241.

CODES

ICD10

Q43.1 Hirschsprung's disease

FAQ

- Q: What is the likelihood that a newborn with a diagnosis of HD will have normal bowel function after surgery?
- A: There is a good likelihood, but it may take a number of years: In a 29-year review of 259 patients, 30.3% achieved normal bowel function by age 5 years, 43.9% by age 10 years, 18.9% by age 15 years, and 6.8% after 15 years of age.
- Q: How will the bowel movements change after surgery and over time?
- A: Patients report 3–5 stools per day following pull-through that decreases to 1–3 stools per day over time at long-term follow-up.
- Q: Are laxatives required after surgery?
- A: In ~20% of children, some sort of laxative therapy or rectal irrigation may be required.

HISTIOCYTOSIS

Michelle L. Hermiston

BASICS

DESCRIPTION

- Histiocytic disorders are derived from mononuclear phagocytic cells and dendritic cells. They are divided into three groups.
  - Dendritic cell disorders (e.g., Langerhans cell histiocytosis [LCH], juvenile xanthogranuloma [JXG], Erdheim-Chester disease)
  - Macrophage-related disorders (e.g., hemophagocytic lymphohistiocytosis [HLH], macrophage activation syndrome [MAS], Rosai-Dorfman disease)
  - Malignant histiocytosis (lymphoma subtype)
- LCH (the focus of this chapter) results from the clonal proliferation of immature myeloid dendritic cells that share similar morphologic expression to skin LCH cells.
- Other names include the following:
  - Histiocytosis X, Hand-Schüller-Christian syndrome, Letterer-Siwe disease, eosinophilic granuloma
  - Hashimoto-Pritzker syndrome: infant dermatologic involvement, often self-limited

EPIDEMIOLOGY

- 2–10 cases per million children
- LCH may occur at any age. Median age is 30 months.
- Single system disease in 55% of patients; multisystem disease is more common in children 1–3 years of age.
- Male-to-female ratio approximately one
- May be more common in whites of northern European descent than African Americans

RISK FACTORS

Genetics

- No evidence that relatives of LCH patients are at increased risk of disease
- Very rare reports of recurrence within families
- Specific HLA alleles associated with disease phenotype in some case series

PATHOPHYSIOLOGY

- Single-system LCH: limited to one organ system; most commonly bone followed by skin
- Multisystem LCH involves two or more organs/systems with or without risk organs.
- Risk organs include hematopoietic system, liver, and/or spleen and portend a worse prognosis. Lungs are no longer considered a risk organ.
- CNS risk lesions: Lesions in the facial or anterior or middle cranial fossa bones are associated with a 3× increased risk of CNS involvement.
- CNS lesions can include mass lesions, pituitary stalk involvement, or neurodegenerative disease.

ETIOLOGY

LCH etiology is incompletely understood. *BRAFV600E* mutations are found in ~60% of cases but are not prognostic. Activation of the RAS/MAPK pathway is common regardless of *BRAF* mutation status. Inflammatory infiltrates and abnormal cytokine production in lesions are common, although role in disease remains unclear.

DIAGNOSIS

HISTORY

- Signs and symptoms:
  - Wide variation in presenting signs and symptoms depending on affected organ systems
  - Single-system skeletal disease may be asymptomatic, with incidental discovery of lesions on radiographs obtained for other reasons (e.g., trauma).
- Swelling, pain, or pathologic fracture from soft tissue or bone lesion
- Proptosis
- Persistent otorrhea
- Early loss of teeth; persistent oral ulcers
- Erythematous or brown papular rash
- Persistent seborrheic dermatitis
- Gait disturbance
- Failure to thrive
- Diarrhea, possibly bloody
- Fever of unknown origin
- Headache
- Abdominal pain
- Jaundice
- Polydipsia or polyuria (diabetes insipidus [DI])
- School/cognitive problems
- Dyspnea or persistent cough
- History of spontaneous pneumothorax

PHYSICAL EXAM

- Growth or pubertal delay
- Skin: brownish-red papules often involving intertriginous areas, seborrheic dermatitis (cradle cap), purpura, petechial rash especially at areas of skin contact (e.g., top of diaper); rash may become ulcerated, crusted, or scaly.
- Ears: otorrhea, hearing loss
- Skeleton: swelling or mass; may be painless or very tender to palpation; skull, axial skeleton, long bones more often affected than hands or feet
- Teeth: gingivitis, "floating teeth," oral ulcers
- Eyes: orbital swelling, cranial nerve palsies
- Lungs: tachypnea, intercostal retractions
- GI: hepatosplenomegaly, ascites, edema, jaundice; stool with blood or mucus
- Neurologic: ataxia, cognitive difficulties

DIAGNOSTIC TESTS & INTERPRETATION

Lab

- Routine diagnostic evaluation
  - CBC with differential to evaluate for marrow involvement
  - Liver function tests (LFTs), prothrombin time (PT), partial thromboplastin time (PTT) to evaluate liver function
  - Morning urine specific gravity; urine and serum osmolality to evaluate for DI
- Other investigations
  - Pulmonary involvement: pulmonary function tests
  - Suspected diabetes insipidus (polydipsia/polyuria): endocrine evaluation including water deprivation test and evaluation of anterior pituitary hormone production
  - Auricular involvement: audiogram; ear, nose, and throat evaluation
- Bone involvement: biopsy of lesions unless diagnosis of LCH already established

Imaging

- Chest radiograph and skeletal survey (bone scan not as sensitive in most patients but may be better for infants; whole body MRI may also be used)
- Liver/spleen ultrasound
- High-resolution chest CT if pulmonary involvement suspected
- If neurologic involvement or signs of DI, MRI of brain with contrast, including detailed evaluation of sella turcica
- Dental radiographs if teeth are involved
- CT/MRI of lytic-appearing lesions often obtained prior to diagnosis to evaluate potential malignancy; classic "punched out" lesions may not require imaging beyond plain films.

Diagnostic Procedures/Other

- Biopsy of lesion to establish diagnosis
- Cytopenias or other high-risk organ involvement: bone marrow aspirate and biopsy
- Liver dysfunction: liver biopsy to evaluate for sclerosing cholangitis
- GI involvement: endoscopic biopsy of small and large intestine
- Pulmonary involvement: bronchoalveolar lavage (BAL) or lung biopsy to evaluate for infection if diagnosis of LCH not already established or if CT appearance is atypical.

Pathologic Findings

- Proliferation of immature myeloid dendritic with surrounding inflammatory infiltrate.
- LCH cells are CD1a and CD207 positive; contain Birbeck granules on electron microscopy.

DIFFERENTIAL DIAGNOSIS

- Broad differential, depending on constellation of presenting symptoms
- Bone/soft tissue lesions
  - Sarcoma (especially osteogenic sarcoma, Ewing sarcoma, or rhabdomyosarcoma)
  - Benign bone lesion (e.g., osteoma, bone cyst)
  - Infection
  - Metastatic tumor (e.g., neuroblastoma, leukemia/lymphoma)
- Skin lesions
  - Seborrheic dermatitis
  - Otitis externa
  - Tinea infection
  - Viral exanthem (especially herpes simplex virus [HSV] in neonates)
- CNS lesions
  - Teratoma or malignant germ cell tumor
  - Craniopharyngioma
  - Primary CNS tumor
  - Neurodegenerative disorder

- Pulmonary involvement
  - Infection
  - Emphysema (e.g., α_1 antitrypsin deficiency)
- Fever, lymphadenopathy (nontender, nonerythematous)
  - Lymphoma
  - Lymphadenitis (especially large DNA viruses)
  - Granulomatous (e.g., fungal, cat-scratch disease) infections
  - Rosai-Dorfman or Castleman disease
  - Rheumatologic disease
  - HLH
- Hepatic involvement
  - Infections
  - Congenital hepatic and storage diseases
  - HLH
  - Tumor infiltration (e.g., leukemia)
  - Primary sclerosing cholangitis
- Cytopenias
  - Leukemia or other tumor infiltration
  - Aplastic anemia
  - HLH
  - Myelofibrosis or storage diseases

TREATMENT

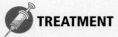

GENERAL MEASURES

- Site and extent of disease determine therapy.
- A multidisciplinary approach is imperative to ensure the best therapy. Patients should be enrolled on a clinical trial whenever possible.
- Duration: 12 months of therapy associated with decrease in reactivation from 50% to 30%
- Type of therapy depends primarily on
  - Number of organ systems affected
  - Number of bone lesions if single system
  - Involvement of "risk organs" associated with morbidity or mortality: liver, spleen, and bone marrow
- Single-system LCH (most often bone, skin)
  - Observation of isolated lesions; often remain stable or spontaneously resolve
  - Local therapy
    - Isolated bone or lymph node: excision or biopsy often curative
    - Confirmed skin-only LCH: topical steroids, nitrogen mustard, or tacrolimus
  - Systemic therapy if multiple or refractory lesions
    - Low-dose chemotherapy for some multifocal bone disease or multiple recurrent single bone lesions; superior results with multiagent regimens
    - Reduces risk of later diabetes insipidus in patients with skull, vertebral, or CNS lesions
- Multisystem LCH
  - Chemotherapy
    - Steroid, vinblastine, plus antimetabolites depending on extent of disease and risk organ involvement
  - Limited response by 6 weeks merits intensification (e.g., 6MP, 2-CdA + AraC)
  - Limited experience with allogeneic stem cell transplantation for very high-risk refractory disease
- Treatment of disease-related morbidity
  - Lifelong intranasal desmopressin acetate often needed for the management of diabetes insipidus; posterior pituitary dysfunction is rarely reversible.
  - Organ transplantation may be necessary for high-risk patients with organ dysfunction.

MEDICATION

- Frontline: corticosteroids and vinblastine; addition of antimetabolites (6-mercaptopurine [6-MP], methotrexate) if multisystem disease and risk organ involvement
- Cladribine has been used in case series for CNS mass lesions. For neurodegenerative disease, case series report variable responses (generally stabilization) to dexamethasone, cytarabine, cladribine, vincristine, IVIg, and retinoic acid.
- Bisphosphonates is being tested for isolated bone lesions.
- Confirmed skin-only disease: topical steroids, tacrolimus, or nitrogen mustard; systemic co-trimoxazole.
- Refractory disease: 2-chlorodeoxyadenosine (2-CDA) ± cytarabine, clofarabine, etoposide,

ADDITIONAL THERAPIES

Radiotherapy rarely used; reserved for refractory or critical bone lesions (e.g., spinal cord compression)

ISSUES FOR REFERRAL

Multidisciplinary care involving several specialties may be required for coordination of chemotherapy and management of orthopedic, endocrinologic, hepatic, hematologic, or pulmonary complications.

SURGERY/OTHER PROCEDURES

- Initial biopsy for diagnosis: often curative for solitary bone lesions even without clean margins
- Excision of isolated bone or lymph node lesions

ONGOING CARE

FOLLOW-UP RECOMMENDATIONS

- Evaluation at regular intervals for recurrence of lesions or new high-risk organ involvement
- Because of variable course, patients should be followed closely at centers with LCH expertise.
- Patients with CNS risk lesions should be monitored for neurodegeneration with detailed neurologic examination, evaluation of school performance, and an annual MRI for 10 years post diagnosis.

Patient Monitoring

- Laboratory and imaging follow-up as described for initial evaluation, with focus on previously affected and high-risk organ systems
- Routine follow-up typically includes history, physical exam, CBC, LFTs, and skeletal imaging.

DIET

Maintain fluid and electrolyte intake if diabetes insipidus is present.

PROGNOSIS

- Prognosis is linked to extent and location of disease. Single-system or bone/skin disease carries low risk of morbidity. Overall survival for patients with high-risk disease is 84%.
- Often, disease will "burn out" by the end of childhood. ~5% of patients will continue to have exacerbations as adults.
- Survival in neonates and younger children with high-risk disease may be poorer. Response to therapy at 6 weeks is the most important prognostic factor.

COMPLICATIONS

- Most common long-term morbidities include orthopedic problems, diabetes insipidus, and neurodegenerative disease.
- Smoking is strongly associated with development of pulmonary disease in LCH patients.
- Chronic disabilities with multisystem disease include pulmonary fibrosis, hepatic fibrosis, deafness, orthopedic problems, short stature, permanent ataxia, neurocognitive deficits, and poor dentition.

ADDITIONAL READING

- Badalian-Very G, Vergilio JA, Fleming M, et al: Pathogenesis of Langerhans cell histiocytosis. *Annu Rev Pathol*. 2013;8:1–20.
- Filipovich A, McClain K, Grom A. Histiocytic disorders: recent insights into pathophysiology and practical guidelines. *Biol Blood Marrow Transplant*. 2010;16(1)(Suppl):S82–S89.
- Gadner H, Grois N, Pötschger U, et al. Improved outcome in multisystem Langerhans cell histiocytosis is associated with therapy intensification. *Blood*. 2008;111(5):2556–2562.
- McClain K. Langerhans cell histiocytosis treatment (PDQ). 2014. http://www.cancer.gov/cancertopics/pdq/treatment/lchistio/HealthProfessional. Accessed February 14, 2015.
- Minkov M, Grois N, McClain K, et al. Langerhans cell histiocytosis: Histiocyte Society evaluation and treatment guidelines. 2009. http://www.histiocytesociety.org/document.doc?id=290. Accessed February 14, 2015.

CODES

ICD10

- C96.6 Unifocal Langerhans-cell histiocytosis
- C96.0 Multifocal and multisystemic Langerhans-cell histiocytosis

FAQ

- Q: Is LCH a cancer?
- A: LCH is not strictly a cancer. It is the abnormal growth of white blood cells that normally help fight infection. Too many are made, and they form a tumor that damages the body. *BRAF* mutations that are associated with several types of cancer are found in approximately half of LCH cases. Similar to true cancers, LCH is frequently treated with chemotherapy.
- Q: Is LCH contagious?
- A: There is no evidence that LCH is caused by an infection or that it is contagious.

HISTOPLASMOSIS

John Arnold • Dylan Kann

BASICS

DESCRIPTION

- Histoplasmosis (also known as Ohio Valley disease, spelunker's lung, cave disease, Darling disease, Appalachian Mountain disease, and reticuloendothelial cytomycosis) is the most prevalent endemic mycosis in United States.
- Dimorphic fungus *Histoplasma capsulatum* var. *capsulatum* in United States (African var. is *duboisii*, which affects skin, LN, and bone)
- Forms include acute, chronic, primary, reactivation, and the affected disease areas (pulmonary, extrapulmonary, disseminated)

EPIDEMIOLOGY

- Endemic in central and southeastern states, classically Ohio and Mississippi River valleys; also prominent in Central America but occasionally in Europe, Asia, and Africa
- Mold form at <35°C (whereas yeast form in tissue above 37°C) grows best in soil environments: warm, moist, and rich in nitrogen (bird/bat guano); found in caves, under roosting trees, abandoned buildings
- Occasional cluster infections usually with soil disruptions (spelunking, building demolition)
- Sporadic cases with some activities: gardening, roofing, installing air-conditioning/heating, cleaning older homes, playing in hollow trees
- Only mammals can be infected (birds don't carry organism).
- No human or animal-to-human transmission except for one case of vertical transmission in infant with co-HIV infection
- Incubation typically 3–17 days but up to 5 months

Incidence

- Total infections: estimated 500,000 per year
- Chronic pulmonary: 1:100,000 cases
- Disseminated: 1:2,000 cases

Prevalence

Skin test reactivity as high as 50–80% by age 18 years in most highly endemic areas

RISK FACTORS

- Males slightly more than females
- Infections more common in 30s–40s but all ages affected
- Disseminated disease risk factors: immature cellular immunity (<2 years of age), large inoculum, acquired immunodeficiency (including TNF-alpha inhibitors), malnutrition

GENERAL PREVENTION

- Avoid areas/dust with likely mold.
- Spray water, oil, or 3% formalin in areas with dust/dirt if work planned.
- Wear cover apparel and face mask able to filter particles >1 millimicron (e.g., N95).
- Prophylaxis for certain populations

PATHOPHYSIOLOGY

- Inhaled mold spores germinate in lungs to yeast form; rarely enter via skin
- Once germinated, some lymphatic and hematologic dissemination even in self-limited disease
- Immune system takes several weeks to respond, involves T lymphocytes, IL-12, IFN-gamma and TNF-alpha; macrophages kill fungus.

ETIOLOGY

Infectious mold spores are microconidia of *H. capsulatum*.

DIAGNOSIS

HISTORY

- Of 5% who develop symptoms, most (60–90%) have pulmonary symptoms and/or flulike illness lasting days to 2 weeks for acute.
  - Most common complaints: headache, fatigue, fever, cough, myalgias, chest pain, which can be pleuritic
  - Pharyngitis, rhinorrhea, and congestion are unusual.
- 5% of symptomatic patients have more prolonged course with additional anorexia, weight loss, arthralgia, and night sweats lasting >2 weeks.
  - "Severe" symptoms: dyspnea and hypoxemia
  - Cavitary form can have TB-like symptoms (e.g., hemoptysis) but rare in children.
- Progressive disseminated histoplasmosis (PDH) (usually <2 years of age or immunocompromised) symptoms: fever, weight loss, hepatosplenomegaly, failure to thrive (in infants)

PHYSICAL EXAM

- For acute pulmonary disease, exam is usually normal, aside from fever and occasionally crackles or decreased breath sounds; wheezing has been reported.
- More severe or diffuse pulmonary disease can present with weight loss, hypoxia, and dyspnea.
- Erythema nodosum (especially adolescent patients)
- Disseminated findings: hepatosplenomegaly, extrapulmonary lymphadenopathy and/or granulomas, oral or skin lesions, adrenal or intestinal masses, multifocal choroiditis, meningitis (60% of PDH of infancy), endocarditis, parotitis, arthritis, signs of DIC
- Other findings could include the following:
  - Pericardial effusion (10% of symptomatic pediatric patients) with potential cardiac rub
  - Pleural effusion
  - Chylothorax
  - Biliary obstruction
  - Superior vena cava syndrome

DIAGNOSTIC TESTS & INTERPRETATION

Lab

- Culture is the definitive method of diagnosis.
  - From sterile site: blood, bone marrow, CSF
  - Can take from 1–6 weeks to grow
  - Culture sensitivity varies with site and host (sputum 10% positive in acute pulmonary, 60% positive in cavitary disease, 90% in BAL from HIV patients).
- Antigen tests using quantitative enzyme immunoassay (often first line)
  - Urine along with blood most common sources for testing (less sensitive but can be done on BAL, CSF)
  - 92% sensitivity: disseminated infection
  - 80% sensitivity: severe pulmonary disease
  - 34% sensitivity: self-limited pulmonary disease
  - 14% sensitivity: chronic pulmonary disease
  - Used to monitor fungal burden
  - Cross-reactivity rarely with *Paracoccidioides brasiliensis*, *Blastomyces dermatitidis*, *Coccidioides immitis*, *Coccidioides posadasii*, and *Penicillium marneffei*
- Serologic: immunodiffusion (ID) and complement fixation (CF) antibody tests
  - Most common test for localized pulmonary disease but often negative in acute period
  - Best tests for chronic meningitis
  - Less sensitive in immunocompromised patients
  - Antibody appears 4–6 weeks after infection, can become negative after 12–18 months
  - Immunodiffusion usually 1st-line serologic test (specific test with only 5% cross-reactivity but only 80% sensitive)
    - Tests for M and H bands; H bands more suggestive of acute infection
    - H bands positive in 23%, M bands positive in 76% of acute pulmonary
  - Complement fixation usually 2nd-line serologic test, as more sensitive but less specific (18% cross-reactivity)
    - Cross-reacts with *Blastomyces*, *Paracoccidioides*, *and Coccidioides*
    - 4-fold increase or single 1:32 or greater is presumptive of active/recent infection.
    - Titers 1:8 and 1:16 unclear significance
- Microscopy
  - Noncaseating granulomas
  - Intracellular yeast form in tissue, blood, bone marrow, or BAL
  - Usually examined with silver stain
- Other lab findings:
  - Mild anemia, elevated ferritin, hypercalcemia, elevated ESR/CRP
  - PDH: pancytopenia, coagulopathy, elevated liver enzymes
  - Meningitis: CSF lymphocytic pleocytosis, protein elevation, and low glucose
- Skin test: not clinically used; only used for epidemiologic studies

Imaging

- CXR
  - Majority are normal in self-limited disease, and 40–50% of cases of PDH are normal.
  - Positive findings can include hilar adenopathy, infiltrates, pleural effusions (5% of children), pericarditis (10% of children), mediastinal granuloma, mediastinal fibrosis (rare in children), mass effect, calcifications.
- Chest CT
  - Miliary nodules and calcifications more easily seen
  - Can be diffuse parenchymal consolidation
- CNS imaging
  - Leptomeningeal enhancement (often basilar), focal brain or spinal cord lesions, strokes, and encephalitis

DIFFERENTIAL DIAGNOSIS

- Pulmonary histoplasmosis
  - Tuberculosis and other mycobacteria
  - Pneumonia (atypical)
  - Other fungal lung infections (blastomycosis, sporotrichosis, and coccidioidomycosis)
  - *Pneumocystis jirovecii* (can mimic PDH symptoms)
  - *Nocardia* and *Actinomyces*
- Mediastinal lymphadenopathy
  - Malignancy
  - Sarcoidosis
- PDH
  - Malignancy
  - Sepsis
  - Opportunistic infections (coinfection is common in immunodeficiency)
  - Hemophagocytic lymphohistiocytosis/macrophage activation syndrome (can be sequelae of PDH as well)
  - Brucella, Q-fever, leishmaniasis

ALERT

- Most children will not require treatment for *H. capsulatum* pulmonary disease.
- Arthritis, pericarditis, and erythema nodosum do not necessitate antifungals.
- Children with PDH should be screened for HIV and immunodeficiency.
- Alert lab of any specimen suspected of *Histoplasma* (lab hazard if grown).

TREATMENT

MEDICATION

- Immunocompetent patients with primary acute uncomplicated (nonsevere) pulmonary histoplasmosis less than 4 weeks' duration do not require treatment.
- Therapy indicated for severe/complicated pulmonary disease, after high inoculum, PDH, infection in immunocompromised
- Pulmonary disease (moderate but >1 month)
  - PO itraconazole 5–10 mg/kg/24 h divided b.i.d. × 6–12 weeks (max 400 mg daily)
- Pulmonary disease (severe)
  - Amphotericin B lipid formulation (unless renal involvement) 3–5 mg/kg/24 h depending on formulation (lipid complex vs. liposomal) or deoxycholate 1 mg/kg daily IV × 1–2 weeks followed by PO itraconazole 5–10 mg/kg/24 h divided b.i.d. (max 400 mg daily) for 12 weeks
  - Methylprednisolone (controversial in children) 1–2 mg/kg daily IV during first 1–2 weeks for patients with worsened hypoxemia or distress
- Disseminated (without HIV infection)
  - Amphotericin B lipid formulation (as above) × 4–6 weeks. Alternative: lipid formulation of amphotericin B (as above) for 2–4 weeks followed by itraconazole PO 5–10 mg/kg/24 h divided b.i.d. for 3–6 months until urine antigen concentration less than 2 mcg/mL
- Disseminated (with HIV infection)
  - Liposomal amphotericin B 5 mg/kg/24 h IV × 2–6 weeks followed by oral itraconazole for at least 1 year to life 5–10 mg/kg/24 h divided b.i.d. (max of 400 mg/24 h)
  - If HAART given for 6 months, CD4 >150 cells/mm^3, antifungal taken for 1 year, and antigen levels low, can consider stopping secondary prophylaxis
- Meningitis
  - Liposomal amphotericin B 5 mg/kg/24 h IV × 4–6 weeks then oral itraconazole 5–10 mg/kg/24 h divided b.i.d. × 12 months and then until resolution of CSF profile; monitor antigen levels.
- Mediastinitis (rare)
  - Amphotericin B × 1–2 weeks then oral itraconazole for 6 months
- Fibrosing mediastinitis (rare)
  - Itraconazole for 3 months
  - May not have any effect on fibrosis
- Pericarditis/rheumatologic manifestations
  - Pericardiocentesis if severe tamponade
  - NSAID (usually indomethacin) for 2–12 weeks
  - Consider oral prednisone (1 mg/kg/24 h).
- Compression by granulomatous disease
  - Consider surgery and corticosteroid with concurrent use of itraconazole.
- Vertical transmission in newborn
  - Amphotericin B (lipid formulation)
- Although the Infectious Diseases Society of America (2007) guidelines state that lipid preparations of amphotericin are "not preferred" in children (except HIV patients), as nonlipid preparations are well tolerated, lipid formulations are most often used due to overall favorable side effect profile.
- Salvage therapy can be done with posaconazole and/or voriconazole; fluconazole is inferior to itraconazole.
- Prophylaxis for CD4 <150 cells/μL, in hyperendemic areas or solid organ transplant recipients, those scheduled to receive TNF inhibitors, or those undergoing intensive chemotherapy with a history of histoplasmosis in the past 2 years: oral itraconazole 5 mg/kg/24 h divided b.i.d. (max 200 mg/24 h)

GENERAL MEASURES

Standard precautions adequate for hospital isolation

INPATIENT CONSIDERATIONS

Patients receiving amphotericin may need prolonged IV access.

ONGOING CARE

FOLLOW-UP RECOMMENDATIONS

- Patient monitoring
  - In PDH, follow antigen levels monthly during therapy and 12 months post therapy
  - Itraconazole blood levels should be measured after >2 weeks of therapy (goal serum level >1 mcg/mL).

PROGNOSIS

- Overall good prognosis except for untreated PDH disease, which is highly fatal
- Self-limited pulmonary patients recover in 2–3 weeks.
- Most treated PDH patients have significant improvement after 2 weeks of IV antifungals.

COMPLICATIONS

- Lymphatic, GI, esophageal, vascular, and biliary obstruction
- Renal stones
- Multifocal choroiditis
- Calcified nodules
- Fibrosis
- Pleural effusion
- Pericarditis
- Chylothorax
- Superior vena cava syndrome
- Macrophage activation syndrome (MAS)

ADDITIONAL READING

- Fischer GB, Mocelin H, Severo CB, et al. Histoplasmosis in children. *Paediatr Respir Rev*. 2009;10(4): 172–177.
- Hage CA, Knox KS, Wheat LJ. Endemic mycoses: overlooked causes of community acquired pneumonia. *Respir Med*. 2012;106(6):769–776.
- Kauffman CA. Histoplasmosis: a clinical and laboratory update. *Clin Microbiol Rev*. 2007;20(1): 115–132.
- Montenegro BL, Arnold JC. North American dimorphic fungal infections in children. *Pediatr Rev*. 2010;31(6):40–48.
- National Institute for Occupational Safety and Health, National Center for Infectious Diseases. *Histoplasmosis: Protecting Workers at Risk*. Washington, DC: U.S. Department of Health and Human Services. http://www.cdc.gov/niosh/docs/2005-109/pdfs/2005-109.pdf. Accessed February 12, 2014.
- Smith JA, Kauffman CA. Pulmonary fungal infections. *Respirology*. 2012;17(6):913–926.
- Wheat LJ, Freifeld AG, Kleiman MB, et al. Clinical practice guidelines for the management of patients with histoplasmosis: 2007 update by the Infectious Disease Society of America. *Clin Infect Dis*. 2007; 45(7):807–825.

CODES

ICD10

- B39.9 Histoplasmosis, unspecified
- B39.4 Histoplasmosis capsulati, unspecified
- B39.2 Pulmonary histoplasmosis capsulati, unspecified

FAQ

- Q: What are the most common clinical presentations of histoplasmosis?
- A: Asymptomatic, mild primary pulmonary disease. Moderate to severe pulmonary, disseminated, and cavitary are uncommon.
- Q: How is histoplasmosis best diagnosed?
- A: Isolation or identification of the organism is definitive. Antigen testing of urine or blood is used for acute infections, especially severe infections. Serologic testing can be helpful but lack sensitivity and specificity. Skin test is not useful.
- Q: Does histoplasmosis need to be treated with antifungal therapy?
- A: For mild primary disease in an immunocompetent patient, no treatment is necessary. More severe or disseminated disease is treated.
- Q: Do patients with histoplasmosis need to be isolated?
- A: Isolation of infected patients is not required.

HODGKIN LYMPHOMA

Elizabeth Robbins

BASICS

DESCRIPTION

B lineage malignant lymphoid neoplasm. Typically presents with painless lymphadenopathy, often cervical (70–80%) or supraclavicular (25%). Mediastinal mass present in 50%. Constitutional symptoms (e.g., fatigue, fever, night sweats, weight loss, cough, pruritus) may or may not be present. Constitutional symptoms sometimes precede development of lymphadenopathy.

EPIDEMIOLOGY

Incidence

- Represents 7% of childhood cancer
- 11.7 cases/million/yr age <20 years
- Most common cancer for ages 15–19 years
- Rarely seen in children < age 5 years
- M > F age <15 years
- F > M age 15–19 years
- Bimodal age distribution in adults: early peak mid/late 20s; late peak > age 50 years

RISK FACTORS

- Few known risk factors include the following:
  - Immune deficiency (e.g., HIV infection)
  - Autoimmune disorders
  - Lower socioeconomic status for childhood form (age 14 years or younger)
  - Higher socioeconomic status for young adult form
- Decreased risk if
  - Multiple older siblings
  - Exposure to common infections in preschool

Genetics

- Familial HL rare, accounting for 4.5% of cases.
- Familial cases may reflect
  - Genetic influences, including inherited immunodeficiency states
  - Environmental factors
  - Exposure to viruses

PATHOPHYSIOLOGY

- Reed-Sternberg cells, a clonal population of large binucleate cells arising from B cells, are the malignant cells in HL. Surface antigen expression includes CD30 but not CD20.
- Only 1% of cells in involved nodes are Reed-Sternberg cells and morphologic variants; the rest are inflammatory cells: lymphocytes, macrophages, fibroblasts, plasma cells, eosinophils.

Classification

Two clinically distinct subtypes of HL recognized:

- Classical HL (90–95% of cases)
  - Nodular sclerosing
  - Mixed cellularity
  - Lymphocyte depleted
  - Lymphocyte rich
- Nodular lymphocyte predominant (5–10% of cases)

ETIOLOGY

- Cause unknown
- Association between Epstein-Barr virus (EBV) infection and HL: 20–50% of patients with classical HL have monoclonal or oligoclonal proliferation of EBV-infected cells.

DIAGNOSIS

HISTORY

- Painless lymphadenopathy slowly increasing in size. Lymphadenopathy often present for weeks to months before presentation. Cervical or supraclavicular sites most common.
- Constitutional ("B") symptoms: 1 or more occur in 20% of children.
  - Fever >38.0°C, not otherwise explained
  - Weight loss >10% within 6 months preceding diagnosis, not explained
  - Drenching night sweats
- Other constitutional symptoms include fatigue, pruritus, cough, and orthopnea.
- Patients with large mediastinal mass may have symptoms of superior vena cava syndrome: dyspnea, facial swelling, cough, orthopnea, headache.

PHYSICAL EXAM

- General appearance: Patients with advanced disease may be tired-appearing and cachectic.
- Fever, if present, is usually intermittent.
- Lymph nodes: Nodes larger than 1 cm are considered abnormal. Cervical, supraclavicular (especially left), and axillary nodes are most common. Other sites include epitrochlear, inguinal, and femoral.
  - Lymph nodes are usually firm, rubbery, nontender, and sometimes matted.
- Lungs: Decreased breath sounds or rhonchi may be noted in patients with large mediastinal mass. Some patients unable to lie flat due to respiratory distress.
- Abdomen: Splenomegaly may be present; hepatomegaly is less common.
- Skin: Pallor due to anemia may be present. Erythematous and excoriated areas may be present in patients with pruritus. Bruises and petechiae rare. Icteric sclera and/or jaundice may be noted in cases with autoimmune hemolytic anemia (rare).

DIAGNOSTIC TESTS & INTERPRETATION

Lab

- No specific lab assay is diagnostic of HL.
- Erythrocyte sedimentation rate (ESR): useful as tumor marker if elevated at diagnosis
- CBC with differential
- Bilateral bone marrow biopsy in selected cases (e.g., patients with B symptoms or advanced disease [Stage III or IV])
- Liver and renal function studies
- Thyroid function (if radiation planned)
- Baseline electrocardiogram, echocardiogram
- Pulmonary function tests (pre-bleomycin)

Imaging

To evaluate extent of disease at diagnosis for staging and to follow response to treatment

- Chest radiograph (posterior-anterior and lateral) to evaluate for mediastinal mass
- CT scan of neck, chest, abdomen, pelvis
- PET or PET/CT: Functional imaging with PET has replaced previous staging modalities such as splenectomy, lymphangiogram, and gallium scan. Used at diagnosis and to follow response to therapy.

Diagnostic Procedures/Other

- Fine needle aspirate or core needle biopsy may occasionally be adequate for diagnosis provided typical Reed-Sternberg cells can be identified.
- Excisional biopsy of lymph node is usually necessary for diagnosis.
- Biopsy tissue studies include the following:
  - Flow cytometry (classic HL usually CD30+)
  - Cytogenetics
  - Culture for aerobic, anaerobic, and acid-fast bacilli if indicated

ALERT

General anesthesia is usually contraindicated in patients with mediastinal mass or tracheal deviation because of the possibility of airway collapse from loss of smooth muscle tone during anesthesia.

- Ann Arbor staging criteria:
  - Stage I—involvement of a single lymph node region (I) or of a single extralymphatic organ or site (I_E)
  - Stage II—involvement of two or more lymph node regions on the same side of the diaphragm (II) or localized involvement of an extralymphatic organ or site and one or more lymph node regions on the same side of the diaphragm (II_E)
  - Stage III—involvement of lymph node regions on both sides of the diaphragm (III), which may be accompanied by involvement of the spleen (III_S) or by localized involvement of an extralymphatic organ or site (III_E) or both (III_{SE})
  - Stage IV—diffuse or disseminated involvement of one or more extralymphatic organs or tissues with or without associated lymph node involvement
  - Modifiers: A/B—presence of one or more B symptoms (see "History") is designated by the suffix B; A denotes absence of B symptoms.

DIFFERENTIAL DIAGNOSIS

- Other malignant process (lymph nodes usually nontender to palpation)
  - Non-HL
  - Soft tissue sarcoma, germ cell tumor
  - Metastatic adenopathy—soft tissue sarcoma, nasopharyngeal carcinoma
- Infection (lymph nodes may be tender to palpation)
  - Epstein-Barr virus
  - Atypical *Mycobacterium*
  - Histoplasmosis
  - Toxoplasmosis
  - Tuberculosis
  - Cat-scratch disease
  - *Staphylococcus aureus*, *Streptococcus*
- Drug reaction (e.g., phenytoin)

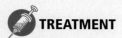

TREATMENT

MEDICATION

- Long-term survival in pediatric patients with HL is >90%. Recent treatment strategies have therefore focused on decreasing intensity of therapy to minimize late effects. Chemotherapy combined with radiation therapy has been the standard approach historically, but HL is increasingly being treated with chemotherapy alone. Response to treatment as measured by PET serves to guide treatment decisions; patients whose disease is no longer PET-avid after 2–4 courses of chemotherapy are often treated with chemotherapy alone.
- Chemotherapy regimens (28-day cycles):
  - ABVD: doxorubicin (Adriamycin), bleomycin, vinblastine, dacarbazine; standard 1st-line regimen for adults
  - COPP/ABV: cyclophosphamide, vincristine (Oncovin), procarbazine, prednisone, doxorubicin (Adriamycin), bleomycin, vinblastine
  - VAMP: vinblastine, doxorubicin (Adriamycin), methotrexate, prednisone
  - BEACOPP: bleomycin, etoposide, Adriamycin, cyclophosphamide, vincristine, prednisone, procarbazine; efficacy similar to ABVD but with more acute toxicities, risk of secondary leukemia, nearly universal infertility

ADDITIONAL THERAPIES

- Radiation therapy
  - Used in combination with chemotherapy
  - Provides effective local control for areas of bulky disease, defined as a mediastinal mass >1/3 the thoracic diameter measured at the dome of the diaphragm on a PA CXR or a large nodal aggregate >6 cm (10 cm by some criteria).
  - Radiation doses and fields have been reduced over the past decade, but late effects including cardiac disease and secondary malignancies including breast cancer are still significant.
- Radiotherapy is commonly employed in the following:
  - Patients with bulky disease (some treated with chemotherapy alone)
  - Patients whose disease is responding poorly to chemotherapy
  - As part of a combined modality treatment strategy with lower dose radiation and less intense alkylator therapy (e.g., Stanford V or recent COG regimens)
  - Salvage therapy for relapsed disease
- Long-term survival ~50% for patients with recurrence. Specific salvage therapy based on remission duration and initial therapy. Typical salvage includes reinduction followed by high-dose chemotherapy and autologous stem cell transplant. Radiation may also be used.

ONGOING CARE

FOLLOW-UP RECOMMENDATIONS

Patient Monitoring

- Patients are monitored for evidence of disease recurrence and for long-term toxicity from chemotherapy/radiation therapy. Two thirds of recurrences occur within the first 2 years of diagnosis.
- Monitoring for disease recurrence includes the following:
  - History, physical exam q 3 months during 1st 2 years off therapy; q 6 months for 3rd, 4th years off therapy; then annually
  - Lab studies including ESR if elevated at diagnosis; CBC
  - Surveillance CT scans q 3–6 months 1st few years off therapy mandated by many protocols; however, some providers follow clinically to avoid radiation exposure and because detecting recurrence by imaging, presumably earlier than clinically, may not result in improved survival. PET scan if recurrence suspected.
  - Periodic CXR: Some providers follow CXR 1st few years off therapy if mediastinal disease.
  - Monitoring for late effects depends on the patient's treatment.
  - Cardiac: periodic echocardiogram, EKG if anthracycline therapy or mediastinal radiation
  - Pulmonary: periodic pulmonary function tests if bleomycin or mediastinal radiation
  - Reproductive: hormonal testing (LH, FSH, estradiol/testosterone) beginning at puberty or by age 12 years
  - Thyroid: annual thyroid function (T_4, TSH) if radiation
  - Secondary malignancies
    - Breast: monthly breast self-exam; yearly mammogram with adjunct MRI beginning 8 years after radiation or age 25 years, whichever is later
    - Thyroid: yearly thyroid exam if radiation
    - Colon: colonoscopy q 5 years beginning age 35 years if radiation
    - Leukemia: yearly CBC, platelets, differential for 10 years after exposure to etoposide, alkylating agents, anthracyclines

PROGNOSIS

- Overall 5-year survival >90% regardless of stage. Prognosis for 5-year disease-free survival depends on stage at diagnosis:
  - >90% for low-stage disease (stage I, II, nonbulky, no B symptoms)
  - 65–90% for advanced disease (stage III, IV)

COMPLICATIONS

- Acute complications of treatment:
  - Chemotherapy
    - Hair loss, nausea, vomiting, cytopenias resulting in infection, bleeding
- Late complications of treatment:
  - See "Cancer Therapy Late Effects" chapter.
  - Chemotherapy
    - Cardiomyopathy, decreased pulmonary function, pulmonary fibrosis, alterations in fertility, secondary leukemia
  - Radiation therapy
    - Breast cancer, other secondary malignant neoplasm, cardiomyopathy, coronary artery disease with myocardial infarction, pericarditis, accelerated atherosclerosis with increased stroke risk, pulmonary fibrosis, hypothyroidism, impaired growth of bones and soft tissue

ADDITIONAL READING

- Cote GM, Canellos GP. Can low-risk, early-stage patients with Hodgkin lymphoma be spared radiotherapy? *Curr Hematol Malig Rep*. 2011;6(3):180–186.
- Kelly KM, Hodgson D, Appel B, et al. Children's Oncology Group's 2013 blueprint for research: Hodgkin lymphoma. *Pediatr Blood Cancer*. 2013;60(6):972–978.
- Meyer RM, Hoppe RT. Point/counterpoint: early-stage Hodgkin lymphoma and the role of radiation therapy. *Blood*. 2012;120(23):4488–4495.
- O'Brien MM, Donaldson SS, Balise RR, et al. Second malignant neoplasms in survivors of pediatric Hodgkin's lymphoma treated with low-dose radiation and chemotherapy. *J Clin Oncol*. 2010;28(7):1232–1239.

CODES

ICD10

- C81.90 Hodgkin lymphoma, unspecified, unspecified site
- C81.91 Hodgkin lymphoma, unsp, lymph nodes of head, face, and neck
- C81.92 Hodgkin lymphoma, unspecified, intrathoracic lymph nodes

HUMAN IMMUNODEFICIENCY VIRUS INFECTION

Hiwot Hiruy • Allison Agwu

BASICS

DESCRIPTION

- HIV-1 and HIV-2 are the etiologic agents of HIV infection and AIDS. Infection is lifelong.
- HIV-1 is more common worldwide, whereas HIV-2 is mainly prevalent in West Africa.
- Typically, an acute phase with flulike symptoms develops 2–4 weeks after acquiring infection, followed by a long asymptomatic period (5–15 years in adults, shorter in children), then the development of nonspecific signs and symptoms (weight loss, adenopathy, hepatosplenomegaly, failure to thrive) and mild clinical immunodeficiency.
- Without treatment, the infected person will experience progressive immunologic deterioration and eventually become susceptible to opportunistic infections and cancers (AIDS).

GENERAL PREVENTION

- HIV infection is almost completely preventable.
- Risk of transmission to newborns of HIV-infected women can be decreased:
  - With antenatal 3-drug regimens, delivery via elective cesarean section for selected cases, and 6 weeks of postnatal zidovudine, perinatal transmission rates are now 2% or less in HIV specialty care sites.
  - All pregnant women should be offered HIV testing at the first prenatal visit. In areas of high incidence, repeat testing should be done at 36 weeks of gestation.

EPIDEMIOLOGY

HIV infection is transmitted via the following:

- Sexual contact
  - Male-to-female transmission more efficient than female to male
  - Anal receptive sex more likely to transmit than vaginal sex
- Exposure to infected blood or bodily fluids
  - Usually parenteral exposure to infected blood (via transfusions or sharing needles)
  - Risk of transmission from an HIV-contaminated needle is 1/300.
- Breast milk
  - Overall risk of breastfeeding is ~15%.
  - In countries where breastfeeding is the norm, up to 30% of perinatally acquired HIV infections occur through breastfeeding.
- Perinatal infection can occur either in utero or during labor and delivery:
  - Of perinatally infected infants, 5–10% are believed infected in utero, whereas ~20% acquire infection around the time of birth.
  - Risk of an HIV-infected mother (not on treatment) giving birth to an infected infant is ~20% (in the absence of breastfeeding), with increased rate of transmission for women with low CD4 counts or higher viral titers. Vaginal delivery, especially with rupture of membranes >8 hours, appears to increase the risk of infant infection.
  - Presence of untreated sexually transmitted infections (STIs), chorioamnionitis, and prematurity all increase the risk of mother-to-child transmission of HIV.
- HIV is not believed to be transmitted by the following:
  - Bites
  - Sharing utensils, bathrooms, bathtubs
  - Exposure to urine, feces, vomitus (except where these fluids may be grossly contaminated with blood, and even then transmission is rare, if it happens at all)
  - Casual contact at home, school, or day care center

DIAGNOSIS

HISTORY

Clinical signs, symptoms, and scenarios in which HIV testing should be performed:

- Infants with maternal HIV status that is unknown or positive
- IV drug use
- Noninjectable drug use
- STIs, especially syphilis
- All adolescents (particularly those endorsing sexual activity), at least annually
- Transfusions before 1986
  - Frequent infections, including recurrent sinopulmonary infections, recurrent pneumonia/invasive bacterial disease:
- Severe acute pneumonia (*Pneumocystis*)
- Recurrent or resistant thrush, especially after 12 months of age
- Congenital syphilis
- Acquired microcephaly
- Progressive encephalopathy, loss of developmental milestones
- History of idiopathic thrombocytopenic purpura/thrombocytopenia
- Failure to thrive
- Recurrent/chronic diarrhea
- Recurrent/chronic parotid gland enlargement
- Generalized lymphadenopathy

PHYSICAL EXAM

- May be normal in the first months of life
- 90% have exam findings by 2 years of age
- Most common findings are generalized adenopathy, hepatosplenomegaly, failure to thrive, recurrent/resistant thrush, (especially after 1 year of age)
- Recurrent or chronic parotitis

DIAGNOSTIC TESTS & INTERPRETATION

Lab

- Enzyme-linked immunosorbent assay (ELISA) antibody screen
  - For children >18 months of age, repeatedly reactive ELISA antibody screen, followed by confirmation with Western blot analysis, is diagnostic of HIV infection.
  - Any positive test should always be repeated before a definitive diagnosis is discussed with family.
  - In 1st year of life, positive HIV ELISA and Western blot antibody tests simply confirm maternal infection because the antibody test is IgG based and maternal anti-HIV antibodies readily cross placenta. Maternal antibodies may remain detectable in the infant until 15 months of age.
- HIV-1/2 antigen/antibody combination point-of-care testing is a qualitative immunoassay that simultaneously detects presence of HIV p-24 antigen and HIV 1/2 antibodies is available for children >13 years of age
  - The test can help identify patients with acute HIV infection, which may have not been identified by antibody testing alone.
  - Note that this test is NOT FDA approved for use in newborns and children younger than 12 years of age.
- HIV RNA or DNA polymerase chain reaction (PCR) DNA testing
  - Most reliable way of diagnosing HIV infection in infancy
  - Both tests have sensitivities and specificities >95% after 2 weeks of age.
- Elevated IgG levels: generally reaches twice the normal values by 9 months of age
- CD4 counts
  - Obtained at diagnosis and every 1–3 months
  - Results need to be evaluated based on age-adjusted normal values. Absolute CD4 counts are elevated in childhood, with normal median values >3,000/mm^3 in the 1st year of life, which then gradually decline with age, reaching values comparable with adult levels (800–1,000/mm^3) by age 7 years.
  - For children <5 years of age, CD4% should be used instead of absolute CD4 count.
- Quantitative viral RNA PCR assays
  - Termed "viral loads," results are reported in a range from undetectable, usually <20 copies/mL (cpm), to upper values of >10 million cpm.
  - Long-term prognosis is closely related to viral loads.
  - Viral loads that remain >100,000 are associated with poor short-term (2- to 5-year) outcomes.
  - Also used as a marker of efficacy of treatment; goal is to suppress viral replication to the undetectable range for as long as possible. 50–80% of pediatric patients presently followed at tertiary sites have an undetectable viral load.
  - Test is done at time of diagnosis (twice) to establish baseline, 1 month after initiating or changing therapies, and approximately every 3 months thereafter.
- Neurologic evaluation, with consideration of psychometric testing (baseline) and subsequently, particularly if abnormal. Neuroimaging is indicated in those with abnormal results.
- Postimmunization antibody levels to assess B-cell function
- Other frequent lab abnormalities include thrombocytopenia, anemia, and elevated liver enzymes.

DIFFERENTIAL DIAGNOSIS

- Neoplastic disease
  - Lymphoma
  - Leukemia
  - Histiocytosis X
- Infectious
  - Congenital/perinatal cytomegalovirus
  - Toxoplasmosis
  - Congenital syphilis
  - Acquired Epstein-Barr virus

- Congenital immunodeficiency syndromes
  - Wiskott-Aldrich syndrome
  - Chronic granulomatous disease

ALERT

Failure to screen for HIV infection during pregnancy results in inability to offer antiretroviral therapy during pregnancy, which may lead to failure of preventing infant infection, as well as the inability to prescribe *Pneumocystis carinii* pneumonia prophylaxis to infected newborns.

TREATMENT

ADDITIONAL TREATMENT

General Measures

- Active immunizations
  - All infected children receive standard childhood immunizations, including the pneumococcal conjugate vaccine.
  - Infected children should receive yearly influenza A/B immunizations and 23- valent pneumococcal vaccine at age 2 years.
  - Symptomatic children should not receive the varicella vaccine, and those with severely low CD4 counts should not receive measles-mumps-rubella vaccination.
- Postexposure passive immunization (immunoglobulin) is recommended for the following:
  - HIV-infected children without history of previous chickenpox or those that did not receive two doses of vaccine who are exposed to chickenpox
  - HIV-infected children with severe immunosuppression and tetanus-prone wound
  - HIV-infected children with severe immunosuppression who are exposed to measles
- Immune enhancement
  - Passive: Studies done before the present era of antiretroviral therapy indicate that monthly gamma globulin infusions somewhat decreased febrile episodes and pneumococcal bacteremia. The children who benefit the most are those not on antibiotic prophylaxis for *P. carinii* pneumonia and/or who have had at least 2 episodes of invasive bacterial infections.
- Prophylaxis: One of the major advances has been the ability to offer prophylaxis against the most common opportunistic infections.

MEDICATION

Antiretroviral therapy

- Specific combination antiretroviral therapy prolongs life, delays progression of illness, promotes improved growth, and improves neurologic outcome.
- There is one report (2013) of a toddler initiated on antiretroviral therapy within hours of life who attained "functional cure," but detectable levels of HIV were found in the child less than one year later. More studies are underway to evaluate early antiretroviral therapy.
- Standard of care now involves the administration of combination therapy (usually 3 or more drugs), termed highly active antiretroviral therapy (HAART). There are now 5 different drug classes and as multiple multiclass combination pills.
- Given the complexities of therapy, antiretroviral therapy should always be prescribed in consultation with a specialist in pediatric/adolescent HIV infection.
- Adherence to prescribed schedules is critical. When patients miss even 10–20% of doses, the durability of response is short.

ONGOING CARE

FOLLOW-UP RECOMMENDATIONS

- Family psychosocial support is critical.
- All infected patients should be comanaged with an HIV specialty care site.
- Patients should be seen every 1–3 months to monitor adherence, immune status (CD4 counts), and virologic suppression (quantitative plasma viral RNA).

PROGNOSIS

Due to HAART, morbidity and mortality have both greatly decreased:

- Median survival is now into adulthood.
- Incidence of new opportunistic infections (AIDS-defining illnesses) has decreased greatly, as have hospital admissions.

COMPLICATIONS

- *P. jiroveci* (previously *P. carinii*) pneumonia
  - Most common early fatal illness in HIV-infected children (peak age 3–9 months) mortality is 30–50%. A high index of suspicion is necessary for prompt diagnosis (by lavage) and initiation of therapy.
  - 40% of new cases of HIV-related pediatric *P. jiroveci* pneumonia involve infants not previously recognized as HIV infected.
- Lymphocytic interstitial pneumonitis
  - Frequently asymptomatic; can lead to slow onset of chronic respiratory symptoms
  - Causes a distinctive diffuse reticulonodular pattern on chest radiographs
  - Usually diagnosed between 2 and 4 years of age; related to dysfunctional immune response to Epstein-Barr virus infection
  - Definitive diagnosis is made by lung biopsy.
  - For symptomatic patients, prednisone is effective.
- Recurrent invasive bacterial infections
  - Prior to the use of pneumococcal conjugate vaccines and HAART, the risk of bacteremia/pneumonia was ~10%/year in HIV-infected children.
  - Pneumococcal bacteremia is the most common invasive bacterial disease.
  - Bacterial pneumonia, sinusitis, and otitis media are common.
- Progressive encephalopathy
  - Diagnosed between 9 and 18 months of age, the hallmark is progressive loss of milestones or neurologic dysfunction.
  - Cerebral atrophy, with or without basal ganglion calcifications, on neuroimaging
- Disseminated *Mycobacterium avium* intracellulare
  - Older children, usually >5 years of age, with severe immunodeficiency (CD4 ≤100)
  - Symptoms include prolonged fevers, abdominal pain, anorexia, and diarrhea.
- *Candida* esophagitis: Older children with severe immunodeficiency usually present with dysphagia or chest pain and oral thrush. Diagnosis indicated by barium swallow, but definitive diagnosis made by biopsy
- Disseminated cytomegalovirus disease
  - Retinitis less common in HIV-infected children than in adults
  - Cytomegalovirus may also cause pulmonary disease, colitis, and hepatitis.
- HIV-related cancers: Non-Hodgkin lymphoma most common cancer, with primary site usually located in the CNS.
- Other organ dysfunction associated with HIV-infection in children: cardiomyopathy, hepatitis, renal disease, thrombocytopenia, idiopathic thrombocytopenic purpura

ADDITIONAL READING

- American Academy of Pediatrics. Human immunodeficiency virus infection. In: Pickering LK, Baker CJ, Kimberlin DW, et al, eds. *Red Book: 2012 Report of the Committee on the Infectious Disease*. 29th ed. Elk Grove Village, IL: American Academy of Pediatrics; 2012.
- Panel on Antiretroviral Therapy and Medical Management of HIV-Infected Children. Guidelines for the use of antiretroviral agents in pediatric HIV infection. http://aidsinfo.nih.gov/contentfiles/lvguidelines/pediatricguidelines.pdf. Accessed September 2013.
- Panel on Treatment of HIV-Infected Pregnant Women and Prevention of Perinatal Transmission. Recommendations for use of antiretroviral drugs in pregnant HIV-1- infected women for maternal health *and* interventions to reduce perinatal HIV transmission in the United States. http://aidsinfo.nih.gov/contentfiles/lvguidelines/PerinatalGL.pdf. Accessed September 2013.
- Rakhmanina N, Phelps BR, Pharmacotherapy of pediatric HIV infection. *Pediatr Clin North Am*. 2012;59(5):1093–1115.

CODES

ICD9

- B20 Human immunodeficiency virus [HIV] disease
- Z21 Asymptomatic human immunodeficiency virus infection status
- R75 Inconclusive laboratory evidence of human immunodef virus

FAQ

- Q: Should HIV-positive mothers breastfeed?
- A: The recommendation for HIV-positive mothers in resource-rich areas is to NOT breastfeed, as breastfeeding poses continued risk of exposure and infection with HIV to the infant. In areas where there are no affordable and safe substitutes of breastfeeding, exclusive breastfeeding is advised.
- Q. What are the recommendations for HIV screening in adolescents?
- A. The Centers for Disease Control and Prevention (CDC) recommend routine HIV testing for individuals aged 13–65 years. As part of anticipatory guidance, the American Academy of Pediatrics recommends offering HIV testing for adolescents aged 16–18 years of age at least once if prevalence of HIV in the area is >0.1%. Continued HIV screening is also recommended for youth with high-risk behavior and those undergoing STI evaluations.

HUMAN PAPILLOMA VIRUS

Elizabeth M. Wallis • Sarah E. Winters

BASICS

DESCRIPTION
- Members of the Papillomaviridae family, the human papillomaviruses (HPV), which cause warts of the skin and mucous membranes
  - Exophytic venereal warts or condylomata acuminata are primarily caused by HPV types 6 and 11.
  - Warts can be found on the external genitalia and the urethra, vagina, cervix, anus, and mouth. HPV types 6 and 11 are also associated with squamous cell carcinoma of the external genitalia.
  - Virus types 16, 18, 31, 33, and 35 typically cause subclinical infection in the anogenital region and have been associated with intraepithelial genital carcinomas.
- HPV can also cause recurrent respiratory papillomatosis (RRP) in infants and young children. RRP primarily impacts the larynx but can also cause lesions anywhere along the respiratory tract.
- Increasing evidence that HPV may play a role in squamous cell carcinomas of the oropharynx

EPIDEMIOLOGY
- General
  - HPV is the most common viral sexually transmitted infection (STI).
  - Genital warts and HPV infection are diseases of young adults 16–25 years of age.
  - Cervical cancer is the 3rd most common female cancer worldwide.
- Genital HPV
  - Peak prevalence among women 18–24 years of age
  - At least 40% of sexually active adolescents are infected with HPV.
  - <1% of adolescents develop genital warts.
  - 500,000 new cases of cervical cancer diagnosed each year internationally
- RRP
  - RRP impacts 4.5 per 100,000 children, mostly those age 2–3 years.
  - 67% of children with RRP are born to mothers who had condyloma during pregnancy.

RISK FACTORS
- Infants
  - Primarily vertical transmission at birth
- Adolescents
  - Behavioral risks, including young age at 1st coitus, multiple partners, cigarette use, and having older male partners
  - Biologic risk in adolescent girls secondary to cervical anatomy

GENERAL PREVENTION
- Vaccination to prevent HPV types 6, 11, 16, and 18. Vaccination is recommended for female and male patients starting at age 11 years and is approved for use for persons aged 9–26 years.
- Condom use may diminish transmission.
- Examine partners; treat those infected.
- Pap smear in adult women to assess for cervical dysplasia
- HPV infection is not a reportable disease.

PATHOPHYSIOLOGY
- Transmission
  - Primarily through sexual contact
  - Can also be acquired during the birth process
  - Transmission from nongenital sites is rare.
- The incubation period is variable and ranges from 3 months to several years.
- The virus is trophic for epithelial cells and infects the basal layer of actively dividing cells.
- Infection results in koilocytosis and nuclear atypia. Genital infections may progress to severe dysplasia and carcinoma in situ (CIS).
- Spontaneous regression of clinical disease occurs in 90% of low-risk types and 75% of high-risk types.
- Recurrence is common.

COMMONLY ASSOCIATED CONDITIONS
- Epidermodysplasia verruciformis
- Other STIs

DIAGNOSIS

HISTORY
- Genital HPV
  - Most patients have no symptoms.
  - Presence of warts, often painless
  - Vaginal, urethral, or anal discharge; bleeding; local pain
  - Dysuria
  - Pruritus
- RRP
  - Infants have hoarse or weak cry, stridor, and failure to thrive.
  - Older children have hoarseness, stridor, dysphonia, and obstructive sleep apnea.

PHYSICAL EXAM
- Genital HPV
  - Warts appear as soft, sessile tumors with surfaces ranging from smooth to rough with many finger-like projections.
  - HPV may also cause flat keratotic plaques that project only slightly with a hyperpigmented surface and are difficult to identify without the addition of acetic acid.
  - Subclinical infection is common, causing many foci of epithelial hyperplasia invisible to the examiner.
  - In males, infection is found on the penis, urethra, scrotum, and perianal areas.
  - In females, infection involves the urethra, vagina, cervix, and perianal area.
  - Diagnosis is made by visual inspection of the anogenital region. Cervical dysplasia is not clinically apparent on exam.
- RRP
  - Often normal exam but, on visualization of trachea, multiple verrucous, polypoid growths on vocal rods, subglottic region, and trachea can be seen.

DIAGNOSTIC TESTS & INTERPRETATION

Lab
- Application of 3–5% acetic acid for 5 minutes causes lesions to appear white and thus more readily apparent and can help with the detection of cervical disease.
- Tissue specimens may show koilocytosis typical for HPV infection.
- Pap smear with liquid cytology to assess for evidence of cervical dysplasia resulting from HPV infection
- Colposcopy aids the diagnosis of cervical lesions.
- Polymerase chain reaction is commercially available for HPV typing and is used in patients >21 years with abnormal Pap smears.

Diagnostic Procedures/Other
- Genital HPV
  - Pap smear or colposcopy to screen for cervical dysplasia
- RRP
  - Direct visualization of the airway through laryngoscopy

DIFFERENTIAL DIAGNOSIS
- Genital HPV
  - Condyloma lata (syphilis infection)
  - Molluscum contagiosum
  - Pink pearly papules or hypertrophic papillae of the penis
  - Lipomas
  - Fibromas
  - Adenomas
- RRP
  - Croup
  - Vocal cord paralysis
  - Other forms of nasal, laryngeal, pharyngeal, or tracheal obstruction

TREATMENT

MEDICATION

Table 1. Treatment for external warts

Medication	Procedure	Side effect
Podofilox 0.5%	Patient applies medicine with a cotton swab b.i.d. for 3 days. After 4 days, it is repeated as necessary for 4 cycles. The area for treatment should not exceed 10 cm^2, and total drug should not exceed 0.5 mL/24 h.	Local
Imiquimod 5% cream	Patient applies cream at bedtime 3 times per week for up to 16 weeks. It is washed off after 6–10 hours.	Local
Podophyllin 10–25%	A practitioner applies a small amount to each wart and allows it to air dry. It is washed off 1–4 hours later. Dose is limited to 0.5 mL per treatment to avoid systemic toxicity. Dose may be repeated once weekly up to 4 doses. External lesions only	Local
Trichloroacetic acid (TCA) 80–90%	The practitioner applies this sparingly to each wart directly. Talc is applied to remove unreacted acid. It is washed off after 4 hours. Can be used on mucosal lesions	Local
Laser surgical excision	Requires special equipment and training; often requires general anesthesia; controlled tissue destruction	Local
Cryotherapy	Liquid nitrogen or cryoprobe is used every 1–2 weeks by a specially trained provider.	Local

ADDITIONAL TREATMENT

General Measures

- To date, no therapy exists that eradicates the virus. Recurrences are likely.
- Most patients require a course of therapy rather than a single treatment.
- Genital HPV
  - Lesions on mucosal surfaces respond better to topical treatments.
  - All available therapies have equal efficacy in eradicating warts, ranging from 22 to 94%, with the significant rate of relapse of 25% within 3 months (see table in "Medication"):
    - Consider size, location, number of warts, previous treatment, and patient preference.
    - Also consider patient preference, expense, and side effects.
    - Patients with extensive lesions should be referred to physicians who routinely treat these lesions.
  - Treatment:
    - External: See table in "Medication."
    - Meatal: cryotherapy or podophyllin
    - Anal: cryotherapy or trichloroacetic acid
    - Vaginal: trichloroacetic acid
    - Cervical: Refer to an expert.
- RRP
  - Primarily surgical excision, may regress after puberty

ONGOING CARE

FOLLOW-UP RECOMMENDATIONS

Patient Monitoring

- Follow-up should continue until the warts have disappeared.
- Latent infection and recurrent disease are common.
- United States Preventive Services Task Force (USPSTF), American Cancer Society (ACS), and American College of Obstetrics and Gynecology (ACOG) recommend initial Pap smear at 21 years of age.
- Pap smears may be indicated in sexually active patients younger than 21 years of age if they have HIV, solid-organ transplantation, or chronic immunosuppression.

PROGNOSIS

Therapy will not eradicate the virus; thus, HPV causes recurrent disease.

ADDITIONAL READING

- Brentjens MH, Yeung-Yue KA, Lee PC, et al. Human papillomavirus: a review. *Dermatol Clin*. 2002;20(2):315–331.
- Gunter J. Genital and perianal warts: new treatment opportunities for human papillomavirus infection. *Am J Obstet Gynecol*. 2003;189(3)(Suppl):S3–S11.
- Hathaway, JK. HPV: diagnosis, prevention, and treatment. *Clin Obstet Gynecol*. 2012;55(3):671–680.
- Workowsi KA, Berman S; Centers for Disease Control and Prevention. Sexually transmitted diseases treatment guidelines, 2010. *MMWR Recomm Rep*. 2010;59(RR-12):1–110.

CODES

ICD10

A63.0 Anogenital (venereal) warts

FAQ

- Q: What treatment is indicated during pregnancy?
- A: Most experts recommend surgical removal if necessary. Podophyllin is absolutely contraindicated.
- Q: Should partners of patients with genital warts be referred for examination?
- A: Recurrence is due to reactivation of the virus; reinfection plays no role. Partner may benefit from an examination to evaluate for the presence of warts and for education and counseling. There is no information regarding prophylaxis to prevent infection, so treatment for this is not indicated. Most partners have subclinical infection. Female partners should follow the routine recommendations for Pap smear screening.
- Q: Are genital warts in children always indicative of sexual abuse?
- A: No. The HPV virus has an incubation period of many months. Thus, warts transmitted to infants at the time of birth may not become clinically apparent for 1–2 years. Whether the incubation period can be longer than this time period remains unknown. Thus, maternal history and, potentially, examination are both important factors. However, all children with anogenital warts should be evaluated by a clinician experienced in child abuse evaluations. It is possible that caregivers may transmit the virus to children through close but nonsexual contact; thus, this history is also important in older children.
- Q: Will young women still need to get Pap smears if they have received the HPV vaccine?
- A: Yes. The vaccine does offer good protection against the strains most commonly associated with genital warts and cervical cancer, 6, 11, 16, and 18. However, these strains are not the only ones that can cause infection or lead to cervical cancer. It is important to continue regular screening to ensure that one has not been exposed to other strains that may cause cervical dysplasia.

HYDROCELE

Sophia D. Delpe • Adam B. Hittelman

BASICS

DESCRIPTION

A hydrocele is the accumulation of fluids around the testicle, within the tunica vaginalis or processus vaginalis.

- Can be communicating, fluid passing from peritoneal cavity into patent processus vaginalis, or noncommunicating, fluid confined within the processus vaginalis (hydrocele of the cord) or tunica vaginalis
- Abdominal-scrotal hydrocele has fluid collection within processus vaginalis, extending into retroperitoneum.
- Reactive hydrocele (noncommunicating) is accumulation of fluid within tunica vaginalis caused by infection, trauma, or other inflammatory conditions.

EPIDEMIOLOGY

- 2–5% of male neonates have hydrocele.
- Male more common than female
  - Female: "cyst" or "hydrocele" in the canal of Nuck. May be communicating or noncommunicating
- Right more common than left
- Majority asymptomatic
- Simple (noncommunicating): commonly seen at birth, frequently bilateral, may be large
  - Majority spontaneously resolve in 12–24 months.
- Persistent hydroceles beyond 24 months and those presenting after birth more likely to be communicating
- Age >12 years old: majority noncommunicating
- Adolescent/adult hydroceles are generally acquired (reactive) and idiopathic in origin.

RISK FACTORS

- Similar to inguinal hernia
- Prematurity, low birth weight, gestational progestin use, connective tissue anomalies, cystic fibrosis, cryptorchidism, posterior urethral valves, and other syndromic disorders
- Trauma or infection
- Lymphatic obstruction (i.e., varicocelectomy, filariasis, pelvic radiation, malignancy

PATHOPHYSIOLOGY

- Communicating hydrocele can become indirect inguinal hernia, with potential for incarceration.
- Noncommunicating hydrocele generally thought to be low clinical concern
- Potential damage in large, tense hydroceles
  - Raised intrascrotal temperature can cause potential testicular harm.
  - Tense hydrocele may cause pressure atrophy.
  - Increased resistive index observed in subcapsular artery.
  - Absent testicular diastolic flow

ETIOLOGY

- Similar to indirect inguinal hernia
- In testicular descent, lip of peritoneum descends with testicle, the processus vaginalis, and covers testicle, tunica vaginalis.
- Patent processus in girls (canal of Nuck) related to descent of round ligament to labia, female equivalent of gubernaculum
- Communicating hydrocele essentially is an indirect inguinal hernia (defined by contents entering through patent processus vaginalis: peritoneal fluid versus fat or visceral organ.
- Related to delayed closure of processus vaginalis
  - Complete closure on both side in 18% of newborns
  - 40% close in first 2 months of life.
  - 60% close by 2 years
  - Patent processus vaginalis commonly associated with undescended testicles
  - Adult autopsy data demonstrate 15–30% patent.
- Reactive (acquired) hydrocele is imbalance between fluid production and absorption.
  - Majority are idiopathic.
    - Defective lymphatic drainage
    - Aspirated fluid similar protein content to lymphatic fluid
  - Varicocelectomy 2nd most common cause
  - Result of inflammation from trauma, testicular torsion, torsion of testicular appendage, epididymo-orchitis

DIAGNOSIS

HISTORY

- Inguinal or scrotal/labial swelling
- Age of onset
  - Birth, after birth, >12 years old
- Laterality
- Fluctuation in size: smaller in morning and larger over day in response to activity and upright position; change with crying/straining
  - May be preceded by constipation, upper respiratory infection, vomiting
- Undescended testicle
- Infection, trauma, torsion
- Pain/discomfort
- History of varicocele or other inguinal surgery

PHYSICAL EXAM

- Palpate scrotal/labial swelling
  - Soft or tense
  - Compressible/reducible
  - Palpate testicle
    - Confirm descent
    - Rule out mass, trauma, infection
  - Bowel contents—rule out hernia.
- Transilluminate scrotum to confirm fluid; not diagnostic

DIAGNOSTIC TESTS & INTERPRETATION

Lab

- Urine analysis and culture if concerns for epididymo-orchitis
- Tumor markers (HCG, α-fetoprotein [AFP]) if concern for testicular mass

Imaging

- Imaging not required in an uncomplicated scrotal hydrocele with palpable testicle.
- Transscrotal ultrasound if testicle difficult to palpate or concerns for concomitant problem
  - Assess testicle for pathology, blood flow, and inflammation/infection.
  - Differentiate bowel loops (hernia) from fluid.
  - Fluid tracking to peritoneal cavity can differentiate communicating versus noncommunicating.
  - Fluid tracking to abdominal component (retroperitoneal collection) demonstrates abdominoscrotal hydrocele.

DIFFERENTIAL DIAGNOSIS

- Indirect hernia
- Varicocele
- Spermatocele/epididymal cyst
- Epididymo-orchitis
- Hematocele
- Scrotal lymphedema
- Nephrotic syndrome

ALERT

If palpation of testicle is limited by tense hydrocele, transscrotal ultrasound is important to assess for testicular location, viability, and potential pathology.

TREATMENT

GENERAL MEASURES

- Conservative management for babies presenting at birth with noncommunicating hydrocele (no fluctuation in size) for 24 months
  - Consider surgical intervention if persistent >24 months.
- Fluid aspiration discouraged in babies due to risk of infection.
- Treatment for communicating hydrocele essentially same as inguinal hernia
  - Some surgeons advocate observation for 6–12 months for potential spontaneous resolution.
- Reactive hydrocele managed conservatively
  - Antibiotics for epididymo-orchitis
  - Surgery reserved for pain or patients self-conscious regarding size/appearance.

SURGERY/OTHER PROCEDURES

- Inguinal approach for communicating hydrocele
  - Concomitant orchiopexy (undescended testicle) or orchiectomy (testis mass) when clinically indicated
- Transscrotal approach for reactive hydroceles in adolescent (>12 years old) and adult
  - Consider surgical intervention if persistent >24 months.
- Transscrotal aspiration, with or without sclerosing agent, reserved for postoperative hydroceles.

ADDITIONAL READING

- Cimador M, Castagnetti M, De Grazia E. Management of hydrocele in adolescent patients. *Nat Rev Urol*. 2010;7(7):379–385.
- Clarke S. Pediatric inguinal hernia and hydrocele: an evidence-based review in the era of minimal access surgery. *J Laparoendosc Adv Surg Tech A*. 2010;20(3):305–309.
- Hall NJ, Ron O, Eaton S, et al. Surgery for hydrocele in children—an avoidable excess? *J Pediatr Surg*. 2011;46(12):2401–2405.
- Merriman LS, Herrel L, Kirsch AJ. Inguinal and genital anomalies. *Pediatr Clin North Am*. 2012;59(4):769–781.
- Mickelson JJ, Yerkes EB, Meyer T, et al. L stent for stomal stenosis in catheterizable channels. *J Urol*. 2009;182(4)(Suppl):1786–1791.

CODES

ICD10

- N43.3 Hydrocele, unspecified
- N43.2 Other hydrocele
- P83.5 Congenital hydrocele

FAQ

- Q: Does this need to be corrected?
- A: Noncommunicating hydroceles can be managed conservatively and commonly will resolve within the first 12–24 months of life. Recommendations for watchful waiting are recommended in this age group. Persistent hydroceles after age 2 years are assumed to be communicating hydroceles. Communicating hydroceles are managed similar to indirect inguinal hernias. Some surgeons advocate monitoring asymptomatic communicating hydrocele for 6–12 months to see if they resolve. Hydroceles progressing to inguinal hernia require surgical intervention. Reactive hydroceles are treated if patient is symptomatic, self-conscious of size, or testicle is difficult to palpate.
- Q: What are the potential consequences of leaving hydrocele untreated?
- A: There are no clear long-term adverse consequences for having noncommunicating hydrocele. Potential concerns raised for testicular growth and function, though, may be correctable with hydrocele repair. Hydrocele may continue to grow in size, causing discomfort and distress. Untreated communicating hydrocele may progress to inguinal hernia.
- Q: Are there risks of a hydrocele developing on the other side?
- A: Similar to inguinal hernia, communicating hydroceles have risk of metachronous development of hydrocele on contralateral side. Inguinal hernia will present on other side 8.5–15% of time, although not clearly defined in communicating hydrocele. Visualization of a contralateral patent processus vaginalis does not always correlate with metachronous development of a contralateral inguinal hernia or communicating hydrocele.
- Q: What are the risks of the surgery?
- A: Risks of the surgery are similar to inguinal hernia repair and include anesthetic risks, injury to testicle or spermatic cord structures (gonadal vessels, vas deferens), injury to ilioinguinal nerve, subsequent atrophy of the testicle, and recurrent hydrocele.

H

HYDROCEPHALUS

Jennifer A. Markowitz

BASICS

DESCRIPTION

- Accumulation of CSF in the ventricles and subarachnoid spaces, leading to their enlargement
- Overall head size may enlarge in response, depending on age and cause.

PATHOPHYSIOLOGY

- Normal pathway of CSF: choroid plexus and interstitial fluid (sources), lateral ventricles, foramina of Monro, 3rd ventricle, aqueduct of Sylvius, 4th ventricle, foramina of Luschka and Magendie, subarachnoid space, arachnoid villi, and venous circulation
- Hydrocephalus results from obstruction to CSF flow, impaired reabsorption, or overproduction of CSF.
- Noncommunicating (obstructive) hydrocephalus results from obstruction within the ventricular system.
- Communicating hydrocephalus usually results from impaired CSF reabsorption or (rarely) overproduction (e.g., due to a choroid plexus papilloma).
- The noncommunicating/communicating distinction has no prognostic significance but has implications for etiology and choice of therapeutic intervention.

ETIOLOGY

- Intraventricular hemorrhage is most commonly due to prematurity but may also occur with trauma. It results in impaired CSF absorption due to meningeal adhesions, granular ependymitis, and clots. Posthemorrhagic hydrocephalus (PHH) occurs in 35% of all neonates surviving intraventricular hemorrhage; its incidence increases with increasing severity of hemorrhage.
- Tumors or cysts near the foramina or the aqueduct or within the ventricular system
- Infection (meningitis, intrauterine infection) can lead to leptomeningeal adhesions and granulations that block reabsorption of CSF.
- Developmental
  - Chiari malformation, type II (associated with myelomeningocele, brain migrational disorders, small posterior fossa, inferior displacement of medulla and cerebellar vermis, kinking of the brainstem, aqueductal stenosis, beaking of the tectum)
  - Dandy-Walker malformation (absence of cerebellar vermis, small cerebellar hemispheres, enlarged posterior fossa, often with cystic 4th ventricle)
  - X-linked and autosomal dominant hydrocephalus; the former is often associated with aqueductal stenosis and mutations in *L1CAM* on Xq28.
  - Sporadic primary aqueductal stenosis
  - Dysmorphic syndromes (e.g., Apert syndrome, Cockayne syndrome, Crouzon syndrome, Pfeiffer syndrome, trisomy 13, trisomy 18, trisomy 21, triploidy)
  - Alexander disease
  - Mucopolysaccharidoses (e.g., type II [Hunter], type VI [Maroteaux-Lamy])
  - Migrational disorders/congenital muscular dystrophies (e.g., Miller-Dieker, muscle-eye-brain disease, Fukuyama congenital muscular dystrophy, Walker-Warburg syndrome)
  - Achondroplasia
  - Neurocutaneous syndromes (e.g., neurofibromatosis type 1, rare)
  - Idiopathic

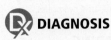

DIAGNOSIS

HISTORY

Presenting concerns:

- Infants: enlarging head, irritability, vomiting, somnolence, poor feeding
- Older children: headache, vomiting, double vision, somnolence

PHYSICAL EXAM

- Vital signs: in advanced acute hydrocephalus, Cushing triad (hypertension, reflex bradycardia, respiratory irregularities): This is not generally seen in infants prior to fusion of the sutures.
- Rapidly increasing head circumference in infants. Fullness of the anterior fontanelle neither sensitive nor specific, but should be noted. May observe splaying of the sutures.
- Mental status: irritability or somnolence in infants, behavioral changes in children (acute or chronic)
- Cranial nerves: "setting sun" sign due to paralysis of upgaze, disconjugate gaze, papilledema, optic atrophy, and visual changes in the chronic setting
- Motor: gait ataxia; spastic paraparesis in chronic hydrocephalus related to pressure on white matter tracts surrounding the ventricles
- Reflexes: increased in chronic hydrocephalus

DIAGNOSTIC TESTS & INTERPRETATION

Imaging

- Head ultrasound
  - Standard screening test for neonates with suspected hydrocephalus or intraventricular hemorrhage
  - Anterior fontanelle must be patent for this test.
  - Demonstrates ventricular size, presence or absence of blood, associated structures, and anomalies
- Unenhanced CT of the brain
  - Mainly used in infants and children whose anterior fontanelles have closed and following shunt procedures
  - Better visualization of 4th ventricle/brainstem and calcifications than with ultrasound; standardized technique that is less operator dependent; better availability in the emergency room setting
- MRI
  - Definitive test for analyzing brain anatomy
  - Can identify posterior fossa developmental malformations such as Chiari and Dandy-Walker
  - Rapid brain MRI protocols for shunt evaluation are replacing CT at some institutions with this capability.
  - MR technique of diffusion tensor imaging may help to estimate local pressure on white matter adjacent to ventricles as a correlate of increased intracranial pressure. The FIESTA sequence (fast imaging employing steady-state acquisition) can show obstruction in the CSF space.

Note: When imaging to diagnose shunt malfunction, it is important to consider the lifetime cumulative radiation exposure for each child and, depending on patient stability, the use of an alternate approach to CT such as rapid brain MRI.

ALERT

Head CT often will not show developmental malformations that may accompany hydrocephalus. MRI is the imaging procedure of choice for elective study.

DIFFERENTIAL DIAGNOSIS

- Other causes of macrocephaly:
  - Familial macrocephaly/"benign external hydrocephalus"
  - Pericerebral effusions
  - Congenital anomalies of intracerebral or extracerebral veins
  - Tumors, intracranial cysts
  - Primary megalencephaly, hemimegalencephaly
  - GM2 gangliosidosis
  - Some leukodystrophies (e.g., Alexander disease, Canavan disease)
  - Head-sparing intrauterine growth retardation (relative macrocephaly)
  - Rapid catch-up growth following prolonged malnutrition
- Other causes of ventriculomegaly, typically with normal head circumference: brain atrophy and chronic ethanol or corticosteroid exposure (reversible)
- Enlargement of the subarachnoid spaces: usually bifrontal, normal to mildly enlarged ventricles. May be seen in children with macrocephaly, who if otherwise normal are diagnosed with "benign external hydrocephalus." Recognize that metabolic and genetic disorders can also present with enlarged subarachnoid spaces (e.g., glutaric aciduria type I, others listed earlier).

TREATMENT

SURGERY/OTHER PROCEDURES

Acute interventions

- Ventricular shunt
  - Indication: progressive or acute symptomatic hydrocephalus
  - Contraindications: active central nervous system infection, active intraventricular hemorrhage, and poor overall prognosis
  - Components: ventricular catheter, reservoir (target of shunt taps), valve, distal catheter
  - Distal sites: Peritoneum is the most common choice; pleura, ureter, venous system, gallbladder, and right atrium are other options.
  - Approach: usually performed as an open procedure; endoscopic procedures available in some centers
  - Complications
    - Shunt failure occurs in 40% of shunts within the 1st year after placement and 50% within the first 2 years. Causes are obstruction, infection, disconnection, or fracture of components; migration of shunt components; overdrainage; and erosion into an abdominal viscus. Presents with symptoms similar to those of acute hydrocephalus
    - Infections occur at a rate of ~8–10% per shunt manipulation, usually during the first 6 months after surgery. Present with low-grade persistent fever and less commonly with erythema of overlying skin. Most common organism is *Staphylococcus epidermidis*; reinfection occurs in 30% of patients harboring this organism.
    - Siphon effect: drop in ventricular pressure on sitting or standing causing headache; newer shunt systems with antisiphon mechanisms are available.
    - Newer shunts have programmable valve mechanisms; one must be cautious when obtaining an MRI in patients with this type of shunt in place, as the magnet may affect valve settings.

ALERT

- Timing of shunt placement is critical and problematic: Sometimes watchful waiting can obviate the procedure, whereas waiting too long may result in brain damage.
- Don't assume hydrocephalus is "cured." Late shunt failure may occur years after placement, often due to fracture of tubing, and can result in death from acute hydrocephalus causing herniation.
- PHH in the neonate may be managed initially with serial lumbar puncture; this has been shown to improve cerebral perfusion in these patients. Most do not require shunt placement. Ultimately, some may require ventriculosubgaleal or ventriculoperitoneal shunts.
- 3rd ventricle fenestration (endoscopic 3rd ventriculostomy):
  - Indications: most effective for obstructive hydrocephalus due to aqueductal stenosis or space-occupying lesions
  - Endoscopic 3rd ventriculostomy combined with choroid plexus cauterization shows benefit for infants, including selected babies with PHH.
  - Complications: overall rate of serious complications 9.4%; these include infection, CSF leak, neurologic deficits, extraparenchymal hemorrhage; rare risk of damage to the basilar artery

ONGOING CARE

FOLLOW-UP RECOMMENDATIONS

- When the etiology or need for shunt placement is unclear, it is important to follow clinical status, head circumference, and ventricular size (by head ultrasound or CT).
- Chronic hydrocephalus is often accompanied by spastic paraparesis, visual problems, and learning problems.
- Most interventions are supportive:
  - Physical therapy, occupational therapy, and orthopedic therapies for spasticity; interdisciplinary cerebral palsy clinics can be critical in providing easy access to these resources.
  - Special education programs may be appropriate for children with severe developmental delay.

ALERT

- It is important for long-term patients in intensive care nurseries to have head circumferences recorded at least twice weekly. Macrocephaly is not always obvious on visual inspection.
- Absence of papilledema does not exclude chronic increased intracranial pressure.

PATIENT EDUCATION

Parent Internet Information: National Hydrocephalus Foundation, http://www.nhfonline.org

PROGNOSIS

Depending on the severity and cause of hydrocephalus, efficacy of treatment, and presence or absence of concomitant neurologic disorders, outcome may vary widely from normal neurologic development to severe impairment or death.

COMPLICATIONS

- Acute hydrocephalus: Herniation syndromes may be fatal.
- Chronic hydrocephalus
  - Macrocephaly
  - Spastic paraparesis may lead to gait and motor problems.
  - Vision loss
  - Developmental delay
  - Precocious puberty due to pressure on the hypothalamus

ADDITIONAL READING

- Air EL, Yuan W, Holland SK, et al. Longitudinal comparison of pre- and postoperative diffusion tensor imaging parameters in young children with hydrocephalus. *J Neurosurg Pediatr*. 2010;5(4):385–391.
- Browd SR, Ragel BT, Gottfried ON, et al. Failure of cerebrospinal fluid shunts: part I: obstruction and mechanical failure. *Pediatr Neurol*. 2006;34(2):83–92.
- Browd SR, Ragel BT, Gottfried ON, et al. Failure of cerebrospinal fluid shunts: part II: overdrainage, loculation, and abdominal complications. *Pediatr Neurol*. 2006;34(3):171–176.
- Drake JM. The surgical management of pediatric hydrocephalus. *Neurosurgery*. 2008;62(Suppl 2):633–640; discussion 640–642.
- Paciorkowski AR, Greenstein RM. When is enlargement of the subarachnoid spaces not benign? A genetic perspective. *Pediatr Neurol*. 2007;37(1):1–7.
- Partington MD. Congenital hydrocephalus. *Neurosurg Clin N Am*. 2001;12(4):737–742, ix.
- Smith MD, Narayan P, Tubbs RT, et al. Cumulative diagnostic radiation exposure in children with ventriculoperitoneal shunts: a review. *Childs Nerv Syst*. 2008;24(4):493–497.
- Warf BC, Campbell JW, Riddle E. Initial experience with combined endoscopic third ventriculostomy and choroid plexus cauterization for post-hemorrhagic hydrocephalus of prematurity: the importance of prepontine cistern status and the predictive value of FIESTA MRI imaging. *Childs Nerv Syst*. 2011; 27(7):1063–1071.

CODES

ICD10

- G91.9 Hydrocephalus, unspecified
- G91.0 Communicating hydrocephalus
- G91.1 Obstructive hydrocephalus

FAQ

- Q: When does an infant need a head ultrasound?
- A: Any infant whose head circumference increases by more than a quartile on the growth chart needs a head ultrasound. Preterm infants below a certain gestational age or birth weight (varies from hospital to hospital) should all receive screening head ultrasounds while in the intensive care nursery.
- Q: When should an infant or child receive an MRI rather than an ultrasound or CT?
- A: Although MRI may be superior in many cases, the logistics of ordering the proper sequences and the need for sedation or anesthesia for long studies (although some institutions now have rapid MR sequences for shunt evaluation) must be strongly considered. Consultation with a neurologist or neurosurgeon is generally advised.
- Q: What is the workup for shunt obstruction and shunt infection?
- A: Symptoms and signs of increased intracranial pressure should lead to a neurosurgical evaluation; the most useful studies include head CT or rapid brain MRI (to assess ventricular size and placement of ventricular catheter) and shunt series (plain films of the entire shunt system to check for disruptions). "Pumping" the shunt reservoir is a procedure with a low positive predictive value for shunt failure. Tapping the shunt to assess pressure must be done with discretion, as repeated taps may disrupt the valve mechanism. Fever is the most important indication for a shunt infection evaluation (shunt tap with CSF cell count, protein, glucose, Gram stain, and culture). Often, patients will be evaluated for both complications.

HYDRONEPHROSIS

J. Christopher Austin • Michael C. Carr

BASICS

DESCRIPTION

- Hydronephrosis: dilation of the renal pelvis (pelviectasis) and calyces (caliectasis) due to excess urine in the collecting system of the kidney
- Hydroureteronephrosis: dilation of the renal collecting system and the ureter to the level of the bladder

EPIDEMIOLOGY

- Incidence of genitourinary abnormalities noted on routine prenatal ultrasound is 0.2%.
- 87% of these are antenatally detected hydronephrosis/hydroureteronephrosis.
- 5% of fetuses with hydronephrosis are due to ureteropelvic junction obstruction.
- Posterior urethral valves and triad syndrome account for 6% of cases.

ETIOLOGY

- Ureteropelvic junction obstruction
  - Intrinsic narrowing or an aperistaltic segment of distal ureter. These are also called megaureters.
- Vesicoureteral reflux
  - In primary reflux (grades I–V depending on the severity), it is due to an insufficient flap valve–type mechanism at the ureterovesical junction.
  - Hydroureteronephrosis is usually seen only with higher grades of reflux (grades III–V) or secondary reflux (reflux in the presence of an abnormal bladder, in which the reflux is often due to high storage or voiding pressures within the bladder). Secondary reflux is not graded.
- Ureterocele
  - Hydroureteronephrosis secondary to obstruction of the ureter from a cystic dilation of the intravesical portion of the distal ureter
  - Most often associated with the upper pole ureter in duplicated collecting system; less frequently associated with a single system
  - Ureterocele is further classified as intravesical (contained completely within the bladder) or ectopic (extending down the bladder neck and often into the urethra).
- Ectopic ureter
  - A ureter that drains into an abnormal location away from the trigone
  - The hydroureteronephrosis can be the upper pole ureter of a duplicated collecting system or a single system.
  - Ectopic ureters can drain at various sites along the lower urinary tract depending on the sex of the child. In boys, they can drain into the bladder neck, prostatic urethra, vas deferens, seminal vesicle, or epididymis. In girls, they can drain into the bladder neck, urethra, introitus, and vagina.
  - The ectopic locations often require passage through the bladder neck or urogenital diaphragm, which produces obstruction of the distal ureter.
- Urolithiasis
  - Obstructing calculi often produce dilation of the urinary tract proximal to its location.
  - Stone disease is rare in infancy except in preterm infants who receive furosemide.
  - The hydronephrosis is usually associated with renal colic.
- Posterior urethral valves
  - Hydroureteronephrosis: nearly always bilateral, produced by outflow obstruction of the bladder from valve leaflets in the prostatic urethra
  - Because both kidneys are affected, there is a significant risk of chronic renal insufficiency and development of end-stage renal disease.
- Triad syndrome
  - Hydroureteronephrosis, often with massively dilated ureters, and a large bladder
  - Also known as prune belly syndrome or Eagle-Barrett syndrome
  - These boys have a triad of hypoplastic abdominal wall musculature (leading to a prunelike appearance), bilateral undescended testes, and a dilated urinary tract.
  - Many have associated urethral atresia, imparting worse renal function prognosis.
  - Exact cause of triad syndrome remains elusive.
  - Significant risk of renal insufficiency in these patients
  - A similar syndrome may occur in girls with a prunelike appearance to the abdomen and anomalies of the urogenital tract; however, it is very rare.

DIAGNOSIS

HISTORY

- Newborns
  - Antenatal hydronephrosis: Presence of hydronephrosis or hydroureteronephrosis
  - If unilateral, severity of hydronephrosis and the status of contralateral kidney
  - If bilateral, presence of bladder wall thickening, bladder enlargement, bladder emptying, or a dilated posterior urethra (keyhole sign) may indicate posterior urethral valves or triad syndrome.
  - If oligohydramnios is present, pulmonary hypoplasia is a concern. The presence of oligohydramnios, increased renal echogenicity, and cystic changes in the kidneys are indicators of poor renal function and dysplasia.
- Older children
  - History of urinary tract infections or gross hematuria
  - General health and growth (poor growth with chronic renal insufficiency or acidosis)
  - Daytime incontinence, poor urinary stream, or symptoms of voiding dysfunction may be an indicator of bladder dysfunction due to posterior urethral valves.
  - History of episodic abdominal (which may not lateralize well), flank, or back pain in the presence of hydronephrosis is often due to symptomatic ureteropelvic junction obstruction (see topic "Ureteropelvic Junction Obstruction").

PHYSICAL EXAM

- Neonate
  - Signs of oligohydramnios (Potter facies, lateral patellar dimples, clubfeet, and other limb deformities) and respiratory distress
  - Palpable abdominal mass
  - Palpable walnut-sized bladder (posterior urethral valves)
  - Patent urachus
  - Ascites
  - Development of abdominal wall musculature (wrinkled prunelike appearance in triad syndrome)
- Older children
  - Presence of abdominal mass
  - Abdominal or flank tenderness

DIAGNOSTIC TESTS & INTERPRETATION

Lab

- Newborn
  - Hydronephrosis or hydroureteronephrosis with a normal contralateral kidney does not require any immediate laboratory testing.
  - If both kidneys are affected or a solitary kidney is affected, there is a need for serial assessments of renal function (serum electrolytes and creatinine).
- Older children
  - Urinalysis to detect hematuria or pyuria. Culture if infection suspected
  - In cases where both kidneys are affected or there is a solitary kidney, renal function should be evaluated.

Imaging

- Infants with antenatally detected hydronephrosis may be evaluated with 3 imaging studies:
  - Renal/bladder ultrasound
  - Voiding cystourethrogram
  - Renal scan
- The timing can be elective for a unilateral lesion with a normal contralateral kidney, but if both kidneys are affected or a solitary kidney is involved, prompt evaluation of the newborn should be undertaken.
- Renal/bladder ultrasound
  - Because of a period of relative oliguria of a newborn in the first 24–48 hours of life, an ultrasound may underestimate the degree of hydronephrosis during this time and thus should be postponed until the infant is at least 48 hours old.
  - This should not preclude evaluating an infant during this time as long as a study is repeated in 4–6 weeks.
  - In cases where both kidneys were affected or there is a solitary affected kidney, the evaluation should not be delayed.
  - Ultrasound of the kidneys should reveal the severity of dilation of the renal pelvis and calyces, changes in the amount and echogenicity of the parenchyma, and presence of cortical cysts.
  - Evaluation of the full bladder is important as well. It will show dilated distal ureters, which may indicate ureterovesical junction obstruction, vesicoureteral reflux, or hydroureteronephrosis from posterior urethral valves or triad syndrome.

- Voiding cystourethrogram
  - Evaluates presence of vesicoureteral reflux
  - Allows grading the severity of reflux as well
  - Bladder shape, presence of diverticulum, and trabeculations may indicate hypertrophy from posterior urethral valves, neurogenic bladder dysfunction, or voiding dysfunction (in older children).
  - Test can be delayed until after discharge from nursery unless there is concern about posterior urethral valves, in which case it should be done in the early postnatal period.
  - The Society for Fetal Urology consensus statement on the evaluation and management of antenatal hydronephrosis states that there is no clear evidence to support or to avoid postnatal imaging for vesicoureteral reflux. The overall incidence of vesicoureteral reflux is up to 30% in children with antenatal hydronephrosis, and currently, it remains unproven whether the identification and treatment of children with vesicoureteral reflux confers any clinical benefit. Without the presence of ureteral dilation on the ultrasound, an argument can be made to defer performing a voiding cystourethrogram study.
- Renal scan
  - Can quantify the differential renal function or the amount each kidney contributes to overall renal function (the normal differential function is 50% ± 5% for each kidney)
  - The 2 most commonly used radionuclides are mercaptoacetyltriglycine-3 (MAG-3) and diethylenetriamine penta-acetic acid (DTPA). MAG-3 is the best choice for infants and babies.
  - In addition to the ability to detect diminished function, if there is poor drainage of the affected kidney, furosemide is given to wash out the radiotracer. The duration for washing out ½ of the accumulated radiotracer ($T_{1/2}$) is often given in the report. A prompt $T_{1/2}$ (<10 minutes) is indicative of a nonobstructed kidney. A slower $T_{1/2}$ may be indicative of obstruction when it is >20 minutes. A 10–20-minute $T_{1/2}$ is indeterminate for obstruction. Many factors affect the $T_{1/2}$, making it less reliable for indicating obstruction. These factors include the hydration status, presence of vesicoureteral reflux, and overall kidney function (very poorly functioning kidneys have a poor response to diuretics).
- IV pyelogram
  - Most useful for evaluating the anatomy of the kidney and the ureters
  - Also useful for evaluating older child with intermittent symptoms of abdominal or flank pain
  - Can be diagnostic of an intermittent ureteropelvic junction obstruction as the cause of the child's pain
- CT scan
  - Most commonly done in cases where the hydronephrosis is symptomatic
  - Noncontrast spiral CT is the most sensitive way to detect stones, as even stones radiolucent on plain films (uric acid) will be detected by CT.
- Magnetic resonance urography is being used more widely in the evaluation of hydronephrosis which avoids the use of ionizing radiation. Refinements in the technique and comprehensive automated functional analysis is now available. Ongoing issues remain concerning the use of sedation and the overall expense of the study which continue to limit its overall applicability.

DIFFERENTIAL DIAGNOSIS

- Cystic renal tumor
  - Most commonly Wilms tumor
  - Distinguished from hydronephrosis by ultrasound or CT scanning
- Multicystic dysplastic kidney
  - Can be difficult to distinguish from severe hydronephrosis with marked parenchymal thinning
  - Renal scan will show no function or perfusion with multicystic dysplastic kidney.

TREATMENT

ADDITIONAL TREATMENT

General Measures

Neonates with hydronephrosis are started on prophylactic antibiotics (1/4 the therapeutic dose given once a day) of amoxicillin. When the baby is 2 months old, the antibiotic can be changed to trimethoprim, trimethoprim/sulfamethoxazole, or nitrofurantoin.

ONGOING CARE

FOLLOW-UP RECOMMENDATIONS

- Ureteropelvic junction obstruction
  - After initial evaluation, infants are usually followed with serial studies, either ultrasound or renal scans, depending on the degree of functional impairment, the severity of the hydronephrosis, and the pattern of drainage on the renal scan.
  - From more information, see topic "Ureteropelvic Junction Obstruction."
- Ureterovesical junction obstruction
  - After initial evaluation, children are followed with serial studies as with ureteropelvic junction obstruction.
  - These lesions are much less common than ureteropelvic junction obstruction, and most of the time, the affected kidneys have normal function and can be followed conservatively.
  - If the function of the kidney is significantly diminished (differential function of 35–40%), surgical treatment of the obstruction is indicated.
- Vesicoureteral reflux
  - Infants with reflux are kept on prophylactic antibiotics.
  - In the absence of breakthrough infections, they are reevaluated annually.
  - If persistent high-grade reflux continues or breakthrough infections are a problem, surgical correction is carried out.
  - For more information, see topic "Vesicoureteral Reflux."
- Ureterocele/ectopic ureter: Because these are obstructive lesions, they are generally treated surgically early in life at the time of diagnosis.
- Posterior urethral valves
  - Full-term infants undergo cystoscopic valve ablation, whereas preterm infants may require a temporary vesicostomy until endoscopic treatment is feasible.
  - These boys require careful follow-up from a pediatric urologist and nephrologist through adolescence.
  - For more information, see topic "Posterior Urethral Valves."
- Triad syndrome: Typically, these boys will undergo bilateral orchiopexy with or without an abdominoplasty depending on the severity of abdominal wall hypoplasia during the first 6–12 months of life.

PROGNOSIS

Perinatal mortality associated with hydronephrosis has ranged from 13–72% but is most strongly correlated with the presence of chromosomal abnormalities, multiple system abnormalities, detection earlier in gestation, oligohydramnios, and evidence of infravesical obstruction.

ADDITIONAL READING

- Darge K, Higgins M, Hwang TJ, et al. Magnetic resonance and computed tomography in pediatric urology: an imagining overview for current and future daily practice. *Radiol Clin North Am*. 2013;51(4):583–598.
- Khrichenko D, Darge K. Functional analysis in MR urography—made simple. *Pediatr Radiol*. 2010;40(2):182–199.
- Nguyen HT, Herndon CD, Cooper C, et al. The Society for Fetal Urology consensus statement on the evaluation and management of antenatal hydronephrosis. *J Pediatr Urol*. 2010;6(3):212–231.

CODES

ICD10

- N13.30 Unspecified hydronephrosis
- N13.39 Other hydronephrosis
- Q62.0 Congenital hydronephrosis

FAQ

- Q: If my baby has hydronephrosis affecting only one kidney, will he need a kidney transplant?
- A: In the absence of oligohydramnios and bilateral hydroureteronephrosis, it would be very rare that a child would develop renal failure requiring transplantation.
- Q: My unborn baby has hydronephrosis in only one kidney, and the other kidney is normal. What are the chances that it is a ureteropelvic junction obstruction?
- A: The chances are ~45% that isolated hydronephrosis is due to a ureteropelvic junction obstruction.
- Q: My male unborn baby has bilateral hydronephrosis but a "normal" bladder. Is there still a chance that he has posterior urethral valves?
- A: Yes. Although it is less likely to be due to posterior urethral valves than if a thick-walled, enlarged, poorly emptying bladder were seen, prenatal ultrasonography is operator dependent. Ultrasound can miss dilated ureters or bladder abnormalities.

HYPERCALCEMIA

Philippe F. Backeljauw

BASICS

DESCRIPTION

Hypercalcemia represents an elevation in ionized and total calcium concentrations.

EPIDEMIOLOGY

- Less common than hypocalcemia
- Less common in children than adults
- Adults: >90% caused by a tumor or hyperparathyroidism (HPT)
- Children: more diverse etiologies dependent on age of presentation

RISK FACTORS

- Family history of hypercalcemia
- Family history of renal stones
- Chronic renal failure
- Immobilization
- Certain genetic syndromes
- Certain malignancies
- History of neck irradiation
- Gestational maternal hypocalcemia

PATHOPHYSIOLOGY

- Increased calcium influx from the intestinal tract or the skeleton
- Increased renal tubule calcium reabsorption

ETIOLOGY

ALERT

The first step in the determination of an etiology of hypercalcemia is measurement of an intact serum parathyroid hormone (intact PTH) concentration.

Hypercalcemia with INCREASED PTH

- Familial isolated primary HPT
  - Autosomal dominant (AD)
  - Parathyroid hyperplasia or adenoma(s)
  - *MEN1, HRPT2, HRPT3* mutations
- Multiple endocrine neoplasia (MEN)
  - MEN1 (AD)
    - MEN1-inactivating mutation
    - Parathyroid tumors in 90%
    - Pancreatic and pituitary tumors
  - MEN2A (AD)
    - RET proto-oncogene mutations
    - Parathyroid tumors in 20%
    - Medullary thyroid carcinoma and pheochromocytoma
- Sporadic parathyroid adenoma
  - *CyclinD1/PRAD1*, MEN1 mutations
- Parathyroid carcinoma (rare)
- Neonatal severe HPT (NSHPT)
  - Homozygous inactivating calcium-sensing receptor (*CaSR*) mutations

Hypercalcemia with NORMAL PTH

- Familial benign hypercalcemia or familial hypocalciuric hypercalcemia (FHH)
  - Heterozygous inactivating CaSR mutations (AD)
  - Typically asymptomatic
  - Mild hypercalcemia
  - PTH usually normal (may be slightly elevated)
  - Fractional calcium excretion <1%

Hypercalcemia with LOW PTH

- Williams syndrome
  - 15% with (transient) hypercalcemia
  - Contiguous gene deletion syndrome involving the gene encoding the transcription factor TFII-I. TFII-I negatively regulates cellular calcium entry. Without TFII-I, transient receptor potential C3 (TRPC3) channels are overexpressed in kidneys and intestine, leading to hypercalcemia.
  - Associated features: supravalvular aortic stenosis, cognitive impairment, "elfin facies"
- Jansen metaphyseal chondrodysplasia
  - Heterozygous mutations in *PTHR1* lead to constitutive activation of PTH/PTHrP receptor.
  - Short-limbed short stature
- Idiopathic hypercalcemia of infancy (Lightwood syndrome)
  - Some cases due to loss of function mutations in *CYP24A1*

Other causes of hypercalcemia (mostly PTH-independent):

- Medications:
  - Thiazides, lithium, vitamin A and D
- Malignancy
  - Local osteolysis (PTHrP, cytokine production, chemotherapy)
  - Humoral hypercalcemia of malignancy (HHM) (PTHrP)
  - Ectopic 1,25(OH)2-vitamin D production (lymphomas)
  - Ectopic PTH production
- Granulomatous disease
  - Sarcoidosis, tuberculosis
  - Increased 1,25(OH)2-vitamin D production due to dysregulated 1-α hydroxylase expression in monocytes/macrophages
- Renal disease
  - Chronic renal failure may lead to secondary and tertiary HPT.
- Endocrine disorders:
  - Thyrotoxicosis, acute adrenal insufficiency, hypophosphatasia
- Inborn errors of metabolism:
  - Blue diaper syndrome (defect in tryptophan metabolism)
  - Congenital lactase deficiency
  - Infantile hypophosphatasia (deficiency of tissue nonspecific alkaline phosphatase)
- Immobilization
  - More common in adolescence
  - Spinal cord injury, quadriplegia
  - May see low serum alkaline phosphatase, hypercalciuria
- Subcutaneous fat necrosis (SCFN)
  - After complicated delivery
  - Often a history of birth asphyxia
  - Excessive 1,25(OH)2-vitamin D production

HISTORY

- Clinical presentation is dependent on age of child, degree of hypercalcemia and the underlying disorder.
- Mild hypercalcemia (10–12 mg/dL)
  - Patients often asymptomatic
  - Failure to thrive
  - Hematuria
  - Nephrolithiasis
  - Nephrocalcinosis
- Moderate hypercalcemia (12–14 mg/dL)
  - Constipation
  - Anorexia
  - Abdominal pain
  - Weakness
  - Hematuria
  - Polyuria
  - Dehydration (in infants)
- Severe hypercalcemia (>14 mg/dL)
  - Nausea, vomiting
  - Dehydration
  - Encephalopathy
  - Psychological changes,
  - Poor feeding, hypotonia, and apnea (in newborns)

PHYSICAL EXAM

- Usually normal—unless syndromic
- Parathyroid mass usually not palpable
- Hypertension
- Dehydration
- Soft tissue calcifications uncommon

DIAGNOSTIC TESTS & INTERPRETATION

Lab

- Confirm hypercalcemia and obtain intact PTH, serum phosphate, and magnesium, plus electrolyte panel.
- Collect urine to measure calcium excretion and examine calcium/creatinine ratio:
  - Normal spot urine calcium creatinine varies by age (<7 months of age, <0.86 mg/mg; 7–18 months of age, <0.60 mg/mg; 19 months to 6 years, <0.45 mg/mg; >6 years to adults, <0.22 mg/mg.
  - In children with low muscle mass, can use urine calcium-to-osmolality ratio instead
- Hypercalcemia + low or inappropriately normal urinary calcium indicate FHH (or NSHPT).
- Hypercalcemia, hypophosphatemia, and hyperphosphaturia, plus increased PTH indicate primary HPT.
- Hypercalcemia, hypophosphatemia, and hyperphosphaturia, with a decreased PTH, indicate HHM if PTHrP is elevated.
- Hypercalcemia/hypercalciuria with normal or increased phosphate point toward other causes (vitamin D or A excess, endocrine disorders, drugs).

Imaging
- Radiography may show soft tissue calcifications in skin, subcutaneous soft tissues, and gastric mucosa
- Radiography may show subperiosteal resorption (distal phalanges), tapering of the distal clavicles, "salt and pepper" appearance of the skull, bone cysts and "brown tumors," called osteitis fibrosa cystica (prolonged hypercalcemia due to HPT).
- Renal ultrasound may show nephrocalcinosis/nephrolithiasis.
- Doppler ultrasound or sestamibi scintigraphy for preoperative assessment of parathyroid adenomas

Diagnostic Procedures/Other
Electrocardiogram may show shortened QTc interval.

ALERT
- In hypoalbuminemia, measured calcium should be corrected for the abnormality in albumin.
- Corrected calcium = measured calcium (in mg/dL) + 0.8 (4.0 − albumin [in g/dL])
- Some prefer to measure ionized calcium in such situations.

TREATMENT

GENERAL MEASURES
- Management depends on the etiology and the severity of hypercalcemia.
- Prompt therapy is needed for severe hypercalcemia (calcium >14 mg/dL).
- In mild/asymptomatic hypercalcemia, no treatment may be needed (FHH).

ALERT
Important to diagnose FHH and distinguish it from other forms of hypercalcemia to avoid unnecessary drug therapy and parathyroid surgeries

GENERAL PRINCIPLES
- Rehydration
- Increase urinary calcium excretion.
- Inhibit bone resorption.
- Decrease intestinal absorption:
  - Depending on cause of hypercalcemia, consider low-calcium diet.

MEDICATION (DRUGS)
- Hydration therapy (saluresis)
  - Isotonic saline 3,000 mL/m^2 over 24–48 hours intravenously
- Promote calciuresis (after hydration):
  - Furosemide 1 mg/kg every 6 hours intravenously
- Decrease bone resorption:
  - For persistent moderate to severe hypercalcemia
  - Acutely: calcitonin 4 units/kg subcutaneously every 12 hours
  - Bisphosphonate therapy (pamidronate 0.5–1 mg/kg intravenously over 4–6 hours)
- Glucocorticoids
  - Inhibit 1-α hydroxylase and reduce intestinal absorption
  - Prednisone 1–2 mg/kg/24 h
- Calcimimetics (cinacalcet) bind the CaSR and suppress PTH secretion:
  - At this time, caution in using cinacalcet in children given pediatric death in a research study using this drug.

SURGERY/OTHER PROCEDURES
- Dialysis: last resort
- Surgery (for primary HPT)

ONGOING CARE

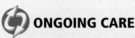

FOLLOW-UP RECOMMENDATIONS
Postsurgical hypocalcemia is common after parathyroidectomy—especially after severe HPT ("hungry bone syndrome"), and requires calcium and phosphate supplementation, and sometimes calcitriol treatment.

PROGNOSIS
- Depends on cause
- Permanent hypoparathyroidism may result from total parathyroidectomy.

ADDITIONAL READING

- Hendy GN, D'Souza-Li L, Yang B, et al. Mutations of the calcium-sensing receptor (CASR) in familial hypocalciuric hypercalcemia, neonatal severe hyperparathyroidism, and autosomal dominant hypocalcemia. *Hum Mutat*. 2000;16(4):281–296.
- Lafferty FW. Differential diagnosis of hypercalcemia. *J Bone Miner Res*. 1991;6(Suppl 2):S51–S59.
- Letavernier E, Rodenas A, Guerrot D, et al. Williams-Beuren syndrome hypercalcemia: is TRPC3 a novel mediator in calcium homeostasis? *Pediatrics*. 2012;129(6):e1626–e1630.
- Schlingmann KP, Kaufmann M, Weber S, et al. Mutations in *CYP24A1* and idiopathic infantile hypercalcemia. *N Engl J Med*. 2011;365(5):410–421.
- Sebestyen JF, Srivastava T, Alon US. Bisphosphonates use in children. *Clin Pediatr*. 2012;51(11):1011–1024.
- Trehan A, Cheetham T, Bailey S. Hypercalcemia in acute lymphoblastic leukemia: an overview. *J Pediatr Hematol Oncol*. 2009;31(6):424–427.
- Wesseling K, Bakkaloglu S, Salusky I. Chronic kidney disease mineral and bone disorder in children. *Pediatr Nephrol*. 2008;23(2):195–207.

CODES

ICD10-CM
- E83.52 Hypercalcemia
- P71.8 Other transitory neonatal disord of calcium & magnesium metab
- E21.3 Hyperparathyroidism, unspecified

FAQ
- Q: When should vitamin D or vitamin A levels be measured?
- A: If there is a history of alternative medicine, over-the-counter drugs, or supplements
- Q: When should one consider bisphosphonate therapy?
- A: In hypercalcemia mainly due to mobilization of calcium from bone (e.g. severe HPT, immobilization, tumor)
- Q: When should one consider glucocorticoids?
- A: In hypervitaminosis D or A and in excessive 1,25(OH)2-vitamin D production

HYPERIMMUNOGLOBULINEMIA E SYNDROME

Rachel G. Robison

BASICS

DESCRIPTION

Hyperimmunoglobulinemia E syndrome (HIES) is a primary immunodeficiency with markedly elevated serum IgE associated with recurrent skin abscesses, pulmonary infections, and eczematoid dermatitis.

EPIDEMIOLOGY

- Rare
- True incidence and prevalence is unknown; affects equal numbers of males and females

RISK FACTORS

Genetics

- Autosomal dominant cases (AD-HIES) are caused by mutations in signal transducer and activator of transcription 3 (STAT3).
- Autosomal recessive cases (AR-HIES) have mutations in the dedicator of cytokinesis-8 gene (*DOCK8*).
- AR-HIES patients differ in phenotype from AD-HIES patients.
- Sporadic cases do occur.

PATHOPHYSIOLOGY

- *STAT3* is integral in secretion and signaling of multiple cytokines involved in proinflammatory and anti-inflammatory responses.
- A failure of Th 17 cell differentiation and failure of IL-17 secretion makes patients susceptible to *Candida* infections.
- Deficiency in IL-11 signaling results in tooth abnormalities and craniosynostosis.
- *DOCK8* deficiency results in failure of dendritic cells to migrate to lymph nodes and affects long-term memory B cells and viral-specific CD8+ T cells.

DIAGNOSIS

HISTORY

- Recurrent infections
  - Skin
    - Abscesses
    - Furuncles
    - Cellulitis
    - Lymphadenitis
  - Sinopulmonary infections
    - Pneumonia with aberrant healing forming pneumatoceles and bronchiectasis
  - Fungal infections: mostly mucocutaneous candidiasis
  - Typical organisms: *Staphylococcus aureus*, *Streptococcus pneumoniae*, *Haemophilus influenzae*
  - Opportunistic infections with *Pneumocystis jiroveci* pneumonia
  - Those with AR-HIES have viral skin infections, including molluscum, warts, and/or recurrent herpes.
- Rash
  - Present in newborn period
  - Can resolve or become eczematoid
- Retention of primary teeth
  - Delayed exfoliation of 3 or more teeth in 70% of patients
- Vascular anomalies
  - Tortuosity, dilation, and aneurysms of medium-sized vessels

PHYSICAL EXAM

- Facial features are noted in late childhood to early adolescence, including:
  - Asymmetric facies
  - Prominent forehead/chin
  - Wide-set eyes
- Dermatitis
- Skeletal anomalies
  - Scoliosis
  - Craniosynostosis
  - Hyperextensible joints
  - Osteopenia leading to resultant bone fractures from minor trauma
- Hard palate anomalies, high-arched palate

DIAGNOSTIC TESTS & INTERPRETATION

Lab

- Total serum IgE of >2,000 IU/mL
  - Elevation may not be present in newborns.
  - Can decline to normal levels in adult years
  - Level does not correlate with disease severity.
- Peripheral eosinophilia
  - Does not correlate with IgE
  - Present in >90% of patients
- Immunoglobulin levels
  - IgG and IgM are usually normal.
  - IgA may be normal or low.
  - IgM is often decreased in AR-HIES.
- Specific antibody response is variable.
- Reduced CD45RO+ memory T cells and memory B cells with normal total lymphocyte counts
- Neutropenia may be present in a subset of patients.

Imaging

CT of the lungs if history of pneumonia to look for bronchiectasis and/or pneumatoceles

DIFFERENTIAL DIAGNOSIS

- Atopic dermatitis
- Wiskott-Aldrich syndrome
- Severe combined immunodeficiency (SCID)
- Omenn syndrome
- Immune dysregulation, polyendocrinopathy, enteropathy X-linked syndrome (IPEX)
- Netherton syndrome

TREATMENT

MEDICATION

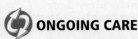

- Prophylactic antibiotics, typically trimethoprim/sulfamethoxazole, for prevention of staphylococcal infection
- Immunoglobulin replacement therapy in the case of concomitant hypogammaglobulinemia
- Consideration of antifungal prophylaxis if recurrent/chronic candida infections

ADDITIONAL TREATMENT

General Measures

- Implement good management of dermatitis with regular hydration and emollient use.
- Control pruritus with antihistamines.
- Dilute bleach baths to decrease staphylococcal skin colonization.
- Promptly and aggressively treat all infections.
- Physical therapy for joint pain related to hyperextensibility

ONGOING CARE

FOLLOW-UP RECOMMENDATIONS

Patient Monitoring

Blood pressure monitoring in patients, especially those with known vascular anomalies, as hypertension is common

COMPLICATIONS

- Parenchymal lung changes from aberrant healing. Pulmonary surgery to correct these is associated with an increased risk of further complications.
- Increased chance of malignancy, most commonly lymphoma

ADDITIONAL READING

- Buckley RH. The hyper-IgE syndrome. *Clin Rev Allergy Immunol*. 2001;20(1):139–154.
- Davis SD, Schaller J, Wedgwood RJ. Job's syndrome: recurrent, "cold", staphylococcal abscesses. *Lancet*. 1966;1(7445):1013–1015.
- Freeman AF, Holland SM. Clinical manifestations of hyper IgE syndromes. *Dis Markers*. 2010;29(3–4): 123–130.
- Paulson ML, Freeman AF, Holland SM. Hyper IgE syndrome: an update on clinical aspects and the role of signal transducer and activator of transcription 3. *Curr Opin Allergy Clin Immunol*. 2008;8(6): 527–533.
- Yong PF, Freeman AF, Engelhart KR, et al. An update on the hyper-IgE syndromes. *Arthritis Res Ther*. 2012;14(6):228–237.

CODES

ICD10

D82.4 Hyperimmunoglobulin E [IgE] syndrome

FAQ

- Q: How do AD-HIES and AR-HIES differ?
- A: Aside from arising from different mutations, AD-HIES has more skeletal and facial anomalies, whereas AR-HIES is more often associated with viral skin infections and has a higher chance of malignancy.
- Q: Will HIES patients show signs typical of infection?
- A: HIES patients may lack classical signs of infection such as warmth and redness. Skin infections have been referred to as "cold" abscesses.
- Q: What are the other names for HIES?
- A: HIES has been referred to as Buckley syndrome, Job-Buckley syndrome, and Job syndrome in the literature. In the initial 1966 case series, Davis and colleagues wrote that the "appearance of these patients and the history of recurrent abscesses and skin infections makes the name 'Job's syndrome' seem suitable." The reference is to the Biblical character Job, who was smote "with sore boils from the sole of his foot unto his crown" (Job, Chapter 2; Verse 7).

H

HYPERINSULINISM

Katherine Lord • Diva D. De León

BASICS

DESCRIPTION

Hyperinsulinism (HI) is a disorder of dysregulated insulin secretion resulting in hypoglycemia. Congenital HI refers to a permanent inborn condition, other forms can be transient.

EPIDEMIOLOGY

Most common cause of persistent or recurrent hypoglycemia in children

Incidence

- Annual incidence estimated at ~1:40,000–50,000 live births in United States.
- May be as high as 1:2,500 in select populations (Saudi Arabians, Ashkenazi Jews)

Genetics

- K_{ATP}HI: inactivating mutations in K_{ATP} channel genes *ABCC8* and *KCNJ11* (on 11p15)
  - Mutations inherited in an autosomal recessive manner result in diffuse involvement throughout the pancreas (diffuse HI).
  - Autosomal dominantly inherited mutations can also rarely cause diffuse HI.
  - Non-Mendelian inheritance: A paternally inherited recessive mutation of K_{ATP} channel gene and a loss of maternal alleles on the imprinted chromosome region 11p15, leads to paternal uniparental disomy; results in focal adenomatous lesion (focal HI)
- Glucokinase-HI: autosomal dominant–activating mutations of glucokinase (*GCK*)
- GDH-HI: autosomal dominant–activating mutations of glutamate dehydrogenase (GDH), encoded by *GLUD1*; known as *hyperinsulinism/hyperammonemia* (HI/HA) syndrome
- SCHAD-HI: autosomal recessive mutations of mitochondrial enzyme short-chain-3-hydroxyacyl-CoA dehydrogenase (SCHAD), encoded by *HADH*
- UCP2-HI: autosomal dominant mutations of mitochondrial carrier uncoupling protein 2 (UCP2), encoded by *UCP2*
- HNF4A and HNF1A-HI: autosomal dominant mutations in transcription factors, *HNF4A* and *HNF1A*. Mutations in *HNF4A* and *HNF1A* also are known to cause familial monogenic diabetes.
- MCT1-HI: autosomal dominant mutations in the regulatory region of *SLC16A1*–encoding monocarboxylate transporter 1 (MCT1)
  - Causes exercise-induced HI

PATHOPHYSIOLOGY

- These mutations result in uncoupling of insulin secretion from the glucose-sensing machinery of the pancreatic β cell.
  - Leads to inappropriate insulin secretion even in the face of low plasma glucose concentrations
  - In the absence of functional K_{ATP} channels, plasma membrane is depolarized leading to opening of voltage-dependent calcium channels and constant insulin secretion.
- In the focal form of the disease (~60% of cases), a cluster of pancreatic β cells are affected, whereas in diffuse HI, all β cells are abnormal.
- In HI/HA syndrome, activating mutations of GDH (an enzyme that regulates amino acid–stimulated insulin secretion) cause dysregulated insulin secretion (particularly after ingestion of protein) and persistently elevated ammonia levels.
- Glucokinase acts as "glucose sensor" of the β cell. Activating mutations result in lower glucose threshold for insulin secretion.
- SCHAD is an inhibitory regulator of GDH. Inactivating mutations of *HADH* result in insulin dysregulation due to loss of GDH inhibition.
- UCP2 is a negative regulator of insulin secretion. Loss-of-function mutations lead to HI.
- In exercise-induced HI, ectopic expression of MCT1 allows transport of pyruvate, elevated during anaerobic exercise, into the β cell; leads to an increased ATP-to-ADP ratio, thus stimulating insulin secretion

ETIOLOGY

- Mutations in 9 genes have been associated with congenital HI: Genes coding for the two subunits of the β cell K_{ATP} channel [SUR1, sulfonylurea receptor (*ABCC8*); Kir6.2, inwardly rectifying potassium channel (*KCNJ11*)]; glucokinase (*GCK*), glutamate dehydrogenase (*GLUD1*), SCHAD (*HADH*), UCP2 (*UCP2*), *HNF4A*, *HNF1A* and monocarboxylate transporter-1 (*SLC16A1*).
- A transient form of HI has been associated with perinatal stress (small for gestational age [SGA] birth weight, maternal hypertension, precipitous delivery, or hypoxia), but the mechanism has not been elucidated.

COMMONLY ASSOCIATED CONDITIONS

HI can be associated with Beckwith-Wiedemann syndrome and congenital disorders of glycosylation (CDG). The underlying mechanism of HI in these disorders is not clear.

DIAGNOSIS

HISTORY

- Symptoms of hypoglycemia in the infant:
  - Poor feeding
  - Hypotonia
  - Lethargy
  - Cyanosis
  - Tachypnea
  - Tremors
  - Seizures
- May have high IV glucose infusion requirements (>10 mg/kg/min)

ALERT

Infants with severe hypoglycemia may be asymptomatic.

PHYSICAL EXAM

- Large for gestational age
  - Suggests K_{ATP}HI
- Small for gestational age
  - Suggests transient HI or CGD
- Macroglossia, umbilical hernia, hemihypertrophy
  - Suggest Beckwith-Wiedemann syndrome
- No midline defects, including normal palate and genitalia
  - Midline defects suggest hypopituitarism as cause of hypoglycemia.

DIAGNOSTIC TESTS & INTERPRETATION

Lab

- Obtain critical sample at time of hypoglycemia (plasma glucose <50 mg/dL).
- Evidence of excess insulin action at time of hypoglycemia:
  - May have detectable insulin
  - Suppressed levels of β-hydroxybutyrate (<0.6 mm) and free fatty acids (< 0.5 mm)
  - Glycemic response to 1 mg glucagon (blood glucose rise >30 mg/dL in 40 minutes)
- Elevated plasma ammonia levels
  - Indicate HI/HA syndrome
- Elevated plasma 3-hydroxybutyrylcarnitine and urinary 3-hydroxyglutarate
  - Indicate SCHAD
- Low cortisol and growth hormone at time of hypoglycemia is not diagnostic of adrenal insufficiency/growth hormone deficiency.
  - Perform appropriate stimulation tests to confirm.

ALERT

Insulin levels may not be elevated or detectable at time of hypoglycemia in some patients with HI. Base diagnosis on other evidence of insulin excess.

Imaging

- ^{18}F-DOPA PET scans at specialized HI centers to identify and to localize focal lesions
- Traditional imaging studies such as US, CT scan, and MRI are not helpful in identifying focal HI lesions.

Pathologic Findings

- Two major forms of pancreatic histology in children with HI due to K_{ATP} channel mutations:
  - Diffuse HI: abnormally enlarged islet cell nuclei found throughout the pancreas
  - Focal HI: discrete area of islet cell hyperplasia surrounded by normal pancreas

DIFFERENTIAL DIAGNOSIS

- Infant of diabetic mother (IDM)
- Beckwith-Wiedemann syndrome
- Neonatal (pan)hypopituitarism
- Congenital disorders of glycosylation
- Children with dumping syndrome after fundoplasty can have severe postmeal hypoglycemia due to excessive insulin secretion after a meal.

TREATMENT

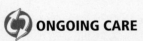

GENERAL MEASURES

- The major goal is prevention of brain damage.
- IV dextrose infusions should be given to stabilize blood glucose acutely.
  - For an acute hypoglycemic event, give a bolus of 2–3 mL/kg of 10% dextrose (0.2–0.3 g/kg).
  - Use dextrose infusion to maintain blood glucose >70 mg/dL.
  - May require central line to administer higher concentrations of dextrose and to avoid fluid overload
- Frequent oral feeds are not sufficient as treatment for hypoglycemia due to HI.

MEDICATION

- Diazoxide, a K_{ATP} channel agonist, at 5–15 mg/kg/24 h PO divided q12h
  - Most K_{ATP}HI patients do not respond.
  - Patients with HI/HA, SCHAD-HI, or transient HI typically respond well.
  - Diuretic may be necessary due to fluid retention.
- Octreotide, a somatostatin analog, at 5–20 mcg/kg/24 h divided q6h or given by continuous IV infusion at 0.08–0.40 mcg/kg/h
  - Tachyphylaxis and hyperglycemia may occur.
  - May increase the risk of necrotizing enterocolitis in neonates
- Glucagon, at 1 mg/24 h by continuous IV infusion, may stabilize blood glucose levels prior to surgery.

SURGERY/OTHER PROCEDURES

- Pancreatectomy in children refractory to medical therapy or in those with focal lesions. Near total pancreatectomy with gastrostomy tube for those with diffuse disease. Resection of pancreatic adenomatous lesion for focal disease
- For focal HI, surgery can be curative.

ONGOING CARE

FOLLOW-UP RECOMMENDATIONS

- Up to 30–44% of patients can have neurodevelopmental abnormalities due to hypoglycemia.
- Patients who undergo near total pancreatectomy are at very high risk of developing diabetes later in life.

Patient Monitoring

- Home blood glucose monitoring, especially with longer fasts or intercurrent illnesses
- Hospitalizations for IV glucose infusions may be necessary during intercurrent illnesses with vomiting or poor oral intake.
- Follow-up fasting studies may be needed to evaluate safety and/or disease regression.
- Diazoxide may cause fluid retention and hypertrichosis.
- Neonates treated with octreotide should be closely monitored for evidence of necrotizing enterocolitis.
- Octreotide can suppress GH secretion, so close observation of linear growth is necessary. Thyroid function tests should also be monitored.
- Evaluation of pancreatic exocrine function after near-total pancreatectomy
- Periodic neurodevelopmental assessments

DIET

- Avoidance of long fasts
- Avoidance of protein loads in those with HI/HA, SCHAD, and K_{ATP}HI, as high-protein diets may stimulate insulin secretion

COMPLICATIONS

- Severe refractory hypoglycemia
- Cognitive deficits
- Seizures
- Coma
- Permanent brain damage
- Glucose intolerance or frank diabetes mellitus after pancreatectomy
- Pancreatic exocrine insufficiency after pancreatectomy

ADDITIONAL READING

- Beltrand J, Caquard M, Arnoux JB, et al. Glucose metabolism in 105 children and adolescents after pancreatectomy for congenital hyperinsulinism. *Diabetes Care*. 2012;35(2):198–203.
- De León DD, Stanley CA. Mechanisms of disease: advances in diagnosis and treatment of hyperinsulinism in neonates. *Nat Clin Prac Endocrinol Metab*. 2007;3(1):57–68.
- Hoe FM, Thornton PS, Wanner LA, et al. Clinical features and insulin regulation in infants with syndrome of prolonged neonatal hyperinsulinism. *J Pediatr*. 2006;148(2):207–212.
- Laje P, States LJ, Zhuang H, et al. Accuracy of PET/CT scan in the diagnosis of the focal form of congenital hyperinsulinism. *J Pediatr Surg*. 2013;48(2):388–393.
- Lord KL, De León DD. Monogenic hyperinsulinemic hypoglycemia: current insights into the pathogenesis and management. *Int J Pediatr Endocrinol*. 2013;2013(1):3.
- Meissner T, Wendel U, Burgard P, et al. Long-term follow-up of 114 patients with congenital hyperinsulinism. *Eur J Endocrinol*. 2003;149(1):43–51.
- Otonkoski T, Jiao H, Kaminen-Ahola N, et al. Physical exercise-induced hypoglycemia caused by failed silencing of monocarboxylate transporter 1 in pancreatic beta cells. *Am J Hum Genet*. 2007;81(3):467–474.
- Palladino AA, Stanley CA. A specialized team approach to diagnosis and medical versus surgical treatment of infants with congenital hyperinsulinism. *Semin Pediatr Surg*. 2011;20(1):32–37.

CODES

ICD10

E16.1 Other hypoglycemia

FAQ

- Q: What is the chance of HI in the sibling of an affected child?
- A: 25% in the autosomal recessive type; 50% in the autosomal dominant type; <1% for siblings of children with focal HI
- Q: How low and for how long can glucose go before brain damage occurs?
- A: The definition of hypoglycemia has been the subject of controversy in pediatrics, but activation of glucose counterregulatory systems occurs when blood glucose levels reach the 65–70-mg/dL range; symptoms of hypoglycemia present at the 50–55-mg/dL level, and cognitive dysfunction occurs when blood glucose levels are in the 45–50-mg/dL range. Taking these data into account, blood glucose concentration should be maintained >70 mg/dL. The duration of hypoglycemia necessary for brain damage to occur is unknown.
- Q: What is the chance that HI will eventually resolve without surgery?
- A: Only ~40–50% of cases are controlled with medication alone. Patients with K_{ATP}HI may be more likely to require surgery, and in those patients with focal disease, surgery can be curative. Perinatal stress–induced HI usually resolves within the first 6 months of life.

H

HYPERLEUKOCYTOSIS

Monica Khurana • Caroline Hastings

BASICS

DESCRIPTION

Hyperleukocytosis is a total white blood cell (WBC) count of $\geq$100,000/μL.

RISK FACTORS

ALERT

Children with trisomy 21 (Down syndrome) have an increased risk of developing transient leukemoid reactions and have an increased risk of developing acute leukemia, more commonly acute lymphoblastic leukemia (ALL).

- Presentation with hyperleukocytosis depends on the type of leukemia.
- Percent with hyperleukocytosis
  - Chronic myeloid leukemia (CML) especially in blast crisis ~100%
  - Acute myeloid leukemia (AML) especially in infants 5–25%
  - ALL (especially with mediastinal mass) 8–13%
- Factors associated with more severe clinical course:
  - Coagulopathy
  - Metabolic derangements
  - Presentation with clinical evidence of central nervous system (CNS) or pulmonary leukostasis

PATHOPHYSIOLOGY

The primary mechanism for symptoms is leukostasis due to increased viscosity and impaired blood flow. Contributory factors other than number of leukemic cells include their shape and size, which increases viscosity, as well as endothelial cell damage, which further impedes microcirculation.

- WBCs lack the concave shape that enables reversible deformability of cellular contents of red blood cells (RBCs) to pass through the microvasculature. As compared to normal WBCs, blasts are much larger with less deformability.
- Myeloblasts are twice the size of lymphoblasts, which are 25% larger than mature neutrophil granulocytes. Monoblasts are larger than myeloblasts. Aggregates of these large, undeformable cells cannot pass through capillaries.
- In addition to increased cell-to-cell adhesions, leukemic blast cells have increased adhesion to the damaged endothelium, which promote additional cell aggregates through endothelial toxin and cytokine release.
- Leukemic cells have a hypersensitive response to cytokines, which may account for clinical leukostasis at lower peripheral blast counts.
- Leukostasis impairs blood flow and exacerbates hypoxemia; as expected, leukemic blasts have increased oxygen consumption due to a high rate of cell division.

DIAGNOSIS

DIFFERENTIAL DIAGNOSIS

- Hyperleukocytosis occurs primarily secondary to malignancy but may be seen with a leukemoid reaction secondary to infection or physiologic stress.
- Malignancy
  - ALL
  - AML
  - CML
  - Transient myeloproliferative disorder (TMPD) is primarily associated with Down syndrome
- Leukemoid reaction
  - Leukemoid reactions are WBC counts more than 50,000/μL and consist of myeloid precursor cells in the peripheral blood at all stages of maturity rather than proliferation of an immature WBC clonal population characteristic of malignancies.
  - Leukemoid reactions reflect a physiologic bone marrow response to cytokine secretion prompted by external stimuli such as infection or inflammation.
  - Nucleated RBCs (also seen in malignancy)

HISTORY

- Symptoms and signs of hyperleukocytosis relate to the organ involved. Clinical evidence of leukostasis is most apparent in the CNS, lungs, retina, and penis.
- CNS
  - Headache
  - Confusion
  - Blurred vision
  - Tinnitus
  - Paresis
  - Nausea/vomiting
- Pulmonary
  - Dyspnea
  - Shortness of breath
  - Chest pain
- Genitourinary (males)
  - Anuria/oliguria
  - Erection
- Retina
  - Decreased visual acuity

PHYSICAL EXAM

- CNS
  - Coma
  - Somnolence
  - Altered mental status
  - Agitation
  - Seizures
  - Papilledema
  - Sluggish pupils
- Pulmonary
  - Hypoxia
  - Tachypnea
- Hematologic
  - Hemorrhage
  - Thrombosis
- Reticuloendothelial system
  - Hepatomegaly
  - Splenomegaly
  - Enlarged lymph nodes
- Genitourinary (males)
  - Priapism

ALERT

- Symptomatic hyperleukocytosis as a result of leukostasis represents an oncologic emergency.
- Confused and/or hypoxic patients are at risk for severe late effects or death and require emergent intervention.

DIAGNOSTIC TESTS & INTERPRETATION

Lab

ALERT

- Confirm presence of leukemic blasts. Automated counting machines may mistake leukemic blasts for atypical/reactive lymphocytes or even monocytes.
- Confirmation may require a manual differential and a pathologist or oncologist to review the peripheral smear.

- Peripheral blood analysis with morphology and flow cytometry aid in immediate diagnosis of acute leukemia.
- Evaluate other cell lines. Concurrent presence of anemia and/or thrombocytopenia supports an underlying marrow disorder and may require inventions such as transfusions.
- Tumor lysis laboratory evaluation includes the following:
  - Electrolytes
  - BUN, creatinine
  - Calcium
  - Phosphorous
  - Magnesium
  - Lactate dehydrogenase (LDH)
  - Uric acid

Imaging

- Obtain CXR, even if asymptomatic.
  - Evaluate for mediastinal mass.
  - Evaluate for pulmonary infiltrates.
- If clinically indicated, obtain MRI or CT.

Procedures

Bone marrow aspirate may be required per clinical trial criteria, which includes cytogenetics for future prognostic/therapeutic decision making.

TREATMENT

- The goal of treatment is to quickly make a correct diagnosis and implement definitive therapy while simultaneously identifying and addressing the potential complications of leukostasis secondary to hyperleukocytosis.
- Leukoreduction refers to interventions that result in a rapid decline of the WBC. Leukoreduction is an absolute indication if a patient shows symptoms or signs of leukostasis. It is a relative indication in an asymptomatic patient with a WBC count ≥100,000–300,000/μL (depending on type of leukemia). Controversy exists about its impact on decreasing morbidity, risk of CNS hemorrhage, or mortality.
- Induction chemotherapy
  - This is the definitive therapy for hyperleukocytosis secondary to malignancy.
  - Initiate chemotherapy as soon as malignant diagnosis is confirmed.
- Management
  - Aggressive hydration at 2–4× maintenance
  - Identify and correct metabolic abnormalities.
    - Tumor lysis syndrome
    - Hyperuricemia, indication for rasburicase
  - Identify and correct coagulopathies.
  - Transfuse for cytopenias.
    - Do not transfuse packed RBCs if hemodynamically stable due to increased blood viscosity.
    - Do not exceed hemoglobin 10 g/dL.
    - Transfuse platelets to maintain platelets >10,000/μL; will not affect blood viscosity
- Cytoreduction
  - Leukapheresis
    - *Benefit*: Each pheresis session decreases the circulating WBC count by 20–50%. During pheresis, FFP may be administered to reduce risk of hemorrhage.
    - *Limitation*: availability of equipment, trained personnel, and anticoagulation
    - *Caution*: Leukapheresis only transiently decreases blast counts until definitive treatment can be initiated.
  - Exchange transfusion, including partial
    - *Benefit*: This technique is preferred over leukapheresis when (1) patient is an infant or <10 kg and (2) there is concurrent severe anemia and/or (3) need for concurrent administration of coagulation factors (i.e., FFP to treat CNS hemorrhage). Partial exchanges minimize volume overload and hyperviscosity.
    - *Limitation*: higher risk of infection
    - *Caution*: Patients are at high risk for tumor lysis syndrome (TLS).
  - Hydroxyurea (HU)
    - *Mechanism of action*: This antimetabolite inhibits ribonucleoside diphosphate reductase, which halts cells in the G_1 phase and interferes with DNA repair.
    - *Dose*: 20–30 mg/kg/day
    - *Benefit*: HU is an oral medication and easily administered. It may be dissolved in water for NGT/OGT administration. Time to peak onset is only 1–4 hours.
    - *Caution*: may also worsen thrombocytopenia

ISSUES FOR REFERRAL

Obtain immediate oncology consult.

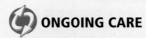

ONGOING CARE

PROGNOSIS

- Patients usually require treatment in a pediatric intensive care unit because they require rapid and continuous monitoring at presentation and during early phase of therapy due to complications of leukostasis and TLS.
- Presence of organ failure or coagulopathy correlates with poor prognosis, specifically death, during induction chemotherapy, despite supportive care.

ALERT

- Early deaths are primarily due to intracranial and pulmonary complications.
- Coagulopathy are most common in AML patients, in particular M3 or M4 subtypes.
- The CNS and lungs are the two most common organs damaged by leukostasis.

ADDITIONAL READING

- Blum W, Porcu P. Therapeutic apheresis in hyperleukocytosis and hyperviscosity syndrome. *Semin Thromb Hemost*. 2007;33(4):350–354.
- Jain R, Bansal D, Marwaha RK. Hyperleukocytosis: emergency management. *Indian J Pediatr*. 2013;80(2):144–148.
- Majhail N, Lichtin A. Acute leukemia with a very high leukocyte count: confronting a medical emergency. *Cleveland Clin J Med*. 2004;71(8):633–637.
- Porcu P, Cripe L, Ng EW, et al. Hyperleukocytic leukemias and leukostasis: a review of pathophysiology, clinical presentation and management. *Leuk Lymphoma*. 2009;39(1–2):1–18.
- Sung L, Aplenc R, Alonzo TA, et al. Predictors and short-term outcomes of hyperleukocytosis in children with acute myeloid leukemia: a report from the Children's Oncology Group. *Haematologica*. 2012;97(11):1770–1773.

CODES

ICD10

- D72.829 Elevated white blood cell count, unspecified
- C91.00 Acute lymphoblastic leukemia not having achieved remission
- C92.10 Chronic myeloid leukemia, BCR/ABL-positive, not having achieved remission

FAQ

- Q: Is there a linear relationship between the WBC count and the presence/severity of clinical disease and complications?
- A: No. Clinically significant hyperleukocytosis usually occurs at WBC ≥200,000/μL or ≥300,000/μL in patients with AML or ALL and CML in blast crisis, respectively; however, symptoms may present with a WBC as low as 50,000/μL.
- Q: Is there a linear correlation between the WBC count and presence of TLS?
- A: Yes. Risk increases as the tumor burden increases. With high WBC counts and rapid cell turnover, the lysis/death of malignant cells release by-products, leading to electrolyte and metabolic abnormalities known as TLS. TLS is more common in ALL patients as compared to AML or CML. Components of TLS include hyperkalemia, hyperphosphatemia, hyperuricemia and hyperuricosuria, and hypocalcemia.
- Q: Because transfusions for other cytopenias increase total blood viscosity, what are the current guidelines for transfusions?
- A: For anemia, if hemodynamically unstable, transfuse to maintain hemoglobin 8–9 g/dL. Do not exceed hemoglobin levels >10 g/dL as increasing hematocrit increases blood viscosity. For thrombocytopenia, transfuse to maintain platelet >20,000/μL because platelet transfusions minimally increases blood viscosity. If CNS hemorrhage is present, maintain platelets at 75,000–100,000/μL.

H

HYPERLIPIDEMIA

Zeina M. Nabhan

BASICS

DESCRIPTION

Hyperlipidemia is an elevation of serum lipids. These lipids include cholesterol, cholesterol esters (compounds), phospholipids, and triglycerides. Lipids are transported as part of large molecules called lipoproteins.

- 5 major families of lipoproteins
  - Chylomicrons
  - Very-low-density lipoproteins (VLDL)
  - Intermediate-density lipoproteins (IDL)
  - Low-density lipoproteins (LDL)
  - High-density lipoproteins (HDL)
- Normal serum lipid concentrations
  - Total cholesterol: 170 mg/dL (borderline, 170–199 mg/dL)
  - LDL cholesterol: <110 mg/dL (borderline, 110–129 mg/dL)
  - HDL cholesterol: ≥35 mg/dL
  - Total triglycerides: 100 mg/dL (borderline, 100–140 mg/dL)
  - More detailed age- and gender-specific values are available (refer to Table 2 of 2008 Clinical report: lipid screening and cardiovascular health in childhood).
- Primary hypercholesterolemia or hypertriglyceridemia: elevation in serum cholesterol or triglyceride as a result of an inherited disorder of lipid metabolism (i.e., familial hypercholesterolemia)
- Secondary hypercholesterolemia or hypertriglyceridemia: elevation in serum cholesterol or triglyceride as a result of another disease process (e.g., diabetes mellitus)

EPIDEMIOLOGY

- The prevalence of homozygous familial hypercholesterolemia (FH) is 1 in 1,000,000; the incidence of the heterozygous state is 1 in 500.
- Unknown causes result in hypercholesterolemia and/or hypertriglyceridemia, occurring in 2% of the population.
- National Health and Nutrition Examination Surveys (NHANES I-III) provides information about pediatric serum cholesterol concentrations.
  - For all children 4–17 years, the 95th percentile for serum total cholesterol is 216 mg/dL and the 75th percentile is 181 mg/dL.
  - Before puberty, average total and LDL cholesterol levels are significantly higher in girls than boys.
  - The mean total cholesterol level for all children from 4 to 11 years old peaks at age 9–11 years and then gradually decreases until mid to late adolescence.

RISK FACTORS

Genetics

- FH: dominantly inherited defect of LDL receptor
- Familial combined hyperlipidemia (FCHL): dominantly inherited lipid disorder, polygenic
- Familial hypertriglyceridemia (FHTG): autosomal recessive disorder due to defects in lipoprotein lipase

GENERAL PREVENTION

- Fat intake is generally unrestricted prior to 2 years of age. After 2 years of age, two complementary approaches are recommended.
- Diet and lifestyle guidelines are to promote:
  - Consuming an overall healthy diet
  - Maintaining a healthy body weight (BMI <85% for children)
- Recommended lipid levels
  - LDL cholesterol <110 mg/dL
  - HDL cholesterol >50 mg/dL in women, >40 mg/dL in men
  - Triglycerides <150 mg/dL
- Normal, age-appropriate BP
- Normal blood glucose level (fasting blood glucose ≤100 mg/dL)
- Remaining physically active
- Avoiding use of and exposure to tobacco products

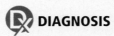

DIAGNOSIS

HISTORY

- Family history of premature heart disease or dyslipidemia
  - Almost all cases of primary hyperlipidemia are of dominant inheritance.
- Smoking
  - Smoking reduces HDL cholesterol levels and increases the risk of vascular disease.
- Use of oral contraceptives
  - Birth control pills have been shown to cause elevations in lipoprotein levels and, when coupled with already elevated lipid levels, can increase the risk of atherosclerosis.
- Diet
  - Children with increased intake of fat, carbohydrates, sugar-added drinks, and fast foods are likely to be overweight/obese.
- Obesity
  - Obese children are more likely to have abnormal serum lipids.

PHYSICAL EXAM

- Eye exam
  - Arcus corneae: deposits of cholesterol, resulting in a thin, white circular ring located on the outer edge of the iris
- Skin exam
  - Tendon xanthomas: thickened tissue surrounding the Achilles and extensor tendons
  - Xanthelasma: yellowish deposits of cholesterol surrounding the eye
  - Palmar xanthomas: pale lines in palmar creases
  - Eruptive xanthomas: characteristic of hypertriglyceridemia; papular yellowish lesions with a red base that occur on the buttocks, elbows, and knees
  - Enlarged tender liver may present in association with fatty liver.

DIAGNOSTIC TESTS & INTERPRETATION

Lab

- Starting age 2–8 years
  - Screen children and adolescents who have:
    - Positive family history of dyslipidemia or premature cardiovascular disease (CVD) (≤55 years old for men, ≤65 years old for women), such as coronary atherosclerosis, documented myocardial infarction (MI)
    - Unknown family history
    - Obesity (BMI ≥95th percentile) or overweight (BMI ≥85th–<95th percentile)
    - Cigarette smoking exposure
    - Hypertension
    - Diabetes mellitus
  - Screen using a fasting lipid profile (FLP): total cholesterol, HDL cholesterol, LDL cholesterol, and triglycerides.
  - If FLP is within normal range, repeat test in 3–5 years.
- Age 9–11 years: NHLBI-AAP recommend universal screening.
  - Screen using either an FLP or nonfasting lipid profile (LP): if done nonfasting and non-HDL >145 mg/dL, then repeat as FLP.
  - Non-HDL = total cholesterol-HDL
- Age 12–16 years
  - Screen children and adolescents with risk factors as with 2–8 years group.

Consider other testing:

- Chemistry panel (glucose, ALT, AST, bilirubin, BUN, creatinine, urinalysis)
  - Screening test for diabetes, liver, and kidney disease
- Thyroid evaluation (thyroxine [total T_4], thyroid stimulating hormone [TSH])
  - Determines the presence of hypothyroidism

ALERT

- Serum total cholesterol is inaccurate when serum triglycerides are >400 mg/dL.
- Hypertriglyceridemia is associated with falsely lowered serum Na.

DIFFERENTIAL DIAGNOSIS

- Hypercholesterolemia
  - Primary hypercholesterolemia (see above)
  - Hypothyroidism
  - Nephrotic syndrome
  - Liver disease (cholestatic)
  - Renal failure
  - Anorexia nervosa
  - Acute porphyria
  - Medications (antihypertensives, estrogens, steroids, microsomal enzyme inducers, cyclosporine, diuretics)
  - Pregnancy
  - Dietary: excessive dietary intake of fat, cholesterol, and/or calories
- Hypertriglyceridemia
  - Primary hypertriglyceridemia (see above)
  - Acute hepatitis
  - Nephrotic syndrome
  - Chronic renal failure
  - Medications (diuretics, retinoids, oral contraceptives)
  - Diabetes mellitus
  - Alcohol abuse
  - Lipodystrophy
  - Myelomatosis
  - Glycogen storage disease
  - Dietary: excessive dietary intake of fat and/or calories

TREATMENT

MEDICATION

- Drug therapy should be considered only for children ≥8 years of age after an adequate trial of diet therapy (for 6–12 months) and if they have one of the following:
  - LDL cholesterol level remains >190 mg/dL
  - LDL cholesterol level remains >160 mg/dL, and there is a family history of premature CVD (≤55 years of age for men, ≤65 for women) or ≥2 other risk factors are present (obesity, hypertension, cigarette smoking).
  - LDL ≥130 mg/dL and have diabetes mellitus
- Physicians caring for overweight and obese children who have lipid disorders should emphasize the importance of diet and exercise rather than drug therapy for most of their patients.
- Statins (first-line drug therapy)
  - Decrease endogenous cholesterol synthesis and increase clearance of LDL from circulation
  - Similar safety and efficacy in the treatment of lipid disorders in children as in adults
  - Side effects include hepatitis and myositis.
- Bile acid–binding resins
  - Bind cholesterol in bile acids in intestine and prevent reuptake into enterohepatic circulation
  - Associated with GI discomfort
  - Very poor compliance in children
- Niacin
  - Lowers LDL and triglycerides while increasing HDL
  - Poorly tolerated in children due to side effects in >50%, including flushing, itching, and elevated hepatic transaminases
- Drugs needing further pediatric studies: cholesterol absorption inhibitors and fibrates

ADDITIONAL TREATMENT

General Measures

- Outpatient management unless secondary hyperlipidemia caused by liver or renal failure, which would necessitate inpatient management of primary illness. Note: The cause of secondary hyperlipidemia should be treated with disease-specific therapy to reduce elevated lipid levels.
- Risk assessment and treatment
  - Population approach
    - General emphasis on healthy lifestyle to prevent development of dyslipidemias
    - Recommendations include increasing intake of fruits, vegetables, fish, whole grains, and low-fat dairy products; reducing intake of fruit juice, sugar-sweetened beverages and food.
  - Individual approach
    - Focuses on patients who are high risk
    - Initial intervention is focused on changing diet, but patients often require pharmacologic intervention.

ADDITIONAL THERAPIES

Activity

- 60 minutes of moderate to vigorous play or physical activity daily
- Reduce sedentary behaviors (e.g., watching TV, playing videogames, using computers)
- Participation in organized sports

ONGOING CARE

FOLLOW-UP RECOMMENDATIONS

Patient Monitoring

- For patients with primary hyperlipidemia who are off medication, follow-up should be performed every 1–2 years with a lipoprotein profile evaluation. For those patients on medication, follow-up should be conducted every 3–6 months.
- For all other patients with risk factors and normal lipid profile, a monitored lifestyle and dietary changes should be strongly recommended at every office visit.

DIET

- Dietary modification is safe in the treatment of hyperlipidemia in children >2 years of age:
  - Restrict saturated fat to <7% daily calories.
  - Restrict dietary cholesterol to 200 mg/day.
  - Limit trans fatty acids to <1% daily calories.
  - Supplemental fiber at goal dose of child's age + 5 g/day (up to 20 g/day)
- For children between 12 months and 2 years who are overweight, obese, or have a family history of dyslipidemia or CVD, the use of reduced fat milk can be considered.

PROGNOSIS

- Familial hypercholesterolemia
  - Homozygotes: coronary artery disease in 1st or 2nd decade of life
  - Heterozygotes: 50% of males develop premature heart disease by age 50 years (females, age 60 years).
- Familial combined hyperlipidemia: occurs in 1–2% of the population and accounts for 10% of all premature heart disease. A reduction of LDL cholesterol by 1% reduces risk by 2%.
- Children and adolescents with high cholesterol levels are more likely than the general population to have high levels as adults.

COMPLICATIONS

- Hypercholesterolemia has been linked to premature coronary artery disease and vascular disease.
- Severe hypertriglyceridemia can cause pancreatitis.

ADDITIONAL READING

- Daniels SR, Greer FR; Committee on Nutrition. Lipid screening and cardiovascular health in childhood. *Pediatrics*. 2008;122(1):198–208.
- Expert Panel on Integrated Guidelines for Cardiovascular Health and Risk Reduction in Children and Adolescents; National Heart, Lung, and Blood Instute. Expert panel on integrated guidelines for cardiovascular health and risk reduction in children and adolescents: summary report. *Pediatrics*. 2011;128(Suppl 5):S213–S256.
- Gidding SS, Dennison BA, Birch LL, et al. Dietary recommendations for children and adolescents: a guide for practitioners: consensus statement from the American Heart Association. *Circulation*. 2005;112(13):2061–2075.
- Kavey RE, Allada V, Daniels SR, et al. Cardiovascular risk reduction in high-risk pediatric patients. A scientific statement from the American Heart Association. *Circulation*. 2006;114(24):2710–2738.
- McCrindle BW, Urbina EM, Dennison BA, et al. Drug therapy of high-risk lipid abnormalities in children and adolescents: a scientific statement from the American Heart Association. *Circulation*. 2007;115(14):1948–1967.

CODES

ICD10

- E78.5 Hyperlipidemia, unspecified
- E78.0 Pure hypercholesterolemia
- E78.1 Pure hyperglyceridemia

FAQ

- Q: When should I screen for dyslipidemia, and what test should I use for screening?
- A: All children between ages 9 and 11 years should be screened for dyslipidemia using a non-FLP. Children between 2–8 years and 12–16 years should be screened using an FLP only if they have risk factors.
- Q: What should my initial management of a child with dyslipidemia include?
- A: The management plan of any child with dyslipidemia is dependent on the age of the child and should include dietary recommendations, a focus on all aspects of heart health, and in selected cases, the use of pharmacotherapy.

HYPERTENSION

Stephanie Nguyen

BASICS

DESCRIPTION
- Hypertension: average systolic and/or diastolic blood pressure (BP) above the 95th percentile for age, gender, and height percentile on at least 3 separate occasions
- Prehypertension: BP between the 90th percentile and 95th percentile or BP ≥120/80 mm Hg in adolescents
- Stage 1 hypertension: BP 95–99% plus 5 mm Hg
- Stage 2 hypertension: BP >99th% plus 5 mm Hg
- Primary (essential) hypertension: hypertension for which there is no underlying cause
- Secondary hypertension: hypertension for which an underlying cause can be identified
- White coat hypertension: elevated BP readings in a medical setting with normal BP on ambulatory blood pressure monitoring (ABPM)
- Masked hypertension: normal BP readings in a medical setting with elevated BP readings on ABPM

EPIDEMIOLOGY
- Primary hypertension is now identifiable in children and adolescents and is associated with overweight status, metabolic syndrome, and family history of hypertension.
- The prevalence of hypertension is increasing due to the epidemic of youth obesity and the metabolic syndrome.
- Hypertension in the pediatric population is estimated to be between 1% and 4%.
- 30% of children with body mass index (BMI) >95% have prehypertension or hypertension.

RISK FACTORS
- Primary hypertension: obesity, sedentary lifestyle, low birth weight, smoking, alcohol use, hyperlipidemia, family history, stress, sodium intake, sleep apnea
- Secondary hypertension: renal or urologic disease, transplant, congenital heart disease, umbilical artery catheterization, urinary tract infection (UTI), diabetes mellitus, elevated intracranial pressure, or medications known to raise BP
- The younger the child and the more elevated BP, the greater likelihood of a secondary cause.

Genetics
- The genetic basis of primary hypertension is polygenic but more likely to develop in individuals when there is a strong family history.
- The genetics of secondary causes depend on the underlying condition, for example
  - Polycystic kidney disease: autosomal dominant, autosomal recessive
  - Neurofibromatosis: autosomal dominant
  - Glucocorticoid-remediable aldosteronism: autosomal dominant

GENERAL PREVENTION
Avoidance of excess weight gain and regular physical activity can prevent obesity-related hypertension.

ETIOLOGY
- Secondary causes
  - Renal: acute glomerulonephritis, chronic renal failure, polycystic kidney disease, reflux nephropathy
  - Renovascular: fibromuscular dysplasia, neurofibromatosis, vasculitis
  - Cardiac: coarctation of the aorta
  - Endocrine: pheochromocytoma, hypo/hyperthyroid, neuroblastoma, glucocorticoid-remediable aldosteronism, Conn syndrome, apparent mineralocorticoid excess, congenital adrenal hyperplasia, Liddle syndrome, Gordon syndrome
  - Neurologic: increased intracranial pressure
  - Drugs: corticosteroids, oral contraceptives, sympathomimetics, illicit drugs (cocaine, phencyclidine)
  - Other: pain, burns, traction
  - Reduced nephron number secondary to premature birth, low birth weight, or postnatal insults are associated with hypertension.

PATHOPHYSIOLOGY
Blood pressure is a product of cardiac output and total peripheral vascular resistance. Increases of either or both of these products lead to hypertension. The various causes of hypertension alter blood pressure through different mechanisms such as volume overload (sodium retention, excess sodium intake), volume distribution, renin-angiotensin excess, sympathetic activation, insulin, and endothelin.

DIAGNOSIS

- Hypertensive emergency: severely elevated BP with evidence of target organ injury (encephalopathy, seizures, renal damage)
- Hypertensive urgency: severely elevated BP with no evidence of secondary organ damage

HISTORY
- Headache, blurry vision, epistaxis, unusual weight gain or loss, chest pain, flushing, fatigue
- UTIs can be associated with reflux nephropathy and hypertension.
- Gross hematuria, edema, and fatigue may suggest renal disease.
- Birth history: umbilical artery catheterization
- Medications: corticosteroids, cold preparations, oral contraceptives, illicit drugs
- Family history: hypertension, diabetes, obesity, familial endocrinopathies, renal disease
- Trauma: arteriovenous (AV) fistula, traction
- Review of symptoms: sleep apnea, obesity

PHYSICAL EXAM
- BP
  - Children >3 years of age should have their BP measured during a health care episode or younger if they have any risk factors for hypertension.
  - Child should be seated quietly for 5 minutes, feet on the floor with the right arm supported at the level of the heart. Routine BPs are measured in the right arm.
  - Use the proper cuff size. The inflatable bladder should completely encircle the arm and cover ~80–100% of the upper arm. A cuff that is inappropriately small will artificially increase the measurement.
  - Elevated BPs obtained by oscillometric devices should be repeated by auscultation.
  - When hypertension is confirmed, BP should be measured in both arms and in a leg. Normally, BP is 10–20 mm Hg higher in the legs. If leg BP is lower than arm, consider coarctation of the aorta.
- Tachycardia in hyperthyroidism, pheochromocytoma
- Body habitus: thin, obese, growth failure, virilized, stigmata of Turner or Williams syndromes
- Skin: café au lait spots, neurofibromas, rashes, acanthosis, malar rash
- Head/neck: moon facies, thyromegaly
- Eyes: funduscopic changes, proptosis
- Lungs: rales
- Cardiovascular: rub, gallop, murmur, femoral pulses
- Abdomen: mass, hepatosplenomegaly, bruit
- Genitalia: ambiguous, virilized
- Neurologic: Bell palsy

DIAGNOSTIC TESTS & INTERPRETATION

Lab
- The laboratory evaluation to determine the cause of hypertension should proceed in a stepwise fashion. In adolescents with stage 1 hypertension, it is reasonable to evaluate for white coat hypertension using ABPM as a first step before other testing.
- Patients should have the following: urinalysis, serum electrolytes, blood urea nitrogen, creatinine, calcium, cholesterol, CBC, ECG, echocardiogram (the most sensitive study to monitor end-organ changes), renal ultrasound, retinal exam
- Further evaluation is based on history, physical exam, and/or to prove secondary causes: voiding cystourethrogram, DMSA renal scan, 3D CT angiogram, MRA, urine or plasma for catecholamines and metanephrines, plasma renin activity, aldosterone levels
- More invasive studies include renal angiogram; renal vein renin concentrations; meta-iodobenzylguanidine (MIBG) scan; renal biopsy; genetic studies to identify rare causes of hypertension

Diagnostic Procedures/Other
- Ambulatory BP monitoring refers to a procedure in which a portable BP device, worn by the patient, records BP over a specified period, usually 24 hours.
- Ambulatory BP monitoring may be helpful in cases in which the diagnosis of hypertension is uncertain (e.g., white coat hypertension) or in assessing the effectiveness of antihypertensive agents. ABPM may also be useful in assessing children at high risk of cardiovascular disease (e.g., diabetes mellitus, labile hypertension).
- Systolic hypertension on ABPM is a better predictor for the development of left ventricular hypertrophy (LVH) when compared to office BP measurements.

DIFFERENTIAL DIAGNOSIS
The initial objective after diagnosing hypertension in children is distinguishing primary from secondary causes. Generally, the younger the child and more elevated the BP measurements, the more likely the cause of hypertension is secondary.

TREATMENT

MEDICATION
- Classes of antihypertensive agents include α- and β-blockers, diuretics, vasodilators (direct and calcium channel blockers), ACE inhibitors, and angiotensin receptor blockers (ARBs).
- Therapy should be initiated with a single drug.
- Avoid multiple medications with the same mechanism of action.
- Elicit a history of adverse effects and adjust medications accordingly.
- Specific classes should be used with concurrent medical conditions: ACE inhibitors or ARBs in children with diabetes and microalbuminuria or proteinuric renal diseases; β-blockers or calcium channel blockers with migraine headaches.
- Certain classes of medication should be avoided in patients with specific conditions, such as asthma and diabetes (β-blockers) and bilateral renal artery stenosis (ACE inhibitors).
- ACE inhibitors are associated with congenital malformations and are contraindicated during pregnancy; calcium channel blockers and β-blockers are alternatives.

ADDITIONAL TREATMENT
General Measures
- If BP is >95th percentile, it should be repeated on 2 more occasions.
- If BP is >99th percentile plus 5 mm Hg, prompt referral for evaluation and therapy should be made.
- If the patient is symptomatic, immediate referral and treatment are indicated.
- Mild primary hypertension may be managed with nonpharmacologic treatment: weight reduction, exercise, sodium restriction, avoidance of certain medications such as pseudoephedrine.
- Pharmacologic therapy should be directed to the cause of secondary hypertension when this is known or for severe, sustained hypertension.
- Medications may be needed in children with mild to moderate hypertension if nonpharmacologic therapy has failed or if end-organ changes, kidney disease, or diabetes is present.

ADDITIONAL THERAPIES
- Regular aerobic physical activity (30–60 minutes at least 5 days a week)
- Limitation of sedentary activities to <2 hours per day
- Patients with uncontrolled stage 2 hypertension should be restricted from high-static competitive sports until the BP is in normal range.

SURGERY/OTHER PROCEDURES
- Dialysis may be needed for hypertension in chronic renal failure.
- Surgical correction of renovascular hypertension and coarctation of the aorta. Percutaneous transluminal angioplasty has been used for renal artery stenosis.

INPATIENT CONSIDERATIONS
Initial Stabilization
- Hypertensive emergencies should be treated with IV BP medications, aiming to decrease the BP by 25% over the first 8 hours and gradually normalizing BP over 24–48 hours.
- Hypertensive urgencies can be treated by either IV or PO antihypertensives depending on symptomatology.

Admission Criteria
- Hypertensive emergencies should be admitted to the ICU if indicated.
- Hypertensive urgencies should be admitted to the hospital.

ONGOING CARE

FOLLOW-UP RECOMMENDATIONS
Patient Monitoring
- The reduction of BP with medication should be gradual to avoid side effects.
- Ongoing monitoring is required for medication side effects, such as exercise intolerance (β-blockers), headaches (vasodilators), renal insufficiency or hyperkalemia (ACE inhibitors), or hypokalemia (diuretics).
- Regular monitoring for development of LVH (echo or ECG) is recommended.
- Patients with white coat hypertension require ongoing monitoring, as they are at risk for developing true hypertension.

DIET
- Dietary increase in fresh vegetables, fresh fruits, potassium, fiber, and nonfat dairy
- Restriction of sodium, calories, saturated fat, and refined sugar
- Low-sodium (DASH) diet: <2.3 g of sodium per day for adolescents

PATIENT EDUCATION
- Diet
  - Increase in fresh vegetables, fresh fruits, fiber, and nonfat dairy
  - Restriction of sodium and calories
- Activity
  - Regular aerobic physical activity (30–60 minutes at least 5 days a week)
  - Limitation of sedentary activities to <2 hours per day
- Prevention
  - Avoidance of excess weight gain, smoking, and alcohol use; regular physical activity

PROGNOSIS
The patient's prognosis depends on the underlying cause of the hypertension. It is excellent if the BP is well controlled.

COMPLICATIONS
- LVH and heart failure
- Renal failure
- Encephalopathy
- Retinopathy

ADDITIONAL READING

- Feld LG, Corey H. Hypertension in childhood. *Pediatr Rev*. 2007;28(8):283–298.
- McCambridge TM, Benjamin HJ, Brenner JS, et al. Athletic participation by children and adolescents who have systemic hypertension. *Pediatrics*. 2010;125(6):1287–1294.
- McCrindle B. Assessment and management of hypertension in children and adolescents. *Nat Rev Cardiol*. 2010;7(3):155–163.
- National High Blood Pressure Education Program Working Group on High Blood Pressure in Children and Adolescents. The fourth report on the diagnosis, evaluation, and treatment of high blood pressure in children and adolescents. *Pediatrics*. 2004;114(2):S555–S576.
- Suresh S, Mahajan P, Kamat D. Emergency management of pediatric hypertension. *Clin Pediatr*. 2005;44(9):739–745.
- Urbina E, Alpert B, Flynn J, et al. Ambulatory blood pressure monitoring in children and adolescents: recommendations for standard assessment. *Hypertension*. 2008;52(3):433–451.

CODES

ICD10
- I10 Essential (primary) hypertension
- I15.9 Secondary hypertension, unspecified
- I15.1 Hypertension secondary to other renal disorders

FAQ
- Q: What is the value of ambulatory BP monitoring?
- A: This device is similar to a Holter monitor and measures BPs over a 24-hour period while the patient is awake and asleep. By reviewing the BPs, one can determine if a significant proportion of readings are elevated and whether or not the normal dip in BP during sleep is seen. Thus, conditions such as white coat hypertension can be verified or discounted.
- Q: What are the indications for invasive studies, such as angiography?
- A: This decision should be individualized and based on the severity of the hypertension, response to medication, the clinical presentation (e.g., neurofibromatosis), and results of other studies. In general, young children and all children with severe, unexplained hypertension should be completely evaluated.
- Q: Can adolescents with elevated BP compete in sports?
- A: Adolescents with hypertension should be encouraged to participate in athletics if their BP is well controlled. The use of stress testing in this population is controversial.
- Q: Do I need to worry about isolated systolic hypertension?
- A: Studies in adults have shown that sustained systolic hypertension may be just as important as diastolic hypertension.

HYPOCALCEMIA

Pisit Pitukcheewanont • Chawkaew Kongkanka

BASICS

DESCRIPTION

- Severity varies from asymptomatic to acute life-threatening condition.
- Etiology is important for appropriate management.
- Neonates
  - Term/premature >1,500 g: total calcium <8 mg/dL (2 mmol/L) if serum protein normal (ionized < 1.1 mmol/L)
  - Premature <1,500 g: total calcium <7 mg/dL (1.75 mmol/L); ionized <0.8 mmol/L
- Children: total serum calcium <8.5 mg/dL (2.1 mmol/L) and ionized calcium <4.5 mg/dL (ionized <1.1 mmol/L).

EPIDEMIOLOGY

- Many normal neonates have serum calcium <8 mg/dL during first 3 weeks of life owing to physiologic transient hypoparathyroidism.
- Parathyroid gland (PTG) immaturity can lead to deficient PTH release and exaggerated fall in calcium during the first 3 days of life.
- Relative immaturity of renal phosphorus handling and PTH response can lead to late neonatal hypocalcemia precipitated by a high-phosphate diet.
- Prevalence of vitamin D deficiency in neonate with mother at risk or maternal vitamin D deficiency is about 52–90%.
- Following total thyroidectomy, 10% develop transient hypoparathyroidism; of these, <50% remain permanently hypoparathyroid.

RISK FACTORS

- Neonate
  - Maternal disorders: diabetes mellitus, toxemia, preeclampsia, hyperparathyroidism, severe vitamin D deficiency
  - Maternal drugs; anticonvulsants, high intake of alkali, magnesium sulfate antacid
  - Prematurity, low birth weight, IUGR, perinatal stress/asphyxia, sepsis
  - Hyperbilirubinemia, phototherapy, citrated blood product use, exchange transfusion
  - Nutrients/drugs; lipid infusion, phosphate therapy, phytate, aminoglycosides, bicarbonate, loop diuretics, glucocorticosteroids, anticonvulsants
  - Osteopetrosis type II
  - Phosphate load; high dietary phosphate (such as cow's milk), phosphate enema, chronic renal insufficiency
  - Hypomagnesemia rarely hypermagnesemia
  - Vitamin D deficiency: malabsorption, renal insufficiency, and liver disease
  - Osteopenia of prematurity
- Hypoparathyroidism
  - Transient neonatal hypoparathyroidism
  - PTG dysgenesis/agenesis
    - Several identified genetic causes including isolated hypoparathyroidism (*GCM2*, *PTH*, *SOX3*), DiGeorge syndrome (*DGS*) (*TBX1*), mitochondrial fatty acid disorders (Kearns-Sayre, Pearson, mitochondrial encephalopathy, lactic acidosis, stroke-like—MELAS)
  - PTH insensitivity
    - Blomstrand chondrodysplasia (*PTHR1*)
    - Pseudohypoparathyroidism type IA (*PHP IA*)
  - Dyshormonogenesis
  - Autoimmune hypoparathyroidism
    - Autoimmune polyglandular syndrome type I (AIRE1)
    - Activating antibodies to the calcium sensing receptor (CaSR)
  - Acquired
    - Postsurgical, PTG radiation destruction
    - PTG infiltrative disease (excessive iron or copper deposition, granulomatous or neoplastic invasion)
  - Enzyme deficiencies
    - Deficiency of 25-hydroxylase (CYP2R1)
    - Deficiency of 25OH-vitamin D_3-1-hydroxylase (CYP27B1)
  - Loss of function vitamin D receptor mutations
- Calcium deficiency
  - Nutritional deprivation
  - Hypercalciuria
- Hypomagnesemia
  - Malabsorption
  - Hypermagnesuria
    - Primary (CLDN16)
    - Bartter syndrome type V (CaSR)
  - Renal tubular acidosis
  - Acute renal failure
  - Chronic inflammatory bowel disease, intestinal resection
  - Diuretics
- Hyperphosphatemia
  - Renal failure
  - Phosphate administration
  - Tumor lysis syndrome
  - Rhabdomyolysis

COMMONLY ASSOCIATED CONDITIONS

- Hypoproteinemia
- Hyperventilation
- Drugs: furosemide, bisphosphonates, calcitonin, anticonvulsants, ketoconazole, antineoplastic agents, citrated blood products
- "Hungry bone syndrome"
- Sepsis, acute pancreatitis, shock
- Organic acidemia

PATHOPHYSIOLOGY

- Calcium is most abundant mineral ion in body; 99% of total body calcium is deposited in bone. Three forms of calcium in serum: protein-bound (50%), complex with serum anions (5%), and ionized form (45%).
- Calcium homeostasis is regulated by many factors: hormones and their receptors (PTH/PTHR, vitamin D/VDR, calcitonin), organs (bone, kidneys, PTGs, intestine, and liver), CaSR (the serum calcium set point), and others such as serum pH.
- Tetany is a manifestation of neuromuscular irritability in patients with hypocalcemia.
- Hypocalcemia may present with seizure or other nonspecific symptoms.

ETIOLOGY

- Abnormal hormonal response
  - Hypoparathyroidism
    - Abnormal PTH production: PTG agenesis/dysfunction, acquired hypoparathyroidism, abnormal PTH secretion
    - Pseudohypoparathyroidism
  - Vitamin D disorder: deficiency/resistance
- Abnormality of calcium-regulating organs
  - Kidneys, bone, intestine
- Abnormal CaSR
  - Gain of function mutation of *CaSR* gene
  - Antibodies to the CaSR
- Other causes of hypocalcemia
  - Phosphate load
  - Calcium sequestration or clearance
  - Decreased ionized calcium

DIAGNOSIS

HISTORY

- In neonates and infants, include relevant maternal history, prematurity, nutrition, IUGR, perinatal illness
- Other nonspecific symptoms; apnea, poor feeding
- Family history of calcium disorders
- Current illness and drug use
- History of neck surgery
- Recurrent infection
- History of seizure
- Muscle cramps
- Paresthesia, a tingling sensation, usually present around the mouth, fingers, and toes

PHYSICAL EXAM

- Neuromuscular irritabilities
  - Tetany, hyperreflexia
    - *Chvostek sign (usually in 1 month to 2 years of age)*: twitching of the orbicularis oris muscle with light tapping at anterior external auditory meatus on the CN VII
    - *Peroneal sign*: dorsiflexion and abduction of the foot on tapping the peroneal nerve on the lateral surface of the fibula just before the knee
    - *Trousseau sign*: carpopedal spasm when BP cuff maintained 20 mm Hg above SBP for 3 minutes
  - Lethargy
  - Muscle weakness
  - Focal or generalized seizure
  - In neonate: laryngospasm, apnea, bradycardia/tachycardia, hypotension, cyanosis, emesis
- Prolonged hypocalcemia
  - Basal ganglia calcification
  - Subcapsular cataracts
  - Papilledema (occasional)
  - Dental enamel hypoplasia, particularly of the primary teeth
- Features associated with genetic syndrome/inherited causes of hypocalcemia
  - Dysmorphic features
  - Hearing loss
  - Congenital heart disease
  - Clinical signs of rickets, alopecia
  - Mucocutaneous candidiasis, ectodermal dysplasia, vitiligo
  - Albright hereditary osteodystrophy (AHO)
  - PHP IA has AHO features: short stature, husky-obese body habitus, shortening of the 3rd–5th metacarpal bones and distal phalanx of the 1st finger (brachydactyly), syndactyly between the 2nd and 3rd toes, round face, flat nasal bridge, short neck, subcutaneous calcifications (heterotopic ossification), cataract, and developmental delay in some patients.

DIAGNOSTIC TESTS & INTERPRETATION

Initial Lab Tests

- Blood: total and ionized calcium, albumin, arterial pH, phosphate, intact PTH, Mg, alkaline phosphatase, creatinine, 25-hydroxyvitamin D; consider 1,25-dihydroxyvitamin D
- Urine: calcium, creatinine

- 12-lead ECG
  - Prolonged QT interval associated with early after-repolarizations and triggered dysrhythmias
  - ECG abnormalities common but serious dysrhythmias infrequent
- If hypoalbuminemia present: correction calculated by: calcium measured + 0.8 [4 − albumin (mg/dL)]
- When serum pH increased (alkalosis), Ca^{2+} bound to protein
- Phosphate is an indirect index of PTH activity; low and high phosphate levels may reflect a raised and a reduced PTH, respectively.
- Hypoparathyroidism: low/subnormal serum calcium and high serum phosphate with normal or inappropriately low serum iPTH after ruled out hypo/hypermagnesemia
- Parathyroid hormone insensitivity
  - In PHP IA, low serum calcium, high serum and urine phosphate, and elevated PTH
  - No increased serum calcium, urinary cyclic AMP or phosphate after rhPTH1-34 (unresponsive to exogenous PTH)
- Hypomagnesemia inhibits PTH secretion and activity.
- Hypermagnesemia suppresses PTH secretion and decreases renal tubular calcium reabsorption.
- Urine calcium/urine creatinine: normal values for spot collections vary by age. For 0–6, 7–12, and >24 months are <0.8, <0.6, and <0.21 mg/mg, respectively.
- Alkaline phosphatase: bone formation marker
- Serum Cr is used to exclude renal failure.
- Vitamin D disorders: low/ subnormal serum calcium, low/normal phosphate with secondary hyperparathyroidism. In vitamin D deficiency, serum 25-hydroxyvitamin D <30 ng/mL. Serum 1,25-dihydroxyvitamin D_3 inappropriately low in patients with severely compromised renal function, hypoparathyroidism, and deficiency of 25OH-vitamin D3-1-hydroxylase.

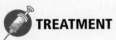

TREATMENT

MEDICATION

Neonatal hypocalcemia

- Asymptomatic neonatal hypocalcemia
  - Increased oral calcium intake, calcium glubionate/carbonate 50–100 mg of elemental Ca/kg/day divided q4–6h if no feeding intolerance (be careful, high osmolality of oral calcium in whom at risk of necrotizing enterocolitis), or 10% calcium gluconate continuous IV infusion for 48 hours. Calcium glubionate is preferable in neonates.
  - Once serum calcium normalizes, can taper supplements
- Symptomatic neonatal hypocalcemia
  - 10% calcium gluconate IV over 10 minutes (elemental Ca 9.3 mg/mL), 18.6 mg elemental Ca (2 mL)/kg/dose (max. 20 mg elemental Ca/kg), diluted 1:1 with 5% dextrose, with cardiac monitoring
  - If severe hypocalcemia with poor cardiac function, *may* give calcium chloride 20 mg/kg via central line over 10–30 minutes
  - Maintenance of 50–100 mg of elemental Ca/kg/day, continuous IV infusion for 48 hours
  - If serum calcium is normal at 48 hours, taper to 50% dose for next 24 hours and then stop/continue depending on etiology; may switch to oral calcium on the last day before stopping or for continued treatment
  - Avoid extravascular extravasation.
- Treatment for specific causes
  - Calcium supplement doses depend on patient requirement and cause of hypocalcemia.
  - Hypomagnesemia: Give 50% (500 mg/mL) $MgSO_4$ 50–100 mg/kg (0.1–0.2 mL/kg) IV/IM q12h for 2 doses with cardiac monitoring. A maintenance dose is 100 mg (0.2 mL)/kg/day PO for 3 days.
  - Phosphate load: Encourage exclusive breastfeeding or use low-phosphate formula (similac PM 60/40, Ca : P = 1.6:1). Phosphate-binding gels are not recommended.
  - Hypoparathyroidism: Supplement 1, $25(OH)_2$ vitamin D_3/calcitriol 20–60 ng/kg/day or 0.5–1 mcg/day PO.
  - Vitamin D deficiency: Supplement vitamin D_2 or D_3 (age 0–1 year) 2,000 IU daily for 6 weeks to achieve level above 30 ng/mL, then maintenance therapy 400–1,000 IU daily.

Hypocalcemia in childhood and adolescence

- Asymptomatic hypocalcemia
  - Likely long-standing; may not require immediate treatment
  - Supplement oral calcium 25–100 mg of elemental Ca/kg/day q4–6h. Calcium citrate may be preferable.
- Symptomatic hypocalcemia
  - Give 10% (100 mg/mL) calcium gluconate 200 mg (2 mL)/kg/dose IV, slow rate over 10 minutes with cardiac monitoring; may repeat dose q6–8h
  - Maintenance by 20–80 mg of elemental Ca/kg/day, continuous IV infusion for 48 hours
  - If hypocalcemia is caused by hypomagnesemia, give 50% (500 mg/mL) $MgSO_4$ 50–100 mg (0.1–0.2 mL)/kg IM with cardiac monitoring.
- Higher supplemental calcium doses required in patient with severe bone demineralization (hungry bone syndrome)
- In hypoparathyroidism: calcitriol 20–60 ng/kg/day PO and calcium 30–75 mg elemental Ca/kg/day q4–6h
- Additional medication: Thiazide (hydrochlorothiazide [HCTZ] 0.2 mg/kg/day) combined with a low-salt diet may increase renal tubular reabsorption of Ca and lower calcitriol requirement.
- Others: Recombinant human PTH therapy in adults can be considered; black box warning in children
- In chronic hypocalcemia, goals are to control symptoms and avoid complications. Maintain serum calcium at the lower end of normal range, Ca × phosphate < 55 (higher products could precipitate calcium phosphate in soft tissue: kidney, lens, and basal ganglia), and urine Ca/urine creatinine < 0.2 to avoid hypercalcemia, hypercalciuria, nephrocalcinosis, and nephrolithiasis, especially in hypoparathyroidism.

ONGOING CARE

FOLLOW-UP RECOMMENDATIONS

Patient Monitoring

- Regular serum and urine monitoring during initial therapy and dose adjustment and 3–6-month interval if stabilized
- Annual renal ultrasound, slit-lamp, and ophthalmoscopic examination are recommended.

PROGNOSIS

Depends on etiology

COMPLICATIONS

Precipitation of calcium–phosphate salts in soft tissues (e.g., kidney, lens, and basal ganglia), hypercalcemia, hypercalciuria, nephrocalcinosis, nephrolithiasis, renal insufficiency

ADDITIONAL READING

- Cusano NE, Rubin MR, McMahon DJ, et al. Therapy of hypoparathyroidism with PTH (1-84). *J Clin Endocrinol Metab*. 2013;98(1):137–144.
- Liamis G, Milionis HJ, Elisaf M. A review of drug-induced hypocalcemia. *J Bone Miner Metab*. 2009; 27(6):635–642.
- Lima K, Abrahamsen TG, Wolff AB, et al. Hypoparathyroidism and autoimmunity in the 22q11.2 deletion syndrome. *Eur J Endocrinol*. 2011;165(2):345–352.
- Malloy PJ, Feldman D. Genetic disorders and defects in vitamin D action. *Endocrinol Metab Clin North Am*. 2010;39(2):333–346.
- Nhan C, Dolev Y, Mijovic T, et al. Vitamin D deficiency and the risk of hypocalcemia following total thyroidectomy. *J Otolaryngol Head Neck Surg*. 2012;41(6):401–406.
- Shoback D. Clinical practice: hypoparathyroidism. *N Eng J Med*. 2008;359(4):391–403.

CODES

ICD10

- E83.51 Hypocalcemia
- P71.1 Other neonatal hypocalcemia
- P71.0 Cow's milk hypocalcemia in newborn

FAQ

- Q: What is the relationship between calcium and phosphate in hypocalcemic setting?
- A: It depends on abnormal hormonal regulation and etiology of hypocalcemia.

Hormonal problems	Serum calcium	Serum phosphate
Parathyroid hormone deficiency/resistant	Low	High
Vitamin D deficiency/resistant	Normal/ low	Normal/ low

- Q: When should parenteral or oral calcium supplement be used?
- A: Every patient can be treated with oral calcium supplement except in acute symptomatic hypocalcemia such as seizure and individuals who temporally hold on enteral feeding or have active malabsorption issue.
- Q: What is the treatment goal of hypocalcemia in children?
- A: Keep serum calcium level in the lower normal range without symptoms of hypocalcemia to reduce the long-term complications, especially nephrocalcinosis.

HYPOGAMMAGLOBULINEMIA

Rachel G. Robison

BASICS

DESCRIPTION

- A disorder of the humoral immune system characterized by deficient or absent immunoglobulins and the inability to produce specific antibody
- Subtypes include primary immunodeficiency and secondary deficiency due to other extrinsic disease (i.e., malignancy).

EPIDEMIOLOGY

Incidence and prevalence depends on underlying defect or cause. Antibody deficiency syndromes represent ~70% of primary immune deficiencies.

RISK FACTORS

Genetic defects have been identified in many cases, which are identified in the "Differential Diagnosis."

DIAGNOSIS

HISTORY

- Recurrent upper and lower respiratory tract infections (otitis media, pneumonia, and sinusitis)
- Infections with encapsulated bacteria such as *Streptococcus pneumoniae*, *Haemophilus influenzae*
- May have diarrhea, infections with *Giardia*
- Chronic cough and chronic rhinitis may be present.

PHYSICAL EXAM

- May be normal if an infection is not present
- Evaluate for growth delay and failure to thrive.
- Patients with X-linked agammaglobulinemia (XLA) may have absent or minimal tonsillar tissue.
- Digital clubbing may be present in cases with history of severe infections.

DIAGNOSTIC TESTS & INTERPRETATION

Lab

- CBC with differential
  - Can rule out associated anemia, thrombocytopenia, and neutropenia
- Quantitative immunoglobulins: IgG, IgM, IgA, and IgE
  - Look for low or absent isotypes.

ALERT

Normal immunoglobulin levels vary by age.

- Qualitative antibody titers specifically to tetanus, *H. influenzae type B*, *S. pneumoniae* postvaccination
  - Absent response after vaccination can identify specific antibody deficiencies.
- Evaluate for presence of isohemagglutinins (primary IgM antibodies to the main blood groups) in unvaccinated children.
- Flow cytometry to evaluate B cell numbers

Imaging

- Chest radiography, CT chest and/or sinus
  - To evaluate for acute disease and if with history of multiple infections, to look for chronic parenchymal changes such as bronchiectasis

DIFFERENTIAL DIAGNOSIS

Primary Defects in Antibody Production

- Selective IgA deficiency
  - Most common cause of hypogammaglobulinemia
  - Low to undetectable levels of IgA with normal other immunoglobulin classes
  - Prevalence of 1/300–1/800 in Caucasians
  - Most are asymptomatic, a proportion may have recurrent infections (upper and lower respiratory infections), risk of giardiasis, and GI infections
  - May develop anaphylactic reactions to blood products due to presence of antibodies to IgA
- Common variable immunodeficiency
  - The second most common cause of hypogammaglobulinemia
    - Peaks in 1st and 3rd decades of life
    - Affects both sexes equally; incidence of 1/20,000–1/100,000
  - Characterized by decreased IgG (2 *SD* below the age-adjusted mean) and impaired humoral response to polysaccharide antigens
  - Risk of development of malignancy such as non-Hodgkin lymphoma, gastric cancer
  - Can be associated with autoimmunity in up to 25% (i.e., rheumatoid arthritis, idiopathic thrombocytopenic purpura, autoimmune hemolytic anemia)
  - Genetic defects have been identified in TACI, ICOS, BAFF-R, and CD19, although only 10% have a family history of disease.
- XLA
  - X-linked mutation in Bruton tyrosine kinase (Btk) gene leading to a defect in B cell maturation
  - Reported in 1/379,000 U.S. births
  - Patients often present with infections after waning of maternal IgG after 3 months of age.
  - Labs reveal low serum immunoglobulin levels and <2% circulating B cells.
  - Patients are susceptible to viral infections such as enterovirus.
  - Autosomal recessive agammaglobulinemia occurs in ~15% without Btk mutations and can occur in females; has a similar phenotype.
- Transient hypogammaglobulinemia of infancy
  - Prolongation of the "physiologic" hypogammaglobulinemia of infancy, which is normally observed during the first 3–6 months of life
    - IgG levels should be at least 2 *SD* below the mean age-matched controls.
    - Typically recover by 9–15 months of age and have normal Ig levels by 2–4 years
    - Must be diagnosed in retrospect after immune recovery and patients should be followed with serial immunoglobulin levels.
  - Etiology remains unknown.
  - Antibiotic prophylaxis and/or immunoglobulin replacement should be considered in those with severe recurrent infections.

- Disorders of immunoglobulin class-switch recombination (Ig-CSR)
  - CD40L mutation: X-linked hyper IgM syndrome (HIGM)
    - Also known as HIGM1
    - Estimated frequency of 1 in 500,000 live male births
    - Due to a mutation in the CD40 ligand gene
    - IgM may be elevated or normal. IgG, IgA, and IgE levels are low to absent.
    - Affects T cell priming and antigen-specific T cell responses, in addition to defective antibody production
    - Chronic diarrhea and failure to thrive are present.
    - In addition, can have opportunistic infections, particularly with *Pneumocystis*, *Cryptosporidium*, and *Histoplasma* organisms
    - May have lymphadenopathy and hepatosplenomegaly on exam
    - Treatment includes allogeneic hematopoietic cell transplantation.
  - Autosomal recessive hyper IgM syndromes (AR-HIGM)
    - Includes mutations in the following:
      - CD40 (HIGM3)
      - Activation-induced cytidine deaminase (AID) (HIGM2): the most common AR-HIGM, AD mutations in AID are also described
      - Uracyl-N-glycosylase (UNG) (HIGM5)
    - CD40 mutations present similarly to X-linked HIGM.
    - AID and UNG mutations have less incidence of opportunistic infections and neutropenia and are associated with lymph node hyperplasia.

Secondary Defects in Antibody Production

- Increased loss: Loss of protein can occur via the kidneys, intestinal tract, lymphatic system, or skin.
  - Protein-losing enteropathy
    - Intestinal lymphangiectasia can be congenital.
    - Post-Fontan procedures with resultant hypogammaglobulinemia
  - Nephrotic syndrome
- Decreased production
  - Malignancy
    - Chronic lymphocytic leukemia
    - Lymphoma
    - Multiple myeloma
  - Medications
    - Sulfasalazine
    - Systemic steroids
    - Phenytoin
    - Carbamazepine
    - Androgen replacement

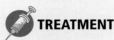

TREATMENT

MEDICATION

- Appropriate antimicrobial therapy at first sign of infection. Prompt initiation of therapy is recommended.
- Select patients may benefit from prophylactic antibiotics.
- Regular replacement therapy with gammaglobulin in either IV or SC forms. Usually 300–600 mg/kg every 3–4 weeks IV or every 1–2 weeks SC.
- Trough levels of 700–800 mg/dL are now preferred compared to previous recommendations of >300 mg/dL.

ONGOING CARE

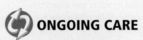

PATIENT MONITORING

Patients on immunoglobulin replacement should have trough IgG levels followed regularly as well as CBCs with differential and metabolic panels to look for hemolytic processes and side effects of replacement.

PROGNOSIS

In most cases (except transient hypogammaglobulinemia of infancy), it requires lifelong therapy.

ADDITIONAL READING

- Conley ME. Genetics of hypogammaglobulinemia: what do we really know? *Curr Opin Immunol*. 2009;21(5):466–471.
- Qamar N, Fuleihan RL. The hyper IgM syndromes. *Clin Rev Allergy Immunol*. 2014; 46(2):120–130.
- Rose ME, Land DM. Evaluating and managing hypogammaglobulinemia. *Cleve Clin Med*. 2006;73(2): 133–144.
- van der Burg M, van Zelm MC, Driessen GJA, et al. New frontiers of primary antibody deficiencies. *Cell Mol Life Sci*. 2012;69(1):59–73.
- Yong PFK, Chee R, Grimbacher B. Hypogammaglobulinaemia. *Immunol Allergy Clin North Am*. 2008; 28(4):691–713.

CODES

ICD10

- D80.1 Nonfamilial hypogammaglobulinemia
- D80.0 Hereditary hypogammaglobulinemia
- D80.2 Selective deficiency of immunoglobulin A [IgA]

FAQ

- Q: When should I check immunoglobulin levels?
- A: Immunoglobulins and antibody responses to vaccinations may be considered in any patient with a history of recurrent sinopulmonary infections.
- Q: I have a 2-month-old male patient with a family history of XLA. His IgG level is normal. Do I need to recheck it in the future?
- A: At 2 months of age, most infants still have maternal IgG present. Levels tend to wane and the infant will start to produce his or her own IgG in the 3–4-month range. Rechecking after this time is recommended.

HYPOPHOSPHATEMIC DISORDERS

Erik A. Imel • Peter J. Tebben

BASICS

DESCRIPTION

Hypophosphatemia is defined by serum phosphorus values below the age-appropriate normal range.

ALERT

- Normal phosphorus concentrations in infants and children are significantly higher than in adults.
- Hypophosphatemia can be missed if an adult normal range is used for pediatric patients.

EPIDEMIOLOGY

Acute hypophosphatemia is a common laboratory finding in the hospital, especially in the intensive care unit (ICU) setting.

ETIOLOGY

- Chronic hypophosphatemia is a common etiology of rickets. It can result from multiple causes, including:
  - Vitamin D deficiency
    - Most common form of rickets
  - X-linked hypophosphatemic (XLH) rickets
    - Most common inherited cause of rickets (prevalence ≈1 in 20,000)
    - Other genetic forms of rickets are less common.
- Isolated dietary phosphate deficiency is rare; dietary phosphate deficiency usually involves generalized malnutrition.

Genetics

Genetic forms are less common than acquired forms and occur due to mutations in:

- *PHEX* (XLH rickets)
- *FGF23* (autosomal dominant hypophosphatemic rickets [ADHR])
- *DMP1* (autosomal recessive hypophosphatemic rickets [ARHR])
- *ENPP1* (ARHR, generalized arterial calcification of infancy [GACI])
- *FAM20C* (autosomal recessive hypophosphatemia, Raine syndrome)
- *SCL34A3* (NPT2c, hereditary hypophosphatemic rickets with hypercalciuria [HHRH])
- *CYP27B1* (1α-hydroxylase deficiency)
- *VDR* (vitamin D receptor)
- *GNAS* (McCune-Albright syndrome, activating mutations of Gsα, sometimes associated with hypophosphatemia)
- Others

RISK FACTORS

- Nutritional
  - Vitamin D deficiency
  - Malnutrition/refeeding syndrome
  - Chronic diarrhea
- Medications affecting phosphate absorption
  - Antacids
  - Sevelamer
  - Lanthanum carbonate
  - Excess calcium salts
- Genetics
  - Primary renal phosphate wasting disorders (see "Differential Diagnosis")
  - Vitamin D metabolism disorders
  - Renal Fanconi syndrome
- Other:
  - Medications affecting renal phosphate transport
  - Treatment of diabetic ketoacidosis
  - Acute respiratory alkalosis
  - Post renal transplant
  - Hungry bone syndrome after parathyroidectomy for hyperparathyroidism
    - Also causes hypocalcemia

PATHOPHYSIOLOGY

- Decreased nutritional intake or malabsorption
- Redistribution of extracellular phosphate into the intracellular compartment
- Increased renal phosphate loss (due to medications, hormonal effects, or primary renal tubulopathy)

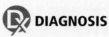

DIAGNOSIS

HISTORY

- Family history of hypophosphatemia or rickets
- Medications
- Known disease affecting phosphate metabolism (see "Differential Diagnosis")
- Nutritional history
  - Vitamin D intake, phosphate sources
  - Anorexia or other malnutrition
  - Parenteral or enteral nutrition formulation
- Duration of symptoms (acute vs. chronic)
- Dental abnormalities
  - Abscessed teeth associated with XLH
- Gastrointestinal symptoms
  - Chronic diarrhea
- Cardiovascular, respiratory, or neurologic symptoms (may accompany acute hypophosphatemia, usually in hospital setting)
- Myalgia or weakness
- Bowed legs, short stature
- Bone pain or stress fractures/pseudofractures
- Precocious puberty, café au lait macules, fibrous dysplasia—due to McCune-Albright syndrome

PHYSICAL EXAM

- Height, rate of growth
- Rachitic features
  - Frontal bossing
  - Delayed closure of fontanelle
  - Rachitic rosary
  - Harrison sulcus (groove corresponding to the rib insertion site of the diaphragm)
  - Widened wrists or ankles
  - Valgus, varus, or windswept deformity of the legs
- Dental abscess
- Muscle weakness
- Café au lait macules (McCune-Albright syndrome)

DIAGNOSTIC TESTS & INTERPRETATION

Lab

Confirm laboratory diagnosis before treating (unless unstable).

- Serum phosphorus concentration—below age-appropriate normal range (ideally fasting)
- Normal ranges by age
  - 0–1 month 4.8–8.2 mg/dL
  - 1–4 month 4.8–8.1 mg/dL
  - 4 months–1 year 4.8–6.8 mg/dL
  - 1–5 years 3.6–6.5 mg/dL
  - 5–10 years 3.4–5.5 mg/dL
  - 10–20 years 2.6–5.2 mg/dL
  - >20 years 2.5–4.9 mg/dL
- Serum calcium
  - Normal in most primary renal phosphate wasting disorders
  - Elevated in primary hyperparathyroidism
  - Low or low normal in vitamin D deficiency rickets
- Parathyroid hormone concentration
  - Can be elevated if chronic hypophosphatemia is due to vitamin D deficiency or to XLH (pre- or posttreatment). Elevations in parathyroid hormone (PTH) concurrent with hypercalcemia indicate primary hyperparathyroidism.
- Alkaline phosphatase
  - Elevated in rickets and many patients with hyperparathyroidism
- Serum creatinine
- 25-hydroxyvitamin D
  - Low in vitamin D deficiency rickets
- 1,25-dihydroxyvitamin D
  - Low in 1α-hydroxylase deficiency
  - Elevated in vitamin D receptor mutations and nutritional phosphate deficiency
  - Low or inappropriately normal in fibroblast growth factor 23 (FGF23)-mediated causes of hypophosphatemia
- Urine phosphorus and creatinine for assessment of tubular maximum phosphate reabsorption per glomerular filtration rate (TmP/GFR or TP/GFR)
  - Should be obtained at same time as serum phosphorus and creatinine
  - TP/GFR = serum phosphorus − (urine phosphorus × serum creatinine/urine creatinine)
  - Normal or high in vitamin D–mediated hypophosphatemia and nutritional deficiency
  - Low in renal phosphate wasting disorders

- FGF23 (a phosphaturic hormone)—may be helpful in renal phosphate wasting disorders
  - Elevated in many forms of inherited rickets (XLH, ADHR, ARHR)
  - Elevated in most patients with tumor-induced osteomalacia (TIO) due to FGF23-secreting tumors
  - Low in nutritional phosphate deficiency or malabsorption or Fanconi syndrome or HHRH

Imaging

- Radiographs to evaluate for signs of rickets
  - Knees and wrists
- Skeletal survey in patients suspected of fibrous dysplasia of bone
  - Bone scan is also very sensitive in evaluating for fibrous dysplasia.
- Rare: other imaging to identify TIO—these rare tumors can be very difficult to localize
  - PET/CT scan, MRI, CT, octreotide scan, whole body sestamibi scan

Diagnostic Procedures/Other

Genetic studies, when appropriate

DIFFERENTIAL DIAGNOSIS

- Nutritional- or absorption-related
  - Low phosphorus intake
  - Premature infants
  - Chronic diarrhea
  - Short bowel syndrome
  - Vitamin D deficiency
    - Nutritional, lack of sun exposure
    - 1α-hydroxylase deficiency
    - Vitamin D receptor mutation
  - Medications
    - Antacids
    - Sevelamer
    - Lanthanum carbonate
    - Excess calcium salts
- Redistribution of phosphate into the intracellular compartment
  - Insulin therapy for diabetic ketoacidosis
  - Acute respiratory alkalosis
  - Refeeding syndrome
  - Hungry bone syndrome (after parathyroidectomy for primary hyperparathyroidism)
- Increased renal phosphate loss
  - Medications (glucocorticoids, diuretics)
  - Primary hyperparathyroidism
  - FGF23-dependent (FGF23 excess)
    - XLH rickets
    - ADHR (may present after childhood with new-onset hypophosphatemia; consider ADHR if considering TIO)
    - ARHR
    - TIO (primarily diagnosed in adults, but cases reported in children)
    - Fibrous dysplasia of bone
    - Postrenal transplant phosphate wasting
  - FGF23-independent
    - Renal Fanconi syndrome
      - Familial
      - Medication-induced
      - Associated with other disorders (cystinosis, multiple myeloma, and others)
    - HHRH (rare—mutations impairing NPT2c)

TREATMENT

MEDICATION

- Acute
  - Oral phosphate supplementation preferred route
  - Intravenous phosphate should be used with caution:
    - High doses require central venous catheter.
    - Can cause severe hypocalcemia: Monitor calcium.
    - Telemetry recommended due to possible arrhythmias
  - Replete vitamin D if needed (this will not acutely increase serum phosphorus levels)
- Chronic
  - If dietary deficiency or malabsorption: oral phosphate and vitamin D repletion
  - If renal phosphate wasting due to an FGF23-mediated cause
    - Phosphate 20–40 mg/kg/day divided in 3–5 doses
      - Start therapy with low doses and then increase gradually to reduce risk of diarrhea.
    - Calcitriol 20–30 ng/kg/day in 2 divided doses (may require higher doses)
  - Non–FGF23-mediated renal phosphate wasting with elevated 1,25-dihydroxyvitamin D (HHRH)
    - Phosphate 20–40 mg/kg/day divided in 3–5 doses

ADDITIONAL TREATMENT

- Chronic hypophosphatemic disorders resulting in skeletal deformity (especially inherited causes) may require surgical intervention to correct valgus or varus deformities of the lower extremities.
  - Adequate medical therapy should be initiated first, as it may reduce the need for surgical interventions.
- Routine dental care
  - Dental abscess common in some genetic forms of hypophosphatemia
- For the rare cases of TIO, complete surgical removal of the offending tumor is curative.

General Measures

- Routine dental care at least twice per year (especially for patients with inherited rickets)
- Audiology evaluation in patient with inherited hypophosphatemic rickets
  - Increased risk of hearing loss

ONGOING CARE

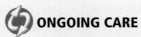

FOLLOW-UP RECOMMENDATIONS

- For chronic hypophosphatemia
  - Frequent laboratory monitoring is mandatory if long-term phosphate and calcitriol therapy is needed (every 3–4 months)
    - Calcium
    - Phosphorus
    - Creatinine
    - Alkaline phosphatase
    - Parathyroid hormone
    - Urine calcium, creatinine, and phosphorus
  - The goal is NOT to normalize serum phosphate in chronic renal phosphate wasting disorders, as this may lead to secondary or tertiary hyperparathyroidism and/or nephrocalcinosis.
  - Periodic radiographic studies
    - Annual renal ultrasound to evaluate for nephrocalcinosis
    - Periodic x-ray of knees/wrists to evaluate response to treatment
      - Improvement in rachitic changes
      - Improvement in varus/valgus deformities

PROGNOSIS

- Hypophosphatemia due to nutritional deficiency
  - Hypophosphatemia resolves with adequate replacement of nutritional deficiencies or discontinuation of phosphate-binding agents.
- Acute hypophosphatemia (typically seen in the hospital setting) can be life-threatening and requires careful monitoring and treatment.
  - Hypophosphatemia resolves when the underlying condition is treated.
- Chronic renal phosphate wasting disorders have a variable response to treatment. Some have radiographic healing of rickets, correction of varus/valgus deformity, and normalization of alkaline phosphatase, whereas others have an incomplete response to therapy.
- Short stature is a common result of chronic hypophosphatemia.
- Hypophosphatemia resolves with removal of the offending tumor in patients with TIO, but long-term monitoring for recurrence is necessary, as hypophosphatemia may recur years later.

ADDITIONAL READING

- Carpenter TO, Imel EA, Holm IA, et al. A clinician's guide to X-linked hypophosphatemia. *J Bone Miner Res*. 2011;26(7):1381–1388.
- Imel EA, Econs MJ. Approach to the hypophosphatemic patient. *J Clin Endocrinol Metab*. 2012;97(3): 696–706.

CODES

ICD10

- E83.39 Other disorders of phosphorus metabolism
- E72.09 Other disorders of amino-acid transport
- E83.31 Familial hypophosphatemia

FAQ

- Q: What is the most important complication of intravenous phosphate administration?
- A: Severe life-threatening hypocalcemia. Infusions of phosphate should be slow and monitored with telemetry.
- Q: Should I measure FGF23 concentrations?
- A: Generally, a diagnosis can be made without FGF23 measurement. FGF23 measurement is only useful if the TP/GFR is low.
- Q: What are dietary phosphate sources?
- A: Phosphate sources are ubiquitous; examples include processed meats, dairy, legumes, nuts, whole grains, citrus, and colas. Phosphates are used as a preservative in processed foods.

H

HYPOPLASTIC LEFT HEART SYNDROME

Laura Mercer-Rosa

BASICS

DESCRIPTION

Hypoplastic left heart syndrome (HLHS) is a continuum of congenital cardiac defects resulting from severe underdevelopment of the structures of the left side of the heart (left atrium, mitral valve, left ventricle, aortic valve, and ascending aorta).

EPIDEMIOLOGY

- 0.16–0.36 per 1,000 live births
- 8% of congenital heart disease (CHD); 3rd most common cause of critical CHD in the newborn
- 23% of all neonatal mortality from CHD
- Male predominance (67%)

RISK FACTORS

Genetics

- Familial inheritance: Sibling recurrence risk ranges from 8% to 21%, with higher recurrence observed when cardiovascular malformations are present in either parent. In addition, rare kinships have a frequency approaching autosomal dominant transmission.

COMMONLY ASSOCIATED CONDITIONS

- Increased mortality when associated with definable genetic disorders, which comprise 10–28% of HLHS patients:
  - Turner syndrome, Noonan syndrome, Smith-Lemli-Opitz syndrome, Holt-Oram syndrome
  - Trisomy 13, 18, 21, or microdeletion syndromes
- Major extracardiac anomalies (diaphragmatic hernia, omphalocele)

PATHOPHYSIOLOGY

- The etiology appears multifactorial, most likely resulting from an in utero reduction of left ventricular inflow or outflow (mechanisms postulated include premature closure of the foramen ovale and fetal cardiomyopathy).
- As a result, the right ventricle (RV) must supply both the pulmonary and systemic circulations (via the ductus arteriosus) before and after birth.
- The reduction in pulmonary vascular resistance that occurs with lung expansion at birth reduces the proportion of RV output to the systemic circulation. If the ductus arteriosus closes, shock occurs.

DIAGNOSIS

HISTORY

- In the current era, HLHS is often diagnosed prenatally.
- Postnatal signs and symptoms:
  - Respiratory distress (tachypnea, grunting, flaring, retractions)
  - Cyanosis
  - Cardiovascular collapse and profound metabolic acidosis when the ductus arteriosus closes

PHYSICAL EXAM

- CHF secondary to pulmonary overcirculation (e.g., tachycardia, hepatomegaly, gallop)
- Normal S_1 and single S_2 (A_2 absent); a murmur of tricuspid regurgitation may be auscultated
- Varying degrees of cyanosis
- Decreased perfusion and weak peripheral pulses

DIAGNOSTIC TESTS & INTERPRETATION

Lab

- Chest radiograph: varying degree of cardiomegaly with increased pulmonary vascular markings (if the atrial septum is intact or highly restrictive, lungs will appear hazy with a pulmonary venous obstructive pattern)
- ECG: right axis deviation (+90 to +210 degrees), RV hypertrophy with a qR pattern in the right precordial leads, decreased left ventricular forces with an rS pattern in the left precordial leads
- Echocardiogram: varying degrees of hypoplasia or atresia of the mitral valve, left ventricle, aortic valve, ascending aorta, and aortic arch; patent ductus arteriosus with right-to-left shunt in systole and diastolic flow reversal; atrial septal defect with left-to-right flow
- Cardiac catheterization: no longer routinely performed; similar findings as with echocardiography

DIFFERENTIAL DIAGNOSIS

- Cardiac: Other causes of circulatory collapse in the neonate include critical aortic stenosis and coarctation of the aorta, cardiomyopathy (infectious, metabolic, or hypoxic), persistent supraventricular tachycardia, obstructive cardiac neoplasms, and large arteriovenous fistulae.
- Noncardiac: neonatal septicemia, respiratory distress syndrome, inborn errors of metabolism

TREATMENT

INITIAL STABILIZATION

During initial resuscitation and stabilization of a newly diagnosed infant:

- Prostaglandin E1 therapy should be initiated as soon as possible to maintain ductal patency.
- Avoid using oxygen despite low pulse oximetry saturation. Increasing FiO_2 will lower pulmonary vascular resistance, preferentially shunting cardiac output away from the systemic circulation toward the lungs, thereby worsening systemic perfusion.
- Should invasive ventilation be required, avoid hyperventilation.
  - Permissive hypercapnea is preferred due to the secondary increase in pulmonary vascular resistance and subsequent improvement in systemic perfusion.
  - Maintain mildly elevated $Paco_2$ levels (40–50 mm Hg).

SUPPORTIVE CARE

- Although surgical intervention has become the medical standard, supportive measures are sometimes offered, especially when multiple noncardiac congenital anomalies exist or when severe multiorgan system damage is present.
- The preoperative goal is to balance the systemic and pulmonary circulations provided by the RV to a Qp/Qs (ratio of pulmonary to systemic blood flow) of ~1:1, usually achieved with a pulse oximetry measurement of 75%.
- Prostaglandin E1 infusion: 0.05–0.1 mcg/kg/min
- Aggressive treatment of hypocalcemia with calcium boluses, avoidance of metabolic acidosis with fluid boluses, consider sodium bicarbonate
- 0.21 FiO_2, goal Pao_2 of 35–40 mm Hg
- Careful use of small amounts of inotropic agents (in cases of sepsis or RV failure). Aggressive use of inotropic agents (alpha effect) may worsen systemic perfusion.

SURGERY/OTHER PROCEDURES

- Palliative surgery is generally performed in 3 stages:
  - Stage I Norwood palliation (performed in the first few days of life or soon after presentation): transection of the main pulmonary artery with anastomosis of the augmented aortic arch to the pulmonary valve stump to form a neoaortic valve and arch, placement of an aorta-to-pulmonary artery shunt (modified Blalock-Taussig shunt), and often an atrial septectomy. The RV provides both systemic and pulmonary blood flows with postoperative saturations of ~75%.
  - Stage I Sano modification: Developed in 2003 as an alternative to the Norwood procedure, the Sano modification replaces the modified Blalock-Taussig shunt with an RV to pulmonary artery conduit, with the RV continuing to supply both pulmonary and systemic circulations.
  - Hybrid procedure: An additional alternative to the Norwood procedure uses both median sternotomy (pulmonary artery banding) and interventional cardiac catheterization (PDA stenting) to provide both systemic and pulmonary blood flow while avoiding cardiopulmonary bypass.
  - Stage II/Hemi-Fontan or bidirectional Glenn (cavopulmonary anastomosis) procedure: involves anastomosis of the superior vena cava to the pulmonary artery, resulting in volume unloading of the RV. All prior shunts are usually removed. The oxygen saturations after this procedure are usually 85–90%.
  - Stage III/Modified Fontan procedure: baffling the inferior vena cava to the pulmonary artery with placement of a small fenestration in the baffle, permitting a small residual right-to-left shunt. The RV is now supplying only systemic blood flow. The oxygen saturations after this procedure are usually 90–95%.
- There are many surgical modifications to these 3 procedures. In addition, these procedures may be performed at different ages based on an institution's experience. Our approach has been to perform the hemi-Fontan operation at 4–6 months of age and the Fontan operation at 18 months to 2 years of age.
- Orthotopic heart transplantation may be performed either as an initial approach or after a stage I palliation.

FOLLOW-UP RECOMMENDATIONS

Admission Criteria

The admission for the first operation usually lasts for about 3–4 weeks after birth. Patients are watched to ensure stable oxygen saturation and weight gain. Nutritional needs often require nasogastric tube feed supplementation.

PROGNOSIS

- Fatal if untreated (95% mortality within the first month of life)
- Improved outcomes may result from early diagnosis and prevention of the presentation as neonatal shock.
- 90% early survival after stage I palliation if treated in a timely fashion at experienced institutions
- 5% mortality at stage II hemi-Fontan (bidirectional cavopulmonary anastomosis) procedure
- Recently, 1% mortality at Fontan operation (with the addition of a fenestration to allow right-to-left shunting)
- Excluding infants who die waiting for a donor organ, the 5-year actuarial survival for either staged palliation (Fontan) or heart transplantation is similar, ~75%.

COMPLICATIONS

Neonatal presentation:

- Circulatory collapse with resultant metabolic acidosis
- Multiorgan system failure (i.e., necrotizing enterocolitis, renal failure, liver failure, CNS injury)

Patient Monitoring

Interval evaluations should include careful consideration of growth parameters, cardiovascular symptoms, and developmental milestones. Examinations should focus on the presence or absence of cyanosis, edema, pleural effusions, diarrhea, ascites, and arrhythmias.

- For patients after staged palliation, frequent echocardiograms and intermittent cardiac catheterizations may be needed to assess for the following:
  - RV dysfunction
  - Residual or recurrent aortic arch obstruction
  - Branch pulmonary artery narrowing
  - Venous collateral formation causing increased cyanosis
  - Protein-losing enteropathy
  - Sinus node dysfunction
  - Atrial arrhythmias
- For patients treated alternatively with heart transplantation, other lifelong issues should be addressed:
  - Graft rejection and/or coronary vasculopathy
  - Infection
  - Hypertension
  - Lymphoproliferative disease
- Follow-up medications:
  - Lifelong subacute bacterial endocarditis (SBE) prophylaxis
  - Furosemide is generally administered until the hemi-Fontan.
  - Afterload reduction (i.e., angiotensin-converting enzyme inhibitors) may be used to reduce the workload on the heart at any stage.
  - Antiplatelet (aspirin) and anticoagulant (Coumadin) therapies are used by most physicians after stage 1 and later in the setting of the low-flow state of the cavopulmonary connection.
- For transplant patients, immunosuppressive regimens are managed differently according to institution preferences.

ADDITIONAL READING

- Alsoufi B, Bennetts J, Verma S, et al. New developments in the treatment of hypoplastic left heart syndrome. *Pediatrics*. 2007;119(1):109–117.
- Grossfeld P. Hypoplastic left heart syndrome: new insights. *Circ Res*. 2007;100(9):1246–1248.
- Mahle WT, Clancy RR, McGaurn SP, et al. Impact of prenatal diagnosis on survival and early neurologic morbidity in neonates with the hypoplastic left heart syndrome. *Pediatrics*. 2001;107(6):1277–1282.
- McClure CD, Johnston JK, Fitts JA, et al. Postmortem intracranial neuropathology in children following cardiac transplantation. *Pediatr Neurol*. 2006;35(2):107–113.
- Pigula FA, Vida V, Del Nido P, et al. Contemporary results and current strategies in the management of hypoplastic left heart syndrome. *Semin Thorac Cardiovasc Surg*. 2007;19(3):238–244.
- Stamm C, Friehs I, Mayer JE, et al. Long-term results of the lateral tunnel Fontan operation. *J Thorac Cardiovasc Surg*. 2001;121(1):28–41.
- Tabbutt S, Dominguez TE, Ravishankar C, et al. Outcomes after the stage I reconstruction comparing the right ventricular to pulmonary artery conduit with the modified Blalock Taussig shunt. *Ann Thorac Surg*. 2005;80(5):1582–1590.
- Tworetzky W, McElhinney DB, Reddy VM, et al. Improved surgical outcome after fetal diagnosis of hypoplastic left heart syndrome. *Circulation*. 2001;103(9):1269–1273.
- Wernovsky G, Ghanayem N, Ohye RG, et al. Hypoplastic left heart syndrome: consensus and controversies in 2007. *Cardiol Young*. 2007;17(Suppl 2):75–86.

CODES

ICD10

- Q24.8 Other specified congenital malformations of heart
- Q96.9 Turner's syndrome, unspecified
- Q87.1 Congenital malform syndromes predom assoc w short stature

FAQ

- Q: What should the differential diagnosis include when an infant with HLHS who's undergone stage I palliation presents with cyanosis and respiratory distress?
- A: Modified Blalock-Taussig shunt thrombosis, anemia, intercurrent lower respiratory tract infection leading to V/Q mismatch, low cardiac output state, sepsis
- Infants with HLHS status post stage I palliation are solely dependent on the modified Blalock-Taussig shunt for pulmonary blood flow. This synthetic tube graft ranges from 3.5 to 4 mm in diameter and is prone to thrombosis, especially during periods of illness, which lead to dehydration (gastroenteritis), poor nutrition, or systemic inflammation.
- Q: Should there be a specific concern if a patient with HLHS who's completed the 3-stage palliation with Fontan procedure presents with complaints of unremitting diarrhea, crampy abdominal pain, ascites, and peripheral edema?
- A: Yes. Protein-losing enteropathy (PLE) is a poorly understood disease process affecting patients with single ventricle after Fontan operation associated with significant morbidity and mortality. PLE is defined as the abnormal loss of serum proteins into the lumen of the gastrointestinal tract and occurs in up to 11% of patients after Fontan palliation. Diuretic therapy and nutritional supplementation are often insufficient management strategies, often requiring the addition of somatostatic analogs (octreotide), sildenafil, and/or the creation of a fenestration in the Fontan circuit to palliate potentially elevated Fontan pressures.

HYPOSPADIAS

Natasha Gupta • Ming-Hsien Wang

BASICS

DESCRIPTION

Hypospadias is one of the most common congenital anomalies of the male external genitalia. It is characterized by a urethral meatus that opens proximally on the ventral surface of the penis or in the scrotum or perineum instead of at the tip of the glans. Classification is based on the position of the external meatus relative to the penile shaft or surrounding structures (distal, middle, proximal). Although the ventral foreskin is incomplete in the vast majority of cases, the megameatus variant is characterized by an intact foreskin.

EPIDEMIOLOGY

- 1/200–1/300 live male births
- Concordance rates among twins: 18–77%
- Megameatus variant: 5% of cases
- Incidence is likely not increasing over time. Although there have been some data suggesting an increasing incidence over time, the majority of published studies in the U.S. population indicate a stable incidence.

RISK FACTORS

- In vitro fertilization
- Maternal exposures to substances such as pesticides, hormones, phthalates, and phytoestrogens that can act as endocrine disruptors during penile development
- Associated with maternal preexisting diabetes mellitus, placental insufficiency, and low birth weight
- More common among Caucasians

Genetics

- Likely polygenic
- Familial clustering: 7% of affected boys have an affected 1st- or 2nd-degree relative.
- Equally maternally and paternally transmitted
- Associated with genetic mutations in several genes involved in the androgen pathway and external genitalia development, including homeobox, fibroblast growth factor, and sonic hedgehog genes

ETIOLOGY

- Due to incomplete fusion of the urethral folds during penile development, which is an androgen-driven process that occurs during weeks 8–16 of gestation
- Likely multifactorial with environmental and genetic interplay
- Defects in urethral development are usually accompanied by foreskin developmental defects (an incomplete ventral foreskin and dorsal hooded foreskin), except in the megameatus variant

COMMONLY ASSOCIATED CONDITIONS

- Usually idiopathic and isolated
- Less commonly associated with some chromosomal abnormalities and ~200 syndromes, including disorders of sexual differentiation (DSD)
- Hypospadias, particularly proximal hypospadias, can be associated with an increased risk of other genitourinary (GU) malformations.
- The most commonly associated GU malformations include the following:
  - Chordee
  - Cryptorchidism
  - Inguinal hernia

DIAGNOSIS

HISTORY

- Important to inquire about the following:
  - Family history of hypospadias, congenital anomalies, or genetic disorders
  - Patient history of genetic disorder and/or DSD
  - GU symptoms
  - Maternal history of fertility treatments
  - Maternal exposures during pregnancy
  - Birth history
  - For older patients
    - Painful erections
    - Infertility or difficulties with intercourse
    - Difficulty urinating while standing
    - Deflected urinary stream

PHYSICAL EXAM

- Assess for hypospadias in all male newborns with complete GU exam, paying particular attention to the following:
  - Any sign of incompletely formed foreskin or dorsal hooded foreskin
  - Any phallus curvature
  - Location of the meatus
  - Presence of rugated scrotum
  - Impalpable testes

DIAGNOSTIC TESTS & INTERPRETATION

Lab

- No tests are needed for isolated hypospadias.
- If testes are impalpable bilaterally with proximal hypospadias, consider workup for DSD.
- Additional workup for DSD as needed based on level of concern

Imaging

- Not usually indicated
- Renal ultrasound or voiding cystourethrogram in cases of proximal hypospadias
- Ultrasound of urinary tract and internal genitalia if hypospadias is present in conjunction with cryptorchidism or nonpalpable testicle(s)

DIFFERENTIAL DIAGNOSIS

DSD such as congenital adrenal hyperplasia or partial androgen insensitivity syndrome

TREATMENT

GENERAL MEASURES

- Preferably refer to pediatric urologist within the first few weeks of life.
- Preoperative stimulation with parenteral testosterone may be required to increase penis size in cases of micropenis to improve surgical outcomes.
- Cases of mild, distal hypospadias may be observed.

ALERT
- For newborn circumcision, retract the foreskin (megameatus variant requires foreskin retraction for detection). If *any* abnormalities noted, abort the circumcision and refer to a pediatric urologist.
- In cases of hypospadias, circumcision is absolutely contraindicated because foreskin is used in hypospadias repair.
- Bilateral impalpable testes and hypospadias during newborn period must be worked-up to rule out DSD.

SURGERY/OTHER PROCEDURES
- Surgical repair
  - Outpatient procedure
  - May be accompanied by chordee repair if needed
  - Performed at age 6 months–1 year to minimize psychological trauma of surgery
  - Complex cases may require staged repair, with stage 1 generally performed at 6 months of age and stage 2 at 1 year of age.
  - Perioperative care may include the following:
    - Antibiotics (no standard course duration)
    - Pain management (generally with a caudal nerve block and acetaminophen with opioid analgesic or ketorolac as needed)
  - Type of repair performed is based on patient's anatomy.
  - Some types of repair may involve temporary urethral stent placement.
- Types of repair include the following:
  - Urethromeatoplasty
  - Meatal advancement and glanuloplasty (MAGPI)
  - Meatal inverted V flap
  - Sleeve technique
  - Flip-flap technique (local flap)
  - Adjacent tissue transfer
  - Glans approximation procedure
  - Thiersch-Duplay
  - Transverse incised plate or Snodgrass procedure
- Most common complications include the following:
  - Urethrocutaneous fistula
  - Urethral diverticulum
  - Urethral or meatal stenosis
  - Dehiscence

ONGOING CARE

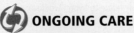

FOLLOW-UP RECOMMENDATIONS
Patient Monitoring
- Surgical dressings are variable and surgeon dependent.
- Postoperative clinic visit (surgeon-dependent)
- If urethral stent is placed, removal usually occurs on postoperative days 5–14 at clinic visit.
- Antibiotics may be continued postoperatively.

PROGNOSIS
Success rate is generally high, although dependent on the type of repair, degree of hypospadias, and patient's overall medical condition.

ADDITIONAL READING

- Kalfa N, Liu B, Klein O, et al. Mutations of CXorf6 are associated with a range of severities of hypospadias. *Eur J Endocrinol*. 2008;159(4):453–458.
- Kalfa N, Liu B, Klein O, et al. Genomic variants of ATF3 in patients with hypospadias. *J Urol*. 2008;180(5):2183–2188; discussion 2188.
- Kalfa N, Philibert P, Baskin LS, et al. Hypospadias: interactions between environment and genetics. *Mol Cell Endocrinol*. 2011;335(2):89–95.
- Madhok N, Scharbach K, Shahid-Saless S. Hypospadias. *Pediatr Rev*. 2009;30(6):235–237.
- Moriyama M, Senga Y, Satomi Y. Klinefelter's syndrome with hypospadias and bilateral cryptorchidism. *Urol Int*. 1988;43(5):313–314.
- van der Zanden LF, van Rooij IA, Feitz WF, et al. Aetiology of hypospadias: a systematic review of genes and environment. *Hum Reprod Update*. 2012;18(3):260–283.
- Wang MH, Baskin LS. Endocrine disruptors, genital development, and hypospadias. *J Androl*. 2008;29(5):499–505.
- White PC, Speiser PW. Congenital adrenal hyperplasia due to 21-hydroxylase deficiency. *Endocr Rev*. 2000;21(3):245–291.
- Zaontz M, Long CJ. Management of distal hypospadias. *AUA Update Series*. 2013;32(Lesson 5):1–51.

CODES

ICD10
- Q54.9 Hypospadias, unspecified
- Q54.1 Hypospadias, penile
- Q54.3 Hypospadias, perineal

FAQ
- Q: Does the patient with hypospadias routinely have other urinary tract abnormalities?
- A: No. Hypospadias is usually an isolated anomaly, and most patients have no other anatomic problems.
- Q: Should a newborn circumcision be performed if there are concerns with the meatal opening?
- A: Circumcision should be delayed, and the patient should be evaluated by a pediatric urologist.
- Q: Are there any medical alternatives to surgical repair?
- A: No. Surgery is the only treatment of hypospadias, but very mild cases may not warrant surgical repair.

HYPOTHYROIDISM, CONGENITAL

Adda Grimberg

For issues related to acquired hypothyroidism, please see the separate chapter on page 16.

BASICS

DESCRIPTION
Primary thyroid failure present at birth

EPIDEMIOLOGY
- Increasing trend in the United States
  - Unclear etiology (definitional issues related to newborn screening vs. true increase from unidentified risk factors)
  - Had been 1 in 3,000–4,000 births, United States and worldwide
  - In 2007, U.S. incidence 1 in 2,370 births
- Male-to-female ratio is 1:2–1:3.
- 80% dysgenesis or agenesis; 20% dyshormonogenesis
- Racial differences: prevalence in African American infants ~1/3 that in whites
- Higher prevalence of congenital hypothyroidism in low-birth-weight (<2,000 g) and macrosomic (≥4,500 g) babies

RISK FACTORS
Genetics
- Dysgenesis is usually sporadic.
  - Familial occurrence in 2%
  - Mutations have been found in the TSH-receptor gene and in the transcription factors *PAX-8*, *TTF-1*, and *TTF-2* (*FOXE1*).
- Dyshormonogenesis is inherited in an autosomal recessive pattern. Most commonly
  - Chromosome 2p: Mutations in the thyroid peroxidase gene result in partial or complete loss of iodide organification.
  - Chromosome 19p: Mutations in the sodium-iodide symporter gene result in an inability to maintain the normal thyroid-to-plasma iodine concentration difference.
- Pendred syndrome (chromosome 7q): Mutations in PDS gene cause the most common syndromal form of deafness; a mild organification defect leads to goiter, usually in childhood.

ETIOLOGY
- Thyroid gland malformation
  - Agenesis: absent thyroid gland
  - Dysgenesis: ectopic (e.g., sublingual) or incorrectly formed (e.g., hemigland) thyroid
- Dyshormonogenesis
  - 15 known defects of thyroxine (T_4) synthesis, including those in iodide transport and iodide organification
- Transient hypothyroidism
  - Maternal ingestion of antithyroid drugs
  - Transplacental transfer of maternal antithyroid antibodies (transient or permanent damage)
  - Exposure to high levels of iodine-povidone, (i.e., Pyodine, Betadine) in neonatal period

COMMONLY ASSOCIATED CONDITIONS
- Down syndrome neonates have lower T_4 (left-shifted normal distribution) and mildly elevated TSH, suggesting a mild hypothyroid state.
- Newborns with congenital hypothyroidism have an increased risk for congenital heart defects, and vice versa (common embryologic developmental program).

DIAGNOSIS

HISTORY
- Symptoms that may relate to hypothyroidism:
  - Prolonged jaundice
  - Poor feeding
  - Constipation
  - Sedate or placid child
  - Poor linear growth
- Family history of thyroid disorders
  - Autoimmune thyroid disease
  - Vague histories of "mild hypothyroidism" not requiring treatment are often found in families with thyroid-binding globulin deficiency.
- Maternal medications
- Birth history
- Results of the newborn screen
- Signs and symptoms:
  - Most children are diagnosed by the neonatal screening program:
    - 5–10% false-negative rate
    - Neonatal screening protocols differ state to state (i.e., may screen TSH, T_4, or both).
    - In severely ill neonates transferred from 1 unit or hospital to another, be sure the state screen has been performed and not overlooked. If missed by the state screening procedure, the symptoms above are seen within the 1st 2 months of life.

PHYSICAL EXAM
- Signs that may relate to hypothyroidism:
  - Hypothermia
  - Large fontanelles (especially posterior) with wide cranial sutures
  - Coarse facial features, including macroglossia
  - Hoarse cry
  - Hypotonia
  - Delayed deep tendon reflex release
  - Distended abdomen
  - Umbilical hernia
- Examine for possible goiter; helpful pearls
  - Inspect the base of tongue for ectopic gland.
  - While supporting the posterior neck and occiput, allow the infant's head to hang back over a parent's arm or exam table. This will extend the neck and allow better visualization of the anterior region.

DIAGNOSTIC TESTS & INTERPRETATION
Lab
- Neonatal screening program (filter card)
  - Methods vary from state to state (screen for T_4 or TSH); primary TSH screening plus serial testing for infants at risk for later rising TSH shown to outperform other strategies.
  - Abnormal results on state screen should prompt *immediate* examination and confirmatory tests.
  - Because of delayed TSH elevations, very low-birth-weight babies and those with congenital cardiac anomalies may need rescreening for diagnosis.
- Confirmatory tests:
  - Serum T_4 and TSH are preferable to a repeated filter screen, which may result in delayed diagnosis and treatment.
  - If abnormalities in binding are suspected, also check thyroid-binding globulin level and free T_4 concentration or triiodothyronine (T_3) resin uptake.
  - Free T_4 is the most sensitive indicator of secondary or tertiary hypothyroidism (hypopituitarism).
- Antenatal tests
  - Fetal goiter can be detected by prenatal ultrasound.
- Reference ranges for 3rd trimester amniotic fluid concentrations of TSH and total and free T_4 are established for diagnosis of fetal hypothyroidism among those with goiters. Otherwise, cordocentesis is needed.

Imaging
- ^{123}I or technetium thyroid scan to define gland anatomy (agenesis, dysgenesis, ectopic gland)
- ^{123}I scan with perchlorate washout to help identify dyshormonogenesis
- ^{123}I scan must be obtained before beginning thyroxine replacement therapy. If this delays treatment, defer scanning until brain growth is complete (2 years of age), when a period off medication is safer.
- Ultrasonography can also evaluate thyroid anatomy (but not dyshormonogenesis) and does not require deferral of treatment.

DIFFERENTIAL DIAGNOSIS
- Developmental
  - Transient hypothyroxinemia in the 1st weeks of life in premature babies
- Metabolic
  - Sick euthyroid syndrome in severely ill neonates
- Secondary or tertiary
  - Panhypopituitarism
  - Congenital isolated central hypothyroidism (a "hot spot" mutation in the TSH-β gene)
  - Central congenital hypothyroidism due to maternal Graves disease during pregnancy (estimated incidence 1:35,000; thought to indicate impaired maturation of the fetal hypothalamic–pituitary–thyroid system from a hyperthyroid fetal environment)
- Genetic
  - Thyroid-binding globulin deficiency (X-linked recessive)
- Environmental
  - Iodine exposure (e.g., delivery by cesarean section, surgery in the neonatal period)
  - Maternal iodine deficiency (American Thyroid Association recommends pregnant and lactating women to take prenatal vitamins containing 150 mcg of iodine daily.)
  - Maternal use of antithyroid drugs or lithium
- Immunologic
  - Transfer of maternal antithyroid and TSH receptor–blocking antibodies

ALERT

False positives

- X-linked thyroid-binding globulin deficiency: low total T_4, normal TSH, and normal free T_4. Diagnose with low thyroid-binding globulin level or high T_3 resin uptake. No treatment is necessary!
- Panhypopituitarism: low T_4 and low or low-normal TSH (i.e., loss of the negative feedback loop). Screen with free T_4. Treat with L-thyroxine as for primary hypothyroidism, and investigate for other pituitary hormone deficiencies.
- Blood specimens obtained before 48 hours of life may have "elevated" TSH as a result of the normal postnatal surge.

False negatives

- Normal newborn screening can be falsely reassuring in babies with congenital central hypothyroidism.

TREATMENT

MEDICATION

Levothyroxine

- Start at 10–15 mcg/kg/24 hr PO once a day. Titer dose to keep T_4 in the upper range of normal.
- TSH levels may not normalize for several weeks even with good T_4 values.
- Starting dose of 50 mcg PO daily (12–17 mcg/kg/24 hr) may provide more rapid normalization (free T_4 by 3 days and TSH by 2 weeks).
- A minority of infants have variable pituitary–thyroid hormone resistance, with relatively elevated serum levels of TSH for their free T_4 that improves with age.
- Duration: lifelong
  – If medication is started without imaging studies and diagnosis is not clear, can stop levothyroxine after completion of early brain growth (2–3 years of age). Reevaluate need for supplementation after a 6-week trial off therapy.

ONGOING CARE

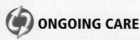

FOLLOW-UP RECOMMENDATIONS

- When to expect improvement:
  – Most children are asymptomatic at diagnosis.
  – Parents may note an increase in activity, improvement in feeding, and increase in urination and bowel movements soon after starting treatment.
- Signs to watch for: Poor growth and low T_4 and elevated TSH values suggest poor compliance or undertreatment.
- Neuropsychological sequelae:
  – IQ scores are predominantly in the normal range, but subtle impairments in language and motor skills and specific learning disabilities may occur despite early treatment.
  – Neurocognitive evaluation and rehabilitation should be provided.
  – Maternal hypothyroxinemia during early gestation can lead to neurodevelopmental delays if not corrected during pregnancy.

DIET

- No restrictions
- Soybean flour (as in some formulas) and iron can decrease gastrointestinal absorption of levothyroxine.
- Pharmacies in recent years have been recommending that levothyroxine be administered on an empty stomach. The Drugs and Therapeutics Committee of the Pediatric Endocrine Society recommended that consistency in administration, coupled with regular dose titration to thyroid function tests, is more important than improving absorption by restricting intake to only times of empty stomach.

PATIENT EDUCATION

- Whether the child has learning disabilities related to hypothyroidism depends on when the diagnosis was made and how quickly treatment was started. There may be an increase in learning disabilities when compared with siblings, even in patients treated within the 1st 4 weeks of life.
- If a dose of levothyroxine is forgotten, it should be given as soon as it is remembered. If it is the next day, 2 doses should be given.
- Levothyroxine is available only in tablet form. The tablet should be crushed between 2 spoons and the powder dissolved in a small amount of formula or breast milk and offered to the baby at the *start* of a feeding to ensure complete ingestion.
- There are no side effects from the medication. The tablet contains only the hormone that the child's thyroid is not making. It is synthetically produced, so there are no infectious risks.

PROGNOSIS

- Excellent, if treatment is started within the 1st 2 weeks of life
- Level of T_4 at birth is an important indicator of long-term sequelae.

COMPLICATIONS

- If untreated:
  – Severe mental retardation (cretinism)
  – Poor motor development
  – Poor growth
- Children with hypothyroidism as part of hypopituitarism do not seem to be as significantly affected by their low thyroid hormone levels as do those with primary hypothyroidism.

ADDITIONAL READING

- American Academy of Pediatrics, Rose SR; Section on Endocrinology and Committee on Genetics, American Thyroid Association, Brown RS, et al. Update of newborn screening and therapy for congenital hypothyroidism. *Pediatrics*. 2006;117(6): 2290–2303.
- Delahunty C, Falconer S, Hume R, et al. Levels of neonatal thyroid hormone in preterm infants and neurodevelopmental outcome at 51/2 years: millennium cohort study. *J Clin Endocrinol Metab*. 2010;95(11):4898–4908.
- Fu J, Jiang Y, Liang L, et al. Risk factors of primary thyroid dysfunction in early infants born to mothers with autoimmune thyroid disease. *Acta Paediatr*. 2005;94(8):1043–1048.
- Grüters A, Krude H. Detection and treatment of congenital hypothyroidism. *Nat Rev Endocrinol*. 2011;8(2):104–113.
- Kempers MJ, Ozgen HM, Vulsma T, et al. Morphological abnormalities in children with thyroidal congenital hypothyroidism. *Am J Med Genet A*. 2009;149A(5):943–951.
- Korzeniewski SJ, Grigorescu V, Kleyn M, et al. Performance metrics after changes in screening protocol for congenital hypothyroidism. *Pediatrics*. 2012;130(5):e1252–e1260.
- Larson C, Hermos R, Delaney A, et al. Risk factors associated with delayed thyrotropin elevations in congenital hypothyroidism. *J Pediatr*. 2003;143(5): 587–591.
- Leung AM, Pearce EN, Braverman LE. Iodine content of prenatal multivitamins in the United States. *N Engl J Med*. 2009;360(9):939–940.
- Nebesio TD, McKenna MP, Nabhan ZM, et al. Newborn screening results in children with central hypothyroidism. *J Pediatr*. 2010;156(6):990–993.
- Ng SM, Anand D, Weindling AM. High versus low dose of initial thyroid hormone replacement for congenital hypothyroidism. *Cochrane Database Syst Rev*. 2009;(1):CD006972.
- Olney RS, Grosse SD, Vogt RF Jr. Prevalence of congenital hypothyroidism—current trends and future directions: workshop summary. *Pediatrics*. 2010;125(Suppl 2):S31–S36.
- Passeri E, Frigerio M, De Filippis T, et al. Increased risk for non-autoimmune hypothyroidism in young patients with congenital heart defects. *J Clin Endocrinol Metab*. 2011;96(7):E1115–E1119.
- Raymond J, LaFranchi SH. Fetal and neonatal thyroid function: review and summary of significant new findings. *Curr Opin Endocrinol Diabetes Obes*. 2010;17(1):1–7.

CODES

ICD10

- E03.1 Congenital hypothyroidism without goiter
- E03.0 Congenital hypothyroidism with diffuse goiter

FAQ

- Q: What are some of the reasons that a normal newborn may have an abnormal thyroid screen?
- A: Blood tests obtained prior to 48 hours of age may have an elevated TSH from newborn surge; some states (for quality control) will ask to have a certain percentage of tests repeated, even though they are normal.

IDIOPATHIC INTRACRANIAL HYPERTENSION (PSEUDOTUMOR CEREBRI)

Daphne M. Hasbani • Sabrina E. Smith

BASICS

DESCRIPTION

Diagnostic criteria of idiopathic intracranial hypertension (IIH) include the following:

- Signs and symptoms of increased intracranial pressure (e.g., headache, vomiting, ocular manifestations, and papilledema)
- Elevated cerebrocranial fluid pressure but otherwise normal CSF
- Normal neurologic exam except for papilledema (occasional abducens or other motor cranial neuropathy)
- Normal neuroimaging study (or incidental findings only)

EPIDEMIOLOGY

- Boys and girls are affected equally in childhood; in adulthood, more women than men are affected.
- IIH has been reported in patients as young as 4 months of age, with a median age of 9 years.

Incidence

Estimated to be 0.5/100,000 cases/year for children younger than 18 years old

RISK FACTORS

Genetics

Sporadic, no clear genetic predisposition, unless related to an underlying hormonal, toxic, or inflammatory condition; no data are available in children.

PATHOPHYSIOLOGY

Pathogenesis unknown but may involve decreased CSF absorption owing to arachnoid villi dysfunction or elevated intracranial venous pressure. For example, obesity may lead to increased intra-abdominal, intrathoracic, and cardiac filling pressure, leading to elevated intracranial venous pressure.

ETIOLOGY

- Numerous precipitants of IIH have been reported. In adolescents, it is clearly associated with obesity and weight gain but not clearly linked to obesity in children <11 years of age. Many weaker associations may be due to chance.
- IIH is often linked to minocycline, tetracycline, sulfnamides, isotretinoin, and thyroid replacements and to corticosteroid withdrawal. It is also linked to vitamin A deficiency or intoxication, chronic anemia, and hypothyroidism.

COMMONLY ASSOCIATED CONDITIONS

- Visual loss due to optic nerve pressure
- Endocrinopathies, exogenous steroids, lead exposure, and therapy involving tetracycline and several other antibiotics may be associated with IIH.

DIAGNOSIS

HISTORY

- Headache
- Blurred vision
- Transient visual darkening
- Stiff neck
- Pulsatile tinnitus
- Dizziness
- Infants and young children may present with irritability, somnolence, or ataxia.
- IIH should be considered in any child with chronic headache or unexplained visual changes.
- Directed history for signs of associated endocrinopathy, exposure to antibiotics or steroids, sinus infection, abnormal clotting, or familial tendency for thrombosis or visual disturbance

PHYSICAL EXAM

- Examination of the fundi is essential.
- Recording baseline visual acuity and visual fields in older children is essential.
- Papilledema is almost always present in older children with IIH.
- Most infants have some degree of papilledema, even with open fontanelles and split sutures.
- 6th cranial nerve (abducens) palsies are common in children with IIH; they were found in 29 of 68 patients in 1 series.
- Facial or other cranial nerve deficits rare

DIAGNOSTIC TESTS & INTERPRETATION

Lab

- CSF exam including opening pressure; cell count, glucose, and protein are essential and should be normal in IIH.
- CBC and thyroid function tests should be obtained because anemia, hypothyroidism, and hyperthyroidism have rarely been associated with IIH.
- The following may be useful in selected cases:
  - ANA test
  - ESR
  - Urine cortisol
  - Serum lead level
  - Serologic testing for Lyme disease

Imaging

Cranial CT or MRI should be normal. MRI is recommended because of superior imaging of brainstem, posterior fossa, and venous sinuses. Magnetic resonance venography is strongly suggested to evaluate for venous sinus thrombosis, which can be difficult to distinguish from IIH.

Diagnostic Procedures/Other

- Lumbar puncture manometry, with the patient in a relaxed lateral decubitus position, should show an opening pressure >280 mm H_2O.
- Goldmann perimeter visual field testing or computerized visual fields are useful in children >5 years of age to document field deficits and monitor response to therapy.

DIFFERENTIAL DIAGNOSIS

Some conditions may cause increased intracranial pressure and be confused with IIH, but the clinical picture and CSF analysis usually permit their distinction.

- Chronic meningitis (e.g., CNS Lyme disease), encephalitis, or cerebral edema (may show minimal changes on neuroimaging with elevated CSF protein levels and little evidence of pleocytosis)
- Cerebral venous sinus thrombosis
- Chronic headache (common) with pseudopapilledema (optic nerve disc drusen)

TREATMENT

MEDICATION

First Line

- For patients with mild to moderate visual loss, acetazolamide, a carbonic anhydrase inhibitor that decreases CSF production, is the drug of choice.
  - The pediatric dosage is 25–100 mg/kg/24 h divided b.i.d.–q.i.d. for the standard form and b.i.d. for the long-acting form (Diamox sequels).
  - The initial adult dose is 250 mg q.i.d. or 500 mg b.i.d., increased to 750 mg q.i.d. or 1,500 mg b.i.d. if tolerated.
- If visual loss, papilledema, and symptoms of pressure resolve, acetazolamide dosage can be tapered after 2 months of therapy.

Second Line

Furosemide can be used if acetazolamide is ineffective or has intolerable adverse effects.

ISSUES FOR REFERRAL

Follow-up and tapering of acetazolamide should be done in conjunction with a neurologist or neuro-ophthalmologist.

SURGERY/OTHER PROCEDURES

- Serial lumbar punctures are not recommended as standard therapy, although the initial puncture can be useful to relieve symptoms quickly.
- Surgical therapy (e.g., optic nerve sheath fenestration, lumboperitoneal shunt) is indicated for progressive visual loss despite medical therapy and may also be considered as an urgent intervention at presentation depending on degree of visual loss. Optic nerve sheath fenestration may be the preferred surgical treatment, especially in children, because of the high failure rates of lumboperitoneal shunting. High-dose IV steroids and acetazolamide therapy may be used while awaiting surgical therapy.
- Recent studies of stenting in adults with transverse sinus stenosis and a pressure gradient on angiography demonstrated some improvement in visual symptoms and papilledema with variable effects on headache. However, this intervention is controversial and may not be technically feasible in children because of the smaller caliber of their vasculature.

INPATIENT CONSIDERATIONS

Initial Stabilization

- The urgency of diagnosis and treatment depends on the severity of visual loss. Recent reports suggest that severe visual loss may progress rapidly, warranting close initial (weekly) tracking of vision and prompt consideration of surgical treatment (see below).
- For patients with no visual loss, removal of possible causative agents may be the only intervention needed, along with treatment of associated conditions (e.g., obesity, anemia, thyroid disease). Consider treatment with acetazolamide (Diamox; see later comment). Headache can be treated symptomatically if needed.

ONGOING CARE

FOLLOW-UP RECOMMENDATIONS

Patient Monitoring

- Initially, patients should have visual acuity, visual fields, and fundi evaluated weekly or biweekly.
- If vision is stable, monthly visits may be adequate for 3–6 months.
- More frequent follow-up is required for any signs of progressive visual loss.
- IIH can recur. In one pediatric series, nearly 1/4 of patients had recurrence.
- Pitfalls: Children are not exempt from permanent visual loss as a consequence of IIH. Ophthalmologic follow-up is important. Occasional patients, especially adolescents, may experience headache weeks or months after resolution of objective signs of IIH (i.e., even though intracranial pressure has returned to normal).
- IIH may be diagnosed erroneously if
  - Pseudopapilledema is mistaken for papilledema. (Pseudopapilledema is apparent optic disc swelling that simulates papilledema but is usually secondary to an underlying benign process. It can be differentiated by an experienced ophthalmologist or neurologist.)
  - CSF abnormalities (i.e., isolated increase in protein) are overlooked.
  - Clinician fails to identify underlying cerebral venous sinus thrombosis.

ADDITIONAL READING

- Avery RA, Licht DJ, Shah SS, et al. CSF opening pressure in children with optic nerve head edema. *Neurology*. 2011;76(19):1658–1661.
- Friedman DI, Jacobson DM. Diagnostic criteria for idiopathic intracranial hypertension. *Neurology*. 2002;59(10):1492–1495.
- Kesler A, Bassan H. Pseudotumor cerebri—idiopathic intracranial hypertension in the pediatric population. *Pediatr Endocrinol Rev*. 2006;3(4):387–392.
- Lim M, Kurian M, Penn A, et al. Visual failure without headache in idiopathic intracranial hypertension. *Arch Dis Child*. 2005;90(2):206–210.
- Soiberman U, Stolovitch C, Balcer LJ, et al. Idiopathic intracranial hypertension in children: visual outcome and risk of recurrence. *Childs Nerv Syst*. 2011;27(11):1913–1918.

CODES

ICD10

G93.2 Benign intracranial hypertension

FAQ

- Q: What are the side effects of acetazolamide?
- A: Side effects of acetazolamide include GI upset, paresthesias, loss of appetite, drowsiness, metabolic acidosis, and renal stones. An alternative is furosemide.
- Q: If IIH occurs on tetracycline, can the patient take penicillin?
- A: Penicillins/cephalosporins have not been reported as a significant cause of IIH.
- Q: Are there any limitations on physical activity?
- A: Activity can be graded entirely according to the child's symptoms.

IDIOPATHIC THROMBOCYTOPENIC PURPURA

Charles Bailey

BASICS

DESCRIPTION

- Idiopathic or immune thrombocytopenic purpura (ITP) is an autoimmune syndrome characterized by the following:
  - Isolated thrombocytopenia (platelet count formally $<100{,}000/mm^3$, typically $<20{,}000/mm^3$)
  - Shortened platelet survival
  - Platelet autoantibodies
  - Increased number of megakaryocytes in the bone marrow
- Primary ITP implies absence of other causes for thrombocytopenia; secondary ITP indicates another diagnosis associated with autoimmune thrombocytopenia.
- Phases of ITP
  - Newly diagnosed (acute) ITP: within 3 months of initial diagnosis
  - Persistent ITP: transient improvement or continued thrombocytopenia for 3–12 months
  - Chronic ITP: persistent thrombocytopenia >12 months after initial presentation

EPIDEMIOLOGY

- Most common acquired platelet disorder in childhood
- Often follows viral syndrome by a few weeks; this may be associated with higher likelihood of spontaneous recovery.
- Males and females are equally affected in childhood ITP (mild male predominance in younger children; female-to-male ratio is 3:1 in adult and chronic ITP).
- Median age at diagnosis is 4 years. Children <1 year or >10 years are more likely to develop chronic ITP.
- >70% of childhood ITP resolves within 6–12 months.
- Risk of severe bleeding is <5% and of intracranial bleeding is ~0.5%.

Incidence

Incidence is 1–10/100,000 children per year (<15 years of age).

PATHOPHYSIOLOGY

- Thrombocytopenia due to increased destruction of antibody-coated platelets in the reticuloendothelial system, particularly the spleen
- Hypothesized that antibodies generated in response to foreign antigen or drug cross-react with platelet membrane glycoproteins (most commonly IIb/IIIa and Ib/IX)
- Other mechanisms of immune dysregulation have been implicated, including possible inhibition of thrombocytopoiesis, limiting ability to compensate for destruction.
- Typical bone marrow aspirate shows increased numbers of immature megakaryocytes.

COMMONLY ASSOCIATED CONDITIONS

- In younger children, primary ITP is the most common presentation of ITP.
- Secondary ITP is seen with autoimmune disorders (e.g., systemic lupus erythematosus [SLE], autoimmune lymphoproliferative syndrome [ALPS]).
- HIV

DIAGNOSIS

HISTORY

- Presents with unusual bruising (with minor or no trauma, or in uncommon locations such as torso, neck, face), petechiae, epistaxis, prolonged bleeding with minor trauma, gingival bleeding, hematuria, or hematochezia
- Acute onset in an otherwise well child
- Not associated with pallor, fatigue, weight loss, or persistent fevers
- A majority of cases are preceded by a viral infection 1–3 weeks before onset (particularly varicella; also Epstein-Barr virus, cytomegalovirus).
- Associated with recent MMR in younger children; possibly hepatitis A vaccine, Tdap in older children
- Ascertain history of other autoimmune diseases (e.g., rheumatologic disorders, thyroid disease, hemolytic anemia).
- Obtain medication history, focusing on drugs with antiplatelet effects or associated with thrombocytopenia (e.g., valproate, heparin).
- Family history is usually negative for bleeding disorders. Ask about family autoimmune disease.
- Screen for bleeding, headache, abdominal or back pain, and any focal neurologic change.

PHYSICAL EXAM

- Clusters of petechiae or large or purple bruises readily apparent on skin or mucosae
- Hematomas or persistent slow bleeding on mucosal surfaces or from minor trauma
- Absence of lymphadenopathy (LAD), hepatosplenomegaly (HSM), masses, bone pain
- Screen for nonobvious bleeding (neurologic and funduscopic exam, abdominal or muscular tenderness); these events are rare.

DIAGNOSTIC TESTS & INTERPRETATION

Lab

- Thrombocytopenia (typically $<20{,}000/mm^3$) with normal WBC and hemoglobin (or mild anemia in proportion to amount of blood loss)
- Mean platelet volume may be increased.
- Peripheral blood smear will be otherwise normal, with no red cell fragmentation, no spherocytes, and no blasts. Review also rules out pseudothrombocytopenia from platelet aggregation.
- Prothrombin time/INR and partial thromboplastin time are normal. Bleeding time will be prolonged, but testing is unnecessary.
- Direct antiglobulin (Coombs) test to exclude coexisting autoimmune hemolysis (Evans syndrome)
- Limited role for antinuclear antibody (ANA) and other immunologic tests in subset of patients at higher risk for other autoimmune disease
- HIV testing if risk factors are identified
- Bone marrow aspirate is needed only if unexplained anemia, abnormal WBC, blasts on peripheral smear, organomegaly, jaundice, or lymphadenopathy is present. It is safe to perform with a low platelet count.
- There is controversy over whether to obtain a marrow aspirate before giving corticosteroids and little evidence to support it.
- Marrow shows normal to increased numbers of megakaryocytes with otherwise normal morphology and cellularity.
- Assays for platelet-associated antibodies (either direct or indirect) are not sensitive and are not routinely indicated.
- Demonstration of platelet-associated IgG may be useful in more complicated patients in whom chronic ITP is a possible diagnosis.

Imaging

As indicated by symptoms, particularly abdominal pain, headache, vision, or focal neurologic change

DIFFERENTIAL DIAGNOSIS

- Consider malignancy if persistent fever, weight loss, adenopathy, bone pain, or organomegaly is present (mild splenomegaly seen in 5–10% of patients with ITP).
- Other destructive thrombocytopenias
  - Secondary ITP: infection, drug induced, post-transfusion purpura, autoimmune hemolytic anemia (when coexistent with ITP is called Evans syndrome), lymphoproliferative disorders, SLE
  - Nonimmunologic: microangiopathic hemolytic anemia (including TTP, HUS), disseminated intravascular coagulation (DIC), Kasabach-Merritt syndrome (hemangioma), cardiac defects (left ventricular outflow obstruction, prosthetic heart valves), malignant hypertension
- Impaired or ineffective production
  - Marrow-infiltrative processes (leukemias, other tumor metastases, myelofibrosis, osteopetrosis, storage diseases)
  - Drug- or radiation-induced thrombocytopenia or aplastic anemia, nutritional deficiency states (iron, folate, vitamin B_{12})
  - Infection-associated suppression: typically viral (e.g., hepatitis, Epstein-Barr virus, HIV, parvovirus B19), also severe or neonatal sepsis
  - Congenital disorders: thrombocytopenia absent radii (TAR) syndrome, dyskeratosis congenita, Fanconi anemia, trisomies 13 and 18, Bernard-Soulier syndrome, Wiskott-Aldrich syndrome, May-Hegglin anomaly, other inherited thrombocytopenias (X linked or autosomal dominant), metabolic disorders (e.g., methylmalonic acidemia)

TREATMENT

- Because severe hemorrhage is rare and ITP resolves spontaneously in 90% of pediatric cases, most patients without severe bleeding will not require treatment.
- Treatment slows antibody-mediated platelet clearance and raises platelet counts acutely but does not alter the long-term course.
- Patients with a platelet count $<10{,}000/mm^3$ are at higher risk for bleeding, but platelet count alone is not an indication for treatment.

- Active toddlers or children at risk for trauma may require treatment when platelet count is $<20{,}000–30{,}000/mm^3$.
- Observation alone is acceptable for older children without serious bleeding and with adequate supervision and assured follow-up; may be preferable to repeated treatment in clinically well children with chronic ITP

MEDICATION

First Line

- IVIG: 94–97% will have an increase in platelet count $>20{,}000/mm^3$ by 72 hours. The usual dose is 0.8–1 g/kg. Response typically peaks after 1 week and lasts 3–4 weeks.
  - Advantages: faster time to platelet increase (24 hours), helps confirm diagnosis
  - Disadvantages: high cost, long infusion time, allergic reactions; 10–30% have evidence of aseptic meningitis with severe headache and stiff neck; headache, nausea, vomiting, or fever more common
  - Scheduled acetaminophen and diphenhydramine for 24 hours after infusion may reduce acute side effects.
  - Subcutaneous administration has been used successfully as an alternative to IV.
- Corticosteroids: 80% respond with platelet counts $>20{,}000/mm^3$ by 72 hours (faster with high-dose pulse therapy). Oral prednisone at 2 mg/kg/24 h tapered over 1–4 weeks is typical.
  - Advantages: ease of dosing, low cost, often longer duration of response
  - Disadvantages: short-term side effects: mood changes, increased appetite and weight gain, hypertension, insulin resistance. Long-term side effects with chronic use: adrenal suppression, osteopenia, growth delay
- Anti-Rh D immunoglobulin—WinRho-SDF (patient must be Rh[+], nonsplenectomized, and not have hemolysis or hemorrhage): 80% respond with platelet counts $>20{,}000/mm^3$ after 72 hours. Dose is 50–75 mcg/kg IV over 3–5 minutes. If hemoglobin (Hb) <10 mg/dL, give 25–40 mcg/kg. 1 mcg = 5 IU of drug. Response lasts ~5 weeks.
  - Advantages: less expensive than IVIG but more costly than steroids; lower rate of allergic side effects (10%) than with IVIG and does not cause aseptic meningitis; amenable to outpatient administration
  - Disadvantages: fever/chills, mild hemolysis (Hb decrease of 1–3 g/dL) in all patients; rare reports of catastrophic hemolysis; subcutaneous route may ameliorate risk.
- Any of these therapies may be repeated if responsive patient later develops recurrent thrombocytopenia.

Second Line

- Rituximab (anti-CD20 monoclonal antibody) induces response in many refractory patients (after median 5 weeks), but duration is often limited (median 12 months).
- Thrombopoietin receptor agonists (e.g., eltrombopag, romiplostim) have been shown in trials to improve platelet counts and bleeding risk in patients with chronic ITP. Cost, concerns about adverse effects including myelofibrosis and thrombosis, and paucity of long-term follow-up data limit use.
- Cytotoxic drugs (e.g., vincristine) or immunosuppression (e.g., cyclosporine A or mycophenolate mofetil) is effective in some patients refractory to other therapy and splenectomy.

ADDITIONAL TREATMENT

General Measures

- Platelet transfusions are generally ineffective because transfused platelets are rapidly destroyed. Role is limited to emergent support for critical hemorrhage.
- Avoid medications that affect platelet function, such as aspirin, ibuprofen, most other NSAIDs, and anticoagulants.
- Educate parents about signs and symptoms of intracranial hemorrhage and GI bleeding.
- Avoid activities with significant fall, collision, or other trauma risk while thrombocytopenic.

SURGERY/OTHER PROCEDURES

Splenectomy: 70–80% respond with complete remission. No reliable presurgical predictors of response have been found; generally deferred until >12 months from diagnosis to allow for spontaneous remission or medical response

- Advantages: response in patients refractory to medical therapy
- Disadvantages: surgical morbidity; risk of sepsis with encapsulated organisms (immunize preoperatively against *Haemophilus influenzae*, pneumococcus, and meningococcus and consider penicillin prophylaxis)

INPATIENT CONSIDERATIONS

Initial Stabilization

Life-threatening hemorrhage: The goal is to stop bleeding rapidly. Platelet transfusion, IVIG, and steroids (after emergent marrow exam, if indicated) should be given concomitantly.

ONGOING CARE

FOLLOW-UP RECOMMENDATIONS

Patient Monitoring

- Platelet count twice weekly when $<20{,}000/mm^3$, weekly when $<50{,}000/mm^3$ or after treatment, except in stable chronic ITP. Increase interval if no symptoms and platelet count $>50{,}000/mm^3$.
- Platelet counts may fall transiently with intercurrent illnesses prior to resolution of ITP.
- Discontinue monitoring when no symptoms and normal platelet count for >3 months.

PROGNOSIS

- Acute ITP: In 3 months, 60% of children will have a platelet count $>100{,}000/mm^3$; at 1 year from diagnosis, 90%. Recurrence is rare.
- Chronic ITP: Platelet count tends to be higher, at $40{,}000–80{,}000/mm^3$. Remissions can occur many years after diagnosis (predicted spontaneous remission rate 61% after 15 years).
- Not yet possible to prospectively distinguish patients with self-limited ITP from those who will persist with chronic ITP
- Patients with chronic ITP should be periodically reevaluated for secondary ITP.

COMPLICATIONS

- The incidence of significant bleeding-related morbidity and mortality is low (<5%).
  - Intracranial hemorrhage is rare (<0.5%).
  - May occur without prior trauma
- Retinal hemorrhage is rare.
- Mucosal bleeding from nose, gums, lower GI tract, or kidneys is not uncommon. Hematemesis and melena are rare.
- Significant menorrhagia may occur.

ADDITIONAL READING

- Eberl W, Dickerhoff R; Pediatric Committee of Society of Thrombosis and Hemostasis Research. Newly diagnosed immune thrombozytopenia—German guideline concerning initial diagnosis and therapy. *Klin Padiatr*. 2012;224(3):207–210.
- Kime C, Klima J, Rose MJ, et al. Patterns of inpatient care for newly diagnosed immune thrombocytopenia in US children's hospitals. *Pediatrics*. 2013;131(5): 880–885.
- Neunert CE, Buchanan GR, Imbach P, et al. Bleeding manifestations and management of children with persistent and chronic immune thrombocytopenia: data from the Intercontinental Cooperative ITP Study Group (ICIS). *Blood*. 2013;121(22):4457–4462.
- Neunert C, Lim W, Crowther M, et al. The American Society of Hematology 2011 evidence-based practice guideline for immune thrombocytopenia. *Blood*. 2011;117(16):4190–4207.

CODES

ICD-10-CM

- D69.3 Immune thrombocytopenic purpura
- D69.41 Evans syndrome

IMMUNE DEFICIENCY

Kathleen E. Sullivan

BASICS

DESCRIPTION

Immunodeficiencies generally represent a defect in host defense. Less common deficiencies represent defects in the regulation of immune function. Congenital and acquired forms exist.

- Defects in antibody production: often characterized by frequent sinopulmonary infections with typical organisms
  - X-linked agammaglobulinemia
    - Onset of symptoms after 6 months of age; sinopulmonary infections with typical bacterial pathogens
    - Markedly decreased immunoglobulins (Ig) and B cells. Tonsils are absent.
  - Hyper-IgM syndromes: several forms
    - Usually present with recurrent bacterial infections in infancy; *Pneumocystis jiroveci* is seen; intermittent neutropenia is common.
    - Decreased IgG, IgE, IgA with normal or increased IgM
  - Common variable immunodeficiency (CVID)
    - Usually presents with recurrent bacterial infections; most commonly arises in the 2nd or 3rd decade (but seen at all ages)
    - Ig levels and function gradually decline; autoimmunity is common.
  - IgA deficiency
    - Most common congenital immunodeficiency (1:500); most are asymptomatic.
    - Symptoms seen at any age; typically sinopulmonary infections; increased risk of allergy, autoimmune disease, and anaphylaxis from blood products
  - Transient hypogammaglobulinemia of infancy
    - A developmental delay of Ig production; function is intact; typically resolves between 1 and 2 years of age
- T-cell defects: most often characterized by persistent viral infections or opportunistic infections
  - Severe combined immunodeficiency (SCID)
    - Most common presentation is a respiratory virus that fails to clear or chronic diarrhea.
    - Failure to thrive, thrush, and *P. jiroveci* pneumonia are also common.
    - Many states now have SCID newborn screening; patients identified have no symptoms.
  - Combined immune deficiencies
    - Several forms
    - Children exhibit increased severity of a broad range of infections, opportunistic infections, and unusual autoimmunity.
  - Chromosome 22q11.2 deletion syndrome
    - See "DiGeorge Syndrome."
  - Chronic mucocutaneous candidiasis
    - Multiple forms of this disorder
    - One form is also called autoimmune polyendocrinopathy candidiasis ectodermal dystrophy (APECED) and has an association with polyendocrinopathies and ectodermal dysplasia.
    - The other types are more likely to have an associated T-cell defect. Infants have extensive or recurrent *Candida* infection; modest predisposition to other infections.
  - IPEX (immunodeficiency, polyendocrinopathy, enteropathy, X-linked syndrome)
    - Diarrhea associated with villous atrophy and a T-cell infiltrate, progressive autoimmune destruction of endocrine organs
    - Infections can be severe but the autoimmune manifestations predominate.
- Neutrophil defects: *Staphylococcus*, *Pseudomonas*; unusual bacterial or fungal infections are characteristic.
  - Autoimmune neutropenia of infancy
    - Most common neutrophil defect of childhood; usually detected at ~6–12 months of age
    - Often resolves by 2 years of age
  - Congenital neutropenia
    - Infections may be skin infections or sinopulmonary.
    - Patients have either persistently absent or markedly low neutrophil counts.
    - Some patients will have 21-day cycles of neutropenia—cyclic neutropenia.
  - Leukocyte adhesion deficiency
    - 10% have delayed separation of the umbilical cord.
    - Most common presentations are recurrent skin ulcers and periodontitis.
    - Spontaneous peritonitis occurs.
  - Chronic granulomatous disease (CGD)
    - Recurrent skin abscesses common, deep hepatic abscesses, and pulmonary infections
    - Typical organisms are *Staphylococcus aureus*, *Burkholderia*, *Serratia*, *Nocardia*, mycobacteria, *Aspergillus*, and *Candida*.
    - Age of onset is usually 1–3 years.
- Innate defects in signaling: typically present with severe bacterial or viral infections in early infancy
  - IRAK4 and MyD88 deficiencies
    - Associated with staphylococcal, streptococcal, or pseudomonal sepsis/meningitis
    - Clostridial infections are also seen.
  - Herpes simplex encephalitis is associated with several gene defects.
- Macrophage activation defects
  - Universally associated with atypical mycobacteria. *Salmonella* is also seen.
  - Biopsies may reveal poorly formed granulomas.
- Complement deficiency
  - Deficiencies of C5–C9 are associated with *Neisseria* infections.
  - Deficiencies of C1, C2, and C4 are associated with lupus and recurrent bacterial infections.
  - C3 deficiency associated with glomerulonephritis and severe recurrent infections.
  - Defects in complement regulatory proteins are associated with atypical hemolytic uremic syndrome (HUS) or hereditary angioedema.
- Immunodeficiency syndromes
  - Ataxia telangiectasia
    - Progressive cerebellar ataxia during infancy; ocular telangiectasias at about 5–15 years of age
    - Recurrent sinopulmonary infections; α-fetoprotein is elevated, IgA and IgG2 are diminished.
  - Wiskott-Aldrich syndrome
    - Clinical triad of eczema, thrombocytopenia, and recurrent infections
    - Ig levels are variable but responses to vaccines often poor; small platelets and thrombocytopenia
  - Hyper-IgE syndrome
    - Recurrent infections of the skin and lungs; *S. aureus* is a major cause of infection, and pulmonary infections typically heal with pneumatoceles.
  - X-linked lymphoproliferative syndrome
    - 4 main types of presentation and 2 genetic types: acute Epstein-Barr virus infection with hemophagocytosis, lymphoma, hypogammaglobulinemia, and aplastic anemia
    - Family history is key to diagnosis.
  - Chédiak-Higashi syndrome
    - Pigmentary dilution, progressive neuropathy, and frequent infections; associated with a hemophagocytic process
    - Neutrophil counts are low and neutrophils have giant inclusions.
  - Familial hemophagocytic lymphohistiocytosis
    - Defect in cytotoxic function; presents with fever, pancytopenia, and hepatosplenomegaly; usually <5 years of age
  - Ectodermal dysplasia with immune deficiency
    - Two forms. Variable ectodermal dysplasia and variable immune deficiency. Ig levels are variable as are responses to vaccines.
    - Susceptibility to mycobacteria, *Pneumocystis*, and common bacterial pathogens
- Secondary immunodeficiencies include the following:
  - HIV infection
  - Malignancy
  - Viral suppression
  - Nephrotic syndrome
  - Protein-losing enteropathy
  - Malnutrition
  - Medications
  - Splenectomy

EPIDEMIOLOGY

Primary immune deficiencies range from the common (1:600) to the very rare (1:1,000,000).

- 1:600 for IgA deficiency in Caucasians
- 1:3,000 for chromosome 22q11.2 deletion syndrome (DiGeorge syndrome)
- 1:20,000 for common variable immune deficiency
- 1:50,000 for SCID
- 1:200,000 for CGD

RISK FACTORS

Genetics

- The immunodeficiencies are generally autosomal recessive, although there are several important exceptions.
- X-linked
  - Properdin deficiency, X-linked agammaglobulinemia, X-linked hyper-IgM, X-linked SCID, X-linked CGD, X-linked lymphoproliferative syndrome (2 types), IPEX, Wiskott-Aldrich syndrome, NEMO deficiency. All of these have autosomal recessive phenocopies or may be seen in females with altered X inactivation.
- Autosomal dominant
  - Hyper-IgE syndrome, chromosome 22q11.2 deletion syndrome, some macrophage activation defects
- Polygenic
  - IgA deficiency and CVID

DIAGNOSIS

DIFFERENTIAL DIAGNOSIS
- Chronic inflammation of mucous membranes such as that due to reflux or allergies can lead to recurrent infections.
- Immunocompromised status due to chemotherapy and immunosuppressive drugs
- Malnutrition
- Intercurrent viral infections such as Epstein-Barr virus and cytomegalovirus
- Medications such as antiseizure drugs and corticosteroids can cause IgA deficiency or hypogammaglobulinemia.
- Inborn errors of metabolism
- Chromosomal syndromes
- Protein loss can be associated with hypogammaglobulinemia.
- HIV infection

HISTORY
- **Question:** Family history?
- *Significance*: X-linked disorders are common.
- **Question:** Number and duration of infections?
- *Significance*: To determine whether the problem is one of clearance or frequency
- **Question:** Types of infections?
- *Significance*: Infections of skin are frequently due to neutrophil problems, whereas recurrent infections of a single site imply an anatomic problem. Opportunistic infections are associated with both neutrophil defects (unusual bacteria and fungi) and T-cell defects (opportunistic viruses).
- HIV risk factors

PHYSICAL EXAM
Examination should be directed at defining organ damage as a result of infection, the presence of any current infections, syndromic features, signs of autoimmune disease, and the characterization of accessible lymphoid organs, liver, and spleen.

DIAGNOSTIC TESTS & INTERPRETATION
- **Test:** IgG, IgA, IgM, IgE levels, and responses to vaccines such as diphtheria and tetanus
- *Significance*: Recurrent sinopulmonary infections with typical organisms are associated with defects in antibody production.
- **Test:** Evaluation of T-cell production and function—T-cell enumeration and lymphocyte proliferation studies
- *Significance*: T-cell defects will often have low T-cell numbers.
- **Test:** Evaluation of neutrophil numbers and function—a CBC with differential, morphologic exam of neutrophils, and a measure of respiratory burst
- *Significance*: Neutrophil disorders typically present with skin abscesses or ulcers or deep infections with *Staphylococcus* or fungi.
- **Test:** Special studies designed to test the function of the toll-like receptor signaling complex
- *Significance*: Innate defects, such as IRAK4, MyD88, and NEMO deficiencies, can be detected.
- **Test:** A CH50
- *Significance*: A CH50 will detect most of the structural component deficiencies. Special studies are needed for defects of the alternative pathway and the regulatory proteins.
- **Test:** CBC with differential; IgG, IgA, and IgM levels; and diphtheria and tetanus titers
- *Significance*: In certain patients, it may be difficult to differentiate between viral processes and bacterial processes. In these cases, a CBC with differential; IgG, IgA, and IgM levels; and diphtheria and tetanus titers are a useful screen to evaluate for the most common immunodeficiencies.

TREATMENT

- Prophylactic antimicrobials
  - Chronic mucocutaneous candidiasis
  - Hyper-IgE syndrome
  - CGD

ADDITIONAL TREATMENT
General Measures
- Suspected SCID requires isolation, cytomegalovirus-negative/irradiated blood products, and a prompt evaluation for hematopoietic stem cell transplant.
- Ig replacement (either IV or SC)
  - X-linked agammaglobulinemia
  - Hyper-IgM
  - CVID
- Probiotics may be useful for antibiotic-associated diarrhea.
- Hand washing to prevent infections
- Prophylactic antibiotics can be useful.

SURGERY/OTHER PROCEDURES
- Hematopoietic stem cell transplantation
  - SCID
  - Wiskott-Aldrich syndrome
  - X-linked lymphoproliferative syndrome
  - Chédiak-Higashi syndrome
  - Familial hemophagocytic lymphohistiocytosis
  - Selected cases of hyper-IgM, CGD, macrophage activation defects
- Thymus transplantation
  - Severe chromosome 22q11.2 deletion syndrome (DiGeorge syndrome)

ONGOING CARE

PROGNOSIS
- Most antibody deficiencies have an excellent prognosis. Transient or developmental deficiencies of IgG or IgG subclasses typically resolve by 2 years of age.
- Some patients with CVID can develop malignancy or autoimmune disease and this defines the prognosis.
- The treatment of neutrophil disorders remains problematic; most children with CGD will not have full life expectancy.
- Patients with T-cell disorders for whom bone marrow transplantation is not performed can do well if the defect is mild and if they do not suffer from autoimmune disease, malignancy, or recurrent infections.

COMPLICATIONS
- Bronchiectasis
- Deafness
- Autoimmune disease
- Lymphoreticular malignancies occur in patients with T-cell disorders.
- Live viral vaccines administered to patients with significant T-cell dysfunction can result in unchecked viremia.
- Oral polio vaccine administered to patients with agammaglobulinemia can cause meningoencephalitis.

ADDITIONAL READING

- Ballow M. Approach to the patient with recurrent infections. *Clin Rev Allergy Immunol*. 2008;34(2):129–140.
- Fischer A. Human primary immunodeficiency diseases. *Immunity*. 2007;27(6):835–845.
- International Union of Immunological Societies. Primary immunodeficiencies: 2009 update. *J Allergy Clin Immunol*. 2009;124(6):1161–1178.
- Slatter MA, Gennery AR. Primary immunodeficiency syndromes. *Adv Exp Med Biol*. 2010;685:146–165.
- www.immunodeficiencysearch.com

CODES

ICD10
- D84.9 Immunodeficiency, unspecified
- D80.9 Immunodeficiency with predominantly antibody defects, unspecified
- D83.9 Common variable immunodeficiency, unspecified

FAQ

- Q: Does a child with thrush require evaluation?
- A: A child with severe thrush in the absence of risk factors should have an evaluation for T-cell dysfunction, HIV, and the possibility of chronic mucocutaneous candidiasis of childhood. Moderate thrush or recurrent simple thrush does not require evaluation unless it is occurring in an older child.
- Q: A newborn in my practice still has his umbilical cord attached at 6 weeks of age. Is that abnormal, and does it require an evaluation for leukocyte adhesion deficiency?
- A: A completely healthy-appearing cord at 6 weeks of age does not require any evaluation. If there is clinical suspicion of leukocyte adhesion deficiency, a CBC can be performed to identify neutrophilia.
- Q: Which immunodeficiencies are associated with absent tonsils and adenoids?
- A: Boys with X-linked agammaglobulinemia and X-linked hyper-IgM have absent tonsils and adenoids.
- Q: Which immunodeficiency is associated with abscesses that are not painful?
- A: Children and adults with hyper-IgE syndrome develop abscesses that are not painful.

IMMUNOGLOBULIN A DEFICIENCY

Nashmia Qamar • Ramsay L. Fuleihan

BASICS

DESCRIPTION

Serum IgA <7 mg/dL and a normal serum IgG and IgM in patients >4 years of age

RISK FACTORS

Genetics

- Exact pattern of inheritance remains unclear; however, the following associations may occur:
  - 22q11 deletion syndrome
  - 18q syndrome
  - Partial deletions in the long or short arm and ring forms of chromosome 18
  - Also associated with HLA-A1, HLA-A2, B8, DR3, DQ2 (8.1), and Dw3
  - Also associated with non–MHC-associated genes involved in autoimmunity including IFIH1 on chromosome 2q24, CLEC16A on chromosome 16

PATHOPHYSIOLOGY

- Failure of B lymphocyte differentiation into plasma cells producing IgA
- Block may be due to
  - Defect in T-helper cells
  - Antigen-presenting cells
  - B cells
  - Lack of effects from various cytokines, including IL-21, IL-4, IL-6, IL-7, or IL-10

COMMONLY ASSOCIATED CONDITIONS

Increased association with the following:

- Atopy
- Sinopulmonary infections
- GI infections (especially *Giardia lamblia*)
- Inflammatory bowel disease (Crohn disease and ulcerative colitis)
- Celiac disease
- Nodular lymphoid hyperplasia
- Malignancy
- Autoimmune illnesses
  - Systemic lupus erythematosus
  - Immune endocrinopathies (e.g., Graves disease, type 1 diabetes)
  - Autoimmune hematologic conditions
  - Chronic active hepatitis

DIAGNOSIS

HISTORY

- Patients with IgA deficiency
  - Can have frequent sinopulmonary infections
  - Can have frequent GI infections
  - Tend to be allergic
  - Have an increased incidence of autoimmune diseases
- ~30% of patients with IgA deficiency are completely healthy.
- Patients with low switched memory B cells exhibit more severe clinical features including pneumonia, autoimmune disease, and bronchiectasis.

PHYSICAL EXAM

- Look for signs of recurrent infection and atopy.
- Allergies are associated with IgA deficiency. Signs include the following:
  - Cobblestoning of the conjunctiva
  - Allergic shiners
- Serous otitis media may be the result of recurrent ear infections or persistent fluid:
  - Increased ear infections can be seen in IgA deficiency.
  - Persistent fluid can be secondary to allergies.
- Pain on palpation of the sinuses
  - Recurrent sinus infections are associated with IgA deficiency.
- Lung examination
  - An increased frequency of pneumonia is associated with IgA deficiency.
- Swollen joints:
  - An increased frequency of autoimmune disease is associated with IgA deficiency.

DIAGNOSTIC TESTS & INTERPRETATION

Diagnostic Procedures/Other

The general goal is to decide whether the patient's complaints are consistent with IgA deficiency (frequent upper respiratory and GI infections or allergies).

- Measure serum IgA level:
  - If the patient is IgA deficient, exclude other conditions associated with IgA deficiency.
  - Serum IgA level: Patient is considered deficient if the serum IgA level is <7 mg/dL.
- Total immunoglobulins
  - If normal, helps rule out X-linked agammaglobulinemia (Bruton), common variable immunodeficiency, and severe combined immunodeficiency
- IgG subclasses:
  - Helps rule out an associated IgG subclass deficiency
- Lymphocyte stimulation to mitogens
  - A functional lymphocyte study
  - If normal, helps rule out common variable immunodeficiency, severe combined immunodeficiency, ataxia telangiectasia, DiGeorge syndrome, and Nezelof syndrome
- Lymphocyte stimulation to *Candida* antigen
  - No response to *Candida* in vivo is consistent with chronic mucocutaneous candidiasis.
- Specific antibody responses to polysaccharide and protein antigens: to evaluate for an associated specific antibody deficiency
- Screening for celiac disease
  - Should include IgG antibodies against gliadin and tissue transglutaminase because IgA isotype may not be detected

DIFFERENTIAL DIAGNOSIS

- Toxic, environmental, drugs
  - Penicillamine and anticonvulsants can induce IgA deficiency.
- Cyclosporine A has been reported to cause permanent IgA deficiency.
- Genetic/metabolic
  - X-linked agammaglobulinemia (Bruton)
  - Common variable immunodeficiency (CVID)
  - Severe combined immunodeficiency
  - Ataxia telangiectasia
  - DiGeorge syndrome
  - Chronic mucocutaneous candidiasis
  - Nezelof syndrome
  - Selective IgG2 deficiency
- Miscellaneous: Patients may be completely healthy, and IgA deficiency may be an incidental finding.

ALERT

Factors that may alert you to request a referral include the following:

- Suggestion that IgA deficiency may be part of a more complex immune deficiency: An allergist/immunologist can assist with an appropriate immunologic evaluation.
- Suggestion of associated autoimmune disease: Evaluation and treatment by a rheumatologist is indicated.
- Patient likely to need a blood transfusion: An allergist/immunologist can help select appropriate blood products.

TREATMENT

ADDITIONAL TREATMENT

General Measures

- There is no specific drug therapy.
- Recurrent infections should be treated aggressively with broad-spectrum antibiotics.
- Antibiotic prophylaxis to prevent recurrent sinopulmonary infections is often indicated.
- IV gammaglobulin is generally not indicated unless there is evidence of an associated specific antibody deficiency.

ALERT

Patients with no detectable IgA may develop antibodies against IgA in transfused blood products. These patients are at risk for allergic reactions including anaphylactic (or anaphylactoid) transfusion reactions on subsequent exposure. It should be noted, however, that life-saving products should not be withheld in emergent situations. In the nonurgent setting, to avoid potential allergic reactions, patients may receive the following:

- Packed RBCs (only if these cells have been washed 3 times)
- Plasma products from IgA-deficient donors
- Autologous banked blood

ONGOING CARE

FOLLOW-UP RECOMMENDATIONS

- Patients should be observed for the following:
  - Sinopulmonary infections
  - GI infections
  - Autoimmune diseases
  - Inflammatory bowel disease
  - Malignancy typically of lymphoid origin
- It is important to manage infectious complications aggressively and to intervene promptly if associated conditions develop.
- It is also known that IgA deficiency may progress to CVID in some cases.

PATIENT EDUCATION

- IgA deficiency can be induced by some anticonvulsants and by penicillamine.
- IgA-deficient patients should wear medical alert bracelets. These patients can have anaphylaxis if administered blood products containing IgA. In an emergency situation, this is important information for the caregivers to know. However, this is not very common and does not occur with the first blood product infusion/transfusion.

PROGNOSIS

Survival into the 7th decade is common. However it is also known that some patients may progress to CVID.

COMPLICATIONS

Increased incidence of the following:

- Sinopulmonary infections
- GI tract infections
- Atopy
- Autoimmune diseases
- Malignancy

ADDITIONAL READING

- Burrows PD, Cooper MD. IgA deficiency. *Adv Immunol*. 1997;65:245–276.
- Janzi M, Kull I, Sjöberg R, et al. Selective IgA deficiency in early life: association to infections and allergic diseases during childhood. *Clin Immunol*. 2009;133(1):78–85.
- Smith CA, Driscoll DA, Emanuel BS, et al. Increased prevalence of immunoglobulin A deficiency in patients with the chromosome 22q11.2 deletion syndrome (DiGeorge syndrome/velocardiofacial syndrome). *Clin Diagn Lab Immunol*. 1998;5(3):415–417.
- Stiehm RE. The four most common pediatric immunodeficiencies. *Adv Exp Med Biol*. 2007;601:15–26.
- Wang N, Hammarström L. IgA deficiency: what is new? *Curr Opin Allergy Clin Immunol*. 2012;12(6):602–608.
- Yel L. Selective IgA deficiency. *J Clin Immunol*. 2010;30(1):10–16.

CODES

ICD10

D80.2 Selective deficiency of immunoglobulin A [IgA]

FAQ

- Q: Should patients with IgA deficiency be monitored for the development of progressive immunodeficiency?
- A: Patients with IgA deficiency should be monitored for progression to CVID, as this is associated with a poorer prognosis and would require treatment with IV gammaglobulin.
- Q: Should IgA-deficient patients wear medical alert bracelets?
- A: Yes. These patients can have anaphylaxis if they are given blood products containing IgA. In an emergency situation, this is important information for the caregivers to know.

I

IMMUNOGLOBULIN A NEPHROPATHY

Maha N. Haddad • Lavjay Butani

BASICS

DESCRIPTION

Primary immune complex–mediated glomerulonephritis

EPIDEMIOLOGY

- Most common chronic glomerulonephritis worldwide
- Prevalence varies considerably across countries; more common in Caucasians and Asians compared to African Americans.
- Because reported prevalence is based on biopsy-confirmed diagnosis and therefore does not account for mild or asymptomatic cases, data grossly underestimate "true" prevalence.
- Represents 2–10% of all biopsy-confirmed primary glomerular diseases in adults in the United States
- No robust epidemiologic data in children

RISK FACTORS

- Typically sporadic
- Familial cases have been described suggesting that genetic factors influence susceptibility to and severity of disease.
- Reported in children with history of perinatal HIV-1 infection
- Increased risk of IgA nephropathy in adult patients with celiac disease, cirrhosis, and HIV infection

PATHOPHYSIOLOGY

- Etiology and pathogenesis remain uncertain.
- Substantial evidence that IgA nephropathy is a systemic immune complex–mediated disease as it recurs after transplantation
- Multiple studies have found abnormal glycosylation patterns of the IgA1 molecule (galactose deficiency), suggesting the following hypotheses:
  - Glycan-specific IgG antibodies form immune complexes with galactose-deficient IgA1.
  - Complexes deposit in the glomerular mesangium.
  - Activated mesangial cells proliferate and excrete extracellular matrix, cytokines, and chemokines with resulting renal injury.
- Majority of patients have elevated galactose-deficient IgA1 in the serum.

DIAGNOSIS

HISTORY

- Clinical presentation varies widely in constellation of signs and symptoms and also in severity.
- Patients may be completely asymptomatic.
- In children, the most common presentation is recurrent gross hematuria.
  - Triggered by acute upper respiratory tract infection in about half of the patients
  - In IgA nephropathy, in contrast to postinfectious glomerulonephritis, the hematuria presents at the same time ("synpharyngitic") or within a few days after the onset of the respiratory illness.
- Other presentations include the following:
  - Microscopic hematuria found on routine urinalysis
  - Hematuria (gross or microscopic) and proteinuria
  - Acute nephritic syndrome (hematuria, proteinuria, edema, impaired renal function, and hypertension). Rarely, this may be rapidly progressive.
  - Nephrotic syndrome: edema, hypoalbuminemia, and nephrotic range proteinuria
- Variable levels of proteinuria are seen.

PHYSICAL EXAM

- Hypertension: usually absent in mild disease; variably present depending on severity
- Edema: found in patients with high levels of proteinuria

DIAGNOSTIC TESTS & INTERPRETATION

Lab

- Urinalysis: RBCs, RBC casts, and protein
- Spot urine protein/creatinine ratio or 24-hour urine collection to quantify proteinuria
- Comprehensive metabolic panel
  - Kidney function tests (blood urea nitrogen and serum creatinine), serum electrolytes, and albumin are normal in mild disease.
  - Variably affected depending on severity
- In patients presenting with rapidly progressive glomerulonephritis, check complement levels, antinuclear antibody (ANA), antineutrophil cytoplasmic antibody (ANCA), and anti–glomerular basement membrane (GBM) antibodies to rule out other diseases.
- Serum IgA levels have very low sensitivity and specificity and are not recommended.

Imaging

Kidney ultrasound findings are nonspecific and either normal or, in more severe cases, may demonstrate increased echogenicity of the renal parenchyma.

Diagnostic Procedures/Other

- Kidney biopsy is required for a definitive diagnosis.
- Hallmark of the diagnosis is the presence, on immunofluorescence staining, of IgA deposits in the mesangium, either alone or with C3 (in children), IgM and IgG, or both (in adults).
- Biopsy is generally not required in mild cases as it does not affect the management or prognosis in the absence of proteinuria.
- Biopsy findings are variable on light microscopy:
  - Main finding is diffuse or focal mesangial proliferation with mesangial expansion.
  - Other possible findings include segmental or global endocapillary hypercellularity with segmental crescents and segmental necrosis.
  - Glomerulosclerosis in advance disease
  - Tubulointerstitium is usually normal with varying degree of atrophy and fibrosis in chronic cases.
  - Electron microscopy: immune complex deposits in the mesangium
  - Several histologic classifications have been developed with the purpose of predicting clinical course, prognosticating, and in guiding therapy.
  - The Oxford classification is one such example, based on a constellation of findings such as mesangial cellularity score, segmental glomerulosclerosis, endocapillary hypercellularity, and tubular atrophy/fibrosis.

DIFFERENTIAL DIAGNOSIS

- Thin basement membrane disease, Alport syndrome, or idiopathic hypercalciuria in mild cases presenting with hematuria
- Other forms of glomerulonephritis must be considered in the setting of a more acute presentation, including the following:
  - Postinfectious glomerulonephritis
  - Lupus nephritis
  - Membranoproliferative glomerulonephritis (MPGN)
  - Pauci-immune glomerulonephritis
  - Other vasculitides
- Henoch-Schönlein purpura nephritis has similar biopsy findings as IgA nephropathy but has additional nonrenal manifestations such as skin rash, abdominal pain, and periarthritis.

ALERT

May be progressive and lead to end-stage renal disease in moderate to severe cases. Refer to a nephrologist if persistent proteinuria, abnormal creatinine, gross hematuria, or hypertension.

TREATMENT

- Weak evidence base and mostly derived from expert opinion
- Varies based on severity of renal impairment, amount of proteinuria, and whether or not the course is rapidly progressive with associated crescents on biopsy. Higher amounts and persistence of proteinuria are associated with greater risk of disease progression.

MEDICATION

- Control of proteinuria and blood pressure
  - Protein excretion 0.5–1 g/1.73 m^2/day: angiotensin-converting enzyme inhibitor (ACEI) or angiotensin receptor blockers (ARBs). Increase dose to effect as long as symptomatic hypotension or hyperkalemia do not develop.
  - Protein excretion >1 g/1.73 m^2/day despite optimum blood pressure control and the use of ACEI or ARB and when GFR is >50 mL/min/1.73 m^2: Consider alternate day oral glucocorticoids for 6 months.
- Rapidly progressive glomerulonephritis and/or crescents on biopsy: intravenous (followed by oral) glucocorticoids, and consider additional immunosuppression such as cyclophosphamide or azathioprine (strength of evidence is poor for immunosuppression other than ACEI/ARB and glucocorticoids)

ADDITIONAL THERAPIES

- Fish oil suggested when proteinuria is persistent >1 g/1.73 m^2/day despite optimal supportive care.
- Mycophenolate mofetil: multiple studies with conflicting conclusions

GENERAL MEASURES

- Clinical presentation: Treat hypercholesterolemia associated with nephrotic syndrome. Address factors that modulate progression of chronic kidney disease—obesity, smoking, hypertension.
- Optimize blood pressure control.

ONGOING CARE

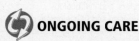

FOLLOW-UP RECOMMENDATIONS

- IgA nephropathy may be a progressive disease. Patients should be monitored periodically for the following:
  - Kidney function tests
  - Level of proteinuria
  - Blood pressure
  - Intensity and frequency of monitoring depends on severity. Patients presenting with microscopic hematuria and minimal proteinuria should be monitored with UA every 6 months to assess for progression of proteinuria.

PROGNOSIS

- Variable depending on severity of clinical presentation and renal histopathologic score
- 15–40% of adult patients with IgA nephropathy eventually progress to end-stage renal disease (ESRD).
- Although some reports suggest that children are more likely to have a benign course and have better prognosis than adults, other studies have reported similar outcomes for adults and children.
- In one series, renal survival rates in Japanese children were 95% at 10 years and 80% at 20 years.
- Patients who present with microscopic hematuria and minimal proteinuria have an excellent prognosis.
- Clinical predictors associated with poor outcome include severe persistent proteinuria, hypertension, and impaired renal function at presentation.
- The strongest predictive factor is the amount of proteinuria.
- Histopathologic features associated with poor outcome include mesangial hypercellularity score, endocapillary hypercellularity, tubular atrophy, and glomerular crescents.

ADDITIONAL READING

- Edström Halling S, Söderberg MP, Berg UB. Predictors of outcome in pediatric IgA nephropathy with regard to clinical and histopathological variables (Oxford Classification). *Nephrol Dial Transplant*. 2012;27(2):715–722.
- Gutierrez E, Zamora I, Ballarín JA, et al .Long-term outcomes of IgA nephropathy presenting with minimal or no proteinuria. *J Am Soc Nephrol*. 2012;23(10):1753–1760.
- Hogg RJ, Fitzgibbons L, Atkins C, et al. Efficacy of omega-3 fatty acids in children and adults with IgA nephropathy is dosage-and size-dependent. *Clin J Am Soc Nephrol*. 2006;1(6):1167–1172.
- Purswani MU, Chernoff MC, Mitchell CD, et al. Chronic kidney disease associated with perinatal HIV infection in children and adolescents. *Pediatr Nephrol*. 2012;27(6):981–989.
- Radhakrishnan J, Cattran DC. The KDIGO practice guideline on glomerulonephritis: reading between the guidelines—applications to the individual patient. *Kidney Int*. 2012;82(8):840–856.
- Ronkainen J, Ala-Houhala M, Autio-Harmainen H, et al. Long-term 19 years after childhood IgA nephritis: a retrospective cohort study. *Pediatr Nephrol*. 2006;21(9):1266–1273.
- Shima Y, Nakanishi K, Hama T, et al. Validity of the Oxford classification of IgA nephropathy in children. *Pediatr Nephrol*. 2012;27(5):783–792.
- Suzuki H, Kiryluk K, Novak J, et al. The pathophysiology of IgA nephropathy. *J Am Soc Nephrol*. 2011;22(10):1795–1803.
- Wang T, Ye F, Meng H, et al. Comparison of clinicopathological features between children and adults with IgA nephropathy. *Pediatr Nephrol*. 2012;27(8):1293–1300.
- Welander A, Sundelin B, Fored M, et al. Increased risk of IgA nephropathy among individuals with celiac disease. *J Clin Gastroenterol*. 2013;47(8):678–683.

CODES

ICD10

- N02.8 Recurrent and persistent hematuria w oth morphologic changes
- N02.5 Recurrent and perst hematur w diffuse mesangiocap glomrlneph
- N02.2 Recurrent and perst hematur w diffuse membranous glomrlneph

FAQ

- Q: Will my child ever outgrow IgA nephropathy?
- A: No. The etiology and pathogenesis of IgA nephropathy remain uncertain. IgA nephropathy is a chronic condition, but sometimes it can go into spontaneous remission. Spontaneous remission is reported to occur in 59% of children with mild disease. More severe cases can also go into remission with medications.
- Q: My child has had a kidney transplant. Can IgA nephropathy recur in the graft?
- A: Yes. Recurrence of the condition can develop in 33% of patients. Depending on the published series, recurrence rates vary between 9 and 66%. However, even if it does come back, it can be controlled/treated with medications.
- Q: My child has microscopic hematuria and proteinuria. He has normal kidney function and blood pressure. His kidney biopsy was consistent with the diagnosis of IgA nephropathy. What is the strongest predictor for progression?
- A: The amount of proteinuria. Children with no or mild proteinuria usually have good long-term prognosis, whereas those with high amounts of protein in the urine are more likely to progress and develop long-term kidney damage.

IMPERFORATE ANUS

Lusine Ambartsumyan

BASICS

DESCRIPTION

- Imperforate anus (IA) is a congenital abnormality in which the bowel fails to perforate or only partially perforates the pelvic muscular floor.
- IA may also perforate the epidermal covering of the pelvic muscular floor (anal membrane).
- Spectrum of anorectal malformations that range in severity from imperforate anal membrane to complete caudal regression
- IA has been classically described as low and high anomalies.
  - In a low lesion, the colon remains close to the skin and there may be a stenosis of the anus, or the anus may be missing altogether, with the rectum ending in a blind pouch.
  - In a high lesion, the colon is higher up in the pelvis, with a fistula connecting the rectum and the bladder, urethra, or the vagina.
- More recently, classification of IA is by type of associated fistula: rectal, bladder, urethra, or vaginal.

EPIDEMIOLOGY

- Prevalence is estimated to be in the range of 1:3,000–1:5,000.
- High lesions are more common in males (2:1).
- Low lesions occur with equal frequency in both sexes.

RISK FACTORS

Genetics

- Can be an isolated defect or part of a syndrome or association
- Syndromic disorders that contain IA are associated with defects on chromosomes 6, 7, 10, and 16.
- Can be associated with trisomy 21 (typically IA without fistula)
- Can be part of omphalocele-exstrophy of the bladder-IA-spinal defects (OEIS) complex or cloacal exstrophy (EC)

PATHOPHYSIOLOGY

- During the 6th week of fetal development, the hindgut comes into contact with the cloacal membrane. The hindgut is divided into a ventral urogenital and dorsal rectal component. By the 8th week, the dorsal 1/2 perforates to the exterior. In IA, the process is arrested during this critical period.
- There is a wide spectrum of anatomic variants of IA; commonly associated with urologic and spinal defects
- Classification of anatomic variants is based on the relationship between the rectum and the puborectalis muscle: supralevator (high) and translevator (low) malformations
- Cloaca is a complex defect, where the rectum, urethra, and the vagina drain into a common channel that communicates with the perineum.
  - A fistula communicating from the rectum to the external opening (perineal fistula) or to the urogenital system is present in 90% of cases.
  - Females: Most common defect is a rectovestibular fistula where the rectum opens into the vestibule.
  - Males: Most common defect is a rectourethral fistula from the rectum to lower posterior urethra (bulbar) or upper posterior urethra (prostatic).

COMMONLY ASSOCIATED CONDITIONS

- Other anomalies are present up to 50% of patients with an IA.
- IA can be associated with vertebral, cardiac, tracheoesophageal fistula, renal, and limb anomalies (VATER or VACTERL).
- Other associated anomalies include urologic, spine/sacrum (hypoplastic sacrum, sacral agenesis, presacral mass, myelomeningocele, tethered cord), gastrointestinal (esophageal/intestinal atresia, malrotation, omphalocele, annular pancreas), gynecologic (duplicate uterus, septate vagina, vaginal atresia), and cardiovascular defects (septal defects).

DIAGNOSIS

HISTORY

- Most children are diagnosed during a routine neonatal examination.
- Failure to pass meconium, a history of constipation, and signs of low intestinal obstruction (abdominal distention and vomiting) should mandate reexam of perianal area.
- Approximately 13–25% may present beyond the neonatal period and have higher morbidity (19–35%) and mortality (4–10%).

PHYSICAL EXAM

- Placement of the anus: lack of or anterior/lateral malposition
- Decreased or abnormal radial corrugations of the anus
- Abnormal rectal caliber
- Poor anal tone or patulous anal opening
- Absent or asymmetric anal wink
- Spinal dimples or tufts
- Flat buttocks, abnormal gluteal crease, lack of midline grove
- Abnormal genitourinary or neurologic examination
- Associated renal, cardiac, vertebral, or limb anomalies.

DIAGNOSTIC TESTS & INTERPRETATION

- Exclusion of associated anomalies
- Classification of the malformation (established after 18–24 hours)

Imaging

- Prone cross-table lateral and invertogram: After sufficient time for a transit of gas (>12 hours after birth), the child is placed in an upside-down position for 5 minutes, after which a lateral view of the pelvis is obtained to identify level of obstruction.
- Lumbosacral films to evaluate for vertebral anomalies and sacral integrity
- MRI of the spine and pelvis should be considered to look for a tethered cord and evaluate the pelvic anatomy.
- Water contrast enema to evaluate the anatomy: rectosigmoid caliber and genitourinary fistulas
- Renal and pelvic ultrasound to evaluate for hydronephrosis, megaureters, and hydrocolpos
- Voiding cystoureterogram and IV pyelogram can be used if urinary tract anomalies are highly suspected.
- Echocardiogram

DIFFERENTIAL DIAGNOSIS

- No disorders can mimic IA.
- Task is to define the location of the termination of the bowel and the opening of the fistula.

TREATMENT

SURGERY/OTHER PROCEDURES

- Surgery should be performed by an experienced surgeon.
- High lesions require an emergent and protective diverting colostomy, followed by pull-through procedure with posterior sagittal anorectoplasty (PSARP) at 3–9 months of age. Colostomy is closed after the anoplasty has healed and any necessary secondary dilations have been completed.

- Laparoscopy-assisted PSARP in conjunction with muscle electrostimulation may be performed in those with complex and high lesions.
- Transanal anorectoplasty was recently shown to have sphincter sparing and results in accurate placement of anus in external canal with good neurologic function.
- After surgery, follow-up with anal dilatation helps minimize the risk of stricture formation and helps the newly constructed canal to become functional.
- Complications of surgery include stricture of the anocutaneous anastomosis, rectourinary fistula, mucosal prolapse, constipation, and incontinence.

ONGOING CARE

PATIENT EDUCATION

- Prognosis for bowel and urine continence depends on type of malformation and sacral integrity.
- Low malformations have greater bowel control, increased incidence of megacolon with subsequent constipation, and "overflow" incontinence.
- High malformations have increased associated defects and poor bowel and urinary control.

PROGNOSIS

- Prognostic factors: type of malformation, sacral integrity, and length of the cloaca common channel
- Sacral integrity is the most important prognostic indicator of bowel control.
- Good prognostic indicators of bowel control:
  - Normal sacral integrity
  - No presacral mass
  - Two well-formed buttocks and midline grove
  - Low anorectal malformations (rectal atresia, rectoperineal fistula, rectobulbar urethral fistula, cloaca with common channel <3 cm, and IA without fistula)
- Poor prognostic indicators of bowel control:
  - Abnormal sacral integrity
  - Myelomeningocele
  - High anorectal malformations (rectoprostatic urethral fistula, rectobladder neck fistula, cloacal exstrophy cloaca, >3 cm common channel, complex defects)
- Experienced centers report
  - ~75% have voluntary bowel movements after age 3 years, of which 50% continue to have intermittent fecal incontinence.
  - In their cohort, ~25% have fecal incontinence despite treatment.
- Continence can be attained in 80–90% of patients who have low lesions.
- <50% of patients with high lesions are continent before school age, but most continue to improve and achieve continence by adolescence.
- Many patients will need regular enemas or comprehensive bowel management program for years to prevent or reduce constipation and fecal incontinence.

ADDITIONAL READING

- Arbell D, Gross E, Orkin B. Imperforate anus, malrotation, and Hirschsprung's disease: a rare and important association. *J Pediatr Surg*. 2006;41(7): 1335–1337.
- Chen CJ. The treatment of imperforate anus: experience with 108 patients. *J Pediatr Surg*. 1999;34(11):1728–1732.
- Di Lorenzo C, Benninga MA. Pathophysiology of pediatric fecal incontinence. *Gastroenterology*. 2004;126(1)(Suppl 1):S33–S40.
- Javid PJ, Barnhart DC, Hirschl RB, et al. Immediate and long-term results of surgical management of low imperforate anus in girls. *J Pediatr Surg*. 1998; 33(2):198–203.
- Keppler-Noreuil K, Gorton S, Foo F, et al. Prenatal ascertainment of OEIS complex/cloacal exstrophy—15 new cases and literature review. *Am J Med Genet A*. 2007;143A(18):2122–2128.
- Khalil BA, Morabito A, Bianchi A. Transanoproctoplasty: a 21-year review. *J Pediatr Surg*. 2010;45(9): 1915–1919.
- Levitt M, Kant A, Peña A. The morbidity of constipation in patients with anorectal malformations. *J Pediatr Surg*. 2010;45(6):1228–1233.
- Levitt M, Peña A. Update on pediatric faecal incontinence. *Eur J Pediatr Surg*. 2009;19(1):1–9.
- Lima M, Tursini S, Ruggeri G, et al. Laparoscopically assisted anorectal pull-through for high imperforate anus: three years' experience. *J Lapoaroendos Adv Surg Tech A*. 2006;16(1):63–66.
- Pakarinen M, Rintala R. Management and outcome of low anorectal malformations. *Pediatr Surg Int*. 2010;26(11):1057–1063.
- Pena A, Hong A. Advances in the management of anorectal malformations. *Am J Surg*. 2000;180(5): 370–376.
- Rintala RJ, Pakarinen MP. Imperforate anus: long- and short-term outcome. *Semin Pediatr Surg*. 2008; 17(2):79–89.

CODES

ICD10

- Q42.3 Congenital absence, atresia and stenosis of anus without fistula
- Q42.2 Congenital absence, atresia and stenosis of anus with fistula

FAQ

- Q: Is IA an isolated defect in my child?
- A: IA is often associated with multiple other anomalies. In particular, renal and vertebral anomalies must be excluded.
- Q: What is the genetic basis for this defect?
- A: IA can be associated with chromosomal anomalies or can be an isolated problem.
- Q: How likely is it that my child will ever be able to be toilet trained successfully?
- A: Successful toilet training will depend on what type of IA defect your child has: Children with high lesions may have more difficulty becoming toilet trained than children with low lesions. All children should improve over time but will need specialist treatment and a comprehensive bowel management program for many years to prevent or reduce constipation and fecal incontinence.

IMPETIGO

Maribeth Chitkara

BASICS

DESCRIPTION

- Impetigo is a superficial skin infection seen frequently in children.
  - It is one of the most common skin and soft tissue infections observed in pediatrics.
  - Pyoderma and impetigo contagiosa are synonyms for impetigo.
- Classification
  - Primary impetigo: direct bacterial invasion of previously normal skin
  - Secondary impetigo: infection at sites of minor skin trauma or underlying conditions
- Types of impetigo
  - Nonbullous impetigo
    - Most common form
    - Lesions begin as papules that progress to vesicles surrounded by erythema.
    - Subsequently, the papules mature into pustules that enlarge and break down to form thick, adherent, golden crusts.
  - Bullous impetigo
    - Vesicles enlarge to form bullae containing clear yellow fluid, which become darker and more turbid.
    - Ruptured bullae leave a honey-colored crust.
  - Ecthyma
    - An ulcerative form of impetigo
    - Lesions extend through the epidermis and deep into the dermis.

EPIDEMIOLOGY

- Location: most frequently in tropical or subtropical regions but also prevalent in northern climates during summer months
- Age: found most commonly in children aged 2–5 years and can spread rapidly through child care centers and schools

RISK FACTORS

- Poverty, overcrowding
- Poor hygiene
- Underlying scabies infection
- Eczema

ETIOLOGY

- *Staphylococcus aureus*: most common etiologic agent. Toxin-producing strains cause cleavage in superficial skin layer.
- Impetigo due to community-associated methicillin-resistant *Staphylococcus aureus* (CA-MRSA) has occurred in a minority of cases.
- Beta-hemolytic streptococci (primarily group A, but serogroups C and G have been implicated in some cases)

DIAGNOSIS

HISTORY

- Patients with impetigo may report a history of minor trauma, insect bites, scabies, herpes simplex virus infection, varicella infection, or eczema before the development of the infection. Lesions are usually present for a few days to weeks before the patient seeks medical attention.
- Lesions may be described as itchy but are usually painless.
- Additional symptoms such as fever, respiratory distress, vomiting, or diarrhea are rare and perhaps indicative of another diagnosis.
- Outbreaks commonly occur in families and child care centers as well as among sports team members.

PHYSICAL EXAM

- Nonbullous impetigo
  - Usually occurs on exposed areas of body, most frequently the face and extremities
  - Lesions first begin as papules or thin-walled vesicles on an erythematous base. The lesions gradually enlarge, may coalesce, and break down over the course of 4–6 days. After rupture, their serum is released, which dries and forms a thick brown, "honey-colored" crust.
  - As the lesions resolve with treatment, the crusts slough from the affected areas and may leave hypopigmented areas.
  - Lymphadenopathy is rare.
- Bullous impetigo
  - Lesions may form on grossly normal or previously traumatized skin.
  - Appear initially as superficial vesicles that rapidly enlarge to form flaccid bullae, filled with clear yellow liquid that gradually becomes more turbid and sometimes purulent.
  - After the lesions rupture, a thin, light brown crust remains.
  - Lymphadenopathy is rare.
- Ecthyma
  - The lesion is a vesicle or pustule overlying an inflamed area of skin that deepens into a dermal ulceration. "Punched-out" ulcers are covered with yellow crust, surrounded by raised violaceous margins.
  - Ecthyma heals slowly and commonly produces a scar.
  - Regional lymphadenopathy may occur, but systemic symptoms are usually absent.

Lab

- Impetigo is a clinical diagnosis, and no laboratory workup is routinely indicated.
- Culture of bullae or purulent fluid may be useful in patients who have failed empiric treatment. Swabs of intact skin are not helpful.
- If MRSA is suspected, a Gram stain and culture of lesion should be considered.
- If systemic symptoms are present, a CBC and blood culture should be considered to evaluate for other possible causes of infection.
- Skin biopsy may be useful if diagnosis is unclear.

DIFFERENTIAL DIAGNOSIS

- Varicella
- Staphylococcal scalded-skin syndrome
- Erythema multiforme
- Herpes simplex virus infection
- Burns (thermal and chemical)
- Contact dermatitis
- Atopic dermatitis
- Tinea corporis
- Insect bites
- Scabies
- Lice

TREATMENT

MEDICATION

- Topical therapy
  - Topical therapy is preferred when there are a limited number of lesions without bullae.
  - Mupirocin
    - 2% ointment or cream
    - Children >2 months old
    - Applied to affected areas three times daily for 5 days
  - Retapamulin
    - 1% ointment
    - Children >9 months old
    - Applied to affected area (up to 2% body surface area [BSA]) twice daily for 5 days
  - Although the components of over-the-counter triple antibiotic ointments (bacitracin, neomycin, polymyxin B) have some activity against the organisms causing impetigo, they are not considered effective for treatment.
- Oral therapy
  - Oral antibiotic therapy should be used for impetigo when the lesions are bullous or when topical therapy is impractical due to the extent or location of lesions.
  - Methicillin-sensitive *Staphylococcus aureus* (MSSA) or beta-hemolytic streptococci
    - Amoxicillin/clavulanic acid 40 mg/kg/24 h PO in 2 divided doses
    - Cephalexin 25 mg/kg/24 h PO in 4 divided doses
    - Dicloxacillin 12.5 mg/kg/24 h PO in 4 divided doses
    - Clindamycin 15–25 mg/kg/24 h PO in 3 divided doses
    - Erythromycin 40 mg/kg/24 h PO in 4 divided doses
  - When MRSA is suspected
    - Clindamycin 15–25 mg/kg/24 h PO in 3 divided doses
    - Trimethoprim-sulfamethoxazole: trimethoprim 8 mg/kg and sulfamethoxazole 40 mg/kg daily PO in 2 divided doses (has activity against MRSA but not against streptococci)

ADDITIONAL TREATMENT

General Measures

- Clipping fingernails short to minimize effects of scratching is recommended.
- Hand washing is important for reducing spread among children, as is covering the lesions.
- Treatment is important for reducing spread of infection to self and others.
- Cleansing and debriding the lesions are unnecessary.
- Crusted lesions can be cleansed gently with soap and water.

ONGOING CARE

FOLLOW-UP RECOMMENDATIONS

- Duration of therapy
  - The duration of antimicrobial therapy should be tailored to clinical improvement; 7 days of treatment is usually adequate.
  - Children should be excluded from out-of-home child care until 24 hours after treatment has been initiated.
- Signs of incomplete therapy
  - Recurrent infection may indicate incomplete therapy, reinfection, or an *S. aureus* carrier state.
  - Development of fever is unusual and may indicate a more serious infection and/or the presence of cellulitis or an abscess.
- Prevention of recurrence
  - Impetigo frequently spreads among close contacts and family members.
    - Patients and family members should wash their hands frequently.
    - Keep clothes and bedding clean.
    - Do not share towels and other personal care items.
  - Underlying skin conditions (e.g., eczema) and infestations (e.g., scabies) should be treated appropriately to decrease the likelihood of the development of impetigo.

COMPLICATIONS

- Cellulitis
- Lymphangitis
- Suppurative lymphadenitis
- Staphylococcal scalded-skin syndrome
- Poststreptococcal glomerulonephritis
  - Most cases are believed to be caused by a preceding streptococcal impetigo rather than streptococcal pharyngitis.
  - Deposition of group A beta-hemolytic streptococci (GABHS) nephrogenic antigens induce immune complex formation in kidneys.
  - Latent period is 3–6 weeks following skin infection.
- Scarlet fever, osteomyelitis, septic arthritis, pneumonia, septicemia, and rheumatic fever have also been observed in patients with impetigo.

PROGNOSIS

The lesions of impetigo usually heal without significant scarring. Overall, the infection is highly curable, but the condition often recurs in young children.

ADDITIONAL READING

- Koning S, van der Sande R, Verhagen AP, et al. Interventions for impetigo. *Cochrane Database Syst Rev*. 2012;1:CD003261.
- Stevens DL, Bisno AL, Chambers HF, et al. Practice guidelines for the diagnosis and management of skin and soft-tissue infections. *Clin Infect Dis*. 2005;41(10):1373–1406.
- Todd JK. Staphylococcal infections. *Pediatr Rev*. 2005;26(12):444–450.

CODES

ICD10

- L01.00 Impetigo, unspecified
- L01.01 Non-bullous impetigo
- L01.09 Other impetigo

FAQ

- Q: Which is the more effective treatment for impetigo—oral or topical antibiotics?
- A: In general, if there are a few localized lesions, topical therapy is preferred. If there is more diffuse involvement, or systemic symptoms, a course of oral antibiotics is recommended.
- Q: Can a child with impetigo attend school or child care?
- A: The child should be excluded from child care until 24 hours after treatment has been initiated. Once the lesions begin to improve, the child may resume his or her activities without restrictions.
- Q: How does one help prevent impetigo from spreading?
- A: Gently wash the affected areas with mild soap and running water, use the antibiotics (topical or oral) as directed, and then cover lesions with bandages. Wear gloves when applying any antibiotic ointment to the patient's lesions and endorse thorough hand washing afterward. Do not share clothes, linens, or towels used by the affected individual until the infection has cleared.

INFANTILE SPASMS

John R. Mytinger

BASICS

DESCRIPTION

- Infantile spasms (IS) are seizures commonly associated with West syndrome—a severe infantile epileptic encephalopathy often with poor developmental outcome.
  - IS are characterized by sudden flexion, extension, or mixed flexion-extension of the neck, trunk, arms, and/or legs.
  - IS can be subtle such as a mild contraction of the abdominal muscles or subtle movements of the head, shoulder, or eyes.
  - IS can occur singly, but the clustering (often on awakening) is a key diagnostic feature.
- IS are commonly dismissed as "normal" movements or misdiagnosed as reflux/colic.
- West syndrome is classically the triad of (1) IS, (2) developmental delay, and (3) hypsarrhythmia—a chaotic, high amplitude EEG background typically associated with multifocal spikes.

EPIDEMIOLOGY

- The onset occurs in the 1st year of life in >90%, typically 3–12 months of age (peak onset 4–8 months, mean 6 months).
- Rarely occurs after 18 months of age

Incidence

The incidence is 2–3.5/10,000 live births.

PATHOPHYSIOLOGY

- Unknown
- In 70–80% of cases, a specific condition is associated with IS; however, this does not necessarily suggest a direct cause-and-effect relationship with IS.

ASSOCIATED CONDITIONS

- Hypoxic-ischemic encephalopathy (HIE)
- Chromosomal disorders such as trisomy 21
- Brain malformation such as holoprosencephaly, malformations of cortical development (such as pachygyria or lissencephaly [including Miller-Dieker syndrome with deletion of 17p13.3], hemimegalencephaly, schizencephaly, heterotopia, and focal cortical dysplasia)
- Stroke
- Intraventricular/intraparenchymal hemorrhage
- Periventricular leukomalacia
- Tuberous sclerosis complex (TSC)
- Other neurocutaneous conditions such as neurofibromatosis type 1 (NF1), incontinentia pigmenti achromians (Hypomelanosis of Ito)
- Disorders of X-linked inheritance such as Aicardi syndrome (consider in girls with agenesis of the corpus callosum and chorioretinal lacunae)
- Hydrocephalus of various causes
- There is an expanding list of IS-associated genes: *ARX, CDKL5, FOXG1, GRIN1, GIN2A, MAGI2, SPTAN1, MEF2C, SLC25A22, STXBP1, SCN1A, SCN2A, GABRB3*, and *ALG13*.
- Trauma (any but often nonaccidental)
- Progressive encephalopathy with edema, hypsarrhythmia, and optic atrophy syndrome
- Infections: meningitis/encephalitis, TORCH
- Inborn errors of metabolism such as Menkes disease, disorders of amino acid metabolism (such as phenylketonuria and maple syrup urine disease), pyruvate dehydrogenase complex deficiency, mitochondrial disorders (such as Leigh syndrome), pyridoxine-dependent seizures, glucose transporter protein type 1 (GLUT1) deficiency, and uncommonly, organic acidurias (such as methylmalonic aciduria)

DIAGNOSIS

HISTORY

- A description of spells including the timing of onset (single IS can precede clustering)
- Prenatal and perinatal history including complications of pregnancy or delivery, gestational and maternal ages, place of birth (for access to newborn screening)
- History of HIE (perinatal, cardiac arrest, near drowning, near-miss SIDS)
- History of miscarriages, early infant death, family members with birth marks or seizures (a family history of IS is rare but can occur)
- Developmental history including any loss of skills (loss of visual tracking or social smile)

PHYSICAL EXAM

- Head circumference, dysmorphisms (such as Down syndrome or Miller-Dieker syndrome), cardiac murmur (rhabdomyoma in TSC), skin abnormalities (hypopigmented macules [may be present at birth in TSC and highlighted by the Wood's lamp] and café au lait spots [in NF1]), hepatomegaly (inborn errors of metabolism)
- Retinal evaluation (for metabolic disease and chorioretinal lacunae in Aicardi syndrome)
- Social smile, tracking, strength (head lag and axial slipping with the child held underarm in vertical suspension), tone, and reflexes

DIAGNOSTIC TESTS & INTERPRETATION

- Although nearly all children with IS have an abnormal EEG background, only 60% have hypsarrhythmia (or one of its variants). Thus, the presence of hypsarrhythmia is *not* required for the diagnosis or treatment of IS.
- The diagnosis is made with a video-EEG to characterize the spell and EEG background.
- An epilepsy protocol brain MRI to determine the etiology is strongly recommended.
- Early diagnosis and effective treatment can improve developmental outcome.
- The diagnostic and posttreatment EEG should include sleep, as the abnormal background is most often present during non-REM sleep.
  - IS begins with an initial phasic contraction lasting 1–2 seconds, sometimes followed by a tonic contraction that can last 2–10 seconds.
  - Most IS are clinically symmetric, but asymmetric spasms can occur and may indicate a focal brain lesion.
  - The EEG background is typically high voltage and disorganized with multifocal spikes.
  - The EEG correlate of IS is often a slow wave or sharp then slow wave followed by an electrodecrement (i.e., voltage attenuation).
- A 100-mg pyridoxine infusion during the EEG to assess for background improvement may help diagnose pyridoxine-dependent seizures.

Lab

- Testing should emphasize those conditions with a specific treatment:
  - Ammonia level
  - Serum lactic acid
  - Biotinidase assay (assess newborn screen)
  - Serum amino acids (assess newborn screen)
  - Copper/ceruloplasmin (for Menkes disease)
  - Consider lumbar puncture (LP) for GLUT1 deficiency (compare CSF to serum glucose).
  - Urine organic acids (uncommon etiology, assess new born screen)
- Any metabolic, chromosomal, genetic, and CSF studies must be considered on an individual basis: karyotype and or microarray analysis (especially with dysmorphisms), IS-associated gene/panel testing, whole exome sequencing.

Imaging

- Epilepsy protocol, brain MRI is recommended.
- Consider PET to assess for or better define a lesion that may be correctable with surgery.

Diagnostic Procedures/Other

Consider LP for neurotransmitter and folate metabolites, tetrahydrobiopterin, and lactic acid.

DIFFERENTIAL DIAGNOSIS

- *Normal movements confused with IS:* Moro reflex and similar-appearing startle/arousal responses; normal sleep myoclonus and hypnagogic/hypnic jerks
- *Nonepileptic movement disorders confused with IS:* benign myoclonus of early infancy; posturing; hyperekplexia; colic and gastroesophageal reflux (Sandifer syndrome)
- *Epileptic syndrome confused with IS:* benign myoclonic epilepsy of infancy

- *Neonatal epileptic encephalopathies that may include or evolve to IS:* early infantile epileptic encephalopathy (Ohtahara syndrome); early myoclonic epilepsy
- *Childhood epileptic encephalopathy that may include or evolve from IS:* Lennox-Gastaut syndrome (LGS)

TREATMENT

MEDICATION

First Line

- Generally accepted 1st-line medical treatments include adrenocorticotropic hormone (ACTH), high-dose oral corticosteroids (HOC), and vigabatrin.
- The etiology may determine the initial treatment: epilepsy surgery (such as tumor, hydrocephalus), ketogenic diet (such as GLUT1 deficiency, pyruvate dehydrogenase complex deficiency), vigabatrin (TSC).
- The approach should focus on an early "all or none" electroclinical remission with early changes in treatment if needed.
  - If no clinical remission by 2 weeks, consider changing treatment.
  - If there is clinical remission, confirm absence of spasms with EEG (at various durations).
  - If spasms noted on EEG, consider modification of treatment.
- ACTH
  - High rates of electroclinical remission have been reported with high-dose regimens (see Baram et al, 1996 for published regimen).
  - However, one study of high-dose (150 U/m^2/day) versus low-dose (20–30 U/day) found no difference in electroclinical remission.
  - Short-course ACTH may limit side effects.
    - Common: weight gain (increased appetite/fluid retention), irritability, poor sleep, hypertension
    - Less common: hyperglycemia, electrolyte abnormalities (hypokalemia), hypertrophic cardiomyopathy, immunosuppression, gastritis/gastric ulcer, reduced bone mineral density, adrenal insufficiency/failure
    - Rare: death most commonly due to immunosuppression with infection
  - Inpatient admission is typically performed for initiation of treatment and caregiver education.
    - Gastric acid suppression to avoid gastritis/gastric ulceration is typical.
    - ≥1 time weekly during treatment: blood pressure, urine glucose, and stool guaiac
    - One time weekly during treatment: electrolytes
    - Treatment of hypertension may be needed (e.g., enalapril or a reduced dose of ACTH).
- High-dose oral corticosteroids
  - High-dose regimens are recommended (see Lux et al, 2004 for published regimen)
  - The side effects, initial hospital admittance, and monitoring are the same as for ACTH.
- Vigabatrin
  - Initially, 50 mg/kg/24 h (divided twice daily) and increased by 50 mg/kg/24 h every 3 days to a maximum dose of 150–200 mg/kg/24 h (divided twice daily)
  - If there is no response in 2 weeks, use an alternative and taper vigabatrin off.
  - With electroclinical remission, the dose can be continued for 6 months and then weaned.
  - Risk of permanent peripheral visual field loss
  - The incidence and degree of retinal injury with short courses of vigabatrin (e.g., 6 months) are unknown but appear to be low.
  - The short-term rates of clinical remission appear to be superior with hormone treatment (ACTH or HOC) compared to vigabatrin, and this may impact later developmental outcome (at least for those with an unknown etiology).

Second Line

- Ketogenic diet: treatment of choice for some conditions and can be effective for others
- Zonisamide (5–15 mg/kg/day divided twice daily)
- Valproic acid: Consider POLG mutation analysis before starting (15–45 mg/kg/day in 2–3 divided doses).
- Oral pyridoxine: Some cases of pyridoxine-dependent seizures require longer treatment trials (e.g., 10 mg/kg/day for several weeks).
- Topiramate: not a 1st-line treatment due to the low-response rates, but commonly used and occasionally effective (10–30 mg/kg/day once daily or divided twice daily)

SURGERY/OTHER PROCEDURES

- Can be effective and should be considered early (generally after failed 1st-line treatment)
  - Examples: functional hemispherectomy for stroke and hemimegalencephaly, shunting of hydrocephalus, and resection of a tumor for focal cortical dysplasia

INPATIENT CONSIDERATIONS

Initial Stabilization

After the ABCs, consider metabolic stabilization and treatment of convulsive seizures if presenting with IS (IS themselves are typically not life-threatening.).

ONGOING CARE

PROGNOSIS

- Prognosis depends on the underlying etiology and associated conditions.
- Best prognosis in those with unknown etiology and normal development before diagnosis
- About 1/3 die early (most from underlying disease and uncommonly from treatment).
- Spontaneous remission of IS can occur (cumulative rate of 25%, 1 year from onset).
- Regardless of treatment, IS typically remits (persisting beyond 7 years of age in only 8%).
- Early, successful, and sustained electroclinical remission, as well as a short time-lag to treatment, is necessary for optimal outcome
- About 1/3 with electroclinical remission will experience a relapse requiring treatment.
- About 1/2 have other seizure types (occurring before, after, or at the time of IS onset).
- 1/5–1/2 will evolve to LGS.
- 1/5–1/4 will have a favorable outcome (normal or slightly impaired intelligence).
- About 1/3 will have autism (common in TSC).
- About 2/5 will have cerebral palsy.

COMPLICATIONS

For hormone treatment: Hold non-live vaccines for 2 months and live vaccines for 6 months.

ADDITIONAL READING

- Baram TZ, Mitchell WG, Tournay A, et al. High-dose corticotropin (ACTH) versus prednisone for infantile spasms. *Pediatrics*. 1996;97(3):375–379.
- Lux AL, Edwards SW, Hancock E, et al. The United Kingdom Infantile Spasms Study comparing vigabatrin with prednisolone or tetracosactide at 14 days: a multicentre, randomised controlled trial. *Lancet*. 2004;364(9447):1773–1778.
- Pellock JM, Hrachovy R, Shinnar S, et al. Infantile spasms: a U.S. consensus report. *Epilepsia*. 2010;51(10):2175–2189.

CODES

ICD10

- G40.822 Epileptic spasms, not intractable, w/o status epilepticus
- G40.824 Epileptic spasms, intractable, without status epilepticus

FAQ

- Q: Should I prescribe an abortive medication for longer clusters of IS?
- A: Generally, No. IS do not typically respond acutely to benzodiazepines.
- Q: My patient has IS and an abnormal EEG but no hypsarrhythmia. Should I treat him?
- A: Yes. Treat the seizures with 1st-line therapy; only 60% will have hypsarrhythmia.
- Q: Caregivers report that IS has resolved with treatment. Do I need the EEG?
- A: Yes. IS can be subtle making them difficult to detect. In addition, you must have evidence of EEG background improvement.

INFLUENZA

Kristen A. Feemster

BASICS

DESCRIPTION

An acute febrile illness characterized by fever, malaise, and respiratory symptoms

EPIDEMIOLOGY

- Although influenza affects people of all ages, the highest morbidity and mortality occur in young children <2 years old, the geriatric population, and those with high-risk conditions.
- Influenza epidemics occur almost exclusively during winter months, peak ~2 weeks after the index case, and last 4–8 weeks.
- Attack rates are highest among school-aged children (range 10–40%).
- An estimated 10–20% outpatient visits among children <5 years old attributable to influenza
- Transmission of influenza virus occurs via large respiratory droplets or contact with contaminated surfaces.
- After an incubation period of 1–4 days, viral shedding starts 24 hours before symptom onset and usually continues for 7 days.
  - Prolonged shedding in young children and immunocompromised individuals

RISK FACTORS

High-risk conditions for severe disease include the following:

- Chronic pulmonary disease (i.e., asthma)
- Hemodynamically significant cardiac disease
- HIV and other immunodeficiencies
- Chronic immunosuppressive therapy
- Hemoglobinopathies (i.e., sickle cell disease)
- Long-term salicylate use
- Chronic renal dysfunction
- Chronic metabolic disease, morbid obesity
- Neuromuscular disorders

GENERAL PREVENTION

- Vaccination
  - Routine influenza vaccination for ALL individuals ≥6 months old
- Prioritize vaccination for those at highest risk for influenza complications and their close contacts, including young children ages 6–59 months, older adults ≥50 years, adults and children with certain chronic diseases and high-risk conditions, long-term care facility residents, American Indians/Alaska Natives, pregnant women, health care professionals, out-of-home caregivers and household contacts of all children <5 years old OR children 5–18 years old with high-risk conditions (see "Risk Factors").
- Vaccine types
  - Trivalent inactivated influenza vaccine (TIV) approved for ages ≥6 months; administered as an intradermal injection
- Quadrivalent influenza vaccines newly available for 2013–2014 season and beyond; include second influenza B strain
  - Inactivated: Fluarix (GlaxoSmithKline) for ages ≥3 years and Fluzone (Sanofi Pasteur) for ages ≥6 months
  - Live-attenuated influenza vaccine (LAIV); for healthy nonpregnant 2–49-year-olds; administered as an intranasal spray
- Trivalent cell culture-based inactivated vaccine (Flucelvax, Novartis) for ages ≥18 years
- Recombinant hemagglutinin vaccine (FluBlok, Protein Sciences) for ages 18–49 years; egg-free
- Special vaccination considerations:
  - There is no preferential recommendation for one vaccine product over another for children who can receive more than one of the available vaccines.
  - Children ≤8 years old receiving seasonal influenza vaccination for the first time should receive 2 doses of vaccine at least 4 weeks apart.
- LAIV not recommended for individuals with high-risk conditions, young children (ages 2–4 years) with history of wheezing in past year, contacts of severely immunocompromised persons (such as contacts of BMT patients in a protected environment), or children receiving chronic aspirin therapy
  - LAIV can be given simultaneously with other live or inactivated vaccines. However, after administration of any live vaccines, a minimum of 4 weeks should pass before administering another live vaccine.
- Contraindications to vaccination: history of severe allergic reaction to any vaccine component or after previous influenza vaccine dose
  - Precautions: Those with history of Guillain-Barré syndrome within 6 weeks of previous influenza vaccination should consult a physician before receiving the vaccine.
- Influenza vaccines can be safely administered to children with history of egg allergy (see http://www.cdc.gov/flu/professionals/acip/ for specific recommendations).
- Postexposure chemoprophylaxis
  - Indicated for high-risk children who are unvaccinated or were vaccinated within 2 weeks of exposure, immunocompromised patients who have a poor vaccine response, or to control outbreaks in institutions housing high-risk people
  - Chemoprophylaxis should begin within 48 hours of exposure to be most effective.

ETIOLOGY

- Orthomyxoviruses influenza types A, B, and C. Influenza C virus has not been reported as a cause of influenza epidemics.
- Influenza A subtypes defined by 2 surface antigens: hemagglutinin and neuraminidase.
  - Currently circulating subtypes include pH1N1 (pmd09) and H3N2.
- Mild variation, or antigenic drift, for both A and B viruses results in seasonal epidemics; antigenic shift occurs only with A viruses and results in pandemics.

DIAGNOSIS

Clinical case definition of influenza-like illness is fever (≥100°F) AND cough and/or sore throat but may look similar to other respiratory illnesses.

- Positive predictive value of these symptoms for influenza lower (~65%) among children <5 years old
- Clinical presentation varies with age:
  - Infants and young children are less likely to present with typical symptoms but may have higher fever and more severe respiratory symptoms.

HISTORY

- Abrupt onset of illness, beginning with chills, headache, malaise, and dry cough
- Subsequent increase in respiratory tract symptoms that can range from mild cough to severe respiratory distress (infants)
- Other symptoms: fever, anorexia, myalgias, sore throat, irritability
- Younger children may have GI complaints including vomiting, diarrhea, and severe abdominal pain.
- Children may also present with otitis media.

PHYSICAL EXAM

- Cough is the predominant respiratory sign. Infants and small children may exhibit a "barky" cough (croup).
- Nasal congestion with conjunctival and pharyngeal injection
- Cervical adenopathy, especially in children
- Neonates may appear septic with apnea, circulatory collapse, or petechiae.
- A generalized macular or maculopapular rash is sometimes observed.

DIAGNOSTIC TESTS & INTERPRETATION

Laboratory testing can confirm diagnosis, provide surveillance data, and help guide treatment and infection control decisions because clinical symptoms alone may not accurately identify all influenza cases. However, during periods of high influenza activity when the likelihood of infection is high and a child has symptoms consistent with influenza, testing may not be indicated.

- Gold standard: RT-PCR or viral culture
  - RT-PCR preferred: most accurate and sensitive; results within 3–8 hours
  - Only viral culture can be used to measure subtype and antiviral resistance of circulating strains but requires 3–10 days.
- Direct immunofluorescent antibody (DFA) and indirect immunofluorescence antibody (IFA) tests have moderate sensitivity (60–70%) and excellent specificity (>95%) and are completed within 2–4 hours.
  - Predictive value greatly affected by prevalence of circulating influenza.
- Rapid antigen testing (RIDT) available for diagnosing influenza A and influenza B. Results available in ~15 minutes but with wide range of sensitivities (22–77% in community settings) which may limit their usefulness.
- A negative test result should not guide management, especially when community prevalence is high.
- Serology: Look for 4-fold rise in serum antibody titers between acute and convalescent samples (at least 10–14 days apart); not helpful for clinical decision making
- Special considerations for laboratory testing:
  - The false-positive rate for DFA, IFA, and rapid antigen testing may be as high as 20% (influenza A) and 40% (influenza B).
  - Nasopharyngeal aspirates rather than swabs may reduce false-positive rate by 5–10%.
  - Tests most sensitive <4 days of symptom onset

Imaging

Chest x-ray

- May be normal despite significant respiratory involvement
- X-rays of patients with lower airway disease are indistinguishable from those in patients with other viral lower respiratory infections.

Ancillary Laboratory Data

- Leukocyte count may be high, low, or normal with a variable differential.

- Arterial blood gas analysis or pulse oximetry to evaluate oxygenation in severe cases of influenza infection. Infants without radiologic evidence of lower respiratory tract infection can experience apnea or rapid decrements in pulmonary function.
- May see elevated creatine phosphokinase (CPK) with benign acute viral myositis. If with myoglobinuria, consider acute viral rhabdomyolysis, which can damage the kidneys. May require hospitalization and hydration.

DIFFERENTIAL DIAGNOSIS

- Viral infections including but not limited to respiratory syncytial virus, parainfluenza, adenovirus
- *Streptococcus pyogenes*, *Mycoplasma pneumoniae*, or *Legionella* spp infection
- Bacterial sepsis in young infants

TREATMENT

MEDICATION

- Antiviral treatment is recommended for any patient who is
  - Hospitalized
  - Has severe or progressive illness
  - At high risk for complications
- Treatment most effective when initiated <2 days after symptom onset but may still reduce morbidity and mortality for hospitalized patients or patients with severe disease if started up to 5 days after symptom onset.
- Treatment of healthy children with suspected or confirmed influenza in the outpatient setting is at the clinician's discretion but should be initiated <2 days after symptom onset.
- Neuraminidase inhibitors: the recommended antiviral medications for both treatment of and chemoprophylaxis against influenza A and B
- Dosage recommendations:
  - Zanamivir is approved for treatment in children ≥7 years and prophylaxis in children ≥5 years of age.
    - Treatment: two 10-mg inhalations b.i.d. × 5 days
    - Prophylaxis: two 10-mg inhalations once per day × 10 days
    - Can cause bronchospasm so should not be used in patients with history of chronic pulmonary diseases such as asthma
- Oseltamivir is approved for treatment in children ≥2 weeks of age and prophylaxis in children ≥1 year of age.
  - Dose depends on age and weight (<1 year: 3 mg/kg/dose; >1 year and <15 kg: 30 mg; 15–23 kg: 45 mg; >23–40 kg: 60 mg; >40 kg: 75 mg), twice per day × 5 days for treatment and once daily × 10 days for prophylaxis
  - May cause nausea and vomiting
- Amantadine hydrochloride and rimantadine: approved for treatment of influenza A in children >1 year of age but NOT recommended for either treatment or prophylaxis due to increasing resistance. Neither effective against influenza B.
- Resistance to neuraminidase inhibitors <1% among currently circulating influenza strains
- Investigational parenteral medications: peramivir and zanamivir
  - For severely ill high-risk patients with suspected or confirmed oseltamivir-resistant infection
  - Available through emergency investigational new drug protocol only
- Consider longer course of therapy if patient remains severely ill after 5 days.
- Preexposure prophylaxis can be considered for very high-risk patients who cannot be protected through other means when there is high risk of exposure to influenza cases.
  - Duration depends on expected duration of exposure, but 4–6 weeks has been well tolerated.
- Chemoprophylaxis should not be given within 14 days after LAIV receipt as the vaccine strains are susceptible to the antiviral medications.

ADDITIONAL TREATMENT

General Measures

- Most patients with influenza infection require supportive oral hydration, antipyresis, and routine decongestant therapy.
- With the exception of young infants, previously healthy children with influenza infection rarely require emergency treatment.
- Humidified air, with oxygen as needed, is helpful to most patients with respiratory symptoms.
- Airway maneuvers, including endotracheal intubation, may be required for severe laryngotracheitis or patients with hypoxia that is unresponsive to high-flow oxygen administration.

ONGOING CARE

FOLLOW-UP RECOMMENDATIONS

When to expect improvement:

- Fever associated with influenza infection usually lasts up to 5 days. Recrudescence of fever does not necessarily signify the onset of a secondary bacterial infection.
- Cough may last up to 2 weeks.
- Lethargy or malaise may persist for up to 2 weeks.
- Influenza A infection usually lasts longer than influenza B or influenza C infection.

COMPLICATIONS

- Secondary bacterial infections including pneumonia (pneumococcal or staphylococcal)
- Otitis media (24%)
- Sinusitis
- Primary progressive viral pneumonia
- Pulmonary hemorrhage
- Acute myositis during convalescence
  - More common with influenza B
  - Marked by extreme muscle tenderness, especially in the calf muscles
- Rhabdomyolysis/myoglobinuria
- Elevated transaminase levels
- Reye syndrome: fatty degeneration of the liver and diffuse encephalopathy; associated with aspirin use during acute illness
  - More commonly associated with influenza B but may also occur with influenza A
- Febrile convulsions
- Drug toxicity: Influenza infection may result in increased serum levels of certain medications that are metabolized by the liver.
- Rare sequelae in severe cases of influenza infection:
  - Focal and diffuse myocarditis
  - Diffuse cerebral edema
  - Mediastinal lymph node necrosis
  - Sudden death
  - Guillain-Barré syndrome
  - Encephalitis

Patient Monitoring

Signs to watch for:

- Clinical signs of secondary bacterial infection
- Deteriorating mental or respiratory status after initial improvement
- Myoglobinuria in the face of muscle pain

ADDITIONAL READINGS

- Chung EY, Huang L, Schneider L. Safety of influenza vaccine administration in egg-allergic patients. *Pediatrics*. 2010;125(5):e1024–e1030.
- Dawood FS, Chaves SS, Pérez A, et al. Complications and associated bacterial co-infections among children hospitalized with seasonal or pandemic influenza, United States, 2003-2010. *J Infect Dis*. 2014;209(5):686–694.
- Dawood FS, Fiore AE, Kamimoto L, et al. Burden of seasonal influenza hospitalization in children, United States, 2003 to 2008. *J Pediatr*. 2010;157(5):808–814.
- Grohskopf LA, Shay DK, Shimabukuro TT, et al. Recommendations of the Advisory Committee on Immunization Practices—United States, 2013-2104. *MMWR* 2013;62(RR07):1–43.
- Fiore AE, Fry A, Shay D, et al. Antiviral agents for the treatment and chemoprophylaxis of influenza: recommendations of the Advisory Committee on Immunization Practices (ACIP). *MMWR*. 2011;60(1):1–24.
- Stebbins S, Stark JH, Prasad R, et al. Sensitivity and specificity of rapid influenza testing of children in a community setting. *Influenza Other Respir Viruses*. 2011;5(2):104–109.

CODES

ICD10-CM

- J11.1 Influenza due to unidentified influenza virus with other respiratory manifestations
- J10.1 Flu due to oth ident influenza virus w oth resp manifest
- J11.00 Flu due to unidentified flu virus w unsp type of pneumonia

FAQ

- Q: When is it safe for a child with influenza to return to day care or school?
- A: Older children with influenza may shed the virus in nasal secretions for up to 7 days from onset of symptoms and younger children even longer. Therefore, older children with influenza may return to school 1 week after onset of symptoms, and infants and toddlers should remain home for 10–14 days.
- Q: Can a child on chronic steroid therapy be immunized against influenza?
- A: In general, children who require maintenance steroid therapy for their underlying illness should still receive influenza immunization. If possible, immunize while the child is on the lowest possible dose of steroids.
- Q: Is chemoprophylaxis an acceptable alternative for protecting children against influenza?
- A: In general, chemoprophylaxis should not be used as a substitute for vaccination. Specific recommendations and indications for chemoprophylaxis can be found at www.cdc.gov/flu/professionals/antivirals/summary-clinicians.htm.

INGUINAL HERNIA

Nora M. Fullington • Jeremy T. Aidlen

BASICS

DESCRIPTION

Inguinal hernia is a protrusion of abdominal contents (intestine, omentum) into, and often through, the inguinal canal.

EPIDEMIOLOGY

- Inguinal hernia is the most frequent problem requiring elective surgical intervention in children.
- Significantly more common in boys (90% of cases)
- Has a familial tendency
- Because of later descent of right testis and subsequently delayed obliteration of right processus vaginalis, inguinal hernia presents more frequently on the right side.
  - Clinical presentation is on the right side in 60% of cases, on the left side in 30%, and bilateral in 10%.
- Frequency varies with age and ranges from 3–5% in full-term babies to 10–30% in preterm infants.

RISK FACTORS

- Prematurity
- Urologic conditions: cryptorchidism, hypospadias, epispadias, bladder exstrophy
- Abdominal wall defects: gastroschisis, omphalocele, Eagle-Barrett syndrome
- Conditions that increase intra-abdominal pressure (e.g., ascites, peritoneal dialysis, ventriculoperitoneal shunt)
- Cystic fibrosis
- Connective tissue disease: Marfan syndrome, Ehlers-Danlos syndrome
- Mucopolysaccharidoses
- Family history

PATHOPHYSIOLOGY

Indirect inguinal hernia

- During the 7th month of male gestation, the testes begin their descent from the peritoneal cavity through the inguinal canal into the scrotum.
- Between the 7th and 9th months of gestation, after the testes reach the scrotum, the path of peritoneum through which the testicle passed (processus vaginalis) begins to obliterate spontaneously, leaving only a small potential space adjacent to the testes (tunica vaginalis).
- In girls, although the ovaries do not leave the abdomen, the round ligament (part of the gubernaculum) travels through the inguinal ring into labium majus. When the processus vaginalis remains open, it is called the canal of Nuck.
- Incomplete obliteration of the processus vaginalis leaves a sac of peritoneum extending all the way from the internal inguinal ring to the scrotum or labium majus, through which an inguinal hernia may develop.

Direct inguinal hernia

- Uncommon in children
- Results from either a congenital or acquired/traumatic weakness or tear in abdominal wall fascia

Other types of inguinal hernias

- Sliding hernia occurs when one wall of the hernia is composed of abdominal viscera (bladder, colon, adnexa).
- Richter hernia results from the herniation of only a part of the bowel wall. If this hernia is incarcerated/strangulated, it may progress to bowel perforation without obstruction.
- Hernia of Littre includes a Meckel diverticulum within the hernia sac.
- Amyand hernia is an inguinal hernia in which the appendix is included within the hernia sac.

DIAGNOSIS

HISTORY

- Most common presentation is complaint of swelling or bulge in the inguinal area.
- Intermittently appearing
  - Present during times of increased intra-abdominal pressure such as crying or straining
  - A picture taken by the caregiver while the hernia is out may be helpful.
- Reducible hernias are not generally painful.
- If bulge is painful, incarcerated inguinal hernia must be suspected, and other etiologies (e.g., testicular torsion) should be excluded.

PHYSICAL EXAM

- Examine the child in the supine and upright positions.
- If the bulge is apparent in the standing position but disappears when the child is supine, presence of a hernia is strongly suggested.
  - Reduction of hernia contents through the inguinal ring is confirmatory.
  - If the bulge is not readily apparent, perform maneuvers that increase intra-abdominal pressure (gently press on his or her abdomen, have him or her cough, or strain or jump around).
- Transillumination
  - Can be an unreliable finding, particularly in babies
  - Some inguinal hernias (which usually do not transilluminate) can be differentiated from hydroceles (which usually do transilluminate).
- Silk glove sign
  - When empty hernia sac is palpated over the cord structures, sensation is similar to rubbing 2 layers of silk together: thick tissue that slides over cord structures
- Tender scrotal mass: Consider incarcerated hernia, testicular torsion, epididymitis, orchitis, or trauma.

DIAGNOSTIC TESTS & INTERPRETATION

Lab

- In cases where incarceration is suspected, such as presentation with a hard, painful, swelling in the groin, CBC and chemistry should be checked. Leukocytosis or acidosis should increase concern for compromised bowel.
- Genetic testing
  - Karyotype is necessary when a testis is discovered during hernia repair in a phenotypic female. Biopsy of the gonad is also typically performed.
  - 1% of full-term females with bilateral inguinal hernias have a disorder of sexual development—complete androgen insensitivity.

Imaging

Diagnosis is usually made with history and physical exam. However, use of scrotal or inguinal ultrasonography is indicated in cases involving:

- Scrotal tenderness
  - Suggestion of torsion (use duplex ultrasound to evaluate blood flow)
  - Scrotal trauma and concern for testicular rupture
- Mass along the spermatic cord or testicular tumor

DIFFERENTIAL DIAGNOSIS

- Lymphadenopathy
- Hydrocele
- Retractile testis
- Undescended testis
- Varicocele
- Testicular tumor

TREATMENT

GENERAL MEASURES

- Try to reduce the hernia with the child in the supine and/or head-down position so that gravity assists the maneuver.
- Many suggest application of pressure to hernia that is directed toward the inguinal canal.
- Gentle traction of the sac away from the canal and toward the contralateral knee is sometimes more effective if constant pressure is applied to the hernia sac contents.
  - The neck of the hernia is elongated by the traction and placed in line with the inguinal canal.
  - As edema is squeezed out, contents slip back into the abdomen.
- It is typical to feel a "pop" at the internal ring once the hernia is completely reduced. This can lead to immediate relief of symptoms.

SURGERY/OTHER PROCEDURES

Inguinal hernia will not resolve spontaneously and must be treated surgically to avoid incarceration.

- Complication rate after elective inguinal hernia repair is low (1–2%).
- Hernia incarceration commonly occurs in the 1st year of life and is associated with markedly increased complication rate at repair (20%). To avoid this risk, repair is recommended soon after diagnosis of an inguinal hernia.
- Surgeons will often wait 24–48 hours after reduction of an incarcerated hernia to operate in order to allow edema to resolve.
- Routine contralateral inguinal exploration in children with unilateral hernia continues to be a topic of debate. Some surgeons perform diagnostic laparoscopy to evaluate for a contralateral patent processus vaginalis at the time of unilateral herniorrhaphy.
- Laparoscopic inguinal hernia repair can be performed safely in children of all ages, with a variety of techniques.

INPATIENT CONSIDERATIONS

There is no consensus regarding the optimal timing for hernia repair in hospitalized infants. The risk of incarceration must be balanced against the potential risks of operative and anesthetic complications.

ONGOING CARE

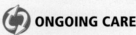

PATIENT EDUCATION

- Preoperative: Parents should consult a physician immediately if signs of incarceration are present (firm or tender lump, pain, or emesis).
- Postoperative: Avoidance of major physical activity for 1 week is recommended.

COMPLICATIONS

- Incarceration: >50% of cases occur within the first 6 months of life.
- Bowel obstruction secondary to incarcerated loop of small intestine
- Strangulation: incarceration with progression to ischemia
- Intestinal infarction can lead to perforation and peritonitis.
- Testicular/ovarian ischemia or infarction. Ovaries are less likely to suffer ischemic insult given narrow vascular pedicle.

ADDITIONAL READING

- Sarpel U, Palmer SK, Dolgin SE. The incidence of complete androgen insensitivity in girls with inguinal hernias and assessment of screening by vaginal length measurement. *J Pediatr Surg*. 2005;40(1):133–136.
- Wang KS; Committee on Fetus and Newborn, American Academy of Pediatrics; Section on Surgery, American Academy of Pediatrics. Assessment and management of inguinal hernias in infants. *Pediatrics*. 2012;130(4):768–773.
- Yang C, Zhang H, Pu J, et al. Laparoscopic vs open herniorrhaphy in the management of pediatric inguinal hernia: a systemic review and meta-analysis. *J Pediatr Surg*. 2011;46(9):1824–1834.

CODES

ICD10

- K40.90 Unil inguinal hernia, w/o obst or gangr, not spcf as recur
- K40.20 Bi inguinal hernia, w/o obst or gangrene, not spcf as recur
- K40.30 Unil inguinal hernia, w obst, w/o gangr, not spcf as recur

FAQ

- Q: When should a pediatric surgeon be consulted for a suspected inguinal hernia?
- A: Inguinal hernias do not resolve and require repair to avoid the complications associated with incarceration and strangulation. A pediatric surgeon should be consulted at the time of diagnosis in order to plan for herniorrhaphy. Additionally, findings suspicious for incarceration or strangulation such as a painful, swollen mass in the inguinal area should result in immediate pediatric surgical consultation as urgent intervention may be required.
- Q: At what age is a patient most at risk for incarceration of an inguinal hernia?
- A: Incarceration of an inguinal hernia most often occurs within the first 6 months of life.

INTELLECTUAL DISABILITY

Rita Panoscha

BASICS

DESCRIPTION

- Intellectual disability (formerly called mental retardation) is characterized by a slow rate of learning or slow cognitive-processing abilities. By definition, there are significant cognitive and adaptive delays first evident in childhood. Significant cognitive delays are defined as 2 standard deviations below the population mean on a standard cognitive or IQ test.
  - Usually indicates an IQ score of <70–75
- Adaptive skills are the functional skills of everyday life, including communication, social skills, daily living/self-care skills, and the ability to safely move about the home and community.
- Intellectual disability is typically subdivided into mild, moderate, severe, and profound categories, depending on the severity of the delays. A more recent definition by the American Association on Mental Retardation (AAMR) puts more emphasis on the level of functioning and the amount of support required by an individual.

ALERT

- Children with behavioral problems may also be masking cognitive delays.
- Hearing impairment may present as a delay in development.
- Children with mild intellectual disability may not be diagnosed as having a problem until they are having difficulties keeping up in elementary school.

EPIDEMIOLOGY

Found in both sexes and all racial and socioeconomic groups

Prevalence

- Prevalence of intellectual disability is generally listed as 2–3% of the population.
- Of the different subcategories of intellectual disability, the mild form is the most prevalent, at 85% of those with intellectual disability.
  - Profound intellectual disability is least prevalent, at ~1% of this group.

GENERAL PREVENTION

- There is no specific prevention, but prevention of some underlying causes may be possible.
- Immunization programs, early detection of metabolic disorders, and education programs for head injury/asphyxia prevention may be useful in some cases.
- Avoidance of alcohol and some drugs during pregnancy may also decrease the likelihood of some specific brain insults.

ETIOLOGY

- The cause of the intellectual disability is usually an insult to the brain or abnormal development of the CNS but is not evident in many cases. The following represent potential causes.
- Genetic/familial/metabolic
  - Fragile X syndrome
  - Trisomy 21 (Down syndrome) and other chromosomal abnormalities
  - Tuberous sclerosis
  - Neurofibromatosis
  - Phenylketonuria (PKU)
  - Other inborn errors of metabolism
- Nervous system anomalies
  - Hydrocephalus
  - Lissencephaly
  - Seizures
- Endocrinologic
  - Congenital hypothyroidism
- Infectious
  - Prenatal cytomegalovirus, rubella, toxoplasmosis, HIV
  - Postnatal bacterial meningitis, neonatal herpes simplex
- Environmental toxins
  - Heavy metal poisoning such as lead
  - In utero drug or alcohol exposure, including fetal alcohol syndrome
- Traumatic
  - Closed-head trauma
  - Asphyxia

COMMONLY ASSOCIATED CONDITIONS

- Associated findings are more common in the more severe forms of intellectual disability.
- Intellectual disability has many associated findings, including seizures, autism, cerebral palsy, communication disorders, failure to thrive, sensory impairments, and psychiatric disorders.
- Behavioral disorders can be seen, including attention-deficit/hyperactivity disorder and self-injurious and self-stimulating behaviors.
- Families often face additional stressors when caring for a child with intellectual disability.

DIAGNOSIS

HISTORY

Complete information regarding the following:

- Pregnancy history
  - Maternal age and parity
  - Maternal complications (including infections and exposures)
  - Medications/drugs used
  - Tobacco or alcohol used, along with quantities
  - Fetal activity
- Birth history
  - Gestational age
  - Birth weight
  - Route of delivery
  - Maternal or fetal complications/distress
  - Apgar scores
- General health
  - Significant illnesses, hospitalizations, or surgeries
  - Accidents or injuries
  - Hearing and vision status
  - Medications used
  - Known exposures to toxins
  - Any new or unusual symptoms
- Developmental history
  - Current developmental achievement in each stream of development
  - Age when developmental milestones were achieved
  - Any loss of skills
  - Where parents think their child is functioning developmentally
- Educational history
  - Type of schooling and services received, if any
  - Any previous educational/developmental testing
- Behavioral history
  - Any perseverative or stereotypical behaviors
  - Interaction skills
  - Attention and activity levels
- Family history
  - Family members with developmental delays, neurologic disorders, syndromes, inherited disorders, or consanguinity

PHYSICAL EXAM

A complete physical exam including growth parameters is needed looking for etiology. Key features to include are the following:

- Observation of interactions and behavior
  - Atypical behaviors and general impressions
- Head circumference
  - Macro- or microcephaly
- Skin exam
  - Neurocutaneous lesions
- Major or minor dysmorphic features
  - Indication of a syndrome or anatomic malformation
- Neurologic exam
  - Assess for cranial nerve deficits, neuromuscular status, reflexes, balance and coordination, and any soft signs.

DIAGNOSTIC TESTS & INTERPRETATION

Lab

Initial lab test

- There is no specific laboratory test battery for intellectual disability.
- Testing must be tailored to the individual situation based on history and physical exam. A high index of suspicion should be maintained for any associated findings and delays in the other streams of development. Listed below are some of the more common studies.

- Genetic testing
  - For any dysmorphic features or a family history of delays or genetic disorder, a karyotype and fragile X DNA testing should be considered, particularly for significant cognitive delays, although the comparative genomic hybridization (CGH) microarray is increasingly recommended as a 1st-line genetic test.
- Metabolic tests
  - Quantitative plasma amino acid, quantitative urine organic acid, lactate, pyruvate, or ammonia levels should be considered if there is any loss of skills or indication of a metabolic disorder.
  - Additional metabolic tests may be indicated depending on symptoms.
- Thyroid function tests
  - Most infants will have had screening for hypothyroidism shortly after birth. This should be rechecked if symptoms indicate.

Imaging

Head MRI: Consider for head abnormalities, significant neurologic findings, loss of skills, or for workup of a specific disorder, such as trauma or leukodystrophy.

Diagnostic Procedures/Other

- When developmental delays are present and intellectual disability is suspected, more formal developmental screening or testing should be done.
- The pediatrician can do some in office developmental screening, but the diagnosis needs to be made based on standardized tests, usually done by a clinical psychologist. Such standardized testing might involve the Stanford-Binet Intelligence Scale, the Wechsler scales, and the Vineland Adaptive Behavior Scales.
- Audiologic testing
  - For any child with speech and language and/or cognitive delays
- EEG
  - An EEG should be considered if there is any concern about seizures.

DIFFERENTIAL DIAGNOSIS

The differential can include several other developmental diagnoses, including the following:

- Borderline cognitive abilities
- Developmental language disorder
- Autism
- Learning disability
- Cerebral palsy
- Significant visual or hearing impairment
- Degenerative disorders

TREATMENT

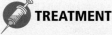

GENERAL MEASURES

- There is no specific cure for intellectual disability. The ultimate goal of all therapies is to help the child reach his or her full potential.
- Therapy should consist of appropriate treatment for any underlying or associated medical condition.
- Early intervention and special education programs are available for an individualized education program based on the child's needs and abilities.
- Behavior management programs or selected use of medications is available for patients with severe behavioral problems.

ISSUES FOR REFERRAL

- A referral is made to a clinical psychologist for the formal diagnosis.
- Subspecialists
  - Referral to other medical specialists may also be indicated.
  - These specialists may include developmental pediatrics, neurology, genetics, or ophthalmology.

ONGOING CARE

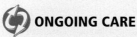

FOLLOW-UP RECOMMENDATIONS

Patient Monitoring

- Children with intellectual disability will need regular pediatric preventive care in addition to management of any underlying medical conditions.
- Ongoing monitoring of the educational programs, to ensure that it is still meeting the child's needs, is important.
- The family will also need ongoing counseling and support in dealing with a child having special needs.

PROGNOSIS

- The prognosis for longevity varies with the associated findings and overall health, but individuals with intellectual disability can live to adulthood and old age.
- An individual's level of functioning is variable depending on the level of retardation, special individual skills, and family or community supports. In general, the following applies:
  - Mild intellectual disability (IQ 55–70): formerly called educable. May be in school with extra help and may achieve roughly a 4th–6th grade level in reading and math. May be employed in an unskilled to semiskilled job. May live in a group home or independently.
  - Moderate intellectual disability (IQ 40–54): may learn to recognize basic words and learn basic skills. May work in a sheltered workshop or with supported employment in an unskilled job. May live with family or in a group home doing much of their own care.
  - Severe intellectual disability (IQ 25–39): may live with family or in a group home or institution. Some may be in a sheltered workshop. May be able to do some daily self-care or chores with supervision.
  - Profound intellectual disability (IQ <25): live with family, in a group home, or in institution. Usually require full-time care.

ADDITIONAL READING

- Battaglia A. Neuroimaging studies in the evaluation of developmental delay/mental retardation. *Am J Med Genet C Semin Med Genet*. 2003;117C(1): 25–30.
- Battaglia A, Carey JC. Diagnostic evaluation of developmental delay/mental retardation: an overview. *Am J Med Genet C Semin Med Genet*. 2003;117C(1):3–14.
- Gropman AL, Batshaw ML. Epigenetics, copy number variation, and other molecular mechanisms underlying neurodevelopmental disabilities: new insights and diagnostic approaches. *J Dev Behav Pediatr*. 2010;31(7):582–591.
- Moeschler JB, Shevell M, American Academy of Pediatrics Committee on Genetics. Clinical genetic evaluation of the child with mental retardation or developmental delays. *Pediatrics*. 2006;117(6):2304–2316.
- Shea SE. Intellectual disability (mental retardation). *Pediatr Rev*. 2012;33(3):110–121.
- Shevell M. Global developmental delay and mental retardation or intellectual disability: conceptualization, evaluation, and etiology. *Pediatr Clin N Am*. 2008;55(5):1071–1084.
- Stankiewicz P, Beaudet AL. Use of array CGH in the evaluation of dysmorphology, malformations, developmental delay, and idiopathic mental retardation. *Curr Opin Genet Dev*. 2007;17(3):182–192.
- Walker WO, Johnson CP. Mental retardation: overview and diagnosis. *Pediatr Rev*. 2006;27(6): 204–211.

CODES

ICD10

- F79 Unspecified intellectual disabilities
- F70 Mild intellectual disabilities
- F71 Moderate intellectual disabilities

FAQ

- Q: Will my child be "normal" by adulthood?
- A: Generally, intellectual disability is considered a lifelong condition. Some individuals, usually with the milder form of intellectual disability, can function well in the community, especially when given added supports.
- Q: Can my child learn?
- A: Except for the most severe forms of intellectual disability, children do learn. This learning may not be as rapid or as extensive as that of a typically developing child.
- Q: But my child looks fine and has had appropriate motor development. How can he be mentally retarded?
- A: Mental retardation or intellectual disability is a slowed rate of cognitive development. Many children with intellectual disability do not have obvious dysmorphic features. Other streams of development, such as gross motor skills, may be reached on time or nearly so, yet the cognitive developmental streams can be significantly delayed.

INTESTINAL OBSTRUCTION

Nora M. Fullington • Jeremy T. Aidlen

BASICS

DESCRIPTION

- Blockage of normal flow of air and other contents through the intestine
  - May be partial or complete, mechanical or functional
  - May arise from intrinsic abnormalities (e.g., meconium ileus, intestinal atresia) or extrinsic abnormalities (e.g., adhesions, bands, or volvulus)
  - May also be caused by neuromotor dysfunction of the gastrointestinal tract (i.e. hypomotility or paralysis of the intestine)
  - Most commonly involves the small bowel
- Untreated, obstruction can lead to intestinal ischemia.

PATHOPHYSIOLOGY

- Pathophysiology depends on the mechanism of the obstruction.
- Functional obstruction (paralytic ileus)
  - Failure of intestinal motor function without mechanical obstruction
    - Common after abdominal surgery, following extensive manipulation of the bowel
    - Other causes: infection (pneumonia, gastroenteritis, urinary tract infection, peritonitis, systemic sepsis), drugs (e.g., opiates, loperamide, vincristine), metabolic abnormalities (hypokalemia, hypomagnesemia, uremia, myxedema, and diabetic ketoacidosis)
- Mechanical obstruction
  - Intestinal dilation proximal to site of obstruction as the bowel fills with intestinal contents and air
  - Common after abdominal surgery following extensive manipulation of the bowel
  - Buildup of intestinal contents results in further distention, nausea, and vomiting.
  - Internal and external losses result in hypovolemia, oliguria, and azotemia.
  - Bacteria proliferate in the small bowel and its contents can become feculent.
  - "Closed loop" obstruction occurs when contents cannot get in or out of an intestinal segment.
- Ischemic obstruction
  - Occurs secondary to occlusion of intestinal blood supply
  - Causes
    - Twisting/kink of feeding blood vessels
    - Increased intramural pressure in the setting of bowel distention can result in decreased perfusion to the affected area.
  - With progression, gangrene, peritonitis, and perforation may occur.
  - Damage to the normal gut barrier may enable bacteria, bacterial toxins, and inflammatory mediators to enter the circulation, causing sepsis.

ETIOLOGY

May be congenital (e.g., atresia, duplication), acquired (e.g., neoplastic, inflammatory), or iatrogenic (e.g., adhesions, radiation stricture)

Etiology varies by age:

- Neonates
  - Intestinal atresia (most common cause in neonates)
  - Obstructive meconium disorders (associated with cystic fibrosis)
    - Meconium ileus
    - Meconium plug syndrome
    - Meconium peritonitis
  - Duodenal atresia (associated with Down syndrome)
  - Annular pancreas
  - Anorectal malformation/Imperforate anus
  - Necrotizing enterocolitis
  - Hirschsprung disease
- Infants
  - Pyloric stenosis (age: 1–2 months)
  - Intussusception (age: 2 months to 2 years)
  - Postoperative adhesions
  - Incarcerated inguinal hernia
  - Hirschsprung disease
  - Duplications
  - Meckel diverticulum
- Older children
  - Postoperative or postinfectious intestinal adhesions (e.g., perforated appendicitis)
  - Inflammatory bowel disease
  - Malrotation with or without midgut volvulus
  - Annular pancreas
  - Meckel diverticulum
  - Superior mesenteric artery syndrome
  - Corrosive injury
  - Foreign body ingestion
  - Juvenile polyposis and related syndromes
  - Distal intestinal obstruction syndrome (cystic fibrosis)
  - Roundworm (*Ascaris lumbricoides*)
  - Gastric and intestinal bezoars
  - Colonic volvulus secondary to aerophagia and constipation (more common in neurodevelopmentally impaired)
  - Cancer-related intestinal obstruction and radiotherapy-induced adhesions

DIAGNOSIS

- Presentation may be acute and dramatic or chronic and subtle. Chronic or intermittent obstruction can be more challenging to diagnose.
- Careful history, physical examination, and consideration of age-related etiology will usually identify the specific cause.

HISTORY

- The classic symptoms of intestinal obstruction include vomiting, abdominal distention, colicky abdominal pain, and failure to pass flatus/stool (vomiting will be bilious if obstruction is distal to ampulla of Vater). Closed loop obstruction may present with pain and retching without emesis.
- Neonates
  - History of maternal polyhydramnios and aspiration of >20 mL gastric fluid after birth may suggest high intestinal obstruction.
  - Failure to pass meconium within 48 hours of birth is suggestive of a distal obstruction.
- Older children
  - Commonly present with pain which can be poorly localized, colicky visceral pain or sharp peritoneal pain
  - Nausea and vomiting: High intestinal obstruction results in bilious emesis; distal obstruction may lead to feculent emesis.
  - Passage of blood or mucus per rectum may be a sign of intestinal ischemia or mucosal sloughing (e.g., intussusception and volvulus).

ALERT

Due to potentially delayed diagnosis and reduced functional reserve, neonates with unrecognized intestinal obstruction deteriorate rapidly, with increased morbidity, mortality, and surgical complications.

PHYSICAL EXAM

- General assessment and vital signs, signs of dehydration, sepsis, or malnutrition
- Palpation typically reveals abdominal distention. It may also reveal the presence of a hernia, a mass suggestive of stool, or intussusception.
- Tenderness denotes inflammation, significant distention, or ischemia and should raise concern for bowel compromise. Guarding and rigidity result from full-thickness bowel wall involvement or perforation/peritonitis.
- Bowel sounds are unreliable. They may be initially increased in hyperperistaltic obstructed loops. They may also become decreased, occasional, or even absent; typically absent sounds with ileus
- Anal inspection excludes anorectal malformation. Rectal examination reveals, at times, a palpable polyp or intussusceptum and blood (overt, occult, or "currant jelly," typical of intussusception).
- Fever, tachycardia, signs of peritonitis, and severe pain that persists after nasogastric decompression may indicate a need for surgical intervention.

DIAGNOSTIC TESTS & INTERPRETATION

Lab

- No laboratory studies are diagnostic, but CBC, electrolytes, and blood gas should be obtained to help optimize supportive treatment.
- Assess for hypochloremic, hypokalemic metabolic alkalosis.
- Bowel infarction may lead to marked leukocytosis, thrombocytopenia, and metabolic acidosis.
- Serum amylase and lipase should be determined to rule out pancreatitis (may be mildly elevated in intestinal obstruction).

Imaging

- Plain abdominal x-rays: supine and erect or decubitus views may identify the classic features: gasless abdomen or air–fluid levels and distended loops of intestine
  - In small bowel obstruction: dilated small bowel, air–fluid levels without gas in the colon
  - Paralytic ileus: distended loops of bowel throughout.
  - Duodenal obstruction: "double-bubble" sign
  - Pneumoperitoneum in perforation
  - Peritoneal calcifications in meconium peritonitis
  - Right lower quadrant ground-glass appearance in meconium ileus
  - High small bowel obstruction or ischemic obstruction (midgut volvulus) may present with normal or nearly normal X-rays.
- Ultrasonography: may identify a mass or phlegmon (e.g., perforated appendix), pyloric stenosis, malrotation (orientation of vessels), intussusception ("target sign" or "Doughnut sign"), or pelvic pathology in adolescents
- CT or MRI: localize the obstruction "transition zone"; diagnosis of strangulation-ischemic segment does not perfuse with contrast; may demonstrate ileus—absence of transition zone, Crohn disease—terminal ileitis or stricture, and neoplasms
- Contrast enema: to confirm/treat intussusception or to evaluate for Hirschsprung; may show "microcolon" of disuse in neonatal small bowel obstruction
- Upper GI series: for malrotation with or without volvulus.
- Water-soluble, low osmolarity materials should be preferred (risk of perforation). Effort should be made to minimize radiation exposure.

ALERT
Evaluation for associated congenital anomalies is mandatory in some surgical conditions, as some are life threatening. The most frequent are cardiac and renal abnormalities.

DIFFERENTIAL DIAGNOSIS

Other causes of abdominal pain and vomiting should be considered and ruled out by history and physical examination:

- Appendicitis
- Torsion of testis or ovary
- Lower lobe pneumonia
- Pancreatitis
- Sickle cell crisis
- Henoch-Schönlein purpura
- Biliary colic
- Lead poisoning
- Acute adrenal insufficiency
- Diabetic ketoacidosis
- Acute intermittent porphyria

ALERT
There is no spontaneous resolution of inguinal hernia. Surgery should be scheduled before incarceration occurs. Inguinal hernias have 10–28% risk for incarceration.

TREATMENT

INITIAL STABILIZATION

- Hold oral intake.
- Decompress the stomach by nasogastric tube.
- Administer IV fluids, correct electrolyte imbalance, and ensure adequate urine output.
- Cultures and broad-spectrum antibiotics (covering gram-negative aerobes and anaerobes) for sepsis or perforation/peritonitis
- Identify etiology of obstruction.

GENERAL MEASURES

- Paralytic ileus is usually self-limiting and resolves with supportive treatment.
- Nasogastric decompression and fluids alone initially for adhesions. Adhesive postoperative obstruction is less likely to resolve without surgery in a child younger than age 1 year old.
- In intussusception, hydrostatic or air enema reduction is successful in 90% of cases.
- Anti-inflammatory medication/steroids for inflammatory obstruction of IBD; persistent strictures may require resection
- Contrast enemas and direct enteral installation of *N*-acetylcysteine for uncomplicated meconium ileus
- Manual reduction of incarcerated inguinal hernias followed by repair
- Colonic volvulus may be treated with endoscopic decompression followed by elective surgery.
- Endoscopic removal of foreign bodies

SPECIAL THERAPY

- Nonoperative management with decompression by nasogastric tube and IV fluids is the 1st-line approach in
  - Early postoperative, partial, and recurrent adhesive obstructions
  - Necrotizing enterocolitis
  - Meconium ileus
  - Duodenal hematomas
  - Superior mesenteric artery syndrome
  - Crohn disease

SURGERY/OTHER PROCEDURES

- Surgery may be required for definitive correction of bowel obstruction.
- Exceptions to this rule may include the above-mentioned conditions managed conservatively.
- In all situations: If no improvement within 12–24 hours, surgery is advisable.
- Additionally, bowel obstruction without a definitive causal diagnosis requires surgery.
- The surgical procedure is individualized according to the specific type, site, anatomy of the obstruction, and associated conditions.
- Laparoscopic surgery can be used for the diagnosis and repair of select intestinal obstructions and for adhesiolysis.

ONGOING CARE

PROGNOSIS

- Varies with different causes of intestinal obstruction, age of the patient, and associated conditions
- Extensive bowel resection or multiple repeat bowel resections can lead to short bowel syndrome, in which a requirement for long-term central access and parenteral nutrition is associated with significant morbidity and mortality.

COMPLICATIONS

- May result from delayed operation
  - Dehydration, azotemia, renal failure
  - Intestinal ischemia with sepsis and shock
  - Bowel perforation and peritonitis
  - Short-gut syndrome

ADDITIONAL READING

- McAteer JP, Kwon S, LaRiviere CA, et al. Pediatric specialist care is associated with a lower risk of bowel resection in children with intussusception: a population-based analysis. *J Am Coll Surg*. 2013;217(2):226–232.
- Reid JR. Practical imaging approach to bowel obstruction in neonates: a review and update. *Semin Roentgenol*. 2012;479(1):21–31.
- Young J, Kim DS, Muratore CS, et al. High incidence of postoperative bowel obstruction in newborns and infants. *J Pediatr Surg*. 2007;42(6):962–965.

CODES

ICD10

- K56.60 Unspecified intestinal obstruction
- P76.0 Meconium plug syndrome
- Q41.9 Congen absence, atresia and stenosis of sm int, part unsp

FAQ

- Q: When should I consult a pediatric surgeon?
- A: If there is concern for bowel obstruction, a pediatric surgical consultation should be obtained early. In some cases, emergency surgery is necessary, whereas other times, it is more reasonable to place an NGT, administer IV fluids, and monitor for gradual resolution of the obstruction by clinical exam and radiographs.
- Q: Why are nasogastric tubes used in the treatment of intestinal obstruction?
- A: Tube decompression of the stomach allows for some symptomatic relief of nausea. In addition, it decreases the amount of fluid in obstructed intestine which may speed recovery. NGT output volume and character can guide management.
- Q: Is my child likely to have recurrent episodes of intestinal obstruction?
- A: It depends on the cause of the obstruction. Conditions associated with recurrence include intussusception, inflammatory conditions, and postoperative adhesions.

INTOEING–TIBIAL TORSION

George D. Gantsoudes

BASICS

DESCRIPTION

- Intoeing, as a presumptive diagnosis, results in numerous orthopedic consultations.
- Causes of intoeing are most frequently one or more of the following: metatarsus adductus, internal tibial torsion, and femoral anteversion.
- Definitions:
  - Version: normal variation in axial alignment
  - Torsion: any variation beyond two standard deviations of normal
- Clear explanation of the difference between physiologic variations and pathologic anatomy will allow the treating physician to effectively manage expectations.

EPIDEMIOLOGY

Very common; one the most common reasons for a "well child" to visit an orthopedist

RISK FACTORS

Genetics

No strong evidence of familial links

PATHOPHYSIOLOGY

- Most are self-limiting issues but when paired together, can cause significant issues.
- Excessive femoral anteversion and external tibial torsion can result in the so-called "miserable malalignment," known to cause significant patellofemoral issues.

ETIOLOGY

- In utero, fetuses are subjected to forces that mold feet and tibiae into adductus and internal torsion, respectively.
- Most children are born with a relatively increased femoral anteversion (approximately 45 degrees).
  - Tends to resolve and "unwind" as the child develops
  - Usually resolves by age 8–10 years to the normal adult anteversion of 10–20 degrees

ASSOCIATED CONDITIONS

May be more common in first-born children (especially metatarsus adductus) as part of the "packaging disorders" such as developmental dysplasia of the hip and torticollis

DIAGNOSIS

HISTORY

- Varies based on age of presentation
- The most common reasons for malalignment visits in the preambulatory infant are either intoeing due to metatarsus adductus, or due to an external hip rotation contracture that all children have, which results in an obligatory and physiologic outtoeing.
- The ambulatory toddler will commonly come in with either intoeing or "bowleggedness" as a complaint.
  - The bowleggedness is almost always physiologic or related to the illusion of genu varum due to the child externally rotating their hips to prevent tripping over their internally rotated feet.
- Intoeing in an older child is most often due to femoral anteversion, which is slightly slow to "unwind."
- The most common complaints are as follows:
  - Frequent tripping
  - Motor delay that is slower than peers or other relatives
  - Family member observation (e.g., an older relative who insists "something is wrong")
- There may be also be an adult family member with similar issues who did not "grow out of it," prompting an early evaluation.

ALERT

Functional limitations (such as tripping and falling frequently) may suggest other diagnoses, such as mild cerebral palsy, especially if abnormal birth history, abnormal developmental milestones, and physical findings consistent with cerebral palsy.

PHYSICAL EXAM

- Goal to rule out significant pathologies that could cause the relatively benign complaints
  - For example, any male child with a history of clumsiness must get a Gower test and deep tendon reflexes to rule out muscular dystrophy.
- If possible, observe the child exploring the room before starting the physical exam. The examiner may gain more information here than at any other point in your exam.
- Watch the child walk and run in the hallway.
  - Ask the child to toe walk, heel walk, and use tandem gait (walk in a straight line touching the heel of one foot to the toes of the other foot) to further explore levels of coordination and function.
  - Look at the foot progression angle (angle formed between axis of foot and axis of forward progression of gait); normally 6–10 degrees of external rotation. An abnormal angle should be explainable by looking at rotation of other parts of leg during gait (hip rotation, thigh-foot angle, and/or foot abnormalities). If something does not add up, ask the child to walk again.
  - Gait can be too complex to observe all at once. If necessary, focus on one level (hips, knees, feet) at a time and have the child walk back and forth numerous times.
  - A "quick hint" is to watch the patella when evaluating the knees; they should always be roughly collinear with the feet.
- All children should have a thorough hip exam to rule out hip dysplasia as a cause.
  - All children have their hip abduction checked; any asymmetry is further evaluated with pelvis x-rays.
  - Children younger than 2 years: Get a Barlow/Ortolani to check for hip instability.
    - Barlow: Adduct hip (thigh toward midline) applying light pressure on knee and direct force posteriorly. Positive sign if femoral head dislocates.
    - Ortolani: Flex hip to 90 degrees, use index fingers to place anterior pressure on greater trochanters, and abduct the legs using thumbs. Positive sign is "clunk" as femoral head relocates in acetabulum.
- The usefulness of a prone hip rotation exam far outweighs that of the supine exam.
- When examining for tibial torsion, there are a few different methods to evaluate the angle.
  - Thigh-foot axis
    - With the patient prone and the knee flexed 90 degrees, measure the difference between the axis of the foot and the axis of the femur.
    - The angle of the foot should be approximately 15 degrees externally rotated.

- Transmalleolar axis
  - With the patella facing the ceiling, the axis between the floor and a line drawn through the malleoli is measured.
  - Twenty degrees external is normal.
- 2nd toe test
  - With the patient prone, the second toe is rotated until it is perpendicular to the floor.
  - The femur is then held in place and the knee is flexed 90 degrees.
  - The angle of the tibia to the vertical should be roughly 20 degrees.
- Metatarsus adductus is assessed by looking at the sole of the foot and drawing a bisecting line from the center of the heel distal. The line should travel through the 2nd and 3rd webspace. The further lateral the bisector line exits the foot, the more severe the adductus.
  - Spontaneous correction of the adducted forefoot is a positive sign and is assessed by gently stroking the lateral border of the foot.
- Assess for limb length differences.
- Asses deep tendon reflexes.

DIAGNOSTIC TESTS & INTERPRETATION

Lab

Never useful for simple torsion

Imaging

- Almost never ordered for run-of-the-mill torsional exams
- Order AP and frog pelvis films if there is a high suspicion of hip dysplasia.
- A standing (or supine) AP limb alignment x-ray can be a useful tool to examine for frontal plane abnormalities; taken from pelvis to ankles
  - Should be standardized at each institution with patellae facing the beam
- In the event of significant torsion, advanced imaging (e.g., CT or MRI) can be ordered to discover the true anatomic axes. This is almost always obtained exclusively as a preoperative tool.

DIFFERENTIAL DIAGNOSIS

- Almost always the diagnosis is that of physiologic alignment.
- The examiner must rule out cerebral palsy, muscular dystrophy, hip dysplasia, etc.

TREATMENT

- The younger child (younger than 8 years) should spontaneously resolve minor internal torsion of the tibia and femur.
- Corrective shoes, Denis-Brown bars, twister cables, stretching, and formal physical therapy no more effective than observation. In addition, there has been some correlation of poor self-esteem in those patients prescribed with braces.
- Observation is the rule.
  - There are no restrictions to activity, in fact the children should be encouraged to be active.
- Recalcitrant torsion in the older patient may be an indication for osteotomy to derotate the limbs, only very rarely recommended.
- Managing family expectations is crucial.
  - It may be helpful to have a handout to give to families, to both explain the issues and to show the frequency with which the diagnosis shows up in the office.
  - Get comfortable with a standard explanation of the normal physiology; use terms that are easy to understand.
  - Families may be reassured by data suggesting positive correlation with intoeing and elite-level sprinting.

ONGOING CARE

PROGNOSIS

- Most patients are discharged with follow-up "as needed" with instructions to return if the problem hasn't improved over a period of 2 years or if the problem acutely worsens.
- Patience is strongly encouraged, as the "unwinding" of the limbs takes years to occur.
- The overall prognosis is excellent.
  - This is a very common reason for an orthopedic visit and a very rare reason to go the operating room.

COMPLICATIONS

Many patients will come in already having seen practitioners (podiatry, physical therapy, chiropractic, orthotists) who will associate torsion with degenerative arthritis and as a cause of more proximal issues (hips, spine). The evidence for this is anecdotal at best.

ADDITIONAL READING

- Craig CL, Goldberg MJ. Foot and leg problems. *Pediatr Rev*. 1993;14(10):395–400.
- Fuchs R, Staheli LT. Sprinting and intoeing. *J Pediatr Orthop*. 1996:16(4):489–491.
- Schoenecker PL, Rich MM. The lower extremity. In: Morrissy RT, Weinstein SL, eds. *Lovell and Winter's Pediatric Orthopaedics*. 6th ed. Philadelphia, PA: Lippincott Williams & Wilkins; 2005:1157–1212.
- Staheli LT. Lower positional deformity in infants and children: a review. *J Pediatr Orthop*. 1990;10(4): 559–563.

CODES

ICD10

Q68.4 Congenital bowing of tibia and fibula

FAQ

- Q: Are special shoes or braces ever indicated for tibial torsion?
- A: Almost never. There is no convincing evidence that any of these treatments truly alter the natural history of the condition. The situation will improve without treatment in most children.
- Q: Why do patients with torsional pathology occasionally have knee pain?
- A: Children may have increased femoral anteversion with associated external tibial torsion (i.e., an external rotation of the tibia that matches and, in effect, balances the internal rotation of the femur). This can be diagnosed by observing the rotational profile and by noting an increased Q-angle of the knee. This situation is sometimes a "setup" for patellofemoral pain.

INTRACRANIAL HEMORRHAGE

Jorina Elbers

BASICS

DESCRIPTION

The pathologic accumulation of blood into the epidural, subdural, subarachnoid, intraparenchymal, or intraventricular space within the cranium due to loss of blood vessel integrity or coagulopathy

EPIDEMIOLOGY

- Intraventricular hemorrhage is rare beyond the newborn period.
- Trauma: common cause of ICH in children
- Arteriovenous malformations (AVMs): most common cause of nontraumatic ICH in children

Incidence

Incidence of hemorrhagic (nontraumatic) stroke is 1.1 per 100,000 person years.

RISK FACTORS

Increased frequency with hereditary disorders of coagulation, congenital heart disease, and polycystic kidney disease associated with intracranial aneurysms

Genetics

Multiple cerebral cavernomas may be associated with autosomal dominant trait with *CCM1*, *CCM2*, and *CCM3*.

GENERAL PREVENTION

- Automobile seat belts
- Bicycle, skating, and skateboarding helmets
- Child abuse prevention
- Diving safety practices
- Preventing falls
- Maintaining safe driving speeds
- Keeping children away from firearms
- Hematologic monitoring for those at risk for hemorrhage due to bleeding disorders

PATHOPHYSIOLOGY

- Epidural hematoma (blood between the dura mater and the skull) is frequently arterial, related to skull fracture; typically middle meningeal artery bleeding following temporal bone fracture; may also arise from dural venous sinus laceration.
- Subdural hematoma (blood between the dura mater and the arachnoid membrane) is frequently venous from trauma causing stretching and tearing of bridging cortical veins or coagulopathy.
- Subarachnoid hemorrhage (blood between the arachnoid membrane and brain): ruptured intracranial aneurysm, AVM, or trauma
- Intraparenchymal hemorrhage: trauma, infections (herpes simplex encephalitis, bacterial endocarditis), coagulopathy, brain tumor, Moyamoya arteriopathy, venous sinus thrombosis, or cerebral infarction (occurs mostly with rupture of medium or smaller branches of major cerebral arteries)
- Intraventricular hemorrhage: may occur in isolation (more frequent in preterm infants <36 weeks gestation) or in a mixed pattern with intraparenchymal or subarachnoid hemorrhage. In term infants, rule out venous sinus thrombosis (especially in patients with accompanying thalamic hemorrhage).
- 4 grades of intraventricular hemorrhage:
  - Grade I: isolated to 1 or both germinal matrices
  - Grade II: intraventricular hemorrhage without ventricular dilatation
  - Grade III: intraventricular hemorrhage with ventricular dilatation (hydrocephalus)
  - Grade IV: intraventricular hemorrhage with ventricular dilatation and extension into the periventricular white matter

ETIOLOGY

- Vascular
  - Congenital vascular anomalies: aneurysm, AVM, cavernous hemangioma, arteriovenous fistula, vein of Galen malformation
  - Developmental/acquired vasculopathy: Ehlers-Danlos syndrome type IV, Moyamoya arteriopathy, sickle cell disease, hypertension (posterior reversible encephalopathy syndrome [PRES]), infective aneurysm, vasculitis (cocaine, inflammatory diseases), cerebral venous sinus thrombosis, hemorrhagic conversion of ischemic stroke, brain tumor
- Hematologic abnormalities: thrombocytopenia, hemophilia, sickle cell disease, liver failure, disseminated intravascular coagulation, iatrogenic (ECMO or anticoagulation therapy)
- Traumatic
  - Accidental injury
  - Nonaccidental injury

ALERT

ICH, especially in young infants and children without an obvious etiology, should raise the suspicion of nonaccidental trauma.

COMMONLY ASSOCIATED CONDITIONS

- Prematurity
- Hemophilia (prevalence of ICH 3–12%)
- Sickle cell disease (250-fold increased risk of ICH)
- Bacterial endocarditis
- Venous infarction
- Arterial infarction
- Alcohol, cocaine, and other sympathomimetics

DIAGNOSIS

HISTORY

- Delivery complications
- Head trauma
- Infection
- Cardiac disease
- High-output cardiac failure
- Patient or family history of coagulopathy
- Drug use
- Cerebral venous sinus thrombosis: dehydration, coagulopathy, polycythemia, sepsis, asphyxia (especially in newborns)
- Arterial aneurysms: polycystic kidney disease, coarctation of the aorta, fibromuscular dysplasia, connective tissue disease
- Vein of Galen malformation: presents as failure to thrive, hydrocephalus, seizures, high-output cardiac failure
- Clinical presentation of ICH: headache (severity, quality, onset, location), neck pain or stiffness, vomiting, irritability, altered level of consciousness ("lucid interval" with epidural hematoma), seizures, visual problems (diplopia, blurred vision), focal neurologic deficits, epistaxis (may occur if skull fracture is present)
  - Posterior fossa bleed: disconjugate gaze, ataxia, and rapid deterioration to coma

ALERT

Increasing intracranial pressure from hemorrhage or hydrocephalus is life threatening.

PHYSICAL EXAM

- Signs of increased intracranial pressure or herniation, such as Cushing triad (hypertension, bradycardia, abnormal respiratory pattern); papilledema; fixed, dilated pupil; ophthalmoparesis
- In infants, increased intracranial pressure may result in a bulging fontanelle, splayed sutures, and increasing head circumference.
- Low-grade fever
- Meningeal signs
- In setting of trauma:
  - Leakage of CSF from the ear or nose
  - Battle sign: bruising over the mastoid process suggestive of basilar skull fracture
  - Raccoon eyes: periorbital ecchymosis suggestive of basilar skull fracture
  - Retinal hemorrhages

DIAGNOSTIC TESTS & INTERPRETATION

Lab

- CBC
- Metabolic profile
- INR, prothrombin time, activated partial thromboplastin time (PT/aPTT)
- Fibrinogen
- Factors VIII, IX, XI
- Von Willebrand factor antigen
- Urine toxicology screen
- Electrocardiogram (for evaluation of cardiac disease or endocarditis)
- Lumbar puncture: Lumbar puncture will show RBCs, reduced glucose, and xanthochromia. Consider spinal fluid evaluation if CT negative.

Imaging

Initial approach

- Rapid CT of the head
  - The most important study to obtain when considering ICH in the differential diagnosis because of its relative convenience, speed, and low false-negative rate
  - Acute intracerebral blood demonstrates increased density; between 1 and 6 weeks becomes isodense with adjacent brain parenchyma. Acute ICH may appear isodense if hemoglobin <8–10 g/dL.

- Epidural hemorrhage: biconvex, lens-shaped hemorrhage, displacing gray–white matter
- Subdural hemorrhage: crescent-shaped hemorrhage; bilateral subdural hemorrhage frequent in nonaccidental injury
- Contrast-enhanced CT: Contrast extravasation within the hematoma may identify patients at high risk of ICH expansion.
- MRI gradient echo and T2 susceptibility-weighted imaging are helpful for acute and remote hemorrhage.

Follow-Up Tests & Special Considerations

- CT/MRI/conventional cerebral angiography and venography: for evaluation of vascular lesions, including congenital vascular anomalies, vasculopathies, venous sinus thrombosis
- Head ultrasound: Intraventricular hemorrhage in infants warrants serial head ultrasound exams to rule out hydrocephalus.

ALERT
Early subarachnoid hemorrhage may not be apparent on initial CT and may require lumbar puncture (if safe to perform) or serial CT evaluation while the patient is under clinical observation.

DIFFERENTIAL DIAGNOSIS

- Ischemic stroke/transient ischemic attack
- Brain tumor
- Headache (migraine, primary thunderclap)
- Metabolic derangements (hyper/hyponatremia, hypoglycemia)
- Encephalitis
- Meningitis
- Seizure with post-ictal Todd paralysis

TREATMENT

MEDICATION

- Correction of coagulopathies (suggested by PT, PTT, platelet abnormalities) should be done promptly and may require hematology evaluation. Therapies include vitamin K, fresh frozen plasma, cryoprecipitate, or platelet infusion. Monitor for fluid overload, especially in patients with cardiac disease.
- Management of elevated blood pressure: Blood pressure should be maintained within normal parameters for age with a target of 50th–95th percentile according to age and height. Nicardipine drip (1 mcg/kg/min) or labetalol (0.2 mg/kg IV push over 2–3 minutes, repeat every 15 minutes PRN)
- Management of seizures: fosphenytoin or levetiracetam 20 mg/kg IV load + maintenance for clinical or electrographic seizures. No evidence for seizure prophylaxis in ICH.
- Acyclovir therapy if herpes simplex type 1 encephalitis is considered
- Recombinant factor VIIa is FDA-approved in children with hemophilia who have systemic bleeding and are resistant to factor VIII therapy.
- Corticosteroids NOT recommended; may result in harmful hyperglycemia

ADDITIONAL TREATMENT

General Measures

- Temperature management: maintain normothermia. Fever associated with worse neurologic outcome in adults
- Maintain normoglycemia and euvolemia
- Urgent neurosurgical consultation
- Management of elevated ICP: head of bed elevated to 30 degrees, maintain adequate analgesia and sedation, consider invasive ICP monitoring and aggressive therapies (mannitol, hypertonic saline, hyperventilation) in consultation with neurosurgery and PICU
- Consider continuous EEG monitoring for seizures.

ADDITIONAL THERAPIES

Physiotherapy, occupational therapy, speech therapy as required

SURGERY/OTHER PROCEDURES

- Elevated intracranial pressure may necessitate surgical hematoma evacuation or decompressive hemicraniectomy.
- Aneurysms or AVMs may require neurosurgical or neurointerventional treatment.

INPATIENT CONSIDERATIONS

Initial Stabilization

- Admission to pediatric/neurointensive care unit
- Urgent management of coagulopathy, hypertension, seizures, elevated ICP as listed earlier

Admission Criteria

- Patients with altered mental status to monitor for elevated ICP
- Patients with focal neurologic deficits for workup and rehabilitation
- Patients with seizures for continuous EEG monitoring and anticonvulsant management
- Patients with hypertension for management
- Patients with coagulopathy for correction
- Patients requiring neurosurgical or neurointerventional management

IV Fluids

Avoid D5 and excessive fluid administration; maintain euvolemia.

ONGOING CARE

FOLLOW-UP RECOMMENDATIONS

Patient Monitoring

Long-term observation for signs of injury: cognitive deficits, focal weakness, seizures

PROGNOSIS

- Children may develop long-term focal or cognitive deficits or seizures.
- Often, good neurologic recovery is possible.
- Predictors of poor neurologic outcome: infratentorial location, GCS ≤7 at admission, aneurysm, age <3 years, underlying hematologic disorder

COMPLICATIONS

- Increased intracranial pressure and brain herniation syndromes
- Hydrocephalus
- Vasospasm secondary to blood and breakdown products of erythrocytes
- Seizures
- Motor, visual, and cognitive deficits
- Death (5–54%, pooled data 25%)

ADDITIONAL READING

- Jordan LC, Hillis AE. Hemorrhagic stroke in children. *Pediat Neurology*. 2007;36(2):73–80.
- Lo WD, Lee J, Rusin J, et al. Intracranial hemorrhage in children. An evolving spectrum. *Arch Neurol*. 2008;65(12):1629–1633.
- Proust F, Toussaint P, Garniéri J, et al. Pediatric cerebral aneurysms. *J Neurosurg*. 2001;94(5):733–739.
- Roach ES, Golomb MR, Adams R, et al. Management of stroke in infants and children: a scientific statement from a special writing group of the American Heart Association Stroke Council and the Council on Cardiovascular Disease in the Young. *Stroke*. 2008;39(9):2644–2691.
- Squier W. Shaken baby syndrome: the quest for evidence. *Dev Med Child Neurol*. 2008;50(1):10–14.

CODES

ICD10

- I62.9 Nontraumatic intracranial hemorrhage, unspecified
- S06.300A Unsp focal TBI w/o loss of consciousness, init
- Q28.2 Arteriovenous malformation of cerebral vessels

FAQ

- Q: What is the annual risk of hemorrhage in children with known AVM?
- A: The estimated annual hemorrhagic risk is 2–4%. In 25% of patients, the hemorrhage is fatal.
- Q: How often should an asymptomatic child at risk for AVM be screened, and with what imaging modality?
- A: Depending on the risk of aneurysm in a given condition, screening with MRA every 1–5 years is reasonable.

INTUSSUSCEPTION

Pradeep P. Nazarey

BASICS

DESCRIPTION

- The invagination or telescoping of a proximal portion of bowel (the intussusceptum) into a distal segment of bowel (the intussuscipiens)
  - Can be unremitting (80%) or transient (20%)
  - 85% are ileocolic; ileoileal and colocolic types also occur.
  - Telescoping of the bowel occurs over a "lead point"—a lesion or defect in the bowel wall.
- Telescoping of the bowel causes diminished venous blood flow and bowel wall edema, which can result in ischemia and obstruction.
  - Over time, arterial blood flow is inhibited and infarction of the bowel wall occurs, which results in hemorrhage.
  - If untreated, possible perforation and death
- Bowel necrosis can occur within 48–72 hours after onset.
- Clinical presentation can vary but usually includes the following:
  - "Paroxysms of pain": episodes of calmness interspersed with fussiness
  - Bilious vomiting
  - "Currant jelly stools" which represent mucosal sloughing

EPIDEMIOLOGY

- 1–4/1,000 live births
- Male-to-female ratio: 2:1
- Generally occurs in patients 3 months to 3 years of age
- Peak age: from 5 to 10 months
- More common in winter months
- The most common abdominal emergency of early childhood and second most common cause of abdominal pain next to constipation
- Increased incidence in children who received the RotaShield rotavirus vaccine (no longer available). Currently available vaccines (RotaTeq or Rotarix) have not been shown to increase the risk.

ETIOLOGY

- Children <3 years: usually idiopathic (95%) or due to an enlarged Peyer patch (from viral infection)
- Children ≥3 years: higher incidence of a pathologic lead point (4%): Meckel diverticulum, polyps, and lymphomas are most common. Other common etiologies include Henoch-Schönlein purpura (HSP), Peutz-Jeghers syndrome, intestinal duplications, inflammatory bowel disease, and other tumors.
- Postoperative(1%): can occur in children who have had large retroperitoneal tumors removed

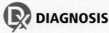

DIAGNOSIS

HISTORY

- Common to have recent history (prodrome) of a viral upper respiratory illness or gastroenteritis
- Classical presentation involves the sudden onset of severe intermittent (colicky) abdominal pain characterized by drawing the legs up to the abdomen and crying.
  - Subsequently, the child may appear asymptomatic between paroxysms of pain that recur in <24 hours.
  - Classical presentation only occurs in 25–30% of patients.
- Young infants may appear listless or lethargic during episodes.
- Nonbilious emesis initially, becomes bilious with progressive obstruction
- Currant jelly stools (sloughed mucosa, blood, and mucous) appear in 50% of cases and should be considered a late finding suggestive of a longer course of the disease prior to presentation.

PHYSICAL EXAM

- Lethargic with intermittent colicky abdominal pain
- Palpable abdominal mass, usually in right upper quadrant, tubular or "sausage" shaped
- Dance sign: absence of bowel contents in right lower quadrant
- Abdominal distention
- Rectal exam: blood-tinged mucous or currant jelly stool
- Symptoms and signs of peritonitis

DIFFERENTIAL DIAGNOSIS

- Infectious
  - Gastroenteritis
  - Enterocolitis
  - Parasites
- Immunologic
  - HSP
- Gastrointestinal
  - GER or GERD
  - Food allergy
  - Inflammatory bowel disease
  - Celiac disease
- Miscellaneous
  - Appendicitis
  - Peutz-Jeghers syndrome
- Obstruction
  - Adhesions
  - Hernias
  - Volvulus
  - Stricture
  - Foreign body
  - Polyp
  - Tumor

DIAGNOSTIC TESTS & INTERPRETATION

Lab

CBC, electrolytes

Imaging

- Abdominal x-ray
  - May show paucity of gas in right lower quadrant, air–fluid levels
  - "Meniscus sign" is indicative of a mass in the colon (25–45%).
- Abdominal ultrasound
  - Primary diagnostic modality
  - Highly sensitive and specific with experienced radiologist
  - "Target sign" with presence of several concentric rings of bowel
  - Can sometimes indicate the pathologic lead point

- Contrast enema
  - Diagnostic and therapeutic with reduction often achieved (95%)
  - Air enema (good chance of success, low risk of perforation,) preferred over barium enema (more effective but higher risk of perforation)

ALERT
- Only 25–30% of patients present with the classical triad of abdominal pain, vomiting, and currant jelly stool, so high clinical suspicion is necessary.
- Patients should always have an IV placed and be undergoing fluid resuscitation prior to imaging or procedures.

TREATMENT

GENERAL MEASURES
- Prompt recognition and reduction is imperative.
- Spontaneous reduction occurs in 5–20%.
- IV insertion, fluid therapy, and surgical consultation should be obtained once diagnosis is entertained.
- Broad-spectrum antibiotics if perforation, peritonitis, or bacterial translocation due to a compromised gastrointestinal mucosa is suspected
- Radiologic, pneumatic reduction with air contrast enema is mainstay of therapy.
- Absolute contraindications to reduction by enema:
  - Peritonitis
  - Shock
  - Perforation
- Multiple attempts may be made at reduction if initially unsuccessful or patient transferred to tertiary care facility after failed attempt.
- Perforation during reduction occurs in <1% of cases, mostly in the transverse colon, and requires immediate operative intervention.

SURGERY/OTHER PROCEDURES
- If patient presents with generalized peritonitis and/or signs of perforation, they should immediately go to the OR.
- Unsuccessful attempts at pneumatic reduction
- Open surgery involves milking the intussusceptum out of the intussuscipiens and rarely involves resection.
- Laparoscopic surgery has gained more traction with better outcomes, cosmesis, and shorter length of stay.

ONGOING CARE

FOLLOW-UP
- Some centers may discharge home immediately or observe after nonoperative reduction.
- Diets can be advanced quickly.

EDUCATION
- Parents should be counseled that a 10% recurrence risk exists after nonsurgical reduction in the first 24 hours.
- Recurrences may require repeat pneumatic reduction and/or ultimate operative intervention.

PROGNOSIS
- Timely diagnosis results in a highly favorable prognosis with no effects on the bowel.
- Recurrences or failed reduction in children >3 years old may require workup for pathologic lead point.

COMPLICATIONS
- Bowel necrosis secondary to local ischemia
- Gastrointestinal bleeding
- Bowel perforation
- Sepsis, shock, death

ADDITIONAL READING

- Daneman A, Navarro O. Intussusception. Part 1: a review of diagnostic approaches. *Pediatr Radiol*. 2003;33(2):79–85.
- Daneman A, Navarro O. Intussusception. Part 2: an update on the evolution of management. *Pediatr Radiol*. 2004;34(2):97–108.
- McCollough M, Sharieff GQ. Abdominal surgical emergencies in infants and young children. *Emerg Med Clin North Am*. 2003;21(4):909–935.
- Pepper VK, Stanfill AB, Pearl RH. Diagnosis and management of pediatric appendicitis, intussusception, and Meckel diverticulum. *Surg Clin North Am*. 2012;92(3):505–539.
- Vesikari T, Matson DO, Dennehy P, et al. Safety and efficacy of a pentavalent human-bovine (WC3) reassortant rotavirus vaccine. *N Engl J Med*. 2006;354(1):23–33.

CODES

ICD10
K56.1 Intussusception

FAQ

- Q: Can my child have a recurrent intussusception?
- A: Yes, if your child has had a nonsurgical reduction via air (or barium) enema. However, the risk is considered low (<10%). If the lead point has been removed surgically, recurrence is very unlikely. The greatest risk for recurrence is in the first 24 hours after reduction.
- Q: What are common ages for presentation with intussusception?
- A: 3 months to 3 years is the age range associated with the greatest risk of intussusception, but it may occur at any age. The prevalence of intussusception being a sign of an underlying pathologic condition rises with age.
- Q: Could an infant have intussusception and not be crying in pain?
- A: Yes. Infants often present without the classical manifestations of intussusception. It is critical to have a high index of suspicion in any infant presenting with acute onset of emesis, especially bilious emesis, and lethargy.

IRON DEFICIENCY ANEMIA

Irina Pateva • Peter de Blank

BASICS

DESCRIPTION

A reduction in hemoglobin production due to an insufficient supply of iron that results in a microcytic, hypochromic anemia

EPIDEMIOLOGY

- Iron deficiency is the most common nutritional deficiency of children.
- Leading cause of anemia among infants and children in the United States
- Most commonly seen in children ages 9 months–3 years and in teenage girls

Prevalence

- Prevalence is variable depending on socioeconomic status, availability of iron-fortified formulas, and prevalence and duration of breastfeeding.
- Prevalence of iron deficiency anemia in United States is generally between 1% and 5% of children.

RISK FACTORS

- Low socioeconomic status
- Certain ethnic groups (e.g., Southeast Asian) may be at increased risk due to dietary practices.
- History of prematurity

GENERAL PREVENTION

- Maintain breastfeeding for the first 5–6 months of life if possible.
  - Breast milk has lower iron concentration than formula, but iron in breast milk is more bioavailable (50% vs. 10%).
- Iron supplementation
  - 1 mg/kg/day for infants who are exclusively breastfed beyond 4 months
  - 2 mg/kg/day by 1 month of life for low-birth-weight and premature infants who are breastfed because of poor iron stores and increased growth rate
  - Iron-fortified formula for the first 12 months of life for infants who are not breastfed
  - Encourage iron-enriched cereal when infants are started on solid food.
- Avoid whole cow's milk during the 1st year of life to prevent occult GI bleeding.
- Screen hemoglobin level at periodic intervals.
  - The American Academy of Pediatrics recommends screening at 12 months, 1–3 years old, and adolescents as well as annually in menstruating females.
  - CDC recommends screening high-risk groups annually between ages 2 and 5 years and all menstruating women every 5–10 years.

PATHOPHYSIOLOGY

- Iron is required for oxygen transport by hemoglobin.
- Iron absorption and distribution is regulated by hepcidin, a peptide hormone secreted by liver, macrophages, and adipocytes.
- Iron is absorbed primarily in the duodenum.
- Iron deficiency develops because of an inadequate supply or increased demand for iron or a combination of these.
- Sequential stages of iron deficiency
  - Depletion of iron stores: reflected by low serum ferritin and absent bone marrow stores
  - Iron-deficient erythropoiesis: Near-normal number of red blood cells (RBCs) produced, but they have abnormal hemoglobin synthesis with wide distribution in RBC size.
  - Iron deficiency anemia: microcytosis evident

ETIOLOGY

- Causes of inadequate supply include dietary deficiency and malabsorption.
  - Dietary deficiency in infants and young children results from introduction of cow's milk prior to age 12 months, exclusive breastfeeding beyond age 6 months without iron supplementation, and excessive cow's milk intake (>24 oz/day).
  - Malabsorption results from surgical resection of intestine or celiac disease.
  - Certain foods impair iron absorption (tannins in tea and coffee, phytates).
- Causes of increased demand include rapid growth and blood loss.
  - Periods of rapid growth include infancy (especially low-birth-weight and premature infants) and adolescence.
  - GI blood loss is most common and includes cow's milk enteropathy (seen in infants), inflammatory bowel disease (IBD), and bleeding from Meckel diverticulum.
- Other etiologies of blood loss include perinatal loss, menorrhagia, pulmonary hemosiderosis, and hematuria.

DIAGNOSIS

HISTORY

- Evaluate dietary intake of iron, including breast- or formula feeding and type of formula (iron fortified or low iron).
- Age at introduction of cow's milk
- Daily intake of cow's milk
- Birth history for prematurity or blood loss
- Lead exposure
- Blood loss from urine, stool, menorrhagia
- Iron deficiency anemia often develops slowly, and no symptoms may be present. When present, signs and symptoms include the following:
  - Irritability and behavioral disturbances
  - Fatigue, exercise intolerance
  - Pallor
  - Headache
  - Pica or pagophagia (chewing ice)

PHYSICAL EXAM

- Often normal
- Pallor, irritability
- Tachycardia, flow murmur if anemia is more severe
- Koilonychia (spoon nails)
- Glossitis or stomatitis

DIAGNOSTIC TESTS & INTERPRETATION

Lab

- Hemoglobin level <2 standard deviations below the age-specific mean defines anemia.
- Low MCV (red cell volume) and MCH (hemoglobin concentration) for age
- High RDW (red cell distribution width)
  - Measures the variation in red cell size
  - Normal is <14.5%.
  - Often increased before anemia is present
- Low serum ferritin (≤12 ng/mL) reflects reduced tissue iron stores.
  - Earliest laboratory abnormality
  - May be normal or increased with concurrent infection or inflammation
  - Higher cutoff improves sensitivity of the test.
  - Ferritin ≤30 ng/mL has sensitivity of 92% and PPV of 83% for iron deficiency anemia versus sensitivity of 25% for ferritin ≤12 ng/mL.
- Low serum iron
- Increased total iron-binding capacity
- Low transferrin saturation; measures the iron available for hemoglobin synthesis
- Increased soluble transferrin receptor (sTfR)
  - Indicator of increased tissue iron demand
  - Also increased in thalassemia syndromes but not in anemia of chronic inflammation
  - sTfR/log(ferritin) <1 suggests anemia of chronic inflammation.
  - sTfR/log(ferritin) >2 suggests iron deficiency anemia.
- Decreased reticulocyte hemoglobin content: This test is an early indicator of iron deficiency because reticulocytes have a short (1–2-day) lifespan before becoming mature red cells.
- Increased free erythrocyte protoporphyrin, a precursor molecule in hemoglobin synthesis; also high in lead poisoning and chronic inflammation
- Thrombocytosis (can approach 1 million/dL)
- Peripheral blood smear with microcytosis, hypochromia, poikilocytosis (varying shapes), pencil forms, and anisocytosis (varying sizes)
- Test for occult blood in stool often positive with GI blood loss
  - However, the test can be positive with oral iron supplementation.
- Iron absorption test can assess adequacy of PO iron supplementation. 3 mg/kg elemental iron should increase serum iron more than 100 mcg/dL within 4 hours of ingestion.

Diagnostic Procedures/Other

Bone marrow examination: shows decreased iron stores by Prussian blue staining; it is the gold standard to determine iron stores but rarely needed to establish diagnosis.

DIFFERENTIAL DIAGNOSIS

- Recent infection
- Lead poisoning
- Thalassemia trait
- Anemia of chronic inflammation (e.g., juvenile rheumatoid arthritis, IBD)
- Sideroblastic anemias

TREATMENT

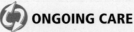

- Iron supplementation
- Family education regarding age-appropriate diet and iron-containing foods
- Specific treatment if underlying condition causing blood loss is found (e.g., hormonal therapy for menorrhagia, medications for IBD)
- May require initial inpatient observation in cases of severe anemia
- Red cell transfusion only if evidence of cardiovascular compromise (rarely indicated)

MEDICATION

First Line

Oral replacement with ferrous iron, 3–6 mg/kg/24 h of elemental iron divided into 2 or 3 doses

- Iron should be given on an empty stomach or with a vitamin C–containing juice to increase absorption. Ascorbic acid increases oral absorption of iron by ~30%.
- Side effects (in 10–20%) include nausea, constipation, GI upset, and vomiting. Iron suspensions can stain teeth temporarily.

Second Line

Parenteral iron formulations are indicated for severe noncompliance or malabsorption or if ongoing loss exceeds absorption capacity. Administration may be associated with pain at injection site or anaphylaxis, less common with newer preparations such as ferric gluconate and iron sucrose.

ISSUES FOR REFERRAL

- Evaluation for source of GI blood loss
- Unexplained recurrence after treatment
- Failure to improve with iron supplementation

INPATIENT CONSIDERATIONS

Admission Criteria

- Active bleeding
- Severe anemia (hemoglobin level <6 g/dL) especially if symptoms or ongoing blood loss
- Tachycardia, S_3 gallop, or other signs of CHF

Nursing

Family education: teaching administration of iron and dietary counseling

Discharge Criteria

- No signs of CHF
- If blood loss, bleeding is controlled
- Stable hemoglobin level
- Parent demonstrates ability to administer oral iron therapy to young children and demonstrates adequate knowledge about dietary modifications.
- Adequate follow-up ensured

ONGOING CARE

FOLLOW-UP RECOMMENDATIONS

Patient Monitoring

- Reticulocyte count increases in 3–4 days.
- Hemoglobin concentration should rise by at least 1 g/dL in 2–3 weeks.
- Continue iron for 2 months beyond correction of anemia to replenish body stores.
- Causes of poor response to oral iron supplementation include the following:
  - Nonadherence (most common)
  - Ongoing blood loss
  - Insufficient duration of therapy
  - High gastric pH
  - Concurrent lead intoxication
  - Other diagnosis: Thalassemia trait and anemia of chronic disease are not iron responsive.

DIET

- Milk should be restricted to <24 oz daily or eliminated in those with milk protein enteropathy.
- Bottle should be discontinued after 12 months.
- Diet should include foods rich in iron: meats, beans, iron-fortified cereal, strawberries, spinach.

PATIENT EDUCATION

- Activity: Usually, no activity restriction is needed. Those with severe anemia resulting in CHF should have limited activity until the anemia is corrected.
- Diet: A diet containing iron-rich foods should be encouraged. Limit milk intake to <24 oz daily.
- Prevention: Prevention of iron deficiency is preferable. Anticipatory guidance about diet, prolonged bottle use, etc., should be given.

PROGNOSIS

- Anemia is readily corrected with iron replacement.
- Developmental delay may be long lasting or irreversible.

COMPLICATIONS

- Impaired cognitive and motor development as well as behavioral changes in infants and toddlers
- Short-term memory impairment and poor exercise performance in adolescents

ADDITIONAL READING

- Baker RD, Greer FR; Committee on Nutrition American Academy of Pediatrics. Diagnosis and prevention of iron deficiency and iron-deficiency anemia in infants and young children (0–3 years of age). *Pediatrics*. 2010;126(5):1040–1050.
- Centers for Disease Control and Prevention. Iron deficiency—United States 1999-2000. MMWR Morb Mortal Wkly Rep. 2002;51(40):897–899.
- Goodnough LT, Nemeth E, Ganz T. Detection, evaluation, and management of iron-restricted erythropoiesis. *Blood*. 2010;116(23):4754–4761.
- Konofal E, Lecendreux M, Deron J, et al. Effects of iron supplementation on attention deficit hyperactivity disorder in children. *Pediatr Neurol*. 2008;38(1):20–26.
- Centers for Disease Control and Prevention
- McCann JC, Ames BN. An overview of evidence for a causal relation between iron deficiency during development and deficits in cognitive or behavioral function. *Am J Clin Nutr*. 2007;85(4):931–945.
- Wu AC, Lesperance L, Bernstein H. Screening for iron deficiency. *Pediatr Rev*. 2002;23(5):171–177.

CODES

ICD10

- D50.9 Iron deficiency anemia, unspecified
- D50.8 Other iron deficiency anemias
- D50.0 Iron deficiency anemia secondary to blood loss (chronic)

FAQ

- Q: What dietary changes can help prevent the recurrence of iron deficiency?
- A: Limit milk to 24 oz/day to improve appetite for iron-containing foods. Heme iron, found in meats, fish, and poultry, is absorbed better than nonheme iron and enhances absorption of nonheme iron. Other foods that have iron are raisins, dried fruit, sweet potatoes, lima beans, chili beans, green peas, peanut butter, and enriched foods. Give iron on an empty stomach along with an ascorbic acid–containing juice to increase absorption. Foods that decrease absorption include bran, vegetable fiber, tannins found in tea, and phosphates. Antacids may also decrease iron absorption.
- Q: What are the side effects of iron therapy?
- A: Iron may cause temporary staining of the teeth, which can be decreased by diluting the iron with a small amount of juice. Iron will also change the color of bowel movements to greenish black. Constipation may occur.
- Q: What are the most important tests to do to establish the diagnosis of iron deficiency?
- A: For patients with a history of dietary deficiency or known blood loss, a CBC that shows a low hemoglobin and MCV and an elevated RDW is very suggestive of iron deficiency. A therapeutic trial of iron without further laboratory testing is an appropriate next step. A rise in the hemoglobin concentration of ≥1 g/dL after 1 month of therapy confirms the diagnosis. Otherwise, further laboratory testing is necessary and other diagnoses should be considered.
- Q: How does a concurrent infection affect the diagnosis of iron deficiency?
- A: Common childhood infections may be associated with a mild microcytic anemia that resembles iron deficiency. Laboratory tests to diagnose iron deficiency may be misleading while a child is acutely ill. Acute infection is associated with a shift of iron from serum to storage sites, causing a decrease in serum iron and an increase in ferritin. It is more helpful to test a child for iron deficiency 3–4 weeks after an acute infection.

IRON POISONING

Carl Tapia • Angela Mazur

BASICS

DESCRIPTION

- Iron poisoning is a common and potentially fatal ingestion.
- Toxicity depends on the amount of elemental iron ingested, although tolerable and lethal concentrations are not firmly established.
- Doses of <20 mg/kg of elemental iron are generally not symptomatic, of 20–60 mg/kg are variably symptomatic, and of >60 mg/kg are severe toxic and potentially fatal.

EPIDEMIOLOGY

- Accounts for about 2–4% of all exposures in children and adolescents
- Many factors contribute to the incidence of iron ingestion:
  - High-iron preparations such as prenatal vitamins are readily available.
  - Many preparations are attractive and candy-like.
  - Caregivers often fail to appreciate the danger of overdose from vitamins and pure iron preparations.
- Although vitamin ingestions are increasing, the incidence of fatal iron ingestions has declined since the 1990s, perhaps due to changes in package labels and child-resistant packaging.

RISK FACTORS

- Birth of a sibling (increased availability of maternal vitamins)
- Among unintentional ingestion, almost all serious mortality and morbidity is in children younger than 5 years of age (ingestion of adult iron formulations).

PATHOPHYSIOLOGY

- Iron directly damages cells, interfering with aerobic respiration. The primary systems affected by iron are the gastrointestinal (GI) tract, including the liver, and the cardiovascular system.
- There are five classic stages of iron poisoning:
  - Stage I (GI phase)
    - Occurs up to 6 hours postingestion
    - Characterized by GI mucosal injury, leading to pain, vomiting, diarrhea, and GI bleeding
    - Metabolic acidosis may be present, and death may be caused by capillary leakage and hypovolemic shock.
  - Stage II (quiescent)
    - 6–24 hours after ingestion
    - Relative stability and temporary resolution of GI symptoms
  - Stage III (recurrence)
    - 24–48 hours after ingestion
    - Recurrence of GI injury leading to bleeding, shock, and acidosis
    - Vasodilation can lead to hypovolemia, and myocardial injury can lead to cardiogenic shock.
    - Coagulopathy is common.
  - Stage IV (hepatotoxicity)
    - Within 48 hours after ingestion
    - May result in liver failure
  - Stage V (late)
    - 2–8 weeks postingestion
    - Gastric injury may result in strictures, leading to vomiting and potentially gastric outlet obstruction.

DIAGNOSIS

HISTORY

- Witnessed or suspected iron product ingestion
- Determine the amount of elemental iron ingested and the time of ingestion.
- The percentage of elemental iron by iron salt is ferrous fumarate, 33%; ferrous chloride, 28%; ferrous sulfate, 20%; and ferrous gluconate, 12%.

PHYSICAL EXAM

ALERT
Strongly consider the diagnosis of acute iron poisoning in a lethargic, hypotensive toddler.

- Evaluate for poor perfusion: hypotension, decreased capillary refill, pallor, tachycardia, and CNS depression (lethargy or coma).
- Evaluate for GI injury: abdominal tenderness and occult or apparent GI bleeding.
- Evaluate for heart injury: distant heart sounds, poor pulses, mottled skin, distended jugular veins, pulmonary edema.

DIAGNOSTIC TESTS & INTERPRETATION

Lab

Initial lab tests

- Blood gas
- Complete blood count
- Glucose, liver function, and coagulation studies
- Renal function
- Electrolytes

Imaging

- Abdominal radiograph
  - May reveal iron pills. The absence of findings does not exclude iron toxicity (liquid preparations and multivitamins are not radiopaque).
  - GI decontamination may be recommended if undissolved tablets are confirmed.

Diagnostic Procedures/Other

- Serum iron level
  - Measure on presentation and every 1–2 hours.
  - The serum iron level peaks at 4–6 hours postingestion and can help determine the severity of overdose. Iron levels 300–500 mcg/dL: usually mild to moderate GI toxicity; 500–1,000 mcg/dL: serious toxicity; greater than 1,000 mcg/dL: severe and life-threatening toxicity
- Total iron-binding capacity (TIBC) not recommended (may be inaccurate in toxicity)

DIFFERENTIAL DIAGNOSIS

- Ingestions
  - Methanol
  - Propylene glycol
  - Ethanol
  - Ethylene glycol
  - Salicylate
  - Toluene
- GI bleeding
  - Trauma
  - Perforation
  - Intussusception
  - Gastritis
  - Esophageal inflammation or tear
  - Vascular malformation
- Other
  - Reye syndrome
  - Serious bacterial infection: sepsis, meningitis
  - Diabetic ketoacidosis

TREATMENT

GENERAL MEASURES

- Asymptomatic patients after 6 hours of ingestion or ingestions of less than 40 mg/kg elemental iron with mild symptoms can be observed at home.
- Symptomatic patients with persistent or severe GI symptoms, or ingestion with greater than 40 mg/kg elemental iron, should be evaluated in a health care facility.

SPECIAL THERAPY

- GI decontamination
  - Whole-bowel irrigation for patients with a significant number of pills on imaging studies
  - Gastric lavage with tap water or normal saline if early after ingestion and suspect a large iron load
  - Activated charcoal is not recommended (iron binds poorly).
  - Syrup of ipecac is not recommended.
  - Rarely, endoscopy or gastrotomy may need to be performed to remove embedded pills.
- Iron chelation with deferoxamine
  - Deferoxamine binds with free iron and is excreted by the kidneys. It is indicated if systemic signs of toxicity or peak iron concentration is greater than 500 mcg/dL.
  - Administered parenterally via continuous infusion at 15 mg/kg/h. (Consultation with a specialist or regional poison control center is recommended.)
  - Chelation can be discontinued with clinical improvement and resolution of metabolic acidosis.
  - Side effects of chelation include hypotension and acute respiratory distress.
  - Although iron cannot be dialyzed, the ferrioxamine complex after chelation can be, and dialysis may be indicated in the setting of acute renal failure.

INPATIENT CONSIDERATIONS

Initial Stabilization

- Evaluate and stabilize shock.
- Intubation should be considered in a lethargic patient to facilitate GI decontamination.

Admission Criteria

- Patients with mild but persistent symptoms after 6 hours or ingestion with greater than 40 mg/kg (recommend consultation with a specialist or poison control center)
- Symptomatic patients with significant toxicity or shock should be treated in an intensive care setting by specialists skilled in management of pediatric ingestions.

Discharge Criteria

Stable hemodynamic status and resolution of metabolic acidosis (recommend consultation with a specialist or poison control center)

ONGOING CARE

FOLLOW-UP RECOMMENDATIONS

Monitor for possible late complications, such as strictures of the GI tract (can occur up to 2 months postingestion).

PATIENT EDUCATION

Encourage families to secure iron-containing vitamins and supplements out of reach of children.

PROGNOSIS

- Iron ingestions rarely result in serious injury.
- Shock and ingestion of elemental iron greater than 1,000 mcg/dL associated with mortality

COMPLICATIONS

- GI and hepatic infarction and necrosis
- Gastric or intestinal scarring and strictures
- Metabolic acidosis
- Shock (hypovolemic, hemorrhagic, cardiogenic)
- Coagulopathy
- Pulmonary edema
- *Yersinia enterocolitica* infection or sepsis (Chelation can encourage bacterial growth.)
- Death

ADDITIONAL READING

- Fine JS. Iron poisoning. *Curr Probl Pediatr*. 2000;30(3):71–90.
- Henretig FMI. Acute iron poisoning. In: Shaw LM, Kwong TC, eds. *The Clinical Toxicology Laboratory: Contemporary Practice of Poisoning Evaluation*. Washington, DC: AACC Press; 2001:401–409.
- Madiwale T, Liebelt E. Iron: not a benign therapeutic drug. *Curr Opin Pediatr*. 2006;18(2):174–179.
- Manoguerra AS, Erdman AR, Booze LL, et al. Iron ingestion: an evidence-based consensus guideline for out-of-hospital management. *Clin Toxicol*. 2005;43(6):553–570.
- Tenenbein M. Unit-dose packaging of iron supplements and reduction of iron poisoning in young children. *Arch Pediatr Adolesc Med*. 2005;159(6):557–560.

CODES

ICD10

- T45.4X1A Poisoning by iron and its compounds, accidental, init
- T56.891A Toxic effect of other metals, accidental (unintentional), initial encounter

FAQ

- Q: Why isn't syrup of ipecac recommended to induce vomiting?
- A: Because the major early signs and symptoms involving the GI tract include vomiting, inducing vomiting may interfere with the clinical assessment. There is also the risk of aspiration in the patient with severe poisoning.
- Q: What is the recommendation regarding observation of a patient for development of symptoms with iron ingestion of an unknown quantity?
- A: Observe for 6 hours. Those who are asymptomatic 6 hours after ingestion are not likely to exhibit systemic illness.
- Q: What is the recommendation regarding nonintentional ingestion of children's vitamins with iron, carbonyl iron formulations, or polysaccharide iron complex formulations?
- A: These ingestions are generally deemed to contain low levels of iron, and the American Association of Poison Control Centers recommends against emergency room referral for nonacute patients with adequate home supervision. Even patients with mild diarrhea and emesis can be safely observed in the home following these ingestions, although consultation with a physician and poison control hotline is still advised.

IRRITABLE BOWEL SYNDROME

Laurie N. Fishman

BASICS

DESCRIPTION
- Irritable bowel syndrome (IBS) is a common functional GI tract disorder where defecation is disordered and associated with abdominal discomfort.
- Characterized by abdominal pain, bloating, diarrhea or constipation
- Symptoms of IBS do not result from inflammatory, infectious, metabolic, or anatomic causes. However, there can be overlap with other conditions.
- Symptoms typically exacerbated by stress or particular foods (i.e., spices, fatty foods, caffeine)

EPIDEMIOLOGY
- 10–15% of the general population is affected by IBS.
- More common in females
- Prevalence estimates vary based on whether the study is community-based or practice-based, as many people do not seek medical care.
- Prevalence is also based on whether Manning, Rome II, or Rome III criteria are used.
- IBS occurs in children and was found to affect 6% of middle school students and 14% of high school students in one community-based study.

RISK FACTORS
- Prior history of bacterial enteritis
- History of abuse or trauma

PATHOPHYSIOLOGY
- IBS considered a disorder of GI function relating to motility, sensation, and/or perception.
- Best model is a biopsychosocial construct with dysregulation of the gut-brain homeostasis affected bidirectionally by both peripheral and central factors.
- The pathogenesis of IBS is believed to be multifactorial and include the following:
  - Abnormal gut motility
  - Genetics
  - Bacterial overgrowth
  - Visceral hypersensitivity
  - Behavioral response
  - Microscopic inflammation
  - Dysregulation of brain-gut axis
  - Malabsorption

DIAGNOSIS

HISTORY
- IBS is not a diagnosis of exclusion.
- Diagnosis is based on careful history with particular attention to characteristics of pain, precipitating factors, and defecation pattern.
- Symptoms that support constipation-predominant IBS (IBS-C) include the following:
  - <3 stools per week
  - Hard or lumpy stools
  - Straining with defecation
- Symptoms that support diarrhea-predominant IBS (IBS-D) include the following:
  - >3 stools per day
  - Loose or mushy stools
  - Urgency
- All IBS types may have the following:
  - Sense of incomplete evacuation
  - Mucus in stools
  - Abdominal bloating
- Symptoms may not only intensify with known stressors (such as school exams), but also with positive experiences (such as parties, amusement park trips, dates, or prom).

DIAGNOSTIC TESTS & INTERPRETATION

Lab
- There is no laboratory testing that confirms IBS. Tests are done solely to rule out other conditions.
- Selective testing:
  - CBC, ESR, or CRP,
  - Stool for occult blood
  - Stool for parasites (*Giardia*)
  - Total IgA, tissue transglutaminase (IgA)
  - Stool lactoferrin or calprotectin
  - Consider albumin.
  - Consider lactose testing.
- More testing needed if "red flags" present the following:
  - Weight loss (over 5–10 lb)
  - Bloody stool
  - Fever
  - Anemia
  - Family history of inflammatory bowel disease or GI cancer

Imaging
There is no imaging that can be used to diagnose IBS. Imaging studies should be performed if indicated to evaluate for other conditions.

Diagnostic Procedures/Other
- In severe IBS, with weight loss and diarrhea resulting in incontinence or nocturnal stooling, colonoscopy may be required to rule out colitis.
- If history and empiric restriction do not lead to clear answer, as to whether lactose intolerance is a contributing factor, can perform lactose breath testing to objectively quantify lactase activity

DIFFERENTIAL DIAGNOSIS
- Giardia infection
- Lactose intolerance
- Fructose intolerance
- Celiac disease
- Inflammatory bowel disease
- Constipation with overflow
- Endometriosis
- Medication effects
- Psychiatric disorder (especially anxiety, depression, posttraumatic stress disorder, or school avoidance)

TREATMENT

- The aims of IBS treatment are to:
  - Improve a global sense of well-being
  - Reduce specific symptoms
- It is important to remind patients that treatment will not cure their IBS.
- Comprehensive treatment consists of the following:
  - Education about IBS
  - Dietary changes
  - Fiber
  - Probiotics/antibiotics
  - Pharmacology
  - Herbal and natural products
  - Complementary techniques
  - Psychological techniques
  - Continued provider relationship

MEDICATIONS
- Antibiotics can be used intermittently for gassiness and bloating symptoms:
  - Neomycin, rifaximin (nonabsorbed)
  - Metronidazole, norfloxacin (systemic)
- Bile acid malabsorption has been postulated as a trigger in IBS-D (even in absence of liver or ileal disease). Potential medications include cholestyramine (Questran), colesevelam
- Symptomatic relief for diarrhea:
  - Consider loperamide (mu opioid receptor agonist).
  - Side effects include constipation.
- Symptomatic relief for constipation:
  - Consider magnesium, polyethylene glycol, senna, or bisacodyl; however, these therapies are not well-studied for this indication.
- Lubiprostone
  - Can be used at 8 mcg b.i.d. for general IBS discomfort or 24 mcg b.i.d. for constipation
  - Nausea is a frequent side effect.
- Linaclotide
  - Guanylate cyclase receptor agonist
  - Recently approved for patients older than 18 years of age with IBS-C
  - Minimal side effects as not absorbed systemically
- Antispasmodics (dicyclomine, hyoscyamine)
  - Can be used on a regular basis or as needed
  - It can be very reassuring to the patient to have a medication available when needed.

- Belladonna/phenobarbital is also described as useful, but is not available in United States.
- Low-dose antidepressants (amitriptyline, citalopram)
  - Can be very useful for the treatment of abdominal pain.
  - It is important to explain the rationale for using these medications to avoid the misperception by the patient that the diagnosis is a psychiatric disease.
- Placebo rates in IBS are often more than 40% in studies. Effectiveness of known placebos for patients with migraine may also be helpful in patients with IBS.

ADDITIONAL TREATMENTS

General Measures

- For patients with mild symptoms of IBS, reassurance, education, and lifestyle changes such as avoiding identified triggers may be adequate for management.
- In patients with more severe or complex symptoms, a multidisciplinary approach including pharmacotherapy and psychosocial intervention may be needed.

COMPLEMENTARY & ALTERNATIVE THERAPIES

- Probiotics
  - Current literature suggests mixed results from clinical trials
  - Different individual and combinations of probiotics strains of *Bifidobacterium*, *Lactobacillus*, and *Saccharomyces* have been used.
  - 3–4 weeks of treatment are considered adequate trial.
- Herbal products
  - Chamomile, in the form of warm tea, can be helpful for spasms.
  - Peppermint, either tea or capsules of peppermint oil, will relax the smooth muscle via the calcium channel. Can cause heartburn
  - Less commonly cited remedies have been reported such as artichoke leaf extract, turmeric, and natural clay powder.

ISSUES FOR REFERRAL

- Psychological therapies such a cognitive behavioral therapy (CBT) and psychodynamic therapy are helpful.
  - Acquiring CBT skills can help lower stress, address comorbid anxiety or depression, and often have lasting effect.
- Hypnotherapy requires trained provider, but has proven benefits lasting 6–12 months.

DIET

- Have patients systematically look at typical dietary triggers:
  - Spicy foods
  - Fatty or fried foods
  - high-sugar foods
  - Beans/legumes
  - Sugar-free gum, candy, or drinks
  - Lactose
- Try gluten withdrawal (after testing to rule out celiac), as some patients can have non-celiac gluten sensitivity.
- In conjunction with a nutritionist, consider trying elimination of FODMAP foods (fermentable oligosaccharides, disaccharides, monosaccharides and polyols)
- Fiber
  - Gradually increase to goal of 10 g (adults) or age +5 g (child)
  - Fiber can help with global symptoms and constipation, less helpful for pain.
  - Soluble fibers (psyllium, ispaghula, calcium polycarbophil) improve symptoms, whereas insoluble (bran, corn) worsen symptoms.
  - Adequate trial of any particular fiber is at least 3–4 weeks, may need to try multiple types.

ONGOING CARE

FOLLOW-UP RECOMMENDATIONS

Patient Monitoring

- The provider–patient relationship is an important component of therapy, and ongoing visits can help monitor symptoms.
- Planned medical follow-up also provides a sense of well-being, helps patients to anticipate flares, and prevent repeated evaluations.

PATIENT EDUCATION

- Establish a positive diagnosis:
  - It is important that patients perceive that their MD "knows they have IBS" rather than the MD has "ruled everything else out so the diagnosis must be IBS."
- Reassurance about overall health
- Explain there are many interventions (diet, medication, techniques) that will improve, although not cure, symptoms.
- Reassure patients that you will not abandon them but continue to help.

COMPLICATIONS

- Patients with moderate to severe IBS can have significantly lower quality of life, absenteeism from school/work.
- IBS can also lead to frequent physician visits, unnecessary medical testing, and high health care costs.

ADDITIONAL READING

- Bijkerk CJ, de Wit NJ, Muris JW, et al. Soluble or insoluble fibre in irritable bowel syndrome in primary care? Randomised placebo controlled trial. *BMJ*. 2009;339:b3154.
- Bijkerk CJ, Muris JW, Knottnerus JA, et al. Systematic review: the role of different types of fibre in the treatment of irritable bowel syndrome. *Aliment Pharmacol Ther*. 2004;19(3):245–251.
- Chogle A, Mintiens S, Saps M. Pediatric IBS: an overview on pathophysiology, diagnosis and treatment. *Pediatr Ann*. 2014;43(4):e76–e82.
- Cristofoi F, Fontana C, Magista A, et al. Increased prevalence of celiac disease among pediatric patients with irritable bowel syndrome: a 6-year prospective cohort study. *JAMA Pediatr*. 2014;168(8):555–560.
- Dom SD, Morris CB, Hu U, et al. Irritable bowel syndrome subtypes defined by Rome II and Rome III criteria are similar. *J Clin Gastroenterol*. 2009;43(3):214–220.
- Halmos EP, Power VA, Shepherd SJ, et al. A diet low in FODMAPs reduces symptoms of irritable bowel syndrome. *Gastroenterology*. 2014;146(1):67–75.
- Spiegel BM, Farid M, Esrailian E, et al. Is irritable bowel syndrome a diagnosis of exclusion? A survey of primary care providers, gastroenterologists, and IBS experts. *Am J Gastroenterol*. 2010;105(4):848–858.

CODES

ICD10

- K58.9 Irritable bowel syndrome without diarrhea
- K58.0 Irritable bowel syndrome with diarrhea

FAQ

- What is the FODMAP diet?
- The FODMAP diet involves the exclusion of foods that are "fermentable," as well as those with "oligosaccharides, disaccharides, monosaccharides, and polyols." Following the FODMAP diet been shown to provide relief for patients with IBS.

JAUNDICE

Kathleen M. Loomes

BASICS

DESCRIPTION

- Jaundice: a yellow or green/yellow hue to the skin, sclerae, and mucous membranes which can be appreciated at serum bilirubin levels >2 mg/dL. Intensity of color is directly related to the serum bilirubin level.
- Unconjugated bilirubin: 80% is due to hemoglobin turnover and 20% is from degradation of hepatic and renal heme proteins. It is a hydrophobic compound that must be carried to the liver by albumin for processing.
- Conjugated bilirubin: conjugated to glucuronic acid in the liver, a water-soluble derivative that helps lipid emulsification and absorption
- Conjugated hyperbilirubinemia (direct hyperbilirubinemia): a conjugated bilirubin of >2 mg/dL or >20% of the total bilirubin

EPIDEMIOLOGY

The most common causes of pathologic jaundice are as follows:

- Newborn period: biliary atresia, idiopathic neonatal hepatitis, α-1-antitrypsin deficiency, infection
- Older child: autoimmune hepatitis, viral hepatitis, Wilson disease, biliary obstruction

DIAGNOSIS

DIFFERENTIAL DIAGNOSIS

- **Unconjugated hyperbilirubinemia**
  - Congenital/anatomic
    - Placental dysfunction/insufficiency resulting in polycythemia (e.g., infants of diabetic mothers)
    - Upper GI tract obstruction (e.g., pyloric stenosis, duodenal web, atresia)
    - Congenital hypothyroidism
  - Infectious
    - Sepsis
  - Trauma/delivery complications
    - Cephalohematoma/bruising
    - Delayed cord clamping, twin–twin transfusion, maternal–fetal transfusion leading to polycythemia
    - Intrauterine hypoxia (secondary to cocaine abuse, high altitude) resulting in polycythemia
    - Induction of labor with oxytocin
    - Prematurity
  - Genetic/metabolic
    - Inherited red cell enzyme, membrane defects (e.g., spherocytosis, glucose-6-phosphate dehydrogenase [G6PD] deficiency, phosphokinase deficiency, elliptocytosis)
    - Hemoglobinopathies (sickle cell anemia, thalassemia)
    - Defect in hepatic bilirubin conjugation (e.g., Crigler-Najjar types I and II, Gilbert)
    - Inborn errors of metabolism
  - Allergic/inflammatory/immunologic
    - Isoimmunization (ABO, Rh, Kell, other incompatibility)
  - Functional
    - Physiologic jaundice
    - Breastfeeding-associated jaundice
    - Swallowed maternal blood
    - Increased bilirubin load due to infant bleeding from a clotting disorder
    - Familial benign unconjugated hyperbilirubinemia in mother and neonate (Lucey-Driscoll syndrome)
- **Conjugated hyperbilirubinemia**
  - Extrahepatic
    - Extrahepatic biliary atresia
    - Choledochal cysts and other abnormalities of the choledochopancreatic ductal junction
    - Spontaneous perforation of the bile duct
    - Bile or mucous plug or biliary sludge
    - Gallstones
  - Infectious etiologies
    - Bacterial: gram-negative sepsis, urinary tract infection
    - Viral: cytomegalovirus; echovirus; herpes simplex virus; rubella; Epstein-Barr virus; HIV; hepatitis A, B, C, D, and E
    - Toxoplasmosis
    - *Pneumocystis carinii*
    - *Entamoeba histolytica*
    - *Mycobacterium tuberculosis*
    - *Mycobacterium avium-intracellulare*
    - Syphilis
  - Toxic, environmental, drugs
    - Post shock or post-asphyxia (ischemic injury to liver)
    - Drugs: acetaminophen, valproate, chlorpromazine, Amanita toxin, and others
    - Hyperalimentation (total parenteral nutrition)
  - Neoplastic
    - Neuroblastoma, hepatic, biliary, pancreatic, duodenal, peritoneal
    - Infiltrative processes such as HLH
    - Langerhans cell histiocytosis
  - Genetic/metabolic
    - Arteriohepatic dysplasia (Alagille syndrome)
    - Progressive familial intrahepatic cholestasis (including FIC1, BSEP, and MDR3 deficiency)
    - Benign recurrent intrahepatic cholestasis
    - Defects in bile acid metabolism
    - Defects in amino acid metabolism
    - Defects in lipid metabolism: Wolman disease, Niemann-Pick disease, Gaucher disease
    - Defects in carbohydrate metabolism: galactosemia, hereditary fructose intolerance, glycogenosis type IV
    - Defects in fatty acid oxidation
    - Defects in mitochondrial DNA and respiratory chain defects
    - α-1-antitrypsin deficiency
    - Cystic fibrosis
    - Wilson disease (older children)
    - Inherited noncholestatic conjugated jaundice syndromes (e.g., Dubin-Johnson and Rotor syndrome)
    - Hereditary cholestasis with lymphedema (Aagenaes syndrome)
  - Inflammatory/immunologic/endocrine:
    - Idiopathic neonatal hepatitis
    - Congenital alloimmune hepatitis
    - Idiopathic panhypopituitarism
    - Autoimmune hepatitis (children and adolescents)
    - Sclerosing cholangitis (children and adolescents, unless neonatal form)

APPROACH TO THE PATIENT

- **Phase 1:** Determine if hyperbilirubinemia is unconjugated or conjugated.
- **Phase 2:** if unconjugated hyperbilirubinemia
  - Obtain CBC and indices.
  - Reticulocyte count
  - Coombs test: If test is positive, the diagnosis is isoimmune; if test is negative, then consider polycythemia, extravascular bleed, or RBC structural or enzyme defects.
- **Phase 3:** if conjugated hyperbilirubinemia
  - Alanine aminotransferase (ALT), aspartate aminotransferase (AST), γ-glutamyltranspeptidase (GGT)
    - PT/PTT/international normalized ratio (INR)
  - Ultrasound of the liver/pancreas/gallbladder and biliary tree
  - Rule out those etiologies of conjugated hyperbilirubinemia that may adversely affect the outcome if diagnosis is delayed (biliary atresia, tyrosinemia, galactosemia, inborn error of bile acid synthesis, hereditary fructose intolerance, panhypopituitarism, and others).

HISTORY

- **Question:** Unexplained itching?
- *Significance*: Cholestatic liver disease (conjugated hyperbilirubinemia)
- **Question:** History of poor school performance, change in mental status, handwriting?
- *Significance*: Wilson disease
- **Question:** History of other family members having prolonged jaundice, hepatic failure, or sudden death in infancy?
- *Significance*: Suggests an underlying inborn error of metabolism such as tyrosinemia, galactosemia, or a fatty acid oxidation defect
- **Question:** History of IV drug abuse or exposure to blood or blood products, especially prior to 1992?
- *Significance*: The patient may have transfusion-associated hepatitis (e.g., hepatitis C).

PHYSICAL EXAM

- **Finding:** Scratch marks?
- *Significance*: Pruritus secondary to cholestasis
- **Finding:** Spider angioma, palmar erythema?
- *Significance*: Chronic liver disease

- **Finding:** Petechiae, purpura, microcephaly, thrombocytopenia?
- *Significance*: Congenital TORCH infection
- **Finding:** Heart murmur?
- *Significance*: Alagille syndrome (peripheral pulmonic stenosis)
- **Finding:** Splenomegaly?
- *Significance*: Suggests acute hemolysis (in unconjugated hyperbilirubinemia) or chronic liver disease and portal hypertension (conjugated hyperbilirubinemia)
- **Finding:** Ascites?
- *Significance*: Suggests portal hypertension
- **Finding:** Acholic stool?
- *Significance*: Severe cholestasis or biliary obstruction

DIAGNOSTIC TESTS & INTERPRETATION

- Percutaneous liver biopsies: Liver pathology—in infants with cholestasis, the most common patterns are giant cell hepatitis, bile duct proliferation, and bile duct paucity. A pattern of duct proliferation, bile plugs, portal expansion, and fibrosis suggests biliary obstruction, most likely biliary atresia.
- Intraoperative cholangiogram is indicated for infants with a liver biopsy suggestive of biliary obstruction and possible biliary atresia. If the cholangiogram is consistent with biliary atresia, the surgeon will perform the Kasai portoenterostomy.
- Total bilirubin with fractionation into unconjugated, conjugated, and delta fractions
- *Significance*: Direct versus indirect hyperbilirubinemia

If unconjugated hyperbilirubinemia, investigation is initiated with the following:

- **Test:** CBC with indices, reticulocyte count, and peripheral blood smear for RBC morphology
- *Significance*: Polycythemia in neonate, hemolysis, or other conditions associated with increased destruction of red cells
- **Test:** Coombs test
- *Significance*: Isoimmune and autoimmune hemolytic anemia
- **Test:** PT/PTT/INR, platelet count
- *Significance*: Coagulopathy associated with hemorrhage that causes an increased bilirubin load

If neonatal conjugated hyperbilirubinemia, investigation is initiated with the following:

- **Test:** Serum aminotransferases (ALT, AST)
- *Significance*: Ongoing liver inflammation
- **Test:** Alkaline phosphatase and GGT
- *Significance*: Biliary tree obstruction, bile duct injury, or cholestasis
- **Test:** PT/INR, PTT, serum albumin, fibrinogen
- *Significance*: Liver synthetic function
- **Test:** Sepsis evaluation (blood and urine and spinal fluid)
- *Significance*: Sepsis can impair conjugation and excretion of bilirubin
- **Test:** Free T_3, T_4, and thyroid-stimulating hormone
- *Significance*: Congenital hypothyroidism
- **Test:** α-1-Antitrypsin serum levels and PI phenotype
- *Significance*: Serum α-1-antitrypsin levels will be low in inherited protease inhibitor deficiency.
- **Test:** Urine dipstick for glucose and reducing substances
- *Significance*: Positive reducing substances are seen in galactosemia and hereditary fructose intolerance.
- **Test:** Urine for bile acid analysis
- *Significance*: Inborn error of bile acid metabolism
- Metabolic workup may be performed depending on clinical setting, including plasma amino acids, urine organic acids, succinylacetone, lactate, pyruvate, and other tests as indicated.
- In an older child presenting with conjugated hyperbilirubinemia, the most common causes are biliary obstruction due to gallstones, viral hepatitis, and autoimmune hepatitis.

Imaging

- Ultrasound
  - A noninvasive method to examine the overall liver appearance, size, and density
  - Allows for examination of the biliary tree and gallbladder to rule out choledochal cysts, sludge/stones, and ductal dilatation indicating possible obstruction
  - Infants with biliary atresia/splenic malformation syndrome may have other findings including polysplenia, asplenia, and preduodenal portal vein with azygous continuation.
- Hepatobiliary scintigraphy (HIDA scan): Tracer secretion into the duodenum excludes biliary atresia or extrahepatic biliary obstruction.

TREATMENT

GENERAL MEASURES

- Treat Crigler-Najjar syndrome promptly with phototherapy and phenobarbital to prevent kernicterus.
- Older children with Wilson disease may present with profound hemolysis and may have predominantly unconjugated hyperbilirubinemia with severe parenchymal liver disease and fulminant liver failure.

ISSUES FOR REFERRAL

- Any infant with jaundice beyond 10–14 days of age should have a fractionated bilirubin sent.
- Any infant with conjugated hyperbilirubinemia should be referred immediately to a pediatric gastroenterologist for further workup.

ADDITIONAL READING

- American Academy of Pediatrics Subcommittee on Hyperbilirubinemia. Management of hyperbilirubinemia in the newborn infant 35 or more weeks of gestation. *Pediatrics*. 2004;114(1):297–316.
- Brumbaugh D, Mack C. Conjugated hyperbilirubinemia in children. *Pediatr Rev*. 2012;33(7):291–302.
- Cohen RS, Wong RJ, Stevenson DK. Understanding neonatal jaundice: a perspective on causation. *Pediatr Neonatol*. 2010;51(3):143–148.
- Kelly DA, Davenport M. Current management of biliary atresia. *Arch Dis Child*. 2007;92(12):1132–1135.
- Mack CL, Feldman AG, Sokol RJ. Clues to the etiology of bile duct injury in biliary atresia. *Semin Liver Dis*. 2012;32(4):307–316.
- Maisels MJ, McDonagh AF. Phototherapy for neonatal jaundice. *N Engl J Med*. 2008;358(9):920–928.
- Watchko JF. Hyperbilirubinemia in African American neonates: clinical issues and current challenges. *Semin Fetal Neonatal Med*. 2010;15:176–182.

CODES

ICD10

- R17 Unspecified jaundice
- P59.9 Neonatal jaundice, unspecified
- P59.0 Neonatal jaundice associated with preterm delivery

FAQ

- Q: Are there any findings in neonatal jaundice that are specifically concerning?
- A: These findings are concerning until proven otherwise:
  - Jaundice before 36 hours of life
  - Persistent jaundice beyond 10 days of life
  - Serum bilirubin concentration $>$12 mg/dL
  - Elevation of direct bilirubin $>$2 mg/dL or 20% of total bilirubin at any time
- Q: Are there any specific factors associated with higher bilirubin levels in neonates?
- A: Factors that have been associated with high serum bilirubin levels are low birth weight, certain ethnic groups (Asian, Native American, Greek), delayed meconium passage after birth, and breastfeeding. G6PD deficiency has also been associated with a higher risk of neonatal jaundice. Factors that have been associated with lower serum bilirubin levels in neonates include maternal smoking and certain drugs such as phenobarbital. Of note, African American neonates have a lower risk of jaundice overall but are overrepresented in the U.S. Kernicterus Registry. This finding is due partially to a higher incidence of G6PD deficiency in males.
- Q: Where does the term "jaundice" come from?
- A: Jaundice is derived from the French word jaune, which means "yellow."

KAWASAKI DISEASE

Rebecca Reindel • Stanford Shulman

BASICS

DESCRIPTION

- Kawasaki disease (KD) is a medium vessel vasculitis of early childhood with a predilection for the coronary arteries, which can result in dilatation, aneurysms, thrombosis, and stenosis.
- No diagnostic test exists, and incomplete presentations are common. Prompt recognition and treatment can reduce risk of coronary artery involvement from 25% to 5%.

EPIDEMIOLOGY

- Worldwide with highest incidence in Japan
- Peak of hospitalizations December–March
- 76% of children with KD are <5 years old.

Incidence

- U.S. hospitalization data (1997–2007) demonstrate an annual incidence of 17.1–20.8/100,000 children aged <5 years.
- KD is more common in boys than girls. In 2006, the hospitalization rate for boys was 24.2/100,000 versus 16.8/100,000 in girls.
- More common in Asian/Pacific Islanders, with highest rates in Japan
  - Ethnic predisposition persists in different geographic locations, with highest incidence in the United States in Asian/Pacific Islander children <5 years of age (30.3/100,000).
  - Rates are higher in black and Hispanic children compared to white children.

Prevalence

5,523 reported cases of KD in the United States in 2006

RISK FACTORS

- Asian/Pacific Islander descent
- Young age

Genetics

- Siblings have 10–30-fold higher risk of KD.
- Genome-wide linkage studies suggest single nucleotide polymorphisms in the *ITPKC* gene confer susceptibility to KD.

PATHOPHYSIOLOGY

- Generalized vasculitis with early neutrophilic infiltrate, with later transition to lymphocyte infiltration, and lastly to luminal myofibroblastic proliferation
- Can very rarely result in destruction of the endothelium through to the adventitia resulting in aneurysms and rupture

ETIOLOGY

- Etiology is unknown.
- Infectious cause suggested by the following:
  - Abrupt onset and resolution of symptoms without recurrence
  - Clusters and epidemics
  - Age of affected patients
  - Seasonal predominance
  - Oligoclonal IgA plasma cells noted in KD tissues, which bind to cytoplasmic inclusion bodies found in affected tissues
- Data suggest that KD is caused by a previously unrecognized ubiquitous RNA virus that causes disease in an immunologically susceptible population.
  - No supporting evidence for multiple proposed etiologic agents: toxic shock toxin, rug shampoo, retrovirus, bocavirus, coronavirus, mercury, EBV/CMV.

DIAGNOSIS

- KD is a clinical diagnosis.
- Current diagnostic criteria: fever for ≥5 days and ≥4 of 5 clinical findings, which need not be present at the same time
  - Extremity changes (erythema of palms, soles, and/or edema of hands, feet)
  - Polymorphous exanthema (frequently in perineal region with early desquamation)
  - Nonexudative bilateral bulbar conjunctivitis (with limbic sparing)
  - Mucosal changes (erythema of lips and oropharyngeal mucosa, strawberry tongue, cracked/swollen lips)
  - Unilateral cervical lymphadenopathy (>1.5 cm in diameter)
- Incomplete KD
  - If patient has characteristics consistent with KD along with fever for ≥5 days with 2 or 3 clinical criteria and CRP ≥3 and/or ESR ≥40, obtain echocardiogram (ECHO). If patient with ≥3 supplemental lab criteria, treat for KD.
  - Supplemental lab criteria for incomplete KD: albumin ≥3, platelets (after 7 days) ≥450,000/μL, WBC ≥15,000/μL, urine ≥10 WBC/HPF, anemia for age, ALT elevation

ALERT
Young infants with KD often present with few, if any, clinical characteristics of KD. Maintain a high index of suspicion for KD in young infants with prolonged fever.

HISTORY

- High-spiking fevers usually greater than 39°C can persist up to 3–4 weeks (mean 11 days).
- In addition to the clinical criteria above, the following complaints are sometimes seen:
  - Irritability
  - Abdominal pain/emesis/diarrhea
  - Refusal to ambulate or pain with ambulation
  - Poor appetite

PHYSICAL EXAM

- Extremity changes with palmar/plantar erythema and/or hand/foot swelling
  - Periungual desquamation of hands and feet within 2–3 weeks of fever onset
  - Beau lines (transverse grooves across nails) within 1–2 months of fever onset
- Polymorphous rash
  - Usually, diffuse maculopapular rash
  - Often, perineal rash with desquamation
  - Also seen: erythema multiforme, erythroderma, urticaria, scarlatiniform
  - Not vesicular or bullous
- Bilateral nonexudative conjunctivitis
  - Bulbar, with limbic sparing
  - Painless
  - Anterior uveitis/iridocyclitis can be seen.
- Mucosal changes
  - Cracked, red, swollen lips
  - Strawberry tongue with erythema and prominent papillae
  - Buccal and pharyngeal mucosa erythema

ALERT
In a patient with ongoing fever and nonsuppurative lymphadenitis despite adequate antibacterial therapy, consider KD.

- Unilateral cervical lymphadenopathy of one or more nodes that are >1.5 cm in diameter
  - Can be misdiagnosed as bacterial lymphadenitis
  - Usually without overlying erythema
  - Least common clinical finding in KD
- Other clinical findings
  - Myocarditis with tachycardia, gallop, innocent flow murmur
  - Shock and hypotension
  - Arthritis and arthralgias (early can be multiple joints, later is usually weight-bearing joints)
  - Urethritis, meatitis
  - Rare findings: transient hearing loss

DIAGNOSTIC TESTS & INTERPRETATION

- No definitive diagnostic test
- The presence of ancillary lab findings can support diagnosis of KD and be helpful in identifying those patients with incomplete KD.

Lab

- Elevated ESR and/or CRP

ALERT
ESR is artifactually elevated after administration of IVIG and therefore not useful in this scenario.

- CBC
  - WBC normal to elevated with left shift
  - Anemia (normocytic/normochromic)
  - Platelets usually normal in the 1st week of illness and increase over the next 2–3 weeks, sometimes to >1,000,000/mm^3
- Chemistries
  - Hypoalbuminemia
  - Hyponatremia
  - Transaminitis and elevated GGT
  - Hyperbilirubinemia
- Aseptic meningitis with CSF pleocytosis
- Sterile pyuria
- Synovial fluid leukocytosis
- Elevated triglycerides and LDL, low HDL

Imaging

- Chest x-ray
  - Interstitial pneumonitis
- ECHO
  - Aneurysms or ectasias of the epicardial coronary arteries that evolve over time
    - Z-score corrects for variations in body surface area among children.
    - Larger aneurysms with higher risk of thrombosis and death
  - Decreased myocardial contractility
  - Mitral or aortic (rare) regurgitation
  - Pericardial effusion
  - Rarely, aneurysms of other medium sized vessels, including iliac and axillary
- Abdominal ultrasound
  - Hydrops of the gallbladder

DIFFERENTIAL DIAGNOSIS

- Viral infections
  - Measles, adenovirus, Epstein-Barr virus
- Bacterial infections
  - Scarlet fever
  - Streptococcal or staphylococcal toxic shock
  - Staphylococcal scalded-skin syndrome
  - Leptospirosis
  - Rocky Mountain spotted fever
  - Cervical lymphadenitis
- Rheumatologic conditions
  - Juvenile idiopathic arthritis, especially systemic onset
- Drug reactions
  - Stevens-Johnson syndrome
- Mercury hypersensitivity

TREATMENT

MEDICATION

- Combination therapy with IV immunoglobulin (IVIG) and aspirin
  - Proven efficacy in reducing coronary artery aneurysms when given by 10th day of illness
  - Clinical benefit to therapy after 10th day, although prevention of coronary aneurysms unclear
  - IVIG dose: 2 g/kg given over 10–12 hours
  - Aspirin dose: 80–100 mg/kg/24 h PO divided q6h until acute-phase reactants normalize and patient defervesces, or until 14th day of illness, at which time the dose is reduced to 3–5 mg/kg *once daily*
- Treatment of refractory KD
  - 5–15% of patients do not respond to the first dose of IVIG.
  - 70–80% of nonresponders will respond to a second dose of IVIG.
  - Limited evidence to support a treatment recommendation for those not responding to 2nd IVIG dose, but salvage therapy with a 3rd dose of IVIG, IV corticosteroids, infliximab, cyclophosphamide, and methotrexate has been reported.
- Corticosteroids as adjunctive therapy
  - Primary adjunctive corticosteroid therapy appears to reduce the incidence of coronary artery disease in a subset of high-risk Japanese patients.
  - Some data support adjunctive corticosteroids for IVIG-refractory patients to reduce coronary artery disease risk.
  - Optimal dose, duration, and formulation of steroid has not been established.
- Antithrombotic therapy for aneurysms
  - Consider addition of antiplatelet therapy or anticoagulation in consultation with cardiology depending on size and extent of aneurysms.

ADDITIONAL TREATMENT

- Surgical therapy for life-threatening aneurysms
  - Coronary artery bypass
  - Heart transplantation (rarely)

General Measures

- Rapid diagnosis and treatment can decrease the risk of coronary artery aneurysms.
- Close follow-up and monitoring for the development of aneurysms after discharge

INPATIENT CONSIDERATIONS

Admission Criteria

Prolonged fever and clinical and laboratory findings suggestive of KD

Nursing

- Frequent vital signs and monitoring during IVIG administration
- Patient education

Discharge Criteria

- Resolution of fever for 24 hours after completion of IVIG administration
- Improvement in clinical symptoms
- Patients should have ECHO completed and interpreted prior to discharge, with additional therapy, monitoring, and prolonged hospital stay as indicated.

ONGOING CARE

FOLLOW-UP RECOMMENDATIONS

- Low-dose aspirin should be continued until follow-up ECHO at 2 weeks and 6–8 weeks after discharge are normal.
- Some centers perform ECHO at 6–12 months after discharge.
- Inflammatory markers and CBC should be followed until normalized.
- More frequent follow-up and monitoring for those with coronary abnormalities; advise to monitor for emesis, irritability, and nonspecific symptoms of myocardial ischemia.

Patient Monitoring

- No coronary abnormalities: routine pediatric care after follow-up ECHOs complete
- Transient coronary arteritis that resolves by 6–8 weeks: low-dose aspirin until ECHO normalizes, follow-up every 3–5 years
- Isolated small- to medium-sized (3–6 mm) aneurysm: low-dose aspirin until regression is documented on annual follow-up ECHOs. Biennial stress test or myocardial perfusion assay for patients 11 years or older. Perform angiography if stenosis or is ischemia suggested.
- One or more large (>6 mm) or giant (>8 mm) aneurysm/multiple smaller or complex aneurysms: long-term antiplatelet therapy or clopidogrel indefinitely, with anticoagulation with warfarin or subcutaneous low-molecular-weight heparin. ECHO and ECG q6 months, stress testing yearly. Angiography 6–12 months after diagnosis and repeated if concerns for myocardial ischemia; no strenuous activity, additional limits on activity based on stress testing
- Evidence of stenosis or obstruction: emergent referral for cardiovascular surgical evaluation and thrombolytic therapy

PROGNOSIS

- The process of resolution of aneurysms is incompletely understood. Some histopathologic changes in the arterial lumen likely persist despite angiographic regression.
- Smaller aneurysms are more likely to resolve than larger aneurysms.
- Resolution of aneurysms (by angiography) is reported in ~50–67% of vessels.
- Improved prognosis with age <1 year, fusiform rather than saccular aneurysm, distal location
- Giant aneurysms with worst prognosis: higher likelihood of thrombosis and stenosis
- Cause of death usually myocardial infarction due to thrombosis
- Long-term implications for cardiovascular health unclear, even when no aneurysms

COMPLICATIONS

- Aneurysmal rupture (very rare)
- Myocardial infarction
- Coronary artery stenosis years after onset
- Rare association with hemophagocytic syndrome
- Recurrence rate <1%, higher in Asian populations

ADDITIONAL READING

- Burns JC, Glode MP. Kawasaki syndrome. *Lancet*. 2004;364(9433):533–544.
- Freeman AF, Shulman ST. Refractory Kawasaki disease. *Pediatr Infect Dis J*. 2004;23(5):463–464.
- Holman RC, Belay ED, Christensen KY, et al. Hospitalizations for Kawasaki syndrome among children in the United States, 1997–2007. *Pediatr Infect Dis J*. 2010;29(6):483–488.
- Kobayashi T, Saji T, Otani T, et al. Efficacy of immunoglobulin plus prednisolone for prevention of coronary artery abnormalities in severe Kawasaki disease (RAISE study): a randomised, open-label, blinded-endpoints trial. *Lancet*. 2012;379(9826):1613–1620.
- Newburger JW, Sleeper LA, McCrindle BW, et al. Randomized trial of pulsed corticosteroid therapy for primary treatment of Kawasaki disease. *N Engl J Med*. 2007;356(7):663–675.
- Newburger JW, Takahashi M, Gerber MA, et al. Diagnosis, treatment, and long-term management of patients with Kawasaki disease. *Pediatrics*. 2004;114(6):1708–1733.
- Pinna GS, Kafetzis DA, Tselkas OI, et al. Kawasaki disease: an overview. *Curr Opin Infect Dis*. 2008;21(3):263–270.
- Rowley A. Kawasaki disease: novel insights into etiology and genetic susceptibility. *Annu Rev Med*. 2011;62:69–77.
- Rowley A, Shulman ST. Pathogenesis and management of Kawasaki disease. *Expert Rev Anti Infect Ther*. 2010;8(2):197–203.

CODES

ICD10

M30.3 Mucocutaneous lymph node syndrome [Kawasaki]

KNEE PAIN, ANTERIOR/PATELLOFEMORAL MALALIGNMENT SYNDROME

Theodore J. Ganley • Matthew Grady

BASICS

DESCRIPTION

- Condition characterized by discomfort at the anterior aspect of the knee that is generally associated with activities, especially those that involve running, jumping, and climbing stairs
- Has also been called "miserable malalignment syndrome"

PATHOPHYSIOLOGY

- Predisposing factors for patellofemoral malalignment syndrome include the following:
  - Femoral anteversion
  - Genu valgus
  - Pes planus
- These three anatomic features have been commonly referred to as a terrible triad contributing to anterior knee pain. Because the entire kinetic chain is linked in function, malalignment at one area can lead to secondary stresses at a distant location.
- Excess femoral anteversion, as well as marked pes planus, can contribute to increased lateral pull on the patella and subsequent patellofemoral pain.
- Further contributing factors include a wider pelvis and a more laterally positioned tibial tubercle, both of which also contribute to altered biomechanics at the knee.
- Weak hip abductors and quadriceps muscles and tight hamstrings, iliotibial band, Achilles tendon, and quadriceps can lead to increased forces across the patellofemoral joint.

DIAGNOSIS

HISTORY

- Pain under and around the kneecap with activities including squatting, sitting for prolonged periods with the knees bent, and going up or down stairs or hills: These activities increase patellofemoral contact stress.
- Recent history of direct trauma to the kneecap: A blunt trauma to the kneecap can cause soft tissue or subchondral contusion that may exacerbate this condition.

PHYSICAL EXAM

- Assess one-legged squat for weak hip abductors—knee will go into valgus.
- Palpate medial and lateral patellar facets for areas of pain due to increased contact forces.
- Cracking noises from the front of the knee with flexion and extension
  - Cracking can be a sign of softening of the undersurface of the patella.
  - Chondromalacia is patellar articular cartilage pathologic change, which ranges from mild cracking attributed to softening to locking and catching attributed to cartilage disruption.
- There is no single angulation or rotation profile that is universal for all anterior knee pain patients. However, many have femoral anteversion, genu valgus, and pes planus. Weak hip abductors and tight hamstrings or quadriceps may also be found.

DIAGNOSTIC TESTS & INTERPRETATION

Imaging

- Anterior and posterior, lateral, Merchant plain radiographs of the knee
  - The Merchant kneecap view shows the shape of the patella within the trochlea.
  - Patients will frequently be found to have lateral patellar tilt, as well as an abnormally shaped patella with excessive elongation of the lateral portion of the patella/lateral patellar facet.
- MRI: not a 1st-line study for patellofemoral syndrome; however, it may be performed to rule out associated pathology in patients with recalcitrant pain and unusual clinical presentations.

DIFFERENTIAL DIAGNOSIS

- Osgood-Schlatter disease
  - Tenderness not at the patella but at the anterior tibial tubercle
  - A self-limiting inflammation of the apophysis that tends to occur in growing teenagers and preteens
  - Irregularity and fragmentation of the apophysis are seen on lateral radiographs.
- Meniscus tear
  - Disruption of the crescent-shaped fibrocartilaginous tissue adjacent to the tibial and femoral articular surfaces
  - Most commonly presents as posteromedial or posterolateral hemijoint tenderness with knee hyperflexion and rotation

- Distal iliotibial band tendonitis
  - Irritation of distal iliotibial band as it rubs over the lateral condyle before attaching on lateral tibia (Gerdy tubercle)
  - Common in runners or those with weak hip abductors
- Prepatellar bursitis
  - An inflammation of the fluid-filled bursa sac beneath the SC tissue and immediately anterior to the patella
  - More common in patients who kneel for extended periods of time and has been called "carpet layer's knee"
  - Swelling and tenderness immediately anterior to the patella; does not primarily present with deeper tenderness in the medial and lateral parapatellar regions found in patellofemoral syndrome

ALERT

Patients with a traumatic effusion, locking, catching, instability to ligamentous stress testing, multiple joint effusions, or night waking should be evaluated for other traumatic or medical conditions.

TREATMENT

GENERAL MEASURES

- A progressive exercise program is the main focus of treatment.
- Strength and flexibility exercises are needed to improve the mechanics of the patellofemoral joint.
- Strengthening should include hip abductors, hip extensors, hamstrings, and the quadriceps muscles.
  - This strengthening can be performed several times each day as a home exercise program or formally with physical therapy in more recalcitrant cases.
- Stretching should include quadriceps, hamstrings, iliotibial band, and tendoachilles stretches as indicated by the physical examination (PE).
- Patients can be advanced from low-resistance exercises such as swimming, stationary bike, and elliptical trainers to higher level running activities.
- Activity restriction in the initial acutely symptomatic stage is instituted to eliminate high-impact sports, including especially those that involve running and jumping.

ADDITIONAL READING

- Collado H, Fredericson M. Patellofemoral pain syndrome. *Clin Sports Med*. 2010;29(3):379–398.
- Flynn J, Lou J, Ganley T. Prevention of sports injuries in children. *Curr Opin Pediatr*. 2002;14(6):719–722.
- Ganley TJ, Pill SG, Flynn JM, et al. Pediatric and adolescent sports medicine. *Curr Opin Orthopaed*. 2001;12:456–461.
- Hart L. Supervised exercise versus usual care for patellofemoral pain syndrome. *Clin J Sport Med*. 2010;20(2):133.
- Murray KJ. Hypermobility disorders in children and adolescents. *Best Pract Res Clin Rheumatol*. 2006;20(2):329–351.

CODES

ICD10

- M25.569 Pain in unspecified knee
- M22.2X9 Patellofemoral disorders, unspecified knee
- M22.40 Chondromalacia patellae, unspecified knee

FAQ

- Q: Is it acceptable to play sports, or is this condition too dangerous?
- A: Patients with a history of patellofemoral syndrome who have regained their strength and flexibility are permitted to return to their activities, provided that they do not have pain and limping during their activities. A history of catching, locking, or knee effusions may be a sign of further biomechanical intra-articular pathology that should be addressed.
- Q: Is bracing indicated?
- A: Some patients with anterior knee pain respond to neoprene sleeves, and those with a component of increased lateral translation may benefit from neoprene sleeves with lateral patellar supports. Bracing, however, is not a substitute for strength and conditioning program.
- Q: Is chondromalacia patella the same as patellofemoral syndrome?
- A: No. Chondromalacia is a classification of the anatomic pathologic changes of the undersurface of the patella. Patellofemoral syndrome is the clinical condition encompassing the patient's history, physical, and radiographic elements of anterior knee pain.

K

LACRIMAL DUCT OBSTRUCTION

Bethlehem Abebe-Wolpaw

BASICS

DESCRIPTION

A congenital blockage identified in infants from failure of canalization, most commonly at the distal portion, of the nasolacrimal duct. Epiphora (constant tearing) is the most common presentation followed by discharge unresponsive to treatment. Less commonly, the blockage is an acquired condition.

EPIDEMIOLOGY

- Most common cause of persistent tearing in infants
- True congenital nasolacrimal duct obstruction affects about 6% of newborns.
- Spontaneous resolution occurs in 90% of cases within 1 year.

RISK FACTORS

Incidence is higher in infants with craniofacial malformations and Down syndrome.

PATHOPHYSIOLOGY

- Congenital obstruction most commonly occurs at the level of the valve of Hasner in the distal portion of the nasolacrimal duct as it enters the nose.
- Types of distal obstruction include an imperforate membrane or cellular debris at the level of the valve, bony obstruction, or narrowing of the inferior meatus.
- Acquired obstructions are rare in children but do occur as a result of chronic inflammation and scar tissue occluding the duct. Causes include infection (i.e., ethmoidal sinusitis), inflammation, malignancy, and trauma.

ETIOLOGY

Canalization of the duct is usually complete by the 7th month of gestation, but a persistent membrane can remain and may represent the embryologic basis of lacrimal duct obstruction.

COMMONLY ASSOCIATED CONDITIONS

- Dacryocystocele (distention of the lacrimal sac) is a rare variant of lacrimal duct obstruction seen in 0.1% of infants with the disorder. There is the typical distal obstruction as well as a proximal obstruction at the junction of the common canaliculus and the lacrimal sac.
- Acute dacryocystitis is strongly suggestive of the presence of obstruction. Unclear whether obstruction is the primary cause leading to secondary infection from accumulation of tears and cellular debris or that dacryocystitis is the primary event with an acquired obstruction from fibrosis and inflammation

DIAGNOSIS

HISTORY

- Congenital obstruction presents in first few weeks of life.
- Symptoms can be either unilateral or bilateral.
- Chronic tearing
- Mucoid discharge
- Crusting on eyelids and eyelashes
- Acquired obstruction is associated wtih chronic eye infections or a history of trauma (i.e., naso-orbito-ethmoidal fractures, lid laceration).

PHYSICAL EXAM

- Discharge and/or crusting on the eyelashes
- Eyelid excoriation
- Compression of lacrimal sac reveals mucoid discharge and/or tears expressed through the punctum.
- Usually absence of conjunctival injection
- Bluish firm mass below the medial canthus suggests presence of dacryocystocele.

DIAGNOSTIC TESTS & INTERPRETATION

Usually, patients are treated without imaging and testing. If symptoms are intermittent and diagnosis is unclear, imaging and tests may be done.

Lab

Bacterial cultures are not a reliable indicator of the presence of obstruction or infection thus is not indicated for diagnostic purposes.

Imaging

- Radionuclide dacryocystography (also known as dacryoscintigraphy) helps evaluate the functioning of the lacrimal system by taking pictures as a radioisotope passes through the lacrimal system.
  - Technically difficult to perform in children so is rarely done
  - Does not allow for visualization of surrounding bony structures
- CT scan is useful for trauma or to assess bony obstruction resulting from craniofacial malformations or presence of dacryocystocele or other masses.

Diagnostic Procedures/Other

- Fluorescein dye disappearance test
  - Preferred tool for diagnosis of congenital obstruction if symptoms are intermittent
  - 90% sensitive and 100% specific for nasolacrimal duct obstruction
  - Fluorescein is placed in the lower conjunctival fornix and the patient is observed for 5 minutes.
  - If there is no obstruction, most of the fluorescein drains into the nose and minimal amounts of fluorescein is noted in the eye.
  - If there is an obstruction, fluorescein will be seen in the eye with an increased tear meniscus with likely overflow of tears onto the cheeks.
- If dacryocystocele is suspected, nasal endoscopy is recommended. Application of a topical decongestant such as oxymetazoline hydrochloride to the nasal mucous membranes enhances visualization.

DIFFERENTIAL DIAGNOSIS

- Neonatal conjunctivitis
- Acute dacryocystitis
- Agenesis or imperforation of the lacrimal puncta or canaliculi
- Excess tear production
  - Congenital glaucoma
  - Corneal abrasion
  - Abnormal eyelid position (entropion, epiblepharon)
  - Trichiasis
  - Foreign body
  - Blepharitis
  - Keratitis
  - Uveitis

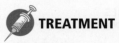

TREATMENT

MEDICATION

Topical ophthalmic antibiotics are used in congenital obstruction when there is an increase in discharge, purulent discharge, or findings consistent with conjunctivitis. Topical antibiotics of choice include erythromycin, tobramycin, sulfacetamide, gentamicin, or fluoroquinolones.

ADDITIONAL TREATMENT

General Measures

- Primary treatment for congenital obstruction is lacrimal sac massage in a downward fashion. Topical antibiotics are added as needed.
- Crigler maneuver can be effective in rupturing the membranous obstruction.
- Probing and irrigation are generally recommended if symptoms persist after 6–12 months of age.
  - Some ophthalmologists prefer to perform the procedure prior to 12 months of age, and some continue with conservative measures until 15–18 months of age.
- Failed probing is usually noted within 6 weeks of procedure with return of symptoms.

- Probing may be repeated, although with increasing age, repeated probing may be less successful.
- Additional procedures may be done at the time of repeat probing that may increase the success rate, including the following:
  - Balloon catheter dilatation. Some experts advocate that this can be considered as a primary treatment in place of probing.
  - Nasal endoscopy allows visualization of the probe entering the nose, helping to avoid false passage.
  - Silicone tube intubation helps prevent formation of granulation tissue and can aid in dilating stenotic segments of the lacrimal outflow system. Tube is left in place for 2–6 months but success has been seen with removal as early as 6 weeks in patients younger than age 2 years.

ISSUES FOR REFERRAL

- Referral to a pediatric ophthalmologist is indicated if symptoms persist beyond 6–12 months of age with the application of conservative measures. Depending on severity and preference of the ophthalmologist, probing is done or conservative measures are continued.
- Early referral is warranted in cases of acute dacryocystitis and dacryocystocele.
- Cases of acquired obstruction should be referred for surgical treatment.

SURGERY/OTHER PROCEDURES

- Dacryocystorhinostomy
  - Indicated when aforementioned procedures have failed and in cases of chronic dacryocystitis, bony obstruction, or dacryocystocele
  - Creates a bypass fistula between the lacrimal sac and the nose to provide an alternate pathway for lacrimal flow
- Primary conjunctivodacryocystorhinostomy
  - Creates a direct bypass tract between the medial canthus and the nose
  - Limited reports on this technique being used in children
- Surgery is typically performed on patients with acquired obstructions and congenital anomalies of the upper lacrimal system.

INPATIENT CONSIDERATIONS

Admission Criteria

- Neonates with dacryocystocele with an associated intranasal cyst obstructing their airway causing significant respiratory distress need to be admitted for airway management.
- Acute dacryocystitis should be admitted for parenteral antibiotic therapy with ophthalmology involved in the plan of care; may need surgery to drain the collection.

ONGOING CARE

FOLLOW-UP RECOMMENDATIONS

Patient Monitoring

- Conservative measures are appropriate for infants with congenital obstruction, although at 6–12 months of age, referral should be considered for possible probing and irrigation.
- Children with a history of lacrimal duct obstruction need close follow-up for anisometropic amblyopia.

PROGNOSIS

- About 90% of cases of congenital obstruction resolve by 12 months of age.
- Success rate of initial probing when performed at 12 months of age is about 80–90%.
- Probing is less successful after age 3 years.

COMPLICATIONS

- Infections such as bacterial conjunctivitis, acute and chronic dacryocystitis, and orbital cellulitis
- Respiratory distress in neonates with dacryocystocele that have an associated intranasal cyst at the valve of Hasner that obstructs their airway
- Anisometropic amblyopia

ADDITIONAL READING

- Arora S, Koushan K, Harvey JT. Success rates of primary probing for congenital nasolacrimal obstruction in children. *J AAPOS*. 2012;16(2):173–176.
- Casady DR, Meyer DR, Simon JW, et al. Stepwise treatment paradigm for congenital nasolacrimal duct obstruction. *Ophthal Plast Reconstr Surg*. 2006;22(4):243–247.
- Dantas RR. Lacrimal drainage system obstruction. *Semin Ophthalmol*. 2010;25(3):98–103.
- Goldich Y, Barkana Y, Zadok D, et al. Balloon catheter dilatation versus probing as primary treatment for congenital dacryostenosis. *Br J Ophthalmol*. 2011;95(5):634–636.
- Kapadia MK, Freitag SK, Woog JJ. Evaluation and management of congenital nasolacrimal duct obstruction. *Otolaryngol Clin N Am*. 2006;39(5): 959–977.
- Schnall BM. Pediatric nasolacrimal duct obstruction. *Curr Opin Ophthalmol*. 2013;24(5):421–424.
- Takahashi Y, Kakizaki H, Chan WO, et al. Management of congenital nasolacrimal duct obstruction. *Acta Ophthalmol*. 2010;88(5):506–513.
- Wong RK, VanderVeen DK. Presentation and management of congenital dacryocystocele. *Pediatrics*. 2008;122(5):e1108–e1112.

CODES

ICD10

- H04.559 Acquired stenosis of unspecified nasolacrimal duct
- H04.539 Neonatal obstruction of unspecified nasolacrimal duct
- Q10.6 Other congenital malformations of lacrimal apparatus

FAQ

- Q: Why not fix the obstruction upon diagnosis?
- A: Studies have shown that about 90% of cases of congenital obstruction resolve by 12 months of age using conservative measures consisting of massage with occasional addition of topical antibiotics for infection that can occur concurrently with obstruction.
- Q: When is the optimal age for probing and irrigation?
- A: This is controversial, although most studies suggest conservative measures are preferred younger than 12 months of age. After 12 months of age, continued conservative measures or probing are selected based on severity of symptoms. Recent studies indicate that probing becomes less successful as a primary treatment in patients around age 3 years. This may be due to factors other than increasing age, including severe symptoms, canalicular stenosis, and nonmembranous obstruction.
- Q: Does probing and irrigation require general anesthesia?
- A: Sometimes probing is performed as an in-office procedure without general anesthesia if done when patient is young, younger than 12 months of age. When child is older than 12 months of age, probing is ideally performed under general anesthesia to ensure procedure is controlled and safe as well as allowing for direct visualization with endoscopy.

LACTOSE INTOLERANCE

Elizabeth J. Hait

BASICS

DESCRIPTION

- Lactose intolerance is defined as the inability to digest the ingested disaccharide lactose secondary to a deficiency of the intrinsic enzyme lactase, resulting in clinical symptoms.
- Lactose is a disaccharide composed of glucose and galactose.
- Lactose is important as a source of energy; it is the major carbohydrate in human and other mammalian milks; promotes the absorption of calcium, phosphorus, and iron; and has a probiotic effect on the gut flora.
- Four types of lactase deficiency
  - Congenital lactase deficiency
    - Extremely rare
    - Presents during the newborn period
    - Will cause severe diarrhea and failure to thrive and risk the newborn's life
  - Primary lactase deficiency (adult-type hypolactasia)
    - Due to relative or absolute absence of lactase
    - Develops during childhood at different ages in different racial groups
    - Most common cause of lactose intolerance
  - Secondary lactase deficiency
    - Results from small bowel injury (acute gastroenteritis, persistent diarrhea, small bowel bacterial overgrowth, chemotherapy)
    - Can present at any age, more common in infancy
  - Developmental lactase deficiency
    - A relative lactase deficiency observed in premature infants <34 weeks' gestation

EPIDEMIOLOGY

Prevalence

- ~70% of the world's population is prone to primary lactase deficiency.
  - The prevalence of primary lactase deficiency in northern Europeans, who have a diet rich in dairy, is 2%.
  - In Hispanic populations, the prevalence of primary lactase deficiency is 50–80%.
  - In Ashkenazi Jewish and African American populations, the prevalence is 60–80%.
  - In Asian populations, the prevalence of primary lactase deficiency is nearly 100%.
- Nearly 20% of children <5 years from Hispanic, Asian, or African American descent have lactase deficiency and lactose malabsorption.
- Caucasian children usually do not develop symptoms until after 5 years of age.

RISK FACTOR

Genetics

- Posttranslational regulatory mechanisms in primary lactase deficiency or adult-type hypolactasia
- Correlation between the genetic polymorphism of mRNA and persistence of lactase activity with early loss at 1–2 years in Thai children and late loss at 10–20 years in Finnish children

PATHOPHYSIOLOGY

- Symptoms depend on the amount of lactose ingested.
- Malabsorbed lactose creates an osmotic load that draws fluid and electrolytes into the bowel lumen, leading to an osmotic diarrhea.
- Nonabsorbed lactose acts as a substrate for intestinal bacteria.
- In the colon, bacteria metabolize lactose, producing volatile fatty acids and gases leading to flatulence, bowel distension, pain, and low pH.

DIAGNOSIS

HISTORY

- Classic symptoms include bloating, gaseousness, colicky abdominal pain, and diarrhea after digestion of lactose-containing meal.
- Dietary intake history provides important information.
- Association with milk ingestion may not be evident.
- Symptoms vary in severity with dose of lactose ingested.
- Detailed history of symptoms:
  - Blood or mucus in the stools, weight loss, poor growth, fat malabsorption, or any extraintestinal symptoms strongly suggest different causes.

PHYSICAL EXAM

- Height and weight should be measured and plotted against age-appropriate norms; any deviation should not be attributed to lactose intolerance alone.
- Abdomen percussion: Abdomen may be distended and tympanitic.
- Blood in the stool must be further evaluated as lactose intolerance does not cause bleeding.

DIAGNOSTIC TESTS & INTERPRETATION

Lab

- Stool-reducing substances and fecal acidity
  - A pH <6.0 or reducing substances >0.5% should be interpreted as positive results.
  - Positive results indicate malabsorption of carbohydrates.
- Lactose hydrogen breath test
  - Noninvasive and highly sensitive
  - A rise of breath H_2 concentration of ≥20 ppm over baseline has been shown to correlate with enzyme deficiency.
  - However, there is poor association between symptoms of lactose intolerance and breath H_2 excretion, which underscores the need for caution in the interpretation of the clinical significance of the breath hydrogen test.

- False-positive test results can occur if inadequate fasting before the test, rapid intestinal transit, toothpaste, smoking, and bacterial overgrowth.
- False-negative results occur with diarrhea, hyperventilation, recent antibiotic exposure, and delayed gastric emptying. In addition, up to 10% of the population is colonized with bacteria unable to produce hydrogen, which can lead to a falsely negative result.

- Lactase activity measurement from endoscopically obtained duodenal tissue biopsies (invasive and expensive)

Pathologic Findings

The small bowel intestinal histology will often be normal in primary lactase deficiency (unless the reason is insult/damage to the small bowel mucosa).

DIFFERENTIAL DIAGNOSIS

- Infection
  - Viral and bacterial infections can cause secondary lactose intolerance due to villous injury.
  - Most common pathogen is rotavirus.
  - Parasitic infections can mimic lactose intolerance (giardiasis).
- Inflammatory conditions
  - Small intestinal Crohn disease
  - Celiac disease
- Congenital
  - Other carbohydrate enzyme deficiencies can mimic lactose intolerance. These include sucrase–isomaltase or glucose–galactose malabsorption.
  - Cystic fibrosis
  - Shwachman-Diamond syndrome (SDS): Primary features include the following:
    - Bone marrow insufficiency
    - Pancreatic insufficiency
    - Skeletal abnormalities
    - Short stature
- Allergic/immune
  - Food protein allergies
  - Oral medications containing lactose: common in tablets

TREATMENT

MEDICATION

- Oral lactase replacement capsules
- Calcium supplements to ensure daily recommended intake levels despite dairy restriction

ADDITIONAL TREATMENT

General Measures

- Removal of lactose from the diet is effective in eliminating symptoms.
- However, it is important to recognize that a milk-free diet is associated with calcium deficiency.
- Predigestion of lactose can be done by the addition of commercially available enzyme supplementation (extrinsic lactase). Multiple products are available over the counter. Liquid preparations, capsules, and chewable tablets can be obtained.
- Acquired deficiencies, particularly those associated with infection, may resolve over time or with specific treatment. Many patients with lactose intolerance do not recover the ability to digest lactose.
- Supplemental probiotics may improve symptoms of lactose intolerance.

ONGOING CARE

DIET

- Lactose-free formula, lactase-containing milk
- Cow milk substitutes (e.g., rice or soy milk)
- Yogurt and aged cheeses, which generally have smaller content of lactose.

PROGNOSIS

- Prognosis of lactase deficiency and clinical intolerance is excellent with lactose reduction or elimination as well as enzyme replacements are possible.
- Lactose intolerance secondary to disease processes should be recognized and treated appropriately.

ADDITIONAL READING

- Heyman MB, Committee on Nutrition. Lactose intolerance in infants, children, and adolescents. *Pediatrics*. 2006;118(3):1279–1286.
- Krawczyk M, Wolska M, Schwartz S, et al. Concordance of genetic and breath tests for lactose intolerance in a tertiary referral centre. *J Gastrointestin Liver Dis*. 2008;17(2):135–139.
- Law D, Conklin J, Pimentel M. Lactose intolerance and the role of the lactose breath test. *Am J Gastroenterol*. 2010;105(8):1726–1728.
- Levitt M, Wilt T, Shaukat A. Clinical implications of lactose malabsorption versus lactose intolerance. *J Clin Gastroenterol*. 2013;47(6):471–80.
- Mattar R, de Campos Mazo DF, Carrilho FJ. Lactose intolerance: diagnosis, genetic, and clinical factors. *Clin Exp Gastroenterol*. 2012;5:113–121.
- Usai Satta P, Congia M, Schirru E, et al. Genetic testing is ready to change the diagnostic scenario of lactose malabsorption. *Gut*. 2008;57(1):137–138.

CODES

ICD10

- E73.9 Lactose intolerance, unspecified
- E73.0 Congenital lactase deficiency
- E73.8 Other lactose intolerance

FAQ

- Q: When is the usual time for presentation of lactose intolerance?
- A: In whites, the age of presentation is after 5 years of age. In African Americans, 2–3-year-old children may present with clinical signs and symptoms. The differential diagnosis must distinguish primary from secondary causes.
- Q: Does lactose intolerance prevent a child from ever eating lactose?
- A: No. The patient can take smaller amounts of lactose in the diet or have the enzyme supplemented.
- Q: Does this problem ever get better?
- A: No. It is a lifelong problem, but seems to become less symptomatic for adults, in light of their individual desire to tolerate symptoms. Secondary lactose intolerance may improve with time or treatment of the primary disorder.

LEAD POISONING

Julie O'Brien • Kent Olson

BASICS

DESCRIPTION

- Lead poisoning is one of the most common pediatric environmental health problems, most often involving systemic intoxication with inorganic lead. Lead poisoning is an older term that is less specific than an actual blood lead level (BLL).
- The Centers for Disease Control and Prevention (CDC) considers an elevated BLL to be ≥5 mcg/dL.
  - This "reference value" is based on the 97.5th percentile for lead levels of children aged 1–5 years collected for the National Health and Nutrition Examination Surveys (NHANES).
  - This replaces the previous "level of concern" terminology for levels ≥10 mcg/dL based on the Advisory Committee on Childhood Lead Poisoning Prevention (ACCLPP) recommendations in light of many studies demonstrating cognitive and behavioral effects at BLL less than 10 mcg/dL.

EPIDEMIOLOGY

A recent national survey estimates that 38 million housing units have lead-based paint (1/3 of all U.S. housing).

- 24 million housing units have hazards from lead-based paint.
- ~83% of American pre-1978 privately owned units contain some lead-based paint.

Prevalence

The prevalence of elevated BLLs and the geometric mean BLLs have decreased significantly in the past 20 years.

- ~450,000 American children aged 1–5 years are estimated to have BLLs of ≥5 mcg/dL.
- Racial income disparities persist due to disparities in housing quality, nutrition, and access to health care.

RISK FACTORS

- Young children with more oral behaviors
- Children with developmental delays/mental retardation
- Children with pica
- Residence in older homes with flaking or deteriorating lead-based paint
- Renovation or remodeling of older homes without lead hazard controls in place
- Recent immigration from countries where ambient lead contamination is high (i.e., where leaded gasoline is still used)
- Use of lead-glazed ceramic pottery
- Use of traditional therapies containing lead (e.g., Azarcon, some Ayurvedic and Chinese medicines)
- Ingestion of lead-containing candies from Mexico

GENERAL PREVENTION

- Primary prevention: removal of potential environmental lead hazards prior to exposure
  - The ACCLPP focuses on primary prevention as it emphasizes that there is no "safe" level of lead and the effects of lead are likely irreversible.
  - Clinicians should provide anticipatory guidance to all parents about lead exposure pathways and the prevention of exposures.
- Secondary prevention: screening for elevated BLLs
  - Minimum screening recommendations: blood lead test for children at 1 and 2 years and for those 36–72 months old who have not had previous screening
  - Screening children immigrating from other countries and screening pregnant and lactating women and their neonates and infants for lead exposure prior to or during pregnancy and lactation
- Tertiary prevention: case management and environmental remediation for children with lead poisoning
- Control measures
  - Abatement of building-based (residential) lead hazards by removal, encapsulation, or enclosure of lead-containing structures
  - Control of environmental lead dust exposure and ingestion by good housekeeping (wet dusting and mopping of household dust); personal hygiene (cleaning of child's hands, toys, personal items, wiping feet on mats prior to entering the home), and hiring certified renovators who are EPA-approved to perform renovations that may disrupt lead-based paint
  - Removal of any other known lead source from the child's environment

PATHOPHYSIOLOGY

- Lead adversely affects many organ systems including neurologic, hematologic, GI, renal, and reproductive.
  - Many toxic effects result from inhibition of enzymes involved in heme biosynthesis, as the electropositive metal binds to negatively charged sulfhydryl groups on active sites of δ-aminolevulinic acid dehydratase (ALAD), ferrochelatase, porphobilinogen synthase, coproporphyrinogen oxidase, and other enzymes.
  - Divalent lead also acts competitively with calcium in various biologic systems.
- Children absorb lead more efficiently from the GI tract and are more likely than adults to ingest lead through hand-to-mouth activities.
- Because the developing, immature CNS is susceptible to toxic effects of lead, the neuropsychologic effects of lead poisoning on fetuses/young children are of particular concern. Even relatively low BLLs are associated with IQ deficits, attention-related behaviors, and poor academic achievement.

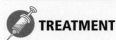

DIAGNOSIS

HISTORY

- It is important to assess for risk factors for exposure, as most children are asymptomatic.
- Etiology/common sources of lead:
  - Ingestion of lead-based paint or contaminated dust or soil through residence in or visitation of older (pre-1980), deteriorated housing
  - A parental occupation or hobby involving lead exposure (e.g., construction or battery plant work, stained glass window or pottery making)
  - Use of remedies, cosmetics, pottery, toys, or consumer products containing lead
  - Ingestion of contaminated water, food, or beverages
- Typical symptoms:
  - Most children are asymptomatic; many clinical manifestations are nonspecific. A cluster of complaints including anorexia, intermittent abdominal pain, constipation, sporadic vomiting, change in mental status (e.g., irritability or lethargy), decreased play activity, and change in developmental status (e.g., regression of developmental milestones) may herald this condition.
- Lead encephalopathy
  - Can present with change in consciousness, ataxia, persistent vomiting, seizures, and coma
  - Often presents after a prodrome of symptoms mentioned above

PHYSICAL EXAM

As patients are generally asymptomatic, physical exam is not generally helpful at lower lead levels.

- Symptomatic and/or encephalopathic patients may have acute GI, neurologic, hematologic, and systemic manifestations.
- Assess for developmental delay.

DIAGNOSTIC TESTS & INTERPRETATION

Lab

- Blood lead test, either venous or capillary (but must be drawn in lead-free tube):
  - Results may be reportable to local health authorities.
  - The test result is a measure only of recent lead exposure and does not indicate total body burden of lead.
  - Capillary testing is associated with more false-positive results. If abnormal, a venous lead should be sent.
  - A confirmed elevated BLL is defined as a child with a venous blood sample ≥5 mcg/dL.
- CBC: to assess for anemia
  - Iron deficiency anemia is often seen concomitantly.
  - Anemia related to lead toxicity is typically normocytic and normochromic; a microcytic, hypochromic anemia may be seen with a mixed etiology.
  - Basophilic stippling is sometimes seen on peripheral blood smear.
- Free erythrocyte protoporphyrin
  - Marker of lead-induced inhibition of heme synthesis
  - Can be useful clinically to follow the recovery from heme synthesis inhibition during management

Imaging

- Abdominal radiograph: Look for radiopaque foreign material suggestive of ingestion of lead paint chips or other lead-containing foreign body, when ingestion of such is suspected in the history or with very high BLLs.
- Long bone radiographs are not recommended for routine screening.

DIFFERENTIAL DIAGNOSIS

Consider lead poisoning as the etiology for the following diagnoses:

- Seizures, altered mental status, and/or coma
- Anemia

ALERT

Failure to diagnose results from the following:

- Delay in checking a blood lead test in the presence of clinical signs, symptoms of lead poisoning, or neuropsychologic disorders
- Failure to inquire about lead exposure possibilities

TREATMENT

Treatment for most individuals is focused on environmental management to prevent further lead exposure. Medications are only required at higher BLLs.

GENERAL MEASURES

- Environmental management
  - Remove children from the lead source(s).
  - Should occur when venous lead levels are recurrently 10 mcg/dL (CDC class IIA) and higher; could be done for lower BLLs as resources allow
- Reduction of lead levels in the household
- Consultation with a qualified lead abatement contractor is advised.

MEDICATION

- Chelation therapy
  - Should complement environmental management in all children with venous levels of ≥45 mcg/dL using parenteral calcium disodium ethylenediaminetetraacetate (Ca-EDTA; calcium disodium versenate) or oral agents such as meso-2,3-dimercaptosuccinic acid (DMSA, succimer, Chemet)
  - Chelation of children with levels <45 mcg/dL is not recommended, as evidence suggests it does not reverse or diminish neuropsychological effects of lead.
  - Outpatient therapy can take place if a lead-safe environment has been identified and compliance is expected.
  - Succimer is given at 10 mg/kg (or 350 mg/m^2) q8h for 5 days, then q12h for 14 more days. Weekly monitoring for neutropenia, platelet abnormality, and increased liver enzymes is recommended.
- Children with symptomatic lead poisoning or with levels of ≥70 mcg/dL should be admitted immediately to a hospital for parenteral chelation with both IM dimercaprol (British anti-Lewisite, BAL) and IV or IM calcium disodium EDTA. Because there are many issues involved with administration of both chelating agents, consultation with a clinician experienced in lead toxicity treatment is advised.
- Children with encephalopathy constitute a medical emergency and should receive the preceding treatment in an intensive care setting with attentive neurosurgical support.
- Ingested lead-containing foreign bodies should be evacuated with whole-bowel irrigation using a polyethylene glycol electrolyte solution.

ISSUES FOR REFERRAL

- Close communication with the local health department is essential before, during, and after admission.
- Referral may be made to early intervention or development assessment programs, social workers, therapists, neurologists, or other specialists, as needed.

INPATIENT CONSIDERATIONS

Admission Criteria

Admit all symptomatic children, those with BLLs ≥70, and those with BLLs ≥45 for which one cannot ensure a lead-safe environment and/or compliance with oral medication.

Discharge Criteria

Consider discharge when symptoms have resolved, BLL has significantly declined, and a lead-safe discharge environment has been identified.

FOLLOW-UP RECOMMENDATIONS

Patient Monitoring

- Prompt environmental follow-up of current lead exposure situations and investigation for additional exposure (e.g., with family moves, visitation of new residences) should occur.
- Follow-up venous lead levels should be performed for those with BLLs ≥5 mcg/dL about every 1–3 months, with less frequent follow-up after levels decline.
- Follow-up venous levels should be performed 1–3 weeks following chelation therapy, with frequent monitoring thereafter until levels have decreased significantly and no new lead exposure is apparent. BLLs will increase from the nadir level immediately after treatment to rebound to a level between this and the pretreatment level.

DIET

- Nutritional support with calcium and iron supplementation should be given if intake is inadequate; deficiencies of these increase lead absorption from the GI tract.
- The recommendation for adequate intake of calcium is 500 mg/day, which can typically be achieved through a regular healthy diet.
  - There is currently no evidence that supplementation of calcium beyond the recommended "adequate intake" is beneficial for children with elevated BLLs.
- Iron repletion should be initiated with 3 mg/kg of elemental iron for those children who are found to be iron deficient.
  - Iron supplementation should be withheld during chelation therapy.
- Additionally, it is recommended to consume at least two servings daily of foods high in vitamin C, such as fruits, vegetables, and juices.

PROGNOSIS

There is an increased risk for long-term neuropsychological sequelae, which increases with lead exposure and absorption that is more intense, of longer duration, and begins at an early age when the CNS is still developing.

- Recurrent episodes of symptomatic lead poisoning increase the risk for permanent sequelae.
- Subtle effects may be missed until school entry.

COMPLICATIONS

- Acute encephalopathy
- Seizures
- Coma
- Death (predominantly owing to cerebral edema)
- Mental retardation
- Cognitive, behavioral, attentional, and neurodevelopmental impairment
- Anemia
- Fanconi syndrome
- Abdominal colic
- Adverse reproductive outcomes

ADDITIONAL READING

- Advisory Committee on Childhood Lead Poisoning Prevention of the Centers for Disease Control and Prevention. *Low Level Lead Exposure Harms Children: A Renewed Call for Primary Prevention*. Atlanta, GA: U.S. Department of Health and Human Services, Centers for Disease Control and Prevention; 2012.
- American Academy of Pediatrics Committee on Environmental Health. Lead exposure in children: prevention, detection and management. *Pediatrics*. 2005;116(4):1036–1046.
- Bellinger DC. Very low lead exposures and children's neurodevelopment. *Curr Opin Pediatr*. 2008;20(2):172–173.
- Binns, HJ, Campbell C, Brown MJ. Interpreting and managing blood lead levels of less than <10 microg/dL in children and reducing childhood exposure to lead: recommendations of the Centers for Disease Control and Prevention Advisory Committee on Childhood Lead Poisoning Prevention. *Pediatrics*. 2007;120(5):e1285–e1298.
- Canfield RL, Henderson CR Jr, Cory-Slechta DA, et al. Intellectual impairment in children with blood lead concentrations below 10 microg/dL per deciliter. *N Engl J Med*. 2003;348(16):1517–1526.
- CDC response to Advisory Committee on Childhood Lead Poisoning Prevention Recommendations in "*Low Level Lead Exposure Harms Children: A Renewed Call for Primary Prevention*."
- Centers for Disease Control and Prevention. *Guidelines for the Identification and Management of Lead Exposure in Pregnant and Lactating Women*. Atlanta, GA: Centers for Disease Control and Prevention; 2010.
- Centers for Disease Control and Prevention. *Preventing Lead Poisoning in Young Children*. Atlanta, GA: Centers for Disease Control and Prevention; 2005.
- Lanphear BP, Hornung R, Khoury J, et al. Low-level environmental lead exposure and children's intellectual function: an international pooled analysis. *Environ Health Perspect*. 2005;113(7):894–899.
- Lanphear BP, Matte TD, Rogers J, et al. The contribution of lead-contaminated house dust and residential soil to children's blood lead levels. *Environ Res*. 1998;79(1):51–68.

CODES

ICD10

- T56.0X4A Toxic effect of lead and its compounds, undetermined, init
- T56.0X1A Toxic effect of lead and its compounds, accidental, init

FAQ

- Q: What is lead abatement?
- A: Lead abatement is removal of a lead hazard from the environment either by replacing it (e.g., installing a new window), enclosing the area with the lead source (e.g., installing paneling), removing the lead-based paint from a surface (burning or dry sanding methods should never be used), or encapsulating the area (placement of a specific coating over the lead-containing surface, which prevents access to the lead hazard).
- Q: Is lead abatement permanent?
- A: Often, lead paint that is chipping or peeling is removed from a home. Any areas with intact lead-based paint may become deteriorated with aging, leading to new lead hazards, although ongoing maintenance and repair may prevent this.
- Q: Why didn't my child's brother and sister get lead poisoning at the same age since they lived in the same house?
- A: Children are different; some do much more hand-to-mouth activity than others, which is the main way that children get lead into their bodies. Also, your home may not have had the same lead dangers (hazards) when the siblings were younger.

LEARNING DISABILITIES

Monica D. Dowling • Jeffrey P. Brosco

BASICS

DESCRIPTION

Learning disabilities (LD) are a group of disorders characterized by unexpected and sustained difficulties acquiring and applying academic skills, including reading accuracy, reading fluency, reading comprehension, written expression, mathematic calculations, and mathematic problem-solving.

- LD comprise one category within the classification of Neurodevelopmental Disorders (NDDs) in the *Diagnostic and Statistical Manual of Mental Disorders*, 5th edition (DSM-V, 2013) and the *International Classification of Diseases, Code Book 10* (ICD-10, 2013).
- Academic achievement must be substantially below the level expected for age and not attributable to intellectual disability (ID), neurologic or motor disorders, lack of schooling, psychosocial factors, economic disadvantage, or major sensory problems.
- LD have neurobiologic and genetic roots.
- Reading disability is the most frequently diagnosed type of LD and is typically characterized by impairments in phonologic processing and/or orthographic coding skills. Children with math disability show procedural, retrieval, and number sense deficits.
- The role of the pediatrician is to advocate for a child with LD, interpret predisposing factors in child's developmental and medical history, and offer scientific interpretation of the range of theories and interventions.
- Early intervention improves outcomes.

EPIDEMIOLOGY

- In 2009–2010, 2.4 million or 5% of total public school enrollees (ages 3–21 years) identified with LD as eligible for special education based on U.S. Department of Education National Center for Education Statistics, 2012.
- The National Institutes of Health (NIH) estimates that as many as 15–20% of Americans are affected by LD.

RISK FACTORS

- LD are familial and moderately heritable.
- Risk loci and genes have been identified for reading and language disorders.
- Aberrant neuronal migration hypothesized as principal pathophysiology
- Genetic contribution increases with a high level of parent education (a bioecologic gene by environment interaction).
- Environmental factors include prematurity, low birth weight, prenatal nicotine or alcohol exposure, infections, and traumatic brain injury.

COMMONLY ASSOCIATED CONDITIONS

- Language disorders
- Speech sound disorders
- Auditory processing disorders
- Developmental coordination disorder
- ADHD/executive function deficits

GENERAL PREVENTION

- High-quality developmentally appropriate preschool experiences
- Early literacy initiatives (e.g., Reach Out and Read)
- Early intervention for speech, language, motor difficulties
- Evidence-based reading curricula and ongoing academic progress monitoring beginning in kindergarten
- Supplemental instruction for children who show early signs of learning problems

DIAGNOSIS

DIFFERENTIAL DIAGNOSIS

- ID
  - Borderline intellectual functioning or mild ID may not be evident in early childhood.
- ADHD
  - Especially when inattentive and distractible symptoms are greater than hyperactive symptoms
  - Comorbidity is approximately half of diagnosed cases of LD.
- Sensory impairments
  - Hearing or vision impairments
  - School screening results should be confirmed by the pediatrician in children with academic problems.
- Neurologic etiologies
  - Absence seizures and other nonconvulsive epileptic disorders
  - Neurodegenerative disorders such as Niemann–Pick disease, adrenoleukodystrophy, ceroid lipofuscinosis, and subacute sclerosing panencephalitis may rarely present as school-age learning problems.
  - CNS trauma
- Genetic syndromes
  - Some genetic syndromes may show subtle dysmorphology that is not noted until learning problems arise. Examples include the following:
    - Sex chromosome aneuploidies
    - Fragile X syndrome
    - Neurofibromatosis
    - Tuberous sclerosis
    - Velocardiofacial/DiGeorge syndrome
- Hypothyroidism
- HIV infection
- Lead intoxication
- Chronic malnutrition
- Iron deficiency
- Iatrogenic interventions
  - Some medications (e.g., antiepileptic drugs) affect cognition.
  - Cancer treatment
- Psychosocial issues
  - Issues related to family stress, peer relationships, illness, school absence, or adolescence may present as academic difficulty.
  - Conversely, behavior problems at home or at school always should prompt evaluation of school functioning.
- Psychiatric comorbidity
  - Adjustment disorders, anxiety, mood disorders, oppositional defiant disorder, conduct disorder, tic disorders, substance abuse, and other behavior problems may precede or follow the presentation of LD.

APPROACH TO THE PATIENT

- Many learning problems respond to appropriate educational interventions, regardless of specific etiology, and failure to respond to intervention is part of the diagnostic process for specific LD.
- It is the role of the educator to (a) monitor academic progress of all students, (b) provide educational intervention and frequent progress monitoring to struggling students, and (c) conduct a psychoeducational assessment of students who do not respond to initial intervention.
- Once a child presents with learning problems, it is the role of the pediatrician to
  - Help the family obtain timely and evidence-based educational interventions. LD Navigator (http://www.ncld.org) provides health care professionals with resources.
  - Identify and treat underlying medical problems.
  - Identify and help treat underlying psychosocial issues:
    - Psychosocial stresses may exacerbate learning difficulties or be a primary etiologic factor.
    - School attendance is a particularly important factor in learning.
  - Identify and treat comorbid psychiatric disorders.

HISTORY

- **Question:** When and how does the child fail in his or her daily academic pursuits?
- *Significance*:
  - LD typically impact only school activities and are often limited to one skill area such as reading or math.
  - Children with ADHD typically show problems in multiple settings (school, home, extracurricular, peers).
  - Children with ID usually have a history of developmental concerns.
- **Question:** Is decline in school performance recent and/or abrupt?
- *Significance*: If abrupt, consider pathophysiologic processes such as vision or hearing impairment, side effect from medication, neurodegenerative disorders (rare), or recent psychosocial issue.

- **Question:** Past medical history, medications, review of systems, psychosocial stresses?
- *Significance*
  - School attendance (illness vs. avoidance)
  - Early development and behavior
  - Family history of learning problems
  - Sleep patterns (apnea, insomnia)

PHYSICAL EXAM

- **Finding:** Subtle dysmorphology?
- *Significance*: May suggest the presence of a genetic syndrome or a pattern of malformation resulting from teratogenic fetal exposures (e.g., alcohol, phenytoin)
- **Finding:** Skin lesions?
- *Significance*: May suggest underlying genetic syndromes such as tuberous sclerosis
- **Finding:** Enlarged tonsils?
- *Significance*: May cause sleep disturbance that affects learning and/or behavior
- **Finding:** Abnormal neurologic examination?
- *Significance*
  - Any focal signs demand additional evaluation
  - Slow rapid alternating finger movements (neuromaturational signs) are often present in children with LD but are generally not helpful clinically.

DIAGNOSTIC TESTS & INTERPRETATION

- Physician
  - Audiology and vision screening
  - Standardized behavior questionnaires (e.g., Teachers and Parent Vanderbilt)
  - Consider other screening tools for depression, anxiety, family dysfunction, parental depression, and substance abuse.
  - Genetic, neurologic evaluation if indicated by history or physical exam
- Educator
  - Teacher-administered measures or computer-administered tests to monitor progress. Standardized achievement tests can be administered yearly to measure current functioning and review progress.
- Psychologist
  - Testing must be performed individually and include intellectual and academic functioning at a minimum.
  - Federal law requires schools to provide comprehensive evaluations on written request by the parents. Specific information for each state is available from the National Dissemination Center for Children with Disabilities (800-695-0285; http://www.nichcy.org).
  - University- and hospital-based centers outside the school system also conduct evaluations of children with LD.
  - For children who do not respond to educational interventions, or if the psychoeducational evaluation is inconclusive, neuropsychologic testing may identify specific cognitive factors that are helpful in developing an effective educational plan.

TREATMENT

- Discourage a "wait and see" approach to decision making.
- Begin evidence-based interventions as soon as problems are evident; children who do not respond require more thorough etiologic workup.
- Academic or attention difficulties may lead to spiraling psychological problems from depression or damaged self-esteem to conduct disorder and school dropout.

GENERAL MEASURES

- Physician
  - Responsible for treatment of underlying medical diagnoses
  - Ensure appropriate treatment of psychological problems with pharmacologic therapy and behavioral therapy (family therapy, social skills training, cognitive-behavioral therapy) as needed.
- School
  - Educational treatment varies with the age and educational level of the child and should follow an approach of increasing intensity as needed.
    - Tier 1: For patients displaying poor academic achievement, begin with extra support (e.g., homework clinic, tutoring) in the regular educational program (assuming culturally and linguistically appropriate instruction).
    - Tier 2: If academic problems disrupt classroom participation and impede progress, refer to school-based child study team and provide intensive assistance as part of general curriculum, such as summer school or specialized materials.
    - Tier 3: If child is >1 year behind or has shown minimal response to Tier 2 interventions, refer for a comprehensive psychoeducational evaluation to identify specialized interventions, typically provided under the umbrella of special education.
  - Specialized instruction is at the center of treatment, often within the regular classroom (inclusion) with supplemental instruction through either a consultant special teacher or a resource room.
  - Children may also benefit from classroom accommodations such as preferential seating, extra time for test taking, word processors and computer applications, text-to-speech programs, calculators, note-takers, and modified instructions.
  - Treatment is most effective when it uses a team approach, including parents, teachers, and other therapists.
  - Grade retention has not been shown to be effective.

ONGOING CARE

Children with LD require continued monitoring of academic progress. Even when the initial learning problems are resolved, later difficulties may arise in writing, note-taking, composition, organization, or with more abstract academic subjects.

PROGNOSIS

- In most cases, prognosis is quite good with treatment, although LD never go away.
- Prognosis varies with intensity, timing, and appropriateness of intervention.
- Early diagnosis and treatment is essential for minimizing impact and to take advantage of typical developmental progression.
- Current brain imaging research shows remedial reading instruction alters brain functioning if provided during critical window of development (younger than age 8–10 years).

ADDITIONAL READING

- American Psychiatric Association. *Diagnostic and Statistical Manual of Mental Disorders, Fifth Edition (DSM-5)*. Arlington, VA: American Psychiatric Association; 2013.
- Catts HW, Nielsen DC, Bridges MS, et al. Early identification of reading disabilities within an RTI framework. *J Learn Disabil*. 2013;20:1–17.
- Olulade OA, Napoliello EM, Eden GF. Abnormal visual motion processing is not a cause of dyslexia. *Neuron*. 2013;79(1):180–190.
- Peterson RL, Pennington BF. Developmental dyslexia. *Lancet*. 2012;379(9830):1997–2007.
- Raskind WH, Peter B, Richards T, et al. The genetics of reading disabilities: from phenotypes to candidate genes. *Front Psychol*. 2013;3:601.
- World Health Organization. *International Statistical Classification of Diseases and Related Health Problems, 10th Revision (ICD-10)*. Geneva, Switzerland: World Health Organization; 1992.

CODES

ICD10

- F81.9 Developmental disorder of scholastic skills, unspecified
- F81.0 Specific reading disorder
- F81.2 Mathematics disorder

FAQ

- Q: What is the evidence that visual training will improve reading?
- A: Despite anecdotal reports of value, there is strong evidence that visual dysfunction is not causal to reading disability; there is insufficient evidence to recommend vision therapy.

L

LEUKOCYTOSIS

Monica Khurana • Caroline Hastings

BASICS

DESCRIPTION

Leukocytosis refers to a total white blood cell (WBC) count above the normal range for age.

RISK FACTORS

- Very low-birth-weight neonates
- Immunodeficiencies or immunocompromised states
- Inflammatory disorders
- Autoimmune disorders

ALERT

Children with trisomy 21 (Down syndrome) have an increased risk of developing transient myeloproliferative disorder (TMD) or leukemoid reactions.

PATHOPHYSIOLOGY

Leukocytosis results from increased marrow production, demargination, prolonged cell survival, and/or defective extravasculation in response to external stimuli or, less commonly, from an underlying marrow disorder.

DIAGNOSIS

DIFFERENTIAL DIAGNOSIS

- Atopy
  - Allergies
  - Asthma
  - Eczema
  - Psoriasis
- Congenital/genetic
  - Down syndrome
  - Hereditary neutrophilia
  - Leukocyte adhesion deficiency (LAD)
  - Sickle cell anemia
- Hemolysis
  - Hemolytic anemia
  - Transfusion reaction
- Infectious
  - Bacterial
    - *Brucella*
    - *Bartonella*
    - *Bordetella pertussis*
    - *Clostridium difficile*
    - *Francisella tularensis*
    - *Haemophilus*
    - *Mycobacterium tuberculosis* (TB)
    - *Neisseria*
    - *Rickettsia*
    - *Streptococcus pneumoniae*
    - *Staphylococcus aureus*
  - Viral
    - Cytomegalovirus (CMV)
    - Epstein-Barr virus (EBV)
    - Hantavirus (Hantavirus pulmonary syndrome)
    - Hepatitis
    - Respiratory syncytial virus
  - Parasitic
    - *Toxocara canis*
    - *Toxoplasma*
    - *Trichinella*
    - *Plasmodium* spp
  - Fungal
    - Coccidioidomycosis
  - Spirochetal
    - *Treponema pallidum*
- Immunologic/inflammatory/reactive
  - Appendicitis
  - Addison disease
  - Asplenia
  - Chronic granulomatous disease
  - Hypereosinophilic syndrome (HES)
  - Inflammatory bowel disease (IBD)
  - Juvenile idiopathic arthritis (JIA)
  - Löffler syndrome
  - Sarcoidosis
  - Smoking
  - Thyrotoxicosis
  - Vasculitis including Kawasaki disease
- Malignancy
  - Acute leukemias
  - Chronic leukemias
  - Lymphomas
  - Solid tumors
- Medications
  - Antiepileptics
  - Beta agonists
  - Corticosteroids
  - Epinephrine
  - Granulocyte or granulocyte–macrophage colony-stimulating factor
  - Heparin
  - Lithium
  - Minocycline
  - Prostaglandin
- Myeloproliferative disorders
  - Polycythemia vera
  - Essential thrombocytopenia
  - Myelofibrosis (but more often associated with cytopenias)
- Poisons
  - Lead
- Stress
  - Anesthesia
  - Anxiety
  - Emotional stress
  - Overexertion
  - Seizures
- Trauma
  - Acute hemorrhage
  - Severe burns
- Nonaccidental trauma

DIAGNOSTIC TESTS & INTERPRETATION

- Step 1: Confirm that the leukocytosis is real.
  - Etiologies of spurious leukocytosis by automated analyzers of whole blood include nucleated or partially lysed RBCs, cryoglobulin or cryofibrinogen, or platelet clumps.
  - Confirmation includes review of peripheral smear via consultation of a pathologist or hematologist.
- Step 2: Obtain a differential of the WBC count.
  - A manual differential may be required.
  - Distinguishing between myeloid and lymphoid or even blasts contributes to identifying the correct etiology.
  - Myeloid leukocytosis include (1) neutrophilia, which commonly results from bacterial infections; (2) monocytosis; (3) eosinophilia, typically reactive; (4) basophilia, which is rare and suggestive of myeloproliferative neoplasms; and (5) increased blasts, concerning for underlying marrow abnormality.
  - Lymphoid leukocytosis results from viral infections.

ALERT

Beware of any differential that has a high percentage of monocytes or atypical lymphocytes, whether machine generated or manual. Leukemic blasts can be mistaken for these cell types.

- Step 3: Distinguish between reactive and clonal populations.
  - Reactive leukocytosis is heterogenous—pleomorphic, polyclonal, and/or large granular cells are present.
  - Neoplasms such as leukemia/lymphoma are homogenous.
  - May need to use flow cytometry with immunophenotyping and/or cell receptor gene rearrangements to rule out malignancy, especially in lymphoproliferative disorders

- Step 4: Evaluate other cell lines.
  - Concurrent presence of anemia and/or thrombocytopenia suggests an underlying marrow disorder such as leukemia.
  - Leukocytosis and thrombocytosis may be associated with iron deficiency anemia, sickle cell anemia, LAD type III, and pregnancy.
- Step 5: Use this information in clinical context.

HISTORY

- Evaluate for history or signs of infection.
  - Acute infection is the most common cause of leukocytosis.
  - Fever is nonspecific and may be present in infectious, inflammatory, rheumatoid, or malignant diseases.
- Obtain thorough past medical history.
  - Down syndrome: TMD occurs in ~10% infants and spontaneously resolves in 1 month, although 20–30% of these patients progress to AML. This is a medical emergency if there is organomegaly with cardiopulmonary compromise.
  - Hereditary neutrophilia: autosomal dominant disorder with heterozygous mutation in the *CSF3R* gene on chromosome 1p34
  - LAD: rare autosomal recessive disorder characterized by recurrent bacterial infections
  - Sickle cell anemia: Leukocytosis likely reflects chronic inflammation and may be associated with increased vaso-occlusive events.
- Comprehensive review of symptoms may indicate malignancy.
  - B symptoms include fever, drenching night sweats, and weight loss of ≥10% over 6 months.
  - Persistent bone pain may indicate leukemia and be initially diagnosed as growing pains or worked up for osteomyelitis or JIA.
- Do not forget to obtain history of travel or unusual exposures.
  - Shigellosis enteritis may be seen after travel to areas with suboptimal sanitation and present with leukocytosis and even seizures.
  - Nursing home residents, incarcerated individuals, and health care professionals are at higher risk for developing and transmitting TB.
  - Reptiles commonly carry *Salmonella* and rodents commonly carry Hantavirus.
- Obtain complete family history.
  - Family histories positive for autoimmune disorders may raise suspicion for IBD, JIA, HES, thyroid disease, vasculitis, etc.

PHYSICAL EXAM

- Cardiopulmonary
  - A careful lung examination is necessary, as pneumonia is a common cause of leukocytosis.
  - A new murmur or gallop may be an early sign of bacterial endocarditis.
- Abdominal/lymph
  - If hepatosplenomegaly and/or lymphadenopathy is present, consider acute viral hepatitis, infectious mononucleosis from either EBV or CMV, malignancy, malaria, or lysosomal storage disease.
- Musculoskeletal/dermatologic
  - Arthritis or joint pain and/or rashes may be one manifestation in a constellation that may suggest JIA, rheumatic fever, or Lyme disease.

Imaging

Although universal vaccination with Prevnar (pneumococcal conjugate vaccine [PCV]) has decreased the incidence of pneumonia, clinicians should still strongly consider chest radiography in young, highly febrile children with leukocytosis and no obvious source of infection.

TREATMENT

GENERAL MEASURES

- Isolated leukocytosis may be monitored without intervention.
- If ill-appearing, age-appropriate empiric antibiotics are indicated.
- Consultation with other subspecialties may be necessary.
- Prognosis depends on diagnosis.

ONGOING CARE

In the setting of bacterial infection with appropriate microbial coverage, anticipate resolution of leukocytosis within 4 days.

ALERT

If malignancy is in the differential, consult hematology/oncology prior to initiating steroids.

ADDITIONAL READING

- Abramson N, Melton B. Leukocytosis: basis of clinical assessment. *Am Fam Physician*. 2000;62(9):2053–2060.
- Cerny J, Rosmarin AG. Why does my patient have leukocytosis? *Hematol Oncol Clin North Am*. 2012;26(2):303–319.
- George TI. Malignant or benign leukocytosis. *Hematology Am Soc Hematol Educ Program*. 2012; 2012:475–484.

CODES

ICD10

- D72.829 Elevated white blood cell count, unspecified
- D72.0 Genetic anomalies of leukocytes
- D72.828 Other elevated white blood cell count

FAQ

- Q: Does the degree of leukocytosis correlate to the severity of infection?
- A: Just as the height of fever does not always correlate to the severity of infection, the same is true for the degree of leukocytosis. Even a normal WBC does not rule out bacteremia.
- Q: What is a leukemoid reaction?
- A: A leukemoid reaction is a physiologic response to a stress or infection and is characterized by a WBC of $\geq 50 \times 10^9$/L with peripheral blood myeloid precursors at all stages of maturity rather than proliferation of an immature WBC clonal population, which is characteristic of malignancies.
- Q: When is an elevated WBC a clinical emergency?
- A: Leukocytosis or hyperleukocytosis is a clinical emergency when the patient is symptomatic from leukostasis. Hyperleukocytosis is a total WBC count of $\geq 100 \times 10^9$/L. Clinically significant hyperleukocytosis usually occurs at WBC $\geq 200 \times 10^9$/L or $\geq 300 \times 10^9$/L in patients with acute myeloid or lymphoblastic leukemia and chronic myeloid leukemia in blast crisis, respectively; however, symptoms may present with a WBC as low as 50×10^9/L. Refer to hyperleukocytosis chapter for more information.

L

LICE (PEDICULOSIS)

Janet Gingold • Linda Fu

BASICS

DESCRIPTION
Infestation of the head, body, or anogenital region by parasitic, wingless insects that feed exclusively on human blood

EPIDEMIOLOGY
- Head lice
  - Spread by head-to-head contact
  - Most common among children 3–12 years old
  - Associated with female gender, warmer weather, crowded living conditions
  - Less common among African Americans
  - Point prevalence estimates range from <1% in some places to >90% in others.
- Body lice
  - Spread by close physical contact with infested persons, clothing, or bedding
  - Associated with poor sanitation, cool climates, homelessness, war, disasters, refugee camps
  - No racial or gender differences
- Pubic lice
  - Usually sexually transmitted
  - Can also spread through contact with clothing or bedding recently used by infested person
  - Most common among young adults

Incidence
- Varies widely with location and living conditions.
- Estimated 6–12 million cases per year in the United States

GENERAL PREVENTION
Humans are the only host for all three types of lice. Recurrences are common and may be prevented by examining and treating close contacts, especially bedmates.
- Head lice
  - Avoid head-to-head contact with infested persons; don't share brushes, hats, or hair ties. Avoid lying on pillows, furniture, or stuffed toys used by infested person within last 2 days.
  - Wash clothing and bedding used by infested person with hot water (≥130°F) and set dryer to highest heat setting. Items may also be dry-cleaned or sealed in a plastic bag for 2 weeks. Vacuum furniture and carpet.
  - Environmental insecticide is not helpful.
  - Treatment of pets is not necessary.
  - "No-nit" school policies do not control head lice transmission and are not recommended.
- Body lice
  - Regularly wash clothes.
  - Avoid using clothing or bedding used by infested person.
- Pubic lice
  - Avoid close body contact or sharing clothes with infested person.
  - Not prevented by condom use

PATHOPHYSIOLOGY
- Bites of louse are painless.
- To facilitate blood meal, lice inject enzymes, anticoagulant, and vasodilators. These provoke host inflammatory response causing pruritus.
- Bites characterized by intradermal hemorrhage and infiltrates of eosinophils and lymphocytes
- Excoriation can introduce secondary infections.
- Vector-borne pathogens (body lice only) can cause chronic bacteremia, angiomatosis, or endocarditis.

ETIOLOGY
- Head lice (*Pediculus humanus capitis*)
  - Adults white-to-gray; 2–4-mm long; 6 legs; no wings. Crawl quickly away from threat or bright light. Cannot jump or fly. If removed from host, will die within 2 days
  - Females lay up to 10 eggs per day over 2–3-week lifespan, attaching egg to base of hair shaft with adhesive.
  - Eggs are very temperature sensitive; hatch in 7–12 days; empty white egg casing remains on hair.
  - Emerging nymphs (instars) die without blood meal within a few hours. Molt 3 times over 9–11 days to become egg-laying adults.
  - Typical infestation includes lice in all stages of development; effect of treatment depends on stage of life cycle.
- Body lice (*P. humanus corporis*)
  - Morphology and life cycle similar to head lice, but adults are slightly larger
  - Live and lay eggs on clothing and only come to the skin to feed 4–5 times per day
  - Able to live longer off host than head lice
  - Eggs hatch in 6–10 days.
- Pubic lice (*Phthirus pubis*)
  - Crab-like appearance, with larger talus adapted to coarser hair; predilection for pubic hair
  - May also infest axillary hair, perianal area, eyelashes, beard, and rarely scalp

COMMONLY ASSOCIATED CONDITIONS
- Body lice
  - May act as a vector for epidemic typhus (*Rickettsia prowazekii*), relapsing fever (*Borrelia recurrentis*), and trench fever (*Bartonella quintana*) or plague (*Yersinia pestis*)
- Pubic lice
  - Commonly occurs with other sexually transmitted infections
  - Although pubic lice on children's eyelashes usually result from close contact with infested parent, must also consider sexual abuse

DIAGNOSIS

HISTORY
- Chief complaint is usually pruritus; however, patients may be asymptomatic.
- May complain of disrupted sleep
- Ask about exposure to others with similar symptoms, crowded living conditions, and previous similar episodes.
- Review details of previous treatments to differentiate improper or incomplete treatment, reinfestation, and resistance to pediculicide.

PHYSICAL EXAM
- General points
  - Definitive diagnosis requires visualization of live lice.
  - Bright light and magnification are helpful.
- Head lice
  - Wet combing slows the movement of lice.
  - Use comb to lift and separate hair to visualize scalp and base of hair shafts.
  - Lice and nits (eggs or empty egg casings) most commonly found behind ears, on back of head, and nape of neck
  - Typical case involves 5–10 live lice.
  - Nits are firmly affixed at a characteristic angle to the hair shaft (vs. dandruff). Nits within 1 cm of scalp suggest active infestation. Nits >1 cm from scalp are likely empty egg cases.
  - May see excoriation, oozing, matted hair, or lymphadenopathy with secondary infection
- Body lice
  - Skin exam may reveal erythematous macules and papules from bites; rarely lice
  - Lice and nits may be found along seams on inside of clothing, especially near axillae, inguinal areas, waistband, or collar.
  - In long-standing infestations, may find epidermal thickening, hyperpigmentation, or scaly plaques
  - With secondary infection, may find adenopathy, fever, and malaise
- Pubic lice
  - Small, crab-shaped lice and nits in pubic hair or perianal region; be sure to also check axillae, beard, and eyelashes.
  - May find brownish clumps of louse fecal matter
  - With heavy infestation, may find maculae cerulea: 0.5–1-mm bluish macules on the lower abdomen, thighs, or buttocks
  - Eyelash infestation may cause blepharitis or conjunctivitis.

DIAGNOSTIC TESTS & INTERPRETATION

Diagnostic Procedures/Other
Diagnosis is made by direct visualization of lice or under magnification. Lice will stick to cellulose tape applied to infested area, and tape can then be affixed to glass slide for microscopy. Lice and nits fluoresce yellow green under Wood lamp.

DIFFERENTIAL DIAGNOSIS
- Seborrheic, contact, or atopic dermatitis
- Impetigo
- Scabies
- Xerosis with excoriation
- Hair casts, hair spray or other debris, other insects

TREATMENT

MEDICATION

Head lice

- General issues:
  - Because of different mechanisms of action, effects on different stages of louse life cycle, and potential adverse effects, careful adherence to manufacturers' instructions regarding pediculicide use is essential (preparation of hair, length of application, posttreatment rinsing, combing, and reapplication).
  - Conditioner or excess water on hair can interfere with efficacy.
  - Use enough product to coat all hair and scalp, especially areas behind ears and along hairline at back of neck. After treatment, use fine-toothed comb to remove visible lice and nits.
  - Recheck head daily for lice and nits for 2–3 weeks.
  - Pediculicides irritate mucous membranes; may be toxic if taken internally
- Permethrin lotion 1% (OTC); 5% (Rx)
  - Initial drug of choice; resistance increasing
  - Minimum age: 2 months
  - 10-minute application to damp hair. Reapply 7–10 days later if live lice persist.
  - Pediculicidal with some ovicidal activity (acts on insect nervous system)
  - Residue on hair kills newly hatching nymphs as they emerge for up to 2 weeks.
- Pyrethrin 1% with piperonyl butoxide (OTC)
  - Resistance varies by geographic location.
  - Minimum age: 2 years
  - 10-minute application to dry hair. Reapply 7–10 days later.
  - Pediculicidal with low ovicidal activity
  - Contraindication: allergy to chrysanthemums or ragweed
- Malathion lotion 0.5% (Rx):
  - Resistance common in United Kingdom but not in the United States where product contains terpineol.
  - Minimum age: 6 years
  - 8–12-hour application to dry hair. Leave uncovered. Reapply 7–10 days later if live lice persist.
  - Pediculicidal and highly ovicidal (organophosphate; cholinesterase inhibitor)
  - Highly flammable: Avoid hair dryers, smoking, and irons during treatment.
- Benzyl alcohol lotion 5% (Rx)
  - Minimum age: 6 months; potential toxicity in younger infants, especially if taken internally
  - 10-minute application to dry hair. Reapply after 7 days.
  - Pediculicidal but not ovicidal (interferes with action of respiratory spiracles)
- Spinosad topical suspension 0.9% (Rx):
  - Minimum age: 4 years
  - 10-minute application to dry hair. Repeat in 7 days if live lice present.
  - Does not require combing for nit removal
  - Pediculicidal and ovicidal (neurotoxic to insects; also contains benzyl alcohol; combination prevents resistance)
- Ivermectin lotion, 0.5% (Rx)
  - Minimum age: 6 months
  - 10-minute application to dry hair. Single treatment; do not reapply.
  - Pediculocidal; not ovicidal but few nymphs survive more than 2 days (acts on ion channels in invertebrate nerve and muscle cells)
- Wet combing alone to remove nits and lice may be helpful when medication is ineffective or as an alternative to pediculicide use.
- Controversial and untested treatments:
  - Occlusion: olive oil, mayonnaise, and petroleum jelly do not asphyxiate lice but may slow their movement and facilitate removal with nit comb
  - Shaving: can be effective but not necessary and may not be cosmetically acceptable
  - Trimethoprim-sulfamethoxazole (oral 10-day course): may enhance cure rate of topical permethrin; not FDA-approved for this use
  - Essential oils (e.g., tea tree oil): may have some activity against lice and eggs but are unregulated and may be toxic
  - Hot air: Several mechanical devices deliver hot air to the scalp to desiccate lice and nits, but efficacy is questionable.
  - Lindane shampoo 1%: no longer recommended due to neurotoxicity and increased resistance

Body lice

- Pediculicides are usually not needed if infested clothing and other fomites are appropriately laundered, treated with pediculicide, or destroyed. Oral ivermectin has been used effectively during epidemics.

Pubic lice

- The same OTC pediculicides are used for head lice and pubic lice; resistance less common
- It is important to treat all infested areas and sexual contacts.
- For eyelash infestation, apply petroleum jelly twice daily for 10 days. Remove nits with tweezers.

ALERT

- Pediculicides are oculotoxic. Do not use on eyelashes or eyebrows. If pediculicide gets in eyes, immediately flush with water.
- Pregnancy risk category varies for pediculicides. Check package insert.

ONGOING CARE

COMPLICATIONS

- Head lice
  - Intense pruritus can disrupt sleep.
  - Stigma associated with infestation can lead to social isolation, teasing, or bullying.
  - Days lost from school or work due to "no-nit" policies impact academic performance and worker productivity.
  - Secondary bacterial infections can result in pyoderma and lymphadenopathy.

ADDITIONAL READING

- Centers for Disease Control and Prevention. Lice. http://www.cdc.gov/parasites/lice. Accessed February 14, 2015.
- Frankowski BL, Bocchini JA; Council on School Health and Committee on Infectious Diseases. Head lice. *Pediatrics*. 2010;126(2):392–403.
- Lebwohl M, Clark L, Levitt J. Therapy for head lice based on life cycle, resistance and safety considerations. *Pediatrics*. 2007;119(5):965–974.
- Meinking TL. Clinical update on resistance and treatment of Pediculosis capitis. *Am J Manag Care*. 2004;10(Suppl 9):S264–S268.
- Tebruegge M, Runnades J. Is wet combing effective in children with pediculosis capitis infestation? *Arch Dis Child*. 2007;92(9):818–820.

CODES

ICD10

- B85.2 Pediculosis, unspecified
- B85.0 Pediculosis due to Pediculus humanus capitis
- B85.1 Pediculosis due to Pediculus humanus corporis

FAQ

- Q: Are people with long hair more likely to get head lice?
- A: No. Longer hair is not associated with greater likelihood of getting head lice. However, removing lice and nits is easier when hair is shorter.
- Q: How long should children with head lice be excluded from school?
- A: The risk of transmission decreases enough to allow children to return to school once they have been treated with a single pediculicide application.
- Q: Given the increase in resistance, should we stop using OTC treatments and use prescription products instead?
- A: Resistance of head lice varies widely by community. Currently, permethrin 1% remains the initial treatment of choice. Prescription products are more expensive and have greater potential for toxicity. Careful adherence to manufacturers' directions and simultaneous treatment of close contacts (especially bedmates) decreases the likelihood of treatment failure and reinfestation.
- Q: How can health professionals allay anxiety and decrease the social stigma of head lice?
- A: Emphasize that head lice infestation is not a sign of poor housekeeping or hygiene. Point out that the benefits of close friendships outweigh the minimal health risks related to head lice. Encourage open communication to facilitate treatment of close contacts.

LONG QT SYNDROME

Ronn E. Tanel

BASICS

DESCRIPTION

Long QT syndrome (LQTS) is characterized by prolongation of the QT interval on the surface electrocardiogram (ECG), syncope, and sudden death as a result of malignant ventricular arrhythmias. The electrical instability is due to an abnormality of ventricular repolarization associated with a cardiac ion channelopathy.

EPIDEMIOLOGY

Prevalence

Prevalence of LQTS is estimated to be approximately 1 in 2,500.

RISK FACTORS

Genetics

- Autosomal dominant (Romano-Ward syndrome)
- Autosomal recessive, sometimes associated with congenital nerve deafness (Jervell and Lange-Nielsen syndrome)
- Genetic linkage analysis studies have demonstrated that >400 genetic mutations among 13 cardiac ion channel genes account for nearly 3/4 of LQTS.
- Genotype-phenotype–based research studies have identified gene-specific electrocardiographic profiles, gene-specific arrhythmia triggers, gene-directed treatment strategies, and gene-specific risk stratification.

GENERAL PREVENTION

- Preventive measures focus on screening for the electrocardiographic abnormality, especially in individuals who appear to be at risk of having the diagnosis.
- Patients who have been diagnosed are advised to avoid exposure to stimulants, medications that are known to prolong the QT interval or provoke ventricular arrhythmias, and situations that may aggravate the cardiac rhythm or induce torsades de pointes.

PATHOPHYSIOLOGY

Two hypotheses have been proposed to explain the pathogenesis of congenital LQTS syndrome:

- An abnormality or imbalance in sympathetic innervation to the heart, which helps explain the findings of sinus bradycardia, abnormal repolarization, adrenergic dependence of arrhythmias, and response to adrenergic antagonist medications associated with the syndrome
- Intrinsic cardiac ion (potassium and sodium) channel defects appear to be the mechanism responsible for cardiac repolarization abnormalities. Because some identified gene mutations that result in congenital LQTS occur at loci that also encode a cardiac ion channel protein, ion channel dysfunction has been proposed as the intrinsic abnormality that is responsible for abnormal repolarization.

DIAGNOSIS

HISTORY

- Notable findings include the following:
  - Palpitations
  - Presyncope
  - Syncope
- These symptoms may be related to provocative stimuli, especially emotional or physical stress. Any use of medications known to prolong the QTc interval should be noted.
- Most importantly, a thorough family history for arrhythmia, syncope, epilepsy, or sudden unexplained death should be obtained.

PHYSICAL EXAM

Findings are usually normal, but bradycardia may be present.

DIAGNOSTIC TESTS & INTERPRETATION

Lab

- The Bazett formula: QTc = QT/(square root of RR interval). Generally, a QTc >480 msec is considered abnormal, although some clinicians allow a slightly longer QTc for infants <6 months of age.
- Some clinicians believe that the QTc should not be corrected at heart rates <60 beats per minute (bpm). The measurement should be taken in lead II without significant sinus arrhythmia.
- Children frequently have a prominent U wave. It should generally be included in the measurement of the QTc if it exceeds 1/2 the amplitude of the T wave.
- A single measured prolonged QTc interval does not confirm the diagnosis of LQTS.
- T-wave alternans on an electrocardiographic recording is diagnostic.
- Since 2004, genetic testing has been available as a commercial diagnostic test. Unfortunately, only up to 3/4 of all genetic causes of LQTS have been identified, so false-negative genetic testing is possible.
- Clinical scoring systems may help stratify patients into high, moderate, and low probability of having the diagnosis, based on symptoms, family history, and ECG findings.

Imaging

ECG

- Atrioventricular block can be seen on the ECG in infants with relatively rapid heart rates and P waves that occur during the prolonged repolarization period (QT interval) of ventricular refractoriness.

Echocardiogram

- The echocardiogram usually demonstrates normal cardiac structure and function.

Diagnostic Procedures/Other

Other tests that may help confirm the diagnosis include the following:

- 24-hour ambulatory Holter monitoring
  - This recording may disclose asymptomatic ventricular ectopy or arrhythmias, T-wave alternans, or variability in the QTc interval during different periods of the day.
- Exercise stress testing may also be helpful in identifying ventricular arrhythmias or prolongation of the QTc interval, particularly during the recovery phase.

DIFFERENTIAL DIAGNOSIS

- Congenital LQTS is most commonly misdiagnosed as vasovagal syncope or a seizure disorder. All patients who have a syncopal event or who are diagnosed with epilepsy should have a baseline screening ECG.
- Sudden infant death syndrome (SIDS) may be related to congenital LQTS. Some studies have demonstrated that mutations of ion channel proteins that cause LQTS have been found in SIDS victims. QT interval prolongation may be subtle, such that ~10% of affected patients may have a normal result on routine ECG and ~40% may have only borderline prolongation of the QT interval.
- Acquired forms of LQTS should be differentiated from the congenital and inherited form. Acquired LQTS may be due to the following:
  - Electrolyte abnormalities: hypokalemia, hypocalcemia, hypomagnesemia, and metabolic acidosis
  - Toxins: organophosphates
  - Central nervous system trauma
  - Malnutrition: anorexia
  - Primary myocardial disease: myocarditis, ischemia, cardiomyopathy
  - Medication
    - Cardiac medications: quinidine, procainamide, disopyramide, sotalol, and amiodarone
    - Antibiotics/antifungals: erythromycin, trimethoprim–sulfamethoxazole, pentamidine, ketoconazole, and fluconazole
    - Psychotropic medications: tricyclic antidepressants, phenothiazines, and haloperidol
    - Antihistamines: terfenadine, astemizole, diphenhydramine
    - Gastrointestinal: cisapride

TREATMENT

MEDICATION

- The primary therapy is β-blockade, most commonly with propranolol or nadolol. Metoprolol and perhaps atenolol are less effective for this diagnosis.
- Class Ib antiarrhythmic medications (e.g., mexiletine) are also used in patients with congenital LQTS, especially in those with documented ventricular arrhythmia.
- Anti-arrhythmic medications generally do not help treat patients with acquired LQTS, but the administration of magnesium sulfate may be beneficial.

ADDITIONAL TREATMENT

General Measures

Patients are usually treated based on symptoms and the clinical severity of the disease.

Additional Therapies

Implantable cardioverter-defibrillators (ICDs) are usually reserved for older children and adolescents who have significant symptoms, documented ventricular arrhythmias, or other significant risk factors for sudden death.

SURGERY/OTHER PROCEDURES

- Occasionally, implantation of a permanent pacemaker is indicated based on the theory that the tachyarrhythmias (e.g., torsades de pointes) are dependent on bradycardia and/or pauses. Rarely, pacemaker implantation may be necessary to support the low heart rate that occurs as a result of β-blocker therapy. Newborns and infants with a very prolonged QT interval, atrioventricular block, and low ventricular rates are historically treated with a pacemaker.
- An ICD may be recommended for patients thought to be at higher risk of developing ventricular arrhythmias.
- Left stellate ganglionectomy is performed to potentially eliminate the hyperactive left sympathetic ganglion output that has been proposed as a mechanism of ventricular arrhythmias. This treatment option is not universally accepted.

INPATIENT CONSIDERATIONS

Initial Stabilization

Most clinicians treat diagnosed asymptomatic children with medications because of a high incidence of sudden death that occurs as the first symptom.

ONGOING CARE

FOLLOW-UP RECOMMENDATIONS

Patient Monitoring

- Follow-up outpatient appointments should review new or recurrent symptoms, including palpitations, near syncope or syncope, and the efficacy and adverse effects of medical therapy.
- ECG may demonstrate a normal or prolonged QTc.
- Follow-up 24-hour ambulatory Holter monitor recordings and exercise stress tests may help assess the adequacy of β-blocker therapy and identify ventricular arrhythmias.
- All family members of the patient should have an ECG as a minimum screening measure.

PROGNOSIS

- Children have a higher incidence of sudden death than adults, which may reflect an inherent bias because adult patients have already survived childhood. The risk of cardiac events is higher in boys before puberty and in women during adulthood.
- Pediatric patients with greatest risk for sudden death are those with QTc $>$600 msec. Gender, environmental factors, genotype, and therapy are other factors that influence the clinical course.
- A particular clinical phenotype may be caused by different genetic substrates, whereas a single gene can cause very different phenotypes, even within the same family, by acting through different pathways.
- Without treatment, mortality is 21% within 1 year from the first syncope. With proper treatment, mortality has been estimated at 1% during 15-year follow-up. β-blocker therapy has been shown to reduce the incidence of sudden death.
- Current research may lead to the development of therapy specific to the precise ion channel defect.

COMPLICATIONS

- Complications, especially in untreated patients, include the following:
  - Ventricular tachyarrhythmias, specifically torsades de pointes
  - Syncope
  - Sudden death
- In patients with the congenital and inherited form of the condition, asymptomatic family members may be affected.

ADDITIONAL READING

- Ackerman MJ. Genotype-phenotype relationships in congenital long QT syndrome. *J Electrocardiol*. 2005;38(Suppl 4):64–68.
- Hedley PL, Jørgensen P, Schlamowitz S, et al. The genetic basis of long QT and short QT syndromes: a mutation update. *Hum Mutat*. 2009;30(11): 1486–1511.
- Morita H, Wu J, Zipes DP. The QT syndromes: long and short. *Lancet*. 2008;372(9640):750–763.
- Priori SG, Napolitano C, Vicentini A. Inherited arrhythmia syndromes: applying the molecular biology and genetic to the clinical management. *J Interv Card Electrophysiol*. 2003;9(2):93–101.
- Priori SG, Schwartz PJ, Napolitano C, et al. Risk stratification in the long QT syndrome. *N Engl J Med*. 2003;348(19):1866–1874.
- Roden DM. Clinical practice. Long-QT syndrome. *N Engl J Med*. 2008;358(2):169–176.
- Schwartz PJ, Crotti L, Insolia R. Long-QT syndrome: from genetics to management. *Circ Arrhythm Electrophysiol*. 2012;5(4):868–877.

CODES

ICD10

I45.81 Long QT syndrome

FAQ

- Q: Should activity be restricted in patients with congenital LQTS?
- A: Because sudden rises in serum catecholamine levels may precipitate symptoms, it is appropriate to restrict competitive and vigorous athletics. Symptomatic patients may require greater restrictions. Documentation of appropriate β-blockade by a lower maximal heart rate at peak exercise on follow-up exercise stress test may be helpful.
- Q: If someone is identified as having LQTS, should family members be evaluated?
- A: Yes, with a high degree of suspicion. Most cases of congenital LQTS are inherited in an autosomal dominant pattern, so that each child of an affected parent has a 50% chance of having the gene. This does not predict severity of symptoms, but parents, all siblings, and children of patients should be examined with an ECG, Holter monitor, and exercise stress test. These studies may help reveal an abnormal QTc interval in suspected family members.

LOWER GI BLEEDING

Michael A. Manfredi

BASICS

DESCRIPTION
- Lower gastrointestinal bleeding (LGIB) is defined as bleeding that occurs distal to the ligament of Treitz.
- Melena and maroon-colored stools can be seen with small bowel bleeding, whereas hematochezia is classically seen with colonic bleeding.
- It is important to recognize that hematochezia can also be a presentation of severe upper gastrointestinal bleeding (UGIB).

EPIDEMIOLOGY
- In a population study of 40,000 admissions to a tertiary care pediatric emergency department, LGIB accounted for 0.3% of all admissions.
- 4.2% of patients with LGIB met criteria for severe life-threatening bleeding.

ETIOLOGY
Causes of LGIB vary by age:
- Neonatal period (birth to 1 month)
  - Allergic colitis
  - Anorectal fissure
  - Necrotizing enterocolitis
  - Enteric infections
  - Upper GI source
  - Duplication cyst
  - Hirschsprung disease enterocolitis
  - Meckel diverticulum
  - Malrotation with volvulus
  - Hemorrhagic disease of the newborn
- Infancy (1 month to 2 years)
  - Allergic colitis
  - Anorectal fissure
  - Enteric infections
  - Intussusception
  - Meckel diverticulum
  - Malrotation with volvulus
  - Lymphonodular hyperplasia
  - Upper GI source
  - Duplication cyst
  - Enterocolitis with Hirschsprung disease
  - Vascular malformation
- Preschool age (2–5 years)
  - Anorectal fissure
  - Enteric infections
  - Polyps
  - Parasites
  - Meckel diverticulum
  - Intussusception
  - Lymphonodular hyperplasia
  - Inflammatory bowel disease
  - Hirschsprung disease enterocolitis
  - Hemolytic uremic syndrome
  - Henoch-Schönlein purpura (HSP)
  - Vascular malformation
  - Volvulus
  - Rectal prolapse/rectal ulcer
  - Child abuse
  - Perianal streptococcal cellulitis
- School age (5–13 years)
  - Anorectal fissure
  - Enteric infections
  - Inflammatory bowel disease
  - Intussusception
  - Meckel diverticulum
  - Polyps
  - HSP
  - Hemolytic uremic syndrome
  - Intestinal ischemia
  - Neutropenic colitis (typhlitis)
  - Parasites
  - Child abuse
  - Vascular malformations
  - Perianal streptococcal cellulitis
- Adolescent (>13 years)
  - Anorectal fissure
  - Enteric infections
  - Inflammatory bowel disease
  - Hemolytic uremic syndrome
  - Intussusception
  - Midgut volvulus
  - Intestinal ischemia
  - Neutropenic colitis (typhlitis)
  - Polyps
  - Vascular malformations
  - Lymphonodular hyperplasia
  - Parasites
  - Hemorrhoids

DIAGNOSIS

APPROACH TO THE PATIENT
General goals of initial evaluation of patient with LGIB: Determine if patient is actively bleeding, an approximate location of the bleeding and cause, as well as presence or absence of hemodynamic instability, which may indicate need for urgent/emergent clinical resuscitation:
- Phase 1: Determine if there is blood or other cause of bright red or black stools.
- Phase 2: Assess patient to determine etiology; follow history, physical, and laboratory.
- Phase 3: Assess and stabilize patient, decide if emergency treatment is needed or if outpatient referral is required.

HISTORY
- Obtain a detailed history and note if any recently ingested foods resemble blood.
- Evaluate the color of blood:
  - Bright red: Site of bleeding is probably in left colon, rectosigmoid, or anal canal.
  - Darker red stool: right colon
  - Melena or maroon: Bleeding is likely proximal to ileocecal valve.
- Location of blood in the stool:
  - Colitis: Blood will be mixed with stool.
  - Anal fissure/constipation: Blood streaks will be seen on the outer aspect of the stool.
- Consistency of the stool:
  - Diarrhea: suggests colitis
  - Hard stool: may be indicative of fissure and constipation
- Other diagnostic clues:
  - Painful stools: may be consistent with anal fissure, local proctitis, or ischemic bowel
  - Painless rectal bleeding: associated with polyps, Meckel diverticulum, nodular lymphoid hyperplasia of colon, intestinal duplication, intestinal submucosal mass (GIST), or vascular anomaly
  - Abdominal pain: inflammatory bowel disease, other causes of colitis, or a surgical abdomen
- Obtain past medical history for any underlying or known GI disease (i.e., previous GI surgery, past history of colitis, Hirschsprung disease, necrotizing enterocolitis).
- Evaluate for history of jaundice, hepatitis, liver disease, neonatal history: suggestive of portal vein thrombosis (sepsis, shock, exchange transfusion, omphalitis, and IV catheters), portal hypertension, and variceal bleeding.
- Familial history
  - Inflammatory bowel disease, intestinal polyps, and bleeding diathesis (e.g., von Willebrand disease, hemophilia)
- Personal medications: in particular, nonsteroidal anti-inflammatory medications, heparin or warfarin. In addition, a history of medications in the house should also be obtained due to possible accidental ingestion in younger children.
- Associated symptoms:
  - Mouth ulcers
  - Weight loss
  - Joint pains
  - Fevers
  - Rash
  - Petechiae
  - Renal insufficiency
  - History of ingestion of uncooked meat (hemolytic uremic syndrome [HUS])
  - Purpuric rash (HSP)

PHYSICAL EXAM
- Hemodynamic stability should be assessed immediately.
  - Heart rate: Tachycardia may be an early sign of intravascular volume depletion.
  - Blood pressure: Hypotension is a late sign and may not be present even with significant blood loss because vasoconstriction maintains BP until decompensation occurs.
  - In the setting of normal blood pressure, obtain orthostatic BP.
  - Capillary refill: Delayed capillary refill suggests intravascular volume depletion.
  - Oxygen saturation: may be decreased due to decreased oxygen carrying capacity
  - Evaluate for signs of shock:
    - Vitals signs listed earlier
    - Cool clammy extremities
    - Poor mentation
- Skin
  - Petechiae or purpura: HSP or coagulopathy
  - Ecchymosis: coagulopathy
  - Hemangiomas: vascular anomaly
  - Spider angioma: liver disease or portal hypertension
  - Caput medusa: liver disease or portal hypertension
  - Palmar erythema: liver disease or portal hypertension
  - Jaundice: liver disease or portal hypertension
- HEENT
  - Freckles on buccal mucosa: Peutz–Jeghers syndrome
  - Telangiectasias on buccal mucosa: (Osler-Weber-Rendu syndrome).
  - Mouth ulcers: Crohn disease
  - Icteric sclera: portal hypertension
- Abdomen
  - Hepatosplenomegaly, ascites: liver disease or portal hypertension
  - Isolated splenomegaly: cavernous transformation of the portal vein
- Rectal examination
  - Evidence of perianal disease: inflammatory bowel disease
  - Polyps: Rectal polyps may be detected on digital exam.
  - Hemorrhoids: chronic constipation, portal hypertension

DIAGNOSTIC TESTS & INTERPRETATION
- NG tube lavage
  - No longer recommended in patients with suspected upper or lower GI bleeding for diagnosis, prognosis, visualization, or therapeutic effect

- Stool guaiac
  - May help to distinguish blood in stool from other blood colored substances (i.e., food coloring)

Lab

- CBC should be measured serially.
  - Initial hemoglobin values may be unreliable because a delay in hemodilution may falsely produce near-normal values.
- Iron deficiency anemia: may indicate anemia of chronic disease
  - Leukopenia, anemia, and thrombocytopenia: Consider chronic liver disease and portal hypertension.
  - Anemia with normal RBC indices: truly an acute cause for bleeding
  - RBC indices indicate iron deficiency anemia: Consider mucosal lesion, that is, chronic blood loss.
  - Thrombocytopenia: Consider hemolytic uremic syndrome.
- Coagulation profile
  - If PT and PTT are abnormal, consider liver disease or disseminated intravascular coagulation with sepsis.
- Liver function tests: abnormal in chronic liver disease
- Renal function tests (BUN, creatinine, urine analysis): abnormal in hemolytic uremic syndrome, HSP, acute bleed
- ESR or C-reactive protein (CRP): abnormal in inflammatory disorders or infectious colitis
- Stool tests:
  - Stool culture (*Salmonella*, *Shigella*, *Campylobacter*, *Yersinia*, *Aeromonas*, *Escherichia coli*, *Klebsiella*)
  - Stool for *Clostridium difficile* toxin A and B
  - Ova and parasites (Amebae)
  - Stool smears for WBCs (not always positive in colitis) and eosinophils (not always positive in allergic colitis)
  - Stool CMV: Consider in immunocompromised patients.

Imaging

- Abdominal x-ray
  - Can be helpful in evaluating surgical abdomen (dilated bowel, air–fluid levels, and perforation), constipation (presence of excessive stool), colitis (edematous bowel, thumb-printing), pneumatosis intestinalis, and toxic megacolon
- Ultrasound
  - Can show bowel wall thickening consistent with inflammatory bowel disease, Meckel diverticulum, intussusception
- Barium tests:
  - Air-contrast enema is diagnostic and therapeutic in intussusception and diagnostic in mucosal lesions (polyps).
  - Upper GI series with small bowel follow-through is helpful in evaluating anatomy and inflammatory bowel disease.
  - CT scan can show evidence of intestinal inflammation and evidence of bowel obstruction.
- Nuclear medicine
  - Meckel scan: Technetium-99m pertechnetate can detect a Meckel diverticulum when it contains gastric mucosa.
  - Bleeding scan: useful in a patient with significant bleeding that precludes endoscopy or in whom endoscopy is nondiagnostic. Technetium-99m–tagged erythrocyte scan detects rapid bleeding at a rate of 0.1–0.5 mL/min; can be performed at 30-minute intervals for up to 24 hours.

Diagnostic Procedures

- Endoscopy
  - Upper endoscopy and colonoscopy is the prime diagnostic and therapeutic tool for upper and lower GI bleeding.
  - Endoscopy can be used to accurately delineate the bleeding site and/or to determine specific cause. It is 90–95% sensitive at locating bleeding site.
  - Upper endoscopy diagnostic in massive UGIB presenting with hematochezia or melena
  - Upper endoscopy and colonoscopy should be performed when the suspicion is high for inflammatory bowel disease.
  - Colonoscopy should be performed when there is a suspicion for polyps.
- Video capsule endoscopy
  - Capsule endoscopy has become 1st-line treatment in adults and children to diagnose obscure causes of GI bleeding in the small intestine.
  - Capsule endoscopy may be limited by ability of the patient to swallow the capsule.
  - The capsule can be placed endoscopically into the small intestine in younger children.
- Enteroscopy
  - Involves the passage of a special endoscope (either by push, single balloon or double balloon) to evaluate the small intestine
  - May be indicated if a lesion is seen on capsule endoscopy that may be amenable to endoscopic therapy
- Angiography
  - Useful in detecting vascular causes of UGIB; can also be therapeutic (i.e., injection of coils into a vascular malformation may occlude it); requires bleeding rate of 0.5–1 mL/min

TREATMENT

GENERAL MEASURES

- Initial management
  - Make patient NPO.
  - Secure stable vascular access (i.e., intravenous line).
  - Obtain blood type, and cross-match RBCs.
  - Stabilize the patient with IV fluids and blood products if necessary (target hemoglobin $\geq$7 g/dL).
  - Target INR <2.5
  - Consult specialists (pediatric surgery and/or pediatric gastroenterologist).
- Disease-specific therapy
  - Anal fissure
    - Treat the underlying constipation (mineral oil, lactulose, MiraLax, high-fiber diet, increased water intake).
    - Local therapy consists of sitz baths, local emollient creams, and steroid suppositories.
  - Polyp: colonoscopy with polypectomy
  - Intussusception: air-contrast enema for confirmation and hydrostatic reduction
  - Parasites: antiparasitic medications
  - Inflammatory bowel disease: referral to pediatric gastroenterologist for therapy

ISSUES FOR REFERRAL

Refer the following patients to a specialist:

- Any patient with significant acute lower GI bleeding after initial stabilization
- Patients with less acute bleeding for whom an easily identifiable cause has not been found or patients with chronic or recurrent lower GI bleeding

SURGERY/OTHER PROCEDURES

In cases of massive or persistent bleeding with no identifiable site, exploratory laparotomy with intraoperative endoscopic evaluation of the entire bowel to identify mucosal lesions may be required.

HOSPITALIZED PATIENTS

Initial Stabilization

Emergency care

- If patient is critical, stabilize with IV fluids and blood products.
- Order laboratory tests: CBC, PT/PTT, disseminated intravascular coagulation screen, liver function tests, blood type, and cross-match
- Monitor patient's vital signs and hemoglobin.
- Make appropriate diagnosis and institute appropriate therapy.

ONGOING CARE

PATIENT MONITORING

- Monitor hemoglobin in the hospital until patient's condition is stable.
- Send stool studies.
- Refer patients with LGIB that is chronic in nature and hemodynamically stable to specialist for further workup.

DIET

- Consider recommendation of an exclusion diet that restricts (milk and/or soy, egg, wheat, other foods) in breastfeeding mothers of infants consuming breast milk with evidence of allergic colitis.
- Introduce hydrolyzed protein formula in formula-fed infants with suspected cow's milk protein allergy.

ADDITIONAL READING

- Boyle JT. Gastrointestinal bleeding in infants and children. *Pediatric Rev*. 2008;29(2):39–52.
- Cohen SA, Klevens AI. Use of capsule endoscopy in diagnosis and management of pediatric patients, based on meta-analysis. *Clin Gastroenterol Hepatol*. 2011;9(6):490–496.
- Fox V. Gastrointestinal bleeding in infancy and childhood. *Gastroenterol Clin North Am*. 2000;29(1):37–66.
- Leung AK, Wong AL. Lower gastrointestinal bleeding in children. *Pediatric Emerg Care*. 2002;18(4):319–323.
- Liu K, Kaffes AJ. Review article: the diagnosis and investigation of obscure gastrointestinal bleeding. *Aliment Pharmacol Ther*. 2011;34(4):416–423.

CODES

ICD10

- K92.2 Gastrointestinal hemorrhage, unspecified
- K92.1 Melena
- K52.2 Allergic and dietetic gastroenteritis and colitis

FAQ

- Q: What is the most common cause of lower GI bleeding?
- A: In all age groups, fissures are the leading cause, followed by infections.
- Q: What is the most common cause of blood mixed in the stool of an infant?
- A: Allergic colitis. This is an indication to recommend a hypoallergenic diet (exclusion diet in mothers of infants who are breastfeeding, extensively hydrolyzed protein formulas in infants receiving formula).
- Q: What common foods cause stools to be red? Black?
- A: Red: raspberries, cranberries, Kool-Aid, artificial coloring in cereal. Black: bismuth, spinach, blueberries, licorice.

LUPUS ERYTHEMATOSUS

Elizabeth Candell Chalom

BASICS

DESCRIPTION

Systemic lupus erythematosus (SLE) is a multisystem autoimmune disease characterized by production of antibodies to various components of the cell nucleus, in conjunction with a variety of clinical manifestations.

EPIDEMIOLOGY

- Age
  - 20% of lupus begins in childhood, but it is very rare younger than 5 years old.
- Female-to-male ratio:
  - Between 3–5:1 (prepubertal) and 9–10:1 (postpubertal)
- SLE occurs about 3 times more often in African Americans than Caucasians. It is also more common in Hispanic, Asian, and Native Americans.

Incidence

- Peak incidence: between ages 15 and 40 years
- Incidence in children is from 10–20 cases/100,000 children per year.

Prevalence

- U.S. estimate: 5,000–10,000 children

RISK FACTORS

Genetics

- Increased frequency in 1st-degree family members of patients with SLE
- 10% of patients have ≥1 affected relative.
- Concordance rate of 25–50% in monozygotic twins and 5% in dizygotic twins
- Some major histocompatibility complex antigens are associated with increased incidence of lupus, such as HLA-DR2 and DR3 in whites and DR2 and DR7 in blacks.

ETIOLOGY

Although exact etiology is unknown, lupus is an autoimmune disease, with genetic, environmental, and hormonal factors playing a role.

DIAGNOSIS

Classification criteria: 4 of the following 11 criteria, developed by the American College of Rheumatology, must be met to classify a patient as having SLE:

- Malar (butterfly) rash
- Discoid rash
- Photosensitivity
- Oral or nasal ulcers
- Arthritis
- Cytopenia
  - Anemia, leukopenia (<4,000/mm^3), lymphopenia (<1,500/mm^3), or thrombocytopenia (<100,000/mm^3)
- Neurologic disease: seizures or psychosis
- Nephritis: >0.5 g/day proteinuria or cellular casts
- Serositis: Pleuritis or pericarditis
- Positive immunoserology (revised 1997): antibodies to double-stranded DNA or Smith nuclear antigen, false-positive serologic test for syphilis, lupus anticoagulant, or antiphospholipid antibodies
- Positive ANA
- Meeting 4 of 11 classification criteria is highly sensitive and specific for diagnosis of SLE.

HISTORY

- History of photosensitivity or malar rash common but not necessary
- Many patients have systemic complaints, such as fever, fatigue, and malaise.
- Many patients complain of joint pain, Raynaud phenomenon, or alopecia.
- Chest pain from pericarditis or pleural effusions may be present.
- Signs and symptoms:
  - Immune complex–mediated vasculitis, which can occur in almost any organ system
  - Cutaneous lesions: very variable; include
    - Erythematous malar or "butterfly" rash
    - Maculopapular rashes (can occur anywhere on body)
    - Periungual erythema
    - Mucosal membrane vasculitis
  - Arthritis: can affect large and small joints; usually symmetric and nonerosive
  - Hematologic pathology includes the following:
    - Hemolytic anemia
    - Anemia of chronic disease
    - Leukopenia
    - Lymphopenia
    - Thrombocytopenia
  - Neurologic symptoms include the following:
    - Headaches
    - Psychosis
    - Depression
    - Seizures
    - Organic brain syndromes
    - Peripheral neuropathies
  - Renal pathology (present in up to 75% children with SLE)
    - Includes mesangial changes and glomerulonephritis (focal, diffuse proliferative, or membranous)
    - First signs of renal disease in lupus patient are often proteinuria and active urinary sediment.
    - Hypertension, nephrotic syndrome, and renal failure can also occur.
  - Serositis: usually seen as pericarditis or pleuritis but peritonitis can also occur
  - Constitutional symptoms are very common: fatigue, weight loss, fever.

PHYSICAL EXAM

- Rash: may be malar, discoid, or vasculitic. Periungual erythema may also be seen.
- Oral or nasal ulcers (usually on hard or soft palate) that are painless and often go unnoticed by patients
- Arthritis of large and small joints
- Pericardial friction rub if patient has pericarditis
- Edema may be present secondary to renal disease.
- CNS changes such as personality changes, psychosis, or seizures

DIAGNOSTIC TESTS & INTERPRETATION

Lab

- ANA
  - Found in >95% of patients with SLE, but a positive ANA can occur in many diseases and in up to 20% of normal population
- Anti–double-stranded DNA and anti–Smith nuclear antigen
  - Very specific to lupus, but not all patients with lupus have these autoantibodies. In many patients, anti-DNA levels vary with activity of disease.
- CBC
  - Anemia, leukopenia, lymphopenia, and/or thrombocytopenia may be seen.
- Urinalysis
  - May show proteinuria or active urinary sediment if there is renal dysfunction
- Complement levels
  - Can fall very low during a lupus flare (C3 and C4)
- PTT
  - Patients may also have prolonged PTT, as result of antiphospholipid (APL) antibodies, often seen in SLE.
  - Patients with APL antibodies are at increased risk for thrombotic events, such as deep venous thrombosis, stroke, and fetal loss during pregnancies.

DIFFERENTIAL DIAGNOSIS

- Systemic-onset juvenile idiopathic arthritis
- Oncologic disease (leukemia, lymphoma)
- Viral or other infectious illness
- Other vasculitic disorders
- Dermatomyositis
- Fibromyalgia
- Drug-induced lupus
- Pitfalls:
  - Avoid overdiagnosis; positive ANA in the absence of clinical signs or symptoms of SLE is not lupus.

TREATMENT

MEDICATION

- NSAIDs
  - May be used for musculoskeletal and mild systemic complaints, although ibuprofen has been noted to cause aseptic meningitis in a small number of patients with SLE.
  - NSAIDs can also exacerbate renal disease in lupus.
- Hydroxychloroquine often used to help control cutaneous manifestations and to help minimize the chance of lupus flares
- Steroids often necessary to control systemic and renal manifestations
- Patients with renal disease often need immunosuppressive agents such as cyclophosphamide (usually given as monthly IV boluses). Mycophenolate mofetil, cyclosporine, or azathioprine may also be used.
- Patients with mainly arthritic symptoms may be treated with weekly methotrexate, PO or SC.
- Patients with antiphospholipid antibodies can be treated with a baby aspirin daily. If they have already had a significant clotting event, they need stronger anticoagulation.
- Angiotensin-converting enzyme (ACE) inhibitors are often used to help prevent renal damage from proteinuria.
- Patients with abnormal lipid profiles that do not respond to diet may need statins.
- Rituximab (anti-CD20 antibody) causes B-cell depletion and is used in SLE, especially for thrombocytopenia.
- Belimumab, a BLyS (B-lymphocyte stimulator) inhibitor, has been approved in adults but not yet in children.
- Antibodies to CD40 and C5 are also being studied
- Plasmapheresis and IVIG have been used as well.

ADDITIONAL TREATMENT

General Measures

Avoid excessive sun exposure and use sunscreen liberally.

ADDITIONAL THERAPIES

For very severe lupus, bone marrow immunoablation or transplantation are options.

ONGOING CARE

PROGNOSIS

- Extremely variable. Renal disease and CNS involvement are poor prognostic signs, whereas systemic complaints and joint findings are not.
- 10-year survival in children presenting with SLE is >90%.

COMPLICATIONS

- End-stage renal disease
- Infections secondary to treatments used to control disease
- Atherosclerosis and myocardial infarctions at a young age
- Libman-Sacks endocarditis, which increases risk of subacute bacterial endocarditis
- Neonatal lupus
  - Neonatal lupus erythematosus (NLE) is due to maternal autoantibodies (usually SS-A or SS-B antibodies) that cross the placenta and can cause rashes, congenital heart block, cytopenias, and/or hepatitis in the newborn.
  - Most symptoms of NLE resolve by 6 months of age, but heart block, if it occurs, is permanent.
  - Many mothers of babies with NLE are asymptomatic and unaware that they have these autoantibodies.
  - The rash, erythema annulare, can begin a few days after delivery or within the first few weeks of life.
  - Topical steroids can minimize skin lesions.
  - Congenital heart block is due to damage of the conducting system of the developing fetal heart.
  - Bradycardia may be noted by 22 weeks' gestation, and CHF with nonimmune hydrops fetalis may ensue.

ADDITIONAL READING

- Brunner HI, Huggins J, Klein-Gitelman MS. Pediatric SLE—towards a comprehensive management plan. *Nat Rev Rheumatol*. 2011;7(4):225–233.
- Gottlieb BS, Ilowite NT. Systemic lupus erythematosus in children and adolescents. *Pediatr Rev*. 2006;27(9):323–330.
- Macdermott EJ, Adams A, Lehman TJ. Systemic lupus erythematosus in children: current and emerging therapies. *Lupus*. 2007;16(8):677–683.
- Silverman E, Eddy A. Systemic lupus erythematosus. In: Cassidy JT, Petty RE, Laxer RM, et al, eds. *Textbook of Pediatric Rheumatology*. Philadelphia, PA: Elsevier; 2011:315–343.
- Yildirim-Toruner C, Diamond B. Current and novel therapeutics in the treatment of systemic lupus erythematosus. *J Allergy Clin Immunol*. 2011;127(2):303–312.

CODES

ICD10

- L93.0 Discoid lupus erythematosus
- M32.9 Systemic lupus erythematosus, unspecified
- L93.2 Other local lupus erythematosus

FAQ

- Q: If a patient has a positive ANA but no clinical signs of SLE, how often should the ANA be followed?
- A: A positive ANA will usually remain positive indefinitely, but it has no real significance in the absence of clinical or other laboratory disturbances. Up to 20% of the normal population may have a positive ANA, so there is no need to repeat the test.
- Q: Can SLE patients with end-stage renal disease obtain renal transplants?
- A: Yes, and SLE usually does not recur in the new kidney.

LYME DISEASE

Elizabeth Candell Chalom

BASICS

DESCRIPTION

Multisystemic illness caused by the spirochete *Borrelia burgdorferi*, carried by the deer tick

EPIDEMIOLOGY

- Can affect people of all ages, but 1/3–1/2 of all cases occur in children and adolescents
- Male/female ratio: 1:1 to 2:1
- Onset most often in summer months
- Although Lyme disease can be found anywhere, the majority of the cases in the United States are found in Southern New England and the mid-Atlantic states. It is also seen frequently in California, Minnesota, and Wisconsin.

Prevalence

Has become most common tick-borne disease in the United States, with 29,959 confirmed cases reported in 2009

RISK FACTORS

Genetics

Chronic Lyme arthritis seems to be associated with increased incidence of HLA-DR4 and less so with HLA-DR2.

PATHOPHYSIOLOGY

B. burgdorferi is injected into skin with saliva during bite of Ixodes tick. Spirochetes first migrate within skin, forming the typical rash, erythema migrans. Spirochetes then spread hematogenously to other organs, including heart, joints, and nervous system.

ETIOLOGY

The tick-borne spirochete *B. burgdorferi*

COMMONLY ASSOCIATED CONDITIONS

The same ticks that transmit Lyme disease can also transmit *Ehrlichia* and *Babesia*, so infections with those spirochetes can occur simultaneously.

DIAGNOSIS

HISTORY

- Tick bite
  - History of tick bite can only be elicited in 1/3 of patients with Lyme disease
  - Most people with tick bites do not develop Lyme disease.
  - Even in endemic areas, risk of developing Lyme disease after tick bite is <5%.
- Rash
  - 50–80% will have or will recall the typical rash
  - Rash is not painful or pruritic but feels warm.
- Other symptoms
  - Many patients will complain of fatigue, headaches, fevers, chills, myalgias, conjunctivitis, and arthralgias early on.
- Joint pain
  - Many patients will complain of painful joints early on and later will develop joint swelling.
- Signs and symptoms
  - Skin: erythema migrans (typical rash)
    - Starts as red macule or papule and then expands to annular lesion up to 30 cm in diameter with partial central clearing
    - The lesion is usually painless and lasts 4–7 days.
  - Musculoskeletal
    - Early on, patient may experience myalgias, migratory joint pain (often without frank arthritis), and painful tendons and bursae.
    - Weeks to months later, 60% of untreated patients will develop monoarticular or pauciarticular arthritis of large joints, especially knees.
    - Joint fluid can have WBC count anywhere from 500–110,000 cells/mm^3 and cells are mostly neutrophils.
  - Neurologic
    - Several weeks after initial rash, 14% of untreated patients will develop neurologic symptoms including aseptic meningitis, cranial nerve palsies (especially facial nerve palsies), mononeuritis, plexitis, or myelitis.
    - Months to years later, chronic neurologic symptoms may occur, including a subtle encephalopathy: memory, mood, and sleep disturbances.
    - Significant fatigue can occur early or late in the course of Lyme disease.
  - Cardiac
    - Several weeks after initial rash, ~5% of untreated patients develop cardiac disease.
    - Most common cardiac lesion is atrioventricular block (primary, secondary, or complete).
  - Pericarditis, myocarditis, or pancarditis can also develop.

PHYSICAL EXAM

- May be completely normal early in course of disease
- Rash of erythema migrans, if seen, is virtually pathognomonic for Lyme disease.
- If patient does not have the rash, no physical finding exists that gives definitive diagnosis of Lyme
- Patient may have arthritis, Bell palsy, a cranial nerve palsy, conjunctivitis, or an irregular heartbeat.

DIAGNOSTIC TESTS & INTERPRETATION

Lab

Initial lab test

- Enzyme-linked immunosorbent assay (ELISA)
  - Can detect antibodies to *B. burgdorferi* several weeks after tick bite. However, it has relatively high false-positive rate and occasionally false-negative results. It remains positive for years after treatment.
- Western blot analysis
  - Much more specific. After 4–8 weeks of infection, ≥5 of the following IgG bands must be present for test to be positive: 18, 21, 28, 30, 39, 41, 45, 58, 66, and 93 kd. During first 2–4 weeks of infection, 2 IgM bands may establish diagnosis, but false-positive IgM blots are common.
- Positive ELISA with negative Western blot:
  - Usually means patient does not have Lyme disease and ELISA was a false-positive, but false-positive IgM blots are common.
- Polymerase chain reaction (PCR)
  - PCR testing may be done with synovial tissue or fluid or with CSF. Positive PCR indicates active disease, but negative result does not rule out Lyme.
  - Urine tests for Lyme disease have been shown to be very inaccurate and should not be used.

DIFFERENTIAL DIAGNOSIS

- Viral arthritis/arthralgias
- Septic arthritis
- Juvenile idiopathic arthritis
- Postinfectious arthritis
- Fibromyalgia syndrome
- Systemic lupus erythematosus
- Pitfalls
  - Incorrect diagnosis: Many patients with vague systemic complaints (fatigue, headaches, arthralgias) are incorrectly diagnosed with Lyme disease, even though their Lyme tests are negative (or ELISA mildly positive and Western blot negative).
  - These patients are then treated with multiple courses of oral antibiotics; if they do not respond, they are often treated with IV antibiotics, sometimes for prolonged periods.
  - This situation delays diagnosing true problem and subjects patients to unnecessary risks of long-term antibiotic use and occasionally of central venous lines.

TREATMENT

MEDICATION

- Oral antibiotics
  - Initial therapy for early Lyme disease
  - Specific therapies
    - Patients >8 years old: doxycycline is drug of choice.
    - Younger children or people who do not tolerate tetracyclines: Amoxicillin or cefuroxime is preferred, but penicillin V is also acceptable.
    - Penicillin-allergic patients: Erythromycin may be used but is less effective.
  - Duration of therapy
    - Patients with only skin rash: 14–21 days of oral antibiotics usually sufficient
    - If other symptoms present: 21–28 days recommended
- IV antibiotics
  - Become necessary for
    - Persistent arthritis unresponsive to oral medications
    - Severe carditis
    - Neurologic disease (other than an isolated 7th-nerve palsy)
  - Specific IV therapies
    - Ceftriaxone: drug of choice
    - Penicillin V: may also be used
  - Duration of therapy: 14–21 days
- Prevention
  - Some studies suggest that a single dose of doxycycline after tick bite will prevent Lyme disease.
  - Protective clothing, tick repellants, and checking daily for ticks are good preventive measures.

ONGOING CARE

PROGNOSIS

- In general, it is much better for children than for adults. Only 2% of children have chronic arthritis at 6 months.
- Most of the cardiac manifestations will disappear with or without treatment in a short time (3–4 weeks) but may later recur. Severe cardiac involvement rarely may be fatal.

COMPLICATIONS

- Chronic arthritis occurs in ~2% of children.
- Other complications arise from treatment, such as
  - Cholecystitis secondary to treatment with ceftriaxone
  - Infections from indwelling catheters used for IV antibiotics
  - Some patients develop what is thought to be a post–Lyme disease syndrome. This syndrome is not well defined and is very controversial. It often consists of arthralgias and fatigue but may include paresthesias and cognitive complaints. Prolonged antibiotics have not been shown to be helpful. Some of these patients present with a fibromyalgia-like syndrome and improve with physical therapy.

ADDITIONAL READING

- Bunikis J, Barbour AG. Laboratory testing for suspected Lyme disease. *Med Clin North Am*. 2002;86(2):311–340.
- Feder HM Jr. Lyme disease in children. *Infect Dis Clin North Am*. 2008;22(2):315–326, vii.
- Hayes E. Lyme disease. *Clin Evid*. 2002:652–664.
- Huppertz HI. Lyme disease in children. *Curr Opin Rheumatol*. 2001;13(5):434–440.
- Nachman SA, Pontrelli L. Central nervous system Lyme disease. *Semin Pediatr Infect Dis*. 2003;14(2):123–130.
- Shapiro ED, Gerber MA. Lyme disease: fact versus fiction. *Pediatr Ann*. 2002;31(3):170–177.
- Steere AC. Lyme disease. *N Engl J Med*. 2001;345(2):115–125.
- Weinstein A, Britchkov M. Lyme arthritis and post-Lyme disease syndrome. *Curr Opin Rheumatol*. 2002;14(4):383–387.

CODES

ICD10

- A69.20 Lyme disease, unspecified
- A69.23 Arthritis due to Lyme disease
- A69.21 Meningitis due to Lyme disease

FAQ

- Q: What does the deer tick look like?
- A: The deer tick is flat, very small (about the size of a pin head), and has 8 legs. The adult male is black, and the female is red and black. They can grow to 3 times their normal size when they are engorged with blood.
- Q: Do all bites from infected deer ticks cause Lyme disease?
- A: No. Even infected ticks will not cause Lyme disease if they are attached to the skin for a short period of time. If the tick is attached for <24 hours, the chances of transmitting the disease are exceedingly low. The longer the tick is attached, the higher the probability of disease transmission.
- Q: Should all patients be retested for Lyme disease after a full course of treatment?
- A: No. Lyme titers and the Western blot will remain positive for years after adequate treatment for Lyme disease. If the patient's symptoms have resolved, there is no point in rechecking the titer. If the patient is still symptomatic, titers and a Western blot may be checked before starting IV antibiotic therapy to look for a rising titer and to be sure the patient truly has Lyme disease. If symptoms remain after IV therapy, other diagnoses should be considered.
- Q: Should patients with nontraumatic Bell palsy be tested for Lyme disease?
- A: Bell palsy is seen in association with Lyme disease infections. It is a reasonable indication for testing for Lyme disease.

LYMPHADENOPATHY

Kiran Patel • Morna J. Dorsey

BASICS

DESCRIPTION
- Term used to describe ≥1 enlarged lymph nodes >10 mm in diameter (for inguinal nodes, >15 mm; for epitrochlear nodes, >5 mm)
- Any palpable supraclavicular and popliteal lymph node is considered abnormal.

EPIDEMIOLOGY
Incidence
Depends on the underlying process that causes lymph node enlargement

Prevalence
Palpable nodes are present in 5–25% of newborns (cervical, axillary, inguinal) and in >50% of older children (all areas except epitrochlear, supraclavicular, and popliteal).

PATHOPHYSIOLOGY
- Lymph nodes are often palpable in normal, healthy children.
  - Normal lymph nodes: generally <10 mm
  - They are present from birth, peak in size between 8 and 12 years of age, and then regress during adolescence.
- Lymph nodes drain contiguous areas.
  - Cervical nodes drain head and neck area (up to 15% of biopsied nodes are malignant).
  - Axillary nodes drain arm, thorax, and breast.
  - Epitrochlear nodes drain forearm and hand.
  - Inguinal nodes drain leg and groin.
  - Supraclavicular nodes drain thorax and abdomen.
- Lymphatic flow from adjacent nodes or inoculation site brings microorganisms to lymph nodes.
- Lymph node enlargement may occur via any of the following mechanisms:
  - Nodal cells may replicate in response to antigenic stimulation (e.g., Kawasaki disease) or malignant transformation (e.g., lymphoma).
  - Lymphocyte proliferation due to immune defect (e.g. primary immunodeficiency disease [PIDD])
  - Large number of reactive cells from outside node (e.g., neutrophils or metastatic cells) may enter node.
  - Foreign material may be deposited into node by lipid-laden histiocytes (e.g., lipid storage diseases).
  - Vascular engorgement and edema may occur secondary to local cytokine release.
  - Suppuration secondary to tissue necrosis (e.g., *Mycobacterium tuberculosis*)
- Many systemic infections (e.g., HIV) cause hepatic or splenic enlargement in addition to generalized lymphadenopathy.

ETIOLOGY
Usually determined by performing a thorough history and physical exam

COMMONLY ASSOCIATED CONDITIONS
Many systemic infections, malignancy, and lymphoproliferative disorders cause hepatic or splenic enlargement in addition to generalized lymphadenopathy.

DIAGNOSIS

HISTORY
- Preceding symptoms (e.g., URI symptoms preceding cervical lymphadenopathy)
- Localizing signs or symptoms (e.g., stomatitis may be associated with submandibular lymphadenopathy)
- Duration
  - Acute (<3 weeks)
  - Subacute (3–6 weeks)
  - Chronic (>6 weeks)
- Constitutional or associated symptoms (e.g., fever, weight loss, or night sweats)
- Exposures
  - Cat exposure (cat-scratch disease)
  - Uncooked meat (Toxoplasmosis)
  - Tick bite (Lyme disease)
- Medications (e.g., phenytoin or isoniazid) or prior treatments
- Travel to or residence in an endemic area should raise suspicion for tuberculosis and Lyme disease.
- History of recurrent, deep seated, or opportunistic infections, family history of PIDD
- Signs and symptoms
  - Localized lymphadenopathy: involves enlarged nodes in any 1 region
  - Generalized lymphadenopathy: involves ≥2 noncontiguous regions secondary to a systemic process, such as EBV infection
  - Supraclavicular nodes seen with malignancy: Right-sided supraclavicular node is associated with mediastinal malignancy; left-sided node suggests abdominal malignancy.

PHYSICAL EXAM
- Complete physical exam is imperative to look for signs of systemic disease such as skin, oropharyngeal, or ocular findings or hepatosplenomegaly.
- The child's weight should also be checked to be sure there has been no weight loss.
- If localized lymphadenopathy is suspected, examine the area that the lymph node drains for pathology. For example, an arm papule may be associated with axillary lymphadenopathy in cat-scratch disease.
- Cervical, axillary, and inguinal nodes, as well as liver and spleen, must be palpated to help determine if signs of systemic disease or infection are present.
- Characterize nodes. Be sure to note the following:
  - Location: Be as exact as possible (see above).
  - Size: specify dimensions.
  - Consistency: soft, firm, solid, cystic, fluctuant, rubbery. Firm, rubbery nodes may be associated with lymphomas, whereas soft nodes are generally palpated with reactive lymphadenopathy.
  - Fixation: normally freely mobile; infection or malignancy may cause adherence to surrounding tissues or nodes.
  - Tenderness: suggests inflammation

DIAGNOSTIC TESTS & INTERPRETATION
Lab
Consider the following tests if ≥1 node is persistently enlarged, has increased in size, has changed in consistency or mobility, or if systemic symptoms are present:
- CBC with differential: Consider with generalized lymphadenopathy, or if malignancy is in differential diagnosis.
- ESR or CRP: increased with infection or inflammation
- Lactate dehydrogenase (LDH), uric acid, and liver enzymes: Consider if history and physical exam raise concern for malignancy or hepatomegaly.
- Throat culture: if concern for group A β-hemolytic streptococcal (GAS) pharyngitis
- EBV/cytomegalovirus (CMV) titers: Consider with persistent generalized adenopathy.
- *Bartonella henselae* titers: Consider with persistently enlarged unilateral node and/or history of cat exposure.
- Purified protein derivative (PPD) testing: Consider with persistently enlarged node (2–4 weeks) or travel to areas where tuberculosis is endemic.
- HIV testing: Consider with persistent generalized lymphadenopathy and failure to thrive.
- Antinuclear antibody (ANA): if other signs of systemic disease to rule out systemic lupus erythematosus (SLE)
- Consider STD testing in adolescents (e.g., RPR).
- Other infectious workup as dictated by history and physical findings (e.g., Lyme titers for bull's eye rash)

Imaging
- Chest radiograph: helpful with supraclavicular nodes, systemic symptoms, or if positive PPD
- Ultrasound: may help differentiate cystic from solid masses
- CT: may help delineate anatomy or extent of the lesion, iliac lymphadenopathy is abnormal

Diagnostic Procedures/Other
- Biopsy should be considered if
  - Nodes are persistently enlarged, especially if accompanied by signs of systemic disease such as hepatosplenomegaly, weight loss, and exanthema.
  - Nodes are fixed to underlying skin.
  - Ulcerations or skin changes are present.
  - Not responsive to conventional therapy
  - Node is supraclavicular, nontender, or increasing in size or firmness.
- Fine-needle aspiration: cost-effective but sometimes nondiagnostic (e.g., unable to assess architecture); may result in fistulous tract
- Open biopsy: often diagnostic but requires general anesthesia

DIFFERENTIAL DIAGNOSIS

Must be carefully differentiated from lymphadenitis, defined as lymph node enlargement with signs of inflammation (including erythema, tenderness, induration, warmth); often treated with antibiotics

- Localized lymphadenopathy
  - Generally occurs as reactive adenopathy in response to local infection
  - Differential diagnosis for localized adenopathy varies depending on affected site.
    - Cervical adenopathy: includes cystic hygroma, branchial cleft cyst, and thyroglossal duct cyst
    - Inguinal adenopathy: lower extremity infection (e.g., osteomyelitis) or perineal disease
- Generalized lymphadenopathy: may be seen in many systemic illnesses
  - Viral infections: EBV, CMV, adenovirus, HSV, HIV, enterovirus, rubella, measles virus, varicella virus, viral hepatitides
  - Bacterial infections: *Staphylococcus aureus*, *B. henselae*, GAS, Salmonella, *Yersinia*, brucellosis, tularemia, *Mycobacterium tuberculosis*, *Mycoplasma pneumoniae*, rickettsiae
  - Primary immunodeficiency diseases: common variable immunodeficiency disease, X-linked lymphoproliferative syndrome, autoimmune lymphoproliferative syndrome, hyper-IgM syndrome
  - Malignancy: lymphoma, neuroblastoma, leukemia
  - Autoimmune disorders: SLE, juvenile rheumatoid arthritis
  - Other infections: parasites (e.g., Chagas disease) or fungal infections
  - Medications can cause drug-induced hypersensitivity syndromes (e.g., DRESS): aromatic anticonvulsants, sulfonamides, allopurinol
  - Miscellaneous: Kawasaki disease, Castleman disease, Kikuchi-Fujimoto disease (histiocytic necrotizing lymphadenitis), Gianotti-Crosti syndrome (papular acrodermatitis), sarcoidosis, lipid storage diseases (Niemann-Pick, Gaucher, Wolman, Faber diseases)

TREATMENT

MEDICATION

Acute lymphadenitis should be treated with antibiotics directed against *Streptococcus* and *Staphylococcus*.

First Line

- Dicloxacillin 50–100 mg/kg/24 h PO in 4 divided doses; max 4 g/24 h *OR*
- Amoxicillin-clavulanic acid 45 mg/kg/24 h PO in 2 divided doses, children >40 kg adult dosing
- Consider using clindamycin 30 mg/kg/24 h PO in 3 divided doses OR trimethoprim-sulfamethoxazole (TMP–SMX) 8–10 mg TMP/kg/24 h PO/IV in 2 divided doses in areas with a high prevalence of methicillin-resistant *Staphylococcus aureus* (MRSA) in the community.
- Penicillin-allergic patients: clindamycin 30 mg/kg/24 h PO in 3 divided doses or: erythromycin 50 mg/kg/24 h PO in 4 divided doses

Second Line

Consider broader antibiotic coverage for *B. henselae* and atypical mycobacterium: oral: azithromycin 10 mg/kg dose on day 1, followed by 5 mg/kg divided once for 4 more days

ADDITIONAL TREATMENT

General Measures

- Treat underlying disease.
- Close observation, unless history and physical suggest malignancy or lymphadenitis

ISSUES FOR REFERRAL

Refer to surgery or otolaryngology if biopsy or excision required.

SURGERY/OTHER PROCEDURES

Excision for special, prolonged cases

ONGOING CARE

FOLLOW-UP RECOMMENDATIONS

Patient Monitoring

- Localized lymphadenopathy: Observe for several weeks or treat with antibiotics if indicated.
- Serial observation if nodes are persistently enlarged

PROGNOSIS

- Depends on underlying diagnosis
- Excellent for reactive lymphadenopathy

COMPLICATIONS

- Lymphadenitis
- Local infection (e.g., cellulitis)
- Lymph node abscess
- Sepsis via hematogenous spread of inadequately contained infection
- Fistula (e.g., with atypical mycobacteria)
- Fibrosis secondary to purulence or lymphadenitis
- Stridor secondary to enlarged cervical lymph nodes
- Wheezing secondary to enlarged parabronchial mediastinal lymph nodes

ADDITIONAL READING

- Albright JT, Pransky SM. Nontuberculous mycobacterial infections of the head and neck. *Pediatr Clin North Am*. 2003;50(2):503–514.
- Bamji M, Stone RK, Kaul A, et al. Palpable lymph nodes in healthy newborns and infants. *Pediatrics*. 1986;78(4):573–575.
- Brook I. Microbiology and antimicrobial management of head and neck infections in children. *Adv Pediatr*. 2008;55:305–325.
- Friedmann AM. Evaluation and management of lymphadenopathy in children. *Pediatr Rev*. 2008;29(2):53–60.
- Gosche JR, Vick L. Acute, subacute, and chronic cervical lymphadenitis in children. *Semin Pediatr Sur*. 2006;15(2):99–106.
- Nield LS, Kamat D. Lymphadenopathy in children: when and how to evaluate. *Clin Pediatr*. 2004;43(1):25–33.
- Rajasekaran K, Krakovitz P. Enlarged neck lymph nodes in children. *Pediatr Clin North Am*. 2013;60(4): 923–936.
- Twist CJ, Link MP. Assessment of lymphadenopathy in children. *Pediatr Clin North Am*. 2002; 49(5): 1009–1025.

CODES

ICD10

- R59.1 Generalized enlarged lymph nodes
- R59.0 Localized enlarged lymph nodes
- P37.1 Congenital toxoplasmosis

FAQ

- Q: When should there be concern about malignancy in a child with lymphadenopathy?
- A: Malignancy should be considered in any child who has lymphadenopathy that does not improve in spite of antibiotic therapy, that has a location of concern (e.g., supraclavicular) or physical exam features of concern (hard, large size [>2 cm]) that persistently enlarges, or if the child shows signs of systemic disease.
- Q: When should a workup of a well child with localized lymphadenopathy be pursued?
- A: As long as the lymph nodes are soft, mobile, and nontender, the lymphadenopathy is likely to be self-limited. If the cause is unclear, then children should be observed for a couple of weeks. Further workup is needed if the nodes persist or enlarge, if the location is worrisome (e.g., supraclavicular), or if there are signs of systemic disease (e.g., hepatomegaly or weight loss).
- Q: When should a child with lymphadenopathy be referred to a specialist?
- A: Most cases of lymphadenopathy in children are self-limited and can be observed for a few weeks and/or treated with antibiotics, if appropriate. Referral to a surgeon should be considered in any child with persistently enlarged lymphadenopathy (>4 weeks) or immediately if there are signs of malignancy. If there is a history of recurrent or opportunistic infections, referral to an immunologist or infectious disease specialist is warranted.

LYMPHEDEMA

Heidi Engel • Bettina Neumann

BASICS

DESCRIPTION

- Lymphedema is a chronic progressive swelling in subcutaneous tissues, typically in an extremity or the genitals, due to protein-rich accumulation of interstitial fluid from disruption of the lymphatic system. It can be of primary or secondary origin.
- Primary lymphedema has 3 forms, all of which stem from a developmental abnormality of lymphatic flow. Not all primary lymphedemas are clinically evident at birth.
  - Congenital lymphedema, due to anomalous development of lymph system
    - Present at birth
    - Lower to upper extremity ratio: 3:1
    - 2/3 of cases are bilateral.
    - May improve with age
  - Lymphedema praecox (65–80% of primary lymphedema)
    - Usually becomes evident at puberty but may appear between infancy and age 35 years
    - 70% unilateral lower extremity (L > R)
  - Lymphedema tarda: presents at age 35 years or older
- Secondary lymphedema is from an acquired abnormality of lymphatic flow, an injury to the lymphatic system.
  - Common causes in children include the following:
    - Postsurgical obstruction
    - Burns
    - Insect bites
    - Infection
    - Scar tissue from radiation
    - Neoplasm
    - Trauma

EPIDEMIOLOGY

- Most lymphedemas in childhood are primary (or idiopathic) lymphedema (96%).
- Congenital lymphedema comprises 10–25% of primary lymphedema cases; lymphedema praecox, 65–80%; and lymphedema tarda, 10%.
- Affected males—most likely congenital and bilateral; affected females—most likely unilateral lymphedema praecox
- Secondary lymphedema is more common in adults and rare in children. In the United States, it is commonly from breast cancer; worldwide, due to filariasis.
- Affects 1.15 of 100,000 in children <20 years

RISK FACTORS

Genetics

- Milroy disease
  - Also known as hereditary lymphedema type IA
  - A rare, autosomal dominant condition that affects lymphatic function
  - Associated with mutations in the *FLT4* gene that encodes vascular endothelial growth factor receptor 3
- Meige disease
  - Hereditary lymphedema type II—familial lymphedema praecox
- Fabry disease
  - A serious, X-linked inborn error of glycosphingolipid catabolism associated with progressive renal failure, cardiovascular disease, neuropathy, and angiokeratosis
- Lymphedema-distichiasis
  - An autosomal dominant condition that presents with lymphedema and double rows of eyelashes
  - The condition is associated with mutations in the *FOXC2* gene.
- Other genetic conditions prone to lymphedema: Down, Turner, Noonan, yellow nail, Klippel-Trenaunay-Weber, and pes cavus

PATHOPHYSIOLOGY

- Abnormal accumulation of interstitial fluid due to the lymphatic load overwhelming the transport capacity of lymph vessels
- Lymph flow occurs under a low pressure system; unlike generalized edema, capillary filtration remains normal in patients with lymphedema.
- Initially, edema is pitting, whereas chronic edema is generally nonpitting as a result of fibrosis.

DIAGNOSIS

HISTORY

- Unilateral, heavy, often aching lower extremity edema in healthy pubertal female strongly suggests lymphedema praecox.
- Heavy, aching pitting edema distal to site of extremity surgery or trauma suggests secondary lymphedema.
- Sites of previous cellulitis, infection, or insect bites can be associated with secondary lymphedema.

PHYSICAL EXAM

- Heavy, aching pitting edema in unilateral limb is suggestive of lymphedema.
- Lymphedema responds to elevation.
- Risk factors include obesity and inflammatory arthritis.
- Primary lymphedema sites: extremities, usually legs, rare in upper limbs; the foot is always involved in lower extremity lymphedema.
- Chronic inflammation leads to fibrosis and nonpitting or "woody" edema with induration.
- Hair loss and hyperkeratosis of the affected limb develop over time.
- Intense sharp pain in affected limb is uncommon and suggests secondary lymphedema due to thrombophlebitis, cellulitis, or reflex sympathetic dystrophy.
- Global edema suggests other disease states.
- Red streaking of extremity, fever, chills, or nodal enlargement suggests development of cellulitis or lymphangitis.
- History and physical exam are primary source for diagnosis.

DIAGNOSTIC TESTS & INTERPRETATION

Lab

Not usually necessary but may be useful to rule out other causes of edema

- Urinalysis for proteinuria as seen with glomerulonephrosis
- Serum total protein and albumin to rule out hypoproteinemia
- Liver function tests to assess functional status
- Pregnancy test

Imaging

Usually unnecessary to make diagnosis but may help to plan or evaluate therapy

- Lymphangiography is no longer used because related dyes caused inflammation and worsening of lymphatic obstruction.
- Radionuclide lymphoscintigraphy, when indicated, is the preferred method of imaging to define anatomy and to evaluate lymph flow and obstruction.
- CT and MRI may be valuable if a malignancy is suspected or to differentiate subcutaneous from adipose swelling.
- Doppler ultrasound may be helpful if deep vein thrombosis is suspected.

DIFFERENTIAL DIAGNOSIS

- Infection
  - Cellulitis
  - Lymphangitis
  - Herpes simplex virus type 2
- Tumors
  - Pelvic mass
  - Multiple enchondromatosis
- Metabolic
  - Cushing disease
  - Hyperthyroidism
  - Lipedema
- Anatomic
  - Venous stasis
  - Deep vein thrombosis
  - Hemihypertrophy
  - Arteriovenous fistula or malformation
  - Popliteal arterial aneurysm
  - Popliteal cyst (Baker cyst)
- Miscellaneous
  - Heart failure
  - Glomerulonephrosis
  - Cirrhosis
  - Hypoproteinemia
  - Reflex sympathetic dystrophy

TREATMENT

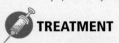

GENERAL MEASURES

- Therapy should be instituted as soon as possible and before fibrosis develops.
- Goals of therapy are to minimize or decrease edema and to prevent infection, fibrosis, and skin changes.
- Compression garments (e.g., Jobst stockings or elastic wraps) is recommended long term but compliance can be a challenge.
- Extremity elevation, especially at night
- Exercise, stay active for a lifetime; muscle contraction assists lymph flow and does not exacerbate swelling.
- Weight control
- Diligent skin care and appropriately fitting shoes to avoid infection
- Manual massage decompression can be helpful for digital edema and for infants who may not tolerate compression garments.
- Automated intermittent pneumatic compression machines shown to facilitate home regimen compliance
- Psychological effects of cosmesis are prominent and should not be overlooked.
- Patient education and support groups can be found through the National Lymphedema Network.

DIET

In children with chylous reflux syndromes, a diet low in long-chain triglycerides may be of benefit.

SPECIAL THERAPY

- Complex decongestive physiotherapy (CDP) is part of a specialized treatment with an initial reductive phase 1 and a maintenance phase 2 provided by a licensed physical therapist or occupational therapist certified in the treatment of lymphedema.
- Treatment is time sensitive and should be instituted as soon as possible to prevent fibrosis developing.
  - Phase 1 consists of manual lymph-drainage therapy, compression therapy specialized bandaging, fitting for appropriate tailored compression garment, and detailed skin and nail care.
  - Phase 2 consists of self-management for drainage techniques, skin care, use and care of compression garments, and exercise advice

MEDICATION

- Diuretics: not generally used in children and adolescents; efficacy for adults is debated
- Prophylactic antibiotic use is indicated for patients with recurrent cellulitis or lymphangitis.

SURGERY/OTHER PROCEDURES

- Microsurgical treatment has been proven to show excellent outcomes in carefully selected patient populations via lymphatic-venous anastomoses or lymphatic-venous-lymphatic anastomoses.
- Traditional surgery has 1 of 2 goals: removal of excess edematous tissue or attempts to restore lymph drainage
  - Both may decrease the rate of infections but have poor cosmetic results.
  - Recommended only for those with uncontrolled swelling with significant disability

ONGOING CARE

PROGNOSIS

- Edema persists throughout life.
- Lymphedema can be staged and monitored via circumferential measurements. Guidelines have been established by the American Physical Therapy Association.
- Natural history: plateau in severity of edema after an initial few years of progression in 50%, slow constant progression in 50%

COMPLICATIONS

- Cellulitis and lymphangitis are the most common complications and are treated with antibiotics; published series showed 24% of cases developed infection and half of these required hospitalization.
- Poor long-term compliance with compression garments due to uncomfortable nature of therapy
- Lymphangiosarcoma (rare)
- Psychological problems
- Physical limitations
- Chronic inflammation and edema ultimately lead to fibrosis and induration of the involved area.

ADDITIONAL READING

- Gary DE. Lymphedema diagnosis and management. *J Am Acad Nurse Pract*. 2007;19(2):72–78.
- Kerchner K, Fleischer A, Yosipovitch G. Lower extremity lymphedema update: pathophysiology, diagnosis, and treatment guidelines. *J Am Acad Dermatol*. 2008;59(2):324–331.
- Mayrovitz HN. The standard of care for lymphedema: current concepts and physiological considerations. *Lymph Res Biol*. 2009;7(2):101–108.
- Rockson SG. Current concepts and future directions in the diagnosis and management of lymphatic vascular disease. *Vasc Med*. 2010;15(3):223–231.
- Schook CC, Mulliken JB, Fishman SJ, et al. Differential diagnosis of lower extremity enlargement in pediatric patients referred with a diagnosis of lymphedema. *Plast Reconstr Surg*. 2011;127(4):1571–1581.
- Zuther JE. *Lymphedema Management: The Comprehensive Guide for Practitioners*. 2nd ed. New York, NY: Thieme; 2009.

CODES

ICD10

- I89.0 Lymphedema, not elsewhere classified
- Q82.0 Hereditary lymphedema
- I97.89 Oth postproc comp and disorders of the circ sys, NEC

FAQ

- Q: Is the swelling going to go away?
- A: No, this is a chronic condition requiring long-term management.
- Q: Could this have been prevented?
- A: No, primary lymphedema is typically due to abnormal embryologic development.
- Q: If the lymph channels have been abnormal since birth, why does the swelling present during adolescence?
- A: No one really knows; hormones may play a role in lymphedema.

LYMPHOPROLIFERATIVE DISORDERS

David T. Teachey

BASICS

DESCRIPTION

- Lymphoproliferative disorders are a class of non-malignant diseases characterized by uncontrolled growth of lymphoid tissues (spleen, bone marrow, liver, lymph nodes).
- Can be congenital or acquired
- Most common in children include
  - Autoimmune lymphoproliferative syndrome (ALPS)
  - Castleman disease (CD)
  - Rosai–Dorfman disease (RDD)
  - EBV-associated lymphoproliferative disorder (ELD)
  - X-linked lymphoproliferative syndrome (XLP)
- Rarer disorders (not discussed in detail)
  - Angioimmunoblastic lymphadenopathy
  - Caspase-8 deficiency syndrome
  - Dianzani autoimmune lymphoproliferative disease
  - Kikuchi-Fujimoto syndrome
  - Lymphomatoid granulomatosis
  - Lymphomatoid papulosis
  - Ocular adnexal lymphoid proliferation
  - RAS-associated leukoproliferative disorder

EPIDEMIOLOGY

All uncommon

RISK FACTORS

Often multifactorial with inherited genetic defect and acquired infection

Genetics

- ALPS (80% of patients have identifiable mutation)
  - 60–70% germline mutation in FAS (*TNFRSF6*)
  - 10% somatic mutation in FAS
  - 2% germline mutation in CASP10
  - <1% germline mutation in FASL
- XLP
  - Majority of cases mutation in *SH2DIA*
  - XLP-like syndrome caused by X-linked inhibitor of apoptosis protein (XIAP) mutations

PATHOPHYSIOLOGY

- ALPS
  - Defective FAS-mediated apoptosis leads to abnormal lymphocyte survival with subsequent lymphoproliferation, autoimmunity, and cancer.
- CD
  - Largely unknown but can be triggered by HHV-8 infection, especially in immunocompromised patients
- ELD
  - EBV triggered lymphoproliferative disorder found in patients on chronic immune suppression typically after organ or bone marrow transplant (PTLD) or with inherited immune deficiency
- XLP
  - Mutation in *SH2D1A* leads to abnormal production of SAP protein in NK and T cells, leading to defective SAP-SLAM signaling and inability to appropriately respond to EBV infection.

DIAGNOSIS

HISTORY

- ALPS
  - Typically presents at young age (average 18 months) with massive lymphadenopathy and splenomegaly
  - Many patients develop secondary autoimmune disease.
  - Most often, autoimmune destruction of blood cells (80% of patients); can be mild to severe
  - Destruction of platelets: See chapter on "Idiopathic Thrombocytopenic Purpura."
  - Destruction of erythrocytes: See chapter on "Autoimmune Hemolytic Anemia."
  - Destruction of neutrophils: See chapter on "Neutropenia."
  - Can have autoimmune involvement of any organ system, similar to systemic lupus erythematosus
  - In young adult years, 10–20% develop lymphoma.
  - Lymphoproliferation can improve or worsen with infection. Often progresses through teenage years and improves in adulthood.
  - Autoimmune disease is less likely to improve with older age.
- CD
  - Two variants
    - Hyaline vascular: presents with enlarged single lymph node or chain of nodes; >90% with no other symptoms; rarely can have fever, weight loss, fatigue
    - Plasma cell: presents with enlarged single lymph node or chain (unicentric) or diffuse adenopathy (multicentric); often with constitutional symptoms (fever, sweats, lethargy, rashes, neuropathy, arthritis)
- RDD
  - Massive, painless bilateral cervical lymphadenopathy with or without other involved nodal groups
  - Fever
  - Snoring common
  - Can have extranodal invasion of almost any organ (25% of patients have extranodal disease) and signs and symptoms depend on involved organ
- ELD/PTLD
  - Can be mild, with lymphadenopathy, fever, and/or diarrhea, or severe, with massive lymphadenopathy, high fever, night sweats, rash, and pruritus, and organ compression from involved nodes
- XLP
  - Can present as fulminant infectious mononucleosis or aplastic anemia or lymphoma or hematophagocytic syndrome
  - Often critically ill in the setting of EBV infection

PHYSICAL EXAM

- ALPS
  - Massive lymphadenopathy (90% of patients): Can compress vital organs including trachea (rare). Most common site of adenopathy is anterior cervical. Nodes are hard but mobile.
  - Splenomegaly (90% of patients)
  - Hepatomegaly (50% of patients)
  - Other physical exam findings as expected with autoimmune destruction of blood cells and/or end-organ autoimmune disease
- CD
  - Hyaline vascular: single enlarged lymph node or chain; most often cervical or mediastinal; may have shotty diffuse nonpathologic adenopathy
  - Plasma cell: single or multiple pathologically enlarged lymph nodes; abdominal nodes most common; hepatosplenomegaly common. Peripheral edema, ascites, and pleural effusions may be present.
- RDD
  - Massive bilateral anterior cervical lymphadenopathy (90% of patients). Other physical exam findings can vary based on extranodal disease.
  - Hepatosplenomegaly (10% of patients)
- ELD/PTLD
  - Similar to other lymphoproliferative disorders (See "Epstein-Barr virus" chapter.)
- XLP
  - Similar to other lymphoproliferative disorders, however, far more acutely ill (see also "Epstein–Barr virus" chapter and Aplastic Anemia" chapter)

DIAGNOSTIC TESTS & INTERPRETATION

Lab

General

- Complete blood and reticulocyte count for anemia, thrombocytopenia, and neutropenia
- Direct antiglobin test (DAT) to check for autoimmune destruction of red blood cells
- Serum chemistries, uric acid, phosphorus to look for cell turnover (usually normal in lymphoproliferative disorders)
- Liver function tests, PT, PTT, and fibrinogen to measure liver function and for coagulopathy
- EBV, PCR and titers, CMV-PCR
- If acutely ill, consider ESR or CRP and ferritin.
- Quantitative immunoglobulins: often elevated in lymphoproliferative disorders

Diagnostic tests for ALPS

- Mandatory criteria
  - (1) Chronic (>6 months) nonmalignant lymphoproliferation (lymphadenopathy) and/or splenomegaly
  - (2) Elevated peripheral blood double-negative T cells (DNTs): T cells that are CD3+, TCR alpha/beta+, CD4−, and CD8−. DNTs are usually rare in peripheral blood (<1% of total lymphocytes or <2.5% of total T cells). DNTs are elevated and often markedly elevated in ALPS. Slight elevation in DNTs can be found in other autoimmune disorders.
- Major (primary) criteria
  - (1) Genetic mutation in ALPS causative gene (germline or somatic) in FAS, FASL, or CASP10
  - (2) In vitro evidence of defective FAS-mediated apoptosis. This assay requires growing blood cells from patient in culture for weeks and exposing to anti-Fas monoclonal antibody to see if T cells are resistant to death. Only performed in a few labs.

- Minor (secondary) criteria
  - (1) Elevated vitamin B_{12} (>1,500 ng/L)
  - (2) Elevated IL-10 (>20 pg/mL)
  - (3) Elevated IL-18 (>500 pg/mL)
  - (4) Elevated sFASL (>200 pg/mL)
  - (5) Classic histopathologic findings on lymph nodes or spleen biopsy
  - (6) Autoimmune cytopenias AND elevated serum IgG
  - (7) Positive family history
- Diagnosis
  - Definitive: both mandatory and one major criteria
  - Probable: both mandatory and one minor criteria (Probable ALPS should be treated the same as definitive ALPS.)

Diagnostic tests for CD
- Castleman syndrome diagnosed by histopathology
- Hypergammaglobulinemia, anemia, high ESR, high IL-6, HHV-8, PCR+

Diagnostic tests for RDD
- RDD diagnosed by histopathology
- Hypergammaglobulinemia, anemia, high ESR, leukocytosis with neutropenia, hematologic autoantibodies

Diagnostic tests for ELD/PTLD
- PTLD after bone marrow graft
- Persistent EBV infection (positive EBV PCR or abnormal seroconversion by titers) in setting of immune suppression or immune compromise
- Diagnosis confirmed with imaging and/or histopathology

Diagnostic tests for XLP
- Persistent EBV infection (positive EBV PCR or abnormal seroconversion on titers)
- Inverted CD4/CD8 ratio
- High IgM and IgA, low IgG
- Defective NK activity
- Secondary hematophagocytic syndrome (elevated ferritin, high triglycerides, low fibrinogen, cytopenias, high fever, splenomegaly, poor NK function, elevated s-IL-2R-alpha, and hematophagocytosis on marrow or node biopsy)
- Diagnosis confirmed by genetic testing for mutations in *SH2D1A* and XIAP genes, and/or SAP protein quantification

Imaging
- CT scans of head, neck, chest, abdomen, and pelvis with IV contrast is important for all lymphoproliferative disorders at initial diagnosis to define extent of disease.
- It is IMPORTANT to obtain plain chest x-ray on initial presentation in patient with diffuse lymphadenopathy before CT scan to ensure a large mediastinal mass is not present. If present, it may be unsafe to lie patient flat and/or sedate for CT scan.
- Most lymphoproliferative disorders are very PET-avid.

Diagnostic Procedures/Other
- ALPS and PTLD can be diagnosed without histopathology; however, most patients have a lymph node biopsy.
- Other lymphoproliferative disorders typically require tissue for diagnosis (biopsy, not fine needle aspirate).
- Consider bone marrow aspirate and/or biopsy to rule out marrow disease or other disease processes.

Pathological Findings
- ALPS: DNTs in lymph node and spleen
- CD: hyaline vascular (shrunken germinal centers with eosinophilic expansion of mantle zones with and vessel hyalinization); plasma cell (extensive plasma cell infiltrate in interfollicular regions)
- RD: emperipoiesis (lymphophagocytosis)—hallmark of disease on biopsy; presence of histiocytes
- XLP/PTLD/ELD: EBER+

DIFFERENTIAL DIAGNOSIS
- Other lymphoproliferative disorders
- Lymphoma
- Infection: EBV, CMV, toxoplasmosis, HIV, TB
- Evans syndrome
- Rheumatologic disease

TREATMENT

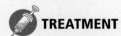

FIRST LINE
- For ALPS: Corticosteroids or IVIG for acute flares
- For CD localized disease
  - Surgical resection or focal radiation. Steroids may be used to shrink lesions prior to surgery.
- For CD multicentric disease
  - Multiagent therapy (vincristine, prednisone, rituximab, cyclophosphamide, doxorubicin)
- For RD
  - May self-resolve (20% of patients)
  - If not, consider prednisone, or vinblastine plus prednisone, or mercaptopurine plus methotrexate, or 2CdA.
- For ELD/PTLD
  - Reduce immune suppression or convert immune suppression to sirolimus if possible
  - Consider rituximab, adoptive transfer of EBV-specific cytotoxic T cells
  - If fails or generalized disease, consider multiagent chemotherapy similar to RDD
- For XLP
  - If hematophagocytosis or aplasia: rituximab, etoposide, steroids, and cyclosporine
  - Hematopoietic stem cell transplant is the only cure.

SECOND LINE
- For ALPS
  - Sirolimus or mycophenolate mofetil for chronic disease
  - Sirolimus (rapamycin): pros: improves autoimmune disease and lymphoproliferation and eliminates DNTs. Cons: drug–drug interactions; requires therapeutic drug monitoring; 10% of patients develop mouth sores (most common in first month).
  - Mycophenolate mofetil (CellCept): pros: No drug–drug interactions, no mouth sores, no therapeutic drug monitoring. Cons: not as effective; does not help lymphoproliferation or lower DNTs; GI upset
  - Recommended treatment: Mild to moderate autoimmune disease start with mycophenolate and transition to sirolimus if poor response or side effects. More severe autoimmune disease or clinically significant lymphoproliferation start with sirolimus.

THIRD LINE
- For ALPS
  - Combination therapy: stem cell transplant
  - Relative contraindications (AVOID, if possible)
    - Splenectomy: high incidence of pneumococcal sepsis even with antibiotic prophylaxis and immunization
    - Rituximab: can lead to lifelong hypogammaglobulinemia (5–10% of patients)

ONGOING CARE

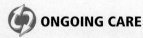

FOLLOW-UP RECOMMENDATIONS
Recommended follow-up imaging varies among institutions. Most physicians will repeat imaging if patient's history changes OR to determine response to therapy.

PROGNOSIS
- Prognosis is good to fair for most lymphoproliferative disorders.
- Prognosis is poor in XLP and advanced CD.

ADDITIONAL READING

- Blaes AH, Morrison VA. Post-transplant lymphoproliferative disorders following solid-organ transplantation. *Expert Rev Hematol*. 2010;3(1):35–44.
- Oliveira JB, Bleesing JJ, Dianzani U, et al. Revised diagnostic criteria and classification for the autoimmune lymphoproliferative syndrome (ALPS): report from the 2009 NIH International Workshop. *Blood*. 2010;116(14):e35–e40.
- Rezaei N, Mahmoudi E, Aghamohammadi A, et al. X-linked lymphoproliferative syndrome: a genetic condition typified by the triad of infection, immunodeficiency and lymphoma. *Br J Haematol*. 2011;152(1):13–30.
- Schulte KM, Talat N. Castleman's disease—a two compartment model of HHV8 infection. *Nat Rev Clin Oncol*. 2010;7(9):533–543.
- Teachey DT, Seif AE, Grupp SA. Advances in the management and understanding of autoimmune lymphoproliferative syndrome (ALPS). *Br J Haematol*. 2010;148(2):205–216.

CODES

ICD10
- D47.9 Neoplasm of uncertain behavior of lymphoid, hematopoietic and related tissue, unspecified
- D89.82 Autoimmune lymphoproliferative syndrome [ALPS]
- D47.Z1 Post-transplant lymphoproliferative disorder (PTLD)

MALABSORPTION

Sabina Sabharwal

BASICS

DESCRIPTION

- Malabsorption is characterized as a syndrome, as opposed to a disease entity, and is defined as any state in which there is a disturbance of digestion and/or absorption of nutrients across the intestinal mucosa.
- The classical symptoms of malabsorption include chronic diarrhea, abdominal distention, and failure to thrive.

EPIDEMIOLOGY

Depends on the underlying disease causing malabsorption

ETIOLOGY

The most common causes of malabsorption in developed countries are as follows:

- Postenteritis syndrome
- Cow's milk protein intolerance
- Giardiasis
- Celiac disease
- Cystic fibrosis
- Inflammatory bowel disease (IBD)

PATHOPHYSIOLOGY

- Depends on the nutrient affected
  - Carbohydrate
    - Monosaccharide: congenital glucose-galactose deficiency, fructose intolerance
    - Disaccharide: lactase deficiency (congenital or acquired), sucrase-isomaltase deficiency
    - Polysaccharide: amylase deficiency (congenital or acquired)
  - Fat
    - Bile salt deficiency: cholestasis, resection of terminal ileum
    - Exocrine pancreatic insufficiency: cystic fibrosis, chronic pancreatitis
    - Inadequate surface area: celiac disease, flat villous lesions
  - Protein
    - Protein-losing enteropathy: intestinal lymphangiectasia, congenital heart failure
    - Exocrine pancreatic insufficiency: cystic fibrosis, Shwachman-Diamond syndrome
    - Inadequate surface area: celiac disease
- According to the place where the alteration occurs
  - Mucosal abnormality
    - Anatomic: post-enteritis syndrome, celiac disease, IBD
    - Functional: disaccharidase deficiencies
  - Luminal abnormality
    - Exocrine pancreatic insufficiency: cystic fibrosis, Shwachman-Diamond syndrome
    - Bile salt insufficiency: biliary cholestatic liver disease, ileal resection
  - Anatomic abnormality
    - Short gut: surgical resection
    - Motility disturbance: intestinal pseudo-obstruction

DIAGNOSIS

HISTORY

- GI symptoms
  - Common in patients with malabsorption syndromes
  - Range from mild abdominal gaseous distention to severe abdominal pain and vomiting
  - Chronic or recurrent diarrhea is by far the most common symptom.
  - Abdominal distention and watery diarrhea, with or without mild abdominal pain associated with skin irritation in the perianal area due to acidic stools, are characteristic of carbohydrate malabsorption syndromes.
  - Fat malabsorption can present with bulky, foul-smelling stools that are oily and thus float in water. Abdominal distention, increased gas, weight loss, and increased appetite are also seen.
  - Periodic nausea, abdominal distention, pain, and diarrhea are common in patients with chronic *Giardia* infections.
  - Vomiting, with moderate to severe abdominal pain and bloody stools, is characteristic of protein sensitivity syndromes.
  - Abdominal pain or irritability (particularly seen in celiac disease)
- Stool characteristics
  - Frequent loose watery stools may indicate carbohydrate intolerance.
  - Bulky, greasy, or loose foul-smelling stools indicate fat malabsorption.
  - In protein malabsorption, stools may be normal or loose.
  - Bloody stools are seen in patients with cow's milk protein allergy, infection, and IBD.
- Other symptoms
  - Failure to thrive caused by malabsorption of carbohydrates, fats, or proteins
  - Anemia, with weakness and fatigue, due to inadequate absorption of vitamin B_{12}, iron, and folic acid
  - Edema, due to decreased protein absorption and hypoalbuminemia
  - Muscle cramping due to decreased vitamin D causing hypocalcemia and decreased potassium levels

PHYSICAL EXAM

- Malabsorption syndromes should be considered during the workup for failure to thrive, malnutrition, poor weight gain, or delayed puberty.
- In particular, they should be suspected in infants with weight loss or little weight gain since birth and in infants with low weight and weight-for-height percentiles.
- Signs of malnutrition, including reduced subcutaneous fat, paleness, angular cheilosis, and muscle weakness
- Abdominal distention, increased bowel sounds
- Rash around mouth and/or anus are commonly seen.

DIAGNOSTIC TESTS & INTERPRETATION

Lab

- Stool analysis
  - The presence of reducing substances and pH <5.5 indicates that carbohydrates have not been properly absorbed.
  - The level of quantitative stool fat and the amount of fat intake in the diet should be measured and monitored for 3 days using special stains; a coefficient of fat absorption is calculated using the following equation:

$$\frac{\text{Ingested fat (g)} - \text{fat in stool (g)}}{\text{Ingested fat (g)}} \times 100$$

– Normal values for the coefficient of fat absorption: >93% in children and adults, >85% in infants, >67% in premature infants
– Moderate fat malabsorption ranges from 60 to 80%.
– Fat absorption of <50% indicates severe malabsorption.
– The presence of large serum proteins in the stool, such as α_1 antitrypsin, indicates leakage of serum protein. A 24-hour stool collection for α_1 antitrypsin (along with a serum level) serves as a screening test for protein-losing enteropathy.
– Exam of the stool for ova and parasites or testing for the stool antigen may reveal the presence of *Giardia* species.
– If bile acid malabsorption is suspected, quantitative conjugated and unconjugated bile acids may be measured in stool, although this test is not commonly available or used.
- Other laboratory studies
  – CBC
    - May reveal anemia in patients with iron, folate, and vitamin B_{12} malabsorption
    - Neutropenia is seen in patients with Shwachman-Diamond syndrome.
  – Total serum protein and albumin levels
    - May be lower than reference range in syndromes in which protein is lost or not absorbed, particularly in protein-losing enteropathy and pancreatic insufficiency
  – With fat malabsorption or ileal resection, fat-soluble vitamin levels in the serum are low.
  – With bile acid malabsorption, levels of LDL cholesterol may be low.
  – Serum calcium may be low due to vitamin D and amino acid malabsorption.
  – Serum vitamin A, E, and carotene may be low due to bile salt deficiency and impaired fat absorption.
  – Other studies must be performed when a specific disease is suspected (e.g., mucosal biopsy for celiac disease, sweat test for cystic fibrosis, or appropriate workup for IBD).
  – Urine analysis should be done to rule out proteinuria in patients with low albumin levels.
  – An upper GI radiographic series and/or a lactulose breath test can be performed to look for small bowel dilation due to bacterial overgrowth.
  – Genetic testing may be performed for identification of inherited malabsorption syndromes.
  – If tissue samples are acquired through a biopsy, ultrastructural analysis may be performed using electron microscopy.

DIFFERENTIAL DIAGNOSIS
- Pancreatic disorders
  – Cystic fibrosis
  – Shwachman syndrome
  – Johanson-Blizzard syndrome
- Chronic cholestasis
  – Biliary atresia
  – Vitamin E deficiency
  – Alagille syndrome
- Infectious diarrhea
  – Giardiasis
  – Cryptosporidiosis
- Mucosal defect
  – Celiac disease
  – Crohn disease
  – Postinfectious diarrhea
- Congenital brush border enzyme deficiencies
  – Glucose-galactose transporter deficiency
  – Sucrase-isomaltase deficiency
  – Microvillus inclusion disease
- Abnormal intestinal lymphatic drainage
  – Primary intestinal lymphangiectasia
  – Secondary intestinal lymphangiectasia

TREATMENT
- Overall, nutritional support is paramount.
- Specific treatment depends on etiology, for example, gluten-free diet for celiac disease, metronidazole for *Giardia* infection, or removal of the offending agent in a case of food intolerance.

ONGOING CARE

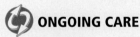

COMPLICATIONS
- Complications of malabsorption vary according to the underlying disease, but malnutrition and its consequences may worsen progressively if the cause is not determined and appropriate treatment prescribed.
- Frequent complications of malabsorption and malnutrition include growth failure, vitamin and micronutrient deficiency (zinc, magnesium, calcium), bone disease, hypoproteinemia and edema, essential fatty acid deficiency, perianal dermatitis, immune dysfunction, and anemia.

ADDITIONAL READING

- Ali SA, Hill DR. *Giardia intestinalis*. *Curr Opin Infect Dis*. 2003;16(5):453–460.
- Crittenden RG, Bennett LE. Cow's milk allergy: a complex disorder. *J Am Coll Nutr*. 2005;24(6)(Suppl): 582S–591S.
- Dodge JA, Turck D. Cystic fibrosis: nutritional consequences and management. *Best Pract Res Clin Gastroenterol*. 2006;20(30):531–546.
- Fasano A, Catassi C. Coeliac disease in children. *Best Pract Res Clin Gastroenterol*. 2005;19(3): 467–478.
- Pietzak MM, Thomas DW. Childhood malabsorption. *Pediatr Rev*. 2003;24(6):195–206.

CODES

ICD10
- K90.9 Intestinal malabsorption, unspecified
- K90.4 Malabsorption due to intolerance, not elsewhere classified
- K90.0 Celiac disease

FAQ
- Q: Why do patients with malabsorption become anemic?
- A: Patients with malabsorption can become deficient in vitamin B_{12}, iron, and folic acid and in turn can become anemic.
- Q: Why do patients with celiac disease develop symptoms of malabsorption?
- A: Celiac disease leads to inflammation of the small bowel mucosa and villous atrophy. In turn, the absorptive capacity of the bowel is decreased.

M

MALARIA

Emily M. Schaaf • Chandy C. John

BASICS

DESCRIPTION

- Malaria is a febrile illness caused by the *Plasmodium* species of protozoan parasites, transmitted by the *Anopheles* mosquito vector.
- 5 *Plasmodium* strains infect humans: *Plasmodium falciparum*, *Plasmodium vivax*, *Plasmodium malariae*, *Plasmodium ovale*, and *Plasmodium knowlesi*. *P. falciparum* and *P. vivax* cause the majority of disease.
- Classic symptoms include stages of chills, followed by high fevers, and then sweating. However, this classic symptom pattern is less likely to be seen in children. Children may manifest initially with only fever as a complaint.

EPIDEMIOLOGY

- High-risk areas of endemic malaria include Africa, parts of Central and South America, Oceania, and tropical regions of Asia.
- *P. falciparum* is the major species in sub-Saharan Africa. Both *P. falciparum* and *P. vivax* are found in India, Southeast Asia, Oceania, and Central and South America, and *P. vivax* is present in some areas of Africa. *P. ovale* is usually found in West Africa.
- *P. falciparum* causes more deaths in children <5 years of age than any other organism.
- WHO reports that 86% of malaria deaths occur in children. Pregnant women are also at high risk.

Incidence

- Worldwide, an estimated 200–300 million cases of malaria occur annually, and 660,000–1.2 million deaths occur from malaria annually.
- ~1,500 cases of malaria are imported into the United States each year. In 2012, almost 2,000 cases of malaria were seen in the United States, the largest number of cases in >40 years.

RISK FACTORS

Genetics

- Sickle cell trait is known to provide protection against malaria.
  - The risk of death of severe *falciparum* malaria is 60–70% less in children with Hb AS than those with Hb AA.
- Thalassemia and G6PD deficiency also provide some protection against malaria.
- Individuals with a Duffy-negative blood type lack receptors for *P. vivax* merozoite invasion and are typically resistant to *P. vivax*, although recently, cases of *P. vivax* in Duffy-negative individuals have been reported.

GENERAL PREVENTION

- Personal protective measures against mosquito bites are extremely important.
  - Remain in well-screened areas.
  - Wear protective clothing, including pants and long-sleeved shirts.
  - Use insect repellents containing DEET.
  - Use insecticide-treated bed nets.
- Chemoprophylaxis is strongly advised for travelers to endemic areas.
  - Chloroquine may be used in areas with chloroquine-sensitive parasites only (5 mg/kg once a week—max 500 mg).
  - In chloroquine-resistant areas, effective options are atovaquone-proguanil (Malarone), mefloquine, or doxycycline.
    - Malarone can be used in all areas but is contraindicated in severe renal impairment and pregnancy.
      - Dosing: 5–8 kg: 1/2 pediatric tablet daily. 8–10 kg: 3/4 pediatric tab daily. 10–20 kg: 1 pediatric tab (62.5/25) daily. 20–30 kg: 2 pediatric tabs daily. 30–40 kg: 3 pediatric tabs daily. ≥40 kg: 1 adult tab (250/100) daily
  - Mefloquine resistance is present in parts of Asia. Contraindications to mefloquine include seizure disorder, major psychiatric illness, or cardiac disease. It is safe in pregnancy and for young infants.
    - Dosing: ≤15 kg: 5 mg/kg weekly. 15–19 kg: 1/4 tablet weekly. 20–30 kg: 1/2 tab weekly. 30–45 kg: 3/4 tab weekly. >45 kg: 1 tab weekly
  - Doxycycline is contraindicated if <8 years of age and in pregnancy. Dosing: 2.2 mg/kg daily (max 100 mg/day)
- Chloroquine and mefloquine are begun 1 week before travel, continued during the period of exposure and for 4 weeks after leaving the endemic region. Malarone is started 2 days prior to travel and continued 1 week after return. Doxycycline is started 2 days before travel and continued for 4 weeks after return.

ETIOLOGY

- Infection is typically transmitted by the bite of the female *Anopheles* mosquito, but it can also be transmitted through contaminated blood transfusions or acquired congenitally.
- The majority of human disease is caused by *P. falciparum* and *P. vivax*.
  - *P. vivax* and *P. ovale* can cause relapsing disease because of the persistent hepatic (hypnozoite) stage of the infection.
  - Asymptomatic carriage for years may occur due to *P. malariae*.
  - *P. knowlesi* is a primate parasite that can cause severe disease in humans.

COMMONLY ASSOCIATED CONDITIONS

- Severe malaria is most commonly caused by *P. falciparum*.
- Severe malaria is defined as parasitemia >5%, shock, acidosis, severe anemia or signs of CNS or other end-organ involvement such as renal failure, pulmonary edema, respiratory distress (acidotic/irregular breathing), impaired consciousness, seizures, hemoglobinuria, DIC, or hypoglycemia.
- Cerebral malaria is a serious consequence of malaria infection, defined as coma in conjunction with *P. falciparum* parasitemia.
  - Occurs most often in children age 3–6 years in Africa but often occurs in adolescents and adults in Southeast Asia
- Severe anemia is common and can be severe, especially with *P. falciparum*. This is due to high parasitemia, hemolysis, and sequestration.
- Respiratory distress has high mortality, particularly if combined with impaired consciousness.
- Blackwater fever is a complication associated with *falciparum* malaria. It occurs due to massive hemolysis with resulting hemoglobinuria and acute renal failure.
- Pulmonary edema, renal failure, distributive shock, and progression to coma or death can occur.
- Hyperreactive malarial splenomegaly is seen with chronic exposure to malaria in endemic areas. High levels of malaria IgM are present, and massive hepatosplenomegaly is seen.
- Splenic rupture may occur due to splenomegaly.
- *P. malariae* can cause nephrotic syndrome.

DIAGNOSIS

HISTORY

- History of travel to malaria endemic region
- Poor compliance with malaria prophylaxis
- Signs and symptoms
  - High fevers, headache, chills, and sweats are classic symptoms.
  - Periodicity of fever depends on the *Plasmodium* species and is less commonly seen in young children and travelers.
  - GI symptoms are common in children. Irritability, anorexia, vomiting, abdominal pain, cough, and arthralgias may be seen.
  - 95% of malaria cases occur within 30 days of return from travel, but malaria may occur as late as months after return.
  - Malaria can cause altered mental status, increased intracranial pressure, seizures, and coma.

ALERT

A high index of suspicion is necessary for the diagnosis of malaria, as failure to diagnose malaria has led to death in some instances. Fever may be the only sign in infants and young children.

PHYSICAL EXAM

- Fever, malaise, ill appearance
- Pallor or jaundice
- Hepatosplenomegaly may be present.
- In severely ill patients, respiratory distress with acidotic, deep breathing may be seen.

DIAGNOSTIC TESTS & INTERPRETATION

Lab

- Hemolytic anemia is commonly seen, with severe malarial anemia most common with *P. falciparum*.
- Thrombocytopenia is common.
- Hypoglycemia may occur with *P. falciparum*.
- Peripheral blood smear
  - Thick and thin peripheral smears are required for definitive diagnosis (thick smears provide better sensitivity if the parasitemia is low; thin smears provide for species identification).

– If initial smears are negative, repeated specimens should be obtained q12–24h over 72 hours to confirm a truly negative result with 3 smears.
– A parasitemia of >5% of red blood cells, altered mental status, or other organ involvement make the diagnosis of severe malaria and require more intensive therapy.
- Rapid diagnostic tests
  – Rapid tests for antigen detection show excellent sensitivity for *Plasmodium* spp., require a small amount of blood for testing, and provide results in <20 minutes.
  – Rapid tests should complement but not replace microscopy testing, as they do not provide an estimate of parasite density.
- PCR
  – PCR is highly sensitive and can be useful for determining the *Plasmodium* species if it is unclear by blood smear. However, it is time-consuming and costly.

DIFFERENTIAL DIAGNOSIS

- Malaria should be considered in any febrile traveler from an endemic area.
- Other causes of fever in travelers should be considered based on the region of travel are as follows:
  – Dengue
  – Typhoid fever
  – Yellow fever
  – Hepatitis A
  – Influenza
  – Measles
  – Leptospirosis
- Common causes of fever such as pneumonia and viral illnesses should also be considered.

ALERT
Consider malaria when a patient with fever has a history of travel.

TREATMENT

MEDICATION

Uncomplicated malaria

- Chloroquine can be used for known chloroquine-susceptible *P. falciparum* and *P. vivax* and for all *P. ovale*, *P. malariae*, and *P. knowlesi* infections.
  – Chloroquine is dosed at 10 mg/kg base PO (max 600 mg), then 5 mg/kg PO at 6, 24, and 48 hours (max 300 mg/dose).
  – Susceptible areas include Central America west of Panama Canal, Haiti, Dominican Republic, and parts of the Middle East.
- For chloroquine-resistant *P. falciparum* or if species is unidentified, options are as follows:
  – Atovaquone-proguanil (Malarone). Malarone (mg atovaquone/mg proguanil) is given as one dose daily for 3 days. 5–8 kg: 2 pediatric tabs (62.5/25) per dose. 9–10 kg: 3 pediatric tabs per dose. 11–20 kg: 1 adult tab (250/100) per dose. 21–30 kg: 2 adult tabs per dose. 31–40 kg: 3 adult tabs per dose. ≥40 kg: 4 adult tabs per dose
  – Artemether-lumefantrine (Coartem). Coartem is given for a 6-dose course. The 2nd dose is given 8 hours after the 1st, and then b.i.d. 5–<15 kg: 1 tablet (20 mg artemether/120 mg lumefantrine) per dose. 15–<25 kg: 2 tabs per dose. 25–<35 kg: 3 tabs per dose. ≥35 kg: 4 tabs per dose
  – Mefloquine. Mefloquine is dosed at 15 mg/kg (max 750 mg) PO, followed by 10 mg/kg (max 500 mg) PO 8–12 hours later.
  – Quinine sulfate (10 mg salt/kg PO t.i.d.) plus doxycycline or clindamycin for 3 days (malaria acquired outside Southeast Asia) or 7 days (malaria acquired in Southeast Asia)
- For chloroquine-resistant *P. vivax*, options are Malarone, mefloquine, or quinine +doxycycline, all in addition to primaquine.
- Primaquine is used for the prevention of *P. vivax* and *P. ovale* relapses, in addition to primary treatment. It should not be used in patients with G6PD deficiency or in pregnancy.

Severe malaria

- Quinidine gluconate, 10 mg salt/kg IV initial dose (max 600 mg) over 2 hours followed by 0.02 mg salt/kg/min infusion + doxycycline or clindamycin
- In 2011, WHO guidelines made artesunate the drug of choice for children with severe malaria worldwide. Artesunate IV is available from the CDC under an investigational protocol for severe malaria in the United States.
- Change to an oral agent once parasite density <1% and the patient can take oral medication. The use of exchange transfusion for patients with hyperparasitemia is controversial, as no controlled trial has shown a clear benefit to this treatment.

INPATIENT CONSIDERATIONS

Admission Criteria

Travelers diagnosed with malaria infection should be managed as inpatients.

ONGOING CARE

PATIENT EDUCATION

- Consultation with a travel clinic is advised prior to travel to a malaria-endemic region.
- Chemoprophylaxis and mosquito bite prevention methods are both essential.

PROGNOSIS

- The prognosis depends on the severity of illness, *Plasmodium* species, underlying health conditions, and age of the patient.
- Infants with *P. falciparum* infection account for most of the mortality due to malaria.
- In African children, highest risk of death occurs in children with impaired consciousness and respiratory distress.
- If treated promptly, even *P. falciparum* malaria will likely respond well to treatment.

COMPLICATIONS

- Cerebral malaria has significant morbidity and mortality and can cause long-term neurocognitive impairment.
- Severe malarial anemia is frequent due to *P. falciparum*. However, death rates with adequate treatment are low.
- Chronic relapses can occur from *P. vivax* and *P. ovale* infections.
- Pregnant women are at higher risk for complications from malaria infection.

ADDITIONAL READING

- Agarwal D, Teach SJ. Evaluation and management of a child with suspected malaria. *Pediatr Emerg Care*. 2006;22(2):127–133.
- Dondorp A, Fanello C, Hendriksen I, et al. Artesunate versus quinine in the treatment of severe falciparum malaria in African children (AQUAMAT): an open-label, randomised trial. *Lancet*. 2010;376(9753):1647–1657.
- Freedman DO. Clinical practice. Malaria prevention in short-term travelers. *N Engl J Med*. 2008;359(6):603–612.
- John CC, Bangirana P, Byarugaba J, et al. Cerebral malaria in children is associated with long-term cognitive impairment. *Pediatrics*. 2008;122(1):e92–e99.
- Kiang KM, Bryant PA, Shingadia D, et al. The treatment of imported malaria in children: an update. *Arch Dis Child Educ Pract Ed*. 2013;98(1):7–15.

CODES

ICD10

- B54 Unspecified malaria
- B50.9 Plasmodium falciparum malaria, unspecified
- B51.9 Plasmodium vivax malaria without complication

FAQ

- Q: What drugs are acceptable choices for treatment of malaria in pregnancy?
- A: Options for uncomplicated malaria treatment in pregnant women in the United States include chloroquine (if sensitive), mefloquine, or quinidine + clindamycin.
- Q: Is there a vaccine available to prevent malaria?
- A: No vaccination is commercially available; however, antimalarial vaccines are currently in clinical trials and are showing some efficacy. The RTS,S subunit vaccine is in large-scale trials at this time.
- Q: How can I determine if the area my patient is traveling to has chloroquine-resistant malaria?
- A: The CDC Web site at www.cdc.gov/malaria has extensive information for travelers, including parasite sensitivity patterns and treatment recommendations. A malaria hotline is also available for clinician questions at 770-488-7788.

MALFORMATIONS OF CORTICAL DEVELOPMENT

Jeffrey Bolton • Annapurna Poduri

BASICS

DESCRIPTION

- Cortical malformations are important in clinical neurology, as they are associated with developmental disorders, motor impairments, and epilepsy.
- Defining the underlying malformation has prognostic value for patient's family, as well as possible genetic counseling implications.
- Classification schemes now emphasize the stage of embryogenesis which is disrupted.
- Disorders of neurulation
  - First key step to development of the CNS is neural tube closure around days 21–26 of gestation. Disruptions to rostral closure may lead to encephalocele or anencephaly.
    - Encephalocele: herniation of the intracranial contents through a midline skull defect; may occur frontal (orbit, nose, or forehead), basal, or occipital
    - Anencephaly: congenital absence of both cerebral hemispheres with preserved forebrain and upper brainstem
- Prosencephalic development
  - The prosencephalon is the precursor to the cerebral hemispheres and deep nuclei. Initial development begins at 4 weeks followed by cleavage occurring in weeks 5–6 and midline development from weeks 7–20.
    - Holoprosencephaly: 3 subtypes: (1) Alobar consists of a single spheroid cerebral structure with a common ventricle, fused thalami and basal ganglion, absent corpus callosum, and hypoplastic or single optic nerve. (2) Semilobar consists of anterior fusion with posterior cleavage and less fusion of deep structures. (3) Lobar is least severe, consisting of near total separation of the hemispheres with fusion in the most rostral and ventral aspects.
    - Agenesis of the corpus callosum (ACC): Corpus callosum fails to develop, ranging from complete to only mild thinning.
    - Septo-optic dysplasia: optic nerve hypoplasia, hypothalamic and pituitary hypoplasia plus midline and forebrain abnormalities (ACC, absent septum pellucidum)
- Neuronal proliferation
  - Neuronal progenitor cells proliferation peaks during the 1st and 2nd month of human gestation leading to rapid cell growth and differentiation into neurons, astrocytes, oligodendrocytes, etc.
    - Hemimegalencephaly: unilateral enlargement of one cerebral hemisphere, with possible abnormal cortical development in the abnormal hemisphere
    - Megalencephaly: brain measuring >2 SD or >98% for age
    - Microcephaly: defined as occipitofrontal head circumference >2 SD below the mean for patient's age
    - Tuberous sclerosis complex (TSC): Multiorgan disease with CNS involvement including cortical tubers (discrete areas of dysplastic cortex, paler and firmer in appearance than normal cortex), subependymal nodules, and subependymal giant cell tumors (SEGA).
    - Neurofibromatosis type I: characterized by café-au-lait spots, Lisch nodules in the eye, and benign and malignant tumors in CNS and PNS
- Migration/organization
  - Neurons migrate from the subependymal zone to cortex between 3 and 5 months of human gestation with gyration and organization peaking by 26–28 weeks.
    - Lissencephaly type I: characterized by thickened cerebral cortex with a smooth surface lacking gyral formation. The underlying cytoarchitecture is abnormal, containing less than the normal six layers.
    - Pachygyria: abnormally formed cortex which contains a few coarse gyri
    - Subcortical band heterotopia: also referred to as "double cortex"; consists of a circumferential symmetric band of cortex located in the white matter just below typical cortex
    - Lissencephaly type II: also known as "cobblestone cortex." Characterized by lissencephaly with protrusions of neurons over the brain surface into the subarachnoid space. On gross inspection, the surface of the brain has a cobblestone appearance.
    - Schizencephaly: consists of a deep cleft extending from cortical surface to the ventricle. The cleft may be lined with polymicrogyria cortex. The cleft may be bilateral or unilateral, with the Sylvian fissure being a common location. Subdivided into open and closed lip, with the former having a wide separation of the cleft wall and the latter having the cleft walls touching.
    - Polymicrogyria: defined as a malformation consisting of multiple small placations of the cortical surface in a festoon-like or glandular formation resulting in cortex with numerous small gyri. It may be subdivided depending on location.
    - Focal cortical dysplasia: consists of areas of cortex with abnormal lamination with ± balloon cells
    - Heterotopias: defined as collections of neurons in the periventricular or subcortical white matter

EPIDEMIOLOGY

- Incidence of malformations varied depending on specific malformation but overall is quite rare.
- The majority of malformations are associated with an increased incidence of epilepsy, ranging from 50–90%.
- Some malformations, such as anencephaly, have been associated with low socioeconomic status.

PATHOPHYSIOLOGY

- Any disruption to the development of the CNS during the prenatal stage may lead to a malformation.
- These disruptions include genetic mutations, metabolic derangements, infections, and toxic/environmental exposures.
- With infectious and toxic etiologies, the timing of the incident is key in determining the resultant malformation.

ETIOLOGY

- Genetic
  - Holoprosencephaly: trisomy 13 and 18; monogenic mutations including 2p21 (*SIX3*), 7q36 (*SHH*), 18q11 (*TGIF*), and 21q22
  - Microcephaly vera: 1q31 (*ASPM*), 8p23 (*MCPH1*), 9q33.2 (*CDKL5RAP2*), 13q12 (*CENPJ*), 19q13.12 (*WDR62*)
  - TSC: *TSC1* 9q34.13 (Hamartin), *TSC2* 16p13 (Tuberin)
  - Neurofibromatosis type I: 17q11 AD mutation of neurofibromin gene
  - Hemimegalencephaly: 1q43 (*AKT3*)
  - Lissencephaly: Miller-Diecker syndrome (lissencephaly, microcephaly, facial dysmorphism, syndactyly) *LIS1* gene 17p13.3
  - Lissencephaly with cerebellar hypoplasia: *Reelin* 7q22
  - X-linked lissencephaly with abnormal genitalia: *ARX* Xp22.13
  - X-linked lissencephaly and subcortical band heterotopia: *DCX* Xq22.3-q23
  - Cobblestone cortex: may be seen in Walker-Warburg syndrome, Fukuyama congenital muscular dystrophy (FCMD), or muscle-eye-brain (MEB) disease
    - Walker-Warburg syndrome and MEB: (*POMT1*) 9q34.13, (*POMGnT1*) 1p33-34, (*FKRP*) 19q13.3, (*LARGE*) 22q12-q13.1
    - FCMD: (*FKTN*) 9q31.2
  - Schizencephaly w/ microcephaly: 19q13.12 (*WDR62*)
  - Polymicrogyria (PMG): known association with 22q11 deletions
  - Bilateral frontoparietal PMG: 16q13 (*GPR56*)
  - Occipital PMG: 9q34.12 (*LAMC3*)
  - Periventricular heterotopia: Xq28 protein filamin A (*FLNA*), autosomal recessive 20q11 (*ARFGE2*)
- Some malformations associated with neurocutaneous syndromes
  - Hemimegalencephaly seen in hypomelanosis of Ito, linear sebaceous nevus syndrome, or Klippel-Trenaunay-Weber syndrome
  - Megalencephaly: Sturge-Weber syndrome, neurofibromatosis, tuberous sclerosis
- Vascular (ischemia or hemorrhage)
  - Microcephaly: may be attributed to chronic placental insufficiency
  - Schizencephaly: often caused by MCA territory prenatal infarcts
  - Polymicrogyria: prenatal hypoxic ischemic injury
- Toxins/exposures
  - Antiepileptic medications (valproic acid [VPA], phenytoin [PHT]): dysraphic states
  - Ethanol, radiation, mercury, retinoids: holoprosencephaly
  - Hyperthermia: encephalocele, anencephaly
  - Maternal diabetes

- Infectious
  - Schizencephaly, microcephaly, anencephaly, polymicrogyria have been associated with various prenatal infections including CMV, toxoplasmosis, rubella, herpes
- Metabolic syndromes
  - Common to see macrocephaly in metabolic disorders, as there may abnormal metabolite accumulation (Canavan, glutaric aciduria, etc.)
  - PMG has been observed in Zellweger syndrome, Refsum disease, and Menkes disease.

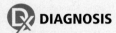

DIAGNOSIS

HISTORY

- A comprehensive family history assessing for members with known syndromes, intellectual disabilities, severe developmental delays, autism, epilepsy, unexplained deaths, frequent miscarriages, or parental consanguinity.
- Close attention should be paid to the pregnancy, inquiring about possible prenatal exposures (ethanol, medications, etc.), infections, or trauma/bleeding.
- Most children with CNS malformations will have developmental delays, thus a detailed developmental history should be obtained.
- Repetitive movements, alterations in consciousness, or other paroxysmal episodes should be asked about as seizures/epilepsy is common in this population.

PHYSICAL EXAM

- At initial presentation, a full physical exam should be performed, paying close attention to head circumference, dysmorphic features, organomegaly, skin findings, and detailed neurologic examination.
- In anencephaly, there is little-to-no overlying skull present. Encephaloceles may be visible as soft, skin-covered protrusions through the skull. In Meckel syndrome, encephalocele is associated with microcephaly, microphthalmia, cleft lip/palate, polydactyly, polycystic kidneys, and ambiguous genitalia.
- Holoprosencephaly may be accompanied by facial anomalies such as absent or malformed nose, single or hyperteloric eyes, in addition to other organ system anomalies such as congenital heart disease, GI, GU, or skeletal defects.
- Skin findings such as hypomelanosis of Ito and linear sebaceous nevus raise concern for hemimegalencephaly.
- Neurofibromatosis type I has characteristic physical findings including macrocephaly, multiple café-au-lait macules, Lisch nodules, axillary/inguinal freckling, and palpable peripheral neurofibromas.
- "Ash-leaf" hypopigmented lesions, facial angiofibromas, and shagreen patches are seen in TSC.
- Miller-Dieker syndrome, associated with lissencephaly, has characteristic facial dysmorphisms including prominent forehead; short upturned nose; thin, protuberant upper lip; and small jaw. Spastic quadriparesis is often noted.

DIAGNOSTIC TESTS & INTERPRETATION

- Many of the malformations can be appreciated on prenatal ultrasound, leading to in utero diagnosis. Many tertiary centers are now able to perform fetal MRI, allowing for a more accurate image of the fetal brain.
- If not diagnosed prenatally, brain MRI should be performed on any patient where there is suspicion for a developmental malformation.
- CT is of little use, as it has low resolution and exposes the child to radiation.
- Once a malformation has been diagnosed via imaging, laboratory investigation should be pursued for known associated genetic etiologies.
- As mentioned prior, many malformations are associated with monogenic variations. Specific genes are available for testing in certain circumstances (e.g., *TSC1* and *2*, *DCX*, and *LIS1)*.
- In the presence of other congenital anomalies, cerebral malformations may be associated with chromosomal changes, thus karyotyping is important in such cases.
- When malformations are known to be associated with metabolic disorders, blood, urine, and CSF should be analyzed.
- When seizures are suspected, video EEG is valuable in assessing for epileptiform activity.

DIFFERENTIAL DIAGNOSIS

- Focal cortical dysplasia may be difficult to distinguish from low-grade glioma on MRI.
- Vascular anomalies and remote infarcts can be mistaken for congenital malformations.

TREATMENT

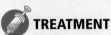

Most cortical malformations are irreversible. Treatment centers around management of comorbid conditions such as epilepsy, spastic quadriparesis, language delay, and other sequelae.

MEDICATION

- Any child with a malformation and epilepsy should be maintained on appropriate antiepileptic medication in conjunction with an experienced neurologist.
- Spasticity may be treated with antispasmodic agents such as baclofen or diazepam.
- In certain cases, such as TSC, novel agents (mTor inhibitors) are being investigated to halt progression of the disease.

SURGERY/OTHER PROCEDURES

- Cortical malformations often result in medically refractory epilepsy. Some patients may benefit from surgical treatment to cure or palliate their epilepsy. This process is done very systematically via an experienced epilepsy surgery center.
- More restricted malformations which lead to medically refractory epilepsy may be amendable to resection and result in seizure freedom or reduction.
- More extensive lesions, such as hemimegalencephaly, may be treated with functional hemispherectomy.

ONGOING CARE

- Long-term prognosis varies depending on underlying malformation. The more extensive/severe the malformation, the more neurologic impairment is present.
- Significantly affected children require multidisciplinary care from a host of pediatric specialists including regular neurology visits.
- Families of children with known genetic etiologies should undergo formal genetic counseling to assess risk for other family members.

ADDITIONAL READING

- Barkovich AJ, Guerrini R, Kuzniecky RI, et al. A developmental and genetic classification for malformations of cortical development: update 2012. *Brain*. 2012;135(5):1348–1369.
- Hehr U, Schuierer G. Genetic assessment of cortical malformations. *Neuropediatrics*. 2011;42(2):43–50.
- Sisodiya SM. Malformations of cortical development: burdens and insights from important causes of human epilepsy. *Lancet Neurol*. 2004;3(1):29–38.

CODES

ICD10

- Q04.3 Other reduction deformities of brain
- Q04.2 Holoprosencephaly
- Q01.9 Encephalocele, unspecified

M

MAMMALIAN BITES

Margaret Wolff • Jill C. Posner

BASICS

DESCRIPTION
Injury to the human skin and/or subcutaneous tissues caused by bite, causing local, and in some cases systemic, effects

EPIDEMIOLOGY
- Animal bites
  - Approximate frequency
    - Dogs: 90–95%
    - Cats: 3–8%
    - Rodents or rabbits: 1%
    - Raccoons and other animals: 1%
  - 90% of the offending animals are well-known to the victim.
  - Children are the most common victims:
    - Boys are twice as likely as girls to be bitten by dogs.
    - Girls are more likely to be bitten by cats.
- Human bites
  - Most common in children ages 2–5 years
  - In older children, bites may occur accidentally during sports activities or intentionally during altercations or abusive situations.

Incidence
- An estimated 4.5 million dog bites and 400,000 cat bites occur annually in the United States.
- The incidence of human bites is unknown due to underreporting.

GENERAL PREVENTION
- Ensure that children receive routine immunizations against tetanus and hepatitis and that family pets are immunized against rabies.
- Encourage children to avoid contact with wild animals and dead animals.

PATHOPHYSIOLOGY
- Injury associated with bite types:
  - Dog
    - Crush and tear injuries
    - May involve bone
  - Cat
    - Puncture-type wounds
    - Penetrate deeper and carry a higher risk of infection
  - Human
    - Generally only violate skin
    - However, penetration into joint and tendon sheath spaces may occur (especially bites overlying the metacarpal-phalangeal areas).
- Infection
  - Rate of infection
    - Dog bites: 3–18%
    - Cat bites: 28–80%
    - Human bites: 15–20%
  - More recent studies have suggested an incidence of infection after dog and cat bites to be closer to 2–3%.
  - Infections are most commonly polymicrobial with both aerobic and anaerobic organisms.
  - Infected dog and cat bites
    - *Pasteurella* species are the most frequent isolates.
    - Dog: *Pasteurella canis*
    - Cat: *Pasteurella multocida* and *Pasteurella septica*
    - Common anaerobes include *Fusobacterium*, bacterioids, *Porphyromonas*, and *Prevotella*.
  - Infected human bites
    - *Streptococcus anginosus*
    - *Staphylococcus aureus*
    - *Eikenella corrodens*
    - *Fusobacterium* species
    - *Prevotella* species

DIAGNOSIS

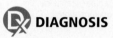

HISTORY
- Animal bites
  - Type of animal
  - Apparent health of the animal
  - Provocation for the attack
  - Location of the bite or bites
  - Availability of animal for undergoing observation (i.e., Is it a known animal as opposed to a stray or wild animal?)
  - Rabies immunization status of the animal
- Past medical history
  - Tetanus immunization status of the child
  - Hepatitis B immunization status of child
  - Is patient immunocompromised or asplenic?

PHYSICAL EXAM
- Carefully assess neurovascular integrity.
- Location of bite
  - If bite is located over a joint, assess for violation of joint capsule.
- Examine entire patient to ensure that all wounds are identified and treated.
- Older wounds
  - Assess for signs of infection such as erythema, induration, purulence, regional adenopathy, and elevated temperature.

DIAGNOSTIC TESTS & INTERPRETATION

Lab
- Blood culture if fever or systemic toxicity is noted
- Aerobic and anaerobic cultures from infected wounds

Imaging
In penetrating injuries overlying bones or joints, consider radiography to evaluate for presence of fracture, foreign body (e.g., tooth), and air within joint.

Diagnostic Procedures/Other
No tests routinely done

TREATMENT

MEDICATION
- Antibiotics: Data are often contradictory. In general:
  - All cat bites should be treated with prophylactic antibiotics, due to high risk of infection with *P. multocida*.
  - Amoxicillin–clavulanic acid PO is drug of choice (50 mg amoxicillin/kg/24 h divided b.i.d. or t.i.d. for 5 days).
  - All human bites should be treated with antibiotic prophylaxis. Amoxicillin–clavulanic acid PO is drug of choice (50 mg amoxicillin/kg/24 h divided b.i.d. or t.i.d. for 5 days).
  - An alternative antibiotic regimen for penicillin-allergic patients is trimethoprim–sulfamethoxazole *plus* clindamycin.
  - Bites to the hand, face, deep puncture wounds, and wounds in immunocompromised patients may be treated empirically.
  - Skin and soft tissue infections requiring hospitalization:
    - Ampicillin/sulbactam IV 150 mg ampicillin/kg/24 h in 4 divided doses

- For penicillin-allergic patients, 3rd-generation cephalosporin
- Antibiotics with poor activity against *Pasteurella* include penicillinase-resistant penicillins, clindamycin, and aminoglycosides.

- Tetanus prophylaxis if indicated
- Rabies prophylaxis if indicated
  - Unknown dog or cat; dogs or cats with unknown immunization status that cannot be observed for 10 days
  - Bites from wild animals, including raccoons, bats, skunks, foxes, coyotes
  - Because bat bites may go undetected, especially by a sleeping child, rabies prophylaxis is recommended after exposure to bats in a confined setting.
  - Rabies is unlikely if the child was bitten by an immunized dog, cat, or other pet (e.g., hamsters, guinea pigs, gerbils).
  - Rabies is unlikely if the child was bitten by a small rodent (squirrels, mice, or rats) or rabbit.
  - The regimen for patients who have not been vaccinated previously should include both human rabies vaccine (a series of 4 doses administered IM on days 0, 3, 7, and 14; immune-compromised patients should receive a 5th dose on day 28) and rabies-immune globulin (20 IU/kg) administered as much as possible into the wound, the remainder given IM at a site distant from the site used for vaccine administration.
- HIV postexposure prophylaxis (PEP)
  - There are case reports describing transmission of HIV by human bites; however, the risk of transmission due to biting is unknown. It is estimated to be extremely small. Bites with saliva containing no visible blood have no associated risk for transmission and, therefore, are not considered exposures.
  - HIV PEP requires a multidrug regimen administered over 28 days that can be associated with significant toxicity.
  - Decisions to initiate PEP are best made in consultation with local experts or by contacting the National Clinicians Post-Exposure Prophylaxis hotline at 888-448-4911.
  - Hepatitis B has been transmitted from nonbloody saliva. Check the vaccination status of the bitten (or biter if necessary) to consider PEP. Unvaccinated children should begin the hepatitis B vaccine series.
  - The transmission rate of hepatitis C via human bites is unknown and no regimen for PEP currently exists.

ALERT

A bite with a break in the skin is considered low risk, and a bite with intact skin is felt to pose no risk.

GENERAL MEASURES

- Wound care:
  - Copious irrigation with normal saline or tap water to remove visible debris
  - Do not use antimicrobial solutions to irrigate.
  - Cleanse, but do not irrigate puncture wounds.
- Human bites over metacarpals (clenched-fist injuries) require orthopedic evaluation for possible surgical exploration and irrigation.
- Debride devitalized tissue.
- The increased risk of infection associated with suturing a potentially contaminated wound must be weighed against the cosmetic effect due to nonclosure:
  - Primary closure of larger wounds or significant facial wounds may be indicated unless wound is old or has evidence of infection.
- Hand wounds may be an exception, due to high propensity for infection.

ISSUES FOR REFERRAL

Local regulations dictate the reporting of animal bites to health departments.

ONGOING CARE

FOLLOW-UP RECOMMENDATIONS

Patient Monitoring

- Signs and symptoms of infection
- All patients with significant bites should receive follow-up 48 hours after bite.

PROGNOSIS

Most injury from animal bites is trivial, but infections, and rarely deaths, do occur.

COMPLICATIONS

Human bites over metacarpals (clenched fist) can penetrate tendon sheaths, become infected, and result in a tenosynovitis.

ADDITIONAL READING

- Havens PL; American Academy of Pediatrics, Committee on Pediatric AIDS. Postexposure prophylaxis in children and adolescents for nonoccupational exposure to human immunodeficiency virus. *Pediatrics*. 2003;111(6):1475–1489.
- Medeiros IM, Saconato H. Antibiotic prophylaxis for mammalian bites. *Cochrane Database Syst Rev*. 2008;(2):CD001738.
- Rupprecht CE, Briggs D, Brown CM, et al. Use of a reduced (4-dose) vaccine schedule for post-exposure prophylaxis to prevent human rabies: recommendations of the advisory committee on immunization practices. *MMWR Recomm Rep*. 2010;59(RR-2):1–9.
- Talan DA, Abrahamian FM, Moran GJ, et al; Emergency Medicine Human Bite Infection Study Group. Clinical presentation and bacteriologic analysis of infected human bites in patients presenting to the emergency departments. *Clin Infect Dis*. 2003;37(11):1481–1489.
- Wu PS, Beres A, Tashjian DB, et al. Primary repair of facial dog bite injuries in children. *Pediatr Emerg Care*. 2011:27(9):801–813.

CODES

ICD10

- S61.459A Open bite of unspecified hand, initial encounter
- S01.85XA Open bite of other part of head, initial encounter
- S61.259A Open bite of unsp finger without damage to nail, init encntr

FAQ

- Q: What are the clinical features of *Pasteurella* infections?
- A: Infections caused by *Pasteurella* tend to progress rapidly, usually over a 12–24-hour period, and are characterized by tenderness and purulent drainage. The rapid progression of these infections tends to distinguish them from wounds that are infected with *S. aureus* and other pathogens.
- Q: Why are cat bites often more severe than dog bites?
- A: Cat bites are associated with puncture-type wounds and are more likely to involve *Pasteurella* infection, which is generally more aggressive than other organisms. However, dog bite infections may also be caused by *Pasteurella*.

MASTOIDITIS

Sadiqa Edmonds Kendi • Frances M. Nadel

BASICS

DESCRIPTION
Infection of the mastoid air cells characterized clinically by protrusion of the pinna and erythema/tenderness over the mastoid process; can range from an asymptomatic illness to a severe life-threatening disease. Acute mastoiditis is defined as the presence of symptoms for less than 1 month.

EPIDEMIOLOGY
- Most patients are between 6–24 months old.
- Male to female ratio of 2:1
- It is unusual to see mastoiditis in young infants because of incomplete pneumatization of the mastoid air cells.

Incidence
- At the start of the 20th century, 20–50% of cases of otitis media developed into coalescent mastoiditis. The routine use of antibiotics for otitis media and aggressive management of treatment failures has decreased incidence to 0.2–0.4%.
- Although some single-site reports have suggested that mastoiditis is on the rise, larger population-based studies demonstrate a stable incidence.

RISK FACTORS
- Age <2 years of age
- Acute otitis media
- Recurrent otitis media

GENERAL PREVENTION
- Appropriate early treatment of otitis media and timely follow-up to identify treatment failures
- Avoid factors that predispose to otitis media, including caretaker smoking and bottle-feeding.
- Early recognition of mastoiditis decreases the risk of intracranial complications.
- Pneumococcal vaccination may help decrease the occurrence of otitis media.

PATHOPHYSIOLOGY
- The mastoid process is the posterior portion of the temporal bone and consists of interconnecting air cells that drain superiorly into the middle ear. Because these mastoid air cells connect with the middle ear, all cases of acute otitis media are associated with some mastoid inflammation.
- Acute mastoiditis develops when the accumulation of purulent exudate in the middle ear does not drain through the eustachian tube or through a perforated tympanic membrane but spreads to the mastoid.
- Acute mastoiditis can progress to a coalescent phase after the bony air cells are destroyed and may then progress to subperiosteal abscess or to chronic mastoiditis.

ETIOLOGY
- Acute mastoiditis is generally caused by an extension of the inflammation and infection of acute otitis media into the mastoid air cells. However, 20–50% of patients may present without evidence of preceding otitis media.
- The bacteria isolated from middle ear drainage or from the mastoid are usually *Streptococcus pneumoniae*, *Streptococcus pyogenes*, *Haemophilus influenzae*, or *Staphylococcus aureus*. However, many patients' cultures are sterile:
  - *S. pneumoniae* is the most frequently isolated cause of mastoiditis in pediatric patients. *S. pneumoniae* resistance to penicillin may be as high as 30%, with the 19A serotype being the most common. With the advent of the 13 valent pneumococcal vaccine (which contains the 19A serotype), the epidemiology may change.
  - *Pseudomonas* infection should be suspected if the child has been on antibiotics recently or has a history of recurrent otitis media.
- Chronic mastoiditis is usually caused by *S. aureus*, anaerobic bacteria, enteric bacteria, and *Pseudomonas aeruginosa*:
  - Chronic mastoiditis is often a multiple-organism infection.
- Unusual agents of chronic mastoiditis include *Mycobacterium tuberculosis*, nontuberculous mycobacteria, *Nocardia asteroides*, and *Histoplasma capsulatum*.
- Cholesteatomas may contribute to the development of mastoiditis by impeding mastoid drainage or erosion of underlying bone.

DIAGNOSIS

HISTORY
- May include a recent or a chronic history of treatment for otitis media
- Sign and symptoms
  - May include fever, otalgia, otorrhea, and postauricular swelling
    - Children who are already on antibiotics may present with more subtle findings.
  - Intracranial extension should be suspected if there is lethargy, a stiff neck, headache, focal neurologic symptoms, seizures, visual changes, or persistent fevers despite appropriate antibiotic treatment.
  - Labyrinthitis initially presents with tinnitus and nausea, which can progress to vomiting, vertigo, nystagmus, and loss of balance.

PHYSICAL EXAM
- The ear may protrude away from the scalp:
  - In children less than 2 years old, the ear protrudes out and is displaced down. In older children, the ear is displaced up.
- The external ear canal may be edematous or sagging.
- The tympanic membrane often is hyperemic, with decreased mobility, or perforated:
  - The tympanic membranes of children on antibiotics may have a normal appearance.
- The mastoid process is tender, with soft tissue swelling:
  - The overlying skin may be warm and erythematous, with posterior auricular fluctuance.
- In chronic mastoiditis, the fever and posterior auricular swelling are often not present and the patient presents with ear pain, persistent drainage, or hearing loss.

DIAGNOSTIC TESTS & INTERPRETATION

Lab
- CBC with differential: nonspecific
  - May be normal or show a leukocytosis with a neutrophil predominance
- ESR/CRP
  - May be elevated in acute mastoiditis but is usually normal in the chronic stage; more often elevated in complicated mastoiditis
- Purified protein derivative (PPD)
  - Should be done if tuberculosis is suspected
- Middle ear aspirate
  - Gram stain and cultures for aerobic and anaerobic bacteria
  - There is some correlation between middle ear bacterial cultures and mastoid cultures.
  - If possible, drainage prior to antibiotic administration is more helpful in making a microbiologic diagnosis.

Imaging
- X-rays
  - Reveal haziness of the mastoid air cells and can show bony destruction in more advanced disease
  - Are unreliable and can be falsely normal, as well as falsely abnormal
- Contrast-enhanced temporal bone and cranial CT
  - Helpful in the confirmation of the diagnosis, identification of coalescence or a subperiosteal abscess, and evaluation for concomitant intracranial complications
  - Intracranial complications are best seen with MRI.

Diagnostic Procedures/Other

Lumbar puncture must be performed in any child with symptoms of meningitis.

DIFFERENTIAL DIAGNOSIS

- Parotitis
- Posterior auricular lymphadenopathy or cellulitis
- Otitis externa or an ear canal furuncle
- Perichondritis of the auricle
- Neoplastic disease
  - Leukemia
  - Lymphoma
  - Rhabdomyosarcoma
  - Langerhans Cell Histiocytosis
- Branchial cleft anomaly
- Tuberculosis

TREATMENT

MEDICATION

- Parenteral antibiotics are chosen based on the most likely organisms, regional bacterial resistance patterns, and the child's condition.
- Intravenous antibiotics are given for at least 7–10 days followed with oral antibiotics for a total duration of 4 weeks of therapy.
- A third- or fourth-generation cephalosporin such as ceftriaxone or cefotaxime or cefepime is often used with or without vancomycin for empiric treatment.
- Subsequent antibiotic choice should be tailored to antimicrobial sensitivities of the ear aspirate.
- If *M. tuberculosis* is suspected, then antituberculosis therapy should be started.

ADDITIONAL TREATMENT

General Measures

Middle ear drainage is essential; therefore, a myringotomy with or without tube placement should be performed early.

SURGERY/OTHER PROCEDURES

- Indications for surgical intervention include the following:
  - Subperiosteal abscess
  - Coalescence
  - Facial nerve palsy
  - Meningitis
  - Intracranial abscess
  - Venous thrombosis
  - Persistent symptoms despite adequate antibiotic treatment
- In the preantibiotic era, mastoidectomy was the treatment of choice for mastoiditis. Currently, this therapy is generally reserved for cases complicated by the aforementioned indications.
- Neurosurgical consultation for treatment of intracranial complications may be necessary.

INPATIENT CONSIDERATIONS

Admission Criteria

Admit for IV antibiotics and for ear, nose, and throat (ENT) evaluation for surgical drainage and to ensure response to antibiotics and to rule out complications.

ONGOING CARE

FOLLOW-UP RECOMMENDATIONS

Patient Monitoring

- If patients respond quickly to parenteral therapy, they can complete a 3- to 4-week course with oral antibiotics and weekly follow-up visits.
- Audiograms should be performed later to screen for hearing loss.

PROGNOSIS

- Mastoiditis has a good prognosis if treated early. However, intracranial extension of mastoiditis can lead to permanent neurologic deficits and death.
- Chronic mastoiditis can lead to irreversible hearing loss.

COMPLICATIONS

- The proximity of the mastoid to many important structures can result in serious complications from extension of infection or as a response to the inflammatory process.
- Complication rates may be as high as 16%.
- Intracranial complications include meningitis and extradural, subdural, or brain parenchymal abscesses.
- Venous sinus thrombophlebitis results from extension of disease to the sigmoid or lateral sinus:
  - Sepsis, increased intracranial pressure, or septic emboli may result.
- Facial nerve palsy is usually unilateral and can be permanent.
- Labyrinthitis, petrositis, or osteomyelitis may result from extension of the infection into adjacent bones.
- Subperiosteal abscess
- Hearing loss can occur from destruction of the ossicles or from labyrinthine damage.
- Bezold abscess is a deep neck abscess along the medial sternocleidomastoid muscle that develops when the infection erodes through the tip of the mastoid bone and dissects down tissue planes.
- Gradenigo syndrome
  - Triad of 6th nerve palsy, retro-orbital pain, and otorrhea

ADDITIONAL READING

- Agrawal S, Husein M, MacRae D. Complications of otitis media: an evolving state. *J Otolaryngol*. 2005;34(Suppl 1):S33–S39.
- Anderson K, Adam H. Mastoiditis. *Pediatr Rev*. 2009;30(6):233–234.
- Bilavsky E, Yarden-Bilavsky H, Samra Z, et al. Clinical, laboratory, and microbiological differences between children with simple or complicated mastoiditis. *Int J Pediatr Otorhinolaryngol*. 2009;73(9):1270–1273.
- Groth A, Enoksson F, Hultcrantz M, et al. Acute mastoiditis in children aged 0-16 years—a national study of 678 cases in Sweden comparing different age groups. *Int J Pediatr Otorhinolaryngol*. 2012;76(10):1494–1500.
- Kaplan SL, Mason EO Jr, Wald ER, et al. Pneumococcal mastoiditis in children. *Pediatrics*. 2000;106(4):695–699.
- Minks DP, Porte M, Jenkins N. Acute mastoiditis—the role of radiology. *Clin Radiol*. 2013;68(4):397–405.
- Pang LH, Barakate MS, Havas TE. Mastoiditis in a paediatric population: a review of 11 years of experience in management. *Int J Pediatr Otorhinolaryngol*. 2009;73(11):1520–1524.
- Pritchett CV, Thorne MC. Incidence of pediatric acute mastoiditis: 1997–2006. *Arch Otolaryngol Head Neck Surg*. 2012;138(5):451–455.
- Psarommatis IM, Voudouris C, Douros K, et al. Algorithmic management of pediatric acute mastoiditis. *Int J Pediatr Otorhinolaryngol*. 2012;76(6):791–796.
- Zanetti D, Nassif N. Indications for surgery in acute mastoiditis and their complications in children. *Int J Pediatr Otorhinolaryngol*. 2006;70(7):1175–1182.

CODES

ICD10

- H70.90 Unspecified mastoiditis, unspecified ear
- H70.009 Acute mastoiditis without complications, unspecified ear
- H70.099 Acute mastoiditis with other complications, unspecified ear

FAQ

- Q: Do all children with mastoiditis need a CT scan of the head if mastoiditis is suspected?
- A: No. In general, if the child with mastoiditis has mild swelling, no fluctuance of the mastoid, and responds to therapy, no CT scan is needed. A patient who appears toxic or fails to respond to appropriate antibiotic therapy or one who may be a surgical candidate should undergo additional imaging studies.
- Q: Should all children with mastoiditis be admitted to the hospital?
- A: Yes. In general, admission with IV antibiotics and ENT evaluation/drainage is warranted to ensure response to antibiotics and rule out complications.

MEASLES (RUBEOLA)

Jeffrey S. Gerber

BASICS

DESCRIPTION

- An exanthematous disease that has a relatively predictable course, making clinical diagnosis possible
- Because it is rare, cases are often initially misdiagnosed as a nonspecific viral exanthema, drug eruption, or Kawasaki disease.
- Patients are contagious from 1 to 2 days before onset of symptoms (3–5 days before rash) until 5 days after the appearance of the rash. The incubation period is generally 8–12 days from exposure to onset of symptoms and ~14 days until the appearance of rash.
- Types of measles include the following:
  - Typical measles (outlined below)
  - Modified measles: occurs in children with partial antibody protection (after postexposure administration of immunoglobulin or in infants <9 months old with transplacental antibodies)
    - Clinically similar to typical measles but is generally mild
    - The patient may be afebrile, and the rash may last only 1–2 days.
  - Atypical measles: caused by a hypersensitivity reaction to measles infection in those who received killed virus vaccine between 1963 and 1967 and are subsequently exposed to wild-type virus

EPIDEMIOLOGY

- Measles is one of the most highly contagious of all infectious diseases.
- Hospital or clinic waiting rooms (especially pediatric emergency department waiting rooms) have been identified as a major risk, accounting for up to 45% of the known exposures. With adequate immunization (2 doses = 99% effective), measles could be eliminated as a disease.
- Although no longer endemic in the United States, networks of intentionally unvaccinated children have led to several recent U.S. outbreaks originating from measles virus imported from abroad.
- Because 20 million cases of measles occur globally per year (>150,000 deaths), it is critical to maintain high levels of vaccination coverage.

Incidence

- Before the 1963 licensure of vaccine, an estimated 3–4 million people acquired measles in the United States each year; by 1983, there were only 0.7 cases per 100,000 population.
- Delays in immunization facilitated large outbreaks in the United States from 1989 to 1991, peaking in 1990 when 27,672 cases were reported, 89 of which were fatal.
- From 2001 to 2012, the median annual number of measles cases reported in United States was 60, peaking in 2011 (22 cases).
- From January to August 2013, 159 U.S. cases were reported, including the largest U.S. outbreak since 1996 (58 cases). The majority of cases occurred in underimmunized individuals and imported from abroad (including U.S. travelers).

GENERAL PREVENTION

- Vaccine recommendations
  - Routine vaccination against measles, mumps, and rubella (MMR) for children begins at 12–15 months of age, with a second MMR vaccination at age 4–6 years.
  - With the recent resurgence of measles, aggressive employee immunization programs should be pursued for all health care workers.
  - Health care workers born after 1956 who have no documentation of vaccination or evidence of measles immunity should be vaccinated at the time of employment and revaccinated ≥28 days later.
- Infection control measures
  - Any inpatient suspected of having measles should be in a negative-pressure respiratory isolation room; health care workers must wear masks, gloves, and gowns (airborne and contact precautions).
  - Isolation is required for 4 days after the 1st appearance of the rash; immunocompromised patients require isolation for the course of the illness.
  - All suspected cases of measles should be reported immediately to the local health department.

PATHOPHYSIOLOGY

Transmission of measles occurs through direct contact with infectious droplets, less commonly by airborne spread.

ETIOLOGY

Measles is an RNA virus (paramyxovirus, genus *Morbillivirus*) with only 1 serotype.

DIAGNOSIS

- The disease involves fever, cough, conjunctivitis, and coryza with an erythematous rash, which has a characteristic progression:
  - The rash appears on the face (often the nape of the neck, initially) and abdomen 14 days after exposure. The rash is erythematous and maculopapular and spreads from the head to the feet, often becoming confluent at more proximal sites.
- Pharyngitis, cervical lymphadenopathy, and splenomegaly may accompany the rash.
- Atypical measles
  - This group of young adults (2nd and 3rd decades of life) may become quite ill, with sudden onset of fever from 103° to 105°F and headache. The rash, unlike typical measles, appears initially on the distal extremities, progressing cephalad.
  - Most patients with atypical measles have pneumonia, often with pleural effusions.
  - Diagnosis depends on clinical recognition and by serologic and molecular (RNA) testing.

HISTORY

- Case definition from the CDC includes the following:
  - Generalized rash lasting ≥3 days
  - A temperature of ≥38.3°C (101°F)
  - Cough, coryza, or conjunctivitis
  - Positive testing or epidemiologic linkage to known case
- The mean incubation period is 10 days (range: 8–21 days).
- The prodrome of measles lasts 2–4 days and begins with symptoms of upper respiratory infection, fever up to 104°F, malaise, conjunctivitis, photophobia, and increasing cough.
- During the prodrome, Koplik spots (white spots on the buccal mucosa) appear on most people.
- Following this prodrome, the rash appears on the face (often initially at the hairline) and abdomen (14 days after exposure). The rash is erythematous and maculopapular and spreads from the head to the feet.
- After 3–4 days, the rash begins to clear, leaving a brownish discoloration and fine scaling.
- Fever usually resolves by the 4th day of rash.

DIAGNOSTIC TESTS & INTERPRETATION

- When measles is suspected, laboratory confirmation is important.
- The course of typical measles follows a predictable pattern; therefore, laboratory studies to confirm infection in known contacts might not be required.

Lab

- Serum measles-specific IgM titer (simplest)
  - Sensitivity may be diminished if assay performed <72 hours from onset of rash; repeat if negative. IgM detectable for at least 1 month from onset of rash
  - A comparison of IgG titers obtained during the acute and convalescent stages can be done. Blood samples must be taken at least 7–10 days apart.
  - Culture or RNA (RT-PCR) testing of nasopharyngeal, throat, blood, or urine

DIFFERENTIAL DIAGNOSIS

With a careful history and physical exam, it is usually possible to diagnose measles. The differential diagnosis includes the following:

- Stevens-Johnson syndrome
- Kawasaki disease
- Other viral exanthem
- Meningococcemia
- Rocky Mountain spotted fever (RMSF)
- Toxic shock syndrome

TREATMENT

GENERAL MEASURES

- No specific therapy; supportive care
- Ribavirin is active in vitro but not approved by FDA for treatment of measles.
- Vitamin A treatment of children with measles in developing countries has been associated with decreases in both morbidity and mortality.
  - The World Health Organization recommends vitamin A for all children with measles worldwide.
  - Vitamin A is given once daily for 2 days:
    - 200,000 IU for children ≥12 months of age
    - 100,000 IU for infants 6–11 months of age
    - 50,000 IU for infants <6 months of age
  - The higher dose may be associated with vomiting and headache for a few hours.
  - For children with signs/symptoms of vitamin A deficiency, a 3rd dose at 4 weeks is indicated.
  - Vitamin A is available in 50,000 IU/mL injectable solution and may be given orally.

ONGOING CARE

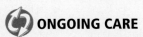

FOLLOW-UP RECOMMENDATIONS

In uncomplicated measles infection, clinical improvement and fading of rash typically occur on the 3rd or 4th day.

PROGNOSIS

- Mortality in the modern outbreak of 1989–1990 occurred in 3 of every 1,000 cases in the United States.
- Case fatality rates are increased in immunocompromised children.

COMPLICATIONS

- Complication rate in 1989–1990 outbreaks that occurred throughout the country was 23% and included diarrhea (9%), otitis media (7%), pneumonia (6%), and encephalitis (0.1%):
  - Encephalitis, which can lead to permanent neurologic sequelae, occurs in 1 of every 1,000 cases reported in the United States.
  - Croup, myocarditis, pericarditis, and disseminated intravascular coagulation (black measles) can also occur.
- In 1990, ~18–20% of patients required hospitalization, many for either dehydration or pneumonia.
- In patients with poor nutrition, most common in developing countries, mortality is higher.
- Subacute sclerosing panencephalitis (SSPE) occurs in 1 per 100,000 children with naturally occurring measles:
  - After an incubation period of several years (mean 10.8), a progressive, usually fatal, encephalopathy develops among unvaccinated children.
  - Patients with SSPE are not infectious.

ADDITIONAL READING

- American Academy of Pediatrics. Measles. In: Pickering LK, Baker CJ, Kimberlin DW, et al, eds. *Red Book: 2012 Report of the Committee on Infectious Diseases*. 29th ed. Elk Grove Village, IL: American Academy of Pediatrics; 2012:489–499.
- Centers for Disease Control and Prevention. Global measles mortality, 2000–2008. *MMWR Morb Mortal Wkly Rep*. 2009;58(47):1321–1326.
- Centers for Disease Control and Prevention. Measles—United States, 2011. *MMWR Morb Mortal Wkly Rep*. 2012;307(22):2363–2365.
- Duke T, Mgone CS. Measles: not just another viral exanthema. *Lancet*. 2003;361(9359):763–773.
- Farizo KM, Stehr-Green PA, Simpsons DM, et al. Pediatric emergency room visits: a risk factor for acquiring measles. *Pediatrics*. 1991;87(1):74.
- Huiming Y, Chaomin W, Meng M. Vitamin A for treating measles in children. *Cochrane Database Syst Rev*. 2005;(4):CD001479.
- Mulholland EK, Griffiths UK, Biellik R. Measles in the 21st century. *N Engl J Med*. 2012;366(19):1755–1757.
- Parker Fiebelkorn A, Redd SB, Gallagher K, et al. Measles in the United States during the postelimination era. *J Infect Dis*. 2010;202(10):1520–1528.
- Perry RT, Halsey NA. The clinical significance of measles: a review. *J Infect Dis*. 2004;189(Suppl 1):S4–S16.
- Rall GF. Measles virus 1998–2002: progress and controversy. *Annu Rev Microbiol*. 2003;57:343–367.
- Sugerman DE, Barskey AE, Delea MG, et al. Measles outbreak in a highly vaccinated population, San Diego, 2008: role of the intentionally undervaccinated. *Pediatrics*. 2010;125(4);747–755.

CODES

ICD10

- B05.9 Measles without complication
- B05.3 Measles complicated by otitis media
- B05.2 Measles complicated by pneumonia

FAQ

- Q: If a health care worker has had a natural measles infection or measles immunization, should one be concerned about infection following exposure?
- A: Those persons born before 1957 who had wild-type measles virus infection are usually immune from reinfection. However, in a report in 1993, 4 health care workers who were previously vaccinated with positive preillness measles antibody levels developed modified measles following exposure to infected patients. Therefore, all health care workers should observe respiratory precautions in caring for patients with measles.
- Q: During an outbreak of measles, should children <12 months of age be vaccinated?
- A: In an outbreak of measles, public health officials may recommend vaccination of infants ages 6–11 months with a single-antigen measles vaccine; children initially vaccinated before their 1st birthday should be revaccinated at 12–15 months of age. A 2nd dose should be administered during the early school years.

MECKEL DIVERTICULUM

T. Matthew Shields

BASICS

DESCRIPTION
- Meckel diverticulum (MD) is the most common congenital abnormality of the GI tract.
- Derives from the omphalomesenteric duct remnants
- The most common clinical presentation in children of MD is painless rectal bleeding.
- Classically characterized by "Rule of 2's"
  - Present in approximately 2% of the population
  - Male-to-female ratio 2:1
  - Within 2 feet of the ileocecal valve
  - Can be up to 2 inches in length
  - Symptoms usually present by 2 years of age.

EPIDEMIOLOGY
- MD as an anomaly occurs in ~2% of the population, but only ~4% of patients with MD develop symptoms over their lifetime.
- MD is more common in patients with other malformations including anorectal atresia, esophageal atresia, omphalocele, and cardiac abnormalities.
- MD is considered to be more common in males, with a male/female ratio of 2:1.
- Males are also more likely to have symptomatic diverticula.

PATHOPHYSIOLOGY
- Diverticula with ectopic tissue are more likely to be symptomatic.
- Ectopic tissue in MD is often of gastric origin; can also be comprised pancreatic, duodenal, or colonic tissue as well
- Bleeding occurs when gastric mucosa is present, resulting in peptic ulcerations of the small bowel downstream from the diverticulum (90% of cases).
- Alkaline secretions from ectopic pancreatic tissue can also cause ulcerations with bleeding.
- Obstruction can occur when the diverticulum acts as a lead point for intussusception, when the diverticulum becomes inflamed with subsequent lumen narrowing, or when the diverticulum induces a volvulus.

ETIOLOGY
- True diverticulum (contains all 3 layers of the bowel wall)
- Originates from the antimesenteric border of the bowel in the region of the terminal ileum and proximal to the ileocecal valve
- Remnant of the omphalomesenteric (vitelline) duct which fails to involute completely during the 5th–6th week of gestation as the placenta replaces the yolk sac as the source of fetal nutrition
- MD accounts for 90% of the vitelline duct anomalies. Other anomalies include the following:
  - Omphalomesenteric fistula
  - Omphalomesenteric cyst
  - Fibrous band

COMMONLY ASSOCIATED CONDITIONS
- MD has also been associated with several other congenital anomalies that include the following:
  - Anorectal atresia (affects 11% of patients with MD)
  - Esophageal atresia (12%)
  - Minor omphalocele (25%)
  - Cardiac malformations
  - Exophthalmos
  - Cleft palate
  - Annular pancreas
  - Some central nervous system malformations
- Malignancies have also been reported in association with MD.
  - Can be present within the diverticulum and can cause obstructive symptoms or can be found incidentally
  - Sarcomas are the most common malignancy associated with MD, followed by carcinoids and adenocarcinomas.

DIAGNOSIS

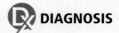

HISTORY
- Rectal bleeding
  - In children, the most common presentation is with painless rectal bleeding, which may range from occult blood to frank bright red blood and hemodynamic instability.
  - The bleeding tends to be self-limiting, because of constriction of the splanchnic vessels secondary to hypovolemia.
  - Bleeding is most commonly seen in children <5 years of age.
- Obstruction
  - Partial or complete small bowel obstruction
  - The clinical symptoms in this setting include recurrent abdominal pain, abdominal distention, nausea, and vomiting.
  - Most common type of presentation in adults and can occur in up to 40% of pediatric patients
  - Intraperitoneal bands, volvulus, or internal herniation may also lead to an obstructive presentation.
- Inflammation/fever
  - Another common presentation for symptomatic MD is inflammation or diverticulitis, which can occur in 12–40% of cases.
  - Patients often present with signs and symptoms consistent with appendicitis, and the diagnosis is made at the time of surgical exploration.
  - In a subset of this group (~1/3), the diverticulum may perforate from infarction or ulceration and lead to a more acute and toxic presentation.

PHYSICAL EXAM
- Physical exam may be normal but will often reflect the type of presenting complication:
  - Bleeding
    - Tachycardia
    - Hypotension
    - Blood in the stool
    - Hyperactive bowel sounds

- Obstruction
  - Abdominal pain
  - Vomiting
  - Bilious emesis
  - Abdominal distention
- Inflammation (i.e., diverticulitis, ruptured diverticulum with peritonitis)
  - Fever
  - Abdominal tenderness
  - Symptoms more consistent with acute abdomen

DIAGNOSTIC TESTS & INTERPRETATION

- The diagnosis of symptomatic MD is difficult to make and requires a high index of suspicion.
- This diagnosis should be considered in any patient with recurrent unexplained abdominal pain, nausea and vomiting, or rectal bleeding.

Lab

- The diagnosis of MD cannot be made with laboratory evaluation or plain radiography alone.
- Laboratory analysis may be helpful to determine the degree of bleeding, with a hemoglobin count and a coagulation profile to rule out an underlying coagulopathy.
- Plain radiographs may show evidence of obstruction but are not diagnostic of MD.

Imaging

- Meckel scan (technetium-99m pertechnetate scan)
  - Evaluates for ectopic gastric mucosa within the diverticulum
  - Sensitivity 85%, specificity 95% in children; considerably lower in adults
  - Cimetidine can be used to increase retention of isotope within ectopic gastric mucosa.
- Mesenteric arteriography
- RBC scan with severe bleeding

Diagnostic Procedures/Other

- Surgery
  - In situations in which the Meckel scan is nondiagnostic or in patients with nonbleeding symptoms (but when there is a high index of suspicion for MD), exploratory laparoscopy may be indicated.
- Capsule endoscopy and balloon enteroscopy can establish the diagnosis but are not routinely used.

DIFFERENTIAL DIAGNOSIS

- Allergic colitis
- Infectious colitis
- Polyps
- Inflammatory bowel disease
- Angiodysplasia
- Constipation/anorectal fissure
- Coagulopathy
- Henoch-Schönlein purpura
- Intussusception
- Lymphonodular hyperplasia
- Intestinal duplication

TREATMENT

The treatment for MD that are symptomatic and identified is surgical removal. Surgery involves diverticulectomy or partial bowel resection.

SURGERY/OTHER PROCEDURES

- Initial management should include supportive care.
- Correct any electrolyte abnormalities.
- Initiate proton pump inhibitor (PPI) for gastrointestinal bleeding (PPI will not affect the results of the Meckel scan).
- Nasogastric tube placement for decompression of bowel obstruction
- Surgical intervention of an incidentally found MD is controversial.
  - If it is found during surgical exploration, intervention depends on the size of the diverticulum, age of the patient, and whether fibrous bands are present.
  - If it is found incidentally during radiologic imaging, symptoms should be monitored closely, but most do not recommend elective surgery.

INPATIENT CONSIDERATIONS

Initial Stabilization

- Bleeding
  - Address issues of anemia and volume status based on vital signs and blood tests.
- Obstruction
  - Evaluate the need for acute management (surgical) and decompression.

ADDITIONAL READING

- McCollough M, Sharieff GQ. Abdominal surgical emergencies in infants and young children. *Emerg Med Clin North Am*. 2003;21(4):909–935.
- Mendelson KG, Bailey BM, Balint TD, et al. Meckel diverticulum: review and surgical management. *Curr Surg*. 2001;58(5):455–457.
- Ruscher KA, Fisher JN, Hughes CD, et al. National trends in the surgical management of Meckel's diverticulum. *J Pediatr Surg*. 2011;46(5):893–896.
- Shalabi RY, Soliman SM, Fawy M, et al. Laparoscopic management of Meckel's diverticulum in children. *J Pediatr Surg*. 2005;40(3):562–567.
- Snyder CL. Current management of umbilical abnormalities and related anomalies. *Semin Pediatr Surg*. 2007;16(1):41–49.
- Tseng YY, Yang YJ. Clinical and diagnostic relevance of Meckel's diverticulum in children. *Eur J Pediatr*. 2009;168(12):1519–1523.
- Uppal K, Tubbs RS, Matusz P, et al. Meckel's diverticulum: a review. *Clin Anat*. 2011;24(4):416–422.

CODES

ICD10

Q43.0 Meckel's diverticulum (displaced) (hypertrophic)

FAQ

- Q: What are various indications for resection of a Meckel diverticulum?
- A: Intussusception, narrowing at base of diverticulum, or presence of ectopic tissue resulting in bleeding
- Q: What is the most common type of ectopic tissue present in Meckel diverticulum?
- A: Gastric
- Q: What is the most common presentation of a Meckel diverticulum?
- A: Intermittent, painless rectal bleeding

M

MECONIUM ASPIRATION SYNDROME

Hussnain S. Mirza • Thomas E. Wiswell

BASICS

DESCRIPTION

Meconium aspiration syndrome (MAS) is a clinical diagnosis defined as respiratory distress in a newborn delivered through meconium-stained amniotic fluid (MSAF) with no other explanation for clinical symptoms. Severity of MAS can be (a) mild: requiring <0.4 FiO_2 for <48 hours; (b) moderate: requiring ≥ 0.4 FiO_2 for >48 hours with no air leak; and (c) severe: requiring assisted ventilation or if associated with persistent pulmonary hypertension of the newborn (PPHN).

EPIDEMIOLOGY

- Incidence of MSAF: 10–15% of all pregnancies
- 2–9% infants born through MSAF develop MAS (0.1–1.8% of all live births).
- MSAF is rare in premature infants and almost nonexistent before 31 weeks' gestation.

RISK FACTORS

- Postmature gestation
- Small for gestational age (SGA)
- Chorioamnionitis
- Fetal hypoxia (in utero aspiration)
- Thick consistency of meconium
- 1 and 5 minutes Apgar <6
- African American or South Asian ethnicity

PATHOPHYSIOLOGY

Meconium aspiration creates ventilation/perfusion (V/Q) mismatch (by the following variable effects on the airways), leading to hypoxemia, hypercarbia, acidosis, and cardiopulmonary failure.

- Mechanical obstruction of airways
  - Complete (atelectasis)
  - Partial (hyperinflation and air leaks due to ball and valve phenomenon)
- Meconium-associated pulmonary inflammation
- Inactivation of existing surfactant
- Decreased production of surfactant
- Meconium-induced lung apoptosis
- Coexisting pulmonary hypertension

DIAGNOSIS

HISTORY

- Term or postterm gestation
- Abnormal fetal tracing
- Evidence of MSAF
- Low Apgar score at 1 and 5 minutes
- Respiratory distress at or shortly after birth

PHYSICAL EXAM

- Meconium staining (vocal cords, skin, nails, and umbilical cord)
- Respiratory distress (tachypnea, retractions, grunting, cyanosis, and flaring)
- Barrel-shaped chest (air trapping or air leak)
- Rales and rhonchi
- Systolic murmur (tricuspid regurgitation) due to pulmonary hypertension
- Preductal oxygen saturation $\geq 10\%$ higher than postductal value
- Signs of encephalopathy, particularly if associated with perinatal asphyxia
- Signs of hypoxemia (cyanosis, poor perfusion, hypotension)
- Rarely, green color urine (meconium metabolites may appear in urine)

DIAGNOSTIC TESTS & INTERPRETATION

Lab

- CBC with differential count
  - Leukocytosis with left shift can help to identify secondary infection or congenital pneumonia; however, a left shift is also common with MAS.
- Peripheral blood culture
  - May help to identify secondary infection, sepsis, or congenital pneumonia
- Arterial blood gas (ABG)
  - Can identify respiratory failure or hypoxemia and guide the need for respiratory support
  - The test is also used to calculate an oxygenation index if the infant is on mechanical ventilation.

Imaging

- Initial chest radiograph
  - Radiographic appearance lags behind clinical symptoms.
  - Frequently, there is no significant association between the extent of radiographic abnormalities and the severity of disease.
  - Initial radiograph can be normal or may have some streaky, linear densities.
- Follow-up chest radiograph
  - As the disease progresses, there can be diffuse patchy densities, hyperinflation, flattening of the diaphragm, pleural effusion, alternating areas of microatelectasis, hyperinflation, and consolidation.
  - Significant air leaks can be noted in 10–30% of infants with MAS.

Diagnostic Procedures/Other

- Pre- and postductal Spo_2 gradient
  - $>10\%$ may be associated with PPHN.
- Oxygenation index (OI)
  - After optimizing mechanical ventilation, OI >40 on two serial ABGs performed 4 hours apart could be an indication for extracorporeal membrane oxygenation (ECMO).
  - $OI = (FiO_2 \times \text{mean airway pressure} \times 100) / Pao_2$
- Echocardiography
  - To rule out congenital heart disease and to evaluate for PPHN

DIFFERENTIAL DIAGNOSIS

- Congenital pneumonia
- Transient tachypnea of newborn (TTN)
- PPHN

TREATMENT

MEDICATION

- IV antibiotics
  - In the early stage of the disease, it is difficult to differentiate between MAS and congenital pneumonia. Many clinicians treat empirically while awaiting the results of cultures.
  - Prophylactic antibiotic treatment does not prevent secondary infection in MAS.
- Surfactant bolus treatment
  - Although not specifically FDA approved for MAS, exogenous surfactant replacement may decrease the need for ECMO.
- Steroid therapy
  - Not recommended for routine treatment of MAS
  - Systemic use of steroids has reportedly been associated with shorter duration of mechanical ventilation and with the improved pulmonary function.
- Inhalational nitric oxide (iNO)
  - iNO is used to treat MAS that is associated with PPHN.

ADDITIONAL THERAPIES

- Oxygen therapy
  - The goal is to keep peripheral Spo_2 between 92% and 98% or Pao_2 between 60 and 80 torr (8–10.7 kPa).
  - Oxygen can be provided via oxyhood or nasal cannula. If >0.6 FiO_2 is required to achieve the above-mentioned goal, consider additional respiratory support.
- Continuous positive airway pressure (CPAP)
  - Due to the possible complications (i.e., air trapping, hyperinflation, and air leaks), many clinicians prefer to avoid CPAP. However, CPAP can be cautiously used if air trapping or air leak is not a major issue.
- Conventional ventilation
  - Used to achieve optimal ventilation and oxygenation. No specific modes have been proven superior.
  - Most clinicians use low positive end-expiratory pressure (PEEP) and prolonged expiratory times in order to prevent hyperinflation, air trapping, and air leaks.
- High-frequency ventilation (oscillator or jet):
  - High-frequency ventilation (HFV) is used as a rescue treatment. No clinical trial has demonstrated clear benefits of HFV over conventional modes in the initial management of MAS. However, in the presence of air trapping or air leaks, jet ventilation may help. Anecdotally, meconium clearance may be increased with high-frequency jet ventilation (HFJV).

- ECMO
  - Indicated for severe respiratory failure manifested by an OI >40 on 2 serial ABGs performed 4 hours apart while on optimal mechanical ventilation
  - Veno-arterial or veno-venous ECMO can be considered in the absence of any vital organ failure, significant congenital anomaly, genetic syndrome, or intraventricular hemorrhage.
- Broncho-alveolar lavage (BAL)
  - BAL with diluted surfactant is an experimental therapy that has been found to produce rapid and sustained improvement in oxygenation, a shorter ventilation course, and decreased need for ECMO.
  - Use of surfactant/dextran mixture for BAL is reportedly helpful in rapid clearance of meconium. However, none of these therapies have been approved for MAS.

GENERAL MEASURES

- ICU care
  - For Spo_2 and continuous cardiopulmonary monitoring, to provide optimal thermal environment, and to ensure minimal handling
- Chest PT is generally not recommended.
- IV fluids
  - Required for maintenance of hydration and prevention of hypoglycemia
  - IV fluid bolus may be required for hypovolemia or hypoperfusion.
- Inotropic therapy
  - May be required to support the systemic perfusion especially if cardiac output is low due to left ventricular (LV) dysfunction (hypoxia or acidosis), severe PPHN, or decreased venous return
- Sedation
  - May be helpful to decrease agitation, optimize ventilation, and minimize right-to-left shunting. However, routine use of muscle relaxants is controversial, as they may increase the risk for atelectasis and V/Q mismatch.
  - Paralysis is generally not recommended.
- Feeding
  - During acute phase of severe illness, enteral feedings are discouraged to protect the underperfused gut from ischemic injury.
- Sodium bicarbonate therapy: generally not recommended

Preventive Measures

- Prevention of fetal hypoxia
  - Optimal obstetric care is the key for prevention of MAS. The decreased incidence of MAS in the last decade has been attributed to the reduction in postterm delivery and aggressive management of abnormal fetal heart tracings.
- Amnioinfusion: not recommended
- Intratracheal suctioning: recommended only for nonvigorous infants born through MSAF
- Oropharyngeal suctioning: not recommended
- Gastric suctioning: No clinical study had assessed this approach.
- Contraindicated procedures:
  - Attempts to prevent deep inspiration prior to oropharyngeal or endotracheal suctioning by mechanical means (e.g., cricoid pressure, manual blockage of the airway, and thoracic compression)

ONGOING CARE

FOLLOW-UP RECOMMENDATIONS

- Long-term consequences include increased bronchial reactivity and wheezing among the survivors of MAS.
- Infants with severe MAS are at risk for delayed development; they should be followed up in the developmental pediatrics clinic for 2–5 years.

PROGNOSIS

- Severity of lung injury is related to the consistency of meconium (thick meconium is high risk for severe disease) and to the degree of hypoxia and acidosis present at birth.
- Generally, 1/3 of infants with MAS need mechanical ventilation, 15–20% develop PPHN, and 10–30% can have air leaks.
- In spite of appropriate management and clinical care, up to 10% of infants with severe MAS may die.

COMPLICATIONS

- Birth depression
  - Occurs in 20–33% of infants born through MSAF
  - These infants can have neurologic manifestations of hypoxic ischemic encephalopathy (HIE) and needs appropriate treatment.
- SIADH
  - More likely to occur among infants with a history of perinatal asphyxia or air leaks
- PPHN
  - Occurs in 15–20% of infants with MAS
  - PPHN in these infants may be caused by (a) pulmonary vasoconstriction secondary to pulmonary inflammation, hypoxia, hypercarbia, and acidosis and (b) pulmonary vascular remodeling as a result of chronic intrauterine hypoxia.
- Secondary lung infection
  - Meconium provides an excellent growth medium for microorganisms. Meconium may also inhibit polymorphonuclear cells.
- Reactive airway disease
  - Up to 50% of infants who survive severe MAS are at risk to develop reactive airway disease in the first 6 months of life.

ADDITIONAL READING

- Kääpä PO. Meconium aspiration syndrome (MAS)—where do we go? Research perspectives. *Early Hum Dev*. 2009;85(10):627–629.
- Mokra D, Calkovska A. How to overcome surfactant dysfunction in meconium aspiration syndrome? *Respir Physiol Neurobiol*. 2013;187(1):58–63.
- Swarnam K, Soraisham AS, Sivanandan S. Advances in the management of meconium aspiration syndrome. *Int J Pediatr*. 2012;2012:359571.

CODES

ICD10

- P24.01 Meconium aspiration with respiratory symptoms
- P24.00 Meconium aspiration without respiratory symptoms

FAQ

- Q: What is the composition of meconium?
- A: Meconium is a variable mixture of intestinal epithelial debris, gastrointestinal secretions, bile, mucus, pancreatic juice, blood, swallowed vernix caseosa, and lanugo.
- Q: What are the recommendations for repeated intratracheal suctioning?
- A: If no meconium is retrieved initially, repetitive suctioning is not required. However, if meconium is retrieved and in the absence of bradycardia, intratracheal suctioning can be repeated.
- Q: How to manage vigorous infants born through MSAF?
- A: Asymptomatic infants should be managed like normal newborns. It is important to clinically observe these infants for any signs of respiratory distress for at least 24 hours prior to discharge.
- Q: What are current therapies being considered for the treatment of MAS?
- A: Meconium-resistant surfactant enriched with high proteins, phospholipids, and polymers (e.g., dextran) is waiting for clinical trials. Research has shown potential benefits of the following drugs in the treatment of MAS; however, none of these treatments are approved for clinical use at this point: antioxidants: superoxide dismutase or *N*-acetylcysteine and angiotensin-converting enzyme (ACE) inhibitors (by suppressing apoptosis).

MEDIASTINAL MASS

Michelle L. Hermiston

BASICS

DESCRIPTION

Space-occupying lesion of the mediastinum

- Anterior mediastinum includes the thymus and other structures anterior to the pericardium.
- Middle mediastinum contains the heart, great vessels, ascending aorta, and aortic arch, as well as lymph nodes.
- Posterior mediastinum contains the tracheobronchial tree, esophagus, descending aorta, and neural structures.

PATHOPHYSIOLOGY

Morbidity is due to compression of adjacent normal structures, particularly large airways, heart, and great vessels.

DIAGNOSIS

DIFFERENTIAL DIAGNOSIS

- Congenital/anatomic
  - Large normal thymus in neonate (anterior)
  - Bronchogenic, pericardial, or foregut cyst (middle)
  - Aortic aneurysm and other vascular anomalies (middle)
  - Thoracic meningocele (posterior)
- Infectious (may cause mediastinal adenopathy and/or pulmonary nodules) (middle/posterior)
  - Tuberculosis
  - Histoplasmosis
  - Aspergillosis
  - Coccidioidomycosis
  - Blastomycosis
- Foreign body in the trachea or esophagus
- Sarcoidosis
- Tumor
  - Benign
    - Thymoma (anterior)
    - Teratoma/dermoid cyst (anterior)
    - Lymphangioma/cystic hygroma (middle/posterior)
    - Hemangioma (middle/posterior)
    - Ganglioneuroma (posterior)
    - Neurofibroma (posterior)
  - Malignant
    - Malignant germ cell tumor (anterior)
    - Hodgkin lymphoma (anterior/middle)
    - Non-Hodgkin lymphoma or leukemia (anterior/middle)
    - Neuroblastoma (posterior)
    - Ganglioneuroblastoma (posterior)
    - Ewing sarcoma or osteogenic sarcoma (anterior/posterior)
    - Pheochromocytoma (posterior)
    - Neurofibrosarcoma (posterior)
    - Rhabdomyosarcoma or pleuropulmonary blastoma (any)

APPROACH TO THE PATIENT

Goal is to quickly establish diagnosis and begin treatment as indicated, as condition may rapidly progress and become life threatening. If malignancy is suspected, the child should be immediately referred to an oncologist.

HISTORY

- **Question:** systemic symptoms (fever, weight loss, night sweats, fatigue)?
- *Significance*: may be associated with infection or malignancy
- **Question:** cough, wheeze, dyspnea on exertion, orthopnea?
- *Significance*: may indicate early airway compromise
- **Question:** face/neck swelling?
- *Significance*: suggests superior vena cava syndrome

PHYSICAL EXAM

Focused attention for signs of respiratory distress or cardiovascular compromise. Check for signs and symptoms noted below.

- **Finding:** edema/suffusion of face and neck, jugular venous distension, conjunctival injection, headache, altered mental status?
- *Significance*: superior vena cava syndrome
- **Finding:** cough (nonproductive), orthopnea or dyspnea, stridor, or wheezing?
- *Significance*: airway compression
- **Finding:** quiet heart sounds, hypotension, narrowed pulse pressure, or pulsus paradoxus?
- *Significance*: cardiac tamponade/diastolic dysfunction secondary to mass effect
- **Finding:** lymphadenopathy or hepatosplenomegaly?
- *Significance*: malignancy or infection. Low cervical, posterior, or supraclavicular adenopathy particularly concerning for malignancy
- **Finding:** pallor, ecchymoses, petechiae, and/or mucosal bleeding?
- *Significance*: suggest anemia and thrombocytopenia, which are seen in malignant conditions also infiltrating the bone marrow
- **Finding:** Horner syndrome
- *Significance*: posterior mediastinal mass, most commonly a neuroblastoma

DIAGNOSTIC TESTS & INTERPRETATION

- **Test:** CBC with differential.
- *Significance*: anemia, thrombocytopenia, and neutropenia noted in malignant diseases infiltrating bone marrow. Circulating blasts frequently noted in leukemia or lymphoma; leukocytosis in infection
- **Test:** lactate dehydrogenase, uric acid, electrolytes, calcium, phosphate, creatinine
- *Significance*: tumor lysis screen
- **Test:** purified protein derivative (PPD) skin test
- *Significance*: tuberculosis
- **Test:** urine vanillylmandelic acid (VMA) and homovanillic acid (HVA)
- *Significance*: elevated in 90% of children with neuroblastoma
- **Test:** alpha-fetoprotein and beta-hCG
- *Significance*: can be elevated in germ cell tumors
- **Test:** other assays for specific pathogens based on history of exposure
- *Significance*: For a patient with a large mass or potential cardiopulmonary compromise, goal is rapid diagnosis using least invasive/painful procedure, to minimize need for sedation/anesthesia.
- **Test:** pulmonary function test
- *Significance*: may be useful to assess pulmonary reserve
- **Test:** bone marrow aspiration/biopsy
- *Significance*: simplest procedure if CBC is suspicious
- **Test:** lymph node biopsy
- *Significance*: if adenopathy at easily accessible site
- **Test:** biopsy of mass
- *Significance*: Consider radiologically guided fine-needle biopsy.

- **Test:** pleurocentesis, pericardiocentesis, or excision of isolated mass
- *Significance*: may have both diagnostic and therapeutic roles
- **Test:** lumbar puncture
- *Significance*: may be combined with other procedures if meningitis or hematologic malignancy is suspected

ALERT

Recumbent positioning, sedation, or positive pressure ventilation may lead to catastrophic respiratory or cardiovascular collapse in patients with partial compromise.

- Imaging of airway and consultation with anesthesia, surgeons, and critical care specialists should be obtained prior to any sedation.
- Procedures may need to be done with local anesthesia only with patient sitting upright.

Imaging

- Chest radiograph (lateral film required) to establish size and location of mass
- CT of the chest (if patient can tolerate semirecumbent positioning)
  - To define size, location, and consistency of mass
  - To assess large blood vessels and airways
- Echocardiogram to assess diastolic filling and vascular patency

TREATMENT

- First line
  - Steroids may be given after diagnosis is established to treat hematologic malignancies or decrease edema/inflammation.
  - If leukemia/lymphoma, diagnostic lumbar puncture should be performed prior to steroid treatment if possible.
  - Additional therapy depends on diagnosis (e.g., chemotherapy, antibiotics).

SPECIAL THERAPY

- Radiotherapy
  - May be indicated for emergent management of malignancies

ADDITIONAL TREATMENT

General Measures

- Close monitoring of cardiorespiratory status
- With cardiorespiratory compromise, avoid positive-pressure ventilation, if feasible.
- Definitive therapy will be based on the diagnosis.

ALERT

- Do not treat a patient with wheezing who has no history of asthma with steroids without obtaining a chest radiograph to confirm that there is no mediastinal mass.
- If symptoms are progressing rapidly or there is evidence of superior vena cava syndrome, tracheal compression, or spinal cord compression, emergent steroids or radiation may be required, following rapid diagnostic procedures if possible.

SURGERY/OTHER PROCEDURES

- May be required for diagnostic biopsy
- Excision may relieve acute compression and may be primary therapy for isolated benign mass.

ONGOING CARE

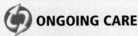

Admission Criteria

- All patients with significant mass, until cardiopulmonary risk defined
- All patients with evidence of significant airway or vascular compression
- All patients with evidence of significant tumor lysis syndrome

Discharge Criteria

Resolution/resection of mass, or clear evidence of cardiopulmonary stability through all activities of daily living (ADLs), including sleep

COMPLICATIONS

- Superior vena cava syndrome
- Tracheal compression
- Spinal cord compression
- Pleural and pericardial effusions
- Secondary infection
- Horner syndrome: ptosis, miosis, and anhydrosis resulting from compression of the cervical sympathetic nerve trunk
- Esophageal narrowing or erosion: may result in feeding difficulty or bleeding
- Tumor lysis syndrome with electrolyte disturbances, kidney failure

ADDITIONAL READING

- Franco A, Mody NS, Meza MP. Imaging evaluation of pediatric mediastinal masses. *Radiol Clin North Am*. 2005;43(2):325–353.
- Gothard JW. Anesthetic considerations for patients with anterior mediastinal mass. *Anesthesiol Clin*. 2008;26(2):305–314.
- Jaggers J, Balsara K. Mediastinal masses in children. *Semin Thorac Cardiovasc Surg*. 2004;16(3):201–208.
- Pizzo PA, Poplack DG, eds. *Principles and Practice of Pediatric Oncology*. 6th ed. Philadelphia, PA: Lippincott Williams & Wilkins; 2011.

CODES

ICD10

- R22.2 Localized swelling, mass and lump, trunk
- Q34.1 Congenital cyst of mediastinum
- D15.2 Benign neoplasm of mediastinum

FAQ

- Q: What should be done if the child is asymptomatic and a mediastinal mass is an incidental finding on chest x-Ray?
- A: Careful history and physical with specific attention to pulmonary, cardiac, and hematologic systems.
  - Vital signs to include temperature and pulse oximetry
  - CBC, differential, ESR, tumor lysis labs
  - PPD, anergy panel if high risk for tuberculosis or initial evaluation is negative
  - CT of chest
  - Referral to oncologist, surgeon, or infectious disease specialist pending above results
- Q: When should an oncologist be consulted?
- A: With any of the following:
  - Rapidly enlarging mass
  - Signs and symptoms of tracheal compression, superior vena cava syndrome, or spinal cord compression
  - Hepatomegaly, splenomegaly, lymphadenopathy, bruises, or petechiae on physical examination
  - Anemia, thrombocytopenia, or leukocytosis suggesting bone marrow involvement
  - Malignant histology demonstrated with biopsy
  - When help is needed in establishing diagnosis

MEGALOBLASTIC ANEMIA

Kieuhoa T. Vo • Elliott Vichinsky

BASICS

DESCRIPTION

- Macrocytosis refers to a blood condition in which red blood cells (RBCs) are larger than normal. It is reported in terms of mean corpuscular volume (MCV). Normal MCV values range from 80 to 100 fL and vary by age and reference laboratory.
- No complications arise from macrocytosis itself as an isolated finding; however, its identification can provide important information regarding the presence of an underlying state.
- In the appropriate clinical setting, MCV values above the upper limit of normal or those that differ significantly from the patient's baseline values may require further clinical and laboratory assessment to determine the underlying cause of macrocytosis.
- Macrocytosis with associated anemia (macrocytic anemia) can be broadly classified as megaloblastic or nonmegaloblastic anemia. This categorization is important and frequently aids in determining the etiology of the anemia.
- Megaloblastic anemia describes an anemic state characterized by the presence of abnormally large RBCs (macro-ovalocytes) and hypersegmented neutrophils in the peripheral blood and bone marrow.

EPIDEMIOLOGY

- The incidence and prevalence is unknown.
- The most frequent causes of megaloblastic anemia are disorders resulting in vitamin B_{12} (cobalamin) or folate deficiency.

RISK FACTORS

- Premature infants
- Malnutrition
- Strict vegetarians without milk, cheese, or egg intake
- Partial or total gastrectomy, ileal resection
- Infants fed goat's milk
- Bone marrow disorders
- *Helicobacter pylori* infection
- Crohn disease
- Zollinger-Ellison syndrome
- Orotic aciduria
- Lesch-Nyhan syndrome
- Exocrine pancreatic disease
- Intestinal tapeworm
- Chronic dialysis
- Therapy with certain anticonvulsants
- Therapy with certain HIV antiretroviral medications
- Therapy with certain chemotherapy agents

PATHOPHYSIOLOGY

- Megaloblastic anemia is a direct result of ineffective or dysplastic erythropoiesis caused by a defect in DNA synthesis that interferes with cellular proliferation and maturation.
- When vitamin B_{12} or folate is deficient, RBC proliferation and maturation result in large erythroblasts with nuclear/cytoplasmic asynchrony. The erythroblasts become large, oval shaped, and contain a characteristic immature, lacy nucleus. These bone marrow features are called "megaloblastic."

ETIOLOGY

- The most common etiologies of megaloblastic anemia are vitamin B_{12} or folate deficiencies.
- Medications are another less common cause of megaloblastic anemia.
- Pernicious anemia is a common cause in adults but rare in children. Pernicious anemia is a type of vitamin B_{12} deficiency anemia and is caused by a decrease in the secretion of intrinsic factor (IF) by gastric parietal cells in the setting of autoimmune atrophic gastritis. IF is a protein essential for absorption of vitamin B_{12} in the ileum.

DIAGNOSIS

HISTORY

- Pallor, fatigue, poor appetite, irritability
- Malabsorption/diarrhea, steatorrhea, weight loss
- Neurologic symptoms primarily seen in vitamin B_{12} deficiency:
  - Paresthesias, altered gait, impaired vision, psychiatric symptoms
- Diet history
  - General malnutrition
  - Personal history of strict veganism
  - Infants with vegan mothers
  - Infants fed goat's milk
- Family history of pernicious anemia or autoimmune diseases
- Surgical history of partial or total gastrectomy, ileal resection, splenectomy
- Drug history
  - Anticonvulsants
  - Chemotherapy agents, particularly antimetabolites
  - HIV antiretrovirals
  - Metformin
  - Aminosalicytes
  - Nitrous oxide, use and abuse

PHYSICAL EXAM

- Pallor, pale conjunctiva
- Glossitis: smooth, tender tongue
- Neurologic findings
  - Muscular weakness
  - Peripheral neuropathy
  - Abnormal position and vibratory sensation
  - Ataxia
  - Positive Babinski test
  - Psychiatric and cognitive changes

DIAGNOSTIC TESTS & INTERPRETATION

Lab

- Complete blood count with differential
  - Decreased hemoglobin
  - Increased MCV
  - Increased red cell distribution width (RDW)
  - May have normal or decreased white blood cell count and platelets depending on degree of megaloblastosis
- Peripheral blood smear
  - Macro-ovalocytes
  - Hypersegmented neutrophils
  - Poikilocytosis: abnormally shaped RBCs
  - Anisocytosis: abnormal variation in size of RBCs
- Reticulocyte count: low
- Increased LDH
- Decreased haptoglobin
- Increased homocysteine levels
- Serum vitamin B_{12} level:
  - $<$100 pg/mL: vitamin B_{12} deficiency
  - 100–400 pg/mL: borderline result; check serum methylmalonic acid (MMA) and homocysteine levels to help differentiate between vitamin B_{12} deficiency and folate deficiency
  - $>$400 pg/mL: vitamin B_{12} deficiency is unlikely; check RBC folate level
- RBC folate level: low in folate deficiency
- If the above testing does not reveal an obvious diagnosis, consider further testing:
  - Comprehensive metabolic panel to look for liver and kidney disease, hemolysis, hematologic malignancies or disorders
  - Thyroid-stimulating hormone to look for thyroid disorders
  - Bone marrow examination

ALERT

Coexistent microcytic anemias due to iron deficiency, thalassemias, and chronic disease can obscure the diagnosis of megaloblastic anemia by lowering the MCV. Hypersegmented neutrophils will still persist in the peripheral blood smear and aid in diagnosis.

Imaging
Diagnostic imaging with a barium study may be needed to rule out gastrointestinal anomalies.

Diagnostic Procedures/Other
- Consider a referral to a hematologist for a bone marrow examination if the diagnosis remains unclear.
- Diagnostic testing for pernicious anemia may include the following:
  - Serum anti-IF antibodies, gastric parietal cell antibodies, pepsinogen (PG) I and II, gastrin
  - Schilling test

DIFFERENTIAL DIAGNOSIS
The differential diagnosis for megaloblastic anemia is large and should include other causes of macrocytic anemia:
- Vitamin B_{12} deficiency
- Folate deficiency
- Bone marrow disorders (e.g., myelodysplastic syndrome)
- Marked reticulocytosis
- Hemolytic anemia
- Hemorrhage
- Severe hyperglycemia
- Chronic alcohol abuse
- Chronic liver disease
- Hypothyroidism
- Splenectomy
- Chronic lung disease with hypoxia
- Heavy smoking
- Pregnancy
- Medications (as listed in "History")
- Arsenic poisoning

TREATMENT

ALERT
It is imperative that vitamin B_{12} deficiency is diagnosed correctly. Treatment of undiagnosed vitamin B_{12} deficiency with folate replacement will not improve the neurologic deficits and may worsen the condition while improving the hematologic parameters.

MEDICATIONS
- Folate deficiency
  - Folic acid 1–5 mg PO daily for 1–4 months or until complete hematologic recovery occurs
  - Long-term treatment is not warranted except in certain cases of malnutrition or ongoing hemolysis.
- Several forms and administration regimens exist for vitamin B_{12} deficiency:
  - Cyanocobalamin 1,000 mcg/day IM or SQ for 2–7 days based on clinical response, followed by 100 mcg weekly for 1 month, then monthly maintenance doses thereafter
  - Hydroxycobalamin 1,000 mcg IM every 1–3 months is also an effective therapy due to its long half-life in the tissues.
  - Oral cyanocobalamin 1,000–2,000 mcg/day for 1 month, followed by 125–150 mcg/day
  - In some cases, nasal and sublingual cyanocobalamin may also be useful in replenishing vitamin B_{12} stores.
  - In the majority of patients (e.g., pernicious anemia), treatment is usually lifelong due to abnormal absorption.

ALERT
Hypokalemia associated with vitamin B_{12} repletion can be life threatening. For severe anemia, a lower initial dose of cyanocobalamin of 0.2 mcg/kg/dose IM or SQ for 2 days followed by the above regimen(s) has been recommended. The clinician should anticipate this complication and provide a potassium supplement if needed.

FOLLOW-UP RECOMMENDATIONS
Patient Monitoring
- Metabolic abnormalities begin to normalize within the first 1–2 days following treatment with parenteral vitamin B_{12}.
- Reticulocytosis occurs about 3–4 days, peaking at 1 week, followed by a rise in hemoglobin within 10 days and a fall in MCV. The hemoglobin will normalize by 8 weeks. A delayed response suggests the presence of an additional abnormality or an incorrect diagnosis.
- Hypersegmented neutrophils disappear at 10–14 days.
- During this period, the patient might note an improved feeling of well-being, long before there are any changes in the degree of anemia.
- Dementia and depression often respond to therapy, whereas other neurologic abnormalities improve gradually over a period of 6 months and may not return to normal.

PROGNOSIS
- In cases of dietary deficiencies, the prognosis is good.
- Inborn errors of metabolism with associated megaloblastic anemia generally has a poor outcome.

COMPLICATIONS
- Patients with severe anemia may have accompanying heart failure because of the anemia itself and myocardial hypoxia. However, due to its insidious onset, this is a rare finding in megaloblastic anemias.
- Neurologic complications from vitamin B_{12} deficiency
- Concomitant folate deficiency can complicate the diagnosis of vitamin B_{12} deficiency.

ADDITIONAL READING

- Aslinia F, Mazza JJ, Yale SH. Megaloblastic anemia and other causes of macrocytosis. *Clin Med Res*. 2006;4(3):236–241.
- Kaferle J, Strzoda CE. Evaluation of macrocytosis. *Am Fam Physician*. 2009;79(3):203–208.
- Wickramasinghe SN. Diagnosis of megaloblastic anaemias. *Blood Rev*. 2006;20(6):299–318.

CODES

ICD10
- D53.1 Other megaloblastic anemias, not elsewhere classified
- D75.89 Other specified diseases of blood and blood-forming organs
- D51.8 Other vitamin B12 deficiency anemias

FAQ
- Q: What are the common dietary sources of vitamin B_{12}?
- A: Red meat, liver, seafood, chicken, dairy products, eggs
- Q: What are the common dietary sources of folate?
- A: Vegetables (especially green, leafy ones), legumes/beans, peanuts, liver. Since 1998, many grain food products have been fortified with folate in the United States and Canada, including breads, cereals, flours, pastas, and rice.

MENINGITIS

Ross Newman • Jason Newland

BASICS

DESCRIPTION

Inflammation of the membranes of the brain or spinal cord, usually caused by viruses or bacteria and, rarely, fungi or parasites

EPIDEMIOLOGY

- Bacterial meningitis
  - Most common agents in children of all ages include *Streptococcus pneumoniae* and *Neisseria meningitidis*.
  - Underlying host factors, age, exposure, and geographic location alter incidence and pathogen.
- Viral meningitis
  - Most common agent in all age groups
  - Most common isolated virus are enteroviruses that tend to occur in outbreaks in summer and early fall.
- Fungal meningitis
  - *Cryptococcus neoformans* is a budding encapsulated yeast-like organism found in soil and avian excreta; associated with immunocompromised patients (especially AIDS), rare cases in healthy children
  - *Candida* species occurs in immunocompromised patients and ill premature infants.
- Tuberculous meningitis
  - *Mycobacterium tuberculosis* (TB) meningitis occurs in 0.5% of untreated primary TB infections.
  - Most common in children aged 6 months to 4 years
  - In ~50% of cases, miliary TB is accompanied by meningitis.

GENERAL PREVENTION

- *Haemophilus influenzae* type b (Hib) vaccine has significantly reduced the incidence of meningitis and other invasive Hib infections by up to 99%.
- 13-valent *S. pneumoniae* protein conjugate vaccine (PCV13) for use in all infants given at 2, 4, 6, and 12–15 months of age
- A tetravalent meningococcal vaccine (MCV4) is recommended for all patients ≥11 years of age and select at-risk populations <11 years. A booster dose is recommended for all patients who receive the first dose of the vaccine between 11 and 15 years of age.

ETIOLOGY

- Bacterial
  - Cause differs depending on age:
    - <1 month old: group B *Streptococcus*, gram-negative pathogens (*Escherichia coli*, *Citrobacter koseri*, *Cronobacter sakazakii*, *Serratia marcescens*, and Salmonella species), *Listeria monocytogenes*, *S. pneumoniae*
    - 1–3 months old: group B *Streptococcus*, *E. coli*, *S. pneumoniae*, Hib
    - 3 months to 5 years old: *S. pneumoniae*, *N. meningitidis*, Hib
    - >5 years old: *S. pneumoniae*, *N. meningitidis*
    - Consider Hib in unvaccinated patients of any age.
- Viral
  - Herpes simplex virus (HSV) in the neonatal population
  - Enteroviruses: ~70 different strains that include polioviruses, coxsackie A, coxsackie B, and echoviruses. Recently discovered enteroviruses are not placed in these 4 groups but are numbered (e.g., enterovirus 68).
  - Other, less common: arboviruses (e.g., West Nile virus), mumps
- Fungal
  - Fungi most commonly isolated include *Candida* species, *Coccidioides immitis*, *Cryptococcus neoformans*, and *Aspergillus* species.
- Aseptic meningitis
  - Agents not easily cultured in the viral or microbiology laboratory can cause meningitis and include *Borrelia burgdorferi* (Lyme disease) and *Treponema pallidum* (syphilis).
- Tuberculous meningitis
- Unusual pathogens more likely in immunocompromised patients

DIAGNOSIS

- Age-specific
- Pain
- Fever
- Nausea and/or vomiting

HISTORY

- Bacterial meningitis
  - Older children may complain of classic meningeal inflammation signs including neck pain, headache, or back pain as well as photophobia, anorexia, and myalgias.
  - Nausea and vomiting are common.
  - In younger children, symptoms are often nonspecific, including fever, hypothermia, irritability, and poor feeding as well as signs of increased intracranial pressure, including seizures and apnea.
  - Attention should be noted to the patient's immunization status, birth history, travel history, trauma, health status, geographic location, and exposure to high-risk contacts.
  - Common chief complaints by the infants' caregivers include the following:
    - Irritable or "sleeping all the time"
    - "Won't take to bottle"
    - "Not acting right"
    - "Cries when moved or picked up"
- Viral meningitis
  - Headache and fever may precede signs of meningitis, such as stiff neck, vomiting, and photophobia.
  - Duration 2–6 days
- Fungal meningitis
  - Cryptococcal meningitis is often indolent, with complaints of worsening headaches and vomiting for days to weeks.
  - Exposure to pigeon or other bird droppings can be a valuable clue.
- Tuberculous meningitis
  - Symptoms are often nonspecific initially, with personality changes, fever, nausea, and vomiting progressing to anorexia, irritability, and lethargy (stage I disease).
  - Stage II disease is characterized by focal neurologic signs (most often involving the cranial nerves III, VI, and VII).
  - Stage III disease is characterized by coma and papilledema.

PHYSICAL EXAM

- Stiff neck in older children. Infants have poor neck muscle tone and this finding is commonly absent.
- Brudzinski and Kernig signs may be present.
  - Brudzinski sign: With the patient supine, flexion of the neck elicits involuntary flexion of the hips or knees.
  - Kernig sign: With the patient supine, the legs are flexed 90 degrees at the hip, extensions of the lower legs are unable to be accomplished beyond 135 degrees.
  - Negative Brudzinski or Kernig sign does not rule out meningitis.
- Younger children may not have nuchal rigidity and Kernig and/or Brudzinski signs.
- Any infant presenting with a sepsis-like picture needs to have meningitis as a consideration.
- Classically, there may be "paradoxical" crying—crying that increases when child is picked up.
- Signs of increased intracranial pressure, including papilledema, asymmetric pupils, bulging fontanelle, diplopia
- Skin exam for erythema migrans from borreliosis (Lyme disease), petechiae, or purpura with invasive meningococcal disease or vesicles in an infant <6 weeks old with HSV

DIAGNOSTIC TESTS & INTERPRETATION

Lab

- CSF analysis (cell count with differential, protein measurement, glucose concentration, and measurement of pressure)
- CSF gram stain and culture
- Blood culture
- CBC, platelet count, electrolytes, BUN, creatinine, serum glucose,
- Consider prothrombin time (PT), partial thromboplastin time (PTT), liver function tests, arterial blood gas

Diagnostic Procedures/Other

- Lumbar puncture
  - Contraindicated with cardiopulmonary compromise, uncorrected coagulopathy, signs of increased intracranial pressure, or focal neurologic findings until head imaging can be obtained
- If no etiology is discovered after the first lumbar puncture and the child is not responding to therapy, repeat lumbar puncture at 36–48 hours.
- Opening pressure: normal is <200 mm H_2O in lateral recumbent position

- Depending on the presentation, age, history, and physical exam findings, some or all of the following tests should be requested for CSF analysis:
  - Cell count with differential and Gram stain
    - Bacterial meningitis is characterized by CSF pleocytosis (>$1.0 \times 10^3/\mu L$) with predominance of neutrophils. Culture is the gold standard for diagnosis.
    - Viral meningitis typically has a lower CSF cell count ($0.05–0.5 \times 10^3/\mu L$) compared to bacterial meningitis with a predominance of lymphocytes.
  - Glucose: Compare with serum glucose; normal is >40 mg/dL or 1/2–2/3 of the serum glucose.
  - Protein: normal is 5–40 mg/dL except in newborns, who may have protein levels of 150–200 mg/dL
    - >1.0 g/dL in bacterial meningitis and normal to slightly elevated in viral meningitis
  - Cultures for bacteria, fungi, virus, and mycobacteria
    - 80% of blood cultures are positive in children with bacterial meningitis.
  - Polymerase chain reaction (PCR) analysis for enterovirus, TB, HSV, Epstein-Barr virus
    - *B. burgdorferi* PCR for CSF samples has a diagnostic yield as low as 17%. Antibody studies for neuroborreliosis are recommended.

DIFFERENTIAL DIAGNOSIS

- Encephalitis
- Toxic encephalopathy
- Epidural abscess
- Cerebral abscess

TREATMENT

GENERAL MEASURES

- Ensure adequate ventilation and cardiac function.
  - Circulation, airway, breathing (CABs)
- Initiate hemodynamic monitoring and support by achieving venous access and treat shock syndrome, if present.
- Prompt initiation of appropriate antimicrobials
  - If a lumbar puncture cannot be obtained or is contraindicated, a blood culture should be obtained and antimicrobials initiated immediately.
- Monitor serum sodium concentrations because syndrome of inappropriate ADH secretion (SIADH) is a frequent complication during the first 3 days of treatment.
- Steroids should be used in the initial therapy of TB meningitis along with anti-TB medication.
- Steroids are indicated for Hib meningitis and can be considered in *S. pneumoniae* meningitis; has been shown to decrease hearing loss and neurologic sequelae but not overall mortality. Consult ID expert for use.
  - If giving steroids, use dexamethasone 0.6 mg/kg/24 h divided into 4 doses and given for 4 days. The first dose should be given before or with the first dose of antibiotic.

MEDICATION

- Antimicrobial agents
  - <1 month of age: ampicillin IV 200–300 mg/kg/24 h divided q6–12h based on postnatal age and weight. If <7 days of age, 200 mg/kg/24 h divided q8h; if >7 days of age, ampicillin 300 mg/kg/24 h divided q6h and cefotaxime IV 200–300 mg/kg/24 h divided q6h
  - >1 month of age: vancomycin IV 60–80 mg/kg/24 h divided q6h; cefotaxime IV 300 mg/kg/24 h divided q6h or ceftriaxone 100 mg/kg/24 h divided q12h (should not be used in infants <2 months of age)
  - Vancomycin IV 60–80 mg/kg/24 h divided q6h should be considered in a patient of any age suspected of *S. pneumoniae*.
  - Alternative therapy for penicillin- or cephalosporin-allergic patients can include carbapenem or a quinolone in addition to vancomycin. Infectious disease specialist input should be considered.
- Fungal meningitis
  - Amphotericin B with or without 5-flucytosine
- Tuberculous meningitis
  - Treatment is generally with 4 drugs for 2 months followed by 2 drugs for 10 months.
  - Initially, treat with isoniazid, rifampin, pyrazinamide, and streptomycin.
- Viral meningitis
  - Enterovirus: supportive care
  - HSV: acyclovir 60 mg/kg/24 h IV divided q8h

ALERT

- Remember that in tuberculous meningitis, up to 50% of children will not react to the 5-tuberculin unit Mantoux tests. Therapy should be started if suspicious; do not rely on the skin testing.
- With the potential for resistant *S. pneumoniae*, vancomycin and cefotaxime or ceftriaxone should be used until antibiotic susceptibility data are available.

ONGOING CARE

FOLLOW-UP RECOMMENDATIONS

- Neonatal HSV meningitis should be evaluated with a repeat CSF HSV DNA PCR at day 21 and therapy extended if the PCR remains positive.
- Prophylaxis in Hib:
  - Oral rifampin (20 mg/kg/dose, maximum 600 mg/24 h for 4 days) should be given to all household contacts if 1 member is <4 years of age and is unvaccinated.
- Prophylaxis in *N. meningitidis*:
  - Oral rifampin (10 mg/kg/dose, maximum 600 mg b.i.d. for 2 days) for all household contacts, day care contacts, and other persons with close contact 7 days prior to onset of illness

Patient Monitoring

- Most children with bacterial meningitis become afebrile by 7–10 days after starting therapy, with gradual improvement in activity with less irritability.
- Evaluation for neurologic sequelae, such as hearing and vision testing, is essential.

PROGNOSIS

- Bacterial meningitis
  - Fatality approaches 100% if untreated.
  - ~500–1,000 deaths each year, or 5–10% of cases
  - Hearing deficits and neurologic damage may occur in up to 30% of children.
- Viral meningitis
  - Prognosis for enteroviral meningitis is good.
- Aseptic meningitis
  - Lyme disease: Prognosis with diagnosis and treatment is good.
- Tuberculous meningitis
  - The long-term prognosis in children with tuberculous meningitis depends on the stage of disease in which treatment is begun.
  - Complete recovery occurs in 94% of those whose treatment was started in stage I but only 51% and 18% for those whose treatment began in stage II or stage III, respectively.

COMPLICATIONS

- Bacterial meningitis
  - Acute complications: SIADH and seizures occur in up to 1/3 of patients, focal neurologic signs occur in 10–15%.
  - Long-term complications: neurocognitive defects, hearing defects (most common morbidity among survivors)
- Viral meningitis
  - Acute complications: SIADH in 10%
  - Long-term complications: Complications from viral meningitis are rare. However, neonates (<1 month of age) may develop severe enterovirus disease and older agammaglobulinemic children may develop chronic enterovirus meningoencephalitis.
- Tuberculous meningitis
  - Acute complications: most common are cranial nerve findings, especially 6th cranial nerve palsy affecting the eyes; hydrocephalus
  - Long-term complications: many, including blindness, deafness, and mental retardation

ADDITIONAL READING

- Brouwer MC, McIntyre P, Prasad K, et al. Corticosteroids for acute bacterial meningitis. *Cochrane Database Syst Rev*. 2013;6:CD004405.
- Kestenbaum LA, Ebberson J, Zorc JJ, et al. Defining cerebrospinal fluid white blood cell count reference values in neonates and young infants. *Pediatrics*. 2010;125(2):257–264.
- Maconochie I, Baumer H, Stewart ME. Fluid therapy for acute bacterial meningitis. *Cochrane Database Syst Rev*. 2008;(1):CD004786.
- Mann K, Jackson MA. Meningitis. *Pediatr Rev*. 2008;29(12):417–430.

CODES

ICD10

- G03.9 Meningitis, unspecified
- G00.9 Bacterial meningitis, unspecified
- A87.9 Viral meningitis, unspecified

FAQ

- Q: Is a lumbar puncture required before starting antibiotics in the patient with suspected meningitis with unstable vital signs requiring resuscitation?
- A: No. In the unstable patient, it is contraindicated to perform a lumbar puncture. Appropriate IV antibiotics should be started. When resuscitated, a lumbar puncture should be performed.

MENINGOCOCCEMIA

Andrew P. Steenhoff

BASICS

DESCRIPTION

- A systemic infection with the bacterium *Neisseria meningitidis*, a gram-negative diplococcus that is relatively fastidious. Despite treatment with appropriate antibiotics, this disease may have a fulminant course (i.e., significant complications within hours of presentation) with a high likelihood of mortality.
- 13 serogroups have been described on the basis of capsular polysaccharide antigens; serotypes B, C, and Y account for most of the cases in the United States. Serogroup Y accounted for 30% of cases between 1996 and 1998.

GENERAL PREVENTION

- Isolation of the hospitalized patient; hospitalized patients require respiratory isolation until 24 hours after initiation of appropriate antibiotic therapy.
- Exposed contacts, including household, day care, and nursery school, should receive the following:
  - Rifampin, 10 mg/kg (maximum 600 mg) PO q12h for 4 doses
  - Contacts <1 month of age should receive rifampin 5 mg/kg PO q12h for 4 doses.
  - Alternatively, ceftriaxone is also effective prophylaxis for contacts ≤15 years of age; a single dose of 125 mg IM is recommended.
  - For contacts >15 years old, ceftriaxone 250 mg IM is recommended. Its safety profile is preferred for pregnant women.
- Medical personnel should receive prophylaxis only if they had close contact with respiratory secretions.
- Vaccines for types A, C, Y, and W-135 are available and produce an immune response in 10–14 days.
- A tetravalent conjugate meningococcal vaccine, MCV4, is licensed for use in people in the age range of 2–55 years. It is recommended in all unimmunized 11–12-year-old adolescents, with a booster dose at age 16 years.
- Serotype B vaccine was recently approved by the FDA and is licensed for use in people 10–25 years of age.
- The Centers for Disease Control and Prevention (CDC) continues to recommend routine adolescent immunization with the exception of persons with a history of Guillain-Barré syndrome (GBS) who are not in a high-risk group for invasive meningococcal disease. An updated fact sheet on GBS and MCV4 is available at http://www.cdc.gov/vaccinesafety/Concerns/gbsfactsheet.html. A study published in 2012 did not support an association between GBS and MCV4 vaccination.

EPIDEMIOLOGY

- The rates of meningococcal disease in the United States have remained stable at 0.9–1.5 cases per 100,000 population per year.
- Children <5 years of age are most often affected, with peak incidence between 3 and 5 months of age.
- During epidemics, more school-aged children may be affected.
- The disease occurs most commonly in winter and spring months.
- Increased disease activity may follow an influenza A outbreak.

RISK FACTORS

- Patients with asplenia, deficiencies of properdin C3, or a terminal complement component (C5–C9), and HIV are at increased risk for invasive and recurrent disease.
- Organism virulence factors, such as differences in the bacterial cell wall lipopolysaccharide, play a role in disease severity. Less virulent organisms are more likely in chronic meningococcemia, which has a favorable prognosis.

Genetics

- Inherited deficiency of terminal complement may be found in 5–10% of patients during epidemics. The frequency increases to 30% in patients with recurrent disease.
- A number of other immune function–related genes associated with either susceptibility or protection from infection have been identified.

PATHOPHYSIOLOGY

- Fulminant disease is signified by diffuse microvascular damage and disseminated intravascular coagulation (DIC); see "Diagnosis" section.
- Death results from effects of endotoxic shock, including circulatory collapse and myocardial dysfunction.

ETIOLOGY

- Colonization and infection of the upper respiratory tract occurs after inhalation of, or direct contact with, the organism, usually in oral secretions.
- Disseminated disease occurs when the organism penetrates the nasal mucosa and enters the bloodstream, where it replicates.

DIAGNOSIS

SIGNS AND SYMPTOMS

- Fever
- Malaise
- Rash
- Petechiae
- Tachycardia
- Delayed capillary fill
- Abnormal mental status
- Bacteremia without sepsis presents with fever, malaise, myalgias, and headache. Patients may clear the infection spontaneously or it may invade meninges, joints, lungs, and so forth.
- Meningococcemia without meningitis occurs after initial bacteremia with systemic sepsis. A rash erupts, which may be nonspecific maculopapular, morbilliform, or urticarial. Progression to petechiae or purpura signifies evolution of disease.
- Fulminant disease can manifest within 1–2 hours of onset of signs or symptoms and is signified by hypotension, oliguria, DIC, myocardial dysfunction, and vascular collapse. Death occurs in 15–20% of these patients.

HISTORY

Time of onset of fever, malaise, and rash

PHYSICAL EXAM

- Physical examination of a child with fever should include careful evaluation of the skin for petechiae and signs of early shock (tachycardia, delayed capillary refill, abnormal mental status, etc.).
- Recognition of abnormal vital signs and lethargy is necessary.
- Nuchal rigidity, lethargy, and irritability should be carefully but expeditiously evaluated.

DIAGNOSTIC TESTS & INTERPRETATION

The organism can be cultured from blood, CSF, and skin lesions.

Lab

- Gram stain of CSF or scraped petechial lesion (pressed against a glass slide) revealing gram-negative diplococci will give a presumptive diagnosis.

- Rapid test for antigen detection
  - Supports diagnosis if found in CSF but not sensitive for serogroup B
- CBC
  - One study showed that 94% of children show abnormalities in 1 or more of the following parameters: abnormalities in absolute neutrophil count ($\leq$1,000/mm^3 or $\geq$10,000/mm^3), immature neutrophil count ($\geq$500/mm^3), and/or immature-to-total neutrophil ratio ($\geq$0.20).

Diagnostic Procedures/Other

Lumbar puncture: antigen detection although culture remains the gold standard

DIFFERENTIAL DIAGNOSIS

- Meningitis due to *N. meningitidis* is indistinguishable from that of other causes, except for 1/3 of children who have a petechial rash.
- Sepsis from other microbial causes (e.g., *Streptococcus*, Rocky Mountain spotted fever, viruses) may have a very similar clinical presentation, including the petechiae or purpuric rash.

TREATMENT

GENERAL MEASURES

- Because of the rapidly progressing nature of meningococcemia in some, patients with acute onset of petechial rash and fever should receive a prompt initial dose of antibiotics (if possible and practical, after blood culture or lumbar puncture).
- Close monitoring of vital signs and clinical status should follow, preferably in an ICU setting.

MEDICATION

- Cefotaxime or ceftriaxone can be initiated as presumptive therapy. After sensitivity is confirmed, penicillin is preferred.
- After isolate is proven sensitive to penicillin, treatment of choice is aqueous penicillin G IV at a dose of 300,000 IU/kg/24 h q4–6h (max, 12 million U/24 h) for 5–7 days.
- In penicillin-allergic patients, 3rd-generation cephalosporins, or chloramphenicol are acceptable alternatives.

ISSUES FOR REFERRAL

Public health officials should be notified of *N. meningitidis* cases.

ONGOING CARE

FOLLOW-UP RECOMMENDATIONS

Patient Monitoring

Patients with bacterial meningitis should have a hearing test as a follow-up.

PROGNOSIS

- Fatality rate of meningococcemia is 15–20%, even when recognized and treated.
- Fatality rate of meningococcal meningitis is 5%. The most severe cases often have a rapid progression from onset of symptoms to death over a matter of hours. At the time of hospital admission, the following signs predict poor survival:
  - Lack of meningitis
  - Shock
  - Coma
  - Purpura
  - Neutropenia
  - Thrombocytopenia
  - DIC
  - Myocarditis

COMPLICATIONS

- Complications may result directly from the infection or be classified as allergic immune complex mediated.
- Meningococcemia may be complicated by myocarditis, arthritis, hemorrhage, and pneumonia; digit or limb amputation, and skin scarring.
- Meningococcal meningitis is most commonly complicated by deafness in 5–10% of survivors.
- Other complications of meningitis include seizures, subdural effusions, and cranial nerve palsies.
- Immunologic complications include arthritis, vasculitis, pericarditis, and episcleritis.

ADDITIONAL READING

- Brouwer MC, Spanjaard L, Prins JM, et al. Association of chronic meningococcemia with infection by meningococci with underacylated lipopolysaccharide. *J Infect*. 2011;62(6):479–483.
- Centers for Disease Control and Prevention. Update: Guillain-Barré syndrome among recipients of Menactra meningococcal conjugate vaccine—United States, June 2005–September 2006. *MMWR Morb Mortal Wkly Rep*. 2006;55(43):1120–1124.
- Demissie DE, Kaplan SL, Romero JR, et al. Altered neutrophil counts at diagnosis of invasive meningococcal infection in children. *Pediatr Infect Dis J*. 2013;32(10):1070–1072.
- Pathan N, Faust SN, Levin M. Pathophysiology of meningococcal meningitis and septicaemia. *Arch Dis Child*. 2003;88(7):601–607.
- Rosenstein NE, Perkins BA, Stephens DS, et al. Medical progress: meningococcal disease. *N Engl J Med*. 2001;344(18):1378–1388.
- Velentgas P, Amato AA, Bohn RL, et al. Risk of Guillain-Barré syndrome after meningococcal conjugate vaccination. *Pharmacoepidemiol Drug Saf*. 2012;21(12):1350–1358.
- Welch SB, Nadel S. Treatment of meningococcal infection. *Arch Dis Child*. 2003;88(7):608–614.

CODES

ICD10

- A39.4 Meningococcemia, unspecified
- A39.3 Chronic meningococcemia
- A39.2 Acute meningococcemia

FAQ

- Q: How long should antibiotic therapy be given to a patient with septic shock?
- A: 7 days
- Q: Is MCV4 meningococcal vaccine indicated for all adolescents?
- A: Yes, MCV4 is now recommended in all previously unimmunized adolescents at the doctor visit from 11 to 12 years or at high school entry, whichever comes first. A booster dose is recommended at age 16 years.
- Q: How does 1 approach MCV4 immunization of adolescents who previously received MPSV4?
- A: If 3–5 years have elapsed since their MPSV4 vaccination, then MCV4 immunization is indicated.
- Q: When should 1 test for complement deficiency?
- A: In patients with recurrent disease
- Q: Which hospital personnel should receive prophylaxis?
- A: Only those with direct exposure to index patient's secretions.

MESENTERIC ADENITIS

Adrienne M. Scheich

BASICS

DESCRIPTION

Mesenteric adenitis is defined as inflammation of the mesenteric lymph nodes. The inflamed nodes are usually clustered in the right lower quadrant (RLQ) small bowel mesentery or are located ventral to the psoas muscle.

EPIDEMIOLOGY

- Age related, most common in patients <15 years of age
- Affects males and females equally
- History of recent sore throat or upper respiratory tract infection found in 20–30% of subjects
- Most common cause of acute abdominal pain in young adults and children
- Self-limiting condition
- Most common cause of inflammatory adenopathy (more common than tuberculosis)
- Mesenteric adenitis in childhood is related to a decreased risk of ulcerative colitis in adulthood.

PATHOPHYSIOLOGY

- Lymph nodes involved are those draining the ileocecal area. Lymph nodes absorb toxic products or bacterial products secondary to stasis.
- Nodes are enlarged up to 10 mm; discrete, soft, and pink; and with time become firm. Calcification and suppuration are rare.
- Cultures of the nodes are negative.
- Reactive hyperplasia: Adenitis results from a reaction to some material absorbed from the small intestine, reaching the intestine from the blood or lymphatic system.
- Hypersensitivity reaction to a foreign protein

ETIOLOGY

- Viral
  - Adenovirus, echovirus 1 and 14, coxsackieviruses, Epstein-Barr virus (EBV), cytomegalovirus (CMV), human immunodeficiency virus (HIV)
- Bacterial
  - Tuberculosis, *Streptococcus* species, *Staphylococcus* species, *Escherichia coli*, *Yersinia enterocolitica*, *Bartonella henselae* (cat-scratch disease)

DIAGNOSIS

Can be difficult to differentiate from acute appendicitis clinically, and many patients may undergo laparotomy before diagnosis

HISTORY

- Abdominal pain
  - Dull ache as well as colicky pain occurs due to stretch on the mesentery.
  - May initially be in the upper abdomen/RLQ or generalized
  - If generalized, eventually becomes localized to RLQ
  - Patients often have difficulty localizing the exact point of the most intense pain, in contrast to appendicitis, where pain is often localized to RLQ.
- Intermittent spasms: Between spasms, the patient feels well.
- Signs and symptoms:
  - Abdominal pain (RLQ)
  - Anorexia and fatigue are common.
  - Nausea and vomiting usually precede abdominal pain.
  - Fever
  - Diarrhea

PHYSICAL EXAM

- Often febrile to >38°C (100.4°F)
- May have associated upper respiratory tract infection symptoms, such as rhinorrhea or hyperemic pharynx
- Presence of peripheral lymphadenopathy
- Abdominal examination
  - Tenderness of the RLQ: may be a little higher, more medial, and less severe than acute appendicitis
  - Point of maximal tenderness may vary from one examination to the next.
  - Voluntary guarding with or without rebound tenderness and without rigidity
- Rectal tenderness

DIAGNOSTIC TESTS & INTERPRETATION

- Mesenteric adenitis is a diagnosis of exclusion.
  - It can only be diagnosed accurately at laparoscopy or laparotomy.
  - Ultrasound or CT scan may demonstrate enlarged mesenteric lymph nodes.
- See "Differential Diagnosis."

Lab

Complete blood count and C-reactive protein may be increased but are not specific.

Imaging

- Abdominal ultrasound
  - Differentiates among acute appendicitis, pelvic inflammatory disease, ovarian pathology, and mesenteric adenitis
- Contrast-enhanced CT scan of the abdomen and pelvis shows enlarged mesenteric lymph nodes, with possible ileal or ileocecal wall thickening, normal appendix
- MRI

Diagnostic Procedures/Other

- Laparoscopic surgery
- Laparotomy

DIFFERENTIAL DIAGNOSIS

- Infection
  - Acute appendicitis: 20% of patients treated for possible acute appendicitis had mesenteric adenitis.
  - Infectious mononucleosis: associated lymphadenopathy more generalized
  - Associated splenomegaly: can screen for positive EBV titers
  - Tuberculosis: associated intestinal involvement, positive purified protein derivative (PPD) test, elevated erythrocyte sedimentation rate (ESR)

– Pelvic inflammatory disease: should be considered in sexually active adolescents, and pelvic exam may be helpful
– Urinary tract infections/pyelonephritis: Urinalysis and urine culture are helpful.
– Abscess: related to missed acute appendicitis or inflammatory bowel disease (IBD)
– *Y. enterocolitica* infection: bloody diarrhea, arthropathy present; stool culture is diagnostic.
– Typhlitis: Transmural inflammation of the cecum is seen in patients with neutropenia
- Tumors
  – Lymphoma: Adenopathy can be more generalized.
  – CT scan of the abdomen and/or laparotomy to confirm the diagnosis
- Trauma
  – Hematomas of the abdominal wall and intestines
  – History of trauma
- Metabolic
  – Acute intermittent porphyria
  – Cyclic episodes of acute abdominal pain and vomiting
  – Appropriate metabolic workup diagnostic
- Congenital
  – Duplication cysts: may present with abdominal pain due to rupture, bleeding, intussusception, or volvulus
  – Meckel diverticulum: may present with diverticulitis or act as a lead point for intussusception
- Miscellaneous
  – Crohn disease: associated mesenteric adenitis and intestinal involvement
  – Intussusception: acute abdominal pain with "currant jelly" stools; barium/air enema is diagnostic and therapeutic.
  – Ovarian cysts: may need abdominal/pelvic ultrasound to differentiate between the two
  – Chronic mesenteric ischemia

TREATMENT

Most patients recover completely without any specific treatment.

ONGOING CARE

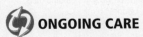

FOLLOW-UP RECOMMENDATIONS

Patient Monitoring

Watch for
- Increasing abdominal pain
- Vomiting
- Fevers
- Toxic appearance
- Severe tenderness that is persistent
- Guarding
- Rigidity
- Decreasing bowel sounds

PROGNOSIS

- Most patients recover completely without any specific treatment.
- When to expect improvement: Acute symptoms may take days to resolve and generally last a few days after the associated viral symptoms have resolved.

COMPLICATIONS

- Suppuration
- Intussusception (enlarged lymph nodes can be a lead point for intussusception)
- Rupture of lymph nodes
- Abscess formation
- Peritonitis
- Death (very rare) from abscess and peritonitis

ADDITIONAL READING

- Carty HM. Paediatric emergencies: non-traumatic abdominal emergencies. *Eur Radiol*. 2002;12(12):2835–2848.
- Frisch M, Pedersen BV, Andersson RE. Appendicitis, mesenteric lymphadenitis, and subsequent risk of ulcerative colitis: cohort studies in Sweden and Denmark. *BMJ*. 2009;338:b716.
- Karmazyn B, Werner EA, Rejaie B, et al. Mesenteric lymph nodes in children: what is normal? *Pediatr Radiol*. 2005;35(8):774–777.
- Lucey BC, Stuhlfaut JW, Soto JA. Mesenteric lymph nodes seen at imaging: causes and significance. *Radiographics*. 2005;25(2):351–365.
- Macari M, Balthazar EJ. The acute right lower quadrant: CT evaluation. *Radiol Clin North Am*. 2003;41(6):1117–1136.
- Macari M, Hines J, Balthazar E, et al. Mesenteric adenitis: CT diagnosis of primary versus secondary causes, incidence, and clinical significance in pediatric and adult patients. *AJR Am J Roentgenol*. 2002;178(4):853–858.
- Toorenvliet B, Vellekoop A, Bakker R, et al. Clinical differentiation between acute appendicitis and acute mesenteric adenitis in children. *Eur J Pediatr Surg*. 2011;21(2):120–123.
- Zeiter DK, Hyams JS. Recurrent abdominal pain in children. *Pediatr Clin North Am*. 2002;49(1):53–71.

CODES

ICD10

I88.0 Nonspecific mesenteric lymphadenitis

FAQ

- Q: Can one differentiate clinically between acute appendicitis and nonspecific mesenteric adenitis?
- A: Yes, but the differences can be subtle. Patients with nonspecific mesenteric adenitis generally cannot localize the exact point of the most intense pain, unlike those with appendicitis, who can localize their pain to the RLQ. Abdominal examination in patients with mesenteric adenitis is characterized by increased tenderness of the RLQ that is a little higher, more medial, and less severe than that in acute appendicitis. Point of maximal tenderness may vary between examinations in patients with nonspecific mesenteric adenitis. There is no rigidity on abdominal examination in patients with nonspecific mesenteric adenitis. However, it is clinically difficult to differentiate the two entities.
- Q: Which investigations can be diagnostic for RLQ pain?
- A: An ultrasound or CT scan of the RLQ can differentiate between acute appendicitis, ovarian pathology, and lymphadenopathy. An upper gastrointestinal series with small bowel follow-through or a magnetic resonance enterography study can be diagnostic for IBD.

METABOLIC DISEASES IN ACIDOTIC NEWBORNS

Leah Fleming • Hilary Vernon

BASICS

DESCRIPTION

- Metabolic acidosis is a common acute presentation of an inborn error of metabolism (IEM), particularly in the presence of elevated anion gap. Acidosis can also be seen as a result of hypoperfusion, congenital heart disease, sepsis, liver failure, toxic ingestion, and diabetic ketoacidosis (DKA).
- IEMs are generally defects of protein, fat, or carbohydrate metabolism or of the mitochondrial respiratory chain that result in either accumulation or deficiency of a metabolite.
- IEMs should be considered early in the workup of a child with metabolic acidosis in order to detect those conditions that are treatable prior to development of permanent neurologic sequelae. Sequelae can be related to duration and severity of exposure. Basic evaluation for IEMs should be undertaken concurrently with other diagnostic evaluations.

ALERT
Infants with IEMs are at increased risk for decompensation and acute presentation in cases of infection, fever, fasting, or other causes of catabolism.

RISK FACTOR

Genetics

Autosomal recessive with exception of pyruvate dehydrogenase deficiency (X-linked dominant), ornithine transcarbamylase (X-linked), and some diseases of the mitochondrial genome(maternally inherited).

GENERAL PREVENTION

- Avoid propofol if possible (anecdotal increase in pancreatitis).
- Avoid prolonged fasting or nutritional deprivation.
- Avoid use of systemic steroids whenever possible.

PATHOPHYSIOLOGY

Metabolic acidosis is often a downstream effect of the primary metabolic abnormality. A block in normal metabolism can result in dysfunction of the mitochondrial respiratory chain, buildup of toxic intermediates, disordered or reduced energy production, buildup of waste nitrogen in the form of ammonia and specific amino acids, and through conjugation of the acids with carnitine, lead to carnitine depletion. These events can lead to multi-organ dysfunction including the following:

- CNS toxicity: edema, neurologic effects of hypoglycemia, toxic encephalopathy
- Cardiac: arrhythmias, left ventricular noncompaction, cardiomyopathy
- Liver: hepatosplenomegaly, elevation of liver function tests, prolonged hyperbilirubinemia
- Hematologic: bone marrow suppression
- Renal: proximal tubule dysfunction, kidney failure (later onset)

ETIOLOGY

Multifactorial. Primary metabolic disease is typically due to a genetic defect that causes a block in metabolism resulting in buildup of toxic intermediates or absence/reduction of necessary downstream products.

COMMONLY ASSOCIATED CONDITIONS

- Maternal HELLP, fatty liver of pregnancy, preeclampsia: associated with specific fetal disorders of fatty acid oxidation
- Metabolic stroke: stroke affecting the basal ganglia (not ischemic or hemorrhagic in character)

DIAGNOSIS

HISTORY

- Pregnancy history: maternal hypertension, elevated liver enzymes, low platelets (HELLP) syndrome; acute fatty liver of pregnancy; preeclampsia; reduced fetal movements; IUGR; fetal bradycardia
- Family history of consanguinity, siblings with unexplained severe childhood illness, sudden infant death syndrome (SIDS), developmental delay, Reye syndrome, or death
- Deterioration after a symptom-free interval (typically at least several days required for toxic metabolic buildup)
  - Classic presentation is of poor feeding, vomiting, and alterations in neurologic status (irritability, hypotonia, encephalopathy).
  - Without treatment, this will progress to lethargy, temperature instability, seizure, coma, and death.
- Diet history including frequency of feeds, vigor, whether breast milk or formula and, if formula, the type of formula (low protein may delay onset of symptoms)
- Fits, cycling movements
- Associations with IEMs
  - Gram-negative sepsis (galactosemia)
  - Cerebral or pulmonary hemorrhage (urea cycle disorder)
  - Severe, prolonged, unexplained hypoglycemia in term neonate (suggests organic acidemia or defect of gluconeogenesis)
  - Mild respiratory alkalosis (hyperammonemia)
  - Ketosis (organic acidemia, congenital lactic acidosis)
  - Coagulopathy, jaundice (mitochondrial, hemochromatosis, fatty acid oxidation disorders, hereditary fructose intolerance, tyrosinemia, galactosemia)

PHYSICAL EXAM

- Vital signs: tachypnea, hypotension. Look for Cushing triad.
- General
  - Dysmorphic features (may be present in mitochondrial and peroxisomal disorders and some fatty acid oxidation disorders)
- HEENT: bulging fontanelle (cerebral edema), maple syrup urine disease (MSUD)
- Eye: cataracts, dislocated lens, corneal clouding, retinal changes
- Skin: jaundice, rashes
- Cardiac
  - Cardiomyopathy (fatty acid oxidation, propionic acidemia), pericardial effusion (congenital disorder of glycosylation), cardiomegaly
- Respiratory: tachypnea, Kussmaul breathing, apnea
- Hepatosplenomegaly (disorders of gluconeogenesis, storage disorders, galactosemia)
- Neurologic: reflexes, tone, seizure
- Odor
  - Sweet: MSUD (urine and ear cerumen)
  - Sweaty feet: isovaleric acidemia
  - Fruity: methylmalonic acidemia, propionic acidemia
  - "Tom Cat" urine odor: multiple carboxylase deficiency
- Growth parameters
  - Typically normal in newborn period but may have IUGR or delayed return to birth weight (BW)

DIAGNOSTIC TESTS & INTERPRETATION

Lab

- Initial evaluation (concurrently with sepsis evaluation)
  - Complete blood count with differential
  - Blood gas including pH and lactate
  - Serum urea, creatinine, glucose, electrolytes (anion gap),AST, ALT
  - Ammonia (place on watery ice, run immediately)
  - Creatine kinase
  - CRP
  - Urinalysis, urine-reducing substance
  - Obtain copy of newborn screen report.
- CSF: if obtained in course of complete sepsis evaluation
  - Consider freezing a tube for later use.
  - May send lactate, lactate-to-pyruvate ratio
- Should be sent for definitive diagnosis:
  - Plasma amino acids (PAA), acylcarnitines, urine organic acids, urine orotic acid (if ammonia is elevated), urine ketones
- Treatment should not be delayed in the case of presumptive IEM.
- In case of death, obtain the following:
  - Urine: deep frozen
  - Blood: EDTA for DNA analysis
  - Skin: sterile, for fibroblast culture; store at 4–8°C
  - Liver, muscle: snap frozen
  - CSF if possible (for amino acids and neurotransmitters)
  - Plasma: heparinized
  - Blood spot: for acylcarnitine profile

Imaging

- Echocardiogram to evaluate for structural heart disease and cardiac function
- Consider head ultrasound (ventriculomegaly seen in pyruvate dehydrogenase complex deficiency)

Diagnostic Procedures/Other

- Ammonia ($>$200 μmol/L) very strongly implies metabolic disease. Up to 65–100 μmol/L is normal in a healthy neonate.

- Calculate anion gap: High anion gap implies excessive acid production or retention.
- If not previously performed, secondary testing should include acylcarnitine profile, free fatty acids and 3-hydroxybutyrate, osmolality, plasma amino acids, lactate and pyruvate ratio, and urine organic acids.
- Ophthalmology exam
- Confirmatory testing is by specific enzyme analysis or genetic testing.

DIFFERENTIAL DIAGNOSIS

In neonates, inborn errors of metabolism present with similar symptoms and can easily be confused with other serious diseases.

- Sepsis
- Birth asphyxia
- Ductal-dependent congenital heart disease
- Neonatal withdrawal syndrome
- Endocrine abnormalities (adrenal insufficiency)
- IEM resulting in metabolic acidosis can be divided into the lactic acidoses, those that cause a ketoacidosis, and the organic acid disorders.
  - Lactic acidosis
    - Pyruvate dehydrogenase deficiency
    - Pyruvate carboxylase deficiency
    - Phosphoenolpyruvate carboxykinase deficiency
    - Defects in tricarboxylic acid cycle enzymes
    - Mitochondrial diseases or other conditions affecting oxidative phosphorylation
    - Severe disorders of gluconeogenesis (e.g., glucose-6-phosphatase deficiency)
    - Multiple carboxylase deficiency, biotinidase deficiency
    - Disorders of fatty acid oxidation
  - Ketoacidosis
    - Disorders of ketone use (e.g., β-ketothiolase deficiency)
    - Ketosis can also occur in lactic acidosis syndromes (above) and organic acidemias (below).
  - Other organic acid disorders
    - MSUD
    - Branched-chain organic acidurias (methylmalonic acidemia, propionic acidemia, isovaleric acidemia)
    - Others: In some cases, other abnormalities (e.g., lethargy, hyperammonemia) may occur prior to severe acidosis.

TREATMENT

GENERAL MEASURES

- Stop feeding.
- Provide 6–10 mg/kg/min dextrose (typically as D10 at twice maintenance).
  - If considering pyruvate dehydrogenase deficiency, use lower dextrose infusion rate, typically D5.
- Admit to intensive care unit.
- Consult biochemical genetics team.
- Consider early continuous venovenous hemodialysis to remove toxin and decrease ammonia. Peritoneal dialysis is less effective but can be used.
- Correct hypothermia, dehydration, electrolyte disturbance, etc.
- Consider sodium bicarbonate.
  - Start at 1 mEq/kg.
  - Often, the patient will require large doses due to ongoing acid production.
- Insulin as needed for iatrogenic hyperglycemia.
- Resume nutritionally complete feeding as soon as possible under guidance of biochemical genetics team. This may include specialized iTPN or formula.

ADDITIONAL THERAPIES

- Nitrogen scavenger such as sodium benzoate and sodium phenylacetate if urea cycle overwhelmed or primary urea cycle disorder
- Carnitine promotes excretion of organic acids. Administer 50 mg/kg/dose IV every 6 hours. Use is controversial in disorders of fatty acid oxidation; not to be used in LCHAD (theoretical arrhythmia risk)
- Specific supplementation
  - Biotin (holocarboxylase deficiency) 10 mg PO/NG
  - Hydroxocobalamin (cobalamin-responsive methylmalonic academia) 1 mg IM
  - Pyridoxine (pyridoxine-dependent seizure)
  - Pyridoxal phosphate (pyridoxine-5′-phosphate oxidase deficiency)
  - Glycine (isovaleric acidemia)
  - Nitisinone (tyrosinemia)
  - Arginine (urea cycle)
  - Thiamine (MSUD, some forms of congenital lactic acidosis) 50 mg PO/NG daily to b.i.d.

ONGOING CARE

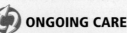

FOLLOW-UP RECOMMENDATIONS

Patient Monitoring

- Refer to a biochemical genetics team for ongoing evaluation and management.
- Generally, patients will require frequent monitoring in the newborn period and throughout life; however, this varies with the diagnosis.
- Specific treatment based on correct diagnosis of IEM

COMPLICATIONS

- Prognosis varies based on disease.
- For some disorders, appropriate treatment dramatically improves morbidity and mortality (especially the fatty acid oxidation disorders and vitamin responsive disorders); for others, there is improved survival but still significant morbidity.
- Long-term complications are becoming better understood with improved survival (e.g., risk of pancreatitis and renal failure in the branch chain acidurias). As in other chronic pediatric illnesses, such as diabetes, recurrent episodes are often triggered by stress, noncompliance, or illness and may increase in frequency during the teen years.
- Severity of neurologic complications increases with frequency and duration of episodes of metabolic decompensation and/or frequency and duration of elevated ammonia. Neurologic complications can include metabolic stroke (basal ganglia), herniation, seizure disorder, and intellectual impairment.
- There may be progressive impairment of the heart, liver, or kidney; chronic bone marrow suppression; as well as effects of malnutrition and hyperglycemia (due to frequent D10 infusions).

ADDITIONAL READING

- Burton BK. Inborn errors of metabolism in infancy: a guide to diagnosis. *Pediatrics*. 1998;102(6): E69–E77.
- Cook P, Walker V. Investigation of the child with an acute metabolic disorder. *J Clin Pathol*. 2011;64(3): 181–191.
- Leonard J, Morris A. Diagnosis and early management of inborn errors of metabolism presenting around the time of birth. *Acta Paediatr*. 2006;95(1):6–14.

CODES

ICD10

- P74.0 Late metabolic acidosis of newborn
- E88.89 Other specified metabolic disorders
- E72.29 Other disorders of urea cycle metabolism

FAQ

- Q: What factors determine developmental outcome in children with inborn errors of metabolism?
- A: The specific diagnosis and patient mutation, how rapidly appropriate therapy is initiated, frequency of decompensating, and compliance with chronic management all contribute to developmental outcome.
- Q: If the newborn screen (NBS) was normal, can the infant still be affected by an IEM?
- A: Many IEMs are not included on the NBS, and there can also be false negatives.
- Q: Do IEMs only affect infants?
- A: No. An individual can present with an IEM at any point in his or her life, depending on the level of enzyme deficiency/threshold for catabolic stress.

METABOLIC DISEASES IN HYPERAMMONEMIC NEWBORNS

Stephan Siebel • Ada Hamosh

BASICS

DESCRIPTION

- Inborn errors of metabolism are inherited defects in biosynthesis, catabolism, or transport of lipids, amino acids, or carbohydrates. The first presentation of an inborn error of metabolism can be at any age, with most cases manifesting during states of metabolic catabolism and/or increased dietary intake of an offending metabolite.
- Clinical findings can range from acute life-threatening crises to milder, nonspecific clinical episodes of malaise, emesis, lethargy, anorexia, or even acute neuropsychiatric abnormalities.
- Some inborn errors of metabolism present with elevated levels of ammonia ($>100\ \mu$M/L). Ammonia is highly neurotoxic, and elevated levels can lead to encephalopathy and death. Maintaining a high degree of clinical suspicion in sick neonates is essential.

EPIDEMIOLOGY

- Incidence and prevalence vary among different types of inborn errors of metabolism. Collectively, approximately 1 in 500 newborns are affected by one of the various inborn errors of metabolism.
- Estimated incidence of urea cycle defects is 1:18,000. Incidence of organic acidemias is 1:1,000 and of medium-chain acyl-CoA dehydrogenase (MCAD) deficiency ranges from 1:4,900 to 1:17,000.

RISK FACTORS

Genetics

Inheritance of most inborn errors of metabolism is autosomal recessive. Ornithine transcarbamylase deficiency (the most common urea cycle defect) is X-linked.

PATHOPHYSIOLOGY

- Nitrogen is an essential building block of amino acids and a major source of ammonia from protein degradation. Ammonia is highly toxic, especially to the central nervous system (CNS). A major mechanism for ammonia detoxification is the urea cycle, which converts ammonia in the liver to water-soluble urea. Urea is then excreted by the kidneys.
- Inborn errors of metabolism causing hyperammonemia interfere with urea cycle function, either directly through primary enzymatic defects of the urea cycle or indirectly, caused by liver failure, decreased production, increased use, or defective transport of a urea cycle intermediate as seen in aminoacidopathies, organic acidemias, fatty acid oxidation defects, and defective carbohydrate metabolism.

ETIOLOGY

Any biochemical defect that alters the amount of ammonia or that interferes with the detoxification of ammonia

DIAGNOSIS

HISTORY

- Evidence of systemic disease: A variety of systemic newborn illnesses, including sepsis, can be complicated by secondary hyperammonemia.
- Family history of poorly explained pediatric death, developmental disability, or neuropsychiatric disorders should raise suspicion for a genetic disorder, such as an inborn error of metabolism. Diagnoses to ask about:
  - Sepsis or recurrent infections (opportunistic organism or no organism identified)
  - Sudden infant death syndrome
  - Cardiomyopathy
  - Uncontrollable seizures
  - Coma
  - Liver failure
- Current diet and feeding schedule: In urea cycle defects, hyperammonemia is exacerbated by protein intake.
- Failure to wake and feed spontaneously is a sign of CNS dysfunction in neonates.
- Perinatal hypoxia can cause temporary liver dysfunction and reduced urea cycle capacity. Relative immaturity of the urea cycle can cause hyperammonemia in premature infants.

PHYSICAL EXAM

- ABCs and vital signs: Cushing triad (apnea, bradycardia, hypertension) should prompt immediate evaluation for elevated intracranial pressure, a complication of hyperammonemia.
- Head, eyes, ears, nose, and throat: macrocephaly, bulging fontanelle (elevated intracranial pressure)
- CVS: dilated or hypertrophic cardiomyopathy in some organic acidemias and fatty acid oxidation defects
- Respiratory: hyperpnea (rapid deep breathing that will lead respiratory alkalosis which is different from the rapid shallow breathing of transient tachypnea of the newborn)
- GI: Hepatomegaly occurs in some of these disorders (argininosuccinate lyase deficiency, fatty acid oxidation, galactosemia).
- Skin: Jaundice is not typical in urea cycle defects but occurs in other inborn errors of metabolism associated with hepatotoxicity.
- Neurologic: extrapyramidal signs, encephalopathy, myoclonic jerks, hyper-/hypotonia, obtundation, and coma

DIAGNOSTIC TESTS & INTERPRETATION

Lab

- Initial labs for a presumptive diagnosis in a patient with hyperammonemia:
  - Dextrose stick
  - Electrolytes, BUN, creatinine
  - CBC, blood culture, serum ketones
  - Blood gas with lactate
  - Liver function tests and PT/PTT
  - Urinalysis for ketones, reducing substances
  - Frequent ammonia levels (q4–12h), obtain as free-flowing samples, placed on wet ice and immediately transport to the lab for processing
  - Review state newborn screen.
- Suspected disorders and follow-up testing:
  - Urea cycle defects: plasma amino acids and urine orotic acid
  - Organic acidemias: urine organic acids, plasma amino acids, and acylcarnitine profile
  - Fatty acid oxidation defects: creatine phosphokinase, urine organic acids, plasma acylcarnitine profile
  - Galactosemia: urine galactitol, red blood cell galactose-1-phosphate uridyltransferase (GALT) activity
  - Open ductus venosus: low urea and glutamine
  - Definitive diagnosis may require enzyme testing or mutation analysis.

Imaging

Brain MRI/CT may show demyelination; circumscribed brain atrophy; cerebellar hypoplasia or aplasia, symmetric and/or fluctuation; and abnormalities of brainstem, basal ganglia, thalamus, and/or hypothalamus, especially in "cerebral" organic acidurias.

DIFFERENTIAL DIAGNOSIS

- Neonatal hyperammonemia not caused by inborn errors of metabolism
  - Sepsis or other severe illness
  - Liver failure (drugs, toxins, others)
  - Transient neonatal hyperammonemia (e.g., open ductus venosus)
  - Perinatal depression/hypoxia
  - Iatrogenic (valproic acid, asparaginase)
- Inborn errors of metabolism
  - Urea cycle defects (*N*-acetylglutamate [NAG] synthetase deficiency, carbamoyl phosphate synthase deficiency, ornithine transcarbamylase deficiency, argininosuccinate synthetase deficiency, argininosuccinate lyase deficiency)
  - Organic acidemias (isovaleric acidemia, propionic acidemia, methylmalonic acidemia, etc.)
  - Fatty acid oxidation defects (medium-chain acyl-CoA dehydrogenase deficiency, etc.)
  - Hyperornithinemia, hyperammonemia, homocitrullinemia (HHH) syndrome

- Pyruvate carboxylase deficiency
- Hepatopathy (due to galactosemia, hereditary fructose intolerance)
- Hyperinsulinism-hyperammonemia syndrome (HIHA; glutamate dehydrogenase deficiency)

TREATMENT

Presumptive treatment should not await a definitive diagnosis but should be based on clinical suspicion and initial labs. Delays in treatment can be fatal and will cause brain damage.

GENERAL MEASURES

- Many patients will require admission to an intensive care unit and may require ventilator support.
- Obtain IV access.
- Promote renal ammonia excretion through increased maintenance fluids.
- Immediately discontinue exogenous protein intake, which exacerbates ammonia production.
- Enhance anabolism with calories from high-rate dextrose infusion (10 mg/kg/min) with insulin (0.1–1 IU/kg/h) and intralipids (0.5–1 g/kg/24 h) (exclude long-chain fatty acid disorder).
- Consider total parenteral nutrition or semi synthetic amino acid formulas during crises.
- Nitrogen-scavenging agents enable ammonia to bind to amino acids which yield products that can be excreted in the urine:
  - Sodium benzoate (250 mg/kg/24 h)
  - Sodium phenylacetate (250 mg/kg/24 h) intravenously when ill, or
  - Sodium phenylbutyrate (400–600 mg/kg/24 h) orally when well. Note that high levels (or serum concentrations) of sodium benzoate and sodium phenylbutyrate can be toxic, >2 mmol/L and >4 mmol/L, respectively. Monitor sodium and potassium levels when using these scavengers.
- Arginine (180–360 mg/kg) or citrulline therapy to supplement residual urea cycle function
- L-carnitine supplementation (100–200 mg/kg/24 h) to support mitochondrial metabolism (unless urea cycle defect is identified as the cause)
- Administration of *N*-carbamyl-L-glutamic acid (Carbaglu) (100–200 mg/kg/24 h) has been shown to reduce ammonia levels in NAG synthetase deficiency, CPS1 deficiency, and the organic acidemias.
- Antiemetics (e.g., ondansetron)
- Metronidazole (10–20 mg/kg/24 h for 10 days every month) to decrease bacterial gut flora as a major source of ammonia and propionate
- Dialysis in severe hyperammonemia (>250 μmol/L) if unresponsive to IV scavengers
- Monitor ammonia, electrolytes, and neurologic status closely during a crisis.

ONGOING CARE

Specific therapies are best carried out under the supervision of a metabolic specialist and a metabolic nutritionist. Goal of every long-term treatment is to achieve a protein-sparing anabolic effect of an optimal diet that limits the episodes of acute crises and promotes adequate growth:

Adjust diet to underlying metabolic defect by restricting metabolites prior to their respective enzymatic block and/or their precursors from the diet, for example:

- Urea cycle defects
  - Restrict natural protein; protein elimination during times of stress during illness/stress; avoid fasting
  - Chronic therapy with nitrogen-scavenging agents
  - Amino acid supplements when indicated (e.g., citrulline in ornithine transcarbamylase deficiency; arginine in citrullinemia, argininosuccinate lyase deficiency)
  - Long-term therapy may involve an orthotopic liver transplant.
- Fatty acid oxidation disorders
  - Low-fat, high-carbohydrate diets with frequent feeds; avoid fasting
- Organic acidemias
  - Protein restriction, semisynthetic amino acid formulas lacking the offending amino acid; protein elimination during times of stress during illness/stress; and avoidance of fasting; intermittent metronidazole in propionic acidemia to eliminate intestinal propionate production; liver and/or kidney transplant
- Provide vitamins, minerals, trace elements, cofactors, and calories in accordance to the Recommended Daily Allowance (RDA) to promote adequate growth and an anabolic state because catabolism may trigger acute crises, especially in urea cycle defects and organic acidemias, to assess adequate nutritional therapy; measure height, weight, and head circumference; and obtain CBC, plasma protein and albumin, plasma amino acids, iron and ferritin, lipid panel, renal and hepatic function test, as well as calcium and phosphorus levels frequently
- Dietary protocol for treatment of intercurrent illness at home
- Emergency letter/protocol and bracelet
- Early treatment of infection
- Routine vaccination

COMPLICATIONS

- Recurrent episodes of hyperammonemia
- Malnutrition → growth retardation, osteoporosis
- Elevated intracranial pressure
- Intellectual disability
- Vision loss due to optic neuropathy
- Nephropathy, cardiomyopathy
- Coma, metabolic strokes, early death

ADDITIONAL READING

- Champion MP. An approach to the diagnosis of inherited metabolic disease. *Arch Dis Child Educ Pract Ed*. 2010;95(2):40–46.
- Ficicioglu C, Bearden D. Isolated neonatal seizures: when to suspect inborn errors of metabolism. *Pediatr Neurol*. 2011;45(5):283–291.
- Häberle J. Clinical practice: the management of hyperammonemia. *Eur J Pediatr*. 2011;170(1):21–34.
- Kasapkara C, Ezgu F, Okur U, et al. N-carbamylglutamate treatment for acute neonatal hyperammonemia in isovaleric academia. *Eur J Pediatr*. 2011;170(6):799–801.

CODES

ICD10

- E88.89 Other specified metabolic disorders
- E72.20 Disorder of urea cycle metabolism, unspecified
- E72.4 Disorders of ornithine metabolism

FAQ

- Q: Can females have ornithine transcarbamylase deficiency?
- A: Ornithine transcarbamylase is an X-linked gene, and females are generally asymptomatic carriers. However, due to "skewed" X inactivation of the OTC, affected female may exhibit symptoms after increased protein intake or states of catabolism.
- Q: Can any of these disorders present outside of the newborn period?
- A: Disease severity depends in large part on a patient's enzyme activity. Therefore, hyperammonemia can occur at any age during a period of metabolic stress.
- Q: What determines developmental outcome in children with inborn errors of metabolism?
- A: Outcome depends on prompt diagnosis, residual enzyme activity, early treatment, and compliance with long-term treatment.

METABOLIC DISEASES IN HYPOGLYCEMIC NEWBORNS

Stephan Siebel • Ada Hamosh

BASICS

DESCRIPTION

- Hypoglycemia is a frequent finding in the neonatal period, which results from the imbalance between carbohydrate intake, endogenous glucose production, and tissue usage.
- Neonates stabilize their serum glucose levels by about 12 hours after birth to 45 mg/dL (2.6 mmol/L). In a healthy state, glucose homeostasis underlays tight regulation through glucose-lowering hormones (insulin) and counterregulatory, glucose-mobilizing hormones (cortisol, growth hormone, and others) by acting on glycolysis, gluconeogenesis, glycogenolysis, and many other metabolic pathways involved in the biosynthesis, catabolism, or transport of carbohydrates, lipids, and amino acids.
- Hence, many inborn errors of metabolism can present with episodes of hypoglycemia during metabolic crises, which can be life threatening if not treated promptly.
- First presentation of an inborn error of metabolism can be at any age, with most cases presenting during times of metabolic stress or transition, as in infancy, illness, and dietary changes. Therefore, it is prudent to quickly establish a tentative diagnosis and initiate treatment in a sick neonate.

EPIDEMIOLOGY

- Incidence of hypoglycemia is estimated at 1–3/1,000 live births.
- Incidence of inherited forms is estimated at 1/50,000 live births in sporadic populations and higher in Ashkenazi Jews.
- The incidence of medium-chain acyl-CoA dehydrogenase (MCAD) deficiency ranges from 1:4,900 to 1:17,000 live births.
- Incidence of familial hyperinsulinism is 1 in 2,500 live births.

Genetics

Almost all inborn errors of metabolism causing hypoglycemia are autosomal recessive. Congenital hyperinsulinism can be autosomal dominant or recessive. Glycerolkinase deficiency is X-linked.

PATHOPHYSIOLOGY

- Through glycolysis and oxidative phosphorylation, glucose is a major source of cellular energy (ATP). Failure to produce ATP is probably the main source of hypoglycemia-associated tissue dysfunction.
- The brain preferentially uses glucose metabolism to produce energy and is particularly sensitive to hypoglycemia.
- A long list of metabolic disturbances in a variety of pathways can result in hypoglycemia.
- Neonates are at particular risk for hypoglycemia because they use glucose more rapidly than adults and have immature ability to obtain energy from other sources (glycogen, muscle protein, adipose tissue).

ETIOLOGY

- Inherited defects in biochemical pathways affecting metabolism of fats, amino acids, or carbohydrates
- Mutations in genes known to be involved in glucose metabolism, for example, congenital hyperinsulinism (*ABCC8*, *KCNJ11*, *GLUD1*, *CAK*, *HADH*, *SLC16A1*, *HNF4A*) and Fanconi-Bickel syndrome (*GLUT2*, *SCLA2*)

DIAGNOSIS

HISTORY

- Family history: Because inborn errors of metabolism are genetic disorders, patients may have a family history of poorly explained pediatric death. Diagnoses to ask about include the following:
  - Sepsis (was an organism identified?)
  - Sudden infant death syndrome
  - Cardiomyopathy
  - Uncontrollable seizures
  - Coma
  - Liver failure
- Unexplained developmental delay or hypoglycemia in older siblings
- First hypoglycemia after introducing different foods (e.g., milk, fruits, etc.)
- Complications with the pregnancy:
  - Maternal diabetes
  - Certain disorders of fatty acid oxidation are associated with fatty liver of pregnancy or HELLP (hypertension, elevated liver enzymes, low platelets) syndrome.
  - Small for gestational age/intrauterine growth retardation/prematurity: may present with transient hypoglycemia
- Results of newborn screen: Children are tested for a variety of inborn errors of metabolism through newborn screening programs. Some of these disorders predispose to hypoglycemia and have specific therapies.
- Current diet and feeding schedule: Timing of hypoglycemia helps form differential diagnosis:
  - Hypoglycemia occurring shortly after feeding (0–4 hours) is suggestive of hyperinsulinism or inability to process carbohydrates (hereditary fructose intolerance).
  - Hypoglycemia between 2 and 10 hours after feeding is concerning for glycogen storage diseases, defects in gluconeogenesis, or counterregulatory hormone deficiencies.
  - Hypoglycemia after fasting (>6 hours) is suggestive of ketotic hypoglycemia, defects in gluconeogenesis, or fatty acid oxidation defects.

PHYSICAL EXAM

- ABCs and vital signs: Tachycardia, irritability, and weakness are commonly seen in hypoglycemia.
- Facies: Decreased interpupillary diameter or other midline anomalies occur in association with abnormalities of the pituitary.
- Skin: Diaphoresis is an effect of the catecholamine surge that accompanies hypoglycemia.
- CVS: cardiomyopathy (fatty acid oxidation defects, glycogen storage disorders, organic acidemias)
- Respiratory: Tachypnea may be the result of either respiratory compensation of metabolic acidosis or hyperammonemia.
- Hepatomegaly
- Occurs in many inborn errors of metabolism causing hypoglycemia and is a key feature in differentiating possible diagnoses.
- May be due to abnormal accumulation of lipid (e.g., in fatty acid oxidation defects) or glycogen (e.g., glycogen storage disease).
- Renal: nephropathy/tubulopathy (organic acidemias, Fanconi-Bickel syndrome)
- GU:
  - Virilization in congenital adrenal hyperplasia
  - Micropenis in hypopituitarism
- Neurologic: Every neonate with a suspected inborn error of metabolism needs a complete neurologic exam to evaluate for level of consciousness, tone, unusual movements, and reflexes. Symptoms of neuroglycopenia include the following:
  - Tremulousness
  - Polyphagia
  - Seizures
  - Irritability
  - Weakness
  - Hypotonia
  - Stupor and coma occur if hypoglycemia is not reversed
- Growth parameters:
  - Infants with Beckwith-Wiedemann syndrome, familial hyperinsulinism, or infants of diabetic mothers may be large for gestational age.
  - Beckwith-Wiedemann syndrome may also present with additional physical stigmata (hemihypertrophy, visceromegaly, macroglossia, abdominal wall defects) and hyperinsulinism.

DIAGNOSTIC TESTS & INTERPRETATION

Lab

The goal of the initial lab evaluation is to make a presumptive diagnosis. In many cases, definitive diagnosis requires specialized and time-consuming tests.

- Initial labs for a presumptive diagnosis in patient with hypoglycemia:
  - Dextrose stick
  - Urine dipstick: glucosuria (glucose transporter defects)
  - Electrolytes, BUN, creatinine, anion gap
  - CBC, blood culture
  - Serum and urinary ketones
  - Arterial blood gas with lactate
  - Liver function tests and PT/PTT
  - Urinalysis for reducing substances: positive in fructose intolerance, galactosemia
  - Plasma ammonia levels (obtained as free-flowing samples without tourniquet): Sample must be placed on wet ice and immediately transported to the lab for processing.
  - Review state newborn screen.
- Suspected disorders and follow-up testing:
  - Familial hyperinsulinism: high insulin levels, low/absent serum/urinary ketones
  - Adrenal insufficiency, hypopituitarism: low cortisol, growth hormone, epinephrine/norepinephrine levels
  - Defects of fatty acid oxidation or ketogenesis: plasma acylcarnitine profile, free fatty acids + 3-hydroxybutyrate/ketones (low)
  - Organic acidemias: urine organic acids, acylcarnitine profile
  - Factitious hypoglycemia/Munchausen syndrome by proxy: elevated C-peptide levels, toxicology screen: sulfonylureas, ethanol
  - Urea cycle defects: plasma amino acids, urine orotic acid
  - Galactosemia: urine galactitol, red blood cell galactose-1-phosphate, uridyltransferase (GALT) activity, total galactose
  - Defects of gluconeogenesis/glycogen storage disease: arterial blood gas with lactate (lactic acidosis), +/− elevated creatine kinase (CK), specific enzyme testing or mutation analysis
  - Prolonged fasting: elevated free fatty acids + 3-hydroxybutyrate
  - Gene testing for specific disorders (Beckwith-Wiedemann syndrome)

DIFFERENTIAL DIAGNOSIS

Hypoglycemia is caused by increased glucose use or decreased glucose availability. Examples of disorders causing each:

- Increased glucose use
  - Sepsis increases metabolic demand and is a leading cause of neonatal hypoglycemia.
  - Familial hyperinsulinism: suspect when required glucose infusion rate (GIR) >10–20 mg/kg/min to maintain normoglycemia
  - Increased insulin production: Beckwith-Wiedemann syndrome
  - Decreased insulin counterregulatory hormones (glucagon, cortisol, growth hormone) due to adrenal insufficiency, hypopituitarism
- Decreased glucose availability/production
  - Infants of diabetic mothers
  - Small for gestational age: low energy stores, immaturity of glucose-regulating pathways
  - Liver failure/disease from ingested carbohydrates: galactosemia, hereditary fructose intolerance
  - Glycogen storage diseases
  - Glycerol kinase deficiency, glycerol intolerance
  - Decreased gluconeogenesis: phosphoenolpyruvate carboxykinase deficiency, fructose-1, 6-diphosphatase deficiency, pyruvate carboxylase deficiency
  - From decreased efficiency of pathways providing alternate energy sources: organic acidemias, fatty acid oxidation defects
- Disorders of glucose transporter:
  - GLUT1 or 2 deficiency
  - SGLT1 or 2 deficiency
- Various toxins or medications interfere with pathways needed to maintain glucose homeostasis, including salicylates, valproate, β blockers, ethanol, and exogenous insulin.

TREATMENT

Presumptive treatment should not await a definitive diagnosis but should be based on clinical suspicion and initial labs.

GENERAL MEASURES

- A well-appearing neonate with a low dextrose stick should be fed immediately. If feeds are contraindicated or not tolerated, obtain IV access.
- In children with associated physical or laboratory findings consistent with an inborn error of metabolism or other serious illness (e.g., vital sign instability, lethargy, acidosis), IV access should be obtained.
- A dextrose bolus (e.g., 5 cc/kg D10) rapidly corrects hypoglycemia in most cases. Infants requiring high glucose infusion rates to maintain normoglycemia are suspicious for hyperinsulinism.

ADDITIONAL THERAPIES

Specific therapies vary according to the diagnosis and are best carried out by metabolic specialists:

- Hyperinsulinism
  - May require continuous glucose administration of 7–10 mg/kg/min (IV or via continuous gastric feeds)
  - Medical therapies including diazoxide and octreotide
  - Pancreatectomy
- Deficiencies in counterregulatory hormones: hormone supplementation
- Galactosemia, hereditary fructose intolerance: Eliminate offending agent from diet.
- Fatty acid oxidation disorders, glycogen storage disease type I, defects in gluconeogenesis: frequent feeds, fasting avoidance, increase caloric intake during stress. Some children may benefit from cornstarch supplementation before bedtime to prevent nocturnal hypoglycemia.

ONGOING CARE

COMPLICATIONS

Recurrent and severe hypoglycemic episodes affect neurocognitive development.

ADDITIONAL READING

- Datye KA, Bremer AA. Endocrine disorders in the neonatal period. *Pediatr Ann*. 2013;42(5):67–73.
- Hoe FM. Hypoglycemia in infants and children. *Adv Pediatr*. 2008;55:367–384.
- Stanley CA. Hypoglycemia in the neonate. *Pediatr Endocrinol Rev*. 2006;4(Suppl 1):76–81.

CODES

ICD10

- P70.4 Other neonatal hypoglycemia
- E88.9 Metabolic disorder, unspecified
- E88.89 Other specified metabolic disorders

FAQ

- Q: Why is hypoglycemia dangerous?
- A: Glucose is a crucial source of rapidly available energy for many tissues, especially the brain. Prolonged hypoglycemia causes CNS damage.
- Q: Why are the critical labs so important?
- A: In some metabolic disorders, the biochemical disturbance is apparent only during hypoglycemic episodes. Collecting this panel of informative labs during an episode greatly increases the chance of making a diagnosis.
- Q: If an infant dies before a diagnosis is made, what can be done to provide information for family members regarding future pregnancies?
- A: A postmortem exam can be helpful. A skin biopsy can yield fibroblasts for genetic and biochemical assays to investigate defects in specific pathways, and a muscle biopsy can be used to investigate mitochondrial disorders. Follow specific protocol for obtaining biopsies.

METABOLIC SYNDROME

Michele Mietus-Snyder • Sheela N. Magge

BASICS

DESCRIPTION

- A systemic disorder of energy regulation associated with ectopic fat deposition, immune activation, insulin resistance, and increased risk for cardiovascular disease (CVD) and type 2 diabetes mellitus (T2DM)
- Recognized by central adiposity, dyslipidemia, hypertension, and abnormal glucose tolerance
- These metabolic parameters change with age, gender, race, and ethnicity, so no established pediatric thresholds have been defined.
- Extrapolation from adult criteria permits diagnosis when ≥3 of the following 5 elements are present (approximate levels):
  - Waist circumference >90th percentile (waist to height ratio >0.6)
  - Low high-density lipoprotein cholesterol (HDL-c) <10th percentile (<40 mg/dL)
  - High triglycerides (TG) >90th percentile (>90 mg/dL to age 9 years, then >110 mg/dL)
  - Hypertension: systolic and/or diastolic BP >95th percentile for age, height, and gender
  - Elevated fasting blood sugar (>99 mg/dL)

EPIDEMIOLOGY

Prevalence

- Uncommon in children of normal weight
- Up to 60% of obese children meet criteria for the metabolic syndrome.
- Rates correlate with visceral, ectopic fat depot.
- Highest rates in Hispanics > non–Hispanic (NH) Whites and ~ Asians > NH Blacks
- More prevalent with age and in males than females

RISK FACTORS

- Prenatal and postnatal stressors
- Family history of T2DM and/or CVD
- Diet high in processed foods, added sugars, and trans fats
- Sedentary lifestyle
- Smoking or passive smoke exposure

Genetics

Sequence and epigenetic modification of genes involved in energy regulation have been implicated in disease progression, including adipose tissue differentiation, insulin signaling, and circadian clock genes as well as the mitochondrial genome.

PATHOPHYSIOLOGY

- Subcutaneous adipose capacity (which varies in individuals for both genetic and environmental reasons) is exceeded.
- Deposition of fat in hypertrophied adipose cells within nonadipose depots, notably visceral, hepatic, and muscular
- Triglyceride-engorged adipocytes trigger major histocompatibility complex (MHC) II response and immune activation. Antigen presentation may be endotoxin from microbial translocation.
- Stimulated monocyte/macrophage infiltration into ectopic adipose depots release TNF alpha, IL-6, and MCP-1
- Chronic low level inflammation
- Mitochondrial dysfunction and excessive intracellular oxidative stress
- Insulin resistance and systemic consequences

ETIOLOGY

- Decreased mitochondrial reserve with age and physical inactivity
- Excessive caloric load, particularly a diet high in refined carbohydrate and/or trans fat
- Genetic and epigenetic predisposition

COMMONLY ASSOCIATED CONDITIONS

- Nonalcoholic fatty liver disease (NAFLD)
- Disordered sleep ± obstructive sleep apnea
- Polycystic ovarian syndrome (PCOS)
- Low vitamin D level

DIAGNOSIS

HISTORY

- Prenatal stress
  - Small or large for gestational age
  - Maternal gestational diabetes or eclampsia
  - Maternal or pregnancy-related overweight
- History of accelerated weight gain
  - Age at which weight gain started (Physiologic insulin resistance of peripubertal years is a common trigger.)
  - Previous difficulty losing weight (difficult to lose weight if hyperinsulinemic)
- Psychosocial stressors: teasing, food insecurity
- Family history: early CVD and T2DM
- Lifestyle
  - Eating behavior
    - Sugared beverage consumption
    - Frequency and content of processed snacks
    - Poor produce and whole grain intake
    - Aberrant eating structure (skipping breakfast, lack of balanced meals)
  - Physical activity
    - Increased hours of screen time
    - Low sports and activity participation
  - Poor sleep hygiene
- Parenting skills
  - Ability to set boundaries
  - Lifestyle role modeling
- Smoke exposure and smoking history
- Signs and symptoms
  - Obese patients with metabolic syndrome are usually asymptomatic but may have
    - Easy and rapid weight gain
    - Excessive hunger, carbohydrate craving
    - Snoring, gasps during sleep (OSA)
    - Fatigue, disinterest in activity
    - Headaches (may be symptom of OSA or pseudotumor cerebri)
    - Thickened, darkened skin in flexures, notably at the nape of the neck and axillae (suggestive of acanthosis nigricans) and skin tags
    - Polydipsia, polyuria, nocturia (concerning for diabetes)
    - Depression, bullying, teasing
    - Abnormal menses, male-pattern hair growth, acne (concerning for PCOS)

PHYSICAL EXAM

A complete physical should be done on all patients. Special attention should be paid to the following:

- Weight, height, and BMI
- Waist circumference and waist to height ratio
- Blood pressure
- Papilledema
- Tanner stage
- Abdominal striae
- Hepatomegaly
- Acanthosis nigricans and skin tags
- Hirsutism, acne
- Affect, mood

DIAGNOSTIC TESTS & INTERPRETATION

Lab

Metabolic screening (preferably fasting specimens) should be done on all obese patients:

- Fasting lipid profile: total cholesterol, HDL-c and TG. Metabolic syndrome is a condition of hypertriglyceridemia not increased cholesterol. LDL-c is typically unremarkable; but in the presence of high TG, LDL particles are smaller and less well cleared so they are more numerous, whereas HDL particles, also smaller, are less stable and decreased in number and thus HDL-c is low.
- Nonfasting lipid profile: non–HDL-c elevation
- Fasting glucose and insulin: Compensatory hyperinsulinism suggests (although not definitive) insulin resistance; homeostasis model assessment – insulin resistance (HOMA-IR) = (fasting insulin × FBG)/405: measure of insulin resistance
- Hemoglobin A1c (HbA1c): may be a helpful indication of chronic caloric overload in nonfasting state; potential screen for diabetes
- Liver function tests (LFTs): ALT and AST elevation are nonsensitive indicators of NAFLD.
- Thyroid function tests: may find very mild elevations of TSH with normal T4
- 25-OH vitamin D level: often low
- 2-hour OGTT: suggested when fasting blood sugar >99 mg/dL, elevated HbA1c (>5.6% but can use clinical judgment), and/or symptoms of diabetes (polydipsia, polyuria, nocturia) to assess for impaired glucose tolerance and T2DM
- Abnormal lab tests should be repeated after a trial of weight management.

Imaging/Additional Studies

- All patients with hypertension should have an ECG to evaluate for LVH; ambulatory BP monitoring can also be useful.
- Patients with elevated ALT or AST (particularly ALT) could have a 2-D echo to assess for hepatic fat infiltration of NAFLD.
- MRI is currently the gold standard for ectopic/visceral fat evaluation.
- A history of disordered sleep and heavy snoring, especially with pauses in breathing, warrants a sleep study (polysomnogram).

DIFFERENTIAL DIAGNOSIS

The full cardiometabolic constellation of findings is unique to this syndrome, but individual features may present in other conditions:

- Hereditary combined dyslipidemia
- Hereditary hypertriglyceridemia
- Essential hypertension
- Type 1 diabetes mellitus
- Lipodystrophies

TREATMENT

MEDICATION

There are no pharmacologic treatments approved for the treatment of metabolic syndrome as a whole. Medications can be used to treat individual components. See "Additional Therapies."

GENERAL MEASURES

Comprehensive behavioral modification through both improved diet and increased physical activity is the first-line treatment for metabolic syndrome. It decreases body weight, improves body composition and insulin sensitivity, and can positively affect CVD risk factors even if weight loss is not achieved due to redistribution of fat from ectopic to subcutaneous depots and/or a favorable shift to lean muscle weight.

- Physical activity: ≥60 minutes per day of moderate to vigorous physical activity (can be in short intervals) defined as a level of effort that increases heart rate and produces heavier than at-rest breathing.
- Diet: upgrade carbohydrate and fat quality
  - Avoid/limit sugar-sweetened beverages, specifically juice and soda. Limit sugar substitutes. Encourage water.
  - Primary dairy beverage for 2–21 years old: low-fat or fat-free unflavored milk
  - Increase fiber intake
    - ≥5 servings of whole fruits and vegetables per day
    - Increase whole grains in diet; avoid grains with <3 g fiber/serving.
  - Limit foods containing high-fructose corn syrup; limit added sugars; aim for total sugar to fiber ratio <5, ideally <3.
  - Fat content
    - Total fat, 25–30% of daily kcal/estimated energy requirement (EER)
    - Saturated fat, 8–10% of daily kcal/EER
    - Avoid trans fat
    - Monounsaturated and polyunsaturated fat (PUFA) up to 20% of daily kcal/EER
    - Favor omega-3 PUFA
    - Cholesterol <300 mg/day
- Sedentary activity/screen time
  - Includes television, video games, texting, or computer not related to school
  - Limit to ≤2 hours per day for children older than 2 years (no screen time if <2 years)
  - No TV in bedroom or screens after bedtime
- Smoking
  - Explicitly counsel about the dangers of smoking and advocate smoking cessation.
  - Counsel to avoid secondhand smoke.

ADDITIONAL THERAPIES

For individual elements of the metabolic syndrome

- Dyslipidemia: ≥10–21 years of age
  - LDL-c will not exceed 190 mg/dL with metabolic syndrome alone.
  - LDL-c >160mg/dL unusual in metabolic syndrome but hypercholesterolemia may coexist (See "Hyperlipidemia" chapter.)
  - LDL-c 130–159mg/dL + 2 high-level risk factors OR 1 high-level + ≥ 2 moderate-level risk factors OR clinical CVD
    - Risk factor algorithm helps identify risk for small dense LDL and a higher LDL particle burden.
    - HMG-CoA reductase inhibitors (statins)—pravastatin or rosuvastatin preferred. Note side effects; needs monitoring.
  - TG ≥110–499, non–HDL-c ≥145 (mg/dL)
    - Restrict refined carbohydrate intake.
    - Consider daily fish oil over-the-counter preparations with ~400 mg DHA + EPA.
  - TG >500–700 mg/dL and >10 years of age
    - Consider adjunct fibrate (off label).
  - TG ≥1,000 mg/dL
    - Not likely in metabolic syndrome alone; rule out primary hypertriglyceridemia
- Hypertension: stage 1 with no response to lifestyle changes × 3 to 6 months and stage 2
  - Rule out primary renal etiology (check U/A, BUN, creatinine, renin)
  - ACE inhibitors, angiotensin receptor blockers, diuretics, and vasodilators are used most commonly in pediatrics. Note side effects and needs monitoring.
- T2DM
  - OGTT: fasting blood glucose ≥126mg/dL or 2-hour ≥200mg/dL or HbA1c ≥6.5%
    - Metformin or metformin XR are the only oral agents approved for the treatment of T2DM in children.
      - To minimize GI distress, titrate up over weeks to 1,000 mg PO b.i.d. with meals.
      - Common side effects: nausea, bloating, diarrhea, and gas, which often resolve within 2 weeks
      - Rare side effects: lactic acidosis, megaloblastic anemia; prophylax with a daily multivitamin
      - Monitor LFTs, creatinine, and Hb/Hct.
      - Discontinue 48 hours prior to contrast administration or surgery.
      - Counsel to use contraceptive methods to avoid pregnancy.
    - Insulin injections—refer to endocrinology
- Prediabetes
  - Impaired fasting glucose: 100–125 mg/dL
  - Impaired glucose tolerance: 2-hour glucose on OGTT, 140–199 mg/dL
  - HbA1c, 5.7–6.4% (debated whether synonymous with prediabetes)
    - Consider OGTT to rule out prediabetes and diabetes.
    - No consensus on the use of metformin in prediabetic states but some evidence of efficacy

ISSUES FOR REFERRAL

- Referral to pediatric lipid specialist for LDL-c ≥130 and/or TG ≥200 (mg/dL)
- Referral to pediatric endocrinologist for diabetes, prediabetes, or PCOS
- Referral to pediatric gastroenterologist for ALT >2 times normal to rule out NAFLD
- Referral to pediatric hypertension specialist for stage 1 hypertension not responsive to lifestyle or stage 2 hypertension
- Consider referral to multidisciplinary pediatric weight management clinic for intensive lifestyle counseling.

SURGERY/OTHER PROCEDURES

Bariatric surgery is a potential weight loss treatment for extreme obesity with cardiometabolic complications in older adolescents with potential for significant insulin sensitization. Refer to a pediatric center experienced in bariatric surgery.

ONGOING CARE

FOLLOW-UP RECOMMENDATIONS

Patient Monitoring

- Ongoing weight management
- Children ≥10 years of age with BMI from 85th–94th percentile: Check lipid profile at least every 2 years; if other risk factors are present, include glucose and LFTs.
- Children ≥10 years of age with BMI ≥95th percentile: Check fasting lipid panel, glucose, and AST/ALT at least every 2 years and other tests as indicated.

PROGNOSIS

Multiple studies have shown that without aggressive intervention, cardiometabolic risk factors track from childhood to adulthood, increasing lifetime risk for T2DM and CVD.

ADDITIONAL READING

- Bremer AA, Mietus-Snyder M, Lustig, RH. Toward a unifying hypothesis of metabolic syndrome. *Pediatrics*. 2012;129(3):557–570.
- D'Adamo E, Santoro N, Caprio S. Metabolic syndrome in pediatrics: old concepts revised, new concepts discussed. *Curr Probl Pediatr Adolesc Health Care*. 2013;43(5):114–123.
- Expert Panel on Integrated Guidelines for Cardiovascular Health and Risk Reduction in Children and Adolescents; National Heart, Lung, and Blood Institute. Expert panel on integrated guidelines for cardiovascular health and risk reduction in children and adolescents: summary report. *Pediatrics*. 2011;128(6):S1–S44.
- Steinberger J, Daniels SR, Eckel RH, et al. Progress and challenges in metabolic syndrome in children and adolescents: a scientific statement from the American Heart Association Atherosclerosis, Hypertension, and Obesity in the Young Committee of the Council on Cardiovascular Disease in the Young; Council on Cardiovascular Nursing; and Council on Nutrition, Physical Activity, and Metabolism. *Circulation*. 2009;119(4):628–647.

CODES

ICD10

E88.81 Metabolic Syndrome

FAQ

- Q: Why is it important to diagnose metabolic syndrome?
- A: Although obesity increases metabolic risk, not everyone who is obese develops complications; those at the greatest cardiometabolic risk need additional screening and intervention.
- Q: Do children with the metabolic syndrome have it when they become adults?
- A: If children with the metabolic syndrome do not use diet and exercise to treat it, they will likely have it as adults.
- Q: Does cardiovascular risk improve if these children lose weight?
- A: Yes, 5–10% body weight loss can result in improvement of CVD risk factors due to preferential weight loss from the ectopic visceral fat depot.

METHEMOGLOBINEMIA

Kevin C. Osterhoudt

BASICS

DESCRIPTION
- Methemoglobin is dysfunctional hemoglobin in which the deoxygenated heme moiety has been oxidized from the ferrous (Fe^{2+}) to the ferric (Fe^{3+}) state.
- Methemoglobinemia is an undue accumulation of methemoglobin within the blood.

EPIDEMIOLOGY
- Toxic methemoglobinemia, resulting from exposure to oxidant chemicals or drugs, is the most common cause of methemoglobinemia among children older than 6 months of age.
- Enteritis-associated methemoglobinemia is the most common cause among children younger than 6 months of age:
  - As many as 2/3 of infants with severe diarrhea have methemoglobinemia.

PATHOPHYSIOLOGY
- Hemoglobin in the allosteric configuration of methemoglobin cannot carry oxygen.
- Methemoglobin increases the oxygen affinity of normal heme moieties in the blood and results in impaired oxygen delivery to tissues.
- NADH-dependent cytochrome b5 methemoglobin reductase is the major source of physiologic reduction of methemoglobin.
- A normally dormant NADPH-dependent methemoglobin reductase is the site of action for antidotal methylene blue therapy.

ETIOLOGY
- Toxic methemoglobinemia
  - Dietary or environmental chemicals: chlorates, chromates, copper sulfate fungicides, naphthalene, nitrates, and nitrites
  - Industrial chemicals: aniline and other nitrogenated organic compounds
  - Drugs: amyl nitrite, benzocaine, dapsone, lidocaine, metoclopramide, nitric oxide, nitroprusside, phenazopyridine, prilocaine, many others
  - Methemoglobinemia is a common iatrogenic complication of drug therapy.
- Enteritis-associated methemoglobinemia is multifactorial in origin:
  - Intestinal nitrate and nitric oxide promotes methemoglobin formation.
  - Innate enzymatic methemoglobin reduction systems may be underdeveloped during infancy.
  - Acidemia further inhibits enzymatic methemoglobin reduction systems.
  - Methemoglobinemia is also reported with nitrite-producing bacterial infections of the intestines or urinary tract.
- Congenital methemoglobinemia (rare)
  - Hemoglobin M: Heterozygotes for autosomal dominant hemoglobin M will exhibit lifelong cyanosis.
  - NADH-dependent methemoglobin reductase deficiency: Homozygotes for this autosomal recessive enzyme will have lifelong cyanosis; heterozygotes may have increased susceptibility to oxidative hemoglobin injury.

COMMONLY ASSOCIATED CONDITIONS
- Heinz body hemolytic anemia
  - Oxidant stress on the globin protein may cause hemolysis.
- Sulfhemoglobinemia
  - Oxidant stress on the hemoglobin porphyrin ring may cause sulfhemoglobinemia.

DIAGNOSIS

HISTORY
- Age of onset
  - New onset of cyanosis in children older than 6 months of age is unlikely to be due to congenital or enteritis-associated methemoglobinemia.
- Source of water
  - Well water may be contaminated with nitrates.
- Drug or chemical exposure
  - May suggest a source of toxic methemoglobinemia
- Diarrhea
  - May suggest enteritis-associated methemoglobinemia

PHYSICAL EXAM
- Cyanosis
  - Cyanosis becomes apparent in the presence of 1.5 g/dL of methemoglobin (in contrast to 4–5 g/dL of deoxyhemoglobin).
- Heart murmur
  - May suggest right-to-left intracardiac shunting rather than methemoglobinemia
- Abnormal lung auscultation:
  - May suggest cyanosis due to pulmonary disorder
- Signs and symptoms
  - Malaise
  - Fatigue
  - Dyspnea
  - Tachycardia
  - Cyanosis

DIAGNOSTIC TESTS & INTERPRETATION
Lab
- Oxygen saturation
  - Oxygen saturation measured by pulse oximetry is artificially low, but oxygen saturation calculated from arterial blood gas is normal (a "saturation gap").
- Co-oximetry
  - Multiple-wavelength co-oximetry is the standard for quantifying methemoglobin in the blood.
- Hemoglobin quantitation
  - The percent methemoglobin concentration must be considered in relation to the total hemoglobin.
  - Anemia may suggest concurrent hemolysis.
- Serum bicarbonate
  - Metabolic acidosis is relatively mild in cases of $<$40% toxic methemoglobinemia.
  - Metabolic acidosis is typically profound in cases of enteritis-associated methemoglobinemia.
- Glucose-6-phosphate dehydrogenase (G6PD) assay
  - G6PD deficiency does not predispose to methemoglobinemia and should not be routinely ordered.
- Hemoglobin electrophoresis
  - Hemoglobin M is rare and does not respond to therapy.
  - This test should not be routinely ordered.

Diagnostic Procedures/Other

- Pulse oximetry may be inaccurate in the setting of methemoglobinemia or methylene blue therapy.
- Blood may have a "chocolate brown" appearance despite exposure to air.

DIFFERENTIAL DIAGNOSIS

- Environmental hypoxia
- Cardiovascular disease
- Pulmonary disease
- Sulfhemoglobinemia
- Factitious skin discoloration

TREATMENT

MEDICATION

- Consider administration of 1% methylene blue.
  - Dose: 1–2 mg/kg IV over 5 minutes, repeated as necessary (caution above 4–7 mg/kg total)
  - Indications: signs of tissue hypoxia, CNS depression, >30% methemoglobinemia
  - Contraindications (relative): known, severe G6PD deficiency
- Methylene blue therapy may be ineffective if
  - Patient is G6PD deficient.
  - Ongoing drug or chemical absorption or biotransformation leads to continuing methemoglobin formation.
  - Sulfhemoglobin is present.
  - Hemoglobin M is present.
  - High doses of methylene blue add to, rather than ameliorate, the oxidant stress.

ADDITIONAL TREATMENT

General Measures

- Acquired methemoglobinemia
  - Administer 100% oxygen.
  - Decontaminate or remove from toxic source of oxidative stress.
  - Alleviate enteritis with IV fluids or elemental formulas.
  - Treat identified bacterial infections.
  - Exchange transfusion is a consideration of last resort.
- Congenital methemoglobinemia
  - No beneficial therapy exists for hemoglobin M.
  - Oral methylene blue or ascorbic acid may provide alternative reduction pathways for patients with NADH-dependent reductase deficiencies.

ONGOING CARE

FOLLOW-UP RECOMMENDATIONS

- Toxic methemoglobinemia
  - Consider consultation with a medical toxicologist.
  - May require environmental investigation
- Enteritis-associated methemoglobinemia
  - Careful formula rechallenge warranted if possibility exists for milk protein allergy or other dietary intolerance
- Congenital methemoglobinemia
  - Consider consultation with a hematologist.

PROGNOSIS

- Toxic methemoglobinemia
  - Full recovery with recognition, removal of oxidant stress, and appropriate therapy
- Enteritis-associated methemoglobinemia
  - Methemoglobinemia may be prolonged and relapsing until enteritis healed.
- Congenital methemoglobinemia
  - Lifelong cyanosis expected

COMPLICATIONS

- >10% methemoglobinemia
  - Cyanosis
- >30% methemoglobinemia
  - Malaise, fatigue, dyspnea, tachycardia
- >50% methemoglobinemia
  - Somnolence, tissue ischemia
- 60% methemoglobinemia
  - Potential lethality

ADDITIONAL READING

- Canning J, Levine M. Case files of the medical toxicology fellowship at Banner Good Samaritan Medical Center in Phoenix, AZ: methemoglobinemia following dapsone exposure. *J Med Toxicol*. 2011;7(2):139–146.
- Osterhoudt KC. Methemoglobinemia. In: Erickson TB, Ahrens WR, Aks SE, eds. *Pediatric Toxicology*. New York: McGraw Hill; 2005:492–500.
- Skold A, Cosco DL, Klein R. Methemoglobinemia: pathogenesis, diagnosis, and management. *South Med J*. 2011;104(11):757–761.

CODES

ICD10

- D74.9 Methemoglobinemia, unspecified
- D74.8 Other methemoglobinemias
- D74.0 Congenital methemoglobinemia

FAQ

- Q: Can methemoglobinemia be diagnosed by the color of the blood?
- A: The "chocolate brown" blood of methemoglobinemia is most easily noted when compared to "control" blood on a white filter paper background. In contrast to deoxygenated blood from patients with cardiopulmonary disease, methemoglobin-darkened blood does not redden on exposure to room air.
- Q: Is methemoglobin responsible for the profound metabolic acidosis often found in diarrheal infants?
- A: Benzocaine-induced methemoglobinemia rarely causes acidosis in infants. In contrast, infants with enteritis-associated methemoglobinemia often have a profound acidemia with a relatively narrow anion gap. Acidosis should be considered a contributing or coexisting factor, rather than a result, of methemoglobinemia among infants with diarrhea.

MICROCYTIC ANEMIA

Tannie Huang • James Huang

BASICS

DESCRIPTION

Microcytic anemia is hemoglobin 2 standard deviations (*SD*) below the mean as well as an abnormally low mean corpuscular volume. Use of age-based norms for both indices is critical.

EPIDEMIOLOGY

- In pediatrics, the most common cause of microcytic anemia is iron deficiency anemia (IDA).
- IDA incidence by age:
  - 1–2 years, 14%
  - Adolescent females, 9%
- Hemoglobinopathies causing microcytic anemia are common in Mediterranean countries, Southeast Asia, China, Africa, and India. Incidence in the United States is currently increasing due to increasing immigration.

RISK FACTORS

Prematurity, breastfeeding, lower socioeconomic class, and overweight infants are more likely to have IDA. Certain ethnic groups such as African Americans and Hispanics have higher rates of iron deficiency. These groups also have a higher incidence of hemoglobinopathies, which can complicate the clinical picture.

PATHOPHYSIOLOGY

- Iron homeostasis in the body is primarily regulated through mechanisms of iron absorption.
- Iron is absorbed through duodenal enterocytes and then transported to the liver. Hepcidin is synthesized by the liver and is the major regulator of iron absorption. The amount of dietary iron that is absorbed is relatively low but varies depending on the patient's iron stores.
- The body loses about 1–2 mg/day of iron through loss of intestinal epithelia. This amount is higher in menstruating females.
- IDA usually develops from absorption that is inadequate to compensate for excretion and the demands required for growth (in children).
- Hemoglobin is made up of two alpha globin chains and two beta globin chains. Abnormalities in the production of these chains can lead to microcytic anemia. Anemia can develop either through inadequate production of one of these chains or through increased clearance of red blood cells (RBC) with mutated globin chains.

ETIOLOGY

- The most common cause of microcytic anemia is iron deficiency.
- Hemoglobinopathies are the next most common cause in childhood. Of the hemoglobinopathies, hemoglobin E and alpha- and beta-thalassemias most commonly cause microcytic anemia.
- Rarely, disorders of heme synthesis such as dyserythropoietic anemias and sideroblastic anemia can be a cause of microcytic anemia.
- Anemia of chronic disease can occasionally be microcytic, although more frequently is normocytic.

DIAGNOSIS

HISTORY

- Age of onset: Iron deficiency is most common in infancy and menstruating females. A teenage male with iron deficiency anemia should be a red flag and an alert to look for ongoing occult blood loss.
- Ethnic background
- Dietary history, including
  - Breast- versus formula-fed in infancy
  - Daily milk consumption of greater than 24 oz is associated with IDA.
  - Lack of red meat consumption
  - Pica
- Lead exposure (often paint in older homes, mini blinds, ceramic dishware, or toys)
- GI symptoms including diarrhea/constipation
- Blood loss (can be from GI, urinary, epistaxis, menstruation, and rarely pulmonary causes)
- Weight loss/fever/malaise or other symptoms of systemic disease
- Family members who have needed transfusions. In pubertal females, a maternal menstrual history may be informative.
- Special questions: Children with behavioral problems, including breath-holding spells, have higher rates of iron deficiency.

PHYSICAL EXAM

- Most children with iron deficiency are well appearing with a normal physical exam. They may be somewhat irritable.
- Frontal bossing or malocclusion of the teeth can be seen in children with thalassemia due to expansion of the bone marrow compartment.
- Pallor is the most common finding.
  - Evaluate in the face, conjunctiva, gums, and nail beds. Palmar crease becomes pale with a hemoglobin less than 7 g/dL.
- Blue sclera can be occasionally observed in iron deficiency. Scleral icterus may be seen in patients with hemoglobinopathies.
- Glossitis may be seen in patients with chronic iron deficiency.
- Cardiovascular examination
  - Auscultate for tachycardia and flow murmurs. However, often, children with chronic IDA may not have tachycardia.
  - Cardiac instability is rare but does occur.
- Splenomegaly: The spleen enlarges in some patients with thalassemia as a site of extramedullary hematopoiesis. This is a rare finding in IDA, although it has been reported.
- Nail abnormalities: Spoon nails (koilonychia) can be seen in long-standing iron deficiency.

DIAGNOSTIC TESTS & INTERPRETATION

- No single test identifies all the causes of microcytic anemia. Children are often identified through routine screening at well-child exams.
- CBC: low hemoglobin level and low mean corpuscular volume for age (lower limit of normal can be estimated by 70+ age in years)
  - Red cell distribution width (RDW) is increased in IDA and normal in thalassemia.
  - RBC count is elevated in thalassemia. Mentzer index: MCV/RBC count in millions: $<$13 points, toward thalassemia; $>$13 points, toward IDA
  - Reticulocyte count: reticulocytopenia in IDA, reticulocytosis in hemoglobinopathies
  - Thrombocytosis is often seen in IDA (can appear prior to microcytosis). In severe, prolonged iron deficiency, thrombocytopenia eventually develops.
  - Peripheral blood smear
    - Hypochromia and bizarre forms in IDA
    - Target cells are seen in patients with thalassemia.
    - Basophilic stippling with lead poisoning

- Iron studies: Ferritin, serum iron, transferrin saturation, and TIBC must be interpreted together. In the face of iron deficiency, the body's iron stores are first mobilized. It is only once these iron stores are depleted that microcytosis develops.
  - Ferritin
    - Decreased in iron deficiency
    - Most sensitive index for iron deficiency. A ferritin of less than 30 is over 90% sensitive and specific for IDA.
    - As a measure of iron stores in the liver, it is one of the earliest indices to change in IDA.
    - May be elevated out of proportion to iron stores because it is an acute-phase reactant and will rise with infection, inflammation, malignancy, or liver disease
    - Can be increased in patients with thalassemia who have not received transfusion because ineffective erythropoiesis leads to increased GI absorption of iron
  - Serum iron
    - Measures transferrin-associated ferric iron and fluctuates with daily iron intake
    - Normal in thalassemia (unless chronically transfused, which leads to increased iron levels)
    - Normal or reduced in infection or inflammatory states
  - TIBC
    - Elevated in IDA but can be normal to decreased in anemia of chronic disease
    - Oral contraceptives can increase TIBC.
    - Liver disease and malnutrition can decrease TIBC.
  - Transferrin saturation
    - Calculated value (serum iron/TIBC × 100)
    - Low in IDA
  - Soluble transferrin receptor
    - Newer test used to determine iron status. It is increased in iron deficiency anemia and also in thalassemia syndromes but not with the anemia of chronic disease.
    - Unlike ferritin, it is not an acute phase reactant and does not increase with inflammation or infection.
    - Should not be used routinely in patients in the evaluation of IDA but only in patients with other illnesses that make the interpretation of ferritin levels difficult
- Lead level and free erythrocyte protoporphyrin (FEP) are both elevated in lead intoxication. Lead poisoning and IDA can exist together.
- Hemoglobin electrophoresis with quantitation

ALERT
Results of hemoglobin electrophoresis are only reliable in patients with normal iron stores. If patients have abnormal iron studies, repeat hemoglobin electrophoresis after adequate period of iron supplementation.

  - Decreased hemoglobin A and increased hemoglobin A2 in beta-thalassemia trait
  - Normal hemoglobin electrophoresis in patients with one (silent carrier) and two (trait) alpha-globin thalassemic mutations
  - Hemoglobin H consists of tetramers of beta globin chains and is seen in patients with three alpha-globin mutations.
- If a patient has been transfused or labs cannot be drawn, labs on the parents may be helpful. A CBC, peripheral smear, and a hemoglobin electrophoresis are usually sufficient.

Diagnostic Procedures/Other
- Bone marrow aspirate is rarely indicated but can be performed if malignancy or disorders of heme synthesis are in the differential.
- Recurrent iron deficiency despite treatment raises suspicion for ongoing blood loss. Hemoccult stools to look for occult GI bleeding, common in children with milk protein allergy. Urinalysis for evidence of renal RBC loss. Pulmonary hemosiderosis can present as recurrent pneumonias.

DIFFERENTIAL DIAGNOSIS
- Iron deficiency
- Hemoglobinopathies
- Chronic lead poisoning
- Anemia of chronic disease
- Sideroblastic anemia

TREATMENT

MEDICATION
- Ferrous sulfate or ferrous gluconate at 6 mg/kg of elemental iron per day in divided doses. Iron salts should be taken with orange juice, as ascorbic acid increases absorption. It should NOT be taken with milk. Milk intake should be stopped completely. Patients on proton pump inhibitors may have decreased absorption.
- Intravenous iron is reserved for patients with malabsorption. Iron sucrose, ferric gluconate, and iron dextran are available in the United States. Anaphylaxis is the primary adverse reaction; iron sucrose and ferric gluconate have lower rates of anaphylaxis.

GENERAL MEASURES
- Many patients are identified on routine well-child screening. Consider therapeutic trial of iron supplementation without further workup if history is suspicious.
- Oral iron supplementation and altered dietary practices improves anemia in almost all patients.
- Parents should be able to report seeing dark black iron in the stool. Iron can cause nausea, GI discomfort, and constipation. Stool softeners can help.
- Transfusion of RBCs is rarely indicated and is only needed in patients with cardiovascular instability.
- Treatment of lead intoxication is achieved through chelation and removal of environmental exposures.
- In patients with microcytic anemia from hemoglobinopathies, but normal iron indices, iron therapy is not indicated.

ONGOING CARE

FOLLOW-UP RECOMMENDATIONS
- Repeat laboratory evaluation can be done in 1 month. Reticulocyte count is the first laboratory value to change and begins to increase within a week after the initiation of iron therapy. Hemoglobin levels take at least 2–3 weeks to respond. MCV is the last index to improve.
- Poor adherence to therapy is the most common cause of treatment failure.
- Children with IDA are more likely to have more difficulties with learning and behavioral problems.
- Children with other hemoglobinopathies should be referred to a hematologist. They do not need further treatment with iron.

ADDITIONAL READING

- Higgs DR, Engel JD, Stamatoyannopoulos G. Thalassemia. *Lancet*. 2012;379(9813):373–383.
- Janus J, Moerschel SK. Evaluation of anemia in children. *Am Fam Physician*. 2010;81(12):1462–1471.
- McCann JC, Ames BN. An overview of evidence for a causal relation between iron deficiency during development and deficits in cognitive or behavioral function. *Am J Clin Nutr*. 2007;85(4):931–945.
- Walters MC, Abelson HT. Interpretation of the complete blood count. *Pediatr Clin North Am*. 1996;43(3):599–622.
- Wang B, Zhan S, Gong T, et al. Iron therapy for improving psychomotor development and cognitive function in children under the age of three with iron deficiency anemia. *Cochrane Database Syst Rev*. 2013;6:CD001444.

CODES

ICD10
- D50.9 Iron deficiency anemia, unspecified
- D58.2 Other hemoglobinopathies
- D50.8 Other iron deficiency anemias

MILIA

Jennifer DiPace • Brooke I. Siegel

BASICS

DESCRIPTION

- Common benign, keratin-filled cysts that present as white pinpoint papules most typically on the face but may occur elsewhere on the body (palate, gingiva, penis)
- Subtypes include primary and secondary milia.
  - Primary: spontaneous
  - Secondary: secondary to trauma, medications, or another disease
- Milia en plaque—rare type of primary milia which typically occurs in the posterior auricular area as an erythematous plaque

EPIDEMIOLOGY

- Congenital milia is the most common form of primary milia.
  - Approx. 40% of newborns have milia.
  - Less common in premature infants
  - No gender or racial predilection
- Secondary milia can occur in all age groups.

RISK FACTORS

- Full-term newborns
- Any bullous condition increases the risk of secondary milia, particularly epidermolysis bullosa and porphyria.

GENETICS

- No known genetic predisposition for primary congenital milia, the most common type of milia encountered in pediatrics
- Milia may be a major feature of rare genetic diseases of the skin (Loeys-Dietz syndrome, oral-facial-digital syndrome type 1, Rombo syndrome, or Bazex-Dupré-Christol syndrome).

GENERAL PREVENTION

There are no known preventative measures for primary milia.

PATHOPHYSIOLOGY

Retention of keratin and sebaceous material within the pilosebaceous duct, eccrine sweat duct, or sebaceous collar surrounding fine vellus hair

ETIOLOGY

- Most commonly spontaneous in newborns
- May be related to trauma or blistering conditions in older children

DIAGNOSIS

HISTORY

- Primary congenital milia
  - Asymptomatic
  - Typically present at birth or in the first few days of life
- Secondary milia
  - Recent trauma or burns
  - History of blistering diseases

PHYSICAL EXAM

- 1–2 mm pinpoint, white, pearly smooth papules without surrounding erythema or inflammation
- Distribution is most often on nose, cheeks, chin, and forehead in congenital milia.
- Other places to consider
  - Oral mucosa: Epstein pearls on midline palate, Bohn nodules at gum margins
  - Glans penis cysts

DIAGNOSTIC TESTS & INTERPRETATION

Diagnostic Procedures/Other

The diagnosis of milia can be made by history and physical exam alone. No further diagnostic testing is needed.

DIFFERENTIAL DIAGNOSIS

Other considerations in the newborn period are as follows:

- Sebaceous gland hyperplasia: secondary to exposure to maternal hormones. Lesions are yellowish, follicular papules typically on nose, cheeks, upper lip, and forehead.
- Neonatal acne: inflammatory, erythematous, papulopustular rash on the face and scalp; usually appears after 1–2 weeks of life, although it may be present at birth
- Erythema toxicum: benign rash in the neonatal period. It is characterized by erythematous macules, often with a central pustule or vesicle.

TREATMENT

- Primary congenital milia require no treatment. Milia are benign, asymptomatic, and self-limiting in this condition.
- Treatment may be indicated in the following settings:
  - Diffuse or persistent milia in older children
  - Milia in areas of trauma or burn leading to cosmetic concern
- Treatment could include topical retinoid or manual extraction.

ONGOING CARE

FOLLOW-UP RECOMMENDATIONS

No specific monitoring or follow-up is necessary in congenital milia.

PROGNOSIS

- Natural history of primary congenital milia is that the majority of cases will resolve spontaneously within 2–4 weeks without scarring or recurrence.
- In infants or children with diffuse or persistent milia, consider further evaluation for genodermatoses. Such conditions include Loeys-Dietz syndrome, oral-facial-digital syndrome type 1, Rombo syndrome, or Bazex-Dupré-Christol syndrome.

COMPLICATIONS

Cosmetic concerns based on location of milia are usually the only complicating factor.

ADDITIONAL READING

- Berk DR, Bayliss SJ. Milia: a review and classification. *J Am Acad Dermatol*. 2008;59(6):1050–1063.
- Leong T, Torres A, Macknet KD Jr, et al. Pronounced secondary milia precipitated by a superficial traumatic abrasion in a 4-year-old boy. *J Pediatr*. 2010;156(5):854.
- Link to images
  - Aby J. Photo gallery, professional education. Stanford School of Medicine Newborn Nursery at Lucille Packard Children's Hospital Web site. http://newborns.stanford.edu/PhotoGallery/Milia1.html. Published 2013. Accessed February 14, 2015.

CODES

ICD10

- L70.2 Acne varioliformis
- L85.1 Acquired keratosis [keratoderma] palmaris et plantaris
- K09.8 Other cysts of oral region, not elsewhere classified

FAQ

- Q: Are milia painful or pruritic?
- A: No. Milia are asymptomatic. If there is pain, pruritus, fever, or other constitutional symptoms, the diagnosis of milia should be reconsidered.
- Q: Are milia contagious?
- A: No, they are not transmitted from person to person. In the case of congenital milia of the newborn, the parent should be reassured that the lesions are not infectious.
- Q: Are milia and miliaria the same condition?
- A: No. Both are benign skin conditions of childhood. However, miliaria is a disorder of the eccrine sweat glands, not of the pilosebaceous duct. Miliaria is characterized by sweat retention and subsequent vesicle formation, usually after prolonged perspiration. Miliaria is thought to occur because of sweat duct obstruction.

MULTICYSTIC DYSPLASTIC KIDNEY

Kelly A. Benedict • Paul Brakeman

BASICS

DESCRIPTION
- Multicystic dysplastic kidney disease (MCDK) is the most severe type of cystic renal dysplasia and is characterized by multiple, noncommunicating cysts which are divided by dysplastic tissue.
- In general, there is no functioning renal tissue in a multicystic dysplastic kidney.
- Involutes over time (usually within the first 5 years)

EPIDEMIOLOGY
- Incidence is 0.3–1 in 1,000 live births.
  - Most cases are detected antenatally.
- Affects boys > girls
- Left kidney > right kidney
  - Usually unilateral but can be bilateral

PATHOPHYSIOLOGY
- Initial growth of the ureteric bud is normal, but renal development halts at a later stage.
- Histology shows disordered renal tissue with areas of undifferentiated mesenchymal cells, abnormal differentiation (i.e., cartilage), rare nephrons

COMMONLY ASSOCIATED CONDITIONS
- Associated anomalies of contralateral GU tract include the following:
  - Vesicoureteral reflux, most common, occurs in ~25%
  - Renal hypoplasia
  - Ureterocele
  - Ureteropelvic junction (UPJ) obstruction
  - Genital anomalies

DIAGNOSIS

HISTORY
Commonly diagnosed by antenatal ultrasound

PHYSICAL EXAM
- Blood pressure at each visit to monitor for hypertension
- Evaluate height and weight
- Neonates: Palpable flank mass may be present.

DIAGNOSTIC TESTS & INTERPRETATION

Lab
- Creatinine
  - If unilateral kidney is normal, serum creatinine should be normal.
  - One strategy is to monitor serum creatinine at 1 month, 18 months, 5 years, and when growth complete to detect reduced function in remaining kidney.
- Urinalysis to check for proteinuria to evaluate for hyperfiltration in remaining kidney.
- Urinalysis and urine culture, if the patient has any symptoms of UTI or unexplained fever

Imaging
- Renal ultrasound
  - To confirm diagnosis of MCDK and evaluate the contralateral kidney
  - Usually no detectable Doppler flow
  - Useful to follow involution of MCDK and hypertrophy of contralateral kidney
  - 50% will have complete involution by 5 years.
  - Should be done after birth and at 1 month, 2 years, 5 years, and 10 years of life
- Voiding cystourethrogram (VCUG)
  - To evaluate for urinary reflux is controversial.
  - Although rate of VUR is high, most is low-grade and would not require prophylactic antibiotics.
  - Patients with febrile UTI should have a VCUG.
- Mercaptoacetyl-triglycine (Mag3) scan
  - To confirm diagnosis and rule out a kidney with severe hydronephrosis

DIFFERENTIAL DIAGNOSIS
Hydronephrotic kidney with poor function

ALERT
If contralateral kidney is abnormal, renal function should be evaluated, and the patient requires ongoing nephrology follow-up.

TREATMENT

MEDICATION
Occasionally, these patients may require antihypertensive medication, an ACE-inhibitor for proteinuria, or urologic evaluation if they suffer from severe VUR or recurrent UTI.

GENERAL MEASURES
- No specific treatment is needed for MCDK.
- Previously, nephrectomy was treatment of choice; however, given low risk of hypertension and malignancy, currently, routine nephrectomy of MCDK is not recommended.

ONGOING CARE

FOLLOW-UP RECOMMENDATIONS

- Blood pressure monitoring
  - Anecdotally, these patients were thought to be at risk for hypertension.
  - However, more recent studies show no increased risk.
- Patients may be at increased risk for developing Wilms tumor in MCDK.
  - Risk 3–10 per 10,000
  - Monitored with periodic renal ultrasound and abdominal exam
- Periodic urinalysis to evaluate for proteinuria and serum Cr to monitor renal function

PROGNOSIS

- Patients with contralateral anomalies are at greater risk for developing chronic kidney disease (CKD).
- Patients with normal contralateral kidneys may have hyperfiltration (~30%) and proteinuria (~10%).
- Risk of developing Wilms tumor
  - May be as high as 3–10 times higher than the general population (1 in 10,000)
  - This estimate is controversial, however, as a systematic review of 1,041 children with unilateral MCDK found no cases of Wilms tumor

ADDITIONAL READING

- Aslam M, Watson AR. Unilateral multicystic dysplastic kidney: long term outcomes. *Arch Dis Child*. 2006;91(10):820–823.
- Mansoor O, Chandar J, Rodriguez M, et al. Long-term risk of chronic kidney disease in unilateral multicystic dysplastic kidney. *Pediatr Nephrol*. 2011;26(4):597–603.
- Onal B, Kogan B. Natural history of patients with multicystic dysplastic kidney—what follow-up is needed? *J Urol*. 2006;176(4, Pt 1):1607–1611.
- Weinstein A, Goodman TR, Iragorri S. Simple multicystic dysplastic kidney disease: end points for subspecialty follow-up. *Pediatr Nephrol*. 2008;23(1):111–116.

CODES

ICD10

- Q61.4 Renal dysplasia
- Q61.3 Polycystic kidney, unspecified

FAQ

- Q: What can be done to preserve contralateral renal function?
- A: Well-controlled blood pressure, treatment of proteinuria, and quick treatment of UTI may decrease the progression of CKD.
- Q: Are patients with MCDK at an increased risk for developing a UTI?
- A: No. Risk of UTI is ~5%, consistent with general pediatric population. However, if a patient with MCDK has a febrile UTI, a VCUG is recommended to evaluate for VUR.
- Q: Can patients with unilateral MCDK live a normal life?
- A: Yes, if the contralateral kidney is normal. Patients should be encouraged to live a healthy lifestyle. If the patient has hypertension or diabetes, they should be tightly controlled.
- Q: How is this different than polycystic kidney disease?
- A: Polycystic kidney disease (PKD) tends to affect both kidneys and is a progressive disorder. Infants with PKD have relatively normal kidneys at birth and cystic disease develops over time. MCDK is not progressive and usually affects one kidney. PKD is an inherited condition, whereas MCDK is usually not inherited.

M

MUMPS/PAROTITIS

Kathleen Gutierrez

BASICS

DESCRIPTION

Centers for Disease Control and Prevention (CDC) clinical case definition for mumps: illness with acute onset of unilateral or bilateral, tender, self-limited swelling of the parotid or other salivary gland, lasting ≥2 days, without other apparent cause

EPIDEMIOLOGY

Incidence

- In the prevaccine era, 90% of all children contracted mumps virus infection by 14 years of age.
- Incidence of this once very common disease has declined dramatically since the advent of universal childhood immunization.
- Outbreaks, however, continue to occur.
- 200–300 cases per year reported in the United States since 2001
- In early 2006, a large epidemic broke out in Iowa and neighboring states:
  - 11 states reported >2,500 cases.
  - Largest epidemic since 1988
  - Median age of patient was 21 years (mostly college students)
  - Led CDC and American College Health Association to recommend 2 doses of MMR vaccine to be a requirement for college entry
- In 2006, 81–100% of children entering United States schools had received 2 doses of mumps vaccine.
- In 2009–2010, an outbreak of mumps occurred in a highly vaccinated population in the northeastern United States. Intense exposure facilitated transmission. Previous vaccination appeared to limit the severity of disease.
- Seroprevalence of antibody to mumps virus in the United States population (1999–2004) is estimated at 90%.

GENERAL PREVENTION

- 2 combination mumps vaccine are used:
  - MMR: Measles, mumps, rubella
  - MMRV: Measles, mumps, rubella, varicella
- A single 0.5-mL SC injection of live mumps vaccine (MMR or MMRV) is recommended at 12–15 months.
- A second vaccination is recommended between 4 and 6 years of age.
- The efficacy of 2 doses of vaccines is estimated at approximately 80–90%.
- Primary vaccine failure and waning vaccine-induced immunity have been reported.
- Some have suggested the need for a 3rd vaccination to mitigate waning immunity. Preliminary studies indicate no increase in adverse effects after a 3rd vaccination.
- The 1st dose of MMR vaccine sometimes causes fever and rash:
  - These symptoms occur 7–12 days after immunization.
  - Measles component is usually the culprit.
- Both MMRV and MMR vaccines, but not varicella vaccine alone, are associated with increased outpatient fever visits and seizures 5–12 days after vaccination in 12- to 23-month-olds, with MMRV vaccine increasing fever and seizure twice as much as the MMR + varicella vaccine.
- Vaccine should not be administered to children who are immunocompromised by disease or pharmacotherapy, as well as to pregnant women.
- If a child has recently received immune globulin, administration of MMR vaccine should be delayed (for 3–11 months depending on the dose of IG).
- Children with HIV infection who are not severely immunocompromised should be immunized with the MMR vaccine.
- 1 attack of mumps (clinical or subclinical) usually confers lifelong immunity.
- Links of the MMR vaccine to autism by Andrew Wakefield MB, BS in a 1998 *Lancet* publication have now been exposed as fraudulent.

PATHOPHYSIOLOGY

- The virus is spread by contact with respiratory secretions.
- The mumps virus enters via the respiratory tract, and a viremia ultimately ensues.
- The virus spreads to many organs, including the salivary glands, gonads, pancreas, and meninges.
- Period of communicability: 7 days before to 9 days after onset of parotid swelling
- Most communicable period: 2–3 days before to 5 days after onset of parotid swelling
- Incubation period: 12–25 days after exposure
- Humans are the only known host for mumps.

ETIOLOGY

- Epidemic parotitis is caused by mumps, an RNA virus in the Paramyxoviridae family.
- Other viral causes of parotitis include Epstein-Barr virus, cytomegaloviruses, influenza, parainfluenza, and enteroviruses
- Parotid enlargement can be an initial sign in HIV-infected children.
- Bacterial cases are usually secondary to *Staphylococcus aureus* (suppurative parotitis).
- Streptococci, gram-negative bacilli, and anaerobic infections are also possible.
- Rare childhood cases may be secondary to an obstructing calculus, foreign body (sesame seed), tumors, sarcoid, Sjögren syndrome, or various drugs (antihistamines, phenothiazines, iodine-containing drugs/contrast media).

COMMONLY ASSOCIATED CONDITIONS

- Salivary adenitis
  - Most common manifestation of mumps
  - 1/3 of cases occur subclinically
- Epididymoorchitis
  - Up to 35% of adolescent mumps cases are complicated by orchitis.
  - Orchitis develops within 4–10 days of the onset of the parotid swelling.
  - Sterility is uncommon.
- Aseptic meningitis
- Pancreatitis
  - Mild inflammation is common.
  - Serious involvement is rare.

DIAGNOSIS

HISTORY

- Prodromal symptoms uncommon but may include the following:
  - Fever
  - Anorexia
  - Myalgia
  - Headache
- Onset usually pain and swelling in front of and below ear
- Swelling
  - Usually starts on one side of the face, then progresses to the other
- Mild fever
  - Usually accompanies parotid swelling
- Dysphagia and dysphonia are common.
- Testicular pain and swelling, along with constitutional symptoms, occurs in postpubertal males usually 1 week after parotid swelling but occasionally simultaneously or alone.
- Epigastric pain and constitutional symptoms with pancreatic involvement
- Fever, headache, and stiff neck with meningitis
- Behavioral changes, seizures, and other neurologic abnormalities are rare.
- Other symptoms are analogous to the particular organ involved.

PHYSICAL EXAM

- Nonerythematous, tender parotid swelling (erythema seen with suppurative parotitis)
- Swelling ultimately obscures the mandibular ramus.
- The ear is displaced upward and outward.
- Importantly, up to 30% of symptomatic cases of mumps are not associated with parotitis.
- Submaxillary and sublingual glands also may be swollen.
- Inflammation may be noted intraorally at the orifice of Stensen duct.
- Presternal edema is occasionally noted.
- Mumps are infrequently associated with truncal rash.
- Tender, edematous testicle in mumps orchitis (usually unilateral)
- Ask the patient if the pain (at the parotid) intensifies with the tasting of sour liquids:
  - Have the patient suck on a lemon drop or lemon juice, and note any discharge from Stensen duct.

DIAGNOSTIC TESTS & INTERPRETATION

Lab

- Uncomplicated parotitis
  - Mild leukopenia with lymphocytosis
- Suppurative parotitis and mumps orchitis
  - Leukocytosis
- Pancreatic involvement
  - Hyperamylasemia and elevated serum lipase
- Salivary adenitis without pancreatic involvement
  - Isolated hyperamylasemia
- Gram stain and culture of pus expressed from Stensen duct is diagnostic in suppurative parotitis.
- CDC lab criteria for mumps diagnosis
  - Isolation of mumps virus from clinical specimens: blood, urine, buccal swab (Stensen duct exudates), throat washing, saliva, or CSF
  - Detection of mumps virus nucleic acid by reverse transcriptase PCR
  - Obtain specimens for culture and PCR as soon as possible after onset of symptoms, particularly in vaccinated individuals.
  - Positive serologic test for mumps IgM

ALERT
Mumps IgM may be negative in MMR-vaccinated individuals who develop mumps disease. A negative IgM test in these patients does not rule out mumps.

  - Significant rise between acute and convalescent titers in mumps IgG levels by any standard assay (complement fixation, neutralization, hemagglutination inhibition, or enzyme immunoassays)

ALERT
Paired acute and convalescent serum titers may not show a rise in IgG levels in MMR-vaccinated individuals with mumps disease.

  - For detailed information regarding collection and interpretation of laboratory studies and mumps case reporting, see http://www.cdc.gov/mumps/.

Imaging

Sialography is useful to evaluate for stones or strictures but is contraindicated in acute infection.

Diagnostic Procedures/Other

Lumbar puncture if meningitis is suspected: CSF pleocytosis (predominately mononuclear)

DIFFERENTIAL DIAGNOSIS

- Mumps parotitis can be distinguished from the other viral causes by clinical presentation along with specialized laboratory studies.
- Cases of tuberculous and nontuberculous (atypical) mycobacterial parotitis are rare but have been reported.
- Salivary calculus can be diagnosed by sialogram.
- Recurrent childhood parotitis, also known as juvenile recurrent parotitis
  - Rare, recurrent swelling of parotids
  - Seen in children 3–6 years old
  - Not associated with suppuration or external inflammatory changes
  - Largely a diagnosis of exclusion
- Cervical or preauricular adenitis
  - May simulate parotitis
  - Close anatomic localization should be diagnostic.
- Infectious mononucleosis and cat-scratch disease are other considerations.
- Drug-induced parotid enlargement occasionally occurs.
- Malignancies of the parotid are extremely rare.
- Sjögren syndrome is rare but reported in children.
- Pneumoparotitis is seen in those with a history of playing a wind instrument, glass blowing, scuba diving, and even general anesthesia.

TREATMENT

GENERAL MEASURES

- Supportive therapy is all that is required in mumps parotitis.
- Antibiotics directed against *S. aureus* should be used in cases of suppurative parotitis.

ONGOING CARE

FOLLOW-UP RECOMMENDATIONS

- Most children have resolution of glandular swelling by ~1 week.
- Disappearance of testicular pain and swelling can be expected 4–6 days after onset.
- Testicular atrophy is common, although infertility is rare.
- Markedly elevated pancreatic enzymes should be monitored until they improve.
- Children should not return to school until at least 5 days after the onset of parotid swelling.
- Isolation: standard precautions; droplet precautions for 5 days after onset of parotid swelling

PROGNOSIS

Complete recovery in 1–2 weeks is the rule.

COMPLICATIONS

- Meningitis
  - >50% have a CSF pleocytosis.
  - This "aseptic meningitis" is usually benign.
- Encephalitis: rarely causes permanent sequelae
- Cerebellitis
- Facial nerve palsy
- Oophoritis, nephritis, thyroiditis, myocarditis, mastitis, arthritis, transient ocular involvement, deafness, and sterility (all rare)

ADDITIONAL READING

- American Academy of Pediatrics. Mumps. In: Pickering LK, ed. *2012 Red Book: Report of the Committee on Infectious Diseases*. 29th ed. Elk Grove Village, IL: American Academy of Pediatrics; 2012:514–518.
- Barskey AE, Schulte C, Rosen JB, et al. Mumps outbreak in Orthodox Jewish communities in the United States. *N Engl J Med*. 2012;367(18):1704–1713.
- Brauser D. Autism and MMR vaccine study: an "elaborate fraud," charges BMJ. Medscape Web site. http://www.medscape.com/viewarticle/735354. Published January 6, 2011. Accessed March 11, 2015.
- Centers for Disease Control and Prevention. Update: multistate outbreak of mumps—United States, Jan 1–May 2, 2006. *MMWR Morb Mortal Wkly Rep*. 2006;55(20):559–563.
- Klein NP, Fireman B, Yih WK, et al. Measles-mumps-rubella-varicella combination vaccine and the risk of febrile seizures. *Pediatrics*. 2010;126(1):e1–e8.
- Kutty PK, Kruszon-Moran DM, Dayan GH, et al. Seroprevalence of antibody to mumps virus in the US population, 1999–2004. *J Infect Dis*. 2010;202(5):667–674.
- MacDonald N, Hatchette T, Elkout L, et al. Mumps is back: why is mumps eradication not working? *Adv Exp Med Biol*. 2011;697:197–220.
- Offit PA. Autism and the MMR vaccine, revisited. Medscape Web site. http://www.medscape.com/viewarticle/735439?src=ptalk. Published January 7, 2011. Accessed March 11, 2015.
- Quinlisk MP. Mumps control today. *J Infect Dis*. 2010;202(5):655–656. doi:10.1086/655395.
- Senanayake SN. Mumps in the United States. *N Engl J Med*. 2008;359(6):654.
- Shacham R, Droma EB, London D, et al. Long-term experience with endoscopic diagnosis and treatment of juvenile recurrent parotitis. *J Oral Maxillofac Surg*. 2009;67(1):162–167.
- Virtanen M, Peltola H, Paunio M, et al. Day to day reactogenicity and the healthy vaccinee effect of measles-mumps-rubella vaccination. *Pediatrics*. 2000;106(5):E62.

CODES

ICD10

- B26.9 Mumps without complication
- B26.89 Other mumps complications
- B26.0 Mumps orchitis

FAQ

- Q: Should immunization be deferred in children with intercurrent illness?
- A: No. Children with minor illnesses, even with fever, should be vaccinated.
- Q: Should vaccination be withheld in children living with immunocompromised hosts?
- A: No. Vaccinated children do not transmit mumps vaccine virus.

MUNCHAUSEN SYNDROME BY PROXY (CHILD ABUSE IN THE MEDICAL SETTING)

John Stirling

BASICS

DESCRIPTION

- Symptoms of illness in a child that are exaggerated, fabricated, or induced by a caretaker. There is usually no underlying health disorder in the child.
- Results in harm to the child victim through repeated interactions with the medical care system, including unnecessary tests, medications, and surgeries
- Known by many names, including the following:
  - "Pediatric condition falsification"
  - "Caregiver-fabricated illness"
  - "Medical child abuse"
  - "Factitious disorder by proxy"
- All refer to harm that befalls children through the actions of a caregiver in a medical setting.
- Symptoms decrease when the child is separated from the perpetrator.

EPIDEMIOLOGY

- Rare, with no typical presentation. The most commonly described symptoms include apnea, seizures, factitious fevers, feeding and GI problems, failure to thrive, behavioral problems, bleeding, and sepsis.
- Presenting symptoms may present along a spectrum of severity from mild to fatal.
- Most victims are <4 years of age, but victims may often be older children.
- Males and females are equally represented.
- Symptoms may be present for years before factitious illness is considered and diagnosed.
- Morbidity is significant; cases may be fatal, especially those involving surreptitious administration of medications, poisoning, or inducing apnea.

ETIOLOGY

- The parent, most commonly the mother, exaggerates, fabricates, or induces the illnesses.
- The term Munchausen syndrome by proxy refers to specific instances where the caregiver is motivated by a desire for self-aggrandizement. As such, it only defines a subset of factitious illnesses.
- Medical providers are advised to concentrate on the specific harm done and the patient's safety rather than on the caregiver's motives.

DIAGNOSIS

HISTORY

Factitious illness should be considered when

- Symptoms and signs described are incongruous with patient's appearance or are seen only when the caregiver is present.
- Diagnostic tests fail to confirm the diagnosis.
- Usual medical treatment is ineffective in alleviating the presenting symptom.
- Caregiver seems unusually knowledgeable or aggressive in suggesting particular medical interventions.
- "Red flags":
  - Frequent moves
  - Siblings who have either died or had unusual medical illnesses
  - Seeking care at a variety of facilities
  - Reluctance to accept less severe diagnoses

PHYSICAL EXAM

- Examinations are usually normal.
- When symptoms have been exaggerated, findings are less than expected (e.g., mild asthma or hyperactive behavior).
- When symptoms have been inflicted, findings are often atypical for the medical condition being considered.
- Failure to thrive or obesity are common.
- Patient may have evidence of additional injuries, including old fractures or scars.

DIAGNOSTIC TESTS & INTERPRETATION

Diagnostic Procedures/Other

- Workup is dictated by the presenting complaint: EEG for seizures, cardiac monitors for syncope, pneumogram for apnea, etc.
- When the workup is consistently normal and symptoms are still described, the differential diagnosis should include factitious disorders.
- If bleeding is the major presentation, identify the blood as the patient's (as opposed to that of the perpetrator or an animal).
- A toxicology screen may be helpful for unusual presentations of poisoning.
- Repeated blood or urine cultures with multiple organisms suggest intentional contamination of the specimen or of the patient.
- Special care must be taken to prevent the caregiver from tampering with diagnostic testing.
- If separating the perpetrator from the patient results in disappearance of symptoms, this "test" may suggest the diagnosis.
- Covert video monitoring of a patient's room may demonstrate the perpetrator harming the child.

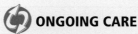

DIFFERENTIAL DIAGNOSIS

Factitious disorders often mimic difficult-to-diagnose diseases:

- Apnea/apparent life-threatening event
- Asthma
- Seizures
- Intermittent fevers
- Genitourinary or GI bleeding
- Unexplained abnormalities in electrolytes
- Feeding problems, chronic diarrhea, or vomiting
- Infections with multiple organisms found in blood or urine culture

ALERT

Diagnosis is often delayed and may take months. There are often impediments:

- Physicians and nursing personnel may be reluctant to suspect the parent because of their own relationship to the family.
- It can be difficult to acknowledge that the child has been harmed by well-intentioned but unnecessary medical procedures or investigations.
- It is often necessary to review records from multiple institutions covering months or years of care. These are often unsuspected and may be difficult to obtain.

TREATMENT

GENERAL MEASURES

- Effective care requires that medical providers work closely with other professionals in the community, both to gather information and to ensure the patient's eventual safety.
- Child protective services, mental health services, and law enforcement agencies each have a role to play. Evaluations must be multidisciplinary.
- A variety of interventions may be appropriate depending on the severity of the presentation, from counseling to foster care to criminal prosecution.

ONGOING CARE

FOLLOW-UP RECOMMENDATIONS

- Long-term follow-up is necessary for both victim and caregiver.
- Watch for recurrence of original presentation, or unusual new symptoms, with special attention to the child's self-image.

PROGNOSIS

- If undiagnosed, morbidity and mortality may be significant.
- Victims are essentially taught to be ill, sometimes with lifelong consequences.
- As there are such diverse presentations, reliable, specific data on long-term morbidity are lacking.

ADDITIONAL READING

- Flaherty E, MacMillin H. Caregiver-fabricated illness in a child: a manifestation of child maltreatment. *Pediatrics*. 2013;132(3):590–597.
- Giurgea I, Ulinski T, Touati G, et al. Factitious hyperinsulinism leading to pancreatectomy: severe forms of Munchausen syndrome by proxy. *Pediatrics*. 2005;116(1):e145–e148.
- Hall DE, Eubanks L, Meyyazhagan LS, et al. Evaluation of covert video surveillance in the diagnosis of Munchausen syndrome by proxy: lessons from 41 cases. *Pediatrics*. 2000;105(6):1305–1312.
- Pankratz L. Persistent problems with the Munchausen syndrome by proxy label. *J Am Acad Psychiatry Law*. 2006;34(1):90–95.
- Roesler TA, Jenny C. *Medical Child Abuse: Beyond Munchausen Syndrome by Proxy*. Elk Grove Village, IL: American Academy of Pediatrics; 2009.
- Schreier H. Munchausen by proxy defined. *Pediatrics*. 2002;110(5):985–988.
- Sheridan MS. The deceit continues: an updated literature review of Munchausen syndrome by proxy. *Child Abuse Negl*. 2003;27(4):431–451.

CODES

ICD10

- F68.12 Factitious disorder w predom physical signs and symptoms
- F68.13 Factitious disord w comb psych and physcl signs and symptoms
- F68.11 Factitious disorder w predom psych signs and symptoms

FAQ

- Q: When should factitious disorders be reported to child abuse authorities?
- A: When there is reasonable suspicion (note: not certainty) that a child is coming to harm due to the actions of a caregiver. When suspicion exists, it is important to involve community agencies in the investigation.
- Q: Is it legal to use video surveillance or to separate the parent from the patient?
- A: Yes, if done properly. When suspicions of factitious illness are high and other laboratory tests are negative, diagnosis may require these measures. Hospital administration and/or risk management should be consulted on how to proceed. Child abuse pediatricians may also provide assistance.

MUSCULAR DYSTROPHIES

Jessica Rose Nance

BASICS

DESCRIPTION

- Muscular dystrophies (MDs) are a heterogeneous group of disorders characterized by a slow degeneration of muscle with consequent weakness and contracture deformity. Cardiac muscle can be involved in some forms.
- MDs with childhood onset can be divided into 5 groups:
  - Dystrophinopathies (i.e., Duchenne MD [DMD], Becker MD [BMD])
  - Limb girdle MDs (LGMDs)
  - Congenital MD (CMD)
  - Facioscapulohumeral MD (FSH-MD)
  - Emery-Dreifuss MD (EDMD)
- Types of MDs can be differentiated by their clinical features (i.e., pattern of muscle weakness, joint contractures), age of onset, genetic test results, and/or muscle biopsy.

EPIDEMIOLOGY

- Dystrophinopathies
  - DMD: 1 per 3,500 boys (most common)
  - BMD: 1 per 30,000 boys
- LGMD (childhood onset): 5–10 per million
- CMD (all types): 1–10 per 100,000
- FSH-MD: 1 per 20,000
- EDMD: 1 per 300,000

RISK FACTOR

Genetics

Genetic testing is clinically available for most MDs:

- Dystrophinopathies (DMD/BMD): X linked
  - DMD exon duplication/deletion in 70% cases
  - DMD point mutation in almost 30% cases
  - New mutations of the dystrophin gene are common, and hence, most cases have no affected relatives despite X-linked recessive inheritance. New mutations in the dystrophin gene are found frequently in the mothers of affected boys.
- LGMD: Most childhood-onset LGMDs are autosomal recessive.
  - Sarcoglycanopathies (LGMD2C–F) make up roughly 70% of childhood-onset LGMDs.
  - LGMD2I (FKRP): 5% childhood-onset LGMDs
- CMD: most autosomal recessive (12 genes)
  - Nonsyndromic (*LAMA2, COL6A1–COL6A3*)
  - Syndromic (e.g., *POMT1, POMGT1, FKRP*)
- FSH-MD: autosomal dominant (*D4Z4* deletion)
- EDMD: X linked (*EMD* or *FHL1* mutations) or autosomal dominant (*LMNA* mutation)

PATHOPHYSIOLOGY

- Deficient or defective muscle fiber proteins causing fiber dysfunction and/or increased membrane fragility
- Muscle biopsy: Increased variability in muscle fiber size (i.e., degenerating, regenerating, and necrotic fibers), split muscle fibers and increased internal nuclei, fibrosis. Immunohistochemistry may note decreased/absent sarcolemmal proteins (e.g., DMD, LGMDs, CMDs).

DIAGNOSIS

HISTORY

- Neonatal hypotonia, feeding difficulty (CMD)
- Gross motor delay/regression
- Global developmental delay (syndromic CMD) or learning disorders (DMD)
- Exercise intolerance/cramping
- Myalgia (BMD, DMD, FSH-MD)
- Seizures: merosin-negative and syndromic CMD
- DMD
  - Onset typically <5 years old with gross motor delays, increasing falls, toe walking, and proximal muscle weakness (e.g., difficulty climbing stairs, rising from floor)
  - Dependence on wheelchair for mobility usually between 8 and 12 years of age
  - Calf pseudohypertrophy is common.
  - Serum creatine kinase (CK) levels are markedly elevated (often >50× normal). Serum transaminases may be elevated (muscle origin).
  - Higher incidence of learning difficulties, ADHD, autism, OCD. Loss of ambulation occurs around 13–16 years old. Incidence of cardiomyopathy increases with age, although respiratory muscle weakness (e.g., ineffective cough, hypoventilation, and eventual respiratory failure) is the cause of death in about 75% of DMD boys.
- BMD
  - Milder version of DMD phenotype; onset typically >8 years old
  - Boys remain ambulatory into their 20s.
  - Higher incidence of myalgia, cramps, and myoglobinuria in BMD (vs. DMD)
  - Rarely, cardiomyopathy may be sole or presenting feature.
- LGMD
  - Proximal muscle weakness (neck flexors, hip flexors, shoulder girdle)
  - Onset and progression highly variable
  - Sarcoglycanopathies (LGMD2C–F) can mimic DMD (including calf pseudohypertrophy).
  - Patients are cognitively normal.
- CMD
  - Hypotonia, gross motor delay, weakness, and feeding difficulty typically noted from birth
  - Two main groups of CMDs: (1) nonsyndromic CMD due to defective structural proteins (e.g., merosin-negative CMD, Ullrich/Bethlem MD) and (2) syndromic CMD due to defective glycosylation (e.g., Fukayama MD, muscle-eye-brain disease, Walker-Warburg syndrome)
    - Most children with nonsyndromic CMD are cognitively normal. Seizures may occur in merosin-negative CMD (20–30%). Ullrich MD shows characteristic proximal contractures and distal joint hyperlaxity (fingers, toes). Bethlem MD shows proximal muscle weakness and distal contractures.
    - Syndromic CMDs show variable severity, often associated with intellectual disability, eye manifestations, and brain anomalies (e.g., neuronal migration disorders, seizures, hydrocephalus).
- FSH-MD
  - Onset typically <20 years old with facial weakness, scapular winging, and humeral (biceps, triceps) weakness
  - Relative sparing of deltoid strength is seen.
  - Rare infantile-onset cases have been reported.
  - Retinal vasculopathy (Coates disease) and sensorineural hearing loss can occur.
  - Cardiac arrhythmia is occasionally noted (<10%).
- EDMD
  - Onset typically in 1st decade
  - Patients initially present with joint contractures (neck, elbow, and ankles) disproportionate to degree of weakness.
  - Muscle weakness and wasting develop in biceps, triceps, spinates muscles, and (later) tibialis anterior and peroneal muscles.
  - Cardiac arrhythmias are common by 2nd decade.
  - Pseudohypertrophy is not seen.

PHYSICAL EXAM

- Facial weakness (FSH-MD)
- Pattern of muscle weakness and atrophy
- Scapular winging (FSH-MD)
- Pattern of joint contractures (EDMD) or joint hypermobility (Ullrich MD)
- Pattern of muscle pseudohypertrophy (e.g., calf muscles in DMD, BMD, LGMD)
- Reflexes normal to mildly decreased (except for joints with contractures). Reflexes are not lost until late in disease course.
- Normal sensory exam
- Scoliosis: rapid progression if nonambulatory
- Gower maneuver (when arising from sitting to standing position, patient must put his hand on his knees and "climb up himself")
- Gait abnormalities (e.g., toe walking, exaggerated lumbar lordosis, Trendelenburg gait)
- Cardiomyopathy (tachycardia, hypotension)
- Respiratory weakness (weak cough)

DIAGNOSTIC TESTS & INTERPRETATION

Lab

- Serum CK
  - Markedly elevated in DMD, BMD, some LGMD, and CMDs (e.g., Fukayama MD)
  - CK may be normal late in disease owing to severe muscle atrophy.
  - CK is typically normal in FSH-MD and some CMDs (e.g., Ullrich MD). Normal to mild CK elevation is seen in EDMD.

Diagnostic Procedures/Other

- Nerve conduction study: Merosin-negative CMD may show mild conduction velocity slowing.
- EMG: nonspecific myopathic changes
- MRI muscle: signal change noted reflecting muscle atrophy and fatty infiltration. May guide site of optimal muscle biopsy. Pattern of muscle involvement maybe helpful in diagnosis.
- MRI brain: Merosin-negative CMD shows diffuse white matter signal abnormalities (typically visible by 6 months old).
- Muscle biopsy can be used to confirm dystrophy (see "Differential Diagnosis"), whereas immunohistochemistry can help in diagnosis of nondystrophic MDs (e.g., LGMD) if DMD genetic testing is normal.

DIFFERENTIAL DIAGNOSIS
- Inflammatory myopathy (e.g., dermatomyositis)
- Metabolic myopathy
- Congenital myopathy
- Anterior horn cell disease (e.g., SMA)
- Polyneuropathy (e.g., CIDP)
- Myotonic dystrophy (different pathology)

TREATMENT

MEDICATION
- Early attention should be directed to prevention of deformity that encumbers function with weakness and prevention of obesity.
- For DMD: Corticosteroids (prednisone [0.75 mg/kg/day] or deflazacort) 0.9 mg/kg/day: Improve muscle strength, prolong independent ambulation (mean = 2.5 years), delay onset of cardiomyopathy and scoliosis, and improve pulmonary function testing. Patients must be monitored for adverse effects of steroid therapy (weight gain, bone demineralization, behavior issues).
- All other MDs: no treatment

ADDITIONAL TREATMENT
General Measures
- Supportive care (e.g., routine immunizations)
- Psychological and/or school support
- Night splinting (DMD, LGMD) to prevent progression of joint contractures
- Physiotherapy: passive stretching
- Orthopedic evaluation: scoliosis surveillance and/or management of joint contractures
- Genetic counseling
- Ophthalmology (retinal) evaluation (FSH-MD), cataract surveillance (DMD patients on steroids)

ADDITIONAL THERAPIES
Several potential therapies for DMD are being studied (e.g., antisense oligonucleotide therapy, DMD nonsense mutation read-through therapy, myostatin inhibitor therapy, stem cell therapy). These therapies remain experimental and are not commercially available in North America or Europe.

ONGOING CARE

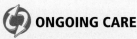

FOLLOW-UP RECOMMENDATIONS
Patient Monitoring
- Respiratory surveillance
  - Baseline pulmonary evaluation (DMD, CMD) with periodic PFT surveillance, incentive spirometry, and/or cough assist devices
  - Monitor for decline in PFT scores (especially FVC) and/or clinical evidence of nocturnal hypoventilation (e.g., morning headache/nausea, daytime somnolence, orthopnea). If noted, obtain sleep study to evaluate for potential need for nocturnal bilevel positive airway pressure (BiPAP).
  - Monitor kyphoscoliosis.
- Orthopedic surveillance
  - When progressive scoliosis is evident, treatment with spinal fusion is indicated to prevent deteriorating quality of life associated with severe deformity.
  - Following loss of ambulation in DMD, affected boys are at high risk for progressive, collapse-type scoliosis and should be screened at 6–12-month intervals until young adult years.
- Cardiology surveillance
  - Cardiomyopathy is well documented for many MDs, necessitating periodic echocardiogram and ECG surveillance studies for DMD, BMD, LGMD1B, LGMD2C–F (20–30% risk), LGMD2I (30–60% risk), merosin-negative CMD, and EDMD.
  - American Academy of Pediatrics (AAP) guidelines recommend DMD patients receive complete cardiac evaluation every 2 years (until age 10 years) and annually thereafter.
  - Cardiac arrhythmia surveillance is required for EDMD, LGMD1B, and FSH-MD (<10% risk); also consider for any MD patient showing echocardiogram evidence of a cardiomyopathy.
  - Cardiac transplantation should be considered for BMD patients with severe cardiomyopathy, particularly if they have relatively minor skeletal muscle involvement.

PROGNOSIS
- DMD: life expectancy into late 20s, death typically from respiratory failure. Life expectancy is improving with advances in care and realistic hope for specific therapies (fueled by these advances).
- BMD: life expectancy into mid-40s, death typically due to cardiomyopathy
- LGMD: variable. Sarcoglycanopathies may show a DMD-like progression. Autosomal dominant LGMD later onset with slow progression
- FSH-MD: Normal life expectancy

ADDITIONAL READING

- American Academy of Pediatrics. Cardiovascular health supervision for individuals affected by Duchenne or Becker muscular dystrophy. *Pediatrics*. 2005;116(6):1569–1573.
- Bonnemann CG. Limb-girdle muscular dystrophy in childhood. *Pediatr Ann*. 2005;34(7):569–577.
- Bönnemann CG, Wang CH, Quijano-Roy S, et al. Diagnostic approach to the congenital muscular dystrophies. *Neuromuscul Disord*. 2014;24(4):289–311.
- Bushby K, Finkel R, Birnkrant DJ, et al. Diagnosis and management of Duchenne muscular dystrophy, part 1: diagnosis, pharmacological and psychosocial management. *Lancet Neurol*. 2010;9(1):77–93.
- Bushby K, Finkel R, Birnkrant DJ, et al. Diagnosis and management of Duchenne muscular dystrophy, part 2: implementation of multidisciplinary care. *Lancet Neurol*. 2010;9(2):177–189.
- El-Bohy A, Wong B. Muscular dystrophies. *Pediatr Ann*. 2005;34(7):525–530.
- Guglieri M, Straub V, Bushby K, et al. Limb–girdle muscular dystrophies. *Curr Opin Neurol*. 2008;21(5):576–584.
- Hermans MCE, Pinto YM, Merkies IS, et al. Hereditary muscular dystrophies and the heart. *Neuromuscul Disord*. 2010;20(8):479–492.
- Kirschner J, Bonnemann C. The congenital and limb-girdle muscular dystrophies: sharpening the focus, blurring the boundaries. *Arch Neurol*. 2004;61(2):189–197.
- Tawil R, Van Der Maarel SM. Facioscapulohumeral muscular dystrophy. *Muscle Nerve*. 2006;34(1):1–15.

CODES

ICD10
- G71.0 Muscular dystrophy
- G71.2 Congenital myopathies

FAQ
- Q: What test should be ordered first in a boy with suspected DMD?
- A: After confirmation that CK is elevated, 1st-line testing is *DMD* duplication/deletion analysis (detects 70% cases). If negative, *DMD* gene should be sequenced. Muscle biopsy is typically reserved for patients with negative genetic testing (i.e., LGMD) or if there is clinical suspicion for inflammatory myopathy (e.g., dermatomyositis). Nerve conduction studies can help differentiate neurogenic disorders (i.e., SMA, polyneuropathy) but show nonspecific myopathic changes in MDs.
- Q: What is the recurrence risk in DMD?
- A: About 2/3 of mothers of males with DMD are carriers. If a female DMD carrier has a son, that boy has a 50% chance of having DMD. If she has a daughter, that girl has a 50% chance of becoming a DMD carrier. Males with DMD or BMD will transmit the mutated gene to all daughters (who become carriers). The sons of DMD males will not be affected (X linked).
- Q: Can female DMD carriers be symptomatic?
- A: Yes. Owing to the random nature of X-chromosome inactivation, roughly 10% of female DMD heterozygotes may develop cardiomyopathy and/or proximal muscle weakness. The AAP recommends female carriers receive a cardiac evaluation in early adulthood and every 5 years after 25–30 years old.

MYASTHENIA GRAVIS

Diana X. Bharucha-Goebel

BASICS

DESCRIPTION

- A neuromuscular (NM) disease presenting with varying weakness that worsens with exercise and improves with rest
- 3 types of myasthenia gravis seen in childhood:
  - Neonatal transient: 10–20% of infants born to mothers with autoimmune myasthenia
  - Congenital myasthenia: rare; <10% of all childhood myasthenia. Weakness usually starts within first 2 years of life; caused by inherited disorder in NM transmission; classified by mutation site (presynaptic, postsynaptic) or by molecular genetics
  - Juvenile myasthenia: autoimmune disorder similar to adult-onset, autoimmune myasthenia gravis; mostly due to production of antibodies against the acetylcholine receptor (AChR). Relatively rare: 1 new diagnosis per million per year; average age of onset 10–13 years, with a female predominance of 2:1 or 4:1

EPIDEMIOLOGY

- Rare: incidence 4–6 per million per year
- Prevalence: 40–80 per million
- Children account for 10–15% of cases of myasthenia gravis annually.

RISK FACTORS

Genetics

- Congenital type: generally autosomal recessive (check consanguinity)
- Occasional family history

PATHOPHYSIOLOGY

- Caused by a disruption in signal transmission from the motor neuron to the muscle. Sensory or cognitive symptoms are absent.
  - The motor nerve terminal lies in close proximity to the end plate, a region of the muscle cell membrane with a high concentration of AChR.
  - Normally, when stimulated, the motor nerve terminal releases acetylcholine that binds receptors, causing muscle contraction. The cleft contains acetylcholinesterase (AChE), an enzyme that breaks down acetylcholine and helps terminate muscle contractions.
- Autoimmune form (juvenile or JMG)
  - Autoantibody blocks AChR activity → increased rate of receptor breakdown → fewer receptors are present → leads to decreased muscle contraction
  - AChR antibody accounts for ~85% of JMG.
  - Thymic pathology is believed to be central to pathogenesis of autoimmune myasthenia; however, thymic pathology (e.g., hyperplasia) is present in less than 1/3 of children who undergo thymectomy.
  - Of JMG patients without elevated AChR antibody, some are positive for antibodies to muscle-specific kinase (MuSK).
  - A small percentage of autoimmune JMG patients do not have an identified antibody.
- Neonatal (transient) myasthenia: Infants are born with weakness and hypotonia.
  - Due to maternal–fetal transmission of antibodies against AChR
  - Severity of maternal symptoms does NOT predict likelihood that infant will be affected. Occasional arthrogryposis (joint contractures) reflects decreased fetal movement in utero.
  - High levels of maternal antibodies against fetal form of AChR pose an increased risk of disease.
  - Previous pregnancy with affected infant places future child at much higher risk.
  - In rare cases, mother is asymptomatic despite placentally transmitted antibody.
- Congenital myasthenic syndromes: group of genetic disorders of NM junction; classified by site of NM transmission defect and more recently by molecular genetics
  - Includes presynaptic defects, synaptic defect (due to end plate AChE deficiency), postsynaptic defects (primary AChR deficiency, primary AChR kinetic abnormality, or perijunctional skeletal muscle sodium channel mutation)

COMMONLY ASSOCIATED CONDITIONS

- In juvenile myasthenia, other autoimmune disorders may occur:
  - Hyperthyroidism in 3–9% of patients
  - Small increase in incidence of juvenile idiopathic arthritis and diabetes
- Some reports suggest increased incidence of seizures in autoimmune myasthenia
- Screening for thymoma at initial diagnosis by chest CT or MRI scan is appropriate:
  - Children appear to have lower incidence of thymic tumor or pathology than adults with autoimmune myasthenia.

DIAGNOSIS

Most patients present with ptosis and diplopia alone or in combination with swallowing difficulties, dysphonia, and generalized weakness.

HISTORY

- Neonatal transient: mother with known autoimmune myasthenia or history of weakness, ptosis, or dysphagia
- Congenital myasthenia
  - Usually presents in first 1–2 years of life (rarely later) with hypotonia, poor feeding, ptosis, and delayed motor milestones
  - Possible family history of similar weakness
  - No response to thymectomy or immunosuppressant medications
- Juvenile myasthenia
  - Gradual onset of fatigable weakness over weeks, months, or even years
  - Symptoms are worse after prolonged activity or late in the day.
  - Intermittent ptosis, diplopia, dysphagia, and dysphonia are common.
  - Ocular myasthenia gravis: a subset of 10–15% of patients with myasthenia who have isolated ptosis and ophthalmoplegia (weakness in extraocular muscles) in absence of systemic or bulbar symptoms

PHYSICAL EXAM

- Neonatal transient: from birth, hypotonic infant with weak suck, weak cry, and ptosis
- Congenital and juvenile myasthenia
  - Weakness of neck flexion
  - Reflexes often preserved
  - Ptosis, ophthalmoplegia, and variable feeding problems often are earliest findings.
  - Generalized weakness in limbs may be asymmetric. Weakness is more pronounced with endurance tasks.
  - Shallow, rapid respirations and/or vital capacity <50% predicted (in older children) suggest impending respiratory failure.
  - Check for scoliosis.

DIAGNOSTIC TESTS & INTERPRETATION

- Juvenile myasthenia
  - Nerve conduction and electromyography studies: Repetitive stimulation of nerve shows diagnostic decremental response due to decreased AChR. May be normal in some patients; normal study doesn't exclude diagnosis.
  - Single-fiber electromyography measures variability in firing rates of 2 muscle fibers innervated by different branches of the same motor neuron. Large variability suggests higher threshold for activation. This test is more sensitive than repetitive nerve stimulation but is technically more challenging and often requires sedation.
  - Edrophonium chloride (Tensilon) is a fast-acting AChE-blocking agent (no longer widely available in the United States).
    - Patients with myasthenia often show immediate, transient improvement in muscle strength after IV infusion.
    - Measurable weakness should be present prior to testing, and a placebo dose of saline should be given initially.
    - Although risk of hyperreactive cholinergic response with muscle weakness and bradycardia is low, atropine should always be available, and vital signs should be closely monitored during test; contraindicated in patients with heart disease
    - Measurable cranial nerve dysfunction, such as ptosis, is often responsive to edrophonium.
    - Children receive 20% of 0.2 mg/kg dose (0.04 mg/kg) of Tensilon over 1 minute; if no response after 45 seconds, the rest of the dose (0.16 mg/kg) is given, up to a maximum of 10 mg. Have atropine and epinephrine readily available.

Lab

- AChR antibody levels (most specific): elevated in ~80% of patients with generalized myasthenia and ~50% of patients with isolated ocular myasthenia

- Second most common antibody is to muscle-specific receptor tyrosine kinase (MuSK-Ab). Antibodies to striated muscle protein and low-density lipoprotein receptor–related protein are also described but are rare.

DIFFERENTIAL DIAGNOSIS

- Generalized botulism
  - In endemic areas, may cause generalized weakness in infants; caused by *Clostridium* toxin that blocks release of acetylcholine from nerve terminal
- Guillain-Barré syndrome or acute inflammatory demyelinating polyneuropathy
  - Frequent cause of rapidly progressive generalized weakness
  - Unlike myasthenia, patients often have sensory symptoms, and areflexia occurs even with minimal weakness.
- Acute spinal cord compression
  - Can present as generalized (but not variable) weakness of extremities
  - Look for sparing of facial and extraocular muscles, a sensory level, bowel or bladder dysfunction, and hyperactive reflexes.
- Organophosphate ingestion: pyridostigmine bromide (Mestinon)
  - Can cause profound weakness
  - Symptoms of parasympathetic hyperactivity are usually present: hypersalivation, miosis, diarrhea, and bradycardia.
  - Penicillamine used to treat autoimmune disorders can induce autoantibodies that bind AChR, causing myasthenia gravis.

TREATMENT

INITIAL STABILIZATION

Treat respiratory failure, a rare but serious complication of juvenile myasthenia gravis.

GENERAL MEASURES

- Neonatal myasthenia
  - Severity of disability should be used to guide aggressiveness of therapy.
  - Respiratory or swallowing impairment: Pyridostigmine syrup, 60 mg/5 mL, 1 mg/kg/dose q4h up to a daily maximum of 7 mg/kg/24 h divided 5–6 doses; 1 mg IM = 30 mg PO dose
- Juvenile myasthenia
  - Most patients benefit from pyridostigmine bromide (Mestinon) given 3–4 times/day. A long-acting formulation prior to bedtime may alleviate obstructive hypoventilation during sleep.
  - Pyridostigmine blocks AChE activity and results in increased acetylcholine.
  - Usual starting dosage is ~1 mg/kg/24 h. Dosage is slowly titrated upward, following symptoms, at several-day intervals to a maximum dose of ~7–8 mg/kg/24 h. Absolute maximum daily dose is 300 mg/day for older children. Common side effects: hypersalivation, blurry vision, and diarrhea.
  - Glycopyrrolate (1 mg PO) may decrease diarrhea.
  - Prednisone
    - Consider in patients with disabling symptoms and inadequate response to pyridostigmine
    - Watch for transient worsening within weeks in up to 50% of patients.
    - Start daily dose at 2 mg/kg, watch for improvement in 3–6 weeks, and taper toward 1.5 mg/kg/24 h on alternate-day schedule for 4 months. Taper slowly thereafter by 5 mg/week.
    - Monitor for side effects, including growth stunting.
    - Calcium every-other-day dosing may limit bone loss from chronic steroids.
  - Rituximab
    - MuSK Ab–positive patients are often refractory to other treatments (Mestinon, steroids, IVIG) with incomplete or short-lived benefit.
    - Rituximab has induced sustained benefit in patients with refractory disease via B-cell depletion in MuSK Ab–positive patients; however, large controlled studies in this population have not been performed.
  - Azathioprine
    - Induces remission in 30%; significant improvement in another 25–60%
    - Useful adjunct to steroids and thymectomy; however, requires 3–12 months for benefits to occur
- Juvenile myasthenics with profound weakness and respiratory failure (myasthenic crisis) should undergo immediate therapy to decrease the number of circulating antibodies:
  - Plasmapheresis or IV immunoglobulin can help within days by decreasing AChR antibodies
  - Steroids diminish antibody production over weeks to months.

SURGERY/OTHER PROCEDURES

Thymectomy

- In adults, 20–60% remission; another 15–30% show marked improvement (somewhat less in pediatric patients)
- Thymectomy earlier in the course of illness appears to produce a higher rate of remission.

ONGOING CARE

- The following medications can exacerbate myasthenia gravis:
  - Corticosteroids may worsen symptoms.
  - Aminoglycosides
  - Ciprofloxacin
  - β-Adrenergic blocking agents, including eye drops
  - Lithium
  - Procainamide
  - Quinidine
  - Phenytoin
- Prolonged recovery after exposure to nondepolarizing NM blocking agents
- Always start new medications cautiously.

PROGNOSIS

- Neonatal transient
  - Self-limited disorder that resolves spontaneously over weeks or months of life as maternal antibodies disappear
  - Infant may require ventilator and nutritional support during first few months of life.
  - Infants with arthrogryposis multiplex congenita (born to mothers with antibodies against the fetal form of AChR) may gain some mobility over time and with passive range-of-motion therapy.
- Congenital myasthenia
  - Prognosis depends on specific defect.
  - Autosomal recessive disorders tend to be more severe than dominant disorders. Weakness shows variable response to cholinesterase inhibitors.
  - Immunosuppressants are not helpful. In general, these are indolent disorders.
  - Ptosis and fatigability resemble the juvenile type but are more stable over time.
- Juvenile myasthenia
  - Most patients do extremely well with treatment; patient selection for early surgery requires experience and may improve outcome.
  - Longitudinal studies suggest rate of spontaneous remission ~2% per year.
  - Patients with generalized weakness slightly less likely to experience remission.
  - Mortality rate from myasthenia is near that of the general population in patients <50 years old.

Patient Monitoring

- Watch for transient worsening of symptoms.
- Monitor for side effects of corticosteroids, including growth stunting.
- Medication effects: GI upset due to AChE inhibitors

COMPLICATIONS

Respiratory failure, nocturnal hypoventilation, visual disturbance, thymic cancer (more common in adults, rare in pediatrics), other autoimmune disorders

ADDITIONAL READING

- Castro D, Derisavifard S, Anderson M, et al. Juvenile myasthenia gravis: a twenty year experience. *J Clin Neuromusc Dis*. 2013;14(3):95–102.
- Harper CM. Congenital myasthenic syndromes. *Semin Neurol*. 2004;24(1):111–123.
- Liew W, Kang PB. Update on juvenile myasthenia gravis. *Curr Opin Pediatr*. 2013;25(6):694–700.
- Lindner A, Schalke B, Toyka VK. Outcome in juvenile-onset myasthenia gravis: a retrospective study with long-term follow up. *J Neurol*. 1997;244(8):515–520.
- Newsom-Davis J. Therapy in myasthenia gravis and Lambert-Eaton myasthenic syndrome. *Semin Neurol*. 2003;23(2):191–198.
- Parent internet information: Myasthenia Gravis Foundation of America, Inc. Living with MG. http://www.myasthenia.org/LivingwithMG.aspx. Accessed March 16, 2015.
- Pineles SL, Avery RA, Moss HE, et al. Visual and systematic outcomes in pediatric ocular myasthenia gravis. *Am J Ophthalmol*. 2010;150(4):453.e3–459.e3.

CODES

ICD10

- G70.00 Myasthenia gravis without (acute) exacerbation
- P94.0 Transient neonatal myasthenia gravis
- G70.01 Myasthenia gravis with (acute) exacerbation

MYOCARDITIS

Bradley S. Marino • John L. Jefferies

BASICS

DESCRIPTION

Myocarditis is defined as inflammation of the myocardium on histologic examination. Cardiovascular complications may be significant and include myocardial dysfunction, arrhythmias, conduction abnormalities, and cardiac arrest.

EPIDEMIOLOGY

- True incidence of acute myocarditis is difficult to estimate because of the wide range in clinical severity, various etiologies, and underdiagnosis.
- More than 50% of pediatric cases seen are in infants <1 year of age.
- Viral myocarditis has a seasonal distribution, which varies according to the viral species.

RISK FACTORS

- Exposure to infectious agents, drugs, toxins, and systemic diseases
- Drug exposure
- Autoimmune disease
- Systemic disease

PATHOPHYSIOLOGY

- Pathophysiology of myocarditis may vary based on cause (see "Etiology").
- Viral myocarditis is best characterized and involves a complex interaction among the virus, host immune response, and environmental factors. Three stages include (1) viral injury and innate immune response, (2) acquired host immune response, and (3) recovery or chronic cardiomyopathy.
- Inflammatory response from innate and acquired immune response may result in significant damage to the myocardium and conduction system.
- Development of autoantibodies may also play a key role in acute and chronic myocardial damage.
- Virus may cause direct damage to the myocardium independent of inflammation, secondary to cleavage of structural proteins.
- Pathogenesis of nonviral myocarditis is poorly understood.
- Regardless of the cause, symptom severity increases with worsening ventricular function and/or with worsening arrhythmias.
- Fulminant myocarditis may be characterized by both severe systolic and diastolic dysfunction.
- Progressive left ventricular systolic dysfunction may lead to hypotension, acidosis, and end-organ dysfunction.
- Left ventricular diastolic dysfunction may result in elevated left ventricular end diastolic pressures, leading to pulmonary venous and arterial hypertension, with concomitant pulmonary edema and right-sided heart failure.

ETIOLOGY

- Causes include infection, toxins, drugs, autoimmune disease, and systemic disease.
- Infectious causes include viral, bacterial, rickettsial, fungal, helminthic, spirochetal, and protozoal infections.
- Viral infection is the most common in developed countries including enteroviruses, erythroviruses, adenoviruses, and herpes viruses. Both RNA and DNA viruses have been implicated. Previously, the enteroviruses, specifically coxsackie B, were commonly seen. However, there has been a shift in the spectrum. Currently, parvovirus B19 is most commonly seen. There are growing reports of certain herpes viruses, specifically HHV6, becoming more prevalent.
- Nonviral infectious causes are far less common but must be considered especially in endemic areas, such as Central and South America where Chagas disease is prevalent.
- Nonviral myocarditis may be secondary to exposure to chemicals (arsenic and hydrocarbons), alcohol, radiation, drugs (chemotherapeutics), drug hypersensitivity, autoimmune disease such as systemic lupus erythematosus, or systemic disease such as Churg-Strauss or sarcoidosis.
- Giant cell myocarditis is a very rare form of myocarditis in children that is associated with autoimmune disease and drug hypersensitivity. These patients respond poorly to typical care and frequently require cardiac transplantation.

DIAGNOSIS

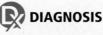

SIGNS AND SYMPTOMS

- Prodromal
  - Antecedent flulike illness
  - Gastroenteritis
  - Rheumatologic symptoms
  - Fever
- Left-sided heart failure
  - Exercise intolerance
  - Easy fatigability
  - Dyspnea
  - Orthopnea
  - Anorexia, loss of appetite/poor feeding, early satiety
  - Emesis (especially in children)
- Right-sided heart failure
  - Abdominal pain/cramping
  - Swelling of abdomen/lower extremities
  - Loose stools

HISTORY

- Duration of symptoms
- Travel history
- Family history

PHYSICAL EXAM

Any of the following may be present:

- Pulmonary
  - Rales
  - Tachypnea
  - Retractions
- Cardiovascular
  - Jugular venous distention
  - Normal to hyperdynamic precordium with or without right ventricular heave
  - Lateral displacement of the point of maximal impulse (PMI)
  - Tachycardia: arrhythmia (atrial and/or ventricular ectopy may be present)
  - Heart sounds: accentuation of second heart sound (secondary to pulmonary artery hypertension), murmur (mitral and/or tricuspid insufficiency), gallop, and/or rub
- Abdomen: hepatomegaly, splenomegaly, ascites
- Extremities
  - Weak pulses
  - Poor capillary refill
  - Cool extremities

DIAGNOSTIC TESTS & INTERPRETATION

- Despite limited sensitivity and specificity, endomyocardial biopsy (EMB), using the Dallas criteria for histopathologic classification, remains the gold standard for confirming the diagnosis of acute myocarditis.
  - These criteria are limited in that they provide information with regard to inflammation but do not assess for the presence of viral pathogens.
  - Current approaches indicate benefit in analyzing the tissue for viral DNA by polymerase chain reaction (PCR).
  - EMB has inherent problems, including sample selection bias, as tissue is only obtained from the right ventricular endocardium and the possible morbidity and mortality associated with an invasive procedure.
- Electrocardiogram findings may be supportive of the diagnosis:
  - Highly variable findings may include sinus tachycardia, low voltage QRS, ST segment depression/elevation, flattening or inversion of the T wave, conduction system disease including complete heart block, prolongation of the QT interval, and arrhythmias (premature atrial contractions/supraventricular tachycardia, or premature ventricular contractions/ventricular tachycardia).

Lab

- Erythrocyte sedimentation rate and C-reactive protein level may be elevated.
- Creatinine kinase MB fraction and troponin T and I levels may be elevated.
- Cultures (bacterial, viral, fungal) of blood, urine, stool, and nasopharyngeal swabs may be considered.
- Viral PCR analysis of tissue including myocardium, blood, or sputum may be considered.
- Acute and convalescent serologic studies may be considered for selected antibody studies.

Imaging

- Chest radiograph
  - Cardiomegaly and varying degrees of pulmonary edema
  - Possible pleural effusions
- Echocardiography
  - Depressed systolic function (may be biventricular with normal to mildly dilated chamber sizes)
  - Depressed diastolic function
  - Focal wall motion abnormalities
  - Valvular insufficiency
  - Pericardial effusion
- Cardiac MRI
  - Assessment of chamber size and systolic function
  - Fibrosis by delayed enhancement
  - Abnormal delayed enhancement and edema as seen by T2 weighting

DIFFERENTIAL DIAGNOSIS

- Severe left-sided obstructive heart lesions
  - Mitral stenosis
  - Valvular aortic stenosis
  - Coarctation of the aorta
- Congenital coronary artery anomalies
  - Anomalous left coronary artery from the pulmonary artery and other coronary variants
- Incessant arrhythmias
  - Incessant supraventricular tachycardia
  - Ventricular tachycardia
- Metabolic disorders including mitochondrial disease
- Drug use
  - Cocaine or other stimulants
- Acquired disease
  - Kawasaki disease
  - Coronary artery disease
- Genetic syndromes
  - Neuromuscular disease
  - Genetically triggered cardiomyopathies

TREATMENT

- Initial management should be based on the clinical presentation. These include the following: bed rest and limited activity (during acute phase).
- Standard medical regimens for acute care should be based on appropriate heart failure therapies and may include the following:
  - Inotropic support should be considered for patients with evidence of low cardiac output. Medication infusions may include milrinone, dopamine, and dobutamine. If epinephrine is required, mechanical support should be considered.
  - Diuretics
  - Afterload reduction may be considered if volume overload exists with preserved cardiac output (e.g., nitroglycerin and nitroprusside).
  - Antiarrhythmics may be used in cases of hemodynamically significant arrhythmias.
  - Mechanical ventilation in patients with respiratory failure secondary to myocardial failure
  - Mechanical support (in patients with rapidly progressing, severe heart failure; used as a bridge to transplantation): left ventricular or biventricular assist devices, extracorporeal membrane oxygenation (ECMO)
  - Rescue therapy: cardiac transplantation
- Standard medical regimens for chronic care should be based on appropriate heart failure therapies and may include the following:
  - Angiotensin-converting enzyme inhibitors (ACEi)
  - β-blockers
  - Angiotensin receptor blockers
  - Diuretics (e.g., spironolactone for ventricular remodeling)
  - Anticoagulation with unfractionated or low-molecular-weight heparin acutely and aspirin and/or Coumadin chronically for patients with severe myocardial depression and ventricular dilation
  - Implantable devices may be considered for patients with conduction system disease (pacemaker) or those at risk for sudden cardiac death (implantable cardioverter-defibrillator).

MEDICATION

- Immunosuppression: High-dose gamma globulin (2 g/kg IV immunoglobulin [Ig] over 24 hours) during the acute phase has been associated with improved recovery of left ventricular function and with a tendency for better survival during the first year after presentation.
- Steroids, azathioprine, calcineurin inhibitors, cyclosporine, cyclophosphamide, and other immunosuppressive medications have all been proposed as effective agents, although insufficient evidence of therapeutic benefit is currently available to recommend routine use.
- Antiviral therapy does not currently have an accepted role in myocarditis management.
- Use of interferon therapy is being widely studied but there continues to be a lack of demonstrable benefit.

ONGOING CARE

FOLLOW-UP RECOMMENDATIONS

Patient Monitoring

- Clinical changes in systolic and diastolic function
- Monitoring for life-threatening arrhythmias
- Effects of the illness on other systems
  - Nutritional status
  - Growth
  - Development
  - Comorbid illnesses

PROGNOSIS

- Prognostic data are limited by the lack of complete ascertainment of all cases of acute myocarditis, with many patients likely exhibiting mild symptoms, which spontaneously resolve.
- Prognosis is often dictated by clinical presentation and underlying etiology. However, if treated appropriately early in the course, outcome can be quite favorable.
- Prognosis is poor in patients with fulminant lymphocytic myocarditis with significant hemodynamic compromise with a mortality of >40% in adults and ~75% in children, without aggressive management strategies.
- Mortality is higher in children presenting in the neonatal period.
- Giant cell myocarditis represents a unique subgroup with a particularly poor prognosis, unless transplanted.

COMPLICATIONS

- Acidosis
- End-organ hypoperfusion and resultant dysfunction
- Pulmonary venous and arterial hypertension
- Pulmonary edema
- Unfavorable ventricular remodeling
- Conduction system disease including heart block
- Arrhythmias

ADDITIONAL READING

- Blauwet LA, Cooper LT. Myocarditis. *Prog Cardiovasc Dis*. 2010;52(4):274–288.
- Bowles NE, Ni J, Kearney DL, et al. Detection of viruses in myocardial tissues by polymerase chain reaction: evidence of adenovirus as a common cause of myocarditis in children and adults. *J Am Coll Cardiol*. 2003;42(3):473–476.
- Foerster SR, Canter CE, Cinar A, et al. Ventricular remodeling and survival are more favorable for myocarditis than for idiopathic dilated cardiomyopathy in childhood: an outcomes study from the Pediatric Cardiomyopathy Registry. *Circ Heart Fail*. 2010;3(6):689–697.
- Jefferies JL, Price JF, Morales DL. Mechanical circulatory support in childhood heart failure. *Heart Fail Clin*. 2010;6(4):559–573.
- Kühl U, Schultheiss HP. Myocarditis in children. *Heart Fail Clin*. 2010;6(4):483–496.
- Moulik M, Breinholt JP, Dreyer WJ, et al. Viral endomyocardial infection is an independent predictor and potentially treatable risk factor for graft loss and coronary vasculopathy in pediatric cardiac transplant patients. *J Am Coll Cardiol*. 2010;56(7):582–592.
- Wilmot I, Morales DL, Price JF, et al. Effectiveness of mechanical circulatory support in children with fulminant and persistent myocarditis. *J Card Fail*. 2011;17(6):487–494.

CODES

ICD10

- I51.4 Myocarditis, unspecified
- B33.22 Viral myocarditis
- I40.9 Acute myocarditis, unspecified

NARCOLEPSY

Jennifer A. Accardo

BASICS

DESCRIPTION
- Lifelong neurologic disorder that often initially manifests in childhood or adolescence and can cause significant functional impairment and disability
- Excessive daytime sleepiness and inappropriate transitions from wakefulness into rapid eye movement (REM) sleep
- Narcolepsy may occur with or without cataplexy.
- Other associated features include hypnagogic hallucinations, sleep paralysis, and nighttime sleep fragmentation.

GENERAL PREVENTION
- Narcolepsy is not preventable.
- Narcolepsy is underrecognized, especially in children.
- Physicians should screen for sleep dysfunction and excessive sleepiness as part of anticipatory guidance.

EPIDEMIOLOGY
- Prevalence in the United States is reported to range from 25 to 50 per 100,000; prevalence may be higher in the Japanese population.
- An estimated 200,000 Americans have narcolepsy, but fewer than 50,000 of these individuals have been diagnosed with the disorder.
- Approximately half of patients with narcolepsy have symptoms before age 15 years and <10% with symptoms <age 5 years, but often, diagnosis may lag 10–15 years after onset of symptoms.
- Cataplexy is present in 50–70% of adult patients and perhaps at least as many pediatric patients but may be initially sporadic or difficult to identify.

RISK FACTORS
- 1st-degree relatives of patients with narcolepsy with cataplexy have a 1–2% risk (which is 10- to 40-fold more than the general population) of developing narcolepsy.
- Both genetic and environmental factors may be involved in the development of narcolepsy.
- There is an association between narcolepsy with cataplexy and histocompatibility leukocyte antigens (HLA) subtypes, specifically DQB1*0602 in 85–95% and DR2 antigens. About 40% of cases of narcolepsy without cataplexy are also DQB1*0602 positive.
- Increased risk of narcolepsy after H1N1 vaccination has been a topic of interest.

PATHOPHYSIOLOGY
- Hypocretin (also known as orexin) is a neuropeptide produced by neurons in the perifornical area of the lateral hypothalamus that is supplied to several areas of the brain that promote wakefulness. It may also inhibit REM sleep. It mediates appetite.
- To better reflect pathophysiology, the American Academy of Sleep Medicine has categorized narcolepsy into type 1 and type 2. Type 1 involves hypocretin deficiency, such as would be detected in cerebrospinal fluid (CSF) via lumbar puncture, or manifested clinically by the presence of cataplexy. Type 2 does not involve hypocretin deficiency, and in the absence of CSF testing would be the presumptive diagnosis for a patient who had not manifested cataplexy. Onset of cataplexy would herald a change in diagnosis from type 1 to type 2.
- Narcolepsy type 1 is caused by selective loss of the hypocretin-producing neurons in the hypothalamic region.
- The association between narcolepsy and specific HLA antigens has suggested autoimmune pathogenesis; however, this has yet to be definitively established.

COMMONLY ASSOCIATED CONDITIONS
- Secondary narcolepsy may be seen with CNS trauma, strokes, brain tumors, and demyelinating diseases, particularly involving the lateral and posterior hypothalamus, midbrain, and the pons.
- Genetic syndromes such as Prader-Willi syndrome, myotonic dystrophy, and Niemann-Pick type C syndrome may be associated with secondary narcolepsy.

DIAGNOSIS

HISTORY
- Excess daytime sleepiness starting with recurrence of naps may be early signs of disease.
- In adults, naps tend to be restorative but are more likely to be described as "unrefreshing" in children.
- Cataplexy, the abrupt loss of muscle tone provoked by laughter or strong emotions such as surprise, sadness, or anger, is almost pathognomonic for narcolepsy. Loss of muscle tone can range from sagging of face, eyelids, or jaw; blurred vision; and knee buckling to complete collapse but with preserved consciousness.
- Hypnagogic (on sleep onset) and hypnopompic (on awakening) hallucinations involve vivid auditory or visual hallucinations during transitions between sleep and wakefulness. Such hallucinations can also be experienced infrequently by normal individuals.
- Sleep paralysis is the inability to move or speak for a few seconds or minutes at sleep onset or offset. Normal individuals can also experience sleep paralysis, often in the context of sleep deprivation.

PHYSICAL EXAM
- Normal in most idiopathic cases; children with narcolepsy are often overweight/obese.
- Vertical gaze palsy, confusion, poor memory, developmental regression, impaired thermoregulation, and signs of endocrine dysfunction may be present in cases of secondary narcolepsy.

DIAGNOSTIC TESTS & INTERPRETATION

Lab
- Levels of CSF hypocretin ≤110 pg/mL (30% of mean control value) are strongly indicative of narcolepsy with cataplexy. CSF testing is usually reserved for complicated or ambiguous cases.
- HLA antigen typing with HLA DQB*0602 and DR2 are strongly associated with narcolepsy with cataplexy but also present in 12–38% of the normal population. A negative result can be helpful in ruling out the condition, and HLA testing should be considered supportive rather than diagnostic.

Imaging
Brain MRI is indicated with sudden onset of sleepiness, recent head injury, or an abnormal neurologic exam.

Diagnostic Procedures/Other

- Overnight polysomnography (PSG) and multiple sleep latency test (MSLT) are considered standard of care for diagnosis.
- MSLT is a protocol consisting of four or five 20-minute nap opportunities 2 hours apart after an overnight PSG to determine mean sleep latency (MSL) and sleep-onset REM periods (SOREMPs) within 15 minutes of falling asleep. PSG is performed to ensure adequate nighttime sleep and exclude other sleep disorders that could cause daytime sleepiness. On MSLT, MSL <8 minutes and ≥2 SOREMPs are diagnostic of narcolepsy. SOREMP at the beginning of the preceding night's PSG can now be substituted for a SOREMP on the MSLT. Two or more SOREMPs tend to be specific for narcolepsy, whereas up to 30% of the general population may have MSL <8 minutes. Other factors influencing sleepiness such as chronic sleep deprivation or sedating medications must provide context for test interpretation.

DIFFERENTIAL DIAGNOSIS

- Chronic insufficient sleep
- Poor sleep hygiene (particularly nighttime electronics use)
- Delayed sleep phase disorder (manifesting as daytime sleepiness)
- Idiopathic CNS hypersomnia (without cataplexy, SOREMPs, or other REM intrusion phenomena in wakefulness or sleep)
- Primary sleep disorders such as obstructive sleep apnea, restless legs syndrome, periodic limb movement disorder
- Kleine-Levin syndrome (cyclical episodes of hypersomnolence, classically also with overeating and hypersexuality lasting days to weeks with normal intervals in between)
- Psychiatric disorders/depression
- Medication side effects, drug/alcohol abuse
- Atonic drop attacks associated with childhood epilepsy syndromes such as Lennox-Gastaut syndrome
- Cataplexy can be associated with Coffin-Lowry syndrome or Norrie syndrome, both rare and involving other deficits including intellectual disability.

TREATMENT

MEDICATION

- Daytime sleepiness
  - Methylphenidate, 5–30 mg/24 h (max 60 mg/24 h). Consider other long-acting formulations such as Concerta, Ritalin LA, Metadate CD, Focalin XR, etc.
  - Dextroamphetamine (Dexedrine) 5–40 mg/24 h (max 60 mg/24 h)
  - Mixed amphetamine salts (Adderall XR) 10–30 mg/24 h
  - Modafinil (Provigil), 100–400 mg/24 h. FDA Pediatric Advisory Committee warning; recommends use only if 1st- and 2nd-line treatments have failed and the benefits outweigh the risks of serious dermatologic and psychiatric side effects
- Cataplexy
  - Sodium oxybate (Xyrem): treats both hypersomnia and cataplexy. Dose is given at bedtime while in bed and again 2½–4 hours later due to profound sedating effects.
  - Venlafaxine (Effexor) starting at 12.5–25 mg
  - Selective serotonin reuptake inhibitors: fluoxetine (Prozac) 5–30 mg/24 h or sertraline (Zoloft) 25–100 mg/24 h
  - Clomipramine (Anafranil) 25–100 mg /24 h
  - Imipramine (Tofranil) 25–75 mg /24 h

ADDITIONAL TREATMENT

- Regular sleep schedule
- Short scheduled naps
- Regular physical exercise

ONGOING CARE

PROGNOSIS

Children with narcolepsy can be expected to have normal life expectancy and normal intellectual functioning. Lifestyle and medication treatments to reduce sleepiness and cataplexy improve academic performance, quality of life, and ability to participate.

ADDITIONAL READING

- Aran A, Einen M, Lin L, et al. Clinical and therapeutic aspects of childhood narcolepsy-cataplexy: a retrospective study of 51 children. *Sleep*. 2010;33(11):1457–1464.
- Dauvilliers Y, Arnulf I, Mignot E. Narcolepsy with cataplexy. *Lancet*. 2007;369(9560):499–511.
- Kotagal, S. Narcolepsy in children. In: Sheldon S, Kryger M, Ferber R, eds. *Principles and Practice of Pediatric Sleep Medicine*. Philadelphia, PA: Elsevier; 2005:171–179.
- Nevsimalova S. Narcolepsy in childhood. *Sleep Med Rev*. 2009;13(2):169–180.

CODES

ICD10

- G47.419 Narcolepsy without cataplexy
- G47.411 Narcolepsy with cataplexy
- G47.429 Narcolepsy in conditions classified elsewhere w/o cataplexy

FAQ

- Q: What is the chance that a sibling of the patient may develop narcolepsy?
- A: There is a 1% possibility that siblings and offspring could be affected.
- Q: Will a patient with narcolepsy be able to drive a car?
- A: Patients with narcolepsy can legally drive, provided they are on the appropriate medications to keep them from falling asleep at the wheel.
- Q: Is there a cure for narcolepsy?
- A: No. Treatment is symptomatic.

NECK MASSES

Nicholas Tsarouhas

BASICS

DESCRIPTION

A mass in the tissues of the neck; cervical adenopathy is defined as a neck node >1 cm.

ETIOLOGY

Varies depending on underlying condition

DIAGNOSIS

To diagnose and appropriately manage neck masses, one must combine the history with a careful examination of the mass. The major task of the differential diagnosis is to distinguish infections from congenital and malignant causes.

HISTORY

- Fever: infection, Kawasaki disease, malignancy, "PFAPA" (periodic fever, aphthous stomatitis, pharyngitis, and cervical adenitis) syndrome
- Intercurrent infection: reactive hyperplasia, mononucleosis, abscess, congenital cyst
- Subacute or chronic cervical lymphadenitis: cat-scratch disease, toxoplasmosis, Epstein-Barr virus (EBV), and mycobacterial infection
- Increasing size: infection, newly infected congenital lesion, malignancy (less common)
- Sore throat: mononucleosis, peritonsillar or retropharyngeal abscess
- Swallowing problems: retropharyngeal or peritonsillar abscess, thyroglossal duct cyst
- Cat contact: cat-scratch disease, toxoplasmosis
- Recurrently infected mass: infected congenital cyst (thyroglossal duct, branchial cleft)
- Mass noticed neonatally: cystic hygroma, hemangioma, sternocleidomastoid tumor of infancy
- Weight loss, cough, chronic constitutional symptoms: malignancy, tuberculosis
- Hypothyroid or hyperthyroid symptoms: thyroglossal duct cyst, thyroidal diseases

PHYSICAL EXAM

- Tender, erythematous, indurated mass may indicate cervical adenitis, infected congenital lesion, or cat-scratch disease
- Nontender, enlarged lymph nodes(s) suggest reactive hyperplasia or malignancy.
- Fluctuant mass may indicate adenitis with abscess or cystic hygroma.
- Drainage suggests adenitis with abscess, atypical mycobacterial disease, infected thyroglossal duct, or branchial cleft cyst.
- Regional adenopathy: reactive hyperplasia, cat-scratch disease, or malignancy
- Exudative pharyngitis: mononucleosis
- Asymmetric soft palate with uvular deviation suggests peritonsillar abscess.
- Pulmonary findings: tuberculosis, malignancy
- Midline mass suggests thyroglossal duct or dermoid cyst or thyroidal disease.
- If mass moves with tongue protrusion, thyroglossal duct cyst may be present.
- Sinus opening may indicate thyroglossal duct, branchial cleft, or dermoid cyst.
- Multiloculated mass that transilluminates suggests cystic hygroma.
- Matted-down mass may indicate malignancy.
- Mass posterior to sternocleidomastoid muscle may be malignancy or infection.
- Inferior deep cervical nodes (scalene and supraclavicular) suggest malignancy.
- Generalized adenopathy suggests malignancy.
- Hepatosplenomegaly may indicate malignancy or infectious mononucleosis.
- Skin discoloration suggests trauma, abscess, or atypical mycobacterial disease.
- A skin papule is a clue to cat-scratch disease.
- Conjunctivitis, oral involvement, extremity changes, rash, and adenopathy, in the context of fever: Suspect Kawasaki disease.
- Torticollis in a neonate suggests sternocleidomastoid (pseudo) tumor of infancy.

DIAGNOSTIC TESTS & INTERPRETATION

- CBC
  - Infections: leukocytosis
  - Mononucleosis: atypical lymphocytosis
  - Kawasaki: thrombocytosis after 1st week
  - Neck malignancies: usually normal initially
- Complete metabolic panel with lactate dehydrogenase (LDH) and uric acid when malignancy is suspected
- "Mono spot" (mononucleosis) test: less reliable in children <4 years old; EBV titers more useful
- Indirect fluorescent antibody titers for *Bartonella*: confirms cat-scratch disease
- Purified protein derivative: negative or weakly positive in atypical mycobacterial infections
- Chest radiograph: important in all evaluations when malignancy is a possibility; adenopathy seen in malignancies and tuberculosis; cavitary lesions and infiltrates in tuberculosis
- Lateral neck radiograph: prevertebral soft tissue space at C2–C3 abnormally wide (>1/2 adjacent vertebral body diameter) in cases of retropharyngeal abscess
- Ultrasound
  - 1st-line imaging modality in neck masses
  - provides immediate, noninvasive information on location, size, and composition of mass (cystic vs. solid)
  - Doppler adds information about vascularity.
- CT or MRI scan: useful in evaluating deep neck infections and complex neck masses
  - CT advantages: more readily available; shorter study; less need for sedation
  - MRI advantages: no ionizing radiation; better soft tissue resolution
- Thyroid scintigraphy: useful when malignancy is a concern
- Gram stain and culture of specimen after needle aspiration or incision and drainage: diagnostic and therapeutic with infections
- Histologic evaluation after fine-needle aspiration or biopsy: diagnostic for malignant versus congenital versus infectious causes

DIFFERENTIAL DIAGNOSIS

- Infectious
  - Reactive hyperplasia: self-limited, enlargement of bilateral minimally tender nodes; usually viral
  - Bacterial lymphadenitis
    - Usually staphylococcal or streptococcal infection of unilateral, tender, swollen, warm, erythematous node
    - Cellulitis–adenitis syndrome in neonates caused by group B *Streptococcus*
  - Cat-scratch disease
    - A usually self-limited, although sometimes protracted, illness (2–4 months)
    - Caused by the gram-negative bacillus *Bartonella henselae*
    - Starts as a papule at a cat-scratch site; progresses to regional adenopathy, 5–50 days later (median, 12 days)
    - Axillary adenopathy is most common; cervical nodes 2nd most common.
    - Adenopathy for weeks to months
  - Tuberculosis: acute or insidious onset of fever and firm, nontender adenopathy in children exposed to adult infected with acid-fast bacillus *Mycobacterium tuberculosis*
  - Atypical mycobacterial disease
    - Infection usually caused by *Mycobacterium avium* complex or *Mycobacterium scrofulaceum* (ubiquitous agents found in the soil)
    - Rapidly enlarging mass of firm, nontender nodes in young children with no known exposure to tuberculosis
    - Nodes often occur with overlying skin discoloration and thinning; some spontaneously drain.
  - Infectious mononucleosis: EBV infection most commonly seen in older children who present with fever, exudative pharyngitis, adenopathy, and hepatosplenomegaly.
  - Toxoplasmosis
    - Parasitic disease caused by *Toxoplasma gondii* which presents with cervical adenopathy, rash, fever, malaise, and hepatosplenomegaly
    - Acquired from contact with cat feces or inadequately cooked meat
  - Retropharyngeal abscess
    - Suppurative adenitis of the retropharyngeal nodes that presents in children <5 years of age
    - These children often have fever, neck stiffness, dysphagia, respiratory distress, drooling, and stridor.
  - Peritonsillar abscess: suppurative sequela of a severe tonsillopharyngitis, usually caused by group A β-hemolytic *Streptococcus* (GABHS); commonly presents in older children and adolescents with trismus, "hot potato" voice, and uvular deviation from a bulging palatal abscess
  - Ludwig angina
    - Rapidly expanding, diffuse inflammation of the submandibular/sublingual spaces
    - May compromise the airway
    - Often occurs with dental infections

- Congenital
  - Branchial cleft cyst: common congenital neck lesion (usually a remnant of the 2nd branchial cleft) which presents as a nontender (unless infected) cyst at the anterior border of the sternocleidomastoid
  - Thyroglossal duct cyst: common congenital neck mass which is a remnant of the embryonic thyroglossal sinus and presents as a nontender (unless infected), mobile, anterior midline mass near the hyoid bone
  - Cystic hygroma (lymphangioma): complex, multiloculated mass of lymphatic tissue, which presents in the 1st year of life as a large, soft, compressible mass in the posterior triangle of the neck; may cause airway obstruction
  - Dermoid cyst: small, firm, nontender mass, usually high in the midline
  - Hemangioma: bluish purple, blanching mass characterized by rapid growth in the 1st year of life, then slow regression
  - Sternocleidomastoid (pseudo) tumor of infancy (congenital muscular torticollis): benign perinatal fibromatosis, often associated with difficult deliveries or abnormal uterine positioning, that results in a hard, immobile, fusiform mass in the sternocleidomastoid
  - Laryngocele: cystic dilation of the laryngeal saccule; presents as an air-filled cyst or as a foreign body sensation with coughing
  - Cervical wattle: benign pedunculated congenital anomaly on lateral neck with a core of elastic cartilage
  - Cervical bronchogenic cyst: cervical neck mass in the anteromedial neck (superior to the sternal notch), resulting from abnormal development of the tracheobronchial tree
  - Thymic cyst: ectopic thymic mass resulting from abnormal development of pharyngeal pouches and branchial clefts
  - Teratoma: malformation of all three germ layers that can cause significant airway obstruction as well as feeding dysfunction
  - Ranula: a mucocele created by obstruction of the sublingual salivary glands; usually a painless, slowly accumulating mass
- Malignant
  - Hodgkin lymphoma: slowly enlarging, unilateral, firm, nontender neck malignancy; usually presents in previously well adolescents
  - Non-Hodgkin lymphoma: presents in young adolescents as a painless, rapidly growing, firm collection of lymph nodes
  - Leukemia: most common tumor associated with cervical adenitis in first 6 years of life
  - Neuroblastoma: commonly presents in infants/young children as a large, nontender abdominal mass; associated with a myriad of signs and symptoms due to its propensity for metastasis
  - Rhabdomyosarcoma: head and neck malignancy that usually presents as a rapidly enlarging mass
  - Melanoma: an increasingly identified cause of neck malignancy in pediatrics
- Thyroid
  - Chronic lymphocytic thyroiditis (Hashimoto thyroiditis): autoimmune childhood goiter that may be eu-, hypo-, or hyperthyroid
  - Thyrotoxicosis (Graves disease): clinically hyperfunctioning thyroid caused by circulating thyroid cell–stimulating antibodies
  - Thyroiditis: painful bacterial infection of the thyroid caused by *Staphylococcus* or *Streptococcus*
- Miscellaneous
  - Kawasaki disease
    - Idiopathic vasculitis distinguished by prolonged fever, conjunctivitis, oral involvement, extremity changes, rash, and unilateral cervical node >1.5 cm
    - Cervical node: least common feature
  - PFAPA syndrome
    - Periodic fever, aphthous stomatitis, pharyngitis, and cervical adenitis
    - Idiopathic, periodic, febrile syndrome most commonly seen in young children
  - Sinus histiocytosis with massive lymphadenopathy (Rosai–Dorfman disease); benign form of histiocytosis that presents as massive, painless enlargement of cervical nodes
  - Hematoma: secondary to trauma
  - Hypersensitivity reaction: secondary to bites, stings, or other allergens
  - Drugs: Notably, phenytoin and isoniazid may be associated with lymphadenopathy.
  - Immunization: Adenopathy may follow DPT or polio immunization.

TREATMENT

GENERAL MEASURES

- Infectious
  - Antibiotics
  - Incision and drainage (I&D) of abscesses
- Congenital
  - Antibiotics if infected
  - ENT referral for surgical excision
- Malignancy: oncology referral for chemotherapy/radiation/excision

ALERT

Corticosteroids should not be given to neck mass patients until malignancy has been excluded, except in dire conditions of airway compromise.

- Thyroidal: endocrine referral for pharmacotherapy
- Miscellaneous
  - Kawasaki disease: IVIG and aspirin therapy to prevent coronary artery aneurysms; cardiology referral for echocardiography
  - PFAPA syndrome: Steroids (a single dose) are efficacious in aborting fever attacks.
  - Sternocleidomastoid tumor of infancy: massage, range of motion, and stretching

ONGOING CARE

Close follow-up is essential for all neck masses; consider referral for biopsy in the following cases:

- Nodes not responding to antibiotics
- Toxic illness/systemic symptoms
- Clinical signs of malignancy (weight loss, peripheral adenopathy, hepatosplenomegaly)
- Firm, nontender nodes fixed to deep tissues
- Nodes posterior to the sternocleidomastoid or in the lower cervical/supraclavicular regions
- Bilateral nodes >2 cm

ADDITIONAL READING

- Al-Dajani N, Wootton SH. Cervical lymphadenitis, suppurative parotitis, thyroiditis, and infected cysts. *Infect Dis Clin North Am*. 2007;21(2):523–541, viii.
- Dulin MF, Kennard TP, Leach L, et al. Management of cervical lymphadenitis in children. *Am Fam Physician*. 2008;78(9):1097–1098.
- Friedman ER, John SD. Imaging of pediatric neck masses. *Radiol Clin North Am*. 2011;49(4):617–632.
- Geddes G, Butterly MM, Patel SM, et al. Pediatric neck masses. *Pediatr Rev*. 2013;34(3):115–124.

CODES

ICD10

- R22.1 Localized swelling, mass and lump, neck
- R59.0 Localized enlarged lymph nodes
- L02.11 Cutaneous abscess of neck

FAQ

- Q: How should nodes respond to therapy?
- A: Consider referral for biopsy if increasing size after 2 weeks, no decrease in size >2–4 weeks, or not back to normal >8–12 weeks.
- Q: Do all external neck abscesses need antibiotic therapy after drainage?
- A: Many experts believe that antibiotics are not always necessary if I&D is done appropriately.
- Q: Is antibiotic coverage for community-acquired methicillin-resistant *Staphylococcus aureus* (CA-MRSA) necessary?
- A: As CA-MRSA is increasingly common, an antibiotic agent with MRSA coverage is indicated; clindamycin is a common choice.

NECROTIZING ENTEROCOLITIS

Susan W. Aucott • Fizan Abdullah

BASICS

DESCRIPTION

Necrotizing enterocolitis (NEC) is a severe acquired GI disorder that occurs in the newborn period and consists of diffuse necrotic injury to the bowel, which can result in perforation or subserosal collections of gas. The entire GI tract is susceptible, but the most frequently involved areas are the distal small bowel and proximal colon. Lesions vary from being diffuse areas of patchy necrosis to more isolated focal disease. Systemic signs and symptoms related to the inflammatory GI injury are accompanied by characteristic radiographic findings of pneumatosis.

EPIDEMIOLOGY

- NEC typically has an onset at 1–3 weeks of life (3–20 days) after the initiation of enteral feedings. The more premature the infant, the longer the child is at risk for developing NEC, with cases reported as late as 3 months of age.
- NEC affects mostly premature infants, but up to 10% of cases occur in term infants.
- The incidence of NEC is variable and ranges from 1 to 7% of all neonatal intensive care unit admissions or 1–3 per 1,000 live births.
- Preterm infants account for the vast majority of total NEC cases; the risk increases with decreasing gestational age and birth weight.
- Prevalence in very-low-birth-weight (VLBW) infants (birth weight <1,500 g) is 7%.
- Highest risk is in infants with birth weights between 500 and 750 g (15%).

RISK FACTORS

- The greatest risk factor for NEC is prematurity. Additional risk factors for both preterm and full-term infants include the following:
  - Cardiovascular instability
  - Respiratory compromise resulting in recurrent or prolonged hypoxia
  - Cyanotic heart disease
  - Polycythemia
  - Exchange transfusions
  - Bowel malformations
  - Perinatal asphyxia
  - Small size for gestational age
  - Maternal preeclampsia
  - Antenatal cocaine abuse
  - Prolonged use of IV antibiotics

GENERAL PREVENTION

- The use of maternal breast milk exclusively has been advocated. Donor breast milk, when maternal breast milk is unavailable, has been shown to decrease the incidence of NEC.
- A rapid rate of feeding advancement (>20 mL/kg/day) may increase the risk of NEC in infants less than 1,500 g. Early initiation of trophic feeds (<10 mg/kg/day) for several days prior to advancing feeding volumes may stimulate maturation of the GI tract with resultant improvement in feeding tolerance.
- The use of probiotics has not been shown consistently to effectively decrease the incidence for VLBW infants. Concern has been raised of an increased risk of sepsis when using probiotics.
- Immunonutrient supplementation with agents such as arginine, glutamine, lactoferrin, and omega-3 polyunsaturated fatty acids is being investigated, but there is currently insufficient evidence to make any recommendations for their use.

PATHOPHYSIOLOGY

- Varying degrees of inflammation early in the course cause superficial mucosal ulcerations and submucosal edema and hemorrhage, leading to transmural coagulation necrosis and perforation in the most severe cases.
- The most common sites for NEC include the terminal ileum, ileocecal region, and ascending colon.
- 50% of infants have both colonic and small intestine disease, with the other 50% divided between isolated ileal and colonic involvement.

ETIOLOGY

- The etiology of NEC is unknown but thought to be a multifactorial process.
- Various factors causing direct and indirect mucosal disruption, which in turn may lead to an increased permeability in the gut of agents that lead to injury, include the following:
  - Hypoxia/ischemia leading to mucosal injury
  - GI tract immaturity
  - Immature host defense
  - Enteral feedings
  - Decreased diversity of bacteria within the GI lumen
- Enteral alimentation
  - Because 95% of infants who develop NEC have been enterally fed, initiation of feedings has been implicated as an important contributor to the etiology of NEC.
  - The composition of the formula (osmolarity), the rate of volume increase, and the immaturity of the mucosa have all been implicated as factors.
- Because of the frequent report of epidemic, cluster-type episodes, a variety of microorganisms has been implicated in the development of NEC, although there is no single causative organism.
  - Blood cultures may be positive in 20–30% of cases, often gram-negative organisms.
- Immaturity of the GI mucosal defense system against invading organisms has been noted in NEC.
- Medications may have a direct mucosal injury.

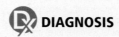

DIAGNOSIS

ALERT

Delay in making the correct diagnosis of NEC and instituting appropriate therapy may lead to a rapid progression of symptoms and often a worse outcome.

PHYSICAL EXAM

- The triad of abdominal distention, bloody stools, and feeding intolerance is frequently seen 8–10 days after initiating enteral feedings.
- The clinical spectrum varies dramatically from non-specific symptoms of feeding intolerance to severe abdominal distention, sepsis, and shock. A staging system ranks the disease into 3 categories based on severity of the clinical signs and symptoms, aiding formulation of individual treatment plans.
  - Stage I (suspected NEC)
    - Temperature instability
    - Apnea
    - Bradycardia
    - Lethargy
    - Cyanosis
    - Glucose instability
    - Increased gastric residuals
    - Emesis (may be bilious)
    - Abdominal distention
    - Heme-positive stools
  - Stage II (definitive NEC): stage I plus
    - Mild metabolic acidosis
    - Mild thrombocytopenia
    - Poor perfusion
    - Severe abdominal distention
    - Absent bowel sounds
    - Abdominal tenderness
    - Grossly bloody stools
    - Possible abdominal wall cellulitis, fullness/mass
    - Ascites
  - Stage III (advanced NEC): stage I and II plus
    - Shock/deterioration of vital signs
    - Metabolic acidosis
    - Thrombocytopenia
    - Disseminated intravascular coagulation (DIC)
    - Significant abdominal tenderness/peritonitis
    - Respiratory compromise
    - Neutropenia

DIAGNOSTIC TESTS & INTERPRETATION

Lab

No single laboratory feature is diagnostic of NEC. Obtaining a blood culture and monitoring serial complete blood counts (CBCs) and blood gases are essential for monitoring patients with NEC to assess for the following:

- Thrombocytopenia
- Acidosis, metabolic
- Anemia
- Neutropenia
- DIC

Imaging

Abdominal radiographs are essential for the diagnosis and staging of NEC:

- Stage I: mild dilatation of bowel loops
- Stage II
  - Dilated loops, which may be fixed
  - Pneumatosis intestinalis (presence of submucosal or subserosal air in the intestinal wall)
  - Possible portal venous gas
- Stage III: likely pneumoperitoneum, free air

DIFFERENTIAL DIAGNOSIS

- Systemic
  - Sepsis with ileus
  - Pneumothorax causing a pneumoperitoneum
  - Hemorrhagic disease of the newborn
  - Swallowed maternal blood
- GI tract
  - Volvulus
  - Malrotation
  - Hirschsprung colitis
  - Intussusception
  - Spontaneous bowel perforation
  - Stress gastritis
  - Meconium ileus
  - Milk protein allergy

TREATMENT

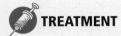

The best therapy for NEC is prevention. When present, early recognition and rapid medical management of infants with NEC are critical to minimize the progression of this aggressive disease.

ADDITIONAL TREATMENT

General Measures

- Length of therapy and reinstitution of feedings are based on the severity of the episode and on clinical, laboratory, and radiologic abnormalities.
- If there are no laboratory or radiographic abnormalities, feedings may be started 24–72 hours after the episode.
- If mild abnormalities are present and the infant is only mildly ill, a 7-day course of therapy is considered.
- When laboratory and radiologic abnormalities include pneumatosis intestinalis, acidosis, and/or thrombocytopenia, a 10- to 14-day course is indicated.

SURGERY/OTHER PROCEDURES

- First-line therapy for NEC is medical management and is successful in 50–75% of infants.
- Surgical intervention is required in 25–50% of all cases.
- Indications include the following:
  - Pneumoperitoneum
  - Cellulitis of the anterior abdominal wall, abdominal mass
  - Suspicion of intestinal infarction with a fixed loop of dilated bowel on radiography
  - Metabolic acidosis secondary to bowel necrosis unresponsive to medical therapy
- The goal of surgery is to remove all necrotic bowel and to preserve as much bowel length as possible. The most widely accepted procedure is laparotomy with resection of gangrenous intestine and exteriorization of all viable ends as stomas.
- Peritoneal drains placed at the bedside were developed as a palliative procedure to decrease surgical morbidity and mortality in infants weighing <1,000 g, decompressing the peritoneal cavity of gas, necrotic debris, and stool. This approach has a higher mortality rate and increased adverse neurodevelopmental outcome than initial laparotomy. However, the majority of pediatric surgeons in the United States believe there is role for peritoneal drainage as a bridge to the more definitive operation.

INPATIENT CONSIDERATIONS

Initial Stabilization

- Therapy is based on the severity and progression of the symptoms.
- Initial management of all patients with suspected or proven NEC
  - NPO status
  - IV fluids
  - Nasogastric (NG) tube placement for decompression
  - IV antibiotics: broad spectrum
  - Total parenteral nutrition (TPN) to ensure adequate nutrition and growth
  - Severely ill patients may require hemodynamic support, acid–base regulation, and respiratory support as clinically appropriate.
- Evaluate every 6 hours to once a day, depending on the severity of the episode:
  - Blood cultures
  - CBC, electrolytes, and blood gas
  - Fluid status
  - Abdominal radiograph

ONGOING CARE

FOLLOW-UP RECOMMENDATIONS

Despite early recognition and intervention, NEC is associated with a significant morbidity and mortality.

DIET

- During acute illness, NPO and TPN
- On resolution of illness, slow reintroduction of feeds is necessary, as the infant is at risk for recurrent NEC.

PROGNOSIS

- Overall mortality for infants with NEC is between 20% and 40% but can be as high as 60% in patients with stage III NEC.
- Infants who survive the acute stage of NEC have a good long-term survival with 80–95% survival to discharge. However, hospitalization is 20 days longer on average than similar infants without NEC.
- Infants recovering from NEC have a 25% risk of microcephaly and serious neurodevelopmental delays.

COMPLICATIONS

- Acute complications that may occur with NEC include GI perforation, DIC, sepsis, shock, fluid and electrolyte imbalance, and respiratory failure.
- Long-term complications occur in 10–30% of infants and include the following:
  - Intestinal strictures
  - Acquired short bowel syndrome if the patient undergoes lengthy surgical resection of bowel
  - Enterocolic fistulas or anastomotic leaks
  - Malabsorption
  - Cholestasis
  - Failure to thrive
- Most common complication (10–35%) is intestinal stricture: occurs mainly in the left colon

ADDITIONAL READING

- Choo S, Papandria D, Zhang Y, et al. Outcomes analysis after percutaneous abdominal drainage and exploratory laparotomy for necrotizing enterocolitis in 4,657 infants. *Pediatr Surg Int*. 2011;27(7):747–753.
- Gordon PV. Understanding intestinal vulnerability to perforation in the extremely low birth weight infant. *Pediatr Res*. 2009;65(2):138–144.
- Lin PW, Stoll BJ. Necrotising enterocolitis. *Lancet*. 2006;386(9543):1271–1283.
- Neu J, Mihatsch WA, Zegarra J, et al. Intestinal mucosal defense system, part 1. Consensus recommendations for immunonutrients. *J Pediatr*. 2013;162(Suppl 3):S56–S63.
- Neu J, Walker WA. Necrotizing enterocolitis. *N Engl J Med*. 2011;364(3):255–264.

CODES

ICD10

- P77.9 Necrotizing enterocolitis in newborn, unspecified
- P77.1 Stage 1 necrotizing enterocolitis in newborn
- P77.2 Stage 2 necrotizing enterocolitis in newborn

FAQ

- Q: What are the most common complications of NEC?
- A: Mortality, poor growth, prolonged hospitalization, and the development of intestinal strictures
- Q: Is NEC preventable?
- A: The development of NEC is not clearly preventable, but cautious feedings in extremely premature infants with gradual advancement and use of breast milk decrease the risk of NEC.
- Q: Is NEC exclusively a process that occurs in the premature infant?
- A: Approximately 10% of cases occur in full-term infants with underlying risk factors.
- Q: How is spontaneous intestinal perforation (SIP) different from NEC?
- A: SIP represents a perforation not associated with pneumatosis, inflammation, or ischemia (all hallmarks of NEC) and occurs in infants that often have not yet been fed. Risk factors include extreme prematurity and early steroid use, particularly in combination with indomethacin in the first week of life.

NEONATAL ALLOIMMUNE THROMBOCYTOPENIA

Anne M. Marsh • Alison T. Matsunaga

BASICS

DESCRIPTION

Neonatal alloimmune thrombocytopenia (NAIT) is one of the major causes of severe thrombocytopenia in the newborn.

- Analogous to ABO/Rh incompatibility but involves platelets instead of RBCs
- Presents with bleeding complications including petechiae, bruising, mucosal bleeding, and/or intracranial hemorrhage (ICH) that can occur in utero

EPIDEMIOLOGY

Incidence is ~1:1,000 to 1:2,000 live births.

GENERAL PREVENTION

The disease cannot be prevented.

PATHOPHYSIOLOGY

Antibody-mediated platelet destruction

ETIOLOGY

Maternal IgG antibodies (Ab), directed against paternally inherited platelet-specific antigens in the fetus, cross the placenta, enter the fetal circulation, and attack fetal platelets.

- HPA-1a (formerly PLA-1) incompatibility is by far the most common cause of NAIT in those of Caucasian ancestry, accounting for ~75% of cases. The disease happens when the mother is HPA-1a negative (HPA 1b/1b) and father is HPA-1a positive (HPA 1a/1a or 1a/1b). If the fetus inherits HPA-1a from father, maternal exposure to HPA-1a–positive fetal platelets during pregnancy causes mother to generate anti–HPA-1a IgG Ab. Anti–HPA-1a Ab crosses the placenta and causes platelet destruction.
- Other common antigens implicated in NAIT include HPA-2, HPA-3, HPA-5, HPA-9, and HPA-15.
- HPA-4 incompatibility accounts for the majority of cases in Asian populations.
- At least 23 other low-frequency antigens have been reported in a small fraction of cases.
- HPA-1a–negative mothers who are HLA-DRB3*0101 positive are far more likely to develop Ab than those who are DRB3 negative.
- The role of HLA platelet antigens in NAIT is unclear.

DIAGNOSIS

HISTORY

- NAIT is suspected in a non–ill-appearing neonate who presents shortly after birth with clinical signs of bleeding and documented thrombocytopenia.
- Maternal history of previous births with thrombocytopenia, NAIT, ICH, or fetal losses?
- Maternal history of thrombocytopenia or ITP?
- Is current maternal platelet count normal?
- Family history of thrombocytopenia or bleeding disorders?
- Symptoms suggestive of an infection in the mother or infant?
- Medications used during pregnancy or in the newborn period

ALERT

Maternal platelet count in NAIT should be normal. Thrombocytopenia in the mother, and/or a history of maternal ITP should prompt you to consider alternative diagnoses such as autoimmune thrombocytopenia (i.e., antibodies directed toward maternal platelets, passively transfer into the fetal circulation, and destroy fetal platelets).

PHYSICAL EXAM

- Most neonates with NAIT are well and nonseptic appearing.
- May have mild easy bruising and bleeding symptoms
- If severely affected, may develop ICH
- Document the following exam findings:
  - General: Evaluate for evidence of a congenital disorder (e.g., dysmorphic features).
  - Head/neck: Exclude presence of full fontanelle and cephalohematoma.
  - Abdomen: Exclude presence of organomegaly and mass.
  - Extremities: Exclude presence of radial-thumb defects.
  - Neurologic exam: Evaluate for irritability, lethargy, seizure, and focal neurologic deficits.
  - Skin: Evaluate for pallor, petechiae, ecchymoses, hemangiomas, and vascular lesions. Evaluate for bleeding from phlebotomy sites, heel sticks, circumcision, and the umbilical cord.
- If congenital anomalies, hepatosplenomegaly, abdominal mass, or skeletal defects are present, consider alternative diagnoses.

DIAGNOSTIC TESTS & INTERPRETATION

Lab

- CBC
- Isolated thrombocytopenia: Platelets are often $<50{,}000/\mu L$ at birth.
- May see anemia if the infant has suffered severe bleeding complications
- Screening coagulation studies
- PT, PTT, thrombin time, and fibrinogen should be normal.
- Maternal platelet count: should be normal
- NAIT testing: HPA incompatibility between mother and child needs to be identified. Testing can be performed on mother and father to avoid collecting blood samples on the infant.
  - Serologic testing: Maternal serum containing platelet-reactive antibodies is tested against a panel of platelet glycoproteins, including HPA-1a, to look for incompatibility.
  - Platelet cross-matching: Maternal serum containing platelet-reactive antibodies is tested against washed paternal platelets to look for incompatibility.
  - Testing also against washed maternal platelets can exclude "autoantibodies" as seen in ITP.
  - Platelet antigen genotyping: DNA-based testing of the platelet glycoprotein genotype of both parents can be performed in only a few laboratories but can reveal potential incompatibilities (i.e., specifically HPA-1 through HPA-6, HPA-9, and HPA-15).

Imaging

Head ultrasound to rule out ICH

DIFFERENTIAL DIAGNOSIS

- Infection
  - Bacterial or viral (e.g., rubella, cytomegalovirus)
- Congenital
  - Thrombocytopenia absent radius
  - Amegakaryocytic thrombocytopenia
  - Wiskott-Aldrich syndrome: X-linked condition with triad of immunodeficiency, eczema, and thrombocytopenia (small platelet size)
  - May-Heglin anomaly: Döhle bodies in WBCs (large platelet size)
- Immunologic
  - Autoimmune thrombocytopenia (i.e., maternal ITP): The degree of thrombocytopenia in autoimmune thrombocytopenia tends to be much less severe than in NAIT.
- Hematologic
  - DIC: increased platelet consumption (e.g., sepsis, NEC)
  - Thrombosis: for example, renal vein thrombosis, catheter-associated thrombosis
  - Hemangioma with Kasabach-Merritt syndrome
- Oncologic
  - Leukemia
  - Neuroblastoma
  - Down syndrome—TMD
- Metabolic
  - Methylmalonic acidemia
  - Isovaleric acidemia

TREATMENT

GENERAL MEASURES

- Daily platelet counts should be obtained until there is documentation of improvement without treatment/intervention.
- Close monitoring for any evidence of bleeding complications, especially ICH
- Avoidance of any invasive procedures (e.g., arterial or lumbar punctures) until platelet count is in a more stable range.
- Platelet count <30,000/μL is generally accepted as a threshold for therapeutic intervention. Much higher thresholds are used if ICH is present.
- Treatment is platelet transfusion (10 mL/kg).

ALERT

All blood products administered should be treated appropriately for a neonate, that is, irradiated, CMV negative, ABO compatible, volume reduced, or washed if indicated.

- Potential sources of platelets for transfusion
  - HPA-1b/1b (i.e., HPA-1a neg) platelets
    - An excellent 1st choice but not always readily available
    - It is *not* appropriate to await HPA-matched platelets for transfusion, especially if the infant has clinically significant bleeding.
  - Random donor platelets
    - Most readily available but not ideal, given that 98% of the population is HPA-1a positive.
    - Will usually elevate the platelet count transiently until a more suitable blood product can be obtained
  - Maternal apheresis platelets
    - Ideal source for platelets but can take days to obtain
    - Do *not* wait for maternal platelets if the infant has clinically significant bleeding.
    - *Important*: Maternal platelets must be washed or volume reduced to remove antibody-containing maternal plasma.
    - Failure to wash or volume reduce maternal platelets may result in prolongation of the fetal thrombocytopenia.
  - HPA-specific platelets
    - If an incompatibility other than HPA-1a is identified, consult your blood bank to see if HPA-specific platelets are available.
- IVIG is another potential therapeutic agent.
- May be used concurrently with platelet transfusions when the platelet count is <30,000/μL, especially when clinical signs of bleeding are present.
- Consider use as monotherapy when the platelet count is 30,000–50,000/μL. Dose of IVIG is 1 g/kg. Multiple doses may be required.

ONGOING CARE

FOLLOW-UP RECOMMENDATIONS

- Given the implications for future pregnancies, NAIT testing should be considered in all infants with thrombocytopenia (<50,000/μL), even if there is another likely etiology.
- If diagnosis of NAIT is confirmed, family counseling regarding management of future pregnancies is strongly recommended. Consultation with a high-risk obstetrician and perinatologist should be made for any future pregnancy at risk for NAIT.

PROGNOSIS

- Overall prognosis is fair to good. Most patients will experience little morbidity or mortality. ICH may lead to very significant morbidity and/or mortality.
- Most cases will resolve in 1–4 weeks.

COMPLICATIONS

- ICH: incidence ~20%, most occur antenatal
- Bleeding from umbilical stump, phlebotomy sites, and/or circumcision
- Petechiae and ecchymoses
- Cephalohematoma
- GI or GU bleeding

ADDITIONAL READING

- Bussel JB, Primiani A. Fetal and neonatal alloimmune thrombocytopenia: progress and ongoing debates. *Blood Rev*. 2008;22(1):33–52.
- Peterson JA. Neonatal alloimmune thrombocytopenia: pathogenesis, diagnosis and management. *Br J Haematol*. 2013;161(1):3–14.
- Symington A, Paes B. Fetal and neonatal alloimmune thrombocytopenia: harvesting the evidence to develop a clinical approach to management. *Am J Perinatol*. 2011;28(2):137–144.

CODES

ICD10

- P61.0 Transient neonatal thrombocytopenia
- D69.42 Congenital and hereditary thrombocytopenia purpura

FAQ

- Q: Can an infant with NAIT safely receive maternal breast milk?
- A: Colostrum and maternal breast milk (MBM) contain immunoglobulins that are passively transferred to an infant. In a pregnancy affected by NAIT, this may include antiplatelet antibodies. The amount of antiplatelet antibodies transferred in MBM is probably minor and there are no reports of adverse consequences in infants with NAIT who have received MBM. The use of MBM in infants with NAIT therefore appears to be safe and should not be discouraged.
- Q: What is the HPA-1a–negative (homozygous HPA-1b/1b) mother's risk of having other affected newborns?
- A: It depends on the genotype of the father.
  - If the father is homozygous for HPA-1a (HPA 1a/1a), all offspring will be heterozygous HPA 1a/1b positive and at great risk for developing NAIT.
  - If the father is heterozygous for HPA-1a (HPA 1a/1b), 50% of offspring will be at risk for developing NAIT.
- Q: Can NAIT happen in a 1st pregnancy?
- A: Unlike hemolytic disease of the newborn due to Rh incompatibility, NAIT can occur even in 1st born offspring. It is important to know that NAIT tends to become more severe with each subsequently affected pregnancy.

N

NEONATAL APNEA

Kalpashri Kesavan • Zankhana Master • Estelle B. Gauda

BASICS

DESCRIPTION

- Apnea of infancy is an unexplained episode of cessation of breathing for 20 seconds or longer or a shorter respiratory pause associated with bradycardia, cyanosis, pallor, and/or marked hypotonia in infants with gestational age (GA) of 37 weeks or more at the onset of apnea.
- Apnea of prematurity (AOP) is a pause of breathing for >15–20 seconds or accompanied by oxygen desaturation (Spo_2 ≤80% for ≥4 seconds) and bradycardia (heart rate <2/3 of baseline for ≥4 seconds) in infants born <37 weeks GA.
- Mechanisms of apnea
  - Central apnea
    - Caused by decreased central nervous system (CNS) stimuli to respiratory muscles
    - No evidence of obstruction to airflow but absent chest wall motion
  - Obstructive apnea
    - Can be due to factors such as pharyngeal instability, neck flexion, nasopharyngeal occlusion
    - Characterized by absent airflow but persistent chest wall motion
  - Mixed apnea
    - Mixed etiology, with obstructive apnea preceding (usually) or following central apnea
- Periodic breathing is a normal neonatal breathing pattern, defined by ≥3 pauses, each ≥3 seconds, with <20 seconds of regular respiration between pauses.

EPIDEMIOLOGY

- Apnea and bradycardia occur in ~2% of all healthy term infants.
- AOP is inversely correlated to GA. It occurs in <10% of neonates 34–35 weeks GA and in almost all neonates <28 weeks GA at birth.

RISK FACTORS

- Prematurity is the most common cause of apnea.
- Risk factors common to both AOP and apnea of infancy are as follows:
  - Age (infant <30 days old at higher risk)
  - Upper respiratory tract infections
  - Gastroesophageal reflux (GER)
  - Anemia
  - Cardiac arrhythmias
  - CNS insult (hemorrhage, seizure, tumors)
  - Immunizations (after DTaP injection)
  - Maternal medications, such as magnesium sulfate, prostaglandins, or narcotics

PATHOPHYSIOLOGY

- Immature respiratory control in neonates
  - Immature chemoreceptors in brainstem and in the periphery (carotid body) may lead to decrease in respiratory drive and apnea.
- Hypoxic ventilatory depression
  - Newborn infants have enhanced sensitivity of respiratory control system to inhibitory neurotransmitters (such as gamma aminobutyric acid [GABA], adenosine, serotonin, and prostaglandin) that can lead to apnea.
- Impaired hypercapnic ventilatory response
  - Prolonging expiratory time (but not increasing frequency or overall tidal volume) may lead to less minute volume as well as uncoordinated movements of respiratory muscles in response to hypercapnia, resulting in apnea.
- Laryngeal chemoreflex
  - Activation of laryngeal chemoreceptors (via superior laryngeal nerve afferents) as seen in GER can result in apnea, bradycardia, and hypotension.
- Sleep state
  - Neonates spend majority of their time in active sleep. Apneas are more common during active sleep when respirations are irregular.
  - Changes in neuromodulatory inputs and generalized inhibition of skeletal muscle activity during sleep are also contributory.
- Congenital central hypoventilation syndrome (CCHS)
  - Alveolar hypoventilation due to abnormality in the central integration of chemoreceptor information as a result of *PHOX2B* mutation

DIAGNOSIS

HISTORY

- Most important part of the evaluation is a thorough and appropriately tailored history.
- Detailed review of the event including time, duration, surrounding circumstances, relation to feeds, appearance of the infant, need for stimulation or resuscitation efforts, and extent
- Thorough details of past medical history including prenatal, birth, and neonatal course; history of prematurity, lung disease, previous apparent life-threatening events (ALTEs)
- Evaluate for recent illness, exposure to infection, feeding difficulties, medications, or vaccines
- Significant family history includes smoke exposure, previous infant deaths, genetic disorders, and cardiac/respiratory disorders.
- Probe for evidence or suspicion of child maltreatment.

PHYSICAL EXAM

- Detailed physical examination, including vital signs, with particular attention to cardiorespiratory and neurologic system is very crucial in determining any underlying condition.
- Examine for signs of child abuse.

DIAGNOSTIC TESTS & INTERPRETATION

ALERT

Initial diagnostic panel for ALTE patients should include CBC with differential, CRP, serum glucose and electrolytes, ABG, urine culture, urine toxicology screen, EKG, respiratory viral panel (RSV, flu, rhinovirus), and pertussis culture.

- Routine screening tests for various etiologies without historical risk factors or suggestive physical exam findings is a very low-yield process.
- Further testing should be based on clinician judgment depending on history and physical exam findings.

Lab

Ammonia, lactate, pyruvate if there are concerns of a metabolic syndrome

Imaging

- Chest x-ray to evaluate for infection or cardiac disease
- Skeletal survey if child abuse is suspected
- Head CT or head ultrasound (if <6 months old) in suspected trauma or elevated intracranial pressure
- Head MRI, if indicated, to evaluate for congenital malformations

Diagnostic Procedures/Other

- EKG/Holter monitoring to evaluate for arrhythmias or conduction problems
- Lumbar puncture if sepsis/meningitis is in the differential diagnosis
- EEG to rule out seizures, especially in case of recurrent ALTE
- A pH probe or modified barium swallow if concerning ALTE is associated with feeding
- Sleep study for evaluation of different types of apnea
- Ophthalmologic exam to identify retinal hemorrhages if child abuse is suspected

DIFFERENTIAL DIAGNOSIS

Immaturity of respiratory control is the primary cause for AOP, but many coexisting factors can potentiate or worsen apnea. Apnea of infancy is uncommon and should warrant a thorough evaluation.

- Infections
  - Respiratory illness: respiratory syncytial virus, pertussis, or pneumonia
  - Sepsis, urinary tract infection, necrotizing enterocolitis, or CNS infection
- Environmental
  - Suffocation, head injury
  - Child abuse
  - Hypothermia or hyperthermia

- Neurologic
  - Seizure
  - Intracranial hemorrhages, CNS malformations
  - Hydrocephalus
  - Neuromuscular disorders
  - CNS tumors
  - Post general anesthesia
- Respiratory
  - Obstructive sleep apnea
  - Nasal obstruction
  - Airway obstruction
  - Foreign body aspiration
  - Breath-holding spells
  - Vocal cord abnormality: laryngotracheomalacia
  - Chest masses/malformations
  - Pneumonia
  - Upper respiratory tract infection
- Metabolic
  - Inborn errors of metabolism
  - Hypoglycemia or electrolyte disturbances
- Cardiovascular
  - Congenital heart disease, patent ductus arteriosus (PDA)
  - Arrhythmias: long QT syndrome, Wolff-Parkinson-White syndrome
  - Cardiomyopathy
  - Myocarditis
- Gastrointestinal
  - GER, feeding hypoxemia
  - Dysphagia or swallowing disorder, intussusception
- Toxin/drugs
- Overdose
  - Sedatives, seizure medications, pain medications
- Hematologic
  - Anemia
- Genetic
  - CCHS
  - Craniofacial anomalies (Pierre Robin sequence)
  - Down syndrome
  - Prader-Willi syndrome

ALERT

Preterm infants with a high frequency of apnea associated with chronic intermittent hypoxia need prolonged respiratory support, take longer to achieve oral feeds, have a greater incidence of retinopathy of prematurity, and have greater risk of adverse neurodevelopmental outcomes.

TREATMENT

MEDICATION

- AOP: Methylxanthines (theophylline and caffeine citrate) are used in hospital settings. Caffeine is preferred due to better absorption, less toxicity, and a wider therapeutic window and half-life that allows once-daily dosing.
- Caffeine citrate (IV or PO) dosing: Loading dose of 20 mg/kg and maintenance dose of 5–8 mg/kg/day. Common side effects include tachycardia, arrhythmia, feeding intolerance, seizures, and diuresis.
- Usually, AOP resolves by 36–40 postmenstrual weeks; however, in more immature infants, born at less than 28 weeks' gestation, apnea may continue until 40–43 weeks postmenstrual age. Once caffeine is discontinued, it is recommended to watch for 5–7 days.

ADDITIONAL TREATMENT

General Measures

- Continuous positive airway pressure (CPAP) splints open the upper airway and improve oxygenation by increasing functional residual capacity. CPAP may be used to treat mixed and obstructive apnea. Positive pressure ventilation may be needed for severe or persistent apnea.
- Patients with a major ALTE should be observed with continuous cardiorespiratory monitoring for a minimum of 23 hours in a hospital setting.
- In case of ALTE where a specific cause was identified, medical or surgical treatment of underlying disorder is indicated.
- Follow-up of the infant with a health care practitioner is recommended within 48 hours after discharge.

ONGOING CARE

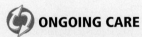

FOLLOW-UP RECOMMENDATIONS

- Infants born before 37 weeks should pass a car seat test prior to discharge after birth.
- Caregivers should be instructed on back-to-sleep, crib safety measure, and avoidance of tobacco smoke exposure and trained in cardiopulmonary resuscitation.
- Home cardiorespiratory monitoring may be considered for infants with chronic lung disease (especially those requiring oxygen supplementation, CPAP, or ventilator). Home monitoring should be used in infants with a tracheostomy or with neurologic, genetic, or metabolic conditions affecting respiratory control. Parents should be appropriately counseled about the purpose, stresses, end point, and proper usage. Parents should be made aware that use of home monitoring does not reduce the risk for sudden infant death.

PROGNOSIS

- Premature infants have 3–5% increased risk for sudden infant death syndrome (SIDS).
- AOP has not been found to be precursor or predictor of SIDS; however, there may be increased risk of SIDS in patients with ALTE.

ADDITIONAL READING

- Chu A, Hageman JR. Apparent life-threatening events in infancy. *Pediatric Ann*. 2013;42(2):78–83.
- Di Fiore JM, Martin RJ, Gauda EB. Apnea of prematurity—perfect storm. *Respir Physiol Neurobiol*. 2013;189(2):213–222.
- Fu LY, Moon RY. Apparent life-threatening events: an update. *Pediatr Rev*. 2012;33(8):361–368.
- Tieder JS, Altman RL, Bonkowsky JL, et al. Management of apparent life-threatening events in infants: a systematic review. *J Pediatr*. 2013;163(1):94–99.
- Zhao J, Gonzalez F, Mu D. Apnea of prematurity: from cause to treatment. *Eur J Pediatr*. 2011;170(9): 1097–1105.

CODES

ICD10

- P28.4 Other apnea of newborn
- P28.3 Primary sleep apnea of newborn
- G47.31 Primary central sleep apnea

FAQ

- Q: Should infants on caffeine for AOP be discharged home?
- A: It is not universal practice that infants with AOP are discharged home on caffeine and home monitoring. It is more common to discharge the infant home 5–7 days after caffeine has been discontinued.
- Q: What should be the end point of home monitoring?
- A: For AOP, if no true events are detected for several weeks and the infant is older than 43 weeks post menstrual age (PMA) and off of all respiratory stimulants for 7 days. For infants who are born at 23–25 weeks, apnea could persist beyond 43 weeks PMA. For monitoring in other cases, it would depend on the frequency and severity of the events.
- Q: What is the role of antireflux medication in the treatment of apnea?
- A: Controversy exists regarding the role of GER in causing apnea in premature infants. Reflux is most likely to trigger apneic events in term infants. Nevertheless, if there is a clear relationship between the apneic event and reflux, then a trial of antireflux medication is recommended. However, if there is no clinical improvement, it should be discontinued.

NEONATAL CHOLESTASIS

Stefany B. Honigbaum • Kathleen B. Schwarz

BASICS

DESCRIPTION

- Neonatal cholestasis is defined as elevated conjugated bilirubin levels that occur in the newborn period. It typically indicates hepatobiliary dysfunction.
- Further studies are needed on any infant who is jaundiced beyond 2 weeks old (or 3 weeks if breastfed).
- Biochemical definition: serum conjugated bilirubin >20% of the total bilirubin concentration or direct bilirubin >2 mg/dL

EPIDEMIOLOGY

- Full-term infants: Most common causes in the 1st month are extrahepatic biliary atresia (EHBA), idiopathic neonatal hepatitis, alpha-1 antitrypsin deficiency, and progressive familial intrahepatic cholestasis (PFIC).
- Premature infants: must consider sepsis and TPN-associated cholestasis
- Incidence of neonatal cholestasis is 1 in 2,500 live births (excluding infants with history of parenteral nutrition).

RISK FACTORS

Genetics

Causes of biliary atresia, neonatal hepatitis, and most other etiologies of neonatal cholestasis remain unknown.

Known genetic causes include the following:

- Alpha-1 antitrypsin deficiency
  - Autosomal codominant expression
  - Mutations in *SERPINA1* gene
  - 10–15% of individuals develop hepatic disease.
  - 2 alleles most commonly associated with liver disease: Z and M
- Alagille syndrome
  - Autosomal dominant, variable expressivity
  - Mutations in *JAG1* and *NOTCH2* gene
- PFIC
  - Group of familial cholestatic disorders: PFIC-1, 2, and 3. Note PFIC 1 and 2 have low GGT values.
  - Autosomal recessive
  - Caused by mutations in *FIC1*, *ATP8B1*, *ABCB11*, and *ABCB4* genes

PATHOPHYSIOLOGY

- Neonatal cholestasis is jaundice secondary to elevated conjugated bilirubin levels in the newborn period.
- Typically, infants are not jaundiced at birth but develop cholestasis within days to weeks of life. In utero, the placenta and maternal liver perform the necessary hepatic functions for the infant. The liver slowly matures throughout the 1st year of life to reach full hepatic metabolism potential.
- Neonatal cholestasis can be caused by a variety of mechanisms of hepatobiliary dysfunction that results in poor bile flow or excretion. In addition, there is inefficient enterohepatic circulation in the newborn period, which contributes to bilirubin accumulation.

ETIOLOGY

Most likely etiologies in <2-month-old infant:

- Obstructive: biliary atresia, gallstones/sludge, inspissated bile, choledochal cyst, neonatal sclerosing cholangitis, congenital hepatic fibrosis/Caroli disease, Alagille syndrome
- Idiopathic: idiopathic neonatal hepatitis
- Infection: UTI, sepsis, cytomegalovirus (CMV), herpes simplex virus (HSV), syphilis, parvovirus B19, adenovirus, enterovirus
- Metabolic/genetic: alpha-1 antitrypsin deficiency, tyrosinemia, PFIC, cystic fibrosis (CF), galactosemia, lipid storage disease, bile acid synthesis defects, mitochondrial hepatopathy, peroxisomal disorders
- Endocrine: hypothyroidism, panhypopituitarism
- Toxic: parenteral nutrition–associated cholestasis, drug-induced
- Miscellaneous: hypoperfusion/shock

COMMONLY ASSOCIATED CONDITIONS

- 10% of infants with biliary atresia also have another major congenital defect (other than laterality defects, see below).
- Biliary atresia splenic malformation (BASM): syndromic form of BA with laterality defects
  - Situs invertus
  - Polysplenia or asplenia
  - Malrotation
  - Congenital heart disease
- Alagille syndrome
  - Syndromic appearance (triangular face, deep set eyes, broad nose)
  - Cardiac anomalies, typically peripheral pulmonary stenosis (PPS)
  - Butterfly vertebrae
  - Ophthalmologic findings: posterior embryotoxon

DIAGNOSIS

HISTORY

- Pregnancy and birth history
- History of consanguinity
- Family history/racial background
- Infectious exposure
- TPN exposure, prolonged history of NPO status
- Presence/absence of extrahepatic manifestations
- Signs and symptoms:
  - Jaundice
  - Hepatomegaly
  - Pale-colored stools
  - Dark-colored urine
  - For specific diagnoses:
    - Alagille syndrome: typical facies, heart murmur
    - Congenital infections: low birth weight, microcephaly, rash, chorioretinitis
    - Metabolic disorders: irritability, hypoglycemia, poor feeding, lethargy

PHYSICAL EXAM

- Jaundice/scleral icterus
- Hepatomegaly
- Splenomegaly
- Cardiac murmurs
- Dysmorphic facial features
- Neurologic abnormalities
- Stool color

DIAGNOSTIC TESTS & INTERPRETATION

Lab

Clinical scenario must be taken into consideration to determine which of the following are appropriate:

- Fractionated serum bilirubin (total and direct)
- ALT, AST, alkaline phosphatase
- Gamma glutamyl transpeptidase (GGT)

- Serum albumin
- Prothrombin time/INR
- Glucose
- CBC
- Urine culture +/− blood culture
- Urine-reducing substances
- Serum alpha-1 antitrypsin level and phenotype
- Serologies: CMV, HSV, enterovirus, hepatitis A and B
- Fat-soluble vitamin levels: A, D, and E
- Cortisol, TSH, T_4
- Infant metabolic screen
- Plasma amino acids, urine organic acids, lactate/pyruvate
- Urine succinylacetone (tyrosinemia)
- Genetic testing for Alagille syndrome, PFIC (1–3), alpha-1 antitrypsin deficiency
- Serum and urine bile acids

Imaging

- Abdominal ultrasound (choledochal cyst, presence of gallbladder)
- Chest x-ray (for butterfly vertebrae with Alagille syndrome)
- Hepatobiliary scintigraphy (HIDA scan) after phenobarbital administrations for 5 days
- X-rays of skull and long bones (for congenital infections and peroxisomal disorders)

Diagnostic Procedures/Other

- Liver biopsy for histology, routine viral culture, immunohistochemistry, and electron microscopy as indicated
- Sweat chloride analysis
- MRCP
- Ophthalmologic exam (for posterior embryotoxin in Alagille syndrome, chorioretinitis)
- Intraoperative cholangiogram
- Echocardiogram (PPS in Alagille syndrome)

DIFFERENTIAL DIAGNOSIS

See "Etiology." The provider must be able to distinguish neonatal cholestasis from physiologic or breast milk jaundice in infancy.

ALERT

Most causes of neonatal cholestasis require expedited diagnosis and intervention:

- Biliary atresia
- Choledochal cyst
- Infection
- Metabolic disorders (e.g., galactosemia)
- Endocrine disorders (e.g., hypothyroidism, hypopituitarism)

TREATMENT

MEDICATION

- Ursodeoxycholic acid (improvement in hepatic function and absorption of fat-soluble vitamins)
- Antihistamines and rifampin (for pruritus associated with cholestasis)
- Antibiotics and antivirals (when appropriate)
- ADEK vitamins (if fat-soluble vitamin deficiencies)

ISSUES FOR REFERRAL

All neonates with cholestasis as defined earlier should have referrals to a pediatric gastroenterologist for further evaluation and management. If the provider suspects biliary atresia or metabolic disease, referral to the appropriate subspecialist should be prompt.

ADDITIONAL THERAPIES

- Consider the need for speech therapy, occupational therapy, or physical therapy when appropriate.
- Nutritional support

SURGERY/OTHER PROCEDURES

- Intraoperative cholangiogram if suspect biliary atresia
- Kasai procedure (hepatoportoenterostomy) for biliary atresia
- Surgical referral for removal of choledochal cyst
- Biliary diversion for severe pruritus associated with Alagille syndrome and PFIC
- Liver transplantation

INPATIENT CONSIDERATIONS

Initial Stabilization

- Sepsis must be identified and treated.
- Coagulopathy (prolonged INR) should be treated with vitamin K.

ONGOING CARE

DIET

- Nutritional support needed. Typically, an elemental formula with high content medium-chain triglycerides is better absorbed in cholestasis.
- Consider need for nasogastric tube feeds.
- Special diets
  - Supplementation with pancreatic enzymes (CF)
  - Galactose-free (galactosemia)

PROGNOSIS

Varies based on underlying diagnosis. Biliary atresia remains the most common indication for pediatric liver transplantation.

COMPLICATIONS

- End-stage liver disease (ascites, coagulopathy) and portal hypertension requiring liver transplantation
- Infection
- Failure to thrive
- Poor bone health
- Developmental delay

ADDITIONAL READING

- Benchimol EI, Walsh CM, Ling SC. Early diagnosis of neonatal cholestatic jaundice: test at 2 weeks. *Can Fam Physician*. 2009;55(12);1184–1192.
- Emerick KM, Whitington PF. Neonatal liver disease. *Pediatr Ann*. 2006;35(4):280–286.
- Moerschel SK, Cianciaruso LB, Tracy LR. A practical approach to neonatal jaundice. *Am Fam Phys*. 2008;77(9):1255–1262.
- Moyer V, Freese DK, Whitington PF, et al. Guideline for the evaluation of cholestatic jaundice in infants: recommendations of the North American Society for Pediatric Gastroenterology, Hepatology and Nutrition. *J Pediatr Gastroenterol Nutr*. 2004;39(2):115–128.

CODES

ICD10

- K83.1 Obstruction of bile duct
- Q44.2 Atresia of bile ducts
- P59.20 Neonatal jaundice from unspecified hepatocellular damage

FAQ

- Q: If my patient has an abnormal HIDA scan, does that mean he/she has biliary atresia?
- A: A HIDA scan can be abnormal in obstructive causes of cholestasis other than biliary atresia. A surgical evaluation via an intraoperative cholangiogram is the gold standard to diagnose biliary atresia.
- Q: What vitamin deficiencies are most common in infants with cholestasis?
- A: Infants with cholestasis often have malabsorption of fat-soluble vitamins (A, D, E, and K) and require supplementation.

NEONATAL ENCEPHALOPATHY

Jennifer C. Burnsed • Frances J. Northington

BASICS

DESCRIPTION

A neonatal neurologic diagnosis notable for depressed level of consciousness with or without seizures. This is a nonspecific term with many etiologies, most commonly hypoxic ischemic encephalopathy (HIE).

EPIDEMIOLOGY

- Most commonly term infants
- Incidence in developed countries 2.5 per 1,000 live births
- 50–80% of cases secondary to HIE

RISK FACTORS

- Variable depending on etiology
- HIE
  - Sentinel event (placental abruption, uterine rupture, cord accident, etc.)
  - Maternal factors: advanced age, obesity, diabetes, severe preeclampsia, infertility treatments, maternal thyroid disease, and placental abnormalities

PATHOPHYSIOLOGY

- Hypoxic ischemic event leading to brain injury with energy failure and ongoing secondary injury, leading to encephalopathy and possibly seizures
- Ongoing injury involves excitotoxic glutamate accumulation in synapses, alterations in cellular calcium management, free radical production and nitrosative/oxidative damage, mitochondrial failure, activation of proteases, and other death cascades, cellular death, with both acute and delayed cytokine production and inflammation.
- Other etiologies include various metabolic disorders, hypoglycemia, kernicterus, nonketotic hyperglycinemia, intracranial infection, perinatal arterial ischemic stroke (PAIS), and sinovenous thrombosis.

DIAGNOSIS

HISTORY

- Sentinel event (uterine rupture, placental abruption, cord accident, cardiorespiratory arrest in delivery room)
- Low Apgar scores
- Advanced resuscitation required in delivery room (intubation, chest compressions, medications)

PHYSICAL EXAM

- Altered level of consciousness (hyperalert or lethargic/obtunded)
- Initial hypotonia
- Weak or absent reflexes
- Decerebrate posturing
- Distal flexion, complete extension
- Abnormal autonomic nervous system:
  - Constricted or unreactive pupils
  - Deviated/dilated pupils
  - Bradycardia
  - Periodic breathing/apnea
- Possible seizure activity: Importantly, seizures may continue but be subclinical (electrical only) after loading dose of an antiepileptic drug (AED).

DIAGNOSTIC TESTS & INTERPRETATION

Lab

- Umbilical cord gas (HIE)
- Glucose (hypoglycemia)
- Electrolytes (metabolic abnormalities)
- Bilirubin (kernicterus)
- Lactate and ammonia (HIE and metabolic abnormalities)
- Plasma amino acids and urine organic acids (metabolic abnormalities)

Imaging

- Head ultrasound (cerebral edema associated with HIE, intracranial hemorrhage)
- MRI with DWI (structural anomalies, stigmata of various encephalopathies, stroke, intracranial hemorrhage)

Diagnostic Procedures/Other

- EEG (seizures, electrographic background—specifically discontinuity, burst suppression patterns)
- Amplitude-integrated EEG (if available)
- Lumbar puncture (cell count for infection, metabolic workup including neurotransmitters)

DIFFERENTIAL DIAGNOSIS

- HIE
- Metabolic disorder
- Intracranial hemorrhage or PAIS
- Hypoglycemia
- Kernicterus
- Nonketotic hyperglycinemia
- Epileptic syndromes/seizure disorder
- Infection (meningitis, encephalitis)

TREATMENT

MEDICATION

- Antiepileptic medications for seizures
  - Phenobarbital or levetiracetam, depending on clinical preference. Multiple other AED are used based on clinical experience and preference.
  - No conclusive data available to guide choice of AED currently. Developing a consensus on treatment with neonatal and neurology consultants is recommended.

ADDITIONAL THERAPIES

- Hypothermia therapy (HT) for moderate to severe HIE (significantly decreased risk of death or moderate to severe disability when treated)
- Criteria for initiation of HT in newborns:
  - <6 hours of age, ≥35 weeks' gestation, and ≥1,800 g
  - Umbilical cord or infant pH ≤7.0 or base deficit ≥16 mmol/L at <1 hour of life AND moderate to severe encephalopathy
  - Umbilical cord or infant pH between 7.01 and 7.15 or base deficit between 10 and 15.9 mmol/L at <1 hour of life AND
    - 10 minute Apgar score <5 OR
    - Need for assisted ventilation at birth with continuation

    AND moderate to severe encephalopathy
  - Moderate to severe encephalopathy (1–3 of the following present in the newborn)
    - Lethargy
    - Stupor/coma
    - Decreased or no activity
    - Distal flexion, complete extension
    - Decerebrate posture
    - Hypotonia or flaccidity
    - Abnormal primitive reflexes: weak/absent/incomplete moro
    - Abnormal autonomic nervous system (constricted or unreactive pupils, deviated/dilated pupils, bradycardia, periodic breathing/apnea)
- Specific management of metabolic disorder or electrolyte/glucose abnormality
  - Time of appearance of symptoms in relationship to birth and presence or absence of a perinatal sentinel event often provides important clues to presence of a metabolic disorder.
  - Immediate recognition and treatment of hypoglycemia, hyponatremia, and hypocalcemia with further investigation into causality and prevention of recurrence
  - Recognition of hyperammonemia is emergent.
  - Lactate/pyruvate ratios, plasma amino acids, urine organic acids, and possibly CSF neurotransmitter levels are often helpful and diagnostic.
  - EEG combined with pyridoxine supplementation can be diagnostic as well.
  - DW-MRI may reveal important diagnostic clues for metabolic encephalopathies.

ONGOING CARE

FOLLOW-UP RECOMMENDATIONS

- Developmental pediatrician
- Pediatric neurologist
- Geneticist (if applicable)

PROGNOSIS

- Widely variable depending on etiology, severity (if HIE), and treatment
- Of patients with moderate to severe HIE treated with hypothermia: at 6–7 years of age, death or an IQ score below 70, 47%; death, 28%; death or severe disability, 41%; moderate or severe disability, 35%; attention–executive dysfunction, 4%; visuospatial dysfunction, 4%
- Perinatal arterial stroke: cerebral palsy (58%), epilepsy (39%), language delay (25%), and behavioral abnormalities (22%)

ADDITIONAL READING

- Badawi N, Kurinczuk JJ, Keogh JM, et al. Antepartum risk factors for newborn encephalopathy: the Western Australian case-control study. *BMJ*. 1998;317(7172):1549–1553.
- Graham EM, Ruis KA, Hartman AL, et al. A systematic review of the role of intrapartum hypoxia-ischemia in the causation of neonatal encephalopathy. *Am J Obstet Gynecol*. 2008;199(6):587–595.
- Jacobs S, Hunt R, Tarnow-Mordi W, et al. Cooling for newborns with hypoxic ischaemic encephalopathy. *Cochrane Database Syst Rev*. 2007;(4):CD003311.
- Raju TN, Nelson KB, Ferriero D, et al. Ischemic perinatal stroke: summary of a workshop sponsored by the National Institute of Child Health and Human Development and the National Institute of Neurological Disorders and Stroke. *Pediatrics*. 2007;120(3):609–616.
- Sarnat HB, Sarnat MS. Neonatal encephalopathy following fetal distress. A clinical and electroencephalographic study. *Arch Neurol*. 1976;33(10):696–705.
- Shankaran S, Laptook AR, Ehrenkranz RA, et al. Whole-body hypothermia for neonates with hypoxic-ischemic encephalopathy. *N Engl J Med*. 2005;353(15):1574–1584.
- Miller SP, Ferriero DM. Hypoxic-ischemic brain injury in the term newborn. In: Swaiman KF, Ashwal S, Ferriero DM, et al, eds. *Swaiman's Pediatric Neurology: Principles and Practice*. 5th ed. Philadelphia: Saunders; 2012:47–58.
- Volpe JJ. Neonatal encephalopathy: an inadequate term for hypoxic-ischemic encephalopathy. *Ann Neurol*. 2012;72(2):156–166.

CODES

ICD10

- P91.60 Hypoxic ischemic encephalopathy [HIE], unspecified
- P91.61 Mild hypoxic ischemic encephalopathy [HIE]
- P91.62 Moderate hypoxic ischemic encephalopathy [HIE]

FAQ

- Q: Is neonatal encephalopathy secondary to HIE always associated with an acute perinatal event?
- A: No. Neonatal encephalopathy may be secondary to an ongoing process in utero and not associated with an acute event. There may be signs prenatally such as decreased fetal movement or abnormalities in fetal heart tracings.
- Q: Does the infant have to be less than 6 hours old to be a candidate for hypothermia therapy?
- A: Yes. Current research has shown that in order to prevent the secondary energy failure and further brain injury, hypothermia should be initiated as soon as possible and within 6 hours of birth. If there is concern for encephalopathy in the delivery room, according to the Neonatal Resuscitation Program, the radiant warmer may be turned off and the infant may be passively cooled until further evaluation can be performed. If applicable, consultation with a referral center that provides hypothermia therapy should be performed as soon as possible. Research trials will determine if there is any value in a more delayed application of the therapy.

NEPHROTIC SYNDROME

Stephanie Clark • Rebecca Ruebner

BASICS

DESCRIPTION

Nephrotic syndrome (NS) is defined by nephrotic-range proteinuria, hypoalbuminemia, edema, and hypercholesterolemia. Nephrotic-range proteinuria is typically found when there is 3–4+ protein on the urine dipstick and is defined as >40 mg/m^2/h or a spot protein-to-creatinine ratio >2 mg protein/mg creatinine.

EPIDEMIOLOGY

- Minimal change nephrotic syndrome (MCNS) is the most frequent cause of NS in younger children:
  - Occurs mainly between 2 and 8 years of age, with a peak at 3 years
  - Boys are more commonly affected than girls (3:2).
  - Atopy and MCNS have an association.
- Focal segmental glomerulosclerosis (FSGS) is the 2nd most frequent cause of NS in childhood:
  - Children with FSGS are more likely than children with MCNS to have steroid-resistant nephrotic syndrome (SRNS).
- Less common than MCNS and FSGS are congenital NS (<3 months) and infantile NS (<1 year).
- Black and Hispanic children have a higher incidence of FSGS than do white and Asian children.
- Prevalence of 16 cases per 100,000 in children <16 years

PATHOPHYSIOLOGY

- Disruption of podocyte architecture composing the glomerular filtration barrier leads to proteinuria, hypoalbuminemia, and subsequently edema.
- Hypercholesteremia occurs due to increased liver production of cholesterol in response to hypoalbuminemia as well as to loss of lipoprotein lipase in urine.
- MCNS Pathology
  - The glomerular tuft and size are normal.
  - Mesangial expansion is absent or minimal.
  - Immunofluorescence is usually negative, although mild staining for C3, IgM, and IgA may occasionally be found.
  - Electron microscopy reveals effacement of the visceral (podocyte) epithelial foot processes, which is reversible.

ETIOLOGY

- Most pediatric cases are primary; 5–10% are secondary to other diseases.
- The most common primary cause of NS in childhood is MCNS. It is characterized by minimal histologic changes on light microscopy and is usually steroid-sensitive nephrotic syndrome (SSNS).
- Other causes of primary NS include FSGS, membranous, and membranoproliferative glomerulonephritis (GN).
- Secondary causes of NS include infections, vasculitis, diabetes, drugs (e.g., NSAIDs), and hereditary disorders.
- Examples of congenital NS include Finnish type, diffuse mesangial sclerosis (DMS), and syphilitic nephrosis.
- NS can also be caused by inherited mutations in proteins involved in the podocyte cytoskeleton, which often results in SRNS and FSGS.

DIAGNOSIS

HISTORY

- Inquire about known atopy or food intolerance.
- Inquire about drug exposure (especially NSAID agents).
- Inquire about any recent infections.
- Signs and symptoms:
  - Fatigue and general malaise
  - Reduced appetite
  - Weight gain and facial swelling
  - Puffy eyes
  - Abdominal swelling or pain
  - Foamy urine
  - Atopy
  - Pitting, dependent edema
  - Fluid accumulation in body spaces (ascites, pleural effusions, scrotal swelling)
  - Mild hypertension (10–20% of patients)

PHYSICAL EXAM

Look for edema in the most dependent area of the child:

- Legs
- Lumbar spine
- Scalp
- Soft ear cartilage
- Scrotum/labia

DIAGNOSTIC TESTS & INTERPRETATION

Lab

Initial lab tests

- The urine dipstick usually shows 2,000 mg/dL (4+) of protein:
  - In small children with NS, the urine dipstick may show <4+.
- Timed or spot urine protein collection
  - 24-hour urine shows >40 mg/kg/day.
  - Spot urine protein-to-creatinine ratio >2 mg/mg.
- Microscopic hematuria is present in 10–20% of cases: The presence of RBC casts is more suggestive of glomerulonephritis.
- Serum creatinine usually normal
- Serum albumin usually <2.5 g/dL
- Total cholesterol elevated, usually >200 mg/dL but can be as high as 500 mg/dL
- Home testing
  - The 1st morning urine is tested for protein with urine dipsticks daily.

Imaging

In complicated cases, renal ultrasound to evaluate for kidney size, parenchymal architecture, and renal venous thrombosis.

DIFFERENTIAL DIAGNOSIS

- Edema
  - CHF
  - Liver failure
  - Protein-losing enteropathy
  - Protein-energy malnutrition (Kwashiorkor)
- NS:
  - MCNS
  - FSGS
  - Membranous GN
  - Membranoproliferative GN
  - Diffuse mesangioproliferative GN

TREATMENT

MEDICATION

First Line

- Corticosteroids are used as 1st-line therapy in suspected MCNS.
  - On presentation: prednisone 2 mg/kg/day for 4–6 weeks (maximum: 60 mg); then prednisone 1.5 mg/kg on alternate days (maximum: 40 mg) and continued for 2–5 months with tapering of the dose.
  - On relapse: prednisone 2 mg/kg/day until urine protein test results are negative or trace for 3 consecutive days; then prednisone 1.5 mg/kg on alternate days for at least 4 weeks.
  - Inadequate duration of corticosteroid therapy is associated with increased risk of relapse

Second Line

- Alkylating agents (cyclophosphamide, chlorambucil)
- Mycophenolate mofetil (MMF)
- Calcineurin inhibitors (cyclosporine A, tacrolimus)
- Rituximab

Supportive Medications

- Diuretics
- ACE inhibitors or angiotensin receptor blockers
- Statins for hypercholesterolemia in persistent NS

ALERT

- Live vaccines are contraindicated while daily corticosteroids or alkylating agents are being given.
- Children in relapse, on corticosteroids, or on alkylating agents and who are nonimmune and exposed to varicella should receive VZIG.
- Albumin and/or furosemide must be used cautiously to prevent pulmonary edema from rapid fluid shifts or intravascular dehydration.

ADDITIONAL TREATMENT

General Measures

- Influenza vaccination yearly
- Full pneumococcal vaccination with PCV13 when needed and 23-valent pneumococcal vaccine
- PPD and chest x-ray at initial presentation prior to starting corticosteroids if risk factors for tuberculosis present

ONGOING CARE

FOLLOW-UP RECOMMENDATIONS

- When to expect improvement:
  - Remission occurs 2–4 weeks after starting corticosteroids in MCNS.
- Signs to watch for:
  - Fever, abdominal pain, oliguria, respiratory distress
- Pitfalls:
  - Recognize situations in which hypovolemia may occur and trigger thrombosis and/or acute kidney injury.
- Monitor for complications of glucocorticoid therapy:
  - Growth failure
  - Cataracts
  - Hypertension
  - Osteopenia
  - Steroid-induced gastritis

DIET

Restrict salt intake while in relapse or on daily corticosteroids.

PATIENT EDUCATION

Educate the family about urine testing, complications, diet, and prognosis.

PROGNOSIS

- The prognosis for MCNS is excellent, with a mortality rate of <1%:
  - 80–90% of MCNS are steroid-sensitive.
  - 20–30% of MCNS will never relapse.
  - 40% of MCNS become steroid-dependent or frequent relapsers.
  - Remaining 30–40% MCNS have infrequent relapses.
- Patients with FSGS, genetic forms of NS, or other secondary causes are more likely to be steroid-resistant and may progress to develop chronic kidney disease.

COMPLICATIONS

- Risk factors for hypovolemia in NS:
  - Severe relapse, GI illness, diuretic use, or sepsis
- Risk factors for thrombosis in patients with NS:
  - Hypovolemia, immobilization, thrombocytosis; urinary losses of protein C, protein S, and antithrombin III
- Risk factors for acute kidney injury in patients with NS:
  - Hypovolemia, bilateral renal vein thrombosis, diuretics, or ACE inhibitors
- Most complications are secondary to steroid therapy and include growth retardation, glaucoma, posterior lens cataracts, obesity, mood changes, hirsutism, osteoporosis, and infection.
- Spontaneous bacterial peritonitis (SBP) is an important and potentially life-threatening complication of NS.
  - Symptoms include fever, abdominal pain, vomiting, and diarrhea.
  - Diagnosis is confirmed by ascitic fluid polymorphonuclear cell count of $\geq$250 cells/mm^3 and positive bacterial culture.
  - Rapid institution of antibiotic therapy is crucial in any patient with NS and suspected SBP.
- Diarrhea and vomiting may result in rapid, severe hypovolemia.
- Vascular thromboses are found with NS in relapse, especially if hypovolemia is present.
  - Sites of thrombosis include lower extremities, IVC, renal veins, cerebral sinuses, and pulmonary emboli.
- Viral infections (measles, varicella) may be life threatening in immunocompromised patients.
- Acute reversible renal failure is an uncommon complication of NS of childhood.

ADDITIONAL READING

- Chesney RW. The idiopathic nephrotic syndrome. *Curr Opin Pediatr*. 1999;11(2):158–161.
- Eddy AA, Symons JM. Nephrotic syndrome in childhood. *Lancet*. 2003;362(9384):629–639.
- Gipson DS, Massengill SF, Yao L, et al. Management of childhood onset nephrotic syndrome. *Pediatrics*. 2009;124(2):747–757.
- Hodson EM, Knight JF, Willis NS, et al. Corticosteroid therapy for nephrotic syndrome in children. *Cochrane Database Syst Rev*. 2000;(4):CD001533.
- Hodson EM, Knight JF, Willis NS, et al. Corticosteroid therapy for nephrotic syndrome in children. *Cochrane Database Syst Rev*. 2003;(1):CD001533.
- Lombel RM, Gibson DS, and Hodson EM. Treatment of steroid-sensitive nephrotic syndrome: new guidelines from KDIGO. *Pediatr Nephrol*. 2013;28: 415–426.
- Robson WLM, Leung AKC. Nephrotic syndrome in childhood. *Adv Pediatr*. 1993;40:287–323.
- Van Husen M, Kemper MK. New therapies in steroid-sensitive and steroid-resistant idiopathic nephrotic syndrome. *Pediatr Nephrol*. 2011; 26(6): 881–892.

CODES

ICD10

- N04.9 Nephrotic syndrome with unspecified morphologic changes
- N04.0 Nephrotic syndrome with minor glomerular abnormality
- N05.1 Unsp neph syndrome w focal and segmental glomerular lesions

FAQ

- Q: Will the MCNS recur?
- A: The clinical course tends to be one of multiple remissions and relapses. Relapses usually improve around the time of puberty.
- Q: Can the NS return in adult life?
- A: Yes. This does occur.
- Q: Is macroscopic hematuria ever found with MCNS?
- A: Gross hematuria suggests a renovascular event or a diagnosis other than MCNS. Microscopic hematuria occurs in ~10–20% of cases.
- Q: What other agents are used to treat NS?
- A: Cyclosporin A, tacrolimus, MMF, cyclophosphamide, and ACE inhibitors/angiotensin receptor blockers are used in children with steroid-dependent or steroid-resistant NS.

NEURAL TUBE DEFECTS

Eric B. Levey

BASICS

DESCRIPTION

Neural tube defects (NTDs): CNS malformations due to abnormalities of neural tube closure during early embryonic development and include anencephaly, encephalocele, and spina bifida (SB)

- Open NTDs: Exposed neural tissue and membranes protrude through a bony defect and lack a skin covering.
  - Due to failure of primary neural tube closure during the 3rd and 4th weeks after fertilization
  - Include anencephaly, craniorachischisis, myelomeningocele, and myeloschisis
- Closed NTDs: theorized to be due to defects of secondary neurulation. Less common than open NTDs and are skin covered.
  - Include some encephaloceles and various types of occult spinal dysraphism (OSD)
- Anencephaly: due to failed closure of rostral neural tube with total or partial absence of cranial vault and cerebral hemispheres
- Encephalocele: partial failure of rostral neural tube closure
  - Abnormal brain tissue protrudes through a skull defect usually covered by skin.
  - 70–80% are occipital, 20% are frontal.
  - 10–20% of occipital defects are meningoceles and contain no brain tissue.
- SB: means "spine split in two" and includes open and closed types
  - Myelomeningocele (MMC): open NTD of the spine, most common type of SB, and characterized by herniation of dysplastic spinal cord and meninges through a posterior vertebral column defect
  - Closed SB: often not diagnosed at birth and often referred to as occult spinal dysraphism.
    - Intact skin over the defect
    - Wide spectrum of defects including lipomyelomeningocele, dermal sinus tracts, diastematomyelia (split cord malformations), myelocystocele, other tumors and cysts of the cord, and congenital spinal cord tethering

EPIDEMIOLOGY

Prevalence

- NTDs affect ~1 in 1,000 established pregnancies worldwide, with significant geographic variation.
- In the United States, birth prevalence has been decreasing due to periconceptional supplementation with folic acid as well as prenatal diagnosis and termination of pregnancy.
- CDC data from 2004 to 2006 showed 0.64 NTDs per 1,000 births (~2,660 cases per year), with 54% classified as SB, 32% anencephaly, and 13% encephalocele.

RISK FACTORS

Most NTDs are due to the interaction of genetic, environmental, and dietary risk factors.

- Variants of multiple genes probably confer some increased genetic susceptibility.
- Maternal nutrition and dietary factors
  - Inadequate maternal folic acid intake
- Maternal diabetes mellitus
- Maternal obesity
- Maternal use of valproic acid (10× risk), carbamazepine, or alcohol during pregnancy
- Maternal exposure to hyperthermia during early pregnancy (e.g., sauna, hot tub, fever)

Genetics

- In most NTD cases, a specific genetic cause is not found.
- Positive family history in ~5% NTD cases
- After 1 child with an NTD, the recurrence rate is 2–5% for subsequent pregnancies.
- A chromosomal or cytogenetic abnormality in ~10% of isolated NTDs, higher percentage in those with multiple congenital anomalies
- NTDs common in trisomy 13 and 18 and can be seen with duplications and deletions.
- Also seen as in single gene disorders or syndromes (e.g., Meckel, Waardenburg, 22q11 deletion syndromes)
- A number of candidate risk factor genes have been studied; the most implicated are those in the folate one-carbon metabolic pathway.
  - A homozygous 677C>T mutation of the methylenetetrahydrofolate reductase (MTHFR) gene in mother or child is associated with ~1.8 times increased risk.

GENERAL PREVENTION

- Periconceptual folic acid supplementation has the potential to reduce NTDs by 50–70%.
- Because many pregnancies are not identified until after neural tube closure occurs, and because more than 50% of pregnancies are unplanned, the CDC recommends that all women of childbearing age receive a minimum of 0.4 mg (400 mcg) of folic acid daily.
- Women at high risk (prior pregnancy with NTD, on valproic acid, etc.) should take high-dose folic acid (4 mg daily), starting 1 month before and through the first 3 months of pregnancy.
- If taking valproic acid, consider switching to alternative medication during pregnancy.

COMMONLY ASSOCIATED CONDITIONS

- Open SB is virtually always associated with some malformation of the brain.
- Most children with MMC have a Chiari II (Arnold-Chiari) malformation, small posterior fossa with elongation of the cerebellum, and herniation through the foramen magnum.
  - Chiari II malformation often causes obstructive hydrocephalus.
  - Historically, about 80% of children with MMC required a CSF shunt.
- Callosal dysgenesis, cortical dysplasia, and subependymal heterotopias are also common.
- MMC is commonly associated with nonverbal learning disabilities and executive dysfunction.
- Open and closed SB: impairments directly due to spinal cord dysfunction:
  - Paraparesis and sensory loss usually correlating with the level of the lesion
  - Neurogenic bladder dysfunction
  - Neurogenic bowel dysfunction
- Congenital foot deformities (club foot) and hip dysplasia are common with NTDs.

DIAGNOSIS

HISTORY

- Anencephaly, occipital encephaloceles, and open forms of SB are usually diagnosed prenatally and are obvious at birth.
- Occult frontal encephaloceles may come to attention because of developmental delays, seizures, or focal neurologic signs.
- OSD can present with progressive neurogenic bowel and bladder dysfunction, lower extremity weakness and/or sensory loss, gait abnormalities, foot deformities, and (rarely) recurrent meningitis.

PHYSICAL EXAM

- Serial head circumferences are (HC) used to monitor infants for progressive hydrocephalus.
  - Macrocephaly strongly suggests increased intracranial pressure (ICP).
  - Normal HC but with increasing percentiles over time may indicate hydrocephalus.
- Dysmorphic features may indicate a syndrome.
- Cranial nerve palsies (strabismus, vocal cord paresis, facial asymmetry), upper extremity (UE) weakness, and abnormal muscle tone can be seen with Chiari II malformation.
- OSD often signaled by a dimple, sinus tract, lipoma, hemangioma, or tuft of hair in the lumbosacral area.
- Functional motor level correlates with ambulatory potential in patients with SB.
- Flaccid paralysis is usually seen below the SB lesion; however, spasticity can be seen.
  - Sensory level may not correspond to motor level.
- Signs of tethered cord syndrome include worsening lower extremity (LE) weakness and spasticity.
- Limb growth may be asymmetric with shorter limb on more affected side (especially in OSD).
- Orthopedic exam should focus on hips, feet/ankles, and spine.
- Skin exam is important for identifying pressure ulcers in areas of impaired sensation.

DIAGNOSTIC TESTS & INTERPRETATION

Lab

- Maternal serum alpha fetoprotein (MSAFP) testing, routinely done at 16–18 weeks gestation, is usually elevated with open NTDs.
- Elevated MSAFP should prompt referral for high-resolution ultrasound.
- Genetic testing including chromosomal microarray often done to look for cause

Imaging

- Prenatal ultrasound
  - Identifies >99% of cases of anencephaly and 90% of cases of MMC
- Postnatal neuroimaging
  - CT: often used to evaluate hydrocephalus: for initial newborn scan and older children when acute shunt malfunction suspected
  - Ultrasound: useful before anterior fontanel closes, especially to monitor hydrocephalus
  - MRI: gold standard for evaluating congenital anomalies of the spine and brain
  - For most patients with MMC, MRI is not necessary in the newborn period.
  - Better for defining the Chiari II malformation and other brain anomalies
  - Spine MRI is used to evaluate tethered cord or syringomyelia.

- Evaluation for suspected OSD
  - Spine ultrasound may be useful for ruling out OSD or tethered cord in newborn or early infant.
  - MRI is used to diagnose and define OSD in infants >6 months of age.
    - Lumbosacral MRI will identify most lesions.
    - However, consider MRI of brain and entire spine to evaluate for higher associated CNS anomalies (e.g., syringomyelia, diastematomyelia, Chiari malformation)
- OSD is common incidental finding on imaging that includes spine (e.g., KUB, upper GI, pelvis x-rays).
  - Isolated SB occulta (a defect of posterior vertebrae) without spinal cord involvement can be found in ~10% of the general population at autopsy.
  - Usually asymptomatic but should be vigilant for signs/symptoms of neurologic involvement
  - Further imaging is usually not necessary.
- Renal imaging is commonly done in children with MMC or other types of SB.
  - Ultrasound of kidneys and bladder is used to evaluate urinary tract in newborns and on regular basis in older children to monitor for hydronephrosis, hydroureter, and stones.
  - Voiding cystourethrogram (VCUG) is used to evaluate bladder emptying and vesicoureteral reflux in newborns and later as needed.
  - Nuclear medicine studies can be useful for evaluating kidney function and scarring from previous pyelonephritis.

Diagnostic Procedures/Other

- Urodynamic studies (cystometrogram) are used to evaluate bladder function and identify those at high risk for hydronephrosis.
- EEG for suspected seizures

TREATMENT

MEDICATION

- Anticholinergic medications (e.g., oxybutynin, tolterodine) are used to relax the spastic bladder and increase capacity.
- Prophylactic antibiotics used when significant vesicoureteral reflux or recurrent urinary tract infections (UTIs)

GENERAL MEASURES

- Route of delivery
  - For most NTDs with vertex presentation, no clear benefit of cesarean delivery
  - Infants who undergo fetal surgery are delivered by cesarean section.
- Clean intermittent bladder catheterization (CIC): commonly used for neurogenic bladder dysfunction
  - For newborns with hydronephrosis, high-grade reflux, or high postvoid residuals
  - Older children for continence
- Latex precautions: avoidance of natural rubber latex to prevent development of latex allergy

ADDITIONAL THERAPIES

- Infants with SB are generally referred to their state's early intervention program.
- Older children typically receive therapy in school but may benefit from additional therapy through the health care system.

SURGERY/OTHER PROCEDURES

- Open encephalocele and SB: neurosurgical closure usually done within first few days of life to prevent infection and protect brain/spinal cord from injury. A moist, sterile dressing is applied to the defect until it is closed.
- Hydrocephalus often develops after an open NTD is closed (stopping leakage of CSF).
- CSF shunts (usually ventriculoperitoneal [VP]) are placed to treat progressive hydrocephalus.
- Fetal closure of MMC has been associated with reduced risk of hydrocephalus and improved developmental and motor outcomes in one prospective randomized trial.
- Fetal surgery for MMC should be considered in select patients prior to 26 weeks' gestation.
- OSD: Neurosurgical exploration and untethering of the spinal cord is usually done after diagnosis.
- Multiple urologic and orthopedic procedures are used to treat the complications of SB. Extensive discussion is beyond the scope of this chapter.

ONGOING CARE

Children with symptomatic SB ideally should be followed in a multidisciplinary SB clinic that includes neurosurgery, urology, and orthopedics as well as a medical generalist (pediatrics, physiatry or neurology) with experience evaluating and treating children with SB.

- Other specialties that are often important:
  - Physical therapy (mobility, LE function)
  - Occupational therapy (ADLs, UE function)
  - Neuropsychology (cognitive function)
  - Social work (coping, adjustment to chronic illness, linkage to resources)
  - Ophthalmology (can identify increased ICP when imaging is equivocal)

PROGNOSIS

- Anencephaly: 75% are stillborn; the remainder do not survive beyond the neonatal period.
- Encephalocele: Prognosis depends on the size of the defect, the amount of brain tissue involved, development of hydrocephalus, and the extent of associated brain malformation.
- MMC
  - Most survive into adulthood.
  - Most have IQ in normal range and almost all of remainder have mild intellectual disability. However, nonverbal learning disabilities and executive dysfunction are very common.
  - Risk of epilepsy ~15%; corresponds to degree of intellectual disability.
- SB (open and closed types)
  - Prognosis for ambulation depends on the level of the lesion:
    - Sacral level: Most are community ambulators without assistive devices.
    - Low lumbar (L4–L5): Most will walk but many require bracing and some require crutches or other assistive devices.
    - Midlumbar (L3): often require bracing of the knee (and sometimes hip) to walk with crutches or a walker.
    - High lumbar (L1–L2) and thoracic: usually walk in therapy only and use wheelchair as primary means of mobility

COMPLICATIONS

- Encephalocele: Hydrocephalus, intellectual disability, motor deficits, and epilepsy are common.
- MMC
  - VP shunt infection or malfunction
  - Symptomatic Chiari II malformation
    - Infants: feeding difficulties/aspiration, hoarse cry or stridor (due to vocal cord paralysis), and central apnea
    - Older children: cranial nerve palsies, occipital headaches, UE weakness, sleep-disordered breathing
  - Syringomyelia
  - Strabismus
- SB (open and closed types)
  - Neurogenic bladder: UTI, hydronephrosis, stones, incontinence, risk of CKD
  - Neurogenic bowel: constipation, impaction, incontinence
  - Orthopedic deformities: scoliosis, hip dysplasia, ankle/foot deformities
  - Tethered spinal cord syndrome
  - Latex allergy
  - Pressure ulcers
  - Osteoporosis and pathologic fractures
  - Deep venous thrombosis
  - Obesity (especially nonambulatory patients)
  - Sexual dysfunction in males

ADDITIONAL READING

- Adzick NS, Thom EA, Spong CY, et al. A randomized trial of prenatal versus postnatal repair of myelomeningocele. *N Engl J Med*. 2011;364(11):993–1004.
- Copp AJ, Stanier P, Greene ND. Neural tube defects: recent advances, unsolved questions, and controversies. *Lancet Neurol*. 2013;12(8):799–810.
- Dennis M, Barnes MA. The cognitive phenotype of spina bifida meningomyelocele. *Dev Disabil Res Rev*. 2010;16(1):31–39.
- Liptak GS, Dosa NP. Myelomeningocele. *Pediatr Rev*. 2010;31(11):443–450.
- Sandler AD. Children with spina bifida: key clinical issues. *Pediatr Clin North Am*. 2010;57(4):879–892.

CODES

ICD10

- Q00.0 Anencephaly
- Q01.9 Encephalocele, unspecified
- Q76.0 Spina bifida occulta

FAQ

- Q: Are neural defects genetic?
- A: Genetic factors are definitely involved, but in most cases, a single genetic cause is not found.
- Q: What is the chance of having another child with a neural tube defect?
- A: Recurrence risk with each subsequent pregnancy is about 2–5%.
- Q: How can someone reduce their risk of having a child with an NTD?
- A: Take 400 mcg of folic acid daily (preferably starting prior to conception) and avoid alcohol and drugs that can increase risk (especially valproic acid).

NEUROBLASTOMA

Lars M. Wagner

BASICS

DESCRIPTION

- Neuroblastoma is a "small round blue cell tumor" of childhood which arises from developing neural crest cells in the sympathetic nervous system.
- The clinical behavior of neuroblastoma is amazingly diverse. Some tumors undergo maturation into benign ganglioneuroma or even spontaneously regress without therapy, whereas others inexorably progress despite intensive treatment.
- Behavior of neuroblastoma tumors can often be predicted by combining clinical features (age, stage) with pathologic/molecular features (histologic characteristics, tumor ploidy, *MYCN* amplification, 1p, and 11q23 status).
- Integrating clinical and molecular features allows for appropriate risk stratification so that treatment can be tailored to the risk of recurrence. Current risk stratification identifies three separate groups of patients with different prognoses and treatment strategies:
  - Low-risk patients: localized tumors and/or favorable clinical and molecular features
  - Intermediate-risk patients: more extensive primary tumor or regional disease or unfavorable clinical and molecular features
  - High-risk patients: patients >18 months with metastatic disease or unfavorable molecular features

EPIDEMIOLOGY

- The median age at diagnosis is 19 months, with 89% of cases diagnosed younger than 5 years of age. Fewer than 5% of patients are diagnosed older than 10 years of age.
- The male:female ratio is 1.1:1.
- The majority of tumors arise in the retroperitoneum, with the adrenal gland being the single most common location.

Incidence

About 800 new cases per year in the United States (10 per million children per year)

Prevalence

- Accounts for 8–10% of all childhood cancer, making it the most common extracranial solid tumor and the most common cancer overall during the first 2 years of life
- Accounts for 15% of all pediatric cancer deaths
- Occurs in 1 per 7,000 live births

RISK FACTORS

Genetics

- Most cases arise spontaneously. One percent are familial (autosomal dominant) and are usually associated with *ALK* mutations.
- Patients with associated congenital central hypoventilation syndrome often have *PHOX2B* mutations.

PATHOPHYSIOLOGY

Tumor growth can cause symptoms in multiple ways:

- Neurologic: nerve or cord compression from paraspinal tumors
- Hypertension: from renal artery distortion or occasionally from excessive catecholamine release
- Pain: from metastatic bone disease
- Pancytopenia: from marrow disease

ETIOLOGY

No known etiology or causative environmental exposures

COMMONLY ASSOCIATED CONDITIONS

May occur along with other disease that have dysregulation of the peripheral nervous system, such as neurofibromatosis type I, Hirschsprung disease, or central congenital hypoventilation syndrome

DIAGNOSIS

HISTORY

- Patients with low-risk disease often appear well and the tumor is discovered incidentally on exam or imaging studies for other reasons.
- High-risk patients often are ill-appearing with obvious symptoms related to tumor location:
  - Abdominal pain or distension
  - Painful bone metastases causing limp
  - Orbital bone metastases causing swelling or discoloration (raccoon eyes)
  - Paraspinal tumors causing weakness, pain, or bowel/bladder symptoms
- Marrow involvement causing pallor and fatigue, petechiae
- Some patients may have paraneoplastic syndromes causing opsoclonus/myoclonus/ataxia related to antineuronal antibodies or excessive diarrhea related to vasoactive intestinal peptide (VIP) secretion.

PHYSICAL EXAM

- Exam findings depend on primary tumor site and extent of dissemination.
- Patients with disseminated disease often have fever and/or worsening nutritional status.
- Patients with abdominal disease may have bulky firm abdominal mass, and hypertension may occur from renal artery distortion or rarely catecholamine release. The liver may be massively enlarged, particularly in patients with stage 4S disease in the 1st year of life.
- Patients with thoracic tumors may have Horner syndrome, and occasionally, respiratory symptoms from airway compression.
- Patients with paraspinal tumors with invasion into the spinal canal may have weakness and/or radicular pain.
- Bone metastases may have associated proptosis, soft tissue swelling, or discoloration from venous stasis.
- Regional or distant nodes may be enlarged, particularly in the supraclavicular region.
- Bluish firm skin nodules may be seen in infants.
- Pallor or petechiae from marrow metastases

DIAGNOSTIC TESTS & INTERPRETATION

Lab

- CBC
  - Decreased hemoglobin, platelets, and/or WBC may indicate marrow involvement.
- Lactic dehydrogenase (LDH)
  - Often elevated with large or metastatic tumors
- Urine catecholamines (homovanillic acid [HVA], vanillylmandelic acid [VMA])
  - Can be done on spot urine samples
  - Elevated in 90% of patients

Imaging

- CT or MRI
  - To evaluate primary tumor site
  - Calcification quite common in neuroblastoma
- Metaiodobenzylguanidine (MIBG)
  - Most specific test for neuroblastoma
  - Uptake seen in primary tumor and metastases in 90% of patients
- Bone scan done if tumor is not avid on MIBG.
- Alternatively, fluorodeoxyglucose-18 positron emission tomography (FDG-PET) scan may also identify tumor in MIBG-negative patients.

Diagnostic Procedures/Other

- Tumor biopsy is usually required, unless there is metastatic tumor in bone marrow coupled with elevated urine HVA/VMA.
  - Tumor tissue usually expresses neuroendocrine markers (synaptophysin, neuron-specific enolase [NSE]) and often contains neuropil.
  - The determination of favorable vs. unfavorable histology is made based on degree of differentiation, presence of stroma, mitotic/karyorrhectic index, and age of patient.
- Neuroblastomas are immature; ganglioneuroblastomas have some maturity but are still malignant, whereas ganglioneuromas are fully mature and benign.
- Bilateral bone marrow aspirates and biopsies help complete staging.
- The International Neuroblastoma Staging System (INSS) is the current staging system:
  - Stage 1: completely resected localized tumor
  - Stage 2: incompletely resected localized tumor (2A) or with regional node involvement (2B)
  - Stage 3: unresectable tumor crossing midline or contralateral regional lymph node involvement
  - Stage 4: dissemination to nodes, bone marrow, liver, skin (except 4S)
  - Stage 4S: <1 year old, with stage 1–2 primary tumor and metastases limited to liver, skin, or bone marrow

DIFFERENTIAL DIAGNOSIS

- Abdominal masses: Wilms tumor, germ cell tumor, hepatoblastoma, abdominal sarcoma, or lymphoma
- Thoracic masses: lymphoma, leukemia, germ cell tumor
- "Small round blue cell tumors of childhood": non-Hodgkin lymphoma, rhabdomyosarcoma, Ewing sarcoma/peripheral neuroectodermal tumor (PNET)

TREATMENT

- Treatment is based on risk stratification using age 18 months, stage, DNA ploidy, favorable vs. unfavorable histology, *MYCN* amplification, and loss of heterozygosity (LOH) 1p/11q.
- Low-risk tumors
  - Treatment is surgery alone, generally without adjuvant chemotherapy.
  - Selected patients with stage 4S disease may never even require surgery and may be closely observed without therapy.
- Intermediate-risk tumors
  - Treatment generally uses 2–8 cycles of outpatient chemotherapy, performing surgical resection when appropriate.
  - Chemotherapy includes carboplatin, etoposide, doxorubicin, and cyclophosphamide.
  - Selected patients may also receive topotecan or cis-retinoic acid.
- High-risk tumors
  - Treatment involves multiple cycles of intense induction chemotherapy, with surgical resection of primary tumor done when appropriate.
  - Treatment is then consolidated with high-dose chemotherapy and autologous peripheral blood stem cell transplant.
  - Following recovery, they receive irradiation to the primary tumor site, as well as any metastatic sites that were slow to respond to induction therapy. Finally, patients receive multiple cycles of cis-retinoic acid coupled with anti-GD2 antibody, which targets the GD2 protein that is ubiquitously expressed on neuroblastoma cells.
  - Chemotherapy used during induction consists of vincristine, doxorubicin, cyclophosphamide, cisplatin, and etoposide. High-dose chemotherapy often involves carboplatin, etoposide, and melphalan. Newer regimens are testing the use of busulfan and melphalan.

ONGOING CARE

FOLLOW-UP RECOMMENDATIONS

Referral to a pediatric oncologist is essential before any diagnostic procedures or therapeutic interventions.

Patient Monitoring

- On therapy
  - Laboratory monitoring for myelosuppression and organ function
  - Disease reevaluation with imaging and bone marrow testing prior to surgery and stem cell transplant
- Off therapy
  - Close follow-up for disease recurrence up to 5 years after completion of therapy, using imaging and urine catecholamine measurement
  - Monitoring for late effects of cancer therapy, especially in young growing children

PROGNOSIS

- Adverse prognostic factors
  - Age >18 months
  - Advanced stage
  - *MYCN* gene amplification
  - Unfavorable histology
  - Diploid tumor genome (primarily infants)
  - LOH at chromosome arms 1p or 11q
- Expected outcomes with current therapy
  - Low-risk disease: >90% 3-year event-free survival
  - Intermediate risk: approximately 85% 3-year event-free survival
  - High-risk: approximately 30–50% 3-year event-free survival

COMPLICATIONS

Treatment-related complications (see "Cancer Therapy Late Effects" chapter)

- Growth delays
- Renal insufficiency
- Hearing loss
- Hypothyroidism
- Second malignancy
- Cardiac dysfunction
- Infertility

ADDITIONAL READING

- Maris JM. Recent advances in neuroblastoma. *N Engl J Med*. 2010;362(23):2202–2211.
- Park JR, Eggert A, Caron H. Neuroblastoma: biology, prognosis, and treatment. *Hematol Oncol Clin North Am*. 2010;24(1):65–86.

CODES

ICD10

- C74.90 Malignant neoplasm of unsp part of unspecified adrenal gland
- C48.0 Malignant neoplasm of retroperitoneum
- C38.3 Malignant neoplasm of mediastinum, part unspecified

FAQ

- Q: Are siblings of children with neuroblastoma at increased risk for neuroblastoma compared with the general population?
- A: No, except in rare families with a known history of neuroblastoma (<1%).
- Q: Can neuroblastoma spontaneously regress?
- A: Yes, but this is usually seen only in children <1 year of age with lower stage disease or in infants with stage 4S disease.
- Q: What are the biggest risks during therapy?
- A: As with all intensive chemotherapy regimens, the risk of infection is high. This is especially true during the autologous stem cell transplant phase.
- Q: What therapy is available to patients who either fail to go into remission or relapse following aggressive therapy?
- A: There is no curative therapy after disease recurrence in high-risk neuroblastoma. However, some patients can have meaningful stabilization of disease with therapeutic MIBG administration or other experimental therapies.

NEUROFIBROMATOSIS-1

Robert Listernick

BASICS

DESCRIPTION
- Neurofibromatosis type 1 (NF-1) is an autosomal dominant tumor suppressor gene disorder.
- NF-1 is diagnosed based on the presence of any 2 of the following National Institutes of Health (NIH) Consensus Conference diagnostic criteria:
  - 6 or more café au lait spots, at least 1.5 cm in diameter in postpubertal individuals or 0.5 cm in diameter in prepubertal individuals
  - Inguinal or axillary freckling
  - 2 or more cutaneous neurofibromas or 1 plexiform neurofibroma
  - 2 or more iris Lisch nodules
  - Optic nerve glioma
  - Osseous lesions, including sphenoid wing dysplasia, dysplasia of a long bone (most commonly tibia)
  - A 1st-degree relative (parent, sibling, or offspring) with NF-1

ALERT
Note: Neurofibromatosis type 2 (NF-2) is a rare distinct autosomal dominant tumor suppressor gene disorder characterized by bilateral vestibular schwannomas as well as schwannomas of cranial and peripheral nerves, meningiomas, and ependymomas. It is caused by mutations in the *NF2* gene, which codes for a protein known as merlin. This chapter focuses on NF-1.

EPIDEMIOLOGY
Incidence
- NF-1: 1 in 3,000 live births
- NF-2: 1 in 33,000 live births

Prevalence
- NF-1: 1 in 4,000–5,000
- NF-2: 1 in 60,000

RISK FACTORS
Genetics
- Autosomal dominant
  - 50% of the cases are inherited; others occur as sporadic mutations.
  - Penetrance is complete; however, expression is variable even between family members who have same mutation.
  - *NF1* gene, which codes for neurofibromin, is located on chromosome 17q11.2
- No known ethnic predisposition
- Course impossible to predict except in two circumstances
  - Deletion of whole *NF1* gene leads to early appearance and large numbers of cutaneous neurofibromas, severe cognitive impairment, and dysmorphic features.
  - 3 base pair in-frame deletion of exon 17 leads to multiple café au lait spots and intertriginous freckling but no other NF-1 manifestations.

DIAGNOSIS

HISTORY
- Growth
  - Accelerated linear growth may be first sign of precocious puberty and presence of optic pathway tumor.
- Vision
  - Optic pathway tumors (OPTs) generally occur before 7 years of age; young children rarely complain of visual loss.
- Development
  - Speech delay, motor incoordination, learning problems, and attention-deficit/hyperactivity disorder (ADHD)
- Headache
  - Common; hydrocephalus due to obstructing tumor may occur.
- Family history
  - 1st-degree relative may have unrecognized NF-1.

PHYSICAL EXAM
- Growth
  - Assess growth chart with attention to accelerated linear growth as early sign of precocious puberty, rarely growth hormone excess.
  - Assess head circumference for macrocephaly.
- Café au lait spots
  - Collections of heavily pigmented melanocytes of neural crest origin in the epidermis
  - 53% of children with NF-1 will have 6 or more by 3 years; 97% by 6 years
- Axillary and inguinal freckling
  - Present in 80% of children by 6 years
- Discrete neurofibromas
  - Benign nerve sheath tumors that appear as discrete masses arising from peripheral nerve
  - Cutaneous neurofibromas protrude just above the skin surface or lie just under the skin often with an overlying violaceous hue.
  - Subcutaneous neurofibromas are generally much harder.
- Plexiform neurofibromas
  - Benign peripheral nerve sheath tumors which involve single or multiple nerve fascicles, often arising from branches of major nerves
  - "Wormy" sensation on palpation often with overlying hyperpigmentation or hypertrichosis
  - Most external plexiform neurofibromas are present at birth or become apparent during the first several years of life.
  - May lead to disfigurement, blindness (secondary to amblyopia, glaucoma, or proptosis), or loss of limb function
  - Thoracic or abdominal plexiform neurofibromas may have no external manifestations but may lead to invasion or compression of vital structures (e.g., ureters, bowel, spinal cord).
- Lisch nodules
  - Best assessed with slit lamp
  - Slightly raised, well-circumscribed melanocytic hamartomas of the iris thought to be virtually pathognomonic of NF-1
  - Increase with age; present in only 30% of children <6 years but >95% of adults
- OPTs
  - Are present in 15% of children with NF-1, although only half are symptomatic and 40% of those will require treatment
  - Complete yearly eye exams mandatory for NF-1 patients <10 years
  - Ophthalmologic signs include afferent papillary defect, optic nerve atrophy, papilledema, strabismus, or defects in color vision.
  - 40% of children who have chiasmal tumors develop precocious puberty.
- Bony dysplasias
  - Sphenoid wing dysplasia may lead to enophthalmos or pulsating exophthalmos.
  - Tibial dysplasia, congenital thinning and bowing; failure of primary union following fracture results in pseudarthrosis.
- Hypertension
  - In children, most commonly due to fibromuscular dysplasia of renal artery
  - Pheochromocytoma rare in children
- Complete neurologic exam
  - Assess for signs of intracranial or intraspinal tumors.
- Scoliosis
  - Assess for idiopathic juvenile scoliosis, short-segment dystrophic scoliosis.

DIAGNOSTIC TESTS & INTERPRETATION

Lab

- *NF1* gene mutation
  - Can be identified in >98% of individuals with clinical diagnosis of NF-1
  - However, gene testing is not necessary in vast majority of cases.
  - Gene testing may be useful for:
    - Very young children who don't meet diagnostic criteria
    - Prenatal testing in familial cases
    - Children with unusual or very mild manifestations of NF-1

Imaging

- "Screening neuroimaging" of asymptomatic children not recommended
- MRI of brain recommended for signs of increased intracranial pressure or focal neurologic deficits, abnormal visual exam, or accelerated growth suggestive of precocious puberty
- Unidentified bright objects ("UBOs")
  - Regions of increased signal intensity on T2-weighted images found in the internal capsule, basal ganglia, cortex, cerebellar hemispheres, optic tract, or brainstem
  - Disappear with age
  - UBOs don't enhance or cause mass effect.
  - Significance unknown; may be associated with cognitive impairment or learning disabilities

Diagnostic Procedures/Other

A biopsy of plexiform neurofibroma looking for malignancy (malignant peripheral nerve sheath tumor) is necessary if there are signs of rapid growth, new onset pain, or neurologic dysfunction.

DIFFERENTIAL DIAGNOSIS

McCune-Albright syndrome has large café au lait spots with irregular margins, polyostotic fibrous dysplasia, and autonomous endocrine hyperfunction (Cushing syndrome, hyperthyroidism, precocious puberty).

TREATMENT

GENERAL MEASURES

- Treatment of neurofibromatosis (NF) is multidisciplinary and should be performed in a multidisciplinary setting.
- All 1st-degree relatives should be examined for the cutaneous manifestations of NF-1 and should undergo slit-lamp examination to ascertain presence of Lisch nodules.
- Available consultants should include experts in orthopedics, oncology, ophthalmology, genetics, endocrinology, surgery, neurosurgery, plastic surgery, and psychiatry.

ONGOING CARE

FOLLOW-UP RECOMMENDATIONS

- Yearly visits allow the physician to identify early NF-1 complications while providing counseling and dissemination of information regarding NF-1.
- All children with NF-1 who are 10 years old and younger should have complete yearly ophthalmologic examinations looking for signs of an optic pathway tumor.
- Blood pressure taken at each visit
- Vigilance/anticipatory care regarding common psychological and developmental issues, such as speech delay, incoordination, ADHD, and learning disabilities
- Early educational assessment and interventions may improve developmental outcome.

COMPLICATIONS

- Cognitive impairment
  - Mean IQ ~95
  - 60% incidence of learning disabilities/ADHD; visual/perceptual disabilities common
- Malignancies
  - Malignant peripheral nerve sheath tumor (5–10% lifetime incidence)
  - Acute myelogenous leukemia
  - Juvenile myelomonocytic leukemia
  - Rhabdomyosarcoma
  - Gastrointestinal stromal tumors
  - Pheochromocytoma
- Skeletal
  - Pseudarthrosis
  - Scoliosis
  - Osteoporosis
- Vasculopathy
  - May involve any arterial vessel
  - Renal artery stenosis, hypertension
  - Moyamoya disease, poststenotic capillary proliferation in cerebral vasculature may lead to cerebral infarct; treatment by encephaloduroarteriomyosynangiosis (EDAMS) procedure.
  - Intermittent claudication of an extremity
- Endocrine
  - Precocious puberty due to chiasmal glioma
  - Pheochromocytoma (rare in children)
  - Growth hormone excess (also rare)

ADDITIONAL READING

- American Academy of Pediatrics Committee on Genetics. Health supervision for children with neurofibromatosis. *Pediatrics*. 1995;96(2, Pt 1):368–372.
- Avery RA, Fisher MJ, Liu GT. Optic pathway gliomas. *J Neuroophthalmol*. 2011;31(3):269–278.
- Feldman DS, Jordan C, Fonseca L. Orthopaedic manifestations of neurofibromatosis type 1. *J Am Acad Orthop Surg*. 2010;18(6):346–357.
- Gutmann DH, Aylsworth A, Carey JC, et al. The diagnostic evaluation and multidisciplinary management of neurofibromatosis 1 and neurofibromatosis 2. *JAMA*. 1997;278(1):51–57.
- Hoa M, Slattery WH III. Neurofibromatosis 2. *Otolaryngol Clin N Am*. 2012;45(2):315–332.
- Lehtonen A, Howie E, Trump D, et al. Behaviour in children with neurofibromatosis type 1: cognition, executive function, attention, emotion, and social competence. *Develop Med Child Neurol*. 2013,55(2):111–125.
- Listernick R, Ferner RE, Liu GT, et al. Optic pathway gliomas in neurofibromatosis-1: controversies and recommendations. *Ann Neurol*. 2007;61(3): 189–198.
- Messiaen L, Yao S, Brems H, et al. Clinical and mutational spectrum of neurofibromatosis type 1-like syndrome. *JAMA*. 2009;302(19):2111–2118.
- North KN, Riccardi V, Samango-Sprouse C, et al. Cognitive function and academic performance in neurofibromatosis 1: consensus statement from the NF1 Cognitive Disorders Task Force. *Neurology*. 1997;48(4):1121–1127.
- Rosser T, Packer RJ. Intracranial neoplasms in children with neurofibromatosis 1. *J Child Neurol*. 2002;17(8):630–637, discussion 646–651.
- Zenker M. Clinical manifestations of mutations in RAS and related intracellular signal transduction factors. *Curr Opin Pediatr*. 2011;23(4):443–451.

CODES

ICD10

- Q85.01 Neurofibromatosis, type 1
- L81.3 Cafe au lait spots

FAQ

- Q: My child has NF-1. What specialists must he see?
- A: Your child should have yearly check-ups with a physician familiar with the issues of NF, ideally in a NF-1 multidisciplinary clinic.
- Q: Does my child with NF-1 need any x-rays?
- A: X-rays or MRI scans need only be done if your child has signs or symptoms suggestive of a particular complication of NF-1.
- Q: Is my child going to die because of NF-1?
- A: Although a very small minority of children with NF-1 has life-threatening complications, almost all individuals with NF-1 live long, productive lives.

NEUTROPENIA

Kristin A. Shimano

BASICS

DESCRIPTION

A decrease in the number of circulating neutrophils (both segmented and band forms), strictly defined as an absolute total neutrophil count (ANC) of <1,500/μL in children older than 1 year of age, <1,000/μL in children younger than 1 year of age, and <5,000/μL in the 1st week of life

- To calculate ANC, multiply the total WBC count by the percentage of segmented neutrophils and band forms.
- For example: WBC count 5,200/μL with 15% segs/polys, 4% bands, 76% lymphocytes, 5% monocytes: ANC = 5,200 × (0.15 + 0.04) = 988
- Severe neutropenia is defined as an ANC <500/μL.

EPIDEMIOLOGY

- Normal values for total WBC counts and ANC vary with age and race.
- Children of some ethnic groups, including African and Middle-Eastern groups, have lower total WBC counts and lower ANCs than do white children.
  - Lower end of normal range for ANC may be 800/μL in 30% of African Americans and does not represent an increased risk for infection.
- Infants have a higher total WBC count and a higher percentage of lymphocytes in their differential counts.
- Prevalence of congenital and idiopathic neutropenia: 2.1 cases per million in the United States
- Incidence of neonatal alloimmune neutropenia: 2 per 1,000 live births

RISK FACTORS

Genetics

- A number of mutations causing severe congenital neutropenia have been identified.
  - Autosomal recessive: Kostmann syndrome (*HAX1*)
  - Autosomal dominant: *ELA2*, *GFL1*, *GATA2*, others
  - X-linked: WASP
- Cyclic neutropenia: autosomal dominant or sporadic (*ELA2*)

ETIOLOGY

- Decreased production of neutrophils
  - Viral suppression
  - Marrow suppression by drugs, chemotherapy, or radiation
  - Nutritional deficiencies
  - Primary disorders of myelopoiesis
- Increased destruction of neutrophils
  - Immune-mediated destruction
  - Increased use (usually with overwhelming infection)
  - Sequestration in the spleen

DIAGNOSIS

HISTORY

- Recent or current viral infection
- Current or recurrent fever, skin abscesses, infections, or oral ulceration
- Temporal pattern of symptoms
- Symptoms of malabsorption, such as diarrhea or failure to thrive
- Delayed cord separation
- Medication use or toxin exposure
- Diet: evidence of nutritional deficiency
- Developmental history
- Ethnicity
- Family history of neutropenia, recurrent infection, or early death; consanguinity
- Results of prior CBC with differential: Prior normal WBC count and ANC essentially rule out severe congenital neutropenia.

PHYSICAL EXAM

- Growth curve
- Oral ulceration or gingival irritation
- Phenotypic abnormalities (thumb anomalies, dwarfism, partial albinism)
- Hepatosplenomegaly or lymphadenopathy
- Bruises, petechiae, pallor
- Birthmarks (café au lait spots)
- Neurologic exam
- Signs of infection
  - Fever (temperature should not be taken rectally)
  - Tachycardia or hypotension
  - Pharyngitis or thrush
  - Cellulitis, perirectal or labial abscesses
  - Signs of local infection (such as inflammation, pus) may be diminished due to lack of neutrophils.

DIAGNOSTIC TESTS & INTERPRETATION

Lab

- Repeat CBC with differential
  - Neutropenia due to viral suppression is extremely common and counts may normalize on repeat exam.
  - Hemoglobin and platelets are important as well; can help determine if this is an isolated neutropenia or pancytopenia
- Serial CBCs, twice weekly for 6 weeks, to rule out cyclic neutropenia
- Evaluation of exocrine pancreatic function if Shwachman-Diamond syndrome is a consideration
- Immunologic evaluation (immunoglobulins, lymphocyte subsets) to rule out immunodeficiency
- Antineutrophil antibodies: can often be detected in autoimmune neutropenia if multiple methods of testing are used; use unclear, however, given imperfect sensitivity and specificity
- Cross-typing maternal serum and paternal neutrophils in evaluation of neonatal alloimmune neutropenia
- Genetic testing for certain disorders

Diagnostic Procedures/Other

- Bone marrow aspirate and biopsy indicated in severe chronic neutropenia, pancytopenia, or when there is other concern for a marrow disorder
- Biopsy may be normal, or may reveal a decrease in the number of myeloid precursors or a maturational arrest of the myeloid line (usually in the later stages), depending on the cause of neutropenia.

DIFFERENTIAL DIAGNOSIS

- Neutropenia associated with infection
  - Viral suppression is a very common cause of transient neutropenia.
  - Viral: hepatitis A and B, parvovirus B19, respiratory syncytial virus (RSV), influenza A and B, rubeola, rubella, varicella, cytomegalovirus (CMV), Epstein-Barr virus (EBV), HIV
  - Bacterial: group B streptococcal disease, tuberculosis, brucellosis, tularemia, typhoid, paratyphoid
  - Other: malaria, visceral leishmaniasis, scrub typhus, sandfly fever
- Drug induced
  - Antibiotics: sulfonamides (trimethoprim/sulfamethoxazole is a common offender), penicillin, chloramphenicol (may be irreversible)
  - Chemotherapy agents: alkylating agents, antimetabolites, anthracyclines
  - Antipyretics: aspirin, acetaminophen (uncommon)
  - Sedatives: barbiturates, benzodiazepines
  - Phenothiazines: chlorpromazine, promethazine
  - Antirheumatic agents: gold, penicillamine, phenylbutazone
- Immunologic
  - Benign neutropenia of childhood: very common cause of chronic neutropenia; immune-mediated; onset usually <2 years of age; typically a benign course with resolution within several years
  - Isoimmune neonatal neutropenia: due to transplacental transfer of maternal antibodies against paternal antigens
  - Manifestation of an autoimmune disease: systemic lupus erythematosus, autoimmune lymphoproliferative syndrome (ALPS), Felty syndrome (neutropenia, splenomegaly, and rheumatoid arthritis), others
- Congenital
  - Severe congenital neutropenia
  - Cyclic neutropenia: regular oscillations in the number of circulating neutrophils (periodicity every 7–36 days; duration of neutropenia, 3–10 days)

- Marrow failure syndromes
  - Shwachman-Diamond Syndrome: neutropenia and exocrine pancreatic insufficiency
  - Part of evolving aplastic anemia: acquired (idiopathic), Fanconi anemia, dyskeratosis congenital, Diamond-Blackfan anemia
- Primary immunodeficiencies
  - Cartilage/hair hypoplasia: neutropenia, dwarfism, abnormal cellular immunity
  - Reticular dysgenesis
  - Chédiak-Higashi syndrome: oculocutaneous albinism, platelet dysfunction, leukocyte inclusions
  - Other abnormalities in T and B lymphocytes
- Bone marrow infiltration
  - Malignancy: leukemia or solid tumors metastatic to bone marrow
  - Osteopetrosis
  - Gaucher disease (lysosomal storage disorder)
- Metabolic
  - Nutritional: malnutrition, copper deficiency, zinc deficiency, megaloblastic anemia secondary to folate or vitamin B_{12} deficiency
  - Inborn errors of metabolism: Barth syndrome (skeletal myopathy, dilated cardiomyopathy, neutropenia), glycogen storage disease I, others
- Miscellaneous
  - Hypersplenism
  - Radiation injury

TREATMENT

MEDICATION

- Granulocyte colony-stimulating factor (G-CSF)
  - Indicated for severe congenital neutropenia and cyclic neutropenia (decreases infections and mortality)
  - May be used in some patients with neutropenia due to other causes

ADDITIONAL TREATMENT

General Measures

- Isolation of hospitalized patient: prudent until the cause of the neutropenia is identified
- "Neutropenic precautions": Standard hand hygiene is sufficient (no need for masks/gowns/gloves).
- Correction of underlying cause of neutropenia (discontinue drug, treat infection, correct nutritional deficiency)
- Treatment of fever and suspected infection when neutropenic: Initially, broad-spectrum antibiotics are indicated; after the diagnosis has been established, this may not always be necessary (i.e., individuals with chronic benign neutropenia).
- Prophylactic antibiotics are not usually beneficial and may predispose to systemic fungal infection.
- Stool softeners may be helpful in the profoundly neutropenic patient at risk for constipation to prevent development of a perirectal abscess.
- No therapy may be required if neutropenia is not severe and there are no serious or recurrent infections (often the case in chronic benign neutropenia).

ADDITIONAL THERAPIES

- Withdrawal of offending drug in drug-induced neutropenia
- Treatment of underlying disorder in many cases of acquired neutropenia
- Stem cell transplant may be indicated in some patients with severe congenital neutropenia or neutropenia due to other causes (such as bone marrow failure syndromes).

ISSUES FOR REFERRAL

- Chronic or profound neutropenia
- History of recurrent unusual or severe infections
- When bone marrow examination is indicated

ONGOING CARE

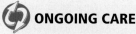

FOLLOW-UP RECOMMENDATIONS

Management of febrile episodes (depends on etiology of neutropenia)

- Prompt evaluation by a physician
- Obtain CBC with differential and blood culture.
- Treat with IV antibiotics.
- Hospitalize if ill-appearing or high-risk for infection.
- Monitor daily CBC with differential.

Patient Monitoring

- CBCs and physical exams at regular intervals while the patient is neutropenic
- Depending on the etiology of the neutropenia, annual bone marrow biopsy surveillance for leukemia or MDS

PROGNOSIS

- Duration of neutropenia depends on diagnosis.
  - Neutropenia resulting from infection or drug-related marrow suppression is usually short lived.
  - Autoimmune neutropenia (benign neutropenia of childhood) typically resolves within 2 years.
  - Congenital neutropenia syndromes may result in chronic lifelong neutropenia.
- Likelihood of infection depends on severity of neutropenia (higher risk if $<500/\mu L$) and cause of neutropenia (higher risk in disorders of neutrophil production).

COMPLICATIONS

- Systemic infections, including pneumonia and sepsis
- Localized infections such as cellulitis, labial abscesses, perirectal abscesses, oral mucosal ulceration, thrush, otitis media, stomatitis, or gingivitis
- Typical pathogens:
  - Bacterial: staphylococci, streptococci, enterococci, *Pseudomonas*, gram-negative bacilli
  - Fungal: *Candida* or *Aspergillus*
- Transformation to leukemia or MDS

ADDITIONAL READING

- Fioredda F, Calvillo M, Bonanomi S, et al. Congenital and acquired neutropenia consensus guidelines on diagnosis from the Neutropenia Committee of the Marrow Failure Syndrome Group of the AIEOP (Associazione Italiana Emato-Oncologia Pediatrica). *Pediatr Blood Cancer*. 2011;57(1):10–17.
- Lehrnbecher T, Phillips R, Alexander S, et al. Guideline for the management of fever and neutropenia in children with cancer and/or undergoing hematopoietic stem-cell transplantation. *J Clin Oncol*. 2012;30(35):4427–4438.
- Walkovich K, Boxer LA. How to approach neutropenia in childhood. *Pediatr Rev*. 2013;34(4):173–184.

CODES

ICD10

- D70.9 Neutropenia, unspecified
- D70.0 Congenital agranulocytosis
- D70.4 Cyclic neutropenia

FAQ

- Q: Do all patients with neutropenia require G-CSF?
- A: No. Patients with severe congenital neutropenia have fewer infections when treated with G-CSF. Patients with benign neutropenia generally do not need G-CSF.
- Q: Can a neutropenic patient receive vaccinations?
- A: Yes, if neutropenia is the only immunologic abnormality
- Q: Should a child with neutropenia be kept in isolation?
- A: No. Neutropenic patients may go to school and do not need to wear masks.

NON-HODGKIN LYMPHOMA

Michelle L. Hermiston

BASICS

DESCRIPTION

- Non-Hodgkin lymphoma (NHL) arises from the malignant proliferation of developing or mature B or T lymphocytes.
- Extent of disease is determined using the Murphy's staging system:
  - Stage I: single tumor (extranodal) or single nodal area, excluding mediastinum or abdomen
  - Stage II: single tumor with regional nodal involvement, 2 or more tumors or nodal areas on the same side of the diaphragm, or a primary GI tract tumor (resected) with or without regional node involvement
  - Stage III: tumors or lymph node areas on both sides of the diaphragm, any primary intrathoracic or extensive intra-abdominal disease (unresectable), or any paraspinal or epidural tumors
  - Stage IV: bone marrow or CNS disease regardless of other sites; marrow involvement defined as 0.5–25% malignant cells

EPIDEMIOLOGY

- 3rd most common childhood malignancy (~12% cancers in individuals <20 years of age in developed countries)
- Number of cases is increasing in adolescents and young adults.
- Male-to-female ratio: 3:1

Incidence

- 10–20 cases per 1 million children/year
- Higher frequency of endemic Burkitt-type in equatorial African countries (10–15 per 100,000 children younger than age 5–10 years)
- Incidence increases steadily with age; in children, usually seen in 2nd decade of life (unusual in those <3 years of age)

RISK FACTORS

Environmental factors

- Drugs: immunosuppressive therapy and diphenylhydantoin
- Radiation: atomic bomb survivors and ionizing radiation
- Viruses: Epstein-Barr virus (EBV) present in >95% of cases of endemic Burkitt versus <20% cases of sporadic; HIV

Genetics

Genetic predisposition: increased risk in patients with immunologic defects (e.g., Bruton agammaglobulinemia, ataxia telangiectasia, Wiskott-Aldrich, severe combined immunodeficiency, X-linked lymphoproliferative syndrome [XLP])

PATHOPHYSIOLOGY

- Unlike adults, low- and intermediate-grade NHL is uncommon in children (~7% of cases).
- NHL in children and adolescent can be divided into 3 major categories according to the National Cancer Institute (NCI):
  - Mature B-cell NHL (Burkitt and Burkitt-like lymphoma, diffuse large B-cell lymphoma [DLBC], primary mediastinal B-cell lymphoma)
    - 50% of childhood NHL
    - Express mature B-cell markers (CD20, surface immunoglobulin [Ig])
    - Terminal deoxyribonucleotidyl transferase (TdT) negative
    - Burkitt lymphoma has characteristic t(8;14), rarely t(8;22) or t(2;8); all chromosomal translocations involve the c-myc proto-oncogene.
    - DLBC usually of the germinal center B-cell phenotype. Unlike adults, the t(14:18) translocation is rare.
  - Lymphoblastic lymphomas (LL)
    - 30% of childhood NHL
    - In children, 90% T-cell and 10% B-cell origin
    - Morphologically identical to acute lymphoblastic leukemia. TdT positive; express early T (CD5, CD7, cytoplasmic CD3) or B (CD19, CD10) cell markers. Bone marrow involvement of >25% blasts is considered leukemia.
    - Early thymic progenitor (ETP) subtype arises earlier in T-cell ontogeny and has a worse prognosis in some studies.
  - Anaplastic large cell lymphoma (ALCL) (mature T-cell or null-cell lymphomas):
    - 10% of childhood NHL
    - Express CD30 (Ki-1)
    - Contain chromosomal rearrangement involving the *ALK* gene (85% t2;5)
- Immunodeficiency-associated NHL usually of B cell origin

DIAGNOSIS

HISTORY

- Mature B cell lymphomas
  - Systemic manifestation (e.g., fever, weight loss, anorexia, fatigue) if disseminated; less likely if tumor localized
  - Abdominal mass with pain, swelling, change in bowel habits, nausea, or vomiting
  - Lump in neck unresponsive to antibiotics
- T-cell LL
  - Mediastinal mass symptoms include cough, hoarseness, dyspnea, orthopnea and chest pain, anxiety, confusion, lethargy, headache, distorted vision, syncope, and/or a sense of fullness in the ears.
  - Marrow involvement: bleeding and/or bruising, bone pain, pallor, fatigue
- B-cell LL
  - Tender or painless swelling in neck, axilla, groin or extremities
  - Symptoms of marrow involvement
- ALCL
  - Painless swelling in neck, axilla, groin
  - B type symptoms: fever, night sweats, weight loss

PHYSICAL EXAM

- Mature B-cell NHL
  - Intra-abdominal mass (90%)
    - Involving ileocecal region, appendix, ascending colon, or a combination
    - Lymphadenopathy may be present in inguinal or iliac region.
    - Hepatosplenomegaly may be present.
    - Acute abdomen with intussusception, peritonitis, ascites, and acute GI bleeding
    - Lymphoma is the most frequent cause of intussusception in children >6 years of age.
  - Other sites: testis, unilateral tonsil hypertrophy, peripheral lymph nodes, parotid gland, skin, bone, CNS, and marrow
  - In endemic Burkitt lymphoma, jaw tumors are the most frequent. Infants often have orbital involvement.
- Lymphoblastic lymphoma
  - T-LL: mediastinal mass (50–70%), possibly pleural effusion present with decreased breath sounds, rales, and cough with or without superior vena cava (SVC) syndrome or superior mediastinum syndrome (SMS):
    - Signs include swelling, plethora, and cyanosis of the face, neck, and upper extremities; diaphoresis; stridor; and wheezing.
  - Lymphadenopathy (50–80%); primarily above diaphragm
  - Abdominal involvement uncommon: likely to involve only liver, spleen, or kidneys
  - Cranial nerve involvement: rare
  - B-LL: firm mass in extremity, enlarged LN
- ALCL
  - Sites: mediastinum, bone, inguinal nodes, skin
  - Bone marrow and CNS involvement: rare at diagnosis

DIAGNOSTIC TESTS & INTERPRETATION

A diagnosis needs to be made expeditiously, as pediatric lymphomas generally have a rapid growth rate.

- Bone marrow aspirate and biopsy may establish the diagnosis without further testing.
- Fluid from ascites in patients with abdominal disease or pleural fluid should be obtained for cytology, immunophenotyping, and cytogenetics.
- Fine-needle aspirate or biopsy of an enlarged lymph node

Lab

- CBC with differential
- Liver and renal function studies
- Tumor lysis labs: serum lactate dehydrogenase (LDH), potassium, calcium, phosphate, uric acid
- Ascitic, CSF, or pleural fluid
  - Cytology
  - Immunophenotyping
  - Cytogenetics

Imaging

- Abdominal ultrasound
- Chest radiographs: posteroanterior and lateral
- CT scan of chest, abdomen, and pelvis
- PET/CT scan
- MRI (especially for bone involvement)

Diagnostic Procedures/Other

- Adequate surgical biopsy
- Bone marrow aspirate and biopsy
- Lumbar puncture with CSF cytology

ALERT

Recumbent positioning, sedation, or positive pressure ventilation may lead to catastrophic respiratory or cardiovascular collapse in patients with partial compromise due to a mediastinal mass. Imaging of airway and consultation with anesthesia, surgeons, and critical care specialists should be obtained prior to any sedation. Procedures may need to be done with local anesthesia only.

DIFFERENTIAL DIAGNOSIS

- Abdominal mass (see chapter)
  - Newborn: hydronephrosis, renal cysts, Wilms tumor, or neuroblastoma
  - Older children: constipation, full bladder, hamartoma, hemangioma, cysts, leukemic or lymphomatous involvement of the liver and/or spleen, Wilms tumor, or neuroblastoma

- Mediastinal mass (see chapter)
  - Anterior: masses of thymic origin, teratomas, angiomas, lipomas, or thyroid tumors
  - Middle: metastatic or infectious lesions involving the lymph nodes, pericardial or bronchogenic cysts, esophageal lesions, or hernias
  - Posterior: neurogenic tumors (e.g., neuroblastoma, ganglioneuroma, neurofibroma), enterogenous cysts, thoracic meningocele, or hernias

TREATMENT

MEDICATION

- Chemotherapy
  - Histology and stage determine therapy
  - Because of a high conversion rate of lymphomas to leukemias, prophylactic CNS treatment is given (except in patients with totally excised intra-abdominal tumor).
  - Duration: mature B cell lymphomas and ALCL, 1–8 months; lymphoblastic lymphomas, 24 months
  - Drugs: cyclophosphamide, vincristine, methotrexate (IV and intrathecal [IT]), prednisone, dexamethasone, daunorubicin, asparaginase, cytarabine, thioguanine, hydrocortisone, doxorubicin, mercaptopurine, etoposide, vinblastine
  - ALCL: crizotinib (a kinase inhibitor that blocks NPM-ALK fusion protein activity)
  - Common side effects: hair loss, myelosuppression with transfusions required, nausea/vomiting
- Immunotherapy
  - Rituximab
    - A chimeric monoclonal antibody to the CD20 antigen, which is almost universally expressed in B-cell NHL
    - Few overlapping side effects with the combination of rituximab and conventional chemotherapeutic agents
    - Whether it improves outcome in children is not known.
  - Brentuximab vedotin
    - Antibody drug conjugate to CD30 that is expressed on all ALCL; currently in clinical trials in children

ADDITIONAL TREATMENT

General Measures

A multidisciplinary approach is imperative to ensure the best therapy.

- Prechemotherapy management
  - Tumor lysis can be present even before initiation of chemotherapy.
  - Allopurinol, hydration, and alkalinization of urine to promote uric acid excretion; may use rasburicase for uric acid >8 mg/dL
  - Monitor uric acid, BUN, calcium, creatinine, potassium, and phosphate levels closely.
- Management of relapse
  - Relapse indicates extremely poor prognosis.
  - No uniform approach to rescue therapy; different chemotherapy combinations may induce a new response.
  - For patients with chemosensitive relapse, salvage therapy followed by high-dose therapy with stem cell support

ADDITIONAL THERAPIES

Radiotherapy

- Adds no therapeutic benefit in children with limited disease; may be indicated in mediastinal DLBCL
- Used occasionally as emergent treatment for SVC obstruction or CNS or testicular involvement
- Cranial radiotherapy given for CNS-positive children with lymphoblastic lymphoma
- Increases short- and long-term toxicity

SURGERY/OTHER PROCEDURES

- Avoid extensive surgery in patients with NHL.
- Performed in mature B-cell NHL if total resection can be achieved
- Additional indications: intussusception, intestinal perforation, suspected appendicitis, or serious GI bleeding

ONGOING CARE

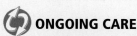

FOLLOW-UP RECOMMENDATIONS

- Patient monitoring weekly to monthly with CBC and physical examination
- Radiologic imaging at intervals during and off therapy

Patient Monitoring

Late effects from therapy:

- Cardiomyopathy from anthracyclines
- Impaired reproductive function or infertility from alkylating agents or radiation
- Second malignant neoplasms from etoposide and alkylators
- Psychological consequences of severe illness

PROGNOSIS

- Important prognostic factors for outcome include tumor burden at presentation.
- Favorable
  - Stages I and II with primary site head and neck (nonparameningeal), peripheral nodes, or abdomen (≥90% 2-year survival)
  - Burkitt: >90% 2-year survival
- Less favorable
  - Stage III or IV disease; ALCL, LL
  - Parameningeal stage II
  - Stage IV with CNS involvement
  - Incomplete initial remission within 2 months (50–80% 2-year survival)

COMPLICATIONS

- Tumor lysis syndrome
  - Combination of hyperuricemia, hyperkalemia, and hyperphosphatemia with hypocalcemia, resulting in uric acid nephropathy that leads to renal failure
- GI obstruction, perforation, bleeding, intussusception
- Inferior vena cava obstruction and venous thromboembolism
- Neurologic (e.g., paraplegia, increased intracranial pressure)
- SVC syndrome and SMS: associated with lymphoblastic lymphomas that invade the thymus and nodes surrounding the vena cava and airways
- Massive pleural effusion
- Cardiac tamponade or arrhythmia

ADDITIONAL READING

- Abramson SJ, Price AP. Imaging of pediatric lymphomas. *Radiol Clin North Am*. 2008;46(2):313–338.
- Bollard CM, Lim MS, Gross TG. Children's Oncology Group's 2013 blueprint for research: non-Hodgkin lymphoma. *Pediatr Blood Cancer*. 2013;60(6):979–984.
- Hochberg J, Waxman IM, Kelly KM, et al. Adolescent non-Hodgkin lymphoma and Hodgkin lymphoma: state of the science. *Br J Haematol*. 2009;144(1):24–40.
- Lones MA, Sanger WG, Le Beau MM, et al. Chromosome abnormalities may correlate with prognosis in Burkitt/Burkitt-like lymphomas of children and adolescents: a report from Children's Cancer Group Study CCG-E08. *J Pediatr Hematol Oncol*. 2004;26(3):169–178.
- Pinkerton CR. Continuing challenges in childhood non-Hodgkin's lymphoma. *Br J Haematol*. 2005;130(4):480–488.
- Pulte D, Gondos A, Brenner H. Trends in 5- and 10-year survival after diagnosis with childhood hematologic malignancies in the United States, 1990–2004. *J Natl Cancer Inst*. 2008;100(18):1301–1309.

CODES

ICD10

- C85.90 Non-Hodgkin lymphoma, unspecified, unspecified site
- C85.10 Unspecified B-cell lymphoma, unspecified site
- C83.70 Burkitt lymphoma, unspecified site

FAQ

- Q: Did I do something to cause this?
- A: No. Most cases are sporadic and not associated with diet, underlying immune dysfunction, or viral illness.
- Q: Is this contagious?
- A: No. Siblings may have slightly higher inherent risk than the general population, but they are not at risk from the affected child.

NONTUBERCULOUS MYCOBACTERIAL INFECTIONS (ATYPICAL MYCOBACTERIAL INFECTIONS)

Rebecca Schein

BASICS

DESCRIPTION

Nontuberculous mycobacteria (NTMB) are mycobacteria other than the *Mycobacterium tuberculosis* complex bacteria (*M. tuberculosis, Mycobacterium africanum, Mycobacterium bovis, Mycobacterium canetti, and Mycobacterium microti*) or *Mycobacterium leprae* capable of causing disease in humans.

- NTMB are classified based on growth rate in culture media as "rapid" or "slow" growers.
- Disease from these infections most commonly presents as cervical lymphadenitis in children.

EPIDEMIOLOGY

- NTMB are ubiquitous in nature and found in soil, food, water, and animals.
- More than 120 species of mycobacteria have been identified.
- Each species has a different level of virulence and many species are associated with specific reservoirs or geographic areas. For example, *Mycobacterium marinum* is found in fish tanks and *Mycobacterium malmoense* is found in Northern Europe.
- Health care–related infections can occur, typically due to rapid-growing *Mycobacterium abscessus* or *Mycobacterium fortuitum*.
- Tap water is a major reservoir for a number of NTMB.

RISK FACTORS

- Cystic fibrosis
- Immune deficiency especially HIV
- Tympanostomy tubes
- Foreign bodies or medical hardware
- Interleukin-12 receptor deficiency

PATHOPHYSIOLOGY

- Rapid growers include the *M. fortuitum* and *Mycobacterium chelonae/abscessus* groups. These rapid growers show significant growth on culture media in 3–7 days.
- Slow-growing mycobacteria take more than 7 days and typically 4–6 weeks to grow in culture.
- Dirty wounds and breaks in oral, respiratory, or gastrointestinal mucosa are the common portals of entry.
- Infection is usually localized near the inoculation site and related regional lymph nodes.
- No evidence of person-to-person spread

ETIOLOGY

- Cervical adenitis is the most common presentation in children 1–5 years of age. In the United States, 80% of these cases are due to *Mycobacterium avium-intracellulare* (MAI).
- In healthy adults, pulmonary disease is the most common illness, typically caused by MAI, *Mycobacterium kansasii, Mycobacterium xenopi, or M. malmoense*.
- Other presentations may include skin and soft tissue infections, bone and joint infections, chronic ear infections, catheter-associated infections, and pneumonia.
- Disseminated disease is seen primarily with MAI in patients with advanced HIV.

DIAGNOSIS

HISTORY

- Travel history and area of residence
- Fever history and systemic complaints
- Length of symptoms—longer history is characteristic.
- Water and animal exposures
- Trauma history
- Recent surgery or hardware

PHYSICAL EXAM

- Lymphadenitis is typically unilateral, minimally tender, anterior cervical, or submandibular.
- Skin disease is usually an ulcer, a localized cellulitis, a draining abscess, or a persistent nodule.
- Pulmonary disease may be associated with fever, weight loss, and fatigue.
  - Mediastinal and hilar lymphadenopathy is common.
  - Lung findings are nonspecific.
- Otitis media in children with tympanostomy tubes presents with chronic drainage unresponsive to antibiotics.
- Disseminated disease is rare; findings include fever, night sweats, abdominal pain, and wasting.

DIAGNOSTIC TESTS & INTERPRETATION

- Definitive diagnosis requires isolation of NTMB in culture.
- Special media and laboratory facilities are required.
- Contamination of nonsterile sites can occur and may require 2 or more cultures to confirm diagnosis.
- Any growth from a draining wound is clinically significant.
- A tuberculin skin test may be positive as cross-reactivity occurs but is not diagnostic.
- PCR for identification of specific NTMB is becoming more readily available and may facilitate quicker diagnosis.

DIFFERENTIAL DIAGNOSIS

- *M. tuberculosis* complex
- Dimorphic fungi: *Histoplasma capsulatum, Coccidioides* species, *Blastomyces dermatitidis, Sporothrix schenckii*
- Malignancy typically leukemia/lymphoma
- *Bartonella henselae*: cat-scratch disease
- Viral or bacterial adenitis

TREATMENT

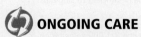

Treatment is variable depending on the site of infection and the specific mycobacterium isolated. In general, complete surgical excision of infected lymph nodes is curative.

MEDICATION

- MAI is treated orally with a macrolide (clarithromycin or azithromycin) plus ethambutol or rifampin. Azithromycin is used as prophylaxis in patients with AIDS.
- Other slow growers such as *M. kansasii*, *M. marinum*, and *Mycobacterium ulcerans* are treated with rifampin-based regimens in combination with ethambutol, macrolides, trimethoprim-sulfamethoxazole, doxycycline, and/or aminoglycosides.
- For rapid growers (*M. fortuitum*, *M. abscessus*, and *M. chelonae*), serious diseases are treated intravenously with an aminoglycoside plus meropenem or cefoxitin depending on susceptibilities. Milder disease or subsequent oral therapy is treated with clarithromycin, doxycycline, trimethoprim-sulfamethoxazole, or ciprofloxacin based on susceptibility testing.
- Combination therapy is indicated in immunocompromised hosts.

SURGERY/OTHER PROCEDURES

- Isolated lymphadenitis is treated with complete surgical excision. Typically, antimicrobials are not beneficial in this situation.
- Any infected hardware should be removed and serious localized disease debrided.

ONGOING CARE

FOLLOW-UP RECOMMENDATIONS

- Medical treatment is typically for a minimum of 3–6 months.
- Follow-up should last 1 year after completion of therapy.

PATIENT EDUCATION

- Chemoprophylaxis for patients with CD4 count <50 cells/μL
- Avoid tap water contamination of central lines.

PROGNOSIS

- For localized disease and adenitis, prognosis is excellent.

COMPLICATIONS

- Chronic draining wounds can occur and treatment is typically long-term antimicrobials in combination with surgical debridement.
- Disseminated disease—occurs in immunocompromised patients

ADDITIONAL READING

- Cruz AT, Ong LT, Starke JR. Mycobacterial infections in Texas children. *Pediatr Infect Dis*. 2010;29(8):772–774.
- Hazra R, Robson CD, Perez-Atayde AR, et al. Lymphadenitis due to nontuberculous mycobacteria in children: presentation and response to therapy. *Clin Infect Dis*. 1999;28(1):123–129.
- Lee WJ, Kang SM, Sung H, et al. Non-tuberculous mycobacterial infections of the skin: a retrospective study of 29 cases. *J Dermatol*. 2010;37(11):965–972.
- Lindeboom JA, Kuijper EJ, Bruijnesteijn van Coppenraet ES, et al. Surgical excision versus antibiotic treatment for nontuberculous mycobacterial cervicofacial lymphadenitis in children: a multicenter, randomized, controlled trial. *Clin Infect Dis*. 2007;44(8):1057–1064.
- Starke JR. Management of nontuberculous mycobacterial cervical adenitis. *Pediatr Infect Dis J*. 2000;19(7):674–675.

CODES

ICD10

- A31.9 Mycobacterial infection, unspecified
- A31.1 Cutaneous mycobacterial infection
- A31.8 Other mycobacterial infections

FAQ

- Q: When should I worry about NTMB?
- A: NTMB should be on the differential for any child with persistent lymphadenitis or a chronically draining wound.
- Q: When should NTMB be considered as a cause of lymphadenitis?
- A: Most lymphadenitis is due to an acute viral or bacterial infection and will improve with time or respond to a short course of antibiotics. NTMB should be suspected in a healthy toddler (age 1–5 years) who presents with a subacute or chronic lymphadenitis. Other considerations should include cat-scratch disease, malignancy, and tuberculosis.
- Q: If infected node is excised, should I treat with antibiotics?
- A: Surgical excision is the treatment of choice of NTMB adenitis. Most studies show that antibiotics are not beneficial after complete surgical excision.

N

NOSEBLEEDS (EPISTAXIS)

Bethlehem Abebe-Wolpaw • Kristina W. Rosbe

BASICS

DESCRIPTION

- Epistaxis: bleeding from the nostril, nasal cavity, or nasopharynx
- Classified as anterior when noted through the nares or posterior when noted through the nasopharynx

EPIDEMIOLOGY

- More than 50% of children aged 6–15 years will experience epistaxis.
- Rarely seen in children younger than age 2 years
- Anterior epistaxis more common in children
- Occurs more frequently in the cold winter months when there is low humidity and when upper respiratory tract infections are more frequent

RISK FACTORS

- Mucosal dryness (also known as rhinitis sicca) is a frequent precursor to episodes of epistaxis as are upper respiratory tract infections.
- Children with allergic rhinitis are more prone to epistaxis.

GENERAL PREVENTION

- Keeping nasal passages moist with the use of humidifiers and saline nasal sprays or ointments (e.g., Vaseline) help reduce mucosal irritation and dryness.
- Ensure fingernails are short and nasal trauma (i.e., nose picking, foreign body) is discouraged
- Use appropriate protective athletic equipment to avoid trauma.

PATHOPHYSIOLOGY

- Blood supply to the nasal cavity contains multiple anastomoses that originate from both the internal and external carotid arteries.
- Kiesselbach plexus located in the anteroinferior aspect of the nasal septum is the most common site of bleeding.
- The thin mucosal surface of the nasal septum and the lateral nasal walls is fragile and thus prone to inflammation and drying.

ETIOLOGY

- Most episodes of epistaxis are due to local inflammation and/or trauma:
  - Upper respiratory infections, allergic rhinitis, rhinosinusitis, nasal vestibulitis, colonization of nasal cavity with *Staphylococcus aureus*
  - Digital trauma, facial trauma, foreign bodies, inhalants/irritants (intranasal corticosteroids, cocaine, heroin)
- In pediatric population, epistaxis is less likely a sign of systemic illness:
  - Bleeding disorders: von Willebrand disease, hemophilia, idiopathic thrombocytopenic purpura, hematologic malignancies
  - Coagulopathy secondary to systemic infection, hepatic disease, renal failure, chronic aspirin or NSAID use
- Local structural/vascular abnormalities
  - Septal deviation, rhinitis sicca, spurs, nasal polyps
  - Telangiectasias (Osler-Weber-Rendu disease)
  - Nasal neoplasms: juvenile angiofibroma, papillomas, hemangiomas

COMMONLY ASSOCIATED CONDITIONS

- Frequently associated with viral upper respiratory infections, allergic rhinitis, nose picking
- More than 90% of children with epistaxis do not have an underlying systemic cause.

DIAGNOSIS

HISTORY

- Frequency and duration
- Laterality of the nosebleed
- Local trauma (nose picking, foreign body)
- Upper respiratory tract infection
- Allergies
- Obstruction
- Discharge
- Medications or drug use
  - NSAIDs, aspirin, anticoagulants, cocaine
  - Alternative medicines: garlic, ginkgo, ginseng
- Personal or family history of bleeding disorders, easy bruising, significant bleeding from minor wounds, frequent or heavy bleeding
- Menstrual history if applicable

PHYSICAL EXAM

- Vital signs
- Use a good light source to perform direct visualization and inspection of nostril, nasal cavity, nasopharynx, and oropharynx.
  - Exam of the nose may be facilitated by application of a topical vasoconstricting agent and/or anesthetic agent to enhance view and slow any current bleeding.
- General exam with particular attention to the skin (bruising, petechiae, purpura, icterus, pallor), lymph nodes, liver, and spleen

DIAGNOSTIC TESTS & INTERPRETATION

- Most episodes are minor and do not require intervention or medical evaluation.
- If history and physical exam are reassuring, diagnostic evaluation is not warranted in healthy children with easily controlled anterior epistaxis.
- If suspicious findings on history or physical exam or child has chronic recurrent epistaxis, laboratory evaluation including complete blood count with platelet count and coagulation panel are indicated.
- Studies suggest that 5–10% of children with chronic recurrent nosebleeds may have mild undiagnosed von Willebrand disease so consider further laboratory tests to include plasma von Willebrand factor (VWF) antigen, VWF activity, and factor VIII activity.
- Persistent unilateral bleeding warrants nasal endoscopy to rule out neoplasm.

DIFFERENTIAL DIAGNOSIS

Epistaxis is a common occurrence in healthy children. A detailed history and physical exam should help identify children with systemic causes for epistaxis, including bleeding disorders and malignancies.

TREATMENT

ACUTE

- Elevate the head.
- Direct pressure, applied by gently squeezing the nostrils, is usually sufficient to stop most nosebleeds.
- Vasoconstricting agents (0.25% phenylephrine, 0.05% oxymetazoline, 1:1,000 epinephrine, or 1–5% cocaine) will help reduce bleeding as well as improve visualization.
- Absorbable hemostatic agents, such as *Floseal*, a bovine-derived gelatin matrix, can also be used for refractory bleeding.
- Parental reassurance is an important, but often neglected, aspect of therapy.

CHRONIC
- Aggressive moisturization including saline irrigation, Vaseline applied with a Q-tip, and sleeping with a humidifier are important for prevention.
- Avoidance of trauma such as repetitive digital manipulation
- Silver nitrate cautery can be performed selectively on prominent vasculature on the anterior septum known as Kiesselbach plexus. This should only be done unilaterally to avoid the risk of septal perforation. If adequate time is given for healing (approximately 1 month), cautery can be performed on the contralateral side.
- For persistent bleeding despite silver nitrate cautery, more powerful cauterization such as Bovie electrocautery can be performed. This procedure is generally not tolerated in patients without general anesthesia.
- In rare cases that do not respond to cautery, vessel embolization by an interventional radiologist or surgical vessel ligation may be required.

ISSUES FOR REFERRAL
Otorhinolaryngologic consultation may be needed for severe nosebleeds or when posterior nasal packing, fracture reduction, surgery, or embolization is required. Nasal endoscopy is now routinely used.

ONGOING CARE

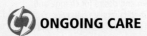

FOLLOW-UP RECOMMENDATIONS
- Nosebleeds are easily controlled and self-limited in most instances.
- Referral to an otorhinolaryngologist is indicated for patients with specific local abnormalities, such as polyps, tumors, or vascular malformations, or severe nosebleeds, recurrent nosebleeds, and/or posteriorly located nosebleeds.
- Identification of systemic illness may require referral to the appropriate specialist.

Patient Monitoring
- Blood clots in the nasopharynx should be removed to enhance visualization.
- Failure to detect a posterior location within the nasal cavity as the source of bleeding may interfere with measures to control bleeding.
- After nasal packing, it is essential to examine the oropharynx to confirm adequate hemostasis.
- Absorbable-type packing should be used, if required, in patients with bleeding disorders. Removable packings are prone to rebleeding on removal.
- Impregnation of nasal packings with antibiotic ointment reduces the risk of toxic shock syndrome.

PATIENT EDUCATION
Families should be given instructions in basic first aid for nosebleeds because minor insults, such as sneezing or excessive manipulation, may cause nosebleeds to recur.

PROGNOSIS
- Uncomplicated epistaxis is most often self-limited or resolves with simple first-aid techniques.
- Refractory or recurrent epistaxis may require more specialized techniques by an otorhinolaryngologist.

COMPLICATIONS
- Usually uncomplicated
- Rare complications: significant blood loss, airway obstruction, aspiration, and vomiting

ADDITIONAL READING

- Bernius M, Perlin D. Pediatric ear, nose, and throat emergencies. *Pediatr Clin North Am*. 2006;53(2):195–214.
- Calder N, Kang S, Fraser L, et al. A double-blind randomized controlled trial of management of recurrent nosebleeds in children. *Otolaryngol Head Neck Surg*. 2009;140(5):670–674.
- Gifford TO, Orlandi RR. Epistaxis. *Otolaryngol Clin North Am*. 2008;41(3):525–536.
- Melia L, McGarry GW. Epistaxis: update on management. *Curr Opin Otolaryngol Head Neck Surg*. 2011;19(1):30–35.
- Qureishi A, Burton MJ. Interventions for recurrent idiopathic epistaxis (nosebleeds) in children. *Cochrane Database Syst Rev*. 2012;9:CD004461.
- Viehweg TL, Roberson JB, Hudson JW. Epistaxis: diagnosis and treatment. *J Oral Maxillofac Surg*. 2006;64(3):511–518.

CODES

ICD10
R04.0 Epistaxis

FAQ
- Q: How should I explain to a child to stop a nosebleed that occurs at home?
- A: The child or parent should apply pressure by compressing the lateral cartilaginous surface of the external nose together for at least 5 minutes. It is important to keep the head elevated but not hyperextended to avoid aspiration of the blood. This can be accomplished either by sitting or standing while bending forward slightly at the waist. Avoid lying down or tilting the head backward. Avoid checking prior to 5 minutes have elapsed to see if bleeding has ceased.
- Q: When should I work-up a patient to ensure there is not an underlying systemic cause for epistaxis?
- A: Most children do not require laboratory evaluation. If the history or physical is concerning or the child has chronic recurrent epistaxis, initial laboratory evaluation may include complete blood count with platelets and coagulation panel. In addition, you can consider checking for von Willebrand disease, as data suggests that up to 5–10% of children with chronic recurrent epistaxis may have a mild form of the disease.

N

OBESITY

Susma Vaidya • Nazrat Mirza

BASICS

DESCRIPTION

Excess adiposity correlates closely with increased health risk for multiple medical and psychological disorders. Body mass index (BMI) is an easily obtained clinical measure to assess for increased body fat and concomitant health risks. BMI is calculated as weight in kilograms divided by height in meters squared. In children, age- and sex-specific percentiles define obesity.

- Children ≥2 years of age
  - BMI 85–94%: overweight
  - BMI 95–98% or BMI ≥30 kg/m^2: obese
  - BMI ≥99%: severe obesity
- BMI reference standards are not available for children <2 years of age. In this age group, overweight is defined as weight-for-length ≥95% for age and sex.

EPIDEMIOLOGY

Prevalence

2009–2010 U.S. National Health and Nutrition Exam Surveys (NHANES) data:

- Younger than age 2 years: 9.7% overweight (≥95 percentile weight-for-length)
- 2–5 years of age: 12.1% obese
- 6–11 years of age: 18% obese
- 12–19 years of age: 18.4% obese
- Higher rates in boys than girls
- Highest rates among Blacks and Hispanics

RISK FACTORS

- Obesity is most often a multifactorial condition with several risk factors:
  - Parental obesity
  - Maternal obesity in pregnancy
  - Maternal history of gestational diabetes
  - Intrauterine growth retardation
  - Rapid weight gain in first 6 months of life
  - Low socioeconomic status
- Genetics
  - Obesity with developmental delay and/or dysmorphic features: Bardet-Biedle, Cohen, Prader-Willi
- Endocrine
  - Obesity with poor linear growth: Cushing syndrome, hypothyroidism

GENERAL PREVENTION

- Encourage exclusive breastfeeding at prenatal visit and support breastfeeding throughout the 1st year of life.
- In formula-fed infants, watch for signs of overfeeding and rapid weight gain in 1st year of life. Educate families on the difference between hunger and oral suck reflex. Avoid rice cereal in the bottle.
- Recognize parental obesity as a significant risk.
- Incorporate early nutrition and activity counseling.
- Careful attention to BMI (and weight-for-length for children <2 years) with intensive counseling for children crossing percentiles.
- Stress importance of portion size and nutrient-rich foods (fruits and vegetables) as infants transition to a solid diet.
- Daily physical activity; limit screen time.

PATHOPHYSIOLOGY

Complex interaction between genetics, hormones, environment, and behavior

- Short-term energy regulation: adaptation of meal size in response to energy needs. Hypothalamic neurons modulate sensitivity of nucleus tractus solitarius (NTS) neurons to satiety signals adjusting for changes in body fat mass.
- Long-term energy regulation: Hypothalamus senses and integrates energy balance signals including hormones such as insulin, leptin, ghrelin, and nutrients such as fatty acids, amino acids, and glucose.
  - Leptin
    - A negative feedback regulator—plays an important role in energy homeostasis.
    - Communicates to hypothalamus changes in energy balance and fuel stored as fat.
    - Increased fat mass results in increased leptin signaling which limits energy intake and supports energy expenditure.
    - Decreased leptin promotes increased food intake, positive energy balance, and fat accumulation.
  - Ghrelin
    - Derived from the stomach, it is the only known peripherally acting orexigenic hormone. It stimulates appetite.
    - All other gut-derived hormones are anorectic and limit food, optimize digestion and absorption, and avoid overfeeding.
  - Adiponectin
    - Insulin sensitizing, anti-inflammatory, and antiatherogenic
    - Increased visceral fat results in reduced levels of adiponectin and increased proinflammatory milieu leading to insulin resistance and endothelial dysfunction. This predisposes to metabolic syndrome, diabetes, and atherosclerosis.

ETIOLOGY

Energy imbalance

- Excessive caloric intake: Calorie-rich foods and beverages consumed preferentially over nutrient-rich foods. Portion size is inappropriately large for age.
- Low-caloric expenditure: excessive sedentary time with TV, computers, video games, and handheld devices; limited daily physical activity

COMMONLY ASSOCIATED CONDITIONS

- Endocrine
  - Type 2 diabetes mellitus
  - Metabolic syndrome
  - Polycystic ovarian syndrome (PCOS)
  - Low vitamin D level
- Cardiovascular
  - Hypertension
  - Dyslipidemia
- Respiratory
  - Sleep apnea
  - Asthma
- Gastrointestinal
  - Nonalcoholic fatty liver disease (NAFLD)
  - Nonalcoholic steatohepatitis (NASH)
  - Gallstones
  - Gastroesophageal reflux (GER)
- Orthopedic
  - Slipped capital femoral epiphysis (SCFE)
  - Blount disease (tibial bowing)
- Skin conditions
  - Acanthosis nigricans
  - Hirsutism
- CNS: pseudotumor cerebri
- Psychiatric
  - Binge-eating disorder
  - Mood disorder: anxiety and depression
  - Low self-esteem

DIAGNOSIS

HISTORY

- Birth history: birth weight, maternal gestational weight gain, gestational diabetes
- Growth history: weight trajectory and age where percentiles were crossed
- Medical and/or social stressors
- Medical history: asthma, medications, obesity comorbidities
- Motivation
  - Parental concern and desire for change and willingness to modify family's behavior
  - Child's concern and motivation (as age appropriate)
- Family history
  - Obesity
  - Diabetes
  - Cardiovascular disease
  - Dyslipidemia
  - Eating disorders
- Dietary history
  - Sugar-sweetened beverages consumed
  - Frequency of fruits and vegetables
  - Frequency and type of snack foods
  - Frequency of fast food
- Eating behavior
  - Family meals
  - TV viewing during meals
  - Recognition of satiety
  - Binge eating with or without loss of control
- Physical activity
  - Total screen time including phone and handheld devices
  - Duration, intensity, and frequency of physical activity
- Sleep duration and pattern
- Previous attempts at weight loss
  - Medication use (prescribed and OTC)
  - Weight loss programs
- Review of systems
  - Headache: pseudotumor cerebri
  - Snoring/pauses in breathing, daytime somnolence: obstructive sleep apnea (OSA)
  - Abdominal pain: reflux, gallstones
  - Joint pains: hip pain (SCFE)
  - Social isolation, emotional eating, behavior difficulties: depression
  - Skin color changes (acanthosis nigricans)
  - Irregular menses/amenorrhea: PCOS
  - Polydipsia, polyuria: diabetes

PHYSICAL EXAM

- Anthropometrics: weight, height, BMI, and BMI percentile
- Blood pressure for age, sex, and height percentile
- General physical findings suggestive of endocrine or genetic condition
  - Short stature
  - Dysmorphic facies
  - Developmental delay
- Head, ears, eyes, nose, throat (HEENT)
  - Papilledema
  - Tonsillar hypertrophy and narrow pharyngeal opening
- Cardiopulmonary
  - Poor aeration, wheezing
  - Heart murmur
- Abdomen
  - Hepatomegaly
  - Abdominal pain
- Genitourinary: Tanner stage
- Musculoskeletal
  - Range of motion at hips
  - Abnormal curvature of lower leg
  - Limp
- Skin
  - Acanthosis nigricans
  - Hirsutism
  - Striae
- Psychological
  - Mood: assess for evidence of depression
  - Bullying, social isolation

DIAGNOSTIC TESTS & INTERPRETATION

Laboratory Tests: Initial

- BMI 85–94%ile without risk factor: fasting Lipid profile
- BMI 85–94%ile age $\geq$ 10 years with risk factors: fasting lipid profile, ALT, AST, fasting glucose
- BMI $\geq$ 95%ile Age $\geq$ 10 years: fasting Lipid profile, ALT, AST, fasting glucose, other tests as indicated by health risks

Abnormal Results

- Lipid panel: Obese children often have elevated LDL and triglycerides and low HDL.
  - High LDL $\geq$130 mg/dL
  - High triglyceride:
    - 0–9 years old $\geq$100 mg/dL
    - 10–19 years old $\geq$130 mg/dL
  - Low HDL $<$40 mg/dL
- ALT value $>$2 times normal or $>$60 IU/L merits gastroenterology consult.
- Fasting glucose $\geq$126 mg/dL or random glucose $\geq$200 mg/dL supports a diagnosis of diabetes and warrants endocrinology consult.
  - HgbA1c $\geq$6.5% suggests possible diabetes.
  - Fasting glucose $\geq$100 mg/dL or HgbA1c $\geq$5.7% and $\leq$6.4% indicates impaired fasting glucose and a prediabetic state.

Diagnostic Procedures/Other

- Polysomnogram: history of snoring with pauses in breathing, narrow pharyngeal airway, or tonsillar hypertrophy (OSA)
- AP and frog-leg views of the hips: knee pain or hip pain, limitation or pain with internal rotation of hip (SCFE)
- Knee and lower extremity radiographs: abnormal curvature of the lower extremities, especially asymmetry (Blount disease)
- Echocardiogram: hypertension (LVH)
- Ambulatory blood pressure monitoring: elevated blood pressure/hypertension
- Abdominal ultrasound: elevated LFTs or abdominal pain (NAFLD, gallstones)
- Head CT: headache and papilledema on ocular exam (pseudotumor cerebri)

TREATMENT

MEDICATION

- Orlistat: an intestinal lipase inhibitor that is the only FDA-approved medication for obesity in children $\geq$12 years
  - Limits nutrient absorption
  - Side effects: abdominal pain, oily stools, flatulence, fat-soluble vitamin deficiencies; self-limited success, poor compliance
  - 5% weight loss, similar to placebo
  - Not recommended for routine use

ADDITIONAL TREATMENT

General Measures

- Prevention and treatment include healthy lifestyle behavior: Goal is to start with small incremental changes in lifestyle.
  - Eliminate consumption of sugar-sweetened beverages including juice and sports drinks.
  - Encourage nonfat milk and water.
  - Increase servings of nutrient-rich foods such as fruits and vegetables with every meal and for snacks.
  - Avoid skipping meals.
  - Reduce eating out or takeout foods.
  - Encourage family meals.
  - Educate families about portion size as soon as solids are started and in early childhood.
  - Advise 1 hour/day of moderate physical activity.
  - Limit screen time to $<$2 hours a day.
- Weight loss goals
  - Weight maintenance may be appropriate in younger children, as BMI will improve with increase in height.
  - Older children and severely obese children can lose up to 2 lb a week.

SURGERY/OTHER PROCEDURES

Bariatric surgery indication

- Adolescents with a BMI $\geq$40 kg/m^2 or BMI $\geq$35 kg/m^2 with concomitant comorbidities such as diabetes and hypertension
- Lack of sustained weight loss on supervised weight-reduction program for 6 to 12 months
- Physical, emotional, and cognitive maturity

ONGOING CARE

FOLLOW-UP RECOMMENDATIONS

- Assess BMI monthly and achievement of dietary and physical activity goals.
- Follow patient more frequently with weight gain and/or refer for nutrition counseling or a weight management program at a tertiary care center.
- Refer to subspecialist with diagnosis of accompanying comorbidities.

PROGNOSIS

- Success is greater in younger children and children with lower BMIs.
- Better success if whole family involved in healthy lifestyle change
- Better success with self-monitoring
- Less success with severe obesity
- Poor prognosis if untreated mental health issues and/or lack of motivation

ADDITIONAL READING

- Barlow SE; Expert Committee. Expert committee recommendations regarding the prevention, assessment, and treatment of child and adolescent overweight and obesity: summary report. *Pediatrics*. 2007;120(Suppl 4):S164–S192.
- Daniels SR. Complications of obesity in children and adolescents. *Int J Obes*. 2009;33(Suppl 1):S60–S65.
- Ogden CL, Carroll MD, Kit BK, et al. *Prevalence of Obesity in the United States, 2009–2010*. Hyattsville, MD: National Center for Health Statistics; 2012. NCHS data brief no. 82.
- Spear BA, Barlow SE, Ervin C, et al. Recommendations for treatment of child and adolescent overweight and obesity. *Pediatrics*. 2007;120(Suppl 4):S254–S288.

CODES

ICD10

- E66.9 Obesity, unspecified
- E66.3 Overweight
- R63.5 Abnormal Weight Gain

FAQ

- Q: How do I broach such a sensitive topic with families?
- A. Review growth charts at every well-child visit and discuss any concerning increase in BMI. Describe in terms of healthy weight and the need to avoid comorbidities which become more likely with increasing BMI.
- Q: How do I counsel a family not interested in making lifestyle changes?
- A: Discuss the risk that an unhealthy BMI poses for the child. Describe small simple changes the family can make to alleviate this risk. Avoid assigning blame. Abnormal lab values may motivate a family to make changes.

OBSESSIVE-COMPULSIVE DISORDER

Holly H. Martin • Manisha Punwani

BASICS

- Obsessive-compulsive disorder (OCD) is a psychiatric illness manifested by recurrent and persistent obsessions and compulsions.
- Obsessions are defined as intrusive, unwanted thoughts, images, or impulses that cause the patient distress, and attempts are made to ignore or suppress these thoughts.
- Compulsions are repetitive actions that patient feels driven to perform in response to an obsession. The behaviors are aimed at preventing or reducing anxiety or distress or preventing some dreaded event or situation.
  - It is not necessary that children recognize these thoughts or behaviors to be excessive or unreasonable.
  - The obsessions or compulsions cause marked distress, are time consuming (>1 hour daily), and cause impairment in daily functioning.
  - Not attributed to physiologic effects of a substance nor are explained by another mental disorder
  - Specified as "with good or fair insight," "with poor insight," "with absent insight/delusional beliefs," or tic-related

EPIDEMIOLOGY

- There are at least 1 in 200—or 500,000—children and adolescents that have OCD. This figure is similar to the number of children who have diabetes.
- OCD can start at any time from preschool to adulthood.
- Although OCD does occur at earlier ages, there are generally two age ranges when OCD first appears. The first range is between ages 10 and 12 years and the second between the late teens and early adulthood.

RISK FACTORS

- Familial heritability pattern
- Moderate genetic component based on twin studies
- Acute streptococcal infection (PANDAS)

COMMONLY ASSOCIATED CONDITIONS

- Depression
- Anxiety disorders
- Tourette syndrome
- Trichotillomania

DIAGNOSIS

HISTORY

- The diagnostic evaluation should entail gathering data through separate interviews with the child/adolescent and the parents.
- Current symptoms should be elicited within attention to severity, duration, and level of functional impairment.
- Core symptoms should be elicited concerning the content of obsessions and the nature of compulsions. These are most frequently checking behaviors, repetition rituals, or a focus on symmetry and organization.
- Sensitivity in assessing violent or sexually intrusive thoughts is necessary, as children may be uncomfortable disclosing these.
- Compulsions may manifest in physical action or in mental repetition.
- Assess the amount of functional impairment by estimating the time spent occupied by obsession and compulsions and how it interferes with their daily lives.
- Explore their level of insight into the irrationality of the symptoms. Diagnostically, children do not have to recognize the symptoms to be excessive. Assess any parental accommodation of the ritualized behaviors, such as excessive cleaning.
- Determine if the onset was acute, severe, and temporally associated with symptoms of a streptococcal infection.

PHYSICAL EXAM

No pertinent findings

DIAGNOSTIC TESTS & INTERPRETATION

Lab

- No pathognomonic laboratory findings
- If onset is acute, severe, and associated with symptoms of a streptococcal infection, consider obtaining an ASO titer.

Diagnostic Procedures/Other

Diagnostic scales: Children's Yale-Brown Obsessive Compulsive Scale (CY-BOCS)

DIFFERENTIAL DIAGNOSIS

- Pervasive developmental disorders
- Delusional disorder
- Obsessive-compulsive personality disorder
- Body dysmorphic disorder
- Anorexia nervosa
- Trichotillomania
- Tourette syndrome
- Schizophrenia
- Sydenham chorea
- Pediatric autoimmune neuropsychiatric disorders associated with strep infections (PANDAS)

TREATMENT

GENERAL MEASURES

There are 2 types of treatment for OCD, psychosocial treatment and pharmacotherapy.

- Cognitive behavioral therapy (CBT) is most effective and well-studied psychosocial treatment:
  - Selective serotonin reuptake inhibitors (SSRIs) are the 1st-line agents for medication management.
  - Start intervention with CBT alone and add medication if treatment response is limited.
- Emphasis is placed on graduated exposure with response prevention.
- Parental education is an important aspect of treatment adherence.

- Pitfalls
  - Failing to use appropriate psychosocial treatments especially school-based modifications
  - Not identifying the extent of the functional impairment
- It is important to recognize
  - The child's fear of the internal thoughts he or she is having
  - The parents' desire to have a "normal" child and thus their tendency to minimize/reassure the child who has concerns

MEDICATION

- SSRIs (1st-line) once-daily oral dosing; initiate 1/2 the starting dose for children with anxiety disorders:
  - Fluoxetine (Prozac) (10–60 mg)
  - Sertraline (Zoloft) (25–200 mg)
  - Fluvoxamine (Luvox) (25–200 mg)
  - Side effects include GI upset, headaches, dizziness, and agitation.

ALERT
A black box warning by the FDA indicates that all antidepressants may increase suicidal thinking and behavior in children and adolescents.

  - Close monitoring is recommended (see next section).
- Tricyclic antidepressants (TCAs) are 2nd-line agents:
  - Clomipramine (Anafranil) (25–250 mg PO once daily)
  - Side effects include dizziness, xerostomia, blurred vision, postural hypotension, tachycardia, sedation, and constipation.

ONGOING CARE

FOLLOW-UP RECOMMENDATIONS

Patient Monitoring

- Monitoring of response to psychosocial treatment should be performed routinely every 2–3 months.
- If medication is initiated, close monitoring on a weekly basis is recommended for the 1st 4 weeks, followed by monthly monitoring.
- CBT is performed on a weekly or twice weekly regimen.
- Monitoring of any emerging comorbidities is suggested.

PROGNOSIS

- OCD is a chronic condition. Treatments have been demonstrated to show significant response, but remission of symptoms is rare.
- Childhood onset is a poor prognostic indicator.

ADDITIONAL READING

- Coskun M, Zoroglu S, Ozturk M. Phenomenology, psychiatric cormorbidity and family history in referred preschool children with obsessive compulsive disorder. *Child Adolesc Psychiatry Ment Health*. 2012;6(1):36.
- March JS; Pediatric OTC Treatment Study Team. Cognitive-behavior therapy, sertraline, and their combination for children and adolescents with obsessive-compulsive disorder: the Pediatric OCD Treatment Study (POTS) randomized-controlled trial. *JAMA*. 2004;292(16):1969–1976.
- O'Neill J, Gorbis E, Feusner JD, et al. Effects of intensive cognitive-behavioral therapy on cingulate neurochemistry in obsessive-compulsive disorder. *J Psychiatr Res*. 2013;47(4):494–504.
- Robinson S, Turner C, Heyman I, et al. The feasibility and acceptability of a cognitive-behavioural self-help intervention for adolescents with obsessive-compulsive disorder. *Behav Cogn Psychother*. 2013;41(1):117–122.

CODES

ICD10

- F42 Obsessive-compulsive disorder
- F63.3 Trichotillomania
- R46.81 Obsessive-compulsive behavior

FAQ

- Q: Is OCD inherited?
- A: Although no specific genes for OCD have been identified, there appears to be familial relationship to its inheritance.
- Q: What causes OCD?
- A: There is no proven cause of OCD. Research suggests that OCD involves problems in communication between the front part of the brain (the orbital cortex) and deeper structures (the basal ganglia).
- Q: Is there a cure?
- A: OCD is a chronic condition, but effective treatments are available.

OMPHALITIS

Jessica P. Clarke-Pounder • W. Christopher Golden

BASICS

DESCRIPTION

Omphalitis, an infection of the umbilical stump, begins in the neonatal period as a superficial cellulitis but may progress to necrotizing fasciitis, myonecrosis, or systemic disease.

EPIDEMIOLOGY

- Episodes of omphalitis are usually sporadic, but rare epidemics occur.
- Mean age of onset is 5–9 days in term infants and 3–5 days in preterm infants.
- Incidence varies from 0.2 to 0.7% of live births in developed countries and up to 21% of live births in developing countries.

RISK FACTORS

- Low birth weight
- Prior umbilical catheterization
- Septic delivery
- Male sex

GENERAL PREVENTION

- There are multiple methods used for umbilical cord care, many of which are acceptable.
- Antimicrobial agents applied to the umbilicus may decrease bacterial colonization and prevent omphalitis, particularly in developing countries.
- Effective methods of umbilical cord care:
  - Clean, dry cord care (AAP/WHO recommended)
  - Triple dye
  - Topical 4% chlorhexidine
  - 70% alcohol solution
- There is significant evidence to support the use of topical 4% chlorhexidine to prevent omphalitis in developing countries, although it does delay time to cord separation.
- There is no evidence that application of an antiseptic to the umbilical cord is better than clean, dry cord care in a hospital setting.

PATHOPHYSIOLOGY

- Potential bacterial pathogens normally colonize the umbilical stump after birth.
- These bacteria invade the umbilical stump, leading to omphalitis.
- Established aerobic bacterial infection, necrotic tissue, and poor blood supply facilitate the growth of anaerobic organisms.
- Infection may also extend beyond the subcutaneous tissues to involve fascial planes (fasciitis), abdominal wall musculature (myonecrosis), and umbilical and portal veins (phlebitis).

ETIOLOGY

- Most cases of omphalitis are polymicrobial.
- The most common organisms include gram-positive cocci (*Staphylococcus aureus*, group A streptococci) and gram-negative enteric bacilli (*Escherichia coli*, *Klebsiella pneumoniae*, and *Proteus mirabilis*).
- Gram-positive organisms predominate; however, antistaphylococcal cord care has led to an increase in colonization and infection with gram-negative organisms.
- Anaerobic bacteria, including *Bacteroides fragilis* and *Clostridium perfringens*, are most likely in cases complicated by necrotizing fasciitis or myonecrosis.
- *Clostridium tetani* and *Clostridium sordellii* are seen primarily in developing countries when cow dung is used in cord care.

COMMONLY ASSOCIATED CONDITIONS

- Leukocyte adhesion deficiency
  - Omphalitis may be the initial manifestation of one of the leukocyte adhesion deficiencies (LADs).
  - LADs are rare, autosomal recessive immunologic disorders affecting leukocyte adhesion to blood vessel walls.
  - Cord separation requires the influx of leukocytes; therefore, this deficiency causes delayed separation and can cause concomitant omphalitis.
  - Infants also may present with leukocytosis, absence of pus formation, impaired wound healing, and recurrent infections localized to the skin and mucosal surfaces.
  - Treatment involves prompt recognition of infection and use of appropriate antibiotics. Severe cases may need hematopoietic stem cell transplantation.
- Neutropenia
  - Omphalitis complicated by sepsis can be associated with neutropenia.
  - Other syndromes of neonatal neutropenia may present initially with omphalitis.
    - Neonatal alloimmune neutropenia: Maternal IgG antibodies cross the placenta and cause immune-mediated destruction of fetal neutrophils bearing antigens differing from mother's.
    - Other causes of neutropenia: autoimmune neutropenias, X-linked agammaglobulinemia, hyper-IgM immunodeficiency syndromes, HIV, glycogen storage disease type IB, or disorders of amino acid metabolism
- Anatomic abnormalities
  - Patent urachus: The urachus, a tubular structure connecting the bladder to the umbilicus, should obliterate by the 5th gestational month. If it remains patent, a continuous, significant amount of urine can drain from the umbilicus.
  - Persistent omphalomesenteric duct: congenital malformation where a communication exists between the umbilicus and the gut. Drainage consists of intestinal secretions.
  - Excessive granulation tissue: results from delayed healing of cord stump. Drainage is serosanguinous and pink.
- Considerations in preterm infants:
  - Preterm infants are more susceptible secondary to immature immune defenses (including the skin) and possible umbilical catheterization.
  - These infants are more likely to present with omphalitis at an earlier age and with low neutrophil counts.

DIAGNOSIS

HISTORY

- Identify risk factors such as prolonged membrane rupture and septic delivery.
- Symptoms such as fever, irritability, lethargy, respiratory distress, or feeding intolerance may indicate systemic dissemination of the infection.
- A history of urine or stool discharge from the umbilicus suggests an underlying anatomic abnormality.
- Family history may reveal individuals with metabolic disorders or recurrent infections.

PHYSICAL EXAM

- Varies with the extent of disease
- Localized infection
  - Abdominal tenderness
  - Periumbilical edema and erythema
  - Purulent or malodorous discharge from the umbilical stump
- Indications of more extensive local disease, such as necrotizing fasciitis or myonecrosis:
  - Periumbilical ecchymoses or gangrene
  - Abdominal wall crepitus
  - Progression of cellulitis despite antimicrobial therapy
- Signs of systemic disease are nonspecific and include thermodysregulation and evidence of multiorgan dysfunction:
  - Fever or temperature instability
  - Tachycardia, hypotension, poor perfusion
  - Respiratory distress
  - Abdominal distention, diminished bowel sounds
  - Cyanosis, petechiae, jaundice
  - Lethargy, hypotonia

DIAGNOSTIC TESTS & INTERPRETATION

Lab

- Umbilical stump Gram stain and culture for aerobic and anaerobic organisms
  - Identify potential organisms and antimicrobial susceptibility patterns. Cultures of umbilical discharge may reflect only colonization of the stump and are not proof of an etiologic role in the underlying process. If myonecrosis is suspected, muscle specimens should be cultured.
- Blood culture
  - Identify systemic dissemination of infection
- CBC with differential
  - Identify neutropenia or leukocytosis
  - An immature-to-total neutrophil ratio >0.2 is suggestive of systemic infection.
  - Thrombocytopenia may be present.
- D-dimers, prothrombin time, partial thromboplastin time, and fibrinogen
  - Indicated for sepsis or disseminated intravascular coagulation

Imaging

Radiographs (case dependent)

- Abdominal radiographs
  - Intestinal ileus may indicate systemic spread of infection; portal venous or intramural air requires immediate surgical consultation.
- Abdominal CT
  - Confirms involvement of fascia and muscle and delineates the extent of infection
  - May identify anatomic abnormalities
- Voiding cystourethrogram
  - Reveals patent urachus

Diagnostic Procedures/Other

Lumbar puncture: for any neonate with signs of focal/systemic illness or a positive blood culture

DIFFERENTIAL DIAGNOSIS

- The characteristic clinical picture of omphalitis allows diagnosis on clinical grounds.
- Determine the presence of associated complications, such as necrotizing fasciitis, myonecrosis, or systemic infection.
- Consider an underlying immunologic or metabolic disorder.

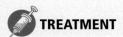

TREATMENT

MEDICATION

Empiric coverage

- Antistaphylococcal agent (oxacillin, vancomycin) plus an aminoglycoside (e.g., gentamicin) or cefepime
- Consider local antibiotic susceptibility patterns when choosing antibiotics, paying particular attention to hospital and community incidence of methicillin-resistant *S. aureus*.
- Add anaerobic coverage (e.g., metronidazole or clindamycin) with necrotizing fasciitis or myonecrosis.
- Duration of therapy is typically 7–14 days.

ADDITIONAL TREATMENT

General Measures

Antibiotics and supportive care

ISSUES FOR REFERRAL

If systemic illness is present, infants may need referral to a tertiary care center and consultation by a pediatric infectious disease specialist or pediatric surgeon.

SURGERY/OTHER PROCEDURES

- Early and complete surgical debridement of affected tissue and muscle is important.
- Delay in diagnosis or surgical intervention allows local progression of infection and worsening systemic toxicity.

INPATIENT CONSIDERATIONS

Initial Stabilization

Emergency care: Immediate evaluation, intravenous antimicrobial therapy, and supportive care are essential to survival.

ONGOING CARE

FOLLOW-UP RECOMMENDATIONS

- Infants developing associated portal venous thrombosis require follow-up for complications owing to portal hypertension.

PROGNOSIS

- The outcome of infants with uncomplicated omphalitis is generally good.
- The mortality rate among all infants with omphalitis, including those who develop complications, is 7–15%.
- The mortality rate is significantly higher (38–87%) with necrotizing fasciitis or myonecrosis.

COMPLICATIONS

- Systemic sepsis (up to 13% of cases)
  - Evidenced by temperature instability, abdominal distension, respiratory distress, and/or hypotension
- Abscess
  - Retroperitoneal, pelvic, cutaneous, hepatic
- Peritoneal complications
  - Peritonitis can occur if the umbilical vein is involved in infection and is evidenced by poor feeding, bilious vomiting, and signs of systemic illness.
  - Portal vein thrombosis or hepatic abscess can occur with transmission via the umbilical vein.
  - Adhesive small bowel obstruction may be seen as a late complication.
- Myonecrosis
  - Infectious involvement of the muscle
  - Requires surgical treatment with resection
- Necrotizing fasciitis (8–16% of cases)
  - Bacterial infection of the subcutaneous fat and superficial and deep fascia
  - Characterized by rapidly spreading infection and systemic toxicity

ADDITIONAL READING

- Anderson J, Philip A. Management of the umbilical cord: care regimens, colonization, infection, and separation. *Neoreviews*. 2004;5:155–163.
- Evens K, George J, Angst D, et al. Does umbilical cord care in preterm infants influence bacterial colonization or detachment? *J Perinatol*. 2004;24(2):100–104.
- Fraser N, Davies BW, Cusack J. Neonatal omphalitis: a review of its serious complications. *Acta Paediatr*. 2006;95(5):519–522.
- Guvenc H, Aygun D, Yasar F, et al. Omphalitis in term and preterm appropriate for gestational age and small for gestational age infants. *J Trop Pediatr*. 1997;43(6):368–372.
- Imdad A, Bautista R, Senen K, et al. Umbilical cord antiseptics for preventing sepsis and death among newborns. *Cochrane Database Syst Rev*. 2013;5:CD008635.
- van de Vijver E, van den Berg TK, Kuijpers TW. Leukocyte adhesion deficiencies. *Hematol Oncol Clin North Am*. 2013;27(1):101–116.

CODES

ICD10

- P38.9 Omphalitis without hemorrhage
- B95.0 Streptococcus, group A, causing diseases classd elswhr
- 95.8 Unsp staphylococcus as the cause of diseases classd elswhr

FAQ

- Q: Do all preterm infants require antiseptic treatment of the umbilical cord?
- A: No. Although preterm infants are at higher risk for omphalitis, there is no evidence to support antimicrobial treatment of the umbilical cord over clean, dry cord care in a hospital setting. If born in a developing country or out of asepsis, antimicrobial cord care is recommended.
- Q: Is omphalitis always restricted to the umbilical stump?
- A: No. Omphalitis can invade the periumbilical skin, the abdominal wall, and the peritoneum. Prompt treatment is necessary to prevent systemic spread of infection.

OSTEOGENESIS IMPERFECTA

Kara J. Connelly • Robert D. Steiner

BASICS

DESCRIPTION

Osteogenesis imperfecta (OI) is a genetic connective tissue disorder affecting primarily bones and soft tissues, characterized by bone fragility and susceptibility to bone fractures.

- Clinical severity is widely varied and dependent in part on the genetic etiology.
- Typical symptoms can include recurrent fractures, bone and/or spine deformities, short stature, blue or grey sclerae (occurring in approximately 80% of cases), dentinogenesis imperfecta (DI; occurring in approximately 40% of cases), and joint hypermobility.

EPIDEMIOLOGY

Incidence

1 in 10,000 births

Prevalence

6–7:100,000 persons

RISK FACTORS

Genetics

- The majority of cases (~85%) are due to autosomal dominant mutations in the genes encoding type I collagen, *COL1A1* and *COL1A2*.
- Traditionally, OI has been classified due to clinical presentation, as initially described by Sillence. However, in the last decade, new dominant and recessive forms caused by mutations in several different genes have been described, which has altered the classification of OI. Modified classification typing is noted in parentheses below:
  - Type I (classic nondeforming OI with blue sclerae): usually normal stature, fractures infrequent, and usually in prepubertal years. No bowing of long bones. Blue sclerae. Early hypoacusia common.
  - Type II (perinatally lethal OI): death usually in perinatal period due to pulmonary hypoplasia. Intrauterine fractures, shortened long bones, and blue sclerae are common.
  - Type III (progressively deforming OI): severely shortened stature, severe deformities of long bones, prevalent vertebral fractures, scoliosis, chest deformities. Characteristic triangular face.
  - Type IV (common variable OI with normal sclerae): DI common, short stature, bowing of long bones, vertebral fractures, scoliosis, and joint laxity. Patients are usually ambulatory. Sclerae are usually normal hue.
  - Other clinical forms of OI
  - OI with calcification in interosseous membranes (type V): autosomal dominant mutations of *IFITM5* gene. Patients can develop hyperplastic calluses in long bones after fracture causing tender, firm swellings over bones. Blue sclerae and DI not common.
  - Type VI: rare form of recessive OI due to mutations in *SERPINF1* gene causing severe matrix mineralization defect. No blue sclerae, DI, or wormian bones. Rhizomelic shortening of extremities.
  - Type VII: recessive mutation of *CRTAP* gene causing rhizomelia, early fractures, and osteopenia
  - Type VIII: absence or severe deficiency of prolyl 3-hydroxylase activity due to mutations in the *LEPRE1* gene
  - Type IX: moderate to severe OI caused by defects in the *PPIB* gene
  - Type X and XI: chaperone defects caused by *SERPINH1* or *FKBP10* mutations. Type XI due to *FKBP10* mutations can cause progressively deforming OI or Bruck syndrome.

PATHOPHYSIOLOGY

- Mutations in *COL1A1* or *COL1A2* cause altered triple-helical collagen structure leading to abnormal collagen fibrils.
  - Procollagen molecules more susceptible to proteolytic degradation
  - Collagen fibrils are disorganized
  - Abnormal osteoid formation
  - Decrease in osteoid seams
- Recessive OI is caused by defects in genes whose products interact with type I collagen leading to many of the same cellular features, although the precise pathomechanisms are as yet incompletely understood.
- Osteoblasts: increased osteoblast cellularity; however, reduction in differentiated cells capable of making mineralized matrix
  - Decreased bone formation during remodeling
- Osteoclasts: increased osteoclast number to remove defective matrix
- Growth retardation: Disruption of balance between bone formation and resorption is more pronounced during periods of rapid linear growth (i.e., childhood, puberty).

ETIOLOGY

- Failure of normal maturation of procollagen to type 1 collagen and failure of normal collagen cross-linking
- Abnormality of collagen production and organization

DIAGNOSIS

HISTORY

- Widely varied; may include recurrent fractures including fractures with little or no predisposing trauma
- May have positive family history, particularly if condition is due to an autosomal dominant mutation

PHYSICAL EXAM

- Severe congenital forms:
  - Intrauterine and perinatal fractures
  - Limbs deformed and short
  - Skull soft
  - Rib deformities and pulmonary hypoplasia leading to respiratory insufficiency
- Mild and moderate forms:
  - General: short stature
  - Head: triangular facies in type III OI
  - Eyes: blue or grey sclerae
  - Ears: hypoacusia (generally develops in adulthood)
  - Teeth: ~50% with DI: deciduous teeth more severely affected than permanent teeth, enamel normal, teeth easily broken but no increase in cavities; malocclusion
  - Spine: kyphoscoliosis; often associated with pectus carinatum or pectus excavatum. Barrel chest deformity common.
  - Pelvis: trefoil pelvis, protrusio acetabuli
  - Extremities: bowing of long bones, coxa vara deformity, cubitus varus, joint hypermobility

DIAGNOSTIC TESTS & INTERPRETATION

Lab

- Serum calcium and phosphorus levels
  - Normal
- Alkaline phosphatase
  - May be elevated after a fracture
- Type I collagen *N*-telopeptide normalized to urinary creatinine (NTx/uCr) highest in type III OI patients
- Diagnosis typically by DNA sequencing of genes implicated in OI from peripheral blood or cultured fibroblasts or analysis of collagen synthesis, structure, and electrophoretic mobility in cultured skin fibroblasts from skin biopsy.

Imaging

- Skull
  - Wormian bones: detached portions of primary ossification centers in adjacent membranous bones; can be seen in other conditions
- Long bones
  - Fractures: varying stages of healing
  - Osteopenia
  - Bowing deformity
  - Metaphyseal ends: honeycomb appearance
  - Acetabular protrusion
  - Popcorn calcifications
- Spine
  - Scoliosis
  - "Codfish vertebrae" due to compression fractures
  - Atlantoaxial subluxation
  - Spondylolisthesis

Diagnostic Procedures/Other

- Once diagnosis is established
  - Formal audiology assessment
  - Dental evaluation if DI
  - Consider screening for basilar impression with CT or MRI in more severe forms.
  - Bone densitometry may be helpful.

DIFFERENTIAL DIAGNOSIS

- In utero
  - Hypophosphatasia
  - Thanatophoric dysplasia
  - Campomelic dysplasia
  - Achondrogenesis
- Infancy and childhood
  - Child abuse
  - Idiopathic juvenile osteoporosis
  - Osteoporosis-pseudoglioma syndrome

– Cole-carpenter syndrome
– Hajdu-Cheney syndrome
– Bruck syndrome
– Hypophosphatasia
– Leukemia
– Osteopenia related to prematurity
– Glucocorticoid-induced osteopenia
– Cushing disease
– Homocystinuria
– Immobilization
– Anticonvulsant therapy
- Hyperplastic callus formation in OI type V may be confused with osteogenic sarcoma.

TREATMENT

MEDICATION

- Antiresorptive agents (bisphosphonates)
  – Currently used in clinical trials and more widely in clinical practice in recent years
  – May improve bone mineral density, pain, and mobility
  – May lessen fracture risk
  – Most common side effects: flulike syndrome during initial treatment; hypocalcemia; delayed osteotomy healing
  – Long-term side effects unknown
  – Theoretically could be associated with atypical fractures and jaw osteonecrosis
- Adequate calcium (varies with age) and vitamin D intake (400–1,000 IU daily)
- Anabolic agents (growth hormone, insulin-like growth factor 1 [IGF-1], parathyroid hormone [PTH]): not considered routine treatment options, note PTH has black box warning now for pediatric indications
- Gene therapy: currently being developed; not yet available

ADDITIONAL TREATMENT

General Measures

- Intramedullary rodding with or without osteotomies: mainstay of care in severe cases
  – Often performed as early as 18 months of age
  – Should weight-bear as soon as possible after surgery
  – Many nonambulatory patients are able to walk after osteotomies.
- Spinal deformities
  – Seen in ~90%
  – Orthoses do not stop progression.
  – Treatment: spinal fusion or halo gravity traction and posterior spondylodesis
- Fracture treatment
  – Bone mineral density can decline after fracture while immobilized.
  – Postfracture physiotherapy critical

INPATIENT CONSIDERATIONS

Initial Stabilization

Emergency care
- For unstable fractures, such as femur fractures, spine instability
- Depends on location of fracture and details of individual situation

ONGOING CARE

FOLLOW-UP RECOMMENDATIONS

Patient Monitoring

Multidisciplinary approach
- Pediatric endocrinologist or geneticist
  – Medical management of OI
- Pediatric orthopedic surgeon
  – Fracture repair, rodding, osteotomies, spinal fusion
- Physiotherapist
  – Postoperative rehabilitation, orthotics, physical therapy to improve mobility and stability of bones and increase muscle strength
- Psychologist/social worker
  – Adjustments and accommodations at school
  – Issues regarding self-esteem

PATIENT EDUCATION

- Techniques for safe handling, protective positioning, and safe movement are taught to parents.
- Physical education at school should be strongly encouraged, but children should not participate in contact sports. An individualized program may be necessary depending on OI severity.

PROGNOSIS

- Largely depends on severity of OI
- In general, the earlier the fractures occur, the more severe the disease.
- Tendency toward improvement after somatic growth is complete in adolescence with relatively lower bone removal and less frequent fractures.
- Future therapeutic options including gene therapy hold promise for improved treatment.

COMPLICATIONS

- Pathologic fractures
- Scoliosis
- Cardiorespiratory problems (restrictive lung disease in severe cases with severe kyphoscoliosis, aortic dilatation, mitral valve prolapse, aortic regurgitation)
- Hearing loss
- Short stature
- Basilar impression: descent of the skull on the cervical spine; may progress to brainstem compression or obstructive hydrocephalus

ADDITIONAL READING

- Bishop N, Adami S, Ahmed SF, et al. Risedronate in children with osteogenesis imperfecta: a randomised, double-blind, placebo-controlled trial. *Lancet*. 2013;382(9902):1424–1432.
- Byers PH, Pyott SM. Recessively inherited forms of osteogenesis imperfecta. *Annu Rev Genet*. 2012;46(1):475–497.
- Glorieux FH, Moffatt P. Osteogenesis imperfecta, an every-expanding conundrum. *J Bone Miner Res*. 2013;28(7):1519–1522.
- Marini JC, Blissett AR. New genes in bone development: what's new in osteogenesis imperfecta. *J Clin Endocrinol Metab*. 2013;98(8):3095–3103.
- Morello R, Bertin TK, Chen Y, et al. CRTAP is required for prolyl 3- hydroxylation and mutations cause recessive osteogenesis imperfecta. *Cell*. 2006; 127(2):291–304.
- Sillence DO. Osteogenesis imperfecta: an expanded panorama of variants. *Clin Orthop Relat Res*. 1981;1(159):11–25.
- Steiner RD, Adsit J, Basel D. COL1A1/2-related osteogenesis imperfecta. GeneTests Web site. http://www.genetests.org. Accessed March 11, 2015.

CODES

ICD10

Q78.0 Osteogenesis imperfecta

FAQ

- Q: What is the typical life expectancy for persons with OI?
- A: Infants with perinatal/lethal (type II) OI do not survive the perinatal period and often die within the first 48 hours of life. For mild and moderate OI, life expectancy is normal. Life expectancy for patients with severe (type III) OI is widely variable and can be shortened by kyphoscoliosis contributing to restricted lung disease.
- Q: How is OI inherited?
- A: OI is often inherited in an autosomal dominant manner. New mutations are not uncommon, and this often provides the explanation for lethal cases of OI in families with no history of OI. More recently, autosomal recessive forms of OI (mainly severe and lethal) have been described.
- Q: How is OI differentiated from child abuse?
- A: Differentiation of OI from child abuse is usually straightforward once the history, physical examination, radiographic findings, and family history are carefully considered. However, in difficult cases, genetic and/or biochemical testing may be useful.

OSTEOMYELITIS

Blanca E. Gonzalez • Virginia M. Pierce

BASICS

DESCRIPTION
- Infection of any bone
- Most commonly occurs in the metaphysis of a long bone (especially the distal femur or proximal tibia)

EPIDEMIOLOGY
- One of the most common invasive bacterial infections in children, accounting for 1% of all pediatric hospitalizations
- 1/3 third occurs in children younger than 2 years of age and ~50% of cases occur in children ≤5 years of age.
- A history of minor trauma to the affected site is common but of unclear significance.
- Boys are more commonly affected than girls (2:1 ratio).

PATHOPHYSIOLOGY
- Hematogenous spread is most common in children (inoculation of bone during an episode of bacteremia). The infecting organism enters the bone via a nutrient artery and then is deposited in the metaphysis due to its rich vascular supply. The organism replicates in metaphyseal capillary loops, causes local inflammation, spreads through vascular tunnels, and adheres to the bone matrix. Increased pressure in the metaphysis allows pus to perforate through the cortex and lift the periosteum.
- In newborns and young infants, rupture of pus into the adjacent joint space is more common because blood vessels connect the metaphysis and epiphysis.
- Local spread from a contiguous focus of infection and direct inoculation (e.g., penetrating injury) are less common mechanisms of infection.

RISK FACTORS
- Sickle hemoglobinopathy
- Primary or acquired immunodeficiency, especially chronic granulomatous disease (CGD), and HIV
- Bone trauma (open fractures, puncture wounds, bites, surgical manipulation)
- Implanted orthopedic devices or indwelling vascular catheters
- Pressure ulcers

ETIOLOGY
- *Staphylococcus aureus* is responsible for 70–90% of osteomyelitis in all age groups, with MRSA an increasingly common problem.
- *Streptococcus pyogenes* accounts for ~10% of osteomyelitis and is more common in preschool and early school–aged children.
- *Streptococcus pneumoniae* causes ~10% of osteomyelitis in children younger than 3 years old, although a decline in pneumococcal infections has been seen with widespread vaccination. Conversely, *S. pneumoniae* remains an important cause of osteomyelitis in children infected with HIV.
- *Kingella kingae*, a gram-negative organism found in the respiratory tract, is an important pathogen in children younger than the age of 3 years, especially in those that attend day care centers.
- Group B *Streptococcus*, gram-negative enterics, and *Candida* spp. are important causative organisms in neonates.
- *Salmonella* spp. can be the cause in children with sickle cell disease and in patients from or traveling to tropical countries.
- *Pseudomonas aeruginosa* is a common cause following puncture wounds to the foot.
- There has been a significant decline in the incidence of *Haemophilus influenzae* type b (Hib) osteomyelitis since immunization with the Hib conjugate vaccine became widespread.
- Other more unusual pathogens may be seen in patients with specific risk factors (e.g., coagulase-negative staphylococci in the presence of prosthetic material, anaerobes after animal or human bites, *Aeromonas* after injuries sustained in fresh water settings).
- In a significant percentage of cases, a definitive causative microorganism is not identified. The use of antibiotic prior to collection of samples, presence of fastidious organisms, low inoculum, or inappropriately collected samples, may be a factor in culture-negative osteomyelitis.
- Infections after open fractures or puncture wounds may be polymicrobial.

DIAGNOSIS

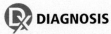

HISTORY
- Persistent, increasing pain and tenderness over the affected bone
- Restricted use of the involved limb (pseudoparalysis may be the only sign in a neonate), refusal to bear weight, or limp
- Fever, malaise, anorexia, irritability
- Children with vertebral and pelvic osteomyelitis may complain of poorly localized pain for several weeks, often resulting in delay in the diagnosis and treatment.
- In some patients, osteomyelitis will have an indolent, subacute presentation with the development of a minimally symptomatic abscess within the bone, eponymously known as a "Brodie abscess."

PHYSICAL EXAM
- Swelling, warmth, and erythema of the soft tissues over the affected bone may be noted.
- Exaggerated immobility/pain with micromotion of an adjacent joint suggests pyogenic arthritis (alternatively or in addition to osteomyelitis).
- Multifocal osteomyelitis may be seen in neonates and in children with *S. aureus* sepsis syndrome.

DIAGNOSTIC TESTS & INTERPRETATION

Lab
- The white blood cell count may be normal or elevated.
- Erythrocyte sedimentation rate (ESR) and C-reactive protein (CRP) levels are usually elevated.
- Blood cultures are positive in ~50% of patients.
- Bone needle aspiration cultures are positive in ~60–70% of cases.
- Some uncommon bacteria causing osteomyelitis are fastidious and difficult to culture; they may require molecular methods to establish the diagnosis (e.g., polymerase chain reaction).

Imaging
- Plain radiographs may show deep soft tissue swelling early in the course of infection and may help to suggest or exclude alternative diagnoses. Evidence of bone destruction and periosteal elevation are not typically seen until 10–14 days after the onset of symptoms.
- MRI is sensitive and specific and offers superior anatomic resolution, making it a more useful modality for surgical planning and for identification of intraosseous, subperiosteal, and soft tissue abscesses.
- Bone scans are especially useful if the site of infection is poorly localized or if there is concern for multifocal osteomyelitis. However, they may be positive in other illnesses that cause osteoblastic activity.

Diagnostic Procedures/Other
- Biopsy or aspiration of the infected bone (or an associated abscess) for Gram stain and culture is useful for determining the etiologic organism. Inoculating a portion of an aspirated sample into a blood culture bottle enhances yield for *K. kingae*.
- If a plan is in place to rapidly obtain a bone culture in a clinically stable patient, it is reasonable to defer initiation of antibiotic therapy until after the culture specimen is secured.
- Biopsy may help differentiate osteomyelitis from noninfectious bone pathology.

DIFFERENTIAL DIAGNOSIS
- Trauma
- Cellulitis
- Soft tissue abscess
- Pyomyositis or fasciitis
- Septic arthritis
- Congenital syphilis
- Aseptic bone necrosis or bone infarction (sickle cell disease)
- Tumor (e.g., Ewing sarcoma, osteoid osteoma, eosinophilic granuloma)
- Acute leukemia, neuroblastoma with bone invasion
- Chronic recurrent multifocal osteomyelitis (CRMO)
- Inflammatory arthritis or juvenile idiopathic arthritis
- Transient synovitis
- Bone cyst

TREATMENT

MEDICATION

- Empiric antibiotics should cover the most likely pathogens considering patient age, history of presentation, physical findings, and underlying medical conditions.
- Empiric therapy should always include an agent directed against *S. aureus*, usually nafcillin, oxacillin, or a 1st-generation cephalosporin. However, in areas where the rate of methicillin resistance among community *S. aureus* isolates exceeds 10%, an antibiotic effective against community-acquired MRSA should be selected (i.e., clindamycin or vancomycin).
- When clindamycin is considered for treatment of an identified MRSA isolate, the D-test (to exclude inducible macrolide, lincosamide, and streptogramin B resistance) should be performed by the clinical microbiology laboratory.
- Clindamycin and vancomycin are also usually effective against *S. pneumoniae* and *S. pyogenes* but are not effective in vitro against *K. kingae*. The latter organism is usually susceptible to most beta-lactam antibiotics (penicillins and cephalosporins).
- In addition to antistaphylococcal coverage, a 3rd generation cephalosporin, such as ceftriaxone or cefotaxime should be used to cover *Salmonella* spp. in patients with sickle cell disease.
- Gram-negative coverage should also be added to the empiric regimen for neonates.
- If the patient recently had a foot puncture wound, coverage for *P. aeruginosa* should be considered.
- If an organism is isolated and susceptibilities determined, antibiotic therapy should be modified based on the susceptibility profile.

ADDITIONAL TREATMENT

- Traditionally, 4–6 weeks of antibiotics have been recommended. Newer data is emerging suggesting that for non-MRSA hematogenous osteomyelitis, 20 days of therapy may be sufficient. However, this may require the use of more frequent dosing schedules as well as higher doses.
- Total treatment duration should be individualized based on the extent of infection, the promptness and completeness of surgical debridement (when indicated), the rate of clinical response, the presence or absence of distant foci of infection, and the patient's underlying risk factors and comorbid conditions.
- If an intraosseous, subperiosteal, or soft tissue abscess is present, surgical debridement may be necessary in addition to antibiotic therapy.
- Surgical debridement is important in the management of osteomyelitis that is secondary to a puncture wound.
- After an initial period of parenteral antibiotic administration, many patients can be transitioned to an oral regimen to complete therapy (assuming the availability of an oral antibiotic with an appropriate spectrum of activity and adequate bone penetration as well as patient ability to adhere to and absorb an oral regimen). This sequential IV–oral approach reduces the risk of complications (e.g., catheter-associated bloodstream infection, catheter malfunction, and thrombosis) associated with the prolonged presence of a central venous catheter.
- The decline in CRP alongside improvement in clinical signs may be a good indicator of when it is safe to transition to oral therapy.
- The treatment of osteomyelitis should be done in consultation with an infectious disease specialist.

ONGOING CARE

FOLLOW-UP RECOMMENDATIONS

- Most children who receive appropriate treatment have no long-term sequelae.
- Inflammatory markers (ESR and CRP) are typically measured serially until they normalize during the course of antibiotic therapy.
- Patients should be followed to ensure medication compliance, adequacy of treatment, side effects of therapy, and continued growth of the involved extremity.

COMPLICATIONS

- Septic arthritis
- Recurrence or progression to chronic osteomyelitis in ~5% of patients
- Disturbances of bone growth, limb length discrepancy
- Arthritis
- Pathological fractures

ADDITIONAL READING

- Arnold J, Cannavino CR, Ross MK, et al. Acute bacterial osteoarticular infections: eight-year analysis of c-reactive protein for oral step-down therapy. *Pediatrics*. 2012;130(4):e821–e828.
- Dodwell E. Osteomyelitis and septic arthritis in children: current concepts. *Curr Opin Pediatr*. 2013;25(1):58–63.
- Gerber JS, Coffin SE, Smathers SA, et al. Trends in the incidence of methicillin-resistant *Staphylococcus aureus* infection in children's hospitals in the United States. *Clin Infect Dis*. 2009;49(1):65–71.
- Gutierrez K. Bone and joint infections in children. *Pediatr Clin North Am*. 2005;52(3):779–794.
- Harik NS, Smeltzer MS. Management of acute hematogenous osteomyelitis in children. *Expert Rev Anti Infect Ther*. 2010;8(2):175–181.
- Kaplan SL. Osteomyelitis in children. *Infect Dis Clin North Am*. 2005;19(4):787–797, vii.
- Pääkkönen M, Peltola H. Bone and joint infections. *Pediatr Clin North Am*. 2013;60(2):425–436.
- Peltola H,Pääkkönen M, Kallio P, et al. Short vs. long-term antimicrobial treatment for acute hematogenous osteomyelitis of childhood. *Pediatr Infect Dis J*. 2010;29(12):1123–1128.
- Yagupsky P. *Kingella kingae*: from medical rarity to an emerging paediatric pathogen. *Lancet Infect Dis*. 2004;4(6):358–367.
- Zaoutis T, Localio AR, Leckerman K, et al. Prolonged intravenous therapy versus early transition to oral antimicrobial therapy for acute osteomyelitis in children. *Pediatrics*. 2009;123(2):636–642.

CODES

ICD10

- M86.9 Osteomyelitis, unspecified
- M86.00 Acute hematogenous osteomyelitis, unspecified site
- M86.10 Other acute osteomyelitis, unspecified site

FAQ

- Q: Can children with osteomyelitis present without fever and with normal CBCs and inflammatory markers?
- A: Fever along with leukocytosis and elevated inflammatory markers (CRP and ESR) are common in children who have acute hematogenous osteomyelitis. However, children with subacute or chronic osteomyelitis and with other forms of osteomyelitis, such as puncture wound osteochondritis, may not exhibit these findings.
- Q: What is the imaging modality of choice in a child suspected of having acute hematogenous osteomyelitis?
- A: MRI is the most sensitive and specific imaging study to detect acute osteomyelitis. Plain films do not reveal periosteal elevation for at least 10–14 days after infection. A bone scan is less specific than MRI and does not reveal extraosseous features of infection.

OSTEOSARCOMA

Sheila Thampi • Steven G. DuBois

BASICS

DESCRIPTION

Osteosarcoma is a malignant tumor of the bone and arises from mesenchymal cells. The malignant cells are usually pleomorphic spindle cells that lay down abnormal bone (osteoid formation).

EPIDEMIOLOGY

- Osteosarcoma is the most common pediatric primary bone cancer and is the 8th most common malignancy of childhood.
- A bimodal distribution is noted with the first peak in adolescence (median, age 16 years) and second peak during the 7th and 8th decade of life.
- Incidence of osteosarcoma parallels skeletal growth and is more frequently noted in tall individuals.
- Males are more commonly affected than females.
- In the United States, there are about 4.4 cases per million children and adolescents.
- Approximately 400 new pediatric cases of osteosarcoma are diagnosed each year in the United States.

RISK FACTORS

- Radiation exposure
- Hereditary retinoblastoma, in which patients with germline *Rb* gene mutation have increased risk of osteosarcoma with or without radiation exposure.
- Li-Fraumeni syndrome, in which patients have germline *TP53* gene mutation and increased risk of a range of sarcomas, among other malignancies
- Rothmund-Thomson syndrome
- Bloom syndrome
- Enchondromatosis
- Hereditary multiple exostoses
- Fibrous dysplasia
- Paget disease of the bone, although less relevant to pediatric populations

PATHOPHYSIOLOGY

- The histologic hallmark of osteosarcoma is the presence of osteoid.
- Most cases of pediatric osteosarcoma are high-grade cancers, although lower grade variants are seen.
- No classic genetic change, although karyotypes are typically highly abnormal
- Major subtypes of osteosarcoma include osteoblastic, chondroblastic, fibroblastic, telangiectatic, and small cell.
- At diagnosis, 80% of patients will have localized disease and 20% will have metastatic disease.
- In 80% of tumors, the metaphysis of long bones will be involved, such as the femur, tibia, and humerus, with distal femur the most common primary site. In 20% of tumors, other sites of involvement will include the pelvis, facial bones, and shoulder blade.
- The most common sites of metastatic disease are lungs and bone. Involvement of regional lymph nodes is rare.

ETIOLOGY

- The etiology of most cases is unknown.
- Abnormal TP53 and/or Rb function implicated in laboratory studies of osteosarcoma
- Radiation exposure is a known cause of osteosarcoma and usually presents 10–20 years after exposure.

DIAGNOSIS

SIGNS AND SYMPTOMS

History

- Pain and palpable mass are the most common clinical symptoms.
- Pain is often described as dull or aching at the tumor site.
- Pain is often initially attributed to an injury in active children or adolescents.
- Symptoms of pain can vary prior to presenting to medical attention but warrant further investigation if present for several weeks to months and if it disrupts sleep.
- Presence of bone metastasis may result in pain at sites distant from the primary tumor.
- Systemic symptoms, such as fever and weight loss, are unusual.

Physical Exam

- Presence of a firm, often tender mass
- Swelling at the tumor location
- Depending on location of the tumor, one can have a loss of function, limp, or decreased range of motion

DIAGNOSTIC TESTS & INTERPRETATION

Lab

- 30% of patients will have an elevated lactate dehydrogenase (LDH).
- An elevated erythrocyte sedimentation rate (ESR) can be seen.
- May see an elevated alkaline phosphatase (AP), particularly with metastatic disease
- Leukocytosis may suggest osteomyelitis.

Imaging

- Conventional x-ray may show
  - Osteolytic and sclerotic lesion
  - Periosteal reaction including Codman sign (shadow from a lifted periosteum), onion-skinning as new layers of periosteum are laid down, and sunburst appearance reflecting calcified bone beyond periosteum
  - Pathologic fracture
- An MRI from joint to joint of involved bone will show full extension of the tumor and involvement of surrounding structures.
- A technetium bone scan will show areas of intense primary tumor uptake and screen for bone metastasis.
- A chest CT should be performed to evaluate for pulmonary metastasis.
- Use of positron emission tomography with [F-18]-fluorodeoxyglucose (FDG-PET) is increasing, as it can characterize size, location of tumor, and can allow for assessment of response.

Diagnostic Procedures/Other

The diagnosis of osteosarcoma is a tissue diagnosis.

ALERT

Biopsy should be performed at the center that will provide definitive treatment for the patient with a suspected primary malignant bone tumor. The placement of biopsy is critical to the planning of surgical local control and inappropriate biopsy could lead to adverse outcomes.

DIFFERENTIAL DIAGNOSIS

- Benign tumors
  - Unicameral bone cyst
  - Aneurysmal bone cyst
  - Osteoblastoma
  - Eosinophilic granuloma
  - Osteochondroma
  - Fibrous dysplasia
- Malignant tumors
  - Ewing sarcoma
  - Chondrosarcoma
  - Fibrosarcoma
  - Metastatic lesions
- Infection
  - Osteomyelitis
  - Septic arthritis
- Trauma: fracture with or without hematoma

TREATMENT

CHEMOTHERAPY

- Prior to the 1970s, overall survival for high-grade osteosarcoma was poor, as treatment primarily consisted of surgical resection allowing for relapse with metastatic disease. With the addition of both neoadjuvant and adjuvant chemotherapy, survival has improved.
- Neoadjuvant chemotherapy (before definitive surgery) allows for treatment of micrometastases and shrinkage of the primary tumor mass prior to resection.

- Neoadjuvant chemotherapy also allows time for complex endoprostheses to be constructed prior to planned limb salvage procedures.
- Response to neoadjuvant chemotherapy (percent of tumor that is necrotic at the time of complete resection) has proven to be an important prognostic factor.
- Most children and adolescents with high-grade osteosarcoma are treated based on or according to cooperative group chemotherapy protocols.
- In North America, the standard backbone of treatment is high-dose methotrexate, doxorubicin, and cisplatin. Treatment duration is usually 12 months, depending on the individual protocol, response to therapy, and tumor extent at diagnosis.
- Clinical trials in patients with newly diagnosed disease have investigated the role of ifosfamide and etoposide. The addition of interferon with chemotherapy did not improve survival.

SURGERY/OTHER PROCEDURES

- Complete surgical resection with wide margins is necessary for cure.
- Surgical options for osteosarcomas of the extremities include the following:
  - Amputation
  - Limb salvage with local resection and reconstruction of the limb
  - Rotationplasty for tumors at the knee
- Surgical resection alone is curative in low-grade osteosarcoma.
- Surgical resection of lung metastases at presentation or at relapse also plays an important role in management.

RADIOTHERAPY

Osteosarcoma is not a radiation-sensitive tumor although radiation has been used for palliative purposes to treat unresectable primary or metastatic lesions.

PHYSICAL THERAPY

Physical therapy is critical after either amputation or limb-sparing procedures.

ONGOING CARE

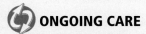

ISSUES FOR REFERRAL

- Children with a suspected malignant bone tumor should be immediately referred to a children's hospital with expertise in these tumors.
- Multidisciplinary teams include pediatric oncologists, orthopedic oncologists, pediatric surgeons, nurses, pharmacists, and social workers.

PROGNOSIS

- Patients with localized disease have an estimated 5-year overall survival of 60–70%, whereas patients with metastatic disease have an estimated 5-year overall survival of 20–30%.
- Key adverse prognostic factors are as follows:
  - Axial primary tumor location
  - Metastatic disease
  - Histologic necrosis <90% after neoadjuvant chemotherapy
  - Inability to achieve wide surgical margins during resection

COMPLICATIONS

Orthopedic

- Surgical site wound infections
- Limb length discrepancy after surgical treatment in growing children
- Phantom leg pain after amputation

Acute Chemotherapy Toxicity

- Myelosuppression
- Ototoxicity and tinnitus
- Mucositis
- Renal dysfunction

Late Effects

- Cardiomyopathy from doxorubicin
- Hearing loss and nephrotoxicity from cisplatin
- Reduced fertility from ifosfamide
- Secondary malignancy from radiation or chemotherapy

Patient Monitoring

- Patients should be followed by a pediatric oncologist with serial imaging of the primary site (MRI and x-rays) and lungs (chest CT or chest x-ray) to monitor for recurrence.
- Patients should be monitored for long-term side effects/complications of therapy, ideally within the context of a survivorship clinic.

ADDITIONAL READING

- Bielack SS, Carrle D, Hardes J, et al. Bone tumors in adolescents and young adults. *Curr Treat Options Oncol*. 2008;9(1):67–80.
- Gill J, Ahluvalia MK, Geller D, et al. New targets and approaches in osteosarcoma. *Pharmacol Ther*. 2013;137(1):89–99.
- Heare T, Hensley MA, Dell'Orfano S. Bone tumors: osteosarcoma and Ewing's sarcoma. *Curr Opin in Pediatr*. 2009;21(3):365–372.
- Longhi A, Errani C, De Paolis M, et al. Primary bone osteosarcoma in the pediatric age: state of the art. *Cancer Treat Rev*. 2006;32(6):423–436.

CODES

ICD10

- C41.9 Malignant neoplasm of bone and articular cartilage, unsp
- C40.20 Malignant neoplasm of long bones of unspecified lower limb
- 40.00 Malig neoplasm of scapula and long bones of unsp upper limb

FAQ

- Q: How can we differentiate between malignant osteosarcoma and benign tumors?
- A: An experienced radiologist can look for defining features on imaging of malignant osteosarcoma that are not found with benign tumors. However, only a biopsy can confirm a diagnosis of osteosarcoma.
- Q: What are long-term survival rates of patients who relapse after treatment?
- A: Unfortunately, patients who relapse after treatment do poorly and long-term survival is poor at 10–20%. Late relapses (>24 months after completion of treatment), surgical resection of relapsed disease, and unilateral lung involvement at relapse appear to be more favorable.
- Q: Do siblings of children with osteosarcoma need to be evaluated?
- A: If there is suspicion for a genetic risk factor (i.e., Li-Fraumeni syndrome), then siblings and families should be evaluated by a geneticist to determine if the risk factor is present. This will provide education for families and siblings. Otherwise, siblings of children with osteosarcoma that are asymptomatic do not need evaluation for osteosarcoma.
- Q: What are the differences between Ewing sarcoma and osteosarcoma?
- A: The two sarcomas are the most common malignant bone tumors in pediatrics and both require multimodal therapy, although the chemotherapy regimens are different. Ewing sarcoma can have both bone or soft tissue involvement and presence of different histologic features will allow differentiation from osteosarcoma.

OTITIS EXTERNA

Melissa Long

BASICS

DESCRIPTION
- Diffuse inflammation of external auditory canal with or without infection
- Also known as "swimmer's ear"
- May be categorized as acute, chronic, or malignant
  - Acute: rapid onset, usually bacterial
  - Chronic: lasting longer than 4 weeks or occurring 4 or more times in 1 year, usually due to nonbacterial causes such as atopic or allergic contact dermatitis from contact with metal, plastic, or chemicals
  - Malignant or necrotizing: extension of infection to osteomyelitis of the base of the skull; more common in immunocompromised patients (e.g., HIV, diabetes)

EPIDEMIOLOGY
- Peaks in children age 5–14 years
- Uncommon in children younger than age 2 years
- Peaks in summer months in temperate climates; occurs year-round in warm/humid climates

Incidence
Annual incidence is 8.1/1,000 in the general population.

Prevalence
Affects 3–5% of the population

RISK FACTORS
- Prolonged exposure to water (e.g., frequent swimming, shampooing, long showers, excessive sweating) leading to impaired natural defense mechanisms in external ear
- Microfissures from trauma
- Debris from dermatologic conditions (e.g., atopic or seborrheic dermatitis)
- Use of external devices (e.g., hearing aids or ear plugs)
- Obstruction of ear canal (e.g., by impacted cerumen, foreign body, sebaceous cyst)
- Chronic otorrhea or purulent otorrhea from otitis media
- Drainage from tympanostomy tubes
- Hairy ear canal
- Anatomic abnormalities
  - Stenosis of ear canal
  - Exostoses (abnormal bone growth within the ear canal)
- Hx of radiotherapy leading to damaged epithelium, desquamation, and diminished cerumen production

GENERAL PREVENTION
- Elimination of predisposing factors when feasible is the key to prevention.
- Avoid exposure to excessive moisture.
  - There are no randomized trials evaluating preventive strategies but you may instruct swimmers to keep their ears as dry as possible by toweling off, tilting the head to assist with drainage, and using a hair dryer to the ear canal on the lowest setting.
  - Some experts also recommend the use of ear plugs and caps, although this is controversial because it may lead to cerumen impaction, predisposing to otitis externa (OE).
  - Use of a 1:1 alcohol-to-vinegar solution before and after swimming and again before bedtime also may decrease the rate of recurrence.
- Avoid trauma to the ear canal—in particular, avoid cotton-tip swabs or other cleaning devices.
- Manage underlying dermatologic conditions.

PATHOPHYSIOLOGY
- The ear canal is lined with apocrine and sebaceous glands that produce cerumen.
- Cerumen serves as a barrier to excessive moisture and may help prevent infection due to lysozyme activity and a slightly acidic pH that helps inhibit the growth of pathogenic bacteria.
- With prolonged exposure to water, cerumen may be washed away and no longer be able to serve this barrier function.
- Too much cerumen can also lead to entrapment of debris and water retention, thus predisposing to infection.
- In certain dermatologic conditions, the integrity of the keratin layer may be affected by excessive desquamation.
- Local trauma to the external canal may also predispose to infection.

ETIOLOGY
- In the United States, bacterial agents are implicated in more than 90% of cases and most commonly include *Pseudomonas aeruginosa* and *Staphylococcus aureus*.
- May be polymicrobial in up to 30% of cases
- Fungal causes due to *Aspergillus niger* and *Candida* species
- Viral infection (in particular, varicella-zoster leading to Ramsay Hunt syndrome) account for a minority of cases.

DIAGNOSIS

HISTORY
- Symptoms are rapid in onset (generally within 48 hours) and include otalgia, pruritus, a sense of fullness, drainage, and occasionally impaired hearing.
- 90% of cases are unilateral.
- May have a low-grade fever but temperature over 101°F (38.3°C) suggests more serious infection and likely extension beyond the external ear canal.
- Ask about potential predisposing factors including swimming, dermatologic conditions, or trauma.
- Important to know status of immune system (e.g., history of diabetes, HIV infection)

PHYSICAL EXAM
- Examine external canal, tympanic membrane (TM), regional lymph nodes, and skin for dermatologic conditions.
- Signs of inflammation include tenderness or pain with manipulation of the pinna and with pressure on the tragus, erythema and edema of the external auditory canal, and otorrhea.
- More severe forms of OE may involve regional lymphadenopathy or frank lymphadenitis, cellulitis extending beyond the external canal, and/or perichondritis.
- May be difficult to visualize TM due to edema and debris
  - Can clear debris with ear curette or suction
  - Avoid lavage until TM is known to be intact.
  - Pneumatic otoscopy can assess for TM mobility for diagnosis of otitis media.
- Although rare in children, consider malignant OE if there is necrosis of the skin of the canal, exposed bone or granulation tissue, severe pain, and/or cranial nerve palsy.
- Consider viral infection (Ramsay Hunt syndrome) if there are vesicular lesions with facial paralysis, loss of taste, and decreased lacrimation on the affected side.

DIAGNOSTIC TESTS & INTERPRETATION

Labs and Diagnostic Procedures
- In uncomplicated OE, testing is generally not indicated.
- Consider bacterial culture of drainage with Gram stain and/or fungal culture in cases of severe illness or treatment failure.
- Consider viral testing if vesicular lesions are present.
- If concerned for malignant OE by history or exam, consider lab work (including erythrocyte sedimentation rate) and imaging (MRI generally preferred over CT scan).

DIFFERENTIAL DIAGNOSIS
- Important to rule out life-threatening causes of otalgia and otorrhea
  - Clear persistent fluid may occur after traumatic head injury, leading to cerebrospinal fluid otorrhea.
  - Purulent otorrhea could be due to acute otitis media associated with mastoiditis, brain abscess, or venous sinus thrombosis.
  - With bloody drainage, must consider traumatic perforation of the TM, barotrauma leading to hemotympanum, or a tumor
- Other infections
  - Furunculosis in the external auditory canal (also known as localized OE)
  - Otomycosis
  - Infected sebaceous cyst
  - Acute otitis media
  - Chronic suppurative otitis media with ruptured TM
  - Drainage through tympanostomy tubes
- Miscellaneous
  - Foreign body
  - Cholesteatoma
  - Contact dermatitis (e.g., to metal, plastics)

TREATMENT

MEDICATION

- For uncomplicated OE, topical antibiotics are the treatment of choice, as they are both effective and well tolerated.
- A 2010 Cochrane review found no difference among topical antibiotic preparations in terms of clinical or microbiologic cure rates. There was also insufficient evidence to suggest that the addition of corticosteroids to topical antibiotic preparations leads to improved outcomes.
- Choice of topical antibiotic therapy should be guided by the following:
  - Effectiveness
  - Consideration of potential adverse effects
  - Patency of the tympanic membrane
  - Expected adherence
  - Risk of developing drug resistance
  - Cost and availability
- Aminoglycoside preparations (e.g., neomycin) should be avoided when the patency of the tympanic membrane cannot be confirmed because of the associated ototoxicity to the middle ear. Note that neomycin can cause an allergic contact dermatitis. Note that neomycin is often combined with polymyxin B for antipseudomonal coverage and hydrocortisone.
- Fluoroquinolone preparations are safe to use in cases of nonintact TM and are dosed once or twice daily, which may increase adherence.
- Tips for medication administration
  - Consider warming the ototopical agent to body temperature prior to administration to decrease likelihood of dizziness from caloric stimulation.
  - Preferable for parent to administer treatment, even for older children
  - Patient should lie with affected ear upward.
  - Drops should fill the canal.
  - Manipulate the pinna/tragus to help disperse the medication.
  - Remain in that position for 3–5 minutes.
  - Leave canal open to dry (do not insert cotton ball).
- Duration of treatment is usually 7–10 days, with expected improvement of symptoms within 3 days and resolution by 6 days.
- For those with symptoms persisting beyond the 7- to 10-day period, treatment should continue until symptoms resolve to a maximum of 14 days, at which point, treatment failure should be considered. At that time, a culture may guide further antimicrobial therapy.
- Oral antibiotics should be considered only in complicated OE (coexisting acute otitis media, lymphadenitis, or facial cellulitis) and in immunocompromised individuals who are at higher risk for developing necrotizing or malignant OE.

ADDITIONAL TREATMENT

General Measures

- Pain management
  - For mild to moderate pain, acetaminophen or ibuprofen and application of heat or cold packs often will suffice.
  - For severe pain, a short course of narcotics may be required because pain may intensify during first 48 hours of treatment.
  - There is no data to suggest that benzocaine otic drops are effective for pain management and in fact they may limit the effectiveness of the topical antibiotic by interfering with its contact with the epithelium of the ear canal.
- Clearing aural debris
  - In moderate to severe cases of OE when thick drainage obstructs the view of the TM, it may be necessary to clear debris with light suction or manual removal.
  - Do not use irrigation until you have confirmed the TM is intact.
  - May need to refer to ear, nose, and throat (ENT) physician for aural toilet under microscopic guidance
- Edema
  - In cases in which edema has progressed to cause >50% narrowing of the canal, a medication wick may be necessary (e.g., ¼-inch ribbon gauze or compressed cellulose) to ensure adequate delivery of antimicrobial therapy directly to the epithelium.
  - Do not use a cotton ball because it could fall apart and pieces could become trapped in the canal.
- The wick may fall out on its own as edema resolves or may be removed by clinician.
- Keep the area dry and refrain from swimming for the duration of treatment or at least until symptoms resolve.
- Refrain from using hearing aids until symptoms resolve.

ISSUES FOR REFERRAL

Referral to an otolaryngologist may be indicated for aural cleaning, severe disease, treatment failure, or suspicion of malignant OE.

ONGOING CARE

FOLLOW-UP RECOMMENDATIONS

- Reevaluate if symptoms do not improve within 48 hours of initiating treatment, progression of symptoms despite treatment, or severe illness.
- Immunocompromised patients should be followed closely due to risk for developing malignant OE.

PROGNOSIS

- Excellent in uncomplicated OE with symptom improvement in 2–3 days and resolution of symptoms in 6 days
- Recurrence is common if steps are not taken to address predisposing factors.

COMPLICATIONS

- Stenosis of the ear canal, cellulitis, lymphadenitis, chondritis, parotitis, chronic OE (rare in children)
- Malignant OE in immunocompromised patients (also rare in children)
- Reaction to antibiotic preparation (pruritus, local reaction, rash, discomfort, otalgia, dizziness, vertigo)

ADDITIONAL READING

- Conover K. Earache. *Emerg Med Clin North Am*. 2013;31(2):413–442.
- Ely JW, Hansen MR, Clark EC. Diagnosis of ear pain. *Am Fam Physician*. 2008;77(5):621–628.
- Kaushik V, Malik T, Saeed SR. Interventions for acute otitis externa. *Cochrane Database Syst Rev*. 2010;(1):CD004740.
- Long M. Otitis externa. *Pediatr Rev*. 2013;34(3):143–144.
- Rosenfeld RM, Brown L, Cannon R, et al. Clinical practice guideline: acute otitis externa. *Otolaryngol Head Neck Surg*. 2006;134(Suppl 4):S4–S23.
- Rosenfeld RM, Schwartz SR, Cannon CR, et al. Clinical practice guideline: acute otitis externa. *Otolaryngol Head Neck Surg*. 2014;150(1)(Suppl):S1–S24.
- Schaefer P, Baugh R. Acute otitis externa: an update. *Am Fam Physician*. 2012;86(11):1055–1061.

CODES

ICD10

- H60.90 Unspecified otitis externa, unspecified ear
- H60.339 Swimmer's ear, unspecified ear
- H60.509 Unsp acute noninfective otitis externa, unspecified ear

FAQ

- Q: How should I clean my child's ear?
- A: The external ear can be cleaned with a washcloth. Cotton swabs or other objects should not be inserted into the ear canal, as they may cause trauma or lead to impaction of cerumen. If there is concern for impacted cerumen causing symptoms such as ear fullness, pain, or hearing loss, then a physician should be consulted for discussion of methods for removal.
- Q: Is there a role for oral antibiotics in the treatment of OE?
- A: In uncomplicated OE where the infection is limited to the external canal, topical antibiotics are sufficient. If infection extends beyond the external canal (e.g., otitis media or cellulitis), then an oral antibiotic is advised.
- Q: How should treatment of OE differ if one cannot visualize the tympanic membrane due to accumulated debris and/or edema?
- A: In cases where the tympanic membrane cannot be confirmed to be intact, do not perform lavage. Debris can be removed by curette in the primary care physician's office or the patient may be referred to an otolaryngologist for removal under microscopic guidance. Choose a topical antimicrobial agent other than an aminoglycoside due to its toxic effects on the middle ear. Depending on the certainty of your diagnosis of OE, consider whether the history suggests a coexisting acute otitis media necessitating presumptive treatment with oral antibiotics.

OTITIS MEDIA

C. Matt Stewart • Rosalyn W. Stewart

BASICS

DESCRIPTION
Otitis media is a general term for middle ear inflammation with or without symptoms. It can be acute or chronic.

- 2 specific diagnoses
  - Otitis media with effusion, middle ear effusion (MEE)
  - Acute otitis media (AOM)
    - Uncomplicated/nonsevere
    - Severe
    - Recurrent

EPIDEMIOLOGY
- Most common condition for which antibacterial agents are prescribed for children in the United States
- Peak incidence between 6 and 12 months of age
- By age 3 years, 50–85% of children have had AOM.

RISK FACTORS
- Age <2 years
- Gender: male > female
- Family history of AOM
- Anatomic differences, craniofacial abnormalities
- Environmental tobacco smoke exposure
- Exposure to large numbers of other children
  - Day care
  - Siblings in home

GENERAL PREVENTION
- Breastfeeding for at least 3–6 months
- Decreased pacifier use after 6 months
- Vaccines
  - Pneumococcal conjugate vaccine
  - Influenza vaccine
- Reduction in secondhand smoke
- Reduction of day care crowding

PATHOPHYSIOLOGY
- Eustachian tube dysfunction leads to MEE. If effusion is not cleared by the mucociliary system, bacteria and viruses have a good environment for growth.
- Severe eustachian tube dysfunction occurs during 66% of upper respiratory infections (URIs) in school-aged children and in 75% of URIs in day care–aged children.

ETIOLOGY
- Nontypeable *Haemophilus influenzae*: 35–50%
- *Streptococcus pneumoniae*: 25–40%
- *Moraxella catarrhalis*: 5–10%
- Viruses: 40–75%
  - High rate of coinfection with bacteria
  - Without bacterial coinfection: 5–22%
- Group A *Streptococcus* (3%)
- *Staphylococcus aureus* (2%)
- Gram-negative organisms such as *Pseudomonas aeruginosa*: 1–2%
  - More common in neonatal AOM

DIAGNOSIS

HISTORY
- Recent abrupt onset of signs and symptoms of middle ear inflammation and MEE
- Ear pain for <48 hours
- New-onset otorrhea not caused by acute otitis externa
- Fever
- Irritability
- Past medical history, including underlying disorders (e.g., cleft palate, Down syndrome), immune deficiency, and previous history of otitis media
- Recent treatment with antibiotics
- Exposure to large numbers of children (school, child care, large family)

PHYSICAL EXAM
- Look for other causes of fever and irritability in children: URIs, pharyngitis, lymphadenitis, meningitis, urinary tract infection, and bone and joint infections.
- Physical exam is best done with pneumatic otoscopy:
  - The patient should be adequately restrained if uncooperative.
  - Cerumen should be removed if view of tympanic membrane (TM) is inadequate.
  - Visualize TM at rest and with gentle positive and negative pressure via pneumatic otoscopy.
- The presence of an MEE is determined by the characteristics of the TM:
  - Contour: normal, retracted, full, or bulging; associated bulla(e)
  - Color: gray, pink, yellow, white, or red; hemorrhagic
  - Translucency: translucent or opaque
  - Mobility: normal, decreased, or absent
- Middle ear inflammation is indicated by the following:
  - Erythema of the TM
  - Otalgia
- MEE is indicated by the following:
  - Bulging of the TM
  - Limited or absent mobility of the TM
  - Air–fluid level behind the TM
  - Otorrhea
- A diagnosis of AOM is suggested if an MEE is present along with ear pain, fever, erythema, fullness, or bulging of TM.
- The concomitant presence of conjunctivitis (otitis media–conjunctivitis syndrome) suggests the presence of *H. influenzae* or a virus as a causative organism.
- AOM should not be diagnosed when pneumatic otoscopy and/or tympanometry do not show MEE.

DIAGNOSTIC TESTS & INTERPRETATION

Diagnostic Procedures/Other
- Tympanometry
  - Easily performed by office personnel
  - Provides information on middle ear pressure and TM compliance
  - Sensitive in detecting MEE but poor positive predictive value
- Tympanocentesis
  - For episodes of AOM that are resistant to antibiotic therapy, tympanocentesis and culture and sensitivity of the middle ear fluid may help guide antibiotic therapy.
- Tympanocentesis or myringotomy may also be required as part of the treatment of suppurative complications.

DIFFERENTIAL DIAGNOSIS
- MEE: TM may appear dull with a diffuse light reflex, fluid bubbles may be visible, and mobility may be decreased.
- Otitis externa
- Auricular lesions like a furuncle or laceration
- Other causes of fever, including viral URIs, pharyngitis, pneumonia, meningitis, UTIs, and bone and joint infections
- Pharyngitis and dental pain may be mistaken for otalgia.

TREATMENT

MEDICATION

Note: AOM management should include pain evaluation and treatment.

- Antibiotic therapy for AOM in children ≥6 months of age with severe signs or symptoms (moderate or severe otalgia or otalgia of 48 hours or temperature ≥39°C [102.2°F])
- Antibiotic therapy for bilateral AOM in children 6–23 months of age without severe signs or symptoms
- Antibiotic therapy or observation with close follow-up if joint decision-making with caregiver for unilateral AOM in children 6–23 months of age without severe signs or symptoms
  - Observation and follow-up and antibiotic therapy if child worsens or fails to improve in 48–72 hours
- Initial treatment
  - Amoxicillin (80–90 mg/kg/24 h PO divided b.i.d.)
    - When child has not received amoxicillin in past 30 days
    - Does not have concurrent purulent conjunctivitis
    - Not allergic to penicillin
- Antibiotic treatment after 48–72 hours of no improvement
  - Amoxicillin-clavulanate (90 mg/kg/24 h amoxicillin and 12.8 mg/kg/24 h clavulanate PO divided b.i.d.)
    - Has received amoxicillin in the last 30 days
    - Concurrent purulent conjunctivitis
    - History of recurrent AOM unresponsive to amoxicillin
- Initial oral antibiotic treatment if penicillin allergy
  - Cefdinir (14 mg/kg/24 h QD or divided b.i.d.)
  - Cefuroxime (30 mg/kg/24 h divided b.i.d.)
  - Cefpodoxime (10 mg/kg/24 h divided b.i.d.)
  - Ceftriaxone (50 mg IM or IV per day for 1 or 3 days)
- Treatment after 48–72 hours of no improvement
  - Ceftriaxone (50 mg IM or IV per day for 1 or 3 days)
  - Clindamycin (30–40 mg/kg/24 h PO divided t.i.d.), with or without 3rd-generation cephalosporin

ADDITIONAL TREATMENT

General Measures

- Do not use prophylactic antibiotics to reduce frequency of episodes of AOM in children with recurrent AOM.
- Adjunctive therapy
  - Fever relief with acetaminophen or ibuprofen
  - Pain may be treated with acetaminophen, ibuprofen, or topical anesthetic drops.

ISSUES FOR REFERRAL

- Consider otolaryngology referral:
  - Tympanostomy tubes for recurrent AOM if
    - 3 episodes in 6 months
    - 4 episodes in 1 year with 1 episode in the preceding 6 months
    - Persistent and/or recurrent otitis with abnormal hearing and/or speech

ONGOING CARE

FOLLOW-UP RECOMMENDATIONS

- Expect symptomatic improvement within 48–72 hours of treatment; may need to switch antibiotic and/or evaluate for complications
- Follow-up exam should be scheduled 3–4 weeks after completion of antibiotic therapy to ensure resolution of AOM.
- If effusion is present, follow up monthly. For persistent effusions of >3 months' duration, a hearing evaluation is recommended.

PROGNOSIS

- Symptoms of acute infection (fever and otalgia) are relieved within 48–72 hours in most patients.
- Treatment failures are more likely with increased severity of disease and younger age.
- Development of another infection within 30 days usually represents a recurrence caused by a different organism rather than a relapse.
  - Recurrences are frequent and more common in younger children and if initial episode is severe.
- 30–70% of treated children will have an effusion at 2 weeks.
  - MEE may persist for weeks to months.

COMPLICATIONS

- Hearing loss
  - Acute conductive hearing loss is common and usually resolves as the effusion resolves.
  - Fluid of long-standing duration may lead to permanent conductive hearing loss.
  - Sensorineural hearing loss may result from spread of infection into the labyrinth.
- TM perforation
- Chronic suppurative otitis media
- Tympanosclerosis
- Cholesteatoma
- Acute mastoiditis
- Petrositis
- Labyrinthitis
- Facial nerve paralysis
- Bacterial meningitis
- Epidural abscess
- Subdural empyema
- Brain abscess
- Lateral sinus thrombosis

ADDITIONAL READING

- Coker TR, Chan LS, Newberry SJ, et al. Diagnosis, microbial epidemiology, and antibiotic treatment of acute otitis media in children: a systematic review. *JAMA*. 2010;304(19):2161–2169.
- Gould JM, Matz PS. Otitis media. *Pediatr Rev*. 2010;31(3):102–116.
- Hoberman A, Paradise JL, Rockette HE, et al. Treatment of acute otitis media in children under 2 years of age. *N Engl J Med*. 2011;364(2):105–115.
- Lieberthal AS, Carroll AE, Chonmaitree T, et al. The diagnosis and management of acute otitis media. *Pediatrics*. 2013;131(3):e964–e999.
- Spiro DM, Tay KY, Arnold DH, et al. Wait-and-see prescription for the treatment of acute otitis media. *JAMA*. 2006;296(10):1235–1241.
- Takata GS, Chan LS, Morphew T, et al. Evidence assessment of the accuracy of methods of diagnosing middle ear effusion in children with otitis media with effusion. *Pediatrics*. 2003;112(6, Pt 1): 1379–1387.

CODES

ICD10

- H66.90 Otitis media, unspecified, unspecified ear
- H65.199 Other acute nonsuppurative otitis media, unspecified ear
- H65.499 Other chronic nonsuppurative otitis media, unspecified ear

FAQ

- Q: When should children with AOM be treated?
- A: Antibiotic therapy for AOM in children ≥6 months of age with severe signs or symptoms. Antibiotic therapy for bilateral AOM in children 6–23 months of age without severe signs or symptoms
- Q: What is the antibiotic of choice for initial therapy of AOM?
- A: The initial therapy is amoxicillin. The antibiotic treatment after 48–72 hours of no improvement is amoxicillin-clavulanate.
- Q: What can be done to prevent the development of AOM in an individual child?
- A: Pneumococcal conjugate vaccine.
  Annual influenza vaccine.
  Encourage breastfeeding for at least 6 months.
  Encourage avoidance of tobacco smoke exposure.

PALLOR

David T. Teachey

BASICS

DESCRIPTION

- Pallor is defined as paleness of the skin and may be a reflection of anemia or poor peripheral perfusion.
- The normal range for hemoglobin is age dependent.
- Anemia can be defined functionally as the inability of hemoglobin to meet cellular oxygen demand.
- Parents often fail to notice pallor of gradual onset.
  - Grandparents or others who see the child less often may be the first to suspect pallor.

RISK FACTORS

- Ages between 6 months and 3 years or adolescent females
  - Peak age ranges for iron deficiency
- Gender
  - Some red cell–enzyme X-linked defects such as glucose-6-phosphate dehydrogenase (G6PD) and phosphoglycerate kinase deficiencies are sex linked.
- Race
  - African: hemoglobins S and C, α- and β-thalassemia trait, G6PD deficiency
  - Southeast Asian: hemoglobin E and α-thalassemia
  - Mediterranean descent: β-thalassemia and G6PD deficiency

Genetics

Familial history: Some of the congenital hemolytic anemias are autosomal dominant.

DIAGNOSIS

- Determine first that the child appears pale, not simply fair skinned. Second, decide if there is a medical emergency associated with circulatory failure. If not, the goal is to investigate the etiology and intervene appropriately.
- Phase 1: Assess for signs of shock.
  - If present, initiate emergency procedures as required to stabilize the patient, such as airway, breathing, and circulation.
- Phase 2: If patient is stable, perform history, physical examination, and CBC with reticulocyte count to establish time of onset of pallor, associated symptoms, and level of anemia.
- Phase 3: Follow specific diagnostic workup based on findings in phase 2.

SIGNS AND SYMPTOMS

- Pallor
- Other signs and symptoms dependent on etiology

HISTORY

- Acute versus chronic onset
  - Helps with differential diagnosis
- Associated symptoms: weight loss, fever, night sweats, cough, and/or bone pain
  - Suggest an underlying systemic illness, such as leukemia, infection, or rheumatologic disorder
- Jaundice, scleral icterus, dark urine
  - Suggest hemolysis
- Age <6 months
  - May represent a congenital anemia or isoimmunization
- Premature infant
  - Increased risk of both iron and vitamin E deficiency
  - Exaggerated hyperbilirubinemia can be the presenting symptom of isoimmune hemolytic or other congenital hemolytic anemia.
- Pica
  - Often associated with plumbism and iron deficiency
- Medications
  - Can cause bone marrow suppression and/or hemolysis
- Milk intake
  - Introduction of cow's milk at <12 months of age is associated with iron deficiency.
  - Drinking a lot of cow's milk (>24 oz/day) puts a toddler at risk for iron deficiency.
- Recent trauma and/or surgery
  - Blood loss can result in iron deficiency.
- Recent infection
  - Can be associated with hemolysis or bone marrow suppression
  - Most common form of mild anemia in childhood
- Family history
  - Familial history of splenectomy and/or early cholecystectomy can be a clue for a previously undiagnosed hemolytic anemia.

PHYSICAL EXAM

- Rapid respiratory rate, decreased BP, weak pulses, slow capillary refill
  - Indications of uncompensated anemia and/or shock
- Frontal bossing and prominence of the malar and maxillary bones
  - Extramedullary erythropoiesis
- Enlarged spleen
  - Hemolytic anemias, malignancy, infection
- Glossitis
  - Vitamin B_{12} deficiency
  - Iron deficiency
- Scleral icterus or jaundice
  - May indicate hemolysis
- Systolic flow murmur
  - Anemia
- Bruits
  - May indicate vascular malformations
- Petechiae and bruising
  - May indicate an associated thrombocytopenia, coagulopathy, or vasculitis
- Dysmorphic features
  - Diamond-Blackfan and Fanconi anemia are associated with other congenital defects, including thumb abnormalities, short stature, and congenital heart disease.

DIAGNOSTIC TESTS & INTERPRETATION

Lab

- CBC with red cell indices
  - Establishes the diagnosis of anemia, distinguishes by size: normocytic, macrocytic, microcytic
- Reticulocyte count
  - Distinguishes between decreased production and increased destruction of red cells
- Coombs test and antibody screen
  - Identifies immune-mediated red cell destruction
  - Can have false positives and negatives
- Peripheral blood smear
  - Specific morphologic findings can be diagnostic.
- Iron studies: iron-binding capacity, serum iron, ferritin, transferrin
  - Iron deficiency anemia or anemia of chronic disease
- Hemoglobin electrophoresis with quantification
  - Hemoglobinopathy
- Lead studies: serum lead, free erythrocyte protoporphyrin
  - Plumbism
- Stool guaiac
  - Occult blood loss

- Osmotic fragility
  - Red cell membrane defects (spherocytosis)
  - Any spherocytic anemia may be positive.
- Quantitative red cell–enzyme assays
  - Inherited RBC enzyme deficiencies
- Serum folate, RBC folate, and serum vitamin B_{12} levels
  - Deficiency

Diagnostic Procedures/Other

Bone marrow aspiration and biopsy: if malignancy or bone marrow failure syndrome suspected

DIFFERENTIAL DIAGNOSIS

- Congenital
  - Hemoglobinopathies: sickle cell syndromes, thalassemia syndromes, other unstable hemoglobins
  - Erythrocyte membrane defects: hereditary spherocytosis, elliptocytosis, stomatocytosis, pyropoikilocytosis, infantile pyknocytosis
  - Erythrocyte enzyme defects: G6PD deficiency, pyruvate kinase deficiency
  - Diamond-Blackfan anemia: congenital pure red cell aplasia (rare)
  - Fanconi anemia: constellation of varied cytopenias, multiple congenital anomalies, abnormal bone marrow chromosomal fragility
- Infectious
  - Septic shock
  - Can get mild anemia after mild infections in childhood (anemia of inflammation)
  - Infection-related bone marrow suppression: parvovirus B19 infection
  - Infection-related hemolytic anemias: Epstein-Barr virus, influenza, coxsackievirus, varicella, cytomegalovirus, *Escherichia coli*, *Pneumococcus* species, *Streptococcus* species, *Salmonella typhi*, *Mycoplasma* species
- Nutritional/toxic/drugs
  - Iron deficiency anemia: common cause of anemia in children, especially those <3 years of age and in female adolescents
  - Plumbism: anemia usually due to coexisting iron deficiency; very high lead levels associated with altered heme synthesis
  - Vitamin B_{12} and/or folate deficiency: results in a megaloblastic anemia
  - Medication-induced bone marrow suppression: chemotherapy; antibiotics, especially trimethoprim-sulfamethoxazole
  - Drug-related hemolytic anemia: antibiotics, antiepileptics, azathioprine, isoniazid, nonsteroidal anti-inflammatory drugs
- Trauma
  - Acute blood loss
- Tumor
  - Leukemia with bone marrow infiltration
  - Metastatic tumors with bone marrow infiltration
- Genetic/metabolic
  - Metabolic derangements: severe electrolyte disturbance, pH disturbance, inborn errors
  - Shwachman-Diamond syndrome: marrow hypoplasia with associated pancreatic insufficiency and associated failure to thrive
- Other:
  - Transient erythroblastopenia of childhood: acquired pure RBC aplasia
  - Aplastic anemia: bone marrow failure syndrome with at least 2 of the 3 blood cell lines eventually affected
  - Systemic diseases: anemia of chronic disease, chronic renal disease, uremia
  - Hypothyroidism
  - Sideroblastic anemia: defective iron use within the developing erythrocytes
  - Autoimmune and isoimmune hemolytic anemias
  - Microangiopathic hemolytic anemias: thrombotic thrombocytopenic purpura (TTP), hemolytic uremic syndrome (HUS), disseminated intravascular coagulation (DIC)
  - Mechanical destruction: vascular malformation, abnormal or prosthetic cardiac valves

TREATMENT

INITIAL STABILIZATION

- Severe anemia of unclear etiology with hemodynamic instability
  - Transfuse with packed RBCs cautiously.
  - In an autoimmune hemolytic process, the child is at risk for a transfusion reaction, and there may be delay in obtaining cross-matched blood.
  - Obtain blood for diagnostic studies before transfusion if possible.
- Circulatory failure without anemia
  - Requires intensive monitoring and access to critical care in an emergency department or intensive care unit
  - Fluid resuscitation and/or inotropic pressor support as needed
- Acute blood loss
  - Treat circulatory failure as described.
  - Transfuse with packed RBCs, platelets, and fresh frozen plasma as needed.
- Malignancies
  - Emergency care should be directed toward treatment of circulatory failure and possible associated infection and then to rapid diagnosis and treatment of the malignancy.
  - Consultation with an oncologist should be sought as soon as possible.

GENERAL MEASURES

- Treat underlying cause.
- Consider packed RBC transfusion if in extremis or severe anemia and low likelihood of recovery in near future.
- Consider emergent plasmapheresis if with microangiopathic hemolytic anemia.
- Consider immunosuppressive medications (corticosteroids, intravenous immunoglobulin (IVIG) if with autoimmune hemolytic anemia.
- Iron deficiency anemia
  - Elemental iron

MEDICATION

Elemental iron for patients with iron deficiency

- 4–6 mg/kg/24 h PO divided b.i.d.–t.i.d.
- Absorbed best with acidic drinks, including orange juice; dairy products decrease absorption.
- Reticulocyte should improve 72 hours after starting iron therapy; the hemoglobin may take a week to rise.
- Iron should be continued for at least 3 months to replenish iron stores.

ONGOING CARE

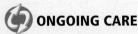

ISSUES FOR REFERRAL

- Severe or unexplained anemia
- Anemias other than dietary iron deficiency or thalassemia trait
- Recurrent iron deficiency
  - May suggest ongoing bleeding or iron malabsorption
- All bone marrow failure or infiltrative processes

ADDITIONAL READING

- Baker RD, Greer FR; Committee on Nutrition, American Academy of Pediatrics. Diagnosis and prevention of iron deficiency and iron-deficiency anemia in infants and young children (0-3 years of age). *Pediatrics*. 2010;126(5):1040–1050.
- Glader BE. Hemolytic anemia in children. *Clin Lab Med*. 1999;19(1):87–111.
- Graham EA. The changing face of anemia in infancy. *Pediatr Rev*. 1994;15(5):175–183.
- Monzon CM, Beaver D, Dillon TD. Evaluation of erythrocyte disorders with mean corpuscular volume (MCV) and red cell distribution width (RDW). *Clin Pediatr*. 1987;26(12):632–638.
- Segal G, Hirsh M, Feig S. Managing anemia in pediatric office practice: part 2. *Pediatr Rev*. 2002;23(4):111–122.
- Sills RH. Indications for bone marrow examination. *Pediatr Rev*. 1995;16(6):226–228.

CODES

ICD10

R23.1 Pallor

PANCREATIC PSEUDOCYST

Amit S. Grover • Menno Verhave

BASICS

- A pancreatic pseudocyst is a peripancreatic (or intrapancreatic) fluid collection associated with a history of pancreatitis, that is surrounded by a well-defined inflammatory wall, and that has no solid component.
  - The term "pseudocyst" is often incorrectly used to define various types of fluid collections associated with pancreatitis. As a result, medical literature on pseudocysts is not consistent in its descriptions or its findings.
  - An important distinction between "fluid collections" associated with pancreatitis is that some consist of fluid alone, whereas others arise from necrosis of pancreatic parenchyma and/or peripancreatic tissues. The latter type of fluid collection involves a solid component (with variable amounts of fluid), which distinguishes them from pseudocysts.
- Types of fluid collections:
  - Acute peripancreatic fluid collection (APFC)
    - A fluid collection that develops in the early phase of interstitial edematous acute (typically mild) pancreatitis
    - Lack a well-defined wall on CT scan
    - NOT associated with necrotizing pancreatitis
    - Remain sterile, and usually resolve without intervention
    - If APFC persists beyond 4 weeks, likely to develop into a pancreatic pseudocyst; although this is considered a rare outcome.
  - Pancreatic pseudocyst
    - Refers specifically to a peripancreatic (or less commonly, an intrapancreatic) fluid collection
    - Surrounded by a well-defined inflammatory wall and containing NO solid material
    - Pancreatic pseudocysts develop more than 4 weeks after the onset of interstitial pancreatitis.
  - Acute necrotic collection (ANC)
    - A collection of BOTH variable amounts of fluid and solid (necrotic) material related to pancreatic and/or peripancreatic necrosis
    - Occur within the first 4 weeks of disease, and can resemble an APFC in the first few days of acute pancreatitis
    - As necrotizing pancreatitis develops and necrosis evolves, solid component become evident.
    - May be multiple and may involve the pancreatic parenchyma alone, the peripancreatic tissue alone, or most commonly both
    - May be infected or sterile
    - Generally associated with more severe sequelae of AP
  - Walled-off necrosis (WON)
    - Collection of varying amounts of liquid and solid material surrounded by a mature, enhancing wall of reactive tissue
    - Represents a mature, encapsulated ANC
    - Develops no earlier than 4 weeks after episode of necrotizing pancreatitis
    - May be multiple and present at sites distant from the pancreas
    - May be sterile or infected

PATHOPHYSIOLOGY

- Pseudocysts occur when there is disruption in the pancreatic ductular system, or its intrapancreatic branches, without any evidence of pancreatic or peripancreatic necrosis.
- This results in the extravasation of pancreatic enzymes evoking an inflammatory response.
- The inflammatory reaction leads to a fluid collection that is rich in pancreatic enzymes (APFC).
- If the duration of the fluid collection is >4 weeks, becomes localized (intrapancreatic or extrapancreatic), and develops a fibrin capsule, it becomes a pseudocyst.
- A pseudocyst does not have a true epithelial lining.
- If there is communication between the pseudocyst and the pancreatic duct, the enzyme level in the fluid remain elevated; if there is no communication, the enzyme level falls with time.

DIAGNOSIS

HISTORY

Acute or chronic pancreatitis

- Suspect pancreatic pseudocyst in patients recovering from acute pancreatitis, or in the patient with chronic pancreatitis, who has recurrent/persistent abdominal pain, a palpable abdominal mass, or persistently elevated serum pancreatic enzymes.

PHYSICAL EXAM

- Abdominal tenderness
- Abdominal mass
- Nausea and vomiting
- Weight loss
- Jaundice
- Abdominal distention
  - Mass/ascites
- In many situations, no clinical signs are seen.
- Clinical signs may be secondary to complications:
  - Jaundice in hepatobiliary obstruction
  - Lower limb edema in compression of inferior vena cava
  - Ascites in peritonitis
  - Pleural effusion

DIAGNOSTIC TESTS & INTERPRETATION

Lab

Serum pancreatic enzyme levels:

- Persistently elevated enzymes in blood can be a clue, but is not an absolute indicator.
- Elevated enzymes in fluid drained from a peripancreatic or intrapancreatic fluid collection with no solid component is consistent with a pancreatic pseudocyst.

Imaging

- CT scan
  - Reveals pseudopancreatic cyst; can also be used to gauge size of pseudocyst and its relationship to adjacent organs
- Ultrasonography
  - Visualizes pancreatic pseudocysts
  - Can be used to follow cyst size over time
- Endoscopic ultrasonography (EUS)
  - Common modality in adult patients and increasingly used in pediatrics
  - Can be used to diagnose presence and size of pseudocyst; can also be used to guide peroral fluid aspiration and drainage
- Endoscopic retrograde cholangiopancreatography (ERCP)
  - Used in some cases to delineate the pancreatic ductular system before drainage to distinguish ductal stenosis, disruption, stones, and other obstructions

DIFFERENTIAL DIAGNOSIS

- Congenital/genetic
  - Congenital cysts
  - Polycystic disease
  - Von Hippel-Lindau disease
  - Cystic fibrosis
- Infections
  - Pancreatic abscess
  - Echinococcal (hydatid) cyst
  - Taenia solium cyst
- Tumor
  - Serous cystadenoma
  - Mucinous cystadenoma
  - Cystic islet cell tumors
  - Teratoma
  - Pancreatoblastoma
  - Cystadenocarcinoma
  - Franz tumor
  - Angiomatous cystic neoplasms
  - Lymphangiomas
  - Hemangioendothelioma
- Miscellaneous:
  - Splenic cyst
  - Adrenal cyst
  - Enterogenous cyst
  - Duplication cysts
  - Endometriosis

TREATMENT

GENERAL MEASURES

- Medical management:
  - Most cases resolve with supportive care.
  - If eating precipitates pain, short-term nasojejunal feedings or parenteral nutrition may be warranted.
  - Follow up with ultrasound or CT scan to make sure there are no complications.
  - >60% have complete resolution by the end of 1 year.
  - Usually, no medications are used for managing pseudocysts.
  - Somatostatin analogue (octreotide) has been reported to be used to decrease fluid collection along with drainage.
  - Antibiotics are used in situations of infected pseudocyst.
- Drainage
  - Most often used in the setting of WON
  - Indications: infection, rupture with cardiopulmonary compromise, biliary and gastric outlet obstruction, persistent symptoms, rapid enlargement, failure of large pseudocysts (>6 cm) to shrink after 6 weeks
  - Modalities:
    - Percutaneous drainage (aspiration or catheter drainage) is done in cases in which the pseudocyst has a less mature wall.
    - Percutaneous aspiration has a high recurrence rate of 63% and failure rate of 54%.
    - Continuous drainage has a recurrence rate of 8% and a failure rate of 19%.
    - Endoscopic procedures are becoming the 1st-line drainage modality, as they are less invasive than surgery.
    - Endoscopic procedures include transmural cystoenterostomies and transpapillary route procedures such as stent placement for pseudocysts that communicate with the main pancreatic duct.
    - Endoscopic procedures in experienced hands report success rates of 82–89%, complication rates of 10–20%, and recurrence rates of 6–18%.

SURGERY/OTHER PROCEDURES

- Reserved for failed endoscopic procedures, difficult to access areas of WON and multiple WONs
- Includes internal drainage (cystogastrostomy, cystoduodenostomy, and Roux-en-Y cystojejunostomy), resection, and external drainage
- Success rate is 85–90%.
- Recurrence rate is 0–17%.
- Mortality rate is between 3 and 5%.

ONGOING CARE

PROGNOSIS

Majority of pseudocysts resolve without intervention.

COMPLICATIONS

- Perforation/rupture
  - Cardiopulmonary compromise secondary to pleural effusion and ascites
  - Peritonitis and ascites, which can be fatal
- Hemorrhage
  - Erosions of vessels lining the cyst cause intracystic bleeding and rapid increase in the cyst size.
  - Bleeding may occur directly into stomach, duodenum (clinically manifesting as GI bleeding), or peritoneal cavity.
- Obstruction
  - Biliary obstruction: jaundice
  - Portal obstruction: portal hypertension
  - Gastric outlet obstruction
  - Inferior vena cava obstruction: peripheral edema
  - Urinary obstruction
  - Colonic obstruction
- Infection of pseudocysts is rare in children compared to adults:
  - Associated with high mortality rate for children and adults
  - Management usually requires surgical drainage.

ADDITIONAL READING

- Law NM, Freeman ML. Emergency complications of acute and chronic pancreatitis. *Gastroenterol Clin*. 2002;32(4):1169–1194.
- Reber HA. Surgery for acute and chronic pancreatitis. *Gastrointest Endosc*. 2002;56(6)(Suppl):S246–S248.
- Sarr MG, Banks PA, Bollen TL, et al. The new revised classification of acute pancreatitis 2012. *Surg Clin North Am*, 2013;93(3):549–562.
- Vidyarthi G, Steinberg SE. Endoscopic management of pancreatic pseudocysts. *Surg Clin North Am*. 2001;81(2):405–410.
- Weckman L, Kylanpaa ML, Poulakkainen P, et al. Endoscopic treatment of pancreatic pseudocysts. *Surg Endosc*. 2006;20(4):603–607.

CODES

ICD10

K86.3 Pseudocyst of pancreas

PANCREATITIS

Amit S. Grover • Menno Verhave

BASICS

DESCRIPTION

- Inflammation within the pancreas characterized by 3 phases: early trypsin activation within acinar cells; followed by surrounding intrapancreatic inflammation; and finally, extrapancreatic inflammation with systemic inflammatory responses
- Classified into acute and chronic
  - Acute pancreatitis (AP)
    - *Variable* presentation, however, most often characterized by acute onset of abdominal pain, nausea, and vomiting with elevation of pancreatic enzymes
    - Nonverbal children may present with irritability; infants may present with lethargy and fever.
    - Often self-limited, with reversible changes, but can progress if not appropriately managed
    - Severe AP is rare in children; however, a high suspicion should always be maintained, as severe disease can progress rapidly and result in significant morbidity and mortality.
  - Chronic pancreatitis (CP)
    - Characterized by irreversible morphologic changes and fibrotic replacement of the pancreatic parenchyma
    - Clinically characterized by recurrent abdominal pain or evidence of exocrine and/or endocrine insufficiency
    - Often the result of a persistent and continued pancreatic inflammation secondary to acute attacks

ETIOLOGY

- Biliary tract disease
  - Gallstones
- Medications
  - L-asparaginase, azathioprine/6-MP, mesalamine, sulfonamides, thiazides, furosemide, tetracyclines, valproic acid, corticosteroids, estrogens, procainamide, ethacrynic acid, and others
- Toxins
  - Alcohol, organophosphates, scorpion poison, snake poison
- Trauma
  - Bicycle handle injuries
  - Motor vehicle collisions
  - Child abuse
  - Postoperative
    - Endoscopic retrograde cholangiopancreatography (ERCP)
- Systemic disease
  - Shock/hypoxemia/SEPSIS
  - Inflammatory bowel disease (IBD)
  - Cystic fibrosis
- Idiopathic
- Less common
  - Infections
    - Bacterial: typhoid, mycoplasma
    - Viral: measles, mumps, Epstein-Barr virus, coxsackie B, rubella, influenza, echovirus, hepatitis A and B
    - Parasites: *Ascaris lumbricoides*, *Echinococcus granulosus*, *Cryptosporidium parvum*, *Plasmodium falciparum*
  - Metabolic diseases:
    - Hyperlipidemia
    - Hypercalcemia
    - Diabetic ketoacidosis
    - Uremia
    - Inborn errors of metabolism
  - Systemic diseases:
    - Hemolytic uremic syndrome
    - Celiac disease
    - Diabetes mellitus
    - Vasculitis: systemic lupus erythematosus (SLE), Henoch-Schönlein purpura, Kawasaki disease
- Rare causes:
  - Autoimmune pancreatitis: Rare condition divided into 2 subtypes.
    - Type I often grouped with IgG4-related disease and systemic manifestations.
    - Type II does not have IgG4 association, however, is more common in younger patients and associated with IBD.
  - Congenital anomalies:
    - Pancreatic divisum
    - Annular pancreas
    - Anomalous pancreaticobiliary junction
    - Biliary tract malformations
    - Duplication cyst of the duodenum/gastropancreatic/common bile duct

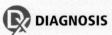

DIAGNOSIS

HISTORY

- Pain
  - Onset, location, and severity can be variable in children.
  - Aggravated by food intake
  - Nonverbal patients (i.e., younger age, developmental delay) may present with increased irritability.
- Vomiting
  - May or may not always be present
  - May be bilious
  - May present as feeding intolerance
- Trauma
  - Even trivial abdominal trauma should be a red flag.
  - Evaluate for evidence of child abuse.
- Family history
  - Hereditary pancreatitis
  - Hypertriglyceridemia (I, IV, or V)
  - CFTR mutations/FH of CF
- Prior history of, or risk factors for, cholelithiasis
- Toxic exposures (i.e., EtOH, pesticides)
- Review of systems:
  - Associated fever may suggest infectious etiology.
  - Diminished urine output raises concern for third-space losses.
  - Shortness of breath raises concern for pulmonary involvement (i.e., effusions).

PHYSICAL EXAM

- General exam
  - Growth parameters (weight and height), vital signs, capillary refill, pulse oximetry, pallor, jaundice, edema, and clubbing
  - Abnormal vital signs (heart rate, respiratory rate, and blood pressure) can be indicative of the systemic inflammatory response syndrome (SIRS), a poor prognostic sign.
  - Clubbing can be an indicator of cystic fibrosis.
- GI
  - Mouth: Presence of aphthous lesions raises possibility of Crohn disease.
    - Inspection: abdominal distention or flank fullness (ascites or pseudopancreatic cyst); bluish discoloration of the flanks (Grey Turner sign) and periumbilical region (Cullen sign) in hemorrhagic pancreatitis
    - Palpation: for liver, gall bladder, spleen, and masses. Patients will have guarding, tenderness, and rebound tenderness, especially in the epigastric region and/or upper abdomen; palpable mass could be a pancreatic pseudocyst.
  - Percussion: dullness and fluid thrill consistent with ascites
  - Auscultation: bowel sounds decreased in ascites or absent in paralytic ileus
- Rectal exam
  - Perianal region for skin tags, fistulas, abscesses, or healed scars, which could be indicative of IBD; perirectal exam for mass, melena, or occult blood
  - Hematochezia can be suggestive of IBD.
- GU
  - Assess urinary output.
  - High specific gravity suggestive of reduced intravascular volume, result of third-space losses
- Respiratory system
  - Pleural effusion and acute respiratory distress syndrome (ARDS)
  - Diffuse respiratory findings could be indicative of cystic fibrosis.
- CNS
  - Stupor or coma

DIAGNOSTIC TESTS & INTERPRETATION

Lab

- CBC
  - Hemoglobin may be decreased in hemorrhagic pancreatitis.
  - Leukocytosis may be present in infectious pancreatitis.
  - Hemoconcentration: elevated HCT
- Basic metabolic panel
  - Hemoconcentration due to third-space losses and intravascular depletion (elevated BUN, Cr)
  - Calcium may be elevated (etiology) or decreased (sequelae).
  - Glucose may be transiently elevated.
  - Bicarbonate may be low secondary to acidosis.
- Liver function tests:
  - Elevated transaminase levels suggest biliary cause.
  - Elevated bilirubin level/GGTP/Alk Phos suggestive of gallstone pancreatitis

- Amylase level
  - 3-fold elevation of amylase levels increases specificity for the diagnosis of pancreatitis.
  - Starts rising 2–12 hours after the insult and remains elevated for 3–5 days
  - Degree of elevation does not have any correlation to the severity or the course of the illness.
  - Other causes of elevated amylase levels include bowel obstruction, acute appendicitis, biliary obstruction, salivary duct obstruction, diabetic ketoacidosis, cystic fibrosis, pneumonia, salpingitis, ruptured ectopic pregnancy, ovarian cyst, cerebral trauma, burns, renal failure, and macroamylasemia.
- Lipase level
  - Lipase levels are more specific than amylase for the diagnosis of pancreatitis.
  - Starts rising 4–8 hours after the insult and remains elevated for 8–14 days
  - 3-fold increase in the level is very sensitive and specific for pancreatitis.
  - Levels do not correlate with severity or with clinical outcome.
  - Other causes of elevated lipase levels include intestinal perforation, intestinal obstruction, appendicitis, mesenteric infarction, cholecystitis, diabetic ketoacidosis, renal failure, and macrolipasemia.
- Urinalysis
  - Urine specific gravity is a simple indicator of intravascular volume.
    - Elevated value can suggest third-space losses, a harbinger for severe disease.

Imaging

- Abdominal x-rays:
  - Sentinel loop: distended small intestinal loop near the pancreas
  - Colon cutoff sign: absence of gas shadow in the colon distal to the transverse colon
  - Multiple fluid levels in paralytic ileus
  - Calcification or stones in pancreas or gallbladder
  - Diffuse haziness: ascites
- Chest x-ray
  - Pleural effusion or ARDS
  - Diaphragmatic involvement
- US abdomen
  - Best initial test
  - Will demonstrate pancreatic size; echogenicity; associated fat stranding; ductal diameter/disruption; and calcifications, cholelithiasis, CBD dilation, ascites, and free fluid within abdomen
  - Limited by obesity and bowel gas
  - Endoscopic US (EUS) is more useful than the transabdominal US study but is difficult in children; used if pancreatic biopsy is indicated
- CT scan
  - May be used if history of trauma to look at extent of injury to pancreas and other intra-abdominal structures
  - Best to show evidence of pancreatic necrosis with AP from any cause, however, not sensitive within the first 48 hours
  - Reveals pathology in the pancreaticobiliary system in most instances
  - Involves exposure to radiation
- Magnetic resonance cholangiopancreatography (MRCP)
  - Good for ductal visualization (especially if secretin stimulated)
  - Can reveal anatomic abnormalities/obstructive lesions, that is, pancreatic divisum
  - Can mitigate need for ERCP, unless there is concern for choledocholithiasis +/− ascending cholangitis
  - Good for distinguishing pseudocyst versus walled-off necrosis
  - No exposure to radiation
- ERCP
  - Indicated in persistent/CP for delineation of pancreatic ducts and for therapeutic interventions (i.e., sphincterotomy or stent placement)
  - Risk of post-ERCP pancreatitis in 10–20% of cases
    - In adults, administration of rectal indomethacin has been shown to reduce this risk.

TREATMENT

FLUID RESUSCITATION

- Aggressive volume resuscitation with isotonic solutions is the cornerstone of therapy for AP.
- Under-resuscitation is associated with increased risk of mortality from AP.
- Targeted approach involving bolus (20 mL/kg), followed by continuous infusion at 1.5–2× maintenance (contraindicated if presence of fluid-sensitive cardiac disease) with serial monitoring q6–8h

MEDICATION

- Antibiotics
  - No evidence to support the routine use of antibiotics in patients with acute necrotizing pancreatitis *unless*:
    - Sepsis is suspected.
    - An extrapancreatic infection (bacteremia, pneumonia, UTI) is present.
    - Patient is on chemotherapy and/or is neutropenic.
- Pain management
  - Effective analgesia should be a priority.
  - Combination of intermittent IV narcotics +/− PCA

ADDITIONAL TREATMENT

Nutrition

- Initially, patient should remain NPO for pancreatic rest.
- New evidence suggests early feeding may not be beneficial.
- Postpyloric feeds can be considered if initial trial of enteral feeding fails.
- If prolonged NPO course and failure of postpyloric feeds, consider parenteral nutrition.

SURGERY/OTHER PROCEDURES

- If gallstone impaction with choledocholithiasis, should consider ERCP + sphincterotomy + stent
- Severe third-spacing can lead to abdominal compartment syndrome, necessitating surgical decompression.
- Development of walled-off necrosis with persistent pain may benefit from necrocystectomy (endoscopic or surgical).

ONGOING CARE

PROGNOSIS

AP is usually a self-limiting disorder in children.

COMPLICATIONS

- Pancreatic edema
- Peripancreatic fat necrosis
- Acute pancreatic fluid collections
- Pancreatic necrosis
- Pancreatic pseudocyst or walled-off necrosis
- Pancreatic ductal strictures
- Pancreatic ductal dilatation
- Systemic complications:
  - Shock and multiorgan failure
- GI and hepatobiliary
  - Paralytic ileus
  - Ascites, peritonitis
  - Stress ulcer
  - Intestinal hemorrhage
  - Portal vein thrombosis/splenic vein thrombosis/obstruction
  - Bile duct obstruction
- Pulmonary
  - Atelectasis, pleural effusion, pneumonitis, ARDS
- Cardiovascular
  - Hypotension/circulatory collapse
  - Pericarditis/pericardial effusion
  - EKG changes
- Sudden death

ADDITIONAL READING

- Bai HX, Lowe ME, Husain SZ. What have we learned about acute pancreatitis in children? *J J Pediatr Gastroenterol Nutr*. 2011;52(3):262–270.
- Banks PA, Bollen TL, Dervenis C, et al. Classification of acute pancreatitis—2012: revision of the Atlanta classification and definitions by international consensus. *Gut*. 2012;62(1):102–111.
- Forsmark CE, Baillie J; AGA Institute Clinical Practice and Economics Committee; AGA Institute Governing Board. AGA Institute technical review on acute pancreatitis. *Gastroenterology*. 2007;132(5):2022–2044.
- Tenner S, Baillie J, DeWitt J, et al. American College of Gastroenterology guideline: management of acute pancreatitis. *Am J Gastroenterol*. 2013;108(9):1400–1415.

CODES

ICD10

- K85.9 Acute pancreatitis, unspecified
- K86.1 Other chronic pancreatitis
- K85.8 Other acute pancreatitis

PANHYPOPITUITARISM

Craig A. Alter • Stacy E. Dodt

BASICS

DESCRIPTION

Technically, "panhypopituitarism" (*pan* meaning "all") requires deficiency of all 8 pituitary hormones; however, the term generally is used for deficiencies of >1 pituitary hormone.

EPIDEMIOLOGY

- Congenital forms affect both sexes equally and are diagnosed early in childhood.
- The epidemiology of acquired or secondary forms depends on the underlying cause.

RISK FACTORS

Genetics

Most cases are not thought to be genetic; however, there are rare autosomal recessive, autosomal dominant, and X-linked forms.

PATHOPHYSIOLOGY

- Pathology is based on specific deficiency or deficiencies.
- Growth hormone (GH): hypoglycemia in newborns and poor growth in patients older than 6–12 months
- Adrenocorticotropic hormone: hypocortisolism
- Thyroid-stimulating hormone (TSH): hypothyroidism
- Luteinizing hormone (LH)/follicle-stimulating hormone (FSH): hypogonadism
- Antidiuretic hormone: diabetes insipidus
- Prolactin: Hyperprolactinemia can accompany hypothalamic causes of hypopituitarism.

ETIOLOGY

- Idiopathic (some may be due to hypophysitis, [inflammation of the pituitary gland])
- Congenital
  - Absence of the pituitary (empty sella syndrome is a risk)
  - Pituitary malformations (ectopic posterior pituitary, hypoplastic infundibular stalk, hypoplastic pituitary)
  - Genetic disorders due to mutations in genes or transcription factors (*POUF1, HESX1, LHX3, LHX4, OTX2, SOX2, SOX3, PTX2, PROP1*, etc.)
  - Familial panhypopituitarism
  - Rathke cleft cyst
- Acquired
  - Birth trauma or perinatal insult
  - Surgical resection of the gland or damage to the stalk
  - Traumatic brain injury
  - Hypophysitis
  - Iron deposition secondary to chronic transfusion therapy (e.g., β-thalassemia)
- Infection
  - Viral encephalitis
  - Bacterial or fungal infection
  - Tuberculosis
- Vascular
  - Pituitary infarction
  - Pituitary aneurysm
- Cranial irradiation
- Tumors:
  - Craniopharyngioma
  - Germinoma
  - Glioma
  - Pinealoma
  - Primitive neuroectodermal tumor (medulloblastoma)
- Histiocytosis
- Sarcoidosis

COMMONLY ASSOCIATED CONDITIONS

- Midline defects such as cleft lip/palate, hypotelorism, single central maxillary incisor
- Septo-optic dysplasia (de Morsier syndrome)
- Holoprosencephaly

DIAGNOSIS

HISTORY

- Birth history
  - Infants with hypopituitarism are usually normal or small for gestational age, in contrast to hyperinsulinemic infants, who are typically large for gestational age.
  - Documented or symptoms of hypoglycemia, which include poor feeding, lethargy, irritability, or seizures
  - Prolonged hyperbilirubinemia: may be first sign of hypothyroidism and/or hypopituitarism
- Complications during pregnancy or delivery:
  - Birth trauma may be associated with pituitary injury.
  - Breech delivery or vacuum extraction has been associated.
- History of surgeries and previous diseases: Congenital hypopituitarism is often associated with midline facial defects, such as a single central incisor, bifid uvula, or cleft palate, which require repair.
- Growth pattern: Plot previous lengths/heights and look for growth pattern. GH deficiency usually manifests as poor linear growth by the end of the 1st year of life.
- Delayed puberty
  - Children with delayed puberty show further growth failure in adolescence.
  - Sense of smell should be assessed to rule out Kallmann syndrome (isolated central hypogonadism and anosmia).
- Increased thirst and urination: Children with hypothalamic disorders may present with symptoms of diabetes insipidus.
- Complaints of headache and/or a visual defect: can be symptoms of a brain tumor. Focal neurologic symptoms are highly suggestive of CNS pathology.

PHYSICAL EXAM

- Height and weight
  - Patients with panhypopituitarism have normal to small size in the newborn period.
  - May have poor linear growth after 6–12 months of life
- Micropenis in male newborns: Neonatal penis should be ≥2.5 cm in length; micropenis suggests gonadotropin and/or GH deficiency.
- Delayed puberty if no breast development by 13 years of age in girls, and no testicular enlargement by 14 years of age in boys.
- May have other anatomic midline defects
- Physical exam pearls:
  - Penile and testicular size: Measure stretched phallic length (from pubic ramus to glans) with patient lying supine and phallus at 90 degrees to the body; use Prader beads to assess testicular volume.
  - Midline defects: Palpate for submucosal cleft palate and look for single central incisor.
  - Visual field testing: Visual field defects suggest a brain tumor.

DIAGNOSTIC TESTS & INTERPRETATION

Lab

- Liver function tests (LFTs): LFTs in newborns with congenital hypopituitarism are often elevated and accompanied by conjugated hyperbilirubinemia, as opposed to simple congenital hypothyroidism, in which unconjugated hyperbilirubinemia exists.
- Thyroid function tests: Total and free T_4 will be low, but TSH may be low, normal, or elevated.
- Serum insulin-like growth factor-1 (IGF-1) and insulin-like growth factor–binding protein-3 (IGFBP-3): may be low, but normal growth factors do not exclude GH deficiency in children with brain tumors. IGF-1 may be low due to poor nutrition.
- GH stimulation tests: should be performed by a pediatric endocrinologist
- Basal serum cortisol: Draw at 8 a.m. in children with a normal diurnal rhythm.
- Cortrosyn stimulation test: more helpful in the diagnosis of primary adrenal insufficiency than secondary (adrenocorticotropic hormone) or tertiary (corticotropin-releasing hormone) deficiency
- Metyrapone or corticotropin-releasing hormone stimulation test
  - Tests for adrenocorticotropic hormone or corticotropin-releasing hormone deficiency
  - Must be performed by a pediatric endocrinologist
- Estradiol, testosterone, ultrasensitive LH and FSH: Measure concentrations in first 6 months of life and again after age 11 years. Best measured in the morning
- Water deprivation test
  - Definitive test for antidiuretic hormone deficiency (diabetes insipidus)
  - Should be performed by a pediatric endocrinologist
- Comments on testing:
  - Measurement of water intake and urine output over 24 hours at home can help diagnosis of diabetes insipidus.
  - Baseline serum tests (prolactin, 8-a.m. cortisol, T_4, free T_4, IGF-1, IGFBP-3, serum and urine osmolality, testosterone, estradiol, ultrasensitive LH and FSH) can all be done in a nonfasting state.
  - Stimulation tests must be performed by a pediatric endocrinologist.

Imaging

- Bone age: typically significantly delayed in GH deficiency and/or hypothyroidism
- MRI with contrast of brain with fine cuts through the hypothalamus and pituitary
  - Look for tumors, but also size of pituitary, infundibulum, and presence of normal "bright spot" in posterior pituitary.
  - Absence of the "bright spot" is highly associated with central diabetes insipidus of any etiology, although can be present in normal infants.
  - Ectopic pituitary consistent with GH deficiency and other anterior pituitary deficiencies.

ALERT

- If adrenocorticotropic hormone deficient, stress dosing of glucocorticoids is necessary.
- Replacing thyroid hormone in a child with untreated adrenal insufficiency can precipitate adrenal crisis.
- A patient with diabetes insipidus who does not have an intact thirst mechanism and access to free water is at high risk for acute hypernatremia.

DIFFERENTIAL DIAGNOSIS

- Hyperinsulinism (HI) in newborns
- Isolated hormone deficiency, such as GH deficiency in newborns
- Constitutional growth delay

TREATMENT

MEDICATION

- Recombinant human GH (rhGH) by SC injection daily: 0.15–0.3 mg/kg/week
- Desmopressin acetate (DDAVP): available in oral and intranasal formulations. Rarely given subcutaneously. Dose is variable.
  - Acute hypernatremia may be managed with DDAVP, IV vasopressin, or fluids alone.
  - Some infants with diabetes insipidus can be managed initially with thiazide diuretics.
- Estrogen/testosterone: started at puberty at low doses and slowly increased over ~2 years to mimic endogenous secretion of sex steroids
  - Infants with micropenis may be given monthly testosterone for 3 doses to aid penile enlargement.
- Estrogen given as topical or oral forms to girls, whereas testosterone initially given as injection to boys every month
- Levothyroxine PO: 25–200 mcg daily, based on weight, age, and free T_4 levels
- TSH levels may not be useful in monitoring therapy for central hypothyroidism, even after treatment is initiated.
- Hydrocortisone
  - Replacement doses if needed: 8–15 mg/m^2/24 h PO, divided b.i.d. or t.i.d.
  - In stress circumstances such as fever, severe illness, vomiting, or surgery, doses increased to 50–100 mg/m^2/24 h PO.
  - If dosed IV, provide a loading dose of 50–100 mg/m^2 IM or IV followed by 50–100 mg/m^2/24 h divided q4h; oral stress doses should be divided q8h.
  - To calculate hydrocortisone dose, estimate body surface area (BSA) using a nomogram or the following formula: BSA (m^2) = square root of (height [cm] × weight [kg]/3,600).
- Duration: long-term therapy: monitored by a pediatric endocrinologist
  - rhGH: in children and adolescents: until growth velocity drops to 2.5 cm/year; puberty is complete.
  - GH-deficient adults may benefit from lifelong rhGH because of the GH impact on body composition, lipid profile, and cardiac function.
  - Patient should again undergo GH provocative testing of rhGH therapy to determine if adult treatment is necessary.
  - DDAVP: for life, as needed to control symptoms of polyuria/polydipsia
  - Sex steroids: Begin around age 12 years; may be continued for lifetime
  - Levothyroxine for life
  - Hydrocortisone: replacement dose based on individual's need; stress dose coverage for life

ONGOING CARE

FOLLOW-UP RECOMMENDATIONS

- Initially, every 3 months by a pediatric endocrinologist
- When pituitary hormones are replaced, expect the following:
  - GH: immediate resolution of hypoglycemia; and improved growth velocity within 3–6 months
  - T_4 levels should normalize within 4–6 weeks.
  - Side effects of GH therapy: headache, vision problems, seizures, changes in activity level, limp, knee or hip pain

PROGNOSIS

- For congenital forms, the prognosis is excellent with endocrine replacement.
- Diabetes insipidus in infants can be challenging to manage.
- For secondary forms, the overall prognosis depends on the primary disease.

COMPLICATIONS

- Hypoglycemia in the newborn period
- Short stature
- Adrenal crisis
- Dehydration/hypernatremia

ALERT

- rhGH therapy can be associated with idiopathic intracranial hypertension (pseudotumor cerebri).
- rhGH deficiency/therapy can also be associated with slipped capital femoral epiphysis (SCFE). Carefully evaluate any limp or knee, or hip pain in patients on rhGH therapy. SCFE mandates orthopedic consultation.
- Diagnosis of panhypopituitarism must be considered in patients with hypoglycemic seizures.
- The family and the patient must understand the importance of taking stress doses of steroid appropriately (e.g., with surgery, vomiting, or febrile illnesses).
- 20% of normal children will fail a single GH provocative test.
- TSH levels are generally not helpful when evaluating pituitary/hypothalamic causes of hypothyroidism. The unbound free T_4 level (by equilibrium dialysis) is the most useful test both to establish the diagnosis and to monitor L-thyroxine replacement therapy.

ADDITIONAL READING

- Ascoli P, Cavagnini. Hypopituitarism. *Pituitary*. 2006;9(4):335–342.
- Di Iorgi N, Napoli F, Maghnie M, et al. Diabetes insipidus—diagnosis and management. *Horm Res Paediatr*. 2012;77(2):69–84.
- Grossman, AB. Clinical review: the diagnosis and management of central hypoadrenalism. *J Clin Endocrinol Metab*. 2012;95(11):4855–4863.
- Jenkins PJ, Mukherjee A, Shalet SM. Does growth hormone cause cancer? *Clin Endocrinol*. 2006;64(2):115–121.
- Nandagopal R, Laverdiere C, Meacham L, et al. Endocrine late effects of childhood cancer therapy: a report from the children's oncology group. *Horm Res*. 2008;69(2):65–74.

CODES

ICD10

E23.0 Hypopituitarism

FAQ

- Q: When do I give stress doses of steroid, and for how long?
- A: Whenever the patient has fever, vomiting, serious illness, or surgery. Continue until 24 hours after stress resolves (e.g., the day after fever breaks or vomiting stops).
- Q: Is it acceptable to replace thyroid hormone while the evaluation of other pituitary hormones is pending?
- A: You must ensure the patient is adrenally sufficient; if not, glucocorticoids must be initiated prior to thyroid hormone replacement.
- Q: Do all state newborn screens detect central hypothyroidism?
- A: No. Many states initially screen for elevated TSH levels.

PARVOVIRUS B19 (ERYTHEMA INFECTIOSUM, FIFTH DISEASE)

Julia Shaklee Sammons

BASICS

DESCRIPTION

Parvovirus B19 (B19) is a small, single-stranded DNA virus of the family *Parvoviridae*. There are three major genetic variants (1–3). B19 is a common infection in humans, most often associated with the childhood exanthem, erythema infectiosum, or fifth disease.

EPIDEMIOLOGY

- B19 infections are ubiquitous worldwide, occurring most often in school-aged children.
- Humans are the only hosts.
- Incubation period is 4–14 days but can be as long as 21 days.
- Modes of transmission
  - Contact with respiratory secretions
  - Percutaneous exposure to blood or blood products (1,011 virions/mm of serum in patients with hereditary hemolytic anemias)
  - Vertical transmission from mother to fetus

Incidence

Attack rates: 15–60% of susceptibles (i.e., seronegative) will become infected upon exposure.

Prevalence

- Seroprevalence of B19 IgG antibodies
  - >5 years old: 2–9%
  - 5–18 years old: 15–35%
  - Adults: 30–60%
  - Elderly: 90%

GENERAL PREVENTION

- B19 transmission can be decreased through routine infection control practices, including hand hygiene and appropriate disposal of contaminated facial tissues.
- For hospitalized children with suspected aplastic crisis, immunocompromised patients with chronic infection and anemia, and patients with papular purpuric gloves and socks syndrome secondary to B19, droplet precautions in addition to standard precautions are recommended.
- No additional preventive measures are needed for normal hosts with rash.
- Due to the potential risks to the fetus from B19 infections, pregnant health care workers should adhere to strict infection control procedures and avoid contact with immunocompromised hosts with B19 infection or those with aplastic crisis.
- Due to high prevalence of B19 in the community, routine exclusion of pregnant women from the workplace where B19 infections are suspected (e.g., schools, day care) is not recommended.

PATHOPHYSIOLOGY

- Parvovirus B19 inhibits erythropoiesis by lytically infecting RBC precursors in the bone marrow.
- It is associated with a number of clinical manifestations, ranging from benign to severe.

COMMONLY ASSOCIATED CONDITIONS

- Erythema infectiosum, or fifth disease, is the most common form of infection caused by B19 and occurs in up to 35% of school-aged children.
- Asymptomatic infection may occur in ~20% of children and adults.
- Transient aplastic crisis secondary to B19 infection may cause severe anemia in patients with hereditary hemolytic anemias or any condition that shortens the RBC lifespan, such as sickle cell disease or spherocytosis.
- Polyarthropathy syndrome (symmetric joint pain and swelling, typically of the hands, knees, and feet) is seen in up to 80% of adults, especially women. Arthralgias and arthritis occur infrequently in children. When present, arthritis in children most often involves the knees.
- Hydrops fetalis may develop after maternal B19 infection with intrauterine involvement (typically within the first 20 weeks of pregnancy).
- Chronic anemia/pure red cell aplasia due to persistent B19 infection has been reported in immunocompromised patients.
- Papular purpuric gloves and socks syndrome (PPGSS) consists of painful and pruritic papules, petechiae, and purpura localized to the hands and feet and is often associated with fever.
- B19 is one of the most common viruses identified in cases of myocarditis, although its role in pathogenesis is unclear.
- Reports of neurologic manifestations (including meningitis, encephalitis, and peripheral neuropathy), hemophagocytic syndrome, hepatitis, and Henoch-Schönlein purpura have also been associated with B19 infection.

DIAGNOSIS

Diagnosis depends on recognition of typical symptoms and the results of laboratory testing.

HISTORY

- Erythema infectiosum (fifth disease)
  - Characterized by an erythematous facial rash with a distinctive "slapped cheek" appearance, often accompanied by circumoral pallor
  - A symmetric, macular, often lace-like rash occurs on the trunk, spreading outward to the rest of the body and extremities. The rash is often pruritic and may intensify with exposure to sunlight, heat, or exercise. It occasionally involves the palms and soles. Rarely, the rash can be papular, vesicular, or purpuric. It may last for ~7 days, but can persist >20 days.
  - A brief, mild prodrome of systemic symptoms, including headache, sore throat, myalgias, and low-grade fevers, often precedes the appearance of rash by 7–10 days.
  - The child is usually well-appearing and remains active and playful.
- Aplastic crisis
  - Prodromal symptoms in B19-infected children with sickle cell disease or other hereditary hemolytic anemias are nonspecific and consist of fever, malaise, and headache. Rash is usually absent.
  - Symptoms are usually self-limited, lasting 7–10 days.
  - Severe anemia, CHF, stroke, and acute splenic sequestration have also been associated.
- Chronic anemia/pure red cell aplasia
  - In immunocompromised patients, B19 infection may persist for months, leading to chronic anemia with B19 viremia.
  - Low-grade fever and neutropenia may accompany anemia.

PHYSICAL EXAM

Fifth disease

- An erythematous facial rash with a "slapped cheek" appearance, often associated with circumoral pallor
- Truncal, macular, lacy-appearing rash spreading to the arms, buttocks, and thighs
  - Often pruritic and may become more intense with exercise or heat exposure
- Occasionally can be found on the palms and soles, and rarely can be papular, vesicular, or purpuric

DIAGNOSTIC TESTS & INTERPRETATION

Lab

- There is no practical in vitro system for isolation or culture of the virus.
- Antibodies
  - Detection of parvovirus B19-specific IgM or IgG antibodies as determined by EIA or radioimmunoassay
  - The presence of B19-specific IgM antibodies is diagnostic in patients with symptoms of erythema infectiosum or aplastic crisis. IgM- and IgG-specific antibodies are detected in 90% of such patients by 3–7 days of illness.
  - B19-specific IgG antibodies persist for life, whereas specific IgM antibodies begin to decrease 30–60 days after onset of illness.
- Polymerase chain reaction (PCR) techniques
  - B19 DNA can be detected by PCR in serum for up to 9 months following the initial viremic phase. B19 DNA has also been shown to persist in solid tissues following primary infection, even in healthy individuals. Thus, identification of B19 DNA does not necessarily signify acute infection.
  - Immunocompromised patients with chronic marrow suppression may be unable to produce B19-specific IgG or IgM antibodies. In such cases, PCR for B19 viral DNA is the diagnostic method of choice.
  - PCR may also be used to detect virus in the fetus.
- Hematocrit and reticulocyte count in patients with aplastic crisis
  - Laboratory studies reveal reticulocytopenia, usually with counts of <1%. During the illness, the patient's hematocrit may fall as low as 15%.

DIFFERENTIAL DIAGNOSIS

B19 infection should be considered in all patients with arthritis or viral exanthems with a consistent history and exam.

TREATMENT

GENERAL MEASURES

- There is no specific antiviral therapy for B19 infection.
- Most patients require supportive care only. However, transfusions may be required for treatment of severe anemia in patients with aplastic crisis.
- IV immunoglobulin (IVIG) therapy has been given with some success to patients with chronic marrow suppression secondary to B19 infection.
- The mainstay of treatment for an infected fetus is delivery, but intrauterine transfusions may be lifesaving.

ONGOING CARE

FOLLOW-UP RECOMMENDATIONS

Expected course of illness

- The rash of erythema infectiosum in a child or adult may last up to 20 days. It may, at times, fade and/or intensify, depending on sunlight exposure, exercise, or body surface temperature changes (e.g., bathing).
- During aplastic crisis secondary to B19, the reticulocyte count usually remains low (often <1%) for ~8 days before spontaneous recovery.

PROGNOSIS

- The prognosis is quite good for all manifestations of B19 infections.
- Most patients recover spontaneously and require only supportive care.

COMPLICATIONS

- Parvovirus B19 during pregnancy
  - 30–50% of pregnant women are susceptible to B19 infection.
  - Fetal loss, intrauterine growth retardation, or hydrops fetalis may result from maternal infection with B19 during pregnancy. Fetal death occurs in 2–6% of cases.
  - B19 has not been proven to cause congenital anomalies.
  - The greatest risk for B19 infection affecting the fetus exists in the first 20 weeks of gestation.
  - The risk of fetal death after exposure, if antibody status is unknown, is <1.5%.
  - There is no indication for elective abortion in cases of maternal infection.
- Arthritis/arthropathy
  - Although most cases of polyarthritis resolve within 2 weeks, persistent symptoms for months to even years (rarely) have been reported.

ADDITIONAL READING

- Douvoyiannis M, Litman N, Goldman DL. Neurologic manifestations associated with parvovirus B19 infection. *Clin Infect Dis*. 2009;48(12):1713–1723.
- Molina KM, Garcia X, Denfield SW, et al. Parvovirus B19 myocarditis causes significant morbidity and mortality in children. *Pediatr Cardiol*. 2013;34(2):390–397.
- Lamont RF, Sobel JD, Vaisbuch E, et al. Parvovirus B19 infection in human pregnancy. *BJOG*. 2011;118(2):175–186.
- Smith-Whitley K, Zhao H, Hodinka RL, et al. Epidemiology of human parvovirus B19 in children with sickle cell disease. *Blood*. 2004;103(2):422–427.
- Young NS, Brown KE. Parvovirus B19. *N Engl J Med*. 2004;350(6):586–597.

CODES

ICD10

B08.3 Erythema infectiosum [fifth disease]

FAQ

- Q: When may children with B19 infection return to school?
- A: Children are contagious only during the prodromal phase of illness, which is often unrecognized. Once the rash appears, they are no longer infectious and may return to school or day care.
- Q: What can be done to reduce risk of fetal infection?
- A: Because B19 infections during pregnancy may result in fetal death, and B19 infections often occur in community outbreaks, fetal risks following maternal exposure to persons with recognized B19 infection are a frequent concern. Risk to the fetus appears to be greatest if the infection occurs prior to the 20th week of gestation. Among pregnant women of unknown antibody status, the risk of fetal death after exposure to B19 is estimated to be <1.5%. Routine exclusion of pregnant women from the workplace when B19 infection is suspected is not recommended. However, pregnant teachers who are at risk for infection may consider a leave of absence during community outbreaks of B19.

PATENT DUCTUS ARTERIOSUS

Alexander Lowenthal

BASICS

DESCRIPTION

- Patent ductus arteriosus (PDA) is the persistence into postnatal life of the normal fetal vascular conduit between the central pulmonary and systemic arterial systems. Normally, the ductus arteriosus (DA) functionally closes within the first 1–3 days of life. Structural closure is usually completed by the 3rd week of life. If the DA remains patent beyond 3 months of life, it is considered abnormal and is unlikely to close spontaneously (spontaneous closure rate 0.6% per year).
- In the infant with a normal left aortic arch, the DA connects the main pulmonary artery (MPA) at the origin of the left pulmonary artery to the descending aorta, distal to the origin of the left subclavian artery.
- Many variations can occur, although they are less common. The main, proximal right, or proximal left pulmonary artery may be connected to virtually any location on the aortic arch or proximal portions of the brachiocephalic vessels.
- 5 distinct clinical conditions are associated with PDA:
  - Isolated cardiovascular lesion in premature infants
  - Isolated cardiovascular lesion in otherwise healthy term infants and children
  - Incidental finding associated with more significant structural cardiovascular defects
  - Compensatory structure in cases of neonatal pulmonary hypertension without congenital heart disease (CHD)
  - Critical compensatory structure in some cyanotic or left-sided obstructed lesions

EPIDEMIOLOGY

- As an isolated defect, PDA is the 6th most common congenital cardiovascular lesion.
  - Represents 5% of all types of CHD
  - 1 per 2,000 live births
  - If "silent" PDA are included, the rate may be as high as 1:500 live births.
- Female-to-male ratio: 2:1

RISK FACTORS

- Prematurity
  - Increases with the degree of prematurity (50–80% in preterm infants <26 weeks' gestation)
  - 60–70% of preterm infants of <28 weeks' gestation receive medical or surgical therapy for a PDA.
- Incidence of PDA varies significantly depending on environmental factors (altitude), management style (e.g., amount of maintenance fluid prescribed, surfactant administration), and presence of coexisting diseases (e.g., respiratory distress syndrome, hypoxemia, fluid overload, necrotizing enterocolitis, sepsis, hypocalcemia).
- Higher rate of PDA in babies with trisomy 21, Wolf-Hirschhorn syndrome (4p deletion), Char syndrome, Carpenter syndrome, Holt-Oram syndrome, and incontinentia pigmenti

PATHOPHYSIOLOGY

- The PDA is derived from the distal portion of the left 6th embryonic arch, connecting the left pulmonary artery to the descending aorta.
  - The PDA is formed by the 8th week of fetal life.
  - It is necessary for fetal circulation throughout the remainder of gestation.
- Fetal blood flows from the MPA to the DA to the aorta, thus bypassing the pulmonary vascular bed and supplying systemic blood flow. With the 1st postnatal breaths, the pulmonary vascular resistance falls abruptly, the DA constricts, and pulmonary blood flow is directed into the lungs.
- With a PDA, excessive blood flow will continue from the aorta into the pulmonary artery, causing increased pulmonary blood flow and volume overloading of the left side of the heart.
- In premature infants and term infants with pulmonary hypertension, delayed closure represents an impaired developmental process, whereas in the healthy full-term infant, PDA probably reflects an anatomic abnormality of the ductal tissue.

ETIOLOGY

- Prematurity
- Rubella infection in the 1st trimester
- Genetic or familial factors
- High altitude
- Idiopathic

DIAGNOSIS

HISTORY

- Premature infants
  - Variable: ranging from asymptomatic to complete cardiovascular collapse
  - Increased ventilatory support, pulmonary hemorrhage, respiratory or metabolic acidosis from low cardiac output, and excessive pulmonary blood flow
  - Tachypnea, feeding intolerance, apnea, bradycardia, necrotizing enterocolitis, and decreased urine output
- Infants and older children
  - Small PDA: usually asymptomatic, with incidental heart murmur found on routine exam
  - Moderate PDA: possible congestive heart failure (CHF), poor feeding, and poor weight gain
  - Large PDA: symptoms as above and recurrent respiratory infections

PHYSICAL EXAM

- Premature infants
  - Tachypnea, rales, tachycardia ($\pm S_3$ gallop)
  - Hyperdynamic precordium and bounding pulses with wide pulse pressure (due to diastolic "runoff" from the aorta to the pulmonary artery)
  - The typical PDA murmur in a premature infant is a pansystolic murmur audible at the left upper or midsternal border.
  - With a large PDA and equalization of pressure between the MPA and the aorta, no murmur may be heard.
  - Hepatomegaly may exist with heart failure (late sign).
- Infants and older children: Findings vary with size of shunt.
  - Small PDA
    - Pansystolic murmur may be heard at the 2nd left intercostal space.
    - Murmur becomes continuous (i.e., extends into diastole), as the pulmonary vascular resistance decreases over the 1st months of life.
  - Moderate or large PDA
    - The murmur is louder, has a harsh quality, and acquires a machine-like quality often being heard posteriorly. In that case, a systolic thrill may be felt at the left upper sternal border.
    - Tachycardia, bounding pulses with a wide pulse pressure, and a mid-diastolic low-frequency rumbling murmur may be audible at the apex with a large PDA.
    - With severe left ventricular failure the classic PDA signs may disappear, but there will be findings consistent with CHF (tachycardia, S_3 gallop at the apex, hepatomegaly, tachypnea, rales).
    - In extreme cases, pulmonary hypertension may occur, with the murmur shortening, the diastolic component disappearing, and S_2 becoming accentuated. At advanced stages of irreversible pulmonary vascular disease, cyanosis begins to appear, often more pronounced in the lower limbs, with reversal of shunting.

P

DIAGNOSTIC TESTS & INTERPRETATION

Imaging

- ECG
  - Usually normal with a small PDA
  - Left atrial enlargement and left ventricular hypertrophy with moderate and large PDA
  - Biventricular hypertrophy in later stages
- Chest x-ray
  - Usually normal with a small PDA, although prominence of main and peripheral pulmonary arteries may be seen
  - In moderate and large PDAs, these findings become more pronounced, along with an enlarged heart. Increased pulmonary vascular markings are proportionate to the left-to-right shunt. Pulmonary edema can be seen if CHF develops. In premature infants with respiratory distress syndrome, there is evidence of deteriorating lung disease with unclear cardiac borders.
- Echocardiogram
  - Delineates the PDA and assesses the size of the left atrium and the left ventricle
  - Doppler techniques assess the ductal flow pattern and may be useful for estimating the pulmonary artery pressure.
- Cardiac catheterization
  - Most often not essential for diagnosis
  - Indicated for suspected concomitant pulmonary hypertension
  - Can be performed for treatment via transcatheter closure techniques

DIFFERENTIAL DIAGNOSIS

- Aortopulmonary window
- Systemic or pulmonary arteriovenous communications
- Ruptured sinus of Valsalva
- Coronary artery fistula
- Truncus arteriosus
- Aortic insufficiency
- Innocent venous hum in older children
- Pulmonary atresia with collaterals
- Ventricular septal defect with aortic regurgitation
- Ventricular septal defect in infancy

TREATMENT

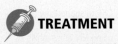

GENERAL MEASURES

- Premature infant
  - Supportive treatment (careful use of oxygen, respiratory assistance, correction of metabolic acidosis)
  - Management of CHF with fluid restriction and diuretics
  - If PDA persists or patient is symptomatic, closure of PDA is indicated.
  - Medical closure: Indomethacin is most often used; ibuprofen is as effective.
    - Contraindications to medical management include renal failure (creatinine $>$1.8 mg/dL), thrombocytopenia (platelets $<$100,000), and associated conditions (necrotizing enterocolitis, intraventricular hemorrhage).
  - Surgical closure is indicated if medical treatment fails or use of indomethacin is contraindicated.
- Infants and older children
  - Medical management of CHF with digoxin, diuretics, and afterload reduction
  - PDA is no longer a stated indication for subacute bacterial endocarditis (SBE) prophylaxis, but clinical practice may vary.
  - Spontaneous closure rate is low, and closure with indomethacin is not usually effective in this group of patients.
  - Closure is indicated whenever a symptomatic or hemodynamically significant PDA exists.
  - For asymptomatic audible PDA, closure can be performed electively and is primarily performed to reduce the risk of endocarditis. Recommendations for closure of an asymptomatic, incidentally found ("silent" ductus) PDA are not standard.
  - Most infants and children can have a PDA safely and effectively closed during cardiac catheterization, obviating the need for a surgical procedure.

SURGERY/OTHER PROCEDURES

Surgical closure of PDA can be achieved by 1 of 3 techniques:

- Open surgical ligation and division: mostly in premature infants
- Video-assisted thoracoscopic ligation: depends on the institution
- Transcatheter occlusion with coils or other devices

ONGOING CARE

PROGNOSIS

- Outcome in treated premature infants is generally good but depends mostly on the degree of prematurity and the presence of associated conditions.
- Outcome in term infants and older children is excellent if no complications have occurred.
- PDA among adults may be associated with significant mortality with or without surgery.
- After closure of PDA, no endocarditis prophylaxis is needed if complete obliteration of flow is achieved. Most cardiologists continue prophylaxis for 6 months after the procedure that closed the PDA if closed by a coil or device.

COMPLICATIONS

- Pulmonary edema and CHF
- Pulmonary hemorrhage
- Pulmonary vascular obstructive disease
- Increased chronic lung disease
- Failure to thrive
- Recurrent respiratory infections
- Lobar emphysema or collapse
- Infective endarteritis
- Thromboembolism of cerebral arteries
- Aneurysm of the ductus
- Intracranial hemorrhage
- Necrotizing enterocolitis
- Renal dysfunction

ADDITIONAL READING

- Anilkumar M. Patent ductus arteriosus. *Cardiol Clin*. 2013;31(3):417–430.
- Clyman RI, Chorne N. Patent ductus arteriosus: evidence for and against treatment. *J Pediatr*. 2007;150(3):216–219.
- Clyman RI, Couto J, Murphy GM. Patent ductus arteriosus: are current neonatal treatment options better or worse than no treatment at all? *Semin Perinatol*. 2012;36(2):123–129.
- Evans N. Current controversies in the diagnosis and treatment of patent ductus arteriosus in preterm infants. *Adv Neonatal Care*. 2003;3(4):168–177.
- Hamrick SE, Hansmann G. Patent ductus arteriosus of the preterm infant. *Pediatrics*. 2010;125(5): 1020–1030.
- Noori S. Pros and cons of patent ductus arteriosus ligation: hemodynamic changes and other morbidities after patent ductus arteriosus ligation. *Semin Perinatol*. 2012;36(2):139–145.
- Ohlsson A, Walia R, Shah SS. Ibuprofen for the treatment of patent ductus arteriosus in preterm and/or low birth weight infants. *Cochrane Database Syst Rev*. 2013;4:CD003481. doi:10.1002/14651858. CD003481.pub5
- Schneider DJ. The patent ductus arteriosus in term infants, children, and adults. *Semin Perinatol*. 2012;36(2):146–153.
- Takami T, Yoda H, Kawakami T, et al. Usefulness of indomethacin for patent ductus arteriosus in full-term infants. *Pediatr Cardiol*. 2007;28(1):46–50.

CODES

ICD10

Q25.0 Patent ductus arteriosus

PELVIC INFLAMMATORY DISEASE

Krishna K. Upadhya • Maria E. Trent

BASICS

DESCRIPTION
- Pelvic inflammatory disease (PID) refers to a spectrum of upper female genital tract inflammatory disorders, including endometritis, salpingitis, tubo-ovarian abscess (TOA), and peritonitis.
- Definitive diagnosis of PID can be made by laparoscopy; however, diagnosis is usually made based on clinical findings.
- Centers for Disease Control (CDC) guidelines state that empiric PID therapy should be initiated in sexually active young women with pelvic or lower abdominal pain, if no other cause for the illness can be identified and the patient has the following:
  - Uterine tenderness, *OR*
  - Adnexal tenderness, *OR*
  - Cervical motion tenderness
- Additional criteria enhance the specificity of the diagnosis of PID, but are not required for the diagnosis:
  - Oral temperature >38.3°C (101°F)
  - Abnormal cervical or vaginal discharge
  - Abundant WBCs on a wet mount of vaginal secretions
  - Elevated ESR or CRP
  - Laboratory-documented evidence of infection with *Neisseria gonorrhoeae* or *Chlamydia trachomatis*
- Definitive diagnostic criteria:
  - Histopathologic evidence of endometritis on endometrial biopsy
  - Transvaginal sonography or MRI showing thickened fluid-filled tubes with or without free pelvic fluid or TOA
  - Laparoscopic abnormalities consistent with PID

EPIDEMIOLOGY
- There are an estimated 750,000 cases of PID annually in the United States.
- In 2011, there were 90,000 initial visits to physician offices for PID:
  - Visits for PID declined between 2002 and 2011.
  - Increased screening and treatment of chlamydia likely led to this decline.
- Cases of PID are disproportionately higher among adolescent girls and racial minorities

RISK FACTORS
- Factors that increase PID risk include the following:
  - Multiple sexual partners
  - Intercourse with a partner who has multiple sexual partners
  - Prior history of sexually transmitted infection (STI) or PID
  - Intercourse without condoms
  - Douching
  - Recent (within past 20 days) insertion of intrauterine device (IUD)
- Cases of PID are highest among the following:
  - Sexually active adolescents and young women younger than age 25 years
  - Women in communities with high prevalence of gonorrhea and chlamydia
  - Patients presenting to STD clinics

GENERAL PREVENTION
- Consistent condom use
- Regular STI screening
- Partner screening for STIs
- Limit number of sexual partners.
- Avoid douching.

PATHOPHYSIOLOGY
- Ascending infection spreading from vagina/cervix to upper genital tract by the following:
  - Migration
  - Sperm transport
  - Refluxed menstrual blood flow
- Up to 75% of cases occur within 7 days of menses.

ETIOLOGY
- Polymicrobial origin
- Many cases are associated with *N. gonorrhoeae* (GC) and *C. trachomatis* (CT).
- *Mycoplasma genitalium* and *Ureaplasma urealyticum* have been associated with laparoscopic PID and infertility.
- Other vaginal, enteric, and respiratory flora associated with PID include the following:
  - *Gardnerella vaginalis*, *Escherichia coli*, *Bacteroides* species, *Haemophilus influenzae*, group B–D streptococci, *Streptococcus pneumoniae*, and group A *Streptococcus*.

DIAGNOSIS

ALERT
- Clinical criteria for PID are designed to have high sensitivity because the consequences for untreated PID are significant.
- If PID is suspected based on clinical presentation and examination, treatment should be initiated prior to results of other supportive testing.

HISTORY
- Should be taken from the patient in a private interview:
  - Confidentiality policies should be reviewed with the patient in advance of history.
- Abdominal or pelvic pain is a common presenting complaint:
  - "Classic" presentation of shuffling gait or "chandelier sign" is rare.
- Some cases may be mild with relatively few symptoms:
  - Subclinical or "silent" PID can result in infertility and chronic pelvic pain.
- Other presenting symptoms may include the following:
  - Vaginal discharge
  - Abnormal vaginal bleeding
  - Dyspareunia
  - Dysuria
  - Right upper quadrant pain
- Complete history should be taken including past medical, gynecologic, gastrointestinal, and urinary history
- Sexual history should be elicited in a sensitive manner; and should include number of partners, new partners, condom use, contraceptive method use, history of sexual assault.

PHYSICAL EXAM
- Evaluate the patient for signs of general discomfort.
- Review vital signs for fever, tachycardia.
- Careful abdominal exam to evaluate for tenderness, rebound, or guarding
  - Evaluate right upper quadrant for tenderness associated with perihepatitis.
- Pelvic exam is essential to PID diagnosis and must be performed for any sexually active female with abdominal pain or genital complaints.
- External genital exam should assess for external lesions, inguinal adenopathy.
- Speculum exam should note vaginal discharge or lesions, signs of cervical friability or discharge.
  - Collect vaginal swabs for pH and wet prep.
  - Collect cervical swabs for STI testing.
  - Collect swab for Gram stain if materials and equipment available.
- Bimanual exam to evaluate for cervical motion tenderness, uterine tenderness, and adnexal tenderness or fullness.

DIAGNOSTIC TESTS & INTERPRETATION

Lab
- Urine β-hCG
- Vaginal pH (pH >4.5 is abnormal)
- Wet mount and KOH (>10 WBC/HPF is suggestive of infection)
- Nucleic acid amplification test for GC, CT, and *Trichomonas vaginalis*
  - If the patient reports sexual assault or abuse at the time of evaluation, bacterial cultures should also be obtained.
- Urinalysis and culture
- Consider collecting CBC, CRP to support the diagnosis.
- Testing for other STIs including HIV and syphilis should also be done.

Imaging
- In patients with adnexal fullness or other signs suggestive of TOA, obtain transvaginal ultrasound.
- Signs of PID on imaging include the following:
  - Thickened or fluid-filled fallopian tubes
  - Free pelvic fluid
  - Tubo-ovarian abscess

Diagnostic Procedures/Other
- Laparoscopy
- Endometrial biopsy
- These tests can provide definitive evidence of PID, but are not routinely used.

DIFFERENTIAL DIAGNOSIS

- Pelvic pain may be the presenting complaint for a variety of disease processes.
- Gynecologic
  - Ectopic pregnancy
  - Intrauterine pregnancy
  - Endometriosis
  - Hemorrhagic ovarian cyst
  - Ovarian cyst
  - Ovarian tumor
  - Ovarian torsion
  - Tubal torsion
  - Septic abortion
  - Vaginal foreign body
  - Hematometrocolpos
  - Chemical irritants
- Urinary
  - Urinary tract infection
  - Acute pyelonephritis
- Gastrointestinal
  - Acute appendicitis
  - Acute cholecystitis
- Heme/vascular
  - Pelvic thrombophlebitis
- Other:
  - Functional abdominal pain
  - Sexual assault
  - Sexual abuse

TREATMENT

ALERT

- All CDC-recommended treatment regimens for PID require 14-day treatment duration.
- Fluoroquinolones not recommended for PID treatment because of GC resistance

MEDICATION

Parenteral treatment regimens:

- Regimen A:
  - Cefotetan 2 g IV every 12 h OR cefoxitin 2 g IV every 6 h PLUS
  - Doxycycline 100 mg PO b.i.d. × 14 days
  - May add metronidazole 500 mg PO b.i.d. × 14 days for severe cases or suspected anaerobes
- Regimen B:
  - Clindamycin 900 mg IV every 8 hours PLUS
  - Gentamicin loading dose IV or IM (2 mg/kg), followed by a maintenance dose (1.5 mg/kg) every 8 hours OR
  - Gentamicin 3–5 mg/kg every 24 hours
  - After 24 hours or clinical improvement, can switch to oral doxycycline 100 mg PO b.i.d. or clindamycin 450 mg PO q.i.d. to complete 14 days of total therapy
- Alternative regimen:
  - Ampicillin/sulbactam 3 g (ampicillin) IV q6h PLUS
  - Doxycycline 100 mg PO b.i.d. × 14 days

Oral treatment regimens:

- Regimen A:
  - Ceftriaxone 250 mg IM (single dose) PLUS
  - Doxycycline 100 mg PO b.i.d. × 14 days
  - May add metronidazole 500 mg PO b.i.d. × 14 days
- Regimen B:
  - Cefoxitin 2 g IM (single dose) PLUS
  - Probenecid 1 g PO (single dose) PLUS
  - Doxycycline 100 mg PO b.i.d. × 14 days
  - May add metronidazole 500 mg PO b.i.d. × 14 days
- Alternate regimen:
  - Other parenteral 3rd-generation cephalosporin PLUS
  - Doxycycline 100 mg PO b.i.d. × 14 days
  - May add metronidazole 500 mg PO b.i.d. × 14 days

ADDITIONAL TREATMENT

General Measures

- Criteria for hospitalization:
  - Surgical emergency
  - Pregnancy
  - Lack of response to outpatient therapy
  - Inability to tolerate or follow outpatient regimen
  - Severe illness (e.g., fever, nausea/vomiting)
  - Suspected or confirmed TOA
- Strong consideration of hospitalization should be given for early and middle adolescents who may require additional supports for optimal management.
- Patients should be counseled to:
  - Abstain from intercourse for at least 14 days.
  - Notify their partners for STI testing and treatment.
  - Use condoms consistently and correctly.
  - Limit number of sexual partners.
  - Consider contraception if not currently using and not desiring pregnancy.
  - Return if worsening symptoms or not able tolerate the prescribed treatment.

ONGOING CARE

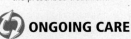

FOLLOW-UP RECOMMENDATIONS

- All patients diagnosed with PID should have follow-up within 72 hours to assess the following:
  - Treatment tolerance/adherence
  - Symptom improvement
- If patients are not improving additional evaluation may be necessary including the following:
  - Bimanual examination
  - Pelvic imaging
  - Hospitalization
- Return for repeat STI testing in 3 months.

PROGNOSIS

- Dependent on treatment adherence and number of episodes of PID
- Women with documented GC or CT infection have higher rates of reinfection within 6 months of treatment.
- Each additional episode of PID increases risk of infertility and chronic pelvic pain.

COMPLICATIONS

- Short-term
  - Perihepatitis (in 15% of patients)
  - Periappendicitis
- Long-term
  - Ectopic pregnancy
  - Infertility (10–15% of cases of PID)
  - Chronic pelvic pain

ADDITIONAL READING

- Goyal M, Hersh A, Luan X, et al. National trends in pelvic inflammatory disease among adolescents in the emergency department. *J Adolesc Health*. 2013;53(2):249–252.
- Haggerty CL, Ness RB. Newest approaches to treatment of pelvic inflammatory disease: a review of recent randomized clinical trials. *Clin Infect Dis*. 2007;44(7):953–960.
- Soper DE. Pelvic inflammatory disease. *Obstet Gynecol*. 2010;116(2, Pt 1):419–428.
- Trent M. Pelvic inflammatory disease. *Pediatr Rev*. 2013;34(4);163–172.
- Trent M, Haggerty CL, Jennings JM, et al. Adverse adolescent reproductive health outcomes after pelvic inflammatory disease. *Arch Pediatr Adolesc Med*. 2011;165(1):49–54.

CODES

ICD10

- N73.9 Female pelvic inflammatory disease, unspecified
- N71.9 Inflammatory disease of uterus, unspecified
- N70.93 Salpingitis and oophoritis, unspecified

FAQ

- Q: My patient has negative testing for GC and CT, should I have her discontinue the medications if she has clinically improved?
- A: No. PID is a polymicrobial infection and the patient's improvement is likely secondary to broad-spectrum antibiotic treatment. The patient should continue antibiotics as prescribed.
- Q: My patient has problems with adherence, could I use directly observed doses of azithromycin in the office?
- A: Although use of azithromycin is not considered a standard and/or recommended therapy by the CDC, one RCT in Brazil successfully used ceftriaxone 250 mg and azithromycin 1 g at baseline and then repeated the dose in 1 week. Although patients had good results, this has not been replicated and the CDC currently recommends that metronidazole 500 mg b.i.d. be administered with azithromycin to improve anaerobic coverage.
- Q: My patient is 6 weeks pregnant. Can she really have PID?
- A: PID is less common during pregnancy given the bactericidal protection afforded by the cervical mucous plug. However, it is possible for sperm to transport bacteria into the uterus during fertilization, infection to occur in the interim between implantation and full establishment of the mucous plug, and early loss of the mucous plug later in pregnancy. Caution should be used in caring for pregnant patients with PID because fetal wastage can occur due to infection. As such, the CDC recommends that these women be hospitalized for initial treatment.

PENILE AND FORESKIN PROBLEMS

Benjamin M. Whittam • Mark P. Cain • Richard C. Rink

BASICS

DESCRIPTION

Penile problems:

- Buried penis
  - Hidden or concealed penis, poor skin fixation at the penoscrotal/penopubic junction resulting in buried or hidden appearance
  - Buried penis may be normal in obese children with large suprapubic fat pad.
- Penile curvature (chordee)
  - Bending of the penis with erection, can be lateral, ventral (most common), or dorsal curve
  - Chordee is usually associated with abnormal foreskin
- Webbed penis
  - Penoscrotal webbing or poor separation of penile skin from scrotum, obscuring penoscrotal angle
- Balanitis
  - Inflammation of the glans
  - Probably overdiagnosed owing to physiologic drainage of smegma or urea dermatitis from failure to retract foreskin during voiding in toilet-trained boys
  - When infections present, there can be significant cellulitis of the penis, edema, and fever.
  - Most commonly caused by gram-positive organisms. Yeast is another causative organism.

Foreskin problems:

- Balanoposthitis
  - Inflammation of glans and prepuce
  - Seen in 4% of uncircumcised boys age 2–5 years
  - See balanitis.
- Phimosis/penile adhesions
  - Physiologic attachment of prepuce to glans, which it protects and gradually separates to allow retraction of the foreskin
  - Ring of fibrotic scar tissue that prevents the foreskin from being retracted
- Paraphimosis
  - When narrow prepuce is retracted behind the glans, constricting penile shaft causing glanular and foreskin edema and preventing replacement of prepuce over glans

Postcircumcision problems:

- Penile adhesions
  - Attachments of the foreskin back to the glans after circumcision
  - Penile skin bridges are dense scar adhesions that cannot be separated.
- Meatal stenosis
  - Urethral meatus narrowing
  - Significant meatal narrowing will produce an upwardly deflected urine stream, which is narrow and strong. In severe cases, straining, and prolonged voiding
- Epidermal inclusion cysts
  - Small, enlarging white lesions growing subcutaneously along the scar from circumcision

RISK FACTORS

Genetics

Epidermal inclusion cysts may occur from congenital rests of skin cells buried during development, but these are rare and occur along the median raphe of the penis or scrotum.

GENERAL PREVENTION

Some penile and foreskin problems may be prevented with proper hygiene and education of the caretakers.

ETIOLOGY

- Buried/webbed penis
  - Scrotal attachments attending along ventral penile surface to varying degrees
  - Penis tethered by abnormal attachments of dartos tissue
- Penile curvature (chordee)
  - Asymmetry in tunica albuginea of corporal bodies and compliance of corpora cavernosa
- Balanoposthitis/balanitis
  - Unclear etiology: possible infection, mechanical trauma, contact irritation, and contact allergies
- Phimosis
  - Probably results from recurrent bouts of irritation of the foreskin from improper hygiene habits such as voiding through the foreskin or repetitive forceful retraction
- Penile adhesions
  - Physiologic adhesions: The prepuce has adhered down to the glans after circumcision.
  - Surgical adhesions (skin bridges): Adherence between the scar of the circumcision and the glans due to healing of the crushed tissue where the foreskin was removed and the glans
- Meatal stenosis
  - Narrowing of the urethral meatus secondary to recurrent irritation of the meatus, likely from rubbing against moist diapers. Occurs almost exclusively in circumcised boys
- Epidermal inclusion cysts
  - Caused by small islands of epithelium buried beneath the skin surface that progressively accumulate desquamated skin cells

DIAGNOSIS

HISTORY

- Issues with newborn circumcision
- Ability to retract foreskin
- Retraction of foreskin in uncircumcised males during voiding
- Penis straight with erection
- Character of urinary stream
- Ballooning of the foreskin with voiding
- Straining to void
- Presence of fever
- Penile discharge
- In older boys, inquire about sexual activity.

PHYSICAL EXAM

- Circumcised males
  - Size and position of meatus
  - Redundancy of preputial skin
  - Presence of adhesions to the glans and whether they involve the scar line between the shaft skin and the inner preputial skin
  - Lesions or erythema of glans or shaft
  - Watch patient void if meatal stenosis is suspected, usually upward deviated stream.
- Uncircumcised males
  - Ability to retract foreskin with gentle retraction
  - Presence of phimotic ring
  - Lesions or erythema of prepuce

ALERT

- Do not try to forcefully retract the foreskin in an infant or young child. It can take 3–5 years before the foreskin can be retracted.
- Do not circumcise infants with a buried or webbed penis, asymmetric foreskin, or those with a significantly deviated penile raphe.
- Never circumcise an infant with an abnormally located meatus (hypospadias, epispadias).
- Always replace the foreskin back over the glans after retraction (for cleaning, voiding, or examination) to prevent paraphimosis.
- Paraphimosis is an emergency. The sooner it is diagnosed, the easier it is to treat and reduce without surgery.

DIAGNOSTIC TESTS & INTERPRETATION

Lab

- In cases of balanitis with drainage, cultures may be taken by spreading foreskin (with hemostat) and sending drainage for culture.
- If urethral discharge is present, culture for gonorrhea and chlamydia in an adolescent male.

TREATMENT

MEDICATION

Balanitis/balanoposthitis

- If child is afebrile, oral antibiotics such as a 1st-generation cephalosporin would be the 1st line of treatment.
- If the child develops fever or there is progression of cellulitis, then treatment with IV antibiotics (cefazolin, clindamycin)

ADDITIONAL TREATMENT

General Measures

- Phimosis
  - Physiologic: no need for intervention
  - Good hygiene practices should be encouraged such as pulling the foreskin back to expose the meatus when voiding and not voiding through the foreskin. The foreskin should always be placed back over the glans after voiding (or any retraction) to prevent paraphimosis.
  - Pamphlets or Web sites that explain the care of the penis for uncircumcised males are helpful to give to the parents.
  - If there is a fibrotic ring of scar tissue preventing the retraction of the foreskin, a trial of betamethasone cream 0.05–0.01% applied to the foreskin t.i.d. for 4–6 weeks with daily gentle retraction may soften the scar tissue enough to resolve the phimosis. According to Orsola et al, use small amounts of cream only in the constrictive ring and do not use occlusive dressings.
  - In cases where conservative measures fail, a circumcision may be indicated.
- Penile adhesions
  - Physiologic: Practices in the past have included separation using anesthetic cream (EMLA). If there is redundancy of the foreskin or a prominent suprapubic fat pad that can tend to hide the penis in infants, adhesions often recur or require constant application of barrier creams or ointments to the penis and manual retraction of the redundant foreskin by the parents to prevent recurrence:
    - In many cases, no treatment is necessary, as the adhesions will break down over a period of years.
    - If there are extensive adhesions with significant redundancy of foreskin, consideration should be given to revision of the circumcision if the adhesions are to be treated.
  - Surgical (skin bridges)
    - These are due to scar tissue formation between the raw cut edge where the foreskin was removed and the glans.
    - As this represents true scarring and not two epithelial surfaces stuck together, the surfaces cannot be simply pulled apart like physiologic adhesions. They will not resolve with time, and if left in place, with growth, penile skin will be transferred to the glans, resulting in discoloration, especially in patients with darker skin tones.
    - These adhesions need sharp division either in the office with EMLA cream anesthesia or under general anesthesia if they are extensive.
- Meatal stenosis
  - When the narrowing at the meatus is producing an upwardly deflected, narrow stream (which can make aiming into the toilet difficult) or is causing straining and prolonged voiding, treatment is indicated.
  - A meatotomy can be done in the office using EMLA anesthesia or as an outpatient surgical procedure.
- Epidermal inclusion cysts
  - These subcutaneous islands of skin cells will progressively enlarge over time.
  - Complete excision is generally curative.
- Balanitis
  - When the inflammation and irritation seem to be from chronic dampness and exposure to urine, treat with barrier creams or ointments.
  - Keeping the area clean and dry will help prevent future episodes.
  - If there are small whitish plaques (not smegma), associated with redness, yeast may be present and an antifungal cream such as 1% clotrimazole can be used to help speed the healing.
  - Antibiotics as necessary (see "Medication")
  - In cases where there is purulent drainage and cellulitis of the penis, which can often be rapidly spreading over 24 hours, treatment with antibiotics is recommended.
  - Genital infections of this nature should be taken quite seriously, and if treatment as an outpatient is attempted, close follow-up (return visit in 24–48 hours) is prudent.

ONGOING CARE

PATIENT EDUCATION

- It is important that all parents of uncircumcised boys teach them proper hygiene habits during toilet training.
- Guidance for parents:
  - Do not forcibly retract the foreskin.
  - Gently clean with warm water during baths and dry after.
  - Retract the skin when voiding in toilet-trained boys.
  - Always place the foreskin back over glans after voiding or retraction of foreskin.

ADDITIONAL READING

- Blalock HJ, Vemulakonda V, Ritchey ML, et al. Outpatient management of phimosis following newborn circumcision. *J Urol*. 2003;169(6):2332–2334.
- Orsola A, Caffaratti J, Garat JM. Conservative treatment of phimosis in children using a topical steroid. *Urology*. 2000;56(2):307–310.
- Van Howe RS. Incidence of meatal stenosis following neonatal circumcision in a primary care setting. *Clin Pediatr*. 2006;45(1):49–54.

CODES

ICD10

- Q55.64 Hidden penis
- Q54.4 Congenital chordee
- Q55.69 Other congenital malformation of penis

FAQ

- Q: The foreskin is stuck down to my son's penis. Does that mean he needs another circumcision?
- A: Not necessarily. If there is minor redundancy and a small physiologic adhesion, then no treatment is needed.
- Q: My uncircumcised son had some thick white drainage from his foreskin. Is that from an infection?
- A: Probably not. The thick white material is probably shed skin cells, which have been slowly separating the foreskin from the glans, this is also known as smegma (Greek for soap).

PERICARDITIS

Meryl S. Cohen

BASICS

DESCRIPTION

Inflammation of the pericardium, usually resulting in the accumulation of fluid in the pericardial space between the visceral (serosal tissue intimately related to the myocardium) and parietal (fibrosal layer composed of elastic fibers and collagen) pericardium. Pericarditis may be serous, fibrinous, purulent, hemorrhagic, or chylous.

EPIDEMIOLOGY

- Infectious pericarditis is more frequently seen in children younger than 13 years of age, with predominance in children younger than 2 years of age.
- Postpericardiotomy syndrome occurs in ~5–10% of children following uncomplicated cardiac surgery, particularly when the atrium has been entered.

PATHOPHYSIOLOGY

- Fine deposits of fibrin develop next to the great vessels, leading to altered function of the membranes of the pericardium, including changes in oncotic and hydrostatic pressure with subsequent accumulation of fluid in the pericardial space.
- Effusion is defined as excessive pericardial contents secondary to inflammation, hemorrhage, exudates, air, or pus.
- In postpericardiotomy syndrome, there appears to be a nonspecific hypersensitivity reaction to the direct surgical entrance into the pericardial space.

ETIOLOGY

- Infectious
  - Viral: coxsackievirus, echovirus, mumps, varicella, Epstein-Barr, adenovirus, influenza, human immunodeficiency virus
  - Bacterial: *Streptococcus*, pneumococcus, *Staphylococcus*, meningococcus, *Mycoplasma*, tularemia, *Haemophilus influenzae type B*, *Pseudomonas aeruginosa*, *Listeria monocytogenes*, *Pasteurella multocida*, *Escherichia coli*
  - Tuberculosis, atypical mycobacterium
  - Fungal: candidiasis, histoplasmosis, actinomycosis
  - Parasitic: toxoplasmosis, echinococcus, *Entamoeba histolytica*, *Rickettsia*
- Rheumatologic/inflammatory
  - Acute rheumatic fever
  - Rheumatoid arthritis
  - Systemic lupus erythematosus
  - Systemic sclerosis
  - Sarcoidosis
  - Dermatomyositis
  - Kawasaki disease
  - Familial Mediterranean fever
  - Inflammatory bowel disease
- Metabolic/endocrine
  - Hypothyroidism
  - Uremia (chemical irritation)
  - Gout
  - Scurvy
- Neoplastic disease
  - Lymphoma
  - Lymphosarcoma
  - Leukemia
  - Sarcoma
  - Metastatic disease to the pericardium
  - Radiation therapy induced
- Postoperative
  - Postpericardiotomy syndrome (after cardiac surgery)
  - Chylopericardium
- Other
  - Trauma
  - Drug-induced (hydralazine, isoniazid, procainamide)
  - Aortic dissection
  - Postmyocardial infarction
  - Idiopathic

DIAGNOSIS

HISTORY

- Dependent on etiology
- Signs and symptoms
  - Most common signs and symptoms:
    - Precordial chest pain
    - Fever
    - Cough
    - Shoulder pain aggravated by changes in position
  - Rapid accumulation of fluid may lead to the following:
    - Respiratory distress/dyspnea
    - Signs of hypotension
    - Change in mental status/loss of consciousness
  - Pain: often relieved if the child sits leaning forward
  - Slow, chronic accumulation may be associated with no symptoms at all until tamponade develops.
  - Other symptoms depend on the etiology of the pericarditis.
- Recent upper respiratory infection or gastroenteritis (viral pericarditis)
- Sepsis or other source of bacterial infection
- Symptoms of rheumatic disease
- Known thoracic neoplasm

PHYSICAL EXAM

- Pericardial friction rub is the pathognomonic finding (typically heard if only a small amount of fluid is in the pericardial space).
- Quiet precordium, tachycardia, hypotension, and muffled heart sounds may be heard when there is a large amount of fluid and/or tamponade.
- Evidence of right-sided heart failure:
  - Peripheral edema, jugular venous distention, and hepatomegaly
- Pulmonary edema: rare because the heart is underfilled, and left atrial pressure, although elevated, does not exceed right atrial pressure
- Pulsus paradoxus: an exaggerated decrease in systolic BP with inspiration
- Kussmaul sign: paradoxical rise in jugular venous pressure during inspiration, often considered diagnostic of tamponade

DIAGNOSTIC TESTS & INTERPRETATION

Lab

Electrocardiogram

- Nonspecific but generally demonstrates low-voltage QRS complexes secondary to dampening of the signal transmitted through the pericardial fluid
- One can also see diffuse ST segment elevation with or without T-wave inversion.
- These findings may be secondary to inflammation of the myocardium.
- Electrical alternans can be seen with large effusions.

Imaging

- Chest x-ray
  - Often shows enlargement of the cardiac silhouette ("water bottle sign"), usually in association with normal pulmonary vascular markings. However, heart size may appear normal in acute pericarditis.
  - Calcification may be seen in constrictive pericarditis.
- Computed tomography (CT)
  - CT can also demonstrate calcification of the pericardium with excellent sensitivity
- Echocardiogram
  - Most sensitive and specific test for pericardial thickening and fluid in the pericardial space
  - In the presence of a large effusion, the heart may appear to swing within the pericardial cavity.
  - In tamponade, diastolic collapse of the right atrium may be seen. Collapse of the left atrium and right ventricle occur in severe cases.
  - Tamponade can be diagnosed using Doppler inflow patterns of the tricuspid and mitral valves. In tamponade, mitral inflow E-wave velocity decreases by more than 30% during inspiration, whereas the tricuspid inflow E-wave velocity increases by more than 50% during inspiration.

Diagnostic Procedures/Other

- Pericardiocentesis is performed when the etiology of the effusion is in question or tamponade has developed.
  - Fluid obtained should be sent to the lab for cell count, cytology, and culture (including bacteria, viruses, *Mycobacterium tuberculosis*, and fungi).
  - Complications include myocardial puncture, coronary artery/vein laceration, hemopericardium, and pneumothorax.
  - Echocardiogram or fluoroscopic guidance is useful for this procedure but is not required if there is impending cardiovascular collapse.
- Pericardial window
  - In cases of chronic pericardial effusion, removal of part or all of the pericardium may be performed (pericardial window).

DIFFERENTIAL DIAGNOSIS

- Acute myocarditis
  - History, physical examination, and laboratory findings of acute pericarditis can be quite similar to those found in acute myocarditis.
  - In addition, myocarditis can be associated with pericardial disease and vice versa.
  - Echocardiogram is an excellent tool to help differentiate between these two entities.
- Restrictive cardiomyopathy
- Other causes of chest pain
- Myocardial infarction

P

TREATMENT

GENERAL MEASURES

- Treatment should be directed toward the etiology of the disease. However, no matter the cause, pericardiocentesis is required if there is an effusion that causes hemodynamic compromise. It may be life-saving in patients with bacterial pericarditis.
- Viral pericarditis usually resolves spontaneously in 3–4 weeks with bed rest and analgesics (NSAIDs).
- Bacterial pericarditis is potentially life threatening and requires immediate decompression of the pericardial space (often with open drainage and pericardial window creation), IV antibiotic therapy for at least 4 weeks, and supportive therapy (i.e., volume expansion, inotropes).
  - *S. aureus* is the most common organism responsible for bacterial pericarditis.
- Rheumatologic causes of pericardial inflammation usually respond to corticosteroids and/or salicylates and rarely require pericardiocentesis.
- Uremic pericarditis usually responds to dialysis, but pericardiotomy (surgical removal of the pericardium) may be necessary in chronic situations.
- Neoplastic pericarditis is addressed by treating the primary disease and performing pericardiocentesis if indicated for diagnostic and/or hemodynamic reasons.
- Hemorrhagic pericarditis with effusion accumulation secondary to trauma should be drained because of the risk of subsequent development of constrictive pericarditis.
- Constrictive pericarditis is treated with complete stripping of the pericardium (pericardiectomy). Often, immediate clinical improvement is not seen because there has been myocardial damage. However, eventual full recovery is the norm.
- Postpericardiotomy syndrome occurs 1–4 weeks after cardiac surgery.
  - Treat with anti-inflammatory drugs, bed rest, and occasionally steroids.
  - Pericardiocentesis is indicated if tamponade develops.

ONGOING CARE

- Most forms of pericarditis resolve on their own, or with anti-inflammatory medication, over the course of several weeks.
  - Follow-up is necessary to ensure that effusions have resolved and to assess for recurrence (up to 15% relapse).
  - Patients with bacterial pericarditis require long-term antibiotic therapy and close follow-up to assess for the development of constrictive pericarditis.
- Signs to watch for include the following:
  - Postpericardiotomy syndrome: All cardiac surgical patients need an evaluation 2–4 weeks after surgery to assess for postpericardiotomy syndrome, with treatment and follow-up as necessary.
  - Signs of low cardiac output and right-sided heart failure indicate impending cardiac tamponade.
  - Constrictive pericarditis may present with a rapidly decreasing cardiac silhouette, calcifications on chest roentgenogram, and signs or symptoms of right-sided heart failure.

PROGNOSIS

- Most children recover fully from pericarditis, even if it is bacterial in etiology.
  - However, there is significant morbidity and mortality associated, especially in young infants, when the diagnosis is delayed and/or when *S. aureus* is the etiologic agent.
- Pericarditis can also recur in as many as 15% of patients.
- Prognosis varies with the cause of pericarditis but generally is related directly to the primary disease.

COMPLICATIONS

- Cardiac tamponade
  - Intrapericardial pressure increases at a rapid rate secondary to decreased compliance of the pericardial membranes, resulting in restriction of ventricular filling and eventual decrease in stroke volume and cardiac output.
  - The compliance of the pericardium is influenced by the disease process itself (i.e., the pericardium is thickened and stiff in bacterial and tuberculous pericarditis).
  - During cardiac tamponade, ventricular end-diastolic, atrial, and venous pressures are all equal.
  - In acute pericarditis, tamponade may occur with small amounts of fluid because of a rapid increase in the intrapericardial pressure. In contrast, large amounts of fluid may be tolerated if the accumulation is a chronic, slow process.
- Constrictive pericarditis
  - Thick, fibrotic, and often calcified pericardium is seen, usually a late result of purulent or tuberculosis pericarditis; it can occur months to years after the initial infection. It can also be seen in oncology patients with direct invasion of tumor into the pericardium or after significant radiation to the chest.
  - Poor compliance of the pericardium leads to diminished diastolic filling of the ventricle. Patients may complain of exercise intolerance and fatigue. Additionally, they may have signs of right heart failure.
  - This entity may be difficult to distinguish from restrictive cardiomyopathy.

ADDITIONAL READING

- Demmler GJ. Infectious pericarditis in children *Pediatr Infect Dis J*. 2006;25(2):165–166.
- Tissot C, Phelps C, Younoszai AK. Restrictive cardiomyopathy and pericardial disease in Echocardiography. In: Lai WW, Mertens L, Cohen MS, et al, eds. *Pediatric and Congenital Heart Disease from Adult*. Oxford, United Kingdom: Wiley-Blackwell; 2009:597–618.
- Towbin JA. Myocarditis and pericarditis in adolescents. *Adolesc Med*. 2001;12(1):47–67.

CODES

ICD10

- I31.9 Disease of pericardium, unspecified
- I30.9 Acute pericarditis, unspecified
- I30.1 Infective pericarditis

FAQ

- Q: How does cardiac tamponade present?
- A: Patients with impending tamponade appear quite ill, with tachycardia, chest pain, and signs of right heart failure including jugular venous distention, hepatomegaly, ascites, and peripheral edema. They may also have signs of poor systemic perfusion secondary to low cardiac output. Chest x-ray may or may not show an enlarged cardiac silhouette, depending on how acutely the process occurs. It takes much less fluid to cause tamponade in an acute process than in a chronic process. Echocardiography is the standard diagnostic tool, and pericardiocentesis is the treatment.
- Q: What is pulsus paradoxus and how does one measure it?
- A: Pulsus paradoxus is an exaggerated response of the systolic BP to the normal respiratory cycle. Normally with inspiration, the systolic BP drops ~5 mm Hg secondary to the increased capacitance of the pulmonary veins from the increased systemic venous return. In tamponade, this response becomes more profound (>10 mm Hg), most likely secondary to diminished filling of the left heart. Pulsus paradoxus can also be seen in patients with severe respiratory distress associated with asthma and emphysema.
- To assess for pulsus paradoxus, measure the systolic BP first in expiration, then allow it to fall to the place where it is heard equally well in inspiration and expiration. A difference of >10 mm Hg is considered abnormal.

PERINATAL BRACHIAL PLEXUS PALSY

Jonathan A. Zelken • Richard J. Redett

BASICS

DESCRIPTION

- The brachial plexus contains sensory and motor nerves to the upper extremities, stemming from the cervical and thoracic spine (commonly C5–T1 roots).
- The brachial plexus contains a consistent pattern of nerves that innervate predictable muscles and skin regions.
- Brachial birth palsy is a proximal stretch, avulsion, or rupture type injury and may involve
  - C5–C6 (Erb palsy), most common, best prognosis
  - C5–C7, less common, worse prognosis
  - C5–T1, least common, flail extremity and worst prognosis

EPIDEMIOLOGY

- There is no predominance of gender, but variations in clinical care, preventive measures, and birth weight may explain estimates of incidence to range from 0.4 to 4 per 1,000 live births.
- Incidence drops from 0.2% with vaginal delivery to 0.02% after cesarean section as there is a probable mechanical basis for the plexopathy.
- Erb palsy is the most commonly encountered plexus injury.

RISK FACTORS

- Large size for gestational age, multiparity, prolonged labor, breech position, difficult delivery—especially when forceps- or vacuum-assisted
- Diabetic mothers and/or neonatal birth weight >4.5 kg
- Although there is no genetic basis per se, previous delivery leading to obstetric palsy is a risk factor.

GENERAL PREVENTION

- Careful positioning of the upper extremity during childbirth and conversion to cesarean section when necessary
- Prevention of long-term disability and contracture can be minimized with exercise of the child's joints and functioning muscles every day beginning at 3 weeks of age.

PATHOPHYSIOLOGY

- Seddon and Sunderland have described classification systems to describe degree of injury.
  - Neuropraxia
    - Mildest form, interruption of conduction, axons continuous
    - Good recovery
  - Axonotmesis
    - Axonal degeneration with loss of axonal continuity
    - Nerve intact. Epineurium and perineurium intact.
  - Neurotmesis
    - Most severe, nerve is completely contused. Axonal discontinuity
    - Nerve may be grossly intact, but epineurium, perineurium, and axons disrupted. Recovery difficult to predict.

ETIOLOGY

- Downward mechanical force on the shoulder during difficult delivery can lead to stepwise stretch injury leading to transient or permanent damage or total avulsion of nerve roots.
- Upward mechanical force, that is, after face delivery, leads to C8–T1 injury (Klumpke).
- Avulsion injury carries the worst prognosis, particularly if proximal to the cell body of the motor nerve (preganglionic), as these injuries cannot spontaneously recover.

ASSOCIATED INJURIES

Horner syndrome, phrenic nerve injury, and long thoracic nerve injury (winged scapula) may be observed and are associated with preganglionic injury and a poor prognosis.

DIAGNOSIS

HISTORY

- In neonates: obstetric history including birth weight, use of assistive devices, multiparity, perinatal difficulties, previous difficult deliveries, etc.
- Despite a prominent association between shoulder dystocia and neonatal brachial plexus palsy injury, some of these injuries occur without any shoulder dystocia.
- In older children: Consider recent infectious processes (viruses), tetanus shots, trauma, and tumor.

PHYSICAL EXAM

- Serial examination is key for predicting recovery.
- Active and passive ROM testing, bulk, deep tendon reflexes (DTRs), autonomic function, and evaluation for phrenic nerve injury and paravertebral muscle weakness are important adjunctive exams.
- Sensory testing may be more challenging because of age and overlap of dermatomes.
- Because of invariability of brachial plexus anatomy, injury patterns yield predictable disabilities.
- Erb palsy
  - Associated with downward force on the head and neck during delivery, leading to upper plexus injuries
  - Shoulder limp, adducted, internally rotated
  - Elbow extended, forearm pronated, wrist and fingers flexed ("waiter's tip" posture)
  - Hand grip and intrinsic function generally preserved. Shoulder and elbow flexion is weak.
  - DTRs: biceps and brachioradialis absent, Moro asymmetric
- Klumpke palsy
  - Risk of injury to the lower brachial plexus results from traction on an abducted arm, as with an infant being pulled from the birth canal by an extended arm above the head.
  - Shoulder intact, elbow flexed, forearm supinated, wrists and fingers extended
  - Hand grip is weak, while shoulder and elbow function may be normal. Horner syndrome can be present.
  - DTRs: triceps absent; Horner sign suggests ipsilateral T1 injury.
- Complete plexus injury ("flail"):
  - Entire extremity and shoulder girdle is flaccid, anesthetic, and areflexic.

DIAGNOSTIC TESTS & INTERPRETATION

- Plain radiographs may demonstrate clavicle injury and shoulder and elbow subluxation and dislocation.
- MRI neurography is generally favored over CT myelography and electromyography (EMG) and is less invasive.
- Previous cases using EMG data to determine whether an injury occurred in utero has been investigated; interpretation of all these modalities may lead to false positives and negatives.
- Somatosensory and motor evoked potentials are less useful as they generally corroborate physical exam findings.

FOLLOW-UP

- Following the diagnosis of brachial plexus palsy, neonates should be followed closely to determine if the injury will resolve spontaneously or will require further treatment.
- Patients should be followed by an experienced multidisciplinary brachial plexus team of therapists, pediatricians, and pediatric surgery subspecialists.

DIFFERENTIAL DIAGNOSIS

- Important to rule out clavicular, shoulder, elbow, and humeral injury as primary cause of limb paresis or weakness
- Central lesions resulting from tumors and strokes, as well as spinal cord lesions, should be considered.
- Congenital contractures and limb deformities can resemble brachial plexus injuries.
- Central paralysis is generally spastic and peripheral (i.e., brachial plexus or lower motor neuron) is flaccid.
- Horner syndrome may be associated with proximal injury.
- Parsonage-Turner syndrome may cause plexus inflammation and symptoms without obvious injury.

TREATMENT

REHABILITATION

- Therapy is paramount in managing symptoms of plexopathy.
- Goals include comfort, optimizing recovery, and assessing improvement.
- Stretching exercises, splints to prevent contracture, joint taping to stabilize shoulder, and sensory awareness activities are commonly used.

GENERAL MEASURES

- Palsies must be observed during the first weeks to months of life.
  - Immobilization of a flaccid limb encouraged very early for pain control
  - After 3 weeks of immobilization and fractures/dislocation have been ruled-out, ROM exercises should commence to prevent deformity and contracture.
- Majority of neonates with obstetric brachial plexus injury will resolve spontaneously.
- Classic Erb palsy has the best prognosis.

- The majority of upper brachial plexus birth injuries are transient.
- Global palsies have a poor prognosis with nonoperative treatment.
- Failure to recover antigravity biceps function by 3–6 months of age is a poor prognostic sign.
- Infants with C5–6 or C5–7 injuries may continue to demonstrate spontaneous improvement up to 9 months of age, thus precluding the need for early surgery.

PROGNOSIS

~75–85% of all patients regain very good to full strength and function, with 1/2 doing so rapidly (the mild group) and 1/2 more slowly (the moderate group).

SURGERY/OTHER PROCEDURES

- Indications for early surgical intervention
  - Pan-plexus ("flail") lesions (generally warrant early intervention as soon as 3 months if no improvement)
  - All brachial plexus injuries should be evaluated by a multidisciplinary team at 3, 6, and 9 months of age. Failure to improve at each examination is usually and indication for surgery. There are several different grading systems, which can be used to assess an infant's healing progress.
- Nonsurgical measures
  - Neuromuscular electrical stimulation can be used as part of an infant's comprehensive therapy to help improve blood flow, preserve muscle bulk and minimize atrophy.
  - Botulinum toxin A therapy to impair preserved muscle groups allow weaker muscle groups to strengthen.
- Primary surgery
  - Surgical outcome is best if performed by 6–12 months and probably not useful if done after 24 months; ongoing care
  - Exploration generally confirms clinical and radiographic findings.
  - Injured nerves generally present as neuromas.
    - Neurolysis to free uninjured nerve from scar versus
    - Excision of neuroma en bloc with interpositional nerve grafting
    - Excision is favored when nerve transmission across the injured site is significantly diminished (<50%) or absent, immobilization of a flaccid limb encouraged very early for pain control
  - Autologous sural nerve is an excellent donor, and it is reversed when interposed to maximize signaling to the CNS
  - When there is insufficient nerve graft, neurotization —attachment of functional motor nerves to distal recipient nerves—is a useful adjunct.
  - Common donor nerves include the spinal accessory, contralateral C7 nerve root, and intercostal nerves.
  - Use of nerve conduits and adjunctive neurotrophic factors is under investigation.

ONGOING CARE

SECONDARY SURGERY

Tendon transfers (generally wait 2–4 years to assess long-term nerve recovery) improve flexibility and functional mobility of affected joints.

- Shoulder: transfer of preserved internal rotators to impaired abductors and external rotators
- Elbow: triceps to biceps repair, pectoralis to biceps repair, latissimus to biceps repair
- Forearm: Biceps rerouting and pronator lengthening can relieve pronation and supination contractures.
- Scapula: contralateral rhomboid, trapezius, and latissimus transfer to anchor and support a winged scapula
- Osteotomies (late presentation)
  - External rotational osteotomy of humerus to improve upper extremity function with fixed, internally rotated shoulder
  - Radius rotational osteotomy to address pronation and supination deformities
- Soft tissue (late presentation)
  - Capsulotomies and joint manipulation under anesthesia can facilitate movement in a contracted joint.
  - Local flaps and tissue transfer can augment a contracted flexor or extensor zone.

ADDITIONAL READING

- Borschel GH, Clark HM. Obstetrical brachial plexus palsy. *Plast Reconstr Surg*. 2009;124(1)(Suppl):144e–155e.
- Chuang DC, Ma HS, Wei FC. A new evaluation system to predict the sequelae of late obstetric brachial plexus palsy. *Plast Reconstr Surg*. 1998;101(3):673–685.
- Chuang DC, Ma HS, Wei FC. A new strategy of muscle transposition for treatment of shoulder deformity caused by obstetric brachial plexus palsy. *Plast Reconstr Surg*. 2008;101(3):686–694.
- Seddon HJ. Three types of nerve injury. *Brain*. 1943;66:237–288.
- Terzis JK, Papakonstantinou KC. Management of obstetric brachial plexus palsy. *Hand Clin*. 1999;15(4):717–736.
- Wolfe SW, Strauss HL, Garg R, et al. Use of bioabsorbable nerve conduits as an adjunct to brachial plexus neurorrhaphy. *J Hand Surg Am*. 2012;37(10):1980–1985.
- Zafeiriou DI, Psychogiou K. Obstetrical brachial plexus palsy. *Pediatr Neurol*. 2008;38(4):235–242.

CODES

ICD10

P14.3 Other brachial plexus birth injuries

FAQ

- Q: My baby was diagnosed with a brachial plexus injury. What are the odds she will recover completely?
- A: Most (roughly 80%) children recover completely. The nerves were stretched and are inflamed, but this should resolve. Babies with more significant injuries causing axonotmesis and neurotmesis may not recover completely or at all.
- Q: My last baby suffered a brachial plexus injury at birth, but since got better. What are the odds my next child will have the same problem?
- A: Your next child has a 14-fold increase in risk for brachial plexus injury compared to the general population.
- Q: My baby is 3 months old and cannot move his left arm? Whom should I call?
- A: A center for brachial plexus injury is ideal. A well-organized team includes physical and occupational therapists, neurologists, and surgeons (neurosurgeon, plastic surgeon, orthopedic surgeon, or combination thereof).
- Q: Could my obstetrician have prevented this?
- A: Likely, not. Although there may be increased risk for shoulder dystocia in some women, it is not a diagnosable problem. Preemptive cesarean section in at-risk women may be unnecessarily risky to mother and fetus.

PERIODIC BREATHING

Richard M. Kravitz

BASICS

DESCRIPTION

- A respiratory pattern consisting of regular oscillations in breathing amplitude
- Typically, a respiratory pattern in which ≥3 apneas lasting ≥3 seconds occur, separated by <20 seconds of respiration

ALERT

Don't confuse periodic breathing with obstructive and/or central apnea.

EPIDEMIOLOGY

- Usually absent in the 1st 48 hours of life
- More frequent during rapid eye movement (REM or active) sleep versus non-REM (quiet) sleep
- Less common in prone versus supine position
- In full-term infants
  - Amount of periodic breathing usually <4% of total sleep time
  - Amount gradually decreases through the 1st year of life.
  - By 1 year of age, the mean amount of periodic breathing is <1% of total sleep time.
- In premature infants
  - Amount of periodic breathing is higher than in full-term infants.
  - Amount correlates inversely with gestational age.

PATHOPHYSIOLOGY

- No common pathologic finding
- Abnormalities, when they exist, are related to the underlying disorder causing the periodic breathing.

ETIOLOGY

- Periodic breathing can be seen in healthy infants, children, and adults.
- Abnormalities, in any component of the breathing control system, may result in an increased amount of periodic breathing.
- Possible etiologies
  - A delay in detecting changes in blood gas values by the chemoreceptors
  - Increased chemoreceptor gain

COMMONLY ASSOCIATED CONDITIONS

- Periodic breathing in infants is associated with the following:
  - Apnea of prematurity or infancy
  - Familial history of sudden infant death syndrome (SIDS)
  - Anemia of prematurity
  - Hypoxemia
  - Hypochloremic alkalosis
- Periodic breathing with adults is associated with the following:
  - Cardiac abnormalities (especially congestive heart failure [CHF])
  - Neurologic dysfunction (meningitis, encephalitis, brainstem dysfunction)
  - Exposure to high altitudes

DIAGNOSIS

HISTORY

- In most cases, parents notice periodicity in the child's respiratory pattern.
- An apparent life-threatening episode (ALTE) might precipitate an evaluation in which periodic breathing is documented.
- In otherwise healthy premature or term infants, there are no other symptoms.

PHYSICAL EXAM

In otherwise healthy premature or term infants, the physical exam is normal.

DIAGNOSTIC TESTS & INTERPRETATION

Imaging

Chest x-ray: usually normal findings

Diagnostic Procedures/Other

- Polysomnography
  - Assesses the extent of periodic breathing episodes
  - Determines if there is accompanying hypoxemia, hypercarbia, or bradycardia with the events
  - Distinguishes between periodic breathing and obstructive and/or central apnea
  - Useful for following response to treatment (i.e., normalization of polysomnography)
- pH probe done in combination with the polysomnogram (if gastroesophageal reflux is suspected): Record for a minimum of 6 hours.
- 2-channel pneumogram
  - Gives less information than polysomnography
  - Can document periodic breathing, but it may miss episodes of obstructive apnea
  - Monitors heart rate and respiratory effort (If oxygen saturation monitoring is desired, an additional channel is required).

DIFFERENTIAL DIAGNOSIS

- Other forms of apnea:
  - Central apnea
  - Mixed apnea
  - Obstructive apnea (or hypopnea)
- Other forms of periodic breathing:
  - Cheyne-Stokes respirations
  - Biot breathing
  - Kussmaul respirations
- Normal irregular respiration seen in infants

TREATMENT

MEDICATION

- Stimulants
  - Caffeine IV or PO (based on caffeine base; multiply dosage by 2 for caffeine citrate salt)
    - Loading dose: 10 mg/kg
    - Maintenance dose: 2.5 mg/kg/24 h
    - Therapeutic level: 5–20 mg/L
  - Theophylline PO (if using aminophylline IV, divided dosage by 0.79)
    - Loading dose: 4–5 mg/kg
    - Maintenance dose: 3–5 mg/kg/24 h divided t.i.d.
    - Therapeutic level: 6–10 mg/L

ADDITIONAL TREATMENT

General Measures

- Therapy should be directed at treating the underlying primary disease:
  - If periodic breathing is associated with apnea, hypoxemia, and/or other sleep disturbances, appropriate treatment of the underlying etiology should be instituted.
  - In cases secondary to CHF, appropriate cardiac interventions need to be instituted.
  - In cases associated with high altitude, treatment options include the following:
    - Acclimation (if tolerated)
    - Descent to lower altitude, then gradual ascent
    - Medication (acetazolamide most commonly used)
- Duration of therapy
  - Depends on the underlying cause of the periodic breathing
  - Treatment does not change the natural course of periodic breathing in otherwise healthy infants.
  - Therapy should continue until the periodic breathing resolves or is no longer clinically significant.

ADDITIONAL THERAPIES

- Supplemental oxygen: useful if periodic breathing is secondary to hypoxemia
- Nasal continuous positive airway pressure (CPAP): very effective in eliminating periodic breathing
- Home monitoring should be considered (although not absolutely indicated) in the following cases:
  - Significant amount of periodic breathing
  - Accompanying apnea
  - Associated hypoxia and/or bradycardia
  - History of a significant ALTE
  - Parental anxiety

ONGOING CARE

FOLLOW-UP RECOMMENDATIONS

- Time to improvement depends on the underlying cause of the periodic breathing.
- Improvement is anticipated as the infant ages.
- When treatment is started, a decrease in the amount of periodic breathing should be seen almost immediately.

PROGNOSIS

- Excellent in otherwise healthy premature or term infants
- Governed by primary process in patients with an underlying cardiac or neurologic disorder

COMPLICATIONS

Relationship between periodic breathing and SIDS is controversial.

ADDITIONAL READING

- Carroll JL, Agarwal A. Development of ventilatory control in infants. *Paediatr Respir Rev*. 2010;11(4):199–207.
- Horemuzova E, Katz-Salamon M, Milerad J. Breathing patterns, oxygen and carbon dioxide levels in sleeping healthy infants during the first nine months after birth. *Acta Paediatr*. 2000;89(11):1284–1289.
- Hunt CE, Corwin MJ, Lister G, et al. Longitudinal assessment of hemoglobin oxygen saturation in healthy infants during the first 6 months of age. *J Pediatr*. 1999;135(5):580–586.
- Miano S, Castaldo R, Ferri R, et al. Sleep cyclic alternating pattern analysis in infants with apparent life-threatening events: a daytime polysomnographic study. *Clin Neurophysiol*. 2012;123(7):1346–1352.
- Poets CF. Apnea of prematurity: what can observational studies tell us about pathophysiology? *Sleep Med*. 2010;11(7):701–707.
- Schechter MS; Section on Pediatric Pulmonology, Subcommittee on Obstructive Sleep Apnea Syndrome. Technical report: diagnosis and management of childhood obstructive sleep apnea syndrome. *Pediatrics*. 2002;109(4):e69.
- Sterni LM, Tunkel DE. Obstructive sleep apnea in children: an update. *Pediatr Clin North Am*. 2003;50(2):427–443.

CODES

ICD10

R06.3 Periodic breathing

FAQ

- Q: What is the risk of the patient dying of SIDS?
- A: The relationship between periodic breathing and SIDS is not clear, although most studies have not found a higher frequency of SIDS among patients with periodic breathing.

PERIORBITAL CELLULITIS

Aaron E. Kornblith • Christine S. Cho

BASICS

DESCRIPTION

- Periorbital or preseptal cellulitis is an acute infection characterized by pain, erythema, and edema to the anterior eyelid and surrounding tissue.
- The infection lies superficial to orbital septum, a thin fascial layer forming the anterior boundary of the orbital compartment.
- In contrast, orbital cellulitis is an infection involving the deeper structures of the orbit and requires emergent intervention.

EPIDEMIOLOGY

- Often occurs in young children, commonly <5 years of age, but can occur at any age
- Periorbital cellulitis is at least three times more common than orbital cellulitis.

RISK FACTORS

Predisposing factors that may lead to infection include skin trauma and lacrimal/eyelid injury.

PATHOPHYSIOLOGY

Often, extension from an external source including trauma (insect bite, recent surgery, foreign body) or adjacent infection (sinusitis, dacryocystitis, hordeola, dental abscess)

ETIOLOGY

- Variable depending on mechanism
  - Most common pathogens are *Staphylococcus aureus* (increasingly methicillin-resistant) and Streptococci species.
  - Anaerobic infections can extend from dental source.
  - *Haemophilus influenza type B* was historically the most common pathogen; consider in unimmunized child younger than 5 years of age.

COMMONLY ASSOCIATED CONDITIONS

Rarely associated with bacteremia; however, consider this condition in children younger than 3 years of age or in immunocompromised patients.

DIAGNOSIS

HISTORY

- Onset, time course of symptom progression, and any predisposing factors
- A history of trauma is suggestive of periorbital cellulitis.
- The presence of pain supports cellulitis, whereas complaints of pruritus are more suggestive of an allergic etiology.
- Diplopia and visual changes are more suggestive of orbital cellulitis.
- Quantify systemic symptoms such as fever and lethargy.
  - These indicate a more severe, disseminated infection.

PHYSICAL EXAM

- Superficial orbital tissues and lids will be edematous, erythematous, warm to the touch, and typically tender on palpation.
  - Often unilateral, the findings can start in one eyelid, but both the upper and lower eyelids are usually involved.
  - May be signs of previous trauma, cutaneous injury, etc.
- Occasionally, the eyelids are so swollen that it is difficult to examine the globe. To do so, place anesthetic eyedrops on the eye and use ocular speculum or fashion a paperclip into a lid retractor to lift the eyelid.
- The globe should be carefully examined.
  - In periorbital cellulitis, the ocular exam is often normal. The sclera is usually white, although patients can have some conjunctival erythema but rarely chemosis.
  - Any change in vision, pupillary function, or limitations in eye motility suggests orbital involvement.
- The presence of proptosis and/or pain with eye movement suggests deep orbital involvement.
- Neurologic findings, such as cranial nerve deficit, are suggestive of deep space involvement.
- Evaluate for signs of fever, respiratory infection, and sepsis.

DIAGNOSTIC TESTS & INTERPRETATION

Lab

- Lab tests are usually not helpful or indicated.
- CBC is warranted only if bacteremia is suspected.
  - Leukocytosis has no value in differentiating periorbital and orbital cellulitis.
- Skin cultures and blood cultures have a low yield.
  - Blood cultures are obtained only when the child is febrile or appears septic.
  - Wound cultures can be obtained if there is an abscess.

Imaging

- Periorbital cellulitis is a clinical diagnosis and radiologic confirmation is only indicated if the diagnosis is unclear. Imaging may be required in the following circumstances:
  - If orbital cellulitis is suspected
  - Cases that do not respond to medical treatment
  - Neurologic symptoms are present.
- Serial CT scanning should be done only if the child is not improving with treatment.

DIFFERENTIAL DIAGNOSIS

- Infectious
  - Early orbital cellulitis, dacryocystitis, stye, severe viral conjunctivitis
  - Orbital cellulitis is an ophthalmologic emergency and requires prompt therapy.
- Allergic
  - Periocular allergic reaction: insect bite, angioedema, contact dermatitis
- Other
  - Periocular trauma
  - Rhabdomyosarcoma
  - Idiopathic orbital inflammatory syndrome (IOIS)
  - Cavernous venous thrombosis
  - Hypoproteinemia

P

TREATMENT

GENERAL MEASURES

- Simple periorbital cellulitis should be empirically treated based on local prevalence of *Staphylococcus* and *Streptococcus* species.
  - Consider MRSA
  - Examples include second-generation cephalosporins or β-lactamase–resistant penicillins.
- There is no evidence to suggest that intravenous are better than oral antibiotics; however, younger children need close observation and/or follow-up.
- For children <1 year of age, strongly consider hospitalization for IV therapy and very close observation.
- Children between the ages of 1 and 5 years should either be hospitalized or arranged for close follow-up after initiating antibiotics.
- Children >5 years of age can usually be treated with an oral regimen as long as they do not appear toxic or have orbital involvement.
- Any patient with symptoms suggestive of deep space involvement or hematogenous involvement should be hospitalized.

MEDICATION

- In nontoxic children, oral antibiotics: amoxicillin/clavulanate, cefalexin, clindamycin (if MRSA is a concern), etc. are started on an outpatient basis; the child should be seen again within 24–48 hours.
- Consider admission for IV antibiotics (clindamycin, ampicillin/sulbactam, etc.) for those patients younger than 1 year of age, ill appearing, have bacteremia, or symptoms suggestive of orbital involvement.

SURGERY/OTHER PROCEDURES

Surgical intervention is usually required when an abscess or a foreign body is present.

ONGOING CARE

- Patients should have close follow-up 24–48 hours after initiating outpatient treatment.
- Patients who do not improve after close follow-up should be admitted for IV antibiotics and imaging.
- Patients should be seen daily until a definite improvement is noted.

PROGNOSIS

Excellent, with minimal incidence of long-term sequelae, unless a complication is encountered

COMPLICATIONS

- Orbital extension (2.5–17%)
- Skin abscess (8%)
- Eyelid necrosis (1–2%)
- Sepsis
- Intracranial extension (2–3%)

Patient Monitoring

- Watch patients closely for signs of orbital extension, bacteremia, or other forms of disseminated infection.
- Neonates and infants can become septic very quickly, so they need to be closely monitored.

ADDITIONAL READING

- Bedwell J, Bauman N. Management of pediatric orbital cellulitis and abscess. *Curr Opin Otolaryngol Head Neck Surg*. 2011;19(6);467–473.
- Donahue SP, Schwartz G. Preseptal and orbital cellulitis in childhood: a changing microbiologic spectrum. *Ophthalmology*. 1998;105(10):1902–1905.
- Foster JA, Katowitz JA. Pediatric orbital and periocular infections. In: Katowitz JA, ed. *Pediatric Oculoplastic Surgery*. New York, NY: Springer-Verlag; 2001:407–420.
- Georgakopoulos CD, Eliopoulou MI, Stasinos S, et al. Periorbital and orbital cellulitis: a 10-year review of hospitalized children. *Eur J Ophthalmol*. 2010;20(6):1066–1072.
- Hauser A, Fogarasi S. Periorbital and orbital cellulitis. *Pediatr Rev*. 2010;31(6);242–249.
- Lessner A, Stern GA. Preseptal and orbital cellulitis. *Infect Dis Clin North Am*. 1992;6(4):933–952.
- Powell KR. Orbital and periorbital cellulitis. *Pediatr Rev*. 1995;16(5):163–167.
- Rutar T, Chambers HF, Crawford JB, et al. Ophthalmic manifestations of infections caused by the USA300 clone of community-associated methicillin-resistant *Staphylococcus aureus*. *Ophthalmology*. 2006;113(8):1455–1462.
- Wald ER. Periorbital and orbital infections. *Pediatr Rev*. 2004;25(9):312–320.
- Vayalumkal JV, Jadavji T. Children hospitalized with skin and soft tissue infections: a guide to antibacterial selection and treatment. *Paediatr Drugs*. 2006;8(2):99–111.

CODES

ICD10

- H05.019 Cellulitis of unspecified orbit
- H00.039 Abscess of eyelid unspecified eye, unspecified eyelid

PERIRECTAL ABSCESS

Naamah Zitomersky

BASICS

DESCRIPTION

- Abscess in the perirectal area
- May be associated with fistula-in-ano
- Classification of the abscess is based on the location in relation to the levator and sphincteric muscles of the pelvic floor.
- Classification by decreasing frequency: perianal, ischioanal, intersphincteric, and supralevator

EPIDEMIOLOGY

- May occur at any age
  - More common in males 2:1
  - In children, more common in those less than 2 years

PATHOPHYSIOLOGY AND ETIOLOGY

- Most often originates from an occluded anal gland with subsequent bacterial overgrowth and abscess formation
- Infection from within the anal glands, penetrates through the internal sphincter, and ends in the intersphincteric space
- Chronic infection and inflammation may result in the formation of fistula-in-ano. This occurs in up to 50% as a result of persistent anal sepsis or an epithelialized tract.

COMMONLY ASSOCIATED CONDITIONS

- Nonspecific anal gland infection
- Crohn disease
- Immune deficiency (e.g., neutropenia, diabetes mellitus, AIDS)
- Perforation by a foreign body
- External trauma
- Tuberculosis
- Chronic granulomatous disease (CGD)
- Tumor (e.g., carcinoma, rhabdomyosarcoma)

DIAGNOSIS

SIGNS AND SYMPTOMS

- General
  - Constant anal or perianal pain that often precedes local findings
  - Localized swelling, erythema, and fluctuance
  - Painful defecation or ambulation
  - Constitutional symptoms (e.g., fever or malaise)
- Perianal abscess
  - Result of distal vertical spread of the infection to the anal margin
  - Presents as tender, fluctuant mass
  - Most common type of perianal abscess
- Ischiorectal abscess
  - Secondary to horizontal spread of infection across the external anal sphincter into the ischiorectal fossa
  - Infection may track across the internal anal sphincter into the anal canal.
  - Presents as diffuse, tender, indurated, fluctuant area
  - Patients may have pain and fever prior to visible swelling.
- Intersphincteric abscess
  - Limited to the intersphincteric space between the internal and external sphincters; therefore, often does not cause perianal skin changes
  - Associated with painful defecation
  - Accounts for only 2–5% of all anorectal abscesses
- Supralevator abscess
  - May arise from two different sources
    - Proximal vertical spread from the gland through the intersphincteric space to the supralevator space
    - Pelvic inflammation or infection (e.g., Crohn disease)
  - Presents with pelvic or anorectal pain, fever, and, at times, urinary retention
  - Rectal exam usually reveals an indurated swelling above the anorectal ring.
  - Imaging may be necessary to establish the diagnosis.
- Horseshoe abscess
  - Secondary to abscessed anal gland located in the posterior midline of the anal canal
  - Due to presence of anococcygeal ligament, the infection is forced laterally into the ischiorectal fossae and is therefore known as "horseshoe."
  - May be unilateral or bilateral
  - Presents with pain

DIAGNOSTIC TESTS & INTERPRETATION

Lab

- CBC
- Abscess culture

Imaging

- Magnetic resonance imaging (MRI)
  - Preferred modality, as it provides excellent spatial and contrast resolution
  - Enables comprehensive evaluation of the entire peritoneum and lower pelvis
- Computed tomography (CT) scan
  - Has limited soft tissue contrast resolution which makes distinguishing perineal musculature and fistula tracts difficult, although organized fluid collections larger than 1 cm are generally seen
  - This modality also uses ionizing radiation, which is less desirable in the pediatric population.
- Ultrasound (US)
  - Endoscopic and transperineal US have been used, but do not always show the full extent of inflammation.
  - Deeper structures may not be visualized, owing to the lack of sound wave penetration.
  - Endoscopic US may be used to diagnose, characterize, and monitor rectal abscesses.

DIFFERENTIAL DIAGNOSIS
- Pilonidal infection
- Bartholin abscess
- Presacral epidermal inclusion cyst
- Hidradenitis suppurativa
- Rectal duplication cyst

TREATMENT

GENERAL MEASURES
- Lack of fluctuation should not delay treatment.
- Abscess should be drained with placement of a seton or drainage catheter.
- Abscess should be cultured at time of drainage to direct therapy in the case antibiotics are needed.
- Antibiotics are reserved for situations in which infection does not appropriately respond to drainage or with adjacent cellulitis, an immunocompromised patient, a patient with abnormal cardiac valves, enteric organism on culture, or in Crohn disease.
- Sitz baths may be helpful with drainage.

SURGERY/OTHER PROCEDURES
- Drainage may be performed either with conservative incision and drainage or with judicious probing for fistulae.
- It is a matter of debate as to whether a fistulotomy or fistulectomy should be performed at the time of drainage for an accompanying fistula.

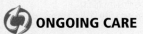

ONGOING CARE
- If abscess recurs, consider other associated conditions (e.g., neutropenia, HIV, diabetes mellitus, Crohn disease, rectal duplication cyst).
- Exploration for fistula-in-ano is recommended to prevent recurrence.

PROGNOSIS
- Prognosis is good if there is early detection and drainage of abscesses.
- Patients typically recover well after surgical drainage without the need for antibiotics.

COMPLICATIONS
- Sepsis
- Fistula formation

SPECIAL CONSIDERATIONS
- Crohn disease should be considered in patients with perirectal abscess with or without fistula-in-ano.
- Signs and symptoms that increase suspicion for Crohn disease include weight loss or poor growth, chronic diarrhea, or abdominal pain.

ADDITIONAL READING

- Caliste X, Nazir S, Goode T, et al. Sensitivity of computed tomography in detection of perirectal abscess. *Am Surg*. 2011;77(2):166–168.
- Chang HK, Ryu JG, Oh JT. Clinical characteristics and treatment of perianal abscess and fistula-in-ano in infants. *J Pediatr Surg*. 2010;45(9):1832–1836.
- Hammer MR, Dillman JR, Smith EA, et al. Magnetic resonance imaging of perianal and perineal Crohn disease in children and adolescents. *Magn Reson Imaging Clin N Am*. 2013;21(4):813–828.
- Huang A, Abbasakoor F, Vaizey CJ. Gastrointestinal manifestations of chronic granulomatous disease. *Colorectal Dis*. 2006;8(8):637–644.
- Lejkowski M, Maheshwari A, Calhoun DA, et al. Persistent perianal abscess in early infancy as a presentation of autoimmune neutropenia. *J Perinatol*. 2003;23(5):428–430.
- Malik AI, Nelson RL, Tou S. Incision and drainage of perianal abscess with or without treatment of anal fistula. *Cochrane Database Syst Rev*. 2010;(7):CD006827.
- Marcus RH, Stine RJ, Cohen MA. Perirectal abscess. *Ann Emerg Med*. 1995;25(5):597–603.
- Niyogi A, Agarwal T, Broadhurst J, et al. Management of perianal abscess and fistula-in-ano in children. *Eur J Pediatr Surg*. 2010;20(1):35–39.
- Rosen NG, Gibbs DL, Soffer SZ, et al. The nonoperative treatment of fistula-in-ano. *J Pediatr Surg*. 2000;35(6):938–939.
- Whiteford MH, Kilkenny J III, Hyman N, et al. Practice parameters for the treatment of perianal abscess and fistula-in-ano (revised). *Dis Colon Rectum*. 2005;48(7):1337–1342.

CODES

ICD10
- K61.1 Rectal abscess
- K60.3 Anal fistula
- K61.3 Ischiorectal abscess

FAQ
- Q: What are complications of this problem?
- A: Fistula formation is seen in up to 50% of patients, with a predilection for males.
- Q: What are the most common organisms of the abscess?
- A: *Staphylococcus* species
- Q: What other disease may perirectal abscess be associated with?
- A: Crohn disease. If there has been exposure, tuberculosis should also be excluded.
- Q: What treatments can be done other than surgery?
- A: Sitz baths and warm compresses may be able to help with smaller more superficial abscess.

PERITONITIS

Sarah S. Lusman

BASICS

DESCRIPTION

- Inflammation of the peritoneal cavity in reaction to infection or chemical irritation by organic fluids (e.g., intestinal contents, bile, blood, or urine)
- Infectious peritonitis can be classified as follows:
  - Primary or spontaneous bacterial peritonitis (SBP), which occurs without an obvious source or a break in the continuity of the intestinal lumen. Pathogens enter the peritoneum via translocation from the intestine; from the circulation; from vaginal, oropharyngeal, or skin flora; or from foreign bodies inserted into the peritoneal cavity.
  - Secondary peritonitis occurs with visceral disruption from bowel perforation, abscess formation, ischemic necrosis, or penetrating abdominal injury.
  - Tertiary peritonitis is recurrent peritonitis after presumed adequate treatment for secondary peritonitis.
- SBP almost always occurs in patients with cirrhosis and ascites.

RISK FACTORS

- End-stage liver disease
- Serum albumin $<$1.5 g/dL
- Low serum levels of complement factors C3 and C4
- Nephrotic syndrome (inability to clear organisms, most common is *Streptococcus pneumoniae*)
- Splenectomy (encapsulated organisms: group A streptococci, *Escherichia coli*, *S. pneumoniae*, *Bacteroides* sp.)
- Peritoneal dialysis
- Presence of gastrointestinal hemorrhage
- Prematurity

GENERAL PREVENTION

- Children with chronic liver disease should receive all recommended childhood vaccinations.
- Children with functional asplenia due to portal hypertension should receive the meningococcal and pneumococcal conjugate vaccines as early as possible.
- Oral antibiotic prophylaxis reduces occurrence of SBP and improves short-term survival in adults with cirrhosis.

PATHOPHYSIOLOGY

- When bacteria or chemicals reach the peritoneal cavity, a local peritoneal and systemic host defense response is initiated:
  - Mechanical clearance of bacteria via lymphatics: Entrance of bacteria and bacterial products into the bloodstream contributes to the systemic response.
  - Phagocytosis and destruction of bacteria
  - Sequestration and walling off of bacteria with delayed clearance by phagocytic cells
  - Initial response is characterized by hyperemia, exudate of fluid into peritoneal cavity, and influx of macrophages followed by neutrophils.
  - Mesothelial cells secrete cytokines after stimulation (interleukins [IL-6, IL-8], tumor necrosis factor-α [TNF-α]). IL-6 stimulates T- and B-cell differentiation, and IL-8 is a selective chemoattractant for neutrophils.
  - Cytokines promote local resolution and compartmentalization through fibrin deposition.
- In SBP, pathogenic bacteria are cultured from peritoneal fluid without any apparent intra-abdominal surgical treatable source of infection. Recognized as a complication in patients with ascites as a result of cirrhosis of any etiology
  - Generalized bacteremia and translocation of organisms from the gut (*E. coli*, *Klebsiella* sp.) into the portal veins or lymphatics or, less likely, directly into the ascitic fluid may account for the source of the infection.
  - Clearance of bacteria from the bloodstream may be impaired in patients with cirrhosis and ascites.
    - Poor clearance is due to diminished phagocytic activity of the hepatic reticuloendothelial system secondary to cellular functional defects or shunting of blood away from the liver.
  - Complement, necessary for the opsonization of bacteria and ultimately clearance by phagocytes, is decreased in the ascitic fluid.
- Infectious organisms include aerobic gram-negative organisms (*E. coli* and *Klebsiella* species) and aerobic gram-positive organisms (*Streptococcus* and *Enterococcus* species).
- In secondary bacterial peritonitis, the underlying bacterial infection tends to be a complex polymicrobial infection with an average of 3 or 4 different isolates.
  - The most common isolates are combinations of *E. coli* and *Bacteroides fragilis*.
  - The most common gram-positive organisms are nonenterococcal streptococci and enterococci.

ETIOLOGY

- Primary peritonitis: liver cirrhosis or other conditions associated with ascites, such as the following:
  - Budd-Chiari syndrome
  - Congestive heart failure
  - Nephrotic syndrome
  - Systemic lupus erythematosus and other vasculitides
  - Rheumatoid arthritis
- The etiology of secondary peritonitis varies with age.
  - Neonates and infants
    - Meconium peritonitis (begins prenatally)
    - Necrotizing enterocolitis
    - Idiopathic gastrointestinal perforation
    - Perforation due to Hirschsprung disease
    - Spontaneous biliary perforation
    - Omphalitis (common in developing countries due to poor umbilical cord care)
    - Perforation of a urachal cyst
  - Children and adolescents
    - Secondary to appendicitis
    - Perforation of Meckel diverticulum
    - Gastric ulcer perforation
    - Pancreatitis
    - Cholecystitis
    - Traumatic or spontaneous perforation of the intestine
    - Intussusception and other bowel obstruction leading to necrosis
    - Neutropenic colitis (typhlitis)
    - Crohn disease with fistula and abscess formation
    - Toxic megacolon
    - Tuberculosis
    - Salpingitis and pelvic inflammatory disease
    - Toxins

DIAGNOSIS

HISTORY

- Dependent on stage, age, and etiology
- Abdominal pain is the most common symptom.
  - Young children may be unable to verbalize pain.
- Fever, chills, vomiting, diarrhea
- $\sim$10% of SBP cases are entirely asymptomatic; presentation may be subtle.
- Infants may present with poor feeding and lethargy.
- Other less common findings include the following:
  - Hypothermia
  - Hypotension
  - Increasing ascites despite diuretics
  - Worsening encephalopathy
  - Unexplained decrease in renal function

PHYSICAL EXAM
- Abdominal distension
- Rebound tenderness
- Decreased bowel sounds
- Evidence of chronic liver disease
- Evidence of ascites

DIAGNOSTIC TESTS & INTERPRETATION
Lab
- Blood
  - Leukocytosis, elevated CRP
  - There may be leukopenia and thrombocytopenia in sepsis.
- Urinalysis to exclude renal diseases which may mimic peritonitis

Imaging
- Abdominal x-ray may show evidence of ileus, obstruction, or perforation.
- Abdominal ultrasound or CT shows ascites, thickening of bowel wall, and abscesses.

Diagnostic Procedures/Other
- Paracentesis is diagnostic and should be performed in all cases of new-onset ascites and when SBP is suspected.
- To improve culture yield, inoculate blood culture bottles with 10 mL of fluid immediately at the bedside. A separate tube is sent for Gram stain.
- Elevated neutrophil count of $\geq$250/mm^3 in ascitic fluid is the most important laboratory indicator of SBP.
- Fluid chemistries: albumin, total protein, glucose, LDH, amylase, bilirubin
- Serum-ascites albumin gradient = serum albumin minus fluid albumin. Difference >1.1 indicates portal hypertension.
- Diagnostic criteria for secondary peritonitis: positive ascitic fluid culture, neutrophil count of $\geq$250/mm^3, and surgically treatable source of infection

TREATMENT

MEDICATION
- Empiric antibiotic coverage should be initiated immediately and directed primarily toward enteric gram-negative aerobes and gram-positive cocci:
  - After the organism is identified, the antibiotic coverage may be optimized.
  - First line: Cefotaxime is drug of choice for SBP in pediatrics.
  - Consider adding metronidazole for secondary SBP.
- Antibiotic resistance is increasing.
  - Quinolones may be used in areas where resistance is low.
  - Second line: carbapenems for severe nosocomially acquired cases

ADDITIONAL TREATMENT
General Measures
- Fluid resuscitation with isotonic saline, 20 mL/kg boluses up to 60 mL/kg, or albumin if large amounts of fluid are required to restore intravascular volume
- Decompression with nasogastric tube
- Patients at significant risk for SBP will benefit from selective intestinal decontamination with fluoroquinolones, trimethoprim-sulfamethoxazole, or rifaximin as an effective preventive measure.

SURGERY/OTHER PROCEDURES
In secondary peritonitis, surgery is the primary management tool:
- Control of the underlying source of infection by closing, diverting, or resecting the affected bowel
- Intraoperative peritoneal lavage and debridement of loculations and abscesses decrease bacterial inoculum and help prevent recurrent sepsis.
- Older studies in adults show benefit of antibiotic peritoneal lavage; controversial, as it may impair the local response and promote adhesions
- Catheters may be placed to drain a well-defined abscess cavity, form a controlled fistula, or provide access for continuous postoperative peritoneal lavage.

ONGOING CARE

PROGNOSIS
- SBP in adults has in-hospital mortality of 10–50%.
  - SBP markedly worsens the prognosis in patients with cirrhosis.
- Recurrence is common: 60% of patients who survive the 1st episode develop 1 or more recurrences.
- Severe secondary peritonitis in adults has a mortality rate of 30–55%.

COMPLICATIONS
- Hypovolemia from reduced fluid intake, vomiting, and third-space fluid extravasation
- Sepsis and multiorgan failure
- Intra-abdominal abscess
- Long-term: adhesions

ADDITIONAL READING

- European Association for the Study of the Liver. EASL clinical practice guidelines on the management of ascites, spontaneous bacterial peritonitis, and hepatorenal syndrome. *J Hepatol*. 2010;53(3):397–417.
- Haecker FM, Berger D, Schumacher U, et al. Peritonitis in childhood: aspects of pathogenesis and therapy. *Pediatr Surg Int*. 2000;16(3):182–188.
- Leonis MA, Balistreri WF. Evaluation and management of end-stage liver disease in children. *Gastroenterology*. 2008;134(6):1741–1751.
- Saab S, Hernandez JC, Chi AC, et al. Oral antibiotic prophylaxis reduces spontaneous bacterial peritonitis occurrence and improves short-term survival in cirrhosis: a meta-analysis. *Am J Gastroenterol*. 2009;104(4):993–1001; quiz 1002.
- Sabri M, Saps M, Peters JM. Pathophysiology and management of pediatric ascites. *Curr Gastroenterol Rep*. 2003;5(3):240–246.
- Wiest R, Krag A, Gerbes A. Spontaneous bacterial peritonitis: recent guidelines and beyond. *Gut*. 2012;61(2):297–310.
- Wong CL, Holroyd-Leduc J, Thorpe KE, et al. Does this patient have bacterial peritonitis or portal hypertension? How do I perform a paracentesis and analyze the results? *JAMA*. 2008;299(10):1166–1178.

CODES

ICD10
- K65.9 Peritonitis, unspecified
- K65.2 Spontaneous bacterial peritonitis
- P78.1 Other neonatal peritonitis

FAQ
- Q: Is peritonitis common in children with ascites?
- A: Despite the frequency of ascites from many different causes, peritonitis occurs rarely. In the setting of children with chronic liver disease and ascites, SBP may occur.
- Q: What are the most useful laboratory aids for this diagnosis?
- A: Paracentesis and analysis of the fluid neutrophil count provides the most useful information regarding the diagnosis of peritonitis. Fluid culture is not required for diagnosis but helps to guide therapy.

PERITONSILLAR ABSCESS

Nicholas Tsarouhas

BASICS

DESCRIPTION

Infectious complication of tonsillitis or pharyngitis resulting in an accumulation of purulence in the tonsillar fossa. Also referred to as "quinsy."

EPIDEMIOLOGY

- Most common deep space infection of head and neck
- Seen most commonly in adolescents but occasionally in younger children

RISK FACTORS

- Tonsillitis
- Pharyngitis

GENERAL PREVENTION

Abscess formation can often be prevented if appropriate antimicrobial therapy is initiated while the infection is still at the cellulitis stage.

PATHOPHYSIOLOGY

- Infectious tonsillopharyngitis progresses from cellulitis to abscess.
- The infection starts in the intratonsillar fossa, which is situated between the upper pole and the body of the tonsil and eventually extends around the tonsil.
- The abscess is a suppuration outside the tonsillar capsule, in proximity to the upper pole of the tonsil, involving the soft palate.
- Purulence usually collects within one tonsillar fossa, but it may be bilateral.
- The pterygoid musculature may become irritated by pus and inflammation, which leads to the clinical finding of trismus.
- Tonsillar and peritonsillar edema may lead to compromise of the upper airway.

ETIOLOGY

- Most of these true abscesses are polymicrobial.
- Group A β-hemolytic streptococci (GABHS)
- α-Hemolytic streptococci
- *Staphylococcus aureus*: Prevalence of methicillin-resistant *S. aureus* continues to increase.
- Anaerobic bacteria play an important role:
  - *Prevotella*
  - *Porphyromonas*
  - *Fusobacterium*
  - *Peptostreptococcus*
- Possible synergy between anaerobes and GABHS
- Gram negatives such as *Haemophilus influenzae* and, more rarely, *Pseudomonas* species may be isolated.

COMMONLY ASSOCIATED CONDITIONS

- Tonsillitis or pharyngitis usually precedes its development.
- Peritonsillar cellulitis is often associated with infectious mononucleosis.

DIAGNOSIS

HISTORY

- Fever and sore throat
  - Most common initial complaints
- Trouble swallowing, pain with opening the mouth (trismus), muffled ("hot potato") voice
  - Classic presenting symptoms
- Unilateral neck or ear pain
  - Other common presenting symptoms

PHYSICAL EXAM

- Unilateral peritonsillar fullness or bulging of the posterior, superior, soft palate
  - Diagnostic finding
- Uvular deviation
  - Classic finding, although it may be absent in the more rare bilateral peritonsillar abscess
- Palpable fluctuance of palatal swelling
  - Calls for urgent aspiration
- Erythematous, edematous pharynx, with enlarged and exudative tonsils
  - Coexisting tonsillopharyngitis is common.
- Cervical adenopathy
  - Common
- Drooling
  - Often present
- Torticollis
  - Sometimes seen

DIAGNOSTIC TESTS & INTERPRETATION

Lab

- WBC count
  - Not a mandatory part of the workup
  - Usually elevated with prominent left shift
- Rapid streptococcal throat antigen studies
  - Helpful to diagnose GABHS infection
- Gram stain and culture of aspirate specimen
  - Confirms causative microorganism
- Monospot/EBV antibody titers
  - Not a mandatory part of the workup
  - Infectious mononucleosis is both in the differential diagnosis and may coexist in some cases of peritonsillar abscess.

Imaging

- Radiographic studies are rarely necessary, as this is clinical diagnosis.
- Intraoral ultrasound or CT (with contrast):
  - Sometimes useful if clinical distinction of peritonsillar cellulitis from peritonsillar abscess is difficult
  - CT scan is most useful if patient cannot open mouth secondary to trismus.
  - CT scan is also important if deep neck extension is suspected.
- MRI
  - MRI may be more precise than CT in detecting multiple space involvement and, of course, is devoid of radiation exposure.
  - Pediatric use is limited by need for longer acquisition time and greater need for patient cooperation.
  - In younger children, the need for sedation for MRI introduces additional logistical challenges and potential airway risks.

DIFFERENTIAL DIAGNOSIS

- Peritonsillar cellulitis
  - Most common diagnostic consideration
  - Also referred to as "phlegmon"
  - Can be distinguished by the lack of classic peritonsillar abscess findings: peritonsillar space fullness, uvular deviation, and trismus
- Retropharyngeal abscess
  - Minimal to no peritonsillar findings
  - Widened prevertebral space on lateral neck radiograph
  - This airway-compromising disease usually occurs in preschool children, not adolescents.
- Epiglottitis
  - This life-threatening airway emergency presents abruptly with fever, stridor, increased work of breathing, and drooling.
  - Usually occurs in toxic-appearing children 3–7 years old
  - Rare entity in children since the advent of the *Haemophilus influenzae* type b vaccine
- Other infectious causes of severe tonsillopharyngitis:
  - EBV (infectious mononucleosis), coxsackievirus (herpangina), *Corynebacterium diphtheriae,* and *Neisseria gonorrhoeae*

TREATMENT

MEDICATION

First Line

- Clindamycin or ampicillin/sulbactam are the most commonly used 1st-line antibiotics, owing to their efficacy versus GABHS, *Staphylococcus*, and anaerobes.
- As methicillin-resistant *S. aureus* isolates continue to increase, clindamycin is becoming more popular as drug of choice.
- Some initiate therapy with high-dose IV penicillin—in the presence of a positive strep antigen or throat culture study.

Second Line

- Nafcillin, oxacillin, and cefazolin are acceptable antibiotic alternatives.
- Steroids
  - Some experts recommend steroids to decrease swelling, pain, and trismus.
  - Most evidence from adult rather than pediatric studies
  - Methylprednisolone, dexamethasone, and prednisone all have been used.

ADDITIONAL TREATMENT

General Measures

Treating an abscess without surgical drainage is inadequate and can have airway-threatening implications.

- Abscesses should be urgently/emergently drained via either needle aspiration or surgical incision and drainage.
- Antibiotic therapy as above
- Steroid therapy recommended by some.
- Appropriate analgesia and adequate hydration should be ensured in all cases.

ISSUES FOR REFERRAL

Peritonsillar abscess: Otorhinolaryngology consultation is imperative both for acute and chronic management.

SURGERY/OTHER PROCEDURES

- As mentioned earlier, either needle aspiration or surgical incision and drainage is mandatory in the acute setting for true abscesses.
- Most surgeons currently prefer interval tonsillectomy after the acute infection has been managed with antibiotics and an acute drainage procedure (needle aspiration or I&D).
- Surgical drainage with tonsillectomy is considered in children not responding to parenteral antibiotics within 24–48 hours.
- Acute or "hot" tonsillectomy (also "quinsy tonsillectomy") is advocated by some.

ONGOING CARE

FOLLOW-UP RECOMMENDATIONS

- Patients may be discharged on oral antibiotics to complete a 10–14-day course when afebrile and peritonsillar swelling has subsided.
- Tonsillectomy should be considered after severe or recurrent peritonsillar abscesses.

PROGNOSIS

- Complete recovery with appropriate therapy.
- Recurrence of the abscess may occur.

COMPLICATIONS

- Upper airway obstruction is the most feared complication.
- Dehydration from decreased oral intake is the most common complication, however.
- Abscesses left untreated can rupture spontaneously into the pharynx, leading to aspiration and pneumonia.
- Other serious complications include parapharyngeal abscess, jugular vein suppurative thrombophlebitis (Lemierre syndrome), cavernous sinus thrombosis, sepsis, brain abscess, meningitis, and dissection into the internal carotid artery.
- Even after appropriate drainage, a small number (10–15%) of peritonsillar abscesses may reform.

ADDITIONAL READING

- Hayward G, Thompson MJ, Perera R, et al. Corticosteroids as standalone or add-on treatment for sore throat. *Cochrane Database Syst Rev*. 2012;10:CD008268.
- Maroldi R, Farina D, Ravanelli M, et al. Emergency imaging assessment of deep neck space infections. *Semin Ultrasound CT MR*. 2012;33(5):432–442.
- Powell J, Wilson JA. An evidence-based review of peritonsillar abscess. *Clin Otolaryngol*. 2012;37(2):136–145.
- Stoner MJ, Dulaurier M. Pediatric ENT emergencies. *Emerg Med Clin North Am*. 2013;31(3):795–808.
- Tagliareni JM, Clarkson EI. Tonsillitis, peritonsillar and lateral pharyngeal abscesses. *Oral Maxillofac Surg Clin North Am*. 2012;24(2):197–204, viii.

CODES

ICD10

J36 Peritonsillar abscess

FAQ

- Q: Are radiographs necessary to make the diagnosis of peritonsillar abscess?
- A: No. The physical examination is diagnostic. A lateral neck radiograph, ultrasound, CT, or MRI are indicated only if the diagnosis is in question or to delineate extent of disease or additional complications.
- Q: Is surgical consultation necessary in cases of peritonsillar abscess?
- A: Yes. Otorhinolaryngology consultation is indicated for both acute as well as chronic management.

PERSISTENT PULMONARY HYPERTENSION OF THE NEWBORN

Jessica Howlett • Jenny Yu

BASICS

DESCRIPTION
Clinical syndrome of severe respiratory failure and hypoxia in a neonate characterized by high systemic pulmonary arterial pressures, tricuspid regurgitation, and intracardiac shunting from right to left when pulmonary vascular resistance fails to decrease after birth

EPIDEMIOLOGY
- Incidence of ~2–6 per 1,000 term live newborns, decreasing incidence with the decreased number of deliveries >41 weeks gestation
- Mostly occurs in full-term newborns, owing to the presence of the muscular layer of arterioles, the risk of uteroplacental insufficiency, and the potential for the passage of meconium in utero, but it can complicate the course of an older premature baby with chronic lung disease.
- Meconium aspiration is the number one cause of persistent pulmonary hypertension of the newborn (PPHN).
- PPHN complicates the course of about 10% of newborns with respiratory failure.

RISK FACTORS
Genetics
- Sporadic in occurrence
- Alveolar capillary dysplasia has been documented to be a rare cause of PPHN. The genetic cause is unknown, but it appears to be familial.
- Surfactant B deficiency has also been implicated, but it is a rare, lethal, autosomal recessive disorder.

PATHOPHYSIOLOGY
- At a neonate's first breath after delivery, the pulmonary vascular resistance normally decreases to redirect ~50% of the cardiac output to the pulmonary circulation. This phenomenon fails to occur in PPHN, hence the previous name of this condition, "persistent fetal circulation."
- Increased pulmonary vascular resistance increases right ventricular afterload, causing a backflow of blood to the right heart. This leads to increased right heart pressures (and subsequent tricuspid regurgitation), which can lead to right ventricular failure.
- Increased pulmonary arterial pressures also cause intracardiac shunting across any patent foramen ovale, ductus arteriosus, or atrioseptal or ventriculoseptal defect that may be present. This shunting causes more deoxygenated blood to go to the left heart and to be pumped to the body. The oxygen saturations postductally are lower than preductally.
- Deoxygenated blood in the left heart can lead to ischemic damage to the heart and right or left ventricular failure.
- If there is no shunting of blood, or the blood cannot get from the right to left heart because of a lack of persistent fetal pathways, a neonate may develop poor systemic perfusion, severe acidosis, shock, right ventricular failure, and even death.
- Any hypoxia, acidosis, or stress that occurs after birth further increases pulmonary vascular resistance.

ETIOLOGY
- Abnormal persistence of pulmonary vasculature constriction after birth secondary to underlying disease: infection, pneumonia, or meconium aspiration
- Secondary to an anatomic abnormality that has caused hypoplastic vasculature: congenital diaphragmatic hernia, oligohydramnios and pulmonary hypoplasia, or alveolar capillary dysplasia
- Idiopathic: The pulmonary vasculature is remodeled due to chronic in utero stress or hypoxia or the maternal use of nonsteroidal anti-inflammatory drugs (NSAIDs) near term. Data is unclear on maternal use of selective serotonin reuptake inhibitors (SSRIs) in the 2nd trimester and PPHN.

COMMONLY ASSOCIATED CONDITIONS
Related to the underlying disease or as a complication of treatment
- Pneumothorax or air leak syndrome
- Chronic lung damage
- Long-term developmental delays
- Cerebral palsy
- Sensorineural hearing loss

DIAGNOSIS

HISTORY
- Pregnancy history
  - Congenital diaphragmatic hernia, congenital pulmonary airway malformation, and congenital heart disease can all be diagnosed with a prenatal ultrasound.
  - History of oligohydramnios, which may be associated with pulmonary hypoplasia in the neonate
- Problems during labor and delivery
  - Events that can cause fetal distress and/or hypoxia: maternal chorioamnionitis, group B streptococcal infection, difficult delivery, or meconium aspiration
- Initial clinical course
  - Infants with PPHN usually present with mild respiratory distress that worsens in the 1st minutes to hours of life, progressing to respiratory failure, labile oxygenation with pre- and postductal saturation differences >5%, hypoxia, and poor perfusion.
- Infants with cardiac disease, congenital pulmonary airway malformation, or congenital diaphragmatic hernia are usually cyanotic and in significant distress from birth.

PHYSICAL EXAM
- The following physical exam findings suggest a diagnosis of PPHN:
  - Significant respiratory distress with tachypnea, nasal flaring, grunting, and retractions and cyanosis
  - Lung sounds may be clear or coarse.
  - Pale, gray color with poor perfusion
  - Tricuspid regurgitation murmur heard at the left lower sternal border or prominent S2
- The following physical exam findings suggest diagnoses other than idiopathic PPHN:
  - Barrel chest shape suggests a pneumothorax or meconium aspiration.
  - Scaphoid abdomen suggests congenital diaphragmatic hernia.

DIAGNOSTIC TESTS & INTERPRETATION
Lab
- CBC with differential: leukocytosis, leukopenia, bandemia, or neutropenia suggests bacterial infection
- Blood culture: should be performed in all cases of PPHN to rule out infection
- Frequent arterial blood gases
  - Help to determine degree of hypoxia, hypercapnia, acidosis, and illness
  - Help manage ventilator support
  - Determine need for extracorporeal membrane oxygenation (ECMO) by calculating the oxygenation index (OI)
- OI
  - OI = (mean airway pressure × FiO_2/PaO_2) × 100
  - Used to express severity of respiratory distress and to determine if neonate is a candidate for ECMO
  - Should be calculated with every blood gas: 3 OIs >40 suggest the need for ECMO.
- Hyperoxia test: While exposed to FiO_2 of 100% oxygen, a PaO_2 >250 mm Hg almost completely rules out cyanotic heart disease.

Imaging
- Chest radiograph
  - In idiopathic disease, usually shows clear lungs
  - Will help diagnose pneumothorax, hyperinflation, meconium aspiration, and atelectasis
  - Assessing cardiac silhouette and pulmonary vascular markings may help rule out some congenital heart disease.
- Echocardiogram (very important)
  - To exclude congenital heart disease
  - To diagnose PPHN with right to left blood flow in the patent ductus arteriosus (PDA) and can estimate pulmonary artery pressure by septal positioning and tricuspid regurgitation
  - To follow cardiac output and function

DIFFERENTIAL DIAGNOSIS
- Congenital
  - Cyanotic congenital heart disease
  - Total anomalous pulmonary venous return
  - Congenital diaphragmatic hernia
  - Congenital pulmonary airway malformation
  - Alveolar capillary dysplasia
- Infectious
  - Pneumonia
  - Sepsis
- Pulmonary
  - Meconium aspiration syndrome
  - Blood or amniotic fluid aspiration
  - Pneumothorax or air leak syndrome
  - Surfactant deficiency (respiratory distress syndrome [RDS])
  - Pulmonary hypoplasia
  - Idiopathic pulmonary hypertension

P

TREATMENT

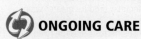

GENERAL MEASURES

- All infants should be transferred to a level III neonatal intensive care unit where high-frequency ventilation (HFV) and inhaled nitric oxide (iNO) are available. If the neonate meets or nearly meets criteria for starting ECMO (OI >40 on 3 different blood gases), then ECMO should be available at the receiving institution.
- Support respiratory status
  - Conventional ventilation or HFV to improve oxygenation and ventilation while minimizing lung damage
  - No set guidelines for ventilator management
  - Most institutions feel that HFV minimizes lung damage when high mean airway pressures (>15 cm H_2O) are needed.
  - Frequent monitoring to keep PaO_2 between 60 and 90 mm Hg, PCO_2 >35–45 mm Hg, and OI below ECMO criteria (OI >40 times 3)
  - Avoid hyperventilation, which has been associated with poor neurodevelopmental outcome.
- Lower the pulmonary vascular resistance and thus promote pulmonary blood flow:
  - Give 100% oxygen.
  - Keep blood gas pH normal (7.3–7.4) while keeping $PaCO_2$ >35–45 mm Hg by ventilator manipulation.
  - Keep systemic BP high (mean BP >45–50 mm Hg) with volume, transfusions, or medications.
  - Treat acidosis with fluid, blood, or bicarbonate infusion.
- Improve O_2 saturation and O_2 tissue delivery:
  - Initially, 100% O_2 should be used to keep the PaO_2 >60–90 mm Hg and the O_2 saturation around >97%. The O_2 can be weaned very slowly (2% per hour).
  - iNO, a pulmonary vasodilator, should be used if the infant is on 100% (FiO_2) O_2 and the OI is >20 on two blood gases.
    - Has been shown to decrease the need for ECMO in term neonates with hypoxic respiratory failure secondary to PPHN, except for those babies with congenital diaphragmatic hernia
    - Wean slowly: If oxygen and iNO are weaned too quickly, the infant can become critically ill because PPHN is a very labile condition.
    - 30% of infants with PPHN do not respond to iNO and will need ECMO.
- Reduce oxygen demand:
  - Sedatives and paralytics may be given to prevent fluctuations in oxygenation during care. Minimize the use of paralytics because they have been shown to increase mortality.
  - Minimize stimulation
- Treat any underlying lung disease with the following, if applicable:
  - Antibiotics
  - Surfactant (especially in meconium aspiration)

ALERT

- Can be difficult to differentiate cyanotic congenital heart disease from PPHN. Infants who fail to improve should be reevaluated for an underlying disease process.
- PPHN is a very labile condition. Neonates can change from being stable to being very sick and emergently needing ECMO.
- ECMO, although lifesaving and with a good survival rate, is not without problems. Side effects include the following:
  - Repeated exposure to blood products
  - Risk of bleeding
  - Potential for long-term neurologic sequelae
  - Long-term risk of having only one patent carotid artery

ONGOING CARE

PROGNOSIS

- PPHN usually resolves either spontaneously or as the underlying parenchymal lung disease improves.
- Survival rate is good even for neonates who receive ECMO. Survival rate and incidence of long-term sequelae depend on underlying disease and severity of illness.
- Survival rate for all causes of PPHN in patients not requiring ECMO is >90%. ~10–20% has sensorineural hearing loss or an abnormal neurologic exam at follow-up.
- For those requiring ECMO, survival rate is 80% for idiopathic disease, 90% for meconium aspiration syndrome, 80% for disease secondary to sepsis, and 50–60% for patients with congenital diaphragmatic hernia. Roughly 20% of these survivors have sensorineural hearing loss or abnormal neurologic examinations at follow-up.

COMPLICATIONS

- Myocardial dysfunction
- Congestive heart failure (CHF)
- Hypoxic ischemic insult

ADDITIONAL READING

- Iacovidou N, Syggelou A, Fanos V, et al. The use of sildenafil in the treatment of persistent pulmonary hypertension of the newborn: a review of the literature. *Curr Pharm Des*. 2012;18(21):3034–3045.
- Konduri GG, Kim UO. Advances in the diagnosis and management of persistent pulmonary hypertension of the newborn. *Pediatr Clin North Am*. 2009;56(3): 579–600.
- Lipkin PH, Davidson D, Spivak L, et al. Neurodevelopmental and medical outcomes of persistent pulmonary hypertension in term newborns treated with nitric oxide. *J Pediatr*. 2002;140(3):306–310.
- Sadiq HF, Mantych G, Benawra RS, et al. Inhaled nitric oxide in the treatment of moderate persistent pulmonary hypertension of the newborn: a randomized controlled, multicenter trial. *J Perinatol*. 2003;23(2):98–103.

CODES

ICD10

P29.3 Persistent fetal circulation

FAQ

- Q: Does iNO improve outcome in newborns with severe PPHN?
- A: Yes. iNO has been shown to decrease the need for ECMO by 40%. Recommended starting dose is 20 ppm. Follow-up studies have shown no difference in long-term disabilities between those babies treated and not treated with iNO. Long-term outcome is mainly determined by the underlying disease and the severity of illness.
- Q: Are there any other potential therapies for treating PPHN?
- A: Yes. Inhaled tolazoline, other smooth muscle relaxants (dipyridamole, zaprinast, and E4021), iloprost, and bosentan have been studied and have been shown to be effective in enhancing the vasodilatory effects of iNO. Sildenafil has been shown to be beneficial but is being used in select cases under special guidance due to concerns for increased mortality in children with pulmonary artery hypertension.

PERTHES DISEASE

Harry K.W. Kim

BASICS

DESCRIPTION

Childhood femoral head osteonecrosis of unknown etiology, which can weaken the femoral head and produce a permanent femoral head deformity in some patients, predisposing them to early arthritis

EPIDEMIOLOGY

- Prevalence varies depending on the region: 0–15 per 100,000 children <15 years of age.
- In the United States and Canada, about 5 per 100,000
- Rare in African Americans
- Most frequent in children 4–8 years old
- 3–5 times more common in boys than girls
- 10–15% develop bilateral disease in asynchronous fashion.

PATHOPHYSIOLOGY

- A partial or complete disruption of blood supply to the femoral head produces a partial or total femoral head osteonecrosis.
  - The greater the femoral head involvement, the worse the prognosis.
  - Bone necrosis and subsequent resorption of necrotic bone weaken the femoral head.
  - Weight bearing worsens the femoral head deformity.
- Chronic hip joint synovitis also develops producing pain and restriction of motion.
- Necrotic femoral head goes through 4 stages of healing over 3–5 years:
  - 1. Stage of avascular necrosis
    - Smaller femoral head epiphysis with increased radiodensity
  - 2. Stage of fragmentation
    - Necrotic epiphysis shows fragmentation.
    - Necrotic bone is resorbed, weakening the head.
    - Most deformity occurs during this stage, which lasts 1–2 years.
  - 3. Stage of reossification
    - New bone begins to fill the epiphysis.
    - Longest stage, lasting up to 3 years
  - 4. Healed
    - Femoral head is completely reossified.
    - Not all heal back in round shape, and deformed femoral heads are at risk for developing arthritis later.

ETIOLOGY

- Unknown
- Unlikely genetic transmission, as <5% have family history
- Many theories:
  - Multifactorial (genetic predisposition with environmental trigger)
  - Hyperactivity and subclinical trauma
  - Type II collagenopathy
  - Thrombophilia (factor V Leiden)
  - Tobacco smoke exposure

COMMONLY ASSOCIATED CONDITIONS

- Delayed bone age
- Hyperactivity
- Genitourinary anomalies (hypospadias, undescended testis, and inguinal hernia)

DIAGNOSIS

HISTORY

- Age at onset of symptoms, location, duration, patient's activity level, and risk factors for osteonecrosis are important.
- Age at onset before 6 years has better prognosis than after 6 years.
- Most common symptoms are limping and pain.
  - Insidious, relatively mild, able to ambulate (unlike septic hip)
  - Commonly complain of knee or thigh pain and NOT hip or groin pain, which may mislead an unsuspecting physician and delay the diagnosis
  - Weeks' to months' duration with waxing and waning of pain and limping
  - Worse during or after sports activities
- Participation in high-impact activities that involve running and jumping may produce greater symptoms and synovitis.
- Known causes of osteonecrosis must be ruled out through history:
  - Previous hip surgery
  - Corticosteroid use
  - Sickle cell disease
  - Neonatal hip sepsis
  - Coagulopathy
  - Gaucher disease
- Obtain family history for Perthes disease, skeletal dysplasias, and early arthritis.

PHYSICAL EXAM

- Because pain can be nonspecific (such as knee or thigh pain), careful exam is required to localize the source of pain.
- Gently check hip and knee passive range of motion with patient recumbent:
  - Patients with Perthes will have limited hip internal rotation and abduction. Knee exam should be normal.
  - The loss of motion may be mild in the early stage and becomes worse during the stage of fragmentation.
  - In severe cases, hip flexion and adduction contractures may be found.
- Assess walking for limping and Trendelenburg gait: head and trunk leaning over to the affected leg as it takes stance.
- Positive Trendelenburg test
  - Have the patient lift one leg off the ground while standing straight.
  - When the weight is on the normal hip, the pelvis is maintained in a horizontal position.
  - When the weight is on the affected hip, the pelvis drops due to the hip abductor muscle weakness.
- Atrophy of thigh muscles and slight shortening of the affected side are late findings.
- Check face, hands, feet, chest, and spine for signs of skeletal dysplasia.

DIAGNOSTIC TESTS & INTERPRETATION

Lab

- Labs are not required.
- May be helpful if infectious, inflammatory, or metabolic conditions mimicking Perthes are being considered.

Imaging

- Diagnosis of Perthes requires imaging.
- Anteroposterior (AP) pelvis and frog-leg lateral views are primarily used.
- Radiographic findings vary depending on the duration and the stage of the disease.
  - Early stage: smaller femoral epiphysis, increased radiodensity, and a widened space between the epiphysis and the medial acetabulum compared to the normal side. In some patients (30%) subchondral fracture or crescent sign can be seen.
  - Fragmentation stage: slight to severe flattening of the epiphysis, which is best seen on a lateral view; fragmented appearance of the epiphysis with radiolucent areas (bone resorption); and lateral extrusion or subluxation of the epiphysis
- MRI, especially gadolinium-enhanced MRI, maybe helpful in the early stage of the disease when the diagnosis is questionable.

DIFFERENTIAL DIAGNOSIS

Perthes is a diagnosis of exclusion. Known causes of osteonecrosis along with other conditions that mimic Perthes must be ruled out.

- Transient or toxic synovitis
- Infection
  - Septic arthritis
  - Subacute osteomyelitis
  - Tuberculosis of hip
- Chondrolysis
- Juvenile rheumatoid arthritis
- Traumatic osteonecrosis secondary to hip fracture or dislocation
- Corticosteroid-associated osteonecrosis: for treatment of leukemia and inflammatory conditions
- Sickle cell disease–induced osteonecrosis
- Iatrogenic osteonecrosis: hip surgery for DDH, hip pinning

- Tumor or tumorlike conditions affecting the proximal femoral epiphysis or acetabulum
  - Osteoid osteoma
  - Chondroblastoma
  - Bone cyst
- Skeletal dysplasias
  - Multiple epiphyseal dysplasia
  - Trichorhinophalangeal syndrome
  - Spondyloepiphyseal dysplasia
- Gaucher disease
- Hypothyroidism
- Hemophilia

TREATMENT

- Treatment principles
  - Restore and maintain good hip motion, especially abduction.
  - Prevent the collapse and lateral extrusion of the femoral epiphysis.
- Initial treatment for symptomatic patients include rest, activity restriction, weight-relief using crutches, walker or wheelchair, gentle range of motion exercises, and NSAIDs.
- In general, patients should be referred and followed by a pediatric orthopedic surgeon with expertise in managing Perthes.
- Early recognition and treatment may prevent or minimize the development of the femoral head deformity.

MEDICATION

- NSAIDs should only be used for a short duration (few days to a week), as prolonged use may inhibit bone formation.
- Supplemental calcium and vitamin D if poor diet and/or inadequate sun exposure.

ADDITIONAL TREATMENT

General Measures

- Based on the age at onset of the disease, the stage of disease, and the extent of head involvement
- Patients with the onset of disease before age 6 years are treated with nonoperative means:
  - Bed rest for few days if motion is severely limited
  - Weight relief of the affected limb using crutches, walker, or wheelchair during the stages of avascular necrosis and fragmentation if severe disease
  - Range of motion exercises
  - Petrie casts (long leg casts with abduction bar) and abduction bracing if unresponsive to aforementioned
- Surgery to keep the femoral head contained within the acetabulum in older age group of patients

ISSUES FOR REFERRAL

Patients with Perthes disease should be referred to a pediatric orthopedic surgeon.

SURGERY/OTHER PROCEDURES

- Surgical treatments such as femoral varus osteotomy or pelvic osteotomy are recommended for patients with the onset of disease after age 8 years and greater than 50% head involvement.
- For 6–8-year-old age group, unclear whether surgical treatment is beneficial.

ONGOING CARE

FOLLOW-UP RECOMMENDATIONS

- Patient should be seen every 3–4 months to assess disease progression and compliance to treatment during the active phase of disease.
- Activity and weight-bearing restrictions generally continue until patient enters the reossification stage.

Patient Monitoring

Examine for the following:

- Worsening of limping and pain
- Loss of hip motion, especially hip abduction
- Radiographic changes: progression of femoral head collapse, lateral extrusion of the femoral epiphysis, and subluxation

PROGNOSIS

- Depends on the following:
  - Age at onset of the disease (onset before age 6 years is better than after age 6 years)
  - Extent of femoral head involvement; poorer prognosis if >50% head involvement
  - Development of poor prognostic radiographic signs: flattening of the lateral part of the epiphysis (lateral pillar C hip), subluxation of the epiphysis, growth disturbance of the proximal femoral physis producing short, broad femoral neck
- Long-term prognosis depends on the shape of the femoral head at skeletal maturity and how well it fits the acetabulum.

COMPLICATIONS

- 1–2 cm limb length discrepancy
- Restricted hip range of motion
- Residual femoral head deformity
- Overriding greater trochanter with lateral impingement and abductor weakness
- Femoroacetabular impingement and labral disease
- Early osteoarthritis

ADDITIONAL READING

- Frick SL. Evaluation of the child who has hip pain. *Orthop Clin North Am*. 2006;37(2):133–140, v.
- International Perthes Study Group: www.perthesdisease.org
- Kim HK. Pathophysiology and new strategies for the treatment of Legg-Calvé-Perthes disease. *J Bone Joint Surg Am*. 2012;94(7):659–669.
- Kim HK. Legg-Calvé-Perthes disease. *J Am Acad Orthop Surg*. 2010;18(11):676–686.
- Saran N, Varghese R, Mulpuri K. Do femoral or salter innominate osteotomies improve femoral head sphericity in Legg-Calvé-Perthes disease? A meta-analysis. *Clin Orthop Relat Res*. 2012;470(9): 2383–2393.

CODES

ICD10

- M91.10 Juvenile osteochondrosis of head of femur, unspecified leg
- M91.11 Juvenile osteochondrosis of head of femur, right leg
- M91.12 Juvenile osteochondrosis of head of femur, left leg

FAQ

- Q: When should I obtain radiographs?
- A: Diagnosis of Perthes requires radiographic confirmation. AP pelvis and frog-leg lateral radiographs should be obtained when a child presents with intermittent thigh, knee, or groin pain that has been present for weeks and has the finding of decreased hip range of motion but normal knee exam.
- Q: Why do patients with Perthes complain of knee or thigh pain instead of hip pain?
- A: Knee, thigh, and hip regions share the same sensory nerve. Thus, pain originating from one site (for instance hip) can be felt by a child as if it is originating from another site (for instance knee). This can cause confusion in localizing the correct source of pain and obtaining appropriate radiographs. Some patients get knee x-rays and MRI before getting hip x-rays because of this. Thus, it is important to examine both the hip and the knee even if a child complains only of knee pain.

PERTUSSIS

Camille Sabella

BASICS

DESCRIPTION

Pertussis (whooping cough), classically caused by *Bordetella pertussis*, is a protracted illness characterized by spasms of cough.

EPIDEMIOLOGY

- Pertussis is one of the most highly communicable diseases with attack rates close to 100% in susceptible individuals exposed at close range.
- Humans are the only hosts of *B. pertussis*.
- Route of spread is via large aerosolized respiratory droplets.
- Spread most commonly occurs during the catarrhal stage and first 2 weeks of cough onset.
- Incubation period 5–21 days.
- Pertussis occurs with seasonal peaks (late summer-autumn) and 3–5-year cycles of increased incidence of disease.
- Adolescents and adults serve as major reservoirs and source of pertussis for infants.

Incidence

- Pertussis infection rates have steadily risen since the early 1980s.
  - This is due to the combination of imperfect vaccines, waning immunity, incomplete vaccination, low transplacental protection for infants, and increased detection and reporting.
- Infants younger than 2 months of age have the highest age-related incidence.
- Rates in adolescents have been steadily increasing and now approach rates in infants.
- Studies have indicated that 10–30% of adolescents and young adults with prolonged cough have pertussis.

GENERAL PREVENTION

- Infection control
  - Isolation of hospitalized patient: droplet precautions for 5 days after starting appropriate antimicrobial therapy or for 3 weeks after the onset of cough, if antibiotics were not given
  - Care of exposed people: Exposed individuals (all household contacts, other close contacts, other children in child care) should receive chemoprophylaxis (same agents and doses as treatment; see the following discussion) to limit secondary transmission, regardless of immunization status. Immunization should be given to all unimmunized and underimmunized children and to adolescents and adults who have not yet received the Tdap booster vaccination.
- Immunizations
  - All pertussis vaccines available in the United States are acellular vaccines in combination with diphtheria and tetanus toxoids.
  - Universal immunization of all children <7 years of age with DTaP vaccine is recommended as per CDC and AAP guidelines.
  - Undervaccinated children ages 7–10 years, all adolescents ages 11–18 years, adults ages 19–64 years, as well as certain adults ages 65 years and older should receive a single dose of Tdap vaccine to help control the rate of infection in infants and young children.

PATHOPHYSIOLOGY

- Tropism and replication are limited to the ciliated epithelium of the respiratory tract.
- Biologically active substances such as pertussis toxin (PT), filamentous hemagglutinin, tracheal cytotoxin, adenylate cyclase, and pertactin are responsible for virulence of the organism, including attachment, ciliostasis, impaired leukocyte function, and local epithelial damage.

ETIOLOGY

- *B. pertussis*, a small, nonmotile, fastidious, gram-negative coccobacillus, causes classic pertussis.
- *Bordetella parapertussis* causes a less protracted cough illness.

DIAGNOSIS

HISTORY

- History of a cough illness in other family members, including older siblings, parents, and grandparents, is important to elicit.
- 3 clinical stages
  - Catarrhal stage (1–2 weeks) with symptoms of an upper respiratory infection
  - Paroxysmal stage (≥2–4 weeks) characterized by paroxysmal cough with increased severity and frequency producing the characteristic whoop during the sudden forceful inspiratory phase; posttussive vomiting is also observed during this stage.
  - The convalescent stage begins and lasts 1–2 weeks, but cough can persist for several months. In the adolescent or adult, long-standing cough of 2–3 weeks is the hallmark symptom. Most patients report a paroxysmal or staccato quality to the cough.
- Apnea is a common manifestation in infants <6 months. The characteristic whoop is typically absent. Short catarrhal stage, gasping, and choking are other manifestations in young infants.
- History of fever is typically absent.

PHYSICAL EXAM

- Normal physical examination between paroxysms is supportive of the diagnosis.
- Conjunctival hemorrhage and petechiae on the upper body may be present.
- Cyanosis, apnea, and bradycardia can be observed during the paroxysmal stage in young infants.
- Fever and signs of lower respiratory tract disease are uncommon.

DIAGNOSTIC TESTS & INTERPRETATION

Lab

- CBC
  - Leukocytosis (15,000–100,000 cells/mm^3 with predominant lymphocytosis is commonly observed at the end of the catarrhal stage and throughout the paroxysmal stage of illness in infants and children; not commonly observed in adolescents and adult
- Culture of *B. pertussis*
  - Achieved using calcium alginate or Dacron swabs of the nasopharynx and plated onto selective media such as Regan-Lowe and incubated for 10 days
  - Most frequently successful during the catarrhal or early paroxysmal stages and is rarely found beyond the 3rd week of illness
  - Specificity 100%; overall sensitivity is 60–70% but can be lower in previously vaccinated individuals if antibiotics have already been given or if beyond the 3rd week of illness.
- Polymerase chain reaction (PCR)
  - Increasingly used; higher sensitivity and more rapid diagnosis than culture in the detection of *B. pertussis* from nasopharyngeal specimens
  - There is no FDA-licensed PCR test available, and there are no standardized protocols or reagents.
- Direct immunofluorescent assays (DFA) of nasopharyngeal specimens are no longer recommended for the diagnosis of pertussis.
- Serology
  - Can be helpful later in the course of the illness
  - No commercially available FDA-approved test available and difficult to interpret in previously immunized individuals
  - In the absence of recent immunization, an elevated serum IgG antibody to PT after 2 weeks of onset of cough is suggestive of recent infection. An increasing titer or a single IgG anti-PT value of approximately 100 IU/mL or greater can be used for diagnosis.

P

Imaging
Chest radiograph: may reveal perihilar infiltrates, interstitial edema, and atelectasis

DIFFERENTIAL DIAGNOSIS
- *B. parapertussis*
- Adenoviruses
- *Mycoplasma pneumoniae*
- *Chlamydia trachomatis*
- Bronchiolitis
- Bacterial pneumonia
- Cystic fibrosis
- Tuberculosis
- Foreign body aspiration
- Reactive airway disease

TREATMENT

MEDICATION
- Azithromycin (PO)
  - 10 mg/kg as a single dose on day 1, then 5 mg/kg/24 h as a single daily dose on days 2–5 is recommended for ages ≥6 months.
  - For infants <6 months of age, dosage is 10 mg/kg/24 h as a single daily dose for 5 days.
  - For adolescents and adults, dosage is 500 mg as a single dose on day 1, followed by 250 mg as a single daily dose on days 2–5.
- Erythromycin PO (40 mg/kg/24 h) in 4 doses for 14 days
  - Erythromycin in infants <4 weeks of age is associated with hypertrophic pyloric stenosis. Thus, azithromycin is the drug of choice for treatment or prophylaxis of pertussis in that age group.
- Clarithromycin PO (15 mg/kg/24 h divided b.i.d for 7 days) can be used in children ≥1 month of age.
- Trimethoprim/sulfamethoxazole in children ≥2 months of age, is an alternative agent, although its efficacy is unproven.

GENERAL MEASURES
- Patients with more severe disease manifestations (apnea, cyanosis, feeding difficulties) or other complications require hospitalization for supportive care:
  - Infants <6 months of age may develop apnea from fatigue secondary to excessive coughing. They need close observation, preferably in the hospital.
- Antibiotics have little effect on the clinical course unless begun early in the disease process (catarrhal phase) but should always be given to prevent spread of the infection.

INPATIENT CONSIDERATIONS
Admission Criteria
- Young infant (<6 months of age) with concern for apnea or fatigue with coughing
- Patients with severe disease manifestations or complications

Discharge Criteria
- No evidence of cardiorespiratory instability
- Able to self-recover from coughing spells

ONGOING CARE

FOLLOW-UP RECOMMENDATIONS
The paroxysmal stage can last up to 4 weeks and the convalescent stage up to several months.

PROGNOSIS
Directly related to patient age
- Highest mortality is observed in infants <6 months of age, with a 0.5–1% risk of death.
- In the older child, prognosis is good.

COMPLICATIONS
- The complications of pertussis are more likely to occur in infants <6 months of age:
  - Apnea
  - Pneumonia, which may be primary or secondary to viruses (adenovirus, respiratory syncytial virus) or bacteria (*Streptococcus pneumoniae*, *Staphylococcus aureus*), occurs in 13–25%; the presence of fever or respiratory symptoms in between cough episodes should raise the possibility of secondary bacterial pneumonia.
  - Other pulmonary complications include atelectasis, pneumothorax, pneumomediastinum, and subcutaneous emphysema.
  - Seizures (2%) and encephalopathy (0.5%) have also been observed in infants with pertussis.
- Complications of pertussis in adolescents and adults include cough syncope, incontinence, rib fractures, and pneumonia.

ADDITIONAL READING

- American Academy of Pediatrics. Pertussis (whooping cough). In: Pickering LK, Baker CJ, Kimberlin DW, et al, eds. *Red Book: 2012 Report of the Committee on Infectious Diseases*. 29th ed. Elk Grove Village, IL: American Academy of Pediatrics; 2012:553–566.
- Centers for Disease Control and Prevention. Updated recommendations for use of tetanus toxoid, reduced diphtheria toxoid and acellular pertussis (Tdap) vaccine from the Advisory Committee on Immunization Practices, 2010. *MMWR Morb Mortal Wkly Rep*. 2011;60(1):13–15.
- Cornia PB, Hersh AL, Lipsky BA. Does this coughing adolescent or adult patient have pertussis? *JAMA*. 2010;304(8):890–896.
- Klein NP, Bartlett J, Rowhani-Rahbar A, et al. Waning protection after fifth dose of pertussis vaccine in children. *N Engl J Med*. 2012;367(11):1012–1019.
- Murray EL, Nieves D, Bradley JS, et al. Characteristics of severe *Bordetella pertussis* infection among infants ≤90 days of age admitted to pediatric intensive care units-Southern California, September 2009–June 2011. *J Pediatr Inf Dis Soc*. 2013;2:1–6.
- Tiwari T, Murphy TV, Moran J. Recommended antimicrobial agents for the treatment and postexposure prophylaxis of pertussis: 2005 CDC guidelines. *MMWR Recomm Rep*. 2005;54(RR-14):1–16.

CODES

ICD10
- A37.90 Whooping cough, unspecified species without pneumonia
- A37.00 Whooping cough due to *Bordetella pertussis* without pneumonia
- A37.01 Whooping cough due to *Bordetella pertussis* with pneumonia

FAQ
- Q: Why is the transmission of pertussis difficult to control in the young infant?
- A: Unfortunately, many physicians do not consider pertussis in adolescents or adults because the symptoms can be nonspecific and often are not severe. They also assume that childhood immunization will protect adults against pertussis. Therefore, delays in antimicrobial treatment are common in adults, owing to the lack of index of suspicion of pertussis by their providers. Finally, there was not a universal recommendation for adolescents and adults to receive pertussis boosters until 2005, even though the immunity protection by pertussis vaccination is limited. It is largely adolescents and adults with pertussis who then spread the disease to young infants and children.
- Q: What is the best way to diagnose pertussis in the young infant?
- A: The diagnosis can be made clinically but requires a high index of suspicion. The diagnosis should be considered based on a history of severe cough in any young infant. At the time of presentation, infants usually appear well and have a normal exam. So, the history provided by the parents of the paroxysmal and severe nature of the course, often associated with gagging, posttussive emesis, and exhaustion, should be taken seriously.

PHARYNGITIS

Daniel E. Felten

BASICS

DESCRIPTION

Pharyngitis specifically refers to inflammation of the pharynx as indicated by erythema and swelling of the structures in the posterior portion of the oral cavity including the tonsillar pillars, the tonsils, the inferior soft palate, the uvula, and the posterior wall. Pharyngitis is usually caused by viral or bacterial infections.

EPIDEMIOLOGY

- Prevalence and etiology of pharyngitis vary based on age of patient and time of year.
- In preschool-aged children, viral agents are most common and exhibit seasonal variation depending on the specific virus.
- Group A *Streptococcus* (GAS) pharyngitis is most common in children between the ages of 5 and 15 years, is very rare in children younger than the age of 3 years, and may occur in outbreaks affecting up to 20% of children at risk.
- Pharyngitis caused by *Neisseria gonorrhoeae* occurs primarily in sexually active adolescents.

ETIOLOGY

- Viral
  - Common causes: adenovirus, Epstein-Barr virus (EBV), influenza A and B, enteroviruses (specifically, coxsackievirus A), herpes simplex virus (especially in adolescents), and echoviruses
  - Uncommon: measles, rubella, cytomegalovirus, human immunodeficiency virus (HIV)
  - Rhinovirus, coronavirus, parainfluenza virus, and respiratory syncytial virus (RSV) may cause sore throat but not usually pharyngitis.
- Bacterial
  - Common: *Streptococcus pyogenes* (group A β-hemolytic *Streptococcus*)
  - Uncommon: *Mycoplasma pneumoniae*, group C or G streptococci, *N. gonorrhoeae* (more likely in sexually active adolescents), *Arcanobacterium haemolyticum*, *Fusobacterium necrophorum* (Lemierre syndrome), *Corynebacterium diphtheriae* (diphtheria), *Chlamydophila pneumoniae*, *Chlamydophila psittaci*, *Yersinia enterocolitica*, *Treponema pallidum* (syphilis), *Francisella tularensis* (tularemia), oral anaerobes (Vincent angina or trench mouth)
- Fungal: *Candida* species (oral thrush)

GENERAL PREVENTION

- Most infectious agents that cause pharyngitis are spread through contact with respiratory droplets or other body fluids, although many can live for some time outside of the body.
- Careful hand washing and avoiding respiratory secretions are key to minimizing transmission.
- Return to school/child care
  - Children diagnosed with GAS pharyngitis should be kept at home for 24 hours after starting antibiotics.
  - Children with pharyngitis due to presumed viral etiology should be fever-free for 24 hours and have symptoms under control prior to return.

RISK FACTORS

- Children who are immunocompromised and children on chronic inhaled corticosteroids who are otherwise immune competent are at risk for candidiasis of the pharynx.
- Adolescents or sexually abused children engaging in oral sex are at risk for pharyngitis due to gonorrhea or HSV.
- Unvaccinated patients or travelers from certain areas are at risk for vaccine-preventable diseases: diphtheria and measles.

DIAGNOSIS

HISTORY

- Typical: sore throat, fever
- Variable
  - Headache, nausea, vomiting, abdominal pain (suggest GAS pharyngitis)
  - Rhinorrhea, cough, hoarseness, stridor, conjunctivitis (suggest viral etiology)
- Rash: scarlatiniform or nonspecific viral
- Sudden onset of fever and sore throat with difficulty swallowing, headache, stomach pain, nausea, vomiting, or scarlatiniform rash support diagnosis of GAS pharyngitis.
- Pharyngitis associated with rhinorrhea, cough, hoarseness, conjunctivitis, diarrhea, or nonspecific rash is more likely to have a viral cause.
- Significant systemic complaints such as fever and malaise are characteristic of EBV or HIV (acute retroviral syndrome).
- History of oral sex suggests possibility of *N. gonorrhoeae* infection.

PHYSICAL EXAM

- Pharynx and oral cavity
  - Exudative tonsillitis suggestive of GAS but also present in EBV, *N. gonorrhoeae*, *Arcanobacterium*, HSV, adenovirus
  - Palatal petechiae suggest GAS.
  - Ulcers on tonsils or tonsillar pillars seen in coxsackievirus, HSV, echovirus
  - Ulceration or inflammation of buccal mucosa or gums seen in HSV, coxsackievirus
- Lymph nodes
  - Tender anterior lymphadenopathy more common in GAS pharyngitis
  - Diffuse LAD, splenomegaly suggests EBV.
- Rash
  - Scarlatiniform rash (diffuse, erythematous, fine-papular, "sandpapery" rash) key feature of scarlet fever from GAS pharyngitis but can be seen with *Arcanobacterium haemolyticum* and in Kawasaki disease
  - Nonspecific, diffuse rash can be associated with viral infection; may be seen shortly after starting antibiotic if underlying etiology is EBV
  - Vesicular lesions on hands, feet, and/or buttocks characteristic of coxsackievirus

DIAGNOSTIC TESTS & INTERPRETATION

Lab

- Rapid antigen detection test (RADT)
  - The diagnosis of GAS pharyngitis should not be made based on clinical features alone but should be confirmed by laboratory testing.
  - Sensitivity varies (55–90%) based on quality of sample obtained. Specificity is more consistent in 95–98% range. Therefore, a good test to rule in GAS, but culture or DNA probe should be used to confirm negative RADTs. Confirmation of positive RADTs is not needed.
  - RADT is not recommended when patients present with symptoms that strongly suggest viral etiology (cough, rhinorrhea, hoarseness, oral ulcers).
  - Testing children <3 years old is not indicated, as those children are at very low risk for acute rheumatic fever (ARF). Testing may be considered in this age group if other risk factors are present such as an older sibling with GAS.
  - Testing of asymptomatic household contacts is not recommended.
- Monospot (heterophile antibody) test
  - Detects presence of IgM for EBV, which appears during the first 2 weeks of illness and gradually disappears over 6 months
  - Atypical lymphocytes may also be seen on WBC differential during the 2nd week of EBV infection. $>10\%$ atypical lymphocytes plus a positive heterophile antibody test is diagnostic of acute infection.
  - Heterophile antibody is often negative in children <4 years of age with EBV, so it should not be used in this age group.
- Testing for certain bacteria (*N. gonorrhoeae*, *A. hemolyticum*, *F. necrophorum*) requires special handling and processing, so must confirm appropriate collection medium and alert the laboratory performing the test if any of these agents is suspected.

DIFFERENTIAL DIAGNOSIS

- Infectious
  - Peritonsillar or retropharyngeal abscess or cellulitis
  - Lemierre syndrome
  - Epiglottitis
  - Kawasaki disease
  - Tularemia
- Ingestions
  - Caustic or irritant ingestions
  - Inhaled irritant
- Tumors
  - Leukemia
  - Lymphoma
  - Rhabdomyosarcoma
- Trauma: vocal abuse from shouting
- Allergy: potnasal drip from allergic rhinitis

- Miscellaneous
  - PFAPA syndrome (periodic fever, aphthous ulcers, pharyngitis, and cervical adenitis)
  - Psychogenic pain (globus hystericus)
  - Vitamin deficiency (A, B complex, C)
  - Dehydration

TREATMENT

GENERAL MEASURES

Treatment is largely supportive for most viral causes of pharyngitis, including pain control and hydration.

MEDICATION

First Line

- Penicillin-resistant GAS has never been documented. Apparent treatment failure (recurrent episode of acute pharyngitis with positive lab tests for GAS) most likely indicates repeat intercurrent viral infection in GAS carrier.
- Oral penicillin V
  - Children: 400,000 U (250 mg) b.i.d. or t.i.d. for 10 days
  - Adolescents/adults: 800,000 U (500 mg) b.i.d. for 10 days or 400,000 U (250 mg) 3–4 times per day for 10 days
- Amoxicillin: 50 mg/kg (max dose 1 g) daily divided b.i.d. for 10 days
  - Once-daily dosing may increase adherence.
- Intramuscular (IM) penicillin G benzathine: ensures compliance, useful in outbreaks
  - Children (>1 month and <27 kg): 600,000 U IM × 1
  - Children (>27 kg) and adults: 1,200,000 U IM × 1
  - Procaine penicillin combinations are less painful.

Second Line

- A 10-day course of a 1st-generation oral cephalosporin is indicated for most penicillin-allergic patients. However, 5–10% of penicillin-allergic patients may also be allergic to cephalosporins, so patients with a type I hypersensitivity to penicillin should not be given a cephalosporin.
- Oral clindamycin 20 mg/kg/24 h (max 1.8 g/24 h) divided t.i.d. may be given to patients with type I hypersensitivity to penicillin.
- Oral azithromycin, clarithromycin, or erythromycin are also acceptable alternatives in penicillin-allergic patients, although cases of ARF have been reported after treatment with these drugs.
  - Azithromycin 12 mg/kg (max 500 mg) daily for 5 days
  - Clarithromycin, 15 mg/kg/24 h divided q12h for 10 days or 500 mg extended-release tablets given once a day for 5 days (studied in adolescents ≥12 years of age)
  - Erythromycin ethylsuccinate, 40–50 mg/kg/24 h in 2–4 divided doses. Resistance is rare in the United States (<5% of isolates).
- Tetracyclines and sulfonamides should not be used due to high rates of resistance.
- In patients with *N. gonorrhoeae* infection
  - 250 mg ceftriaxone IM (>45 kg); 125 mg ceftriaxone IM (<45 kg)
  - Coinfection with *C. trachomatis* is unusual in pharyngitis caused by *N. gonorrhoeae*; however, treatment is recommended: azithromycin 1 g PO in adolescents. In younger children, should confirm infection
- In patients with EBV
  - Antibiotics should not be given; in particular, if amoxicillin or ampicillin is given, a high proportion of patients will develop a nonallergic rash.
  - Short-course corticosteroids may be beneficial but can also have significant adverse effects; should only be used in patients with marked tonsillar inflammation and impending airway obstruction. Usual prednisone dose is 1 mg/kg/24 h for 7 days with subsequent tapering.

SURGERY/OTHER PROCEDURES

Tonsillectomy for recurrent pharyngitis is not recommended but may be considered in the rare patient who has frequent symptomatic episodes of pharyngitis in whom no alternative explanation to GAS pharyngitis is found (e.g., recurrent viral infections in a GAS carrier). Benefit is relatively short-lived.

ONGOING CARE

PATIENT MONITORING

- Most cases of pharyngitis are self-limited; however, patients are at risk for dehydration if PO intake is limited by pain.
- Caregivers should be cautioned to monitor fluid intake and urine output and to return for reassessment if oral intake and/or urine output drops significantly.

COMPLICATIONS

- Streptococcal pharyngitis
  - Suppurative complications include peritonsillar abscess, cervical lymphadenitis, and mastoiditis.
  - Most significant nonsuppurative complication is ARF. This can be prevented if adequate antibiotic treatment is provided within 10 days.
  - Another nonsuppurative complication is post-streptococcal glomerulonephritis.
- Lemierre syndrome: spread of *F. necrophorum* from peritonsillar abscess caused by GAS to jugular vein causing thrombophlebitis, bacteremia, and thromboembolism
- Pediatric autoimmune neuropsychiatric disorder associated with streptococcal infection (PANDAS): controversial association that has not been demonstrated in prospective studies

ADDITIONAL READING

- Leckman JF, King RA, Gilbert DL, et al. Streptococcal upper respiratory tract infections and exacerbations of tic and obsessive-compulsive symptoms: a prospective longitudinal study. *J Am Acad Child Adolesc Psychiatry*. 2011;50(2):108–118.
- Logan LK, McAuley JB, Shulman ST. Macrolide treatment failure in streptococcal pharyngitis resulting in acute rheumatic fever. *Pediatrics*. 2012;129(3):e798–e802.
- Shulman ST, Bisno AL, Clegg HW, et al. Clinical practice guideline for the diagnosis and management of group A streptococcal pharyngitis: 2012 update by the Infectious Diseases Society of America. *Clin Infect Dis*. 2012;55(10):e86–e102.

CODES

ICD10

- J02.9 Acute pharyngitis, unspecified
- J02.0 Streptococcal pharyngitis
- B08.5 Enteroviral vesicular pharyngitis

FAQ

- Q: Is there any benefit to starting therapy while waiting for culture results?
- A: Immediate therapy probably shortens the symptomatic period. However, waiting for culture is appropriate because the goal of treatment is to minimize progression to ARF, and treatment within 10 days of onset of symptoms is effective.
- Q: Should all patients with sore throat be swabbed for RADT and/or strep culture?
- A: No. Most cases of sore throat are not due to GAS. However, clinical exam alone is insufficient to diagnose strep throat. Patients with symptoms that highly suggest a viral etiology (rhinorrhea, congestion, cough, conjunctivitis) should not be tested for GAS, as a positive result would most likely indicate carrier status rather than GAS pharyngitis.
- Q: Should contacts of patients with documented GAS pharyngitis be tested for GAS?
- A: Contacts who have recent or current clinical symptoms of GAS infection should undergo appropriate testing. However, carrier rates of contacts are quite high, up to 50% for siblings and 20% for other contacts, so routine testing of asymptomatic contacts is usually not indicated except during outbreaks or when contacts are at increased risk of developing sequelae of infection.

PHIMOSIS AND PARAPHIMOSIS

Kara N. Saperston • Michael DiSandro

BASICS

DESCRIPTION
- Phimosis is the inability to retract the prepuce (foreskin) after puberty due to a narrow preputial opening.
- Infants and prepubertal children rarely have true phimosis but rather a normal physiologic phimosis.
- Paraphimosis is the entrapment of the prepuce in a retracted position.

EPIDEMIOLOGY
- The incidence of phimosis is 0.4 cases per 100 boys per year.
- Phimosis affects 0.6 boys prior to their 16th birthday.

RISK FACTORS
- Phimosis
  - Forced retraction of the prepuce
  - Lichen sclerosis
- Paraphimosis
  - Prolonged retraction of the prepuce

PATHOPHYSIOLOGY
- Phimosis
  - As the constriction of the phimosis worsens, urine is trapped in the foreskin and ballooning of the prepuce occurs. In severe cases, urine will fill the entire prepucial space and extend down the shaft.
- Paraphimosis
  - Prolonged retraction of the prepuce around the glans causes edema of the prepuce and the glans. The edema makes it harder to correct the phimosis and causes significant pain for the child.

GENERAL PREVENTION
Boys should be instructed to return the foreskin to covering the glans after cleaning to prevent paraphimosis.

DIAGNOSIS

HISTORY
- Phimosis
  - Parent may report ballooning of the prepuce during voiding.
  - Parent may report having to squeeze the prepuce to clear all the trapped urine.
- Paraphimosis
  - Parent will report cleaning the penis during a diaper change, pulling the foreskin back, and then being unable to return it to its normal position covering the glans.
  - Child may pull the foreskin back and then be unable to return the foreskin to its normal position.

PHYSICAL EXAM
- Phimosis
  - Gentle attempt to retract the foreskin to evaluate the size of the preputial opening
  - A child who cannot retract foreskin after onset of puberty has phimosis.
  - Dry, white patchy areas of the foreskin indicate lichen sclerosis and seen with phimosis 50% of the time.
- Paraphimosis
  - Tender penis with marked edema of the prepuce (foreskin)
  - Tight collar around the glans
  - Long duration of the retracted skin will compromise the blood supply of the prepuce and glans.
  - There are case reports of gangrene.
    - Consider calling child protective services if there is gangrene.

DIAGNOSTIC TESTS & INTERPRETATION

Lab
Not needed

Imaging
Not needed

Diagnostic Procedures/Other
Not needed

DIFFERENTIAL DIAGNOSIS
- Physiologic phimosis
  - A child who has not gone through puberty will have a normal physiologic phimosis. This will change as he nears puberty and the foreskin will be easier to retract over time.
  - There may be small lumps of white material under the glans that are desquamated skin cells that are not infection and slowly work their way out of the preputial cavity. This desquamated skin helps with skin separation.

ALERT
Early (before puberty), forced retraction of the foreskin before the foreskin is naturally ready to retract may cause phimosis.

TREATMENT

MEDICATION

- Phimosis
  - Topical steroids t.i.d. for 6 weeks; use a small bead size amount
    - Fluticasone propionate, 0.05%
    - Betamethasone propionate, 0.1%
    - Triamcinolone cream
  - This also treats lichen sclerosis.
    - Topical tacrolimus is 2nd-line treatment for lichen sclerosis.
- Paraphimosis
  - Should be considered an emergency
  - Sedation and reduction by applying pressure to the glans and prepuce

ADDITIONAL THERAPIES

- Phimosis
  - Circumcision
    - Performed when medical treatment fails
- Paraphimosis
  - Dorsal slit is performed if compression fails.
    - Dorsal incision of the prepuce: under sedation

GENERAL MEASURES

- Phimosis
  - Refer to pediatric urologist if patient fails 2 months of medical management.
- Paraphimosis
  - Refer to pediatric urologist immediately if unable to return the foreskin to covering the glans without sedation.
  - Keep the patient in the ER, as sedation will most likely be necessary.

ONGOING CARE

FOLLOW-UP RECOMMENDATIONS

- Phimosis
  - Follow-up in 2 months after use of steroids
- Paraphimosis: If foreskin is back in normal position:
  - Follow up with pediatric urologist in 2 weeks.
  - There should be no retraction of the foreskin in that time frame.
  - Consider use of topical steroids to avoid development of severe phimosis.

PROGNOSIS

- Phimosis
  - Use of steroids is successful 70–90% of the time.
- Paraphimosis
  - High risk of development of severe phimosis
  - May require circumcision in the future

ADDITIONAL READING

- DeVries CR, Miller AK, Packer MG. Reduction of paraphimosis with hyaluronidase. *Urology*. 1996; 48(3):464–465.
- Gausche M. Genitourinary surgical emergencies. *Pediatr Ann*. 1996;25(8):458–464.
- Edwards S. 2001 National guideline on the management of balanitis. http://www.pdfdrive.net/2001-national-guideline-on-the-management-of-balanitis-bashh-e7997290.html. Accessed February 15, 2015.

CODES

ICD10

- N47.1 Phimosis
- N47.2 Paraphimosis

FAQ

- Q: Can a child have phimosis as a newborn?
- A: Physiologic phimosis (inability to retract the foreskin) is normal in prepubertal children. It occurs because of incomplete separation of skin between the glans and the inner prepuce. It does not require treatment.

PHOTOSENSITIVITY

Leslie Castelo-Soccio

BASICS

DESCRIPTION

Adverse or abnormal reaction of the skin to sunlight

EPIDEMIOLOGY

- Variable for each disorder
- Photosensitivities with onset in childhood include albinism, hydroa aestivale, hydroa vacciniforme, the porphyrias (e.g., erythropoietic, erythropoietic protoporphyria, hepatoerythropoietic), and genetic disorders (e.g., xeroderma pigmentosa, Hartnup disease, poikiloderma congenitale, Bloom syndrome, and Rothmund Thomson and Cockayne syndromes).
- Photosensitivities that occur frequently in adults but can occur in childhood are vitiligo, chemically induced photosensitivities, polymorphous light eruption, connective tissue disease, and pellagra.

RISK FACTORS

- Family history
- Disease
- Exposure to toxins

Genetics

- Genetic disorders include the porphyrias and others as previously listed:
  - The various porphyrias have variable inheritance patterns, whereas most of the other genetic disorders are inherited in an autosomal recessive pattern.
  - There is a positive familial history in many cases of polymorphous light eruption.

PATHOPHYSIOLOGY

Findings are diverse for the different disorders and rarely diagnostic.

ETIOLOGY

- Combination of sunlight with some abnormality in the skin such as loss of pigment, a chemical agent, a metabolic product, another skin disorder, a genetic disease, or an unknown factor produces a cutaneous abnormality.
- Specific wavelengths of the radiant energy emitted by the sun and reaching the earth are usually responsible for each photosensitivity disorder, most commonly ultraviolet B (UVB, 290–320 nm), ultraviolet A (UVA, 320–400 nm), and visible light (400–800 nm).

DIAGNOSIS

HISTORY

- Age of onset of rash
- Occurrence
  - Season: spring and summer
  - Relation to sun exposure: time frame, effect of sun through glass
- Oral medications
  - May be related to oral contraceptives, tetracyclines (doxycycline in particular), sulfa drugs, iodines/bromides, or phenytoin
- New topical agents (e.g., perfumes, lemons, limes, sunscreens, etc.):
  - Photosensitivity may occur on neck or places where agents were placed on skin.
- Rash
  - Accentuation of the rash on the nose, cheeks, and forehead with sparing of the eyelids and the submental portion of the chin
  - There is often a sharp cutoff in the nuchal area at the collar line.

PHYSICAL EXAM

- Distribution
  - Distribution of lesions is the main sign of photosensitivity reactions.
  - Lesions are prominent on sun-exposed skin such as the face, pinnae of the ears, the V of the neck, the nuchal area, and the dorsa of the hands.
  - Often, sparing of the philtrum, the area below the chin, the eyelids, and other covered areas is seen.
  - In phytophotodermatitis, linear or bizarre shapes can occur, including, as an example, hand prints if a caregiver has been squeezing limes and then picks up a child and the child is then exposed to sunlight.
- Lesion characteristics
  - Vary with the particular disease and can include the following:
    - Papules
    - Vesicles
    - Plaques (polymorphous light eruption)
    - Sunburn (chemical reaction to a systemic agent)
    - Linear areas of hyperpigmentation (chemical reaction to a topical agent)
    - Skin cancers (xeroderma pigmentosum)
    - Vesicles (porphyria)
  - In some cases, scarring can also be seen related to severe burns (porphyria).

DIAGNOSTIC TESTS & INTERPRETATION

- Phototesting
  - Using an artificial source of light can confirm the presence of certain photosensitivities. Procedures are of 2 types:
    - The 1st is exposure of skin to increasing doses of UVA and UVB to determine the erythema response (present at lower exposures than usual) and possibly reproduce lesions in certain diseases.
    - The 2nd is photopatch testing in which photoallergic chemicals are applied under patches in duplicate, and 1 set is subsequently exposed to UVA. Patients who have photoallergic contact dermatitis develop a reaction under only the exposed patch of the agent causing the problem.

Lab

Initial lab tests

- Genetic tests (optional): Find labs that perform genetic tests at www.genetests.org and enter disease name:
  - Cell culture: evaluates DNA repair for xeroderma pigmentosum or shows chromosomal breaks in Bloom disease
  - Measurement of specific amino acid and indole excretion patterns in Hartnup disease
  - Measurements of antinuclear antibodies are helpful in connective tissue diseases.
- Biochemical tests
  - Helpful for the diagnosis of the porphyrias, with elevated levels of various porphyrins specific to each type in the urine, blood, or stool
- Screening for connective tissue diseases should be done where appropriate.
- Screening for niacin deficiency

DIFFERENTIAL DIAGNOSIS

- Photosensitivity resulting from pigment loss
  - Albinism
  - Vitiligo
- Idiopathic photosensitivity
  - Polymorphous light eruption
  - Solar urticaria
- Chemically induced reactions
  - Topical agents
    - Perfumes
    - Plant-associated phytophotodermatitis (e.g., lemons, limes, celery, parsnips, carrots, dill, parsley, figs, meadow grass, giant hogweed, mangos, wheat, clover, cocklebur, buttercups, shepherds purse, and pigweed)

- Blankophors (e.g., optical brighteners in detergents)
- Sunscreens
- Topical retinoids (e.g., tretinoin, adapalene, tazarotene)
- Systemic agents
  - Tetracyclines, sulfonamides, nalidixic acid, griseofulvin, phenothiazines, oral hypoglycemic agents, amiodarone, quinine, isoniazid, and thiazide diuretics
- Metabolic disorders
  - Porphyrias: disorders of hemoglobin synthesis producing various porphyrins that are photosensitizers
- Genetic disorders: see "Genetics"
- Cutaneous diseases aggravated by sunlight
  - Connective tissue diseases

TREATMENT

GENERAL MEASURES

- Protection against sun exposure
  - Avoiding the sun, particularly between 10 a.m. and 3 p.m., and wearing protective clothing is important.
  - Sunscreens are helpful for those sensitive to UVB.
    - Sunscreens should be water resistant and reapplied q2h.
    - Sun protection factor (SPF; ratio of minimal erythema dose of sunscreened skin to minimal erythema dose of unprotected skin) >30
    - Sunscreens are less effective for blocking UVA and therefore less effective in helping patients with sensitivities to longer wavelengths.
  - Sunscreens that contain both UVA- and UVB-blocking capabilities offer better protection than most. These include sunscreens containing avobenzone, titanium dioxide, and zinc oxide.
    - Avobenzone has a relatively short lifespan but is now available in a chemically stabilized form known by the trade names Helioplex and Active Photobarrier Complex.
    - Mexoryl is another long-acting broad-spectrum sunscreen that has especially good UVA protection.
  - Opaque formulations such as zinc oxide and titanium dioxide block UV and visible light but may be less cosmetically appealing; however, new formulations made from microfine particles of titanium dioxide or zinc oxide make it more appealing.
  - Patients with severe photosensitivities may have to avoid any significant light exposure.
  - Most patients require chronic protection against sun exposure. However, the problem is generally more acute in spring and summer months.
- Removal of the offending agent is necessary in chemically induced photosensitivities:
  - Any severe and acute eruptions may require a short course of oral prednisone.
- Antimalarial agents have been used for polymorphous light eruption, lupus erythematosus, solar urticaria, and porphyria cutanea tarda and require the experience of a specialist.

ISSUES FOR REFERRAL

If possible, it is important to accurately document the specific wavelength of light and the degree of photosensitivity to accurately advise the patient. This requires phototesting by a specialist.

ONGOING CARE

FOLLOW-UP RECOMMENDATIONS

Patient Monitoring

Skin exams for skin cancers routinely with frequency dependent on type of photosensitivity; for example, more monitoring for genetic causes such as xeroderma pigmentosa

PATIENT EDUCATION

Education regarding significance of using sunscreen

PROGNOSIS

With the exception of chemically induced photosensitivities, most of the conditions are chronic.

ADDITIONAL READING

- Chantorn R, Lim HW, Shwayder TA. Photosensitivity disorders in children: part I. *J Am Acad Dermatol*. 2012;67(6):1093.e1–1093.e18.
- Chantorn R, Lim HW, Shwayder TA. Photosensitivity disorders in children: part II. *J Am Acad Dermatol*. 2012;67(6):1113.e1–1113.e15.
- Kuhn A, Ruland V, Bonsmann G. Photosensitivity, phototesting and photoprotection in cutaneous lupus erythematosus. *Lupus*. 2010;19(9):1036–1046.
- Segal AR, Doherty KM, Leggott J, et al. Cutaneous reactions to drugs in children. *Pediatrics*. 2007;120(4):e1082–e1096.
- Ten Berge O, Sigurdsson V, Brijinzeel-Koomen CA, et al. Photosensitivity testing in children. *J Am Acad Dermatol*. 2010;63(6):1019–1025.

CODES

ICD10

- L56.8 Oth acute skin changes due to ultraviolet radiation
- L59.8 Oth disrd of the skin, subcu related to radiation

FAQ

- Q: What is the best sunscreen to use?
- A: It depends on your particular problem. If you are sensitive to UVB, use a sunscreen with the highest SPF. If you are sensitive to UVA, sunscreens containing avobenzone, titanium dioxide, or zinc oxide are best.
- Q: I have heard that sunscreens with an SPF >15 are not necessary. Is this true?
- A: This is definitely not true for patients with photosensitivities who have abnormal responses to light and require excessive protection. Even for the healthy person, it is often not true. An SPF of 15 suggests that someone may receive 15 times more sun exposure with the sunscreen applied than without and not become sunburned. Some physicians have suggested that this is more than anyone should need. However, this number is calculated by testing in a controlled laboratory. Normal outdoor conditions, such as wind, reflection from water and sand, perspiration, and water exposure can significantly decrease the effectiveness of the sunscreen.
- Q: What is "sun allergy"?
- A: This is a lay term for polymorphous light eruption, one of the most common photosensitivities, presenting with papules, vesicles, and plaques 1–2 days after sun exposure. It usually recurs every spring, and most patients learn to avoid sun exposure. However, ironically, it can improve with slow, gradual sun exposure.
- Q: Can I become allergic to sunscreens?
- A: Certain active agents in sunscreens can produce an allergic response in rare individuals. If the rash recurs with each use, switch to another sunscreen with different ingredients. If the problem continues, consult a specialist for evaluation.

PINWORMS

Terry Kind • Hope Rhodes

BASICS

DESCRIPTION

- Infection by a small, white nematode (roundworm), typically *Enterobius vermicularis*
- Pinworms may also be caused by *Enterobius gregorii* in Europe, Africa, and Asia.

EPIDEMIOLOGY

- Considered the most common helminthic infection of humans (the only known natural host) and the most common worm infection in the United States.
- Occurs in school-aged children (5–10 years) and preschool children predominantly
- Does occur in adults, usually in those caring for infected children. Some individuals may be predisposed to having either heavy or light worm burdens.
- Independent of socioeconomic status

Prevalence

- U.S. infection rates: 5–15%
- Among children, people caring for infected children, and people who are institutionalized, prevalence can reach 50%.
- Occurs worldwide but is more prevalent in temperate climates

GENERAL PREVENTION

- Decontaminate the environment by washing underclothes, bedclothes, bedsheets, and towels.
- Maintain good hand hygiene, including hand washing and proper toileting.
- Keep fingernails short and avoid nail biting.
- Treat family members and close contacts.

PATHOPHYSIOLOGY

- *E. vermicularis* eggs are ingested and hatch in the human's stomach and duodenum. Then the larvae migrate to the ileum and cecum. Adult worms copulate in the cecum.
- The pregnant female pinworm migrates from the cecum to the anus ~5 weeks later and deposits eggs on the perianal skin (at which point the female pinworm usually dies). Thousands of eggs are laid, which may result in hundreds of worms.
- Pruritus is caused by the perianal deposition of eggs and a mucosal mastocytosis response. Other GI symptoms, such as anorexia or abdominal pain, may occur because of the mucosal inflammatory response.
- Granulomas may form if dead worms and eggs invoke an inflammatory response in ectopic locations such as the peritoneal cavity, vulva, cervix, uterus, and fallopian tubes.

ETIOLOGY

- Ingestion of organism via fecal–oral transmission
- Can be spread directly, hand-to-mouth, or via fomites found on toys, bedding, clothing, toilet seats, and baths

DIAGNOSIS

HISTORY

- Prior pinworms or sibling with pinworms
  - Eggs can survive for several days in the environment, and the incubation period can be 1–2 months.
  - Spread can occur between family members.
- Daytime itching
  - Pinworm infections usually cause perianal itching during the night or just before waking in the morning.
  - Daytime perianal or perivulvar itching or irritation is likely due to other causes.
- Fevers, diarrhea, or vomiting
  - Pinworms are highly unlikely to cause systemic symptoms (except in rare cases where they migrate aberrantly).
- Visible worms at night
  - Pinworms may be seen 2–3 hours after the child has gone to sleep. Female worms are 8–13 mm, and males are 2–5 mm.
  - They may be visible as small, white worms in the perianal area at night.

PHYSICAL EXAM

- Exam may be normal, and the child may be well-appearing.
- May have self-inflicted, perianal excoriation
- Pinworms may be visible perianally.
- Infection is characterized by perianal pruritus that occurs at night or just before waking.
- Difficulty sleeping, decreased appetite, and/or abdominal pain may occur.

DIAGNOSTIC TESTS & INTERPRETATION

Lab

- Stool or urine samples for ova or parasites
  - Generally not helpful or recommended
  - Very few ova present in stool (even more rare in urine)
- Blood count for eosinophilia
  - Generally not helpful or recommended
  - Eosinophilia is not observed because usually there is no tissue invasion.

Diagnostic Procedures/Other

- Transparent tape, Scotch tape test
  - In the morning, prior to the child awakening and before defecation or washing, the adhesive side of transparent tape is applied to the perianal area.
  - After removal, the tape is applied to a glass slide and examined under light microscopy for pinworm ova. Several samples may be necessary to see the pinworms.

DIFFERENTIAL DIAGNOSIS

- Infection
  - Other parasites (e.g., *Strongyloides stercoralis*)
  - Nonparasitic vulvovaginitis (due to bacterial, fungal, or viral causes)
- Dermatologic
  - Contact or irritative diaper dermatitis
  - Hidradenitis suppurativa
  - Irritative vulvovaginitis secondary to soaps, bubble baths, or lotions
  - Anal fissures (usually cause pain rather than itching)
- Miscellaneous
  - Behavioral: self-stimulation (normal)
  - Sleep disorders not owing to nocturnal pruritus
  - Hemorrhoids

TREATMENT

MEDICATION

Single-drug and single-dose therapy with one of the following agents:

- Mebendazole, 100 mg (available as a chewable tablet) PO once, may repeat in 2 weeks if symptoms still present
- Pyrantel pamoate, 11 mg/kg (maximum 1 g) PO once, may repeat in 2 weeks
- Albendazole, 400 mg PO once, may repeat in 2 weeks
- Experience is limited in children <2 years of age. Consider risks and benefits before use.
- Caution in treating pregnant individuals with anthelminthic medications because mebendazole, pyrantel pamoate, and albendazole are all category C and are not recommended in pregnancy.

ADDITIONAL TREATMENT

General Measures

- Reinfection is common especially if not all close contacts are treated.
- Treat all symptomatic contacts, and consider treating close household contacts, especially if repeated infections have occurred.
- Reinfection can occur if eggs remain on bed linen or clothing.
- Infection may be asymptomatic and transmitted to others.
- Autoreinfection can occur if eggs remain under the nails.

ONGOING CARE

FOLLOW-UP RECOMMENDATIONS

Patient Monitoring

Watch for signs of reinfection.

PATIENT EDUCATION

- National Library of Medicine's health information site: http://www.nlm.nih.gov/medlineplus/pinworms.html
- Centers for Disease Control and Prevention site: http://www.cdc.gov/healthywater/hygiene/disease/pinworms.html

PROGNOSIS

- Reinfection is common.
- With appropriate treatment, symptoms resolve within a few days.
- Any chronic symptoms are likely due to recurrence rather than chronic infection because the life cycle of the adult worm is short, with eggs being laid by the adult worm within 5 weeks.

COMPLICATIONS

- Intestinal
  - Appendicitis (uncommon)
  - Bacterial superinfection of perianal excoriations
  - Granuloma formation
- Extraintestinal
  - Urethritis
  - Vulvovaginitis
  - Pelvic inflammatory disease

ADDITIONAL READING

- American Academy of Pediatrics. Pinworms infection *(Enterobius vermicularis)*. In: Pickering LK, Baker CJ, Kimberlin DW, et al, eds. *Red Book: 2012 Report of the Committee on Infectious Diseases*. 29th ed. Elk Grove Village, IL: American Academy of Pediatrics; 2012.
- Arca MJ, Gates RL, Groner JI, et al. Clinical manifestations of appendiceal pinworms in children: an institutional experience and a review of the literature. *Pediatr Surg Int*. 2004;20(5):372–375.
- Burkhart CN, Burkhart CG. Assessment of frequency, transmission, and genitourinary complications of enterobiasis (pinworms). *Int J of Dermatol*. 2005;44(10): 837–840.
- Elston DM. What's eating you? *Enterobius vermicularis* (pinworms, threadworms). *Cutis*. 2003;71(4):268–270.
- Grencis RK, Cooper ES. *Enterobius*, *Trichuris*, *Capillaria*, and hookworm including *Ancylostoma caninum*. *Gastroenterol Clin North Am*. 1996;25(3):579–597.
- Stermer E, Sukhotnic I, Shaoul R. Pruritus ani: an approach to an itching condition. *J Pediatr Gastroenterol Nutr*. 2009;48(5):513–516.

CODES

ICD10

B80 Enterobiasis

FAQ

- Q: Could the child have acquired pinworms from a pet dog or cat?
- A: No. Household pets are not involved in the life cycles of pinworms.
- Q: When can an infected child return to day care?
- A: After receiving the 1st treatment dose, the child can return to school or day care. It is prudent to bathe the child and to trim and scrub his or her nails prior to school reentry.
- Q: Is it necessary to reevaluate and retest a child once treated?
- A: No. However, reinfection is common.
- Q: Can pinworm eggs survive on bedding, toilet seats, or clothing?
- A: Yes. Eggs can remain infectious in an indoor environment for up to 3 weeks.
- Q: Does pinworm infection cause nocturnal bruxism?
- A: There is no proof of any causal relationship.
- Q: How do the anthelminthic medications work?
- A: They inhibit microtubule function and cause glycogen depletion in the adult worms.

PLAGUE

Gordon E. Schutze

BASICS

DESCRIPTION

Plague is an enzootic disease transmitted by fleas from wild rodents and caused by *Yersinia pestis*. Humans and their pets can enter this cycle, resulting in human plague. Human plague has 3 main forms: bubonic, septicemic, and pneumonic; rarely presents as meningeal, pharyngeal, ocular, or gastrointestinal (GI) plague

EPIDEMIOLOGY

- Worldwide: enzootic in Africa, Asia, and Americas. Since 2000, 95% of the 22,000 cases reported to the World Health Organization have been from countries in sub-Saharan Africa.
- In the United States, most cases occur in Arizona, New Mexico, California, Colorado, Oregon, and Nevada.
- In the United States, most cases occur in spring/summer.
- 51 cases of plague occurred in the United States from 2004 to 2011.
- 20% of U.S. cases with identified mode of transmission are acquired through direct contact with *Y. pestis*–infected animals, not via flea bite.
- No cases of person-to-person transmission of pneumonic plague have been reported in the United States since 1924.
- Untreated bubonic plague: >50% fatal
- Untreated pneumonic plague: nearly 100% fatal

GENERAL PREVENTION

- Reduce rodent shelter and food sources in the immediate vicinity of the home by storing grain and animal food in rodent-proof containers.
- Flea disinfestation of cats and dogs, especially in endemic areas
- Hospital isolation precautions
  - Patients with bubonic or septicemic plague and no evidence of pneumonia: standard precautions; add droplet precautions for first 24 hours of therapy until chest radiograph persistently clear.
  - Patients with pneumonic plague: standard and droplet precautions. Continue droplet precautions until patient has completed 48 hours of appropriate antimicrobial therapy.
- Postexposure management
  - All persons with exposure to known or suspected plague source in last 6 days
    - Daily surveillance for fever or symptoms of disease for 7–10 days
    - Offer prophylaxis.
    - Initiate treatment if becomes ill
- Persons with close (<2 m) contact with a patient with pneumonic plague should receive antimicrobial prophylaxis, but isolation is not necessary.
- Chemoprophylaxis ≥8 years
  - Doxycycline (PO), *OR*
  - Ciprofloxacin (PO) at treatment doses for 7 days from last exposure (see "Medications" for dosing)
- Chemoprophylaxis <8 years: ciprofloxacin (PO)
- Notify state public health authorities of cases of suspected and proven *Y. pestis* infection.
- Vaccination is no longer available and is not considered useful to prevent plague from an enzootic source.

PATHOPHYSIOLOGY

- Skin portal of entry
  - *Y. pestis* is transmitted from fleas to humans via the regurgitation of the organism into the bite during the flea's blood meal (*Y. pestis* blocks foregut, causing regurgitation).
  - Rodents, ground squirrels, cats, prairie dogs, marmots, rabbits, and occasionally dogs harbor infected fleas and are reservoirs of infection (enzootic).
  - Direct skin inoculation of organisms from infected animal tissue or blood occurs through breaks in the skin (e.g., cat scratch, skinning quarry).
  - Lymphatic spread of infection to the regional lymph nodes creates a localized inflammatory response (bubo, bubonic).
  - Subsequent hematogenous spread of the organism to other organs results in high levels of circulating bacterial endotoxin (septicemic plague).
  - By hematogenous spread to lungs, both bubonic and septicemic plague can cause secondary pneumonic plague.
- Respiratory portal of entry
  - Primary pneumonic plague: acquired via inhalation of respiratory tract droplets from a human or animal (e.g., cat) with pneumonic plague
- Incubation period
  - 2–8 days for bubonic or septicemic plague
  - 1–6 days for pneumonic plague

ETIOLOGY

Plague is caused by *Y. pestis*, a pleomorphic, bipolar-staining, gram-negative coccobacillus.

DIAGNOSIS

HISTORY

- A thorough travel history (especially to enzootic areas) is imperative to raise the index of suspicion for diagnosing plague.
- Environmental history should include epizootic deaths (die-offs) of rodents, ground squirrels, or prairie dogs in the patient's locale.
- In enzootic areas, a sick household cat or dog is an additional risk factor.
- Signs and symptoms
  - Bubonic plague
    - Initial symptom: pain in the groin or axillae prior to lymph node swelling
    - Lymphadenitis (usually inguinal > axillary > cervical)
    - Fever, chills, prostration
  - Septicemic plague
    - Tachycardia and hypotension
    - Abdominal symptoms
    - Hemorrhage
    - Fever, chills, prostration
  - Bubonic or septicemic plague may progress to secondary pneumonic plague.
  - Pneumonic plague
    - Cough, dyspnea
    - Systemic manifestations
    - Fever, chills, shock
    - Rapidly progressive and often fatal

PHYSICAL EXAM

- Tachycardic, hypotensive, tachypneic, and toxic-appearing
- Flea bite lymphadenitis classically affects inguinal nodes; cat-associated plague affects mostly axillary or cervical nodes secondary to handling infected cat.
- GI: Abdominal pain, nausea, and diarrhea are common, secondary to inflammatory mediators.
- Neurologic: weakness, delirium, and coma, owing to the effects of the endotoxin of *Y. pestis*
- Heme: disseminated intravascular coagulation
- Renal: glomerular parenchymal damage
- Rare: meningitis, endophthalmitis, endocarditis, and pleuritis

DIAGNOSTIC TESTS & INTERPRETATION

Lab

- Total WBC count
  - Usually 10,000–20,000, but may be as high as 100,000, with immature neutrophils.
- Perform Gram, Wayson, Giemsa, or fluorescent antibody staining on specimen (blood, bubo, CSF, sputum) to look for gram-negative, bipolar-staining organisms.
- *Y. pestis* culture (Notify receiving lab.)
  - Suspect bubonic plague: needle aspiration of the bubo for stain and culture. Puncture center of bubo with a sterile syringe and inject 1 mL of nonbacteriostatic, sterile saline. Withdraw aspirate vigorously until blood-tinged liquid appears in syringe.
  - Suspect pneumonic plague: sputum for stain and culture
  - Blood cultures are usually positive, even with bubonic plague, and should always be done prior to therapy.
    - Slow-grower; may be misidentified as *Yersinia pseudotuberculosis* or *Acinetobacter* sp.
- Serology
  - Single positive acute serology *OR*
  - At least a 4-fold increase in antibody titers by passive hemagglutination test between acute and convalescent sera taken 4–12 weeks apart
- Comprehensive testing and notification to state public health lab and CDC

Diagnostic Procedures/Other

Pitfalls

- Patients who present with a nonspecific febrile illness, tachycardia, and tachypnea, rather than lymphadenitis, are at higher risk for delayed diagnosis and serious sequelae (e.g., septicemic plague, death).
- Failure to consider septicemic plague in the appropriate epidemiologic setting and withholding appropriate antibiotics or using an empiric β-lactam regimen
- Failure to treat suspected bubonic plague with antibiotics while awaiting culture results when needle aspiration of the bubo shows no organisms on direct stain.

DIFFERENTIAL DIAGNOSIS

- Diagnosis of plague follows a high index of suspicion and a thorough review of the patient's lifestyle, travel history, and recent activities. The appearance of septicemia and endotoxin-mediated shock includes a large differential diagnosis that includes sepsis owing to other bacteria or viruses as well as distributive shock resulting from toxic ingestion or anaphylaxis.
- Infection
  - Streptococcal and staphylococcal infections (especially between the toes) can result in tender inguinal lymph nodes, fever, shock.
  - Cat-scratch fever (*Bartonella henselae*) can present with a history of cat scratch or bite, regional lymphadenitis, and fever.
  - Hantavirus in humans has a clinical presentation similar to septicemic and pneumonic plague and occurs in many of the plague-enzootic areas.
  - Rickettsial diseases: *Rickettsia*, *Orientia*, *Coxiella*, *Ehrlichia*, *Anaplasma* (e.g., Rocky Mountain spotted fever [*Rickettsia rickettsii*] and relapsing tick fever due to *Borrelia* sp. may mimic septicemic or pneumonic plague)
  - Recent reports of plague-like illnesses have been associated with infections by other organisms such as *Burkholderia pseudomallei* (melioidosis) and *Francisella tularensis* (tularemia).

TREATMENT

MEDICATION

- Use IV/IM forms for acute disease.
- For children, gentamicin or streptomycin administered intramuscularly or intravenously appear to be equally effective.
- Gentamicin, equally effective as streptomycin in recent study (IV): peds: 2.5 mg/kg/dose q8h. Adult: 5 mg/kg/dose q24h
- Streptomycin traditionally has been the drug of choice (IV/IM): peds: 20–30 mg/kg/24 h divided q12h. Adult: 15 mg/kg/dose q12h to max 1 g q12h
- Meningitis or severe disease: Consider adding chloramphenicol (IV): 12.5–25 mg/kg/dose q6h (max 4 g/24 h). Monitor for toxicity.
- Alternatives
  - Doxycycline: peds (IV/PO): 2.2 mg/kg q12h up to adult dose as the max dose. Adult: 200 mg IV × 1, then 100 mg IV/PO q12h. Some experts recommend adding it to gentamicin for severe disease.
  - Ciprofloxacin: peds (IV/PO): 30 mg/kg/24 h (max 1 g/24 h) divided q12h. Adults: 400 mg IV q12h; 500 mg PO q12h
- Continue antibiotic therapy for 7–10 days or until several days after lysis of fever.
- Severely ill patients may require a substantially longer course of therapy.
- Foci (e.g., abscess) are infectious until sufficient appropriate antimicrobial therapy is given.

ADDITIONAL TREATMENT

General Measures

For septic patients in shock, initial attention should be given to airway management and fluid resuscitation, then antibiotics.

ONGOING CARE

FOLLOW-UP RECOMMENDATIONS

Resolution of symptoms should begin in the first 3 days after initiation of therapy; however, the rate of clinical improvement depends on the initial severity of illness.

Patient Monitoring

None; most recover without sequelae.

COMPLICATIONS

- Hematologic (disseminated intravascular coagulation)
- Renal (glomerular and parenchymal damage)

ADDITIONAL READING

- Butler T. Plague into the 21st century. *Clin Infect Dis*. 2009;49(5):736–742.
- Centers for Disease Control and Prevention. Plague. www.cdc.gov/plague/. Accessed February 2, 2015.
- Gage KL, Dennis DT, Orloski KA, et al. Cases of cat-associated human plague in the western US, 1977–1998. *Clin Infect Dis*. 2000;30(6):893–900.
- Koirala J. Plague: disease, management, and recognition of act of terrorism. *Infect Dis Clin North Am*. 2006;20(2):273–287.
- Raoult D, Mouffok N, Bitam I, et al. Plague: history and contemporary analysis. *J Infect*. 2013;66(1):18–26.

CODES

ICD10

- A20.9 Plague, unspecified
- A20.0 Bubonic plague
- A20.7 Septicemic plague

FAQ

- Q: Can one determine the risks of being exposed to plague during international travel?
- A: Yes. The CDC provides a service that contains updated information for international travel exposures at www.cdc.gov/travel.
- Q: Does persistent fever during treatment for plague warrant altering the antibiotic regimen?
- A: No. Fever can persist for up to 2 weeks despite appropriate 1st-line antibiotic therapy for *Y. pestis*. However, an evaluation for a focus of infection requiring drainage is recommended under these circumstances.
- Q: What is a bubo?
- A: "Bubo" (plural: buboes) comes from the Greek word for groin. A bubo is a painful, swollen lymph node.

PLEURAL EFFUSION

Richard M. Kravitz

BASICS

DESCRIPTION

Accumulation of fluid in the pleural cavity

PATHOPHYSIOLOGY

- Normally 1–15 mL of fluid in the pleural space
- Alterations in the flow and/or absorption of this fluid lead to its accumulation.
- Mechanisms that influence this flow of fluid:
  - Increased capillary hydrostatic pressure (i.e., congestive heart failure [CHF], overhydration)
  - Decreased pleural space hydrostatic pressure (i.e., after thoracentesis, atelectasis)
  - Decreased plasma oncotic pressure (i.e., hypoalbuminemia, nephrosis)
  - Increased capillary permeability (i.e., infection, toxins, connective tissue diseases, malignancy)
  - Impaired lymphatic drainage from the pleural space (i.e., disruption of the thoracic duct)
  - Passage of fluid from the peritoneal cavity through the diaphragm to the pleural space (i.e., hepatic cirrhosis with ascites)
- 2 types of pleural effusion:
  - Transudate: Mechanical forces of hydrostatic and oncotic pressures are altered, favoring liquid filtration.
  - Exudate: Damage to the pleural surface occurs that alters its ability to filter pleural fluid; lymphatic drainage is diminished.
- Stages associated with parapneumonic effusions (infectious exudates):
  - See Appendix, Table 3.
  - Exudative stage
    - Free-flowing fluid
    - Pleural fluid glucose, protein, lactate dehydrogenase (LDH) level, and pH are normal.
  - Fibrinolytic stage
    - Loculations are forming.
    - Increase in fibrin, polymorphonuclear leukocytes, and bacterial invasion of pleural cavity are occurring.
    - Pleural fluid glucose and pH falls while protein and LDH levels increase.
  - Organizing stage (empyema)
    - Fibroblasts grow.
    - Pleural peal forms.
    - Pleural fluid parameters worsen.

DIAGNOSIS

HISTORY

- Underlying disease determines most systemic symptoms.
- Patient may be asymptomatic until the amount of fluid is large enough to cause cardiorespiratory compromise/distress.
- Dyspnea and cough are associated with large effusions.
- Fever (if infectious etiology)
- Pleuritic pain (pneumonia may cause irritation of the parietal pleura, causing pleural pain; as the effusion increases and separates the pleural membrane, the pain may disappear)

PHYSICAL EXAM

- Decreased thoracic wall excursion on the ipsilateral side
- Fullness of intercostal spaces on the ipsilateral side
- Trachea and cardiac apex displaced toward the contralateral side (may produce a mediastinal shift that can reduce venous return and compromise the cardiac output)
- Dull or flat percussion on the ipsilateral side (suggesting the presence of consolidation of pleural effusion)
- Decreased tactile and vocal fremitus
- Decreased whispering pectoriloquy
- Pleural rub during early phase (may resolve as fluid accumulates in the pleural space)
- Decreased breath sounds

DIAGNOSTIC TESTS & INTERPRETATION

- Cytologic exam of pleural fluid
  - Fresh and heparinized specimen should be refrigerated at 4°C (39.2°F) until it can be processed.
  - Fixatives should not be added.
- Pleural fluid parameters to be routinely measured include the following (Appendix, Table 4):
  - pH
  - LDH
  - Protein
  - Glucose
    - Note: Glucose of <40 mg/dL suggests a parapneumonic, tuberculosis, malignant, or rheumatic etiology to the effusion.

Lab

Initial lab tests

Serology values to follow the degree of inflammation and the response to therapy:

- Erythrocyte sedimentation rate (ESR)
- C-reactive protein (CRP)

Imaging

- Chest radiograph
  - Anteroposterior projection can show >400 mL of pleural fluid.
  - Lateral projection can show <200 mL of pleural fluid.
  - Lateral decubitus film to evaluate for free-flowing pleural fluid can show as little as 50 mL of pleural fluid.
- Ultrasound
  - Reveals small (3–5 mL) loculated collections of pleural fluid
  - Useful as a guide for thoracentesis
  - Aids in distinguishing between pleural thickening and pleural effusion
- CT scan
  - Clearly reveals effusions/empyemas, abscess, or pulmonary consolidations
  - Useful for defining the extent of loculated effusions

Diagnostic Procedures/Other

- Thoracentesis
  - Indicated whenever etiology is unclear or if the effusion causes symptoms (e.g., prolonged fever or respiratory distress)
- Pleural biopsy
  - If thoracentesis is nondiagnostic
  - Most useful for diseases that cause extensive involvement of the pleura (i.e., tuberculosis, malignancies)
  - Confirms neoplastic involvement in 40–70% of cases

DIFFERENTIAL DIAGNOSIS

- Transudate
  - Cardiovascular
    - CHF
    - Constrictive pericarditis
  - Nephrotic syndrome with hypoalbuminemia
  - Cirrhosis
  - Atelectasis
- Exudate
  - Infection
    - *Staphylococcus aureus* (increasing incidence of methicillin-resistant species)
    - *Streptococcus pneumoniae* (increasing incidence of penicillin-resistant species)
    - *Haemophilus influenzae* (decreasing incidence since introduction of *H. influenzae* type b [Hib] vaccine)
    - Group A *Streptococcus*
    - Anaerobes
    - Gram-negative enterics
    - No identified organisms (all cultures sterile)
    - Tuberculous effusion
    - Viral effusions (adenovirus, influenza)
    - Fungal effusions: most not associated with effusions; *Nocardia* and *Actinomyces* are most commonly seen.
    - Parasitic effusions
  - Neoplasm: seen mostly in leukemia and lymphoma; uncommon in children
  - Connective tissue disease
    - Rheumatoid arthritis
    - Systemic lupus erythematosus
    - Wegener granulomatosis
  - Pulmonary embolus
  - Intra-abdominal disease
    - Subdiaphragmatic abscess
    - Pancreatitis
  - Sarcoidosis
  - Esophageal rupture

- Hemothorax
- Chylothorax
- Drugs
- Chemical injury
- Postirradiation effusion

TREATMENT

MEDICATION

- Antibiotics
  - Used when effusion is caused by a bacterial infection
  - Specific antibiotics dictated by organism identified
  - If effusion is sterile, broad-spectrum antibiotics are indicated to cover for the usually seen organisms.
  - Clinical improvement usually begins within 48–72 hours of therapy.
  - Continue IV antibiotics until afebrile.
  - Complete remainder of therapy on oral antibiotics.
- Duration of antibiotic therapy depends on the infectious organism and the degree of illness:
  - Total duration is controversial.
  - Usually, at least 2–4 weeks of total IV and PO

ADDITIONAL TREATMENT

General Measures

- Supportive measures:
  - Maintain adequate
    - Oxygenation
    - Fluid status
    - Nutritional balance
  - Antipyretic agents when febrile
  - Pain control
- Treat the underlying disease:
  - Antibiotics for infections
  - Cardiac medications for CHF
  - Chemotherapeutic agents for malignancies
  - Anti-inflammatory agents (i.e., steroids) for connective tissue diseases
  - Medium-chain triglycerides and low-fat diet for chylothorax
- Effective drainage of pleural fluid
  - Thoracentesis
  - Chest tube drainage
  - Surgical drainage
- Duration of chest tube drainage
  - Discontinue when patient is asymptomatic (afebrile, no distress) and drainage <50 mL/h
  - Thick, loculated empyema requires prolonged drainage (and possibly a video-assisted thoracic surgery [VATS] procedure if effusion not improving).

COMPLEMENTARY & ALTERNATIVE THERAPIES

- Thoracentesis
  - For diagnosis purposes
    - To distinguish between a transudate and an exudate
    - For culture material (if infection is suspected)
    - For cytology (if malignancy is suspected)
  - For relief of dyspnea or cardiorespiratory distress
- Chest tube thoracostomy
  - Reduce reaccumulation of fluid.
  - Drain parapneumonic effusion (before loculations develop which will prevent fluid drainage).
- Intrapleural fibrinolytics
  - Adjunct to aid in drainage of complicated (i.e., multiloculated empyema) pleural effusions
  - Streptokinase, urokinase, and tPA are the agents of choice.

SURGERY/OTHER PROCEDURES

- VATS
  - Alternative to more invasive procedures (e.g., open thoracotomy/decortication)
  - Debridement through pleural visualization and lysis of adhesions/loculations
  - Useful when
    - Initial drainage is delayed
    - Loculations prevent adequate drainage by chest tube alone
    - Patient is failing more conservative therapy
- Pleurectomy
  - Chylothorax
  - Malignant effusions
- Pleurodesis
  - For recurrent effusions
  - Chemical agents frequently used include talc, tetracycline, doxycycline, and quinacrine.
  - Surgical methods include the following:
    - Mechanical abrasion
    - Pleurectomy via VATS
    - Open thoracotomy route
  - In cases of malignant effusion:
    - Sclerosing procedures are usually ineffective.
    - Chest tube drainage can create a pneumothorax because the lung is incarcerated by the tumor.

ONGOING CARE

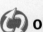

FOLLOW-UP RECOMMENDATIONS

- Clinical improvement usually within 1–2 weeks
- With empyemas, the patient may have fever spikes for up to 2–3 weeks after improvement is noted.

DIET

When the effusion is a chylothorax:

- Medium-chain triglycerides
- Nutritional replacement
- At least 4–5 weeks on this regimen

PROGNOSIS

Depends on underlying disease process:

- Properly treated infectious cause: excellent prognosis
- Malignancy: poor prognosis

COMPLICATIONS

- Hypoxia
- Respiratory distress
- Persistent fevers
- Decreased cardiac function
- Malnutrition (seen in chylothorax)
- Shock (secondary to blood loss in cases of hemothorax)
- Trapped lung

ADDITIONAL READING

- Beers SL, Abramo TJ. Pleural effusions. *Pediatr Emerg Care*. 2007;23(5):330–334.
- Buckingham SC, King MD, Miller ML. Incidence and etiologies of complicated parapneumonic effusions in children. *Pediatr Infect Dis*. 2003;22(6):499–504.
- Calder A, Owens CM. Imaging of parapneumonic pleural effusions and empyema in children. *Pediatr Radiol*. 2009;39(6):527–537.
- Doski JJ, Lou D, Hicks BA, et al. Management of parapneumonic collections in infants and children. *J Pediatr Surg*. 2000;35(2):265–268; discussion 269–270.
- Heffner JE. Discriminating between transudates and exudates. *Clin Chest Med*. 2006;27(2):241–252.
- Krenke K, Peradzynska J, Lange J. Local treatment of empyema in children: a systematic review of randomized controlled trials. *Acta Paediatr*. 2010;99(10):1449–1453.
- Merino JM, Carpinterol I, Alvarez T, et al. Tuberculous pleural effusion in children. *Chest*. 1999;115(1):26–30.
- Proesmans M, De Boeck K. Clinical Practice: Treatment of childhood empyema. *Eur J Pediatr*. 2009;168(6):639–645.
- Rocha G. Pleural effusions in the neonate. *Curr Opin Pulm Med*. 2007;13(4):305–311.

CODES

ICD10

- J90 Pleural effusion, not elsewhere classified
- J86.9 Pyothorax without fistula
- J91.0 Malignant pleural effusion

FAQ

- Q: When will the chest radiograph findings become normal?
- A: They may take up to 6 months (or longer) to return to normal appearance.
- Q: When will the pulmonary function tests normalize?
- A: Depending on extent of effusion, they may take up to 6–12 months.

PNEUMOCYSTIS JIROVECI (PREVIOUSLY KNOWN AS *PNEUMOCYSTIS CARINII* PNEUMONIA)

Danna Tauber

BASICS

DESCRIPTION

Opportunistic lung infection caused by *Pneumocystis jiroveci* (PJ). This organism is currently considered a primitive fungus based on DNA sequence analysis. It has two developmental forms (the cysts contain sporozoites that become trophozoites when excised).

- Although previously known as *Pneumocystis carinii* pneumonia (PCP), the acronym PCP is still in use and refers to *Pneumocystis* pneumonia.
- PCP occurs almost exclusively in the immunocompromised host.
- PCP is an AIDS-defining illness. It is the most common opportunistic life-threatening lung infection in infants with perinatally acquired human immunodeficiency virus (HIV) disease.
- PJ causes a diffuse pneumonitis characterized by fever, dyspnea at rest, tachypnea, hypoxemia, nonproductive cough, and bilateral diffuse infiltrates in the roentgenogram. It is a severe condition frequently leading to respiratory failure, necessitating intubation and mechanical ventilation.
- Chemoprophylaxis against this microorganism has proven successful. Therefore, early identification of the HIV-infected mother becomes essential.
- Despite advances in therapy, the infection continues to be associated with significant morbidity and mortality.

EPIDEMIOLOGY

- Ubiquitous in mammals worldwide, particularly rodents
- Growth on respiratory tract surfaces
- Mode of transmission is unknown:
  - Airborne person-to-person transmission is possible, but case contacts are rarely identified.
  - Environmentally acquired
- Asymptomatic infection appears early in life; >70% of healthy individuals have antibodies by age 4 years.
- Primary infection is likely to be the mechanism in infants. Reactivation of latent disease with immunosuppression was proposed as an explanation for disease later in childhood; however, animal models of PCP do not support this proposition.
- PCP in the HIV patient can occur at any time but usually presents during the 1st year of life. The highest incidence is between 3 and 6 months of age.

RISK FACTORS

- Immunocompromised host
  - Children with congenital or acquired immunodeficiency syndrome (AIDS) and recipients of suppressive therapy in the treatment of malignancies or after organ transplantation are at high risk.
  - In leukemic patients, the incidence of PCP has been directly related to the degree of immunodeficiency resulting from chemotherapy.
  - Epidemics of PCP were reported in premature and malnourished infants and children in resource-limited countries and during times of famine.

PATHOPHYSIOLOGY

- In the immunodeficient child, the pathologic changes occur predominantly in the alveoli. Cysts and trophozoites are seen adhering to the alveolar lining cells or in the cytoplasm of macrophages.
- As infection progresses, the alveolar spaces are filled with a pink, foamy exudate containing fibrin, abundant desquamative cells, and a large number of organisms. Alveolar septal thickening with mononuclear cell infiltration is also seen.

DIAGNOSIS

HISTORY

- In malnourished host
  - Subacute onset with nonspecific manifestations
    - Poor feeding, weight loss, and restlessness
    - Chronic diarrhea
    - Usually without fever
    - After 1–2 weeks, the patient develops progressive tachypnea, respiratory distress, and cough.
- In sporadic or immunocompromised host
  - This form has a more abrupt onset, sometimes even fulminant:
    - Fever (>38.5°C)
    - Nonproductive cough
    - Dyspnea at rest
- These subtypes are characterized by general clinical guidelines. Symptoms may be superimposed and can be seen in infants, children, and adolescents.

PHYSICAL EXAM

- Fever and significant tachypnea are characteristic.
- Hypoxemia: early in the course of disease and disproportionate to the auscultatory findings
- Rapidly progressive respiratory distress with cyanosis: respiratory failure early in course
- Absence of crackles is a common initial finding.
- Chest auscultation can reveal decreased breath sounds, crackles, and rhonchi.
- Coryza and wheezing have infrequently been reported.

DIAGNOSTIC TESTS & INTERPRETATION

Diagnostic Procedures/Other

- Arterial blood gas
  - pH is usually increased.
  - Reduced PaO_2 in room air (<70 mm Hg)
  - Alveolar–arterial oxygen gradient (>35 mm Hg)
- Chest radiograph
  - Most common radiologic presentation is diffuse bilateral alveolar infiltrates:
    - Initially a perihilar distribution that spreads to the periphery
    - Apices are the least affected.
    - Interstitial infiltrates and air bronchograms can be seen.
    - Rapid progression to whole lung consolidation
- Presence of hilar or mediastinal adenopathy may indicate another process such as *Mycobacterium tuberculosis*, *Mycobacterium avium-intracellulare*, fungal infections, cytomegalovirus, or lymphoma.
- Other tests:
  - Lactate dehydrogenase (LDH) can be elevated in patients with AIDS and PCP, but this finding is nonspecific.
  - WBC count is usually normal.

Pathologic Findings

- Definitive diagnosis can be obtained by demonstration of PJ in pulmonary specimens:
  - Induced sputum
  - Bronchoalveolar lavage (BAL) usually through flexible bronchoscopy (90% sensitivity)
  - Open lung or transbronchial biopsy
- Staining
  - Cysts stain with methenamine-silver, toluidine blue-O stains, calcofluor white, and fluorescein monoclonal antibody
  - Sporozoites and trophozoites are identified with Giemsa stain, modified Wright-Giemsa stain, and fluorescein-conjugated monoclonal antibody stain.
  - Polymerase chain reaction assays of BAL fluid or induced sputum is available and more sensitive for detecting PJ than microscopic methods but is not USFDA approved for diagnosis.

DIFFERENTIAL DIAGNOSIS

- Viral infections
  - Common viral respiratory pathogens
  - Cytomegalovirus
  - Epstein-Barr virus
- Bacterial infections
  - *M. tuberculosis*
  - *M. avium-intracellulare*
- Other:
  - Lymphocytic interstitial pneumonitis

TREATMENT

MEDICATION

First Line

- Minimum duration of therapy is 2 weeks; 3 weeks of therapy recommended in patients with AIDS.
- Antibiotics
  - Trimethoprim-sulfamethoxazole (TMP-SMX) is the drug of choice:
    - TMP (15–20 mg/kg/24 h) and SMX (75–100 mg/kg/24 h) IV/PO divided q6h
    - Oral therapy is reserved for patients with mild illness who do not have malabsorption or diarrhea.

Second Line

- Minimum duration of therapy is 2 weeks; 3 weeks of therapy recommended in patients with AIDS.
- Pentamidine isethionate
  - 3–4 mg/kg/dose IV (or IM) given in a single daily dose
  - Used in patients who cannot tolerate TMP-SMX or are unresponsive after 5–7 days of therapy
  - If clinical improvement is seen after 7–10 days of IV pentamidine, consider oral regimen to complete the 21-day course.
- Atovaquone
  - 1–3 months and >24 months of age: 30 mg/kg/24 h PO divided into 2 doses
  - 4–24 months of age: 45 mg/kg/24 h PO divided into 2 doses
  - Maximum dose: 750 mg b.i.d.
- Dapsone plus trimethoprim
  - Dapsone: 2 mg/kg PO daily to a maximum of 100 mg daily
  - Trimethoprim: 15 mg/kg/24 h PO divided into 3 doses
- Primaquine plus clindamycin
  - Primaquine: 0.3 mg/kg PO daily to a maximum of 30 mg PO daily
  - Clindamycin: 40 mg/kg/24 h PO divided into 4 doses to a maximum of 600 mg q6h

ADDITIONAL TREATMENT

General Measures

- Supply oxygen as necessary to keep PaO_2 >70 mm Hg.
- Mechanical ventilation must be considered if PaO_2 is <60 mm Hg on FiO_2 of 0.5.
- Corticosteroids
  - May be beneficial in HIV patients with moderate to severe PCP
  - Not systematically evaluated in children
  - Consider when PaO_2 is <70 mm Hg or the alveolar–arterial oxygen gradient is >35 mm Hg.
  - In patients >13 years of age, suggested dose is prednisone 40 mg PO b.i.d. for days 1–5, 40 mg PO once daily for days 6–10, and 20 mg PO once daily for days 11–21 with tapering. Doses of methylprednisolone or prednisone at 1 mg/kg given b.i.d.–q.i.d. for 5–7 days with a taper over the next 5 days have been suggested.

ADDITIONAL THERAPIES

- Chemoprophylaxis indications: During high-risk periods, PCP can be effectively prevented in the immunodeficient host by chemoprophylaxis in the following groups:
  - HIV exposed: 4–6 weeks to 4 months
  - HIV infected or indeterminate: 4–12 months
  - HIV infected: 1–5 years if $CD4^+$ T-lymphocyte count is <500 cells/μL or <15%
  - HIV infected: ≥6 years if $CD4^+$ T-lymphocyte count is <200 cells/μL or <15%
  - Severely symptomatic HIV patients or those with rapidly declining CD4 counts
  - HIV patients who have had previous PCP illness
  - Children who have received hematopoietic stem cell transplants (HSCTs)
  - All HSCT recipients with hematologic malignancies (e.g., leukemia, lymphoma)
  - All HSCT recipients receiving intense conditioning regimens or graft manipulation
    - Prophylaxis is initiated at engraftment and administered for 6 months; longer than 6 months in children receiving immunosuppressive therapy or with chronic graft-versus-host disease
- Drug regimen for prophylaxis
  - TMP-SMX is the drug of choice.
    - 150 mg/m^2 body surface area per day of TMP or 750 mg/m^2 body surface area per day of SMX PO divided into 2 doses on 3 consecutive days per week
    - TMP-SMX can also be given 7 days a week when prevention against other bacterial infections is sought.
  - For patients who cannot tolerate TMP-SMX
    - Dapsone (>1 month of age): 2 mg/kg (maximum 100 mg) PO daily or 4 mg/kg (maximum 200 mg) PO weekly
    - Aerosolized pentamidine (>5 years of age): 300 mg via Respirgard II nebulizer inhaled monthly
    - Atovaquone at age 1–3 months and >24 months: 30 mg/kg (max 1,500 mg/dose) PO daily; at age 4–24 months: 45 mg/kg (max 1,500 mg/dose) PO daily

ONGOING CARE

FOLLOW-UP RECOMMENDATIONS

- After 5–7 days of treatment
- If no improvement, TMP-SMX should be replaced with pentamidine.
- Standard precautions are required. Isolation from other immunodeficient patients is recommended.

PROGNOSIS

- 5–40% mortality in treated patients
- Near 100% mortality if patient is untreated
- ~35% of patients will have recurrence unless lifetime prophylaxis is instituted.

COMPLICATIONS

- High rate of respiratory failure necessitating intubation and mechanical ventilation (~60%)
- HIV-infected patients have a higher rate (40%) of adverse reactions to TMP-SMX than the general population. Rash is most common, with fever, neutropenia, anemia, renal dysfunction, nausea, vomiting, and diarrhea occurring as well.
- Prophylactic medication protects the patient as long as the drug is administered. However, this does not eradicate PJ.

ADDITIONAL READING

- King SM. Evaluation and treatment of the human immunodeficiency virus-1–exposed infant. *Pediatrics*. 2004;114(2):497–505.
- Miller RF, Huang L, Walzer PD. Pneumocystis pneumonia associated with human immunodeficiency virus. *Clin Chest Med*. 2013;34(2):229–241.
- Mofenson LM, Brady MT, Danner SP, et al; Centers for Disease Control and Prevention. Guidelines for the prevention and treatment of opportunistic infections among HIV-exposed and HIV-infected children. *MMWR Recomm Rep*. 2009;58(RR-11):1–166.
- Morris A, Wei K, Afshar K, et al. Epidemiology and clinical significance of pneumocystis colonization. *J Infect Dis*. 2008;197(1):10–17.

CODES

ICD10

B59 Pneumocystosis

FAQ

- Q: Which are the most common side effects of pentamidine?
- A: They include hypoglycemia, impaired renal or liver function, anemia, thrombocytopenia, neutropenia, hypotension, and skin rashes. These side effects can be expected in 50% of patients.
- Q: How frequently is prophylaxis failure seen?
- A: Adequate TMP-SMX treatment has only a 3% failure rate.
- Q: How are adverse reactions to TMP-SMX during PCP therapy managed?
- A: Continuation of treatment, if the reactions are not severe, is recommended.

PNEUMONIA–BACTERIAL

Erica S. Pan • Shannon Thyne

BASICS

DESCRIPTION

Pneumonia is an infection of the lungs involving the alveoli and distal airways.

EPIDEMIOLOGY

Incidence

- Highest incidence in children <5 years of age (annual incidence 3–4%)
- Viral pneumonias still generally comprise a large proportion of pediatric pneumonia.

RISK FACTORS

- Immune deficiency
  - Immunocompromised status
  - Sickle cell anemia
- Increased aspiration risk
  - Altered mental status
  - Tracheoesophageal fistula
  - Cerebral palsy
  - Seizure disorder
- Compromised lung function/anatomy
  - Cystic fibrosis
  - Congenital pulmonary malformations
  - Bronchopulmonary dysplasia
  - Asthma

ETIOLOGY

- Etiology of bacterial pneumonia differs by age:
  - Neonates: group B *Streptococcus*, enteric gram-negative rods (e.g., *Escherichia coli*), *Listeria monocytogenes, Haemophilus influenzae, Bordetella pertussis*
  - 1–3 months: neonate organisms + *Staphylococcus aureus, Streptococcus pneumoniae, Chlamydia trachomatis*
  - 4 months to 4 years: *Streptococcus pneumoniae, Staphylococcus aureus, H. influenzae*
  - >5 years of age: *Streptococcus pneumoniae, H. influenza, Staphylococcus aureus, Mycoplasma pneumoniae, Mycobacterium tuberculosis*
- Etiology can also differ based on risk factors:
  - Aspiration as etiology increases the risk for oral flora including anaerobes such as *Bacteroides* and *Peptostreptococcus*.
  - Ventilator-dependent patients are at increased risk for *Pseudomonas* or *Klebsiella* infections and infection with other gram-negative rods.
  - Cystic fibrosis increases the risk for *Pseudomonas* and other more unusual organisms.

DIAGNOSIS

HISTORY

- Fever and/or chills
- Rapid breathing is a sensitive but nonspecific finding in bacterial pneumonia.
- Difficulty breathing or shortness of breath is common (can be associated with difficulty feeding in infants).
- Poor feeding or apnea in young infants
- Cough is often seen in bacterial pneumonia. *B. pertussis* pneumonia often presents after a catarrhal phase with a paroxysmal cough and post-tussive vomiting.
- Pleuritic chest pain
- Abdominal pain and/or vomiting: most often seen with lower lobe pneumonia.
- Irritability, lethargy, and/or malaise
- Birth history, including maternal infections (e.g., *C. trachomatis* can be transmitted to an infant through a mother's genital tract at delivery)
- Immunization status: In a fully immunized child, *H. influenzae* type b, *B. pertussis*, and *S. pneumoniae* infections are less common.
- Recent history of upper respiratory tract infection (URI) or RSV can predispose to bacterial pneumonia.
- History of repeated bacterial infections may suggest immunodeficiency or cystic fibrosis (both are risk factors for bacterial pneumonia).
- Exposure to contacts with pertussis, tuberculosis, or history of recent travel
- Travelers, health care workers, and persons working in prisons or institutional settings are at greater risk for tuberculosis.

PHYSICAL EXAM

- Most common findings: oxygen saturation <95%, elevated respiratory rate, nasal flaring, fever, and ill appearance
- General examination can range from mildly ill appearing to toxic in appearance.
- Infants may have a paucity of exam findings disproportionate to their appearance and tachypnea.
- Patients may be dehydrated or in shock.
- Most children with bacterial pneumonia have fever.
- Patients with atypical bacterial pneumonia and pertussis are sometimes afebrile.
- Tachypnea or increased work of breathing: nasal flaring, grunting, and/or retracting
- Decreased oxygen saturation; therefore, oxygen saturation should be obtained by pulse oximetry in children with tachypnea or other signs of distress.
- Localized rales, crackles, rhonchi, decreased breath sounds, or wheezing
- With increasing consolidation, dullness to percussion and decreased breath sounds may be noted.
- In patients who are actively wheezing, it may be difficult to distinguish rales from other auscultated sounds.

DIAGNOSTIC TESTS & INTERPRETATION

- Not indicated for patients with uncomplicated pneumonia
- In toxic-appearing infants, blood, urine, and CSF cultures (i.e., a sepsis workup) should be considered.
- Viral testing for RSV, influenza, and other respiratory viruses if readily available can help exclude viral diagnoses in children who are candidates for outpatient therapy.

Lab

- Blood culture
  - Not indicated in healthy, immunized children with uncomplicated pneumonia
  - Rarely leads to identification of pathogen causing pneumonia
  - Should be obtained in children not responding to antibiotic therapy or moderate to severe pneumonia requiring hospitalization
  - Bacteremia has been noted in up to 30% of patients with pneumococcal pneumonia.
- Elevated peripheral WBC or range 15,000–40,000/mm^3 is associated with bacterial pneumonia or even higher WBC in pertussis but should not be relied upon to distinguish etiology of pneumonia.
- Testing for *M. pneumoniae* may be considered to guide antibiotic therapy if with signs or symptoms of atypical bacteria.
- Acute-phase reactants such as ESR, CRP, or others may provide useful information for clinical management in serious disease but cannot distinguish between viral and bacterial etiologies
- Purified protein derivative (PPD) test or an interferon-gamma release assay (e.g., quantiFERON) should be obtained in all patients in whom *M. tuberculosis* is suspected.

Imaging

- Chest radiograph (CXR), upright
  - A CXR is not required for diagnosis if clinical symptoms and examination findings are consistent with uncomplicated pneumonia.
  - A CXR (PA and lateral) is recommended if pneumonia is suspected but clinical findings are unclear, if the patient has hypoxemia or significant respiratory distress, if a pleural effusion is suspected, or if the patient is not responding to treatment.
  - Characteristic CXR patterns include "alveolar or lobar infiltrate" with air bronchograms. "Round" infiltrates may be seen with *S. pneumococcus*. "Diffuse" interstitial infiltrates and hyperinflation may be seen with atypical pneumonia such as *M. pneumoniae* or chlamydial pneumonias.
  - More commonly, CXR cannot be reliably used to distinguish between viral and bacterial disease.
  - An infiltrate may not be seen (negative CXR) if the disease is diagnosed early or if the patient is dehydrated.
- CXR, lateral decubitus: more sensitive than an upright radiograph in detecting pleural effusions or foreign body aspiration
- CT scan: not recommended as 1st-line imaging for suspected pneumonia. CT is mainly used as adjunct imaging for patients who are worsening (not improving) despite treatment or have complications.

Diagnostic Procedures/Other

If diagnosis is unclear, consider the following:

- Tracheal aspirates for Gram stain and culture if intubation necessary
- In immunocompetent children, bronchoscopy, bronchoalveolar lavage, percutaneous lung aspiration, or lung biopsy should be reserved for severe pneumonia if initial tests are not diagnostic.

DIFFERENTIAL DIAGNOSIS

- Infectious
  - Sepsis
  - Viral pneumonia
    - Infants: cytomegalovirus (CMV), metapneumovirus, herpes simplex virus (HSV)
    - From 1 to 3 months: CMV, respiratory syncytial virus (RSV), metapneumovirus
    - From 4 months to 4 years: RSV, adenovirus, influenza, metapneumovirus
  - Bronchiolitis
  - URI
  - Croup (laryngotracheobronchitis)
  - Fungal infection (if immunodeficiency or exposure history)
  - Parasitic infection (if immunodeficiency or exposure history)

- Pulmonary
  - Asthma
  - Atelectasis
  - Pneumonitis (i.e., chemical)
  - Pneumothorax
  - Pulmonary edema
  - Pulmonary hemorrhage
  - Pulmonary embolism
- Congenital
  - Pulmonary sequestration
  - Congenital pulmonary airway malformation
- Genetic: cystic fibrosis
- Tumors
  - Lymphoma
  - Primary lung tumor
  - Metastatic tumor
- Cardiac: CHF
- GI: gastroesophageal reflux disease
- Miscellaneous
  - Foreign body aspiration
  - Sarcoidosis

TREATMENT

MEDICATIONS

Outpatient: empiric treatment

- Nontoxic, uncomplicated pneumonias in patients older than 3–6 months of age and anticipated to comply with antibiotic therapy may be managed as outpatients.
- Infants and preschool children (<5 years old)
  - Amoxicillin 80–100 mg/kg/24 h (max 3 g/24 h) PO divided q8–12h
- School-aged children (≥5 years old)
  - Amoxicillin 80–100 mg/kg/24 h (max 3 g/24 h) PO divided q8–12h
- Consider for additional coverage of atypical bacterial pathogens
  - Azithromycin 10 mg/kg/dose (max 500 mg) PO × 1 day then 5 mg/kg/dose (max 250 mg) PO once daily × 4 days
  - May consider clarithromycin 15 mg/kg/24 h (max 1 g/24 h) PO divided q12h or doxycycline 4.4 mg/kg/24 h (max 200 mg/24 h) PO divided by 2 doses in patients 7 years of age or older.
- If specific pathogen is known or suspected, use appropriate antibiotic therapy.
- For patients with more severe disease, may consider combining β-lactam antibiotic and macrolide

INPATIENT CONSIDERATIONS

- Patients with moderate to severe pneumonia as defined by respiratory distress and hypoxemia (<90%), infants younger than 3–6 months of age, children and infants with pneumonia caused by a pathogen with increased virulence (e.g., community-associated MRSA), and failed outpatient therapy should be hospitalized
- Intubation and positive pressure ventilation, if clinically indicated
- Empiric antibiotic treatment
- All ages
  - Ampicillin 200–400 mg/kg/24 h (max 12 g/24 h) IV divided q6h (or penicillin 250,000 U/kg/24 h [max 24 million U/24 h] IV divided q6h)
  - Ceftriaxone 50–100 mg/kg/24 h (max 2 g/24 h) IV divided q12–24h or cefotaxime 200 mg/kg/24 h (max 12 g/24 h) IV divided q8h
- If atypical pathogens suspected, may add macrolide or use as alternative: azithromycin IV or PO using the same initial empiric dosage regimen from above
- For seriously ill patients, add vancomycin 15 mg/kg/dose IV q6–8h.
- For antistaphylococcal coverage, add vancomycin 15 mg/kg/dose IV q6–8h or clindamycin 30 mg/kg/24 h IV/PO divided q8h.
- May also consider macrolides or clindamycin as alternative for cephalosporin-allergic patients

ONGOING CARE

FOLLOW-UP RECOMMENDATIONS

Patient Monitoring

- Children on appropriate therapy should show improvement within 48–72 hours.
- If worsening or not responding to treatment, consider repeated or additional diagnostic studies. For example, persistent fever may be due to loculated pleural fluid or an empyema.
- For additional antibiotic guidance for children not improving, consider pediatric infectious disease consultation.
- CXR may be abnormal for up to 10 weeks after successful treatment. Consider follow-up CXR only if indicated for severe disease, clinical progression, or suspected complications (e.g., effusion, empyema).
- For children with recurrent bacterial pneumonia, consider an underlying anatomic or immunologic disorder (e.g., abnormal antibody production, cystic fibrosis, tracheoesophageal fistula, pulmonary sequestration).

COMPLICATIONS

- Pleural effusion
- Empyema
- Lung abscess
- Pneumatoceles
- Pneumothorax
- Bacteremia/sepsis

ADDITIONAL READING

- Bradley JS, Byington CL, Shah SS, et al. The management of community-acquired pneumonia in infants and children older than 3 months of age: clinical practice guidelines by the Pediatric Infectious Diseases Society and the Infectious Diseases Society of America. *Clin Infect Dis*. 2011;53(7):e25–e76.
- Kabra SK, Lodha R, Pandey RM. Antibiotics for community acquired pneumonia in children. *Cochrane Database Syst Rev*. 2006;(3):CD004874.
- Lee GE, Lorch SA, Sheffler-Collins S, et al. National hospitalization trends for pediatric pneumonia and associated complications. *Pediatrics*. 2010;126(2):204–213.
- McIntosh K. Community-acquired pneumonia in children. *N Engl J Med*. 2002;346(6):427–437.
- Ranganathan SC, Sonnappa S. Pneumonia and other respiratory infections. *Pediatr Clin North Am*. 2009;56(1):135–156.

CODES

ICD10

- J15.9 Unspecified bacterial pneumonia
- J15.3 Pneumonia due to streptococcus, group B
- J15.5 Pneumonia due to Escherichia coli

FAQ

- Q: What are the indications for admission and inpatient treatment of pneumonia in children?
- A: Failure of outpatient therapy, moderate to severe pneumonia as defined by respiratory distress and hypoxemia, infants younger than 3–6 months of age, children and infants with pneumonia caused by a pathogen with increased virulence (e.g., community-associated MRSA)
- Q: What is the appropriate duration of therapy for bacterial pneumonia?
- A: Empiric treatment courses of 10 days have been studied the most, although shorter courses may be effective in uncomplicated disease. Pneumonias caused by some pathogens (e.g., CA-MRSA) may require longer duration.
- Q: What is the most common causative organism of pulmonary abscess, and what is the appropriate treatment?
- A: *S. aureus* is the most common causative organism. Treatment includes IV vancomycin, IV or PO clindamycin, or PO linezolid. If MSSA is confirmed cefazolin, nafcillin, or cefuroxime may be used.
- Q: Which children are most likely to have systemic complications from community-acquired pneumonia? Local complications?
- A: An analysis of inpatient data from pediatric hospitals from 1997 to 2006 suggests that children <1 year of age are more likely to have systemic complications (e.g., sepsis, acute respiratory failure), whereas patients aged 1–5 years are more likely to have local complications (e.g., empyema, abscess).
- Q: What are risk factors for invasive pneumococcal disease?
- A: Conditions associated with invasive pneumococcal disease include congenital immune deficiency (e.g., B- or T-lymphocyte deficiencies) asplenia/functional hyposplenism, complement deficiency, diseases associated with immunosuppressive therapy or radiation therapy (including malignancies), and solid organ transplantation and chronic cardiac disease.

PNEUMOTHORAX

Richard M. Kravitz

BASICS

DESCRIPTION

Abnormal collection of free air or gas in the pleural space

EPIDEMIOLOGY

Depends on the underlying lung disease

Incidence

- Spontaneous pneumothorax
  - Male > female (1.4 to 10.1:1)
  - Peak incidence: 10–30 years
- Pneumothorax with cystic fibrosis (CF)
  - For overall CF population: 3.5–8%
  - CF patients >18 years: 16–20%
  - Risk factors for pneumothorax:
    - More severe disease
    - Decreased pulmonary function (i.e., forced expiratory volume in 1 second [FEV_1] <30–50%)
    - Colonization with *Pseudomonas aeruginosa*, *Burkholderia cepacia*, or *Aspergillus*

RISK FACTORS

- Asthma
- CF
- Pneumonia
- Collagen vascular diseases

PATHOPHYSIOLOGY

- Air can enter the pleural space via the following:
  - Chest wall (i.e., penetrating trauma)
  - Intrapulmonary (i.e., ruptured alveoli)
- Usually, collapse of the lung on the affected side seals the leak.
- If a ball valve mechanism ensues, however, air can accumulate in the thoracic cavity, causing the development of a tension pneumothorax (a medical emergency).

ETIOLOGY

- Spontaneous (secondary to rupture of apical blebs)
- Mechanical trauma
  - Penetrating injury (i.e., knife or bullet wound)
  - Blunt trauma (i.e., auto accident)
- Barotrauma
  - Mechanical ventilation
  - Cough (if severe enough)
  - Vaginal birth
- Iatrogenic
  - Central venous catheter placement
  - Bronchoscopy (especially with biopsy)
- Infection: most common organisms
  - *Staphylococcus aureus*
  - *Streptococcus pneumoniae*
  - *Mycobacterium tuberculosis*
  - *Bordetella pertussis*
  - *Pneumocystis jiroveci*
- Airway occlusion
  - Mucus plugging (asthma)
  - Foreign body
  - Meconium aspiration
- Bleb formation (i.e., idiopathic, secondary to CF)
- Malignancy
- Catamenial

DIAGNOSIS

HISTORY

- May be asymptomatic (pneumothorax discovered on chest film obtained for other reasons)
- Cough
- Shortness of breath
- Dyspnea
- Pleuritic chest pain that is usually sudden in onset and localized to apices (referred pain to shoulders)
- Respiratory distress
- Underlying medical problems which increases risk for pneumothorax
- Activity prior to developing symptoms that might have caused the pneumothorax:
  - Heavy lifting
  - Increased coughing

PHYSICAL EXAM

- May be normal
- Decreased breath sounds on the affected side
- Decreased vocal fremitus
- Hyperresonance to percussion on the affected side
- Tachypnea
- Tachycardia
- Shortness of breath
- Respiratory distress
- Shifting of the cardiac point of maximal impulse away from the affected side
- Shifting of the trachea away from the affected side
- Subcutaneous emphysema
- Cyanosis
- Scratch sign (heard through the stethoscope): A loud scratching sound is heard when a finger is gently stroked over the area of the pneumothorax.

DIAGNOSTIC TESTS & INTERPRETATION

- EKG
  - Diminished amplitude of the QRS voltage
  - Rightward shift of the QRS axis (if left-sided pneumothorax)

Lab

- Arterial blood gas
  - Po_2 can frequently be decreased.
  - Pco_2
    - Elevated with respiratory compromise
    - Decreased from hyperventilation
- Pulse oximetry
  - Useful for assessing oxygenation

Imaging

- Chest radiograph
  - Radiolucency of the affected lung
  - Lack of lung markings in the periphery of the affected lung
  - Collapsed lung on the affected side
  - Possible pneumomediastinum with subcutaneous emphysema
- Chest CT
  - Useful for finding small pneumothoraces
  - Can help distinguish a pneumothorax from a bleb or cyst
  - Helpful for locating small apical blebs associated with spontaneous pneumothoraces

Diagnostic Procedures/Other

- Pitfalls:
  - Not considering the diagnosis in otherwise healthy patients
  - Confusing the symptoms with those of an underlying lung disease
  - Inserting a needle into a cyst or bleb (can cause a tension pneumothorax with rapid respiratory compromise)

DIFFERENTIAL DIAGNOSIS

- Pulmonary
  - Congenital lung malformations
    - Cysts (i.e., bronchogenic cysts)
    - Cystic adenomatoid malformation
    - Congenital lobar emphysema
  - Acquired emphysema
  - Hyperinflation of the lung
  - Postinfectious pneumatocele
  - Bullae formation
- Miscellaneous
  - Diaphragmatic hernia
  - Infections (i.e., pulmonary abscess)
  - Muscle strain
  - Pleurisy (i.e., pleuritis)
  - Rib fracture

TREATMENT

GENERAL MEASURES

- Stabilization of the patient
- Evacuation of the pleural air
  - Should be done urgently if a tension pneumothorax is suspected
  - In small asymptomatic pneumothoraces, observation of the patient is indicated.
- Treat the underlying condition predisposing for the pneumothorax:
  - Antibiotics for any underlying infection
  - Bronchodilators and anti-inflammatory agents for asthma attacks
- Oxygen
  - Used to keep $Sao_2 \geq 95\%$
  - Breathing 100% oxygen
    - Can speed the intrapleural air's reabsorption into the bloodstream, hastening lung reexpansion
    - Useful for treating smaller pneumothoraces, especially in neonates

SURGERY/OTHER PROCEDURES

- Needle thoracentesis: useful for evacuation of the pleural air in simple, uncomplicated spontaneous pneumothorax
- Chest tube drainage
  - Used for evacuation of the pleural air in recurrent, persistent, or complicated pneumothoraces and cases with significant underlying lung disease
  - Chest tube should be left in (usually 2–4 days) until
    - Most air is reabsorbed
    - No reaccumulation of air is seen on sealing of the chest tube

- Surgical removal of pulmonary blebs
  - Blebs have a high rate of rupturing with resultant pneumothorax.
  - In patients with established pneumothoraces, the blebs should be removed or oversewn to prevent reoccurrence of the pneumothorax (blebs have a high rate of reoccurrence if not repaired).
  - Thoracotomy versus video-assisted thoracoscopic surgery (VATS)
- Pleurodesis
  - Used to attach the lung to the intrathoracic chest wall to prevent reoccurrence of a pneumothorax
  - Useful in cases of recurrent pneumothorax or if the pneumothorax is unresponsive to chest tube drainage (i.e., CF, malignancy)
  - Mechanism of action: The surface of the lung becomes inflamed and adheres to the chest wall via the formation of scar tissue.
  - 2 commonly used methods:
  - Surgical pleurodesis:
    - Mechanical abrasion of part of the lung or pleurectomy
    - Advantages: very effective; low reoccurrence rate; site specific (limits affected area)
    - Disadvantages: requires surgery and general anesthesia; contraindicated if patient is unstable
  - Chemical pleurodesis
    - Chemicals are used to cause inflammation.
    - Chemicals commonly used: talc, tetracycline, minocycline, doxycycline, quinacrine
    - Advantages: requires no surgery or general anesthesia
    - Disadvantages: less effective than surgery; generalized inflammation (rather than site-specific; makes future thoracic surgery more difficult; painful)

ONGOING CARE

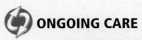

FOLLOW-UP RECOMMENDATIONS

Symptomatic relief within seconds of the air being evacuated

Patient Monitoring

Sign to watch for: inability to remove the chest tube without reaccumulation of air (suggestive of a bronchopulmonary fistula; requires surgical exploration if no improvement in 7–10 days)

PROGNOSIS

- Depends on the underlying cause of the pneumothorax
- If simple, spontaneous pneumothorax, recovery is excellent
- CF: Development of pneumothorax associated with increased morbidity and mortality (median survival after 1st pneumothorax is 4 years).

COMPLICATIONS

- Pain
- Hypoxia
- Respiratory distress
- Tension pneumothorax
  - Hypoxia
  - Hypercarbia with acidosis
  - Respiratory failure
- Pneumomediastinum with subcutaneous emphysema
- Bronchopulmonary fistula

ADDITIONAL READING

- Baumann MH. Management of spontaneous pneumothorax. *Clin Chest Med*. 2006;27(2):369–381.
- Briassoulis GC, Venkataraman ST, Vasilopoulos AG, et al. Air leaks from the respiratory tract in mechanically ventilated children with severe respiratory disease. *Pediatr Pulmonol*. 2000;29(2):127–134.
- Dotson K, Johnson LH. Pediatric spontaneous pneumothorax. *Pediatr Emerg Care*. 2012;28(7):715–723.
- Dotson K, Timm N, Gittleman M. Is spontaneous pneumothorax really a pediatric problem? A national perspective. *Pediatr Emerg Care*. 2012;28(4):340–344.
- Flume PA, Strange C, Ye X, et al. Pneumothorax in cystic fibrosis. *Chest*. 2005;128(2):720–728.
- Johnson NN, Toledo A, Endom EE. Pneumothorax, pneumomediastinum, and pulmonary embolism. *Pediatr Clin North Am*. 2010;57(6):1357–1383.
- Noppen M. Management of primary spontaneous pneumothorax. *Curr Opin Pulm Med*. 2002;9(4):272–275.
- Sahn SA, Heffner JE. Spontaneous pneumothorax. *N Engl J Med*. 2000;342(12):868–874.
- Ullman EA, Donley LP, Brady WJ. Pulmonary trauma emergency department evaluation and management. *Emerg Med Clin North Am*. 2003;21(2):291–313.

CODES

ICD10

- J93.9 Pneumothorax, unspecified
- J93.11 Primary spontaneous pneumothorax
- S27.0XXA Traumatic pneumothorax, initial encounter

FAQ

- Q: Can a pneumothorax reoccur?
- A: Reoccurrence depends on the underlying cause of the pneumothorax. Spontaneous pneumothorax reoccurrence rates:
  - Observation alone: 20–50%
  - If thoracentesis performed: 25–50%
  - If chest tube drainage performed: 32–38%
  - Overall reoccurrence rate: 16–52%
- Chemical pleurodesis reoccurrence rates:
  - Tetracycline: 25%
  - Talc: 8–10%
- Surgical pleurodesis reoccurrence rates:
  - VATS: 13%
  - Thoracotomy: 3%
  - Thoracotomy with pleurectomy: 0–4%
- CF reoccurrence rates:
  - If no drainage attempted: 68%
  - Thoracentesis alone: 90%
  - Chest tube drainage alone: 72%
  - Chemical pleurodesis:
    - Tetracycline: 42–86%
    - Quinacrine: 12.5%
    - Talc: 8%
  - Surgical pleurodesis: thoracotomy with pleurectomy: 0–4%

POLYARTERITIS NODOSA

David D. Sherry

BASICS

DESCRIPTION

An inflammatory process of small- and medium-sized muscular arteries resulting in dysfunction of affected organs

EPIDEMIOLOGY

Incidence

Extremely rare in childhood

Prevalence

Prevalence equal in boys and girls

PATHOPHYSIOLOGY

Necrotizing arteritis of small- and medium-sized arteries resulting in segmental fibrinoid necrosis

ETIOLOGY

- Idiopathic
- Postinfectious (streptococcal, hepatitis B)

DIAGNOSIS

HISTORY

- Persistent constitutional symptoms
- Bilateral calf pain
- Abdominal pain
- Weight loss
- Unexplained fever
- Headache
- Arthralgia/myalgia
- Rashes
- Seizures
- Weakness

PHYSICAL EXAM

- Check skin for the following:
  - Livedo reticularis
  - Splinter hemorrhages
  - Erythema nodosum
  - Necrotic digits
- Assess BP and pulses.
- Neurologic exam for findings consistent with neuropathy (mononeuritis multiplex)
- Ophthalmologic exam for cotton wool spots
- Check testes for tenderness or swelling.
- Check muscles for tenderness, especially calves.

DIAGNOSTIC TESTS & INTERPRETATION

Lab

Initial lab tests

- ESR
  - Usually extremely elevated; leukocytosis and thrombocytosis are seen.
- Urine analysis
  - Proteinuria and hematuria can be present.
- Creatinine and BUN levels
  - May be elevated
- Antinuclear antibodies and rheumatoid factor
  - Usually negative
- Muscle enzymes (creatine kinase, lactate dehydrogenase, aspartate aminotransferase, and aldolase levels)
  - Muscle involvement is common, especially in those with calf pain.
- Antineutrophil cytoplasmic antibodies (ANCAs)
  - Detectable in some; usually perinuclear (p), rarely cytoplasmic (c) staining patterns; ANCA is more commonly associated with other vasculitides:
    - pANCA pattern usually caused by anti-myeloperoxidase (MPO) antibodies; also seen in microscopic polyangiitis
    - cANCA pattern usually caused by anti-proteinase 3 (PR3) antibodies; also seen in granulomatous with polyangiitis (Wegener granulomatosis)

ALERT

The detection of ANCA, previously thought to be highly specific for vasculitis, now appears to be less so. Hence, it remains important to confirm the diagnosis of polyarteritis nodosa with biopsy or angiography.

- Hepatitis B serologies
  - Hepatitis B has been associated in some series of patients with polyarteritis nodosa.
- Streptococcal titers
  - Polyarteritis nodosa may develop after streptococcal infections.

Imaging

- MRI of tender muscles
  - Short T_1 inversion recovery (STIR) images may show edema, so a directed biopsy can be done to avoid false-negative muscle biopsy.
- MRA, CT angiography, or angiography
  - Can demonstrate vessel wall stenoses and aneurysm

Diagnostic Procedures/Other

Biopsy of affected tissue/organ: usually skin, kidney, nerve, testicle

DIFFERENTIAL DIAGNOSIS

- Infection
  - Bacterial endocarditis
  - Brucellosis
  - Influenza B (calf pain)
- Tumors
  - Left atrial myxoma
  - Burkitt lymphoma
- Metabolic
  - Homocystinuria (thromboembolic events)
- Congenital
- Immunologic
  - Systemic necrotizing vasculitis
  - Systemic lupus erythematosus
  - Kawasaki disease
  - Systemic juvenile idiopathic arthritis
  - Granulomatosis with polyangiitis (Wegener granulomatosis)
  - Takayasu arteritis
  - Cryoglobulinemia
  - Antiphospholipid antibody syndrome
  - Thrombotic thrombocytopenic purpura
- Psychologic
  - Munchausen syndrome (factitious skin lesions)
- Miscellaneous
  - Degos disease (malignant atrophic papulosis)

TREATMENT

MEDICATION
- Corticosteroids are mainstay.
  - Usually start at dose of 1–2 mg/kg/24 h and adjust based on response.
  - May initially give methylprednisolone 30 mg/kg up to 1 g/24 h IV once daily for 3 days
- Immunosuppressives such as methotrexate, azathioprine, and cyclophosphamide may be necessary.
- Hypertension should be managed aggressively.

ADDITIONAL TREATMENT
General Measures
- Medication
- Diet
- Caution
  - Do not initiate therapy before efforts to establish the diagnosis.

ONGOING CARE

FOLLOW-UP RECOMMENDATIONS
- Initiation of steroid therapy may bring response in 1–2 weeks; however, management of specific organs affected during acute stage is essential.
- May require long-term therapy

Patient Monitoring
- Watch for the following:
  - Rising creatinine and BUN levels
  - Abdominal pain
  - Uncontrolled hypertension
- Home testing
  - May wish to have patients monitor BP periodically if renal involvement suspected

DIET
- If renal system involved, diet low in sodium and potassium
- Possible conflicts with medications

PROGNOSIS
- May be extremely poor over the long term
- Risk is high for renal failure, hypertension, stroke, myocardial infarction, bowel infarction, and death.
- Owing to low incidence/prevalence, precise data are not available.
- Cutaneous polyarteritis nodosa is relatively benign.

COMPLICATIONS
- Hypertension
- Renal failure
- Digital necrosis
- Intestinal infarction
- Stroke

ADDITIONAL READING

- Eleftheriou D, Dillon MJ, Tullus K, et al. Systemic polyarteritis nodosa in the young: a single centre experience over thirty-two years. *Arthritis Rheum*. 2013;65(9):2476–2485. doi:10.1002/art.38024
- Kawakami T. A review of pediatric vasculitis with a focus on juvenile polyarteritis nodosa. *Am J Clin Dermatol*. 2012;13(6):389–398.
- Khubchandani RP, Viswanathan V. Pediatric vasculitides: a generalists approach. *Indian J Pediatr*. 2010;77(10):1165–1171.
- Morgan AJ, Schwartz RA. Cutaneous polyarteritis nodosa: a comprehensive review. *Int J Dermatol*. 2010;49(7):750–756.
- Ozen S, Anton J, Arisoy N, et al. Juvenile polyarteritis: results of a multicenter survey of 110 children. *J Pediatr*. 2004;145(4):517–522.
- Ting TV, Hashkes PJ. Update on childhood vasculitides. *Curr Opin Rheumatol*. 2004;16(5):560–565.

CODES

ICD10
M30.0 Polyarteritis nodosa

FAQ
- Q: When should I consider polyarteritis nodosa in the differential?
- A: There are 5 major clues to polyarteritis nodosa: (1) prolonged constitutional symptoms without a diagnosis, (2) multisystem disease, (3) an unusual patient for the presenting symptom (myocardial infarction in a teen), (4) a rash that looks vasculitic, and (5) bilateral calf pain in a sick child.
- Q: What is the difference between polyarteritis nodosa and systemic necrotizing vasculitis?
- A: Polyarteritis nodosa has a strict definition. Many children who clearly have vasculitis of the small- and medium-sized arteries do not fit precisely into the description of polyarteritis nodosa. In most ways, the search for organ involvement and therapy is the same.
- Q: Who should manage the patient with polyarteritis nodosa?
- A: Usually, one discipline provides comprehensive management plan (either the pediatrician or rheumatologist). Subspecialist(s) of the affected organ systems provide management guidelines for specific organ issues.

POLYCYSTIC KIDNEY DISEASE

Kelly A. Benedict • Paul Brakeman

BASICS

DESCRIPTION

- Polycystic kidney disease (PKD) is a heritable disorder with diffuse cystic involvement of both kidneys without other dysplastic elements. The term PKD is generally used to describe 2 genetically distinct syndromes:
  - Autosomal dominant polycystic kidney disease (ADPKD)
    - Saccular, epithelial-lined, fluid-filled cysts of various sizes are derived from all segments of the nephron.
    - Cysts progressively enlarge and become disconnected from the tubule of origin.
    - Usually not clinically apparent until the 3rd or 4th decade of life
    - ~2–5% of patients have early-onset disease.
  - Autosomal recessive polycystic kidney disease (ARPKD)
    - Fusiform dilations arise from the collecting ducts and maintain contact with the nephron of origin.
    - Associated hepatic abnormalities are obligatory such as biliary dysgenesis and periportal fibrosis (congenital hepatic fibrosis), with portal hypertension.
    - Affects both the kidneys and the liver in approximately inverse proportions

EPIDEMIOLOGY

- ADPKD
  - One of the most common human genetic disorders; the most common renal inherited disease
  - A major cause of end-stage renal disease (ESRD) in adults
  - Frequency: 1 in 400–1,000
- ARPKD
  - Incidence of 1 in 20,000–40,000 live births
  - Exact incidence unknown owing to perinatal deaths in severe cases

RISK FACTORS

Genetics

- ARPKD
  - Mutations in the polycystic kidney hepatic disease 1 gene (*PKHD1*, chromosome 6)
- ADPKD
  - Type I ADPKD accounts for 85–90% of cases of ADPKD and is caused by mutations in the *PKD1* gene (chromosome 16).
  - Large genomic deletions may encompass *PKD1* and *TSC2* genes, resulting in early-onset ADPKD with tuberous sclerosis.
  - Type II ADPKD is caused by mutations in the *PKD2* gene (chromosome 4) and accounts for 10–15% of the cases.
- Other
  - Presymptomatic genetic screening for ADPKD is not recommended.
  - Normotensive women with ADPKD usually have uncomplicated pregnancies.
  - Higher risk for maternal/fetal complications if there is preexisting hypertension

PATHOPHYSIOLOGY

- ADPKD is produced by decreased functional polycystins:
  - Polycystin-1 is a membrane mechanoreceptor-like protein that forms multiprotein complexes at focal adhesions, cell–cell junctions, and cilia. It is involved in cell polarity, proliferation, cell–matrix interactions, and secretion.
  - Polycystin-2 is a divalent cation channel involved in calcium signaling and intracellular calcium homeostasis and is likely critical for cytoskeletal organization, cell adhesion, migration, and proliferation.
- ARPKD is produced by loss of functional fibrocystin/polyductin:
  - Fibrocystin/polyductin is an integral membrane receptor with extracellular protein-interaction sites that transduce intracellular signals to the nucleus.
  - Proteins affected in cystic kidney disease localize to cilia on epithelial cells.
  - Cilia are critical for cell architecture, proliferation, apoptosis, and polarity.

ETIOLOGY

- ADPKD is generally an adult-onset, systemic disorder with cystic and noncystic manifestations. Cysts occur in the kidneys and other epithelial organs (e.g., seminal vesicles, pancreas, and liver):
  - Polycystic liver disease is the most common extrarenal manifestation.
  - Intracranial aneurysms occur in ~8%.
  - Mitral valve prolapse is the most common valvular abnormality (demonstrated in up to 25% of affected individuals).
  - Colonic diverticula in 80% with ESRD
- ARPKD is a renal and hepatic developmental disorder. The hallmark of ARPKD liver disease is congenital hepatic fibrosis and dilation of intrahepatic bile ducts (Caroli disease).
  - Severely affected infants may have the oligohydramnios sequence at birth, and associated pulmonary hypoplasia and respiratory complications convey a high mortality risk.

DIAGNOSIS

HISTORY

- ADPKD
  - Detailed family history is essential.
  - Most common presenting complaint in adults is pain.
  - Hypertension, gross hematuria, nephrolithiasis, and UTIs are common.
- ARPKD
  - Oligohydramnios sequence
  - Postnatal respiratory insufficiency
  - Renal insufficiency
  - Hypertension (may be severe)
  - Hepatobiliary manifestations (cholestasis, cholangitis, liver failure, portal hypertension, hypersplenism) evolve in older patients.
- Signs and symptoms
  - ADPKD
    - Older children are often asymptomatic but may present with hypertension, abdominal pain, abdominal mass, gross hematuria after trauma, proteinuria, UTI/cyst infection, renal calculi, or decreased renal function.
  - ARPKD
    - Presentation variable
    - Severely affected infants have "Potter" oligohydramnios sequence.
    - Pulmonary hypoplasia/respiratory insufficiency is a major cause of neonatal mortality.
    - Renal insufficiency with neonatal survival
    - Hepatobiliary complications later in course (portal hypertension, hematemesis, hepatosplenomegaly hypersplenism with pallor, petechiae)

PHYSICAL EXAM

- Clinical spectrum variable, particularly in ARPKD
- Hypertension
- Abdominal pain; tenderness at flank or costovertebral angle
- Flank mass or palpable kidneys
- Hepatosplenomegaly, varices, jaundice/icterus, abdominal ascites in ARPKD

DIAGNOSTIC TESTS & INTERPRETATION

Lab

- Metabolic panel to include BUN, creatinine, electrolytes
- Calcium, phosphorus
- Liver function tests
- CBC
- Urinalysis
- Note: Hyponatremia is often present in the neonatal period in ARPKD.

Imaging
- Ultrasonography is the preferred screening method and should include liver and Doppler to evaluate for portal hypertension in ARPKD.
- ARPKD
  - Kidneys enlarged with increased echogenicity and loss of corticomedullary differentiation
  - The liver may be normal in infants and young children. Over time, it becomes enlarged and hyperechoic. Dilated intrahepatic biliary ducts may be seen.
  - Prenatal ultrasound after 24–30 weeks' gestation may show hyperechoic enlarged kidneys, oligohydramnios, and absence of bladder filling.
- Ultrasound diagnostic criteria for ADPKD
  - $<$40 years should have at least 2 cysts in 1 of the kidneys and 1 cyst in the other kidney or 3 cysts in a single kidney.
  - $\geq$40 and $\leq$59 years of age should have at least 2 cysts in each kidney.
  - $>$60 years should have at least 4 cysts in each kidney.
- CT scan with contrast
  - Has limited use in young children owing to exposure to ionizing radiation.
  - It is mostly used in adults with ADPKD because it can distinguish between solid and liquid renal masses.
- MRI with gadolinium
  - Heavy-weighted T2 MRI is the most sensitive method currently available.
  - Can be used in both conditions
  - Particularly useful to evaluate liver involvement in ARPKD
  - Avoid gadolinium in patients with advanced chronic kidney disease.

DIFFERENTIAL DIAGNOSIS
- Multicystic dysplastic kidney (MCDK)
- Glomerular cystic kidney disease (GCKD)
- Acquired cystic disease may occur in patients with ESRD.
- Genetic syndromes with cystic renal dysplasia, including, but not limited to the following:
  - Meckel syndrome
  - Jeune syndrome
  - Ivemark syndrome
  - Zellweger syndrome
  - Bardet-Biedl syndrome
  - Tuberous sclerosis

TREATMENT

MEDICATION
- Hypertension is common in PKD. Patients respond well to diuretics, ACE inhibitors, or calcium channel blockers. ACE inhibitors or angiotensin-receptor blockers are 1st line.
- In patients with PKD and nephrolithiasis, thiazide diuretics may be used for hypercalciuria, and potassium citrate supplements if hypocitraturia is found.
- Pyelonephritis in patients with PKD may lead to infected cysts. The treatment should include antibiotics that penetrate into the cysts (quinolones, trimethoprim) if cephalosporins and aminoglycosides fail to eradicate the infection.

ADDITIONAL TREATMENT
General Measures
- No currently approved targeted treatments to cure or slow progression
- Medical management is supportive.
- Pain is the most common symptom in ADPKD and can be difficult to treat.

ADDITIONAL THERAPIES
Activity: Patients with PKD should not participate in high-contact athletics in which the abdomen may be traumatized repeatedly. Strenuous static exercise should be avoided in hypertensive patients.

ONGOING CARE

FOLLOW-UP RECOMMENDATIONS
A pediatric nephrologist should be involved in the care of children with PKD.

DIET
In both conditions, dietary changes depend on the degree of renal failure. Sodium restriction is indicated in cases of hypertension and/or edema. Caffeine should be avoided in cases of ADPKD.

PATIENT EDUCATION
- Emotional support and education of patients with PKD and their families can be obtained through the Polycystic Kidney Foundation (http://www.PKDcure.org) and the PKD Alliance (http://www.arpkdchf.org).
- Genetic counseling is indicated in these disorders and genetic testing may help families understand future risks.

PROGNOSIS
- ADPKD
  - The probability of being alive and not having ESRD is about 77% at age 50 years, 57% at age 58 years, and 52% at age 73 years. Median onset of ESRD is 53 years (PKD1) versus 69 years (PKD2).
  - Cystic expansion occurs at a consistent rate per individual, although it is heterogeneous in the population.
  - Larger kidneys are associated with more rapid disease progression.
  - PKD1 mutation is more severe because more cysts develop earlier, not because they grow faster.
- ARPKD
  - Neonatal onset is fatal in up to 50% of infants because of pulmonary hypoplasia with associated respiratory failure.
  - Patients who survive the neonatal period have up to an 80% 10-year survival.

ADDITIONAL READING

- Arts HH, Knoers NV. Current insights into renal ciliopathies: what can genetics teach us? *Pediatr Neph*. 2013;28(6):863–874.
- Dell KM. The spectrum of polycystic kidney disease in children. *Adv Chronic Kidney Dis*. 2011;18(5):339–347.
- Sweeney WE Jr, Avner ED. Diagnosis and management of childhood polycystic kidney disease. *Pediatr Nephrol*. 2011;26(5):675–692.
- Torres VE, Harris PC. Strategies targeting cAMP signaling in the treatment of polycystic kidney disease. *J Am Soc Nephrol*. 2014;25(1):18–32.

CODES

ICD10
- Q61.3 Polycystic kidney, unspecified
- Q61.19 Other polycystic kidney, infantile type
- Q61.2 Polycystic kidney, adult type

FAQ
- Q: What can be done to slow the progression of renal insufficiency in ADPKD?
- A: Well-controlled BP and rapid treatment of UTIs may decrease the progression of renal failure.
- Q: Should asymptomatic older siblings of an infant with ARPKD be evaluated?
- A: Yes. An older child may have congenital hepatic fibrosis with minimal renal involvement.
- Q: Should one screen ADPKD-affected family members for the presence of cerebral vessel aneurysms if other family members have berry aneurysms?
- A: Although routine screening is not recommended, intrafamilial clustering of aneurysms has been reported and it may be advisable to screen children with MRI or cranial CT in a family with aneurysms.

POLYCYSTIC OVARY SYNDROME

Selma Feldman Witchel

BASICS

DESCRIPTION

- Polycystic ovary syndrome (PCOS) is a heterogeneous familial disorder characterized by hyperandrogenism, chronic anovulation, and infertility. Hirsutism, polycystic ovaries, obesity, insulin resistance, and hyperinsulinemia may be present but are not required for diagnosis.
- The 1990 NIH consensus meeting criteria for the diagnosis of PCOS were chronic anovulation, hyperandrogenism, and exclusion of other disorders. The 2006 Rotterdam criteria expanded the diagnostic features to include polycystic ovary morphology on US. The Androgen Excess-PCOS Society criteria emphasized the importance of hyperandrogenism.
- Using adult criteria to diagnose PCOS may be inappropriate for adolescent girls because irregular menses and multifollicular ovaries are common during adolescence.

EPIDEMIOLOGY

- Very common endocrine disorder affecting approximately 6–8% of reproductive-aged women
- Onset often during the peripubertal years
- May be preceded by premature adrenarche

Genetics

- Multifactorial polygenic familial disorder
- More prevalent in 1st-degree relatives of affected women
- A few genes associated with PCOS have been identified and replicated in women of European and Chinese ancestry. These genes include fibrillin-3 (*FBN-3*), DENN/MADD domain containing 1A (*DENND1A*), FSH receptor (*FSHR*), and LH receptor (*LHCGR*) variants.

PATHOPHYSIOLOGY

- PCOS is associated with follicular growth arrest. Most follicles arrest at the small antral stage prior to selection of a dominant follicle, giving rise to the typical pattern of multiple small follicles forming a ring in the ovary. Failure to select a dominant follicle leads to chronic anovulation.
- Characterized by a paradox regarding insulin sensitivity. Muscle, liver, and adipose tissue manifest insulin resistance, whereas the adrenal, ovary, and perhaps, the hypothalamus retain insulin sensitivity. The insulin resistance leads to increased insulin secretion by pancreatic beta cells to maintain euglycemia. The elevated insulin concentrations amplify LH- and IGF-1–stimulated theca cell androgen production and decrease SHBG production leading to increased free testosterone concentrations. Obesity exacerbates insulin resistance, intensifies PCOS symptomatology, and increases the risk for development of type 2 diabetes (T2D).
- Prenatal and childhood factors appear to influence the development of insulin resistance consistent with the hypotheses regarding early developmental origins of PCOS. Infants born small for gestational age (SGA) who experience fetal growth restriction followed by significant postnatal catch-up growth show increased insulin resistance prior to the onset of puberty.
- PCOS symptoms tend to improve with age as demonstrated in a 20-year follow-up of young women with PCOS. These women demonstrated decreased androgen concentrations and decreased ovarian volumes without any significant change in BMI or insulin sensitivity.

ETIOLOGY

- The precise etiology or initiating events remain to be elucidated. Likely, there are several potential mechanisms that initiate the perpetual cycle involving neuroendocrine abnormalities, excessive ovarian (and adrenal) androgen secretion, and metabolic dysfunction.
- LH hypersecretion is commonly observed in women with PCOS. For some, this might represent an intrinsic neuroendocrine abnormality. However, in most instances hyperandrogenism is responsible for LH hypersecretion. Amelioration of the LH hypersecretion by flutamide, an androgen receptor blocker, supports the relationship of hyperandrogenism and LH hypersecretion. One potential mechanism identified in adolescent girls is decreased hypothalamic sensitivity to progesterone.
- Although the molecular mechanisms responsible for insulin resistance and hyperinsulinemia in PCOS remain to be better characterized, post insulin receptor signal transduction is impaired. The compensatory hyperinsulinemia promotes ovarian (adrenal) androgen secretion. Adipose tissue dysfunction may provoke insulin resistance, but aberrant adipocyte function may also represent a consequence of hyperinsulinemia. Improved insulin sensitivity brought about by weight loss or metformin improves the symptomatology associated with PCOS.

COMMONLY ASSOCIATED CONDITIONS

- Obesity
- Insulin resistance
- Impaired glucose tolerance
- T2D
- Endometriosis
- Metabolic syndrome
- Dyslipidemia
- Hypertension
- Increased risk for cardiovascular disease
- Nonalcoholic fatty acid liver disease
- Sleep apnea
- Depression and impaired quality of life

DIAGNOSIS

SIGNS AND SYMPTOMS

- Irregular menses
- Infertility
- Hyperandrogenism
- Hirsutism
- Polycystic ovaries on US
- Exclusion of other disorders such as nonclassical congenital adrenal hyperplasia
- Obesity and insulin resistance may occur but are not required for diagnosis.

HISTORY

- Age at onset and sequence of pubertal development
- Menstrual history
- Infertility and reproductive history
- Signs and symptoms of androgen excess, for example, hirsutism, acne, male pattern baldness
- Family history of PCOS, hyperandrogenism, and fertility

PHYSICAL EXAM

- Increased terminal hair growth in androgen-dependent areas (hirsutism)
- Acne
- Obesity
- Acanthosis nigricans

DIAGNOSTIC TESTS & INTERPRETATION

- Hormone determinations:
  - Testosterone and free testosterone
  - Sex hormone–binding globulin
  - 17-hydroxyprogesterone
  - Androstenedione
  - DHEAS
  - LH and FSH
  - Prolactin
  - Thyroid function studies (T_4, TSH)
  - HgbA1c
  - Antimüllerian hormone (AMH)
- Stimulation and tolerance tests:
  - Oral glucose tolerance test to assess for impaired glucose tolerance, impaired fasting glucose tolerance, or diabetes
  - Consider referral to endocrinologist for ACTH stimulation test to exclude the diagnosis of 21-hydroxylase deficiency and other disorders of steroidogenesis.
  - Euglycemic and hyperinsulinemic clamp studies can be performed to assess insulin sensitivity. These tests are generally reserved for research purposes.
- Imaging studies:
  - Ovarian US to assess ovarian volume and follicle number. For the postpubertal girl, revised criteria suggest that a total ovary threshold count of 26 follicles provided the optimal compromise between sensitivity and specificity to distinguish polycystic from normal ovaries.
  - Pelvic MRI: ovarian volume and the number of ovarian follicles

DIFFERENTIAL DIAGNOSIS

- Nonclassic congenital adrenal hyperplasia
- Cushing syndrome
- Androgen-secreting tumors
- Hyperprolactinemia
- Thyroid dysfunction
- Exogenous androgen use

TREATMENT

GENERAL MEASURES

- Treatment should to be individualized to best address the needs of each patient. Common goals include reduced symptoms of hyperandrogenism, regular menses and ovulation, fertility, and decreased risk for comorbidities.
- Lifestyle. Lifestyle intervention to promote weight loss and regular exercise is extremely beneficial.
  - Pharmacologic
  - Oral contraceptives
  - Metformin
  - Spironolactone
  - Antiandrogens
  - Statins
  - Monthly progestins

SURGERY/OTHER PROCEDURES

Ovarian wedge resection was used in the past. This treatment is no longer advocated.

ONGOING CARE

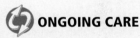

COMPLICATIONS

- One systemic review of 35 studies concluded that women with PCOS have a 2.5-fold increased prevalence of impaired glucose tolerance, 2.5-fold increased prevalence of metabolic syndrome, and 4-fold increased prevalence of T2D.
- Women with the most extreme degrees of androgen excess and insulin resistance demonstrate increased risks for impaired oocyte development and may experience high rate of miscarriages.
- During pregnancy, risk of developing gestational diabetes, pregnancy-induced hypertension, and preeclampsia are increased.
- Possible cancer risk
- Quality of life concerns and issues

ADDITIONAL READING

- Abbott DH, Bacha F. Ontogeny of polycystic ovary syndrome and insulin resistance in utero and early childhood. *Fertil Steril*. 2013;100(1):2–11.
- Bates GW, Legro RS. Long term management of polycystic ovarian syndrome (PCOS). *Mol Cell Endocrinol*. 2013;373(1–2):91–97.
- Blank SK, McCartney CR, Chhabra S, et al. Modulation of gonadotropin-releasing hormone pulse generator sensitivity to progesterone inhibition in hyperandrogenic adolescent girls—implications for regulation of pubertal maturation. *J Clin Endocrinol Metab*. 2009;94(7):2360–2366.
- Carmina E, Campagna AM, Lobo RA. A 20-year follow-up of young women with polycystic ovary syndrome. *Obstet Gynecol*. 2012;119(2, Pt 1):263–269.
- Carmina E, Oberfield SE, Lobo RA. The diagnosis of polycystic ovary syndrome in adolescents. *Am J Obstet Gynecol*. 2010;203(3):201.e1–201.e5.
- Chang RJ, Cook-Andersen H. Disordered follicle development. *Mol Cell Endocrinol*. 2013;373(1–2):51–60.
- Dumesic DA, Richards JS. Ontogeny of the ovary in polycystic ovary syndrome. *Fertil Steril*. 2013;100(1):23–38.
- Eagleson CA, Gingrich MB, Pastor CL, et al. Polycystic ovarian syndrome: evidence that flutamide restores sensitivity of the gonadotropin-releasing hormone pulse generator to inhibition by estradiol and progesterone. *J Clin Endocrinol Metab*. 2000;85(11):4047–4052.
- Goodarzi MO, Dumesic DA, Chazenbalk G, et al. Polycystic ovary syndrome: etiology, pathogenesis and diagnosis. *Nat Rev Endocrinol*. 2011:7(4):219–231.
- Lujan ME, Jarrett BY, Brooks ED, et al. Updated ultrasound criteria for polycystic ovary syndrome: reliable thresholds for elevated follicle population and ovarian volume. *Hum Reprod*. 2013;28(5):1361–1368.
- McGee WK, Bishop CV, Bahar A, et al. Elevated androgens during puberty in female rhesus monkeys lead to increased neuronal drive to the reproductive axis: a possible component of polycystic ovary syndrome. *Hum Reprod*. 2012;27(2):531–540.
- Moran LJ, Misso ML, Wild RA, et al. Impaired glucose tolerance, type 2 diabetes and metabolic syndrome in polycystic ovary syndrome: a systematic review and meta-analysis. *Hum Reprod Update*. 2010;16(4):347–363.
- Moran LJ, Pasquali R, Teede HJ, et al. Treatment of obesity in polycystic ovary syndrome: a position statement of the Androgen Excess and Polycystic Ovary Syndrome Society. *Fertil Steril*. 2009;92(6):1966–1982.
- Mutharasan P, Galdones E, Peñalver B, et al. Evidence for chromosome 2p16.3 polycystic ovary syndrome susceptibility locus in affected women of European ancestry. *J Clin Endocrinol Metab*. 2013;98(1):E185–E190.
- Stepto NK, Cassar S, Joham AE, et al. Women with polycystic ovary syndrome have intrinsic insulin resistance on euglycaemic-hyperinsulaemic clamp. *Hum Reprod*. 2013;28(3):777–784.
- Welt CK, Styrkarsdottir U, Ehrmann DA, et al. Variants in *DENND1A* are associated with polycystic ovary syndrome in women of European ancestry. *J Clin Endocrinol Metab*. 2012;97(7):E1342–E1347.
- Xie GB, Xu P, Che YN, et al. Microsatellite polymorphism in the fibrillin 3 gene and susceptibility to PCOS: a case-control study and meta-analysis. *Reprod Biomed Online*. 2013;26(2):168–174.

CODES

ICD10

- E28.2 Polycystic ovarian syndrome
- L68.0 Hirsutism

FAQ

- Q: Can I still get pregnant if I have this syndrome?
- A: Those patients who desire to become pregnant can be treated with ovulation-inducing agents and benefit from treatment by reproductive endocrine specialists.
- Q: I've noticed increased facial hair recently. Is there anything I can do about this?
- A: Yes. Oral contraceptives and spironolactone may be helpful. Cosmetic methods may be necessary to remove coarse hair growth.
- Q: Will my daughter inherit this disorder?
- A: Daughters and sisters of affected women have a higher chance of developing PCOS than daughters and sisters of unaffected women.

POLYCYTHEMIA

Benjamin J. Huang • Tannie Huang

BASICS

DESCRIPTION

Polycythemia (sometimes referred to as erythrocytosis) is defined as an absolute increase in red blood cell (RBC) mass, most commonly suspected in the context of an elevated hemoglobin, hematocrit, or RBC count. Use of age- and gender-based norms are critical, as they fluctuate throughout childhood. Polycythemia can be categorized as follows:

- Primary polycythemia: defect within erythroid progenitors, resulting in overproduction of RBCs. Serum erythropoietin (EPO) levels are usually low.
- Secondary polycythemia: stimulation of erythrocyte production by an increased level of EPO, which is either elevated appropriately in response to hypoxia or elevated inappropriately due to an EPO-producing tumor or exogenous administration
- Relative polycythemia: elevated hemoglobin, hematocrit, or RBC count without a true increase in RBC mass, often caused by decreased plasma volume

EPIDEMIOLOGY

Primary polycythemias are very rare in children:

- Myeloproliferative neoplasms, including polycythemia vera (PV): Vast majority of cases occur in older adults, but cases of childhood PV have been described.
- Primary familial and congenital polycythemia (PFCP): very rare but presents early during infancy or childhood

The incidence and prevalence of secondary polycythemias depend on the respective underlying conditions.

RISK FACTORS

Genetics

- PFCP: autosomal dominant
- Chuvash polycythemia: autosomal recessive
- 2,3-diphosphoglycerate (DPG) mutase deficiency: autosomal recessive

GENERAL PREVENTION

There are no preventive measures for conditions of primary polycythemia. Treatment of underlying conditions, such as correction of congenital heart disease, will prevent the development of secondary polycythemia.

PATHOPHYSIOLOGY

- Primary polycythemias
  - PV: myeloproliferative neoplasm arising from a clonal population of abnormal hematopoietic progenitor cells with EPO-independent proliferation. EPO levels are usually low. The mutation *JAK2* V617F is found in the vast majority of cases.
- PFCP: Erythroid progenitors are hypersensitive to EPO. Some families have a mutation in the EPO receptor (EPO-R).
- Secondary polycythemias
  - High altitude: compensation for low atmospheric oxygen pressure
  - Chronic pulmonary disease or hypoventilation: compensation for inadequate oxygenation
  - Cyanotic heart disease and arteriovenous malformations: right-to-left cardiac or extracardiac shunting, resulting in desaturation of arterial blood
  - High oxygen-affinity hemoglobinopathies: mutation in either alpha or beta globin chains leading to increased oxygen affinity and decreased oxygen delivery to tissues
  - 2,3-DPG mutase deficiency: rare defect that leads to deficiency of 2,3-DPG. Because 2,3-DPG promotes the release of oxygen from hemoglobin, deficiency leads to decreased oxygen delivery to tissues.
  - Methemoglobinemia: elevated levels of Fe^{3+} hemoglobin, which has an increased affinity for oxygen compared to Fe^{2+} hemoglobin
  - Carboxyhemoglobinemia: Carbon monoxide binds to hemoglobin preferentially compared to oxygen.
  - Hypoxia-sensing pathway defects: Mutations in the genes von Hippel Lindau (VHL) are common in certain ethnic groups (Chuvash polycythemia). Hypoxia-inducible factor 2 (HIF2) and proline hydroxylase (PHD2) have also been described.
  - EPO-producing tumors: renal cell carcinoma, hepatocellular carcinoma, hemangioblastoma, pheochromocytoma, and uterine fibroids

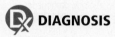

DIAGNOSIS

HISTORY

- Age of onset
  - Neonates who are born to mothers with preeclampsia or diabetes, are small for gestational age, undergo delayed cord clamping, or have certain chromosomal abnormalities (e.g., Down syndrome) are at increased risk for polycythemia during the neonatal period.
- Gender
- Weight: Obesity is associated with obstructive sleep apnea.
- Dehydration
  - Diuretic use or abuse
  - Severe diarrhea
- Hyperviscosity
  - Headache, dizziness, syncope, transient blindness, history of thrombosis
- Symptoms concerning for congenital heart disease or chronic pulmonary disease:
  - Cyanosis
  - Decreased exercise tolerance
  - Shortness of breath
  - Dyspnea on exertion
- Pruritus
  - Seen with polycythemia vera
- Sleep history
  - Snoring, nocturnal apnea, mouth breathing, excessive daytime sleepiness, behavioral problems concerning for obstructive sleep apnea
- Living situation
  - High altitude
  - Older house with fuel-burning heaters
  - Cigarette exposure
- Social history
  - Smoking (tobacco or marijuana)
  - Drug use including steroids, EPO, diuretics
- Family history
  - High hematocrit, hyperviscosity, or need for phlebotomy
  - Family members with similar symptoms may also indicate concurrent exposure to carbon monoxide

PHYSICAL EXAM

Signs and symptoms:

- Cyanosis
- Plethora
- Clubbing
- Cardiac murmurs or bruits
- Dehydration
- Splenomegaly

ALERT

- Fingerstick hematocrit: Squeezing the finger to collect a specimen may give a falsely elevated hematocrit.
- Capillary hematocrit: often higher than venous hematocrit
- Dehydration during blood draw may result in relative polycythemia due to decreased plasma volume.
- PaO_2 is only interpretable with an arterial blood gas.

DIAGNOSTIC TESTS & INTERPRETATION

Lab

- Many patients may be asymptomatic with polycythemia noted on routine screening.
- Initial workup should include the following:
  - CBC with differential: Polycythemia may be associated with abnormalities in other lineages. Leukocytosis and thrombocytosis may be noted in myelodysplastic disorders.
  - Arterial blood gas with co-oximetry: PaO_2 may be low in cardiopulmonary diseases. Co-oximetry allows for evaluation of carboxyhemoglobin and methemoglobin levels. Half-life of carboxyhemoglobin is 4 hours, so testing should be timed to accurately reflect exposures.
  - BUN, serum creatinine, and urinalysis to evaluate renal function
  - Serum EPO: may be helpful in distinguishing primary from secondary polycythemia but significant overlap in EPO levels between the two categories

- Further investigation
  - Hemoglobin dissociation curve P50: the partial pressure of oxygen at which hemoglobin is 50% saturated (must be performed on fresh whole blood samples)
  - Hemoglobin electrophoresis: Normal results do not rule out the presence of high oxygen-affinity hemoglobin, as many can comigrate with normal hemoglobins.
  - Molecular genetic analysis of globin genes
  - 2,3-DPG level
  - Testosterone level
  - Genetic testing for *JAK2* V617F mutation
  - RBC mass measurement using isotope dilution methods
  - Erythroid progenitor studies for erythroid burst-forming units (BFU-E) that grow independent of EPO

Imaging

- Chest radiograph: initial evaluation for chronic pulmonary disease
- Abdominal ultrasound: evaluation for abdominal tumors

Diagnostic Procedures/Other

- EKG and echocardiogram: for clinical findings concerning for congenital heart disease
- Polysomnography sleep study: for clinical findings consistent with sleep apnea
- If myeloproliferative neoplasm is suspected, bone marrow aspirate and biopsy with cytogenetics should be performed. Analysis of erythroid progenitors through colony-forming assays.

DIFFERENTIAL DIAGNOSIS

- Primary polycythemia
  - Polycythemia vera
  - Primary familial and congenital polycythemia
- Secondary polycythemia
  - High altitudes
  - Chronic pulmonary disease
  - Hypoventilation: obstructive sleep apnea, neuromuscular disorders, severe obesity (Pickwickian syndrome), or congenital central hypoventilation syndrome
  - Right-to-left cardiac shunts
  - Arteriovenous malformations
  - High oxygen-affinity hemoglobinopathies
  - 2,3-DPG mutase deficiency
  - Methemoglobinemia
  - Carbon monoxide poisoning
  - EPO-producing tumors: renal cell carcinoma, hepatocellular carcinoma, hemangioblastoma, pheochromocytoma, uterine fibroids
  - Status-post renal transplant
  - Exogenous testosterone or EPO: competitive athletes
  - Cobalt poisoning: Homemade beer may contain cobalt.
- Neonatal polycythemia
  - Preeclampsia or gestational hypertension
  - Small for gestational age
  - Gestational diabetes
  - Delayed cord clamping
  - Placental transfusion
  - Twin-to-twin transfusion
- Relative polycythemia
  - Cigarette smoking
  - Dehydration

TREATMENT

MEDICATION

Primary polycythemia should be managed by a hematologist. Certain medications, such as hydroxyurea and interferon alpha, may be considered.

ADDITIONAL TREATMENT

General Measures

- Most asymptomatic patients with secondary polycythemia require no additional therapy other than management of their underlying condition.
- Due to the long-term leukemic potential of many chemotherapy agents, many pediatric patients with primary polycythemia are managed with phlebotomy only. Low-dose aspirin may be considered to reduce thrombosis risk.
- In neonatal polycythemia, partial exchange transfusion should be considered based on symptoms and degree of polycythemia.

ISSUES FOR REFERRAL

Unexplained cyanosis, symptoms concerning for hyperviscosity, or persistent elevation in hematocrit that is not related to dehydration or neonatal etiologies

ONGOING CARE

FOLLOW-UP RECOMMENDATIONS

Patient Monitoring

Periodic laboratory follow-up depending on the etiology of polycythemia. Monitor for the following:

- Headache, dizziness, or syncope
- Decreased exercise tolerance, shortness of breath, or dyspnea on exertion
- Stroke or thrombosis

PROGNOSIS

Depends on underlying condition:

- Polycythemia vera: guarded as may progress to acute leukemia
- High oxygen-affinity hemoglobinopathies: good
- Other secondary polycythemias: depend on underlying condition (e.g., poor prognosis for Eisenmenger syndrome due to progressive pulmonary hypertension and cor pulmonale)

COMPLICATIONS

From hyperviscosity:

- Decreased exercise tolerance, dyspnea on exertion, transient visual disturbances, and mental status changes
- Stroke or other thrombosis

ADDITIONAL READING

- Cario H, McMullin MF, Pahl HL. Clinical and hematological presentation of children and adolescents with polycythemia vera. *Ann Hematol*. 2009;88(8):713–719.
- Messinezy M, Pearson TC. The classification and diagnostic criteria of the erythrocytoses (polycythemias). *Clin Lab Haematol*. 1999;21(5):309–316.
- Ozek E, Soll R, Schimmel MS. Partial exchange transfusion to prevent neurodevelopmental disability in infants with polycythemia. *Cochrane Database Syst Rev*. 2010;(1):CD005089.
- Prchal JT. Polycythemia vera and other primary polycythemias. *Curr Opin Hematol*. 2005;12(2): 112–116.
- Sarkar S, Rosenkrantz TS. Neonatal polycythemia and hyperviscosity. *Semin Fetal Neonatal Med*. 2008;13(4):248–255.
- Tefferi A. Polycythemia vera and essential thrombocythemia: 2012 update on diagnosis, risk stratification, and management. *Am J Hematol*. 2012;87(3):285–293.

CODES

ICD10

- D45 Polycythemia vera
- D75.1 Secondary polycythemia
- P61.1 Polycythemia neonatorum

FAQ

- Q: What are common causes of polycythemia in the pediatric population?
- A: Secondary polycythemias. In particular, neonates and patients with cyanotic heart disease commonly present with polycythemia.
- Q: What are common causes of relative polycythemia?
- A: Dehydration and heavy cigarette smoking have been associated with decreased plasma volume and relative polycythemia.
- Q: When should a child with polycythemia be referred to a pediatric hematologist?
- A: The child should be referred to a pediatric hematologist if there are symptoms concerning for hyperviscosity or if the elevation in hematocrit is persistent and not clearly due to dehydration or neonatal etiologies.

POLYPS, INTESTINAL

Steven Liu

BASICS

DESCRIPTION

- Intestinal polyps are abnormal tissue growths protruding from the intestinal mucosa into the lumen.
- Most commonly solitary lesions (juvenile polyps) but may also be multiple in number
- May be associated with various polyposis syndromes
- Classified by gross appearance
  - Pedunculated: mushroom-like and attached to mucosa with a narrow stalk
  - Sessile: elevated, flat lesions broadly attached to mucosa
- Types of polyps:
  - Hamartomas
  - Adenomatous
- Polyposis syndromes
  - Juvenile polyposis syndrome (>3–5 juvenile polyps)
    - Juvenile polyposis of infancy
    - Juvenile polyposis coli (colonic involvement only)
    - Generalized juvenile polyposis
  - Peutz-Jeghers syndrome
  - Familial adenomatous polyposis (FAP)
  - Other polyposis syndromes

EPIDEMIOLOGY

- Juvenile polyps are the most common childhood polyps:
  - Account for >90% of polyps seen in children
  - 1–2% of asymptomatic children are estimated to have juvenile polyps.
  - Typically present between 2 and 5 years of age
  - Twice as common in boys than girls
  - >5 juvenile polyps should raise a suspicion for juvenile polyposis syndrome.
- Average age at onset of adenomatous polyps in FAP is 16 years.

Prevalence

- Juvenile polyposis syndrome: 1 in 100,000 to 1 in 160,000
- Peutz-Jeghers syndrome: 1 in 25,000 to 1 in 300,000
- FAP: 1 in 5,000 to 1 in 17,000

RISK FACTORS

Family history of polyposis syndrome

Genetics

Different genes and inheritance patterns with various polyposis syndromes:

- Juvenile polyposis syndrome
  - Autosomal dominant with variable penetrance
  - Mutations in *SMAD4* and *BMPR1A* genes, involved in transforming growth factor-β (TGF-β) signal transduction
- FAP
  - Autosomal dominant
  - Mutation in adenomatous polyposis coli (*APC*) tumor suppressor gene
- Peutz-Jeghers syndrome
  - Autosomal dominant
  - Mutations in *STK11/LKB1* tumor suppressor gene are associated.
- Cowden syndrome and Bannayan-Riley-Ruvalcaba syndrome (BRRS)
  - Autosomal dominant
  - Associated with mutations in *PTEN* gene

PATHOPHYSIOLOGY

Mutations in tumor suppressor genes likely lead to dysregulation of cell proliferation and apoptosis in polyposis syndromes.

COMMONLY ASSOCIATED CONDITIONS

- Juvenile polyposis syndrome, Cowden syndrome, and BRRS all have juvenile polyps as part of their manifestations.
- Peutz-Jeghers syndrome is characterized by multiple GI pedunculated hamartomatous polyps.
- FAP and Turcot syndrome are characterized by multiple adenomatous polyps.

DIAGNOSIS

HISTORY

- Family history of polyps or polyposis syndromes is essential to obtain.
- Presence and amount of blood in stool
- Signs and symptoms:
  - Frequently asymptomatic
  - Painless rectal bleeding is typical presentation.
  - Iron deficiency anemia
  - Prolapsing rectal lesion
  - Abdominal pain or obstruction from intussusception
  - Diarrhea

PHYSICAL EXAM

- Digital rectal exam may identify rectal polyp.
- Pigmentation of skin and mucous membranes consistent with Peutz-Jeghers syndrome
- Mucocutaneous lesions such as facial trichilemmoma, oral fibromas, and acral keratosis are seen in Cowden syndrome.
- Mental retardation, macrocephaly, lipomatosis, hemangiomas, and genital pigmentation are seen in BRRS.

DIAGNOSTIC TESTS & INTERPRETATION

Lab

- Stool test for occult blood may be positive.
- CBC can assess degree of anemia and also for baseline hemoglobin before polypectomy.
- PT/PTT should be considered before polypectomy due to risk of bleeding.
- Genetic testing can be considered if a polyposis syndrome is suspected.
- Use of urine and tissue matrix metalloproteinases (MMPs) as biomarkers for the presence of polyps is being researched.

Imaging

Radiologic studies are not the most effective methods of identifying polyps but can be used:

- Barium enema may identify colonic polyps.
- Upper GI with small bowel study may locate presence of small bowel polyps.
- Use of CT and MR colonography has been studied mainly in adults.

Diagnostic Procedures/Other

- Full colonoscopy with polypectomy is the preferred test to perform.
- Flexible sigmoidoscopy may miss polyps in proximal colon:
  - 32% of juvenile polyps are located proximal to splenic flexure.
  - 12% of patients with juvenile polyps only have polyps located proximal to splenic flexure.
- Video capsule endoscopy and balloon enteroscopy may be useful to identify small bowel polyps.

Pathologic Findings

- Polyp pathology cannot be determined by gross visualization, hence polyps must be removed for histologic exam.
- Juvenile polyps
  - Hamartomatous but occasionally capable of adenomatous changes
  - Potential of malignancy in a solitary juvenile polyp is extremely low but is increased in juvenile polyposis syndrome.
- Peutz-Jeghers syndrome
  - Hamartomatous
  - Microscopically have hyperplasia of the smooth muscle layer, extending in an arborizing, tree-like manner
  - Relatively low potential of GI malignancy but increased potential in other organs such as breast, pancreas, ovary, testicle, and uterus
- FAP
  - Adenomatous polyps
  - Lifetime risk for colorectal cancer is 100%.
  - Increased association with hepatoblastoma, periampullary carcinoma, and desmoid tumors

DIFFERENTIAL DIAGNOSIS

- Because juvenile polyps often present with rectal bleeding, the differential diagnosis for lower GI bleeding should be considered:
  - Anal fissure
  - Meckel diverticulum
  - Infectious enterocolitis
  - Inflammatory bowel disease
  - Intussusception
  - Vascular malformation
  - Hemorrhoids
  - Hemolytic uremic syndrome
  - Henoch-Schönlein purpura
  - Rectal trauma
  - Neoplasm

TREATMENT

MEDICATION

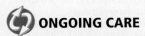

Administration of some NSAIDs (such as sulindac and celecoxib) may slow progression or reduce the number of adenomatous polyps.

ADDITIONAL TREATMENT

General Measures

Full colonoscopy with polypectomy is an essential diagnostic and therapeutic tool. Removal of GI polyps can help to control symptoms and reduce the risk of malignancy.

ISSUES FOR REFERRAL

Patients suspected of having a polyp or polyposis syndrome should be referred to a gastroenterologist for evaluation. Patients with polyposis syndromes should be referred to a tertiary care center for genetic counseling.

SURGERY/OTHER PROCEDURES

- When adenomatous polyps are identified in FAP, prophylactic colectomy should be considered.
- Colectomy should also be considered in other polyposis syndromes with innumerable polyps or polyps showing premalignant changes.
- The main surgical options include a subtotal colectomy with ileorectal anastomosis (IRA) or a proctocolectomy with ileal pouch–anal anastomosis (IPAA).

ONGOING CARE

FOLLOW-UP RECOMMENDATIONS

- For solitary juvenile polyps, follow up with stool guaiac check and CBC 6 months after polypectomy. Repeat colonoscopy is indicated with any abnormalities.
- For polyposis syndromes, screening recommendations differ depending on the syndrome:
  - Typically involve surveillance colonoscopies every 1–3 years depending on findings
  - Asymptomatic children with an *APC* mutation for FAP should have annual colonoscopies starting at 10–12 years of age.
  - Published guidelines for follow-up of patients with various polyposis syndromes are available.

ADDITIONAL READING

- Barnard J. Screening and surveillance recommendations for pediatric gastrointestinal polyposis syndromes. *J Pediatr Gastroenterol Nutr*. 2009;48(Suppl 2):S75–S78.
- Chow E, Macrae F. Review of juvenile polyposis syndrome. *J Gastroenterol Hepatol*. 2005;20(11):1634–1640.
- Erdman SH, Barnard JA. Gastrointestinal polyps and polyposis syndromes in children. *Curr Opin Pediatr*. 2002;14(5):576–582.
- Giardiello FM, Trimbath JD. Peutz-Jeghers syndrome and management recommendations. *Clin Gastroenterol Hepatol*. 2006;4(4):408–415.
- Gupta SK, Fitzgerald JF, Croffie JM, et al. Experience with juvenile polyps in North American children: the need for pancolonoscopy. *Am J Gastroenterol*. 2001;96(6):1695–1697.
- Merg A, Howe JR. Genetic conditions associated with intestinal juvenile polyps. *Am J Med Genet C Semin Med Genet*. 2004;129C(1):44–55.
- Thakkar K, Fishman DS, Gilger MA. Colorectal polyps in childhood. *Curr Opin Pediatr*. 2012;24(5):632–637.

CODES

ICD10

- K63.89 Other specified diseases of intestine
- D12.6 Benign neoplasm of colon, unspecified
- Q85.8 Other phakomatoses, not elsewhere classified

FAQ

- Q: What is the potential of developing cancer from a polyp?
- A: Risk of neoplasia depends on the type of polyp:
  - Patients with solitary juvenile polyps have essentially no increased risk of colorectal carcinoma.
  - Patients with juvenile polyposis syndrome have been reported to have up to a 65% chance of developing GI cancer, with the risk of malignancy commencing from age 20 years.
  - Patients with Peutz-Jeghers syndrome have been reported to have almost a 50% chance of developing cancer in the intestinal tract or other organ systems.
  - Patients with FAP have a 100% lifetime risk of developing colorectal cancer.
- Q: Is a flexible sigmoidoscopy sufficient for the detection of polyps?
- A: No. Approximately 37% of patients with juvenile polyps have polyps proximal to the splenic flexure, and 12% of patients have only proximal colon polyps. A flexible sigmoidoscopy would not identify these polyps, making it necessary to perform a full colonoscopy.
- Q: What is your management recommendation for a patient with painless rectal bleeding that stops on its own?
- A: It is widely believed that pedunculated polyps will autoamputate after outgrowing their blood supply, although there is no objective evidence supporting this. If there is no family history of a polyposis syndrome, the patient can be followed with stool guaiac checks and a CBC in 6 months. If there is a family history, then referral to a gastroenterologist for full colonoscopy is indicated.
- Q: How many polyps can patients have?
- A: Patients with juvenile polyposis syndrome often have 50–200 polyps distributed throughout the colon. Patients with FAP may have a few to over a thousand polyps in the colon.
- Q: When does endoscopic surveillance typically begin for children with FAP?
- A: It is generally recommended that annual endoscopic surveillance begin between 10 and 12 years of age in patients with an *APC* mutation.

PORTAL HYPERTENSION

Rose C. Graham

BASICS

DESCRIPTION

- Definition: elevation of portal blood pressure greater than 10 mm Hg
  - May be pre-, intra-, or posthepatic in origin
  - A major cause of morbidity and mortality in children with chronic liver disease

PATHOPHYSIOLOGY

- An increase in portal resistance and increased portal blood flow are the main pathogenic factors initiating the process of portal hypertension:
  - Other factors contribute to increased portal blood flow and pressure including hyperdynamic circulation, expanded intravascular volume, systemic arteriolar vasodilatation, decreased splanchnic arteriolar tone, and humoral factors (i.e., nitric oxide).
- Decompression of the high venous pressure through portosystemic collaterals leads to all the major sequelae of portal hypertension:
  - Splenomegaly
  - Varices (esophageal, gastric)/GI bleeding
  - Hemorrhoids
  - Caput medusa (periumbilical varices)
  - Ascites
  - Hepatic encephalopathy
  - Hepatopulmonary syndrome

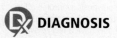

DIAGNOSIS

HISTORY

- History of umbilical catheterization
- History of hepatitis, abdominal trauma, clotting disorder, contraceptive pills, underlying medical problem such as cystic fibrosis, tyrosinemia, Wilson disease
- Ingestion of excessive amounts of vitamin A
- Hematemesis or melena: Upper GI tract bleed from varices may be the 1st sign of long-standing silent liver disease or previously undiagnosed portal vein thrombosis.

PHYSICAL EXAM

- Splenomegaly
- Hepatomegaly may or may not be present.
- Ascites (distension, fluid wave)
- Hemorrhoids
- Prominent vascular pattern on the abdomen (caput medusa)
- Digital clubbing
- Telangiectasia
- Palmar erythema
- Growth failure

DIAGNOSTIC TESTS & INTERPRETATION

Lab

- CBC and smear: detect hypersplenism, GI tract blood loss, and chronic liver disease
- PT/INR and PTT: detect coagulation defects
- Hepatic function panel includes liver enzymes (alanine aminotransferase [ALT], aspartate aminotransferase [AST]), albumin (measure of hepatic function), alkaline phosphatase, and γ-glutamyl transferase (GGT; may be elevated with cholestasis and bile duct injury).
- Additional laboratory testing to determine the cause of underlying liver disease, depending on clinical scenario (see chapter on "Cirrhosis" for more details)

Imaging

- Abdominal ultrasound with Doppler to evaluate
  - Liver size and echogenicity
  - Biliary anatomy
  - Spleen size
  - Renal cysts
  - Presence of ascites
  - Vessel diameter
  - Direction of blood flow
  - Presence of esophageal varices
- Esophagogastroduodenoscopy (EGD) to identify the presence of esophageal varices. EGD is also useful for determining if variceal rupture is the cause of GI tract bleeding.

Diagnostic Procedures/Other

- Liver biopsy: identify the underlying cause of the portal hypertension
- Hepatic venous wedge pressure gradient correlates and selective angiography are not used in pediatrics because of a lack of well-documented pediatric measurements and lack of a favorable risk–benefit ratio.

DIFFERENTIAL DIAGNOSIS

- Prehepatic causes:
  - Portal vein thrombosis with cavernous transformation (increased risk with umbilical vein catheterization, sepsis, dehydration, hypercoagulable state)
  - Splenic vein thrombosis
- Intrahepatic causes:
  - Hepatocellular disorders: viral hepatitis, α_1-antitrypsin deficiency, chronic hepatitis, autoimmune hepatitis, Wilson disease, glycogen storage disease, tyrosinemia, schistosomiasis, peliosis hepatitis, vitamin A toxicity
  - Biliary tract disorders: extrahepatic biliary atresia, ductal plate malformation/congenital hepatic fibrosis, intrahepatic cholestasis syndromes, primary sclerosing cholangitis, choledochal cyst, cystic fibrosis
- Posthepatic causes:
  - Budd-Chiari syndrome: occlusion of suprahepatic inferior vena cava or hepatic veins by congenital web, tumor, or thrombus
  - Congestive heart failure
  - Veno-occlusive disease of hepatic venule

TREATMENT

MEDICATION

- β-Blockade: Nonselective β-blockers, such as propranolol, have been shown to be effective in preventing both initial and recurrent variceal bleeds in adults. Data are limited on use of β-blockers in children with portal hypertension to prevent primary or secondary variceal bleeds. Use in children for this indication is empiric and mainly based on adult data:
  - Mechanisms include lowering portal blood flow and thus portal pressure by both β_2-blockade, which increases splanchnic tone, and β_1-blockade, which decreases cardiac output.
  - Propranolol, specifically, may also decrease collateral circulation.
  - β-Blocker effect on decreasing cardiac output may blunt an adaptive cardiovascular response (elevated heart rate) in the event of a hemorrhage; these medications should not be used in patients with asthma or diabetes.
  - Owing to lack of sufficient prospective data, routine use of β-blockers in children for primary or secondary prevention of variceal bleeding cannot be recommended.
- Diuretic therapy (spironolactone +/− chlorothiazide) when ascites is present

ADDITIONAL TREATMENT

General Measures

Chronic management of varices:

- Surveillance endoscopy and primary prophylaxis in pediatric patients with portal hypertension who have not had a 1st variceal bleed are controversial; however, they may be recommended in select patients.
- Long-term care of patients with portal hypertension who have had a variceal bleed depends on the underlying cause of the portal hypertension and may include secondary prophylactic endoscopic band ligation or sclerotherapy, portosystemic shunts, and liver transplantation.

ADDITIONAL THERAPIES

- Endoscopic sclerotherapy: reduces rebleeding episodes and long-term mortality when initiated after 1st bleed; unclear whether effective primary prophylaxis; in general, supplanted by endoscopic band ligation, except for small children
- Endoscopic band ligation is preferred, as it carries fewer complications compared with sclerotherapy. Endoscopic band ligation is not feasible in small patients.

SURGERY/OTHER PROCEDURES

- Portosystemic shunts
  - May be helpful in the setting of prehepatic causes of portal hypertension to reduce portal pressure. The Rex shunt (mesenteric-left portal bypass) has been used successfully in the setting of cavernous transformation of the portal vein.
  - Does not improve long-term survival in patients with intrahepatic disease
  - Complications may include thrombosis and worsening of hepatic encephalopathy.
  - Transjugular intrahepatic portosystemic shunt (TIPS) procedure may be an effective bridge to liver transplantation in pediatric patients with progressive liver disease and recurrent variceal bleeds.
  - Data in pediatric patients are limited.
- Liver transplantation
  - The current approach at most institutions is liver transplantation for those patients with life-threatening bleeds not amenable to β-blockade or endoscopic therapies.

INPATIENT CONSIDERATIONS

Initial Stabilization

- Acute management of variceal bleed
  - Vital signs: Remember that hemodynamic instability can be masked by β-blockers.
  - Fluid resuscitation: two large-bore IV catheters or intraosseous needles, give crystalloid initially, then RBC transfusion with goal hemoglobin of around 10 g/dL
  - Nasogastric tube placement: Lavage with room temperature saline or sterile water until clear; leave tube in place for evaluation and removal of continued or recurrent bleeding.
  - Correction of coagulopathy: Parenteral vitamin K, fresh frozen plasma, platelet transfusion if platelets $<50{,}000/\mu L$
  - IV antibiotics: Acute variceal hemorrhage increases the risk of spontaneous bacterial peritonitis in the setting of ascites.
  - IV proton pump inhibitor or histamine receptor antagonist to decrease risk of bleeding from ulcers or erosions
  - Pharmacotherapy to control active bleeding
    - Octreotide (somatostatin analog) decreases splanchnic blood flow via its inhibition of intestinal vasoactive peptide secretion. In turn, portal blood pressure is decreased. Somatostatin can be used but has a shorter half-life compared with octreotide.
    - Vasopressin decreases splanchnic blood flow via its vasoconstriction effects, but its use is limited owing to systemic vasoconstriction and a poor side effect profile. Nitroglycerin, a venodilator, has been used in conjunction to decrease side effects. This combination is not preferred.
  - Lactulose to prevent hepatic encephalopathy in patients with cirrhosis
  - Endoscopy (after stabilization) to determine source of hemorrhage (variceal rupture or other, such as gastric ulcer) and perform therapeutic procedures such as sclerotherapy or band ligation for varices or electrocautery or clip placement for ulcer
  - Direct tamponade: Sengstaken-Blakemore tube for severe uncontrollable hemorrhage, but high rate of complications
  - Interventional radiology: variceal embolization, TIPS
  - Surgical intervention: portosystemic shunt, esophageal devascularization, and/or transection; in general, last resort

ALERT

- The site of bleeding needs to be identified and managed appropriately: Not all GI bleeding in a patient with portal hypertension is an upper GI tract source (i.e., hemorrhoids); nasogastric lavage will help to determine if the problem is from the upper tract.
- Be careful not to overestimate the hemoglobin because equilibration may not have taken place at the time of presentation with an acute bleed.

ONGOING CARE

FOLLOW-UP RECOMMENDATIONS

- Patients are followed closely for hepatic decompensation.
- Growth failure, recurrent life-threatening bleeds not controllable with prophylactic intervention, refractory ascites, and poor quality of life are indications for liver transplantation.

DIET

Sodium restriction when ascites is present

PROGNOSIS

- The disease course and prognosis depend on the underlying cause.
- Acute variceal bleeding is associated with a 6-week mortality of up to 30% in adults. The mortality rate in children is much lower.
- Variceal bleeding associated with prehepatic causes of portal hypertension such as portal vein thrombosis typically becomes less problematic as the child ages; these patients will most likely not require a shunt and may be managed with endoscopic therapy.
- Patients with congenital hepatic fibrosis also do very well because the underlying disease is not progressive and bleeding may be easily managed with endoscopic therapy.
- Progressive liver disease has a worse prognosis and often requires liver transplantation.

COMPLICATIONS

- Hemorrhage from varices may present as hematemesis, hematochezia, or melena.
- Hypersplenism
- Malabsorption due to congestion of the intestinal mucosa
- Abnormal sodium retention
- Ascites: Presence of ascites increases risk of spontaneous bacterial peritonitis.
- Hepatorenal syndrome
- Hepatopulmonary syndrome (intrapulmonary right-to-left shunting) leads to hypoxemia, shortness of breath, exercise intolerance, and digital clubbing.
- Pulmonary hypertension can be a life-threatening complication of portal hypertension.

ADDITIONAL READING

- El-hamid NA, Taylor RM, Marinello D, et al. Aetiology and management of extrahepatic portal vein obstruction in children: King's College Hospital experience. *J Pediatr Gastroenterol Nutr*. 2008;47(5):630–634.
- Gugig R, Rosenthal P. Management of portal hypertension in children. *World J Gastroenterol*. 2012;18(11):1176–1184.
- Ling SC. Advances in the evaluation and management of children with portal hypertension. *Semin Liver Dis*. 2012;32(4):288–297.
- Schneider BL, Abel B, Haber B, et al. Cross-sectional multi-center analysis of portal hypertension in 163 children and young adults with biliary atresia. *J Pediatr Gastroenterol Nutr*. 2012;55(5):567–573.

CODES

ICD10

- K76.6 Portal hypertension
- K72.90 Hepatic failure, unspecified without coma
- K76.81 Hepatopulmonary syndrome

FAQ

- Q: What is my child's long-term prognosis?
- A: Disease prognosis of portal hypertension depends on the underlying cause. Variceal bleeding associated with prehepatic causes of portal hypertension such as portal vein thrombosis typically becomes less problematic as the child ages and may be managed with endoscopic therapy.
- Q: Are there any medications I should avoid?
- A: Avoid aspirin and NSAID-containing products such as ibuprofen.

POSTERIOR URETHRAL VALVES

Andrew A. Stec

BASICS

DESCRIPTION

A posterior urethral valve (PUV) is an embryologic remnant of tissue in the urethra that causes obstruction of the lower urinary tract during fetal development; this obstruction results in short-and long-term structural abnormalities and physiologic dysfunction in the genitourinary system (kidney, ureter, bladder, and urethra).

EPIDEMIOLOGY

- Most common cause of lower urinary tract obstruction in males
- The incidence is estimated to be between 1:3,000 and 1:8,000 live male births.
- Approximately 24–45% of children born with PUV will exhibit renal insufficiency during childhood.
- PUV accounts for up to 17% of the cases of children with end-stage renal failure.

RISK FACTORS

Genetics

- Majority of cases are isolated and occur sporadically.
- Rarely, cases have been reported in siblings.

PATHOPHYSIOLOGY

- Multiple theories exist as to the embryologic origin of PUV.
- Male urethral development is usually complete by 14 weeks' gestation; PUV formation is presumed to occur prior to this point.
- Possible embryologic origin of PUVs include (1) presence of an obstructing membrane in the posterior urethra, (2) overgrowth or abnormal folding during normal urethral development, (3) abnormal integration of the Wolffian ducts into urethral development, or (4) abnormal persistence of the urogenital membrane.
- PUVs exist in a spectrum of severity, likely related to the timing and degree of obstruction during development.
- The valve is a leaflet or membrane of thin connective tissue that extends from the anterior urethral lip to the verumontanum posteriorly, obstructing the normal flow of urine through the urethra. This results in an elongated urethra and upstream dilation in the urinary system.
- PUVs are commonly associated with intrinsic renal dysplasia. Studies have demonstrated that dysplastic renal parenchyma at time of birth is permanent.
- Commonly associated pathophysiologic findings in children with PUV include (1) hydroureteronephrosis, (2) dilated bladder with trabeculations and/or diverticulum, and (3) vesicoureteral reflux.
- PUVs may result in early or late bladder dysfunction with decreased compliance and increased voiding pressure that affect both the storage and expulsion of urine as well as expose the upper tract of the urinary system to increased pressure, which leads to worsening renal function over time.

COMMONLY ASSOCIATED CONDITIONS

- Genitourinary: hydroureteronephrosis, vesicoureteral reflux, bladder wall thickening and diverticulum, obstructive urinary symptoms, urinary ascites in cases of bladder rupture, perirenal urinoma in cases of renal collecting system rupture
- Varying degrees of renal insufficiency may also be present in patients from birth through adulthood.
- PUV has been associated with other congenital anomalies of the genitourinary tract: prune belly syndrome, imperforate anus, and congenital heart disease.

DIAGNOSIS

HISTORY

- PUVs generally present in four ways:
  - Fetal diagnoses by ultrasound (US)
  - Neonates with respiratory distress, abdominal distension, metabolic abnormalities
  - Infants with febrile UTI/sepsis/poor urinary stream
  - Delayed presentation in children with UTI or voiding difficulties
- Fetal presentation (diagnosis on ultrasound)
  - Dilated, thick-walled bladder
  - Bilateral and in some cases unilateral hydroureteronephrosis
  - "Keyhole sign": dilated posterior urethra at the base of the bladder
  - Decreased amniotic fluid/oligohydramnios
- Neonatal presentation
  - Tachypnea/respiratory distress
  - Poor feeding/failure to thrive/abdominal distension
  - Lethargy/acidosis and azotemia
  - Cardiovascular compromise and arrhythmia/hyperkalemia
  - Delayed or infrequent voiding
- Infant/toddler presentation
  - Failure to thrive
  - Abdominal distension
  - Fever of unknown origin
  - Febrile UTI
  - Urosepsis
- Delayed presentation
  - UTI
  - Abnormal or weak urinary stream
  - Urinary complaints such as hesitancy, incomplete emptying, dysuria, straining
  - Urinary incontinence, sometimes with palpable bladder
  - Polyuria and urinary frequency secondary to renal concentrating defect

PHYSICAL EXAM

A palpable bladder is the most common physical exam finding. In infants, abdominal distension may be present from severe bladder distension and hydroureteronephrosis or urinary ascites. Hyperpigmented perigenital skin may also be noted from severe incontinence and urine irritation of the skin.

DIAGNOSTIC TESTS & INTERPRETATION

Lab

- Urinalysis: UTI, proteinuria, low specific gravity
- Metabolic panel: elevated creatinine, azotemia, acidosis, hyperkalemia, hyponatremia, renal tubular acidosis (RTA) (type IV)
- CBC: elevated WBC in face of UTI; anemia in renal insufficiency

Imaging

- Renal and bladder US: dilation of posterior urethra (keyhole sign), distended/thick-walled bladder with possible diverticuli, hydroureteronephrosis, echogenic or dysplastic renal parenchyma
- Voiding cystourethrogram (VCUG): diagnostic study. Shows dilated posterior urethra with abnormal runoff of urine in the posterior urethra, capacious bladder with possible trabeculations or diverticulum, vesicoureteral reflux
- KUB: ground-glass appearance in cases of bladder rupture and urinary ascites

Diagnostic Procedures/Other

Operative cystoscopy: visual evaluation of urethra, and bladder provides definitive diagnosis

DIFFERENTIAL DIAGNOSIS

- Prune belly syndrome
- Vesicoureteral reflux
- Urethral stricture disease (congenital and acquired)
- Anterior urethral valves
- Urethral atresia
- Primary ureterovesical junction (UVJ) obstruction (megaureter)
- Severe voiding dysfunction
- Polyuria
- Megacystis–megaureter syndrome
- UTI

TREATMENT

GENERAL MEASURES

Supportive

- Insertion of a urethral catheter or feeding tube in the neonate to bypass obstruction
- Confirm placement of catheter in the bladder by ultrasound, as small catheters may coil in the posterior urethra and drain some urine, giving the false impression of being located within the bladder.
- Correction of electrolyte abnormalities with careful observation for postobstructive diuresis
- Monitoring of fluid status
- Antibiotics for any evidence of a UTI; treat UTI as complex
- Consultation with a pediatric urologist

SURGERY/OTHER PROCEDURES

- Resection of the valve (ablation) is the definitive treatment of the primary lesion; typically performed cystoscopically (through the urethra).
- In utero drainage of the fetal bladder is performed at some centers. Typically performed on patients with good urine parameters to mitigate pulmonary dysfunction from oligohydramnios. No significant improvement found in long-term renal outcome compared to valve ablation after delivery.
- If the infant is premature or the urethra is too small for the cystoscope, a vesicostomy may be required.
- Supravesical diversion (of the kidney or ureter) is sometimes performed in select patients who fail to improve after bladder decompression; associated with poorer long-term bladder function.
- Following valve ablation, the posterior urethra should have decreasing dilation on VCUG. Improvement in hydroureteronephrosis and vesicoureteral reflux (if it resolves spontaneously) will occur more slowly.

ONGOING CARE

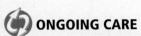

FOLLOW-UP RECOMMENDATIONS

- Lifelong follow-up is required, as renal insufficiency and bladder dysfunction can occur at any time during infancy, childhood, puberty, or adulthood.
- Pediatric urology follow-up is required for future reconstructive procedures and monitoring of bladder function, reflux, and hydronephrosis.
- Pediatric nephrology follow-up is recommended for long-term monitoring and mitigation of renal dysfunction.
- Delayed urethral obstruction is possible due to urethral stricture or incomplete initial valve resection.
- Patients with persistent incontinence, those who develop incontinence, or those with incomplete bladder emptying may require urodynamic evaluation to evaluate the bladder function/physiology and tailor therapy.

Patient Monitoring

- Careful follow-up through adulthood should be performed.
- Visits should include the following:
  - Imaging (US) to evaluate renal, ureteral, and bladder anatomy
  - Assessment of bladder function (incontinence, UTI, incomplete emptying)
  - Blood pressure monitoring
  - Serial creatinine
  - Urinalyses to asses for proteinuria
  - Assessment of overall linear growth

PROGNOSIS

- Oligohydramnios during pregnancy is a predictor of worse long-term renal outcomes. The earlier it occurs during pregnancy, typically more severe issues are noted.
- Pulmonary hypoplasia (with concomitant renal dysfunction) accounts for the highest mortality in infants.
- Overall, the prognosis for severe PUV has improved over the past few decades, owing to earlier recognition and improved management of pulmonary hypoplasia and fluid and metabolic derangements.
- The rate of improvement in renal function after the valvular obstruction is relieved is more indicative of prognosis than initial creatinine at presentation.
- A creatinine level of <0.8 mg/dL around 1 year of age has the best long-term renal prognosis in patients treated in infancy.
- A nadir creatinine level <1.0 mg/dL may still be associated with eventual renal failure as the child ages; monitoring is warranted in all cases.
- Patient may progress to renal failure and require renal transplantation at any point during childhood or adulthood. An abnormal creatinine at 2 years of age carries higher likelihood of end-stage renal progression during adolescence or puberty.
- Children who develop proteinuria have bilateral renal dysplasia and/or bladder dysfunction and are more likely to eventually develop renal insufficiency and hypertension.

COMPLICATIONS

- Intrauterine oligohydramnios in severe cases may result in Potter syndrome and pulmonary hypoplasia.
- Renal dysplasia and parenchymal damage may lead to progressive renal failure, including associated issues, such as anemia, acidosis, fluid and electrolyte abnormalities, and failure to thrive.
- UTIs and vesicoureteral reflux are commonly associated with PUV.
- Urinary incontinence may result from overactive bladder (uninhibited contractions), incomplete emptying (bladder noncompliance), and polyuria.

ADDITIONAL READING

- Chertin B, Cozzi D, Puri P. Long-term results of primary avulsion of posterior urethral valves using a Fogarty balloon catheter. *J Urol*. 2002;168(4):1841–1843.
- Eckoldt F, Heling KS, Woderich R, et al. Posterior urethral valves: prenatal diagnostic signs and outcome. *Urol Int*. 2004;73(4):296–301.
- Hodges SJ, Patel B, McLorie G, et al. Posterior urethral valves. *ScientificWorldJournal*. 2009;9:1119–1126.
- Holmes N, Harrison MR, Baskin LS. Fetal surgery for posterior urethral valves: long-term postnatal outcomes. *Pediatrics*. 2001;108(1):E7.
- Krishnan A, de Souza A, Konijeti R, et al. The anatomy and embryology of posterior urethral valves. *J Urol*. 2006;175(4):1214–1220.
- Radhakrishnan J. Obstructive uropathy in the newborn. *Clin Perinatol*. 1990;17(1):215–239.
- Roth KS, Carter WH Jr, Chan JC. Obstructive nephropathy in children: long-term progression after relief of posterior urethral valve. *Pediatrics*. 2001;107(5):1004–1010.
- Yiee J, Wilcox D. Management of fetal hydronephrosis. *Pediatr Nephrol*. 2008;23(3):347–353.

CODES

ICD10

- Q64.2 Congenital posterior urethral valves
- Q64.39 Other atresia and stenosis of urethra and bladder neck
- N28.89 Other specified disorders of kidney and ureter

FAQ

- Q: What can be done for children with long-term bladder dysfunction and incontinence?
- A: Patients should be on a comprehensive bowel and bladder regimen due to increased incidence of voiding dysfunction. Additionally, more advance bladder management including intermittent catheterization and pharmacotherapy may be required.
- Q: Are patients with PUVs good candidates for renal transplantation?
- A: PUV patients have a 5-year transplanted kidney survival rate of around 50%, likely resulting from poor bladder function. Therefore, aggressive bladder management and long-term follow-up are prudent in these patients.
- Q: What is "valve-bladder syndrome"?
- A: A valve-bladder is a bladder that is noncompliant and stores urine at high pressure, increasing the incidence of renal damage. It is thought to occur in approximately 20% of PUV patients.
- Q: What is VURD syndrome in PUV patients?
- A: Vesicoureteral reflux and unilateral renal dysplasia (VURD) occurs in 13% of PUV patients. A single renal unit has renal dysplasia and severe reflux, thereby allowing the high bladder pressures in PUV to be transmitted to a single kidney, sparing the contralateral (nonrefluxing) kidney from damage.

PREBIOTICS

Gigi Veereman • Andi L. Shane

BASICS

DESCRIPTION

- Prebiotics are nondigestible carbohydrates that promote growth of favorable intestinal microbiotia (probiotic microorganisms) by selective fermentation. Prebiotics may occur naturally or may be manufactured. Naturally occurring prebiotics include human milk oligosaccharides; many are substrates for bifidobacteria. Manufactured prebiotics that mimic this effect are therefore called "bifidogenic."
- The following manufactured nondigestible carbohydrates were shown to be bifidogenic when added to standard infant formula:
  - Galacto-oligosaccharides (GOS) and long-chain fructo-oligosaccharides (lc-FOS from plants or sucrose); also called fructans
  - Some prebiotics are found in foods including chicory, cereals, agave, and milk, although may not be present in levels that would result in fermentation and a change in host microbiota. Additional processing or synthesis is required in these to achieve prebiotic activity.
  - Candidate prebiotics include lactulose, polysaccharides, oligosaccharides, and polyols.

PATHOPHYSIOLOGY

- Prebiotics such as FOS and GOS are selectively fermented resulting in a change in the composition or activity of the microbiota. Fermentation in colon → increased bacteria → increased water binding → increased stool weight → softer stools → increased stool frequency. Butyrate may increase peristalsis, decrease intestinal transit time and reduce bloating, flatulence, and constipation.
- Prebiotics may impact the immune system directly.
- In vitro studies
  - Proposed mechanisms of indirect prebiotic action include gas and short-chain fatty acid production, pH changes, and promotion of fecal bacterial growth. Direct effects include binding of the prebiotic to microbe receptors.
- Animal studies
  - Prebiotics exert their effects by enhancing intestinal barrier function. They also promote the growth of ileal lactobacilli through the production of lactic acid and decreasing intestinal pH.
  - Prebiotics increase calcium, magnesium, and iron absorption; growth; and bone mass in rats and pigs.
- Clinical studies
  - Prebiotics exert their effects in the colon. They must retain the ability to be active through intestinal transit and changes in gastrointestinal pH. Most prebiotics interact with bifidobacteria and lactobacilli without altering other bacteria.
  - Stool bulk and intestinal transit time are frequently measured clinical markers of prebiotic effect.
  - Immune function including cytokine levels and antibody function are biomarkers that are measured to assess prebiotic effect.
  - FOS and long-chain inulin (50/50) increased bone mineral density and content in adolescents.
- Clinical studies on effectivity
  - Variability in subjects including age, nutrition, and health status must be considered when interpreting results.
  - Reduced symptoms, decreased infections, and enhanced immune responses are health outcomes measured in clinical studies with prebiotics.
  - Human feeding trials to assess change in microbiota optimally monitor response to prebiotic intake.
- Challenges to applying clinical studies in clinical practice
  - The body of evidence on some clinical effects is highly variable.
  - Prebiotic effects are specific to a particular product or combination of products.
  - Prebiotic effects are modulated by resident flora and by direct effects on the immune system
  - Effects depend on base line, on host: Pooling results is difficult.

TREATMENT

DOSING

- Optimal prebiotic intake ranges from 2 to 20 g per day, depending on desired effect and prebiotic ingredient.
- Prebiotic ingredients may be added to or be contained in cereals, breads, yogurts, sauces, and drinks.
- Regular intake of prebiotic or prebiotic-containing foods is necessary for sustained effect.
- Prebiotic formulations
  - GOS
    - Not widely studied as single prebiotic
    - Major compound of prebiotic combination products
    - No known safety concerns

- sc-FOS
  - Not widely studied as single prebiotic
  - Some safety concerns and questionable benefits
- Sc-FOS:lc-FOS
  - Not widely studied combination
  - No safety concerns
- GOS:lc-FOS (9:1)
  - Best studied prebiotic mixture
  - Initial safety concerns shown not to be relevant.
  - Long history of safe use; benefits questioned
- GOS:sc-FOS (9:1)
  - Not widely studied as a prebiotic mixture
  - No safety concerns
- GOS:polydextrose (PDX) (1:1)
  - Several studies with this prebiotic mixture
  - Initial safety concerns addressed.
  - Good history of safe use

- Safety, growth, and tolerance
  - Adding prebiotics to infant formula may create an osmotic effect resulting in softer stools.
  - A theoretical risk for dehydration has not been observed with usual dosing.
  - Increased intake of prebiotics may result in bloating and diarrhea that resolves with decreased consumption.

CLINICAL APPLICATIONS

- Inflammatory bowel disease (IBD)
  - Consumption of the prebiotic fructan may reduce inflammatory markers in persons with IBD.
- Irritable bowel syndrome (IBS)
  - Low-dose consumption of prebiotics may reduce symptoms of IBS.
- Stool consistency
  - Consumption of infant formulas supplemented with bifidogenic prebiotics including GOS, fructans, and oligosaccharides may result in a microbiota and stooling pattern similar to that of infants who consume human milk.
- Other effects
  - Daily prebiotic intake, especially of fructans, may reduce appetite, increase gut peptide levels, and improve glucose tolerance.
  - Changes in the microbiota were noted.

ADDITIONAL READING

- Ashley C, Johnston WH, Harris CL, et al. Growth and tolerance of infants fed formula supplemented with polydextrose (PDX) and/or galactooligosaccharides (GOS): double-blind, randomized, controlled trial. *Nutr J*. 2012;11:38.doi:10.1186/1475-2891-11-38.
- Binns N. *Probiotics, Prebiotics, and the Gut Microbiota*. Brussels, Belgium: International Life Sciences Institute; 2013.
- Holscher HD, Faust KL, Czerkies LA, et al. Effects of prebiotic-containing infant formula on gastrointestinal tolerance and fecal microbiota in a randomized controlled trial. *JPEN J Parenter Enteral Nutr*. 2012;36(1)(Suppl):95S–105S.
- Mugambi MN, Musekiwa A, Lombard M, et al. Synbiotics, probiotics or prebiotics in infant formula for full term infants: a systematic review. *Nutr J*. 2012;11:81.doi:10.1186/1475-2891-11-81.
- Veereman-Wauters G, Staelens S, Van de Broek H, et al. Physiological and bifidogenic effects of prebiotic supplements in infant formulae. *J Pediatr Gastroenterol Nutr*. 2011;52(6):763–771.
- Westerbeek EA, Hensgens RL, Mihatsch WA, et al. The effect of neutral and acidic oligosaccharides on stool viscosity, stool frequency and stool pH in preterm infants. *Acta Paediatr*. 2011;100(11):1426–1431.
- Xia Q, Williams T, Hustead D, et al. Quantitative analysis of intestinal bacterial populations from term infants fed formula supplemented with fructo-oligosaccharides. *J Pediatr Gastroenterol Nutr*. 2012;55(3):314–320.

FAQ

- Q: What is the difference between prebiotics and probiotics?
- A: Probiotics are external microorganisms that are consumed to result in a health benefit. Prebiotics have actions that complement those of probiotics but are separate from those of probiotics. A prebiotic is fermented, stimulating the growth and activity of microorganisms, resulting in a health benefit.
- Q: What are synbiotics?
- A: Synbiotics are combinations of the beneficial effects of prebiotics and probiotics. The probiotic organism may play a role in the fermentation of the prebiotic. The probiotic may in turn create a more favorable environment for the proliferation of the probiotic.
- Q: Where can I buy prebiotics?
- A: Naturally occurring prebiotics occur in foods such as chicory, cereals, agave, and milk. However, prebiotic intake may be optimized by consuming foods with labels that indicate that the food contains FOS, inulin (a type of FOS), GOS, or TOS (transgalacto-oligosaccharides).

PRECOCIOUS PUBERTY

Jennifer C. Kelley • Andrew C. Calabria

BASICS

DESCRIPTION

- In most populations, the mean age of onset of puberty is 10.5 years in girls and 11.5 years in boys.
- The first sign of puberty in girls is most commonly breast development (thelarche), followed by pubic hair development (pubarche), and then menarche, which generally occurs 2–3 years after thelarche; in boys, the first sign is usually testicular enlargement, followed by pubarche and penile growth.
- Precocious puberty has traditionally been defined as physical signs of sexual development before age 8 years in girls and age 9 in boys (2.5–3 standard deviations below the mean age of onset of puberty).
- Recent guidelines propose lowering the age considered to be normal for sexual development in girls to as young as age 6 years in black girls and age 7 years in white girls. These new guidelines have not been universally adopted.
- When evaluating precocious puberty, the entire clinical picture, including rate of pubertal progression and the presence of any neurologic symptoms, must be considered.

EPIDEMIOLOGY

- Occurs in ~1 in 5,000 children
- Precocious puberty is up to 10 times more common in girls than boys.
- Racial differences observed in girls: African-American girls may enter puberty 1 year sooner on average than Caucasian girls. Racial difference not present in males.
- Increased incidence in internationally adopted children and in children born premature or small for gestational age
  - In girls: 80–90% of central precocious puberty are idiopathic.
  - In boys: Precocious puberty is more likely to be associated with underlying pathology.
  - ~50% of affected boys have idiopathic central precocious puberty.

Genetics

- Genetic causes include the following:
  - Familial male precocious puberty (testotoxicosis): sex-limited, autosomal dominant inheritance of luteinizing hormone (LH) receptor activating mutation
  - McCune-Albright syndrome: sporadic, postzygotic, somatic mutation in the stimulatory subunit of G-protein receptor; precocious puberty more common in girls

PATHOPHYSIOLOGY

- Central precocious puberty can be associated with CNS disorders.
- Peripheral precocious puberty
  - Arises from peripheral sex hormone sources, including gonadal and adrenal disorders, abdominal or pelvic tumors, or exogenous sex steroids
  - Can progress to central precocious puberty due to maturation of the hypothalamic–pituitary axis by sex steroids

ETIOLOGY

- Central precocious puberty (gonadotropin-releasing hormone [GnRH] dependent)
  - Associated with gonadotropin (LH and/or follicle-stimulating hormone [FSH]) levels that are elevated beyond the normal prepubertal range. Results from activation of hypothalamic–pituitary–gonadal axis.
  - Physical changes are typically those of normal puberty for a child of that sex.
- Peripheral sex hormone effects (peripheral precocious puberty or GnRH-independent; less common)
  - Gonadotropin-independent elevation of sex steroids arising (i) directly from gonads and/or adrenals, (ii) through stimulation of gonads by GnRH-independent mechanism, or (iii) from an exogenous source
  - Physical changes reflect predominant excess hormones (estrogenic or androgenic) and are often markedly discordant from normal pubertal development.

DIAGNOSIS

SIGNS AND SYMPTOMS

- Careful chronology: physical changes, growth spurt, onset of menses
- Neurologic, visual, or behavioral changes suggest a CNS lesion.

HISTORY

- Family history of early puberty (e.g., menarche before age 10 years) or hyperandrogenic disorders (e.g., congenital adrenal hyperplasia)
- Presence of exogenous sex steroid medications or creams in the home

PHYSICAL EXAM

- Plot accurate height (using wall-mounted stadiometer), weight, and growth velocity. Growth acceleration within the past year may be strong evidence for puberty.
- Careful inventory of early estrogenic and androgenic effects
- Estrogenic effects
  - Girls: careful staging of breasts and color of vaginal mucosa
  - Boys: gynecomastia in prepubertal child (gynecomastia is common and normal part of puberty in pubescent male.)
- Androgenic effects
  - Girls: careful staging of pubic hair, clitoromegaly
  - Boys: careful staging of testicular volume (with Prader gonadometer or by measuring testicular length), penile size, and pubic hair
- Examine skin for acne and café au lait spots.
- Perform comprehensive neurologic evaluation to assess for possible CNS pathology.

DIAGNOSTIC TESTS & INTERPRETATION

Lab

- Labs should be selected based on inventory of estrogenic and/or androgenic effects and drawn in early morning.
- Estrogenic effects
  - Girls: FSH and LH (ultrasensitive, pediatric, immunochemiluminometric [ICMA] or electrochemiluminescent [ECL]) (LH is most accurate) and estradiol
  - Boys: ultrasensitive LH and FSH, estradiol, human chorionic gonadotropin (hCG) level
- Androgenic effects
  - Total testosterone by assay designed to measure low concentrations, adrenal steroids including 17-hydroxyprogesterone (17-OHP) to evaluate for late-onset congenital adrenal hyperplasia and dehydroepiandrosterone sulfate (DHEA-S) to exclude or confirm adrenarche, and ultrasensitive LH to evaluate for central puberty
- Other tests
  - Prolactin: may be elevated with CNS tumors
  - Thyroid-stimulating hormone (TSH) and free thyroxine (T_4)
  - Avoid lower yield tests, such as total estrogens, nonultrasensitive LH, free testosterone levels (more helpful in adolescent girls with testosterone levels above 30 ng/dL), and other adrenal steroids such as 17-hydroxypregnenolone and DHEA.
- Provocative stimulation tests should be done when the aforementioned tests are abnormal or equivocal:
  - GnRH test (typically leuprolide stimulation) for central precocious puberty; prepubertal GnRH response is predominantly FSH, whereas pubertal response is predominantly LH.
  - Adrenocorticotropic hormone (ACTH) stimulation test for adrenal abnormalities. Exogenous corticosteroid therapy will interfere with ACTH test but does not interfere with GnRH test of pituitary–gonadal axis.

Imaging

- Bone age x-ray of left hand and wrist: if advanced, further studies, guided by history and physical examination, warranted. If not advanced, or if only early breast or pubic hair development (but not both), premature thelarche or premature adrenarche, respectively, most likely diagnoses.
- MRI of head: In the absence of specific clues to CNS disease, the probability of an intracranial abnormality depends primarily on age of onset of puberty, rate of progression, and the sex of the child. MRI is almost always done in boys because they are less likely than girls to have idiopathic precocious puberty.
- Ultrasound of gonads/adrenals: as indicated by examination and studies. Evaluates for tumors in both sexes; in girls, ultrasound can also evaluate ovarian/uterine maturity.

ALERT
- Obese children often have advanced bone ages.
- Palpation of breast tissue (buds) can be difficult due to adiposity.

DIFFERENTIAL DIAGNOSIS

- Causes of central precocious puberty:
  - Often idiopathic (girls >> boys)
  - Any cause of peripheral precocious puberty
  - CNS tumors
    - Hypothalamic hamartoma: most common CNS mass causing precocious puberty; benign (nonprogressive) congenital malformation of GnRH-secreting neurons
    - Hypothalamic–chiasmatic glioma: often associated with neurofibromatosis
    - Astrocytoma
    - Ependymoma
  - Post-CNS trauma or damage
    - Surgery
    - Radiation: may occur after 18-Gy exposure
    - Hydrocephalus/other CNS malformations
    - Infections: brain abscess, meningitis, encephalitis, granuloma. Lesions may result in stimulation or lack of inhibition of GnRH-secreting area of the hypothalamus, resulting in early pituitary activation.
- Mimickers of central precocious puberty:
  - hCG-secreting tumors (pineal gland or liver): Ectopic hCG activates testicular LH receptors.
  - Severe, acquired hypothyroidism: Elevated TSH may cross-stimulate gonadal FSH and/or LH receptors.
- Causes of peripheral sex hormone effects:
  - Tumors (gonadal and adrenal)
  - Environmental: exogenous estrogens (creams and oral forms) and/or exogenous androgens (anabolic steroids or testosterone formulations)
  - Congenital adrenal hyperplasia: Poorly controlled congenital adrenal hyperplasia can activate the hypothalamic–pituitary–gonadal axis in either gender.
  - McCune-Albright syndrome: triad of precocious puberty, café au lait spots, and polyostotic fibrous dysplasia
  - Familial male precocious puberty (testotoxicosis)
  - Refeeding after severe malnutrition during early development (such as adopted children who had kwashiorkor)
- Incomplete pubertal development
  - Premature thelarche
  - Premature adrenarche
  - Premature menarche

TREATMENT

MEDICATION

- Central precocious puberty: GnRH agonists are the treatment of choice. Adjunctive therapy with growth hormone may be needed to optimize final adult height.
- Calcium supplementation may assist bone mass accretion during GnRH agonist therapy.
- Peripheral sex hormone effects: aromatase inhibitors and antiandrogens (spironolactone or ketoconazole), glucocorticoids for congenital adrenal hyperplasia

ONGOING CARE

- When to expect improvement:
  - Depends on cause. For example, sexual changes of McCune-Albright syndrome are due to autonomously functioning ovarian cysts, which regress variably over time.
  - Treatment of central precocious puberty with a GnRH agonist usually results in cessation of menses within 2 months, slowing or nonprogression of pubertal changes over 4–6 months, and decreased rate of bone age acceleration within 12 months.
- Typically, GnRH agonists such as leuprolide (Lupron) are administered in a depot form every 28 days. Some children require shortening of the interval, often prompted by incomplete pubertal suppression. A longer acting formulation of leuprolide is sometimes used as an every 3-month injection. A 12-month duration implantable formulation (histrelin) is also available.
- The length of treatment is highly individualized but typically continues until the age of normal pubertal onset.

PROGNOSIS

- With treatment, improvement in predicted height may be achieved. Earlier treatment results in improved final height, but most children do not reach target height predicted by mid-parental height measurements.
- Treatment may decrease psychosocial distress.
- Long-term effects of central precocious puberty and GnRH agonists on fertility have not been fully elucidated.

COMPLICATIONS

- Short stature
- Psychosocial stresses of early puberty

ADDITIONAL READING

- Carel JC, Eugster EA, Rogol A, et al. Consensus statement on the use of gonadotropin-releasing hormone analogs in children. *Pediatrics*. 2009; 123(4):e752–e762.
- Carel JC, Léger J. Clinical practice. Precocious puberty. *N Engl J Med*. 2008;358(22):2366–2377.
- Herman-Giddens ME, Slora EJ, Wasserman RC, et al. Secondary sexual characteristics and menses in young girls seen in office practice: a study from the Pediatric Research Office in Settings network. *Pediatrics*. 1997;99(4):505–512.
- Kaplowitz PB. Treatment of central precocious puberty. *Curr Opin Endocrinol Diabetes Obes*. 2009;16(1):31–36.
- Kaplowitz P, Oberfield SE. Reexamination of the age limit for defining when puberty is precocious in girls in the United States: implications for evaluation and treatment. Drug and Therapeutics and Executive Committees of the Lawson Wilkins Pediatric Endocrine Society. *Pediatrics*. 1999;104(4, Pt 1):936–941.
- Nathan BM, Palmert MR. Regulation and disorders of pubertal timing. *Endocrinol Metab Clin North Am*. 2005;34(3):617–641.
- Oostdijk W, Rikken B, Schreuder S, et al. Final height in central precocious puberty after long term treatment with a slow release GnRH agonist. *Arch Dis Child*. 1996;75(4):292–297.

CODES

ICD10

- E30.1 Precocious puberty
- E22.8 Other hyperfunction of pituitary gland
- E30.8 Other disorders of puberty

FAQ

- Q: If my child is treated with a GnRH agonist, will he or she go through puberty when we stop the medication?
- A: Yes. Children on GnRH agonist treatment proceed through normal puberty when the medication is stopped. Effects on fertility have not been fully studied long-term.
- Q: If my child already has some pubertal changes, can they be reversed?
- A: If GnRH agonists are used, menses will cease and breast tissue and pubic hair will often partially or completely regress.

PREMATURE ADRENARCHE

Jennifer C. Kelley • Andrew C. Calabria

BASICS

DESCRIPTION

- Appearance of pubic hair younger than age 8 years in girls and age 9 years in boys
- Recent data suggest that the age of normal sexual development onset in girls is younger than previously recognized, but lowering of the traditionally accepted limits remains subject to debate.
- Axillary hair, acne, and apocrine sweat gland secretion are not always present with premature adrenarche.
- No other signs of sexual development are exhibited. Presence of breast development in girls or testicular enlargement in boys suggests precocious puberty and not premature adrenarche.
- Occurs independently of hypothalamic–pituitary–gonadal axis activation

Genetics

Often sporadic. Familial patterns suggesting recessive and dominant inheritance have been described.

PATHOPHYSIOLOGY

- Concentrations of adrenal steroids such as dehydroepiandrosterone (DHEA) and dehydroepiandrosterone-sulfate (DHEA-S) increase earlier than typically seen in normal puberty.
- Adrenal zona reticularis normally begins to increase androgen secretion at age 7–8 years.

DIAGNOSIS

HISTORY

- Careful attention to presence of any other signs of sexual precocity as well as rate of progression
- Family history of pubertal development, infertility, irregular menses, hirsutism, polycystic ovarian syndrome, and premature male-pattern balding
- Birth weight that is small for gestational age (SGA) may predispose children to development of premature adrenarche.
- Obesity has been associated with an increased incidence of premature adrenarche.
- Girls with premature adrenarche are at increased risk for the development of polycystic ovarian syndrome.

PHYSICAL EXAM

- Linear growth velocity may be increased.
- The presence of pigmented, curly hairs in the pubic area is consistent with androgenic effect from adrenal steroids.
- In girls, clitoromegaly suggests congenital adrenal hyperplasia or androgen-secreting tumors.
- The finding of acanthosis nigricans suggests that insulin resistance and the risk of developing ovarian hyperandrogenism (polycystic ovarian syndrome) are present.

ALERT

Be careful to differentiate between true pubic hair (curly and short) and dark lanugo hair (straight, long, fine). An extra light source may be helpful.

DIAGNOSTIC TESTS & INTERPRETATION

Lab

- If predominantly androgenic effects are present, the most useful initial tests are as follows:
  - Total testosterone by pediatric assay
  - Adrenal steroids including 17-hydroxyprogesterone (17-OHP) to evaluate for late-onset congenital adrenal hyperplasia and DHEA-S to exclude or confirm adrenarche
  - Pediatric luteinizing hormone (LH), also listed as immunochemiluminometric (ICMA), electrochemiluminescent (ECL), or ultrasensitive, to evaluate for central puberty
- Adrenal steroids are often elevated for chronologic age but normal for pubertal stage (usually Tanner 2 or 3). However, testosterone and 17-OHP should be in prepubertal range.
- Additional hormone measurements are often lower yield. These include hormones to evaluate for estrogenic effects (e.g., estradiol) when these effects (e.g., thelarche) are not present, adult LH or testosterone assays, and free testosterone levels (more helpful in adolescent girls with testosterone levels above 30 ng/dL and with concerns for hyperandrogenism/polycystic ovarian syndrome [PCOS]). Other adrenal steroids, such as 17-hydroxypregnenolone and DHEA, are typically less useful as 1st-line tests.
- Gonadotropin-releasing hormone (leuprolide) stimulation test: not routinely recommended but would have a normal prepubertal response
- Children with systemic signs of virilization (such as a significantly advanced bone age) or elevated adrenal steroids (17-OHP) should have adrenocorticotropic hormone (ACTH) stimulation testing to exclude congenital adrenal hyperplasia and other hyperandrogenic syndromes.

Imaging

- Bone age may be advanced by 1–2 years but correlates with height age.
- Abdominal ultrasound, CT scan, or MRI should be considered if signs of significant virilization are present or if rapid progression has occurred; look for intracranial or intra-abdominal masses, especially if androgens are markedly elevated.

DIFFERENTIAL DIAGNOSIS

- For infants with isolated pubic hair: idiopathic pubic hair of infancy
- Congenital: late-onset (nonclassic) congenital adrenal hyperplasia
- Tumors: Androgen-secreting tumors can arise in the gonads or adrenal glands.
- Miscellaneous:
  - Central precocious puberty
  - Familial male precocious puberty (testotoxicosis)
  - Exogenous male hormone exposure

TREATMENT

GENERAL MEASURES

- No treatment
- Reassure parents and children that this is a benign process.
- Reassess every 6 months to look for signs of virilization and pubertal progression.

ONGOING CARE

- Regression does not occur.
- Watch for other signs of puberty, such as breast development, testicular enlargement (≥4 mL), or growth acceleration, that suggest onset of true precocious puberty.
- Increasing virilization suggests nonclassic congenital adrenal hyperplasia or early polycystic ovarian syndrome.
- Acanthosis nigricans or signs of insulin resistance have been reported in girls with a history of premature adrenarche.
- Monitor for glucose intolerance or early type 2 diabetes. Fasting glucose and insulin levels or oral glucose tolerance test may be checked if suspicion is high (e.g., obesity, acanthosis nigricans, polyuria, polydipsia).

PROGNOSIS

- Undergo puberty appropriately with normal fertility
- Development of ovarian or adrenal hyperandrogenism during adolescence (also known as "polycystic ovarian syndrome") is more common in some girls with a history of premature adrenarche. Insulin resistance, a common finding in ovarian hyperandrogenism, has been reported in some children and adolescents with a history of premature adrenarche.
- Final adult height is not affected.

COMPLICATIONS

- Can be the first sign of true precocious puberty (i.e., development of breast tissue and advancement of bone age) and thus warrants careful observation
- Boys with premature adrenarche and precocious puberty are more likely than girls to have an underlying CNS disorder.

ADDITIONAL READING

- Auchus RJ, Fainey WE. Adrenarche–physiology, biochemistry and human disease. *Clin Endocrinol (Oxf)*. 2004;60(3):288–296.
- Herman-Giddens ME, Slora EJ, Wasserman RC, et al. Secondary sexual characteristics and menses in young girls seen in office practice: a study from the pediatric research office in settings network. *Pediatrics*. 1997;99(4):505–512.
- Ibanez L, Jimenes R, de Zegher F. Early puberty-menarche after precocious pubarche: relation to prenatal growth. *Pediatrics*. 2006;117(1):117–121.
- Kaplowitz P. Clinical characteristics of 104 children referred for evaluation of precocious puberty. *J Clin Endocrinol Metab*. 2004;89(8):3644–3650.
- Kaplowitz P, Oberfield SE. Reexamination of age limit for defining when puberty is precocious in girls in the United States: implication for evaluation and treatment. Drug and Therapeutics and Executive Committees of the Lawson Wilkins Pediatric Endocrine Society. *Pediatrics*. 1999;104(4, Pt 1):936–941.
- Kousta E. Premature adrenarche leads to polycystic ovarian syndrome? Long-term consequences. *Ann N Y Acad Sci*. 2006;1092:148–157.
- Midyett LK, Moore WV, Jacobson JD. Are pubertal changes in girls before age 8 benign? *Pediatrics*. 2003;111(1):47–51.
- Nebesio TD, Eugster EA. Pubic hair of infancy: endocrinopathy or enigma? *Pediatrics*. 2006;117(3):951–954.
- Neville KA, Walker JL. Precocious pubarche is associated with SGA, prematurity, weight gain, and obesity. *Arch Dis Child*. 2005;90(3):258–261.
- Oberfield SE, Sopher AB, Gerken AT. Approach to the girl with early onset of pubic hair. *J Clin Endocrinol Metab*. 2011:96(6):1610–1622.

CODES

ICD10

E27.0 Other adrenocortical overactivity

FAQ

- Q: Is there a dietary cause of excess adrenal hormones?
- A: No.
- Q: Does premature adrenarche mean puberty will be early?
- A: The onset of puberty in these children is within the normal range and should follow the familial pattern.
- Q: Can anything be done to reverse the changes?
- A: This is a benign process that does not require treatment. Antiandrogen drugs are available but are not recommended. Girls are at increased risk for the development of polycystic ovarian syndrome, but most children do not have long-term sequelae of premature adrenarche.

PREMATURE THELARCHE

Patricia Vuguin

BASICS

DESCRIPTION

- Breast development in girls <8 years of age without evidence of sexual hair development, vaginal mucosa estrogenization, linear growth acceleration, rapid bone maturation, adult body odor, or behavioral changes
- Exaggerated thelarche, a variant of isolated breast development, occurs without axillary or pubic hair, but with some acceleration of growth and bone maturation, and increased uterine size.
- Data suggests that African American girls may develop pubertal changes as early as 6 years of age and Caucasian girls as early as 7 years of age. However, caution should be used when evaluating children because signs of puberty at these younger ages may not be considered normal and may be due to pathologic conditions.

EPIDEMIOLOGY

- 60–85% of cases are noted between 6 months and 2 years of age.
- There is no one identifiable group of girls who develops early thelarche.
- Note: Breast enlargement in a male infant or young (prepubertal) boy should be concerning.

PATHOPHYSIOLOGY

- Transient increases in follicle-stimulating hormone levels causing follicular ovarian development
- Low levels of estrogen secretion by normal follicular cysts
- Increased sensitivity of breast tissue to low levels of estrogen
- Delay in inhibition of the "minipuberty" of infancy
- Exposure to exogenous estrogen (e.g., cosmetic and hair products, infant formulas containing soy, and xenoestrogens)

DIAGNOSIS

HISTORY

- Careful assessment of onset and progression of breast tissue
- Careful assessment of growth (growth velocity changes in height percentiles)
- Family history of early puberty and or early menses
- Exogenous exposure to estrogens (foods, creams, etc)

PHYSICAL EXAM

- Palpate carefully to distinguish fat from true breast tissue.
- Areolar hyperpigmentation and/or enlargement is usually not present.
- Galactorrhea is not present.
- Look carefully for other signs of puberty:
  - Menstrual blood
  - Dull, gray-pink, or rugose vaginal mucosa (vs. prepubertal appearance: shiny, bright red, and smooth)
  - Pubic or axillary hair or any other sign of androgen excess
- Inspect skin for birthmarks suggestive of McCune–Albright syndrome (café au lait spots in a coast of Maine pattern).
- Evaluate height and assess growth velocity.
- Evaluate for signs of hypothyroidism: goiter, short stature.

DIAGNOSTIC TESTS & INTERPRETATION

Lab

- No test is specific.
- Serum follicle-stimulating hormone, inhibin B, and estradiol may be slightly higher than age-matched controls but are not consistently elevated.
- In isolated premature thelarche, serum ultrasensitive luteinizing hormone level is prepubertal.

Imaging

- Bone age is not significantly or is very mildly advanced (<1 year ahead of chronologic age).
  - Bone age estimates the extent of estrogenic stimulation because estrogen promotes bone maturation.
  - Advanced bone age implies significant estrogen effect, suggesting the need for evaluation of true precocious puberty.
  - Exception: Prepubertal obese girls often have advanced skeletal maturation.
- Pelvic ultrasonography
  - May demonstrate presence and regression of small ovarian cysts (1–15 mm) and a prepubertal-size uterus

DIFFERENTIAL DIAGNOSIS

- Tumors: benign lipomas
- Congenital
  - Neonatal breast hyperplasia in newborn boys or girls that appears shortly after birth and is caused by gestational hormones
  - This form of breast development is normal and usually regresses.
- Severe acquired hypothyroidism
  - High levels of thyroid-stimulating hormone may cross-stimulate gonadal follicle–stimulating hormone and/or luteinizing hormone receptors.
- Gonadotropin-independent estrogen production
  - McCune–Albright syndrome: triad of precocious puberty, café au lait spots, and polyostotic fibrous dysplasia due to gain of function mutations of G proteins
  - Ovarian or adrenal tumors
- True precocious puberty

ALERT

- Must distinguish fat from breast tissue in obese girls
- Caution should be used when evaluating 6–7-year-old girls because signs of puberty at these younger ages may not be considered normal.
- It is a concern if a male infant outside of the newborn period or a young prepubertal boy shows breast enlargement.
- Removal of a breast bud will result in failure of that breast to develop during adolescence.

TREATMENT

GENERAL MEASURES

- Observation
- Reassurance for benign processes

ONGOING CARE

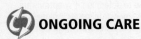

- Regression often occurs by 2 years but may occur up to 6 years after onset.
- No specific characteristics that can assist with prediction of which girls with premature thelarche will go on to have precocious puberty.
- Evidence of pubertal progression should prompt additional evaluation by an endocrinologist:
  - Rapid increase in size of breast tissue
  - Growth acceleration
  - Development of other secondary sexual characteristics
  - Vaginal bleeding

PROGNOSIS

- No known effects on growth, timing of menarche, fertility, or increase risk of breast cancer.
- Onset after age 2 years may be associated with increased risk of progression to precocious puberty.

COMPLICATIONS

May be the first sign of true precocious puberty or may be associated with other pathologies (e.g., tumors, hypothyroidism, and McCune-Albright syndrome)

PATIENT EDUCATION

- Many newborn male and female infants have breast buds as a result of exposure to maternal estrogen in utero; this resolves quickly.
- Asymmetric breast development is quite common in the early stages of pubertal development.
- Malignant tumors of the breast during childhood are extremely rare.
- Any removal of breast tissue prior to or during puberty must be avoided.

ADDITIONAL READING

- Crofton PM, Evans NEM, Wardhaugh B, et al. Evidence for increased ovarian follicular activity in girls with premature thelarche. *Clin Endocrinol (Oxf)*. 2005;62(2):205–209.
- Diamantopoulos S, Bao Y. Gynecomastia and premature thelarche, a guide for practitioners. *Pediatr Rev*. 2007;28(9):e57–e68.
- Haber HP, Wollmann HA, Ranke MB. Pelvic ultrasonography: early differentiation between isolated premature thelarche and central precocious puberty. *Eur J Pediatr*. 1997;154(3):182–186.
- Herman-Giddens ME, Slora EJ, Wasserman RC, et al. Secondary sexual characteristics and menses in young girls seen in office practice: a study from the Pediatric Research Office in Settings network. *Pediatrics*. 1997;99(4):505–512.
- Kaplowitz P, Oberfield SE, Drug and Therapeutics and Executive Committees of the Lawson Wilkins Pediatric Endocrine Society. Reexamination of age limit for defining when puberty is precocious in girls in the United States: implication for evaluation and treatment. *Pediatrics*. 1999;104(4, Pt 1):936–941.
- Klein K, Mericq V, Brown-Dawson JM, et al. Estrogen levels in girls with premature thelarche compared with normal prepubertal girls as determined by an ultrasensitive recombinant cell bioassay. *J Pediatr*. 1999;134(2):190–192.
- Lebrethon MC, Bourguignon JP. Management of central isosexual precocity: diagnosis, treatment, outcome. *Curr Opin Pediatr*. 2000;12(4):394–399.
- Midyett LK, Moore WV, Jacobson JD. Are pubertal changes in girls before age 8 benign? *Pediatrics*. 2003;111(1):47–51.
- Pasquino AM, Pucarelli I, Passeri F, et al. Progression of premature thelarche to central precocious puberty. *J Pediatr*. 1995;126(1):11–14.
- Salardi S, Cacciari E, Mainetti B, et al. Outcome of premature thelarche: relation to puberty and final height. *Arch Dis Child*. 1998;79(2):173–174.
- Stanhope R. Premature thelarche: clinical follow-up and indication for treatment. *J Pediatr Endocrinol Metab*. 2000;13(Suppl 1):827–830.
- Stanhope R, Brook CC. Thelarche variant: a new syndrome of precocious sexual maturation? *Acta Endocrinol (Copenh)*. 1990;123(5):481–486.
- Styne DM. New aspects in the diagnosis and treatment of pubertal disorders. *Pediatr Clin North Am*. 1997;44(2):505–529.
- Traggiai C, Stanhope R. Disorders of pubertal development. *Best Pract Res Clin Obstet Gynaecol*. 2003;17(1):41–56.

CODES

ICD10

E30.8 Other disorders of puberty

FAQ

- Q: Does premature thelarche predispose the child to later abnormalities in pubertal development?
- A: If onset occurs after age 2 years, the girl may be more likely to enter puberty earlier. However, most girls with premature thelarche will have normal pubertal development and fertility.

PREMENSTRUAL SYNDROME

Ann B. Bruner

BASICS

DESCRIPTION

- Premenstrual syndrome (PMS), also called luteal phase disorder, is characterized by psychological and physical symptoms that occur cyclically and consistently during the second half of the menstrual cycle, which negatively impact usual activities of daily living and remit after the onset of menstruation.
- PMS is diagnosed through prospective symptom charting with symptoms present beginning at approximately day 13 of the cycle and resolving within 4 days of menses for 2 consecutive cycles.
  - At least 1 of the following symptoms must occur within 5 days of menses onset: breast tenderness, bloating/weight gain, headache, swelling of hands/feet, aches/pains, mood symptoms (depression, anger, irritability, anxiety, social withdrawal), poor concentration, sleep disturbance, or change in appetite.
- Premenstrual dysphoric disorder (PMDD) is the extreme variant of PMS; defined in *DSM-5* as severe psychological symptoms causing significant dysfunctions in activity, which are not an exacerbation of symptoms of a chronic condition; have occurred in most cycles in the previous year; and are confirmed through prospective daily ratings of at least 2 symptomatic cycles
- Criteria for PMDD: at least 5 symptoms among the following, present in the final week before menses, and improving within a few days of onset of menses, with at least 1 of the symptoms being among the first 4:
  - Depressed mood: feeling sad, hopeless, or self-deprecating
  - Anxiety or tension: feeling tense, anxious, or "on edge"
  - Affective lability: fluctuating emotions interspersed with frequent tearfulness
  - Irritability or anger: increased interpersonal conflicts
  - Decreased interest in usual activities, which may be associated with withdrawal from social relationships
  - Difficulty concentrating
  - Feeling fatigued, lethargic, or lacking in energy
  - Marked changes in appetite, which may be associated with binge eating or craving certain foods
  - Hypersomnia or insomnia
  - A subjective feeling of being overwhelmed or out of control
  - Physical symptoms such as breast tenderness/swelling, headaches, bloating or weight gain, arthralgias, or myalgias

EPIDEMIOLOGY

Prevalence

- Up to 75% of women experience some PMS symptoms at some time.
- Clinically significant PMS occurs in 3–8% of women.
- 2% of women have symptoms that interfere with their usual activities (PMDD).
- 14–88% of adolescent girls have moderate to severe PMS; one study demonstrated a 5.8% prevalence of PMDD in young women ages 14–24 years.

RISK FACTORS

- Age
  - More severe symptoms of PMDD may be seen in younger women.
- Culture
  - PMS/PMDD appear to be more prevalent in Western cultures, possibly due to differences in socialization and symptom expectations.
- Stress
  - PMS and PMDD may be associated with high levels of day-to-day stress and/or a history of stressful events, including sexual abuse.

Genetics

Genetic factors may play a role in the development of PMS/PMDD: Twin studies show a 93% concordance rate in monozygotic twins, with only a 44% rate in dizygotic twins.

PATHOPHYSIOLOGY

- Occurrence of symptoms is related to ovarian function/ovulation:
  - PMS does not occur before menarche, during pregnancy, or after menopause.
  - PMS can occur after hysterectomy but not after bilateral oophorectomy.
  - Symptoms not observed during anovulatory cycles
- Research suggests altered cyclic interactions between sex hormones (particularly progesterone produced by corpus luteum), prostaglandins, and neurotransmitters including serotonin, γ-aminobutyric acid (GABA), and endogenous opioids.
- Women with PMS do not have abnormal serum concentrations of estrogen or progesterone or hormonal imbalance; women with PMS seem to have abnormal responses to normal variations in sex hormones.

ETIOLOGY

Etiology unknown but presumed to be multifactorial

DIAGNOSIS

HISTORY

- Many women report that their PMS symptoms are not taken seriously.
- Complete medical history, including use of medications or illicit substances, cigarettes, dietary evaluation
- Gynecologic history: age at onset of pubertal development, menstrual pattern, sexual activity, contraceptive use, dysmenorrhea
- Psychiatric history: mental health disorders, medications
- Family history: mental health and substance use/abuse
- Psychosocial history: living situation, school/vocational activities and goals, hobbies, peers
- Complete review of systems including both physical symptoms (fatigue, breast tenderness/swelling, bloating, edema, weight gain, headache, arthralgias, myalgias, pelvic discomfort, changes in bowel habit, reduced coordination) and emotional/psychological symptoms (depression, mood lability, irritability, tension, anxiety, tearfulness, restlessness, reduced concentration, fatigue, altered libido, altered appetite/eating habits, altered sleep)
- Chronologic review to determine if symptoms are recurrent with most menstrual cycles, isolated to luteal phase of cycle, and remit with onset of menses

PHYSICAL EXAM

- There are no specific physical findings of PMS.
- Enlarged thyroid gland: may suggest hypothyroidism and need to evaluate for thyroid disease
- Virilization (hirsutism, clitoromegaly): may suggest hyperandrogenism and need to evaluate for adrenal disease, including Cushing syndrome, or other hormonal disorders such as polycystic ovarian syndrome
- Pallor: may suggest anemia
- Orthostatic hypotension: may suggest neurally mediated hypotension

DIAGNOSTIC TESTS & INTERPRETATION

Premenstrual Assessment Form (PAF), Prospective Record of the Impact and Severity of Menstruation (PRISM), or Calendar of Premenstrual Experiences (COPE): Prospective symptom calendars can help establish diagnosis and provide information about symptom patterns (recurrence and relation to menses). Differences in symptom severity between the follicular and luteal phases (before and after ovulation) may be most diagnostic.

Lab

- CBC: Rule out anemia.
- Thyroid-stimulating hormone (TSH) assay: Rule out thyroid disease.

DIFFERENTIAL DIAGNOSIS

- Psychiatric
  - Mood disorder, including major depression, dysthymia, bipolar disorder, postpartum depression, anxiety disorder
  - Substance abuse
  - Physical, sexual, or emotional abuse
  - Somatization disorder
  - Eating disorder
- Endocrinologic
  - Thyroid disease
  - Cushing disease
  - Diabetes mellitus

- Gynecologic
  - Dysmenorrhea (primary or secondary)
  - Pregnancy
  - Endometriosis
  - Hormonal contraceptive use
  - Perimenopause
- Immunologic/hematologic
  - Anemia
  - Fibromyalgia
  - Systemic lupus erythematosus (SLE)
  - Chronic fatigue syndrome
- Neurologic
  - Migraine headache
  - Neurally mediated hypotension

TREATMENT

GENERAL MEASURES

- Treatment goals include reducing both symptom frequency and severity and the impact of symptoms on patients' activities.
- Patient education, counseling, and reassurance may be all that is needed for women with milder symptoms.
- Many pharmacologic and nonpharmacologic modalities have not been formally evaluated.

Diet

- Research supports reducing caffeine and alcohol intake and suggests that reductions in salt and refined sugars may also be beneficial.
- Meta-analyses of research to date have shown that some supplements are beneficial in reducing symptom frequency and severity, including calcium carbonate (1,200 mg/day), pyridoxine/vitamin B_6 (50 mg/day), and possibly magnesium (400 mg/day).
- Many herbal therapies are in use, including evening primrose oil, chaste berry, black cohosh, ginkgo, and St. John's wort. However, there is no strong evidence to support their use in PMS.

Activity

- Increasing physical activity, ensuring adequate and regular sleep, and maintaining a healthy diet are important first steps.
- Mind/body therapies are frequently used including individual psychotherapy, relaxation techniques, guided imagery, yoga, massage, biofeedback, and group therapy; to date, there is no strong evidence to support their use in PMS.

MEDICATION

First Line

- Many menstrually associated symptoms can be managed with nonsteroidal anti-inflammatory drugs (NSAIDs).
- NSAIDs (e.g., naproxen sodium 275–550 mg b.i.d.) relieve the majority of physical symptoms: premenstrual/menstrual cramping, headaches, and myalgias/arthralgias.
- Side effects include gastrointestinal upset and renal dysfunction.

Second Line

SSRIs are first line for PMDD and severe PMS, especially those with predominantly psychological symptoms. SSRIs have been shown to improve mood, decrease irritability, ameliorate physical symptoms such as bloating and breast tenderness, and improve psychosocial function. Continuous and intermittent (during luteal phase) dosing can be used, and symptom amelioration can occur during the first cycle of treatment. Intermittent use includes administration during the last 14 days of the menstrual cycle or treatment begun at expected date of symptom onset:

- Fluoxetine (20–60 mg/24 h), sertraline (50–150 mg/24 h), paroxetine (10–30 mg/24 h), and citalopram (5–20 mg/24 h) are some of the most commonly used SSRIs for PMS/PMDD; side effects include gastrointestinal upset, insomnia, tremor/agitation, fatigue, dry mouth, and sexual dysfunction. SSRIs recently received a U.S. FDA black box warning concerning an increased risk of suicidality among depressed children and adolescents; the warning was for the treatment of depression, not PMS/PMDD.
- Hormonal contraceptives (i.e., low-dose oral contraceptive pills, contraceptive patch) suppress ovulation; formulations with drospirenone may be more effective against hormonally mediated symptoms such as breast swelling/tenderness and bloating.
- Spironolactone (50 mg b.i.d.) is effective for breast tenderness and bloating; potassium levels must be monitored, and spironolactone is contraindicated in patients with abnormal renal function.
- Calcium carbonate 500–600 mg b.i.d. has been shown to decrease PMS symptoms.

ONGOING CARE

- Frequent follow-up and the use of a prospective menstrual/symptom calendar are important.
- After the diagnosis of PMS is established, and after recommending appropriate lifestyle changes (and possibly NSAIDs), the patient should be reevaluated after 3 months. If there has not been substantial improvement, secondary pharmacologic therapies (SSRIs) may need to be considered. When SSRIs are prescribed as 1st-line therapy for patients with more severe PMS or PMDD, response to SSRIs and any adverse reactions should be assessed at follow-up and dosage adjusted as needed.

ISSUES FOR REFERRAL

A gynecologist/reproductive endocrinologist can assist in the management of severe PMS/PMDD: Other pharmacologic agents that are used include gonadotropin-releasing hormone (GnRH) analogues, danazol, estrogen implants, and androgens.

COMPLICATIONS

Psychological morbidity includes difficulty with interpersonal relationships (family and friends) and school absence/failure.

ADDITIONAL READING

- American Psychiatric Association. *Desk Reference to the Diagnostic Criteria From DSM-5*. Arlington, VA: American Psychiatric Association; 2013.
- Borenstein J, Chiou CF, Dean B, et al. Estimating direct and indirect costs of premenstrual syndrome. *J Occup Environ Med*. 2005;47(1):26.
- Claman F, Miller T. Premenstrual syndrome and premenstrual dysphoric disorder in adolescence. *J Pediatr Health Care*. 2006;20(5):329–333.
- Halbreich U. The etiology, biology, and evolving pathology of premenstrual syndromes. *Psychoneuroendocrinology*. 2003;28(Suppl 3):55–99.
- Halbreich U, Bornestein J, Pearlstein T, et al. The prevalence, impairment, impact, and burden of premenstrual dysphoric disorder (PMS/PMDD). *Psychoneuroendocrinology*. 2003;28(Suppl 3):1–23.
- Rapkin AJ, Akopians AL. Pathophysiology of premenstrual syndrome and premenstrual dysphoric disorder. *Menopause Int*. 2012;18(2):52–59.
- Steiner M, Pearlstein T, Cohen L, et al. Expert guidelines for the treatment of severe PMS, PMDD, and comorbidities: the role of SSRIs. *J Womens Health (Larchmt)*. 2006;15(1):57–69.
- Vigod SN, Ross LE, Steiner M. Understanding and treating premenstrual dysphoric disorder: an update for the women's health practitioner. *Obstet Gynecol Clin North Am*. 2009;36(4):907–924.

CODES

ICD10

N94.3 Premenstrual tension syndrome

FAQ

- Q: Can adolescent girls have PMS and PMDD?
- A: The incidence of PMS and PMDD in adolescents is not well established. Although ≤50% of cycles are anovulatory during the first 1–2 years after menarche, younger patients experience many PMS symptoms, and menstrual problems are some of the most common reasons for school absence. Most experts believe that PMS/PMDD will not develop until a regular ovulatory pattern is established, ~2–3 years after menarche.
- Q: Is family history important?
- A: Genetic factors may play a role in the development of PMS/PMDD; twin studies show a 93% concordance rate in monozygotic twins, with only a 44% rate in dizygotic twins.
- Q: Are there any common comorbidities?
- A: The symptoms of PMS/PMDD are also seen with depression, anxiety, and other mood disorders. Psychiatric symptomatology can fluctuate, and symptoms may change in relation to the menstrual cycle. Careful and thorough history taking and prospective symptom diaries can help differentiate PMS/PMDD from another mental health disorder.

PRIMARY ADRENAL INSUFFICIENCY

Jennifer M. Barker

BASICS

DESCRIPTION

Deficiency in the secretion of cortisol and/or aldosterone by the adrenal glands

EPIDEMIOLOGY

- Age
  - Adrenal insufficiency associated with congenital adrenal hyperplasia (CAH) presents in the newborn period.
  - Adrenal hypoplasia congenita presents in infancy or early childhood.
  - Adrenocorticotropic hormone (ACTH) unresponsiveness presents in late infancy or the toddler period.
  - Adrenoleukodystrophy typically presents late in the 1st decade of life with neurologic symptoms. Signs and symptoms of adrenal insufficiency in persons with adrenoleukodystrophy may first present at any age.
  - Addison disease is rare in children and usually presents between the ages of 20 and 50 years. In the pediatric population, it is most often seen in late childhood and adolescence.
- Sex
  - CAH and ACTH unresponsiveness affect both sexes equally.
  - Adrenal hypoplasia congenita, an X-linked disorder, predominantly affects boys
  - Adrenoleukodystrophy, an X-linked disorder, predominantly affects boys.
  - Addison disease is more common in girls.

RISK FACTORS

Genetics

- CAH: autosomal recessive inheritance associated with a gene defect in 1 of multiple adrenal steroidogenic enzymes, most commonly *CYP21A2* for the 21-hydroxylase gene
- Adrenal hypoplasia congenita: X-linked mutation in *DAX1* gene
- ACTH unresponsiveness: autosomal recessive ACTH receptor defect
- Adrenoleukodystrophy
  - X-linked recessive disorder of very-long-chain fatty acid metabolism due to *ABCD1* gene mutation
  - An autosomal recessive form of the disease exists, with presentation during infancy.
- Addison disease
  - Autoimmune adrenal insufficiency may be isolated or part of autoimmune polyglandular syndrome (APS) type 1 or 2. Mutations in the *AIRE1* gene have been identified as the cause of APS type 1. An association exists between idiopathic Addison disease and human leukocyte antigen (HLA)-B8 and DR3.

PATHOPHYSIOLOGY

- CAH: a group of enzymatic disorders of steroid metabolism, of which 21-hydroxylase deficiency is the most common (Appendix, Table 13)
- Adrenal hypoplasia congenita: a defect in adrenal organogenesis
- ACTH unresponsiveness
  - Inherited defect in the ACTH receptor, resulting in isolated glucocorticoid deficiency with hypoglycemia in infancy and hyperpigmentation
- Adrenoleukodystrophy
  - Inherited disorders of impaired peroxisomal degradation of very-long-chain fatty acids, resulting in adrenal insufficiency and progressive neurologic deterioration
- Addison disease
  - Primary hypoadrenalism due to bilateral destruction of the adrenal cortices; this can be due to autoimmune destruction (isolated or associated with APS), tuberculosis, hemorrhage, fungal infection, neoplastic infiltration, or AIDS.
- Waterhouse-Friderichsen syndrome: bilateral adrenal gland hemorrhage classically associated with fulminant meningococcemia but also reported with *Staphylococcus aureus* and *Streptococcus pneumoniae*

COMMONLY ASSOCIATED CONDITIONS

- Deficiencies of other hormones, including aldosterone and adrenal sex steroids
- Adrenal hypoplasia congenita is associated with hypogonadotropic hypogonadism.
- APSs are associated with other autoimmune disorders:
  - APS type 1: mucocutaneous candidiasis, hypoparathyroidism
  - APS type 2: autoimmune thyroid disease, type 1 diabetes
  - Both types can also present in conjunction with multiple other autoimmune disorders (e.g., primary ovarian or testicular insufficiency, celiac disease, pernicious anemia, vitiligo, autoimmune hepatitis).

DIAGNOSIS

HISTORY

Symptoms of primary adrenal insufficiency are nonspecific and similar to those found in many disease processes. Symptoms may be present for years prior to diagnosis. The electrolyte picture of adrenal insufficiency can be seen in renal disorders, obstructive uropathy, and isolated aldosterone deficiency:

- Weakness and fatigue
- Anorexia, weight loss
- Headache
- Nausea, vomiting, diarrhea, abdominal pain
- Orthostatic symptoms
- Muscle or joint pains
- Emotional lability
- Salt craving
- Hyperpigmentation
- Decreased axillary or pubic hair in females due to lack of adrenal androgens
- Amenorrhea in females
- Unexplained hypoglycemia, decreasing insulin requirements and decreasing HgbA1c in patients with type 1 diabetes

PHYSICAL EXAM

- Hyperpigmentation, especially on lip borders, buccal mucosa, nipples, and over skin creases (associated with elevated ACTH)
- Weight loss
- Hypotension or orthostatic hypotension
- Evaluate for other signs of autoimmune disease (e.g., thyromegaly, vitiligo).
- Pubertal staging
- Signs of virilization in females

DIAGNOSTIC TESTS & INTERPRETATION

Diagnostic Procedures/Other

- Specific
  - Newborn screening (NBS) for 21-hydroxylase deficiency identifies infants with CAH prior to presentation with adrenal crisis. Abnormal NBS results require follow-up with serum 17-hydroxyprogesterone, plasma renin activity, and/or electrolytes depending on clinical scenario.
  - Random elevated ACTH with low cortisol may be sufficient to diagnose primary adrenal insufficiency.
  - Cosyntropin (Cortrosyn) stimulation test: Administer cosyntropin (synthetic ACTH) 250 mcg IV and measure cortisol at baseline, 30 and 60 minutes.
    - A normal response is a final cortisol >18 mcg/dL. An insufficient cortisol response is diagnostic of adrenal insufficiency.
    - A baseline ACTH >200 pg/mL with inadequate cortisol is seen in primary adrenal insufficiency.
  - Serum adrenal antibodies may be positive in autoimmune Addison disease.
  - Very-long-chain fatty acids are elevated in adrenoleukodystrophy.
  - Low gonadotropin and sex steroid levels suggesting hypogonadotropic hypogonadism may be seen with adrenal hypoplasia congenita.
  - Adrenal steroid precursors will be elevated in CAH.
- Nonspecific
  - Electrolytes
    - Hyponatremia: result of the mineralocorticoid defect and glucocorticoid deficiency; combination of sodium loss from kidneys, and the inability to excrete a water load
    - Hyperkalemia and acidosis: chronic mineralocorticoid deficiency with the inability to excrete potassium and acid
    - Hypercalcemia: most likely a result of increased calcium absorption due to the lack of glucocorticoid effect on the gut
    - Hypoglycemia: Glucocorticoids have permissive effects on gluconeogenesis.
    - Renin levels are elevated when a mineralocorticoid deficiency is present.

DIFFERENTIAL DIAGNOSIS
- CAH
- Adrenal hypoplasia congenita
- ACTH unresponsiveness
- Adrenoleukodystrophy
- Autoimmune adrenal cortical destruction
- Infectious adrenal cortical destruction
  - Tuberculous
  - Fungal
  - HIV
- Adrenal hemorrhage
- Neoplastic adrenal infiltration

ALERT
- Differential above only covers primary forms of adrenal insufficiency; secondary/tertiary forms may also need to be considered (ACTH/CRH deficiency). For these children, evaluation for other pituitary hormone disorders often warranted (see Panhypopituitarism).
- Replacing thyroid hormone in a child with untreated adrenal insufficiency can precipitate adrenal crisis.

TREATMENT

MEDICATION
- Acute adrenal crisis
  - Hydrocortisone (HC): stress dosage of hydrocortisone: 100 mg/m^2 IV/IM followed by 100 mg/m^2/24 h of hydrocortisone divided q4–6h. Decrease to a physiologic replacement dosage when acute illness has resolved.
  - Mineralocorticoid replacement: Florinef 0.1 mg daily when able to take PO
- Chronic adrenal insufficiency
  - Hydrocortisone 10–12 mg/m^2/24 h PO divided as t.i.d. Increase the dose to 30–50 mg/m^2/24 h for stress of fever, illness, or vomiting. Lower doses may sometimes be used, particularly for forms of adrenal insufficiency other than CAH.
  - For major stress (surgery, significant illness), give hydrocortisone 50–100 mg/m^2 IV/IM followed by 50–100 mg/m^2/24 h IV divided q4–6h. IM hydrocortisone is recommended for emergency home use. In some cases, equivalent doses of prednisone or dexamethasone may be used.
  - Florinef 0.1 mg PO daily
  - May require sodium supplementation (especially infants)

INPATIENT CONSIDERATIONS
Initial Stabilization
- Acute adrenal crisis
  - An intercurrent illness or surgical procedure may provoke an episode of hypotension, tachycardia, and shock.
  - Electrolytes reveal decreased serum sodium, elevated potassium, metabolic acidosis, and a decreased or normal glucose.
  - Serum should be drawn and saved to aid in diagnosis, but emergent treatment should not be delayed for a diagnostic ACTH stimulation test.
- Treatment
  - 5% dextrose in normal saline solution (D5NS) for volume repletion and treatment of salt wasting and hypoglycemia
  - HC or other glucocorticoid
  - Mineralocorticoid replacement

IV Fluids
D5NS for volume repletion and treatment of salt wasting

ONGOING CARE

FOLLOW-UP RECOMMENDATIONS
Acute adrenal crisis usually improves rapidly with the administration of fluids and glucocorticoids. Once the acute phase of illness has resolved, steroids can be resumed at physiologic replacement doses.

Patient Monitoring
- Clinical status
- Reduction in hyperpigmentation
- Electrolytes, ACTH, and renin levels
- Screen for polyautoimmune disorders.
- Growth
- Very-long-chain fatty acid levels and neurologic function in adrenoleukodystrophy
- Pubertal development

PATIENT EDUCATION
- Stress dosing
- Importance of seeking medical attention for significant illness, persistent vomiting, or the inability to take fluids by mouth
- MedicAlert bracelet

PROGNOSIS
- Long-term prognosis of isolated adrenal insufficiency is good, provided adequate hydrocortisone is administered, particularly in times of illness.
- Risk for early mortality related to inappropriately treated adrenal crisis
- Adrenoleukodystrophy carries a poor prognosis.

COMPLICATIONS
- If not diagnosed and/or treated properly, a significant physical stress such as surgery or illness may result in a life-threatening adrenal crisis.
- CAH can cause virilization/ambiguous genitalia in female infants with the disease and can cause salt-wasting crises in infants of both sexes.
- Pubertal delay or hypogonadotropic hypogonadism is seen with adrenal hypoplasia congenita due to *DAX1* mutations.
- Unrecognized ACTH unresponsiveness is associated with recurrent hypoglycemia, seizures, mental retardation, and death.
- Adrenoleukodystrophy results in severe neurologic impairment and death.
- Autoimmune adrenal insufficiency is commonly associated with additional autoimmune disease that can complicate treatment

ADDITIONAL READING

- Achermann JC, Meeks JJ, Jameson JL. Phenotypic spectrum of mutations in DAX-1 and SF-1. *Mol Cell Endocrinol*. 2001;185(1–2):17–25.
- Adem PV, Montgomery CD, Husain AN, et al. *Staphylococcus aureus* sepsis and the Waterhouse-Friderichsen syndrome in children. *N Engl J Med*. 2005;353(12):1245–1251.
- Falorni A, Minarelli V, Morelli S. Therapy of adrenal insufficiency: an update. *Endocrine*. 2013;43(3):514–528.
- Hsieh S, White PC. Presentation of primary adrenal insufficiency in childhood. *J Clin Endocrinol Metab*. 2011;96(6):E925–E928.
- Husebye ES, Perheentupa J, Rautemaa R, et al. Clinical manifestations and management of patients with autoimmune polyendocrine syndrome type 1. *J Intern Med*. 2009;265(5):514–529.
- Selva KA, LaFranchi SH, Boston B. A novel presentation of familial glucocorticoid deficiency (FGD) and current literature review. *J Pediatr Endocrinol Metab*. 2004;17(1):85–92.
- Shulman DI, Palmert MR, Kepm SF. Adrenal insufficiency: still a cause of morbidity and death in childhood. *Pediatrics*. 2007;119(2):e484–e494.
- Vaidya B, Pearce S, Kendall-Taylor P. Recent advances in the molecular genetics of congenital and acquired primary adrenocortical failure. *Clin Endocrinol*. 2000;53(4):403–418.
- White PC, Bachega TA. Congenital adrenal hyperplasia due to 21 hydroxylase deficiency: from birth to adulthood. *Semin Reprod Med*. 2012;30(5):400–409.

CODES

ICD10
- E27.1 Primary adrenocortical insufficiency
- Q89.1 Congenital malformations of adrenal gland
- E71.529 X-linked adrenoleukodystrophy, unspecified type

FAQ
- Q: What are the indications for stress dosing and how rapidly can the stress hydrocortisone dose be tapered?
- A: Patients will require stress dosing of hydrocortisone for surgical procedures, fever (>37.7°C [100°F]), vomiting, diarrhea, and particularly vigorous exercise. The stress dose is typically given for 24 hours, after which the usual dose is resumed. Should it be necessary to administer the stress dosage for a more prolonged period, the dosage can usually be tapered rapidly to physiologic dosage, once the patient's clinical condition has improved.

PRION DISEASES (TRANSMISSIBLE SPONGIFORM ENCEPHALOPATHIES)

Jason Y. Kim

BASICS

DESCRIPTION

- Transmissible spongiform encephalopathies (TSEs) or prion diseases are a family of progressive neurodegenerative diseases of humans and animals that cause irreversible cumulative brain damage and are uniformly fatal.
  - Prions
    - The infectious agents that cause TSE
    - The term *prion* was coined to denote "a small proteinaceous infectious particle resistant to inactivation by most procedures that modify nucleic acids."
  - Prion proteins (PRP)
    - Normal cellular glycoproteins (PRP^C) encoded by the *PRNP* gene
    - Are found on neurons and white blood cells
- The infectious particles that cause TSEs are protease-resistant conformers of PRP^C (PRP^{RES} or PRP^{SC} for protease-resistant or scrapie-causing PRPs, respectively).
- Human TSEs include Creutzfeldt-Jakob disease (CJD), the more recently identified variant CJD (vCJD), kuru, Gerstmann-Sträussler-Scheinker syndrome, and fatal familial insomnia syndrome.
- Six TSEs in animals have been described: bovine spongiform encephalopathy (BSE, also known as mad cow disease), scrapie in sheep and goats, feline spongiform encephalopathy, transmissible mink encephalopathy, exotic ungulate encephalopathy, and chronic wasting disease of cervids.

EPIDEMIOLOGY

- CJD
  - CJD is the most prevalent form of TSE in humans and occurs as either a sporadic or a familial disease.
  - ~85% of cases are sporadic because there is no family history and no known source of transmission. Sporadic CJD occurs throughout the world at a rate 1/1,000,000 people.
  - Familial CJD (fCJD) cases are associated with a gene mutation in PRNP and account for ~10–15% of cases. fCJD shows an autosomal dominant inheritance, with >50 mutations in PRNP identified.
  - ~1% of CJD cases are iatrogenic, resulting from accidental transmission of the causative agent via contaminated surgical equipment, as a result of cornea or dura mater transplants, or administration of human-derived pituitary growth hormones.
  - No evidence confirms person-to-person transmission among family members via direct contact, droplet, or airborne spread.
  - Disease is characterized by progressive dementia, myoclonus, visual or cerebellar disturbance, pyramidal/extrapyramidal dysfunction, and/or akinetic mutism.
  - Classic sporadic CJD most often occurs between the ages of 50 and 70 years and affects both sexes equally; whites have about a 2-fold higher rate than blacks.
  - Death usually occurs within 1 year of onset of symptoms.
- vCJD
  - New form of CJD, first reported in 1994; has unique clinical features
  - In contrast to CJD, affects younger patients including adolescents (average age, 29 years) and has a longer duration of illness with median of 14 months as opposed to 4.5 months with CJD
  - Strong epidemiologic evidence links vCJD to BSE:
    - BSE is a TSE that affects cattle; it was first reported in the United Kingdom. The most likely route of exposure is through bovine-based foods derived from BSE-infected cattle.
    - Highest incidence of vCJD is seen in the United Kingdom, the country with the largest potential exposure to BSE.
    - 3 cases of vCJD have been confirmed in the United States, although each were likely to have been contracted outside the United States.
- Clinical features, found early in the illness, include the following:
  - Prominent psychiatric symptoms (e.g., depression, schizophrenia-like psychosis) and ataxia
  - Other neurologic signs (e.g., paresthesia/dysesthesia, chorea, dystonia, myoclonus, and akinetic mutism) develop as the disease progresses.
- Recently, clinical criteria for the diagnosis of vCJD were validated in the United Kingdom by autopsy-/biopsy-proven cases compared to noncases.
- Fatal familial insomnia (FFI)
  - An autosomal dominant disorder, caused by mutation at codon 178 of PRNP, also identified in fCJD. If there are homozygous alleles at codon 129 encoding methionine in conjunction with the codon 178 mutation, FFI ensues. If codon 129 encodes valine in conjunction with the codon 178 mutation, then fCJD develops.
  - Clinical features include insomnia, dysautonomia, ataxia, myoclonus, and late dementia.
  - Pathology reveals minimal vacuolization and no plaques.
- Gerstmann-Sträussler-Scheinker syndrome
  - A disorder with autosomal dominant inheritance
  - Clinical features include ataxia and dementia.
  - Pathology reveals amyloid plaques.

PATHOPHYSIOLOGY

- TSE arises when exogenous or endogenous PRP^{RES} cause PRP^C to misfold into the abnormal protease-resistant form associated with TSE.
- Progressive accumulation of PRP^{RES} in the CNS disrupts function, leading to vacuolization and cell death. There is no host-adaptive immune response beyond microglial cell activation involved in the pathologic process.
- Neuropathologic findings include neuronal loss, atrophy, vacuolization or spongiform change, reactive astrogliosis, and cell death.
- PRP^{RES} also accumulate in the reticular endothelial system, mucosa-associated lymphoid tissues, and areas of chronic inflammation throughout the body.

ETIOLOGY

- Prions are infectious proteins lacking nucleic acids that are believed to cause TSE.
- Infection arises when normal protease-sensitive host proteins, involved in neuronal function, undergo spontaneous misfolding to yield the abnormal protease-resistant form associated with infectivity.
- Newly formed host PRP^{RES} recruit neighboring cellular PRP^C and convert it to the infectious conformer. The exact molecular and cellular mechanisms surrounding propagation of PRP^{RES} remains unknown.
- Although the presence of PRP^C is necessary for the migration of PRP^{RES} to the RES, the mechanism for migration to the CNS remains unknown.
- Prions reproduce by recruiting neighboring normal cellular PRP and stimulating its conversion to the infectious form.
- Whether PRP^{RES} reproduce without any genetic material, thus bypassing the central dogma is still hotly debated.
- Not all scientists believe the prion hypothesis, and some have argued that the causative agent is virus-like and possesses nucleic acids although none has ever been isolated from TSE pathologic specimens.

DIAGNOSIS

HISTORY

- Evidence of a familial form of TSE
- Potential iatrogenic exposures such as administration of human-derived pituitary growth hormones, implantation of dura mater or corneal grafts from humans, epilepsy surgery, or other CNS surgery involving stereotactic electrodes
- Duration of symptoms >6 months
- Afebrile illness
- In vCJD, progressive neuropsychiatric symptoms including:
  - Depression, anxiety, apathy, withdrawal, or delusions
  - Painful sensory symptoms including pain and/or dysesthesia
  - Ataxia
  - Myoclonus, chorea, or dystonia
  - Dementia

PHYSICAL EXAM

- Afebrile
- Abnormal mental status exam with defects in memory, personality, and other higher cortical functions, or psychosis
- Neurologic signs include unsteady gait and the presence of involuntary movements.
- Late findings include mutism and complete immobility.

DIAGNOSTIC TESTS & INTERPRETATION

Lab

- Most laboratory tests are of little value in the diagnosis of TSE. Exam of CSF fluid may reveal a mild elevation of protein, but otherwise the cerebrospinal fluid is normal.
- EEG
  - In CJD, generalized slowing is seen early in the disease with progression to periodic burst of biphasic or triphasic sharp-wave complexes.
  - In vCJD, the EEG does not show the waveforms characteristic of sporadic CJD.
  - Although EEG abnormalities are seen in most patients, these findings are not specific.

Imaging

- MRI
  - In patients with vCJD, abnormally high T2 signal in the bilateral pulvinar regions of the thalamus may be seen.
  - In CJD, hyperintense signals in the basal ganglia are often seen.
  - In later stages of CJD and vCJD, imaging studies such as MRI or CT scan reveal generalized atrophy with large ventricles.

Diagnostic Procedures/Other

- Diagnosis of TSE in humans can be confirmed only following pathologic exam of the brain.
- Microscopic exam of patients with all types of human TSEs reveals spongiform change accompanied by neuronal loss and gliosis.
- Amyloid plaques or immunohistochemical demonstration of abnormal PRP in the brain may also be seen.
- "Florid" plaques (amyloid plaques encircled by holes or vacuoles resulting in a daisy-like appearance) are consistently present in patients with vCJD.
- Tonsil biopsy revealing accumulation of PRP^{RES} may be helpful in confirming suspected cases of vCJD.

DIFFERENTIAL DIAGNOSIS

- Neurodegenerative disorders—mostly seen in older adults with the exception of Alpers disease
  - Alzheimer disease
  - Parkinson disease
  - Frontotemporal dementia
  - Pick disease
  - Alpers disease (progressive cerebral hemiatrophy)
  - Amyotrophic lateral sclerosis
  - Huntington disease
  - Spinocerebellar ataxia
- Psychiatric disorders—especially when considering vCJD as a diagnosis
  - Depression
  - Schizophrenia
  - Drug-induced psychosis
- Encephalitis, infectious
- Sydenham chorea
- Subacute sclerosing panencephalitis
- Progressive multifocal leukoencephalopathy
- Toxic encephalopathy
- Inborn errors of metabolism
- Hashimoto thyroiditis
- CNS vasculitis
- CNS tumors

TREATMENT

GENERAL MEASURES

- No treatment is effective in slowing or stopping the progression of disease. Appropriate supportive care should be provided. Prognosis for patients with human TSEs is uniformly poor.
- Several compounds and methods have undergone testing in cell-free, tissue, and animal models of TSE. Some decrease the rate of PRP^{RES} accumulation and allow animals to reach their expected lifespan. None reverses the damage seen in the CNS after plaques have formed.
- Infection control
  - Standard universal precautions are indicated for infection control.
  - Strict isolation is not necessary.
  - Caution should be used in obtaining cerebrospinal fluid and handling tissues obtained at autopsy.
  - Equipment contaminated by high-risk tissue should be soaked in $\geq$1 N sodium hydroxide solution for at least 1 hour and then autoclaved at 134°C for at least 1 hour.

ADDITIONAL READING

- Aguzzi A, Heikenwalder M. Pathogenesis of prion diseases: current status and future outlook. *Nat Rev Microbiol*. 2006;4(10):765–775.
- Glatzel M, Soeck K, Seeger H, et al. Human prion disease: molecular and clinical aspects. *Arch Neurol*. 2005;62(4):545–552.
- Hewitt PE, Llewelyn CA, Mackenzie J, et al. Creutzfeldt-Jakob disease and blood transfusion: results of the UK Transfusion Medicine Epidemiological Review study. *Vox Sang*. 2006;91(3):221–230.
- Holman RC, Belay ED, Christensen KY, et al. Human prion diseases in the United States. *PLoS One*. 2010; 5(1):e8521.
- Johnson RT. Prion diseases. *Lancet Neurol*. 2005; 4(10):635–642.
- Kretzschmar HA. Diagnosis of prion diseases. *Clin Lab Med*. 2003;23(1):109–128.
- Prusiner SB. Shattuck lecture—neurodegenerative diseases and prions. *N Engl J Med*. 2001;344(20): 1516–1526.
- Whitley RJ, MacDonald N, Asher DM. American Academy of Pediatrics. Technical report: transmissible spongiform encephalopathies: a review for pediatricians. Committee of Infectious Diseases. *Pediatrics*. 2000;106(5):1160–1165.

CODES

ICD10

- A81.9 Atypical virus infection of central nervous system, unsp
- A81.00 Creutzfeldt-Jakob disease, unspecified
- A81.81 Kuru

FAQ

- Q: Is transmission of TSEs from human blood possible?
- A: There have been 3 verified cases of vCJD attributed to transfusion of blood products in the United Kingdom. There have been no cases of transfusion-related vCJD in the United States.
- Q: Is our food supply safe?
- A: No cases of BSE have been recognized in North America. The incidence in the United Kingdom has been low and is not increasing rapidly. Measures have been taken by the World Health Organization and the U.S. Food and Drug Administration (FDA) to reduce the risk of TSE, including a ban on the use of ruminant tissues in animal feed and surveillance systems to detect TSE in animals and to prevent any part or product of an animal with suspected TSE to enter the human or animal food chain. The FDA has banned biologic agents of bovine origin produced in countries at risk of BSE. There have been 3 cases of vCJD in U.S. citizens, but each case was likely contracted outside the United States (United Kingdom and Saudi Arabia).

PROBIOTICS

Andi L. Shane • Dan Merenstein

BASICS

DESCRIPTION

- Probiotics are defined by the World Health Organization as "live microorganisms, which when administered in adequate amounts, confer a health benefit to the host."
- The presence of "live cultures" does not make a product a probiotic. The microorganism has to be present in adequate amounts to provide specified health benefit, which can vary, depending on the microorganism. The optimal dosing varies with probiotic product, indication, and host.
- Specific probiotic strains are generally regarded as safe. The Center for Food Safety and Applied Nutrition (CFSAN) provides guidelines for the manufacture of probiotic products, but clinicians must carefully evaluate the probiotic agent selected.
- Levels of evidence to support use of a probiotic depend on the formulation and indication (food, supplement, or drug) and the consumer (clinician, patient, healthy individual, and regulatory authority).
- Several formulations of probiotic products are available both in single-strain and multistrain preparations:
  - Probiotic organisms may be consumed as fermented dairy products or as supplements in the form of a capsule, tablet, liquid, or powder formulation.
- Commonly used probiotic supplements contain single organisms, including the following strains:
  - *Bifidobacterium bifidum* strain YIT 4002
  - *Lactobacillus rhamnosus* ATCC 53103
  - *Lactobacillus delbrueckii* subsp. *bulgaricus*
  - *Streptococcus salivarius* subsp. *thermophilus*
- Yeast, including *Saccharomyces boulardii*, is an alternative to bacterial probiotic formulations.
- Multistrain probiotics incorporate a combination of organisms in varying quantities.

PATHOPHYSIOLOGY

- Probiotics are hypothesized to exert their primary effects on the gut by reestablishing the intestinal microbiota balance, competing for receptor sites in the intestinal lumen, and competing with pathogens for nutrients.
- The proposed immunomodulatory functions of probiotics include enhancing host immune defenses via strengthening tight junctions between intestinal enterocytes, increasing immunoglobulin A production, stimulating cytokine production, and producing substances (e.g., arginine, glutamine, and short-chain fatty acids) thought to secondarily act as protective nutrients.

DIAGNOSIS

- The selection of a single-strain versus a multistrain probiotic product, or a bacterial probiotic versus a yeast probiotic, should be based on the underlying indication, host factors, and whether the probiotic is administered for treatment or prophylaxis.
- The following *selected* probiotics have been shown to be efficacious for the treatment and/or prevention of the following gastrointestinal conditions:
- Efficacy with one probiotic strain or species does not imply that other strains will be equally efficacious. Host factors, dosing, and indication must be considered in formulating recommendations.

Probiotic	Indication
L. rhamnosus GG	Infectious diarrhea, especially of viral etiology
S. boulardi	Antibiotic-associated diarrhea
Combination therapy with lactobacilli, bifidobacteria, streptococci, *S. boulardii*	*Clostridium difficile*–associated diarrhea
Lactobacillus reuteri DSM 17938	Colic

TREATMENT

DOSING GUIDELINES

- The unit of dosing for oral probiotic supplements is the colony-forming unit (CFU).
- Currently, there are no established dosing guidelines based on pharmacokinetic data for children.
- Studies have used oral doses of 1–10 billion CFUs per dose, with administration frequency ranging from 3 times daily to weekly.
- Practitioners have used 1/2 of the adult dose for children of average weight and 1/4 of the adult dose for infants.
- The optimal dosing regimen with respect to timing of antimicrobials and probiotic supplements is not known. Currently, available data suggest that temporal separation of probiotic and antimicrobial is not essential for efficacy.

ONGOING CARE

FOLLOW-UP RECOMMENDATIONS

- The American Academy of Pediatrics (AAP) issued a clinical report summarizing the evidence for use of probiotics and supports their use on a case-by-case basis in children who may benefit from supplementation.
- Probiotics have been shown to be efficacious in randomized, double-blind, placebo-controlled studies for the following indications:
  - Decreasing the duration of infectious diarrheal episodes in hospitalized children, childcare attendees, and children with enteric viral infections in resource-poor areas
  - Reducing the mortality and morbidity of necrotizing enterocolitis (NEC), a devastating condition in neonates
  - Reducing antibiotic-associated diarrhea in children receiving oral and intravenous antibiotics
  - Treating and preventing pouchitis, inflammation of a surgically created distal small bowel reservoir, and irritable bowel syndrome in children and adults (multistrain probiotic)
  - Reducing the risk of developing *C. difficile*–associated diarrhea and associated symptoms in children and adults when probiotics and antibiotics are coadministered.

- Probiotic applications currently being evaluated include the following:
  - Maintenance of remission in persons with ulcerative colitis
  - Treatment and prevention of atopic disease including rhinitis and asthma
  - Improving tolerance of *Helicobacter pylori* eradication therapy
  - Prevention of genitourinary infections, such as urinary tract infections and candidiasis
  - Prevention of dental caries
- Future investigations to evaluate the efficacy and safety of probiotics in large-scale, multicenter trials; to monitor the potency and composition of probiotic formulations; to develop in vitro and in vivo systems to understand the molecular mechanisms of action; and to understand the balance among infection, immunity, and probiotics are in progress.
- The selection of a probiotic for pediatric use requires an understanding of the indication, the optimal formulation (single strain vs. multistrain), delivery system, and the host.

Patient Monitoring

- Currently available probiotic formulations are viable microorganisms and therefore have the potential to cause invasive infections in hosts who may have compromised mucosal epithelia.
- Probiotics should be used with caution in children with major risk factors or multiple minor risk factors:
  - Major risk factors include immune compromise or prematurity.
  - Minor risk factors include the presence of a central venous catheter, impaired intestinal epithelial barrier, administration of a probiotic by jejunostomy, concomitant administration of a broad-spectrum antibiotic which may reduce the effectiveness of the probiotic organism, and the presence of cardiac valvular disease.
  - An extremely low incidence of bacteremia has been observed with widespread use of probiotics in Finnish adults.
- To date, there have not been any adverse effects attributable to probiotic consumption in pregnant women consuming a probiotic supplement to prevent atopic dermatitis in their infants.
- HIV-infected adults taking a probiotic supplement to prevent diarrhea and improve tolerance of antiretroviral agents have not experienced adverse effects attributable to the probiotic supplement.

ADDITIONAL READING

- Alfaleh K, Anabrees J, Bassler D, et al. Probiotics for prevention of necrotizing enterocolitis in preterm infants. *Cochrane Database Syst Rev*. 2011;(3):CD005496.
- Binns N. *Probiotics, Prebiotics, and the Gut Microbiota*. Brussels, Belgium: International Life Sciences Institute Europe; 2013.
- Deshpande GC, Rao SC, Keil AD, et al. Evidence-based guidelines for use of probiotics in preterm neonates. *BMC Med*. 2011;9:92.
- Goldenberg JZ, Ma SSY, Saxton JD, et al. Probiotics for the prevention of *Clostridium difficile*-associated diarrhea in adults and children. *Cochrane Database of Syst Rev*. 2013;5:CD006095. doi:10.1002/14651858.CD006095.pub3.
- Thomas DW, Greer FR; Committee on Nutrition: Section on Gastroenterology, Hepatology, and Nutrition of the American Academy of Pediatrics. Clinical report: probiotics and prebiotics in pediatrics. *Pediatrics*. 2010;126(6):1217–1231.

FAQ

- Q: What is the best way to consume probiotics?
- A: Probiotic organisms may be found in fermented foods and yogurt products. Some patients might benefit from probiotic supplements over consumption of probiotic-containing foods. Both supplements and foods may offer beneficial doses of probiotic organisms.
- Q: What is the difference between probiotics and prebiotics?
- A: Probiotic supplements contain live microorganisms, whereas prebiotic supplements are substances that promote the growth of probiotic organisms. The most common prebiotic supplements are fructo-oligosaccharides and galacto-oligosaccharides, which are present in human milk and other naturally occurring food products.
- Q: What factors should a clinician consider when recommending use of a probiotic supplement?
- A: Dose, duration, how administered, the host, and the indication. Probiotic therapy should be considered similarly to an antibiotic regimen, tailoring the therapy and course to the individual.
- Q: What is the standard dose for a probiotic supplement?
- A: There are no uniform dosing recommendations for probiotics. The optimal dose depends on the indication, the host, and the species and strain of the probiotic being used. Many probiotic products include suggested dosing on their packages.

PROTEIN-ENERGY MALNUTRITION

Robert D. Karch

BASICS

DESCRIPTION

- The World Health Organization (WHO) defines malnutrition as "the cellular imbalance between the supply of nutrients and energy and the body's demand for them to ensure growth, maintenance, and specific functions."
- A comprehensive definition of pediatric malnutrition has recently been proposed, which incorporates the chronicity, etiology, and severity of malnutrition, as well as the pathogenic mechanism of nutrient imbalance, association with inflammatory state, and impact on functional outcomes such as growth, development, neurocognition, lean body mass, muscle strength, and immune function.
- This novel definition of pediatric malnutrition considers the etiology of energy, protein, and/or micronutrient imbalance as either "illness-related malnutrition" (secondary to disease/injury) or "non–illness-related malnutrition" (secondary to environmental/behavioral factors). Malnutrition may also be classified as either acute (shorter than 3 months in duration) or chronic (longer than 3 months in duration).
- The term "protein-energy malnutrition" (PEM) describes a general state of undernutrition and deficiency of multiple nutrients and energy.
- There are three clinical presentations of severe PEM: kwashiorkor, marasmus, and marasmic kwashiorkor.
  - Kwashiorkor results from relative protein deficiency in the setting of adequate energy intake and is characterized by hypoproteinemia, pitting edema, varying degrees of wasting and/or stunting, dermatosis, and fatty infiltration of the liver.
  - Marasmus results from both energy and protein deficiency and is characterized by wasting, fatigue, and apathy.
  - Marasmic kwashiorkor is caused by acute or chronic protein deficiency and chronic energy deficit and is characterized by edema, wasting, stunting, and mild hepatomegaly.
  - The distinction between kwashiorkor and marasmus is frequently blurred, and many children present with features of both conditions.
- Severe PEM covers a broad clinical spectrum ranging from frank kwashiorkor to severe marasmus when the body's protein and energy requirements are not adequately met.
- Cicely Williams introduced the name "kwashiorkor" in 1935 in a classic description of her observations of the Ga tribe on the Gold Coast of Africa (currently Ghana).
- "Kwashiorkor" in the Ga language is translated as "the disease of the deposed child (deposed from the breast) when the next baby is born."

RISK FACTORS

- In developed nations, symptoms of kwashiorkor have been described in chronic malabsorptive conditions such as cystic fibrosis.
- In the United States, a few cases of kwashiorkor unrelated to chronic illness have been described.
- Consumption of a protein-deficient milk alternative, sugar water, or fruit juice can be due to poor caregiver knowledge about nutrition, a perceived milk or formula intolerance or adherence to food fads.
- Consumption of a low-protein health food milk alternative, such as rice milk, secondary to a history of chronic eczema and perceived milk intolerance, has occurred in the United States.

EPIDEMIOLOGY

- Malnutrition underlies 55% of childhood mortality worldwide.
- Kwashiorkor may occur at any age but is seen most frequently in children 1–3 years of age.
- Kwashiorkor is seldom seen in the 1st year of life. It is usually seen in the 2nd year or beyond, when a toddler is fully weaned or only partially breastfed and may have a low intake of dietary protein.

PATHOPHYSIOLOGY

- Temperature regulation is impaired, leading to hypothermia in a cold environment and hyperthermia in a hot environment.
- Increase in total-body sodium and decrease in total-body potassium
- Hypophosphatemia is associated with malnutrition and can result in high mortality, especially upon refeeding.
- Protein synthesis is reduced, particularly albumin, transferrin, and apolipoprotein B. Decreased ability to transport fat leads to fatty infiltration of the liver.
- Gluconeogenesis is reduced, which increases risk of hypoglycemia during infection.
- Reduced cardiac output leads to low blood pressure, compromised tissue perfusion, and a reduction in renal blood flow and glomerular filtration rate.
- Diminished inspiratory and expiratory pressures and vital capacity
- Reduction of gastric and pancreatic secretions
- Reduced intestinal motility
- Intestinal mucosa atrophy resulting in malabsorption of carbohydrates, fats, fat- and water-soluble vitamins
- Low circulating insulin levels
- Growth hormone secretion is increased, whereas somatomedin activity is reduced.
  - Glucagon, epinephrine, and cortisol levels are increased.
  - Serum T_3 and T_4 levels are reduced.
- Immune system
  - T-cell immune function is diminished in malnutrition, thereby increasing susceptibility to infection.
  - Serum immunoglobulins are typically normal or increased, although the humoral immune system may be less protective.
  - Delayed wound healing may be seen owing to nutritional deficiencies.

ETIOLOGY

- There are two principal theories regarding the etiology of kwashiorkor: the classical theory of protein deficiency and the newer theory of free radical damage.
- Both theories emphasize different aspects of the environment: in the classical theory, nutrients, and in the free radical theory, oxidative stresses.
- The classical theory of protein deficiency was supported by Williams' original description of kwashiorkor developing in children who were weaned onto starchy gruels after being deposed from the breast and being cured by milk.
- The free radical theory of kwashiorkor proposes that kwashiorkor results from an imbalance between the production of toxic free radicals and their safe disposal. Inadequate diet leads to a state of impaired antioxidant defense.
- The free radical theory attempts to explain the entire spectrum of clinical findings in kwashiorkor by implicating a wide range of nutritional deficiencies, as well as environmental oxidative stressors (noxae):
  - Important noxae include infections and exogenous toxins such as aflatoxin and its metabolites.
  - Aflatoxin, from the fungus *Aspergillus flavus*, has been found in greater concentrations in the serum and urine of children with kwashiorkor than in controls.
  - There is a hierarchy of causes of PEM operating at different levels and interacting with one another; from food scarcity, infection, malabsorption, and neglect, to poverty and social disadvantage, to drought, war, or civil disturbance.
- The multiplicity of causes of PEM necessitates a multidisciplinary approach to its treatment and prevention.

DIAGNOSIS

HISTORY

- Dietary history:
  - Diet before current illness episode
  - Adequacy of protein and total calories
  - Food and fluids taken in past few days
  - Assess whether parents and children adhere to special diets or whether health food milk alternatives, such as rice milk, are given.
- Determine duration and frequency of emesis or diarrhea.
- Loose stools with evidence of malabsorption are common. Stools may be watery and/or tinged with blood.
- Any death of siblings
- Cultural beliefs and practices regarding infant and childhood feeding
- Growth records: Decreased growth velocity commensurate with poor protein intake.

PHYSICAL EXAM

- Weight and length/height
  - Growth failure always occurs to some extent.
  - Wasting is also typical, although it may be masked by the presence of edema.
- Midarm muscle circumference (MAMC) can be used as an indicator of lean body mass and is a useful screening tool in mass settings.
- Triceps skinfold thickness (TSF) can be used to monitor changes in body fat and provides a useful estimate of energy stores.
- Hypothermia or hyperthermia
- General appearance
  - Affected child is usually apathetic and irritable.
  - Child is usually unsmiling and prefers to remain in one position.
- There is some degree of edema in all cases of kwashiorkor:
  - Peripheral edema usually begins in the feet and ascends up the legs.
  - Pitting of the skin above the ankle is diagnostic.
  - The hands and face may become edematous.
  - Facial edema gives the characteristic "moon facies."
  - Hair lacks luster, and color may change to brown or reddish-brown.
  - Hair is easily pluckable.
  - Bands of discolored hair, representing periods of malnutrition, are termed the "flag sign."

- Dermatosis often develops in areas of friction or pressure.
- Hypo- or hyperpigmented patches may appear, which subsequently desquamate in scales or sheets, exposing atrophic ulcers resembling burns.

- Additional clinical signs of PEM:
  - Signs of B-vitamin deficiency, such as perioral lesions
  - Signs of vitamin A deficiency, such as xerosis and/or xerophthalmia
  - Pale, cold, and cyanotic extremities: decreased vascular volume secondary to decreased protein concentration
  - Abdomen is frequently protuberant secondary to poor peristalsis, leading to distended stomach and intestinal loops.
  - Respiratory: Look for signs of pneumonia or heart failure.
  - Enlargement of liver and jaundice may also be seen.

DIAGNOSTIC TESTS & INTERPRETATION

Lab

- Serum protein
- Prealbumin and serum transferrin may be useful in determining severity of kwashiorkor.
- Retinal binding protein may be reduced.
- Hemoglobin and hematocrit are usually low.
- Ratio of nonessential to essential amino acids in plasma is elevated in kwashiorkor and usually normal in marasmus.
- Increased serum elevation of free fatty acids
- Low serum and urine carnitine levels
- Stool exam to rule out infectious cause of chronic diarrhea
- Chest radiograph and PPD to rule out TB

DIFFERENTIAL DIAGNOSIS

- Nephrotic syndrome
- Hookworm anemia
  - May cause edema alone; commonly seen in association with kwashiorkor
  - It is not associated with the kwashiorkor-related dermatologic findings.
- Chronic dysentery
- Protein-losing enteropathy (PLE)
- Pellagra
  - Dermatosis of pellagra and kwashiorkor are similar; however, the dermatosis of pellagra is often seen in sun-exposed areas, not in areas such as the groin, as commonly seen in kwashiorkor.
  - Kwashiorkor dermatosis is often described as "flaky paint" dermatosis.

TREATMENT

- WHO guidelines:
  - Prevent and treat the following:
    - Hypoglycemia
    - Hypothermia
    - Dehydration
    - Electrolyte imbalances
    - Infection
    - Micronutrient deficiencies
  - Provide special feeds for the following:
    - Initial stabilization
    - Providing catch-up growth
    - Providing loving care and stimulation
  - Where guidelines have been fully implemented, mortality has been reduced by at least half.

ADDITIONAL TREATMENT

General Measures

- Whenever possible, a dehydrated child with malnutrition should be rehydrated orally or by nasogastric tube.
- IV infusion should be avoided except for when it is essential (e.g., severe dehydration and shock).
- Hypoglycemia is an important cause of death in the 1st 2 days of treatment.
- Suspected hypoglycemia should be treated with oral rehydration salts solution (ORS) or 10% glucose by mouth or nasogastric tube.
- Severely malnourished children have high levels of sodium and are deficient in potassium. Standard WHO ORS does not meet the special electrolyte requirements of the severely malnourished child.
- ReSoMal is a modified ORS that contains less sodium and more potassium than the standard WHO ORS and is the recommended ORS for severely malnourished children.

ALERT

Rapid and inappropriate refeeding of malnourished individuals may result in the refeeding syndrome, which is manifested as hypophosphatemia. Hypomagnesemia and hypokalemia may also be associated. Cardiac dysfunction, edema, and neurologic changes, due to shifts in fluid and electrolytes following aggressive introduction of nutrients, are associated with the refeeding syndrome.

ONGOING CARE

PROGNOSIS

- Treatment corrects the acute signs of the disease, but catch-up growth in height may never be achieved.
- Mortality rate in kwashiorkor can be as high as 40%, but adequate treatment can reduce it to <10%.
- Some of the factors that indicate poor prognosis:
  - Age <6 months
  - Infections
  - Dehydration and electrolyte abnormalities
  - Persistent tachycardia, signs of heart failure
  - Total serum protein <3 g/100 mL
  - Elevated serum bilirubin
  - Severe anemia with hypoxia
  - Hypoglycemia and/or hypothermia

COMPLICATIONS

Several longitudinal studies have demonstrated associations between early childhood stunting and later cognitive function and academic attainment.

ADDITIONAL READING

- Behrman JR, Hoddinott J, Maluccio JA, et al. What determines adult cognitive skills? Impacts of preschool, schooling and post-school experiences in Guatemala. http://repository.upenn.edu/psc_working_papers/3/. PSC working paper series 06-03. Published October 27, 2006. Accessed March 1, 2015.
- Carvalho NF, Kenney RD, Carrington PH, et al. Severe nutritional deficiencies in toddlers resulting from health food milk alternatives. *Pediatrics*. 2001;107(4):E46.
- De Onís M, Monteiro C, Akre J, et al. The worldwide magnitude of protein-energy malnutrition: an overview from the WHO Global Database on Child Growth. *Bull World Health Organ*. 1993;71(6):703–712.
- Giannopoulos G, Merriman L, Rumsey A, et al. Malnutrition coding 101: financial impact and more. *Nutr Clin Pract*. 2013;28(6):698–709.
- Golden MHN, Ramdath D. Free radicals in the pathogenesis of kwashiorkor. *Proc Nutr Soc*. 1987;46(1):53–68.
- Grover Z, Ee LC. Protein energy malnutrition. *Pediatr Clin North Am*. 2009;56(5):1055–1068.
- Liu T, Howard RM, Mancini AJ, et al. Kwashiorkor in the United States: fad diets, perceived and true milk allergy, and nutritional ignorance. *Arch Dermatol*. 2001;137(5):630–636.
- Mehta N, Corkins M, Lyman B, et al. Defining pediatric malnutrition: a paradigm shift toward etiology-related definitions. *JPEN J Parenter Enteral Nutr*. 2013;37(4):460–481.

CODES

ICD10

- E46 Unspecified protein-calorie malnutrition
- E40 Kwashiorkor
- E41 Nutritional marasmus

FAQ

- Q: What are the signs and symptoms of kwashiorkor, and how do these change over the course of the clinical spectrum of severe protein-energy malnutrition; from kwashiorkor to marasmus?
- A: Signs and symptoms of kwashiorkor:
  - Growth failure, wasting
  - Edema that is peripheral in onset and ascending
  - Hair changes including color change, "flag sign," and easy pluckability; "flaky paint" dermatosis of skin
  - In addition to earlier signs and symptoms, child may also develop vitamin A and B deficiency, decreased peripheral circulation, and decreased peristalsis with distended bowel loops. Hepatomegaly/splenomegaly may also be observed. The child is at higher risk for developing other conditions such as pneumonia or congestive heart failure.
- Q: What are some common causes of severe undernutrition in the United States that may present as kwashiorkor?
- A: Chronic malabsorptive conditions (e.g., cystic fibrosis) and consumption of protein-deficient milk substitutes such as rice milk, fruit juices, etc.

PROTEINURIA

Stephanie Nguyen

BASICS

DESCRIPTION

- Protein may be found in the urine of healthy children.
- The term proteinuria is used to indicate urinary protein excretion beyond the upper limit of normal (100 mg/m^2/day or 4 mg/m^2/h in children and 150 mg/day in adults).
  - Nephrotic range proteinuria >1,000 mg/m^2/day or 40 mg/m^2/h
  - Nephrotic syndrome: nephrotic-range proteinuria with edema and hypoalbuminemia (<2.5 g/dL)
  - Microalbuminuria: elevated urinary excretion of albumin (30–300 mg/g albumin/creatinine ratio or 30–300 mg/day). Currently, it is only used to indicate kidney disease in those with diabetes mellitus.
- Classification
  - Persistent or fixed proteinuria
    - Urinary dipstick ≥1+ in the first morning urine specimen on ≥3 samples >1 week apart
    - Requires prompt referral to nephrology
  - Transient proteinuria
    - Proteinuria absent on subsequent urine examinations
    - It is not usually associated with clinically significant underlying renal disease.
    - Often associated with high fever, cold stress, dehydration, and exercise
  - Orthostatic or postural proteinuria
    - Elevated protein excretion when the patient is upright that normalizes when patient is supine
    - The most common cause of fixed or transient proteinuria in childhood and adolescence
    - Proteinuria rarely exceeds 1 g/m^2/day.
    - Benign condition

PATHOPHYSIOLOGY

- Normally, ~50% urinary proteins are derived from tissue proteins and proteins from cells lining the urinary tract (i.e., Tamm-Horsfall protein).
- Proteinuria may be the result of glomerular proteinuria or tubular proteinuria.
- Glomerular proteinuria
  - An increased permeability of the glomeruli to the passage of plasma proteins
  - Normally may range from <1 to >30 mg/day
  - Large amounts of glomerular proteinuria may be found in the context of edema and hypoalbuminemia (nephrotic syndrome).
  - If there is hypertension, abnormal glomerular filtration rate, and hematuria, there may be nephritis as well.
- Tubular proteinuria
  - Decreased reabsorption of low-molecular-weight proteins by the proximal renal tubules
  - Rarely >1 g/day and is not associated with edema.
  - The major marker is urinary beta-2-microglobulin.
  - It may be associated with other defects of proximal tubular function (e.g., renal tubular acidosis [RTA], glucosuria, phosphaturia, aminoaciduria) and tubular interstitial processes.

DIAGNOSIS

The American Academy of Pediatrics (AAP) no longer recommends screening urinalysis for asymptomatic children due to high false-positive rate, low cost-effectiveness, and lack of treatable disease.

HISTORY

- **Question:** Changes in the aspect of the urine?
- *Significance*: Foamy or colored (red, tea-colored)
- **Question:** Recent illness?
- *Significance*: Pharyngitis and upper respiratory infections
- **Question:** Frequent episodes of fever?
- *Significance*: Lymphoma, malignancies, vasculitides
- **Question:** Medications or herbal/folk remedies?
- *Significance*: Toxins
- **Question:** Illicit drug use and risk factors for STD in adolescent and adults?
- *Significance*: HIV, syphilis, hepatitis
- **Question:** Urinary tract infection in the past?
- *Significance*: Reflux nephropathy
- **Question:** Family history of renal, rheumatologic diseases or hearing loss?
- **Question:** Fatigue, general malaise, reduced appetite?
- **Question:** Weight changes?
- **Question:** Facial swelling (in the morning) and lower limb swelling (in the afternoon)?
- **Question:** Symptoms related to rheumatologic conditions (skin rash, joint pain, joint stiffness)?
- **Question:** Cough, shortness of breath?

PHYSICAL EXAM

- General
  - Hypertension
  - Growth and development
- HEENT
  - Periorbital edema
  - Malar rash
- Chest
  - Pericardial or pleural effusions
- Abdomen
  - Ascites
  - Hepatosplenomegaly
  - Abdominal masses/organomegaly
- Genitalia
  - Scrotal edema
  - Ambiguous genitalia (Denys-Drash syndrome)
- Skin
  - Purpuric or petechial rash (leukemia, lymphomas)
  - Pallor (malignancies, chronic renal failure, hemolytic uremic syndrome [HUS])
  - Angiokeratomas (Fabry disease)
- Extremities
  - Pitting edema
  - Arthralgias/arthritis
- Dystrophic nails

DIAGNOSTIC TESTS & INTERPRETATION

- Dipstick testing
  - Always to be performed in a first morning urine sample
  - Instruct patient to urinate before bedtime and to collect urine as soon as he or she awakens and before ambulation.
  - A negative or trace result in a concentrated urine specimen (specific gravity >1.020) is normal.
  - 1+ protein may be normal in very concreted samples (specific gravity >1.030).
- Spot urine protein and urine creatinine (urine protein/creatinine ratio):
  - Always to be performed in a first morning urine sample
  - Simplest method to quantitate proteinuria
  - Normal values
    - <0.2 mg/mg in children >2 years of age
    - <0.5 mg/mg in children 6–24 months old
- 24-hour collection of urine for protein
  - Indicated for quantification of proteinuria and to confirm the diagnosis
  - Normal range: <100 mg/m^2/day or <4 mg/m^2/h

- Serum albumin
  - To assess for hypoalbuminemia, nephrotic syndrome
- Serum BUN and creatinine levels
  - Impaired renal function suggests inflammation, infection, or obstruction.
- Serum electrolytes and phosphorous levels
  - To screen for RTA
- Evaluation for glomerulonephritis (GN)
  - Proteinuria with edema, hematuria, hypertension, and/or impaired renal function
  - Streptococcal serology (ASO titer, streptozyme): acute postinfectious GN
  - Complement studies (C3,C4): hypocomplementemic GN—immune complex mediated (lupus nephritis, postinfectious GN, membranoproliferative GN)
  - Antinuclear antibody (ANA) titer or anti–double-stranded DNA, hypocomplementemic or signs of systemic vasculitis: vasculitis (lupus)

ALERT
- Most patients with proteinuria will have orthostatic proteinuria that is identified by a first morning urine sample testing negative for protein while samples collected while upright test positive for protein.
- It is important to check the urine sediment for red cell casts; this indicates a glomerular involvement and requires additional studies for nephritis and chronic renal disease.

DIFFERENTIAL DIAGNOSIS

- Idiopathic nephrotic syndrome
  - Minimal change nephrotic syndrome
  - Mesangial proliferation
  - Focal segmental glomerulosclerosis
  - Membranous nephropathy
- Nephrotic syndrome due to genetic causes
  - Finnish-type congenital nephrotic syndrome
  - Familial focal segmental glomerulosclerosis
  - Diffuse mesangial sclerosis
  - Denys-Drash syndrome (nephropathy, Wilms tumor, and genital abnormalities)
- Chronic kidney disease
- Acquired glomerular disease
  - Idiopathic glomerulonephritis
  - Lupus-associated nephritis
  - IgA nephropathy
  - Systemic vasculitides
  - Subacute bacterial endocarditis
  - Diabetes mellitus
  - Hypertension
  - HUS
  - Hyperfiltration secondary to nephron loss (with or without sclerosis)
- Genetic disorders
  - Nail-patella syndrome
  - Alport syndrome
  - Fabry disease
  - Glycogen storage disease
  - Cystic fibrosis
  - Hurler syndrome (mucopolysaccharide type-1)
  - α-1-antitrypsin
  - Mitochondrial disorders (usually tubular proteinuria)
  - Gaucher disease
  - Dent disease (X-linked nephrolithiasis)
  - Cystinosis
  - Wilson disease
- Oncologic/hematologic
  - Sickle cell disease
  - Renal vein thrombosis
  - Leukemia
  - Lymphoma
- Infectious
  - Poststreptococcal glomerulonephritis
  - HIV-associated nephropathy
  - Hepatitis B and C virus infection
  - Malaria
  - Syphilis (can present as congenital nephrotic syndrome)
  - Pyelonephritis
- Drugs/toxins
  - Bee sting
  - Food allergens
  - Antibiotic-induced interstitial nephritis
  - Penicillamine
  - Gold salts
  - NSAIDs
  - Heavy metals (e.g., mercury, lead)
- Miscellaneous
  - Tubular interstitial nephritis
  - Acute tubular necrosis
  - Reflux nephropathy
  - Hypothyroidism
- Congestive heart failure

ADDITIONAL READING

- Gipson DS, Massengill SF, Yao L, et al. Management of childhood onset nephrotic syndrome. *Pediatrics*. 2009;124(2):747–757.
- Hogg RJ, Portman RJ, Milliner D, et al. Evaluation and management of proteinuria and nephrotic syndrome in children: recommendations from a pediatric nephrology panel established at the National Kidney Foundation Conference on proteinuria, albuminuria, risk, assessment, detection, and elimination (PARADE). *Pediatrics*. 2000;105(6):1242–1249.
- Quigley R. Evaluation of hematuria and proteinuria: how should a pediatrician proceed? *Curr Opin Pediatr*. 2008;20(2):140–144.

CODES

ICD10

- R80.9 Proteinuria, unspecified
- R80.2 Orthostatic proteinuria, unspecified
- R80.1 Persistent proteinuria, unspecified

FAQ

- Q: When to refer to nephrology?
- A: Patients with one of the following: fixed proteinuria, associated hypertension, associated hematuria, clinical evidence of nephritis, and patient with family history of renal diseases with proteinuria
- Q: When are imaging studies indicated?
- A: Patients with abnormal renal function, hematuria, or nephrolithiasis. The best initial study is renal and bladder ultrasound.

PRUNE BELLY SYNDROME

Shamir Tuchman

BASICS

DESCRIPTION
- Rare congenital disorder characterized by the triad of
  - Deficiency of abdominal musculature
  - Bilateral cryptorchidism
  - Dilated, anomalous development of the bladder and upper urinary tract
- Presents with a broad spectrum of severity, from mild hydroureter with an enlarged bladder and normal renal function to severe renal dysplasia and pulmonary hypoplasia
- Also known as Eagle-Barrett syndrome

EPIDEMIOLOGY
- Incidence: 1/35,000–50,000 live births
- Most patients are detected during the neonatal period or prenatally during maternal ultrasound.
- Prune belly syndrome is much more common in males (>95%). Females with urethral atresia may be affected.

RISK FACTORS
Genetics
- The genetic basis of prune belly syndrome remains unclear.
- Most patients have normal karyotypes.
- Most cases are sporadic, although rare cases in sibs have been reported.
- Genetic analysis of rare inherited forms have revealed homozygous mutations in the muscarinic acetylcholine receptor gene (*CHRM3*) and heterozygous mutations in α-smooth muscle actin (*ACTA2*), with sporadic forms rarely having mutations in hepatocyte nuclear factor 1β transcription factor (HNF1β).

PATHOPHYSIOLOGY
The bladder in prune belly syndrome is large, irregularly shaped, and thick walled. Many patients have poor urinary flow and high residual volumes:
- Ureters are usually markedly dilated, tortuous, and elongated. Peristalsis is ineffective, and the distal ureters are most severely affected. Vesicoureteral reflux is present in over 75% of cases.
- Renal involvement is variable; the most severe dysplasia occurs in patients with extensive dilation of the urinary tract. Dysplastic changes are usually symmetric.
- Usually, the bladder neck is wide and the prostatic urethra is dilated and triangular.

ETIOLOGY
The cause of prune belly syndrome remains unclear. Two theories have been proposed:
- The triad of congenital defects may result from a primary mesodermal defect in development with congenital deficiency of smooth muscle in the bladder, ureter, and renal pelvis.
- Outflow obstruction of the bladder in utero may result in dilation of the bladder and upper urinary tract with subsequent renal injury. The expanded bladder may block the route of the descending testicles and may cause abdominal distention and abdominal wall muscle atrophy.

COMMONLY ASSOCIATED CONDITIONS
Many patients have associated anomalies:
- GI anomalies
  - Affect up to 25% of patients (e.g., imperforate anus, malrotation, gastroschisis, omphalocele, bowel atresia, and increased risk of volvulus)
- Musculoskeletal anomalies
  - talipes equinovarus, congenital hip dislocation, pectus excavatum, scoliosis, hemivertebrae
- Respiratory
  - Affect upward of 60% of patients (e.g., pulmonary hypoplasia, chronic respiratory tract infections due in part to impaired coughing, reactive airway disease, respiratory difficulty after general anesthesia)
- Genital anomalies in females
  - genital sinus, urethral atresia, vesicovaginal fistula, vaginal atresia, and bicornuate uterus
  - Ovaries in affected female patients are typically normal.
- Cardiac anomalies
  - Affect up to 25% of patients (e.g., patent ductus arteriosus [PDA], atrial septal defect [ASD], ventricular septal defect [VSD], tetralogy of Fallot [TOF])
- Other genetic conditions
  - Children with trisomy 21 (Down syndrome) have an 11-fold increased risk of prune belly syndrome compared with other children.

DIAGNOSIS

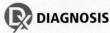

HISTORY
In patients with mild involvement of the abdominal wall that is not detected in the neonatal period, evaluation of UTIs may reveal the dilated urinary tract.

PHYSICAL EXAM
- Abdominal wall is characterized by multiple wrinkles and redundant skin.
- A large, distended bladder creates a suprapubic mass.
- Ureters and kidneys are readily palpable.
- Intestinal loops and peristalsis may be observed.
- Testes are undescended.
- Myopathy results in difficulty in sitting up from a supine position.
- Abnormal gait secondary to congenital hip dislocation and abdominal muscular hypoplasia
- Chronic constipation from abdominal muscular hypoplasia

DIAGNOSTIC TESTS & INTERPRETATION
Lab
- Serum levels of creatinine and BUN may be elevated.
- Renal failure may result in anemia and elevated levels of potassium, phosphorus, hydrogen ion, and uric acid; tubular dysfunction may result in decreased concentrations of sodium and bicarbonate.

Imaging
- Ultrasound will demonstrate dilatation and redundancy of the upper urinary tract.
- When considering a voiding cystourethrogram, assess possible risk of introducing infection into dilated, poorly draining urinary tract.
- Renal function and drainage of the dilated tract can be assessed by radioisotope renal scan or an excretory urogram.

Diagnostic Procedures/Other
Initial evaluation should include assessment of renal function.

DIFFERENTIAL DIAGNOSIS
- Distinctly abnormal findings of physical exam of the affected infant results in an early, accurate diagnosis in most cases.
- Pseudo–prune belly syndrome (e.g., prune belly syndrome uropathy, normal abdominal wall exam, and incomplete or absent cryptorchidism)

P

TREATMENT

SURGERY/OTHER PROCEDURES

- Many clinicians advocate minimal surgical intervention (e.g., conservative approach), based on lack of functional obstruction and that the dilated system has a low pressure owing to the deficient smooth musculature. If renal function deteriorates, urinary tract dilation progresses, the patient has evidence of mechanical obstruction such as urethral atresia, or the patient develops recurrent UTIs despite antibiotic prophylaxis, cutaneous vesicostomy is recommended to facilitate drainage.
- Other physicians advocate extensive early surgical remodeling. Possible procedures include, as indicated:
  - Internal urethrotomy, reduction cystoplasty
  - Excision of the redundant ureter with reimplantation of the remaining segment
  - Cutaneous ureterostomy
  - Pyelostomy
- Reconstruction of the abdominal wall has yielded good cosmetic results but only questionable improvements in physical function.
- Bilateral orchiopexy is indicated, ideally within the 1st year of life.
- Circumcision to prevent UTI has been advocated, but no large trials to document its effectiveness in prune belly syndrome have been published to date.

INPATIENT CONSIDERATIONS

Admission Criteria/Initial Stabilization

- Basic principles of supportive care and management of renal failure apply.
- Antibiotics in the neonatal period and antibiotic prophylactic of indefinite duration are indicated to prevent infection.

ONGOING CARE

FOLLOW-UP RECOMMENDATIONS

Regardless of how patients are managed, affected patients require long-term follow-up, with meticulous attention to renal function, pulmonary function, bladder drainage, and urine bacteriology.

PROGNOSIS

- Patients with the most severe renal dysplasia and pulmonary hypoplasia (e.g., sequelae of severe, early oligohydramnios) succumb as neonates.
- Associated with a mortality rate of up to 20% in the neonatal period
- ~25% of patients with prune belly syndrome who survive the neonatal period will progress to end-stage renal disease (ESRD).
- Those with a milder form do not require urinary tract surgery; renal function is usually stable and prognosis is excellent.
- For patients with moderate involvement, the degree of renal dysplasia and insufficiency determines outcome. In addition, upper urinary tract stasis, poor bladder emptying, vesicoureteral reflux, and bacteriuria are factors that may combine to worsen the long-term prognosis.

COMPLICATIONS

- Pulmonary hypoplasia
- Frequent UTIs secondary to upper urinary stasis, vesicoureteral reflux, and bacteriuria
- Sequelae of progressive renal insufficiency

ADDITIONAL READING

- Hassett S, Smith GHH, Holland AJA. Prune belly syndrome. *Pediatr Surg Int*. 2012;2(3)8:219–228.
- Jennings RW. Prune belly syndrome. *Semin Pediatr Surg*. 2000;9(3):115–120.
- Noh PH, Cooper CS, Winkler AC, et al. Prognostic factors for long-term renal function in boys with the prune-belly syndrome. *J Urol*. 1999;162(4):1399–1401.
- Strand WR. Initial management of complex pediatric disorders: prune-belly syndrome, posterior urethral valves. *Urol Clin North Am*. 2004;31(3):399–415, vii.
- Tonni G, Ida V, Alessandro V, et al. Prune-belly syndrome: case series and review of the literature regarding early prenatal diagnosis, epidemiology, genetic factors, treatment, and prognosis. *Fetal Pediatr Pathol*. 2013;31(1):13–24.
- Woodard JR, Zucker I. Current management of the dilated urinary tract in prune belly syndrome. *Urol Clin North Am*. 1990;17(2):407–418.
- Woolf AS, Stuart HM, Newman WG. Genetics of human congenital urinary bladder disease. *Pediatr Nephrol*. 2014;29(3):353–360.
- Woods AG, Brandon DH. Prune belly syndrome. A focused physical assessment. *Adv Neonatal Care*. 2007;7(3):132–143.

CODES

ICD10

Q79.4 Prune belly syndrome

FAQ

- Q: Are patients with prune belly syndrome candidates for renal transplantation?
- A: Yes. However, special pretransplantation consideration should be given to patients with dilated tracts to optimize bladder function.
- Q: How does the urinary tract function in older children?
- A: A tendency for bladder tone and ureteral peristalsis to improve with age has been noted.
- Q: Are such patients infertile?
- A: Normal sexual activity has been described. However, there are no reports of fertility, and the patients usually have azoospermia.
- Q: What is the usual cause of morbidity in the newborn period?
- A: Respiratory failure.

PRURITUS

Anubhav Mathur • Ilona Frieden

BASICS

DESCRIPTION

Pruritus, or itch, is one of the most frequent dermatologic complaints. It is an unpleasant sensation characterized by the reflexive behavior to scratch and is a symptom associated with numerous inflammatory and infectious skin diseases. However, generalized and persistent pruritus without or with minimal skin changes may be a presenting feature of a variety of systemic diseases.

PATHOPHYSIOLOGY

- Itch-specific peripheral nerves are unmyelinated afferent C-fibers.
- Pruritus depends on the complex interplay of neuroinflammatory modulators among peripheral nerves, keratinocytes, and leukocytes as well as CNS processing.
- There are numerous mediators of pruritus, although histamine is the prototypical pharmacologic target for many patients.

ETIOLOGY

- Dermatologic: arising from skin disease
- Systemic: arising from noncutaneous organ systems including metabolic causes, drugs, and multifactorial disorders
- Neurogenic: arising from disorders of the central or peripheral nervous system
- Psychogenic: arising from primary psychiatric disorders
- Mixed: coexistence of more than one etiology of pruritus
- Idiopathic: pruritus of uncertain etiology

DIAGNOSIS

HISTORY

- Acute versus chronic (>6 weeks) pruritus
- Location: generalized, scattered spots, or localized
- Severity of symptoms
- Presence or absence of a preceding or concurrent rash
- Family members or close contacts with a similar complaint
- Environmental exposures: pets/other animals, poison oak or ivy, skin care products, soaps, shampoos, length and frequency of bathing/showering
- Medications (topical or systemic) or recreational drugs
- History of hematologic, hepatobiliary, renal, metabolic, neurologic, neoplastic, and psychiatric diseases
- Complete review of systems: particularly important for those without obvious skin findings

PHYSICAL EXAM

- Define and differentiate primary morphologies from secondary changes.
- Determine the location of the rash and areas of sparing.
- Evaluate for evidence of secondary cutaneous infections.

APPROACH TO THE PATIENT

- Most children with pruritus have a primary dermatologic disease.
- Common conditions include atopic dermatitis, allergic reactions to insect bites (so-called papular urticaria), fungal infection, scabies, hives, and dermatographism.
- To develop a differential diagnosis, it is helpful to subdivide patients into 1 of 4 groups as below:
  - Generalized pruritus with definite skin disease
  - Generalized pruritus without definite skin disease (minimal or nonspecific skin lesions)
  - Localized pruritus with definite skin disease
  - Localized pruritus without definite skin disease (minimal or nonspecific skin lesions)
- To identify common patterns of pruritus, consider the questions listed below:
- **Question 1:** Are the findings characteristic of atopic dermatitis, the most common skin disease in children?
  - Does the patient have a history of severe cradle cap or chronic/intermittent rash involving the face, antecubital or popliteal fossae, ankles, or wrists?
  - Atopic dermatitis is very common and typically has distinctive sites of predilection.
- **Question 2:** Are there specific or nonspecific (scratching/rubbing induced) skin lesions present?
  - If there are multiple morphologies, consider scabies.
  - If minimal or mostly secondary skin changes are present but pruritus is severe, consider either scabies or a systemic cause (see below).
- **Question 3:** Does the patient have clustered pink excoriated papules on the ankles, mid torso, or legs?
  - This finding may represent bugbite reactions, which are a common cause of pruritus in children.
  - These reactions disproportionately affect young children and may not be evident in their parents/guardians or even siblings.
- **Question 4:** Does the patient have acute onset of rash with tiny vesicles or linear streaks of erythema on the face, arms, or legs?
  - Poison oak/ivy is common and presents as an acute eczematous or vesiculobullous reaction.
- **Question 5:** Does the patient have well-defined erythematous and scaling rash involving the scalp, extensor elbows, knees, umbilicus, or gluteal cleft?
  - These findings suggest psoriasis. Although less common in children than atopic dermatitis, and usually less itchy, it has distinct sites of involvement with characteristic morphology.
  - Family history of psoriasis is common in patients who develop it in childhood.
- **Question 6:** Does the patient have a chronic pruritic scaly rash around the umbilicus?
  - Chronic allergic contact dermatitis from metals, especially to nickel, may present as an isolated itchy rash around the umbilicus due to a belt buckle or pant button.
  - For patients who wear earrings, ear lobes may be affected, providing a diagnostic clue.
  - Many patients with nickel dermatitis have fine papules scattered on the arms and legs (so-called id reaction) or may have preexisting atopic dermatitis.
- **Question 7:** Does the patient have any itchy rash involving the cheeks and nose with a rash on the dorsal forearms, sparing the volar arms?
  - This pattern may present photosensitivity and suggests possible polymorphous light eruption or actinic prurigo.
- For patients with a definite dermatologic cause for pruritus, treat the underlying cause.
- Consider nondermatologic causes (listed below) for patients with severe generalized pruritus and nonspecific skin lesions—exclude scabies/infestation, dermatographism, and atopic dermatitis.
- Localized pruritus with minimal or nonspecific skin lesions may suggest neuropathic itch, which is rare in children.

DIFFERENTIAL DIAGNOSIS

- Dermatologic Diseases
  - Inflammatory skin diseases
    - Dermatitis (atopic including nummular morphology, allergic contact, irritant contact, other)
    - Urticaria
    - Dermatographism
    - Psoriasis
    - Lichen planus
    - Mastocytosis
    - Dermatitis herpetiformis
    - Bullous pemphigoid
    - Epidermolysis bullosa pruriginosa
    - Polymorphous light eruption

- Cutaneous infections and arthropod reactions
  - Scabies
  - Tinea/dermatophyte infection
  - Pediculosis
  - Flea bites
  - Mite reactions
  - Bedbug bites
  - Papular urticaria
  - Other arthropod reactions
- Neoplastic
  - Cutaneous lymphomas

- Systemic Diseases
  - Endocrine
    - Thyroid and parathyroid disease
    - Diabetes mellitus
  - Infections
    - HIV
    - Hepatitis B and C
    - Systemic parasitic infections
  - Hematologic
    - Polycythemia vera/aquagenic pruritus
    - Iron deficiency anemia
    - Lymphomas
    - Leukemias
    - Hypereosinophilic syndrome
    - Myelodysplastic syndromes
  - Biliary diseases leading to cholestasis
  - Renal disease: uremic pruritus in chronic kidney disease
  - Malignancies
    - Solid tumors
    - Carcinoid syndrome
- Neurologic Diseases
  - CNS malignancies or infections
  - Multiple sclerosis
  - Peripheral nerve injuries from compression or irritation
  - Radiculopathy
  - Polyneuropathy
- Psychiatric Diseases
  - Psychogenic excoriations
  - Delusions of parasitosis
  - Somatoform disorders

DIAGNOSTIC TESTS & INTERPRETATION

- Diagnostic testing is rarely required or helpful, as most children with pruritus have a primary dermatologic cause that can be clinically diagnosed.
- In patients with generalized pruritus without an obvious primary skin disease, the following studies should be considered based on clinical suspicion of the underlying cause for pruritus.
- Labs
  - CBC with differential, TFTs, PTH, HgbA1c, AST, ALT, alkaline phosphatase, total bilirubin, BUN, creatinine, HIV 1, HIV 2, ELISA, HBsAg, hepatitis C serology, iron studies
- Imaging
  - Abdominal ultrasound, chest x-ray, CNS imaging with MRI
- Light microscopy (from skin scrapings)
  - KOH prep for dermatophyte infections and mineral oil examination for scabies. Note: must only be done with proper training
- Pathology
  - Skin biopsy specimens for hematoxylin and eosin (H&E) and direct immunofluorescence may be helpful in confirming the suspected dermatologic diagnosis.

TREATMENT

- Treatment is directed to the underlying cause.
- Supportive measures:
  - Gentle skin care measures, including the use of nonsoap cleansers and gentle emollients
  - Loose cotton clothing
  - Sedating antihistamines in select cases
  - Topical corticosteroids and/or topical calcineurin inhibitors in select cases
- Phototherapy
  - Certain inflammatory conditions including psoriasis and some cases of severe atopic dermatitis may benefit from narrow band ultra violet B (NBUVB) therapy.
  - Patients with certain systemic causes of pruritus such hepatobiliary or renal pruritus may benefit from NBUVB.

ISSUES FOR REFERRAL

- Severe cases of inflammatory or cutaneous infectious diseases
- Identification of or suspicion for a noncutaneous cause for pruritus

ADDITIONAL READING

- Cassono N, Tessari G, Vena GA, et al. Chronic pruritus in the absence of skin disease: an update on pathophysiology, diagnosis and treatment. *Am J Clin Dermatol*. 2010;11(6):399–411.
- Charlesworth EN, Beltrani VS. Pruritic dermatoses: overview of etiology and therapy. *Am J Med*. 2002;113(Suppl 9A):25S–33S.
- Greaves MW. Pathogenesis and treatment of pruritus. *Curr Allergy Asthma Rep*. 2010;10(4):236–242.
- Paller AS, Mancini A. *Hurwitz Clinical Pediatric Dermatology*. 4th ed. New York: Saunders; 2011.

CODES

ICD10

- L29.9 Pruritus, unspecified
- F45.8 Other somatoform disorders
- L23.9 Allergic contact dermatitis, unspecified cause

FAQ

- Q: Which antihistamines work the best to treat itch?
- A: Although evidence is conflicting, sedating antihistamines such as hydroxyzine tend to work better than nonsedating ones for itch.
- Q: How does scratching affect pruritus?
- A: Scratching disrupts the skin barrier. By irritation or secondary infection, inflammatory mediators in the skin (such as histamine) can worsen pruritus, leading an "itch-scratch-itch" cycle.
- Q: What is gentle skin care?
- A: Gentle skin care is the concept of keeping the skin moist with emollients including creams or ointments, thereby "repairing" the skin barrier. Application of an emollient, particularly after bathing, will help to keep the skin moist and reduce pruritus in patients with several inflammatory skin diseases.

PSITTACOSIS

Nicholas Tsarouhas

BASICS

DESCRIPTION

- An acute febrile disease characterized by pneumonitis and other systemic symptoms
- The name is derived from the Greek for parrot, *psittakos*; thus, psittacosis is often referred to as "parrot disease."
- Also known as *ornithosis*

EPIDEMIOLOGY

- Birds are the major reservoir of the psittacosis pathogen.
- Nearly all domestic and wild birds may spread this infection.
- Psittacine birds (parakeets, parrots, and macaws) are a major source of disease in the United States, but pigeons and turkeys are also common culprits.
  - Infecting agent is present in bird nasal secretions, urine, feces, feathers, viscera, and carcasses.
  - Inhalation of aerosols of feces, urine, and secretions of infected birds is the most common route of infection.
  - Handling of plumage, bird bites, and mouth-to-beak contact are known to spread infection.
  - Birds may be healthy or sick.
- Most reported cases (70%) are the result of exposure to pet caged birds (especially parrots, parakeets).
- Most common mammalian source of infection is sheep.
- Occupational hazard of workers in poultry plants, pet shops, zoos, farms
- Rarely transmitted person to person

Incidence

- Only 100–200 total cases reported in United States each year
- Very rare disease in young children

RISK FACTORS

Close human contact with birds and, in some cases, sheep

GENERAL PREVENTION

- Epidemiologic investigation is indicated in all suspected cases.
- Birds suspected to be infected should be killed, transported, and analyzed by qualified experts.
- Potentially contaminated living areas where bird was kept should be disinfected and aired.
- Pathogen is susceptible to most household disinfectants (rubbing alcohol, Lysol, bleach).

PATHOPHYSIOLOGY

- Inhalation of aerosolized organisms into the respiratory tract
- Incubation period 5–14 days; may be longer
- Spreads via bloodstream to lungs, liver, and spleen
- Lymphocytic inflammatory alveolar response

ETIOLOGY

- Infection produced by *Chlamydophila psittaci*, an obligate intracellular parasitic bacterium
- Morphologically, antigenically, and genetically different from *Chlamydia* species

COMMONLY ASSOCIATED CONDITIONS

Pneumonitis (with a severe headache) is a common presentation.

DIAGNOSIS

HISTORY

- Mandatory to question parents about exposure of the patient to any type of bird—wild or domestic
- Signs and symptoms
  - Abrupt onset of symptoms
  - Fever, headache, cough, weakness, chills, muscle aches, and joint pain
  - Nonproductive cough
  - Vomiting, confusion, and photophobia are less common findings.

PHYSICAL EXAM

- Ill-appearance, tachypnea, rales, and splenomegaly are common.
- A relative bradycardia is found in some cases.
- Less common findings
  - Rash
  - Meningismus
  - Pharyngeal injection
  - Cervical adenopathy
  - Hepatomegaly
  - Mental status changes

DIAGNOSTIC TESTS & INTERPRETATION

Lab

- Routine laboratory studies are rarely helpful.
- Isolation of the organism is diagnostic.
- Complement fixation titers (see "FAQ")
- Microimmunofluorescence studies and polymerase chain reaction assays are more specific than complement fixation studies.
- Complement fixation titers do not, however, distinguish between the chlamydial infections (*Chlamydia trachomatis*) and the various chlamydophilal infections (*Chlamydophila psittaci*, *Chlamydophila pneumoniae*, and *Chlamydophila pecorum*).

Imaging

- Chest x-rays are abnormal in 90% of hospitalized cases.
- Chest x-rays often demonstrate diffuse interstitial infiltrates but may also have unilateral lower lobe consolidation.

DIFFERENTIAL DIAGNOSIS

- Psittacosis should be considered in a patient with fever of unknown origin or atypical pneumonitis.
- Differential diagnosis includes the following:
  - *Mycoplasma pneumoniae*
  - *C. pneumoniae*
  - *Legionella* spp.
  - *Coxiella burnetii* (i.e., Q fever)
  - Tuberculosis
  - Viral pneumonitis
  - Fungal pneumonitis
  - Pneumococcal pneumonia

P

TREATMENT

MEDICATION

First Line

- Tetracycline (40 mg/kg/24 h) or doxycycline (100 mg b.i.d.) in children ≥8 years of age
- Erythromycin (40 mg/kg/24 h) in children <8 years of age
- Antibiotics should be continued for at least 10–14 days after defervescence.

Second Line

Azithromycin is an additional option.

ONGOING CARE

PROGNOSIS

- Although complete recovery is the rule (even without antibiotic use), fatality rates as high as 15–20% have been reported.
- Resolution of fever and most other systemic symptoms can be expected within 48 hours of antibiotic therapy.
- Untreated patients may have severe pulmonary symptoms for 1–3 weeks.

COMPLICATIONS

- Hepatitis
- Anemia
- Thrombophlebitis
- Pulmonary embolus
- Adult respiratory distress syndrome
- Arthritis
- Keratoconjunctivitis
- Endocarditis
- Myocarditis
- Pericarditis
- Encephalitis: agitation, delirium, confusion, stupor

ADDITIONAL READING

- American Academy of Pediatrics. Chlamydial infections: *Chlamydophila* (formerly *Chlamydia*) *psittaci* (psittacosis, ornithosis). In: Pickering LK, Baker CJ, Kimberlin DW, et al, eds. *Red Book: 2012 Report of the Committee on Infectious Diseases*. Elk Grove Village, IL: American Academy of Pediatrics; 2012.
- Case records of the Massachusetts General Hospital. Weekly clinicopathological exercises. Case 16-1998. Pneumonia and the acute respiratory distress syndrome in a 24-year-old man. *N Engl J Med*. 1998;338(21):1527–1535.
- Cunha BA. The atypical pneumonias: clinical diagnosis and importance. *Clin Microbiol Infect*. 2006;12(Suppl 3):12–24.
- National Association of State Public Health Veterinarians. Compendium of measures to control *Chlamydophila psittaci* infection among humans (psittacosis) and pet birds (avian chlamydiosis), 2010. www.nasphv.org/Documents/Psittacosis.pdf. Accessed January 30, 2015.
- Rohde G, Straube E, Essig A, et al. Chlamydial zoonoses. *Dtsch Arztebl Int*. 2010;107(10):174–180. doi:10.3238/arztebl.2010.0174.

CODES

ICD10

A70 Chlamydia psittaci infections

FAQ

- Q: How is a clinical case confirmed?
- A: A clinically compatible illness with fever, chills, headache, cough, and myalgia with (1) isolation of *C. psittaci* from respiratory tract specimens or blood or (2) 4-fold or greater increase in immunoglobulin G (IgG) by complement fixation (CF) or microimmunofluorescence (MIF) against *C. psittaci* between paired acute- and convalescent-phase serum obtained at least 2–4 weeks apart. A "probable case" of psittacosis requires a clinically compatible illness and either (1) supportive serologic test results (e.g., *C. psittaci* immunoglobulin M [IgM] ≥32 in at least 1 serum specimen obtained after onset of symptoms) or (2) detection of *C. psittaci* DNA in a respiratory tract specimen by polymerase chain reaction assay.
- Q: Does the source bird usually exhibit signs of disease?
- A: No. The bird is often asymptomatic; it may, however, show some signs of illness (e.g., anorexia, ruffled feathers, depression, or watery green droppings).

PSORIASIS

Leslie Castelo-Soccio

BASICS

DESCRIPTION

Skin disease characterized by a chronic relapsing nature and, most commonly, clinical features of scaly, erythematous papules and plaques with thick white scale, usually involving elbows, knees, and scalp (i.e., psoriasis vulgaris). Variants include guttate, erythrodermic, and pustular psoriasis.

EPIDEMIOLOGY

- No gender predilection
- Onset of psoriasis is bimodal, commonly presenting in the 3rd decade with a smaller 2nd peak of onset in the 6th decade; however, it can present at any age, with a mean age of onset in children of 8.1 years.
- Earlier onset is associated with more severe disease.

Prevalence

Psoriasis is universal in occurrence, but prevalence varies in different populations. The average prevalence in the United States is ~1–3%.

RISK FACTORS

Genetics

- Although psoriasis has a strong genetic influence, mode of transmission is not defined. It is likely multifactorial with more than one gene involved and is modified by environmental influence.
- 1/3 of patients with psoriasis report a relative with the disease.
- In family studies, 8.1% of children develop psoriasis when 1 parent is affected.
- When both parents have psoriasis, the affected percentage increases to 41%.
- In twin studies, 65% of monozygotic twins are concordant for the disease, whereas only 30% of dizygotic twins are concordant.

PATHOPHYSIOLOGY

- Plaque-type psoriasis is characterized by a thickened parakeratotic epidermis with an absent granular layer above dermal papillae containing dilated tortuous capillaries.
- Collections of polymorphonuclear leukocytes extend from the dermal papillae into the epidermidis stratum corneum (i.e., Munro microabscesses).
- A mixed perivascular infiltrate is confined to the papillary dermis.

ETIOLOGY

The pathogenesis is unknown. Well-defined trigger factors include the following:

- Trauma to normal skin, producing psoriasis in the area (i.e., isomorphic response, sometimes called the Koebner phenomenon)
- Infections (e.g., upper respiratory infections, *Streptococcus pyogenes*, human immunodeficiency virus)
- Stress
- Winter in colder climates in Northern Hemisphere
- Some drugs (i.e., systemic corticosteroids, lithium, NSAIDs, and antimalarials)

COMMONLY ASSOCIATED CONDITIONS

Leukocytosis and hypocalcemia are associated with pustular psoriasis.

DIAGNOSIS

HISTORY

- 1st appearance of eruption
- Area involved
- Recent illness, particularly sore throat
- Recent medications, particularly systemic steroids
- Any appearance of lesions with trauma to skin
- Joint pain
- Previous treatments and response
- Improvement with sun exposure
- Family history of psoriasis
- Signs and symptoms
  - Thick, flaky scales on skin
  - Psoriasis vulgaris
    - In psoriasis vulgaris, sharply demarcated erythematous plaques with white scale are located most commonly on the elbows, knees, scalp, lumbar area, and umbilicus, but they can cover any surface and large areas of the body.
    - Intertriginous regions are often involved, but scale is absent.
  - Guttate psoriasis
    - Form that more often presents in children and young adults as small papules (0.5–1.5 cm), with limited scale over the trunk and proximal extremities
    - Frequently associated with streptococcal infection
  - Erythrodermic psoriasis
    - Erythema with variable scale involving the majority of the body accompanied by chills is characteristic of erythrodermic psoriasis.
  - Generalized pustular psoriasis
    - Most serious variant
    - Sterile pustules as large as 23 mm arising on erythematous skin over large areas of the body. Usually, such appearance is accompanied by high fever.
  - A chronic and localized variant of pustular disease, however, involves only the palms and soles.
    - Note: Classic plaque psoriasis is easily diagnosed, but variants and less virulent cases require careful exam for physical clues.
- Nails are frequently involved, with pinpoint pits, hyperkeratosis, and oil spots.
- Areas where disease is hidden are the retroauricular portion of the scalp and the perianal region.
- Swollen or deformed joints suggest associated psoriatic arthritis.

PHYSICAL EXAM

- A complete cutaneous exam is necessary.
- Removal of scale on plaques produces bleeding points, a feature known as the Auspitz sign.
- The Koebner phenomenon may produce linear or geometric lesions corresponding to areas of trauma.

DIAGNOSTIC TESTS & INTERPRETATION

Lab

- An elevated uric acid level is a common finding.
- *S. pyogenes* infection is frequent in guttate disease, and throat culture is appropriate.
- Other laboratory values are generally within normal ranges. However, in more severe variants, anemia, elevated ESR, and decreased albumin levels may be found.

DIFFERENTIAL DIAGNOSIS

- Classic plaque psoriasis is easily diagnosed. Variants of psoriasis, including guttate, erythrodermic, and pustular disease, are more difficult to recognize.
- The differential diagnosis varies with the type of psoriasis and includes the following:
  - Nummular eczema
  - Cutaneous T-cell lymphoma
  - Tinea corporis
  - Pityriasis rosea
  - Pityriasis lichenoides et varioliformis acuta
  - Secondary syphilis
  - Atopic dermatitis
  - Drug eruption
  - Candidiasis
  - Seborrheic dermatitis

TREATMENT

GENERAL MEASURES

- Phototherapy
  - UVB
    - Administered on average 2–3 times weekly in a booth with bulbs that emit the appropriate wavelength of UV radiation
    - Effective for guttate and plaque psoriasis
    - Average treatment time: 3 months, with gradual increases in time of exposure. Sunscreen should be used on the face.
    - Narrow-band UVB represents a form of monochromatic UVB, using 311-nm

wavelengths; appears to be a somewhat more effective form of delivering UVB phototherapy using booth or handheld device
  - PUVA (psoralen and UVB)
    - PUVA and oral medications (e.g., methotrexate, acitretin) should be reserved for severe cases and carefully monitored by a dermatologist.

ALERT

Possible conflicts with other drugs: Photosensitizing medication (e.g., tetracyclines, sulfa derivatives, phenothiazines, griseofulvin, among others) should be avoided with phototherapy.

- Topical
  - Topical corticosteroids
    - Mid- to high-potency topical corticosteroid ointments are applied twice daily.
    - Mid-potency preparations (e.g., 0.025% fluocinolone ointment, 0.1% triamcinolone acetonide) are preferred in children.
    - Low-potency corticosteroids (e.g., 1% and 2.5% hydrocortisone) are used on the face and intertriginous regions to prevent atrophy.
    - Agents can also be found in oils or solutions.
  - Anthralin
    - Anthralin, applied for 30 minutes and carefully washed off
    - Irritation and staining are common, so that the face and intertriginous regions cannot be treated with this approach.
  - Calcipotriene
    - Calcipotriene ointment is a vitamin D_3 derivative.
    - It is applied twice daily, avoiding the face and intertriginous regions.
    - Maximum weekly dosage in adults is 100 g.
    - Rare cases of hypercalcemia have been reported.
    - Combination steroid/calcipotriene products exist.
  - Tazarotene gel
    - A topical retinoid
    - Can be irritating when used as monotherapy
    - Often combined with topical steroids as adjunctive therapy applied once daily or twice daily
  - Coal tar
    - A weak therapeutic agent as monotherapy
    - More effective when combined with UVB phototherapy
    - Used in various shampoo preparations as well as in solution that can be added to the bath
  - Systemic agents
    - May be considered when the psoriasis is especially severe or when joint symptoms are prominent.
    - Methotrexate
    - Isotretinoin or acitretin
    - Cyclosporine
    - Biologic agents such as etanercept
    - Systemic corticosteroids should be avoided because withdrawal from steroids may be accompanied by a pustular psoriasis flare.

ISSUES FOR REFERRAL

- Pustules, a significant increase in degree or extent of erythema, or fever may require hospitalization and systemic therapy.
- Erythrodermic psoriasis may require hospitalization.
- Adult and pediatric patients with psoriasis have an increased prevalence of cardiovascular disease and metabolic syndrome. Patients should be monitored for blood pressure, glucose, weight, and lipids to decrease risk.

Initial Stabilization

- Therapy is delivered by topical medications, phototherapy, or systemic medications.
- Localized disease is treated with topical and more diffuse disease with phototherapy.
- Systemic medications for resistant cases
- Except in severe cases, therapy for children should be limited to topical medication and UVB phototherapy.

ONGOING CARE

FOLLOW-UP RECOMMENDATIONS

- Topical therapy is administered chronically, with breaks to minimize side effects.
- Remissions may occur in summer with sun exposure.
- The average treatment course with UVB therapy is 3 months and may be followed by an average remission period of 5 months.

PROGNOSIS

- Once psoriasis appears, it generally persists throughout life.
- Spontaneous remissions of variable length and frequency occur but are unpredictable.
- Response depends on potency of medication and frequency of treatment.
- Improvement with topical medication is obvious at 2 weeks and usually peaks at 2 months.
- Scrubbing by the patient to remove scales also irritates the disease.
- Psychological aspects of the disease, particularly in children, should be addressed.

ADDITIONAL READING

- Au SC, Goldminz AM, Loo DS, et al. Association between pediatric psoriasis and the metabolic syndrome. *J Am Acad Dermatol*. 2012;66(6):1012–1013.
- Gelfand JM, Mehta NN, Langan SM. Psoriasis and cardiovascular risk: strength in numbers, part II. *J Invest Dermatol*. 2011;131(5):1007–1010.
- Marqueling AL, Cordoro KM. Systemic treatments for severe pediatric psoriasis: a practical approach. *Dermatol Clin*. 2013;31(2):267–288.
- Oka A, Mabuchi T, Ozawa A, et al. Current understanding of human genetics and genetic analysis of psoriasis. *J Dermatol*. 2012;39(3):231–241.
- Shah KN. Diagnosis and treatment of pediatric psoriasis: current and future. *Am J Clin Dermatol*. 2013;14(3):195–213.

CODES

ICD10

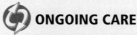

- L40.9 Psoriasis, unspecified
- L40.0 Psoriasis vulgaris
- L40.4 Guttate psoriasis

FAQ

- Q: Will my disease get worse?
- A: It is impossible to predict the course of any patient's disease because it is influenced by both heredity and everyday factors in the environment. Although there is no cure, with treatment, the disease can be kept under control. Remissions do occur and may be for prolonged periods of time.
- Q: When my disease is in remission, what can I do to prevent it from returning?
- A: Avoiding trauma and keeping skin moist are important. In the summer, controlled sun exposure is helpful. You may have to continue other treatments at less frequent intervals. Any cases of sore throat should be cultured and treated if streptococcal disease is present.
- Q: Will my other children get psoriasis?
- A: If neither parent has psoriasis, the chances are <10% that another child will develop the disease; if 1 parent is affected, the chances increase to 15%; if both parents are affected, the chances are 50%. Therefore, unless both parents are affected, it is more likely that other children will not get psoriasis.
- Q: Does stress make psoriasis worse?
- A: Some studies have suggested that flare-ups of psoriasis are associated with increased stress. It is difficult to evaluate whether stress is the cause or the result of the disease. Do all you can to reasonably relieve stress, but do not focus on this as the cause of your psoriasis.

PUBERTAL DELAY

Angela P. Mojica • Lucy D. Mastrandrea

BASICS

DESCRIPTION

- Pubertal delay is the absence of secondary sexual characteristics (testicular enlargement in boys or breast development in girls) by an age >2–2.5 standard deviations (*SD*) than the population mean.
  - In the United States, this is considered to be ~13 years of age for girls and 14 years of age for boys.
  - Development of pubic hair is usually not considered in the definition because adrenarche (adrenal gland maturation) may occur independently of gonadarche.
- Pubertal delay may also occur if progression through puberty stalls or takes more than 4 years between first signs of puberty and completion.
- Most cases of pubertal delay can be ascribed to constitutional delay of growth and puberty (CDGP); however, missing the presentation of an underlying disease should be avoided.
- CDGP
  - Likely an extreme normal variant of pubertal development
  - Enter puberty late and usually reach normal adult height
  - More common in boys than in girls
  - Strong familial component

GENERAL PREVENTION

- Perform pubertal staging at regular intervals.
- Examination of growth charts at routine visits can alert providers to potential problems or changes in growth.
- Begin conversations about pubertal development with both patients and parents in late childhood. Realistic expectations regarding timing can avoid undue stress and unnecessary testing.
- Children with chronic health conditions should receive counseling regarding the effect their illness may have on their puberty. For example, children with cystic fibrosis generally have delayed puberty.

EPIDEMIOLOGY

- Approximately 2.5% of healthy teens will meet criteria for pubertal delay.
- CDGP explains 90–95% of pubertal delay.
- 50–75% of patients with CDGP have a positive family history.
- In contrast to boys, pubertal delay in girls more frequently represents underlying pathology
- Malnutrition is a risk factor for delayed puberty.

GENETICS

- Pubertal timing is highly influenced by genetic factors. This is evidenced by high correlation within ethnic groups, families, and between monozygotic twins.
- 50–80% of variation in timing can be explained by genetics.
- CDGP
  - Inheritance is often consistent with an autosomal dominant pattern.
  - No specific causative gene mutations have been identified.
- Hypogonadotropic hypogonadism is associated with mutations in single genes including *GNRHR*, *KAL-1*, *FGFR-1*, and *GPR54*.
- GPR54 (a G protein–coupled receptor) and its ligand (kisspeptin) play an important role as a signal for gonadotropin-releasing hormone (GnRH) release. Mutations in the *GPR54* gene have been found in patients with isolated hypogonadotropic hypogonadism but not in those with CDGP.
- Pubertal delay as a result of underlying medical conditions is influenced by the pathophysiology of each disorder.

ETIOLOGY

Deficiency of gonadal sex steroids, estrogen in girls or testosterone in boys, is the underlying cause of delayed puberty. Several pathways to the common etiology exist:

- Hypogonadotrophic hypogonadism: delayed puberty as a result of a deficiency in secretion of GnRH or gonadotropin secretion
  - Functional: delay or transient decrease in GnRH or gonadotropin secretion; describes CDGP, hypothyroidism, chronic illness
  - Permanent: irreversible deficiency of GnRH, such as in Kallmann syndrome or panhypopituitarism
- Hypergonadotrophic hypogonadism: gonadal failure as seen in Turner syndrome, Klinefelter syndrome, and anorchia

DIAGNOSIS

HISTORY

- A thorough history of past medical conditions, past growth patterns, and family history is essential.
- Family history of childhood growth patterns and age at pubertal onset of the parents (late menarche in the mother or delayed completion of adult height in the father)
- A complete review of systems to uncover an underlying chronic disorder, such as inflammatory bowel disease, thyroid disorder, celiac disease, or eating disorder, is necessary.
- Bilateral cryptorchidism or a small penis at birth and hyposmia or anosmia may suggest hypogonadotropic hypogonadism.
- A history of chemotherapy or radiotherapy may indicate primary gonadal failure.
- Request and examine a long-term growth chart:
  - CDGP will generally exhibit a consistent low percentile of growth throughout childhood, with linear growth deceleration in the peripubertal period. Growth rate is within the prepubertal normal range.
  - Gonadotropin or gonadal causes will generally present with normal growth in childhood, but no increase in growth rate during the expected pubertal spurt.
- Obtain history of progression of secondary sex characteristics:
  - Adolescents with complete gonadal or gonadotropin deficiencies will not enter puberty unless initiated by exogenous hormones; those with CDGP will progress at a normal rate after initiation of puberty.
  - In CDGP, both adrenarche and gonadarche occur later than average.
  - In isolated hypogonadotropic hypogonadism, adrenarche usually occurs at a normal age.
- Medication history may be useful (e.g., use of glucocorticoids or cytotoxins).
- Assess nutrition history to evaluate for chronic malnutrition or eating disorder.

PHYSICAL EXAM

A thorough physical exam is essential. Pay particular attention to the following elements:

- Thyroid examination
- Neurologic and funduscopic examinations to check for intracranial pathology
- Genital examination and sexual maturity rating (Tanner staging)
  - Breast exam for girls
  - Pubic hair
  - Penis/testicle exam for boys
  - Internal gynecologic examination for girls with amenorrhea may be indicated.
- The first sign of puberty in boys is when testicular length is >2.5 cm (4-cc volume).
- The first sign of gonadarche in girls is breast development.
- In girls, determine whether there is marked discordance between pubic hair and breast development (androgen insensitivity).
- Assess for physical signs of Turner syndrome or Klinefelter syndrome.

DIAGNOSTIC TESTS & INTERPRETATION

Lab

- Initial workup: routine screening tests for chronic or systemic disease
  - CBC
  - ESR
  - Electrolytes, renal function
  - Thyroid-stimulating hormone
  - Gonadotropin level—follicle-stimulating hormone (FSH) and luteinizing hormone (LH)
    - Low levels suggest prepuberty or hypothalamic-pituitary failure.
    - High levels suggest gonadal failure or absence.
    - LH is a better marker of pubertal initiation than FSH.

- In delayed puberty, an FSH value above the upper limit of the normal range for the assay is a sensitive and specific marker of primary gonadal failure.
- If hypergonadotropic, obtain karyotype:
  - XX is suggestive of ovarian failure.
  - XO or abnormal X chromosome is indicative of Turner syndrome or gonadal dysgenesis.
  - XXY is indicative of Klinefelter syndrome.
- Inhibin B—baseline levels may facilitate discrimination between constitutional delay and permanent hypogonadotropic hypogonadism.
- If all of the aforementioned studies are normal, and there is no evidence to support CDGP, reevaluate for cryptic chronic illness (including prolactinoma), substance abuse, eating disorder, or ongoing psychosocial stress until puberty progresses or the underlying cause of delay becomes clear.
- No test reliably distinguishes CDGP from isolated hypogonadotropic hypogonadism.
- Eventual pubertal progression confirms CDGP.

Imaging

- Bone age
  - An essential step in primary workup
  - Plain film of the epiphyseal growth centers in the left hand.
  - Epiphyses change in response to growth hormone, thyroxine, and steroids of adrenal or gonadal origin.
  - Bone age should be reviewed by a practitioner who is experienced in interpreting such radiographs.
  - Comparison to chronologic age can help to differentiate CDGP from organic disorders. A bone age that is >2 years delayed from chronologic age is consistent with CDGP. However, this degree of delay is not specific and can be found with other hypogonadotropic causes of delayed puberty or in gonadal failure.
- Pelvic ultrasound
  - Can be useful in locating intra-abdominal testicular structures or in determination of the presence or absence of müllerian structures
  - Indicated when testes are not palpated in patients with a male phenotype or when müllerian structures cannot be confirmed on physical examination in patients with a female phenotype.
- MRI of the brain/pituitary
  - Useful in assessing pituitary or hypothalamic structures, mass lesions, pathologic calcifications, or increased intracranial pressure if a central cause of delayed puberty is suspected.
- Full neuroendocrine testing
  - Warranted in patients with hypothalamic-pituitary tumors causing hypogonadotropic hypogonadism
- Imaging in patients with the Kallmann syndrome commonly shows olfactory bulb and sulcus aplasia or hypoplasia.

DIFFERENTIAL DIAGNOSIS

- Increased serum gonadotropins (LH/FSH)
  - Congenital
    - Chromosomal abnormalities
    - Turner syndrome (gonadal dysgenesis)
    - Klinefelter syndrome
    - Disorders of sex development
  - Acquired
    - Primary gonadal failure
    - Cytotoxic chemotherapy or radiotherapy
    - Autoimmune gonadal failure
    - Vanishing testes syndrome
    - Trauma
- Normal or low serum gonadotropins
  - CDGP
  - Congenital
    - Gene defects (e.g., Kallmann syndrome)
    - Syndromes (Prader-Willi syndrome)
  - Acquired
    - CNS tumors/traumatic brain injury
    - Hypothalamic amenorrhea (strenuous exercise, eating disorders)
    - Chronic illness
    - Malnutrition
    - Primary hypothyroidism
    - Hyperprolactinemia
    - Drug-associated (psychotropics)

ALERT

- No test can make a definitive diagnosis of CDGP.
- Consultation with a specialist or experienced laboratory personnel is recommended before obtaining pituitary stimulation tests, as they may require special conditions.

TREATMENT

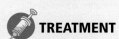

GENERAL MEASURES

Most patients with pubertal delay do not require pharmacotherapy but may benefit from psychological and social support.

MEDICATION

- In cases of presumed CDGP, estrogen/testosterone therapy can be used to affect hypothalamic maturation, thereby initiating endogenous puberty.
- Referral to an endocrinologist or adolescent specialist is usually recommended before the initiation of hormonal therapy to aid in diagnosis and management.

ONGOING CARE

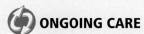

In cases of permanent hypogonadism because of gonadal absence, failure, or gonadotropin deficiency, long-term hormonal therapy is necessary.

ADDITIONAL READING

- Joffe A, Blythe MJ. Abnormalities of growth and development. *Adolesc Med State Art Rev*. 2009;20: 434–441.
- Nathan BM, Palmert MR. Regulation and disorders of pubertal timing. *Endocrinol Metab Clin N Am*. 2005;34(3):617–641, ix.
- Palmert MR, Dunkel L. Clinical practice. Delayed puberty. *N Engl J Med*. 2012;366(5):443–453.
- Pinyerd B, Zipf WB. Puberty—timing is everything! *J Pediatr Nurs*. 2005;20(2):75–82.
- Reiter EO, Lee PA. Delayed puberty. *Adolesc Med*. 2002;13(1):101–118, vii.
- Rosen DS, Foster C. Delayed puberty. *Pediatr Rev*. 2001;22(9):309–315.
- Palmert MR, Dunkel L. Clinical practice. Delayed puberty. *N Engl J Med*. 2012;366(5):443–453.

CODES

ICD10

- E30.0 Delayed puberty
- E28.39 Other primary ovarian failure
- E23.0 Hypopituitarism

FAQ

- Q: As ~95% of pubertal delay is constitutional or physiologic, when can I avoid an expensive workup and just observe the patient?
- A: Only the spontaneous onset of puberty confirms the diagnosis of constitutional delay. Anxiety from delayed puberty may preclude waiting. To make a presumptive diagnosis of CDGP, pathology must be ruled out:
  - Physical examination, including genital anatomy and sense of smell, must be normal.
  - There should be no signs or symptoms consistent with chronic disease.
  - History, including nutritional history and review of systems, must be negative.
  - Screening blood work must be negative.
  - Growth is slow for age, but height and growth rate are within prepubertal range.
  - A delay in bone age is characteristic but not diagnostic of CDGP.
- Q: When should patients with pubertal delay be seen by an endocrinologist or adolescent specialist?
- A: Often, the initial workup of pubertal delay can be completed by the primary care provider. For complex stimulation tests, or if help is needed in interpreting test results, referral to an experienced specialist is warranted. If a specific chronic disease is suspected as the underlying cause, then referral should be made to the appropriate subspecialist.

PULMONARY EMBOLISM

Akinyemi O. Ajayi

BASICS

DESCRIPTION
Occlusion of a pulmonary vessel by a thrombus

EPIDEMIOLOGY
- Pulmonary embolism is seen more frequently in adults and tends to occur in postsurgical situations, especially when patients have been bedridden.
- ~10% of adults who present with an acute pulmonary embolus die within 1 hour of onset.
- Increasing incidence is secondary to increased central catheter use.
- Mortality rate can be as high as 30% if diagnosis is delayed.
- The incidence of new cases of pulmonary embolism presenting to a large, urban pediatric emergency department was 2.1 cases per 100,000 visits.

RISK FACTORS
- In children
  - Presence of a central venous catheter
  - Lack of mobility
  - Congenital heart disease
  - Ventriculoatrial shunt
  - Trauma
  - Solid tumors or leukemia
  - After-surgical procedures (especially reparative intervention for scoliosis repair)
  - Hypercoagulable condition
- In adults: most commonly due to the presence of a deep vein thrombosis, usually in the legs or pelvis

PATHOPHYSIOLOGY
- Thromboemboli may develop anywhere in the systemic venous system.
- Pulmonary embolism is characterized by the triad of hypoxemia, pulmonary hypertension, and right ventricular failure.
  - Diminished pulmonary perfusion causes a ventilation–perfusion mismatch, resulting in hypoxemia.
  - Hyperventilation occurs secondary to stimulation of proprioceptors in the lung.
  - Hypercapnia is seen with severe occlusion of the pulmonary artery (often not seen with smaller emboli).
- Pulmonary infarction is uncommon due to the presence of collateral pulmonary and bronchial arteries along with the airways providing additional sources of oxygen to the tissues.
- Death occurs with 85% obstruction of the pulmonary artery.

ETIOLOGY
Blood clots appear as a result of deep vein thrombosis or other disease states.

DIAGNOSIS

ALERT
Failure to make the diagnosis is the most common mistake.
- Pulmonary embolism must be suspected in critically ill children who have a central venous catheter in place and subsequently develop sudden respiratory failure.
- Because the symptoms of severe lung disease and pulmonary embolism are similar, the diagnosis might be missed if the index of suspicion is low.

SIGNS AND SYMPTOMS
- Pulmonary embolism should be suspected in children who present with the following:
  - Pleuritic chest pain
  - Shortness of breath
  - Hemoptysis
  - Cough
  - Acute respiratory distress
  - Apprehension or anxiety
  - Syncope
  - Cardiovascular shock
- Symptoms may be nonspecific and indicative of other disorders.

HISTORY
Ask about chest symptoms: The clinician must have a high index of suspicion and recognize risk factors to establish the correct diagnosis.

PHYSICAL EXAM
- Findings on physical examination are nonspecific.
- General
  - Fever
  - Diaphoresis
  - Nervousness or apprehension (altered mental status is uncommon)
- Cardiovascular
  - Increased intensity of the pulmonic component of S_2
  - Tachycardia
  - Gallop rhythm
  - New murmur
- Pulmonary
  - Tachypnea
  - Rales
  - Cyanosis (present with 65% obstruction of the pulmonary artery)
  - Pleuritic chest pain
  - Dyspnea
  - Cough
  - Hemoptysis
  - Wheezing (uncommon)
- Extremities
  - Deep venous thrombosis is frequently found in the adult population.
  - Phlebitis
  - Edema

DIAGNOSTIC TESTS & INTERPRETATION

Lab
- In general, blood tests are nonspecific and of no significant value in making the diagnosis of a pulmonary embolus.
- Arterial blood gases
  - Decreased Pao_2 and $Paco_2$
  - Increased alveolar–arterial (A–a) gradient

Imaging
- Electrocardiogram
  - Useful in ruling out other conditions
  - May show sinus tachycardia or nonspecific ST-T wave changes
- Echocardiogram
  - Useful for identifying
    - Abnormalities of cardiac anatomy
    - Thrombi on catheter tips
  - If emboli are seen on echocardiogram, mortality rate is 40–50%. Additionally, if signs of right ventricular dysfunction are noted (e.g., right ventricular dilatation, abnormal right ventricular wall motion, or increased tricuspid regurgitation jet velocity), risk of poor outcome is greater.
- Spiral computed tomography (CT)
  - New diagnostic modality
  - Greater sensitivity than ventilation–perfusion scan in the diagnosis of pulmonary embolism due to the ability to image abnormal pulmonary pathology
- Chest x-ray
  - May be abnormal in 70% of patients with pulmonary embolus
  - Most frequent findings:
    - Parenchymal infiltrates
    - Atelectasis
    - Pleural effusions: seen in 33% of cases, mostly unilateral
    - Hampton hump (pyramidal shape pointing toward the hilum)
- Ventilation–perfusion scan
  - Results of a ventilation–perfusion scan performed to rule out a pulmonary embolus are reported in 1 of 5 categories, ranging from high probability to normal.
  - An abnormal ventilation–perfusion scan with normal ventilation and decreased perfusion in the appropriate clinical setting is 90% specific for a pulmonary embolus.
  - A normal result on ventilation–perfusion scan does not completely rule out pulmonary embolus, although if the patient is at low risk, a pulmonary embolus is highly unlikely.
- Pulmonary angiography
  - Most sensitive and specific test
  - Not done as frequently in children as in adults because of complications associated with the procedure

P

- With the introduction of newer, improved catheters and safer contrast solutions, this test can now safely be performed in the pediatric population.
  - Indicated for cases
    - Intermediate-probability ventilation–perfusion scans
    - High-probability scans in patients who are poor candidates for anticoagulation, hemodynamically unstable, or require an embolectomy

Diagnostic Procedures/Other

- Pulmonary function testing
  - Results are nonspecific.
- Evaluation of the lower extremities
  - Diagnosing deep vein thrombosis via the following
    - Impedance plethysmography
    - Doppler technology
    - Venography

DIFFERENTIAL DIAGNOSIS

- Cardiac
  - Cardiac tamponade
  - Constrictive pericarditis
  - Restrictive cardiomyopathy
- Pulmonary
  - Chronic cough
  - Status asthmaticus
  - Pneumonia with empyema
  - Pneumothorax

TREATMENT

GENERAL MEASURES

Initial Stabilization

- Stabilize patient before anticoagulation or thrombolytic therapy is begun:
  - Improve oxygenation.
  - Correct acidosis.
  - Stabilize blood pressure.
  - Analgesia for severe pleuritic chest pain. Avoid prescribing opiates in cases of cardiovascular collapse.
- Goal of therapy is anticoagulation and/or thrombolysis.
- In patients with an intermediate or high suspicion, begin anticoagulation before investigations.

MEDICATION

- Anticoagulation therapy to prevent further thrombus formation
  - Heparin
    - Bolus dose: 100–200 U/kg
    - Maintenance dose: 10–25 U/kg/h
    - Keep partial thromboplastin time (PTT) at 55–60 seconds.
    - Should be given for 7–10 days
  - Warfarin
    - Warfarin should be started 24–48 hours after heparin therapy is begun.
    - Maintenance dose: 2.5–10 mg/24 h
    - Keep prothrombin time (PT) twice normal and maintain the international normalized ratio (INR) between 2 and 3.
    - Should be continued for 36 months
- Thrombolytic therapy
  - Agents available
    - Urokinase
    - Tissue plasminogen activator (TPA): same efficacy as streptokinase and lower incidence of allergic reactions
  - Indications
    - Hemodynamically unstable
    - Large embolus
- Low-molecular-weight heparin has been used as prophylaxis or as treatment for preexisting conditions in both adults and children.
  - A synthetic, nonthrombocytopenic heparin pentasaccharide with pure antifactor Xa activity is currently being tested.
- Ticlopidine and clopidogrel have been used successfully to prevent thrombotic strokes and arterial thrombotic syndromes.
- Contraindications to anticoagulation therapy
  - Active internal bleeding
  - Recent cerebrovascular accident
  - Major surgery
  - Recent gastrointestinal bleed

SURGERY/OTHER PROCEDURES

- Embolectomy
  - Indicated when hemodynamic instability persists; reserved for patients who have failed thrombolytic therapy or in whom medical treatment is contraindicated
  - Late results are excellent if the patient has not suffered from a perioperative cardiac arrest, which is associated with early mortality.
- Percutaneous caval filtration
  - Indicated if commencement or continuation of anticoagulation is strongly contraindicated or if full anticoagulation has failed to prevent recurrent emboli
  - This should be considered in patients undergoing venous thrombolysis because up to 20% may develop embolization during treatment.

ONGOING CARE

Patients receiving warfarin therapy should have the usual follow-up for those receiving an anticoagulant.

PROGNOSIS

- If treated promptly, prognosis is good.
- If treatment is delayed, especially if the patient is hemodynamically unstable, prognosis is poor.

ADDITIONAL READING

- Agha BS, Sturm JJ, Simon HK, et al. Pulmonary embolism in the pediatric emergency department. *Pediatrics*. 2013;132(4):663–667.
- Biss TT, Brandao LR, Kahr WH, et al. Clinical features and outcome of pulmonary embolism in children. *Br J Haem*. 2008;142(5):808–818.
- Fedullo PF, Tapson VF. Clinical practice. The evaluation of suspected pulmonary embolism. *N Engl J Med*. 2003;349(13):1247–1256.
- Goldhaber SZ, Elliott CG. Acute pulmonary embolism: part I: epidemiology, pathophysiology, and diagnosis. *Circulation*. 2003;108(22):2726–2729.
- Kruip MJ, Leclercq MG, van der Heul C, et al. Diagnostic strategies for excluding pulmonary embolism in clinical outcome studies. A systematic review. *Ann Intern Med*. 2003;138(12):941–951.
- Meister B, Kropshofer G, Klein-Franke A, et al. Comparison of low-molecular-weight heparin and antithrombin versus antithrombin alone for the prevention of symptomatic venous thromboembolism in children with acute lymphoblastic leukemia. *Pediatr Blood Cancer*. 2008;50(2):298–303.
- Monagle P. Diagnosis and management of deep venous thrombosis and pulmonary embolism in neonates and children. *Semin Thromb Hemost*. 2012;38(7):683–690.
- Patocka C, Nemeth J. Pulmonary embolism in pediatrics. *J Emerg Med*. 2012;42(1):105–116.
- Snow V, Qaseem A, Barry P, et al. Management of venous thromboembolism: a clinical practice guideline from the American College of Physicians and the American Academy of Family Physicians. *Ann Fam Med*. 2007;5(1):74–80.
- Zierler BK. Ultrasonography and diagnosis of venous thromboembolism. *Circulation*. 2004;109(12) (Suppl 1):I9–I14.

CODES

ICD10

I26.99 Other pulmonary embolism without acute cor pulmonale

FAQ

- Q: Is it safe for children on warfarin to play contact sports?
- A: The general recommendation is that no contact sports should be allowed while children are on warfarin therapy because of the increased risk of bleeding.

PULMONARY HYPERTENSION

Richard M. Kravitz

BASICS

DESCRIPTION
Increased pulmonary vascular resistance

EPIDEMIOLOGY
Incidence
Incidence in children is unknown.

PATHOPHYSIOLOGY
- Structural alterations in pulmonary vessel architecture (remodeling)
- Smooth muscle hypertrophy
- Extension of blood vessel's smooth muscle into smaller vessels
- Inflammation

ETIOLOGY
- Hypoxemia-induced pulmonary hypertension
- Chronic lung disease
  - Cystic fibrosis
  - Bronchopulmonary dysplasia
  - Interstitial lung disease
  - Diaphragmatic hernia with secondary pulmonary hypoplasia
- Upper airway obstruction
  - Tonsillar and/or adenoid hypertrophy
  - Obesity
- Hypoventilation
  - Neurologically mediated process
  - Secondary to muscular weakness
- High pulmonary blood flow secondary to left-to-right shunting (seen in congenital heart disease)
  - Patent ductus arteriosus
  - Atrial septal defect
  - Ventricular septal defect
- Left-sided cardiac disorders that increase pulmonary venous pressure
  - Left ventricular failure
  - Mitral valve stenosis
  - Obstructed anomalous pulmonary veins
- Occlusion of pulmonary vessels
  - Sickle cell disease
  - Veno-occlusive disease
  - Thromboembolism
- Pulmonary vasculitis
  - Systemic lupus erythematosus
  - Rheumatoid arthritis
  - Scleroderma
- Persistent pulmonary hypertension of the newborn
- Idiopathic cases (primary pulmonary hypertension)

DIAGNOSIS

HISTORY
- Dyspnea (usually earliest complaint reported)
- Fatigue
  - Seen early in course of illness with exercise or exertion (but not at rest)
  - Seen at rest in the later stages of the illness or in severe cases
- Exercise intolerance
- Feeding intolerance
- Failure to thrive
- Excessive sleeping
- Diaphoresis
- Chest pain
- Syncope
- Palpitations (late finding)
- Signs and symptoms pitfalls:
  - Signs and symptoms of pulmonary hypertension are not specific and can easily be missed.
  - Consider obstructive sleep apnea as a possible cause of pulmonary hypertension (ask about snoring if suspecting pulmonary hypertension in the absence of overt cardiac or pulmonary disease).

PHYSICAL EXAM
- Typically governed by the signs and findings related to underlying lung or heart disease
- Tachypnea
- Arrhythmias
- Narrowed splitting of S_2 heart sound
- Increased P_2 heart sound
- Presence of S_3 and/or S_4 heart sounds
- Murmur of pulmonary or tricuspid insufficiency; tricuspid insufficiency more common
- Jugular venous distention
- Peripheral edema
- Hepatomegaly

DIAGNOSTIC TESTS & INTERPRETATION
Lab
Arterial blood gases
- Measurement of Po_2 assesses degree of hypoxia.
- Evaluation of Pco_2 determines presence or absence of hypoventilation.

Imaging
Chest x-ray
- Will vary according to the underlying disorder and extent of pulmonary hypertension
- Degree of pulmonary hypertension correlates poorly with chest x-ray findings.
- In primary pulmonary hypertension
  - Cardiomegaly
  - Enlarged pulmonary artery
  - Peripheral lung appears underperfused ("pruning" of pulmonary vessels).

Diagnostic Procedures/Other
- EKG
  - Can be normal if cor pulmonale has not yet developed
  - If cor pulmonale present, EKG can demonstrate
    - Right QRS axis deviation
    - Right ventricular hypertrophy
    - Right atrial hypertrophy
- Echocardiogram with Doppler flow
  - Increased pulmonary artery pressure
  - Right ventricular hypertrophy
  - Paradoxical movement of the intraventricular septum
  - Pulmonic and tricuspid valve regurgitation
  - Right-to-left shunting via an open foramen ovale
- Cardiac catheterization
  - Most accurate measurement of pulmonary artery pressure is accomplished by right heart catheterization.
  - Criteria for pulmonary hypertension in children:
    - Mean pulmonary arterial pressure >25 mm Hg (at rest)
    - Mean pulmonary arterial pressure >30 mm Hg (with exercise)
    - Pulmonary vascular resistance >3 U/m^2
    - Systolic pulmonary artery pressure >1/2 systolic systemic pressure
- Pressures should be measured before and after various vasodilators to assess potential reversibility of pulmonary hypertension.
- Caution: In patients with severe disease, catheterization is associated with increased risk of complications.

DIFFERENTIAL DIAGNOSIS
- Pulmonary
  - Asthma
  - Cystic fibrosis
  - Chronic obstructive pulmonary disease
  - Emphysema
  - Pulmonary arteriovenous malformations
- Miscellaneous
  - Congestive heart failure (CHF)
  - Noncardiogenic pulmonary edema
  - Fatigue
  - Syncope

TREATMENT

MEDICATION

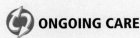

- Oxygen
  - Acts as a vasodilator
  - Keep $Sao_2 \geq 95\%$
  - Supplemental oxygen may prove useful even with normal resting Sao_2 (supplemental oxygen will cover for desaturations associated with exertion, exercise, or illness).
  - Caution: Supplemental oxygen can sometimes cause hypercapnia by blunting the hypoxia-driven respiratory drive.
- Anticoagulation therapy (i.e., Coumadin)
  - Prevents clot formation in the narrowed pulmonary vessels
  - Helpful even in the absence of thromboembolic disease
- Vasodilators
  - Methods of action
    - Decreases pulmonary arterial pressures
    - Improves right-sided cardiac function
  - Available agents
    - Oxygen
    - Calcium channel blocker (i.e., nifedipine)
    - Nitric oxide (continuous inhalation)
    - Prostacyclin (continuous IV infusion) (i.e., epoprostenol)
    - Endothelin receptor antagonist, PO (i.e., bosentan)
    - Phosphodiesterase inhibitor PO (i.e., sildenafil)
  - Caution: Vasodilators should be used under close supervision because of their effect on systemic BP (systemic hypotension can be a significant problem).

ADDITIONAL TREATMENT

General Measures

- Provide for patient stabilization.
- Treat the primary disease process.
- Treat underlying hypoxia (supplemental oxygen).
- Treat underlying hypoventilation:
  - Useful for correcting hypoxia and hypercarbia secondary to hypoventilation
  - Available methods:
    - Noninvasive positive pressure ventilation (bilevel ventilation)
    - Mechanical ventilation (tracheostomy with mechanical ventilation)

SURGERY/OTHER PROCEDURES

- Tonsillectomy and/or adenoidectomy if obstructive sleep apnea is the underlying etiology
- Atrial septostomy may be considered when inadequate right-to-left shunting is present with syncopal episodes and/or right-sided heart failure
- Transplantation (lung or heart-lung transplantation): reserved for patients with refractory, severe pulmonary hypertension

ONGOING CARE

PROGNOSIS

- Depends on underlying disease, but generally poor
- In cases of primary pulmonary hypertension, improvement of pulmonary hypertension with administration of vasodilators during initial catheterization is associated with a better survival rate than if no response occurs.
- 10–40% mortality in treated patients
- Near 100% mortality if patient is untreated
- Treatment can be lifelong unless the primary cause of the pulmonary hypertension can be corrected.
- In acute pulmonary hypertension, response to most treatment modalities is almost immediate.
- Oxygen has been shown to reverse hypoxia-related remodeling of the airways after 1 month of therapy.

COMPLICATIONS

- Chronic hypoxia
- Exercise intolerance
- Right-sided heart failure (cor pulmonale)
- Death

ADDITIONAL READING

- Barst RJ, Ertel SI, Beghetti M, et al. Pulmonary arterial hypertension: a comparison between children and adults. *Eur Respir J*. 2011;37(3):665–677.
- Berger RMF, Bonnet D. Treatment options for paediatric pulmonary arterial hypertension. *Eur Respir Rev*. 2010;19(118):321–330.
- Chatterjee K, De Marco T, Alpert JS. Pulmonary hypertension: hemodynamic diagnosis and management. *Arch Intern Med*. 2002;162(17):1925–1933.
- Hawkins A, Tulloh R. Treatment of pediatric pulmonary hypertension. *Vasc Health Risk Manag*. 2009;5(2):509–524.
- Klings ES, Farber HW. Current management of primary pulmonary hypertension. *Drugs*. 2001;61(13):1945–1956.
- Mourani PM, Sontag MK, Younoszai A, et al. Clinical utility of echocardiography for the diagnosis and management of pulmonary vascular disease in young children with chronic lung disease. *Pediatrics*. 2008;121(2):317–325.
- Oishi P, Datar SA, Fineman JR. Advances in the management of pediatric pulmonary hypertension. *Respir Care*. 2011;56(9):1314–1339.
- Ravishankar C, Tabbutt S, Wernovsky G. Critical care in cardiovascular medicine. *Curr Opin Pediatr*. 2003;15(5):443–453.
- Rosenzweig EB, Widlitz AC, Barst RJ. Pulmonary arterial hypertension in children. *Pediatr Pulmonol*. 2004;38(1):2–22.
- Schulze-Neick I, Beghetti M. Issues related to the management and therapy of paediatric pulmonary hypertension. *Eur Respir Rev*. 2010;19(118):331–339.
- Simonneau G, Galie N, Rubin LJ, et al. Clinical classification of pulmonary hypertension. *Am J Coll Cardiol*. 2004;43(12)(Suppl S):5S–12S.
- Widlitz A, Barst RJ. Pulmonary arterial hypertension in children. *Eur Respir J*. 2003;21(1):155–176.
- Yeh TF. Persistent pulmonary hypertension in preterm infants with respiratory distress syndrome. *Pediatr Pulmonol*. 2001;(Suppl 23):103–106.

CODES

ICD10

- I27.2 Other secondary pulmonary hypertension
- I27.0 Primary pulmonary hypertension
- P29.3 Persistent fetal circulation

FAQ

- Q: How many hours per day should supplemental oxygen be used?
- A: Studies have shown decreased mortality in patients using oxygen 24 hours per day compared with patients using supplemental oxygen for only part of the day.
- Q: Should the dosage of oxygen be adjusted during the day according to the patient's activity?
- A: Increasing supplemental oxygen should be considered for activities that require increased oxygen consumption (i.e., exercise, eating, and sleeping).
- Q: Can an echocardiogram replace the need for a cardiac catheterization?
- A: No. Although an abnormal echo can confirm the presence of pulmonary hypertension, it does not inform one of its severity or the (acute) response to therapy. Furthermore, a normal study does not rule out pulmonary hypertension (especially mild cases).

PURPURA FULMINANS

Victoria E. Price • Anthony Chan

BASICS

DESCRIPTION

- Hematologic emergency characterized by dermal hemorrhagic necrosis and disseminated intravascular coagulation (DIC)
- Associated with a congenital or acquired protein C and/or protein S deficiency
- Life-threatening condition that requires prompt diagnosis and judicious replacement therapy to decrease morbidity and mortality

EPIDEMIOLOGY

- Neonatal purpura fulminans related to homozygous protein C deficiency: 1 in 2–4 million births
- Clinical protein C deficiency: 1 in 20,000 individuals
- Homozygous protein S deficiency is exceptionally rare.
- Predicted prevalence of severe protein C deficiency is 1 in 40,000–250,000 individuals. Significantly less seen in practice, likely due to associated high rate of fetal loss and perinatal mortality

RISK FACTORS

Genetics

- Deficiencies of protein C and protein S are autosomally inherited with variable penetrance.
- Over 150 different genetic mutations of protein C have been described, leading to both qualitative and quantitative defects of the proteins.
- Homozygous protein C or S deficiency and compound heterozygous states are associated with severe deficiency, <1% normal activity level.
- Neonatal purpura fulminans is associated with a severe protein C or S deficiency.
- Coinheritance with other thrombophilias may also contribute to the risk of developing purpura fulminans.
- Heterozygous protein C and S deficiency are associated with a lifetime increased risk of venous and arterial thrombosis.

PATHOPHYSIOLOGY

Common features of purpura fulminans:

- DIC: Endothelial injury from bacterial endotoxin or other trigger may initiate secretion of inflammatory cytokines or activation of coagulation and complement proteins.
- Purpura: due to perivascular hemorrhage
- Dermal vascular thrombosis: formation of microthrombosis in blood vessels of the skin, leading to hemorrhage in the skin (purpura), necrosis of skin, and gangrene

ETIOLOGY

- Acquired causes:
  - Severe acute bacterial infections: *Neisseria meningitidis* most common
  - Postinfectious fulminans: most commonly associated with varicella and *Streptococcus* infections. Caused by cross-reacting IgG antibodies that increase protein S clearance from the circulation. Consider in an otherwise well child with new-onset purpura fulminans and DIC.
  - Warfarin (Coumadin)-induced skin necrosis
  - DIC
  - Antiphospholipid antibodies
  - Cardiac bypass
  - Severe liver dysfunction
  - Galactosemia
  - Severe congenital heart disease
- Inherited protein C pathway defects
  - Predisposes to a reduced capacity to inhibit thrombin formation and therefore a hypercoagulable state
- Inherited defect of coagulation presenting as neonatal purpura fulminans
  - Protein C slows ("brakes") the coagulation cascade at two steps: by degrading activated factor V and activated factor VIII.
  - Also plays a role in inflammatory cascade
  - Protein S is a cofactor for protein C.

DIAGNOSIS

HISTORY

- Current bacterial sepsis: fever, weakness, dizziness, nausea, vomiting, onset of petechial rash
- Recent history of febrile illness
- Medications (e.g., warfarin)
- Family history suggestive of hypercoagulable state
- History of consanguinity
- Thromboses at an early age, such as stroke, deep vein thrombosis, pulmonary embolism
- Family members taking warfarin (Coumadin) or low-molecular-weight heparin or other anticoagulant
- Previous affected child with purpura fulminans or hypercoagulable state

PHYSICAL EXAM

- Signs of sepsis:
  - Fever
  - Hypotension
  - Tachycardia
  - Poor perfusion
  - Cool extremities
  - Decreased pulses
  - Shock
- Nonblanching purpura
- Acral purpura and necrosis: Check fingers, nose, toes, and penis for black areas.
- Skin lesions initially appear dark red and then become purple-black. Lesions may be mistaken as bruising.
- Bullae may form over purpuric skin.
- Skin lesions occur at previous sites of trauma (e.g., intravenous cannula insertion).
- Pain, ischemia, and edema of extremities or internal organ dysfunction may result from deep vein thrombosis or arterial thrombosis, depending on location and severity.
- Severe protein C deficiency is associated with cerebral vessel thrombosis, vitreous hemorrhage, and retinal detachment. These complications may occur in utero.
- Physical exam trick: Depress the purpuric area with a glass slide to determine whether it blanches.

DIAGNOSTIC TESTS & INTERPRETATION

Lab

Screening:

- CBC
  - Platelet count may be low.
  - Hemoglobin may be low.
- Smear screen: thrombocytopenia, schistocytes (evidence of microangiopathic hemolysis)
- Prothrombin time and international normalized ratio (INR): prolonged as in DIC
- Partial thromboplastin time: prolonged as in DIC
- Fibrinogen: decreased with consumption and fibrinolysis
- D-dimer: increased fibrinolysis as in DIC

Etiologic:

- Prior to initiation of treatment, collection of citrated plasma sample for functional activity assays for an accurate diagnosis. Confirm the assay that is used (chromogenic vs. functional), as the results may be discrepant.
- Protein C and S activity levels are undetectable in homozygotes.
- Antigen levels may be helpful if interfering factors (e.g., factor V Leiden mutation, antiphospholipid antibodies, direct thrombin inhibitors) are present.
- Genetic testing of the child and family to confirm diagnosis. Initiation of treatment should not depend on the return of these results.
- Protein C activity in patient, parents, and siblings
- Protein S antigen (total and free) in patient, parents, and siblings
- False positives: Protein C and S levels may decrease because of consumption during a thrombotic episode that is not related to an underlying congenital deficiency. Low measurements often need to be repeated at baseline after recovery. Protein C and S levels may be below adult normal ranges for the first 3–6 months of life in healthy infants. Pediatric reference ranges should be used.
- Test for antiphospholipid antibodies: usually lupus anticoagulant or anticardiolipin antibody
- Factor V Leiden mutation assay

Imaging

To document presence and extent of suspected large vessel thrombosis: The most useful imaging strategy depends on location and clinical situation:

- Ultrasound with Doppler flow study
- CT scan
- MRI: better for visualization of vessels
- Angiography: most invasive; requires vascular injury for access
- Imaging is potentially useful to
  - Distinguish thrombosis from other pathology
  - Assess clot size prior to anticoagulant or thrombolytic therapy

DIFFERENTIAL DIAGNOSIS

- Infection
  - *N. meningitidis*, most common infectious cause of purpura fulminans
  - Streptococci
  - *Haemophilus* species

- Staphylococci
- Gram-negative bacteremia: *Escherichia coli*, *Klebsiella*, *Proteus*, *Enterobacter*
- Rickettsia: Rocky Mountain spotted fever
- Varicella
- *Plasmodium falciparum*

- Environmental
  - Warfarin-induced skin necrosis: 1 in 500–1,000 individuals starting warfarin therapy develop necrosis in subcutaneous fat.
  - Thought to be caused by relative depletion of anticoagulant protein C (a vitamin K–dependent factor) during the initial phase of warfarin effect
- Malignancy: myeloid leukemia
- Congenital: inherited deficiencies of protein C and protein S
  - Only severe, homozygous, or compound heterozygous (<1% activity) deficiencies of proteins C and S are associated with purpura fulminans.
  - Milder, heterozygous deficiencies of protein C and protein S as well as other prothrombotic defects all give rise to hypercoagulable states but usually not neonatal purpura fulminans.
  - Patients with 1 or more risk factors for thrombosis may be more likely to develop purpura fulminans with an environmental stimulus.
- Immune mediated: heparin-induced thrombocytopenia: Antibody to heparin–platelet complex causes platelet activation, thrombocytopenia, and microthrombosis, including dermal vessels.
- Postinfectious purpura fulminans: autoimmune-mediated protein S and C deficiency
- Antiphospholipid antibody syndrome: Predisposition to thrombosis can include skin necrosis.
- Miscellaneous
  - Thrombotic thrombocytopenic purpura
  - Paroxysmal nocturnal hemoglobinuria
  - Henoch-Schönlein purpura

TREATMENT

GENERAL MEASURES

- If classical signs of purpura fulminans, therapy should be commenced emergently.
- Treat underlying cause.
- Anti-infective agents depending on underlying cause
- Manage DIC based on clinical and laboratory findings.

MEDICATIONS

- There is no protein S concentrate available. Fresh frozen plasma (FFP) 10–20 mL/kg every 12 hours or cryoprecipitate is used as replacement therapy.
- Protein C replacement therapy: FFP 10–20 mL/kg every 6–12 hours until protein C concentrate available. 1 mL/kg of FFP will increase plasma protein C concentrate by 1 IU/dL. Aim for trough protein C level of 10 IU/dL.
- Protein C concentrates (human plasma derived): initial dose of 100 U/kg followed by 50 U/kg every 6 hours. Aim protein C trough level of 50 IU/dL.
- Recombinant activated Protein C is no longer available.
- Anticoagulation therapy:
  - Start with replacement therapy in the case of severe protein C or S deficiency. Start with unfractionated heparin (UFH) or low-molecular-weight heparin (LMWH). Warfarin should only be started after a few days of UFH/LMWH and overlap to avoid warfarin-induced skin necrosis.
- Maintenance therapy for congenital protein C or S deficiency: prophylaxis with warfarin alone (INR target 2.5–3.5) or protein C concentrate 30–50 IU/kg every 1–3 days with warfarin therapy (INR target 1.5–2.5).
- LMWH has been used for maintenance anticoagulation therapy (target anti-Xa 0.5–1.0 U/mL). The role of other new anticoagulants has not been defined.
- Venous access is challenging. Long-term subcutaneous administration of protein C concentrate is reported.

ONGOING CARE

FOLLOW-UP RECOMMENDATIONS

Patient Monitoring

- When to expect improvement: related to underlying cause of purpura fulminans
- Signs to watch for:
  - Spread of purpura
  - Hypotension
  - Gangrene
- Treatment during the acute phase should continue until all lesions have resolved.
- Referral to ophthalmologist for management and follow-up of ocular lesions
- Monitor INR weekly on maintenance therapy.
- D-dimer can be used as a marker for adequate replacement therapy and anticoagulation. An increasing D-dimer may be the first sign of recurrent purpura fulminans.

DIET

Patients on warfarin therapy may need to avoid foods with high vitamin K content, especially if there is variation in the dose of warfarin required to maintain adequate anticoagulation.

PROGNOSIS

- Related to underlying cause of purpura fulminans
- Overall, poor for homozygous deficiencies of proteins C and S
- Report of cure of protein C deficiency by liver transplantation

COMPLICATIONS

- Skin necrosis and gangrene
- Scarring
- Acral amputations, from tips of digits to whole limbs
- Small and large vessel thrombosis
- Death

ADDITIONAL READING

- Chalmers E, Cooper P, Forman K, et al. Purpura fulminans: recognition, diagnosis and management. *Arch Dis Child*. 2011;96(11):1066–1071.
- de Kort EH, Vrancken SL, van Heijst AF, et al. Long-term subcutaneous protein C replacement in neonatal severe protein C deficiency. *Pediatrics*. 2011;127(5):e1338–e1342.
- Goldenberg NA, Manco-Johnson MJ. Protein C deficiency. *Haemophilia*. 2008;14(6):1214–1221.
- Leclerc F, Leteurtre S, Cremer R, et al. Do new strategies in meningococcemia produce better outcomes? *Crit Care Med*. 2000;28(Suppl 9):S60–S63.
- Patha N, Faust SN, Levin M. Pathophysiology of meningococcal meningitis and septicaemia. *Arch Dis Child*. 2003;88(7):601–607.
- Price VE, Ledingham DL, Krumpel A, et al. Diagnosis and management of neonatal purpura fulminans. *Semin Fetal Neonatal Med*. 2011;16(6):318–322.

CODES

ICD10

- D65 Disseminated intravascular coagulation
- P54.5 Neonatal cutaneous hemorrhage

FAQ

- Q: What is the risk of a 2nd affected child with protein C or S deficiency?
- A: If the diagnosis is confirmed by family studies that show both parents to be carriers of the deficiency and the affected child to be homozygous, there is a 25% chance that each subsequent infant would have purpura fulminans and a 50% chance that each child would be a carrier. However, other hypercoagulable states have been described that may be risk factors for purpura fulminans.
- Q: Should a child with purpura fulminans be followed by a specialist?
- A: Generally yes, with a pediatric hematologist, to assist in acute management of purpura, establishment of diagnosis, and management of long-term anticoagulation.

PYELONEPHRITIS

Michael H. Hsieh

BASICS

DESCRIPTION

Acute pyelonephritis (upper urinary tract infection [UTI]) is a clinical diagnosis that can feature fever, a positive urine culture, and urinary symptoms (e.g., dysuria, frequency/urgency, and/or flank pain). Histologically, acute pyelonephritis results in acute renal parenchymal (interstitial) inflammation secondary to bacterial invasion.

EPIDEMIOLOGY

- UTIs are more likely to involve the upper renal tracts in children <3 years of age.
- UTIs are more common in females, except in uncircumcised males <3 months of age.

Incidence

Cumulative incidence of UTI during the first 6 years of life:

- 6.6% for girls
- 1.8% for boys

Prevalence

- 5–7% of febrile infants <8 weeks of age
- 1% of all school-aged children
- 1–3% of girls between 1 and 5 years of age
- 0.03% in school-aged boys

RISK FACTORS

- Previous history of UTI
- Sibling with a history of UTI
- Female sex
- Indwelling urinary catheter
- Structural abnormalities of the kidneys and lower urinary tract
- Vesicoureteral reflux (VUR): present in ~30–40% of children with febrile UTIs
- The majority (>95%) of VUR associated with febrile UTIs is low to moderate grade (grades I–III). Although, there is a stronger statistical association of febrile UTI with high-grade (grade >IV) VUR.
- Uncircumcised boys <3–6 months of age

PATHOPHYSIOLOGY

Specific factors related to development of pyelonephritis:

- Host related
  - Anatomic abnormalities (e.g., obstruction)
  - Functional abnormalities (e.g., bladder and bowel dysfunction, VUR)
- Pathogen related
  - Adherence factors (P and type 1-fimbriae, adhesins)
  - Virulence factors (e.g., lipopolysaccharide, capsular antigen)
  - Formation of antibiotic- and immune clearance–resistant intracellular bacterial pods within urothelium
- Adhesion of bacteria to uroepithelium induces cytokine release and a subsequent inflammatory response.
- Patchy infiltration of the medullary parenchyma by polymorphonuclear leukocytes and lymphocytes leads to degradation of extracellular matrix, tubular disruption, and interstitial edema.
- Parenchymal scarring may result as a consequence of the infection.

ETIOLOGY

- Enterobacteriaceae: *Escherichia coli* most frequent cause (90% of initial infections and in up to 66% of recurrent infections); *Proteus, Klebsiella, Enterobacter* spp. also implicated
- Gram-positive organisms cause 10–15% of cases: *Staphylococcus aureus, Staphylococcus epidermidis, Staphylococcus saprophyticus, Enterococci* spp.
- Other organisms: *Pseudomonas, Haemophilus influenzae, Streptococcus* group B

COMMONLY ASSOCIATED CONDITIONS

- Struvite kidney stones: associated with urease-producing bacteria (e.g., *Proteus* sp.)
- Anatomic or physiologic abnormality of the collecting system: found in up to 50% of infants with pyelonephritis

DIAGNOSIS

HISTORY

- Fever may be the only presenting complaint.
- In the neonate, inquire caregivers about vomiting, lethargy, poor feeding, irritability, fever, hypothermia, trembling, and jaundice.
- Older children are more likely to present with flank pain, dysuria, frequency, urgency, and incontinence.
- Important factors that predispose to the development of UTI that should be specifically inquired about:
  - Constipation
  - Incorrect toilet training
  - Perineal skin irritation
  - Antibiotic exposure
  - Uncircumcised males
  - Previous UTIs
  - Investigations already performed
  - A family history of UTIs or reflux nephropathy
  - A history of structural abnormalities of the kidneys and/or lower urinary tract
  - Symptoms suggestive of bladder and bowel dysfunction, such as that the bladder always feels full, infrequent use of the toilet, double-voiding, and urgency incontinence
  - Previous surgery or trauma to the back
- Lower motor milestones
- Signs and symptoms:
  - Fever
  - Chills
  - Flank pain
  - Urinary symptoms: dysuria, frequency, urgency

PHYSICAL EXAM

- Findings may be nonspecific.
- Fever, irritability, rigors, lethargy
- Flank tenderness
  - Gentle posterior punch test will reveal tenderness at the costovertebral angle.
  - May be related to underlying renal tract abnormality, such as hydronephrosis; cystic kidney disease; spina bifida, apparent or occult (as evidenced by a dimple); pilonidal sinus; or hemangioma
- Bimanual palpation of kidneys to assess tenderness and size
- Careful neuromuscular exam of lower limbs and back to evaluate for the presence of neurologic abnormalities associated with neurogenic bladder
- Assess rectal tone.

DIAGNOSTIC TESTS & INTERPRETATION

Lab

- Collect urine using sterile methods (e.g., midstream in toilet-trained children, catheter or suprapubic aspiration for infants).
- Urine dipstick for measurement of leukocyte esterase and nitrites as a rapid screen for UTI
- WBC casts on urine microscopy are diagnostic.
- As a screening test, an unspun clean-catch urine specimen with bacteria on stained microscopic exam correlates (80–90%) with culture results exceeding 100,000 colonies/mL.
- Urine for culture and sensitivity: A positive culture result is defined by the growth of a single pathogenic organism of 100,000 colonies/mL in a clean-catch specimen, ≥1,000 colonies/mL in a catheter-acquired specimen, or any growth in a suprapubic specimen.
- CBC with an elevated WBC count
- Erythrocyte sedimentation rate (ESR) and C-reactive protein (CRP) levels are often increased.
- Serum procalcitonin is an emerging biomarker of pyelonephritis.

Imaging

- Renal ultrasound to rule out obstruction and assess renal size and parenchyma if no previous imaging obtained
- Voiding cystourethrogram (VCUG) to rule out anatomic anomalies including obstruction (e.g., posterior urethral valves) and VUR
- ^{99m}Tc-dimercaptosuccinic acid (DMSA) test can be done to confirm the presence of acute pyelonephritis and to look for renal scarring. This is a sensitive and specific test that some clinicians believe to be the imaging study of choice for diagnosing acute pyelonephritis and renal scarring.
- MRI is an emerging imaging modality for pyelonephritis that avoids ionizing radiation.

Diagnostic Procedures/Other
- Imaging evaluation of the urinary tract after a UTI should be individualized based on the child's age, sex, and clinical presentation.
- All children <24 months of age should have an ultrasound.
- It is controversial whether to routinely perform a VCUG in children aged 2 months–2 years with a 1st febrile UTI.
- After the urine is sterile, a VCUG can be performed; there is no need to wait 4 weeks.
- Administer antibiotic prophylaxis before VCUG.

ALERT
- False-positive test results:
  - May be due to nonsterile collection techniques (bagged urine specimen) or allowing urine to stand unrefrigerated
- False-negative test results:
  - The rapid test for nitrites requires urine to stay in the bladder for several hours and is therefore not useful in infants who do not store urine in the bladder.
  - Precollection antibiotic exposure

DIFFERENTIAL DIAGNOSIS
- Cystitis
- Sterile pyuria
  - Vulvovaginitis
  - Balanitis
  - Systemic viral illness
  - Postvaccination
  - Pregnancy
  - Appendicitis
  - Cystic renal disease
  - Tuberculosis
- Lower lobe pneumonia

TREATMENT

MEDICATION
- Initiate broad-spectrum antibiotics. Children who appear toxic, are dehydrated, are <2 months of age, or vomiting should receive IV antibiotics until afebrile for at least 24 hours, then change to an oral formulation.
- In total, 7–14 days of oral and/or IV antibiotic therapy are required.
- Consider low-dose antibiotic prophylaxis until an imaging evaluation is completed for patients with 1st time UTIs.
- Children with frequent symptomatic recurrences of UTI and those with high-grade vesicoureteric reflux may benefit from long-term antibiotic prophylaxis.
- Antibiotics such as co-trimoxazole (Bactrim), amoxicillin–clavulanate (Augmentin), and the 2nd-generation cephalosporins are appropriate initial therapy depending on local resistance patterns.
- Familiarity with local antibiotic patterns of resistance is particularly important in treating hospital-acquired infections.
- Antipyretics (e.g., acetaminophen)

ALERT
- Removing struvite or other infected calculi during active infection may precipitate bacteremia/urosepsis.
- High index of suspicion is required for pyelonephritis associated with cystic renal disease, as urine cultures may be negative when the infection is intracystic.

INPATIENT CONSIDERATIONS
IV Fluids
- May be necessary when children are hospitalized with fever and vomiting to maintain hydration and urine output.
- Underlying anatomic or functional urinary collecting system abnormality should be evaluated/treated by a urologist.

ONGOING CARE

FOLLOW-UP RECOMMENDATIONS
Patient Monitoring
Requirements for testing: Educate caregivers in the symptoms and signs of UTI.

PROGNOSIS
- Fever usually resolves in 3–5 days.
- Ongoing fever or persistent flank pain requires further evaluation to exclude a drug-resistant organism, kidney stone, kidney abscess, or urinary tract obstruction.
- Diagnosis and treatment of any underlying bladder and bowel dysfunction and constipation are required for successful management of UTIs in children.
- Outcome of acute pyelonephritis is usually good but may result in parenchymal scarring.
- Pyelonephritis associated with struvite renal stones requires removal of the infectious stones after antibiotic treatment is completed.
- Risk factors for renal damage include obstruction, reflux with dilation, young age, delay in treatment, number of episodes of pyelonephritis, and bacterial virulence factors.

COMPLICATIONS
- Acute:
  - Reduced concentrating ability, hyperkalemic renal tubular acidosis (transient mineralocorticoid resistance)
  - Bacteremia: highest risk in young infants (23% of children <2 months of age)
  - Perinephric abscess formation
- Chronic:
  - Focal renal scarring, hypertension, proteinuria, azotemia, xanthogranulomatous pyelonephritis

ADDITIONAL READING

- Agarwal S. Vesicoureteral reflux and urinary tract infections. *Curr Opin Urol*. 2000;10(6):587–592.
- Bloomfield P, Hodson EM, Craig JC. Antibiotics for acute pyelonephritis in children. *Cochrane Database Syst Rev*. 2003;(3):CD003772.
- Greenbaum LA, Mesrobian HG. Vesicoureteral reflux. *Pediatr Clin North Am*. 2006;53(3):413–427.
- Hewitt IK, Zucchetta P, Rigon L, et al. Early treatment of acute pyelonephritis in children fails to reduce renal scarring: Data from the Italian Renal Infection Study Trials. *Pediatrics*. 2008;122(3):486–490.
- Hoberman A, Charron M, Hickey RW, et al. Imaging studies after a first febrile urinary tract infection in young children. *N Engl J Med*. 2003;348(3):195–202.
- Keren R, Carpenter M, Greenfield S, et al. Is antibiotic prophylaxis in children with vesicoureteral reflux effective in preventing pyelonephritis and renal scars? A randomized, controlled trial. *Pediatrics*. 2008;122(6):1409–1410.
- Martinell J, Hansson S, Claesson I, et al. Detection of urographic scars in girls with pyelonephritis followed for 13–38 years. *Pediatr Nephrol*. 2000;14(10–11):1006–1010.
- Raszka WV Jr., Khan O. Pyelonephritis. *Pediatr Rev*. 2005;26(10):364–369.
- Subcommittee on Urinary Tract Infection. Urinary tract infection: clinical practice guideline for the diagnosis and management of the initial UTI in febrile infants and children 2 to 24 months. *Pediatrics*. 2011;128(3):595–610.
- Weir M, Brien J. Adolescent urinary tract infections. *Adolesc Med*. 2000;11(2):293–313.

CODES

ICD10
- N12 Tubulo-interstitial nephritis, not spcf as acute or chronic
- N10 Acute tubulo-interstitial nephritis
- N11.9 Chronic tubulo-interstitial nephritis, unspecified

FAQ
- Q: Should a DMSA scan be used to help diagnose acute pyelonephritis?
- A: Routine use of the DMSA scan to diagnose acute pyelonephritis is controversial because disagreement exists about the therapeutic implications of a positive test result, and such routine testing is expensive. Children with hypertension and previous UTIs require a DMSA scan to look for renal cortical scarring.
- Q: Does renal parenchymal scarring occur *without* reflux?
- A: Yes. The causal relationships among reflux, acute pyelonephritis, and renal parenchymal scarring are complex.

PYLORIC STENOSIS

Pradeep P. Nazarey

BASICS

DESCRIPTION

Hypertrophy of the muscular layers of the pylorus with elongation and thickening, leading to projectile nonbilious emesis and gastric outlet obstruction

EPIDEMIOLOGY

- Usually presents between the 3rd and 10th week of life
- Male-to-female ratio 4:1, with first-born males more affected.
- More common in Caucasians

Incidence

~2–4 per 1,000 live births in Western populations

PATHOPHYSIOLOGY

- Marked muscle hypertrophy and hyperplasia primarily involving the circular layer and hyperplasia of the underlying mucosa
- Growth of abnormally contorted and thickened nerve fibers and/or lack of neural elements
- Net result is either partial or complete obstruction of the pyloric channel.

ETIOLOGY

- No definitive causative factors have been identified despite considerable research.
- Genetic predisposition evidenced by variability among races, male preponderance, and genetic syndromes with pyloric stenosis
- Children of affected fathers are affected 3–5%, whereas affected mothers are associated with a 7–20% incidence.
- Several growth factors and gastrointestinal (GI) peptides, including gastrin and elevated acid levels, as well as increases in substance P, EGF, TGFα, and IGF-1, have been implicated.
- Erythromycin estolate given for postexposure prophylaxis for pertussis may cause strong gastric and pyloric contractions that induce hypertrophy. Lactating mothers exposed to erythromycin show babies with increased incidence of pyloric stenosis.
- Decreases in nerve differentiation, reduced density of neural elements, and deficiency of nitric oxide–induced muscle relaxation have been implicated.

COMMONLY ASSOCIATED CONDITIONS

Increased occurrence of esophageal atresia and malrotation was noted in 5% of infants with pyloric stenosis.

DIAGNOSIS

HISTORY

- Emesis
  - Otherwise healthy full-term infant that initially vomits intermittently
  - Over time (approximately 2 weeks), frequency slowly progresses to emesis with nearly every feeding.
  - Emesis becomes forceful or projectile.
  - Color of vomitus will resemble the feeds and is nonbilious.
- Infants look well appearing but act hungry.
- There may be a history of prescription of antireflux medications or formula changes that have no effect on symptoms
- Parents describe a decrease in the frequency of wet diapers.
- As dehydration progresses, infants will become less vigorous and increasingly lethargic.

PHYSICAL EXAM

- Dehydration
  - Infants may have decreased skin turgor, flat fontanelles, and dry mucous membranes.
  - Infants are usually tachycardic and may be hypotensive.
- Abdominal exam
  - Visible peristalsis may be appreciated just after the infant feeds, which is seen as a waveform proceeding from the left upper quadrant toward the pylorus in the right upper quadrant.
  - A palpable, hard, mobile, and nontender mass in the epigastrium to the right of the midline, referred to as an "olive" (palpable 45–75% of cases)
  - Palpation should be attempted after the stomach has been emptied and with the infant quiet and comfortable and can take time.

DIAGNOSTIC TESTS & INTERPRETATION

Lab

- Hypochloremia and metabolic alkalosis
- Hypokalemia
- 2–5% of infants have indirect hyperbilirubinemia associated with jaundice.

Imaging

- Ultrasound
  - Primary modality for diagnosis
  - Ultrasonography identifies the hypertrophic pyloric musculature and identifies wall thickness and channel length.
  - Can see "shoulder sign," which is bulging of hypertrophic muscle into lumen of antrum
  - To confirm the diagnosis, muscle thickness should be >3 mm and pyloric length >15 mm.
- GI studies
  - An upper GI study may be an adjunct if qualified ultrasonographer is unavailable.
  - Can see "string sign" of contrast going through narrowed pyloric channel

DIFFERENTIAL DIAGNOSIS

- Gastroesophageal reflux
- Gastroenteritis
- Milk protein allergy
- Anatomic considerations
  - Malrotation
  - Webs
  - Pyloric atresia
  - Duplications

TREATMENT

INPATIENT CONSIDERATIONS

Initial Stabilization

- Early identification of electrolyte abnormalities and correction with appropriate IV fluids
- Bolus with 10–20 mL/kg of NS
  - Followed by initiation of maintenance fluids of D.45NS + 2 mEq KCl/100 mL at 6 mL/kg/h
  - Goal urine output is >2 mL/kg/h
- Surgery is definitive treatment but is not emergent or urgent. Electrolyte anomalies and alkalosis must be corrected prior to OR.
- Postop feedings usually resume within 4–6 hours after surgery, with spitting up or vomiting common.
- Discharge within 1–2 days

SURGERY/OTHER PROCEDURES

- Pyloromyotomy (Ramstedt procedure): longitudinal incision and spreading of the antropyloric muscle either through an RUQ or umbilical incision
- Laparoscopic pyloromyotomy is safe, feasible, has been gaining traction, and is favored by many surgeons over an open approach.

ONGOING CARE

FOLLOW-UP RECOMMENDATIONS

Vomiting may persist for several days after surgery.

ALERT

- Do not fail to appreciate that alkalosis must be corrected prior to surgery to prevent difficulty with extubation as well as risks of postop apnea and death.
- Infants should undergo aggressive fluid resuscitation.

PROGNOSIS

Morbidity and mortality rates are low; surgery is curative with virtually no recurrence.

COMPLICATIONS

- Dehydration
- Electrolyte abnormalities, primarily hypochloremic, hypokalemic metabolic alkalosis that results from loss of hydrochloric acid and fluid caused by persistent vomiting
- Postoperative complications
  - Incomplete pyloromyotomy
  - Difficult extubation after surgery
  - Postoperative apnea
  - Mucosal injury; may lead to leak and sepsis if not immediately recognized and repaired

ADDITIONAL READING

- Hernanz-Schulman M. Pyloric stenosis: role of imaging. *Pediatr Radiol*. 2009;39(Suppl 2):S134–S139.
- Pantelli C. New insights into the pathogenesis of infantile pyloric stenosis. *Pediatr Surg Int*. 2009; 25(12):1043–1052.
- Pandya S, Heiss K, Hypertrophic pyloric stenosis. *Surg Clinic North Am*. 2012;92(3):527–539.
- Sola J, Neville H. Laparoscopic vs. open pyloromyotomy: a systematic review and meta-analysis. *J Pediatr Surg*. 2009;44(8):1631–1637.

CODES

ICD10

Q40.0 Congenital hypertrophic pyloric stenosis

FAQ

- Q: What is the best initial imaging study to help make the diagnosis?
- A: An abdominal ultrasound is the best initial imaging study to obtain, as the pylorus can be well visualized.
- Q: Why is so much chloride lost?
- A: The chloride loss occurs with the loss of gastric acid, which contains hydrochloric acid.
- Q: What plan should I follow when replacing electrolytes?
- A: Correct the deficiency of fluids with 1.5–2× maintenance fluid volumes. Correct chloride loss with normal saline, and correct potassium loss with potassium chloride.

RABIES

Sergio E. Recuenco

BASICS

DESCRIPTION

Fatal acute viral encephalomyelitis transmitted from animals to humans through bites or exposure to saliva or nervous tissue from a rabid animal. Only mammals are able to contract and transmit the disease.

EPIDEMIOLOGY

- An estimated 55,000 deaths are due to rabies every year in the world, most of them in Asia and Africa. Many of the affected countries do not have proper surveillance systems for rabies.
- Only 1–3 human cases reported annually in the United States. Imported cases infected overseas add 1–3 more cases annually.
- The dog is the main animal reservoir in most of world. In the United States and most developed countries, canine rabies had been eliminated.
- Wildlife such as bats, raccoons, skunk, and foxes are main reservoirs in North America, with frequent spillover to cats, dogs, and other domestic animals.
- All of the continental United States is enzootic for bat rabies, whereas transmission among terrestrial reservoirs occurs in specific geographic regions such as the Eastern United States (raccoon); south central, north central areas, and the state of California (skunk); south west (fox); Alaska (Arctic fox); and Puerto Rico (mongoose).
- Hawaii is considered rabies-free.

Incidence

- From 2003 to 2013, there were 24 cases of rabies acquired in the United States, 19 of these were associated with bat rabies strains, 3 with raccoon rabies, 1 with mongoose rabies, and 1 of unknown origin.
- 30% of the cases were 18 years old or below.
- A total of 5 rabies cases were due to organ transplant.
- The real burden of human rabies exposure in the United States is unknown, but 36,000 individuals are estimated to receive postexposure prophylaxis (PEP) every year across the country.
- Wildlife accounts for 92% of all animal rabies cases; raccoons continue as the most frequent species (32%), followed by bats (27%), skunks (25%), foxes (6%), and other wildlife (2%).

RISK FACTORS

- Travel to areas where canine rabies is endemic
- Recent scratch or bite from known animal reservoir species including bats or other wildlife; exposure from an unvaccinated domestic animal (e.g., cat, dog) without the ability for appropriate management
- Transmission from transplanted corneas, vessels, and solid organs has occurred.
- Working with animals (e.g., veterinarians) or working in a laboratory with the virus
- Outdoor occupations and recreational activities that increase contact with high-risk species
- Mass exposures to potentially rabid animals (e.g., bats, cats) may occur in summer camps, county fairs (e.g., rabid goat), petting zoos (e.g., rabid sheep), schools, and public events.

GENERAL PREVENTION

- Targeted to humans and domestic animals
- Immunoprophylaxis: Preexposure rabies prophylaxis (Pre-EP) is offered to those at high risk (e.g., veterinarians, animal handlers, trappers, travelers to high-risk regions).
- Avoid unnecessary contact with wild animals in the United States and overseas.
- Pets should be vaccinated and kept updated on their immunizations.

PATHOPHYSIOLOGY

- Except for rare cases, the rabies virus enters the body through a bite that breaks the skin and introduces infected saliva:
  - From there, the virus gains access to muscle, where it is sequestered.
  - The virus then enters the peripheral nerves, where it moves centripetally to the CNS at a rate of ~3 mm/h.
  - Once in the CNS, infection spreads rapidly throughout many areas of the brain.
  - Neurologic manifestations progress rapidly from sensorial alterations to coma.
  - Leads to autonomic instability, the mechanisms of which are still poorly understood, which leads to acute death
- Average incubation period is 2–3 weeks to 2–3 months and, in rare cases, is suspected to be several to many years, with the longest documented incubation being 8 years.

ETIOLOGY

The 14 known members of the *Lyssavirus* genus, rhabdovirus family (rabies virus, Lagos bat virus, Mokola virus, Duvenhage virus, Aravan virus, Irkut virus, Khujand virus, European bat lyssavirus types 1 and 2, West Caucasian bat virus, Australian bat lyssavirus, Shimoni bat virus, Ikoma virus, and Bokeloh virus) are suspected to be capable of causing human rabies death. Lyssaviruses are single-stranded RNA viruses, and all except Mokola had been associated with bats. Most cases are due to the rabies virus, with rare cases due to the other lyssaviruses.

DIAGNOSIS

HISTORY

- Behavior of animal: Although signs of rabies in animals vary greatly, atypical behavior for the animal is the norm (e.g., passive animals become aggressive, nocturnal animals roam in daylight).
  - Excessive salivation and lack of coordination may be present.
- Probably due to long incubation periods, some human rabies cases lack a history of animal contact probably because the contact may have seemed trivial at the time (i.e., from a small bat).
- Assessment for postexposure prophylaxis considers risk of rabies in the species, clinical presentation of the exposing animal, route and severity of exposure, and availability of the animal for observation or testing.
- Signs and symptoms
  - Prodrome: 2–10 days with vague and insidious symptoms (e.g., sore throat, malaise, anxiety, change of behavior, hallucinations, fever). Other prodromal symptoms observed are itching, pain, or tingling at the site of the bite.
  - Acute neurologic phase: furious (80%) versus paralytic (20%) rabies
    - Furious rabies: agitation, hyperactivity, bizarre behavior, nuchal rigidity, sore throat, and hoarseness. The pathognomonic sign is hydrophobia and, at times, aerophobia.
    - Paralytic rabies: Initial finding is flaccid paralysis in the limb that was bitten; subsequently spreads to other limbs. Cranial nerve involvement can give complete lack of facial affect.
    - Coma: Onset follows acute neurologic phase; may persist up to 2 weeks and is followed by death almost universally

PHYSICAL EXAM

- Although neurologic findings can vary, cranial nerve paralysis (e.g., palate, vocal cords) is common. Therefore, hoarseness and stridor may occur.
- Meningismus is also fairly common, along with involuntary movements. Beyond this, findings depend on type of presentation (furious vs. paralytic).
- Imaging (e.g., MRI, CT) is unremarkable or unspecific.

DIAGNOSTIC TESTS & INTERPRETATION

Lab

- Existing diagnostic methods for rabies virus infection are not useful before the onset of clinical signs. However, after signs appear, human antemortem laboratory diagnosis is possible with a set of 4 samples: serum, CSF, skin biopsy of at the hairline at the back of the neck, and fresh saliva. All 4 samples need to be taken on the same day and shipped express on dry ice. The following standard methods are used to rule out rabies:
  - Reverse transcription PCR for rabies RNA detection in saliva and skin
  - Direct fluorescent antibody test (DFA) on cryostat sections of the skin biopsy
  - Virus-neutralizing antibody detection in CSF and serum with RFFIT
  - Indirect fluorescent antibody test on CSF and sera to detect IgM and IgG that may bind to rabies virus antigens present in infected cell culture
- Postmortem diagnosis is made by DFA and PCR in samples from brainstem, cerebellum, and sometimes other samples.

DIFFERENTIAL DIAGNOSIS

- Other causes of encephalitis to consider: herpes simplex virus, enterovirus, West Nile virus, and other arbovirus encephalitis; Rocky Mountain spotted fever and other rickettsial encephalitis; Japanese encephalitis; Guillain-Barré syndrome; limbic encephalitis; tetanus; acute disseminated encephalitis; *Bartonella* encephalitis
- Other conditions can mimic rabies: delirium tremens, cocaine overdose, amphetamine overdose, and acute psychosis
- Case reports of rabies wrongly diagnosed as cerebral malaria exist in countries with high malaria risk.

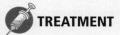

TREATMENT

MEDICATION

- Immunization: Both passive and active immunization should be initiated concurrently when an exposure is identified. Local or state health departments can advise about the risk of specific animal exposures.
- Passive
  - Human rabies immune globulin (HRIG) derived from the plasma of volunteers hyperimmunized with rabies vaccine
  - The present recommendation for HRIG vaccination is 20 IU/kg instilled locally into the tissue at the site of the bite.
    - Remaining HRIG can be given IM, avoiding the arm in which the rabies vaccine (RV) is administered.
    - In cases of multiple wounds, to ensure that all wounds receive an injection of HRIG, dilution in saline (2–3-fold) is acceptable.
    - HRIG is only administered the day 0 of the PEP schedule simultaneously to the first dose of RV. In case not available at the same time of first dose of RV, still can be administered until day 7; after that, it is not necessary.
- Active
  - Two RVs are licensed in the United States: human diploid cell rabies vaccine (HDCV) and purified chick embryo cell vaccine (PCEC).
  - For Pre-Ep, the recommended schedule is 1 mL of RV IM dose in the deltoid area on days 0, 7, and 21 or 28. No HRIG is used.
  - For PEP, the current schedule in the United States is 1 mL of RV IM in the deltoid region on days 0, 3, 7, and 14. For immunocompromised patients, an additional dose on day 28 is given. The anterolateral thigh can be used in infants or young children.
- Discontinue the vaccine series if fluorescent antibody testing of the brain of the biting animal is conducted and result is negative, or if it is a cat, dog, or ferret healthy after a period of 10 days of observation after the bite.

INPATIENT CONSIDERATIONS

Initial Stabilization

Local wound care immediately after bite

- The 1st step in preventing infection is washing out the virus mechanically or inactivating it before it has a chance to attach to and enter susceptible cells.
- The wound should be flushed with copious amounts of soap and water or saline solution.
- For puncture wounds, insertion of a catheter (i.e., angiocatheter) and irrigation with fluid by means of an attached syringe should be performed. If irrigation is too painful, infiltration of the area with local anesthetic can help.

For symptomatic patients after incubation period

- Request antemortem rule out rabies tests.
- Palliative and supportive care should be made available in an intensive care unit.
- Consider experimental therapies (e.g., induced coma) in selected patients (e.g., early rabies confirmation, young age).

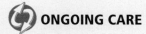

ONGOING CARE

PROGNOSIS

- After the patient CNS is infected with the rabies virus, prognosis is poor. There is no medical therapy available once the encephalitis onset, and after that, PEP is no longer indicated.
- Without PEP before clinical presentation, the disease is fatal with very rare survivors.
- 10% of patient survival had been observed following intensive care and induced coma (see www.mcw.edu/rabies) attempted in about 50 of cases. Three of 7 survivors using this regimen are still alive; the other patients survived the acute illness but died of complications during rehabilitation.

ADDITIONAL READING

- Dyer JL, Wallace R, Orciari L, et al. Rabies surveillance in the United States during 2012. *J Am Vet Med Assoc*. 2013;243(6):805–815.
- Feder HM Jr, Petersen BW, Robertson KL, et al. Rabies: still a uniformly fatal disease? Historical occurrence, epidemiological trends, and paradigm shifts. *Curr Infect Dis Rep*. 2012;14(4):408–422.
- Manning SE, Rupprecht CE, Fishbein D, et al. Human rabies prevention—United States, 2008: recommendations of the Advisory Committee on Immunization Practices. *MMWR Recomm Rep*. 2008;57(RR-3):1–28.
- National Association of State Public Health Veterinarians, Inc. Compendium of animal rabies prevention and control, 2011. *MMWR Recomm Rep*. 2011;60(RR-6):1–17.
- Warrell MJ. Current rabies vaccines and prophylaxis schedules: preventing rabies before and after exposure. *Travel Med Infect Dis*. 2012;10(1):1–15.
- World Health Organization. WHO expert consultation on rabies. Second report. *World Health Organ Tech Rep Ser*. 2013;(982):1–139.

CODES

ICD10

- A82.9 Rabies, unspecified
- Z20.3 Contact with and (suspected) exposure to rabies

FAQ

- Q: Does a wild squirrel or rabbit bite necessitate rabies prophylaxis?
- A: In general, rodents (e.g., squirrels, rats, mice, hamsters, gerbils, etc.), lagomorphs (e.g., rabbits and hares), and marsupials are not known to serve as natural rabies reservoirs. They should not be considered rabid unless they exhibit unusual behavior.
- Q: Is there any evidence of human-to-human spread?
- A: No. However, health care workers or others exposed to a patient with known or suspected rabies should receive vaccination if they have suffered a bite wound or if mucosal surfaces or open wounds have been exposed to the patient's body fluids.
- Q: Are there any countries that require "routine rabies vaccination"?
- A: Yes, Nepal. Recently, Peru and Ecuador started mandatory vaccination programs restricted to very high-risk areas in Amazonia.
- Q: What if a severe allergic reaction occurs during postexposure rabies prophylaxis?
- A: The reaction should be treated at the time as you would any systemic anaphylactic reaction. PEP should continue after that using a different RV and taking additional precautions. The two RVs licensed in the United States (PCECV, HDCV) are interchangeable if indicated.
- Q: If a bat is found in the house, should the family members receive immunoprophylaxis?
- A: If a bat is found in the room of a sleeping person, previously unattended child, or mentally compromised person, it should be tested. If the bat escapes, prophylaxis should be considered case by case. The injury inflicted by a bat bite or scratch may not be obvious.

RECTAL PROLAPSE

Joel Friedlander

BASICS

DESCRIPTION

There are three types of rectal prolapse:

- Complete: Full thickness of rectum prolapses through anus (2 layers of rectum with an intervening peritoneal sac, which may contain small bowel).
- Incomplete/mucosal: prolapse limited to only 2 layers of mucosa
- Concealed: internal intussusception of upper rectum into lower, with no extrusion into the anus

EPIDEMIOLOGY

- Most cases occur in children <4 years of age around time of toilet training; equal incidence in boys and girls
- In older children and adults, strong (6-fold) female predilection
- Common in developing countries, perhaps because of poor nutrition and parasitic infection; less common in the Western world

RISK FACTOR

- Cystic fibrosis
  - Typically presents between 6 months and 3 years of age in patients with cystic fibrosis (CF)
  - Incidence is 20%.
  - Presentation in children with CF >5 years of age is rare.

ETIOLOGY

Exact etiology uncertain, but the following are usually related findings and predisposing conditions:

- Excessive straining with bowel movements from constipation and toilet training (hips and knees flexed) is the most common cause in the Western world.
- Diarrhea; may be more of a cause in tropical and subtropical countries
- Infections: hookworms and other parasitic infections
- Malnutrition; can cause loss of the ischiorectal fat pad
- Complication of past surgery, such as imperforate anus repair
- Complete prolapse is rare in children, but when it occurs, it may be related to poor fixation of rectum to sacrum and to weak pelvic and anal musculature.
- CF
- Ulcerative colitis
- Hirschsprung disease
- Ehlers-Danlos syndrome
- Meningomyelocele
- Pertussis
- Rectal polyp
- Pneumonia
- Anorexia
- Rectal neoplasm

Genetics

- Inheritance patterns depend on associated underlying etiologies.
- No known inheritance pattern for idiopathic rectal prolapse.

DIAGNOSIS

HISTORY

- Signs and symptoms:
  - Protrusion of rectal layers through anus, usually found during defecation or attempted defecation
  - Although the history of rectal prolapse may be evident, it is often difficult to elicit on examination, and by the time the patient is seen after a prolapse at home, it may already be spontaneously reduced. Thus, the assumption of the diagnosis may have to rest primarily on the parental history.
  - Although usually benign, rectal prolapse is distressing to both the parents and the child.
- Assess for symptoms of CF, risk factors for CF, or for symptoms of other associated conditions (infection, malnutrition, etc.).
- Suggest pictures to be taken by family when it occurs.
- Often reduces spontaneously; if not, can instruct parents to attempt reduction manually
- Rectal prolapse may cause some discomfort during bowel movements.
- Trauma to the recurrently prolapsed mucosa may lead to ulceration and mucus discharge.

PHYSICAL EXAM

- Usually, prolapse is not seen on examination while the patient is at rest, unless it is irreducible (dark or bright red mass protruding from child's anus without discomfort).
- May see poor anal tone and/or large anal orifice, especially within hours after the prolapse
- In complete rectal prolapse, concentric mucosal rings can be seen, whereas incomplete (mucosal) prolapse reveals radial folds.
  - If clinician sees >5 cm of rectum emerging, it is most likely a complete prolapse.
  - Asking the patient to strain may allow the mucosa to prolapse. However, this may be challenging in young patients.
- If prolapsed mucosa visualized, insert a finger around the prolapsing apex of the intussusception, between it and the lining of the anal canal.
- Will appear different from a polyp, which is generally plum-colored and does not involve the entire anal circumference

DIAGNOSTIC TESTS & INTERPRETATION

Lab

- Sweat test
  - All children with rectal prolapse should have a sweat test to rule out CF.
  - Complete CF genetic testing can be considered but is more costly.
- Stool cultures for bacterial and parasitic infestations
- Other tests for the aforementioned conditions as clinically indicated

Imaging

- Evacuation proctography
  - A barium enema is given, and movement of barium is observed under fluoroscopy during defecation.
  - This study may reveal an internal prolapse not easily recognizable on physical examination.
  - This study is not commonly used in children because full cooperation is essential.
- Consider AP/lateral lumbosacral imaging to evaluate for spinal fusion anomalies.

DIFFERENTIAL DIAGNOSIS

- Tumors
- Prolapsing rectal tumor
- Trauma
- Sexual abuse (e.g., result of anal penetration)
- Metabolic
- CF: From 10 to 50% of patients diagnosed with CF, >4 years of age have experienced rectal prolapse (either at the time of the diagnosis or as a past event), but few individuals with rectal prolapse have CF.
- Anatomic abnormality (such as absence of Houston valves in infants)
- Solitary rectal ulcer syndrome: An uncommon benign condition usually affecting older children that involves rectal bleeding on defecation is common.
- Prolapsing polyp
- Large hemorrhoids
- Colonic intussusception
- Constipation
- Ehlers-Danlos syndrome
- Hirschsprung disease
- History of imperforate anus
- Pertussis/pneumonia
- Ulcerative colitis
- Meningomyelocele

TREATMENT

MEDICATION

- Stool softeners (i.e., docusate, polyethylene glycol) to relieve constipation or medication with the associated condition
- In patients with CF, optimization of pancreatic enzyme supplementation. Associated with significant improvement in rectal prolapse in this population

ADDITIONAL TREATMENT

General Measures

- Rectal prolapse in children <4 years of age has strong tendency to resolve spontaneously over time (90%).
- Patients who develop rectal prolapse at >4 years of age have less certain prognosis.
- Patients who present with a prolapsed rectum should undergo manual reduction in a prone position:
  - Parents should be provided with gloves and lubricant and taught how to reduce the prolapse.
  - The prolapsed bowel may be grasped with lubricated gloved fingers and pushed back in with gentle steady pressure.
  - If the bowel has become edematous, firm steady pressure for several minutes may be necessary to reduce the swelling and allow for reduction.
  - Digital rectal examination should always follow this procedure to verify complete reduction.
  - If the prolapse immediately recurs, it may be reduced again and the buttocks taped together for several hours.
- The prolapse will resolve more successfully and quickly if the patient is treated for constipation:
  - This should include both dietary manipulations (e.g., increased fiber, hydration) and improved defecation methods.
  - It also will usually require the use of supplemental aids such as laxatives (polyethylene glycol).
- A small child should try to defecate with his or her hips at 90 degrees, his or her buttocks at toilet seat level, and on an appropriately sized toilet.
- In the rare case of stool infection with diarrhea as the underlying etiology, the appropriate therapy for that infection should be instituted.

SURGERY/OTHER PROCEDURES

Numerous (>130) approaches have been attempted and advocated with varying degrees of enthusiasm, suggesting that none is perfect. Across all procedures, including as follows, efficacy is higher in older patients >4 years old:

- Perianal sutures: poor results and high complication rate
- Delorme procedure: Rectal mucosa is excised, and underlying rectal muscle is plicated with sutures.
- Laparoscopic suture rectopexy: Rectal wall is exposed and then sutured to the fascia of the sacral promontory; 5% full thickness recurrence rate
- Abdominal rectopexy: Rectum is mobilized and attached to the sacrum by prosthetic material. Although the procedure provides good results, it has a high complication rate of constipation (>50%).
- Anterior resection rectopexy: resection of the sigmoid loop and upper rectum; good results, but again, high complication rate
- Perineal resection: perineal rectosigmoidectomy with a coloanal anastomosis; good results
- Circumferential injection procedures (90–100% success rate): injection of phenol, oil, hypertonic saline, dextrose 50% solution (500 g/L), or ethyl alcohol to promote adhesion and stabilization of the rectum
- Lockhart–Mummery operation (near 100% success): Mesh pack is placed temporarily in the retrorectal space (8–10 days) to promote adhesions that stabilize rectum.

INPATIENT CONSIDERATIONS

Initial Stabilization

Palliative

- Reassurance of patient and/or family and caregivers
- Teaching around techniques of manual reduction
- Education regarding pros and cons of surgery, which may appear to offer more definite solution, but are not without risk and may lead to further complications. In most cases, it may be more prudent to allow time and medical management to solve the problem.

ONGOING CARE

FOLLOW-UP RECOMMENDATIONS

Ongoing Treatment

- Treatment of constipation should continue indefinitely, or until the child has demonstrated regular bowel habits on a high-fiber diet on his or her own without evidence of prolapse for at least several months.
- Intermittent parental observation to ensure child is avoiding straining with defecation

DIET

- Increase consumption of liquids.
- Add larger amounts of fiber to diet (goal: 5 g + age in years = total g/day fiber intake).

PROGNOSIS

- With proper medical management, there is an excellent prognosis, defined as resolution without surgery.
- May require months to years on a good dietary and behavioral regimen

COMPLICATIONS

- In some older patients who may also have an overactive external sphincter, the need to generate high rectal pressures to defecate, together with the rectal prolapse, may cause venous congestion and solitary rectal ulcer syndrome.
- Repetitive trauma to mucosa can produce proctitis.
- Surgical complications of repair
- Frequent recurrence

ADDITIONAL READING

- Akkoyun I, Akbiyik F, Soylua SG. The use of digital photos and video images taken by a parent in the diagnosis of anal swelling and anal protrusions in children with normal physical exam. *J Pediatr Surg*. 2011;46(11):2132–2134.
- Antao B, Bradley V, Roberts JP, et al. Management of rectal prolapse in children. *Dis Colon Rectum*. 2005;48(8):1620–1625.
- Chan WK, Kay SM, Laberge JM, et al. Injection sclerotherapy in the treatment of rectal prolapse in infants and children. *J Pediatr Surg*. 1998;33(2):255–258.
- Laituri CA, Garey CL, Fraser JD, et al. 15-year experience in the treatment of rectal prolapse in children. *J Pediatr Surg*. 2010;45(8):1607–1609.
- Potter DD, Bruny JL, Allshouse MJ, et al. Laparoscopic suture rectopexy for full-thickness anorectal prolapse in children: an effective outpatient procedure. *J Pediatr Surg*. 2010;45(10):2103–2107.
- Sajid MS, Siddiqui MR, Baig MK. Open vs laparoscopic repair of full-thickness rectal prolapse: a re-meta-analysis. *Colorectal Dis*. 2010;12(6):515–525.
- Siafakas C, Vottler TP, Andersen JM. Rectal prolapse in pediatrics. *Clin Pediatr (Phila)*. 1999;38(2):63–72.

CODES

ICD10

K62.3 Rectal prolapse

FAQ

- Q: What should I do if my child has a rectal prolapse but I cannot reduce it?
- A: You should wrap the prolapse in moist towels and bring your child to the emergency department. Physicians there will try to reduce it. Rarely, if a prolapse is irreducible and left for a period of time, it can cause bowel ischemia and may require surgery.
- Q: My child has rectal prolapse and now he is supposed to have a sweat test to determine whether he has CF. Is this very likely?
- A: No. Although it is important to rule out this disease, most patients with rectal prolapse do not have CF. However, many children with CF suffer from rectal prolapse.
- Q: My child, who has rectal prolapse, is in day care. How will I know if he is having the prolapse?
- A: You should inform someone in the school (a teacher or guardian) of his condition, and he or she should check the child for prolapse after a bowel movement. Although, if present, it usually resolves spontaneously, the teacher should inform you so you can do a manual reduction, if necessary.

REFRACTIVE ERROR

Leah G. Reznick

BASICS

DESCRIPTION

- Refractive errors are abnormalities in the optical components of the eyes that cause light not to be focused on the retinal plane. In order for a person to have clear vision, light entering the eye must precisely focus on the retina.
  - Uncorrected refractive errors blur vision in one or both eyes.
  - If left untreated in children, uncorrected refractive errors may cause permanent vision loss from amblyopia and strabismus (see "Amblyopia" and "Strabismus").
- Refractive errors are measured in diopter units.
- Refractive errors can be classified in three groups based on the optic effects (Appendix, Figure 1):
  - Myopia (near-sightedness): Objects are focused in front of the retinal plane. Near vision is clearer and distance vision is more blurry. Optical correction is with concave lenses (negative power).
  - Hyperopia (far-sightedness): Objects are focused behind the retinal plane and optical correction contains convex lens (plus power).
  - Astigmatism: Unequal curvature of the cornea causing the cornea to be more curved in one direction than another (aspherical). The shape of the cornea is more like a football than a basketball in astigmatism.
    - Images are blurred at near and far distances.
    - Astigmatism can occur concomitantly with myopia and hyperopia.
- Other terms related to refractive error include the following:
  - Emmetropia: No refractive error. Objects are focused on the retinal plane.
  - Anisometropia: Unequal refractive error between the two eyes that increases the risk of amblyopia
- Accommodation: the changing of the shape of the eye's lens to focus clearly at near or all of the time in hyperopes

EPIDEMIOLOGY

Prevalence of refractive errors varies during childhood as the optical components change with development. At birth, usual median refractive error is low hyperopia, approximately +2.00 diopters. In adults, the median is emmetropia; approximately 30% require optical correction.

Prevalence

- In children aged 5–17 years, the prevalence of visually significant refractive error varies on type.
  - Myopia = 0.7–5.0%
  - Hyperopia = 4.0–9.0%
  - Astigmatism = 0.5–3%
- The prevalence and type of refractive error varies among ethnic groups. For example, people of Native American, Chinese, and Japanese descent have an increased prevalence of myopia.

RISK FACTORS

Genetics

- Both genetic and environmental factors are important in refractive status. ~60% of myopia can be predicted by parental degree of refraction.
- There is an increased prevalence of visually significant refractive errors in individuals with prematurity, autism, and cerebral palsy.
- Some genetic syndromes or medical problems associated with refractive errors include the following:
  - Myopia is associated with Stickler, Marfan, Down, and Ehlers-Danlos syndromes.
  - Hyperopia is associated with Senior-Loken syndrome, WAGR (Wilms tumor, aniridia, genitourinary malformations, mental retardation) syndrome, and Down syndrome.
  - Astigmatism is associated with Down syndrome, craniofacial abnormalities, and albinism.
  - Environmental factors associated with refractive error include prematurity, eye surgery, and trauma.

GENERAL PREVENTION

- Early detection and correction of refractive errors is important to prevent amblyopia and strabismus. A child should be able to perform a visual acuity examination by age 4 years.
- Children with significant refractive errors are often asymptomatic. All children should be screened for visual acuity in each eye.
- Glasses may not improve vision alone because of amblyopia (maldevelopment of the brain's ocular cells). Patients with suspected amblyopia should be rechecked even if wearing glasses.

PATHOPHYSIOLOGY

- The three most important determinants of refractive error include the cornea, lens, and axial length of the eye. The cornea and lens bend light to meet the retina in order to create a sharply focused image. The optical power of the cornea and lens must match the actual eye length (distance from cornea to retina). If the cornea and lens do not bend light to hit the retina, there is a refractive error and can blur the vision.
- Small amounts of hyperopia are normal for children. With small hyperopic errors, a child's eye can easily bring objects into clear focus by adjusting the shape of the lens (accommodation). These children have no problems seeing at far or near distances.
- With larger amounts of hyperopia (greater than +3.50 diopters), a child's vision may be blurred at distance and near because accommodation may be limited or cause esotropia (see "Strabismus").
- The refractive components evolve as the eye develops over childhood. The cornea, lens, and eye length should simultaneously develop to lead to emmetropia. Factors determining the normal and abnormal growth of eye are not completely understood.
- There are likely genetic and environmental factors determining the growth of the eye. There may be an association with increased level of education and increased incidence of myopia. Epidemiologic data suggest that increased amount of time spent outdoors protects against the development of myopia.

COMMONLY ASSOCIATED CONDITIONS

Refractive errors are frequently associated with other ocular conditions.

- Anisometropia is associated with nasolacrimal duct obstruction.
- Myopia is associated with childhood glaucoma, deprivation amblyopia, retinopathy of prematurity, retinal dystrophies, coloboma, and retinal detachments.
- Hyperopia is associated with esotropia, Leber congenital amaurosis, and aphakia (absence of lens).
- Astigmatism is associated with ptosis, coloboma, glaucoma, retinopathy of prematurity, lid hemangioma, nystagmus, and limbal dermoid.

DIAGNOSIS

SIGNS AND SYMPTOMS

- Blurred vision
- Headache
- Squinting
- Torticollis
- Strabismus

HISTORY

- Age of onset of vision loss
- History of headaches, squinting, or subjective vision problems
- Associated ocular abnormalities, trauma, injury, or surgery
- History of strabismus, amblyopia
- History of prematurity, genetic disorders
- Family history of strabismus, amblyopia, congenital cataract, ocular or systemic genetic disease

PHYSICAL EXAM

- Age appropriate vision screening is the most effective diagnostic tool for detecting refractive errors.
- Vision must be tested with each eye separately (patch or occluder over one eye).
- In children younger than 3 years of age:
  - Monocular testing for fixing and following will determine visual behavior for each eye.
  - Brückner (simultaneous red reflex) examination with the direct ophthalmoscope can objectively identify high refractive errors (distorted or darkened red reflex) or anisometropia (asymmetric brightness of red reflex).
- In children age 3 years or older:
  - Subjective visual acuity should be testing with matching or identifying optotypes on a vision chart (Allen figures, HOTV, Lea, or Snellen).
  - A failed vision screening or untestable vision after 2 attempts warrants a referral to an eye care provider.
- Vision screenings are important at regular intervals throughout childhood to prevent vision loss.
- Strabismus is frequently a secondary sign of refractive error in children and can be detected by cover test, Hirschberg corneal light reflex test, or Brückner test.
- Photoscreening, which uses the principle of red reflex testing, is also effective in detecting high or asymmetric refractive errors.

DIFFERENTIAL DIAGNOSIS

- Decreased binocular or monocular vision can be caused by a number of structural abnormalities of the eye as well as decreased cortical visual development. In any child with vision loss, refractive error needs to be evaluated as the cause or one of many factors contributing to decreased vision.
- True refractive error needs to be measured by only after instilling cycloplegic eye drops with retinoscopy (objective technique to measure refractive error). Without these drops, a child's lens will accommodate (change shape) and give a false amount of refractive error.

TREATMENT

GENERAL MEASURES

- Refractive errors are treated by corrective lenses. Young children typically use glasses and teenagers may use contact lenses.
- The following guidelines for prescribing glasses have been developed to improve visual acuity and reduce the risk of amblyopia and strabismus.
  - Myopia: >3.00 diopters for age 2–3 years and >1.00 diopter or more in school-age children
  - Hyperopia: +4.50 diopters or more for age 2–3 years, +3.00 diopters or more in school-age children, or +1.50 diopters or more anisometropia
  - Astigmatism: >2.00 diopters in age 2–3 years or >1.50 diopters in school-age children
- If hyperopic correction is needed for treatment but is not well accepted by the child, a brief period of cycloplegia with topical atropine can increase usage of glasses.
- In suspected amblyopia, vision should be retested to measure visual improvement after glasses have been worn for several weeks
- Hyperopic patients may develop esotropia when their glasses are taken off. Full-time glasses usage will prevent loss of vision and depth perception when children have accommodative esotropia.

ONGOING CARE

Because refractive error depends on the eye's shape and the eye's shape changes as a child grows, the refractive error will evolve over time. Because this process is dynamic, children require at least an annual vision evaluation and refraction to assess whether they need a change in their glasses. They also need to be evaluated for amblyopia and strabismus.

PROGNOSIS

If a child has a significant refractive error, his or her visual acuity will likely improve with optical correction. Refractive error rarely leads to significant functional limitations for daily activities and school. If refractive errors accompany other vision problems such as amblyopia or strabismus, other treatments may be needed to improve visual acuity. Special frames for athletic activities should be considered for children if standard glasses are interfering with those activities.

COMPLICATIONS

In children, the most significant complications of uncorrected refractive errors are strabismus and amblyopia.

- Accommodative esotropia
  - For children with moderate to high hyperopia, their eyes will normally accommodate (change shape of lens) to bring objects into focus.
  - This accommodative process may involuntarily cause overconvergence of the eyes and thus esotropia.
  - Small amounts of convergence normally occur with accommodation so that both eyes can be looking at a near target. But in children with accommodative esotropia, they cannot control the degree of convergence and develop esotropia when focusing at both distance and near.
- Refractive amblyopia is poor cortical visual development resulting from a poorly focused image in one or both eyes.
  - Anisometropia (unequal refractive error) is the most frequent cause of unilateral amblyopia (~35%). The brain learns to see well from the eye that has the least amount of refractive error but does not develop equal vision from the eye that has a higher refractive error.
- Bilateral high refractive errors may cause bilateral amblyopia from chronically poor visual input from both eyes.
- High myopia (>5 diopters) can lead to retinal thinning and eventual retinal detachment. It is also associated with increased risk of glaucoma and cataracts as an adult.

ADDITIONAL READING

- American Academy of Ophthalmology. *Preferred Practice Pattern: Refractive Errors*. San Francisco: American Academy of Ophthalmology; 2013.
- American Academy of Ophthalmology Pediatric Ophthalmology/Strabismus Panel. *Preferred Practice Pattern Guidelines. Pediatric Eye Evaluations*. San Francisco: American Academy of Ophthalmology; 2012.
- Bell AL, Rodes ME, Kellar LC. Childhood eye examination. *Am Fam Physician*. 2013;88(4):241–248.
- Paysse EA, Williams GC, Coats DK, et al. Detection of red reflex asymmetry by pediatric residents using the Brückner reflex versus the MTI photoscreener. *Pediatrics*. 2001;108(4):E74.
- Thorn F. Development of refraction and strabismus. *Curr Opin Ophthalmol*. 2000;11(5):301–305.
- Wen G, Tarczy-Hornoch K, McKean-Cowdin R, et al. Prevalence of myopia, hyperopia, and astigmatism in non-Hispanic white and Asian children: multi-ethnic pediatric eye disease study. *Ophthalmology*. 2013;120(10):2109–2116.

CODES

ICD10

- H52.7 Unspecified disorder of refraction
- H52.10 Myopia, unspecified eye
- H52.209 Unspecified astigmatism, unspecified eye

FAQ

- Q: Will my child always need glasses?
- A: Not necessarily. As children grow, the shape of the eyes change. Because the need for glasses depend on the eye's shape, it is unclear whether the child will continue to need glasses to have normal vision as his or her eye develops. If optical correction remains necessary, contact lenses and refractive surgery are also possible in older children or adults.
- Q: Will wearing glasses weaken my child's eyes?
- A: No. Glasses change the way light enters the eye to focus on the retina and optimize vision. Glasses do not weaken the eyes or vision. Glasses are important to prevent amblyopia and permanent vision loss.
- Q: If my child wears glasses and his or her vision improves, can my child stop wearing glasses?
- A: In the majority of children, they will need to continue to wear glasses to clarify the blur from their refractive error. The glasses are improving their visual acuity.
- Q: Is my child too young for glasses?
- A: If a child needs glasses to improve his or her visual acuity, then a child is never too young to wear them. Small frames are designed for children as young as a few months. If glasses improve vision, a child usually quickly accepts correction.
- Q: My child can see well. Why does he need glasses?
- A: Some children with hyperopia can see charts well, but the accommodation (i.e., focusing) necessary to overcome the refractive error may cause eye strain, fatigue, and esotropia. Others may need glasses for unilateral refractive error and seem to see well with both eyes open. In these children, wearing correction may treat or prevent problems even though they may seem to see well without correction.
- Q: Everyone in my family has needed glasses for myopia in childhood. Is there anything we can do for my child that will prevent the development of myopia?
- A: Unfortunately, few environmental factors have been clearly identified to affect the development of myopia. Reading, particularly at an early age; excessively close visual targets (holding books or toys too close to the face); and light exposure during nighttime have been suggested as factors in myopia development. Increased hours spent outdoors may prevent myopic progression. Avoiding long periods of reading, avoiding intensive near work, using a reasonable reading distance (i.e., 16–18 inches), and avoiding use of night-lights may reduce some environmental stimuli.

RENAL ARTERY STENOSIS

Danielle Soranno • Michelle Denburg

BASICS

DESCRIPTION

Narrowing of 1 or both renal arteries and/or their more distal branches, resulting in decreased perfusion, increased renin release, increased vascular resistance, and systemic hypertension

EPIDEMIOLOGY

- Hypertension in infants and young children is often secondary to some identifiable cause. Of those with secondary hypertension, most have intrinsic renal disease (e.g., renal scarring, dysplasia, chronic nephritis).
- Up to 5% of adults with hypertension have renal artery stenosis (RAS).
- RAS accounts for ~10% of secondary hypertension in children. Its importance clinically is not its frequency but its potential curability.

RISK FACTOR

- Any condition associated with thromboembolic events (such as a complication of an umbilical artery catheter in newborns)
- Renal trauma including renal artery surgery (e.g., transplantation)
- Extrinsic compression of the renal artery (e.g., Wilms tumor, neuroblastoma, or pheochromocytoma).

GENERAL PREVENTION

Reduce risk factors, such as thromboembolic events, which can lead to renal artery narrowing.

PATHOPHYSIOLOGY

Arterial narrowing leads to diminished perfusion of the affected kidney, leading to signals in the juxtaglomerular apparatus, which lead to renin release and results in increased vascular resistance and blood pressure (BP).

ETIOLOGY

- Majority are caused by fibromuscular dysplasia (FMD), a noninflammatory vascular disease of unknown etiology.
  - Primarily affects females and affects up to 4 in 100 adults
  - The renal vasculature is the most common arterial bed affected.
  - FMD can concurrently affect other vascular beds including carotid, vertebral, and intracranial vascular beds.
- Arterial narrowing by atheroma is common in adults but rare in children.

COMMONLY ASSOCIATED CONDITIONS

- RAS may occur in many other conditions, including congenital anomalies (e.g., renal artery hypoplasia), neurocutaneous disorders (neurofibromatosis [type 1], tuberous sclerosis), vasculitis (Wegener, polyarteritis nodosa, Kawasaki disease, Takayasu arteritis, moyamoya disease), syndromes (Williams, Marfan, Alagille), and infections (e.g., congenital rubella and fungal infection [immunocompromised hosts]).
- Nephrotic syndrome may accompany renal artery stenosis and is probably secondary to it.
- RAS has been associated with multicystic dysplasia in the contralateral kidney.

DIAGNOSIS

HISTORY

- Ask about prior BP determinations, family history of hypertension, previous renal disease, symptoms of hypertension, and preexisting conditions associated with renal artery stenosis.
- Signs and symptoms:
  - Symptoms of hypertension in infants are not specific and include irritability, poor feeding, and vomiting.
  - In children, symptoms include headache, nausea/vomiting, visual disturbance, dizziness, and seizure.
  - Many affected children remain asymptomatic and 1/3 of children with RAS are diagnosed incidentally.

PHYSICAL EXAM

- BP assessment
  - Consider RAS in a child with very high BP readings (i.e., at or above the 99th percentile).
  - Obtain multiple, manual BP readings using an appropriate-size cuff in the right upper extremity with patient relaxed at baseline heart rate and compare to the BP nomogram for age, sex, and length/height percentile.
  - Avoid using automated devices (oscillometers).
  - Most accurate readings are obtained with either a mercury column or an aneroid sphygmomanometer.
- Determine the BP in all extremities. A gradient from the upper to lower extremities should prompt evaluation for aortic coarctation or midaortic syndrome.
- Examine the skin for lesions suggestive of vasculitis or neurocutaneous disorder (e.g., café au lait macules).
- Assess the child's facies and habitus for features of associated syndromes.
- View the optic fundi for hypertensive vascular changes.
- Auscultate the lower back and abdomen for the presence of a bruit (suggesting turbulent flow).
- In infancy, signs of heart failure may be present.

DIAGNOSTIC TESTS & INTERPRETATION

ECG or echocardiogram to assess for left ventricular hypertrophy and function

Lab

- BUN and creatinine to evaluate for renal insufficiency
- Electrolytes to assess possible hyperaldosteronism with hypokalemia and metabolic alkalosis. Hyponatremia may sometimes occur.
- ESR or CRP to screen for vasculitis

Imaging

- The definitive diagnostic test remains the selective renal arteriogram. If the diagnosis is made, angioplasty may be part of the same procedure. Angiography should not be delayed in any child in whom the diagnosis is strongly suspected.
- Renal ultrasound with Doppler to identify a smaller kidney and/or increased resistance to flow is simple and not invasive, but it is neither sensitive nor specific. Length discrepancy of >1 cm in children can increase suspicion for RAS.
- Contrast-enhanced CT or MR angiography also is not completely diagnostic and is not therapeutic.
- Nuclear renal scans using dimercaptosuccinic acid (DMSA) or MAG-3 enhanced with captopril (and more recently angiotensin receptor blockers [ARB]) also are not diagnostic for all children.
- Diagnostic accuracy of various imaging studies including with magnetic resonance angiography (MRA), computed tomography angiography (CTA)

Technique	Sensitivity (%)	Specificity (%)
Ultrasound	73–85	71–92
DMSA with ACE	52–93	63–92
CTA	64–94	62–97
MRA	64–93	72–97

DIAGNOSTIC PROCEDURES/OTHER

- Avoid excessive investigation in children whose BP is minimally or episodically elevated and therefore in whom the diagnosis of renal artery stenosis is less likely.
- Selective renal vein renin determinations suggest unilateral stenosis if the affected side is 1.5 times the contralateral (normal) side. However, the procedure is invasive and requires catheterization of the femoral vein.
- Random renin determinations have little value and may be misleading. If obtained, renin levels should be interpreted in the context of the urine sodium concentration.

Pathologic Findings

- FMD is a segmental sclerotic process involving smooth muscle hyperplasia of the media layer of the artery. It is unilateral in 75%.
- Stenosis is usually distal in the renal artery, sometimes involving intrarenal branches.
- The stenotic area(s) of the artery may be associated with distal aneurysms.
- In neurofibromatosis, arterial narrowing is at the vessel's ostium and usually involves the intimal layer.

DIFFERENTIAL DIAGNOSIS

- RAS should be suspected and investigated in children with severe, progressive, and/or difficult-to-manage hypertension.
- The differential diagnosis consists of other causes of significant hypertension, including increased intracranial pressure, coarctation of the aorta, midaortic syndrome, rapidly progressive glomerulonephritis, vasculitis, and pheochromocytoma.

TREATMENT

Treat children who are symptomatic immediately (e.g., severe headaches, seizures, blurred vision, facial palsy).

MEDICATION

- Hypertension accompanying RAS is often difficult to control and may worsen over time. Multiple medications given in high doses are common until the diagnosis is made and angioplasty can be done.
- Because RAS results in increased renin levels, renin-angiotensin blockade with ACE inhibitor therapy (e.g., enalapril, lisinopril) and/or angiotensin receptor blockers (ARBs, e.g., losartan) is often effective. In children where bilateral renal artery stenosis is known or suspected, ACE inhibitor and ARB therapy must be avoided to prevent acute renal failure. 50% of children will have bilateral disease. Renal function should be checked before and after initiation of ACE inhibition or ARB therapy.
- If BP is easy to control on monotherapy, may consider medical management alone rather than angioplasty.
- β-Blockers, calcium channel blockers, diuretics, and direct vasodilators (e.g., minoxidil, hydralazine) are all possibly effective.

ADDITIONAL TREATMENT

General Measures

- If renal artery stenosis is suspected, begin the diagnostic evaluation and pharmacotherapy together.
- If BP is very high, use bed rest until BP is better controlled.

ISSUES FOR REFERRAL

- Cardiology follow-up for echo changes, if indicated
- Ophthalmologic follow-up for resolution of vascular changes, if indicated

SURGERY/OTHER PROCEDURES

- Actual surgery on the stenotic renal artery has been replaced by angioplasty, which has been successfully carried out in very young infants. Stents are occasionally used.
- Surgery must sometimes be performed, especially in children with neurofibromatosis where the stenosis is frequently at the renal artery's ostium.

INPATIENT CONSIDERATIONS

Initial Stabilization

- If symptomatic, use potent, rapidly acting medications such as labetalol or nicardipine.
- Be prepared to have difficulty adequately controlling the BP using a single medication.

Admission Criteria

- Children who present with a BP at or above the 99th percentile
- Children who appear to have symptomatic hypertension
- Children with progressive renal insufficiency

Nursing

- Obtain BP levels frequently and carefully.
- Notify MD if high or low limits exceeded.
- Monitor intake of salt, I&O, and weight.

Discharge Criteria

BP in the 90–95th percentile

ONGOING CARE

FOLLOW-UP RECOMMENDATIONS

- The child's BP must be followed closely, both before and after the angioplasty. Response to angioplasty may be immediate but may require continued antihypertensive therapy at some level for weeks to months.
- Medical therapy should be monitored closely. Until correction, the need for progressively higher doses and/or additional medications is common.
- Disposition
  - Close follow-up by the primary care provider, mainly for monitoring BP, and a specialist comfortable with the evaluation and treatment of childhood hypertension.
  - Patient and/or family must be familiar with medication, exercise program, and diet.

Patient Monitoring

- Long-term follow-up of the BP is most important. If on no medications, the BP should be checked monthly, preferably somewhere the child is comfortable and the correct cuff is employed. Begin to space visits after 6 months.
- Checking renal growth on serial renal ultrasounds is important (e.g., at 6 months postangioplasty and then yearly). If the child is fully grown, check ultrasound at 6 months.
- Check renal function annually.

DIET

Limit salt intake.

PROGNOSIS

Long-term outcome of percutaneous angioplasty is excellent; most children require no long-term antihypertensive medications. Percutaneous angioplasty is less successful in neurofibromatosis than in other causes of RAS.

COMPLICATIONS

- Rate of restenosis of the renal artery, either ipsilateral or contralateral, is 22–39%.
- When renal artery stenosis causes severe hypertension, it may cause encephalopathy, severe headache, seizures, or stroke.
- If untreated, chronic hypertension may cause end-organ damage, including heart and kidney.
- Angiography may lead to contrast-induced renal failure. The procedure may also cause injury to the kidney and/or renal artery.
- Rare cases of subarachnoid hemorrhage secondary to coexisting intracranial aneurysm may occur.

ADDITIONAL READING

- Konig K, Gellerman J, Querfeld U, et al. Treatment of severe renal artery stenosis by percutaneous transluminal renal angioplasty and stent implantation: review of the pediatric experience: apropos of two cases. *Pediatr Nephrol*. 2006;21(5):663–671.
- Olin JW, Gornik HL, Bacharach JM, et al. Fibromuscular dysplasia: state of the science and critical unanswered questions : a scientific statement from the American Heart Association. *Circulation*. 2014;129(9):1048–1078.
- Rountas C, Vlychou M, Vassiou K, et al. Imaging modalities for renal artery stenosis in suspected renovascular hypertension: prospective intraindividual comparison of color Doppler US, CT angiography, GD-enhanced MR angiography, and digital substraction angiography. *Ren Fail*. 2007;29(3):295–302.
- Sethna CB, Kaplan BS, Cahill AM, et al. Idiopathic mid-aortic syndrome in children. *Pediatr Nephrol*. 2008;23(7):1135–1142.
- Shahdadpuri J, Frank R, Gauthier BG, et al. Yield of renal arteriography in the evaluation of pediatric hypertension. *Pediatr Nephrol*. 2000;14(8–9):816–819.
- Spyridopoulos T, Kaziani K, Balanika AP, et al. Ultrasound as a first line screening tool for the detection of renal artery stenosis: a comprehensive review. *Med Ultrason*. 2010;12(3):228–232.
- Tullus K. Renal artery stenosis: is angiography still the gold standard in 2011? *Pediatr Nephrol*. 2011;26(6):833–837.
- Vade A, Agrawal R, Lim-Dunham J, et al. Utility of computer tomographic renal angiogram in the management of childhood hypertension. *Pediatr Nephrol*. 2002;17(9):741–744.
- Zhu G, He F, Gu Y, et al. Angioplasty for pediatric renovascular hypertension: a 13-year experience. *Diagn Interv Radiol*. 2014;20(3):285–292.

CODES

ICD10

- I70.1 Atherosclerosis of renal artery
- Q27.1 Congenital renal artery stenosis
- I15.0 Renovascular hypertension

RENAL TUBULAR ACIDOSIS

Elaine Ku • Anthony A. Portale

BASICS

DESCRIPTION

- Renal tubular acidosis (RTA) is characterized by hyperchloremic metabolic acidosis in the setting of normal or near-normal glomerular filtration rate (GFR).
- The acidification defect can be localized to the proximal tubule (type II RTA) resulting in incomplete bicarbonate reabsorption, or the distal tubule (type I or type IV RTA) resulting in impaired net acid secretion.
- Type I and II RTA are associated with hypokalemia; type IV is associated with hyperkalemia.
- Timing of onset and severity of presentation are variable, depending on the underlying cause of the acidification defect.
- Type I RTA is associated with nephrocalcinosis, osteopenia, rickets and sometimes hearing loss.
- Four different types of RTA are recognized:
  - Type I (classic, hypokalemic, distal)
  - Type II (proximal)
  - Type III (characteristics of both proximal and distal RTA, rare inherited disorder associated with mental retardation, osteopetrosis, and cerebral calcification)
  - Type IV (hyperkalemic, distal)
    - Associated with aldosterone deficiency or resistance to its renal effect

EPIDEMIOLOGY

RTA is a rare disorder. Increased prevalence is observed in areas where consanguinity is common.

ETIOLOGY

- Genetic causes of proximal RTA:
  - Mutation in carbonic anhydrase II
  - Mutation in sodium bicarbonate cotransporter
- Genetic causes of distal RTA:
  - Mutation in anion exchanger 1 (AE1) in alpha-intercalated cell
  - Mutation in H^+-ATPase
  - Mutation in carbonic anhydrase II
- Genetic causes of Fanconi syndrome/proximal RTA:
  - Lowe syndrome
  - Dent disease
  - Cystinosis
  - Tyrosinemia
  - Galactosemia
  - Hereditary fructose intolerance
  - Wilson disease
  - Fanconi-Bickel syndrome
  - Mitochondrial disorders
- Acquired causes of proximal RTA:
  - Drugs:
    - Ifosfamide
    - Cisplatin/oxaliplatin
    - Valproic acid
    - Carbonic anhydrase inhibitor (e.g., acetazolamide)
    - Topiramate
    - Aminoglycosides
    - Antiretroviral therapy (tenofovir)
- Acquired causes of distal RTA type I:
  - Autoimmune disorders
  - Drugs:
    - Lithium toxicity
    - Amphotericin
    - Ifosfamide
- Acquired causes of distal RTA type IV:
  - Aldosterone resistance/deficiency
    - Diabetic renal disease
    - Obstructive uropathy
    - Adrenal insufficiency
  - Drugs:
    - Nonsteroidal anti-inflammatory medications
    - Heparin
    - Potassium-sparing diuretics
    - Angiotensin-converting enzyme inhibitor or angiotensin receptor blocker
    - Calcineurin inhibitors (e.g., tacrolimus or cyclosporine)
    - Trimethoprim
    - Pentamidine

PATHOPHYSIOLOGY

- With ingestion of a typical Western diet, healthy adults generate ~1 mEq/kg net acid per day and infants and children ~2–3 mEq/kg/day.
- Under physiologic conditions, the proximal tubule is responsible for reclaiming 85–90% of filtered bicarbonate.
  - Bicarbonate reclamation in the proximal tubule is achieved by a sodium–hydrogen ion antiporter, which secretes hydrogen ion into the urine resulting in generation of bicarbonate within the cell. Cellular bicarbonate is then transported into the bloodstream via an Na-HCO_3 transporter on the basolateral membrane.
- The distal tubule normally reclaims the remaining 10–15% of filtered bicarbonate and secretes a net amount of acid, both via hydrogen ion secretion.
  - In the distal tubule, hydrogen ion secretion occurs primarily via H^+-ATPase.
  - Secreted hydrogen ions are buffered in the urinary lumen primarily by ammonia and excreted as ammonium ions.
- In proximal RTA, mutations in the basolateral sodium bicarbonate cotransporter or in carbonic anhydrase prevent adequate bicarbonate reclamation in the proximal tubule.
  - Unreclaimed bicarbonate enters the distal nephron, which has limited capacity for bicarbonate reclamation, resulting in bicarbonaturia and non–anion gap metabolic acidosis (usually serum bicarbonate does not decrease below 16 mEq/L).
- In distal RTA, mutations in the basolateral anion exchanger or the H^+-ATPase prevent bicarbonate transport into the bloodstream and hydrogen ion secretion into the lumen, respectively, resulting in impaired net acid secretion and non–anion gap metabolic acidosis.
- Proximal RTA can be associated with Fanconi syndrome in which there is general proximal tubular dysfunction leading to bicarbonaturia, glucosuria, phosphaturia, and tubular proteinuria.
- Distal RTA type I is associated with urine pH >5.5
- Distal RTA type IV is associated with either low aldosterone levels or aldosterone resistance and presents with hyperkalemic non–anion gap metabolic acidosis.

DIAGNOSIS

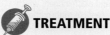

HISTORY
- Failure to thrive in infants and children
- Polyuria
- Constipation
- Anorexia
- Symptoms of hypokalemia:
  - Muscle weakness
  - Constipation
- Kidney stones
- Intellectual disability
- Propensity for fractures

PHYSICAL EXAM
- Constitutional: failure to thrive
- Head: frontal bossing
- Ears: deafness (associated with some forms of RTA)
- Neurologic: developmental and cognitive delay
- Skin: decreased turgor, prolonged capillary refill

DIAGNOSTIC TESTS & INTERPRETATION
- Serum electrolytes
  - To identify metabolic acidosis with normal anion gap, and hypokalemia or hyperkalemia
  - Magnesium level (can be low in Fanconi syndrome)
  - Phosphorus level (can be low in Fanconi syndrome)
- Serum creatinine: to evaluate GFR
- Urine electrolytes
  - Urine anion gap, calculated as (urine sodium + urine potassium − urine chloride): typically >10 in distal RTA (type I or IV)
  - Urine phosphorus: Fractional excretion is high in Fanconi syndrome, resulting in hypophosphatemia.
- Urinalysis
  - Urine pH is high in distal RTA, often >6.8 and can be elevated or normal in proximal RTA.
  - Look for glucosuria in setting of normal serum glucose.
- Urine spot for calcium/creatinine ratio: Look for hypercalciuria (normal values are age-dependent).
- 24-hour urine collection for citrate (typically low)

Imaging
- Renal ultrasound: Evaluate for nephrocalcinosis and kidney stones.
- Long bone films to look for signs of rickets or osteopenia

DIFFERENTIAL DIAGNOSIS
- Renal insufficiency (earlier stages)
- Diarrhea
- Urinary diversion via bowel conduits
- Acetazolamide use

TREATMENT

MEDICATION
- Alkali supplementation given as sodium or potassium bicarbonate or citrate (typically requires 5–8 mEq/kg/24 h in distal RTA and 5–15 mEq/kg/24 h in proximal RTA)
- Thiazide diuretics (in proximal RTA) to induce volume depletion which can be sensed by the proximal tubule, resulting in increased proximal tubular reabsorption of bicarbonate
- Mineralocorticoid supplementation (for those with select causes of type IV RTA)

ADDITIONAL TREATMENT

General Measures
- Vitamin D supplementation as needed
- Phosphorus supplementation as needed (if concurrent Fanconi syndrome)

ONGOING CARE

FOLLOW-UP RECOMMENDATIONS
- Frequent monitoring of serum electrolytes
- Close follow-up of linear growth
- Renal ultrasound to monitor for evidence or progression of nephrocalcinosis

PROGNOSIS
- Can rarely progress to chronic kidney disease over time depending on etiology of RTA (as in cystinosis) or if associated with nephrocalcinosis
- May be associated with development of nephrolithiasis

ADDITIONAL READING

- Batlle D, Haque SK. Genetic causes and mechanisms of distal renal tubular acidosis. *Nephrol Dial Transplant*. 2012;27(10):3691–3704.
- Haque SK, Ariceta G, Batlle D. Proximal renal tubular acidosis: a not so rare disorder of multiple etiologies. *Nephrol Dial Transplant*. 2012;27(12):4273–4287.
- Karet FE. Mechanisms in hyperkalemic renal tubular acidosis. *J Am Soc Nephrol*. 2009;20(2):251–254.

CODES

ICD10
N25.89 Other disorders resulting from impaired renal tubular function

FAQ
- Q: Can RTA be diagnosed in the setting of renal failure?
- A: No. Typically, RTA is diagnosed in the setting of relatively preserved renal function. Renal function associated with non–anion or anion gap acidosis typically occurs when GFR is <30 mL/min/1.73 m^2.
- Q: Does a urine pH <5.5 exclude RTA?
- A: A low urinary pH excludes distal RTA but could still be consistent with a proximal RTA. However, urine pH as tested on urine dipsticks or formal urinalysis can be unreliable depending on duration between time of sample delivery and analysis.
- Q: What are the available forms of alkali supplementation?
- A: Alkali supplementation is best provided as a combination of sodium and potassium citrate or bicarbonate (except in distal RTA type IV, in which potassium alkali is avoided).

RENAL VENOUS THROMBOSIS

Daniel Ranch

BASICS

DESCRIPTION

- Most common non–catheter-related thromboembolism in the neonatal period
- May also be associated with nephrotic syndrome, hypercoagulable states, and oral contraceptive use
- May present with a clinical triad of flank mass, gross hematuria, and thrombocytopenia

EPIDEMIOLOGY

- Most commonly seen in the newborn period
- Slight male predominance
- In neonates, most cases are unilateral, with the left kidney more frequently affected.

Incidence

- Not well-defined due to lack of data
- Ranges from 0.5 to 2.3 per 100,000 live births

Prevalence

Accounts for 16–20% of thromboembolic events in newborns

RISK FACTORS

- Maternal diabetes mellitus
- Birth asphyxia
- Dehydration/blood loss
- Polycythemia
- Cyanotic heart disease
- Hypercoagulable states
- Nephrotic syndrome
- Venous catheter
- Sepsis
- Oral contraceptive use
- Renal transplant recipient

Genetics

- ~50% of affected neonates have at least 1 hereditary prothrombotic risk factor.
- Factor V Leiden, protein C/S, and *MTHFR* mutations and lupus anticoagulant

GENERAL PREVENTION

- Maintaining a high index of suspicion in patients at risk (i.e., infant of diabetic mother, child with nephrotic syndrome)
- Counseling regarding the importance of adequate fluid intake and avoidance of dehydration, especially in newborn infants
- Prophylactic anticoagulation may be indicated in certain populations, although conclusive data is lacking.

PATHOPHYSIOLOGY

- Thrombus formation is initiated by endothelial cell injury from hypoxia or other insults.
- In neonates, non–catheter-related renal vein thrombosis is believed to originate in the arcuate or interlobular veins, as evidenced by early ultrasound findings.
- Thrombosis may extend to the main renal veins and inferior vena cava.
- Neonates also have decreased levels of protein C, protein S, antithrombin, and plasminogen, which may make them more susceptible to thrombosis.
- Lower renal blood flow may also predispose neonates to venous thrombosis.
- In older children, thrombosis may be associated with nephrotic syndrome, hypercoagulable states, or cyanotic heart disease.
- Renal venous thrombosis can result in renal enlargement, decreased renal venous flow, and increased arterial resistive indices.
- Adrenal hemorrhage and left varicocele may also result from renal venous thrombosis.

DIAGNOSIS

HISTORY

- More than half of neonatal cases present within 3 days of birth and almost all within the 1st month of life.
- Macroscopic hematuria is seen in about half of affected infants.
- The classic triad of flank mass, gross hematuria, and thrombocytopenia is present in less than 25% of patients.
- Signs and symptoms:
  - Palpable flank mass
  - Abdominal/flank pain
  - Hematuria
  - Dehydration/shock
  - Edema
  - Fever
  - Hypertension
  - Varicocele

PHYSICAL EXAM

- Palpable enlarged kidney can be found in about half of neonates.
- Abdominal/flank tenderness
- Periorbital/peripheral edema
- Left varicocele
- Hypertension

DIAGNOSTIC TESTS & INTERPRETATION

Lab

- Urinalysis
  - Macroscopic or microscopic hematuria
  - Proteinuria
- Complete blood count
  - Thrombocytopenia is seen in about half of affected neonates.
  - Hemolytic anemia may be present on peripheral blood smear.
- Coagulation tests
  - Prothrombin time and partial thromboplastin time may be prolonged.
  - Fibrin split products may be elevated.
  - Plasma fibrinogen levels may be decreased.
  - Tests for hypercoagulable states, such as factor V Leiden or lupus anticoagulant, should be performed.
- Renal function tests
  - Increased blood urea nitrogen (BUN) and/or creatinine may be present due to acute kidney injury.
  - Electrolyte abnormalities may exist depending on the underlying disease and degree of renal insufficiency.

Imaging

- Ultrasonography
  - Pathognomonic echogenic streaks may be seen with early clot formation.
  - Progresses to renal enlargement and increased parenchymal echogenicity
  - Later findings include loss of corticomedullary differentiation and calcified thrombi in the renal veins.
- Doppler ultrasound
  - Demonstrates decreased or absent renal venous flow
  - May see increased arterial resistive indices

DIFFERENTIAL DIAGNOSIS

- Renal tumors (Wilms, mesoblastic nephroma)
- Pyelonephritis/renal abscess
- Hematoma
- Cystic kidney disease
- Obstructive uropathy
- Thrombotic microangiopathy (hemolytic uremic syndrome [HUS], thrombotic thrombocytopenic purpura [TTP])

TREATMENT

MEDICATION

- The American College of Chest Physicians *Evidence-Based Clinical Practice Guidelines for Antithrombotic Therapy in Neonates and Children* (9th edition) recommend the following:
  - For unilateral renal vein thrombosis (RVT) in the absence of renal impairment or extension into the inferior vena cava (IVC), either (1) supportive care with radiologic monitoring for extension of thrombosis (if extension occurs, anticoagulation is suggested) or (2) anticoagulation with unfractionated heparin (UFH)/low-molecular-weight heparin (LMWH) or LMWH in therapeutic doses rather than no therapy. If anticoagulation is used, a total duration of between 6 weeks and 3 months rather than shorter or longer durations of therapy.

– For unilateral RVT that extends into the IVC, anticoagulation with UFH/LMWH or LMWH for a total duration of between 6 weeks and 3 months
– For bilateral RVT with evidence of renal impairment, anticoagulation with UFH/LMWH or initial thrombolytic therapy with tissue plasminogen activator (tPA) followed by anticoagulation with UFH/LMWH
– However, the overall evidence supporting these recommendations is weak. Also, no recommendations exist for patients with unilateral RVT and renal impairment or patients with prothrombotic risk factors.

ADDITIONAL TREATMENT

General Measures

- Treatment of the underlying disease process, if present
- Management of acute kidney injury (i.e., fluid imbalance, electrolyte abnormalities, hypertension)

ISSUES FOR REFERRAL

Patients with renal venous thrombosis should be evaluated by a nephrologist and hematologist.

SURGERY/OTHER PROCEDURES

- Surgery is rarely indicated, except possibly for malignancy-related cases or refractory hypertension or infection.
- Local thrombolytic therapy via an angiocatheter has been reported for severe IVC thrombosis and bilateral RVT causing renal failure.

INPATIENT CONSIDERATIONS

Initial Stabilization

Supportive therapy for the underlying process, correction of fluid/electrolyte imbalance, and pain control

Admission Criteria

- Admission for treatment of an underlying cause, if present
- Renal impairment
- Pain management
- Thrombolytic therapy

ONGOING CARE

FOLLOW-UP RECOMMENDATIONS

Patient Monitoring

Long-term monitoring for development of hypertension, renal atrophy, or chronic renal insufficiency

PROGNOSIS

- Treatment with anticoagulants may not change renal outcomes.
- RVT has a low mortality rate but may result in significant complications.
- Patients require long-term follow-up to screen for development of hypertension, renal atrophy, proteinuria, or renal insufficiency.
- Hypertension develops in ~20% of patients with neonatal RVT.
- Chronic kidney disease has been reported to develop in up to 71%.
- However, end-stage renal disease is uncommon and is more commonly associated with bilateral RVT.
- Death is uncommon and is usually related to the underlying disease process.
- Certain findings may be linked to worse outcomes, such as the following:
  – Kidney size >6 cm at presentation
  – Decreased overall renal perfusion by Doppler ultrasound
  – Subcapsular bleeding
  – Patchy hypoechogenicity or
  – Irregular pyramids

COMPLICATIONS

- Hypertension
- Renal atrophy
- Proteinuria
- Renal insufficiency

ADDITIONAL READING

- Brandao LR, Simpson EA, Lau KK, et al. Neonatal renal vein thrombosis. *Semin Fetal Neonatal Med*. 2011;16(6):323–328.
- Goldenberg NA. Long-term outcomes of venous thrombosis in children. *Curr Opin Hematol*. 2005; 12(5):370–376.
- Lau KK, Stoffman JM, Williams S; Canadian Pediatric Thrombosis and Hemostasis Network. Neonatal renal vein thrombosis: review of the English-language literature between 1992 and 2006. *Pediatrics*. 2007;120(5):e1278–e1284.
- Messinger Y, Sheaffer JW, Mrozek J, et al. Renal outcome of neonatal renal venous thrombosis: review of 28 patients and effectiveness of fibrinolytics and heparin in 10 patients. *Pediatrics*. 2006;118(5):e1478–e1484.
- Monagle P, Chan AK, Goldenberg NA; American College of Chest Physicians. Antithrombotic therapy in neonates and children: *Antithrombotic Therapy and Prevention of Thrombosis*, 9th ed: American College of Chest Physicians Evidence-Based Clinical Practice Guidelines *Chest*. 2012;141(2) (Suppl):e737S–e801S.

CODES

ICD10

I82.3 Embolism and thrombosis of renal vein

FAQ

- Q: Which population is most susceptible to renal vein thrombosis?
- A: Neonates have the highest risk, especially those with a history of maternal diabetes mellitus, birth asphyxia, or dehydration.
- Q: What is the classic presentation of renal vein thrombosis?
- A: Flank mass, gross hematuria, and thrombocytopenia. However, this "triad" is present in less than 25% of patients, so a high degree of suspicion must be maintained.
- Q: How is renal vein thrombosis diagnosed?
- A: Renal Doppler ultrasound can show renal enlargement, increased echogenicity, or absent renal venous flow.
- Q: What are the current treatment recommendations for renal vein thrombosis?
- A: Supportive therapy and monitoring is recommended, except for bilateral involvement, IVC extension, or evidence of renal impairment. The role of anticoagulation is otherwise still controversial.

RESPIRATORY DISTRESS SYNDROME

Julie M. Nogee • Lawrence M. Nogee

BASICS

DESCRIPTION

Respiratory distress syndrome (RDS) is an acute, developmental lung disease affecting primarily premature infants. Disease is characterized by alveolar collapse due to a lack of pulmonary surfactant owing to lung immaturity that results in increased work of breathing, hypoxemia, and respiratory acidosis. The term hyaline membrane disease (HMD) is often used synonymously.

EPIDEMIOLOGY

- RDS is the most common lung disease in premature infants, affecting approximately 60–80,000 infants per year in the United States.
- Risk increases with the degree of prematurity; nearly 100% of infants born at <26 weeks' gestation affected.
- For near-term infants delivered operatively without benefit of labor, the risk of developing RDS increases roughly 2-fold for every week <39 weeks' gestation.

RISK FACTORS

- Prematurity
- Low birth weight
- Maternal diabetes
- Delivery without labor
- Absence of antenatal steroid administration
- Male gender
- Caucasian race
- Perinatal depression

PATHOPHYSIOLOGY

- Insufficient or dysfunctional surfactant results in alveolar instability and atelectasis, causing hypoventilation and ventilation–perfusion mismatch, leading to hypoxemia and respiratory acidosis.
- The lack of surfactant in conjunction with pulmonary immaturity also leads to transudation of fluid and alveolar edema.
- Surfactant inactivation from transudation of proteins or other substances into the alveolus
- Increased work of breathing generates high negative intrathoracic pressures to overcome alveolar collapse. Retractions result from the highly compliant newborn rib cage combined with poorly compliant lungs.
- Expiratory grunting is due to glottic closure at the end of expiration to prevent end-expiratory atelectasis and maintain functional residual capacity.
- Infants with a well-developed pulmonary arterial muscular bed can develop secondary pulmonary hypertension, with hypoxemia leading to pulmonary vasoconstriction.

GENERAL PREVENTION

- Prevention of prematurity
- Maternal antenatal steroids

DIAGNOSIS

HISTORY

- Gestational age, birth weight
- Lack of antenatal steroids
- Delivery history: matevrnal diabetes, perinatal asphyxia, route of delivery, absence of labor, 2nd-born twin
- Resuscitation: need for supplemental oxygen, positive pressure, intubation, surfactant

PHYSICAL EXAM

- Assessment of color (cyanosis), grunting, nasal flaring, accessory muscle usage
- Vital signs (including respiratory rate to assess for tachypnea) and pulse oximetry (to assess for hypoxemia)
- Pulmonary exam, including shallow or decreased breath sounds, symmetry of breath sounds, and inspiratory rales

DIAGNOSTIC TESTS & INTERPRETATION

Lab

- Blood gases (BGs): Arterial BGs allow for accurate determination of pH, $Paco_2$, and Pao_2 to avoid hyperoxia as well as hypoxemia.
- Capillary BGs obtained from appropriately warmed extremities can provide accurate determinations of pH and Pco_2, but poor perfusion to the extremity or inadequate warming may result in inaccurate determinations.
- Oxygenation may be determined noninvasively through pulse oximetry.

Imaging

- Chest radiography
  - Classic findings include hypoinflation, diffuse reticulogranular or "ground-glass" appearance, and air bronchograms.
  - Lateral films may be helpful for determination of air leak.
- Other imaging modalities (CT, ultrasound) are generally unnecessary for the diagnosis and management of RDS but may be indicated if there is suspicion for other pulmonary pathology.

DIFFERENTIAL DIAGNOSIS

Common

- Transient tachypnea of the newborn (TTN)
- Infection (sepsis, pneumonia)
- Air leak (may also be a complication of RDS)
- Meconium aspiration syndrome

Unusual

- Pulmonary hypoplasia
- Congenital heart disease
- Primary ciliary dyskinesia
- Genetic surfactant dysfunction

TREATMENT

GENERAL MEASURES

Diet

Sufficient glucose infusion to prevent hypoglycemia. Hydration and nutrition for expected increased caloric needs with early initiation of IV nutrition while working to establish enteral nutrition

Supportive Care

- Radiant warmer or incubator for warmth
- Blood pressure support with volume expansion and/or pressors to maintain perfusion and normal blood pressure for gestational age

MEDICATION

- Exogenous surfactant
  - Both modified mammalian-derived surfactants and synthetic surfactants have been shown to reduce morbidity and mortality from RDS.
  - Exogenous surfactant is delivered directly into the trachea through the endotracheal tube and thus currently requires that the infant be intubated, although alternative delivery methods are being explored.
  - Timing of surfactant
    - Prophylactic: as soon as infant is stabilized, usually less than 15 minutes of life, based on the risk for RDS without demonstrating that the infant has disease. Prophylaxis is usually reserved for those infants at highest risk for RDS, such as <26 weeks' gestation.
    - Rescue: after the diagnosis of RDS is established; usually after first hour and before 48 hours of life
    - Additional doses are considered for persistently high FiO_2 requirements (FiO_2 >0.3–0.4) or for ongoing need for mechanical ventilation. Consultation with a neonatologist is recommended.

ALERT

- Occasionally, the surfactant material may clog the endotracheal tube, causing acute airway obstruction with resultant hypercapnia and hypoxemia, necessitating suctioning or removal and replacement of the endotracheal tube.
- Surfactant therapy can also result in acute improvements in pulmonary compliance. Monitor physical exam, Spo_2, blood gasses, and tidal volumes to avoid inadvertent overventilation.

- Caffeine citrate
  - Used for apnea of prematurity and may be helpful in RDS if it is able to minimize the duration of mechanical ventilation

ADDITIONAL THERAPIES

- Continuous positive airway pressure (CPAP)
  - Can be delivered via nasal prongs or mask either using a ventilator, dedicated apparatus, or through "bubble CPAP"
  - CPAP prevents end-expiratory atelectasis and can be started in the delivery room.

- Humidified high-flow nasal cannula (HFNC)
  - May achieve CPAP benefit with easier handling of the patient and less risk of pressure necrosis of nasal septum
  - Pressure delivery variable
- Mechanical ventilation
  - May be required for infants with significant respiratory acidosis and hypoxemia. Can be initiated following intubation for surfactant delivery
  - High-frequency ventilation (oscillatory or jet) may be valuable in very severe cases or with air leak (jet).

ONGOING CARE

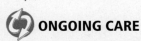

FOLLOW-UP RECOMMENDATIONS

- Very low-birth-weight and extremely low-birth-weight infants should receive follow-up in specialty clinics that can provide for their specialized needs, including neurodevelopmental, pulmonary (for those with bronchopulmonary dysplasia [BPD]), and ophthalmology (for those with retinopathy of prematurity).
- Immunizations are extremely important preventive measures to prevent subsequent respiratory morbidity and mortality. See chapter on "Bronchopulmonary Dysplasia" for recommendations for passive immunization against respiratory syncytial virus with palivizumab (Synagis).

PROGNOSIS

Natural history: disease severity worsens over the first 24–72 hours, with improvement occurring after 5–10 days of age. With antenatal steroids, CPAP, newer modes of mechanical ventilation, and surfactant replacement therapy, more rapid improvement is often seen, and mortality from RDS is rare. Outcome is usually related to the degree of prematurity and its related complications.

COMPLICATIONS

Air-leak: pneumothorax, pneumomediastinum, pulmonary interstitial emphysema, pneumopericardium

ALERT

- Emergency treatment of pneumothorax: Acute tension pneumothorax can occur as a complication of RDS and its management and can be life threatening, even in larger or term infants. Needle aspiration may provide temporary stabilization, and chest tube placement may be necessary.

- Pulmonary hemorrhage: typically occurs between 1 and 3 days of age with sudden respiratory deterioration and pink or red frothy fluid or bright red blood in the endotracheal tube. Associated with diffuse opacification of the lung fields and marked decrease in pulmonary compliance.
- Complications related primarily to prematurity that are often associated with RDS:
  - Patent ductus arteriosus: Pulmonary edema and high-output congestive heart failure may develop as a consequence of left-to-right shunting through the ductus.
  - Bronchopulmonary dysplasia: a chronic disease of multifactorial etiology involving abnormal lung development and abnormal repair following lung injury due in part to RDS as well as edema, infection, and other factors causing inflammation

ADDITIONAL READING

- Engle WA. Surfactant-replacement therapy for respiratory distress in the preterm and term neonate. *Pediatrics*. 2008;121(2):419–432.
- Finer NN, Carlo WA, Walsh MC, et al. Early CPAP versus surfactant in extremely preterm infants. *N Engl J Med*. 2010;362(21):1970–1979.
- Jobe AH. What is RDS in 2012? *Early Hum Dev*. 2012;88(Suppl 2):S42–S44.
- Morley CJ, Davis PG, Doyle LW, et al. Nasal CPAP or intubation at birth for very preterm infants. *N Engl J Med*. 2008;358(7):700–708.
- Sweet DG, Carnielli V, Greisen G, et al. European consensus guidelines on the management of neonatal respiratory distress syndrome in preterm infants—2013 update. *Neonatology*. 2013;103(4):353–368.
- Tita AT, Landon MB, Spong CY, et al. Timing of elective repeat cesarean delivery at term and neonatal outcomes. *N Engl J Med*. 2009;360(2):111–120.

CODES

ICD10

P22.0 Respiratory distress syndrome of newborn

FAQ

- Q: Should all babies with a diagnosis of RDS be started on antibiotics?
- A: It is important to consider sepsis/pneumonia in all infants with a diagnosis of RDS, particularly infection with group B *Streptococcus* (GBS). Risk factors to be considered include maternal GBS colonization, evidence of chorioamnionitis, intrapartum antibiotic use, and route of delivery. Antibiotics may sometimes be held if the risk factors for sepsis are low compared to those for RDS, such as in a baby delivered electively by caesarean section for maternal indications. However, as congenital pneumonia can radiographically appear identical to RDS, it is often common practice to screen for sepsis in all infants with RDS by performing blood cultures and looking for other laboratory evidence of infection including complete blood counts with differentials and acute-phase reactants such as C-reactive protein, and start empiric antibiotic therapy with ampicillin or penicillin in combination with an aminoglycoside. Duration of antibiotics is typically 48 hours depending on results of blood cultures as well as the clinical picture and other laboratory data. Therapy may be narrowed if a specific organism is identified.
- Q: What is the most worrisome acute complication of RDS?
- A: Acute air leak (primarily tension pneumothorax) can be life threatening, even in near-term or full-term infants with RDS, and such infants should be cared for in centers that are prepared to properly handle this emergent situation in a timely fashion (i.e., availability of a provider who can perform an emergent needle aspiration and chest tube placement). In smaller infants, pulmonary hemorrhage can also be life threatening.
- Q: Because the risk of a baby developing RDS for a baby born at 26 weeks' gestation is so high, should such babies automatically receive prophylactic surfactant?
- A: Not necessarily. Early prospective, randomized, placebo-controlled studies did demonstrate that mortality from RDS was reduced with prophylactic surfactant in preterm infants ≤26 weeks' gestation. However, those studies were conducted in an era before widespread use of antenatal steroids and early use of CPAP. Recent prospective, randomized trials of different approaches to extremely low-birth-weight infants in the delivery suite have demonstrated that such infants treated with early and continued CPAP alone may have outcomes comparable to those immediately intubated and treated with surfactant replacement therapy.
- Q: As some surfactant preparations are prepared from cow lungs, is there an increased risk that babies receiving such surfactants will develop a milk protein allergy?
- A: It is very unlikely that surfactant treatment with preparations derived from animal lungs increases the risk of immune responses. The two proteins in replacement surfactants are present in low amounts and are extremely hydrophobic and unlikely to generate an immune response given the limited number of surfactant doses (usually maximum of 4) administered. They are also not structurally related to proteins found in human milk, and their amino acids sequences are highly conserved between species, such that it is unlikely that they would be seen as foreign antigens by the baby's immune system.

RESPIRATORY SYNCYTIAL VIRUS (SEE ALSO: BRONCHIOLITIS)

David K. Hong • Alan R. Schroeder

BASICS

DESCRIPTION

- An enveloped, nonsegmented RNA virus of the family Paramyxoviridae and in the subfamily Pneumovirinae along with human metapneumovirus. There are 2 subgroups, A and B, differentiated by the major attachment G protein, a large surface glycoprotein. The fusion or F protein is relatively homologous between the 2 subgroups.
- It is the most common cause of bronchiolitis, a lower respiratory tract disease that primarily affects the small airways.

EPIDEMIOLOGY

- Incubation period is 2–8 days.
- Virus is detected in secretions 4 days prior to clinical symptoms. Typically shedding of infectious virions is 3–8 days but can be as long as 3–4 weeks in immunocompromised.
- Transmission occurs by direct contact of nasopharyngeal or ocular mucosa with infected secretions or fomites.
- Nosocomial spread can occur because the virus can survive on surfaces and hands for several hours.
- In the United States, epidemics typically occur between November and April and last for roughly 18–20 weeks.
- In tropical climates, respiratory syncytial virus (RSV) seasons are less predictable and can circulate year-round.
- One antigenic strain predominates during any given epidemic, but both subtypes can circulate concurrently.

Incidence

- Peak incidence is the first 2 years of life. 20–30% of infected infants develop lower respiratory tract disease.
- Annual rate of RSV-associated hospitalization is roughly 3/1,000 in children <5 years of age and 17/1,000 in children <6 months of age.

Prevalence

- 50% of children are infected by their 1st birthday. 100% of children are infected by age of 2 years.
- Reinfection can occur during the same RSV season and is common during the first few years of life.
- Subsequent infections are typically milder.

RISK FACTORS

Those at greatest risk for severe infection include:

- Children <1 year of age, especially those <6 months of age
- Children born prematurely (<35 weeks gestation)
- Children with underlying cardiopulmonary disease (e.g., chronic lung disease of prematurity, congenital heart disease)
- Those with primary immune deficits
- Patients on immunosuppressive medications (e.g., transplant patients, oncology patients)

GENERAL PREVENTION

- There is currently no RSV vaccine. A formalin-inactivated RSV vaccine tested in the 1960s caused enhanced illness after reexposure to wild-type RSV likely due to an overexuberant immune response.
- Because RSV can survive on surfaces, strict hand washing can minimize nosocomial spread.
- Contact isolation with routine usage of gowns and gloves has been shown to decrease RSV nosocomial spread.
- Patients with RSV infection should be isolated in private rooms.
- Palivizumab, a humanized monoclonal antibody directed against the highly conserved F protein of RSV, is the only product available for the prevention of RSV infection in certain high-risk children.
  - Children who should receive palivizumab:
    - Children <2 years of age who receive medical therapy for chronic lung disease
    - Infants with a history of prematurity (birth at <32 weeks gestation)
  - Children for whom palivizumab should be considered:
    - High-risk premature infants born between 32 and 35 weeks' gestation
    - Infants with congenital heart disease, congenital airway abnormalities, or neuromuscular disease
  - Palivizumab is given IM (15 mg/kg) every 30 days for 5 doses usually from November to April.
  - Specific recommendations are available from the American Academy of Pediatrics (AAP) Committee on Infectious Diseases and Committee on Fetus and Newborn.

PATHOPHYSIOLOGY

- The G protein is the major surface glycoprotein responsible for attachment of virus to cells.
- The F protein aids in viral entry in to cells and is responsible for fusion of adjacent cells to form a syncytia.
- Infection is initiated in nasopharynx and then can move to the lower respiratory tract.
- Infection of smaller airways leads to edema and necrosis of epithelial cells and infiltration of inflammatory cells, resulting in airway obstruction and air trapping.
- Severe RSV infection has been associated with recurrent wheezing later in life. It is unclear whether RSV infection causes subsequent wheezing or if patients predisposed to severe wheezing are more likely to have severe RSV disease.

DIAGNOSIS

HISTORY

- Initial symptoms include copious nasal discharge, cough, and fever.
- Cough is the most common symptom typically progressing over 1–2 days.
- Concerning findings on history:
  - Apnea, severe coughing with possible cyanotic episodes
  - Poor oral intake
  - Decreased urine output (e.g., fewer wet diapers)
  - Trouble breathing

PHYSICAL EXAM

- Profuse rhinorrhea
- Acute otitis media or otitis media with effusion
- Signs of dehydration (dry mucus membranes, delayed capillary refill time)
- Conjunctivitis
- Varying levels of respiratory distress:
  - Mild: suprasternal retractions, mild tachypnea
  - Moderate: subcostal or intracostal retractions
  - Severe: severe retractions, grunting, RR >60, lethargy
- Air trapping resulting in hyperexpansion of lungs can lead to a barrel-shaped chest, palpable liver, or spleen below the costal margin.
- Pulse oximetry may reveal hypoxemia.

DIAGNOSTIC TESTS & INTERPRETATION

Lab

- A definitive diagnosis of RSV can be made by viral culture but requires up to 5 days.
- Rapid diagnostic antigen assays from nasopharyngeal specimens are used for RSV detection, usually with a sensitivity of 80–90%:
  - Enzyme immunoassay
  - Immunofluorescent assay
- Reverse transcriptase-polymerase chain reaction (RT-PCR) assays are commercially available and may have superior sensitivity to rapid antigen testing. However, these assays detect viral RNA that may persist in nasal secretions after patient is no longer shedding infectious virus.
- Because concurrent serious bacterial infections are not common, complete blood counts or blood cultures are not indicated.
- Given reported 3% incidence of concurrent urinary tract infections (UTIs), urinalysis and urine culture can be considered for infants with persistent fever.

Imaging

- Chest x-rays should not be routinely obtained in children with RSV.
- Often reveals hyperinflation, increased bronchial markings, and areas of atelectasis/infiltrates, findings which may not alter the treatment plan or may in some cases lead to unnecessary antibiotics.

DIFFERENTIAL DIAGNOSIS

- Infection
  - Influenza virus
  - Parainfluenza virus
  - Human metapneumovirus
  - Adenovirus
  - Coronaviruses
  - *Mycoplasma pneumoniae*
- Environmental: foreign body in upper airway
- Tumors: mass compressing upper airway
- Congenital: laryngomalacia or tracheomalacia

TREATMENT

MEDICATION

- β-Adrenergic agents: Bronchodilators should not be used routinely. However, there are some data to suggest that they may lead to transient improvement in respiratory scores in some patients, but no data that suggests that this impacts hospitalization rates or length of stay.
- Racemic epinephrine: Racemic epinephrine has been demonstrated to reduce hospital admission rates compared to placebo and to shorten length of stay when compared to albuterol.
- Select patients may benefit from a trial of bronchodilators, but this remains controversial. Careful attention should be paid to the clinical exam before and after administration to support their ongoing use.
- Corticosteroids are not useful in bronchiolitis and should not be used.
- Ribavirin: has in vitro antiviral activity against RSV, but ribavirin aerosol treatment for RSV infections should not be used routinely in the treatment of children with bronchiolitis. There may be some benefit in severely ill patients such as immunocompromised patients with severe disease.
- Antibiotics are rarely indicated because concurrent bacterial disease (lung or blood) is uncommon in patients with RSV bronchiolitis. However, 3% of patients with bronchiolitis and fever have urine culture findings consistent with UTI.
- There is limited evidence that nebulized hypertonic saline (3%) may reduce length of hospital stay and improve clinical symptoms.

ADDITIONAL TREATMENT

General Measures

- Supportive care: hydration therapy and supplemental oxygen as needed if oxygen saturation persistently falls below 90%
- Cardiorespiratory monitoring and pulse oximetry should be used for infants at risk for apnea and hypoxemia.
- In severe cases, respiratory support with continuous positive airway pressure (CPAP) or mechanical ventilation is required.

INPATIENT CONSIDERATIONS

Initial Stabilization

Apnea or severe respiratory distress with impending respiratory failure may require intubation and mechanical ventilation.

ONGOING CARE

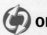

FOLLOW-UP RECOMMENDATIONS

- Lower respiratory tract symptoms usually arise 2–3 days after initial symptoms.
- Symptoms usually peak from 5 to 7 days, but 20% of children can have symptoms for 3 weeks.
- Recurrent apneic episodes are rare, and home monitoring is usually not indicated.
- Fever commonly resolves over 2–3 days.

Patient Monitoring

Signs to watch for:

- Increased respiratory rate and increased work of breathing
- Lethargy, altered mental status
- Signs and symptoms of dehydration (dry mucous membranes, decreased urine output)

PROGNOSIS

- Most children have a mild to moderate disease course requiring only supportive care.
- Approximately 1–3% of children will require hospitalization. Most children recover with no sequelae.
- Infants born prematurely or with underlying cardiopulmonary disease are at increased risk for more severe and longer duration of disease.
- Reinfections occur throughout life with an incidence of about 5% per year.
- There are some data to suggest that patients with severe RSV bronchiolitis may have more episodes of recurrent wheezing in the 1st year of life. It is unclear whether severe RSV infection causes long-term airway hyperresponsiveness.

COMPLICATIONS

- Dehydration
- Apneic episodes in young infants (can occur in all causes of bronchiolitis, not just RSV)
- Hypoxemia
- Hypercarbia
- Respiratory failure
- Pneumonia, rarely bacterial
- Croup
- Acute otitis media
- Asthma

ADDITIONAL READING

- American Academy of Pediatrics. Respiratory syncytial virus. In: Pickering LK, Baker CJ, Kimberlin DW, et al, eds. *Red Book: 2012 Report of the Committee on Infectious Diseases*. 29th ed. Elk Grove Village, IL: American Academy of Pediatrics; 2012:609–618.
- American Academy of Pediatrics Subcommittee on Diagnosis and Management of Bronchiolitis. Diagnosis and management of bronchiolitis. *Pediatrics*. 2006;118(4):1774–1793.
- Hall CB, Weinberg GA, Iwane MK, et al. The burden of respiratory syncytial virus infection in young children. *N Engl J Med*. 2009;360(6):588–598.
- Zhang L, Mendoza-Sassi RA, Wainwright C, et al. Nebulized hypertonic saline solution for acute bronchiolitis in infants. *Cochrane Database Syst Rev*. 2008;(4):CD006458.

CODES

ICD10

- B97.4 Respiratory syncytial virus causing diseases classd elswhr
- J21.0 Acute bronchiolitis due to respiratory syncytial virus
- J20.5 Acute bronchitis due to respiratory syncytial virus

FAQ

- Q: How did my child get this illness?
- A: RSV bronchiolitis is caused by respiratory syncytial virus, an extremely common virus which is passed from one person to another by contact with nasal secretions and through airborne transmission of droplets.
- Q: For how long is my child contagious?
- A: Viral shedding occurs for 24 hours prior to the onset of clinical symptoms and for up to 21 days from the onset of symptoms.
- Q: Will my child develop asthma because of the wheezing that is occurring now?
- A: There is an association between severe RSV bronchiolitis and recurrent wheezing episodes during the 1st year of life. However, it is not clear whether RSV causes asthma later in life.
- Q: How do I prevent my child from being infected with RSV?
- A: Unfortunately, there is no vaccine against RSV. In high-risk infants (infants born prematurely with chronic lung disease, congenital heart disease) palivizumab can be administered during RSV season to prevent severe lower respiratory tract disease.

RETINOBLASTOMA

Sheila Thampi • Paul Stewart

BASICS

DESCRIPTION

Retinoblastoma is a malignant tumor of the retina. Due to current treatment options, survival rates are high in developed countries. Primary management focuses on the best treatment approach to spare the child's life, while secondary goals focus on sparing vision and reducing risk of secondary malignancies.

EPIDEMIOLOGY

- Retinoblastoma is the most common intraocular malignancy in children.
- Hereditary retinoblastoma commonly presents with bilateral disease or multiple tumors in unilateral disease
- Median age at diagnosis for unilateral disease is 24 months and less than 12 months for bilateral disease.
- 25% of patients will present with bilateral disease.
- No association with race, gender, or laterality of eye involvement
- The greatest disease burden is found in countries with the largest populations and high birth rates such as Asia and Africa.

Incidence

- In the United States, there are about 4 cases per million children per year, with a higher incidence in children younger than age 5 years.
- Approximately 300 new pediatric cases of retinoblastoma are diagnosed each year in the United States.
- Retinoblastoma represents 3% of all pediatric malignancies.

RISK FACTORS

- Hereditary retinoblastoma, in which patients have a germline *Rb* gene mutation
  - 25–45% of all retinoblastoma cases are hereditary.
- Family history of retinoblastoma in parents or siblings warrants early screening and continued follow-up to monitor for development of disease.

PATHOPHYSIOLOGY

- Tumor development requires loss of function of the *RB1* gene, which resides on chromosome 13.
- Constitutional loss of one *RB1* allele predisposes a patient to cancer. Loss of the second allele or other mutations of retinal cells will initiate formation of retinoblastoma.
- Sporadic or nonhereditary retinoblastoma has no germline *RB1* mutation but instead requires biallelic inactivation of the *RB1* gene in a single retinal cell.
- There are 3 common growth patterns:
  - Intraretinal (growth only in the retina)
  - Endophytic (inner surface of retina to vitreous)
  - Exophytic (outer surface of retina to subretinal space)
  - Tumor cells that break off from the primary mass will invade the vitreous and grow independently in the vitreous.
- Children with loss of *RB1* with large chromosomal deletions of surrounding genes are at risk for developmental anomalies such as facial dysmorphism and mental and/or motor impairment.
- Initial classification of tumor extent is imperative for assessment of prognosis and outcomes.
- International Classification of Retinoblastoma (ICRB), also known as the ABC classification system, is predictive of treatment success following systemic chemotherapy and focal laser treatment. However, the older Reese-Ellsworth classification system is still commonly used.
  - ICRB groups eyes from less advanced disease, group A, to most advanced disease, group E.
  - ICRB predicts high-risk retinoblastoma seen in group D or E eyes.
- High-risk features on histology include tumor invasion of the optic nerve and massive choroidal invasion. High-risk features will lead to metastases in about 24% of patients if not treated with systemic chemotherapy as compared to 4% of those treated with systemic chemotherapy.
- Patients with bilateral retinoblastoma are at risk for involvement of the pineal gland, termed trilateral retinoblastoma.

ETIOLOGY

Mutations in the *RB1* gene lead to predisposition of retinal tumors.

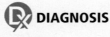

DIAGNOSIS

HISTORY

Parents often report noticing a white color in the pupil on photographs, eye(s) turning in or outward, and poor vision.

PHYSICAL EXAM

- Most common presenting signs include the following:
  - Leukocoria
  - Strabismus
  - Poor vision (poor tracking)
- Proptosis is worrisome for more advanced disease.
- Associated bone pain should be evaluated for metastatic disease.

DIAGNOSTIC TESTS & INTERPRETATION

Lab

- CBC to look for leukopenia, anemia, or thrombocytopenia
  - CBC should be evaluated to determine bone marrow involvement.
  - If cytopenias are noted, then evaluation of the bone marrow is indicated.
- Extraocular spread noted on imaging warrants evaluation of the cerebrospinal fluid.
- Chromosome analysis should be performed, particularly in patients with bilateral eye involvement or developmental delay.

Imaging

- Brain and orbit MRI can aid in distinguishing between retinoblastoma and Coats disease and will assess for trilateral disease. CT scan can provide information regarding tumor calcification but due to radiation is used less frequently.
- Ophthalmic ultrasonography can demonstrate retinal masses and calcifications.
- A technetium bone scan will show areas of intense primary tumor uptake and screen for bone metastasis and should be performed if concern for metastasis noted on exam.

Diagnostic Procedures/Other

- A biopsy is not performed due to risk for dissemination.
- The diagnosis of retinoblastoma is based on ophthalmologic exam.
- An experienced pediatric ocular oncologist should perform the exam under anesthesia (EUA).
- Early involvement of pediatric oncology should be initiated.

DIFFERENTIAL DIAGNOSIS

- Coats disease
- Persistent fetal vasculature
- Vitreous hemorrhage
- Congenital cataract
- Coloboma
- Toxocariasis
- Astrocytic hamartoma
- Retinopathy of prematurity

TREATMENT

CHEMOTHERAPY

- Systemic chemotherapy is currently the most common form of treatment for retinoblastoma, as it allows preservation of the globe and prevention of systemic metastasis.
- Systemic chemotherapy is combined with local retinal therapy for adequate treatment.

- Systemic chemotherapy may prevent development of trilateral retinoblastoma.
- Most common chemotherapeutic agents used for retinoblastoma include carboplatin, etoposide, and vincristine (CEV).
- Intra-arterial chemotherapy (IAC) is a newer modality for treatment of retinoblastoma and provides direct retinal chemotherapy via the ophthalmic artery.
- Less commonly used approaches to deliver chemotherapy include periocular or intravitreal injections.

RADIOTHERAPY

- Retinoblastoma is a radiosensitive tumor.
- Radiation therapy can be provided by external beam therapy or plaque therapy (brachytherapy) and is a useful method to preserve vision.
- Use of radiation is generally avoided due to risk of secondary malignancies, particularly in children with hereditary retinoblastoma.

SURGERY/OTHER PROCEDURES

- Local retinal therapy with cryotherapy or laser photocoagulation is an important modality of treatment.
- Enucleation, removal of the eye, provides definitive treatment for retinoblastoma. Advanced eyes (group E) are usually managed with enucleation to prevent metastatic spread. Unilateral cases with less advanced disease also are frequently managed with enucleation.

PHYSICAL THERAPY

- Physical therapy is not commonly required for children with retinoblastoma.
- Occupational therapy or speech therapy can help children cope with loss of vision or hearing changes that develop due to side effects of chemotherapy.

ONGOING CARE

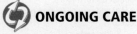

ISSUES FOR REFERRAL

- Children suspected to have retinoblastoma should be immediately referred to a children's hospital with expertise in these tumors. Prompt evaluation by an ocular oncologist is required for early diagnosis.
- Multidisciplinary teams include ocular oncologists, pediatric oncologists, nurses, pharmacists, and social workers.
- Children with bilateral retinoblastoma should be referred to a pediatric geneticist for genetic testing for *RB1* mutations.

PROGNOSIS

- Five-year overall survival in the United States is excellent at 96.5%.
- All forms of metastatic spread: Leptomeningeal disease, trilateral or pineal involvement, and distant metastases require aggressive therapy and still result in poor overall survival.

COMPLICATIONS

- Surgical
  - Surgical site wound infections after enucleation
  - Complications associated with orbital implants (infection, bleeding, conjunctival erosion, wound dehiscence)
- Acute systemic chemotherapy toxicity
  - Myelosuppression
  - Ototoxicity
  - Infections
  - Renal dysfunction
  - Peripheral neuropathy
- Radiation
  - Skin erythema
  - Risk of cataract development
  - Vascular endothelium damage
  - Vitreous hemorrhage
  - Facial and temporal bone hypoplasia
  - Secondary malignancy
- IAC toxicity
  - Myelosuppression
  - Redness or swelling of the eyelid
  - Vitreous hemorrhage
  - Choroidal atrophy
  - Rare risk of stroke or blindness
- Late effects
  - Hearing loss and nephrotoxicity from carboplatin
  - Secondary malignancy from radiation or chemotherapy (i.e., etoposide).

Patient Monitoring

- Patients should be followed regularly by an ocular oncologist for EUAs to monitor for reoccurrence.
- Patients should be followed by a pediatric oncologist with serial MRI of the brain and orbit and additional imaging based on sites of disease at presentation.
- Patients should be monitored for long-term side effects/complications of therapy, ideally within the context of a survivorship clinic.

ADDITIONAL READING

- Abramson DH, Schefler AC. Update on retinoblastoma. *Retina*. 2004;24(6):828–848.
- Dimaras H, Kimani K, O Dimba EA, et al. Retinoblastoma. *Lancet*. 2012;379(9824): 1436–1446.
- Shields CL, Fulco EM, Arias JD, et al. Retinoblastoma frontiers with intravenous, intra-arterial, periocular, and intravitreal chemotherapy. *Eye*. 2013;27(2): 253–264.

CODES

ICD10

- C69.20 Malignant neoplasm of unspecified retina
- C69.21 Malignant neoplasm of right retina
- C69.22 Malignant neoplasm of left retina

FAQ

- Q: Are children with retinoblastoma at risk for developmental delays?
- A: Children who carry *RB1* gene mutations should be followed closely for developmental delays with speech and/or motor skills. Children with deletions in chromosome 13 have been described to have an array of developmental delays in association with retinoblastoma.
- Q: Do siblings of children with retinoblastoma need to be evaluated?
- A: Given the high possibility of hereditary *RB1* mutations, children of siblings or parents with retinoblastoma should be evaluated at an early age and followed by an ophthalmologist.
- Q: Do I need to worry about other cancers in my child who has retinoblastoma?
- A: Children with the hereditary form of retinoblastoma (*RB1* gene mutation, bilateral disease, or family history) are at increased risk for other cancers such as osteosarcoma.
- Q: Is my child with retinoblastoma blind?
- A: The size and location of the tumor(s) will determine your child's vision. Advanced retinoblastoma (group D or E) is more likely to have total retinal involvement and poor vision.

RETINOPATHY OF PREMATURITY

Michael X. Repka

BASICS

DESCRIPTION

Retinopathy of prematurity (ROP) is an abnormal pattern of retinal vascularization of preterm infants leading in some cases to permanent visual loss and blindness as well as many other eye problems.

EPIDEMIOLOGY

- ROP is the leading cause of blindness among children in the developed world:
  - 0.2% of all infants born in the United States
  - 20% of infants born <1,500 g
- 1,300 develop severe disease requiring treatment annually in the United States.
- Birth weight and ROP (incidence of ROP stage 1 or greater)
  - <750 g: 90%
  - 750–<1,000 g: 78%
  - 1,000–1,250 g: 47%
  - >1,250 g:<1%
- Gestational age and ROP (incidence of any ROP stage 1 or greater with BW <1,251 g)
  - ≤27 weeks: 83%
  - 27–31 weeks: 55%
  - ≥31 weeks: 29%

RISK FACTORS

- Gestational age
- Hyperoxia
- Hypoxia
- Acidosis
- Hypercarbia
- Apnea
- Bradycardia
- Nutritional deficiencies
- Ambient light
- Intraventricular hemorrhage
- Lower birth weight
- Lower gestational age
- Multiple gestation
- Born at another facility and transferred

PATHOPHYSIOLOGY

- Normal retinal vascularization begins at the optic disc at about 16 weeks postmenstrual age and is typically completed at about term.
- Preterm delivery exposes the actively growing vessels to unusual conditions. These alter production of vascular endothelial growth factors. In some cases, the vascular growth stops and then resumes normally, whereas in other cases, the retinal blood vessels grow abnormally off the surface of the retina.
- The timing for development of acute ROP is related to postmenstrual age and not chronologic age or birth weight. It is rare to see any disease prior to 32 weeks postmenstrual age. Fewer than 10% of babies smaller than 1,250 g birth weight will have disease sufficiently severe to have treatment.

DIAGNOSIS

HISTORY

- All infants with birth weight less than 1,500 g or gestational age less than 30 weeks are at risk.
- Other children with significant oxygen exposure are also referred for retinal evaluations.
- Each nursery needs a protocol to identify and document the infants needing examinations, both initial and follow-up. Reasons for exam deferral should be included in the medical record.

ALERT

A common error in ROP management is failure to perform exams on the required schedule. The most vulnerable time for this lapse is during a transition to another unit or another facility or after discharge to home.

PHYSICAL EXAM

- Requires a retinal examination with pupillary dilation, binocular indirect ophthalmoscopy, sterile eyelid speculum, and scleral depression
  - Topical anesthesia may be used.
  - Pupillary dilation is obtained using 1% phenylephrine/0.2% cyclopentolate solution (Cyclomydril) administered as a single drop to each eye, repeated in 5–10 minutes.
    - Administer at least 30 minutes and preferably 1 hour prior to the exam.
    - The dilating eye drops are associated with delay in gastric emptying.
    - Careful monitoring is needed following the drop administration and the eye examination.
    - Bradycardia and emesis are common following mydriatic eye drop administration and eye examination.
- The results of the examination should be recorded in a manner defined by the International Classification of Retinopathy of Prematurity. A retinal drawing is suggested:
  - Zone I: posterior circular area of the retina centered on the optic disc with a radius twice the distance from disc to fovea
  - Zone II: peripheral ring of retina extending from zone I to anterior edge of the nasal retina and estimated temporally
  - Zone III: temporal retina beyond zone II
- Diagnostic retinal examinations and/or imaging should commence unless the infant is too unstable.
  - At 31 weeks for those infants born at 26 weeks postmenstrual age or earlier
  - By 4 weeks postnatal age for infants >26–30 weeks postmenstrual age
- Exams typically are ordered every 2 weeks.
- Additional examinations may be requested by neonatology for infants outside the consensus birth weight and postmenstrual age criteria.
- Subsequent examinations are determined by the ophthalmologist.
  - Exams typically ordered every 2 weeks
  - When there is prethreshold disease, weekly or even more frequent exams are conducted.
  - When there is zone III disease, the exam interval may be lengthened.
  - Exams continue until retinal vascularization into zone III is recorded.
  - If VEGF inhibitors have been used for treatment, the exams may need to be extended substantially past term. Exams continue until retinal vascularization into zone III is recorded.
- ROP is typically symmetric, with similar exams in both eyes seen in 85% of infants.
- Eye examinations performed in the office setting may require monitoring depending on the infant's medical status.

DIAGNOSTIC TESTS & INTERPRETATION

Imaging

- Wide-field digital camera with images of posterior pole, as well as superior, inferior, nasal, and temporal retinas, allows documentation and review of the findings as well as consultation.
- The images are reviewed either in real-time or using store-forward technology for evidence of referral-warranted ROP, at which time indirect ophthalmoscopy must be performed to determine if the patient has reached the treatment threshold or be monitored.
- Some facilities are using telemedicine as a substitute, rather than a supplement, for a clinical exam.
  - Skilled nursery personnel are needed to handle the camera and obtain useful images.
  - Plan for image review and urgent treatment referral when needed.

Diagnostic Procedures/Other

- Ophthalmic ultrasonography
  - If difficult to obtain adequate indirect ophthalmoscopy, B-mode ultrasound of the eye can be useful to determine progression of ROP to retinal detachment and to monitor the detachment.

DIFFERENTIAL DIAGNOSIS

- Norrie disease
- Incontinentia pigmenti
- Familial exudative vitreoretinopathy
- Trauma
- Stickler syndrome
- Cyanotic congenital heart disease in rare cases
- Idiopathic

TREATMENT

SURGERY/OTHER PROCEDURES

- Each nursery needs a policy in place for where and how treatment is to be performed.
  - Treatment should be performed within 48 hours if at all possible.
- Treatment is recommended when a particular stage of disease called type 1 occurs. Type 1 is ROP in zone I or II with PLUS characteristics (dilation and tortuosity of retinal arteries and veins), any stage in zone I, and stage 2 or 3 in zone II. Ideally, the treatment is completed within 48 hours, depending on the stability of the infant.
- Standard care treatment of ROP is ablation (destruction) of the peripheral nonvascularized retina using a laser incorporated into a binocular indirect ophthalmoscope.
  - Requires airway management, topical eye drop anesthesia, and either sedation or general anesthesia
  - 25% have unfavorable visual outcomes at 6 years.
  - 9% have unfavorable structural outcomes at 6 years.
  - 83% of treatments performed in infants ≤27 weeks' gestation
- Cryotherapy of the peripheral retina that has not been vascularized (anterior) has been shown to be effective compared to observation.
  - Used less frequently today because of pain, tissue damage, and difficulty treating more posterior disease
  - Improves the chance of favorable structural outcomes at age 15 years from 48 to 70%
- Vitreoretinal surgery including vitrectomy is performed after retinal ablation or intravitreal injection has failed and the infant has progressed to stage 4 or 5 ROP (retinal detachment).
  - Rarely associated with visual outcome of 20/200 or better (16%)
  - Retinal reattachment in about 30%

MEDICATION

- Oxygen restriction: Restriction of oxygen to 85–89% saturation measured by pulse oximetry has been associated with a reduction in the risk of severe ROP but was associated with an increased mortality rate.
- Oxygen supplementation: In the Stop-ROP trial, supplemental oxygen for infants with prethreshold disease appeared to reduce the rate of progression but was associated with increased risk for pulmonary disease.
- Vascular endothelial growth factor (VEGF) inhibitors (e.g., bevacizumab)
  - Intravitreal injection of a small dose of one of these drugs is currently of great interest.
  - In a clinical trial, a single dose of bevacizumab was more effective than laser ablation for zone I disease.

ONGOING CARE

FOLLOW-UP RECOMMENDATIONS

- Infants with treated ROP and more severe stages of ROP without treatment typically require lifelong ophthalmologic monitoring.
  - Substantially increased risk for the development of multiple eye conditions
    - Retinal detachment
    - Strabismus
    - Amblyopia
    - Myopia
    - Glaucoma
    - Optic nerve atrophy
    - Cerebral visual impairment
- Infants with prethreshold ROP have moderately increased risk of the ophthalmic conditions mentioned above. Referral managed with typical practice.
- A history of treatment for ROP is correlated with a high risk of disability on motor, communication–social, self-care, and continence scales on the Wee-FIM (Functional Independence Measure for Children).

PROGNOSIS

- If ROP treatment was required, visual outcomes reported at 15 years:
  - 25% with 20/20–20/40
  - 50% with 20/20–20/200
  - 33% with less than 20/200

ADDITIONAL READING

- Early Treatment for Retinopathy of Prematurity Cooperative Group, Good WV, Hardy RJ, et al. Final visual acuity results in the Early Treatment for Retinopathy of Prematurity study. *Arch Ophthalmol*. 2010;128(6):663–671.
- Fierson WM; American Academy of Pediatrics Section on Ophthalmology, American Academy of Ophthalmology, American Association for Pediatric Ophthalmology and Strabismus, et al. Policy statement: screening examination of premature infants for retinopathy of prematurity. *Pediatrics*. 2013;131(1):189–195.
- International Committee for the Classification of Retinopathy of Prematurity. The International Classification of Retinopathy of Prematurity revisited. *Arch Ophthalmol*. 2005;123(7):991–999.
- Mintz-Hittner HA, Kennedy KA, Chuang AZ, et al. Efficacy of intravitreal bevacizumab for stage 3+ retinopathy of prematurity. *N Engl J Med*. 2011;364(7):603–615.
- Palmer EA, Hardy RJ, Dobson V, et al. 15-year outcomes following threshold retinopathy of prematurity: final results from the multicenter trial of cryotherapy for retinopathy of prematurity. *Arch Ophthalmol*. 2005;123(3):311–318.
- The natural ocular outcome of premature birth and retinopathy. Status at 1 year. Cryotherapy for Retinopathy of Prematurity Cooperative Group. *Arch Ophthalmol*. 1994;112(7):903–912.

CODES

ICD10

- H35.109 Retinopathy of prematurity, unspecified, unspecified eye
- H35.119 Retinopathy of prematurity, stage 0 unspecified eye
- H35.129 Retinopathy of prematurity, stage 1 unspecified eye

FAQ

- Q: Does intrauterine growth retardation (IUGR) affect the chance for development of ROP?
- A: The chance for development of ROP in an infant with IUGR is more related to the postmenstrual birth age rather than the birth weight. However, in as much as the IUGR infant is sick, that could increase the risk over infants of similar postmenstrual age at birth.
- Q: When should a missed exam be made up?
- A: In most cases, it is safe to wait a week unless there has been recent evidence of stage 2 or worse disease in which case the exam should be completed as soon as the infant is stable for the dilated exam.
- Q: Does acute ROP ever need to be retreated?
- A: Following ablative therapy, about 10% of eyes will need additional treatment to untreated areas of the retina if the PLUS disease has not begun to diminish. This typically occurs about 10–14 days. The rate for retreatment after VEGF inhibitor therapy is not yet well established.

R

RETROPHARYNGEAL ABSCESS

Camille Sabella

BASICS

DESCRIPTION
A relatively rare but potentially life-threatening infection occurring in the potential space between the posterior pharyngeal wall and prevertebral fascia

EPIDEMIOLOGY
Children <6 years of age are most at risk, with 50% of the cases occurring in those <48 months of age.

Incidence
Most large children's hospital centers report 1–5 cases per year.

PATHOPHYSIOLOGY
- Most infections result from pharyngitis or supraglottitis and occur because of suppuration of the retropharyngeal lymph nodes, which lie in 2 paramedial chains and drain various nasopharyngeal structures and sinuses.
- These lymph gland chains disappear in childhood; thus, retropharyngeal abscesses are most common in infancy and early childhood.
- Cellulitis of the retropharyngeal area leads to formation of a phlegmon, which matures into an abscess.
- Other sources of infection in this space, often seen in older children and adolescents, include penetrating trauma of the posterior pharynx (e.g., foreign object aspiration, dental procedures, attempts at intubation).
- Extension of infection into this space can arise from vertebral body osteomyelitis or a dental abscess.

ETIOLOGY
- Infectious: Cultures frequently reveal multiple organisms.
- The predominant organisms isolated include the following:
  - *Streptococcus* (group A and others)
  - *Staphylococcus aureus*
  - Various anaerobic species (e.g., *Bacteroides*, *Peptostreptococcus*, *Fusobacterium*)
- Many of the isolates are β-lactamase producers.

DIAGNOSIS

HISTORY
- Symptoms may be present from hours to days before correct diagnosis is established. Many patients will have been taking oral antibiotics for presumed pharyngitis/sinusitis.
- Ask about neck trauma, especially penetrating injuries, recent surgery (especially dental), and history consistent with aspiration of a foreign object.
- Physicians must maintain a high index of suspicion. The presentation of a retropharyngeal abscess can be subtle, with the most frequent initial diagnostic impression usually epiglottitis or severe pharyngitis.
- Signs and symptoms:
  - Most frequent symptoms include sore throat, decreased oral intake, muffled voice, drooling, stiff or painful neck, fever, dysphagia, and stridor.
  - Fever
  - Stridor (seen in up to 50% of children in 1 study but only 5% in a more recent series)
  - Drooling
  - A tender cervical neck region/mass and restricted range of motion
  - Classic diagnostic finding of a bulging posterior pharyngeal wall; may be absent or difficult to appreciate in an ill, apprehensive child

PHYSICAL EXAM
- Classic presentation is the young child who develops fever, neck stiffness, torticollis, neck mass, and acute cervical lymphadenitis.
- Infants and children often appear ill, but the manifestations are subacute and may be subtle.
- Other findings may include the following:
  - Muffled voice
  - Drooling
  - Fever
  - Dysphagia
  - Stridor

DIAGNOSTIC TESTS & INTERPRETATION

Lab
CBC may reveal an elevated total leukocyte level, with a significant left shift.

Imaging
- Lateral neck x-ray
  - Widening of retropharyngeal space and at times an air–fluid level
  - Negative plain neck film does not rule out retropharyngeal abscess.
- CT scan (contrast-enhanced) of the neck
  - Superior to plain film
  - Can usually differentiate abscess from local cellulitis/adenitis, although the sensitivity and specificity of this study for defining abscess vs. cellulitis are less than 70%

DIFFERENTIAL DIAGNOSIS

- Pharyngitis
- Peritonsillar or lateral wall abscess
- Epiglottitis/supraglottitis
- Penetrating foreign body
- Cervical osteomyelitis

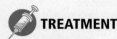

TREATMENT

MEDICATION

- Start empiric broad-spectrum antibiotics, active against *Staphylococcus aureus*, *Streptococcus pyogenes*, other non–group A streptococci, and anaerobic organisms.
- Ampicillin-sulbactam or clindamycin are good initial choices. Vancomycin may be added for suspected methicillin-resistant *S. aureus* infections in a child with severe infection.
- Antibiotics may be tailored based on microbiologic and susceptibility data.

ADDITIONAL TREATMENT

General Measures

- Urgent consultation with an otolaryngology surgical team is warranted for airway management and possible surgical drainage; a team experienced in pediatric airway management is critical.
- Recent data suggest that up to 50% of patients can be successfully managed without surgical intervention.
- Patients with a well-defined abscess on admission CT are most likely to require surgical intervention.
- Patients treated with antibiotics alone must be followed closely for signs of worsening clinical status.

ISSUES FOR REFERRAL

After diagnosis is confirmed, urgent consultation with experienced surgical staff who have expertise in management of a pediatric airway is mandatory.

INPATIENT CONSIDERATIONS

Initial Stabilization

Emergency therapy requires maintaining patent airway; be wary of sudden spontaneous drainage of the abscess, with catastrophic aspiration.

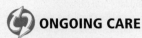

ONGOING CARE

PROGNOSIS

Excellent with appropriate antibiotics, expectant care, and surgery, if needed, at optimal time

COMPLICATIONS

- Spontaneous rupture with aspiration of infected material, with subsequent asphyxia or overwhelming pulmonary infection
- Hemorrhage from extension into local arteries and/or venous thrombosis from involvement of major neck vessels
- Extension of the infection inferiorly can occur, leading to mediastinitis, a subdiaphragmatic or psoas abscess.

ADDITIONAL READING

- Chang L, Chi H, Chiu NC, et al. Deep neck infections in different age group of children. *J Microbiol Immunol Infect*. 2010;43(1):47–52.
- Daya H, Lo S, Papsin BC, et al. Retropharyngeal and parapharyngeal infections in children: the Toronto experience. *Int J Pediatr Otolaryngol*. 2005;69(1):81–86.
- Elsherif AM, Park AH, Alder SC, et al. Indicators of a more complicated clinical course for pediatric patients with retropharyngeal abscess. *Int J Pediatr Otorhinolaryngol*. 2010;74(2):198–201.
- Grisaru-Soen G, Komisar O, Aizenstein O, et al. Retropharyngeal and parapharyngeal abscess in children—epidemiology, clinical features and treatment. *Int J Pediatr Otorhinolaryngol*. 2010;74(9):1016–1020.
- Loftis L. Acute infectious upper airway obstructions in children. *Semin Pediatr Infect Dis*. 2006;17(1):5–10.
- Page NC, Bauer EM, Lieu JEC. Clinical features and treatment of retropharyngeal abscess in children. *Otolaryngol Head Neck Surg*. 2008;138(3):300–306.

CODES

ICD10

J39.0 Retropharyngeal and parapharyngeal abscess

FAQ

- Q: What is the age group most at risk of having a retropharyngeal abscess?
- A: They are most common in preschool children; the paramedical chains of lymph nodes in the retropharyngeal area regress during childhood and adolescents. Thus, prior to their regression, these nodes filter lymph from the nasopharynx and paranasal sinuses and are responsible for retropharyngeal abscesses.

REYE SYNDROME

Jayaprakash A. Gosalakkal

BASICS

DESCRIPTION

- Acute encephalopathy and fatty degeneration of the liver which may be idiopathic or secondary
- "Classic" Reye syndrome is associated with aspirin (acetylsalicylic acid) therapy, whereas Reye-like syndromes are due to metabolic disorders or other etiologies.
  - Acute, noninflammatory encephalopathy that is documented clinically by (a) an alteration in consciousness and, if available, (b) a record of the CSF containing $\leq$8 leukocytes/mm^3 or a histologic specimen demonstrating cerebral edema without perivascular or meningeal inflammation
  - Liver enlargement documented by either (a) a liver biopsy or an autopsy considered to be diagnostic of Reye syndrome or (b) a 3-fold or greater increase in the levels of the serum glutamic-oxaloacetic transaminase (SGOT), serum glutamic-pyruvic transaminase (SGPT), or serum ammonia
  - No more reasonable explanation for the cerebral and hepatic abnormalities

EPIDEMIOLOGY

- Peak incidence age 6 years
- Most children range from 4 to 12 years of age.
- Association with ingestion of aspirin-containing medicines by children with varicella or influenza B
- In 1982, the U.S. Surgeon General issued an advisory on the use of salicylates and Reye syndrome.
- Reye-like illness is often associated with fatty acid oxidation defects and other inborn errors of metabolism.

Incidence

- Peak incidence of 555 cases in children in the United States in 1980
- From 1994 to 1997, there were no more than 2 cases of Reye syndrome annually.
- Reye-like illness due to metabolic causes should be suspected now in all cases with this presentation.

PATHOPHYSIOLOGY

- Mitochondrial injury of unknown etiology in a viral-infected host results in dysfunction of oxidative phosphorylation and fatty acid oxidation.
- Mitochondrial toxins, usually salicylates, exacerbate the condition when ingested after mitochondrial injury.
- Multiple factors may sometimes be involved, including complex metabolic problems affecting the mitochondria.
- Postmortem
  - Liver: grossly yellowish-white due to increased triglyceride levels; foamy cytoplasm with increased microvesicular fat, decreased glycogen
  - Brain: marked edema with increased intracellular fluid and loss of neurons
  - Abnormal-looking mitochondria can be detected in many tissues.
  - Multiple organ involvement may be present in fatty acid oxidation or other defects.

DIAGNOSIS

HISTORY

- Prodromal illness: upper respiratory infection (73%)—influenza B, influenza A, and varicella
- Abrupt-onset vomiting within 47 days of initial illness
- Natural history: neurologic deterioration in which delirium may progress to seizures, coma, or death
- Underlying history of inborn errors of metabolism or family history of conditions like medium-chain acyldehydrogenase deficiency should be sought.

PHYSICAL EXAM

- Slight liver enlargement without jaundice
- Absence of focal neurologic signs
- Neurologic exam varies with stage of disease:
  - Stage 0: alert, wakeful
  - Stage 1: difficult to arouse, lethargic, sleepy
  - Stage 2: delirious, combative, with purposeful or semipurposeful motor responses
  - Stage 3: unarousable, with predominantly flexor motor responses, decorticate
  - Stage 4: unarousable, with predominantly extensor motor responses, decerebrate
  - Stage 5: unarousable, with flaccid paralysis, areflexia, and pupils unresponsive
  - Stage 6: treated with curare or equivalent drug and therefore unclassifiable
- Organomegaly may be present in Reye-like illness.

DIAGNOSTIC TESTS & INTERPRETATION

Lab

- Ammonia test: Result may be normal at the onset of vomiting. Serum level >45 g/dL suggests higher mortality.
- CSF: normal except for elevated intracranial pressure
- Hypoglycemia is often present.
- Ketonemia may be present.

Imaging

EEG: characteristic of metabolic encephalopathy with generalized slow-wave abnormalities

Diagnostic Procedures/Other

- Liver and muscle function testing: elevated levels of transaminases, creatinine kinase, lactate dehydrogenase, and ammonia; increased PT
- Metabolic workup: Abnormalities of organic and amino acids may be present if symptoms are caused by a metabolic disorder.
- Cultured fibroblasts for fatty acid oxidation defects

DIFFERENTIAL DIAGNOSIS

- It is important to distinguish between so-called classic Reye syndrome, associated with aspirin (acetylsalicylic acid) therapy, and Reye-like syndromes, often due to metabolic disorders and other causes as mentioned subsequently. All cases who present with Reye syndrome should be investigated for metabolic disorders.

- Metabolic diseases: In a report by Hou et al., Reye-like syndrome was secondary to hereditary organic acidemias (n = 13), urea cycle defects (n = 4), mitochondrial disorders (n = 3), fulminant hepatitis (n = 2), tyrosinemia (n = 1), and valproate-associated hepatotoxicity (n = 1). In the United Kingdom, 12% of Reye syndrome cases between 1981 and 1996 were subsequently reclassified as metabolic disorders.
- CNS infections (e.g., meningitis, encephalitis)
- Toxins
- Drug ingestion (e.g., salicylates, valproate)

ALERT
Failure to recognize early and control or prevent cerebral edema is associated with increased mortality.

TREATMENT

GENERAL MEASURES

Vitamin K, fresh frozen plasma, and platelets as needed for treatment of secondary coagulopathy

INPATIENT CONSIDERATIONS

Initial Stabilization

- Should be tailored based on severity of presentation
- IV glucose to counteract effects of glycogen depletion
- Fluid restriction in patients with cerebral edema (1,500 mL/m^2/day), along with mannitol to increase serum osmolality and induce cerebral dehydration

ONGOING CARE

FOLLOW-UP RECOMMENDATIONS

Cerebral function at presentation is the best predictor of outcome. Evaluate for metabolic diseases if not done already.

PROGNOSIS

- Most patients suffer only mild illness without progression.
- Patients with milder disease (stages 0, 1, 2) tend to recover completely.
- Patients with stage 3 disease are equally likely to recover completely or die.
- Patients with stage 4 or 5 disease usually do not survive.

COMPLICATIONS

- Elevated intracranial pressure secondary to cerebral edema
- Cardiovascular collapse
- Overall mortality of 31%

ADDITIONAL READING

- Belay ED, Bresee JS, Holman RC, et al. Reye's syndrome in the United States from 1981 through 1997. *N Engl J Med*. 1999;340(18):1377–1382.
- Chow EL, Cherry JD, Harrison R, et al. Related articles, reassessing Reye syndrome. *Arch Pediatr Adolesc Med*. 2003;157(12):1241–1242.
- Duerksen DR, Jewell LD, Mason, AL et al. Co-existence of hepatitis A and adult Reye's syndrome. *Gut*. 1997;41(1):121–124.
- Glasgow JF, Middleton B. Reye syndrome—insights on causation and prognosis. *Arch Dis Child*. 2001; 85(5):351–353.
- Gosalakkal JA, Khamoji V. Reye syndrome and Reye like syndrome. *Pediatr Neurol*. 2008;39(3):198–200.
- Green CI, Blitzer MG, Shapira E. Inborn errors of metabolism and Reye's syndrome: differential diagnosis. *J Pediatr*. 1988;113(1, Pt 1):156–159.
- Hou JW1, Chou SP, Wang TR. Metabolic function and liver histopathology in Reye-like illnesses. *Acta Paediatr*. 1996;85(9):1053–1057.
- Schrör K. Aspirin and Reye syndrome: a review of the evidence. *Paediatr Drugs*. 2007;9(3):195–204.
- van Bever HP, Quek SC, Lim T. Aspirin, Reye syndrome, Kawasaki disease, and allergies: a reconsideration of the links. *Arch Dis Child*. 2004;89(12):1178.

CODES

ICD10

G93.7 Reye's syndrome

FAQ

- Q: Is Reye syndrome fatal?
- A: ~30% of children will die, usually due to cerebral edema. Mortality rates are best predicted by neurologic state at the onset of presentation.
- Q: How can the neurologic findings of Reye syndrome be differentiated from those of meningitis?
- A: Aside from elevated intracranial pressure, the lumbar taps of patients with Reye syndrome are at best unremarkable. Elevated leukocyte count is not seen in these cases.
- Q: What additional recommendations are suggested for children on chronic aspirin therapy?
- A. When annual influenza vaccine supply is limited, according to the CDC, vaccination efforts should focus on delivering vaccination to specific subpopulations, including children "receiving long-term aspirin therapy and who therefore might be at risk for experiencing Reye syndrome after influenza virus infection."

RHABDOMYOLYSIS

Erica Winnicki • Farzana Perwad

BASICS

DESCRIPTION

- Rhabdomyolysis is defined as skeletal muscle breakdown resulting from injury.
- Injury may result from many causes including trauma, infection, medications or inherited disorders
- Classic presentation is with a triad of myalgia, weakness, and dark urine.
- Characterized by elevated creatinine kinase (CK) and myoglobinuria
- Release of intracellular contents from damaged muscle cells may cause severe electrolyte disturbances including life-threatening hyperkalemia, hyperphosphatemia, and hypocalcemia.
- The resulting myoglobinuria can cause obstruction of renal tubules and pigment-induced acute kidney injury (AKI), the most serious complication of rhabdomyolysis.

EPIDEMIOLOGY

- Rhabdomyolysis is more common in adults than children, where it is commonly due to illicit or prescription drugs or due to trauma.
- Rhabdomyolysis may be a common clinical problem in a catastrophic disaster (e.g., an earthquake).
- Rhabdomyolysis accounts for 7–10% of cases of AKI in the United States.

RISK FACTOR

Genetics

Many unusual causes of rhabdomyolysis, including muscle enzyme deficiencies, muscular dystrophy, and disorders of mitochondrial metabolism, are heritable disorders.

ETIOLOGY

- There are numerous potential causes of rhabdomyolysis, which can be sporadic or recurrent, traumatic, or nontraumatic.
- Muscle trauma is a common cause in both adults and children. This may occur from crush or compression injury (crush syndrome), compartment syndrome, or electric shock.
- The most common cause in children is infection, specifically viral infections. Some of the associated infections include viral (influenza A and B, Epstein-Barr virus, cytomegalovirus, human immunodeficiency virus), certain bacterial infections (*Legionella* species, group A beta-hemolytic streptococci, *Salmonella*), and protozoa (Malaria).
- Exertion-related rhabdomyolysis may be a common cause for young athletes. Specifically, exercise which is novel, intense, or prolonged, and especially in the presence of extremely hot weather may cause rhabdomyolysis. Seizure, tetany, and alcohol withdrawal syndrome are other causes of exertion-related rhabdomyolysis.
- Certain inherited disorders should be considered with recurrent rhabdomyolysis. Myopathies involving muscle enzyme or energy substrate deficiencies include disorders of lipid metabolism (e.g., carnitine palmitoyltransferase II deficiency), disorders of glycogenolysis (e.g., phosphorylase kinase deficiency, McArdle disease), disorders of glycolysis (lactate dehydrogenase deficiency), and mitochondrial deficiency disorders. Usual triggers for rhabdomyolysis in such conditions are fasting, exertion, or viral illness.
- Rhabdomyolysis is more likely to occur after exertion in association with the dystrophinopathies, which include all forms of muscular dystrophy.
- Illicit drug use including alcohol (alcohol withdrawal syndrome), cocaine, heroin, amphetamines, phencyclidine (PCP), and ecstasy
- Causative prescription medications include lipid-lowering drugs (statins, fibrates) and antipsychotic medications (mostly due to neuroleptic malignant syndrome).
- Prolonged immobilization or loss of consciousness leading to muscle hypoxia. Certain metabolic and electrolyte disorders may result in rhabdomyolysis. These include hypokalemia, hypophosphatemia, hypocalcemia, and hyperosmolar states such as diabetic ketoacidosis.
- Body temperature changes (hyperthermia and hypothermia) may cause rhabdomyolysis.
- Malignant hyperthermia is a rare inherited condition that results in hyperthermia, muscle breakdown, and subsequent rhabdomyolysis on receiving halogenated hydrocarbon–containing anesthetics or muscle relaxants such as succinylcholine.
- Neuroleptic malignant syndrome is a rare neurologic disorder characterized by hyperthermia, rhabdomyolysis, and autonomic changes in patients receiving neuroleptic or antipsychotic medications.
- Other implicated toxins include snake bite, spider venom and vespid venoms, quail, and some mushrooms.
- The list of causes of rhabdomyolysis above is not exhaustive. Any child with sudden onset of muscle pain, tenderness, or weakness should be suspected of having rhabdomyolysis, and any child with dark urine suspected of myoglobinuria.
- The insult may lead to muscle cell destruction with release of intracellular contents including proteins and electrolytes and sequestration of fluids by damaged muscle leading to severe hypovolemia.
- Rhabdomyolysis leads to AKI by direct toxicity of myoglobin to the renal tubules, renal tubular obstruction, and renal ischemia from hypoperfusion.
- Rhabdomyolysis has also been associated with diverse conditions, including status asthmaticus, diabetes mellitus, and thyroid disease. It may also occur in Kawasaki disease, hemolytic uremic syndrome, and adrenal insufficiency, associations which are rare but must not be missed.

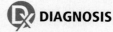

DIAGNOSIS

HISTORY

- Prior history of any illness or insult associated with rhabdomyolysis should be sought. Rhabdomyolysis may follow certain illnesses (e.g., influenza), insults (e.g., crush injury, severe exertion), and medications (e.g., statins).
- Symptoms of muscle pain or weakness may result from rhabdomyolysis and help suggest diagnosis if present.
- Signs of reddish-brown discoloration of the urine may be present.

PHYSICAL EXAM

- Palpate muscles for tenderness and, less commonly, swelling or fullness.
- Test for motor strength.
- Elicit reflexes to exclude neuropathy.
- Examine skin and mucous membranes for signs of vasculitis.
- Look for signs suggestive of child abuse.
- Examine for signs of a concomitant precipitating illness.
- The clinical picture is generally consistent with volume depletion given the sequestration of fluids in injured muscle tissue.

Lab

- Serum CK level, specifically the CK-MM isoenzyme, which is found in skeletal muscle, will be elevated to greater than 4–5 times the upper limit of normal. CK levels usually rise within 12 hours of the injury and peak within 2–3 days. If the CK levels continue to rise, it should raise suspicion for ongoing muscle damage or development of compartment syndrome.
- Serum electrolytes including calcium and phosphorus must be measured given the potential for severe derangements. Abnormalities may include hyperkalemia, hyperphosphatemia, and/or hypocalcemia. There may be metabolic acidosis with a wide anion gap in those conditions associated with lactate production.
- Creatinine level may be elevated out of proportion to that of BUN, secondary to conversion of liberated muscle creatine to creatinine.
- CBC and smear should be obtained because many of the metabolic disorders causing rhabdomyolysis cause a hemolytic anemia as well.
- Patients with rhabdomyolysis are at increased risk for disseminated intravascular coagulation (DIC) secondary to thromboplastin released from the injured myocytes. Therefore, PT/INR, PTT, platelets, and fibrinogen levels should be obtained.
- Serum uric acid may be elevated from release of purines from muscle cells and may contribute to renal tubule obstruction.

- Other muscle enzyme levels (myoglobin, aldolase, lactate dehydrogenase, AST, ALT) will be elevated secondary to muscle injury but are not necessary for diagnosis.
- Urinalysis
  - Urine may appear brown and test positive for blood on dipstick without red blood cells on microscopy.
  - Granular pigmented casts are common. Low fractional excretion of sodium (<1%) is found in those with AKI.
- Myoglobin in is not generally measured; however, urine myoglobin can be quantitatively measured using an immunoassay. Serum CK levels are more sensitive to assess the degree of ongoing rhabdomyolysis.
- Other tests:
  - EKG may reveal changes associated with acute hyperkalemia, such as peak T waves, prolongation of PR, absent P wave with prolonged QRS interval, or even ventricular tachycardia/fibrillation in severe untreated hyperkalemia.
  - Metabolic and genetic testing if recurrent or otherwise suspected metabolic myopathy

Imaging
Imaging is not generally required for the diagnosis. Note that use of radiocontrast in imaging studies as part of diagnostic evaluation can worsen acute kidney injury.

Other Diagnostic Procedures
Muscle biopsy: necessary to diagnose metabolic myopathies; should wait several weeks after the clinical event to perform. A biopsy will demonstrate immunohistochemical features of a myopathy. Immunoblotting is helpful in evaluating the dystrophinopathies.

DIFFERENTIAL DIAGNOSIS
- Consider other causes of discolored urine such as hematuria and beet ingestion.
- Consider other causes of muscle pain and/or weakness: viral illnesses, Lyme disease, suppurative myositis, Guillain-Barré syndrome, collagen vascular diseases.

TREATMENT

INITIAL STABILIZATION
Aggressive repletion of fluids should be initiated promptly. If an underlying cause is identified, it should be corrected or removed.

General Measures
- Early fluid resuscitation is essential to prevent worsening kidney function. Vigorous hydration with crystalloid IV fluids should be followed by adequate maintenance fluids (e.g., 2–3 times maintenance) to provide brisk urine flow (e.g., >2 mL/kg/h or >200 mL/h).
- Alkalinization of the urine is not clearly superior to fluids alone, although risks of alkalinization are minimal.
- Use of diuretics, including furosemide (a loop diuretic), are controversial and use should be limited to fluid-replete patients. Use of mannitol is not clearly beneficial and may actually worsen AKI.

MEDICATION
- Administration of sodium bicarbonate (along with fluids) to correct or prevent acidosis is reasonable. Correction of acidosis is also beneficial in the management of hyperkalemia (potassium is shifted intracellularly).
- With alkalinization, monitor closely for worsening hypocalcemia.
- Use of diuretics is controversial; consider use in fluid-replete patients with AKI to maintain urine output and avoid volume overload (e.g., furosemide 1–2 mg/kg/dose IV). Furosemide will also maximize potassium elimination by the kidney.
- Additional treatment for severe hyperkalemia may be necessary and incudes IV calcium gluconate, sodium bicarbonate, insulin and glucose, beta-2-agonist drugs, and Kayexalate.
- Correct hypocalcemia only if symptoms are present or in the setting of severe hyperkalemia in order to prevent the complication of calcium-phosphate deposition and late hypercalcemia.
- Conventional hemodialysis does not remove myoglobin effectively; continuous venovenous hemofiltration may be more effective. Indications for dialysis include acute renal failure with the following:
  - Severe hyperkalemia refractory to medical management or rapidly rising potassium
  - Severe metabolic acidosis resistant to medical management
  - Volume overload/respiratory distress secondary to pulmonary edema

ONGOING CARE

Close monitoring of labs with serial measurements of CK levels, creatinine, and electrolytes is essential. The patient's fluid status should be monitored closely, and volume repletion should be continued until urine is clear and negative for blood. The patient should also be watched closely for signs of ongoing muscle injury, compartment syndrome, or DIC.

PROGNOSIS
- Prognosis is generally good, with acute kidney injury being the major life-threatening complication.
- Prompt cessation of rhabdomyolysis may be expected when the inciting cause is corrected or resolved.
- Although most children recover promptly, severe muscle injury may cause prolonged muscle weakness and warrant follow-up by physical and occupational therapy.
- With resolution of myoglobinuria, acute kidney injury is expected to be reversible.

COMPLICATIONS
- Electrolyte release from muscle can lead to severe hyperkalemia, hyperphosphatemia, and secondary hypocalcemia.
- Electrolyte derangement may result in cardiac arrhythmias.
- AKI occurs in 13–50% of patients. Risk factors for AKI include higher CK level (>3,000), concurrent administration of nephrotoxic agents, and volume depletion.
- Compartment syndrome may result from muscle swelling.
- Use of bicarbonate may precipitate symptomatic hypocalcemia.
- Use of calcium therapy for severe hyperkalemia or symptomatic hypocalcemia may result in calcium-phosphate deposition or exacerbate late hypercalcemia.
- Failure to discontinue IV fluids if oligoanuric renal failure develops could produce iatrogenic fluid overload.

ADDITIONAL READING

- Bosch X, Poch E, Grau J. Rhabdomyolysis and acute kidney injury. *N Engl J Med*. 2009; 361:62–72.
- Elsayed EF, Reilly RF. Rhabdomyolyis: a review, with emphasis on the pediatric population. *Pediatr Nephrol*. 2010;25(1):7–18.
- Talving P, Karamanos E, Skiada D, et al. Relationship of creatinine kinase elevation and acute kidney injury in pediatric trauma patients. *J Trauma Acute Care Surg*. 2013;74(3):912–916.

CODES

ICD10
- M62.82 Rhabdomyolysis
- T79.5XXA Traumatic anuria, initial encounter

R

RHABDOMYOSARCOMA

Amit J. Sabnis • Steven G. DuBois

BASICS

DESCRIPTION

- A soft tissue cancer with features of skeletal muscle differentiation. Prognostic classification of rhabdomyosarcoma (RMS) currently depends on the following:
  - Anatomic site of disease (stage)
  - Extent of resection and spread (group)
  - Underlying histology (alveolar vs. embryonal or other variants, e.g., botryoid)

EPIDEMIOLOGY

- The most common pediatric soft tissue sarcomas (tumors of mesenchymal origin)
- Accounts for ~5% of childhood cancer
- Boys at slightly increased risk compared to girls (incidence by gender of 1.5:1)
- Peaks in children <7 years of age, with another smaller peak in late adolescence
- Median age at diagnosis is 5 years.

Incidence

- 4.5 cases per 1 million children per year
- U.S. annual incidence of about 350 cases per year

RISK FACTORS

- Radiation exposure, including a possible connection to in utero exposure
- High birth weight associated with embryonal rhabdomyosarcoma in one study.

Genetics

- About 90% of cases are sporadic.
- Several predisposing conditions:
  - Li-Fraumeni (autosomal dominant)
    - *TP53* mutation leads to cancer predisposition through loss of DNA damage signaling.
    - Increased risk for soft tissue sarcomas, osteosarcoma, adrenocortical carcinoma, choroid plexus carcinoma, leukemias, breast cancer, and other cancers
  - Beckwith-Wiedemann syndrome (sporadic)
    - Improper epigenetic regulation of 11p15 leads to an overgrowth syndrome.
    - Increased risk of a range of embryonal cancers early in life, including Wilms tumor, hepatoblastoma, and RMS
  - Neurofibromatosis type I and Costello syndrome (autosomal dominant)
    - Mutational activation of *HRAS* (Costello) or loss of the RAS-negative regulator *NF1* (neurofibromatosis) leads to unchecked RAS signaling and increased risk for RMS.

GENERAL PREVENTION

- No standard approach because most cases are sporadic
- Avoidance of radiation in patients with known predisposing syndromes (e.g., Li-Fraumeni syndrome)

PATHOPHYSIOLOGY

- Alveolar rhabdomyosarcomas (ARMS; about 20% of cases) carry translocations t(2;13) or t(1;13) resulting in the fusion transcription factors *PAX3-FOXO1* or *PAX7-FOXO1*.
  - Alveolar histology and presence of *PAX3-FOXO1* is a poor prognostic factor.
  - Animal models combining expression of *PAX3-FOXO1* and loss of either *TP53* or *CDKN2A* recapitulate ARMS.
- Embryonal rhabdomyosarcomas (ERMS; about 60% of cases) commonly carry mutations in the *RAS* pathway as well as loss of heterozygosity at 11p15.
  - Animal models of ERMS target activating *Ras* mutations to myogenic progenitor cells.
  - The botryoid subtype of ERMS includes submucosal tumors with a favorable prognosis.
- The remainder of cases include pleomorphic or anaplastic histologies and also harbor a poor prognosis.

COMMONLY ASSOCIATED CONDITIONS

- Syndromes listed in "Genetics" have the highest association.
- CNS and genitourinary (GU) anomalies (Chiari malformations, horseshoe kidneys, etc.) in one autopsy-based report

DIAGNOSIS

HISTORY

- Often presents as a firm mass that may be painless
- Additional symptoms relate to location of primary mass:
  - Orbital (10%): unilateral proptosis, ophthalmoplegia, visual changes
  - Head and neck—parameningeal (16%): sinus pressure, nasal congestion, hypophonation, discharge from the nose or ear, unilateral hearing loss, ophthalmoplegia
    - Parameningeal tumors with intracranial extension can present with headache, vomiting, and cranial nerve palsies.
  - Head and neck—nonparameningeal (10%; includes scalp, buccal mucosa, face): asymmetric facies, palpable mass
  - Extremities (20%): palpable mass, often tender or inflamed
  - Genitourinary (25%): bloody or mucous vaginal discharge, prolapse of tissue through vagina or urethra, hematuria, urinary retention, constipation, firm testicular mass

PHYSICAL EXAM

- Exam findings correlate with sites, as described earlier under "History."
  - Orbital: proptosis; tumor may be visible beneath everted palpebrum
  - Head and neck: visibly asymmetric facies. Tumors arising in the sinuses or pharynx may be visible in the oral or nasal cavity.
  - Extremities: palpable mass, often tender or inflamed. Lymph nodes commonly involved.
  - Genitourinary: Prolapsed tissue may be visible through urethra (bladder primary) or vagina (vaginal primary); firm scrotal mass (paratesticular primary)
- Abnormal neurologic exam raises suspicion for intracranial extension.
- Evidence of cytopenias (petechiae, pallor) raises suspicion for bone marrow metastases.
- Enlarged lymph nodes suggest regional nodal spread, common in extremity RMS.

DIAGNOSTIC TESTS & INTERPRETATION

Lab

- CBC
  - To provide an estimate of marrow involvement
  - To help rule out a hematopoietic malignancy
- Electrolytes including calcium and magnesium, liver function tests, and blood urea nitrogen (BUN)/creatinine prior to initiating therapy
- Tumor lysis labs (uric acid, lactate dehydrogenase [LDH] and phosphate in addition to chemistries above) may be helpful if other malignancies are diagnostic considerations.

Imaging

- MRI (preferred) or CT scan of primary site
- Chest CT to rule out pulmonary metastases (most common site of metastatic disease)
- Abdominal and pelvic CT to evaluate for nodal metastases in paratesticular tumors
- ^{99m}Tc bone scan and/or PET scan to evaluate for bone metastasis

Diagnostic Procedures/Other

- Surgical biopsy, performed by an experienced surgeon with a high index of suspicion for malignancy and with appropriate precautions to prevent tumor spill

ALERT

Testicular masses should not be biopsied but rather resected along with the spermatic cord through an inguinal approach. It is vital that the performing surgeon is aware of the potential diagnosis of RMS.

- Bilateral bone marrow biopsies to evaluate for metastatic disease in the bone marrow
- Lumbar puncture for CSF cytology if intracranial extension is a possibility (parameningeal tumors)
- Echocardiogram to ensure normal cardiac function before administering anthracyclines

Pathologic Findings

- Small round blue cells are characteristic, although may see spindle cell elements.
- All RMS are considered high-grade tumors.
- Immunohistochemical stains include positivity for desmin and myogenin, negativity for CD45, CD99, and synaptophysin.
- Diffuse myogenin staining suggests ARMS.
- Fluorescence in situ hybridization (FISH) probes for *FOXO1* translocations may help identify ARMS.

DIFFERENTIAL DIAGNOSIS

- Other small round blue cell tumors
  - Ewing sarcoma (CD99+)
  - Neuroblastoma (synaptophysin+)
  - Non-Hodgkin lymphoma (CD45+)
- Other cancers
  - Non-RMS soft tissue sarcomas
  - Germ cell tumors (especially GU masses)
  - Rhabdoid tumor
- Nonmalignant masses
  - Trauma
  - Benign growths (lipoma, rhabdomyoma)
  - Abscess or other infectious process

TREATMENT

MEDICATION

- The backbone of RMS chemotherapy in North America is cycles of vincristine and actinomycin D, with or without cyclophosphamide (also known as "VA" or "VAC").
  - VA can be given as outpatient therapy.
  - Cyclophosphamide is omitted for low-risk patients.
- Additional agents under investigation for high risk or relapsed patients include doxorubicin, ifosfamide, etoposide, and camptothecins (e.g., irinotecan).
- Experimental protocols include insulin-like growth factor 1 receptor (IGF-1R) monoclonal antibodies.
- Supportive care regimens include *Pneumocystis carinii* pneumonia (PCP) prophylaxis, myeloid growth factors (e.g., granulocyte colony-stimulating factor [G-CSF]) to shorten neutropenia, antiemetics, and laxatives.

ADDITIONAL TREATMENT

General Measures

- Therapy usually lasts approximately 1 year.
- Patients require surgery and/or radiation therapy for local control.
- Cytotoxic chemotherapy has significant short- and long-term toxicities (see "Complications").
- The majority of children are treated at pediatric oncology centers to provide
  - Access to the most recent cooperative group clinical trials
  - A multidisciplinary team of pediatric oncologists, surgeons, radiation oncologists, pathologists, pharmacists, nutritionists, and social work support

ADDITIONAL THERAPIES

- In North America, radiation therapy is used for local control in all cases, except completely resected ERMS.
- Any nonresected sites of metastatic disease are also typically treated with radiation.

ISSUES FOR REFERRAL

- Referral to an experienced pediatric oncology center is strongly encouraged.
- A pediatric oncologist should be consulted whenever the diagnosis of RMS is suspected, prior to any invasive procedures.
- Pediatric oncology consultation should also be encouraged for young adults with RMS.

SURGERY/OTHER PROCEDURES

- Surgeons assist in pretreatment staging and in determining a patient's clinical group based on extent of initial surgery.
- Given radiosensitivity of RMS, avoid surgical procedures that will result in significant loss of function.
- If deemed resectable without significant loss of function, the goal should be complete excision with negative margins.

INPATIENT CONSIDERATIONS

- Admit patients with severe cytopenias, threat to vision or airway due to mass effect, or for expedited workup if unable to access care.
- Diagnostic workup can often be performed on an expedited outpatient schedule.

ONGOING CARE

FOLLOW-UP RECOMMENDATIONS

- Patients seen regularly by pediatric oncology
- After completion of therapy, follow-up with pediatric oncology is every 3 months for the 1st year, then the interval between visits can be gradually increased.
- Patients should continue to receive annual preventive health visits with their primary medical doctor (PMD).
- Vaccinations are deferred during cytotoxic therapy due to limited efficacy, although annual influenza vaccines are recommended.

PATIENT EDUCATION

- Patients' families are reminded that fevers are medical emergencies in children receiving chemotherapy.
- Patients' families are advised of signs/symptoms that might suggest recurrent disease.

PROGNOSIS

- Overall survival is approximately 70%, with significant differences based on risk group.
- Current risk stratification in North America includes the following:
  - Stage (based on anatomic site of disease, size, and regional node involvement)
    - Orbital, nonparameningeal head and neck, vaginal, and biliary tract are favorable.
    - Extremity and parameningeal sites are unfavorable.
  - Clinical group (extent of residual disease remaining after initial surgery)
    - Gross residual disease is unfavorable (except in orbital disease).
    - Metastatic disease is very unfavorable.
  - Histology
    - ARMS is never classified as low risk.
- 5-year event-free survival is estimated to be
  - >90% for low-risk disease
  - 70–80% for intermediate-risk disease
  - <30% for high-risk disease

COMPLICATIONS

- RMS therapy is intensive and has numerous secondary effects.
- Acute toxicities:
  - Marrow suppression, requiring blood and platelet transfusions and raising the risk of life-threatening sepsis
  - Severe nausea and vomiting
  - Mucosal injury with pain and poor PO intake
  - Neuropathic pain, extremity weakness, and constipation due to vincristine
  - Risk of hemorrhagic cystitis (rare) with cyclophosphamide
  - Hepatic sinusoidal obstructive syndrome
- Late effects (see "Cancer Therapy Late Effects" chapter):
  - Infertility (related to cyclophosphamide or ifosfamide)
  - Cardiomyopathy (related to doxorubicin)
  - Secondary malignancies (e.g., leukemia from chemotherapy or sarcomas in radiation field)
  - Radiation vasculopathy (increased risk of stroke in patients with CNS radiation, hypertension in those with renal radiation)
  - Long-term monitoring in a Cancer Survivorship program is recommended.

ADDITIONAL READING

- Hayes-Jordan A, Andrassy R. Rhabdomyosarcoma in children. *Curr Opin Pediatr*. 2009;21(3):373–378.
- Huh WW, Skapek SX. Childhood rhabdomyosarcoma: new insight on biology and treatment. *Curr Oncol Rep*. 2010;12(6):402–410.
- Malempati S, Hawkins DS. Rhabdomyosarcoma: review of the Children's Oncology Group (COG) Soft-Tissue Sarcoma Committee experience and rationale for current COG studies. *Pediatr Blood Cancer*. 2012;59(1):5–10.
- Van Gaal JC, De Bont ES, Kaal SE, et al. Building the bridge between rhabdomyosarcoma in children, adolescents, and young adults: the road ahead. *Crit Rev Oncol Hematol*. 2012;82(3):259–279.

CODES

ICD10

- C49.9 Malignant neoplasm of connective and soft tissue, unsp
- C49.0 Malignant neoplasm of connective and soft tissue of head, face and neck
- C49.5 Malignant neoplasm of connective and soft tissue of pelvis

FAQ

- Q: Are other children in the family at risk for developing rhabdomyosarcoma?
- A: Familial risk for developing RMS is rare, outside of syndromes addressed in "Genetics."
- Q: Does a patient's age influence outcome?
- A: Patients <1 and >10 years of age have poorer outcomes than the majority of RMS patients, who are diagnosed between those ages.

RHEUMATIC FEVER

David Hehir

BASICS

DESCRIPTION
- A postinfectious inflammatory disease caused by rheumatogenic strains of group A β-hemolytic *Streptococcus* (GABHS)
- Acute rheumatic fever (ARF) results in a wide range of disease, from mild joint involvement to chronic carditis.
- The most significant socioeconomic impact is caused by its most severe form, rheumatic heart disease (RHD). Although rarely fatal in the acute phase, RHD may result in significant disability and shortened lifespan. Therefore, the elimination of RHD is a main goal of the World Health Federation.

EPIDEMIOLOGY
- Occurs following pharyngitis with rheumatogenic GABHS strains
- GABHS strains causing skin infections have been associated with ARF in tropical and underdeveloped areas of the world.
- Initial episode seen primarily in patients 5–15 years of age
- No racial or ethnic predilections

Incidence
- Historically, untreated GABHS infection results in ARF in 0.1–0.3% of cases, with attack rates as high as 3% in endemic areas.
- Decrease in incidence due to increased use of antibiotics, improved environmental factors such as overcrowding, and changing virulence patterns of GABHS strains

Prevalence
- 12 million people are affected by ARF worldwide, with 400,000 cases of RHD.
- RHD accounts for 25–40% of all cardiac disease worldwide.

RISK FACTORS

Genetics
No specific genetic risk factor identified, although numerous studies have demonstrated an association of ARF with specific human leukocyte antigen (HLA) alleles.

PATHOPHYSIOLOGY
- GABHS triggers a complex inflammatory host response, affecting the heart, joints, brain, blood vessels, and subcutaneous tissue.
- Classic example of molecular mimicry, in which the host produces antibodies to certain GABHS M proteins, which are similar in structure to host proteins such as myosin, resulting in autoimmune tissue damage
- Aschoff nodules are proliferative lesions noted in the myocardium that may persist for months to years after initiation of disease.

ETIOLOGY
Immune-mediated inflammatory reaction to specific rheumatogenic strains of GABHS

DIAGNOSIS

HISTORY
Diagnosis is based on the modified Jones criteria (updated 1992):
- Evidence of recent GABHS infection **PLUS** 2 major **OR** 1 major and 2 minor criteria
- Major criteria (% affected)
  - Polyarthritis (70%): migratory arthritis of major joints; more common in adults
  - Carditis (50%): 85% of those with carditis have mitral regurgitation, and 54% have aortic valve involvement. Symptoms range from asymptomatic murmur to fulminant heart failure; carditis is more common and more severe in children.
  - Sydenham chorea (15%): abnormal behavior and/or involuntary, purposeless movements
  - Erythema marginatum (10%): evanescent, pink rash with serpiginous borders
  - Subcutaneous nodules (2–10%): painless nodules over extensor surfaces of large joints, the occiput, and/or vertebral processes
- Minor criteria
  - Fever
  - Arthralgia (mild pain without objective findings): can only be considered without finding of arthritis
  - Elevated acute-phase reactants: ESR, C-reactive protein
  - Prolongation of the PR interval on ECG
- Exceptions to the Jones criteria include the following:
  - Sydenham chorea alone
  - Subclinical carditis (echocardiogram evidence of RHD) in the absence of other criteria should be treated as ARF.
  - Jones criteria not useful with recurrence; World Health Organization (WHO) recommends treating recurrence in a patient with RHD history and presence of any new major or minor criterion.

PHYSICAL EXAM
- Cardiac
  - Murmur of valvulitis: holosystolic mitral regurgitant murmur, Carey-Coombs apical mid-diastolic murmur, or a basal diastolic murmur of aortic insufficiency (major criterion)
  - Pericardial friction rub: pericardial effusion
- Musculoskeletal
  - Pain, limited motion, erythema, warmth of 2 or more large joints: arthritis (major criterion)
- Neurologic
  - Choreiform movements (must be differentiated from tics, athetosis, and hyperkinesis)
  - Sydenham chorea (major criterion)
- Dermatologic
  - Evanescent, pink rash with pale centers and serpiginous borders on the trunk and proximal extremities: erythema marginatum (major criterion)
  - Firm, painless nodules over the extensor surface of large joints, occiput, and/or spinous processes: subcutaneous nodules (major criterion)

DIAGNOSTIC TESTS & INTERPRETATION

Lab
- Specific tests: No specific diagnostic test is available.
- Nonspecific tests
  - Throat culture: neither sensitive nor specific; false negative in up to 2/3 of affected patients or false positive in patients who are colonized
  - Elevated or rising streptococcal antibody titers, antistreptolysin O, anti-DNase B, and antihyaluronidase may be helpful.
  - ESR and C-reactive protein elevation

Imaging
- ECG: prolonged PR interval (minor criterion), junctional rhythm, transient arrhythmias, ST-T wave changes
- Chest radiograph: Cardiomegaly may indicate carditis or pericardial effusion. Pulmonary edema may reflect left heart failure due to valvulitis.
- Echocardiogram: Assess valve involvement, ventricular dilatation, function, and pericardial effusion.

DIFFERENTIAL DIAGNOSIS
- Carditis
  - Viral
  - Bacterial
  - Rickettsial
  - Parasitic
  - *Mycoplasma* myocarditis
  - Kawasaki disease
- Arthritis
  - Poststreptococcal reactive arthritis (PSRA)
  - Serum sickness
  - Septic arthritis (e.g., gonococcal)
  - Lyme disease
- Collagen vascular disease
  - Juvenile rheumatoid arthritis (small joints, not migratory, and not relieved promptly with aspirin)
  - Systemic lupus erythematosus
  - Bacterial endocarditis
- Chorea
  - Congenital choreoathetosis
  - Brain tumors
  - Huntington chorea
  - Wilson disease
  - Pediatric autoimmune neuropsychiatric disorders associated with streptococcus (PANDAS)
- Hematologic disorders with joint involvement
  - Sickle cell anemia
  - Leukemia
- Congenital heart defects: previously undiagnosed valvular heart disease
- Mitral valve prolapse with regurgitation

TREATMENT

MEDICATION

First Line

- Anti-inflammatory
  - Aspirin 60–100 mg/kg/24 h PO divided q6–8h; may be reduced when fever and acute-phase reactants have normalized for 6–8 weeks
- Antibiotics in ARF
  - Penicillin V potassium
    - Children: 250 mg 2–3 times/day for 10 days
    - Adolescents, adults: 500 mg 2–3 times/day for 10 days
- Secondary prophylaxis
  - Penicillin G benzathine IM (600,000 U for weight <27 kg or 1,200,000 U for weight >27 kg) every 3–4 weeks

Second Line

- Anti-inflammatory
  - Prednisone 2 mg/kg/24 h for 2 weeks, then taper
- Antibiotics in ARF
  - Erythromycin, amoxicillin, 1st-generation cephalosporin
- Secondary prophylaxis
  - Penicillin V potassium 250 mg b.i.d.
  - Erythromycin, sulfadiazine

ADDITIONAL TREATMENT

General Measures

- Primary prevention: appropriate and early treatment of GABHS pharyngitis
- Interventions to address poverty, crowding, and housing challenges
- Treatment of ARF
  - Antibiotics: full course of penicillin or equivalent to eradicate active infection; does not alter course of carditis
  - Anti-inflammatory: High-dose aspirin is standard; steroids may help for severe carditis but remain controversial.
  - Cardiac support: aggressive support of cardiac function and use of systemic afterload reduction for severe disease
  - Surgical valvuloplasty or valve replacement may be necessary in severe cases.
  - Bed rest: controversial; recommended at times for severe cases
- Secondary prevention of recurrence
  - Ideally administered as penicillin G benzathine as a monthly IM injection, but oral daily penicillin or erythromycin is acceptable in areas of low prevalence.
  - Duration is based on clinical presentation and degree of cardiac involvement:
    - ARF without cardiac involvement: 5 years or until age 18 years, whichever is longer
    - ARF with mild or resolved carditis: 10 years or until age 25 years, whichever is longer
    - ARF with severe carditis or cardiac surgery: lifelong
- Treatment of chorea
  - Usually supportive
  - Phenobarbital and haloperidol are most commonly used; chlorpromazine, diazepam, or valproic acid also used

ISSUES FOR REFERRAL

Patients with new murmurs or clinical evidence of heart failure should be referred to a cardiologist.

INPATIENT CONSIDERATIONS

Initial Stabilization

- Full treatment of streptococcal pharyngitis infection and cardiac support if heart failure present
- Treatment phases include primary prevention, management of ARF, and secondary prevention of recurrence.

ONGOING CARE

FOLLOW-UP RECOMMENDATIONS

- Patients without carditis
  - Close follow-up is needed for 2–3 weeks to assess patient's condition for development of acute carditis.
  - Long-term pediatric follow-up is needed to diagnose patients with indolent carditis.
  - Long-term follow-up is needed to evaluate patients who develop chorea.
  - Prophylaxis should be stressed even in patients without carditis.
- Patients with carditis
  - Cardiology follow-up is needed to assess development or evolution of RHD.
  - Symptoms of worsening heart failure suggest progression of valvular or myocardial disease, recurrent ARF, or endocarditis.
  - Secondary prophylaxis and bacterial endocarditis prophylaxis should be stressed.

PROGNOSIS

- ARF recurrence rate as high as 36% without prophylaxis
- Chorea may last weeks to months and has a similarly high recurrence rate.
- Carditis may resolve spontaneously (70–80%) or progress. Severity of the initial carditis is a major determinant of progression.

COMPLICATIONS

Long-term complications related to evolution of RHD

- Mitral stenosis
- Mitral regurgitation
- Aortic stenosis
- Aortic regurgitation
- Chronic heart failure

ADDITIONAL READING

- Carapetis JR, McDonald M, Wilson NJ. Acute rheumatic fever. *Lancet*. 2005;366(9480):155–168.
- Cilliers AM, Manyemba J, Saloojee H. Anti-inflammatory treatment for carditis in acute rheumatic fever. *The Cochrane Library*. 2006;4:1–37.
- Kerdemelidis M, Lennon DR, Arroll B, et al. The primary prevention of rheumatic fever. *J Paediatr Child Health*. 2010;46(9):534–548.
- Lawrence JG, Carapetis JR, Griffiths K, et al. Acute rheumatic fever and rheumatic heart disease: incidence and progression in the Northern Territory of Australia, 1997 to 2010. *Circulation*. 2013;128(5):492–501.
- Van Driel M, De Sutter AI, Keber N, et al. Different antibiotic treatments for group A streptococcal pharyngitis. *The Cochrane Library*. 2013;4:1–49.

CODES

ICD10

- I00 Rheumatic fever without heart involvement
- I09.9 Rheumatic heart disease, unspecified
- M06.9 Rheumatoid arthritis, unspecified

FAQ

- Q: Does a negative throat culture rule out ARF?
- A: No. Throat cultures may be negative in 2/3 of patients.
- Q: Is there a vaccine available that is effective in preventing ARF?
- A: Not at present. Given that >90 antigenic strains of group A *Streptococcus* have been identified; vaccines development is focused on strains with the greatest virulence.
- Q: What genetic factors predispose to ARF?
- A: Patients with certain HLA-DR antigens are predisposed to ARF. The specific antigen/allele varies with the ethnic group.
- Q: Can ECG evidence of carditis alone be used to diagnose rheumatic fever?
- A: An ECG finding of carditis in the absence of a murmur does not fulfill the Jones criteria. However, many experts would agree to treat subclinical carditis as ARF, especially in areas of high prevalence.

RHINITIS, ALLERGIC

Esther K. Chung • Karen P. Zimmer

BASICS

DESCRIPTION

- Inflammation of the nasal and sinus mucosae, associated with sneezing, swelling, increased mucus production, and nasal obstruction; may be classified as seasonal, perennial, or a combination
  - Seasonal: periodic symptoms, involving the same season for at least 2 consecutive years; most often due to pollens (e.g., trees, grass, weeds) and outdoor spores
  - Perennial: occurring at least 9 months of the year; may be more difficult to detect because of overlap with other infections; may be due to multiple seasonal allergies or continual exposure to allergens (e.g., dust mites, cockroaches, molds, and animal dander)
  - Perennial, with seasonal exacerbations
- The Allergic Rhinitis and Its Impact on Asthma (ARIA) World Health Organization expert panel prefer the classification for allergic rhinitis of intermittent or persistent, with subclassifications of mild, moderate, or severe.

EPIDEMIOLOGY

Prevalence

Most common allergic disease; affecting approximately 40 million Americans; affects 40% of children and 15%–30% of adolescents

RISK FACTORS

Genetics

Increased incidence in families with atopic disease. If 1 parent has allergies, each child has approximately a 30% chance of having an allergy; if both parents have allergies, each child has a 70% chance of having an allergy.

GENERAL PREVENTION

- Minimize exposure to dust mites: Consider removing carpets, upholstered furniture, and curtains; washing bedding in hot water frequently, at least every 1–2 weeks; use pillow and mattress covers.
- Minimize exposure to animal dander.
- Minimize exposure to all animals; consider using solutions containing tannic acid, which will denature animal allergens; shampoo pets frequently if pets cannot be removed from the household; use air vent filters.
- Minimize exposure to pollens: Keep windows closed, use air-conditioning and avoid leaf raking or lawn mowing.
- Minimize exposure to molds: Keep houseplants out of the bedroom; avoid spending time in the basement, keep humidity at 35–50%.
- Early introduction of complementary foods—particularly cereals, fish, eggs—prior to a year of age was inversely associated with allergic rhinitis.

ETIOLOGY

- Indoor allergens: house dust mite, cockroaches, animal dander, cigarette smoke, hair spray, paint, molds
- Pollens: tree pollens in early spring, grass in late spring and early summer, ragweed in late summer and autumn
- Multiple environmental factors
- Changes in air temperature

COMMONLY ASSOCIATED CONDITIONS

- Asthma
- Allergic conjunctivitis
- Atopic dermatitis (eczema)
- Urticaria
- Otitis media with effusion
- Sleep, taste, and/or smell disturbance
- Nasal polyps
- Mouth breathing
- Snoring
- Adenoidal hypertrophy and sleep apnea
- Decreased appetite
- Delayed speech

DIAGNOSIS

HISTORY

- Typical symptoms: Patient often reports bilateral stuffy nose, sneezing, itching, runny nose, noisy breathing, snoring, cough, halitosis, and repeated throat clearing. Sensation of plugged ears and wheezing may occur.
- Red and itchy eyes
- Symptom occurrence: seasonal, perennial, or episodic
- Exacerbating factors including pollen, animals, cigarette smoke, dust, molds
- Family history of atopic disease such as asthma or atopic dermatitis
- Any related illnesses: Asthma, urticaria, eczema, ear infections, and delayed speech are commonly associated conditions.

PHYSICAL EXAM

- Allergic shiners
  - Dark discoloration beneath the eyes due to obstruction of lymphatic and venous drainage, chronic nasal obstruction, and suborbital edema
- Dennie-Morgan lines
  - Creases in the lower eyelid radiating outward from the inner canthus; caused by spasm in the muscles of Müller around eye due to chronic congestion and stasis of blood
- Allergic salute
  - A gesture characterized by rubbing the nose with the palm of the hand upward to decrease itching and temporarily open the nasal passages
- Allergic crease
  - Transverse crease near the tip of the nose, secondary to rubbing
- Nasal mucosa may appear pale and/or edematous; mucoid or watery material may be seen in the nasal cavity; check for nasal polyps and septal deviation.

DIAGNOSTIC TESTS & INTERPRETATION

- Audiometry and tympanometry when indicated
- Sweat test if cystic fibrosis is suspected or if nasal polyps are present

Lab

- Nasal cytology
- Specimen of nasal discharge to check for the presence of eosinophils. Have the patient blow his or her nose into a piece of nonporous paper or collect discharge with a cotton swab and transfer the discharge to a glass slide. >10% eosinophils are considered positive for nasal eosinophilia. Note: Use of intranasal steroids may reduce the number of eosinophils found in nasal discharge.
- Radioallergosorbent tests (RAST)
  - In vitro test to measure allergen-specific IgE; expensive; useful in patients who have diffuse atopic dermatitis. The ImmunoCAP system (Pharmacia Diagnostics) is the preferred method for specific IgE testing; uses a single blood sample to identify levels of specific IgE to a number of common respiratory allergens (available as a profile specific to the region of the country where the patient resides), food antigens (food allergy profile), or both (childhood allergy profile)
- Total IgE: elevated in allergic rhinitis; not routinely indicated but may come as part of specific IgE testing; >100 kU/L is considered elevated.
- CBC: may show eosinophilia; not routinely indicated
- Skin testing
  - Skin prick test: percutaneous, qualitative test in which antigen concentrate is placed on the skin of the volar surface of the arm or upper back, and a needle is inserted; high negative predictive value; the skin reaction is graded subjectively from 0 to 4.
  - Intradermal test: qualitative test in which antigen is introduced intradermally (0.02 mL with a 26–30-gauge needle); more sensitive than the prick test and often used if prick test is negative or equivocal; the degree of swelling and erythema is graded from 0 to 4.
  - Caution: Skin tests may be difficult to interpret in patients with diffuse eczema and dermatographism.
  - Although positive allergen-specific IgE testing or skin prick testing denote sensitization to an allergen, these positive tests must be interpreted in the context of the clinical presentation.

Diagnostic Procedures/Other

Rhinoscopy to assess the nasal turbinates and to look for nasal polyps

DIFFERENTIAL DIAGNOSIS

- Infection
  - Viral upper respiratory tract infection
  - Bacterial sinusitis
- Environmental
  - Foreign body
  - Temperature
  - Odors
- Tumors
  - Nasal polyps
  - Dermoid cyst
  - Nasal glioma
- Congenital
  - Cystic fibrosis
  - Choanal atresia
  - Ciliary motility disorder (e.g., immotile cilia syndrome)
  - Septal deviation
  - Primary atrophic rhinitis
- Immunologic
  - Sarcoidosis
  - Granulomatosis with polyangiitis (Wegener granulomatosis)
  - Systemic lupus erythematosus
  - Sjögren syndrome
- Allergic
  - Nonallergic perennial rhinitis
  - Idiopathic (vasomotor) rhinitis
  - Drug-induced rhinitis
  - Food-induced rhinitis
- Miscellaneous
  - Rhinitis medicamentosa
  - Rhinitis associated with pregnancy/other hormonal rhinitis
  - Hypothyroidism
  - Idiopathic neonatal rhinitis

TREATMENT

MEDICATION

- Improve mucociliary flow.
  - Steam inhalation
  - Normal saline drops
  - Bicarbonate spray
  - *N*-acetylcysteine (orally or inhaled)
  - Oral guaifenesin
- Antihistamines: competitively blocking histamine (H_1) receptors; suppress itching, ocular symptoms, sneezing, and rhinorrhea; not very effective against nasal congestion
- Intranasal 2nd-generation antihistamine
  - Azelastine: age ≥5 years; 137 mcg per spray; 1 spray per nostril twice a day. Safety and effectiveness of this dose have been established for children older than 5 years, but the efficacy has not yet been established in the pediatric population and is extrapolated from adult data.
- 2nd-generation antihistamines: tend not to cross the blood–brain barrier and therefore do not have CNS side effects such as drowsiness
  - Loratadine (Claritin): FDA-approved for children as young as 2 years of age. Dose: ages 2–5 years, 5 mg/day PO; ages 6 years or older, 10 mg/day PO
  - Desloratadine (Clarinex): FDA-approved for children ≥6 months of age. Dose: 6–12 months, 1 mg/day PO; 12 months–5 years, 1.25 mg/day PO; 6–12 years, 2.5 mg/day PO; >12 years, 5 mg/day PO
  - Cetirizine HCl (Zyrtec): FDA-approved for children as young as 6 months of age. Dose: age 6 months–5 years, 2.5 mg = 1/2 tsp/day (1 mg/mL banana–grape-flavored syrup) PO with maximum dose of 5 mg/day (must be divided into 2.5 mg b.i.d. for children <2 years of age). Age ≥6 years, 5–10 mg/day
  - Levocetirizine (Xyzal): dose: age 6 months–5 years: 1.25 mg/day (1/2 tsp = 2.5 mL); ages 6–11 years: 2.5 mg/day (half tab or 1 tsp = 5 mL) PO; age ≥12 years: 5 mg/day (1 tab or 2 tsp = 10 mL) PO
  - Fexofenadine HCl (Allegra): ages 2–11 years: 1 tsp = 5 mL (30 mg/5 mL) or 30-mg tab b.i.d.; age ≥12 years, 60 mg b.i.d. or 180 mg/24 h PO
- 1st-generation antihistamine side effects include drowsiness, performance impairment, and paradoxical excitement; anticholinergic (e.g., dry mouth, tachycardia, urinary retention, and constipation): diphenhydramine (Benadryl) 5 mg/kg/day PO divided q.i.d.
- Intranasal steroids: blunt early-phase reactions and block late-phase reactions; may not be fully effective until several days to 2 weeks after initiation of therapy; must be used regularly and best when administered lying down with the head back
  - Beclomethasone (Vancenase, Beconase): for use in children ≥6 years of age
  - Flunisolide (Aerobid): for use in children ≥6 years of age
  - Fluticasone propionate (Flonase 0.05%): for use in children ≥4 years of age
  - Budesonide (Rhinocort): for use in children ≥6 years of age
  - Triamcinolone acetonide (Nasacort): for use in children ≥2 years of age
  - Mometasone furoate monohydrate (Nasonex): for children ≥2 years of age
- Intranasal antihistamines: azelastine hydrochloride (Astelin; approved for children ≥5 years; 5–11 years: 1 spray each nostril b.i.d.; ≥12 years: 2 sprays each nostril b.i.d.) and olopatadine (Patanase; approved for children ≥6 years; 6–11 years: 1 spray per nostril b.i.d.; 12 years and older: 2 sprays per nostril b.i.d.) are FDA-approved for use in seasonal allergic rhinitis.
- Topical cromolyn (Nasalcrom): mast cell stabilizer; minimal side effects; does not provide immediate relief (may take 2–4 weeks to see clinical effect): for use in children ≥2 years of age
- Oral decongestants: Alpha-1 and -2 agonists (e.g., ephedrine, pseudoephedrine, and phenylephrine) act to cause vasoconstriction, decreased blood supply to the nasal mucosa, and decreased mucosal edema. Cardiovascular and CNS side effects include tremors, agitation, hypertension, insomnia, and headaches.
- Topical decongestants: Sympathomimetics such as short-acting phenylephrine (Neo-Synephrine) and long-acting oxymetazoline (Afrin) may be useful for a few days to open nasal passages to allow for delivery of topical steroids; side effects include drying of the mucosa and burning. Use for more than a few (3–5) days may result in rebound vasodilatation and congestion (rhinitis medicamentosa).
- Combined oral decongestants and antihistamines: numerous preparations on the market
- Leukotriene receptor antagonist (montelukast [Singulair]): for use in children ≥6 months of age. Dose for 6 months to 23 months, one packet 4-mg granules; 2–5 years, 1 granule packet (4 mg) or 4-mg chewable tab daily; 6–14 years, 5-mg chewable tab daily; age ≥15 years, 10-mg tab daily
- Immunotherapy: also referred to as hyposensitization or desensitization; consists of a series of injections with specific allergens, with increasing concentrations of allergens, once or twice weekly; recommended for patients who have not responded to pharmacologic therapy
  - Effective and long lasting. After several months to years of treatment, total serum IgE levels decrease, and the intensity of the early-phase response is reduced.
  - Side effects include urticaria, bronchospasm, hypotension, and anaphylaxis.

ADDITIONAL TREATMENT

General Measures

Avoidance therapy: Identify and eliminate known/suspected allergens.

SURGERY/OTHER PROCEDURES

- Removal of allergic polyps
- Inferior turbinate surgery to reduce the size of the turbinate and relieve obstruction
- Endoscopic sinus surgery to relieve obstruction

ONGOING CARE

FOLLOW-UP RECOMMENDATIONS

Patient Monitoring

Fever, prolonged or severe headache, dizziness, pain, or purulent discharge should suggest a diagnosis other than allergic rhinitis alone

PROGNOSIS

Generally good: Complete recovery occurs in 5–10% of patients.

COMPLICATIONS

- Chronic sinusitis
- Recurrent otitis media
- Hoarseness
- Loss of smell
- Loss of hearing
- High-arched palate and dental malocclusion from chronic mouth breathing

ADDITIONAL READING

- Brożek JL, Bousquet J, Baena CE, et al. Allergic rhinitis and its impact on asthma (ARIA) 2010 revision. http://www.whiar.org/docs/ARIAReport_2010.pdf. Accessed September 4, 2013.
- Nwaru BI, Takkinen HM, Niemela O, et al. Timing of infant feeding in relation to childhood asthma and allergic diseases. *J Allergy Clin Immunol*. 2013;131(1):78–86.
- Phan H, Moeller ML, Nahata MC. Treatment of allergic rhinitis in infants and children: efficacy and safety of second-generation antihistamines and the leukotriene receptor antagonist montelukast. *Drugs*. 2009;69(18):2541–2576.
- Radulovic S, Calderon MA, Wilson D, et al. Sublingual immunotherapy for allergic rhinitis. *Cochrane Database Syst Rev*. 2010;(12):CD002893. doi:10.1002/14651858.CD002893.pub2.
- Sicherer SH, Wood RA; American Academy of Pediatrics Section on Allergy and Immunology. Allergy testing in childhood: using allergen-specific IgE tests. *Pediatrics*. 2012;129(1):193–197.
- Turner PJ, Kemp AS. Allergic rhinitis in children. *J Paediatr Child Health*. 2012;48(4):302–310.
- Wallace DV, Dykewicz MS, Berstein DI, et al. The diagnosis and management of rhinitis: an updated practice parameter. *J Allergy Clin Immunol*. 2008;122(2)(Suppl):S1–S84.

CODES

ICD10

- J30.9 Allergic rhinitis, unspecified
- J30.1 Allergic rhinitis due to pollen
- J30.89 Other allergic rhinitis

FAQ

- Q: How does one minimize exposure to dust mites?
- A: Keep household temperature low; maintain humidity at ~40–50%; wash linens weekly at hot temperatures; use a microfilter when vacuuming; place mattress and box spring in tightly woven casing; use air-conditioning; use high-efficiency particulate air filter units.
- Q: How often are nasal polyps associated with cystic fibrosis?
- A: In up to 40% of children, nasal polyps are associated with cystic fibrosis. <0.5% of children with asthma and rhinitis have nasal polyps.
- Q: When used on a daily basis, are intranasal steroids safe?
- A: Yes. It is generally accepted that inhaled steroids are safe. Growth suppression has been reported in children using certain intranasal steroids; however, this effect does not appear to be an effect of all intranasal steroids. Importantly, one should use the lowest effective dose of intranasal steroids when treating allergic rhinitis.

RICKETS/OSTEOMALACIA

Alison M. Boyce • Laura L. Tosi

BASICS

DESCRIPTION

- Osteomalacia refers to impaired bone mineralization, caused primarily by deficiencies in vitamin D and/or calcium.
- In children, osteomalacia leads to growth plate abnormalities, termed rickets.

EPIDEMIOLOGY

- The prevalence of rickets and osteomalacia is very high in many parts of the world.
- Reported with increasing frequency in the United States since the 1980s

GENERAL PREVENTION

- Vitamin D supplements should be given to breastfed infants and high-risk individuals.
- In the United States and Canada, cow's milk, infant formula, and cereals are fortified with vitamin D.

PATHOPHYSIOLOGY

Rickets arises due to decreased availability of phosphorus and calcium to mineralize the skeletal matrix, leading to growth plate disorganization and accumulation of undermineralized osteoid. This results in growth plate expansion, bone weakening, and skeletal deformities.

ETIOLOGY

Primary causes include the following:

- Nutritional
  - Insufficient vitamin D and/or calcium intakes (common)
  - Insufficient phosphorus intake (rare)
- Deficient sunlight exposure
- Malabsorption
  - Celiac disease
  - Cystic fibrosis
  - Liver disease
- Renal tubular defects
  - Cystinosis
  - Fanconi syndrome
  - Renal tubular acidosis
- Abnormalities in vitamin D metabolism
  - Anticonvulsant use
  - Liver disease
- Genetic forms (see "Table 1.")

RISK FACTORS

- Infants born to vitamin D–deficient mothers
- Low birth weight and/or prematurity
- Breastfeeding without vitamin D supplementation
- Poor nutrition
- Increased skin pigmentation
- Higher latitudes and winter months
- Use of sunscreens
- Malabsorption
- Renal tubulopathies

DIAGNOSIS

HISTORY

- Inadequate nutrition
  - Prolonged breastfeeding without vitamin D supplementation
  - Low dietary calcium intake
  - Strict vegan diet without adequate calcium
  - Premature infants taking unfortified formula
  - Parenteral hyperalimentation
- Low levels of sunlight exposure
- Symptoms of malabsorption:
  - Steatorrhea, abdominal pain, weight loss
- Symptoms of renal tubular dysfunction:
  - Nephrolithiasis, polyuria
- Bone pain
- Delayed gross motor development
- Generalized muscular weakness
- Irritability
- Fractures following minimal trauma
- Dental abscesses
- Anticonvulsant use
- Family history of rickets

PHYSICAL EXAM

- Growth deceleration
- Widening at the wrists, knees, and/or ankles
- Bowing of the extremities (varus or valgus deformities)
- Skull abnormalities
  - Anterior fontanelle widening and/or delayed closure
  - Frontal bossing
  - Craniotabes (softening of the skull)
- Chest deformities
  - Prominent costochondral junctions ("rachitic rosary")
  - Pectus carinatum
  - Horizontal groove along the lower ribs ("Harrison groove")
- Scoliosis
- Hypotonia
- Waddling gait

DIAGNOSTIC TESTS & INTERPRETATION

Initial Labs

- 25-vitamin D
  - Major circulating form, and most sensitive indicator of vitamin D stores
  - Sometimes reported as D_2 (plant derived) and D_3 (animal derived) forms
  - $D_2 + D_3$ = total available 25-vitamin D
- Serum calcium, phosphorous (make sure age-appropriate norms for phosphorus are used by lab), and alkaline phosphatase
- Intact parathyroid hormone
- Urine calcium, creatinine, and urinalysis
- If rarer forms of rickets being considered: 1,25-vitamin D, urine phosphorus

Imaging

- Radiographic findings:
  - Widening, cupping, and/or fraying of the growth plates
  - Expansion of anterior ribs at the costochondral junctions
  - Bowing of the long bones
  - Osteopenia
- Knee or wrist films may be used diagnostically, and to monitor treatment response

DIFFERENTIAL DIAGNOSIS

- See Table 1 for ways to differentiate forms of rickets.
- Metaphyseal chondrodysplasia
- Blount disease
- Chronic recurrent multifocal osteomyelitis
- Neurofibromatosis type 1
- Renal osteodystrophy (combines features of rickets, osteomalacia, secondary hyperparathyroidism, and osteoporosis)

TREATMENT

GENERAL MEASURES

Treatment depends on the underlying etiology.

ADDITIONAL THERAPIES

- Treatment of vitamin D deficiency: high dose repletion with cholecalciferol (D_3) or ergocalciferol (D_2) over 8–12 weeks (goal total of ~200,000–400,000 IU)
  - Infants and children <5 years of age: 2,000 IU daily
  - Children 5 years of age–adult: 4,000–5,000 IU daily, or 14,000 to 50,000 IU weekly

Table 1. Biochemical features of rickets/osteomalacia

	Ca	Phos	Alk phos	iPTH	25-(OH)D	1,25-(OH)$_2$D	Urine Ca/Cr	TRP
Nutritional/insufficient sunlight	N or ↓	↓	↑	↑	↓	↑	↓	↑
Malabsorption	N or ↓	↓	↑	↑	↓	↑	↓	↑
Renal tubular defects	N or ↓	↓	↑	↑	N	↑	↑	N or ↓
Altered vitamin D metabolism	N or ↓	↓	↑	↑	↓	↑	↓	↑
Genetic forms of rickets								
X-linked, AD, and AR hypophosphatemic rickets	N	↓	↑	N or ↑	N	N or ↑	N or ↓	↓
1α-hydroxylase deficiency	↓	↓	↑	↑	N	↓	↓	↑
Vitamin D receptor mutations (Vitamin D resistance)	↓	↓	↑	↑	N	↑	↓	↑
Hereditary hypophosphatemic rickets with hypercalciuria	N or ↓	↓	↑	↑	N	↑	↑	↓
Hypophosphatasia	N or ↑	N or ↑	↓	N or ↓	N	N or ↓	N or ↑	N

Ca, calcium; Phos, phosphorus; Alk phos, alkaline phosphatase; iPTH, intact parathyroid hormone; 25-(OH)D, 25-vitamin D; 1,25-(OH)$_2$D, 1,25-dvitamin D; Ca/Cr, calcium/creatinine ratio; TRP, tubular reabsorption of phosphorus ([1 − (U phos × P Cr/U Cr × S Phos)] × 100, normal 85–95%); N, normal; AD, autosomal dominant; AR, autosomal recessive

Table 2. Dietary reference intake for calcium and vitamin D

	Calcium			Vitamin D		
Age	Estimated Average Requirement (mg/day)	Recommended Dietary Allowance (mg/day)	Upper Level Intake (mg/day)	Estimated Average Requirement (IU/day)	Recommended Dietary Allowance (IU/day)	Upper Level Intake (IU/day)
0–6 months	200	200	1,000	400	400	1,000
6–12 months	260	260	1,500	400	400	1,500
1–3 years	500	700	2,500	400	600	2,500
4–8 years	800	1,000	2,500	400	600	3,000
9–18 years	1,100	1,300	3,000	400	600	4,000
19–30 years	800	1,000	2,500	400	600	4,000

Adapted from Ross C, Abrams S, Aloia J, et al. Dietary Reference Intakes for Calcium and Vitamin D. Washington, DC: The National Academies Press; 2011.

- Following repletion, transition to daily maintenance dose (see "Table 2").
- Supplement with 30–75 mg/kg elemental calcium divided t.i.d. to prevent hungry bone syndrome (hypocalcemia and hypophosphatemia during healing).
- Higher doses of vitamin D often required in patients with malabsorption, altered vitamin D metabolism, and/or obesity
- Optimal serum 25-vitamin D concentrations are controversial, however concentrations >20 ng/mL (50 nmol/L) sufficient to prevent rickets in otherwise healthy children.

ISSUES FOR REFERRAL

- Consider endocrinology referral for infants, children with hypocalcemia, severe disease, suspected genetic forms of rickets, and/or lack of radiographic evidence of healing by 3 months.
- Nephrology referral for management of tubular dysfunction
- Orthopedic referral for patients with severe bowing

INPATIENT CONSIDERATIONS

Admission Criteria

- Rickets can generally be managed in the outpatient setting, however inpatient admission may be considered if:
  - Severe hypocalcemia with tetany or seizures
  - Lack of response to therapy (suspected non-adherence)

Discharge Criteria

- Stable laboratory values
- Normalization in mental status and neurology exam improvement

ONGOING CARE

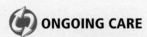

FOLLOW-UP RECOMMENDATIONS

Patient Monitoring

- Monitor serum calcium, phosphorus, alkaline phosphatase, PTH, and spot urinary calcium/creatinine ratio every 2–4 weeks. Note: Alkaline phosphatase may rise initially with treatment and then decrease gradually.
- Consider follow-up imaging after completion of high-dose vitamin D repletion.
- Patients who continue high-dose vitamin D for longer than prescribed may be at risk for hypercalcemia.

PATIENT EDUCATION

Ensure appropriate vitamin D and calcium intake to prevent recurrence (see "Table 2").

PROGNOSIS

- Rickets generally resolves with appropriate treatment.
- If radiographs and/or biochemical parameters not improving, consider the possibility of poor adherence, other forms of rickets, or alternative diagnoses.

COMPLICATIONS

- Failure to thrive, poor motor development
- Bowing and skeletal deformity
- Fractures
- Hypocalcemic tetany and seizures

ADDITIONAL READING

- Holick MF, Binkley NC, Bischoff-Ferrari HA, et al. Evaluation, treatment, and prevention of vitamin D deficiency: an Endocrine Society clinical practice guideline. *J Clin Endocrinol Metab*. 2011;96(7):1911–1930.
- Prentice A. Vitamin D deficiency: a global perspecive. *Nutr Rev*. 2008;66(10)(Suppl 2):S153–S164.
- Ross C, Abrams S, Aloia J, et al. *Dietary Reference Intakes for Calcium and Vitamin D*. Washington, DC: The National Academies Press; 2011.
- Shaw NJ, Mughal MZ. Vitamin D and child health part 1 (skeletal aspects). *Arch Dis Child*. 2013;98(5):363–367.
- Weisberg P, Scanlon K, Li R, et al. Nutritional rickets among children in the United States: review of cases reported between 1986 and 2003. *Am J Clin Nutr*. 2004;80(6)(Suppl):1697S–1705S.

CODES

ICD10

- E55.0 Rickets, active
- E55.9 Vitamin D deficiency, unspecified
- E58 Dietary calcium deficiency

FAQ

- Q: What is the best way to diagnose rickets?
- A: Laboratory evaluation and x-rays are the best ways to make the diagnosis. Radiographic findings are best seen at the distal radius and ulna, and/or the distal femur and proximal tibia.
- Q: What are the recommendations for vitamin D supplementation in infants and children?
- A: The American Academy of Pediatrics recommends the following:
  - All breastfed infants should receive 400 IU daily.
  - Nonbreastfed infants ingesting <500 mL/day of vitamin D–fortified formula or milk should receive 400 IU daily.
  - Children who do not get regular sunlight exposure or do not consume at least 500 mL/day of vitamin D–fortified milk should receive 600 IU daily.
- Q: How is rickets/osteomalacia different from osteoporosis?
- A: Osteoporosis in children is defined by a combination of decreased bone mass coupled with fracture. Although bone density is reduced, bone matrix is generally normally mineralized. In rickets/osteomalacia, the primary defect is impaired mineralization of the underlying bone matrix. Osteoporosis and rickets/osteomalacia both result in an increased fracture risk; however, osteoporosis does not generally lead to growth plate and long bone deformities.

RICKETTSIAL DISEASE

Gordon E. Schutze

BASICS

DESCRIPTION

- Disorders caused by the Rickettsiae family of organisms including those which cause Rocky Mountain spotted fever and other similar tick-borne illnesses, the typhus group, and the organisms that cause ehrlichiosis and anaplasmosis
- All organisms are obligate intracellular gram-negative bacteria and therefore are difficult to grow in culture.
- The diseases caused by each group of organisms are similar, encompassing a syndrome including fever, rash, headache, and capillary leak; all are transmitted via an insect vector.

GENERAL PREVENTION

- Fleas, ticks, and mites should be controlled in endemic areas with the appropriate insecticides.
- Clothing to cover the entire body should be worn in tick-infested areas. In the case of a recognized bite, ticks should be removed from human skin properly, with care not to expel the contents of the tick's stomach into the site of the bite.
- In areas where louse-borne typhus is epidemic, periodic delousing and dusting of insecticide into clothes are recommended.
- Paradoxic effect of rodenticides:
  - Fleas and mites seek alternate hosts (i.e., humans) when mice or rats are not present.
  - Therefore, rodenticides should not be the only preventive measure taken in endemic areas.
- Except for scrub typhus, all rickettsial diseases produce long-term immunity to the etiologic organisms within the same group.

PATHOPHYSIOLOGY

Spotted fever, typhus, ehrlichiosis, and anaplasmosis groups cause vasculitis as a result of organisms invading the endothelial cells of small blood vessels or white blood cells. This manifests as rash in cutaneous tissues and systemic illness due to capillary leak throughout other organs.

ETIOLOGY

- Spotted fever group rickettsia and the agents of ehrlichiosis and anaplasmosis (*Ehrlichia* and *Anaplasma species*) are transmitted to humans by ticks.
- Rickettsialpox and scrub typhus are transmitted by mites associated with mice.
- Epidemic typhus is a louse-borne illness, and endemic typhus, also known as murine typhus, is transmitted by fleas.
- The rickettsial diseases that occur in the United States are Rocky Mountain spotted fever, murine typhus, rickettsialpox, epidemic typhus, ehrlichiosis, and anaplasmosis.

DIAGNOSIS

HISTORY

- In general, rickettsial disease should be considered as a diagnosis in a patient with fever, headache, and rash. Progression of rash can be particularly helpful in considering the diagnosis.
- Signs and symptoms:
  - Spotted fever group
    - Illness often begins with fever, myalgia, and headache.
    - Rash occurs 3–5 days following onset of symptoms and is typically described as centripetal, beginning on hands and feet and moving toward the trunk. Rash is variable and may not always follow this pattern.
    - Other symptoms include headache, neurologic changes, hypotension, hyponatremia, and consumptive coagulopathy.
    - Fulminant RMSF may cause cardiovascular collapse.
  - Rickettsialpox
    - Similar to spotted fever group, although less severe and with fewer systemic symptoms; rash often includes an inoculation eschar.
  - Typhus group
    - Epidemic typhus is transmitted by the human body louse and causes fever, headache, and rash that can progress to pulmonary symptoms, neurologic disease, and death.
    - Endemic typhus is transmitted by fleas associated with rodents and causes symptoms similar to epidemic typhus, although with a less prevalent rash.
    - Scrub typhus is also similar but causes marked neurologic symptoms including mental status changes.
  - Ehrlichiosis/anaplasmosis
    - Spectrum of illnesses including human monocytotropic ehrlichiosis and human granulocytotropic anaplasmosis that cause fever, headache, and myalgias similar to the spotted fever group.
    - Rash is less common as compared to spotted fever and occurs in <50% of patients in ehrlichiosis and very few in anaplasmosis.

PHYSICAL EXAM

- All rickettsial diseases cause fever and the majority cause rash.
- These 3 findings suggest illness caused by the spotted fever group:
  - Hypotension, cardiovascular instability
  - Hepatosplenomegaly
  - *Tache noire* (French for black spot): The earliest finding in the spotted fever group, this lesion originates at the site of the infecting bite and may form eschar with regional lymphadenopathy related to the eschar. The lesion is usually found on the head in children and on the legs in adults; present in 30–90% of cases.
- These 3 findings suggest illness caused by the typhus group:
  - Impaired level of consciousness
  - Pulmonary and renal involvement
  - Brill-Zinsser disease is actually a recrudescence of a previous infection with epidemic (louse-borne) typhus caused by *Rickettsia prowazekii*; can occur years after the initial infection and is usually less severe than the initial episode of louse-borne typhus.
- These findings suggest ehrlichiosis:
  - Acute febrile illness characterized by headache and myalgia
  - Rash in ~50%; spares palms, soles, and face
  - Thrombocytopenia, leukopenia (lymphopenia), hyponatremia, and elevated liver function tests
- These findings suggest anaplasmosis:
  - Acute febrile illness characterized by headache and myalgia
  - Thrombocytopenia, leukopenia (neutropenia), hyponatremia, and elevated liver function tests

DIAGNOSTIC TESTS & INTERPRETATION
Lab
- Serologic testing is the standard for laboratory diagnosis of rickettsial disease because the organisms are obligate intracellular bacteria and do not grow in culture.
- Serologic tests are available for all rickettsial organisms. There is some cross-reactivity among similar organisms.
- Serologic testing is often negative at the onset of illness and requires a convalescent (paired) sample done 2–3 weeks later for comparison. If the convalescent titer is 4-fold or greater than the acute, it is considered positive.
- Polymerase chain reaction (PCR) tests are rarely done in clinical labs and have significant inaccuracy given the similarities in genomes of these organisms.
- The Weil-Felix agglutination test has poor sensitivity and specificity and is not used in the United States.

DIFFERENTIAL DIAGNOSIS
- Before rash appears, constitutional symptoms associated with the spotted fevers result in a broad differential diagnosis. After rash appears, the diagnoses are more limited.
- Infectious:
  - Measles
  - Meningococcemia
  - Secondary syphilis
  - Coxsackievirus (e.g., hand-foot-and-mouth disease)
  - Infectious mononucleosis
  - Enteroviral infection
- Environmental (poisons)
- Drug hypersensitivity reaction (i.e., toxicodermatosis)
- Tumors: leukemia with thrombocytopenia
- Immunologic: idiopathic thrombocytopenia purpura
- Miscellaneous:
  - Leukocytoclastic angiitis
  - Erythema multiforme/Stevens-Johnson syndrome

TREATMENT

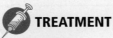

MEDICATION
- The 1st-line antibiotic treatment for all rickettsial diseases is doxycycline. Therapy is most effective if instituted within the 1st week of illness.
- Antibiotics should be given for 7–14 days.
  - Studies have shown that there is little risk of tooth staining in children <8 years old who receive doxycycline.
  - In the case of rickettsial disease, the benefit of giving doxycycline far outweighs the risk of adverse effects.

INPATIENT CONSIDERATIONS
Initial Stabilization
- Fluid resuscitation and respiratory support as indicated
- Antimicrobial therapy should be instituted as soon as the diagnosis is suspected and should not be delayed while awaiting serologic confirmation.
- Patients may require blood product transfusion in the case of consumptive coagulopathy or severe thrombocytopenia.

ONGOING CARE

PROGNOSIS
Improvement in the patient's clinical status usually takes place within 1–2 weeks after therapy starts, depending on the severity of illness. This improvement may also be delayed if treatment is begun after the 1st week of illness.

COMPLICATIONS
- Venous thrombosis
- Disseminated intravascular coagulation
- Cardiac injury including endocarditis
- Severe disease is more common in patients with glucose-6-phosphate dehydrogenase (G6PD) deficiency, cardiac insufficiency, or immunodeficiency.

ADDITIONAL READING

- Demma LJ, Holman RC, McQuiston JH, et al. Epidemiology of human ehrlichiosis and anaplasmosis in the United States, 2001–2002. *Am J Trop Med Hyg*. 2005;73(2):400–409.
- Dumler JS, Dey C, Meier F, et al. Human monocytic ehrlichiosis: a potentially severe disease in children. *Arch Pediatr Adolesc Med*. 2000;154(8):847–849.
- Pickering LK, Baker CJ, Kimberlin DW, et al, eds. *Red Book: 2012 Report of the Committee on Infectious Diseases*. 29th ed. Elk Grove Village, IL: American Academy of Pediatrics; 2012:620 -622.
- Purvis JJ, Edward MS. Doxycycline use for rickettsial disease in pediatric patients. *Pediatr Infect Dis J*. 2000;19(9):871–874.

CODES

ICD10
- A79.9 Rickettsiosis, unspecified
- A77.0 Spotted fever due to Rickettsia rickettsii
- A75.9 Typhus fever, unspecified

FAQ
- Q: Should my child receive antibiotics if he is bitten by a tick in an area endemic to rickettsial disease?
- A: There is no role for prophylaxis against rickettsial diseases for patients who have suffered tick bites.
- Q: Are there differences between typhoid and typhus?
- A: Typhoid, or typhoid fever, is a separate entity from typhus. Typhoid is an enteric infection caused by *Salmonella typhi* and is unrelated to the rickettsial diseases.
- Q: If I contract a rickettsial illness, can I get that illness or a similar illness again?
- A: With the exception of scrub typhus, infection with a rickettsial organism confers immunity to other rickettsia within the same group.

ROCKY MOUNTAIN SPOTTED FEVER

Carolyn A. Paris • George Anthony Woodward

BASICS

DESCRIPTION

- Life-threatening, small vessel vasculitis
- Caused by infection with *Rickettsia rickettsii*, an obligate intracellular gram-negative coccobacillus, transmitted by *three species of* ticks in the United States
- Member of spotted fever subgroup of rickettsial diseases
- Seasonal endemic disease but may occur in other areas and throughout the year
- Classic symptoms of fever, headache, and rash following tick exposure are often not present.

EPIDEMIOLOGY

- Most common rickettsial disease in the United States
- Seasonal: April–September accounts for 90% of cases.
- Geographic
  - Restricted to countries of western hemisphere
  - Cases reported from all states except Alaska, Hawaii, and Maine
  - Occurs most often in southern Atlantic and south central regions: 1994–2003, >50% of cases in North Carolina, South Carolina, Tennessee, Oklahoma, Arkansas
  - Less often seen in Rocky Mountain states
  - Also occurs in southern Canada, Mexico, and Central and South America
- Single isolated cases most common in United States; clusters are reported infrequently in United States (4.4% familial) but are more typical in certain endemic areas (e.g., Brazil).
- Up to 2/3 of patients are <15 years old.

Incidence

- Annual incidence: 7 cases per million people (2002–2007); the highest recorded level in >80 years of national surveillance
- Cyclic fluctuations in incidence; 250–1,200 cases reported per year
- More often reported in American Indians, whites, males, and children; incidence highest in 5–9-year-olds
- Fatal outcome reported in 23% of untreated, and 5% of treated, cases
- Geographic variations in case fatality occur, likely due to different levels of pathogenicity, host factors, and delayed recognition in less endemic regions.
- 15% reported deaths in children <10 years of age

Prevalence

4–22% of children show significant antibody titers in endemic areas, likely representative of subclinical disease.

RISK FACTORS

R. rickettsii–infected tick exposure or rural environment or occupation increasing forest exposure in endemic region

GENERAL PREVENTION

- Avoid tick-infested areas; limit skin exposure with long, light-colored clothing, tucked-in socks, or boots; inspect frequently.
- Use tick repellants or impregnated clothing.
  - DEET most effective
  - Essential oils that offer natural alternatives considered safe (soybean, lemon eucalyptus, citronella, and clove)
- Remove ticks promptly.
  - Do not crush; may increase transmission
  - Avoid direct contact; remove with tweezers or gloved fingers close to skin.
  - Apply steady upward traction until tick's grip is released.
  - Clean wound.
  - Matches, petroleum jelly, nail polish, and rubbing alcohol are not effective for removal.
- Vaccine not available in the United States; may not prevent disease but does prevent deaths

PATHOPHYSIOLOGY

- Transmission usually occurs from tick bite (reservoir):
  - Usually >4 hours of attachment needed to transmit disease (often 24 hours)
  - Can occur by transfusion or aerosol route
- Incubation period 2–14 days, average 7 days
- *R. rickettsii* spreads through the lymphatic system, causing a small vessel vasculitis that affects all organs, especially skin and adrenals; increased vascular permeability and focal areas of endothelial proliferation
- Causes hyponatremia, hypoalbuminemia, edema, and hypotension
- Immunity is conferred following disease.

ETIOLOGY

Wood tick (*Dermacentor andersoni*) in Rocky Mountain states and southwest Canada; dog tick (*Dermacentor variabilis*) in east central region and areas of Pacific coast; *Rhipicephalus sanguineus* in Arizona and northern Mexico; *Amblyomma cajennense* and *Amblyomma aureolatum* in Central and South America

COMMONLY ASSOCIATED CONDITIONS

- Patients with glucose-6-phosphate dehydrogenase (G6PD) deficiency account for a disproportionate number of deaths.
- Serious biologic weapon threat due to virulence causing severe disease; difficulty establishing diagnosis; low levels of immunity; agent available in nature; high infectivity; and feasibility of propagation, stabilization, and dispersal; thus development of a cross-protective vaccine against all *Rickettsia* is desirable for biodefense as well as for travel medicine.

DIAGNOSIS

HISTORY

- History: classic triad of fever, headache, and rash seen in ~50% of cases
- Abdominal pain common mainly in children
- Symptoms usually appear 2–8 days after tick bite.
- Gradual fever onset to >40°C (104°F), often unresponsive to antipyretics
- Headache: intense, retrobulbar or frontal, persistent and difficult to treat; young children may not describe
- Cough, dyspnea
- Nausea, vomiting, abdominal pain, diarrhea
- Tick bite is reported in only 50–60% of cases.

PHYSICAL EXAM

- Fever and rash present in 85% of patients.
- Skin
  - Rash: usually appears by illness days 2–3, may be >6th day; 10–15% never develop rash so absence should not delay therapy.
  - Usually small, irregular, erythematous blanching macules, become maculopapular then petechial and confluently hemorrhagic
  - Usually on wrists and ankles first, spreads within hours to trunk, neck, and face; may involve palms, soles, and scrotum
    - May appear first on trunk or diffusely; can progress to necrosis of ears, nose, scrotum, fingers, or toes
    - Difficult to detect in people with dark skin
- CNS: meningismus, restlessness, irritability, apprehension, confusion, delirium, lethargy, stupor, coma, ataxia, opisthotonos, aphasia, papilledema, seizures, cortical blindness, central deafness, spastic paralysis, cranial nerve palsy
- Cardiac: CHF, myocarditis, arrhythmias, hypovolemic vascular collapse
- Pulmonary: pneumonitis, dyspnea, pulmonary edema, hypoxemia, pleural effusions, alveolar infiltrates
- GI: diarrhea, hepatomegaly, splenomegaly, anorexia, jaundice, mild pancreatitis
- Ocular: conjunctivitis, venous engorgement, papilledema, cotton wool spots, retinal hemorrhages, retinal artery occlusion, uveitis
- Other: edema, myalgias (especially calf or thigh), parotitis, orchitis, pharyngitis

DIAGNOSTIC TESTS & INTERPRETATION

Presumptive diagnosis based on signs, symptoms, exposure history, and epidemiologic considerations rather than laboratory aids

Lab

- Nonspecific
  - CBC: anemia (30%), thrombocytopenia (from consumptive coagulopathy); normal or low leukocytes days 4–5, subsequent leukocytosis associated with secondary bacterial disease; bandemia common
  - Electrolytes: hyponatremia
  - Elevated BUN, creatinine, liver function tests, bilirubin, creatine kinase
  - Screen for disseminated intravascular coagulation (rare), prolonged prothrombin time, decreased fibrinogen (consumption).
  - Arterial blood gases: acidosis
  - Hypoalbuminemia
  - CSF: usually clear (leukocyte count <10), may see pleocytosis in 1/3 and increased protein in 1/2 of patients
- Specific serologic tests
  - No early specific laboratory tests; serologic data reliable by days 10–12 of illness; negative results do not exclude diagnosis.
  - All test results normalize with early intervention.

- Indirect immunofluorescence assay (IFA)
  - Best and most widely available method
  - 2 serum samples obtained weeks apart showing 4-fold increase in IgG and IgM anti–*R. rickettsii* antibody titers
  - Positive 6–10 days after onset of disease, sensitivity increases to 94% with convalescence serum sample from days 14 to 21 days; specificity 100%
- PCR, immunohistochemical staining, and culture are best done on biopsy specimen (of rash site or at autopsy) due to low circulating organism levels.
- Routine hospital blood cultures will not detect; available only at specialty labs
- Weil-Felix test: oldest specific test but nonspecific and insensitive; no longer recommended

Imaging

Chest radiograph, ECG, and echocardiogram are recommended. Distinctive features on MR images (brain and spinal cord) may lead to early diagnosis; CT findings are less often present.

DIFFERENTIAL DIAGNOSIS

Measles, meningococcemia, ehrlichiosis, typhoid fever, leptospirosis, rubella, scarlet fever, disseminated gonococcal disease, infectious mononucleosis, secondary syphilis, rheumatic fever, enteroviral infection, immune thrombocytic purpura, thrombotic thrombocytopenic purpura, immune complex vasculitis, drug hypersensitivity reaction, murine typhus, rickettsialpox, and recrudescent typhus

ALERT

Do not exclude diagnosis even if there is no history of tick bite, no rash present, and/or results of serologic tests are negative. Treatment should be started presumptively and postponement of therapy while awaiting laboratory confirmation or presence of rash.

TREATMENT

MEDICATION

Treatment should be initiated based on clinical and epidemiologic information, as laboratory confirmation may not be available during acute illness. All agents are rickettsiostatic (hinder replication), not rickettsicidal, so host can eradicate disease. Treat until there is evidence of clinical improvement and at least 3 days without fever; standard duration is 5–10 days.

First Line

- Doxycycline (usual tetracycline antibiotic) is the drug of choice at any age:
  - Adults: 100 mg q12h PO/IV
  - Children under 45 kg (100 lb): 4.4 mg/kg/24 h PO/IV divided b.i.d.
  - Also treats ehrlichiosis (similar presentation)
  - Side effects: less likely to stain teeth than tetracycline; contraindicated for pregnancy, although can be considered even in pregnancy if the mother's life is in danger and the theoretical concerns on the fetus is discussed
- Chloramphenicol (alternative during pregnancy)
  - Adult: 50–100 mg/kg/24 h IV divided q6h (max 4 g/24 h)
  - Child >1 month of age: 50–100 mg/kg/24 h IV divided q6h (max 4 g/24 h)
  - Side effects: peripheral neuropathy, aplastic anemia, "gray baby syndrome" with high dosage, possible association with leukemia, hemolytic anemia with G6PD
  - Not as effective as tetracyclines, or against ehrlichiosis; higher mortality rate in those treated with chloramphenicol than tetracyclines; consider only rarely such as during pregnancy.

Second Line

- Quinolones (ciprofloxacin, pefloxacin), macrolide (clarithromycin) with in vitro effect, no clinical evidence of efficacy
- Corticosteroids
  - May be helpful in severe cases, although no controlled studies published
  - Not advised for mild or moderately ill patients

ADDITIONAL TREATMENT

General Measures

- Treat empirically if clinical suspicion.
- Platelets as indicated for thrombocytopenia
- Vitamin K (IM) for prolonged clotting time
- Manage hyponatremia with fluid restriction; avoid sodium supplements.
- Albumin if indicated
- Report to state health department.

INPATIENT CONSIDERATIONS

Initial Stabilization

Volume, electrolyte support as indicated

ONGOING CARE

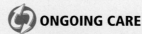

FOLLOW-UP RECOMMENDATIONS

Expect improvement in 24–36 hours and defervescence in 2–3 days with treatment, especially if initiated <5 days after onset of symptoms.

PROGNOSIS

- Related to early recognition of disease and initiation of appropriate therapy
- Case fatality 2–4% if treated <6 days from onset of symptoms
- Case fatality 15–22.9% if treated >6 days from onset of symptoms
  - Higher mortality if <4 years, G6PD deficiency, CNS involvement, renal failure, jaundice, cardiovascular collapse, hepatomegaly, thrombocytopenia, DIC, GI symptoms, inappropriate antibiotics, late rash, absence of headache, or male gender
  - Death usually between 8th and 15th days (fulminant cases with death in 5–6 days)

COMPLICATIONS

- Uncommon with early, appropriate treatment
- Neurologic sequelae
  - Behavioral disturbances, learning disabilities (more common), emotional lability, hyperactivity, memory loss, seizures
- Dermatologic sequelae
  - Gangrene of extremities, end organs, skin necrosis
  - Skin rash usually heals without sequelae.
- Hematologic sequelae: DIC
- GI sequelae
  - Hepatic dysfunction
  - Hypoalbuminemia from hepatic dysfunction, protein loss from damaged vessels
- Cardiac sequelae: can have persistent cardiac findings, CHF, cardiovascular collapse
- Metabolic sequelae: hyponatremia from water shift to intracellular spaces, sodium loss in urine
- Renal sequelae: acute tubular necrosis

ADDITIONAL READING

- Akgoz A, Mukundan S, Lee TC. Imaging of rickettsial, spirochetal, and parasitic infections. *Neuroimaging Clin N Am*. 2012;22(4):633–657.
- Buckingham SC, Marshal GS, Schutze GE, et al. Clinical and laboratory features, hospital course, and outcomes of Rocky Mountain spotted fever in children. *J Pediatr*. 2007;150(2):180–184, 184.e1.
- Centers for Disease Control and Prevention. Rocky Mountain spotted fever (RMSF). http://www.cdc.gov/ncidod/dvrd/rmsf/index.htm. Accessed March 27, 2015.
- Chen LF, Sexton DJ. What's new in Rocky Mountain spotted fever? *Infect Dis Clin North Am*. 2008;22(3):415–432, vii–viii.
- Dantas-Torres F. Rocky Mountain spotted fever. *Lancet Infect Dis*. 2007;7(11):724–732.
- Openshaw JJ, Swerdlow DL, Krebs JW, et al. Rocky Mountain spotted fever in the United States, 2000–2007: interpreting contemporary increases in incidence. *Am J Trop Med Hyg*. 2010;83(1):174–182.
- Shapiro R. Prevention of vector transmitted diseases with clove oil insect repellent. *J Pediatr Nurs*. 2012;27(4):346–349.
- Walker DH. The realities of biodefense vaccines against *Rickettsia*. *Vaccine*. 2009;27(Suppl 4):D52–D55.

CODES

ICD10

A77.0 Spotted fever due to Rickettsia rickettsii

FAQ

- Q: In which patients should Rocky Mountain spotted fever be considered in the differential diagnosis?
- A: Anyone with a fever during the spring and summer who has been in an endemic area, regardless of presence of rash or history of tick bite. Nonspecific symptoms (e.g., GI, respiratory, rashes) may lead to misdiagnosis and thus delay therapy.
- Q: Should a child with a tick bite receive antibiotic prophylaxis when a tick is discovered?
- A: There is no evidence that prophylaxis is necessary or efficacious in preventing disease. To contract disease, one must be bitten by a tick that carries the disease (low risk), the tick must transmit the *Rickettsia* (low risk, usually requires >6 hours of attachment), and the *Rickettsia* must be pathogenic if inoculated (low risk).

ROSEOLA

Ross Newman • Jason Newland

BASICS

DESCRIPTION

Roseola infantum is a common illness in preschool-aged children characterized by fever lasting 3–7 days followed by rapid defervescence and the appearance of a blanching maculopapular rash (usually on the 4th day of illness) lasting only 1–2 days.

EPIDEMIOLOGY

- Roseola affects children from 3 months to 4 years of age. The peak age is 7–13 months.
- 90% of cases occur in the first 2 years of life.
- No gender predilection
- Roseola can occur throughout the year; outbreaks have occurred in all seasons.

GENERAL PREVENTION

- The virus that causes roseola infantum is usually transmitted via respiratory secretions or fecal–oral spread. Good hand hygiene is recommended.
- Outbreaks in hospitals have been reported, and standard infection control precautions are recommended.

PATHOPHYSIOLOGY

- Incubation period is 5–15 days.
- The typical pattern of rash that appears as the fever disappears may represent virus neutralization in the skin.

ETIOLOGY

- A major cause of roseola is human herpesvirus 6 and 7 (HHV-6 and HHV-7).
  - HHV-6 was first associated with roseola infantum in 1988.
  - HHV-6 and HHV-7 account for 20–40% of unexplained febrile illness in emergency department visits by febrile infants 6 months to 2 years of age.
  - Almost all children will acquire a primary infection and be seropositive for HHV-6 by the age of 4 years.
  - ~30% of children infected with HHV-6 will present with the classic manifestations of roseola.
- Roseola-like illnesses have been associated with a number of different viruses, including enterovirus (coxsackievirus A and B, echoviruses), adenoviruses (types 1, 2, 3), parainfluenza virus, and measles vaccine virus.

DIAGNOSIS

HISTORY

- Diagnosis is clinical, based on classic features.
- Affected children generally do not look sick.
- Fever, typically >39.5°C, lasting 3–7 days
- Mild cough and acute rhinitis may be present.

PHYSICAL EXAMINATION

- Rash
  - Erythematous, blanching, maculopapular
  - First appears on trunk, spreads to face and extremities
  - Appears for 1–2 days after fever resolves
- Other findings:
  - Lymphadenopathy
  - Eyelid edema
  - Bulging fontanelle can occur occasionally.

DIAGNOSTIC TESTS & INTERPRETATION

Lab

- Not helpful in diagnosis
  - Polymerase chain reaction (PCR) tests are available for detecting HHV-6 and HHV-7 but generally not needed.
- CBC
  - Occasionally, leukopenia with lymphocytosis is noted.
  - Thrombocytopenia is likely secondary to viral bone marrow suppression.

DIFFERENTIAL DIAGNOSIS

- Roseola has a distinctive presentation but does resemble other viral exanthems.
- Antibiotic-associated rash in a child taking oral antibiotics when rash develops after defervescence
- Rubella and enteroviral infections
- Viral exanthems in preschool-aged children are sometimes called roseola even when fever is concomitant with rash.

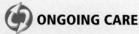

ONGOING CARE

PROGNOSIS

Most children with roseola infantum recover without sequelae.

COMPLICATIONS

- Seizures
  - Most common complication of roseola
  - Between 10 and 15% of children have a generalized tonic–clonic seizure associated with fever.
- Aseptic meningitis with <200 cells, primarily mononuclear cells, have been reported.
- Encephalitis
- Thrombocytopenic purpura

ADDITIONAL READING

- American Academy of Pediatrics. Human herpesvirus 6 (including roseola) and 7. In: Pickering LK, Baker CJ, Kimberlin DW, et al, eds. *Red Book: 2012 Report of the Committee on Infectious Diseases*. 29th ed. Elk Grove Village, IL: American Academy of Pediatrics; 2012.
- Jackson MA, Sommerauer JF. Human herpesviruses 6 and 7. *Pediatr Infect Dis J*. 2002;21(6):565–566.
- Leach CT. Human herpesvirus-6 and -7 infections in children: agents of roseola and other syndromes. *Curr Opin Pediatr*. 2000;12(3):269–274.
- Stoeckle MY. The spectrum of human herpesvirus 6 infection: from roseola infantum to adult disease. *Annu Rev Med*. 2000;51:423–430.
- Vianna RA, de Oliveira SA, Camacho LA, et al. Role of human herpesvirus 6 infection in young Brazilian children with rash illnesses. *Pediatr Infect Dis J*. 2008;27(6):533–537.

CODES

ICD10

- B08.20 Exanthema subitum [sixth disease], unspecified
- B08.21 Exanthema subitum [sixth disease] due to human herpesvirus 6
- B08.22 Exanthema subitum [sixth disease] due to human herpesvirus 7

FAQ

- Q: When can a child with roseola return to day care?
- A: As soon as fever subsides; there is no infectious risk of spread afterward. The child may return to day care even with the rash visible.
- Q: Will there be long-term sequelae in the child who has a seizure associated with roseola?
- A: In general, these seizures are typical febrile seizures that hold only a slightly higher risk than the general population for long-term neurologic sequelae (e.g., epilepsy).

ROTAVIRUS

John Bower

BASICS

DESCRIPTION

Rotavirus is a leading cause of gastroenteritis in the United States and worldwide. Characterized by frequent watery stools, illness ranges from mild diarrhea to disease complicated by severe dehydration, especially in young children.

EPIDEMIOLOGY

- Rotavirus is a major cause of diarrheal disease and accounts for 5% of all deaths in children <5 years of age worldwide.
- The peak age for infection is between 6 and 24 months of age. Nearly all children acquire the virus by 5 years of age.
- In temperate climates, rotavirus activity peaks during the cold weather months but can appear year round in warmer climates.
- Transmission occurs primarily by the fecal–oral route.
- Rotavirus is highly contagious. This is due to several factors.
  - The virus has a very low inoculum of infection, requiring as few as 10 infectious particles to cause disease.
  - A high density of virus is shed into the stool during acute illness and for 1–3 days before and after diarrhea.
  - There is prolonged survival of the virus on a variety of environmental surfaces.
- The incubation period is 1–3 days.
- Prior to the rotavirus vaccine, U.S. children <5 years of age with diarrhea had a hospitalization rate of 52/10,000 person-years and an ED visit rate of 185/10,000 person-years.
- After the rotavirus vaccine was introduced in 2006, the hospitalization rate for all children <5 years with diarrhea fell by nearly 50% and ED visits by 25%.

RISK FACTORS

- Young infants, especially preterm infants, are at higher risk for severe dehydration and gastrointestinal complications.
- Immunocompromised patients, particularly with primary immunodeficiencies and hematopoietic stem cell transplantation are at higher risk for complications and prolonged shedding.

GENERAL PREVENTION

- Proper hand hygiene and cleaning of contaminated surfaces is essential to reducing person-to-person transmission.
- Contact precautions for hospitalized patients
- Two live oral vaccines are licensed in the US:
  - Live human/bovine reassortant pentavalent rotavirus (RV5). Given as a 3-dose series.
  - Live human attenuated monovalent rotavirus (RV1). Given as a 2-dose series.

PATHOPHYSIOLOGY

- Rotavirus infects and replicates within the enterocytes of the small bowel. Several factors appear to contribute to secretory diarrhea.
  - The nonstructural protein (NSP4) acts as an enterotoxin that triggers secretory diarrhea by increasing Cl^- secretion and decreasing Na^+ absorption.
  - Malabsorption develops due to disruption of microvilli and decreased surface transport of digestive enzymes.
  - NSP4 appears to activate the enteric nervous system, which activates a secretory state that further contributes to intestinal fluid loss.

ETIOLOGY

- Rotavirus is an 11-segment double-stranded RNA virus with 7 different antigenic groups (A–G).
- Types A, B, and C are responsible for most human infections, with group A being the most common.
- Group A rotavirus is further divided into multiple serotypes based on 2 outer capsid viral proteins: VP7 (G) and VP4 (P).

DIAGNOSIS

HISTORY

- Stools are watery and often foul-smelling.
- Gross blood or mucus is usually absent—their presence more often suggests a bacterial pathogen.
- Diarrhea usually lasts 3–8 days.
- Stool frequency can range from several to 20 episodes per day.
- Vomiting accompanies diarrhea 85% of the time. Vomiting often precedes diarrhea and resolves in 1–2 days.
- Fever can exceed 102°F in 1/3 of patients.
- Two thirds of patients present with diarrhea, vomiting, and fever.
- Family members often have a history of current or recent diarrhea.

PHYSICAL EXAM

Relevant physical findings are targeted to assess for potential dehydration.

DIAGNOSTIC TESTS & INTERPRETATION

Lab

- Serum electrolytes, BUN, and creatinine are important in evaluating for dehydration and electrolyte abnormalities secondary to diarrhea.
- Rapid tests for rotavirus
  - By EIA or latex agglutination
  - Have an overall sensitivity of 80% and specificity of 99%
  - Sensitivity is highest in the first 4 days of illness.
- Rapid PCR testing is becoming increasingly available for rotavirus, including multiplex assays that incorporate other common agents of viral gastroenteritis.
- Fecal leukocyte and stool guaiac testing is not helpful.
- Two thirds of hospitalized children have mild elevations in their transaminases.

DIFFERENTIAL DIAGNOSIS

- Viral pathogens occur in 80–90% of patients with secretory diarrhea. Besides rotavirus, common gastrointestinal viruses include the following:
  - Norovirus
  - Sapovirus
  - Astrovirus
  - Enteric adenovirus
- Bacterial infections may present with secretory diarrhea.
  - *Salmonella*
  - *Shigella*
  - *Campylobacter*
  - *Aeromonas*
  - *Clostridium difficile*
  - *Yersinia*
- Parasitic infections:
  - *Giardia*
  - *Cryptosporidium*
  - *Cyclospora*
  - *Isospora*

TREATMENT

MEDICATION

- Antimotility agents are generally avoided for all forms of infectious diarrhea in children.
- Several studies suggest that supplementation with a specific probiotic strain, *Lactobacillus rhamnosus* GG, during acute rotavirus gastroenteritis might decrease the duration of diarrhea (mean duration decrease: approximately 1 day).

INPATIENT CONSIDERATIONS

Initial Stabilization

- Provide appropriate intravenous, nasogastric, or oral fluids for volume replacement and correction of electrolyte abnormalities due to diarrhea.
- Monitor fluid balance and serum electrolytes.
- Place patients in contact precautions.

ONGOING CARE

COMPLICATIONS

- Hypernatremia and metabolic acidosis occur more often with rotavirus gastroenteritis than other forms of viral gastroenteritis and may become severe enough to require intensive care management.
- Gram-negative sepsis can occur secondary to mucosal injury.
- Rotavirus gastroenteritis has been associated with necrotizing enterocolitis in preterm infants.
- Diarrhea may be more severe and protracted in immunocompromised hosts.

ADDITIONAL READING

- Bernstein DI. Rotavirus overview. *Pediatr Infect Dis J*. 2009;28(3)(Suppl):S50–S53.
- Cortes JE, Curns AT, Tate JE, et al. Rotavirus vaccine and health care utilization for diarrhea in U.S. children. *N Engl J Med*. 2011;365(12):1108–1117.
- Cox E, Christenson JC. Rotavirus. *Pediatr Rev*. 2012;33(10):439–445; quiz 446–447.
- Curns AT, Steiner CA, Barrett M, et al. Reduction in acute gastroenteritis hospitalizations among US children after introduction of rotavirus vaccine: analysis of hospital discharge data from 18 US states. *J Infect Dis*. 2010;201(11):1617–1624.
- Dennehy PH. Treatment and prevention of rotavirus infection in children. *Curr Infect Dis Rep*. 2013;15(3):242–250.
- Kaiser P, Borte M, Zimmer KP, et al. Complications in hospitalized children with acute gastroenteritis caused by rotavirus: a retrospective analysis. *Eur J Pediatr*. 2012;171(2):337–345.
- Madhi SA, Cunliffe NA, Steele D, et al. Effect of human rotavirus vaccine on severe diarrhea in African infants. *N Engl J Med*. 2010;362(4):289–298.
- Tate JE, Burton AH, Boschi-Pinto C, et al. 2008 estimate of worldwide rotavirus-associated mortality in children younger than 5 years before the introduction of universal rotavirus vaccination programmes: a systematic review and meta-analysis. *Lancet Infect Dis*. 2012;12(2):136–141.

CODES

ICD10

A08.0 Rotaviral enteritis

FAQ

- Q: How long are children contagious following rotavirus infections?
- A: In most children, rotavirus shedding ceases within 7 days of the diarrhea resolving. However, asymptomatic shedding can persist in some children for up to several weeks—and in some cases longer. Young infants with severe diarrhea and immunocompromised patients are more likely to have persistent asymptomatic rotavirus shedding and may pose a risk for spread in the day care and hospital setting.
- Q: Is there a risk for intussusception with rotavirus vaccine?
- A: Postlicensure data for the RV5 and RV1 vaccines do point to a slightly higher risk for intussusception following administration of the first two doses of rotavirus vaccine. This infrequent complication; however, is far outweighed by the vaccine's substantial benefits in reducing hospitalization and death, and its worldwide use is strongly recommended.

SALICYLATE POISONING (ASPIRIN)

Kevin C. Osterhoudt

BASICS

DESCRIPTION

- May occur with acute or chronic overdosage of the following:
  - Acetylsalicylic acid (aspirin)
  - Methyl salicylate (oil of wintergreen)
  - Bismuth subsalicylate (Pepto Bismol)
  - Salicylic acid (a keratolytic)
  - Other salicylate-containing drugs
- The potentially toxic acute oral dose of acetylsalicylic acid is >150 mg/kg.

EPIDEMIOLOGY

- Analgesics are the most common drugs implicated in human exposures reported to U.S. poison control centers.
- Salicylate preparations constitute ~9% of all analgesic poisoning exposures reported to poison control centers.

PATHOPHYSIOLOGY

- Ingested drug is absorbed in stomach and proximal intestine.
- With therapeutic aspirin dosing, serum levels peak in 1–2 hours (standard preparations) or 4–6 hours (enteric coated).
- After oral overdose, absorption may be prolonged and erratic.
- Acetylsalicylate ingestion may produce gastritis and may trigger centrally mediated vomiting.
- After overdose, the elimination half-life of salicylate becomes prolonged.
- As blood pH falls, the proportion of nonionized salicylate rises, and more salicylate shifts into tissues, including brain.
- Toxic salicylate exposures uncouple mitochondrial oxidative phosphorylation and increase oxygen consumption.
- Direct stimulation of the medullary respiratory center leads to hyperventilation and respiratory alkalosis.
- Multiple metabolic derangements produce a wide anion gap metabolic acidosis.
- Dehydration and electrolyte shifts are common.
- Low cerebral glucose concentrations may exist despite normal serum glucose concentrations.
- Pulmonary and/or cerebral edema may occur.

COMMONLY ASSOCIATED CONDITIONS

- Aspirin is often marketed in combination with other pharmaceuticals, which may complicate drug overdose situations.
- Adolescents frequently overdose on more than 1 drug preparation.
- Therapeutic use of acetylsalicylic acid among children with influenza has been associated with the occurrence of Reye syndrome.

DIAGNOSIS

HISTORY

- Aspirin poisoning mimics many illnesses, and chronic overdosage often results in delayed diagnosis.
- Enteric coating may lead to significantly delayed drug absorption.
- Timing of ingestion allows for proper consideration of the risks versus benefits of gastrointestinal decontamination.
- Tinnitus frequently associated with serum salicylate levels >25 mg/dL

PHYSICAL EXAM

- Hyperpnea indicates primary central hyperventilation and/or compensation for metabolic acidosis.
- Hyperpyrexia: Presence of "fever" may confuse salicylism with infection.
- Hypoxia: Pulmonary edema complicates therapy of aspirin overdose.
- Hypotension indicates severe dehydration, likely complicated by metabolic acidosis and salicylate-mediated myocardial inefficiency.
- Encephalopathy: CNS depression or seizures represent grave toxicity.

DIAGNOSTIC TESTS & INTERPRETATION

Lab

- Serum electrolytes: A wide anion gap metabolic acidosis is common, and hypoglycemia or hyperglycemia may occur.
- Arterial blood gas: may show mixed respiratory alkalosis/metabolic acidosis
- Salicylate level: Serum salicylate levels >60–100 mg/dL (acute) or 30–40 mg/dL (chronic) portend serious toxicity.
- Urine pH: allows monitoring of adequacy of urinary alkalinization
- Acetaminophen level: Acetaminophen may be a coingestant.
- Ferric chloride test: A few drops of 10% ferric chloride will turn brown or purple in 1 mL of urine that contains salicylate.

ALERT

- Respiratory acidosis suggests central nervous system depression and is an ominous sign.
- Salicylate levels after chronic or acute-on-chronic overdose correlate poorly to clinical condition.
- Serial salicylate levels may be necessary to rule out ongoing drug absorption.

DIFFERENTIAL DIAGNOSIS

- Gastroenteritis
- Pneumonia
- Metabolic disease
- Ketoacidosis
- Sepsis
- Meningitis/encephalitis

TREATMENT

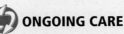

GENERAL MEASURES

- Fluids/alkalinization
  - Intravascular volume should be repleted with intermittent boluses of 10–20 mL/kg of isotonic crystalloid.
  - Altered mentation may imply CNS hypoglycemia and should be treated with dextrose.
  - Acidemia should be treated with sodium bicarbonate to limit salicylate distribution to the brain. Serum pH of 7.5 is reasonable goal.
  - With significant poisoning, an IV infusion of 5% dextrose with 100–150 mEq/L of sodium bicarbonate and 20–40 mEq/L of potassium chloride should be initiated at 1.5–2 times maintenance requirements. Titrate fluid volume to produce urine output of 2–3 mL/kg/h. Titrate alkalinization to produce urine pH between 7.5 and 8, which greatly increases the urinary elimination of salicylate via "ion-trapping" effect.
- Hemodialysis indications
  - Acute serum salicylate level >100 mg/dL
  - Chronic serum salicylate level >60 mg/dL
  - Severe acidosis or severe electrolyte disturbance
  - Renal failure
  - Pulmonary edema
  - Persistent neurologic dysfunction
  - Progressive clinical deterioration

ALERT

- Hypokalemia may interfere with the ability to achieve urinary alkalinization.
- Sedating a salicylate-poisoned patient may lead to respiratory depression and clinical deterioration.
- Endotracheal intubation is dangerous and, if performed, must be accompanied by sodium bicarbonate IV bolus and hyperventilation to prevent worsening acidemia and salicylate distribution to the brain.
- Hemodialysis equipment must be carefully primed to prevent worsening hypovolemia and cardiovascular collapse.
- If hemodialysis is performed, adjust dialysate to maintain alkalemia.
- Pulmonary edema and/or cerebral edema may complicate fluid management.

INPATIENT CONSIDERATIONS

Initial Stabilization

GI decontamination

- Activated charcoal 1 g/kg (maximum 75 g) may be administered if aspirin is judged to be present in the stomach or proximal intestine.
- Many authorities suggest a 2nd charcoal dose 2–4 hours after the 1st or if salicylate levels continue to rise.
- Whole-bowel irrigation may reduce drug absorption after large overdoses.

ONGOING CARE

FOLLOW-UP RECOMMENDATIONS

- Drug administration education should be offered to victims of chronic overdose.
- Mental health services should be provided to victims of intentional overdose.

PROGNOSIS

- Chronic therapeutic misuse often leads to delayed diagnosis and has the most serious prognosis.
- Single acute ingestion of >300 mg/kg acetylsalicylic acid should be considered life threatening.

COMPLICATIONS

- Nausea and vomiting
- Dehydration
- Metabolic acidosis
- Electrolyte abnormalities
- Disorientation, coma, seizures
- Noncardiogenic pulmonary edema
- Renal failure
- Cerebral edema and death

ADDITIONAL READING

- Chyka PA, Erdman AR, Christianson G, et al. Salicylate poisoning: an evidence-based consensus guideline for out-of-hospital management. *Clin Toxicol (Phila)*. 2007;45(2):95–131.
- Glatstein M, Garcia-Bournissen F, Scolnik D, et al. Sudden-onset tachypnea and confusion in a previously healthy teenager. *Ther Drug Monit*. 2010;32(6):700–703.
- Pearlman BL, Gambhir R. Salicylate intoxication: a clinical review. *Postgrad Med*. 2009;121(4): 162–168.
- Stolbach AI, Hoffman RS, Nelson LS. Mechanical ventilation was associated with acidemia in a case series of salicylate-poisoned patients. *Acad Emerg Med*. 2008;15(9):866–869.

CODES

ICD10

- T39.014A Poisoning by aspirin, undetermined, initial encounter
- E87.2 Acidosis
- T39.011A Poisoning by aspirin, accidental (unintentional), init

FAQ

- Q: What amount of the candy-scented oil of wintergreen is toxic to a toddler?
- A: Oil of wintergreen may contain as much as 98% methyl salicylate. 1 mL of methyl salicylate is the equivalent of 1,400 mg of aspirin. Therefore, 1 teaspoon of oil of wintergreen represents a very serious "aspirin" overdose.
- Q: Is there a prognostic nomogram for aspirin poisoning similar to that used for acetaminophen overdose?
- A: The Done nomogram is applicable only to ingestion of non–enteric-coated aspirin by children with normal mentation and normal blood pH, and the validity of its prognostication is suspect. Its use is not widely recommended.

SALMONELLA INFECTIONS

John Bower

BASICS

DESCRIPTION

Salmonella isolates are broadly divided into the following: 1) nontyphoidal serotypes, with illness ranging from uncomplicated gastroenteritis to meningitis; and 2) typhoidal serotypes, responsible for typhoid and paratyphoid fever (collectively called enteric fever).

EPIDEMIOLOGY

- *Salmonella* is a leading cause of foodborne infection in the United States and worldwide.
- Reservoirs
  - Nontyphoidal *Salmonella* serotypes are commonly found in agricultural products, particularly cattle, poultry, and eggs. Less common sources include produce, dairy products, and processed foods. Humans may asymptomatically shed the bacteria for weeks, even months. Reptiles are another well-recognized reservoir for infection.
  - Typhoidal serotypes are found only in humans with acute or chronic infection.
- Transmission
  - Spread occurs via the fecal–oral route. Food and water contamination is the most common mechanism of exposure, followed by direct contact with contaminated surfaces and live animals.
  - *Salmonella* generally requires a high-bacterial inoculum to cause infection.
- Age/season: *Salmonella* infections are most common in children younger than 4 years of age and during the summer months.

RISK FACTORS

- Young infants (especially those <3 months of age), children with sickle cell disease (SCD), human immunodeficiency virus (HIV), malignancy, and other immunocompromised conditions are at high risk for extraintestinal complications from nontyphoidal *Salmonella* gastroenteritis.
- Travel to underdeveloped countries

GENERAL PREVENTION

- Proper cleaning of food preparation surfaces and careful hand hygiene, particularly when handling foods at risk for *Salmonella* contamination
- Foods that frequently harbor *Salmonella*, such as meat, poultry, and eggs, require thorough cooking.
- Children <5 years old, and all those with high-risk conditions, should avoid contact with reptiles (e.g., lizards, snakes, turtles).
- Vaccines for typhoid fever have an efficacy of 50–80% and are recommended for the following: 1) travel to endemic areas and 2) close contacts of carriers. Available vaccines include the following:
  - Ty21a, live vaccine for children ≥6 years of age; given PO every other day for 4 doses
  - ViCPS, inactivated vaccine for children ≥2 years of age; given as a single IM dose

ETIOLOGY

Salmonella is classified into 2 species: *Salmonella enterica* and *Salmonella bongori*. Species are further divided into 1 of over 2,500 serotypes.

- Common nontyphoidal serotypes include the following: *Salmonella enterica* ser Enteritidis, *Salmonella enterica* ser Typhimurium, *Salmonella enterica* ser Newport, and *Salmonella enterica* ser Heidelberg.
- Typhoidal serotypes include the following: *Salmonella enterica* ser Typhi and *Salmonella enterica* ser Paratyphi.

COMMONLY ASSOCIATED CONDITIONS

Following infection of the intestinal epithelium, *Salmonella* strains present with a variety of clinical manifestations.

- Acute gastroenteritis is the most common illness involving nontyphoidal serotypes:
  - Diarrhea is often watery but can be inflammatory with varying amounts of mucus and/or blood.
  - The incubation period is 12–48 hours, and illness usually resolves within 3–5 days. Asymptomatic shedding is common with a mean duration of 5 weeks—longer in infants.
- Transient bacteremia (nontyphoidal)
  - Bacteremia occurs in up to 5% of infected immunocompetent children and in 10% or more of high-risk patients. Young infants are generally at higher risk for bacteremia.
  - The most common serotypes associated with bacteremia include *Salmonella* Enteritidis, *Salmonella* Heidelberg, and *Salmonella* Typhimurium.
  - Bacteremia can result in localized extraintestinal infection.
- Localized extraintestinal infection (nontyphoidal)
  - Local infections occur in 3–5% of otherwise healthy bacteremic children and in up to 30% of high-risk bacteremic patients.
  - Infections include meningitis, septic arthritis, osteomyelitis, and pneumonia.
  - Infants <3 months of age are at higher risk for meningitis.
- Enteric fever (typhoid and paratyphoid fever)
  - The most important serotypes are *Salmonella* Typhi, followed by the less frequent and milder Parathypi strain.
  - Incubation is usually 7–10 days but can be 3–60 days.
  - The clinical course is often insidious with progression of disease over 3–4 weeks. Week 1–2: Fever, headache, myalgia, abdominal pain, and listlessness are common. Diarrhea occurs in less than half of patients, and constipation is common. Week 2–3: Fever increases, and rose spots (maculopapular rash) may appear. Splenomegaly and respiratory symptoms may develop. Week 3–4: Fever gradually improves, however, serious complications, such as intestinal perforation, may develop at this time.

DIAGNOSIS

HISTORY

- Exposure history: nontyphoidal
  - Recent contact with farm animals (e.g., fairs and petting zoos) or reptiles. Reptiles may pose a risk even without direct contact.
  - Recent travel to underdeveloped regions of the world
  - Close contacts with recent gastroenteritis
  - Consumption of raw milk or undercooked eggs
- Exposure history: typhoidal
  - Travel to underdeveloped countries or close contact to persons recently living in, or visiting, endemic regions.
- Clinical history: nontyphoidal
  - Vomiting appears in half of infected children.
  - Fever (up to 39°C) and abdominal pain are common complaints.
  - Stools with mucus and/or blood should raise suspicion for *Salmonella* as well as other common bacterial intestinal pathogens. Blood in the stool appears in less than 1/3 of patients with *Salmonella*.
  - Signs or symptoms indicative of sepsis, meningitis, osteomyelitis, or septic arthritis—especially in young infants and other high-risk patients—should raise suspicion for *Salmonella*.
  - A positive blood culture with a gram-negative rod may precede the diagnosis of *Salmonella* gastroenteritis.
- Clinical history: typhoidal
  - Half of infected patients present with constipation. Only 1/3 of children have diarrhea.
  - Fever ranges from 39° to 40°C and worsens through the first and second week of illness.
  - Rash and mental status changes may be present.
  - In children <5 years, enteric fever may appear as a nonspecific viral illness.

PHYSICAL EXAM

- Nontyphoidal infections
  - Examine for signs of dehydration.
  - Children with uncomplicated bacteremia may be clinically indistinguishable from nonbacteremic patients.
  - Fever can be absent in children with bacteremia, especially young infants.
  - Examine for localized signs of infection in bone and joints.
  - Very young infants with *Salmonella* may present with a normal exam, including those with meningitis.
  - When possible, directly inspect stool for gross blood and mucus.
- Enteric fever
  - Patients with high fever may exhibit a relative bradycardia.
  - A coated tongue may be noted.
  - Hepatomegaly and splenomegaly are common.
  - 2–4 mm maculopapular lesions (rose spots) appear in up to 25% of patients.
  - Rales and rhonchi can be present.

DIAGNOSTIC TESTS & INTERPRETATION

Lab

- Testing involves the following:
  - Basic blood chemistries may reveal dehydration and electrolyte imbalances.
  - WBC counts vary widely and are generally not helpful in diagnosis.
  - Bilirubin and serum transaminases may be elevated with enteric fever.
  - Stool culture is the most sensitive test for nontyphoidal gastrointestinal infection. Preliminary culture results reveal nonlactose fermenting, H_2S-producing colonies.
  - Fecal leukocyte and stool guaiac tests have limited sensitivity and specificity for diagnosing bacterial gastroenteritis.
  - Blood cultures are positive in up to 5% of nontyphoidal infections and 60–80% of patients with enteric fever.
  - Bone marrow aspirations are positive in 80–95% of patients with typhoid fever.
  - Routine bacterial culture of urine, CSF, or bone or joint aspirates should be obtained when clinically indicated.

DIFFERENTIAL DIAGNOSIS

- Illnesses that appear similar to nontyphoidal *Salmonella* infection
  - Acute gastroenteritis caused by *Shigella*, *Escherichia coli*, *Campylobacter*, and *Yersinia* is indistinguishable from *Salmonella*.
  - *Clostridium difficile* causes watery and inflammatory diarrhea, especially in children >2 years of age.
  - Norovirus, rotavirus, *Cryptosporidium*, and *Giardia* are common causes of watery diarrhea.
  - Allergic colitis
  - Inflammatory bowel disease
  - Bone and joint infection due to *Staphylococcus aureus*, group A strep, pneumococcus, and *Kingella*
- Enteric fever from *Salmonella* may appear similar to the following:
  - Appendicitis
  - Brucellosis
  - Dengue fever
  - Malaria
  - Nonspecific viral illness

TREATMENT

MEDICATION

- Antimicrobials are not indicated for uncomplicated nontyphoidal gastroenteritis, and their use has been associated with prolonged carriage.
- Antimicrobial therapy is indicated for the following:
  - High-risk patients with nontyphoidal gastroenteritis pending blood culture results. These include the following: 1) infants <3 months of age; 2) children with HIV, SCD, and 3) those with malignancy and/or receiving immunosuppressive therapy.
  - Patients with known or suspected nontyphoidal bacteremia or localized infection
  - Patients with known or suspected enteric fever
- Antimicrobial choice
  - Ceftriaxone or cefotaxime is the preferred drug for empirical therapy of nontyphoidal and typhoidal infections while awaiting blood culture and sensitivity results.
  - If shown to be susceptible, amoxicillin or trimethoprim/sulfamethoxazole (TMP/SMX) may be used in high-risk patients with uncomplicated nontyphoidal gastroenteritis and negative blood cultures.
  - Antimicrobial selection should be based on culture results when available. High rates of resistance occur with ampicillin and TMP/SMX.
  - Quinolones are generally active but not approved for patients <18 years of age.
- Corticosteroids may provide benefit to critically ill patients with enteric fever.

INPATIENT CONSIDERATIONS

Initial Management

- Patients with dehydration and electrolyte abnormalities require appropriate volume replacement.
- Antimotility agents are generally avoided for all forms of infectious diarrhea in children.
- Consult orthopedics for management of suspected bone and joint infections.
- Administer antimicrobials only for specific clinical indications.

ONGOING CARE

FOLLOW-UP RECOMMENDATIONS

- Acute nontyphoidal gastroenteritis
  - Encourage appropriate oral rehydrating fluids and monitor for signs and symptoms of dehydration.
  - Monitor for invasive complications, especially among high-risk patients.
  - Apprise patients and/or families of the risk for prolonged asymptomatic shedding.
  - Instruct patients and families in proper hand hygiene.
- Enteric fever
  - Fever can persist up to 7 days after starting appropriate antimicrobial therapy.
  - Monitor for serious complications such as intestinal bleeding, even after the patient appears to be improving.
  - Monitor for evidence of relapse.
  - Instruct patients and families in proper hand hygiene.

ALERT

- Serious complications of enteric fever can present as the patient appears to be improving.
- Even with appropriate therapy, patients with enteric fever may relapse 2–3 weeks after the initial fever resolves.

PROGNOSIS

- Noninvasive nontyphoidal gastroenteritis is typically a self-limiting infection.
- Individuals often shed the organism for weeks, and a small number of patients may continue to shed for >1 year.
- Relapse of typhoid fever occurs in 4–20% of patients up to 3 weeks after the fever resolves.

COMPLICATIONS

- Dehydration is the most common complication caused by acute gastroenteritis.
- Nontyphoidal *Salmonella* gastroenteritis may be complicated by the following:
  - Bacteremia, especially in high-risk patients
  - Osteomyelitis and septic arthritis. Patients with sickle cell disease are particularly susceptible.
  - Meningitis. The course is frequently severe and may be associated with abscess formation and relapse.
  - Other infectious complications include pneumonia, pyelonephritis, and pericarditis.
- Enteric fever complications include intestinal perforation and hemorrhage, cholecystitis, hepatitis encephalopathy, pneumonia, myocarditis, shock, and disseminated intravascular coagulation.

ADDITIONAL READING

- Bar-Meir M, Raveh D, Yinnon AM, et al. Non-Typhi *Salmonella* gastroenteritis in children presenting to the emergency department: characteristics of patients with associated bacteraemia. *Clin Micrbiol Infect*. 2005;11(8):651–655.
- Bhutta ZA. Current concepts in the diagnosis and treatment of typhoid fever. *BMJ*. 2006;333(7558):78–82.
- Cheng LH, Crim SM, Cole, CR, et al. Epidemiology of infant salmonellosis in the United States, 1996-2008: a Foodborne Diseases Active Surveillance Network Study. *J Ped Infect Dis*. 2003;2(3):232–239.
- Christenson JC. *Salmonella* infections. *Pediatr Rev*. 2013;34(9):375–383.
- Geme JW III, Hodes HL, Marcy SM, et al. Consensus: management of *Salmonella* infection in the first year of life. *Pediatr Infect Dis J*. 1998;7(9):615–621.

CODES

ICD10

- A02.9 Salmonella infection, unspecified
- A02.0 Salmonella enteritis
- A01.00 Typhoid fever, unspecified

FAQ

- Q: When can children infected with *Salmonella* return to day care or school?
- A: In general, infants and children with nontyphoidal *Salmonella* infection may return to day care or school 24 hours after their diarrhea has resolved. Repeat stool cultures are not recommended because asymptomatic shedding is common, and the risk of spread is low. Health officials may recommend documenting a negative stool culture if there are obvious concerns regarding a child's hygiene. Children with *S*. Typhi infection who are ≥5 years of age and asymptomatic for over 24 hours, may attend school without repeating stool cultures. For children <5 years of age with *S*. Typhi, it is generally required that the child be asymptomatic and have 3 negative stool cultures before returning to day care. Most health departments adopt this approach.

SARCOIDOSIS

Peter Weiser • Randy Q. Cron

BASICS

DESCRIPTION

A multisystem chronic granulomatous disease that has two distinct variants often differentiated by age of onset

EPIDEMIOLOGY

- More common in the southeastern part of the United States
- Early-onset sarcoidosis/Blau syndrome
  - Disease occurs before age 4 years as arthritis, uveitis, and dermatitis.
- Adult-type disease
  - Diagnosed in adolescence as Löfgren syndrome with erythema nodosum, polyarthritis, and hilar adenopathy
  - However, marked pulmonary involvement may also occur in older adolescents.
  - CNS involvement (rare): seizures, cranial neuropathy, hypothalamic dysfunction

RISK FACTORS

Genetics

- Blacks are more commonly affected than whites; specific genetic tendencies not identified.
- Early childhood cases of arthritis, uveitis, and dermatitis may result from mutation of the *CARD15/NOD2* gene—either spontaneous or hereditary (AD)—familial form, the latter also known as Blau syndrome. Some of the mutation-negative patients have systemic/visceral involvement.

ETIOLOGY

- Unknown (possibly infectious)
- Resembles pulmonary borreliosis
- Possible association with substantial dust inhalation (e.g., collapse of World Trade Center towers in New York)

PATHOPHYSIOLOGY

T-cell–mediated disease resulting in noncaseating epithelioid giant cell granulomas in affected organs

DIAGNOSIS

HISTORY

Prolonged malaise, fever, weight loss, rash, painful arthritis, swollen lymph nodes, chronic cough, and hematuria (can be microscopic) may be initial complaints.

PHYSICAL EXAM

- Peripheral lymphadenopathy is most common manifestation.
- Conjunctival injection
- Bilateral parotid gland enlargement and hepatosplenomegaly may be present.
- The arthritis, usually in the ankles, is extremely tender and boggy.
- Rash is diffuse, erythematous, and macular or plaque-like. It can also be erythema nodosum.

DIAGNOSTIC TESTS & INTERPRETATION

Lab

- CBC
  - Mild anemia, leukopenia, lymphopenia
- Erythrocyte sedimentation rate (ESR) elevated
- Angiotensin converting enzyme (ACE) level
  - Can be elevated
  - Produced in many granulomatous diseases but is useful in cases in which index of suspicion is high
  - Not a perfect screening test; however, can follow levels in response to treatment
  - False positives: may be elevated in
    - Miliary tuberculosis
    - Biliary cirrhosis
- Lysozyme level elevation
  - May be more sensitive than ACE level for detecting sarcoidosis
  - May be useful to follow disease activity in proven cases, if ACE levels cannot be used
  - False positives: may be elevated in
    - Lymphoma
- Serum calcium and creatinine levels
  - Important in baseline evaluation
- Urine test for blood
  - Seen in patients with hypercalciuria
- Synovial effusion is typically mildly inflammatory.
- Biopsy of affected organ, such as peripheral lymph node, parotid gland, skin, conjunctivae, minor salivary gland, or synovium (demonstrating noncaseating granuloma), is helpful and many times diagnostic.

Imaging

- Chest radiography
  - May demonstrate hilar adenopathy
- Gallium scan
  - Demonstrates uptake diffusely in lungs (extremely sensitive test)

ALERT

Uveitis may be occult; slit-lamp ophthalmologic evaluation is important.

DIFFERENTIAL DIAGNOSIS

- Infection
  - Tuberculosis
  - Bacterial sepsis
  - Mumps
  - HIV
  - Gonorrhea
  - Lyme disease
  - Pulmonary mycoses
- Tumors
  - Leukemia
  - Neuroblastoma
  - Lymphoma
- Immunologic
  - Oligoarticular juvenile idiopathic arthritis (for early-onset type)
  - Systemic juvenile idiopathic arthritis
  - Systemic lupus erythematosus
  - Sjögren disease

– Dermatomyositis
– Behçet disease
– Crohn disease
- Immunodeficiency
  – Common variable immunodeficiency
- Skin
  – Granuloma annulare
  – Erythema nodosum due to *Streptococcus*, hepatitis B, or inflammatory bowel disease (IBD)

ALERT
- Pitfalls in diagnosis include not considering IBD arthritis with erythema nodosum.
- Granulomatous skin lesions can occur in both.
- Gene mutations in *CARD15/NOD* occur in both IBD and Blau syndrome, albeit at different regions of the same chromosome.

TREATMENT

Medications are used to treat active disease with clinical symptoms.
- Pitfalls include overtreating asymptomatic lymphadenopathy and not detecting hypercalciuria.

MEDICATION
- Corticosteroids may provide rapid improvement; NSAIDs/analgesics for symptom relief.
- In cases of chronic disease, immunosuppressive medications such as methotrexate can be used in addition to corticosteroids.
- The tumor necrosis factor inhibitors, specifically antibodies like infliximab and adalimumab show promising preliminary results and should be considered especially in uveitis.
- In cases of hypercalciuria/hypercalcemia, consider hydration and furosemide.
- Cyclophosphamide for neurosarcoidosis.

ONGOING CARE

FOLLOW-UP RECOMMENDATIONS
Patient Monitoring
- Referral to rheumatologist indicated, also regular ophthalmologic assessment
- Signs to watch for:
  – Climbing creatinine
  – Shortness of breath
  – Persistent uveal tract inflammation
  – Neurologic deficit

PROGNOSIS
- Variable in early onset. Severe organ involvement and joint and eye damage can occur—needs close follow-up.
- Löfgren syndrome can resolve after a couple of years.
- More than 40% of older children with adult-type disease have persistent pulmonary changes, but only a few will have pulmonary symptoms.

COMPLICATIONS
- In children, usually related to uveitis or from hypercalciuria resulting in renal injury. Lung, CNS, and ocular involvement can bring long-term defects.
- In older adolescents, pulmonary problems, such as restrictive lung disease, as well as severe growth delay, may occur.

ADDITIONAL READING

- Baumann RJ, Robertson WC Jr. Neurosarcoid presents differently in children than in adults. *Pediatrics*. 2003;112(6)(Pt 1):e480–e486.
- Iannuzzi MC, Rybicki BA, Teirstein AS. Sarcoidosis. *N Engl J Med*. 2007;357(21):2153–2165.
- Lindsley CB, Petty RE. Overview and report on international registry of sarcoid arthritis in childhood. *Curr Rheumatol Rep*. 2000;2(4):343–348.
- Rose CD, Wouters CH, Meiorin S, et al. Pediatric granulomatous arthritis: an international registry. *Arthritis Rheum*. 2006;54(10):3337–3344.
- Shetty AK, Gedalia A. Childhood sarcoidosis: a rare but fascinating disorder. *Pediatr Rheumatol Online J*. 2008;6:16.

CODES

ICD10
- D86.9 Sarcoidosis, unspecified
- D86.0 Sarcoidosis of lung
- D86.86 Sarcoid arthropathy

FAQ
- Q: Why is therapy in childhood sarcoidosis more aggressive compared with adults?
- A: These may be 2 distinct granulomatous diseases. Early-onset sarcoidosis is a very aggressive and destructive disease requiring chronic therapy rather than a relatively short course of steroids.

SCABIES

Jessica Nash

BASICS

DESCRIPTION

- Scabies is a parasitic infection caused by the mite *Sarcoptes scabiei*, which infects the stratum corneum of the skin and results in an intense pruritic rash.
- Crusted scabies is a subtype categorized by a more intense pruritus and rash with a heavier burden of mites.
  - Previously called "Norwegian scabies"
  - More common in immunocompromised (i.e., HIV, long-term steroid use) and debilitated patients with sensory neuropathies and paralysis
- Nodular scabies is a rare clinical subtype presenting with red to brown nodules secondary to hypersensitivity reaction to mites and their by-products.

EPIDEMIOLOGY

- Results from close personal and prolonged contact with another human infected with mites
- Occurs worldwide and is endemic in many countries
- Scabies affects all people from different ethnicities, social economic levels, and gender.

Incidence

Varies worldwide, with cyclical fluctuations for new cases; estimates are 1–15 new cases per 1,000 people per year.

Prevalence

Estimated 300 million cases worldwide

GENERAL PREVENTION

- Avoid direct skin-to-skin contact with a person who has scabies and with the clothing/bedding used by a person who has scabies.
- Ensure that any close contacts that have been exposed are treated even if asymptomatic because symptoms can take up to 30 days to develop.
- Everyone in the household should be treated at the same time.
- All bedding and clothing used in the prior 3 days by a person with scabies needs to be washed with hot water and dried in a hot dryer for at least 10 minutes or should be dry-cleaned.
- Furniture and carpets in the household of an infected person should be vacuumed.
- Anything that cannot be washed should be isolated from humans for at least 2 days or, more conservatively, for up to 3 weeks.

PATHOPHYSIOLOGY

- The mite of scabies is a parasite that burrows into the skin and lays eggs. They travel anywhere between 0.5 and 5.0 mm a day. The larvae hatch from the eggs in 2–3 days and become adults and then the cycle repeats.
- Papules are not due to the mite itself but due to a hypersensitivity reaction to the mites' saliva, eggs, and feces.
- If the individual has never been exposed, there is an incubation period which can be between 4 and 6 weeks before symptoms manifest.
- Those with prior exposure and thus sensitized can have milder symptoms that occur within 1–4 days.
- Crusted scabies subtype has thousands to millions more mites, making infectivity easier even at less contact. The mite is the same as with classic scabies.

ETIOLOGY

S. scabiei var *hominis* adult female mite is about 0.3-mm long with eight legs and barely visible with the naked eye.

DIAGNOSIS

HISTORY

- Patients usually present with a history of rash that is intensely pruritic and worse at night because mite activity increases at night based on temperature of the human body.
- Rash present on hands and wrist and may also be in genital area.
- Children younger than 2 years of age may present with a vesicular rash on face and other regions of body not typical in older children and adults.
- Other family members or household contacts with a similar rash given contact with infected person is needed for transmission.

PHYSICAL EXAM

- Usually presents with a papular erythematous rash
- One pathognomonic sign is the burrow line, a linear, wavy, S-shaped mark which occurs as the mite burrows into the skin; can be difficult to see because scratching can obliterate the burrow, but it helps with diagnosis if visualized
- To better identify burrows, can use a washable marker on the skin, then remove markings with water or alcohol. The ink will remain within the burrow, making it easier to see.
- Common sites of rash are interdigital web spaces of hands and feet. Papules can be present in flexor region of wrist, extensor region of elbows, axillary folds, genital region, and periareolar regions of breast.
- Presentation differs in young children versus older children and adults.
  - Children younger than 2 years of age usually have a more widespread distribution that also includes face, neck, palms, and soles.
  - Rash in young children also can be more vesicular.

DIAGNOSTIC TESTS & INTERPRETATION

Lab

- Direct visualization
  - Potassium hydroxide preparation of a skin scraping
  - Use a blade to scrape skin, isolate the mite from scrapings, and view scrapings under microscopy.
  - Look for mites and mite fecal matter.
- Visualization of the burrows can be made easier using the "burrow ink test."
  - Use ink to mark areas where scabies are suspected, then wipe away the surface ink with alcohol pad.
  - If ink tracks into the mite burrow, making a grossly visible zigzagged line, the test is positive.
- In atypical cases, skin biopsy can be formed.
- Other more specialized tests are under development such as antigen detection, PCR of skin scrapings, or intradermal tests.

DIFFERENTIAL DIAGNOSIS

- Contact dermatitis
- Atopic dermatitis
- Insect bites
- Drug rash
- Infantile acropustulosis
- Impetigo
- Papular urticaria
- Viral exanthem

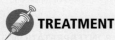

TREATMENT

MEDICATION

- Permethrin 5% cream
  - Drug of choice for children and infants >2 months of age
  - Is neurotoxic to the mite
  - The cream is applied from neck to toe, paying special attention to interdigital regions; skinfolds of wrist, elbow, and inguinal creases; and under nails.
  - In young children, include the entire head and neck as well because these aren't spared in this age group.
  - Rinse cream off the body 8–14 hours after application.
  - Often, one retreatment 1 week after initial treatment is needed. Some recommend retreating once 4 days later (instead of waiting 7 days).
- Crotamiton 10% cream
  - Not commonly used
  - Not approved in children
  - Apply from chin to toe and reapply 24 hours later. Then remove by a cleansing bath 48 hours after the last application.
- Sulfur 5–10% cream
  - Can be used for infants younger than 2 months and pregnant lactating woman
  - Must be reapplied daily for 3 days
- Ivermectin
  - Oral antiparasitic agent
  - Not recommend for women who are pregnant or lactating
  - Safety profile for children is unknown.
  - Not FDA approved for treatment of scabies
- Mild to moderate topical steroids
  - Note, topical steroids have no efficacy in treating the mite infection but can be helpful for the intense pruritus during and just after the scabies infection.
- Lindane 1%
  - Not commonly used due to concern for systemic toxicity
  - American Academy of Pediatrics (AAP) *Redbook* (2012) states that "because of safety concerns and availability of other treatments, lindane should not be used for treatment of scabies."
  - Side effects can include seizures, headache, and vertigo.

ONGOING CARE

FOLLOW-UP RECOMMENDATIONS

Patient Monitoring

- Treatment failure occurs but is usually due to incomplete treatment of all contacts at the same time.
- Recommend follow-up 2 weeks after treatment to ensure no new burrows, new papules, or new vesicles have developed, which would most likely indicate inadequate application of treatment.

PROGNOSIS

Prognosis is great with early identification and treatment.

COMPLICATIONS

- Secondary bacterial skin infection
- Post scabies pruritus: Pruritus that occurs for weeks after treatment should not be confused with treatment failure.

ADDITIONAL READING

- American Academy of Pediatrics. Scabies. In: Pickering LK, Baker CJ, Kimberlin DW, et al, eds. *Red Book: 2012 Report of the Committee on Infectious Diseases*. 29th ed. Elk Grove Village, IL: American Academy of Pediatrics; 2012.
- Chosidow O. Clinical practice: scabies. *N Engl J Med*. 2006;354(16);1718–1727.
- Golant AK, Levitt JO. Scabies: a review of diagnosis and management based on mite biology. *Pediatr Rev*. 2012;33(1):e1–e12.
- Heukelbach J, Feldmeier H. Scabies *Lancet*. 2006;367(9524):1767–1774.
- Leone P. Scabies and pediculosis pubis: an update of treatment regimens and general review. *Clin Infect Dis*. 2007;44(Suppl 3):S153–S159.
- Mounsey KE, McCarthy JS. Treatment and control of scabies. *Curr Opin Infect Dis*. 2013;26(2):133–139.
- Strong M, Johnstone P. Interventions for treating scabies. *Cochrane Database Syst Rev*. 2007;(3):CD000320.

CODES

ICD10

B86 Scabies

FAQ

- Q: What do I do with the clothes or cloth items that cannot be washed at this time?
- A: Store them in a plastic bag and put them away for 3 days because the mite cannot live more than 3 days without a human host. Couches and carpet should be vacuumed.
- Q: When will my child no longer be contagious?
- A: If treated properly, children are no longer contagious after one treatment. Although your child may still have pruritus, he or she is no longer considered contagious and can return to school.
- Q: When will the rash resolve?
- A: The rash may take 3–4 weeks to resolve after treatment and should not be considered a treatment failure unless a new rash develops.

SCARLET FEVER

Emily C. Borman-Shoap • John S. Andrews

BASICS

DESCRIPTION

- Scarlet fever or "scarlatina" is a manifestation of infection with *Streptococcus pyogenes* (group A β-hemolytic *Streptococcus*) that is characterized by an erythematous "sandpaper" rash. It results from infection with a strain of *S. pyogenes* that elaborates streptococcal pyrogenic exotoxin (SPE).
- Typically occurs in the setting of streptococcal pharyngitis but may occur with group A streptococcal skin or wound infections
- Associated SPE A, B, C, and F. SPE A is associated with more virulent disease.
- Similar syndrome may also be seen in infection with certain enterotoxin-producing strains of *Staphylococcus aureus*, known as staphylococcal scarlet fever.

GENERAL PREVENTION

- Prompt treatment leads to fewer secondary cases of streptococcal disease.
- Some experts recommend chemoprophylaxis with penicillin in children with repeated documented episodes occurring at short intervals.
- Control measures, including hygiene advice and exclusion of infected students for 24 hours while initiating penicillin treatment, were ineffective in a school outbreak.

EPIDEMIOLOGY

- Equal prevalence in boys and girls
- Most common between ages 3 and 15 years, possibly related to the requirement for prior sensitization and toxin-specific immunity
- Little seasonal variation, although some increased prevalence in winter and spring
- Incubation period is 2–5 days for strep pharyngitis and may be up to 10 days for strep skin infections.

Incidence

Peak incidence during the first few school years

Prevalence

By age 10 years, 80% of children have developed toxin-specific antibodies.

PATHOPHYSIOLOGY

- Susceptible individuals are thought to lack toxin-specific immunity. This is supported by results of the Dick test, in which a small amount of toxin introduced intradermally produces local erythema in susceptible individuals but no reaction in those with toxin-specific immunity.
- Rash and other toxic manifestations of scarlet fever have been attributed to the development of hypersensitivity to the toxin, which requires prior exposure to the toxin.
- Toxin production depends on lysogeny of the infecting *Streptococcus* by a temperate bacteriophage.
- Histologic examination of affected skin shows dilated blood and lymphatic vessels and engorged capillaries, most prominently around hair follicles.
- Acute, edematous polymorphonuclear inflammatory reaction is seen microscopically within affected tissues.
- Epidermal inflammatory reaction is usually followed by hyperkeratosis, which accounts for scaling during defervescence.

DIAGNOSIS

HISTORY

- Sudden onset of fever up to 40.5°C, sore throat, headache, nausea, vomiting, and toxicity are classic symptoms for group A streptococcal disease.
- Texture of rash (e.g., feels like sandpaper) is more important than appearance.
- Characteristic rash typically occurs 12–48 hours after onset of fever.
- Patient may complain of abdominal pain or muscle aches before onset of rash as well as aching in extremities or back.
- There may be close contacts with streptococcal infection.

PHYSICAL EXAM

- Fine maculopapular (sandpaper texture) rash on erythematous background: usually begins on the trunk and spreads to involve almost the entire body within hours to days. Although the rash seen with scarlet fever is generally fine and sandpaper-like, larger papules and petechiae may be seen.
- Rash may be more easily detected by palpation than visual inspection
- Pastia line: accentuation of erythema in flexor creases (antecubital, axillary, inguinal)
- Circumoral pallor: Area around mouth appears pale in comparison to flushed cheeks.
- Rash blanches with pressure and ultimately desquamates: Desquamation occurs within 7–21 days from onset of illness.
- Systemic toxicity: may indicate incorrect diagnosis
- Dorsum of tongue: has white coat early in illness with edematous red papillae. White covering desquamates and reveals swollen, red, and mottled strawberry tongue.
- Other findings:
  - Pharynx and tonsils are beefy red and may contain exudate.
  - Hemorrhagic spots on interior pillar of tonsils and soft palate
  - Large, tender anterior cervical nodes

DIAGNOSTIC TESTS & INTERPRETATION

Lab

- Rapid streptococcal antigen tests: effective as screening tests; 70–90% sensitivity and >95% specificity. Positive rapid tests do not require culture confirmation.
- Throat culture: the gold standard with best sensitivity (>90%) for group A β-hemolytic streptococci. A culture should be performed when rapid test is negative.
- White blood cell count: usually elevated, although may be elevated in viral pharyngitis as well. Low count would be rare with streptococcal infection.
- Eosinophilia (up to 30%): common in the recovery phase
- Dick test: of historic interest; no longer used clinically
- Pitfalls
  - A positive throat culture may be evidence only of carriage in some cases of acute pharyngitis that are actually viral (e.g., Epstein-Barr virus).
  - Milder disease is becoming more common and is easier to miss. Rash may involve only the bridge of the nose, face, shoulders, and upper chest. Circumoral pallor and severe exudative pharyngitis are being seen less frequently.

DIFFERENTIAL DIAGNOSIS

- Viral exanthems (measles, rubella, erythema infectiosum)
- Drug eruptions
- Staphylococcal scalded skin syndrome
- Toxic epidermal necrolysis
- Toxic shock syndrome (streptococcal or staphylococcal)
- Kawasaki disease
- Uncommon entities:
  - Infection with *Arcanobacterium hemolyticum*
  - Mercury poisoning (acrodynia)
  - Atropine intoxication
  - Boric acid poisoning
  - Rifampin overdose

TREATMENT

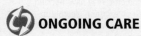

GENERAL MEASURES

- Identical to therapy for streptococcal pharyngitis
- Therapy started as late as 9 days after illness onset should be effective in preventing acute rheumatic fever.
- May withhold treatment until throat culture result is available
- Immediate therapy probably shortens symptomatic period.

MEDICATION

Penicillin or amoxicillin remain the drugs of choice to treat streptococcal pharyngitis. Resistance to penicillin has never been documented in the United States.

- Oral penicillin V potassium (10 days)
  – Children: 250 mg twice or 3 times daily
  – Adolescents: 250 mg 4 times daily or 500 mg twice daily
- Oral amoxicillin (10 days)
  – 50/mg/kg once daily (max 1,000 mg/dose)
  – Alternate 25 mg/kg/dose (max 500 mg/dose) twice daily
- Intramuscular penicillin G benzathine
  – Equally effective as oral penicillin
  – Dose: 600,000 U for children <14 kg (<30 lb); 900,000–1,200,000 U for children 14–27 kg; and 1,200,000 U for children >27 kg and adults
  – Ensures compliance (only one dose needed)
  – Benzathine/procaine penicillin combinations are less painful.

The following medications are options for penicillin-allergic patients:

- Oral cephalexin (10 days)
  – 20 mg/kg/dose twice daily (max 500 mg/dose)
- Oral cefadroxil (10 days)
  – 30 mg/kg/dose once daily (max 2 g/dose)
- Oral azithromycin (5 days)
  – 12 mg/kg/dose once daily (max 500 mg/dose)
- Oral clarithromycin (10 days)
  – 7.5 mg/kg/dose twice daily (max 500 mg/dose)

Tetracyclines and sulfonamides should not be used because of resistance of group A streptococci.

ONGOING CARE

- Fever and symptoms usually resolve within 24–48 hours of antibiotic treatment.
- Nonsuppurative complications occur after the acute streptococcal infection has resolved.
  – Acute rheumatic fever occurs an average of 18 days after untreated infection. Treatment must be initiated within 9 days of onset to prevent this complication
  – Acute postinfectious glomerulonephritis occurs an average of 10 days after infection. The risk of glomerulonephritis is not reduced by treatment with antibiotics.

PROGNOSIS

Overall prognosis is excellent.

- Few patients suffer suppurative complications.
- Risk of developing acute rheumatic fever in untreated streptococcal infections is about 3% under epidemic conditions (0.3% in endemic situations).
- Acute postinfectious glomerulonephritis is uncommon. Risk may be as high as 10–15% following infections with certain nephritogenic strains.

COMPLICATIONS

- Patients with scarlet fever may experience hyperkeratosis. Peeling of the affected skin may also occur 2 weeks after the acute infection.
- Other complications worth noting may occur following any primary manifestation of group A streptococcal infection and are not specific to scarlet fever.
  – Streptococcal toxic shock syndrome is a toxin-mediated complication of streptococcal infection that may be life threatening.
  – Suppurative complications of streptococcal pharyngitis include the following:
    ○ Cervical adenitis
    ○ Peritonsillar abscess
    ○ Retropharyngeal abscess
    ○ Sinusitis
    ○ Otitis media
    ○ Mastoiditis
    ○ Meningitis
    ○ Brain abscess
    ○ Thrombosis of intracranial venous sinuses
  – Nonsuppurative complications include acute rheumatic fever and postinfectious glomerulonephritis

ADDITIONAL READING

- Chiappini E, Regoli M, Bonsignori F, et al. Analysis of different recommendations from international guidelines for the management of acute pharyngitis in adults and children. *Clin Ther*. 2011;33(1):48–58.
- Lamden KH. An outbreak of scarlet fever in a primary school. *Arch Dis Child*. 2011;96(4):394–397.
- Luk EY, Lo JY, Li AZ, et al. Scarlet fever epidemic, Hong Kong, 2011. *Emerg Infect Dis*. 2012;18(10): 1658–1661.
- Shaikh N, Swaminathan N, Hooper EG. Accuracy and precision of the signs and symptoms of streptococcal pharyngitis in children: a systematic review. *J Pediatr*. 2012;160(3):487–493.e3.
- Shulman ST, Bisno ST, Clegg HW, et al. Clinical practice guideline for the diagnosis and management of group A streptococcal pharyngitis: 2012 update by the Infectious Diseases Society of America. *Clin Infect Dis*. 2012;55(10):e86–e102.

CODES

ICD10

- A38.9 Scarlet fever, uncomplicated
- J02.0 Streptococcal pharyngitis

FAQ

- Q: Should household contacts have throat cultures performed?
- A: Obtain cultures only from symptomatic household contacts.
- Q: Is there any indication for throat culture in asymptomatic individuals (e.g., household contact of infected individual or test of cure in treated individual)?
- A: No. Throat culture of close contacts of highly vulnerable individuals (e.g., those with recurrent rheumatic fever) may be indicated.
- Q: Is culture confirmation of strep infection necessary to make the diagnosis of scarlet fever?
- A: No. Although laboratory evidence of strep infection is supportive, scarlet fever is a clinical diagnosis.
- Q: Should posttreatment throat cultures be performed?
- A: Only in symptomatic individuals and patients at risk for acute rheumatic fever.
- Q: Can scarlet fever occur in the absence of pharyngitis?
- A: Yes. Scarlet fever has been reported after group A streptococcal skin infections
- Q: Can scarlet fever recur?
- A: Yes. There have been documented reports of recurrent scarlet fever.
- Q: Have there been documented child care outbreaks of scarlet fever?
- A: Yes. Outbreaks have been traced to single strains in this setting.
- Q: How soon can children return to school or child care?
- A: When they are afebrile and after at least 24 hours of antibiotic therapy

SCLERODERMA

Peter Weiser • Randy Q. Cron

BASICS

DESCRIPTION

- Scleroderma means "hard skin." It can be systemic or localized.
- Systemic sclerosis (SSc) or progressive systemic sclerosis (PSS)
  - Diffuse cutaneous SSc: affects skin and internal organs (lungs, GI tract)
  - Limited cutaneous SSc, also known as CREST: a variant form of SSc characterized by calcinosis, Raynaud phenomenon, esophageal dysmotility, sclerodactyly, telangiectases
- Localized
  - Morphea
  - Linear scleroderma
  - En Coup de Sabre/Parry-Romberg syndrome

EPIDEMIOLOGY

- Systemic
  - Age of onset: 30–50 years; very rare in children
  - Sex ratio
    - <7 years, male = female
    - >7 years, female > male (3:1)
    - 15–44 years, female > male (15:1)
- CREST
  - Earlier age of onset than SSc
  - Almost nonexistent in children
  - Female > male

Incidence

- Systemic: 0.27 per million annually
- CREST: affects ~1/2 of patients with systemic disease
- Localized: approximately 10× more common than SSc in childhood

PATHOPHYSIOLOGY

- Systemic involvement
  - Vasculopathy: based on high association with Raynaud phenomenon; vascular injury leading to fibrotic changes as a part of overcorrection
  - Serum factors: overexpression of endothelin, a potent vasoconstrictor with profibrotic activity
  - Immune dysfunction: autoimmunity directed against connective tissue antigen such as laminin or type IV collagen, platelet-derived growth factor receptors stimulating fibrosis
- Localized form
  - Alteration of normal glycosylation and hydroxylation of collagen
  - May represent distinct early and late processes
    - Early: increased hydrophilic glycosaminoglycan; increased T cells, macrophages, and plasma cells; mast cell hyperplasia
    - Late: increased collagen content; collagen is embryonic with narrow fibrils and immature cross-banding; atrophy of rete pegs, epithelial tissue projecting into underlying connective tissue

DIAGNOSIS

HISTORY

- Thickening of skin
- Tightness of joints
- Discoloration of skin
- Often insidious onset
- Morning stiffness
- Heartburn, dysphagia, reflux, cough with swallowing

Signs and symptoms:

- SSc
  - Diagnostic criteria (1 major criterion or 2 minor criteria required)
  - Major: sclerodermatous changes (tightness, thickening, induration) proximal to metacarpophalangeal or metatarsophalangeal joints
  - Minor: sclerodactyly-sclerodermatous changes limited to digits (unable to pinch skin over the digit), digital pitting, bibasilar pulmonary fibrosis not due to primary lung disease
  - CREST
    - More severe calcinosis
    - Distal symptoms more severe
    - Associated with anti-centromere antibody
    - Occasional evolution into another connective tissue disease such as mixed connective tissue disease (MCTD) or systemic lupus erythematosus (SLE)
- Localized
  - Fibrosis limited to skin, subcutaneous (SC) tissue, and muscle
  - Systemic features including Raynaud phenomenon and visceral involvement are extremely rare except in Parry-Romberg.
  - Forms:
    - Morphea: ≥1 oval or round indurations that become hard and whitish early on, have active inflammatory border with violaceous color. Various forms: plaque or guttate (limited number of lesions); generalized (extensive); nodular (SC)
  - Linear: ≥1 linear areas affecting SC tissue, muscle, and bone; can cross joint lines and also affect limb growth
  - En Coup de Sabre: involves face or scalp; may be associated with seizures
  - Parry-Romberg syndrome: form of linear scleroderma; congenital dysplasia of SC tissue; neurologic changes such as transient ischemic attacks (TIAs) in brain matter under lesion, without its direct extension into the skull

PHYSICAL EXAM

- Findings in SSc:
  - Skin
    - Stage 1: Edema—tense, nonpitting; perhaps warm or tender but often asymptomatic
    - Stage 2: Sclerosis—waxy, hard texture; bound to SC structures, back of digits, face (loss of forehead wrinkles, reduced mouth orifice)
    - Stage 3: Atrophy—shiny appearance, hypopigmented or hyperpigmented, calcium deposits in SC tissue
    - Telangiectasias: macular dilatations that fill slowly, unlike spider telangiectasias
    - Loss of SC tissue pulp of the fingers and ulcerations on fingertips with prolonged healing in SSc
  - Raynaud phenomenon
    - Primary phenomenon or Raynaud disease: not associated with underlying disease; milder; 75% are female.
    - Secondary Raynaud phenomenon: associated with underlying disease such as SSc, SLE, Sjögren syndrome, MCTD, dermatomyositis, and polymyositis; more serious. Present in ~90% of SSc patients.
    - Triple phase: blanching of digits with sharp border to normal-colored skin (arterial vasoconstriction) followed by cyanosis (venostasis) then erythema; tingling/numb sensation of the digits (reflex hyperemia to vasodilatation)
    - Usually fingers; also toes, nose, ears, and tongue; often spares thumb
  - Calcinosis, especially over extensor joint surfaces in systemic form only
  - Pitfalls
    - Failure to recognize limited mouth opening in SSc
    - Failure to evaluate periungual nailfold changes with Raynaud phenomenon: capillary dropout and dilated loops; occasional redundant cuticular growth and digital pitting
  - Musculoskeletal
    - "Creaking" of thickened tendons
    - Contractures, especially proximal interphalangeal joints and elbows
    - Associated arthritis
    - Muscle inflammation in ~30% of cases
  - GI
    - Mucosal telangiectasias of mouth
    - Decreased incisor distance/mouth opening secondary to skin tightness of the lips
    - Sicca syndrome with parotitis
    - Loosening of teeth secondary to periodontal membrane disease
    - Esophageal disease: esophagitis, occasional ulceration or stricture
    - Large-bowel disease less common
  - Cardiac
    - Primary cause of morbidity
    - Possibly due to Raynaud phenomenon of coronary arteries and pulmonary artery hypertension
    - Myocarditis possible
  - Pulmonary
    - Interstitial fibrosis with gradual obliteration of vascular bed and resulting cor pulmonale
    - Parenchymal disease is almost universal; frequently asymmetric; may have hacking cough, dyspnea on exertion, pleural rub.
    - Combined pulmonary vascular and pulmonary parenchymal disease
    - Primary pulmonary vascular disease with right ventricular failure
  - Renal: due to decreased renal plasma flow, proteinuria, hypertension, renal crisis
  - CNS: cranial nerve involvement, especially sensory branch of trigeminal nerve
  - Sicca syndrome
    - Xerostomia (dry mouth)
    - Keratoconjunctivitis sicca (dry eyes)

DIAGNOSTIC TESTS & INTERPRETATION

Lab

There are no specific diagnostic tests.

- Nonspecific tests
  - Systemic form
    - Antinuclear antibody (ANA): often positive
    - Hemoglobin: 25% have anemia due to chronic disease or vitamin B_{12} and folate deficiencies resulting from chronic malabsorption in sclerodermatous gut.

- Eosinophilia: present in 50%
- Sclero-70 (Scl-70 or topoisomerase 1) antibodies: present in 26% of adults; more common with diffuse disease than with peripheral vascular disease
- Anti-centromere antibody: present in 22%, almost exclusively with CREST
- Muscle biopsy

– Localized forms
- Eosinophilia: present in 25–50% during active disease
- ANA: positive in 37–67%

Imaging

- Chest radiograph
  - Bibasilar pulmonary fibrosis
  - Rib notching
  - Calcifications (in CREST)
- High-resolution chest CT
  - Ground-glass attenuation
  - Honeycombing
- Bone radiograph
  - Acro-osteolysis: resorption of tufts of distal phalanges, especially with severe Raynaud phenomenon
  - Periarticular or SC calcification (15–25% patients)
  - Bony erosions

Diagnostic Procedures/Other

- For sicca syndrome
  - Schirmer test for dry eyes
  - Lip biopsy
  - Rose bengal staining of cornea
- ECG
  - 1st-degree block
  - Right and left bundle-branch block
  - Premature atrial contractions (PACs) and premature ventricular contractions (PVCs): nonspecific T-wave changes, ventricular hypertrophy
- Pulmonary function tests
  - Restrictive lung disease: present in 34% of patients with SSc
  - Earliest changes are decreased forced vital capacity (FVC) and small airway disease.
  - Decreased diffusing capacity of the lung for carbon monoxide (DLCO): present in 18% of patients with SSc at the time of diagnosis

Pathologic Findings

- Histologic
  - Skin: loss of SC fat, increased amount of fibroblasts
  - Muscle: increased collagen and fat; negative immunofluorescence
  - Esophagus: Atrophic muscle replaced by fibrous tissue more commonly affects smooth muscle of lower 2/3 of esophagus.
- Esophageal manometry and pH probe: decreased or absent peristalsis of distal esophagus—distal dilatation, hiatal hernia, stricture
- Dilatation of second and third part of duodenum and proximal jejunum

DIFFERENTIAL DIAGNOSIS

- Graft-versus-host disease (GVHD)
- Phenylketonuria
- Borrelia infection: acrodermatitis chronica atrophicans
- Porphyria cutanea tarda
- Scleredema
- Stiff skin syndrome (mucin deposition in the dermis, hardening of the subcutaneous tissue with normal-looking epidermis)
- Eosinophilic fasciitis

TREATMENT

MEDICATION

Disease modification: Many agents have been tried; however, there are few controlled trials, and no proven treatment exists. Medications include the following:

- Localized
  - Imiquimod, calcitriol ointment, psoralen ultraviolet A light (PUVA) therapy, methotrexate, mycophenolate mofetil, cyclosporine
- Systemic
  - Colchicine: inhibits fibroproliferative process
  - Immunosuppressives
    - Steroids, chlorambucil, methotrexate, mycophenolate mofetil, cyclosporine, cyclophosphamide, rituximab
- Pitfall: Avoid excessive use of immunosuppressive therapy late in disease when inflammatory component has resolved.

ADDITIONAL TREATMENT

General Measures

- Supportive care: Avoid trauma and excessive cold; keep extremities warm AND dry.
- Management of Raynaud phenomenon:
  - Avoid beta-blockers, caffeine, and stimulating ADHD medications.

ADDITIONAL THERAPIES

- Physical therapy
  - Helps retard development of contractures and muscle atrophy
  - Pitfall: insufficient physical therapy resulting in permanent joint contractures

ONGOING CARE

FOLLOW-UP RECOMMENDATIONS

Patient Monitoring

- Localized forms
  - Physical exam for joint mobility, muscle bulk, and growth
  - Difficult to follow slow disease progression, thus photography of lesions every 3–6 months is recommended
- Systemic forms
  - Physical exam for digital ulcerations, joint mobility, muscle bulk, and growth
  - Yearly pulmonary function tests
  - Yearly barium swallow
  - ECHO

PROGNOSIS

- In localized forms, natural course includes several phases:
  - Initial: inflammation
  - Late: sclerosis
  - Occasional regression over 3–5 years
- Contractures and limb size difference can persist with linear scleroderma.
- Systemic form is progressive and ultimate prognosis depends on severity of skin tightness, joint contracture, and visceral involvement.
- Mortality with SSc
  - Males > females
  - Non-whites > whites
- Most common cause of death in pediatric patients with SSc is secondary to cardiac, renal, and pulmonary complications.

COMPLICATIONS

- Localized
  - Skin thickening
  - Joint contractures
  - Leg length discrepancies
  - CNS bleed in Parry-Romberg

ADDITIONAL READING

- Fain ET, Mannion M, Pope E, et al. Brain cavernomas associated with en coup de sabre linear scleroderma: two case reports. *Pediatr Rheumatol Online J*. 2011;9:18.
- Fitch PG, Rettig P, Burnham JM, et al. Treatment of pediatric localized scleroderma with methotrexate. *J Rheumatol*. 2006;33(3):609–614.
- Foeldvari I. Methotrexate in juvenile localized scleroderma. *Arthritis Rheum*. 2011;63(7): 1779–1781.
- Foeldvari I. Update on pediatric systemic sclerosis: Similarities and differences from adult disease. *Curr Opin Rheumatol*. 2008;20(5):608–612.
- Herrick AL, Ennis H, Bhushan M, et al. Incidence of childhood linear scleroderma and systemic sclerosis in the UK and Ireland. *Arthritis Care Res*. 2010;62(2):213–218.
- Martini G, Foeldvari I, Russo R, et al. Systemic sclerosis in childhood: Clinical and immunologic features of 153 patients in an international database. *Arthritis Rheum*. 2006;54(12):3971–3978.
- Zulian F. New developments in localized scleroderma. *Curr Opin Rheumatol*. 2008;20(5):601–607.

CODES

ICD10

- M34.9 Systemic sclerosis, unspecified
- M34.1 CR(E)ST syndrome
- L94.0 Localized scleroderma [morphea]

FAQ

- Q: Is a biopsy necessary?
- A: Biopsy is often useful to confirm diagnosis and assess degree of inflammation.
- Q: Is the sclero-70 antibody useful?
- A: Not for diagnosis; it is positive only in a subset of individuals with the systemic form and, therefore, useful for predicting more severe disease.

SCOLIOSIS (IDIOPATHIC)

Scott McKay • Jennifer A. Talarico • John P. Dormans

BASICS

DESCRIPTION

- Scoliosis: lateral curvature of spine exceeding 10 degrees on PA full-spine radiograph (with rotation of spine); curves <10 are termed spinal asymmetry; considered idiopathic only after other causes have been excluded
- Kyphosis: anteriorly concave curvature of vertebral column

EPIDEMIOLOGY

- Female-to-male ratios:
  - 1.4:1 for curves 11–20 degrees
  - 5.4:1 for curves >20 degrees

Prevalence

- Generally considered 1.5–3% for curves ≥10 degrees
- 0.3–0.5% for curves >20 degrees

RISK FACTORS

Genetics

Positive familial history for idiopathic scoliosis in 30% (not predictive of severity)

- Under active investigation: GWAS and whole exome sequencing studies
- Several candidate genes have been identified.

ETIOLOGY

By definition, unknown; listed are some theories, none proven in isolation:

- Genetic
  - Positive familial history for scoliosis in 30% (not predictive of severity)
- Connective tissue disorder
  - Associated with several connective tissue disorders (including Marfan syndrome, Ehlers-Danlos syndrome, etc.)
  - Alterations in connective tissue of the spine, paraspinous muscles, and platelets
  - May be related to osteopenia (decreased bone mineral density) of vertebral bodies
- Neurologic (equilibrium system)
  - Abnormalities noted in vestibular, ocular, proprioceptive, and vibratory functions
- Hormonal
  - Lower levels of melatonin secreted from pineal body in those with adolescent idiopathic scoliosis
  - Growth hormone: more of an influential factor than an etiologic factor in studies
  - Vertebral growth abnormalities
  - Asymmetric growth rates between the right and left sides of the spine

COMMONLY ASSOCIATED CONDITIONS

- Connective tissue disorders, including Marfan syndrome and Ehlers-Danlos syndrome
- Neurofibromatosis
- Neuromuscular conditions, including cerebral palsy, spina bifida, spinal muscular atrophy, Friedreich ataxia, etc.
- If any of these conditions are present, the diagnosis is no longer idiopathic.

DIAGNOSIS

HISTORY

- Onset: Consider when first noted, by whom, rate of worsening, previous treatment, patient recent growth, the physical change of puberty, associated signs or symptoms, familial history, etc.
- Patients with idiopathic scoliosis usually should not have pain, although they might have a discomfort or mild pain.
- Back pain in scoliotic patients must be investigated thoroughly and taken seriously.
- If night pain, consider tumor such as osteoid osteoma.

PHYSICAL EXAM

- General inspection to look for skin changes such as café au lait spots, pigmentation, or other signs of neurofibromatosis; also dysraphic signs (e.g., hairy patches, midline hemangioma, skin dimpling)
- Assess for skeletal maturity, hyperelasticity, contracture, congenital anomalies.
- Assess for deformity; asymmetry of spine, shoulders, waist, and trunk, including decompensation; abnormalities of thoracic kyphosis or cervical or lumbar lordosis; disfigurement of the torso; or rib rotation.
- Adams forward bend test used to look for rib or paraspinous elevations
- Assess for leg length discrepancy, congenital anomalies, and neurologic abnormalities (including abnormal abdominal reflex).
- Special finding:
  - Crankshaft phenomenon
    - Progression of curve size and rotation following posterior spinal fusion in a young child, result of continued anterior spinal growth
    - Patient is Risser 0, open triradiate cartilages, <10 years old, and prior to occurrence of peak height velocity (time of maximum spinal growth).
    - Consider anterior fusion in addition to posterior fusion.
- Physical exam tricks:
  - Measure angle of trunk rotation with scoliometer.
  - Abnormal abdominal reflex may suggest intraspinal pathology, including syrinx.
- Perform Adams forward bend test after the pelvis is leveled by inserting appropriately sized block underneath the short leg in patients with scoliosis and leg length discrepancy.

DIAGNOSTIC TESTS & INTERPRETATION

Pulmonary function testing is useful preoperatively for more severe curves.

Lab

Usually not helpful unless to rule out associated metabolic conditions

Imaging

- Plain standing posterior–anterior and lateral scoliosis films on long 3-foot radiograph cassette or 3-D low-dose radiation system
- One must look for soft tissue and congenital bony abnormalities (Wedge vertebrae, bars, hemivertebrae).
- Curve is measured using Cobb method.
- The status of the triradiate cartilage and Risser classification of iliac apophysis ossification are indicators of maturity.
- The triradiate cartilage usually closes before the iliac apophysis appears (Risser 0).
- Risser sign is defined by the amount of calcification present in the iliac apophysis and measures the progressive ossification from anterolaterally to posteromedially.
  - A Risser grade of 1 signifies up to 25% ossification of the iliac apophysis, proceeding to grade 4, which signifies 100% ossification.
  - A Risser grade of 5 means the iliac apophysis has fused to the iliac crest after 100% ossification.
  - Risser grade (0–5) gives an estimate of how much skeletal growth remains and is correlated with risk of curve progression.
- MRI is not routinely necessary for adult idiopathic scoliosis without back pain.
- 7% prevalence of intraspinal abnormalities are found in left thoracic curves, so MRI maybe indicated.
- Curve patterns are classified according to King or Lenke classifications.
- Renal ultrasound is used for evaluation of patient with congenital scoliosis (look for associated renal abnormalities).

DIFFERENTIAL DIAGNOSIS

- Adolescent idiopathic scoliosis (11–17 years)
- Juvenile idiopathic scoliosis (4–10 years)
- Infantile idiopathic scoliosis (0–3 years)
- Congenital scoliosis—due to bony abnormalities of the spine that are present at birth (failure of formation or segmentations of vertebrae)
- Scoliosis associated with neurofibromatosis
- Scoliosis associated with tumors (e.g., osteoid osteoma)

- Neuromuscular scoliosis (e.g., cerebral palsy, spina bifida, muscle disorders)
- Postural scoliosis (e.g., from leg length discrepancy)
  - No rib hump or rotation
  - Does not have fixed deformities
  - Disappears with forward bending
  - Long curve
  - No progression

TREATMENT

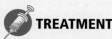

GENERAL MEASURES

- Treatment
  - Concepts for treatment are based on severity of deformity and on likelihood of progression.
- Observation
  - Curves <25 degrees
    - Immature patients (Risser 0, 1, 2) should be reevaluated in 4–6 months.
    - Skeletally mature patients (Risser 4 or 5) usually do not require ongoing follow-up unless special circumstances exist.
  - Curves 25–45 degrees in skeletally mature patients
    - Risser 4 or 5 patients are usually reevaluated in 6 months to 1 year.
    - Mature patients are usually reevaluated yearly.

ADDITIONAL THERAPIES

- Brace treatment
  - Curves 25–45 degrees (Risser 0, 1) and 30–45 degrees (Risser 2 or 3)
    - Brace on initial evaluation.
  - Curves ≥25 degrees (in Risser 0–3 patient) that have demonstrated >10 degrees progression during period of observation
    - Continue brace treatment until maturity (2 years postmenarchal and Risser 4 in females, Risser 5 in males).
- Brace types
  - Thoracolumbosacral orthosis (TLSO): success reported when used >16–18 hours daily; significantly improved outcome when compared with natural history
  - Cervicothoracolumbosacral orthosis (CTLSO): seldom needed except for higher thoracic or cervical curves
  - Nighttime bending brace

SURGERY/OTHER PROCEDURES

- Recommended when curves exceed 45–50 degrees
  - Exception: Balanced thoracic and lumbar curves <55 degrees may be observed for progression.
- Thoracic curves and double major curves
  - Posterior segmental fixation instrumentation remains current state of the art.
  - Anterior spinal instrumentation for selected curves
- Isolated thoracolumbar and lumbar curves
  - Anterior spinal fusion using solid rod segmental constructs

ONGOING CARE

FOLLOW-UP RECOMMENDATIONS

Patient Monitoring

- Watch for back pain associated with idiopathic scoliosis (may indicate other diagnosis):
  - Present in 23% at time of initial evaluation (additional 9% during follow-up)
  - Of those with back pain, only 9% found to have identifiable cause such as spondylolysis, Scheuermann, syrinx, disc herniation, tumor, tether cord.

PROGNOSIS

- Overall, good for most patients
- Risk of curve progression related to patient's maturity (Risser sign, menarcheal status) and to size of curve
- Curves <20–25 degrees have low risk of progression, even if patient is immature.
- Curves 25–45 degrees have higher risk of progression, particularly in skeletally immature patients.
- Curves >45–50 degrees have much higher risk of progression, regardless of maturity.

COMPLICATIONS

Natural history:

- Reduced pulmonary function for patients with thoracic curves >60 degrees
- Progression of lumbar curves >50 degrees in adult life with degenerative disc disease and pain in some
- Cosmetic and emotional issues
- Complications of brace use include skin irritation, discomfort, and noncompliance.
- Surgical complications are usually more severe, including infection, instrumentation loosening or breakage, neurologic damage, paralysis, or death.

ADDITIONAL READING

- Dormans JP. Establishing a standard of care for neuromonitoring during spinal deformity surgery. *Spine*. 2010;35(25):2180–2185.
- Hresko MT. Clinical practice. Idiopathic scoliosis in adolescents. *N Engl J Med*. 2013;368(9):834–841.
- El-Hawary R, Chukwunyerenwa C. Update on evaluation and treatment of scoliosis. *Pediatr Clin North Am*. 2014;61(6):1223–1241.
- Sponseller PD, Flynn JM, Newton PO, et al. The association of patient characteristics and spinal curve parameters with Lenke classification types. *Spine*. 2012;37(13):1138–1141.
- Sucato DJ. Management of severe spinal deformity: scoliosis and kyphosis. *Spine*. 2010;35(25): 2186–2192.

CODES

ICD10

- M41.9 Scoliosis, unspecified
- M40.209 Unspecified kyphosis, site unspecified
- M40.56 Lordosis, unspecified, lumbar region

FAQ

- Q: How long do you observe a patient with spinal asymmetry before ordering a radiograph?
- A: It depends on the presence or absence of abnormalities on the physical exam. If any of the signs mentioned here are seen or significant back pain is present, a radiograph or referral is indicated. The scoliometer is also a useful tool in screening patients.
- Q: How long do you observe a patient with spinal asymmetry before referral to an orthopedic surgeon?
- A: Consider referral if
  - Cobb angle
    - >20 degrees
    - Progression of more than 5 degrees
- Q: If a child presents with scoliosis and back pain that occurs especially at night and is promptly relieved with nonsteroidal anti-inflammatory drugs, what diagnosis is suggested?
- A: Scoliosis associated with osteoid osteoma.

SEBORRHEIC DERMATITIS

Jennifer DiPace • Saskia Gex

BASICS

DESCRIPTION
- Seborrheic dermatitis (SD) is a multifactorial skin disease influenced by both host and environmental factors.
- Involves sebaceous areas of the body
  - Including the scalp, face, back, chest, and intertriginous areas
  - Characterized by greasy, yellow, scaly erythematous lesions
- Usually a self-limited condition in infants but can be a chronic, relapsing condition in adolescents and adults

EPIDEMIOLOGY
- Trimodal distribution: infants, adolescents, and adults >50 years of age
- Highest prevalence in first 3 months of life
- Affects approximately 10% of the general population and up to 70% of infants in the first 3 months of life
- No sex predilection in infants; however, in adolescents and adults, males are affected more commonly than females.
- Seasonal pattern: Prevalence of disease increases in winter months.
- Strong association between *Malassezia* species, a common commensal organism, and SD

RISK FACTORS
- There are no known genetic factors that contribute to disease.
- Hormonal effects: exposure to maternal estrogen in infancy and surge of androgens in puberty
- Immunocompromised status
  - Impaired cellular immunity may contribute to pathogenesis of disease.
  - Prevalence of SD in immunocompromised patients is significantly higher than in general population.

GENERAL PREVENTION
There are no known preventive measures.

PATHOPHYSIOLOGY
- Androgens stimulate sebaceous glands, causing production of more sebum.
- *Malassezia*
  - A lipophilic yeast that is normally found in sebum-rich areas of the skin
  - Can break down skin sebum lipids, producing potentially inflammatory fatty acids
- In response to the inflammatory fatty acids, keratinocytes produce proinflammatory cytokines.

ETIOLOGY
Not completely known, although it was thought that yeast, androgens, and the local host immune response play a role in SD development.

DIAGNOSIS

HISTORY
- Older children and adolescents: Ask about onset of puberty symptoms.
- Typically not pruritic
- Children and adolescents: Ask about symptoms and signs of immunocompromise such as frequent infections, failure to thrive, and chronic diarrhea.
- HIV and tuberculosis (TB) history

PHYSICAL EXAM
- Infants: "cradle cap"
  - Yellow, greasy adherent scales on the scalp
  - Lesions may also occur on the forehead, eyebrows, eyelids, postauricular area, and nasolabial folds.
  - No excoriations
  - No hepatosplenomegaly
- Adolescents and adults
  - Mild: dry, flaking scalp or face in areas of facial hair; no surrounding inflammation
  - More severe SD: patchy, orange/yellow, greasy plaques in scalp, nasolabial folds, postauricular area, intertriginous areas, or other regions of increased sebaceous gland activity
  - Blepharitis with erythema and scaling of the eyelid margins may also occur.
  - No excoriations
  - No hepatosplenomegaly

DIAGNOSTIC TESTS & INTERPRETATION

Lab
Primarily a clinical diagnosis; there are no specific tests for seborrhea.

Diagnostic Procedures/Surgery
Skin biopsy should be reserved for unusual or refractory cases of SD.

Pathologic Findings
- Skin biopsy findings
  - Predominance of neutrophils in the scale crust at the margins of follicular ostia
  - Yeast cells sometimes are visible within keratinocytes on special stains, but hyphae should not be present in SD.

DIFFERENTIAL DIAGNOSIS
- SD can be confused with infectious conditions of the skin, malignancy, or inflammatory disorders.
- Dermatophyte infections
  - *Tinea capitis*, *tinea faciei*, and *tinea corporis* are also scaling lesions. The lesions are scaly but not typically greasy or plaque-like.
  - Microscopic evaluation of lesion can differentiate it from SD by the presence of hyphae in dermatophyte infection.
- Malignancy/Langerhans cell histiocytosis (LCH)
  - LCH may present with a scaly erythematous lesions in the same distribution as SD.
  - Unlike SD, LCH may have the presence of small reddish-brown crusted papules or vesicles.
  - In addition, there may be organ system involvement such as hepatosplenomegaly.
  - LCH is refractory to typical treatment for SD.
- Immunologic
  - Atopic dermatitis
    - May present on the face of infants but typically spares the nasolabial folds
    - May also involve the extensor aspects of the extremities
    - Usually is pruritic
  - Psoriasis vulgaris
    - Typically presents as sharply defined plaques, bright red in color with thick silver scales
    - Unlike SD, children with psoriasis may have nail changes such as nail pitting and onycholysis.

TREATMENT

- Treatment depends on presentation and age of patient.
- For infants, SD usually has a benign and self-limited course. Medications may not be necessary for the treatment of infant SD.
- Physical measures such as the application of emollients followed by the removal of scalp scales with a comb may improve symptoms.
  - Examples of emollients include mineral oil, baby oil, or petroleum jelly.
  - There have been some studies to suggest that the use of organic oils such as olive oil or vegetable oil may provide an excellent media for *Malassezia* overgrowth, potentially worsening SD.
  - Frequent shampooing with a nonmedicated shampoo may also be beneficial.

MEDICATION

- For infants who do not respond to conservative therapy or for older children/adults, medications will likely be necessary.
- Classes of drugs that should be considered are keratolytic, antifungal, and anti-inflammatory medications. At the current time, there is no evidence to support the use of one class of drug versus another.
- Keratolytics: Massage into scalp 2–3 times per week, leave on 5 minutes, then rinse.
  - Salicylic acid
    - Shampoo or lotion
  - Coal tar
    - Shampoo
    - Decreases sebum production
  - Pyrithione zinc
    - Most commonly used as a shampoo
    - Also has antifungal properties
- Antifungals
  - Selenium sulfide
    - Antifungal and keratolytic effect
    - Shampoo. Massage 5–10 mL of shampoo into wet scalp, leave on scalp 2–3 minutes, then rinse thoroughly.
    - Usually, 2 applications each week for 2 weeks will provide control.
  - Azoles: ketoconazole
    - 1% or 2% gel, lotion, or shampoo
    - Shampoo should be used twice per week (at least 3 days between doses) for up to 8 weeks. Caution: may cause eye irritation
    - Gel or lotion should be used twice daily for up to 2–4 weeks.
  - Ciclopirox: 1% shampoo
    - Can be used in children >16 years old
    - Massage into scalp, then rinse.
    - Use 2 times per week (at least 3 days between doses) for up to 4 weeks.
- Anti-inflammatory therapies
  - Corticosteroids
    - Shampoo, foam, ointment, creams, or lotions
    - There are multiple options; treatment will depend on severity of inflammation and age of patient.
    - Ointments should be considered for more severe cases because skin absorption is improved.
    - Foams can be used in hairy areas because of ease of application.
  - Calcineurin inhibitors: tacrolimus ointment
    - Can be used in children >2 years of age
    - Fungicidal and anti-inflammatory properties
    - Apply thin layer of 0.03% ointment to affected area twice daily until symptoms resolve or up to 6 weeks.

COMPLEMENTARY & ALTERNATIVE THERAPIES

- Tea tree oil 5% has been demonstrated to be effective in treating scalp seborrhea.
- Other alternative nutritional therapies that have been considered are probiotics and omega-3 essential fatty acids. However, there are no sufficient data on effectiveness or safety in children.

ONGOING CARE

PATIENT EDUCATION

- Response to treatment will likely occur in the first 2 weeks of therapy; however, long-term intermittent therapy may be required. Adolescents with SD may have a chronic course.
- The intermittent use of an antifungal shampoo can be used to prevent relapses.

PROGNOSIS

- The infantile form will typically self-resolve by the end of the 1st year of life.
- Older children and adolescents may have a more chronic, relapsing course.
- If SD doesn't respond to therapy within approximately 6 weeks, consider alternative diagnoses or underlying conditions such as immunodeficiency.

ADDITIONAL READING

- Berk T, Scheinfeld N. Seborrheic dermatitis. *P T*. 2010;35(6):348–352.
- Cohen S. Should we treat infantile seborrheic dermatitis with topical antifungals or topical steroids? *Arch Dis Child*. 2004;89(3):288–289.
- Dessinioti C, Katsambas A. Seborrheic dermatitis: etiology, risk factors, and treatments: facts and controversies. *Clin Dermatol*. 2013;31(4):343–351.
- Gupta AK, Madzia SE, Batra R. Etiology and management of seborrheic dermatitis. *Dermatology*. 2004;208(2):89–93.
- Gupta AK, Nicol K, Batra R. Role of antifungal agents in the treatment of seborrheic dermatitis. *Am J Clin Dermatol*. 2004;5(6):417–422.
- Sarchell AC, Saurajen A, Bell C, et al. Treatment of dandruff with 5% tea tree oil shampoo. *J Am Acad Dermatol*. 2002;47(6):852–855.
- Schwartz RA, Janusz CA, Janniger CK. Seborrheic dermatitis: an overview. *Am Fam Physician*. 2006; 74(1):125–132.
- Siegfried E, Glenn E. Use of olive oil for the treatment of seborrheic dermatitis in children. *Arch Pediatr Adolesc Med*. 2012;166(10):967.

CODES

ICD10

- L21.9 Seborrheic dermatitis, unspecified
- L21.0 Seborrhea capitis
- L21.1 Seborrheic infantile dermatitis

FAQ

- Q: Is there a laboratory test to diagnose SD?
- A: There are no specific laboratory tests. It is a clinical diagnosis. If the diagnosis is unclear or refractory to treatment, consider a skin biopsy.
- Q: Are there seasonal changes in the course of SD?
- A: Some patients report worsening of symptoms in the winter months. Sunlight may improve patients' symptoms. UV therapy is a treatment option for extensive SD.
- Q: Does SD cause permanent hair loss?
- A: SD may cause some hair loss acutely. However, patients can be reassured that it does not cause permanent hair loss.

SEIZURES—FEBRILE

Rohini Coorg • Liu Lin Thio

BASICS

DESCRIPTION

Febrile seizure: seizure in ≤60-month-old child accompanied by a fever (≥100.4°F or 38°C by any method) but without central nervous system infection or prior unprovoked seizure (American Academy of Pediatrics [AAP] guidelines use 6 months as the lower age limit, whereas International League Against Epilepsy uses 1 month)

2 types:

- Simple: febrile seizures that are generalized, last <15 minutes, *AND* do not recur in 24 hours
- Complex
  - Febrile seizures that are focal (including postictal weakness), last ≥15 minutes, *OR* occur >1 time in 24 hours
  - Febrile status epilepticus: 1 febrile seizure or series of febrile seizures without full recovery in between lasting ≥30 minutes

EPIDEMIOLOGY

- Age
  - Most febrile seizures occur between 6 months and 3 years of age.
  - Peak age is about 18 months.
- Type
  - 65–70% are simple febrile seizures.
  - 20–35% are complex febrile seizures.
  - ~5% are febrile status epilepticus.
- Timing of seizure
  - ~20% before or <1 hour of fever onset
  - ~60% 1–24 hours after fever onset
  - ~20% >24 hours after fever onset

Prevalence

- Most common childhood seizure
- Febrile seizures occur in 2–5% of children in the United States and Western Europe, 9–10% of children in Japan, and 14% of children in Guam.

RISK FACTORS

Positive family history of febrile seizures

Genetics

Usually multifactorial or polygenic inheritance

GENERAL PREVENTION

Antipyretics do not reduce the recurrence risk of simple febrile seizures.

PATHOPHYSIOLOGY

- Elevated temperatures in developing brain may increase neuronal excitability.
- Fever increases cytokines that may enhance neuronal excitability.
- Genetic factors
- Hyperventilation from fever causes a respiratory alkalosis that may promote seizures.

ETIOLOGY

- Any viral or bacterial infection
  - Human herpesvirus 6 and 7
  - Influenza A
- Vaccines
  - MMR(V) and DPT
  - Both increase the risk of febrile seizures but not epilepsy.
  - Benefits greatly outweigh any risk, and families should be encouraged to vaccinate.
- Shigellosis

COMMONLY ASSOCIATED CONDITIONS

- Generalized epilepsy with febrile seizures plus (GEFS+)
  - Febrile seizures beyond 6 years of age or afebrile seizures of varying types ranging from mild to severe
  - Multiple genes identified including *SCN1A, SCN2A, SCN1B, GABRG2, GABRD, and PCDH19*
- Febrile infection–related epilepsy syndrome (FIRES)
  - Catastrophic epileptic encephalopathy of unknown etiology that begins with a febrile illness and refractory status epilepticus
  - Has high morbidity and mortality

DIAGNOSIS

HISTORY

- Obtain detailed description of spell to determine if it was a seizure.
  - Circumstances in which spell occurred
  - Duration
  - Focal features suggest seizure
  - Postictal weakness suggests seizure
- Ask about prior seizures/spells.
  - Prior afebrile seizure suggests epilepsy.
  - Prior febrile seizures supports diagnosis.
  - Prior nonepileptic spells
- Determine cause of fever/illness
  - Duration
  - Height of fever
  - Symptoms: rhinorrhea, diarrhea
- Ask about new neurologic symptoms such as headache or change in gait that would require further evaluation.
- Ask about toxic ingestions.
- Identify seizure risk factors from past medical history.
  - Perinatal complications
  - Prior brain insult: trauma, meningitis
  - Developmental delay
- Medications including antibiotics
- Identify seizure risk factors from family history.
  - Febrile seizures
  - Epilepsy

PHYSICAL EXAM

- Identify fever source.
  - Vital signs, including temperature
  - Assess anterior fontanelle, sutures, and head circumference for increased intracranial pressure, which may occur with meningitis or space-occupying lesion.
  - Assess for signs of meningitis such as nuchal rigidity.
  - Examine ears and throat for infection.
  - Examine skin for rashes and other signs of infection.
  - Examine heart and lungs for infection.
  - Assess for trauma.
- Detailed neurologic exam
  - Assess skin for neurocutaneous syndromes.
  - Assess mental status.
  - Assess for subtle signs of seizure such as myoclonus or nystagmus.
  - Examine cranial nerves. Include funduscopic exam for papilledema.
  - Examine gait, motor system, sensation, coordination, and deep tendon reflexes for abnormalities and asymmetries.

DIAGNOSTIC TESTS & INTERPRETATION

Simple Febrile Seizure

Recommendations from the 2011 AAP Guideline for neurologically healthy infants and children

Lab

- Serum electrolytes, calcium, phosphorus, magnesium, glucose, and complete blood count are not recommended solely for determining the cause of the seizure.
- Consider studies to determine fever source.
- Lumbar puncture
  - Perform when symptoms/signs of meningitis or intracranial infection are present
  - Consider lumbar puncture if
    - 6–12-month-old infant has deficient or unknown immunization status for *Haemophilus influenzae* type b or *Streptococcus pneumoniae*
    - Pretreated with antibiotics

Imaging

Not indicated

Electroencephalogram

- Not indicated
- Not predictive of febrile seizure recurrence or development of epilepsy

Complex Febrile Seizures

There is no AAP Guideline.

Lab

- Consider studies to identify fever source and as clinically indicated.
- Indications for lumbar puncture are similar to indications for lumbar puncture for simple febrile seizure but strongly consider for all, especially those with altered mental status.

Imaging

- Acute brain imaging usually unnecessary, especially if the only complex feature is multiple seizures. Recommend acute MRI (CT acceptable) if with persistently altered mental status, persistent focal neurologic findings, or symptoms/signs of increased intracranial pressure.
- Recommend routine brain MRI if not done acutely especially for focal seizure, focal exam findings, or focal EEG abnormality.

Electroencephalogram

- Recommend stat EEG if concerned about nonconvulsive status epilepticus.
- Recommend routine EEG, especially for abnormal neurologic development or exam. Epileptiform abnormalities or focal slowing may increase risk for developing epilepsy.

Febrile Status Epilepticus

No AAP Guideline. See "Status Epilepticus" chapter.

Lab

- Recommend studies to treat correctable causes of seizures (e.g., hypoglycemia, hyponatremia) and to identify fever source.
- Lumbar puncture
  - Perform for any suspicion of meningitis or intracranial infection but strongly consider for all especially if first episode or if mental status is altered.
  - It is important to note that febrile status epilepticus *rarely* causes a CSF pleocytosis.

Imaging

- Recommend acute brain imaging (MRI preferred but CT acceptable), especially if first episode with abnormal mental status or focal neurologic findings.
- Recommend routine brain MRI if not done acutely; may show hippocampal injury that may increase risk for developing epilepsy

Electroencephalogram

- Recommend stat EEG if concerned about nonconvulsive status epilepticus.
- Recommend routine EEG; may show temporal slowing or attenuation that correlates with hippocampal abnormality on MRI

DIFFERENTIAL DIAGNOSIS

- Acute symptomatic seizure
  - Infection
    - Meningoencephalitis: primary diagnostic consideration; bacterial or viral; consider HSV.
    - Other infection such as gastroenteritis causing hypernatremic dehydration
    - Benign convulsions with mild gastroenteritis
  - Toxic/metabolic
  - Stroke
  - Trauma
- Epilepsy
- Nonepileptic spell
  - Febrile delirium
  - Chills
  - Breath-holding spells

TREATMENT

MEDICATION

- Abortive: consider rectal diazepam (0.5 mg/kg) for febrile seizures ≥5 minutes; may cause drowsiness and ataxia; rarely causes respiratory depression
- Preventive
  - In certain clinical circumstances, for parental anxiety, may use oral diazepam (0.33 mg/kg every 8 hours) to the patient during a febrile illness until afebrile for 24 hours; may cause drowsiness and ataxia
  - Daily phenobarbital, valproate, or primidone prevents febrile seizures, but risks outweigh benefits.

ADDITIONAL TREATMENT

General Measures

- See "Status Epilepticus" chapter for treating febrile status epilepticus.
- Treat infection

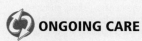

ONGOING CARE

PROGNOSIS

- Febrile seizure recurrence
  - 50% of children <12 months of age at time of first simple febrile seizure have recurrent febrile seizures.
  - 30% of children >12 months of age at time of first febrile seizure have a second.
  - Of children with a second febrile seizure, 50% experience a third.
- Risk for developing epilepsy:
  - 6–7% for all febrile seizures
  - 2–7.5% for simple febrile seizures
  - 10–20% for complex febrile seizures
- Mortality
  - 0.85% for all febrile seizures
  - 0% for simple febrile seizures
  - <1.6% for complex febrile seizures with all deaths from febrile status epilepticus
- No evidence that simple febrile seizures increase risk of neurologic or cognitive deficits.

ADDITIONAL READING

- Chugath M, Shorvon S. The mortality and morbidity of febrile seizures. *Nat Clin Pract Neurol*. 2008;4(11):610–621.
- Dubé CM, Brewster AL, Baram TZ. Febrile seizures: mechanism and relationship to epilepsy. *Brain Dev*. 2009;31(5):366–371.
- Shinnar S, Glauser TA. Febrile seizures. *J Child Neurol*. 2002;17(Suppl 1):S44–S52.
- Subcommittee on Febrile Seizures, American Academy of Pediatrics. Clinical practice guideline-febrile seizures: guideline for the neurodiagnostic evaluation of the child with a simple febrile seizure. *Pediatrics*. 2011;127(2):389–394.
- Subcommittee on Febrile Seizures, American Academy of Pediatrics. Febrile seizures: clinical practice guideline for the long-term management of the child with simple febrile seizures. *Pediatrics*. 2008;121(6):1281–1286.

CODES

ICD10

- R56.00 Simple febrile convulsions
- R56.01 Complex febrile convulsions

FAQ

- Q: What should parents be told?
- A: Good neurodevelopmental outcome for simple febrile seizures but relatively high risk for recurrence.
- Q: Can a child die from a febrile seizure?
- A: No reported mortality from simple febrile seizures or short complex febrile seizures. Small mortality with febrile status epilepticus.
- Q: Can a febrile seizure cause brain damage?
- A: Simple febrile seizures do not. Febrile status epilepticus may.
- Q: What should the parents do when the child has a seizure?
- A: Stay calm. Place child in safe place. Turn child on side to keep airway clear. Do not restrain. Do not put anything in mouth. Time seizure. If seizure lasts 5 minutes, call 911 and administer abortive medication such as rectal diazepam if available.
- Q: What precautions should the parents take?
- A: Common sense steps such as no unsupervised baths or swimming and no climbing above head height. Always wear helmet when riding bike or doing other activity with wheels. No driving all-terrain vehicles.

SEIZURES, PARTIAL AND GENERALIZED

Kristen L. Park • Kelly G. Knupp

BASICS

DESCRIPTION

Seizures arise from abnormal electrical discharges in the cerebral cortex that lead to alterations of consciousness, behavior, motor activity, sensation, or autonomic function. Epilepsy is defined as 2 or more seizures without acute provocation. Seizures are classified as focal, generalized, and unknown.

- Focal seizure types
  - Without impairment of consciousness (either with observable motor or autonomic components or involving subjective sensory or psychic phenomena only)
  - With impairment of consciousness (dyscognitive)
  - Evolving to a bilateral, convulsive seizure
- Generalized seizure types
  - Tonic–clonic, absence, myoclonic, clonic, tonic, atonic
- Unknown seizure types: epileptic spasms

EPIDEMIOLOGY

Incidence

Epilepsy affects 0.5–1% of all children (birth through 16 years). 120,000 children seek care annually in the United States for a seizure. Between 20,000 and 45,000 children/year are diagnosed with epilepsy, highest risk is in the 1st year of life.

Prevalence

4–10 per 1,000 children in developed countries have epilepsy.

ETIOLOGY AND PATHOPHYSIOLOGY

- Genetic
- Structural/metabolic
  - Brain tumor
  - Malformations of cortical development
  - Neurocutaneous syndromes
  - Prior cerebral insult
  - Metabolic disorders
- Unknown cause

Genetics

- Epilepsy is both polygenic and multifactorial.
- The risk of epilepsy with an affected primary relative increases from the population risk (1–2%) to 2–5%.
- Single-gene epilepsy syndromes with defined genetic loci: autosomal dominant nocturnal frontal lobe epilepsy, benign familial neonatal convulsions, severe myoclonic epilepsy of infancy
- Other epilepsy syndromes (benign rolandic, childhood absence, juvenile myoclonic epilepsy) are heterogeneous.
- Epilepsy may also be a feature of other genetic and metabolic disorders such as trisomy 21, Angelman syndrome, and Menkes disease.

COMMONLY ASSOCIATED CONDITIONS

- The incidence of childhood-onset epilepsy associated with intellectual disability and cerebral palsy is 15–38%.
- Epilepsy occurs in 8–28% of children with autism.
- ADHD, depression, and anxiety are more common in children with epilepsy than in the general population.

DIAGNOSIS

HISTORY

- Age, family history of seizures, developmental status, birth history
- Health at seizure onset: febrile, ill, sleep deprivation, trauma, toxins, ingestion, head injury
- Current medications and change in antiepileptic medication
- Other neurologic signs: confusion; encephalopathy; weakness; sensory deficits; and change in vision, behavior, balance, or gait
- Detailed history of symptoms during seizure
  - Aura: subjective sensations
  - Behavior: preceding and during seizure
  - Change in consciousness or responsiveness
  - Vocal: cry, gasp, speech
  - Motor: head or eye turning, jerking, posturing, stiffening, automatisms (purposeless repetitive movements such as picking at clothing, lip smacking)
  - Respiration: cyanosis, change in breathing pattern, apnea
  - Autonomic: pupillary dilation, drooling, incontinence, pallor, vomiting, tachycardia
- Symptoms after seizure: amnesia, confusion, sleepiness, transient focal weakness (Todd paresis), headache

PHYSICAL EXAM

- Vital signs: ABCs need to be checked immediately and recurrently, fever, tachycardia, bradycardia, or hypertension
- Signs of head trauma or child abuse: retinal hemorrhages, papilledema, presence of fractures, bruises of different ages
- Head circumference/abnormal head growth
- Signs of systemic infection: meningismus, purpura
- Skin examination: café au lait or ash leaf spots, facial hemangioma (suggesting neurocutaneous disorders)
- Neurologic examination: pupillary reactivity, mental status, focal motor weakness
- Seizures: If there is a question of continuing seizures, proceed with recommendations for "Status Epilepticus."

ALERT

- Attention to adequate airway and breathing and need for oxygenation or ventilatory support is the primary focus.
- If the child continues to have a seizure or has recurrent seizures, an abortive benzodiazepine should be administered either rectally or IV.

DIAGNOSTIC TESTS & INTERPRETATION

Lab

- Testing should be based on clinical history.
  - In general, a standard laboratory evaluation (electrolytes, CBC, liver enzymes, calcium, and magnesium) did not show unsuspected abnormalities or contribute to the diagnosis or management in several clinical studies.
  - An exception was hyponatremia (<125 mEq/L) found to be associated with seizures in 70% of infants younger than 6 months of age in one clinical study.
- Toxicology screening should be considered in any child in whom there is a question of drug exposure or substance abuse.
- Blood glucose (fingerstick can be obtained quickly)
- Antiepileptic drug (AED) levels if indicated; few of the newer AEDs have relevant or rapidly available serum levels but may be useful for documenting adherence to a medication regimen.

Imaging

- Neuroimaging: Evidence-based reviews showed low yields of acute CT or MRI in children presenting with seizures without focal signs or deficits. Current recommendations are as follows:
  - MRI is generally the preferred modality.
  - Emergent neuroimaging should be performed in any child with focal deficit not returning to baseline within several hours.
  - Nonurgent MRI is recommended based on clinical scenario and EEG findings.

Diagnostic Procedures/Other

- EEG
  - Indicated urgently if there is concern that child may be continuing to seize
  - Nonurgent EEGs are indicated for first afebrile seizure.
- Lumbar puncture
  - Not routinely recommended
  - Should be considered for meningeal signs, infants <6 months of age, or persistent alteration of consciousness
  - If intracranial hypertension, mass lesion, or hydrocephalus is suspected, defer lumbar puncture until after neuroimaging.

DIFFERENTIAL DIAGNOSIS

- Nonepileptic events
  - Syncope
  - Breath-holding spells
  - Hyperventilation

- Nonepileptic events
  - Movements related to gastroesophageal reflux (Sandifer syndrome)
  - Sleep disorders: benign sleep myoclonus, night terrors, somnambulism, narcolepsy–cataplexy
  - Migraine/headache syndromes, especially complicated migraine
  - Nonepileptic movements: startle disease, shuddering spells, paroxysmal dyskinesias, tics, drug-induced dystonia
  - Behavioral: stereotypies, self-stimulatory behaviors, inattention/ADHD

TREATMENT

MEDICATION

- The choice of AED for long-term management of epilepsy depends on the specific seizure type and epilepsy syndrome. Monotherapy is always preferred.
- Many formulations (liquid, sprinkle caps, and extended-release) are available and should be individualized to the patient. For teenagers, extended-release forms may be recommended for compliance.
- Focal seizures (any type)
  - Oxcarbazepine 20–40 mg/kg/24 h
  - Levetiracetam 20–60 mg/kg/24 h
  - Lamotrigine: dosing varies with valproate
  - Topiramate 4–10 mg/kg/24 h
  - Valproate: 15–50 mg/kg/24 h
  - Zonisamide 2–10 mg/kg/24 h
- Genetic generalized epilepsies
  - Ethosuximide 15–40 mg/kg/24 h: initial AED for absence seizures
  - Levetiracetam
  - Topiramate
- Acute treatment of seizures
  - Benzodiazepines should be given for prolonged seizures (>5 minutes) or acute repetitive seizures.
    - Rectal diazepam (0.3–0.5 mg/kg/dose), intranasal/buccal midazolam (0.2 mg/kg/dose), or oral/buccal lorazepam (Intensol, 0.05–0.1 mg/kg/dose, needs refrigeration) can be administered by parents/caregivers.
  - Fosphenytoin 20 mEq/kg IM/IV
  - Phenobarbital 10–20 mg/kg IV
  - Levetiracetam 20 mg/kg IV
- Patients refractory to AED treatment: other options—ketogenic diet, vagus nerve stimulator, surgical resection

ALERT

- Hyponatremic seizures: serum sodium <120 mEq/dL in infants with gastroenteritis; slow sodium correction indicated
- Apnea and hypoventilation from excessive administration of benzodiazepines, phenobarbital for seizures. Monitor ventilation and oxygenation; avoid large doses.

ADDITIONAL TREATMENT

General Measures

- Chronic AED therapy is not indicated after acute symptomatic seizures or after a single unprovoked seizure in a child with normal neurologic examination and EEG.
- Chronic AED therapy may be considered after 1st seizure symptomatic of an acute, structural brain lesion (i.e., brain tumor).

ISSUES FOR REFERRAL

In general, patients who have not responded to 2 seizure medications should be evaluated by a neurologist who specializes in epilepsy.

ALERT

A 2-fold risk of increased suicidality has been associated with AED use, with an FDA black box warning on product labeling. Monitoring for suicidal ideation and mood changes is warranted in all patients taking AEDs.

ONGOING CARE

PATIENT EDUCATION

- Injuries: Rarely, serious injury occurs with brief seizures from loss of consciousness and resultant falls.
- Daily precautions: Few restrictions are needed with the exceptions of driving (see state laws) and dangerous sports.
- Supervision around water is strongly advised; showering is generally safer than bathing.
- Helmets should be worn with all wheeled toys; avoid top bunk beds or locked bedrooms and unprotected heights.
- Sudden unexplained death in epilepsy patients (SUDEP) should be mentioned to all patients at appropriate times.
- Families should be instructed in seizure first aid: roll patient on the side, place nothing in the mouth, ensure safe environment.

PROGNOSIS

- In a child who is neurologically normal with an unprovoked seizure, the risk of recurrence is 24% in 1 year and 45% in 14 years.
- If there is evidence of prior neurologic insult, the risk is 37% in 1 year.
- If the patient has 2 seizures separated by >24 hours, risk is 70% in 1 year.
- The EEG is the most significant predictor of recurrence: 15% risk in 1 year in a child with a normal EEG and 41% with an abnormal EEG.

COMPLICATIONS

- Brain damage
  - From brief seizures: no convincing evidence
  - From prolonged seizures (>30 minutes): Brain injury may occur secondary to hypoxia.
  - Untreated or poorly controlled epilepsy: increased risk of intractable epilepsy and SUDEP
- Status epilepticus
  - Incidence of 18–20/100,000/year in childhood
  - Mortality in children between 3 and 6%
  - Recurrence risk for status epilepticus is approximately 16% within the first year.
- Patient monitoring: depends on treatment and as mentioned earlier

ADDITIONAL READING

- Arthur TM, deGrauw TJ, Johnson CS, et al. Seizure recurrence risk following a first seizure in neurologically normal children. *Epilepsia*. 2008;49(11):1950–1954.
- Epilepsy Foundation. Answer place: parent information on the Internet. http://www.epilepsyfoundation.org/answerplace. Accessed February 2, 2015.
- Glauser TA, Cnaan A, Shinnar S, et al. Ethosuximide, valproic acid, and lamotrigine in childhood absence epilepsy. *N Engl J Med*. 2010;362(9):790.
- Hamiwka LD, Wirrell ED. Comorbidities in pediatric epilepsy: beyond "just" treating the seizures. *J Child Neurol*. 2009;24(6):734–742.
- Hirtz D, Ashwal S, Berg A, et al. Practice parameter: evaluating a first nonfebrile seizure in children: report of the quality standards subcommittee of the American Academy of Neurology, the Child Neurology Society, and the American Epilepsy Society. *Neurology*. 2000;55(5):616–623.

CODES

ICD10

- R56.9 Unspecified convulsions
- G40.209 Local-rel symptc epi w cmplx prt seiz,not ntrct,w/o stat epi
- G40.309 Gen idiopathic epilepsy, not intractable, w/o stat epi

FAQ

- Q: How do I know my child has epilepsy?
- A: The term "epilepsy" is applied to children with 2 or more seizures without an acute cause.
- Q: Will my child always have epilepsy?
- A: The likelihood of outgrowing epilepsy depends on the syndrome. In many cases, anticonvulsants can be discontinued if the child has been seizure free for 2 years.
- Q: Why does my child have epilepsy?
- A: There are many different reasons to have epilepsy, including genetic, trauma, and other abnormalities of the brain. About 40% of people with epilepsy never have an identified etiology.

SEPARATION ANXIETY DISORDER

Julie O'Brien • Renée Marquardt

BASICS

DESCRIPTION

Separation anxiety disorder (SAD) is defined as developmentally inappropriate fear and anxiety about being away from home and/or apart from the individuals to whom a child is most attached.

- This diagnosis should be distinguished from developmentally appropriate worries, fears, and responses to stressors.

EPIDEMIOLOGY

- Prevalence estimates range from 3.5 to 5.1%.
- Incidence is slightly higher in females than males.
- The mean age of onset is from 4.3 to 8.0 years, but the disorder can present at any age.

ETIOLOGY

Studies show that there are genetic and environmental precursors to the development of SAD:

- A temperament of behavioral inhibition in which a child tends to approach unfamiliar situations with distress, restraint, and avoidance has been shown to be associated with development of anxiety disorders.
- Early development of stranger anxiety
- Insecure attachment between parent and child
- Increased parental anxiety
- Parenting style of being excessively controlling and overprotective
- Exposure to negative life events or stressors
- Genetic predisposition with family history of anxiety or depression

COMMONLY ASSOCIATED CONDITIONS

Comorbid conditions are present in up to 80% of children with SAD, most commonly including the following:

- Depression
- Simple phobia
- Social phobia
- Generalized anxiety disorder
- Obsessive compulsive disorder
- Alcohol abuse in adolescence

DIAGNOSIS

- Anxiety with separation is a normative part of development, typically beginning around 6 or 7 months of age, peaking around 18 months and decreasing after 30 months.
  - Normal separation anxiety at 6–7 months manifests as shyness and anxiety with strangers.
  - At 12–18 months of age, children may have sleep disturbances, nightmares or nocturnal panic attacks, and oppositional behavior.
- SAD is distinguished by anxiety that becomes maladaptive, interfering with normal functioning or becomes overly frequent, severe, and persistent.
- *DSM-IV* criteria are as follows:
  - Developmentally inappropriate and excessive anxiety concerning separation from home or from those to whom the individual is attached as evidenced by 3 (or more) of the following:
    - Recurrent excessive distress when separation from home or major attachment figures occurs or is anticipated
    - Persistent and excessive worry about losing, or about possible harm befalling, major attachment figures
    - Persistent and excessive worry that an untoward event will lead to separation from a major attachment figure (e.g., getting lost or being kidnapped)
    - Persistent reluctance or refusal to go to school or elsewhere because of fear of separation
    - Persistently and excessively fearful or reluctant to be alone or without major attachment figures at home or without significant adults in other settings
    - Persistent reluctance or refusal to go to sleep without being near a major attachment figure or to sleep away from home
    - Repeated nightmares involving the theme of separation
    - Repeated complaints of physical symptoms (such as headaches, stomachaches, nausea, or vomiting) when separation from major attachment figures occurs or is anticipated
    - Duration of disturbance is at least 4 weeks.
    - Onset is before age 18 years.
    - Disturbance causes clinically significant distress or impairment in social, academic, or other important areas (occupational).

HISTORY

- Ask parents about the specific behaviors/complaints of the child at separation, including protests (tantrums/pleading negotiating), fearfulness, or somatic complaints.
  - Somatic complaints such as stomachaches and headaches are most typical.
- Ask caregivers what situations are impacted. Settings can include the following:
  - Separation for school or social/extracurricular activities
  - When the caregiver leaves the home
  - Being separated within the home (e.g., in another room from caregiver)
  - Bedtime
- Ask if sleep is impacted; specifically, ask about nightmares.
  - Children with SAD often have nightmares about separation, death, kidnapping, or serious accident.
- Ask if school attendance is impacted.
  - Avoidance behaviors such as procrastination during the morning routine before school or refusing to leave the side of a parent is common.
  - School refusal has been reported to occur in approximately 75% of children with SAD.
- Ask about duration.
  - Transient separation fears are common. In SAD, symptoms must last more than 4 weeks.
- Ask about possible stressors.
  - Symptoms may be precipitated by a stressor in some cases.
- Ask about impact.
  - Interferes with normative development in a number of ways such as difficulty attending school, participating in extracurricular activities, and attending sleepovers
  - Bedtime separation anxiety may result in sleep disruption to child and family.

PHYSICAL EXAM

There are no pertinent findings on physical exam.

DIAGNOSTIC TESTS & INTERPRETATION

- There are no pertinent findings on lab work.
- There is no standard tool for diagnosis.
- There are a variety of scales that can help in the diagnosis, including the Separation Anxiety Assessment Scale, which has both child and parent versions.

DIFFERENTIAL DIAGNOSIS

SAD should be distinguished from normal, developmentally appropriate separation anxiety. Additionally, one should consider possible life stressors or abuse. Alternate anxiety disorders include the following:

- Generalized anxiety disorder
  - Distinguished by anxiety that is generalized and often presents in later adolescence
  - In children, this tends to manifest as excessive concern over the quality of school or athletic performance at school, concern about punctuality, or overzealous in seeking of approval from authority figures.
- Social anxiety
  - Presents as fear or avoidance of social situations in general or specific situations (e.g., eating in public)
- Specific phobias
  - Occur when anxiety is due to a specific object or situation; unlike in adults, children may not recognize their anxiety/fear of the specific item as excessive

TREATMENT

Initial treatment should include psychoeducation for the caregiver (who will need to implement changes with the child) and cognitive behavioral techniques for the child.

- Psychoeducation for the caregiver includes explanations of the following:
  - The normative nature of anxiety
  - Caregiver response to child's protests and fears can inadvertently reinforce the child's separation behaviors.
- Specific advice to caregivers:
  - Do not prolong a good-bye:
    - Be brief.
    - Let the child know when you will return.
    - Reassure the child that you know that he/she will be ok.
  - Do not let the child see you are upset at the separation.
  - Do not overdo the reunion.
  - If a child is having extreme difficulties:
    - Start with smaller separations.
    - Use incentives and positive reinforcement for success (e.g., sticker charts or points).
    - Gradually build to larger separations.
- Anxiety workbooks can be used by the caregiver at home to provide activities for relaxation and reducing stress.
- Caregivers may need treatment for anxiety if their own anxiety seems to be contributing to the child's behavior.
- Cognitive behavioral therapy (CBT) with the child is aimed at helping the child evaluate the accuracy of his or her fears and learn helpful self-talk.

MEDICATION

Psychopharmacology should generally be used for separation anxiety only if nonmedication treatment is insufficient or if there are additional comorbid anxiety diagnoses that are significantly impairing and psychosocial treatments are simultaneously being pursued.

- Selective serotonin reuptake inhibitor (SSRIs) medications are the primary choice for anxiety disorders in children.
- Young children (<10 years of age) are at increased risk of side effects with SSRI medications.
  - As a result, slow dosing and frequent monitoring is needed.
  - Side effects include GI upset, headaches, dizziness, and agitation.
- SSRI medications have an FDA black box warning due to an increase in suicidal thinking and behavior in children and adolescents; monitoring recommendations need to be followed.

ISSUES FOR REFERRAL

If improvement is not seen within a month after providing education and guidance to caregiver, a referral to a mental health provider is indicated.

- A referral should be made to a mental health provider before medications would be considered for SAD.
- Treatment is usually brief for uncomplicated SAD. Therapy 1–2 times per week may last 6–12 weeks.

ONGOING CARE

FOLLOW-UP RECOMMENDATIONS

- If impairing symptoms continue for more than a month, a higher level of intervention may be indicated.
- If medications are started for anxiety in children, monitoring on a weekly basis is needed for at least 4 weeks after the medication is started or increased and monthly thereafter. (See FDA guidelines for specific medications.)

PROGNOSIS

Outcomes are good with intervention.

- Children with SAD are at higher lifetime risk for other mental health conditions, particularly panic disorders.
- SAD can continue through childhood and into adulthood; early identification and intervention is important to minimize morbidity.

ADDITIONAL READING

- Brewer S, Sarvet B. Management of anxiety disorders in the pediatric primary care setting. *Pediatr Ann*. 2011;40(11):541–547.
- Eisen AR, Schaefer CE. *Separation Anxiety in Children and Adolescents: An Individualized Approach to Assessment and Treatment*. New York: The Guilford Press; 2005.
- Ost L-G, Treffers P. Onset, course and outcome for anxiety disorders in children. In: Silverman W, Cambridge P, eds. *Anxiety Disorders in Children and Adolescents: Research, Assessment and Intervention*. Cambridge, United Kingdom: Cambridge University Press; 2001.
- DSM-IV

CODES

ICD10

F93.0 Separation anxiety disorder of childhood

FAQ

- Q: How do I know if it is developmentally normal separation anxiety?
- A: When separation anxiety arises after the age of 6 years, it warrants intervention if it lasts for more than 4 weeks and/or is markedly impacting expected activities. Before the age of 6 years, separation fears are more common but warrant intervention if impairment in normal functioning is seen.
- Q: Can a teenager have SAD?
- A: Yes. SAD can affect a child of any age and can even persist into adulthood.
- Q: What type of mental health provider can treat SAD that does not respond to primary care intervention?
- A: Any master's or doctorate level mental health provider with experience in anxiety disorders in children and behavioral techniques such as CBT.

S

SEPSIS

Joanna E. Thomson • Craig H. Gosdin

BASICS

DESCRIPTION

- Systemic inflammatory response syndrome (SIRS): nonspecific inflammatory response, defined as at least 2 of the following 4 criteria (one of which must be either abnormal temperature OR leukocyte count):
  - Temperature >38.5 or <36°C
  - Tachycardia (mean HR >2 *SD*s above normal for age)
  - Tachypnea (mean RR >2 *SD*s above normal for age)
  - Leukocytosis, leukopenia, or >10% bands
- Infection: suspected or proven infection or clinical syndrome associated with high probability of infection
- Sepsis: SIRS in the presence of infection
- Severe sepsis: sepsis accompanied by evidence of altered end organ perfusion (cardiovascular dysfunction OR acute respiratory distress syndrome [ARDS] OR 2 or more other organ dysfunctions)
- Septic shock: sepsis with cardiovascular dysfunction (hypotension, need for vasoactive drug to maintain normal BP, or any combination of unexplained metabolic acidosis, increased arterial lactate, oliguria, prolonged capillary refill, and core-to-peripheral temperature gap)

EPIDEMIOLOGY

Incidence

- Estimated overall annual incidence of 0.6 cases per 1,000 children but varies by age
  - Infants <1 year of age: 2.5 per 1,000 children
  - Age 1–4 years: 0.5 per 1,000 children
  - Age 5–14 years: 0.2 per 1,000 children
  - Age 15–19 years: 0.4 per 1,000 children

Prevalence

Sepsis is among the most common (10–25%) medical diagnoses on admission to PICUs.

RISK FACTORS

Sepsis may occur in previously healthy children, but it is a particular concern for children with chronic underlying conditions that render them immunosuppressed or vulnerable to invasive infections.

- Neutropenia (neutrophils $<1{,}000/mm^3$, especially $<500/mm^3$)
- Primary or acquired immunodeficiency (e.g., AIDS, severe combined immunodeficiency)
- Malignancy
- Organ transplant recipients
- Chronic use of high-dose systemic steroids
- Indwelling central venous catheters or other invasive devices (e.g., urinary catheter)
- Hyposplenism, either surgical or functional (e.g., sickle cell anemia)
- Neuromuscular disease (e.g., static encephalopathy)
- Extensive burns
- Multiple trauma injuries
- Prematurity
- Unimmunized/underimmunized children
- Severe malnutrition

GENERAL PREVENTION

- Routine vaccination for *Haemophilus influenzae* type b (Hib), *Streptococcus pneumoniae*, and *Neisseria meningitidis* particularly in high-risk patients (e.g., asplenia)
- Antibiotic prophylaxis for household or day care exposure to confirmed cases of Hib or *N. meningitidis*
- Prompt evaluation of fever in immunosuppressed patients
- Aseptic technique for insertion and care of vascular catheters, minimizing duration of use

ETIOLOGY

- Microbial invasion of the bloodstream or release of microbial products/toxins into the bloodstream; stimulates host defense, resulting in activation of proinflammatory mediators and systemic inflammation
- Pathogens vary with age, host immune status, and setting (community or hospital).
- Neonates
  - Group B *Streptococcus*
  - *Escherichia coli*
  - *Staphylococcus aureus*
  - *Listeria monocytogenes*
  - *Enterococcus* spp.
  - Herpes simplex virus
  - Enterovirus
- In neonates with a history of hospitalization, instrumentation, or mechanical ventilation, also consider
  - Coagulase-negative staphylococci
  - Gram-negative bacilli
  - *Candida* spp.
- Otherwise healthy older infants and children
  - *Streptococcus pneumoniae*
  - *N. meningitidis*
  - *Staphylococcus aureus*
  - Group A *Streptococcus*
  - *Salmonella* spp.
  - Rickettsiae
  - Influenza
- Patients with underlying immune defects are also susceptible to a broad range of additional organisms.

DIAGNOSIS

Requires high suspicion; fever and tachycardia are nonspecific and hypotension is generally a late sign.

HISTORY

- See "Risk Factors"
- Duration of illness before presentation
  - Abrupt onset of symptoms more typical of invasive bacterial infection
- Change in behavior may be initial sign of systemic infection.
  - Irritability, lethargy, and poor feeding are especially important in infants and young children.
- Decreased urine output

PHYSICAL EXAM

All patients with suspected sepsis should have a full set of vital signs (e.g., temperature, pulse, respiratory rate, BP, pulse oximetry).

- Temperature
  - Fever is the hallmark of an infection but may be absent; infants may demonstrate hypothermia.
- General
  - Ill or toxic appearing
- HEENT and neck exam
  - Dehydration: sunken fontanelle, dry mucous membranes, sunken eyes
  - Meningismus or bulging fontanelle
  - Mucocutaneous bleeding
- Cardiovascular exam
  - Tachycardia or bradycardia
  - Hypotension
  - Cold shock: delayed capillary refill; diminished pulses; mottling; and cool, clammy extremities
  - Warm shock: flash capillary refill; bounding pulses; and warm, dry extremities
- Respiratory exam
  - Hypoxia and/or cyanosis
  - Apnea or tachypnea
  - Retractions, flaring or grunting
  - Poor air flow
- Abdominal exam
  - Distension
  - Hepatomegaly, splenomegaly
- Skin exam
  - Presence of petechiae and purpura (associated with meningococcemia and disseminated intravascular coagulation)
  - Pallor
- Neurologic
  - Abnormal mental status (somnolence, confusion, agitation, irritability)
  - Seizures
  - Abnormal reflexes or tone

DIAGNOSTIC TESTS & INTERPRETATION

Lab

Patients with suspected sepsis should have

- Blood culture
  - Prior to starting antibiotics when possible
  - Culture yield is related to sample volume.
- CBC with differential
  - Leukocytosis with increased band count or leukopenia may be present.
- Electrolytes, glucose, ionized calcium
  - Metabolic acidosis
  - Hypoglycemia or hyperglycemia
  - Hypocalcemia
- BUN, creatinine:
  - May reflect dehydration
  - Evaluate for acute kidney injury
- Liver function tests
  - Evaluate for end organ injury
- Arterial blood gas (ABG) and lactate
  - Metabolic acidosis and/or hypoxemia
  - Elevated lactate due to inadequate tissue perfusion
- PT, PTT, fibrinogen, fibrin degradation products, platelets, peripheral smear
  - Screen for DIC: elevated PT, PTT, INR; decreased fibrinogen; increased fibrin degradation products
- Urinalysis and urine culture
  - Potential source of infection
- Lumbar puncture (when hemodynamically stable)
  - Required for diagnosis of meningitis
- Inflammatory biomarkers (e.g., CRP, procalcitonin) may be helpful.
- Culture other potential sources of infection: abscess, wounds, indwelling devices, sputum, tracheal aspirate
- Diagnostic testing for other potential causative organisms (e.g., HSV, enterovirus, influenza)

Imaging

- Chest x-ray
- Head CT may be necessary if with altered mental status in presence of coagulopathy.

DIFFERENTIAL DIAGNOSIS
- Congenital heart disease
- Myocarditis, pericarditis, cardiomyopathy
- Cardiac dysrhythmia
- Myocardial infarction
- Pulmonary embolus
- Congenital adrenal hyperplasia
- Thyrotoxicosis, hypothyroidism
- Inborn errors of metabolism
- Hypoglycemia
- Diabetic ketoacidosis
- Severe anemia
- Methemoglobinemia
- Neoplasm
- Hemophagocytic lymphohistiocytosis
- Macrophage activation syndrome
- Dehydration
- Pyloric stenosis
- Necrotizing enterocolitis
- Malrotation/volvulus
- Intussusception
- Pancreatitis
- Infant botulism
- Toxic ingestion/poisoning
- Trauma (accidental or nonaccidental)

TREATMENT

GENERAL MEASURES
- Ensure a patent airway (consider endotracheal intubation).
- Provide supplemental oxygen and assist ventilation (e.g., bag-valve-mask device) as needed.
- Obtain large-bore peripheral intravenous access (consider central venous line or intraosseous line).
- Hemodynamic support
  - Early fluid resuscitation is imperative.
  - Volume resuscitation: bolus 20 mL/kg of normal saline, repeat as needed; consider blood after 60–80 mL/kg of crystalloid
  - Inotropic agents: If hemodynamic instability persists despite fluid resuscitation, start dopamine (begin at 5 mcg/kg/min, titrate up to 20 mcg/kg/min as needed). If fluid refractory/dopamine-resistant shock, start epinephrine for cold shock or norepinephrine for warm shock to normalize BP and restore perfusion.
- Broad-spectrum intravenous antibiotics to cover likely causative pathogens should be initiated promptly. Consider patient age, immune status, need for penetration into certain tissues (e.g., CNS), and whether the infection was community- or nosocomially acquired in empiric choice. In general, bactericidal drugs should be used.
  - Neonates ≤4 weeks: ampicillin and gentamicin or ampicillin and cefotaxime. Add acyclovir to either regimen if herpes simplex virus infection is suspected.
  - Infants and children ≥4 weeks: cefotaxime or ceftriaxone (no meningitis); vancomycin and cefotaxime or ceftriaxone (with meningitis)
  - Patients with immunosuppression and/or central venous catheters: vancomycin plus aminoglycoside plus advanced-generation cephalosporin (e.g., cefepime)
  - Patients with an intra-abdominal focus of infection: carbapenem; ticarcillin-clavulanate or piperacillin-tazobactam; ceftriaxone, cefotaxime, or cefepime plus metronidazole; ampicillin plus gentamicin plus metronidazole or clindamycin
- Correct hypoglycemia and hypocalcemia.
- Corticosteroids: stress-dose hydrocortisone for catecholamine-resistant hypotension and in patients at risk for adrenal insufficiency
- Drainage or eradication of focus of infection

ALERT:
- Rapid recognition of sepsis is critical. Provide adequate initial volume resuscitation; early reversal of shock is associated with improved outcomes.
- Continuous monitoring and reassessment of the patient are essential.

INPATIENT CONSIDERATIONS
Admission Criteria
- Patients with sepsis should be admitted for close monitoring.
- Patients with severe sepsis or septic shock should be admitted to an ICU (e.g., requiring >60 mL/kg fluid resuscitation).

ONGOING CARE

FOLLOW-UP RECOMMENDATIONS
Patient Monitoring
- Admit all patients with suspected sepsis to the hospital; consider ICU admission.
- Continuous BP monitoring for the development of refractory shock
- Serial vital signs and physical exams to monitor response to therapy
- Monitoring for complications of sepsis and the development of multiple organ dysfunction syndrome (MODS)
  - Chest radiograph and serial ABGs for evidence of acute lung injury/ARDS
  - Urine output, BUN, creatinine for acute kidney injury
  - Serial coagulation studies (PT/PTT) and platelets for development of DIC
  - Serial blood glucose levels for hypo- or hyperglycemia
  - Serial liver function tests for evidence of hepatic dysfunction
  - Serial neurologic examinations for evidence of CNS dysfunction
- Upon pathogen identification, antibiotic therapy can be narrowed appropriately.

PROGNOSIS
- Case fatality rates have improved from nearly 50% to ~10%. With implementation of clinical practice guidelines focused on early reversal of shock, several studies have reduced in-hospital mortality rates to ~4–8% for patients with severe sepsis.
  - Mortality is higher in children with chronic illnesses than in previously healthy children.
  - Development of ARDS or MODS is associated with increased mortality.

COMPLICATIONS
- Sepsis is one of the leading causes of pediatric mortality and accounts for 7% of deaths.
- The most common complications are those resulting from hypoperfusion of vital organs or from organ injury incurred by the uncontrolled systemic inflammatory response:
  - Acute lung injury
  - Acute kidney injury
  - DIC
  - Hypoglycemia
  - ARDS
  - MODS

ADDITIONAL READING

- Bateman SL, Seed PC. Procession to pediatric bacteremia and sepsis: covert operations and failures in diplomacy. *Pediatrics*. 2010;126(1):137–150.
- Brierley J, Carcillo JA, Choong K, et al. Clinical practice parameters for hemodynamic support of pediatric and neonatal septic shock. *Crit Care Med*. 2009;37(2):666–688.
- Butt W. Septic shock. *Pediatr Clin North Am*. 2001;48(3):601–625, viii.
- Buttery JP. Blood cultures in newborns and children: optimising an everyday test. *Arch Dis Child Fetal Neonatal Ed*. 2002;87(1):F25–F28.
- Carcillo JA. Pediatric septic shock and multiple organ failure. *Crit Care Clin*. 2003;19(3):413–440.
- Cazaja AS, Zimmerman JJ, Nathens AB. Readmission and late mortality after pediatric sepsis. *Pediatrics*. 2009;123(3):849–957.
- Rivers E, Nguyen B, Havstad S, et al. Early goal-directed therapy in the treatment of severe sepsis and septic shock. *N Engl J Med*. 2001;345(19):1368–1377.

CODES

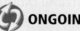

ICD10
- A41.9 Sepsis, unspecified organism
- R65.10 SIRS of non-infectious origin w/o acute organ dysfunction
- R65.20 Severe sepsis without septic shock

FAQ
- Q: What are the early clinical signs of sepsis?
- A: Vital sign changes such as tachycardia, tachypnea, along with respiratory distress/hypoxia and central nervous system alterations can be early signs of sepsis.

SEPTIC ARTHRITIS

Joanna E. Thomson • Erin E. Shaughnessy

BASICS

DESCRIPTION

Microbiologic infection and inflammation of the usually sterile joint space

EPIDEMIOLOGY

- Most common age: toddler and school age (2–6 years)
- Predominant sex: male (2:1 female)
- Most common location: lower extremities (hip, knee, and ankle) and large joints (hip, shoulder, elbow)

PATHOPHYSIOLOGY

- Entry of bacteria into joint space
  - Hematogenous spread (seeding during transient bacteremia) most common
  - Direct inoculation (penetrating trauma or during surgery)
  - Extension from bone infection (mainly in children <1 year old when vessels cross from metaphysis to epiphysis)
- In response to cytokines, influx of inflammatory cells, and release of proteolytic enzymes
- Leads to destruction of synovium and cartilaginous structures

ETIOLOGY

- Most common causes by age:
  - Neonates: group B *Streptococcus*, *Staphylococcus aureus*, *Escherichia coli*, and *Candida albicans*
  - Older children: *Staphylococcus aureus*, group A *Streptococcus*, *Kingella kingae* in toddlers, *Haemophilus influenzae*
- Also consider
  - *Salmonella*: in patients with sickle cell
  - *Neisseria gonorrhoeae*: in sexually active teens and neonates
  - *Neisseria meningitidis*
  - *Mycobacterium tuberculosis*
  - Rubella
  - Parvovirus
  - Hepatitis B or C
  - Mumps
  - Herpesviruses (Epstein-Barr virus, cytomegalovirus, herpes simplex virus, varicella-zoster virus)
  - Fungal etiologies (e.g., coccidioidomycosis)

COMMONLY ASSOCIATED CONDITIONS

- Sickle cell disease: *Salmonella*
- Immunocompromised patients: *Mycoplasma*, *Ureaplasma*, *Klebsiella*, or *Aspergillus* infection

DIAGNOSIS

HISTORY

- Systemic symptoms:
  - Fever (occurs within the first few days of illness in 75% of patients)
  - Malaise
  - Poor appetite
- Joint symptoms:
  - Pain: worsening, does not wax and wane
  - Limp
  - Inability to bear weight, refusal to move joint, positional preferences
  - Typically monoarticular
  - Consider hip involvement when the patient complains of knee or thigh pain.

PHYSICAL EXAM

- Ill appearing
- Joint
  - Warm, swollen, erythematous
  - Held in "position of comfort" maximizing intracapsular joint volume (e.g., hip held flexed, abducted, externally rotated)
  - "Pseudoparalysis": refusal to move the affected extremity
  - Pain throughout entire range of motion (even passive motion)
- Presentation may be delayed and without external findings in deep joints (hip and shoulder).
- In the frightened or uncooperative child, it is possible to have the parent perform an examination for tenderness and range of motion while observing from a distance.

DIAGNOSTIC TESTS & INTERPRETATION

Lab

- Synovial fluid analysis is critical for diagnosis:
  - WBC count: >50–100,000/mm^3 with >75% neutrophils
  - Glucose: <50% that of the serum
  - Gram stain: reveals organism in ~50% of cases
  - Culture: reveals organism in ~75% of cases (except for gonorrhea)
    - Emerging polymerase chain reaction (PCR) technology may allow higher yield and faster identification of causative organisms.
  - Inoculation of joint fluid into blood culture bottle facilitates recovery of *K. kingae*.
    - Real-time PCR for *K. kingae* toxin from joint fluid provides higher yield than routine Gram stain or culture alone.
- Other supportive blood tests:
  - WBC count: neither sensitive nor specific
  - Erythrocyte sedimentation rate (ESR): elevated (>30 mm/h) in 95% of cases
  - C-reactive protein (CRP): increased (>1.0 mg/dL). In one study, a CRP <1.0 mg/dL had a negative predictive value of 87%.
  - Blood cultures: positive in ~40% of cases, sometimes yield pathogen when joint cultures are negative
- Serology for *Borrelia burgdorferi* or PCR of joint fluid may be helpful in differentiating between bacterial arthritis and Lyme disease.

Imaging

- Radiography
  - May show widening of joint space and/or displacement of normal fat pads
- Ultrasound
  - Delineates amount of fluid within joint capsule
  - Increased blood flow with color Doppler is associated with infection. Bilateral effusions suggest transient synovitis.
  - Useful in guiding needle aspiration (especially of deep joints such as the hip)
- MRI and bone scan
  - Should not delay aspiration or antibiotic management
  - MRI: early detection of joint fluid; also will reveal adjacent bone abnormalities to suggest osteomyelitis
  - Bone scan: reveals increased uptake in the perimeter of the joint during the "blood pool" phase of the study
  - Such imaging should be considered to identify concomitant osteomyelitis in patients <4 years of age, involvement of the shoulder, or symptoms >6 days.

DIFFERENTIAL DIAGNOSIS

- Infectious
  - Osteomyelitis with or without contiguous spread to proximal joint
  - Infectious and postinfectious reactive arthritides: *N. meningitidis*, group A *Streptococcus*, *Salmonella*, *Mycoplasma*, *Campylobacter*, *Shigella*, *Yersinia*, *Chlamydia*
  - Cellulitis causing decreased range of motion of joint secondary to inflammation
  - Psoas abscess or retroperitoneal abscess
  - Tuberculous arthritis
  - Lyme arthritis (*B. burgdorferi*)
  - Septic bursitis
- Tumors
  - Osteogenic sarcoma (long bone pain spreading to joint space)
  - Leukemia/lymphoma
- Trauma
  - Occult fracture in proximity to growth plate
  - Ligamentous injury (sprain)
  - Foreign body synovitis
  - Traumatic knee effusion/hemarthrosis
- Immunologic/rheumatic
  - Toxic (transient) synovitis: most common mimic; must examine joint aspirate to differentiate from septic arthritis
  - Acute rheumatic fever
  - Systemic lupus erythematosus
  - Juvenile rheumatoid arthritis
  - Henoch-Schönlein purpura
  - Reactive arthritis syndrome (after GI or chlamydial infection): arthritis, uveitis, urethritis

– Behçet syndrome (iridocyclitis, genital, and oral ulcerations)
– Serum sickness
– Inflammatory bowel disease
- Musculoskeletal
  – Knee: apophysitis (e.g., Osgood-Schlatter disease), patellofemoral pain syndrome, osteochondritis dissecans
  – Hip: slipped capital femoral epiphysis
- Algorithm to differentiate septic arthritis and transient synovitis of the hip: Absence of all 4 factors is strongly associated with absence of septic arthritis.
  – Fever
  – ESR >20 mm/h
  – CRP >1.0 mg/dL
  – WBC >11,000 cells/mL
  – Joint space fluid apparent on plain radiograph

ALERT
- Clinical examination in conjunction with a history of acute onset should raise suspicion for septic arthritis, even in the face of "negative" laboratory screening tests. Analysis of the synovial fluid is necessary for diagnosis.
- Some children, especially neonates and young infants, will not manifest signs of systemic disease early in the course of the illness.

TREATMENT

MEDICATION
- Should be initiated immediately after blood and fluid cultures obtained
- Target empiric antibiotic therapy toward common organisms in age group; may be aided by Gram stain results
  – Typical 1st line: antistaphylococcal penicillin or 1st-generation cephalosporin
  – In areas of methicillin-resistant *Staphylococcus aureus* (MRSA) high prevalence (>15%), consider vancomycin or clindamycin as 1st-line treatment.
- Consider addition of 3rd-generation cephalosporin:
  – In neonates (alternatively could add gentamicin)
  – If gram-negative organism on Gram stain
  – If no organisms on Gram stain
  – High suspicion for *K. kingae*
  – In sexually active adolescents for coverage of *N. gonorrhea*
  – In patients with sickle cell for coverage of *Salmonella*
- Narrow coverage once organism is identified and susceptibilities known
- Duration of therapy depends on organism:
  – *Staphylococcus aureus*: 3 weeks
  – *Streptococcus pneumoniae, K. kingae*, and *N. meningitidis*: 2–3 weeks
  – Longer courses may be necessary for unusual organisms and in complicated courses.
  – May be able to transition to oral antibiotics after short course of intravenous therapy if improving exam and labs
- Pain management with analgesics
- Intra-articular injection of antibiotics is not recommended.

INPATIENT CONSIDERATIONS
Initial Stabilization
- Orthopedic emergency: Drainage of infection should occur as soon as possible.
- Antibiotic administration immediately after joint aspiration is performed
- Indications for open surgical drainage and/or irrigation
  – Hip involvement
  – Shoulder involvement (controversial)
  – Thick, purulent, loculated, or fibrinous exudate unable to pass through 18-gauge needle
  – Lack of improvement within 3 days
- Immobilization of extremity
- Pain management

ONGOING CARE

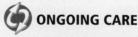

FOLLOW-UP RECOMMENDATIONS
Patient Monitoring
- Follow-up with orthopedic surgery.
- Physical therapy may be useful.
- When to expect improvement:
  – Symptoms typically improve with 2 days of appropriate antibacterial therapy.
  – CRP typically peaks on day 2 of therapy and quickly normalizes within 7–10 days.
- Concerning signs:
  – Continued pain, fever, or lack of improvement of range of motion after 3–4 days of appropriate antibiotic treatment
  – Rising ESR or CRP in the face of antibiotic treatment
  – Severe cases of septic arthritis may require serial drainage and debridement.

PROGNOSIS
- Depends on duration of illness prior to institution of appropriate therapy
  – If antibiotic therapy not instituted within first 4 days of illness, increased incidence of residual joint dysfunction

COMPLICATIONS
- Permanent limitation of range of motion due to tissue destruction and scarring
- Growth disturbance if the epiphysis is involved (leg length discrepancy)
- Avascular necrosis of femoral head (due to increased pressure within joint interrupting blood flow)

ADDITIONAL READING

- Caird MS, Flynn JM, Leung YL, et al. Factors distinguishing septic arthritis from transient synovitis of the hip in children: a prospective study. *J Bone Joint Surg Am*. 2006;88(6):1251–1257.
- Ceroni D, Cherkaoui A, Ferey S, et al. *Kingella kingae* osteoarticular infections in young children: clinical features and contribution of a new specific real-time PCR assay to the diagnosis. *J Pediatr Orthop*. 2010;30(3):301–314.
- Kocher MS, Mandiga R, Murphy JM, et al. A clinical practice guideline for treatment of septic arthritis in children: efficacy in improving process of care and effect on outcome of septic arthritis of the hip. *J Bone Joint Surg Am*. 2003;85-A(6):994–999.
- Liu C, Bayer A, Cosgrove SE, et al. Clinical practice guidelines by the Infectious Diseases Society of America for the treatment of methicillin-resistant *Staphylococcus aureus* infections in adults and children. *Clin Infect Dis*. 2011;52(3):e18–e55.
- Montgomery CO, Siegel E, Blasier RD, et al. Concurrent septic arthritis and osteomyelitis in children. *J Pediatr Orthop*. 2013;33(4):464–467.
- Pääkkönen M, Kallio MJ, Kallio PE, et al. Sensitivity of erythrocyte sedimentation rate and C-reactive protein in childhood bone and joint infections. *Clin Orthop Relat Res*. 2010;468(3):861–866.
- Pääkkönen M, Peltola H. Bone and joint infections. *Pediatr Clin North Am*. 2013;60(2):425–436.
- Sultan J, Hughes PJ. Septic arthritis or transient synovitis of the hip in children: the value of clinical prediction algorithms. *J Bone Joint Surg Br*. 2010;92(9):1289–1293.

CODES

ICD10
- M00.9 Pyogenic arthritis, unspecified
- M00.859 Arthritis due to other bacteria, unspecified hip
- M00.861 Arthritis due to other bacteria, right knee

FAQ
- Q: What is the optimal management of the child with suspected septic arthritis of the hip?
- A: Aspiration of the hip joint is indicated. If purulent fluid is found or analysis of the fluid is suspicious for infection, open drainage of the joint is indicated and must be performed to prevent long-term joint damage. This is a surgical emergency.

SERUM SICKNESS

Denise A. Salerno

BASICS

DESCRIPTION

- Serum sickness
  - Type III hypersensitivity reaction that occurs 7–21 days after injection of foreign protein or serum (usually in the form of antiserums)
  - Immune complexes deposit in the skin, joints, and other organs.
  - Clinical syndrome consists of skin rash, itching, fever, malaise, proteinuria, vasculitis, and joint pain.
- Serum sickness–like reactions
  - Characterized by fever, rash, lymphadenopathy, and arthralgia
  - Occur 1–3 weeks after drug exposure
  - Immune complexes, vasculitis, and hypocomplementemia are *absent*.
  - This type of reaction, most commonly associated with medications, is commonly referred to as serum sickness as well.
  - More common than true serum sickness because equine serum antitoxins have been replaced with human antitoxin sera
- Clinically, these entities present and are treated in the same manner.

EPIDEMIOLOGY

- Limited information is available regarding the incidence of adverse drug reactions in children; generally believed to occur less frequently in children than in adults.
- >90% of serum sickness cases are drug-induced.
- <5% of serum sickness cases are fatal.

RISK FACTORS

Genetics

People with a genetic predisposition to produce IgE are more susceptible.

GENERAL PREVENTION

- No known way to prevent first occurrence
- Take careful history of previous allergic reactions.
- Skin testing prior to antiserum administration will prevent anaphylaxis but not serum sickness.
- When the need for antiserum arises, consider prophylactic antihistamines.

PATHOPHYSIOLOGY

- Serum sickness—type III immune complex, antigen–antibody complement reaction
  - Antibodies form 6–10 days after the introduction of foreign material.
  - Antibodies interact with antigens, forming immune complexes that diffuse across the vascular walls.
  - They become fixated in tissue and activate the complement cascade.
  - C3a and C5a are produced, resulting in increased vascular permeability and activated inflammatory cells.
  - Polymorphonuclear cells and monocytes cause diffuse vasculitis.
- Serum sickness–like reaction
  - Abnormal inflammatory reaction in response to defective metabolism of drug by-products

ETIOLOGY

- Common causative agents:
  - Horse antithymocyte globulins
  - Human diploid-cell rabies vaccine
  - Streptokinase
  - Hymenoptera venom
  - Penicillins
  - Cephalosporins (especially cefaclor)
  - Sulfonamides
  - Hydralazine
  - Thiouracils
  - Metronidazole
  - Naproxen
  - Dextrans
- Case-reported agents:
  - Minocycline
  - Amoxicillin
  - Infliximab
  - Bupropion
  - H1N1 vaccination

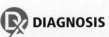

DIAGNOSIS

HISTORY

- Suspect in any patient who has been taking any new drug during the past 2 months and who has an unexplained vasculitic rash.
- Presentation and evolution of rash
  - Typically, the rash first appears on the sides of the fingers, hands, and feet before becoming widespread.
- Previous history of a similar rash
  - Was it associated with any medications in the past? The rash and symptoms of serum sickness will occur sooner on repeat exposure.
- Exposure history
  - Has patient had any drug or antitoxin exposure in the past month?
  - Especially exposures to penicillins, cephalosporins, sulfonamides, hydralazine, thiouracils, streptokinase, metronidazole, naproxen, monoclonal antibodies, or dextrans?
- Timing of the rash and exposure
  - Try to differentiate from simple drug rash; timing of rash after exposure is important in differentiating the two entities.
  - Hypersensitivity reactions occur closer to the time of administration of the offending agent.
- Pruritus is often present.
- Fever
  - Present in 10–20% of cases
  - Usually mild
- Arthritis or arthralgia
  - Present >50% of the time
  - Usually involves the metacarpophalangeal and knee joints
- Associated abdominal pain
  - Some cases may have visceral involvement.
- History of hematuria
  - There can be modest renal involvement, usually presenting as proteinuria and microscopic hematuria.
  - Case reports of renal failure
- Neurologic symptoms
  - Peripheral neuropathy, brachial plexus involvement, and Guillain-Barré syndrome have been reported associations.

PHYSICAL EXAM

- Erythematous purpuric rash starts at the sides of the feet, toes, hands, and fingers and then becomes more widespread.
- Erythema multiforme, maculopapular, purpuric, or urticarial type rash
- Mild to severe fever
- Generalized lymphadenopathy; may be localized to lymph nodes that drain the injection site
- Splenomegaly, occasionally
- Edema of the face and neck
- Joint swelling and tenderness

DIAGNOSTIC TESTS & INTERPRETATION

Lab

- Not extremely helpful in establishing diagnosis because no abnormality is universally present. Diagnosis usually apparent by classic findings and history of foreign protein or drug exposure:
  - Urinalysis: may show proteinuria and/or hematuria
  - Complement levels variably reduced before returning to normal
  - Leukocytosis or leukopenia with or without eosinophilia
  - Erythrocyte sedimentation rate may be slightly elevated.
  - Skin biopsy of rash with direct immunofluorescent (not routinely recommended as part of workup) shows deposits of IgM and C3 complement in capillary walls.

DIFFERENTIAL DIAGNOSIS

- Erythema multiforme
- Mononucleosis
- Systemic lupus erythematosus
- Rocky Mountain spotted fever
- Henoch-Schönlein purpura

- Hypersensitivity syndrome reaction
- Drug-induced pseudoporphyria
- Acute generalized exanthematous pustulosis
- Granulomatosis with polyangiitis (Wegener granulomatosis)
- Pitfalls
  - A history of fever, rash, and arthralgias is commonly seen with many infectious childhood illnesses. One must always consider a broad set of differential diagnoses.
  - Symptoms may be so minimal that patient does not seek medical attention.
  - Often misdiagnosed as simple drug allergy

TREATMENT

GENERAL MEASURES

- Stop suspected medication/antigen immediately.
- Topical steroids to relieve itching
- Antihistamines to inhibit the action of vasoactive mediators
- Antipyretics for fever
- NSAIDs to relieve joint pain
- Oral corticosteroids for severe cases
  - Recommended to administer and taper over 10–14-day period
  - Shorter course may result in relapse, and recurrent symptoms are more difficult to alleviate.
- Admit if symptoms are severe or diagnosis is unclear.
- Future avoidance of triggering agent if identified

ONGOING CARE

FOLLOW-UP RECOMMENDATIONS

When to expect improvement:

- Usually self-limited illness that resolves in a few days to weeks
- If symptoms persist for more than 1 month, reconsider the diagnosis.

PATIENT EDUCATION

- An initial episode of serum sickness cannot be prevented.
- Future episodes can be prevented by avoiding the causative medication (and class of medications) if it has been identified.

PROGNOSIS

Excellent. Most cases are mild and transient with no long-term sequelae.

COMPLICATIONS

- Shock
- Digital necrosis
- Guillain-Barré syndrome (rare)
- Generalized vasculitis (rare)
- Peripheral neuropathy (rare)
- Glomerulonephritis (rare)
- Acute flaccid paralysis (case report)
- Increased risk of anaphylaxis with repeat exposure to precipitating substance
- Fatality (rare, usually due to continued administration of antigen)

ADDITIONAL READING

- Bettge AM, Gross G. A serum sickness-like reaction to a commonly used acne drug. *JAAPA*. 2008;21(3):33–34.
- Bonds RS, Kelly BC. Severe serum sickness after H1N1 influenza vaccination. *Am J Med Sci*. 2013: 345(5):412–413.
- Guidry MM, Drennan RH, Weise JW, et al. Serum sepsis, not sickness. *Am J Med Sci*. 2011;341(2): 88–91.
- McCollom R, Elbe DH, Ritchie AH. Bupropion-induced serum sickness-like reaction. *Ann Pharmacother*. 2000;34(4):471–473.
- Roujeau J, Stern RS. Severe adverse cutaneous reactions to drugs. *N Engl J Med*. 1994;331(19): 1272–1285.
- Tolpinrud B, Bunick C, King B. Serum sickness-like reaction: histopathology and case report. *J Am Acad Dermatol*. 2011;65(3):e83–e85.

CODES

ICD10

- T80.69XA Other serum reaction due to other serum, initial encounter
- T80.62XA Other serum reaction due to vaccination, initial encounter
- T80.61XA Oth serum reaction due to admin blood/ products, init

FAQ

- Q: My child broke out all over her body with an itchy rash and hives a few days after taking cefaclor. Was this serum sickness?
- A: It is more likely that she is allergic to cefaclor. The difference is that drug allergies are type I IgE-mediated hypersensitivity reactions that occur very soon after drug exposure in a previously sensitized individual. Serum sickness is a type III antibody–antigen immune complex and complement amplified hypersensitivity reaction that occurs 1–3 weeks after an initial exposure.
- Q: If my child has had serum sickness, is she at risk for getting it again?
- A: Yes, if she receives the same medication or related medications again. The symptoms will occur more quickly, usually in 2–4 days, and may be more severe.
- Q: Can the vaccines that my doctor recommends for my child give my child serum sickness?
- A: It is possible but very rare. There have been a few reports of serum sickness–like reactions occurring after receiving vaccines submitted to the Vaccine Adverse Event Reporting System (VAERS).
- Q: Is there any way to prevent my child from getting serum sickness?
- A: Unfortunately, there is no way to predict if your child will have a serum sickness–like reaction to a particular medication. It is extremely important to be aware of your child's exact allergies to medications and to inform all health care providers caring for your child.
- Q: My oldest child had serum sickness after taking cefaclor. Is it true that all my children should now avoid taking cefaclor?
- A: No. There is no known genetic predisposition to serum sickness. Your other children do not need to avoid the medication that caused serum sickness.
- Q: How is the Arthus reaction different from serum sickness?
- A: The Arthus reaction is also a type III hypersensitivity reaction but causes only a local reaction. This phenomenon was first described in 1903 by the French physiologist Nicolas Maurice Arthus. The Arthus reaction is a local vasculitis caused by formation of antigen–antibody complexes in local vessel walls, which then activate the inflammation process. The reaction occurs within hours after an individual is injected intradermally with an antigen against which he or she has been actively immunized.
- Q: My child was diagnosed with serum sickness 1 year ago. He still gets episodes of rash, fever, and joint pain every now and then. How can this be cured?
- A: Serum sickness is a self-limited disease, and as long as the offending agent is stopped, your child will completely recover. If there are continuing symptoms and your child is no longer taking the offending agent, then other causes for these symptoms need to be considered.
- Q:My child's best friend was recently diagnosed with serum sickness. Do I need to be concerned?
- A: No. Serum sickness in not contagious.

SEVERE ACUTE RESPIRATORY SYNDROME (SARS)

Nicholas Tsarouhas

BASICS

DESCRIPTION

- WHO clinical criteria (2003):
  - Suspect severe acute respiratory syndrome (SARS) case:
    - A person presenting after November 1, 2002, with high fever (>38°C), and
    - Cough or difficulty breathing, and
    - Close contact with SARS patient or travel criteria to SARS area (see "History")
  - Probable SARS case:
    - A suspect case with radiographic pneumonia or respiratory distress syndrome
    - A suspect case with confirmatory laboratory studies (see "Lab")
    - A suspect case with autopsy findings
- CDC clinical criteria (2003):
  - Early illness
    - 2 or more constitutional symptoms—fever, chills, rigors, myalgia, headache, diarrhea, sore throat, or rhinorrhea
  - Mild to moderate illness
    - Temperature >100.4°F (>38°C)
    - 1 or more lower respiratory findings—cough, shortness of breath, or difficulty breathing
  - Severe illness
    - Clinical criteria of mild to moderate illness, and
    - 1 or more of the following—radiographic evidence, acute respiratory distress syndrome, or autopsy findings
- Clinical criteria for SARS must be interpreted in the context of the prevailing epidemiologic laboratory criteria as published by the WHO and the CDC.

EPIDEMIOLOGY

- SARS time line
  - November 2002: A series of severe idiopathic respiratory illnesses begin occurring in Southeast Asian countries (China, Hong Kong, Vietnam, and Singapore).
  - February 2003
    - The Chinese Ministry of Health notifies the WHO that 305 cases of acute respiratory syndrome of unknown etiology have occurred in Guangdong province in southern China.
    - SARS outbreak in Toronto
  - March 2003
    - CDC activates emergency operations center with first confirmed death of SARS patient.
    - CDC implicates a coronavirus as the causative SARS agent.
  - May 2003: Deaths dramatically rise—7,761 cases, 623 deaths, 31 countries
  - June 2003: Reported cases slow—over 8,000 cases, >770 deaths, 32 countries
  - July 2003: WHO declares the SARS epidemic over.
  - Since July 2003, no further epidemics, but brief reemergence from accidental laboratory exposures in Singapore, Taiwan, and Beijing and from recurrent animal-to-human transmissions in Guangzhou in late 2003 and early 2004
- First emergence of an important human pathogen in the 21st century
- Final statistics of epidemics:
  - Worldwide: >8,000 cases, nearly 800 deaths, >30 countries affected
  - United States: 134 suspected cases, 19 probable cases, 8 confirmed cases, no deaths, 17 states affected

RISK FACTORS

- Transmission
  - Direct or indirect contact of mucous membranes with infectious respiratory droplets or fomites, thus simple masks and good hand hygiene are important.
  - Period of infectivity: most likely during period with active symptoms (fever, cough)
  - Incubation period 2–14 days but may be as long as 21 days; mean 6 days
  - All cases can be traced to contact with individuals from Asian countries or community, spread from an individual whose illness could be traced to Asia.
  - There have been no suspected SARS cases among casual contacts of the U.S. cases.
  - Many health care workers were infected after providing care to SARS patients.
  - No evidence that SARS is transmitted from asymptomatic individuals
  - However, health care workers who developed SARS may have been a source of transmission within health care facilities during early phases of illness, when symptoms were mild and not recognized as SARS.
  - There is no evidence that SARS can be spread after recovery from the disease.
  - Pediatric population
    - Children pose a lower risk of transmission than do adults; only 1 reported case of transmission of SARS from pediatric patient.
    - Vertical transmission of SARS coronavirus (SARS-CoV) from infected mothers to their newborns has not been observed.
    - None of the newborns had clinical, laboratory, or radiologic evidence suggestive of SARS-CoV infection.

GENERAL PREVENTION

- As there is no specific treatment, public health and infection control measures including contact tracing and quarantine of close contacts are paramount.
- Hospital infection control precautions:
  - Hospitalized patients meeting SARS case definition should be placed in a negative-pressure, single examination room.
  - Protective equipment appropriate for standard, contact, and airborne precautions (e.g., hand hygiene, gown, gloves, and N95 respirator) in addition to eye protection are recommended for health care workers to prevent transmission of SARS in health care settings.
- Pediatric patients with potential SARS exposure:
  - Children who have been exposed to an ill individual who is suspected of having SARS, or children who have traveled to an area where SARS is occurring, should be evaluated based on the following:
    - If well, parents should self-monitor the child's condition for fever or respiratory tract illness. Attendance at child care or school is not restricted.
    - If the child is not well, parents should contact their physician and the child should be isolated at home.
    - If the child is not well and is experiencing breathing difficulty, he or she should be hospitalized. Health care workers should be informed before the admission so SARS precautions can be initiated.
  - Children who have been exposed to individuals who are not ill but have traveled to areas where SARS is occurring do not require isolation.
- Vaccine
  - No effective human vaccine has been developed.
  - Safety concerns exist for vaccine production workers.

PATHOPHYSIOLOGY

The virus attaches to human receptor cells and initiates a nonspecific acute lung injury response leading to diffuse, severe alveolar damage.

ETIOLOGY

- SARS-CoV, a previously unrecognized single-stranded RNA coronavirus
- Coronaviruses are a common cause of mild to moderate upper respiratory infections in humans and have occasionally been linked to pneumonia.
- Many believe that the virus originated in an animal species in China, then mutated in such a way that it was able to attach itself to human receptor cells.

DIAGNOSIS

HISTORY

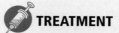

- Recent travel
  - Travel (including transit in an airport) within 10 days of onset of symptoms to an area with recently documented or suspected transmission of SARS is an important epidemiologic criterion for diagnosis.
  - At the height of the SARS epidemic, these areas included China, Hong Kong, Singapore, Taiwan, Toronto, and Hanoi.
- Recent contact with a SARS patient
  - Close contact within 10 days of onset of symptoms with a person known or suspected to have SARS infection is another important epidemiologic criterion.
- The clinical presentation of SARS in children >12 years of age is similar to that of adults.
- Constitutional symptoms, such as fever, chills, rigors, headache, malaise, myalgias, and diarrhea, are common in older patients.
- A meta-analysis (Stockman et al.) of 6 pediatric series of 135 SARS cases noted the following symptom prevalence: fever (98%), cough (60%), and nausea or vomiting (41%).
- Respiratory symptoms
  - At the onset of illness, most cases have mild respiratory symptoms.
  - After 3–7 days, a dry, nonproductive cough begins, often with dyspnea.

PHYSICAL EXAM

- Fever generally heralds the start of the illness.
- Tachypnea, increased work of breathing, or rales are common in adults.
- Adult patients generally present with some evidence of respiratory distress or hypoxemia.
- Importantly, however, although some children present with cough or difficulty breathing, many have remarkably normal examinations.

DIAGNOSTIC TESTS & INTERPRETATION

Lab

- Detection of SARS coronavirus: confirmatory laboratory criteria for the diagnosis of SARS:
  - Antibody by enzyme-linked immunosorbent assay (ELISA) or indirect fluorescent-antibody assay (IFA)
  - RNA by reverse transcriptase-polymerase chain reaction (RT-PCR) assays
  - Viral culture
- SARS virus may be detected in blood, throat, nasopharyngeal aspirates, and stool samples.
- CBC: Hematologic abnormalities are common in children with SARS.
  - Leukopenia (lymphopenia or neutropenia)
  - Thrombocytopenia
- Liver enzymes: Elevated transaminases seen.
- Raised serum lactate dehydrogenase is also seen.

Imaging

- The characteristic feature of pulmonary SARS-CoV infection is patchy airspace consolidation predominantly located at the periphery of the lungs and in the lower lobes.
- Normal chest radiographs also possible.

DIFFERENTIAL DIAGNOSIS

- Bacterial infections
  - *Pneumococcus*
  - *Staphylococcus*
  - *Legionella*
  - *Mycoplasma*
  - *Chlamydophila pneumoniae*
- Viral infections
  - Middle East respiratory syndrome (MERS)
  - Avian influenza A(H7N9) infection (bird flu)
  - Influenza A and B
  - Respiratory syncytial virus
  - Ebola viral infection

ALERT

- Even during an epidemic of SARS, other diseases should still be considered.
- Microbiologic studies should still be performed to confirm or rule out other infectious diseases.

TREATMENT

INPATIENT CONSIDERATIONS

Initial Stabilization

- There is no proven effective treatment.
- CDC currently recommends that patients with SARS receive the same treatment and supportive care that would be used for any patient with serious community-acquired atypical pneumonia of unknown cause.
- Steroids, interferon, convalescent plasma, ribavirin, oseltamivir, and other antivirals have been used without consistent success.

ONGOING CARE

PROGNOSIS

- Patients 12 years of age and younger
  - Milder disease
  - Fewer ICU admits
  - Decreased need for supplemental oxygen
  - No reported pediatric deaths
- Overall fatality rate: 9.5% (all adults)
  - Highest: 27% (Taiwan)
  - Lowest: 0 (United States)

COMPLICATIONS

- Overall, in 10–20% of cases, the respiratory illness was severe enough to require mechanical ventilation.
- In children, only 5% required admission to an ICU, and <1% required mechanical ventilation.

ADDITIONAL READING

- Braden CR, Dowell SF, Jernigan DB, et al. Progress in global surveillance and response capacity 10 years after severe acute respiratory syndrome. *Emerg Infect Dis*. 2013;19(6):864–869.
- Cheng VC, Chan JF, To KK, et al. Clinical management and infection control of SARS: lessons learned. *Antiviral Res*. 2013;100(2):407–419.
- Li AM, Ng PC. Severe acute respiratory syndrome (SARS) in neonates and children. *Arch Dis Child Fetal Neonatal Ed*. 2005;90(6):F461–F465.
- Momattin H, Mohammed K, Zumla A, et al. Therapeutic options for Middle East respiratory syndrome coronavirus (MERS-CoV)—possible lessons from a systematic review of SARS-CoV therapy. *Int J Infect Dis*. 2013;17(10):e792–e798.
- Stockman L, Massoudi MS, Helfand R, et al. Severe acute respiratory syndrome in children. *Pediatr Infect Dis J*. 2007;26(1):68–74.

CODES

ICD10

- J12.81 Pneumonia due to SARS-associated coronavirus
- B97.21 SARS-associated coronavirus causing diseases classd elswhr

FAQ

- Q: Is the clinical presentation and course different in children?
- A: Fortunately, younger children tend to have a shorter and milder course, consisting mainly of low-grade fever, cough, and rhinorrhea. Adolescents, conversely, follow a more severe course, similar to that of adults.
- Q: What constitutes close contact with a SARS patient?
- A: Close contact includes having cared for or lived with a person known to have SARS or having a high likelihood of direct contact with respiratory secretions and/or body fluids of a patient known to have SARS.

SEVERE COMBINED IMMUNODEFICIENCY

M. Elizabeth M. Younger • Howard M. Lederman

BASICS

DESCRIPTION

Severe combined immunodeficiency (SCID) is a primary immunodeficiency characterized by functional defects in both the humoral and cellular immune systems. Most babies present with lymphopenia. Even the suspicion of SCID constitutes a pediatric emergency. Untreated, SCID is universally fatal, usually within the 1st year of life.

EPIDEMIOLOGY

Most patients present in the 1st year of life as immunity from maternal antibody wanes.

Incidence

- Estimated to be 1 in 100,000 births but may be underreported because of early infant mortality
- Highest in regions where consanguineous marriages take place
- SCID due to Artemis defects occurs in 1 in 2,500 births in the Navajo and Apache populations because of a founder mutation.

Genetics

- At least 13 known genetic defects that cause SCID
- Approximately 50% of cases are X-linked (mutation in the IL2 gamma chain); the others are autosomal recessive or de novo mutations.
- Classified by the lymphocytes subsets affected (e.g., T− B+ NK+, T− B− NK+, etc.)

ETIOLOGY

Caused by mutations in genes required for T-cell growth and development, purine salvage pathway function (e.g., adenosine deaminase), and expression of histocompatibility (HLA) antigens.

DIAGNOSIS

HISTORY

- Failure to thrive
- Chronic diarrhea
- Chronic thrush or candidal diaper rash
- Frequent and/or severe infections with common pathogens
- Rotaviral infection after immunization
- Opportunistic infections
- Consanguinity
- Family history of SCID or unexplained infant deaths

PHYSICAL EXAM

- Emaciated or wasted appearance
- Atypical morbilliform rash
- Absence of lymphoid tissue (small or absent tonsils and lymph nodes)
- Evaluation for infection
  - Thrush or diaper dermatitis
  - Manifestations of graft-versus-host disease (skin rash, conjunctivitis, hepatitis, diarrhea) secondary to transplacental alloreactive maternal T cells or T cells from unirradiated blood products

DIAGNOSTIC TESTS & INTERPRETATION

- CBC with differential to assess for lymphopenia: should suspect SCID if absolute lymphocyte count (ALC) <3,000 per microliter in the neonatal period or if ALC is < 1,000 per microliter in any child <3 years of age
- Lymphocyte subsets: All populations are generally decreased, but T cells are almost always severely decreased.
- Serum immunoglobulins (IgG, IgA, IgM): usually low or absent, but IgG may be normal in first 4 months of life because of placental transfer
- T-cell receptor excision circles (TRECs) are part of newborn screening from Guthrie cards (now legally mandated by many states in the United States).
  - Identifies lymphopenia in the newborn
  - TRECs are absent in infants with SCID.
  - TRECs may be reduced in premature infants.
- Lymphocyte proliferation assay: Cells do not proliferate to antigenic stimulation.
- Appropriate cultures to identify pathogens
- Identification of causative mutation is necessary to allow for genetic counselling.

DIFFERENTIAL DIAGNOSIS

- HIV infection
- DiGeorge (22q11 deletion) syndrome
- Iatrogenic lymphopenia (e.g., steroid therapy)
- Other primary immunodeficiency (e.g., X-linked agammaglobulinemia, ataxia telangiectasia)

TREATMENT

- The only curative treatment is stem cell transplant.
  - Success rates >70% have been reported and increase to 96% when the transplant is done before the age of 3 1/2 months.
  - Preconditioning is generally not required because of the lack of T-cell function, but reduced intensity conditioning is often done to ensure engraftment.
- In patients with adenosine deaminase (ADA)–deficient SCID, for whom there is no identical stem cell match, enzyme replacement therapy with pegylated ADA (Adagen) can be given.

ONGOING CARE

- Pre-transplant supportive care
  - Pneumocystis prophylaxis with trimethoprim/sulfamethoxazole
  - Immunoglobulin replacement therapy (intravenous every 3–4 weeks, subcutaneously every 1–2 weeks)
  - Aggressive and early treatment of infections
  - Nutritional support
  - Avoidance of crowds and persons with symptoms of infection (fever, cough, etc.)
  - Routine immunization is unnecessary, as patients are unable to mount antibody responses.
  - Live viral vaccines are absolutely contraindicated.
  - If blood transfusion is required, only irradiated, CMV negative blood products should be used.
- Nontransplant treatment
  - Gene therapy trials are ongoing for patients with ADA-deficient and X-linked SCID.
- Post transplant care
  - Close monitoring for signs of graft-versus-host disease, engraftment failure, infection
  - Immunoglobulin replacement therapy may still be required if B-cell reconstitution is absent or impaired.
  - Genetic counseling for parents

COMPLICATIONS

- Pre- or posttransplant graft-versus-host disease
- Engraftment failure
- Omenn syndrome caused by clonal autoreactive T cells, resembling graft-versus-host disease seen in patients with *RAG1* or *RAG2* mutations
- Increased risk for lymphoreticular cancers
- Radiation sensitivity in patients with SCID caused by DNA repair syndromes (Artemis, Ligase-4, DNA-PKcs, Cernunnos)
- Growth failure and hearing impairment in patients with ADA-deficient SCID

ADDITIONAL READING

- Buckley RH. Transplantation of hematopoietic stem cells in human severe combined immunodeficiency: long-term outcomes. *Immunol Res*. 2011; 49(1–3): 25–43.
- Cavazzana-Calvo M, Fischer A, Hacien-Bey-Abina S, et al. Gene therapy for primary immunodeficiencies: part I. *Curr Opin Immunol*. 2012;24(5):580–584.
- Chinen J, Notarangelo LD, Shearer WT. Advances in basic and clinical immunology in 2012. *J Allergy Clin Immunol*. 2013; 131(3):675–682.
- Puck JM. Laboratory technology for population-based screening for severe combined immunodeficiency in neonates: the winner is T-cell receptor excision circles. *J Allergy Clin Immunol*. 2012; 129(3):607–616.

CODES

ICD10

- D81.9 Combined immunodeficiency, unspecified
- D81.1 Severe combined immunodeficiency w low T- and B-cell numbers
- D81.2 Severe combined immunodef w low or normal B-cell numbers

FAQ

- Q: What should I do if I am notified that a newborn screen has identified a low number of TRECs?
- A: As a precaution while the child is being evaluated, prevent the infant's exposure to sick contacts and public places or places with large crowds (day care centers, malls, churches, large family gatherings). Consider the need for pneumocystis prophylaxis and immunoglobulin replacement therapy while the evaluation proceeds. Send blood for enumeration of T-cell subsets (CD4 and CD8), B-cells (CD19), and NK cells (CD 16/56) and refer the child to a clinical immunologist.
- Q: What vaccines should be given to a child with SCID or suspected SCID?
- A: Children with SCID do not benefit from immunizations, and live viral vaccines of any type (rotavirus, MMR, varicella, and BCG) are absolutely contraindicated.
- Q: What is the chance of another child in the family being affected with SCID?
- A: The answer to this question depends of the cause of SCID. If a child has X-linked SCID, then there is a 50% chance of SCID in any male child born to the mother. In other forms of SCID, the risk is 25% for any male or female. It is crucial that a genetic diagnosis is made for each case of SCID so that families can be given accurate information about recurrence risk, they can be offered prenatal testing, and other affected children can be identified as soon as possible after birth.
- Q: Is there gene therapy for SCID?
- A: There are active *research* protocols for treating children with X-linked SCID and children with ADA deficiency. These protocols are still investigative and not standard therapy. Bone marrow transplantation remains the standard of care at this point.

S

SEXUAL ABUSE

Mitchell A. Goldstein

BASICS

DESCRIPTION

Sexual abuse is the involvement of children in sexual activities that they cannot understand, for which they are not developmentally prepared, to which they cannot give informed consent, and/or that violate societal norms.

- Ranges from oral, genital, or anal contact; fondling; child pornography; prostitution; exhibitionism; and voyeurism
- Twenty-five percent of perpetrators are parents, and 30% are non-parental relatives.
- Most children sexually abused will have no discernible physical injury.

EPIDEMIOLOGY

- ~150,000 substantiated cases/year; most likely underestimates the incidence as these include only those cases reported
- Prevalence rates between 10 and 30%. The National Violence Survey reported 27% of adult women and 16 % adult men reported sexual abuse during childhood.

RISK FACTORS

- Peak age of vulnerability: 7–13 years of age
- Girls are victimized more than boys, although abuse of boys is underreported.
- Single-parent households, domestic violence, parental substance abuse and mental illness
- Children who experience other types of abuse are also more likely to be victimized sexually.
- Race and socioeconomic status do not appear to be risk factors for child sexual abuse.
- Risk factors for revictimization: younger aged children; more severe maltreatment; families with mental health and substance abuse problems and violence histories

DIAGNOSIS

HISTORY

- Diagnosis is made based on the child's history because abnormal physical findings or lab tests are infrequent.
- Attempt to limit the number of interviews.
- Interview should be detailed enough to know whether a report to child protection or law enforcement is needed.
- If the medical provider is the first person to which the child has disclosed, then that person is an "an outcry witness,", and that disclosure can be used in court testimony.
- Answers from the children that are obtained for the medical diagnosis and treatment may be admitted into evidence.
- The interview should be conducted with the child separate from family members.
- Ask open-ended, nonleading questions.
- Use developmentally appropriate language.
- Specific questions important to the triage of the child include the following:
  - Identity of alleged perpetrator/relationship to child
  - Time of last possible contact
  - Specific types of sexual contact
  - Review of systems including genital pain, bleeding, dysuria, constipation, painful bowel movements, and behavioral changes

PHYSICAL EXAM

- Serves to ensure the overall health of a child after an abusive event and to document any injuries or other forensically relevant evidence
- Most exams are normal.
- An emergency exam is indicated if the most recent assault was within 72 hours or if the patient has complaints of pain, dysuria, or bleeding. Beyond 72 hours, the exam can be scheduled at the local child advocacy center.
- A speculum should not be used for a prepubertal sexual abuse exam unless there is acute bleeding and its origin must be determined.
  - Use of the techniques of labial separation and labial traction (gently grasping the posterior portion of the labia majora and pulling laterally, down, and toward the examiner) allows for the best visualization of the hymenal edges.
  - Normal hymenal configurations: annular, crescentic, and fimbriated
  - Newborn hymen: thickened, pale, and redundant
  - Prepubertal hymen: thin, less redundant, with sharp well-defined edges.
  - Postpubertal hymen: thickened, pale, and redundant
- A few physical findings are diagnostic of abuse:
  - Presence of semen or sperm on the victim
  - Pregnancy
  - Acute genital/anal injuries without an adequate accidental explanation (bruising, lacerations, complete hymenal transaction between 4 and 8 o'clock along hymenal rim)
  - Syphilis and *Neisseria gonorrhoeae* infection (excluding perinatal infection).
  - Chlamydia if the child is older than 3 years of age
  - Trichomoniasis in a child older than 1 year of age
- Many genital findings are unlikely to be related to abuse:
  - Normal variants including intravaginal ridges, hymenal mounds, linea vestibularis, diastasis ani
  - Perineal redness
  - Labial adhesions
  - Anal fissures
  - Venous pooling in perianal area
- Any finding on exam thought to be abnormal or diagnostic of child sexual abuse should be reviewed with a child abuse expert for confirmation.

DIAGNOSTIC TESTS & INTERPRETATION

Initial Lab Tests

- Forensic evidence collection
  - Standard rape kit if the last contact was 72 hours or less
  - Always obtain consent.
  - In prepubertal children, recovery of useful forensic evidence is rare beyond 24 hours.
  - Some experts support forensic evidence recovery up to 5 days from the contact in pubertal children.
  - Most positive forensic evidence comes from clothing and linens.
- Sexually transmitted illness (STI) screening: Universal screening is not appropriate unless the victim is a sexually active adolescent.
  - AAP and CDC guidelines recommends STI testing when
    - Child discloses contact that may have involved genital secretions.
    - Child's symptoms or physical exam suggest presence of STI.
    - Abuser is felt to be at risk for STI.
    - Community prevalence of STI is high.
    - Family member is infected with an STI.
    - Patient or family member requests testing.
  - Testing for *N. gonorrhoeae* and *Chlamydia trachomatis* may be performed with vaginal/urethral culture or nucleic acid amplification techniques (NAATs).
  - Cultures have historically been the gold standard method for diagnosing STIs in prepubertal children. NAATs have proven to be sensitive and specific for *N. gonorrhoeae* and *C. trachomatis* infection in this age group.
  - NAATs are not approved for rectal or pharyngeal specimens.
  - NAATs have a higher sensitivity than culture.
  - If an NAAT is done, then important not to treat empirically because if the NAAT is positive, the clinician will want to repeat with another NAAT or culture to reconfirm.
- Trichomoniasis in a child 1 year of age or older is diagnostic of child sexual abuse; can be tested for by wet prep, culture, or PCR
- Screen for syphilis (STT/RPR) and hepatitis B in any case, which meets other screening recommendations.
- HIV screening should also be considered.

Special Considerations

- Genital warts are not diagnostic of child sexual abuse. Neonatal transmission is common and human papilloma virus (HPV) may remain latent for several years. Children who present after age 3–5 years should have a complete medical evaluation for sexual abuse.
- Herpes simplex infections in the genital area are most commonly (but not always) caused by sexual contact. Most mouth infections are caused by HSV-1 and most genital infections are caused by HSV-2, but this distinction is not absolute.

Follow-Up Lab Tests

- Any positive NAAT needs to be repeated with a different NAAT for confirmation prior to empiric treatment.
- Any positive STT/RPR should be confirmed with a treponemal test.
- If serologic testing for HIV, HBV, and syphilis is negative acutely, they should be repeated at 6 weeks, 3 months, and 6 months.

DIFFERENTIAL DIAGNOSIS

- Sexualized behaviors
  - Normal behaviors for age (e.g., masturbation)
  - Exposure to sexual activity (e.g., media)
- Abnormal GU exam
  - Normal variations in hymenal anatomy (e.g., septate, cribriform, imperforate)
  - Normal variations in perineal anatomy (e.g., hymenal mound, intravaginal ridge, vestibular bands)
  - Linea vestibularis: white streaks that run from inferior hymenal border to posterior commissure
  - Failure of midline fusion: presence of mucosal surface between fossa navicularis and anus that commonly resolves at puberty
  - Irritant, contact, and seborrheic dermatitis
  - Labial adhesions
  - Lichen sclerosis et atrophica: thinned white atrophic skin in figure-of-8 appearance which may have bruising or petechiae
  - Ureterocele
  - Urethral prolapse
  - Pearly pink papules in males

- Balanitis in males
- Phimosis or paraphimosis in males
- Accidental trauma, including straddle and impaling injuries
- Accidental tourniquet of genitals by hair

- Abnormal anal exam
  - Diastasis ani: absence of muscle fibers in middle of external anal sphincter
  - Anal skin tags
  - Anal dilatation from constipation or sedation
  - Group A streptococcal perianal cellulitis
- Urethral discharge/bleeding
  - Foreign body
  - UTI
  - Nonspecific vulvovaginitis
  - Group A *Streptococcus*
  - *Haemophilus influenzae*
  - *Staphylococcus aureus*
  - *Mycoplasma hominis*
  - *Gardnerella vaginalis*
  - *Shigella flexneri* (discharge commonly bloody)
- Genital ulcers
  - EBV, HSV
  - Behçet disease
  - Inflammatory bowel disease
- Genital irritation
  - Pinworms
  - Scabies
  - *Candida albicans*
  - Trauma

TREATMENT

MEDICATION

- Prophylactic antibiotics
  - Recommended following sexual abuse/assault in adolescents and adults to prevent *N. gonorrhoeae*, *C. trachomatis*, and *Trichomonas vaginalis*
  - Not recommended in prepubertal victims because of the low likelihood of STI and the importance of establishing the diagnosis
- HIV postexposure prophylaxis (PEP)
  - Recommend consultation with pediatric infectious disease specialist before initiating PEP.
  - High-risk exposures: disclosure of penile anal or penile vaginal penetration by known HIV positive perpetrator
  - Moderate-risk exposures: disclosure of penile anal or penile vaginal penetration and the HIV status of perpetrator is unknown but there is no anogenital trauma but multiple assailants were involved; perpetrator is from a high-risk population; or there is coexisting infection in perpetrator or victim
  - PEP is not recommended in disclosures that do not involve anal, vaginal, or oral penetration; oral penetration without ejaculation
- *N. gonorrhoeae* treatment according to CDC guidelines
  - Adolescents: ceftriaxone 125 mg IM once or cefixime 400 mg PO once
  - Prepubertal child: ceftriaxone 125 mg IM once
- *C. trachomatis* treatment according to CDC guidelines
  - Adolescents: azithromycin 1 g PO one time or doxycycline 100 mg PO b.i.d. × 7 days
  - Prepubertal child
    - Weight less than 45 kg: erythromycin 50/mg/kg/day divided into 4 daily doses for 14 days
    - Weight greater than 45 kg but less than 8 years: azithromycin 1 g PO × 1; age greater than 8 years: azithromycin 1 g PO one time or doxycycline 100 mg PO b.i.d. × 7 days
- Syphilis treatment according to CDC guidelines: parenteral penicillin G; dose depends on stage of disease and child age
- Trichomoniasis treatment: metronidazole 2 g PO once
- Hepatitis B vaccination for unimmunized patients
- Hepatitis B immune globulin for patients with recent sexual contact with known positive perpetrator
- Consider pregnancy prevention (e.g., emergency hormonal contraceptive) for adolescents after ensuring the patient is not pregnant.
- Tetanus booster for patients with acute, serious genital or other injuries.

ADDITIONAL TREATMENT

General Measures

Cases of child sexual abuse require a multidisciplinary approach that includes medical, social services, law enforcement, and states attorney expertise.

Admission Criteria

- Consider in children with injuries that require operative care
- Consider in cases where the clinician wants to ensure protection of the child and external forces preclude that assurance
- Consider in cases where there is a significant mental health concern

ONGOING CARE

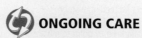

FOLLOW-UP RECOMMENDATIONS

Patient Monitoring

Most children should be followed by a mental health provider.

PROGNOSIS

Varies greatly depending on specifics of abuse sustained and available support systems

COMPLICATIONS

- Posttraumatic stress disorder
- Depression
- Domestic violence and revictimization
- Substance abuse
- Chronic pelvic pain
- Males are more likely to have concerns about sexual orientation.

ADDITIONAL READING

- Adams JA. Medical evaluation of suspected child sexual abuse: 2011 update. *J Child Sex Abuse*. 2011;20(5):588–605.
- Berenson AB, Chacko MR, Wiemann CM, et al. A case-control study of anatomic changes resulting from sexual abuse. *Am J Obstet Gynecol*. 2000; 182(4):820–834.
- Christian CW. Timing of the medical evaluation. *J Child Sex Abuse*. 2011;20(5):505–520.
- Gavril AR, Kellogg ND, Nair P. Value of follow-up examinations of children and adolescents evaluated for sexual abuse and assault. *Pediatrics*. 2012;129(2):282–289.
- Hammerschlag MR. Sexual assault and abuse of children. *Clin Infect Dis*. 2011;53(Suppl 3):103–109.
- Kellogg N; American Academy of Pediatrics Committee on Child Abuse and Neglect. The evaluation of sexual abuse in children. *Pediatrics*. 2005;116(2):506–512.
- Workowski KA, Berman S; Centers for Disease Control and Prevention. Sexually transmitted diseases treatment guidelines. *MMWR Recomm Rep*. 2010;59(RR-12):1–110.

CODES

ICD10

- T74.22XA Child sexual abuse, confirmed, initial encounter
- T76.22XA Child sexual abuse, suspected, initial encounter

FAQ

- Q: How could there have been penetration with a normal physical examination?
- A: The vast majority of child sexual abuse exams are completely normal even with a history of penetration. The healing properties of genital tissues are quick and complete; past injuries are often difficult to detect on physical exam.
- Q: What should I do if I examine a patient with no history of sexual abuse and detect an anatomic abnormality that I think is suggestive of sexual abuse?
- A: Always have exams confirmed by a child abuse expert in your area, as nuances of exams can be hard to discern.
- Q: If child abuse evaluations rarely reveal any abnormalities, why should I subject my patient to such an invasive evaluation?
- A: The vast majority of sexual abuse medical evaluations are normal, but in the small percentage that are abnormal, the information derived can be important medically and forensically. Importantly, the exams allow for detection of other medical conditions which may have gone unnoticed secondary to lack of medical access. Exams also serve to reassure families and children that they are healthy.
- Q: Is an STI diagnosed in a prepubertal patient always indicative of abuse?
- A: No. All STIs may be transmitted vertically (from mother to infant). The incubation periods of different infections vary, so they are expressed at different ages accordingly. Gonorrhea and syphilis are considered diagnostic of sexual abuse outside of congenital infection. *Chlamydia*, herpes simplex virus 2, and *Trichomonas* are probably due to sexual abuse and should be reported for evaluation. *Condyloma acuminata* is probably related to sexual abuse in school-aged and older children but may be transmitted to younger children innocently during toileting or diaper changes.

S

SHORT STATURE

Himala Kashmiri • Susanne M. Cabrera

BASICS

DESCRIPTION

- Short stature is height <2 standard deviations (*SD*) below mean or <3rd percentile for age and sex of the normal population.
- Growth failure defined as height <2 *SD* below midparental height (MPH) or height velocity (HV) <10th percentile for age resulting in downward crossing of height percentiles
- The majority of children with short stature are essentially healthy. True growth failure is typically pathologic and requires evaluation.
- Failure to thrive (FTT) is failure of appropriate weight gain (decreased weight to height ratio). May be accompanied by poor linear growth.

RISK FACTORS

- Poor nutrition, systemic chronic illness, and psychosocial factors can contribute to clinical presentation of short stature or growth failure.
- A family history of short stature or delayed growth and puberty are well-established risk factors for childhood short stature.

PATHOPHYSIOLOGY

- Adequate nutrition and weight gain play major roles in linear growth during childhood.
- Throughout infancy and childhood, growth hormone (GH) and thyroid hormone exert major influences on normal growth.
- Pulsatile GH release stimulates insulin-like growth factor 1 (IGF-1) secretion from liver and other tissues to promote growth at growth plates.
- The pubertal growth spurt is largely mediated by androgen and estrogen activity at the growth plate as well as enhanced GH release.
- Chronic illnesses can cause growth failure.
- Glucocorticoid excess inhibits growth through downregulation of the GH/IGF-1 axis and suppressed osteogenesis.

DIAGNOSIS

HISTORY

- **Question:** Have length/height and weight been charted appropriately on a growth curve?
- *Significance*: Interpretation of growth depends on *precise* and *accurate* measurements that account for both year and month of age.
- **Question:** Is the child short for his or her MPH?
- *Significance*: Height can only be judged to be inappropriate in the context of the genetic potential as determined by MPH:
  - For boys: [father's height (cm) + (mother's height [cm] + 13)] divided by 2
  - For girls: [(father's height [cm] − 13) + mother's height (cm)] divided by 2
  - MPH target range (± 2 *SD*) is +/− 10 cm.
  - If the child's height percentile is decreased relative to the MPH range, evaluation may be warranted.
- **Question:** Height velocity (HV)?
- *Significance*: A normal HV is reassuring, whereas a reduced HV, *regardless of absolute height*, can earlier detect a growth-slowing disorder.
  - The HV for an interval of at least 6 months (to minimize seasonal variation or measurement error) should be annualized and plotted on an HV curve.
  - Normal HV is >4 cm/year in children and >8 cm/year during pubertal growth spurt.
- **Question:** Birth measurements and gestational age?
- *Significance*: Intrauterine growth restriction (IUGR) and/or small for gestational age (SGA) can be associated with possible maternal disorders, genetic disorders, and intrauterine drug exposure or stress that later impact growth.
- **Question:** Postnatal history including hypoglycemia or prolonged jaundice?
- *Significance*: Birth trauma, prolonged jaundice, and postnatal hypoglycemia can be associated with hypopituitarism.
- **Question:** Family history of short stature or delayed puberty?
- *Significance*:
  - Short stature in family members may suggest a heritable growth disorder.
  - Consider a diagnosis of constitutional delay of growth and puberty.
- **Question:** Social situation?
- *Significance*: Psychosocial stressors affect growth and development.
- **Question:** Dietary and feeding history?
- *Significance*: Low daily intake, difficulty feeding, or inefficient use of calories may point to malabsorptive disorders, anorexia.
- **Question:** Developmental milestones?
- *Significance*: delays may signal associated syndrome, chromosomal or metabolic disorder.
- **Question:** Chronic illness or any prior hospitalization, surgery, or head trauma?
- *Significance*: Growth failure may be the only sign of disease such as rheumatoid arthritis, celiac disease, or inflammatory bowel disease (IBD). Previous hospitalizations, trauma, or surgery may be a sign of underlying or acquired pathology. Head trauma may cause hypopituitarism.
- **Question:** Any medication use?
- *Significance*: Use of oral or inhaled steroids as well as stimulant medications can lead to short stature or HV deceleration.
- The history should be completed by obtaining a full review of systems, specifically inquiring about general development, headache, emesis, vision change, anorexia, fatigue, weight change, bowel irregularities, pubertal development, exercise tolerance, polyuria and polydipsia, activity pattern, sleep hygiene.
- Although boys are more frequently referred for short stature, girls are more likely to have a pathologic reason for short stature.

PHYSICAL EXAM

- **Finding:** Low upper to lower segment ratio?
- *Significance*: suggests scoliosis
- **Finding:** Abnormal trunk-to-arm span ratio?
- *Significance*: suggests skeletal dysplasia
- **Finding:** Low weight-to-height ratio?
- *Significance*: FTT, malnutrition, psychosocial deprivation, stimulant medication, chronic systemic illness, or metabolic disorders
- **Finding:** Proportionate/high weight-to-height ratio?
- *Significance*: If normal/near normal HV, then familial short stature, genetic syndrome, SGA, constitutional delay, mild chronic disease, prior resolved growth-attenuating disorder, or acquired growth limitations. If associated with low HV, suggests endocrine disorder, chronic disease, or growth-affecting medications
- **Finding:** Dysmorphic features?
- *Significance*: Primary growth disorders
- **Finding:** Mid-facial hypoplasia, cherubic appearance, truncal fat deposition?
- *Significance*: suggests GH deficiency
- **Finding:** Goiter, edema, slow relaxation of deep tendon reflexes, hair loss, dry skin?
- *Significance*: hypothyroidism
- **Finding:** Abdominal distention or tenderness and gluteal wasting?
- *Significance*: malabsorption and celiac disease
- **Finding:** Webbed neck, increased carrying angle, shield chest, lymphedema?
- *Significance*: Turner or Noonan Syndrome
- **Finding:** Microphallus?
- *Significance*: hypogonadism, GH deficiency
- **Finding:** Abnormal funduscopic or cranial nerve exam? Midline abnormalities?
- *Significance*: CNS pathology ± associated hypopituitarism
- **Finding:** Signs of neglect or abuse?
- *Significance*: psychosocial dwarfism
- **Finding:** Round face, hypocalcemia, short 4th and 5th metacarpals, and mental retardation?
- *Significance*: pseudohypoparathyroidism
- **Finding:** Hypertension, virilization, moon face, buffalo hump, thick violaceous striae
- *Significance*: glucocorticoid excess
- **Finding:** Delayed pubertal maturation?
- *Significance*: Turner syndrome, constitutional delay, hypogonadism, hypothyroidism, IBD, chronic renal disease
- **Finding:** Leg bowing, widening of wrists, rachitic rosary, frontal bossing?
- *Significance*: rickets, malabsorption

DIAGNOSTIC TESTS & INTERPRETATION

- **Test:** X-ray study of the left hand and wrist
- *Significance*: bone age (BA) determination (not reliable in kids <2 years of age)
- **Test:** IgA and anti-tissue transglutaminase IgA
- *Significance*: celiac disease

- **Test:** CBC with differential
- *Significance*: anemia, infection, malignancy, or chronic inflammatory conditions
- **Test:** C-reactive protein (CRP) and/or erythrocyte sedimentation rate (ESR)
- *Significance*: infection, inflammatory conditions
- **Test:** Complete metabolic panel
- *Significance*: Screen for renal/liver disorders, malnutrition, calcium disorders.
- **Test:** Urinalysis
- *Significance*: diabetes, renal/metabolic issue
- **Test:** Thyroxine and TSH
- *Significance*: hypothyroidism
- **Test:** Karyotype or targeted gene testing
- *Significance*: Turner syndrome in girls, *SHOX* mutation, or other chromosomal disorders
- **Test:** IGF-1 and IGFBP-3 concentrations, compared to pubertally matched norms
- *Significance*: Proxy measurements for GH secretory reserve and screen for GH deficiency. Not reliable <3 years of age and can be falsely low in poor nutrition states.

DIFFERENTIAL DIAGNOSIS

- Extremes of normal growth:
  - Familial short stature
    - Normal exam, no systemic illness
    - Consistent short stature with normal HV
    - Normal BA, onset of puberty
    - Adult height is short, close to MPH.
  - Constitutional short stature/delay of growth
    - Family history common
    - Normal exam, no systemic illness
    - Proportionately short; height percentile below MPH
    - Decelerating HV during first 3 years of life with normal to near-normal HV until puberty, when delays in pubertal timing lead to decreased HV compared to peers
    - Delayed BA and pubertal maturation
    - Adult height commensurate with MPH.
  - Idiopathic short stature
    - Categorizes otherwise normal patients who cannot be diagnosed with a variant of normal growth or other short stature cause
    - Predicted adult height is >2 *SD* below MPH.
    - Height is $<$3rd percentile $\pm$ delayed BA.
- Primary growth disorders: disorders intrinsic to skeletal system, BA normal
  - Skeletal dysplasia/defects: may lead to disproportionate short stature. Skeletal involvement can be subtle.
    - Skeletal radiographs with typical findings
    - Common forms: achondroplasia, hypochondroplasia, dyschondrosteosis (Leri-Weill and other *SHOX* mutations)
  - Syndromes
    - Usually associated with other abnormalities
    - Clinical findings may be subtle (mosaicism)
    - Common forms: trisomies (13, 18, 21), Turner or Noonan syndrome, Prader-Willi, DiGeorge, neurofibromatosis type 1
  - IUGR and SGA
    - Often due to maternal, fetal, or placental problems and/or exposures, or idiopathic
    - SGA infants have relative GH resistance seen as elevated GH with low IGF-1 levels.
    - 10% of SGA don't have catch-up growth with height $SD < -2$ by 2 years and need endocrine evaluation.
  - Primordial dwarfism: inherited intrinsic defect leading to prenatal and postnatal growth failure
- Secondary short stature
  - Malnutrition
    - Most common cause internationally
    - Poor nutrition (caloric, vitamin, mineral)
    - Especially <2 years of age
  - Chronic illness: Poor growth can be presenting symptom.
    - Hematopoietic (anemia, sickle cell)
    - Cardiovascular (congenital heart defect)
    - Pulmonary (severe asthma, cystic fibrosis)
    - GI/liver (IBD, celiac disease, malabsorption syndromes, chronic liver disease)
    - Renal (renal tubular acidosis, Fanconi syndrome, uropathy, congenital anomalies)
    - Metabolic (poorly controlled diabetes mellitus, storage disorders, disorders of calcium and phosphorous metabolism)
    - Infectious/Immunologic (HIV)
  - Iatrogenic
    - Medications: glucocorticoids, stimulants
    - Treatment of childhood malignancy, irradiation, chemotherapy
  - Psychosocial growth retardation
    - Emotional deprivation
    - Anorexia
    - Depression
  - Endocrine
    - GH or IGF-1 deficiency/resistance, hypogonadism, hypothyroidism, Cushing syndrome, short stature from earlier accelerated bone maturation (e.g., precocious puberty, hyperthyroidism, congenital adrenal hyperplasia)
    - Among secondary short stature, endocrine causes are *least* frequent.

TREATMENT

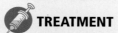

ADDITIONAL TREATMENT

General Measures

Evaluation warranted if HV low for age or growth pattern deviates significantly from the MPH target.

- In the majority of short children, history and exam are unrevealing, and tests yield equivocal or normal results. These children are then considered to have idiopathic short stature.
- Observation is reasonable for familial short stature or constitutional delay.
- In cases of malnutrition, restoration of adequate nutrition results in HV acceleration.
- In cases of endocrinopathies, replacement of the deficient hormone (thyroid hormone for hypothyroidism, GH for GH deficiency, hydrocortisone for adrenal insufficiency) or removal of excess hormone (glucocorticoids) will normalize the HV.
- Children with short stature or poor predicted adult height, who do not have true GH deficiency, may receive different treatment options depending on costs, risks, physician practice, extent of family's concern, and presence of associated psychosocial stressors (e.g., teasing by peers).

ISSUES FOR REFERRAL

- Critical to obtain accurate measurements plotted appropriately to assess growth
- Referrals should be guided by abnormal laboratory evaluations or clinical suspicion (i.e., nephrology referral for elevated creatinine, pulmonary referral for clubbing).
- Endocrine referral warranted if slow HV, growth plateau, delayed bone age with short stature/growth failure, or suggestive labs.
- If poor weight gain, consider nutritional deficiency, malabsorption syndromes. Initial referral to gastroenterologist appropriate.
- The evaluation of growth failure or short stature best done in outpatient setting.

ADDITIONAL READING

- Allen DB, Cuttler L. Clinical practice. Short stature in childhood—challenges and choices. *N Engl J Med*. 2013;368(13):1220–1228.
- Oostdijk W, Grote FK, de Muinck Keizer-Schrama SM, et al. Diagnostic approach in children with short stature. *Horm Res*. 2009;72(4):206–217.
- Rose S, Vogiatzi M, Copeland K. A general pediatric approach to evaluating a short child. *Pediatr Rev*. 2005;26(11):410–420.

CODES

ICD10

- R62.52 Short stature (child)
- E34.3 Short stature due to endocrine disorder
- E23.0 Hypopituitarism

FAQ

- Q: Does short stature portend worse psychosocial outcomes?
- A: This has not been found when studied in the general population. The degree of parent and child distress from short stature is also filtered by referral bias, as those who seek care have the highest degree of concern and anxiety.
- Q: How much height does a child with idiopathic short stature gain from treatment with recombinant growth hormone?
- A: 1.2–2.8 inches in final adult height, at a cost of \$10,000–\$60,000 per patient per year. Height gains are much better in other conditions such as true GH deficiency and Turner syndrome, but the cost remains steep.
- Q: What is a reasonable strategy for constitutional delay of growth and puberty?
- A: Observation and reassurance alone are frequently all that is needed. In males of pubertal age (13–14 years), however, a course of low-dose intramuscular testosterone may be considered to "jump start" pubertal changes and the corresponding growth spurt.

SHORT-BOWEL SYNDROME

Christina Bales • Judith Kelsen

BASICS

DESCRIPTION

Malnutrition, malabsorption, and/or fluid and electrolyte loss after extensive small-bowel resection

PATHOPHYSIOLOGY

- Markedly decreased mucosal surface area due to resection
- Loss of trophic hormones
- Loss of peptide hormones that regulate motility
- Abnormal transit
- Malabsorption of protein, fat, carbohydrate, vitamins, electrolytes, and trace elements, depending on site of resected intestine
  - Patient can lose as much as half of intestine if the duodenum, distal ileum, and ileocecal valve (ICV) are present.
  - If the ICV is gone, patients may not be able to tolerate even a 25% loss of intestine without the help of parenteral nutrition (PN).
- Normal bowel length: 150–200 cm, 26 weeks' gestation; 200–300 cm at birth in full-term infant; 600–800 cm, adult
  - Infants have low intestinal reserve; do not tolerate resection as well as do adults.
  - However, long-term prognosis is often better because of hypertrophy and hyperplasia of the intestine.
- Gastric acid hypersecretion occurs soon after intestinal resection but is transient.
- Bowel adaptation can occur over time. Increased surface area due to bowel dilatation, villous hypertrophy, and bowel lengthening can occur. Stimulation of luminal contents is needed for bowel growth, and factors such as glutamine, short-chain fatty acids, tropic hormones, and growth factors may be important for bowel growth.

ETIOLOGY

- Infants: intestinal resection for necrotizing enterocolitis
- Congenital anomalies include intestinal atresias, gastroschisis, omphalocele, and meconium ileus.
- Malrotation may result in volvulus with bowel resection secondary to ischemic injury.
- Older children: neoplasms and radiation enteritis
- Intestinal resection secondary to Crohn disease, trauma, pseudoobstruction syndrome

DIAGNOSIS

HISTORY

- Defecation pattern: number, size, nature (watery, bulky, foul smelling), presence of blood and mucus
- Ostomy output: consistency (watery, viscous, thick), volume (≥50 mL/kg/day often leads to dehydration and electrolyte imbalance)
- Weight loss or gain; gaining length/height
- Abdominal distention and flatulence
- Intense perianal rashes related to stool acidity and malabsorption of carbohydrates
- Abdominal pain and characteristics
- Vomiting and characteristics
- Diet history: appetite, oral intake, tube feeds, PN
- Central line–associated bloodstream infection (CLABSI) history (if receiving PN)
- Medication history
- Surgical history

PHYSICAL EXAM

- Weight, length, and head circumference measurements (if applicable); obtain previous growth chart if available
- Signs of vitamin deficiencies in exam of mouth, lips, skin, hair, and skeleton and in assessment of healing difficulties
- Signs of liver disease (icterus, hepatomegaly, splenomegaly, dilated abdominal veins)
- Signs of vascular thrombosis (extremity swelling, dilated veins in neck region)
- Abdominal exam: surgical scars, ostomies, distention, bowel sounds
- Rectal exam: consistency of stool, heme positivity, perianal rash

DIAGNOSTIC TESTS & INTERPRETATION

Lab

- Blood tests
  - CBC: Check for anemia, mean corpuscular volume.
  - Electrolytes: Check for losses and adequacy of replacement.
  - Minerals: calcium, phosphorus, magnesium, iron, zinc; check for losses and adequacy of replacement therapy
  - Albumin and prealbumin: Check for protein stores and nutritional status.
  - Liver evaluation: Alanine aminotransferase (ALT), γ-glutamyl transpeptidase (GGT), and bilirubin may be elevated in PN-associated liver disease (PNALD).
  - Vitamin levels
    - Vitamin A, 25-hydroxy vitamin D, vitamin E, RBC folate, and vitamin B_{12}; check for adequacy
    - An elevated methylmalonic acid (MMA) level is a more sensitive marker of B_{12} deficiency but may also be elevated in small-bowel bacterial overgrowth.
    - Prothrombin time/international normalized ratio (PT/INR) indirectly measures vitamin K deficiency. PIVKa (the protein induced in vitamin K absence) is a more sensitive marker of vitamin K deficiency.
  - Carnitine: Check status if on long-term PN and presence of liver disease.
  - Breath tests: lactose and lactulose breath test to check for lactase deficiency and bacterial overgrowth, respectively
- Stool tests
  - Stool for pH and reducing substances: Check for carbohydrate malabsorption.
  - Stool smear for fat (Sudan stain—qualitative): Check for excessive fat loss.
  - Stool for blood: Check for mucosal damage.
  - Stool elastase: measure of pancreatic insufficiency. May be falsely depressed if watery stools (dilutional effect)
- Tests of absorption
  - D-xylose absorption test and lactose breath test to check for carbohydrate malabsorption
  - 72-hour quantitative fecal fat collection along with concomitant diet record
  - Carotene levels to check for fat absorption
  - 24-hour stool collection for α-1-antitrypsin clearance to check for protein absorption

Imaging

Upper GI series with small-bowel follow-through and barium enema to evaluate length, caliber, and location of remaining bowel

Diagnostic Procedures/Other

Endoscopy

- Upper endoscopy: Look for presence of inflammation that may be contributing to malabsorption; obtain and culture duodenal aspirates to assess for bacterial overgrowth.
- Lower endoscopy: Look for presence of colitis, especially eosinophilic colitis. Evaluate caliber and quality of anastomosis site if in colon.

DIFFERENTIAL DIAGNOSIS

- Infants: necrotizing enterocolitis, volvulus, atresia (jejunal and ileal), gastroschisis, perforated meconium ileus, congenital short-bowel syndrome, aganglionosis of the intestine
- Older children: midgut volvulus (due to malrotation), Crohn disease, adhesions causing intestinal obstruction, strictures, trauma

TREATMENT

MEDICATION

- Supplementation of deficient vitamins (E, D, K, B_{12}, folic acid) calcium, magnesium, iron, and zinc
- H_2-receptor antagonists and proton pump inhibitors decrease gastric acid hypersecretion and reduce gastric secretory volume (particularly in the postoperative period).
- Antidiarrheal drugs codeine, diphenoxylate, and anticholinergic drugs (e.g., loperamide) to decrease motility (caution in patients with slow transit or bacterial overgrowth)
- Ion-exchange resins: Cholestyramine binds intraluminal dihydroxy bile acids to prevent bile acid–induced diarrhea.
- Octreotide/somatostatin: decreases gastric, pancreatic, and intestinal secretions; slows GI motility. Use with caution, though, as may reduce splanchnic blood flow.
- Bacterial overgrowth: Commonly used oral antibiotics are metronidazole, trimethoprim-sulfamethoxazole, ciprofloxacin, vancomycin, and gentamicin.
- Prokinetic agents: Reglan to treat delayed gastric emptying. Use with caution given potential side effects.
- Ethanol lock therapy has demonstrated some preliminary success in reducing CLABSI. Therapy may be associated with an increased risk of venous thrombosis. Randomized control trials in the pediatric short-bowel population are needed.

- Miscellaneous
  - Sucralfate to treat bile reflux
  - Probiotics to treat bacterial overgrowth
  - Ursodiol for cholestasis
  - Polycitra for electrolyte losses
  - Dietary fiber to enhance absorption; caution in infancy and in patients with bacterial overgrowth

SURGERY/OTHER PROCEDURES

- Surgery is useful in patients who develop strictures and partial obstruction or in those who have very short intestine length with one or more significantly dilated segments distal to the duodenum.
- Intestinal interpositions (isoperistaltic or antiperistaltic) historically are used to delay gastric emptying, slow intestinal transit, and increase absorption but have largely fallen out of favor.
- Intestinal lengthening and tapering procedures, including the Bianchi and serial transverse enteroplasty (STEP) procedures, increase absorptive surface area.
- In patients with extremely short intestines and PN dependency, small-bowel transplantation or multivisceral transplantation is considered. Factors favoring consideration: advanced liver disease, recurrent prolonged hospitalizations, life-threatening bloodstream infections, and loss of central venous access sites.

ONGOING CARE

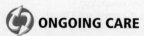

FOLLOW-UP RECOMMENDATIONS

Patient Monitoring

- Signs to watch for:
  - Vomiting, diarrhea, weight loss, severe fluid and electrolyte abnormalities, sepsis, bowel dilatation, intestinal obstruction
- Major cause of death: sepsis and cholestatic liver disease

DIET

- Fluid and electrolyte therapy: extremely important in the acute phase immediately after bowel resection. In the chronic phase, it is important to keep up with ongoing losses, especially when enteral feeds are started.
- Oral diet
  - For patients who are able to avoid PN or tube feeds, a low-lactose diet may be well tolerated.
  - Low-oxalate diets are helpful in preventing oxalate stones.
  - In general, a high-calorie diet regardless of carbohydrate and fat composition should be the mainstay of treatment.
- Enteral feeds: more successful in the patient with less extensive resection, intact ICV, and colon in continuity. In extensive loss, feeds are initiated after electrolytes are stabilized.
  - Feeds started very slowly, often started with elemental diet to facilitate absorption and for concern for allergic injury.
  - Enteral feeds stimulate intestinal adaptation. Before 1 year of age, formula should have low osmolality: higher fat content than carbohydrate.
  - After 1 year of age, there is no advantage of elemental formulas over intact formulas with respect to tolerance, unless small-bowel damage is present.
- Development of oral skills and oral feeding should be encouraged when possible, as introduction of solid foods with maturity slows transit and improves enteral capacity.
- PN: important in the acute phase postoperatively, when nutrition must be maintained in the face of paralytic ileus; indispensable in the chronic phase when full enteral feeds cannot be instituted.
  - Balanced solutions of protein, glucose, and fat should be administered.
  - Prophylactic measures to prevent PN-induced liver damage should be instituted (e.g., prevention of overfeeding, early introduction of enteral feeds, cycling of PN when patient is stable, limitation of IV fat emulsion).
  - If cholestasis is present, it may be necessary to modify amount of trace elements in PN.
  - Need permanent central access to deliver concentrated PN solutions
- IV fish-based oil emulsion (composed of omega-3 polyunsaturated fatty acids) has been studied as a preventive measure against PN-associated liver disease with promising results.

PROGNOSIS

- Contingent on site and amount of bowel resected
- Adaptation is better after jejunal resection than after ileal resection.
- More extensive resection (<40 cm of residual bowel in neonatal period) and loss of the ICV portend a worse prognosis.
- Duration of PN is inversely related to prognosis.
- Most progress is made in the 1st year after bowel resection. Children who are PN dependent at 5 years of age may be unlikely to wean from PN.
- Severe PN-associated liver disease portends a poor prognosis.

COMPLICATIONS

- Fluid and electrolyte loss, resulting in diarrhea, dehydration, and metabolic acidosis
- Calcium and magnesium deficiency, resulting in bone disease and osteoporosis
- Carbohydrate malabsorption
- Fat malabsorption
- Vitamin A deficiency: increased susceptibility to infections
- Vitamin D deficiency: rickets
- Vitamin E deficiency: peripheral neuropathy, hemolysis
- Vitamin K deficiency: prolonged clotting time, bruising
- Vitamin B_{12}: macrocytic anemia and leukopenia
- Folic acid: macrocytic anemia
- Iron deficiency: microcytic anemia
- Copper deficiency: pancytopenia
- Zinc deficiency: poor wound healing, diarrhea, poor vertical growth
- Essential fatty acid deficiency: increased susceptibility to infection, decreased energy stores
- Gallstones: due to disturbed enterohepatic circulation of bile salts and lithogenic bile formation
- Renal stones: due to fat malabsorption and increased oxalate absorption
- Failure to thrive
- TPN-dependent liver disease: cholestasis, end-stage cirrhosis, and portal hypertension
- Carnitine deficiency: contributes to development of steatosis
- Sepsis
- Small-bowel bacterial overgrowth and D-lactic acidosis due to stasis, causing encephalopathy, ataxia, and other neurologic symptoms

ADDITIONAL READING

- Cober PM, Killu G, Brattain A, et al. Intravenous fat emulsions reduction for patients with parenteral nutrition-associated liver disease. *J Pediatr*. 2012;160(3):421–427.
- Cole CR, Kocoshis SA. Nutrition management in infants with surgical short bowel syndrome and intestinal failure. *Nutr Clin Pract*. 2013;28(4): 421–428.
- Duro D, Kamin D, Duggan C. Overview of pediatric short bowel syndrome. *J Pediatr Gastroenterol Nutr*. 2008;47(Suppl 1):S33–S36.
- Mercer DF, Hobson BD, Gerhardt BK, et al. Serial transverse enteroplasty allows children with short bowel syndrome to wean from parenteral nutrition. *J Pediatr*. 2014;164(1):93–98.
- Pieroni KP, Nespor C, Ng M, et al. Evaluation of ethanol lock therapy in pediatric patients in long-term parenteral nutrition. *Nutr Clin Pract*. 2013;28(2):226–231.
- Puder M, Valim C, Meisel JA, et al. Parenteral fish oil improves outcomes in patients with parenteral nutrition associated liver injury. *Ann Surg*. 2009; 250(3):395–402.
- Rudolph JA, Squires R. Current concepts in the management of pediatric intestinal failure. *Curr Opin Organ Transplant*. 2010;15(3):324–329.

CODES

ICD10

K91.2 Postsurgical malabsorption, not elsewhere classified

FAQ

- Q: What are the favorable prognostic factors in short-bowel syndrome?
- A: Greater length of residual small bowel, jejunal versus ileal resection, maintenance of the ICV, and lack of PN-associated liver disease. Neonates demonstrate better bowel adaptation than do adults.
- Q: Are elemental formulas better than intact formulas in the management of patients with short-bowel syndrome?
- A: Limited case series suggest that elemental formulas may be associated with a shorter duration of PN dependence than intact formula, which may be related to a higher incidence of food allergy in the short bowel population. However, elemental formulas have a higher cost and higher osmolarity, which may exacerbate diarrhea. Animal studies suggest that intestinal adaptation is improved with nutrient complexity, suggesting that elemental formula may be inferior to intact protein formula in this regard.

SICKLE CELL DISEASE

Keith Quirolo

BASICS

DESCRIPTION

Sickle cell disease (SCD) is a hemoglobinopathy caused by a one base pair change leading to an amino acid change in the beta globin gene at the sixth position: glutamic acid to valine. The mutation allows the polymerization of hemoglobin in the red cell.

PATHOPHYSIOLOGY

- Disruption of the red cell membrane: leading to increased adhesion to vascular endothelium, activation of cytokines leading to activation of platelets and leukocytes, activation of the coagulation system leading to a hypercoagulable state and ultimately to vaso-occlusion. Red cells release red cell membrane as microparticles.
- Red cell hemolysis: release of free hemoglobin, methemoglobin production, increased plasma ferric iron leading to oxidative stress, decreased nitric oxide leading to decreased production of cyclic GMP causing vasoconstriction, inflammation, and platelet activation

EPIDEMIOLOGY

- The incidence of SCD is 1 in 500 African Americans, 1 in 36,000 Hispanics, with a lesser frequency in other ethnic groups. The incidence of sickle cell trait in African Americans is 1 in 14.
- There are 70,000–100,000 affected individuals with SCD in the United States.

RISK FACTOR

Genetics

- SCD is autosomal recessive.
- Combinations leading to the disease state when inherited with hemoglobin S: SS, SC, S beta zero thalassemia, S beta plus thalassemia, S $D^{\text{Los Angeles}}$, and S O^{Arab} are examples.

DIAGNOSIS

HISTORY

- At diagnosis:
  - In the US, usually diagnosed on newborn screening
  - Often asymptomatic in early infancy (<6 months) due to protective effects of residual HbF production.
  - Family history
  - History of irritability/pain
  - History of pallor
- Subsequent to diagnosis
  - SCD genotype
  - History of:
    - Surgery
    - Transfusion (red cell phenotype)
    - Hospitalizations (particularly ICU)
    - Pain (sites and usual therapy)
    - Stroke and/or transcranial Doppler (TCD) abnormalities
    - Acute chest syndrome
  - Baseline hemoglobin and pulse oximetry
  - Current medication and therapy

PHYSICAL EXAM

- Pallor of anemia with flow murmur
- Scleral icterus
- Splenomegaly, hepatomegaly
- Respiratory effort, decreased breath sounds, or wheeze: obstructive lung disease
- Decreased range of motion: hip and shoulder avascular necrosis
- Neurologic examination: stroke
- Developmental assessment

DIAGNOSTIC TESTS & INTERPRETATION

Lab

- Diagnostic
  - All states have newborn screening.
  - F: thalassemia major
  - FA: normal hemoglobin
  - FAS: A > S: sickle cell trait
  - FSA: S > A: SCD, S beta plus thalassemia
  - FS: hemoglobin S: sickle cell anemia or sickle beta zero thalassemia
  - FSC: hemoglobin SC disease
  - FSV: sickle hemoglobin with variant hemoglobin
  - Alpha gene mapping
    - Alpha thalassemia trait influences the phenotype.
  - Beta gene analysis
    - Beta thalassemia and beta variants
- Monitoring
  - CBC: Degree of anemia depends on genotype, leukocytosis, elevated platelet count, low mean corpuscular volume (MCV) with beta and alpha thalassemia, elevated MCV with hydroxyurea therapy, elevated reticulocyte count corresponding to degree of anemia.
  - Hemoglobin electrophoresis: hydroxyurea and transfusion therapy
  - Chemistry panel: elevated lactate dehydrogenase (LDH), unconjugated bilirubin, aspartate aminotransferase (AST)
  - Vitamin D 25-OH level
  - TCD annually: stroke risk, 2–16 years
  - Brain MRI/MRA: abnormal TCD or neurologic findings
  - Echocardiogram: pulmonary hypertension
  - Pulmonary function testing: obstructive lung disease
  - Ophthalmology: retinopathy
  - Neurocognitive testing: stroke or school delay

TREATMENT

GENERAL MEASURES

- Infection prophylaxis with oral penicillin 125 mg b.i.d. starting by 2 months of age, 250 mg b.i.d. at 36 months
- Pneumococcal vaccine (23-valent at 2 and 5 years of age)
- Meningococcal vaccine
- Recommended routine immunizations
- Folic acid and vitamin D supplementation as indicated
- Parent teaching for fever, splenic sequestration, anemia, stroke, acute chest, and home pain management
- Hospital pain management plan

ADDITIONAL TREATMENT

- Hydroxyurea: Patients who have two or more acute events leading to hospitalization a year or more frequent pain events not leading to hospitalization are considered for treatment.
  - Beginning doses are between 15 and 20 mg/kg/24h If needed, increase dose by 5 mg/kg/24h every 2–6 months up to a maximum of 35 mg/kg/24h or 2,500 mg/24h (whichever is less).
  - Monitor initially at 2 weeks and 1 month.
  - Without toxicity, monitor every 2 months.
- Red cell transfusion can prevent complications, morbidity, and are lifesaving.
  - Phenotypically matched red cells (for ABO, D, C, c, E, e, Kell) decreases alloimmunization.
  - Optimum hemoglobin is 9–10 g/dL, higher levels increase viscosity, decrease oxygenation.
  - Percentage of hemoglobin S should be <30% in acute disease, for stroke and stroke prevention.
  - With elevated hemoglobin or when a low percent S is indicated, exchange transfusion is required.
  - Transfusion iron overload: All patients are monitored and treated with oral chelation.
- Progenitor cell transplant is the only cure for SCD.
  - Full siblings: HLA typing for the patient and the prospective donor
  - Cord blood collection for full siblings
  - Consultation with a transplant physician familiar with transplantation for sickle cell anemia

INPATIENT CONSIDERATIONS

- Fever
  - Patients with SCD and fever are presumed septic.
    - History, physical exam, CBC with reticulocytes, blood culture, chest x-ray, urine culture, and other cultures as indicated
    - Parenteral antibiotic: (ceftriaxone) until culture negative
    - Children younger than the age of 3 years, admitted to hospital
    - Older children and adolescents with a benign examination, no pulmonary infiltrate, or urinary tract infection: ceftriaxone follow-up in 24 hours
- Acute chest syndrome
  - Defined as a new pulmonary infiltrate frequently accompanied by hypoxia, pain, fever, and severe anemia
  - Treat for fever (above).
  - Type and cross
  - Transfusion for severe anemia, progressive infiltrate, hypoxia
  - Add microlide antibiotic.
  - Oxygen to maintain O_2 saturation 95%.
  - Fluid overload can exacerbate pulmonary disease, monitor I and O.
  - Incentive spirometry q2h
- Pain (vaso-occlusive episode)
  - Severe pain is a medical emergency.
  - Hydration: 1.5 maintenance, avoid fluid overload.
  - Incentive spirometry: q2h
  - Pain assessment on pain scale
  - Analgesics
    - Mild pain: NSAIDs and mild oral opioids (20% will not metabolize codeine normally)
    - Moderate pain: may need parenteral therapy with opioids and ketorolac
    - Severe pain: admission with patient-controlled analgesia (PCA) parenteral opioids, may need antihistamine, ketorolac, H_2 blocker with ketorolac
  - Pain assessment after administration of medications
  - Adjunctive therapy: heating pad, visualization, distraction, other therapy
- Acute anemia
  - Parvoviral infection
    - History of decreased energy, pallor
    - Exam with tachycardia, pallor
    - CBC with reticulocyte count: anemia with reticulocytopenia
    - Type and cross
    - Transfusion for severe anemia or cardiovascular compromise
    - Parvoviral B19 titers
    - Isolation precautions
- Splenic sequestration
  - History of decreased energy, pallor
  - Exam with splenomegaly
  - CBC with reticulocyte count: anemia with reticulocytosis
  - Slow transfusion for severe anemia or cardiovascular compromise: Spleen releases red cells increasing hemoglobin and viscosity.
  - Splenectomy for life-threatening or repeated episodes: Immunize prior to splenectomy.
- Stroke
  - Diagnosis by history and physical examination
  - Treatment should not be delayed for imaging.
  - Evidence suggests initial exchange transfusion, to hemoglobin of 9–10 g/dL, percent hemoglobin S of less than 30%, leads to improved long-term outcome.
  - All patients should have brain MRI and MRA urgently and be evaluated by neurology and physical therapy.
  - Eventually, all patients should have neuropsychological testing.
  - Chronic transfusion for life
- Intracranial hemorrhage
  - Initially present with headache only
  - CT scan is diagnostic.
  - More common in adolescents
  - History of cerebral vascular disease
  - Neurosurgical consultation
  - Exchange transfusion is indicated.
  - Prognosis is poor if not aggressively treated.
  - Chronic transfusion for life
- Stroke risk
  - Abnormal TCD
  - Time average maximum mean velocity: 200 cm/s or greater
  - Transfusion to hemoglobin of 10 g/dL
  - MRI–MRA for cerebral vascular disease or ischemic brain injury
  - Transfusion for life with or without findings on MR
- Priapism
  - Diagnosis: unwanted erection with pain lasting for longer than 1 hour
  - Medical emergency
  - Initial management: pain management, intravenous hydration
  - Treatment with subcutaneous terbutaline has been used.
  - Definitive treatment: is aspiration and instillation of pseudoephedrine

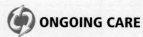

ONGOING CARE

PROGNOSIS

The prognosis for children with sickle cell disease has improved dramatically due to hydroxyurea therapy, increased use of blood transfusion, and screening. Transition to adult care is a priority.

- Chronic complications:
  - Cholecystitis
  - Avascular necrosis (hip and shoulder)
  - Obstructive pulmonary disease
  - Pulmonary hypertension
  - Renal disease (proteinuria)
  - Hyposthenuria (enuresis, dehydration)
  - Retinopathy (increased: SC disease)
  - School failure due to hospitalization
  - Cerebral vascular disease/infarcts

ADDITIONAL READING

- Ballas SK. New era dawns on sickle cell pain. *Blood*. 2010;116(3):311–312.
- Bernaudin F, Verlhac S, Arnaud C, et al. Impact of early transcranial Doppler screening and intensive therapy on cerebral vasculopathy outcome in a newborn sickle cell anemia cohort. *Blood*. 2011;117(4):1130–1140.
- Howard J, Malfroy M, Llewelyn C, et al. The Transfusion Alternatives Preoperatively in SCD (TAPS) study: a randomised, controlled, multicentre clinical trial. *Lancet*. 2013;81(9870):930–938.
- Thornburg CD, Files BA, Luo Z, et al. Impact of hydroxyurea on clinical events in the BABY HUG trial. *Blood*. 2012;120(22):4304–4310.

CODES

ICD-10

- D57.1 Sickle-cell disease without crisis
- D57.3 Sickle-cell trait
- D57.40 Sickle-cell thalassemia without crisis

FAQ

- Q: When can I stop penicillin prophylaxis?
- A: Most morbidity and mortality from infections in sickle cell anemia occur in the first 5 years of life. The risk of pneumococcal sepsis decreases with age but continues to be a significant risk of morbidity and mortality. Patients with surgical splenectomy need penicillin prophylaxis for life.
- Q: Are phenotypically matched red cells necessary for transfusion?
- A: Historically, the incidence of red cell alloimmunization is 30% for patients with SCD who do not receive phenotypically matched red cells. By providing phenotypically matched red cells, the rate of alloimmunization is significantly decreased.

SINUSITIS

Esther K. Chung • Julia Belkowitz

BASICS

DESCRIPTION
- Sinusitis is inflammation of the mucous membranes lining the paranasal sinuses.
- The term is most commonly used to describe bacterial rhinosinusitis, which is a clinical diagnosis made by the presence of upper respiratory tract symptoms that have not improved in 10 days or have worsened after 5–7 days. Diagnosis of sinusitis should be considered based on persistence and/or severity of symptoms.
- Classification based on duration of symptoms:
  - Acute: persistent nasal and sinus symptoms for 10–30 days; worsening or new onset of nasal discharge, daytime cough, or fever after initial improvement; or concurrent high fever and purulent nasal discharge for the first 3–4 days of an acute upper respiratory tract infection (URI)
  - Subacute: clinical symptoms for 30–90 days
  - Chronic: symptoms lasting >90 days
  - Recurrent: acute sinusitis with complete resolution of 10 days between episodes; 3 episodes in 6 months or 4 episodes in 1 year
- Classification by severity of illness:
  - Persistent: >10–14 days but <30 days; nasal discharge and/or daytime cough
  - Severe: temperature of ≥39°C (102.2°F) with concurrent purulent nasal discharge for ≥3 days and/or facial pain, headache, or periorbital edema

GENERAL PREVENTION
- Avoid allergen exposure and treat allergies if present.
- Improve mucociliary clearance by increasing ambient humidity with a humidifier.

PATHOPHYSIOLOGY
- Normal sinus function depends on patency of paranasal sinus ostia, function of the ciliary apparatus, and secretion quality.
- A buildup of secretions is due to ostial obstruction, reduction in ciliary function, and overproduction of secretions.
- Viral URIs and/or allergic rhinitis often precede an acute bacterial infection.

ETIOLOGY
- Viral pathogens (e.g., rhinovirus, parainfluenza virus) have been recovered in respiratory isolates, but their significance is unknown.
- Most illnesses of short duration (<7 days) are thought to be from viral infections and should not be treated with antibiotics.
- Chronic sinusitis often secondary to allergic rhinitis, cystic fibrosis, environmental pollutants, or gastroesophageal reflux
- Bacterial pathogens: with an increasing prevalence of penicillin resistance
- Most common pathogens:
  - *Haemophilus influenzae*, nontypeable
  - *Streptococcus pneumoniae*
  - *Moraxella catarrhalis*
- Other pathogens:
  - Group A streptococci
  - Group C streptococci
  - Peptostreptococci
  - Other *Moraxella* species
  - *Streptococcus viridans*
  - *Eikenella corrodens*
  - *Staphylococcus aureus*
  - *Pseudomonas aeruginosa* (in patients with cystic fibrosis)
  - Anaerobic organisms
  - Polymicrobial
  - Fungal pathogen: *Aspergillus*

DIAGNOSIS

HISTORY
- Previous sinusitis, previous antibiotic use, allergies, child care attendance
- Key symptoms to differentiate from viral URI:
  - Duration of symptoms >10 days or worsening of symptoms after initial improvement
  - Onset of fever, especially with a duration of ≥3–4 days, facial pain, purulent discharge at onset
- Some or all of the following may be present:
  - Nasal discharge: consistency, color. In older patients, nasal discharge may not be the primary complaint, but concurrent rhinitis is a common feature.
  - Postnasal drainage, nasal congestion
  - Fever
  - Recent history of a URI
  - Sore throat from mouth breathing due to nasal obstruction
  - Cough present during the day; may be worse at night
  - Malodorous breath
  - Hyposmia/anosmia
  - Maxillary dental pain
  - Facial swelling
  - Ear pressure or fullness
  - Headache and facial pain are uncommon in young children with sinusitis but may be seen in older children and adolescents.
  - Fatigue
  - Irritability
  - Snoring
  - Hyponasal speech

PHYSICAL EXAM
- Fever may be present.
- Nasal-sounding voice may be present.
- Malodorous breath may be noted but is not a specific indicator of sinusitis.
- Purulent drainage in the nose and/or oropharynx may be appreciated.
- Nasal mucosa may be erythematous, pale, and/or boggy, but these are nonspecific findings.
- Frontal, maxillary, and ethmoid areas may be tender to palpation/percussion.
- Headache and/or facial pain may change with position, increasing in intensity as the patient leans forward.
- Transillumination is not a reliable aid in diagnosis.
- Proptosis, eye swelling, and impaired extraocular movements suggest orbital infection.

DIAGNOSTIC TESTS & INTERPRETATION

Lab
- Gold standard is culture from sinuses via direct aspiration/ endoscopy; not indicated for diagnosis of acute, uncomplicated sinusitis
- For chronic or recurrent sinusitis, consider
  - Sweat chloride test to rule out cystic fibrosis
  - Immunoglobulin levels, IgG subclass levels, complement levels, and testing for human immunodeficiency virus (HIV) infection
  - Mucosal biopsy to assess ciliary function

Imaging
- Imaging is not recommended in uncomplicated cases of sinusitis.
- Sinus radiographs are of limited value with the exception of the Waters (occipitomental) view for identifying maxillary sinusitis.
  - Plain radiographs do not adequately identify ethmoid sinusitis.
  - Findings suggestive of sinusitis include complete sinus opacification, mucosal thickening ≥4 mm, and air–fluid levels.
- CT scan with contrast of the paranasal sinuses: useful in complicated, recurrent, and chronic sinusitis and/or history of polyposis
- CT scan of the head with contrast: indicated when sinusitis is accompanied by signs of increased intracranial pressure, meningeal irritation, proptosis, toxic appearance, limited extraocular movements, or focal neurologic deficits or in patients being considered for sinus-related surgery
- MRI of the sinuses: reserve for complicated cases and in immunocompromised patients in which fungal infection is suspected; will show mucosal thickening and fluid
- MRI with contrast of the head, as an alternative or adjunct to CT with contrast, when intracranial complications are suspected
- Pitfalls
  - Sinus radiographs may be abnormal in asymptomatic children or those with mild URIs.
  - Studies have shown a relatively high incidence of sinus abnormalities on CT scan in asymptomatic children, especially in infants <12 months of age. The significance of opacified sinuses in asymptomatic children is not well understood.
  - Up to 1/3 of patients with symptoms of chronic sinusitis may have normal CT scans.

DIFFERENTIAL DIAGNOSIS
- Infection: viral URI with or without mucopurulent rhinitis
- Environmental: allergic rhinitis
- Drug-induced: rhinitis medicamentosa
- Tumors
  - Nasal polyps
  - Hypertrophied adenoids
  - Neoplasms
- Trauma: foreign body (e.g., bead, cotton, tissue paper)
- Congenital
  - Septal deviation
  - Unilateral choanal atresia
  - Dysmotile cilia syndrome
- Dental disorder
- Other: vasomotor rhinitis

TREATMENT

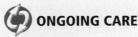

GENERAL MEASURES

- New guidelines support the option of observing children with persistent symptoms, but not those with worsening or severe symptoms, for 3 days before treating with antibiotic therapy.
- If orbital or CNS infection is suspected by history and examination, antibiotics should be started immediately, and emergency CT studies should be performed.
- Pitfalls
  - Diagnosis of sinusitis is being made with increasing frequency and may result in overtreatment, given that up to 50% will have spontaneous resolution.
  - With widespread antibiotic use, there are increasing numbers of resistant organisms.

MEDICATION

- Antibiotics
  - Appropriate drug choice depends on local resistance patterns.
  - High-risk children include age <2 years, hospitalization, antibiotic use within 3 months of diagnosis, and child care attendance.
  - 1st-line treatment: amoxicillin 45 mg/kg/day or 80–90 mg/kg/24 h of amoxicillin if high risk, local pneumococcal resistance >10%, severe symptoms or comorbidity, divided twice daily with a max of 2 g/dose
  - For non–type I penicillin allergy (late or delayed, >72 hours) or type I allergy (anaphylaxis) in children age 2 years and older, cefdinir (14 mg/kg/day), cefpodoxime (10 mg/kg/day), or cefuroxime axetil (30 mg/kg/24 h divided twice daily) may be used.
  - For type I penicillin allergy in children age <2 years, consider clindamycin combined with cefixime to cover resistant bacteria.
  - Macrolides and trimethoprim-sulfamethoxazole are not recommended due to high resistance rates.
  - Duration of treatment should be for 10 (minimum) to 28 days (and until 7 days beyond symptom resolution).
  - Consider changing antibiotic coverage and/or obtaining a culture if symptoms do not improve after 3–5 days of antibiotics, especially in a hospitalized patient.
  - Complicated sinusitis (CNS or orbital involvement) or children with toxic appearance: IV antibiotics and hospitalization; ceftriaxone (100 mg/kg/24 h in 2 doses) or ampicillin-sulbactam (200–400 mg ampicillin component/kg/day in 4 divided doses); cefotaxime 100–200 mg/kg/day divided every 6 hours or, if no other alternative, levofloxacin 10–20 mg/kg/day divided every 12–24 hours
  - If a hospitalized, ill child is not improving on the IV antibiotics listed above, consider adding vancomycin (60 mg/kg/24 h divided into 4 doses) for penicillin-resistant *S. pneumoniae* +/− metronidazole (30 mg/kg/24 h divided into 4 doses) for anaerobic coverage.
  - Chronic sinusitis: consider broad-spectrum antibiotic (amoxicillin/clavulanate [80–90 mg/kg/24 h of amoxicillin divided in 2 doses]) for at least 3 weeks and use of adjuvants such as saline irrigation or intranasal steroids; consider culture if no resolution after 1 week of treatment.
- Other pharmaceuticals:
  - Decongestants and antihistamines are not recommended due to side effects and lack of evidence of clinical improvement with use.
  - Mucolytics, such as guaifenesin, may improve mucous clearance.
  - Topical nasal steroids: may reduce and prevent mucosal swelling, which can lead to ostial occlusion, in patients with allergic rhinitis
- Other treatments:
  - Humidifier: may improve mucociliary clearance
  - Normal saline: Although there is no evidence to support its efficacy in acute sinusitis, saline irrigation and or spray is used by some for symptom relief; increases humidity and enhances mucociliary transport; vasoconstricts and improves drainage and ventilation

SURGERY/OTHER PROCEDURES

- Maxillary sinus aspiration: if unresponsive to multiple antibiotics, severe facial pain, and orbital or intracranial complications; should be performed by a trained ear, nose, and throat (ENT) specialist
- Surgery: performed as a last resort after medical therapy attempted and in patients with orbital or CNS complications

ONGOING CARE

PROGNOSIS

- Spontaneous resolution in up to 50% of patients
- Usually improves within 72 hours of initiation of antibiotics
- Excellent for those who are otherwise healthy

COMPLICATIONS

- Periorbital cellulitis
- Orbital cellulitis
- Orbital abscess
- Subperiosteal abscess
- Meningitis
- Intracranial abscess
- Optic neuritis
- Cavernous or sagittal sinus thrombosis
- Epidural, subdural, and brain abscess(es)
- Osteomyelitis of the maxilla
- Osteomyelitis of the frontal bone (Pott puffy tumor)

PATIENT MONITORING

- Immediate referral is indicated if there are CNS symptoms, periorbital edema, visual changes, facial swelling, extraocular muscle involvement, or proptosis.
- Radiographic soft tissue changes may last for up to 8 weeks; therefore, reimaging is of limited value.
- Referral to an otolaryngologist (ENT specialist) when sinusitis is chronic and not responsive to medical therapy, recurrent, complicated, or when there is polyposis

ADDITIONAL READING

- Brook I. Acute sinusitis in children. *Pediatr Clin North Am*. 2013;60(2):409–424.
- Chow AW, Benninger MS, Brook I, et al. IDSA Clinical practice guidelines for acute bacterial sinusitis in children and adults. *Clin Infect Dis*. 2012;54:1041–1045.
- DeMuri GP, Wald ER. Clinical practice. Acute bacterial sinusitis in children. *N Engl J Med*. 2012;367(12):1128–1134.
- Leo G, Triulzi F, Incorvaia C. Diagnosis of chronic sinusitis. *Pediatr Allergy Immunol*. 2012;23(Suppl 22):20–26.
- Setzen G, Ferguson BJ, Han JK, et al. Clinical consensus statement: appropriate use of computed tomography for paranasal sinus disease. *Otolaryngol Head Neck Surg*. 2012;147(5):808–816.
- Shaikh N, Wald ER, Pi M. Decongestants, antihistamines and nasal irrigation for acute sinusitis in children. *Cochrane Database Syst Rev*. 2012;9:CD007909. doi:10.1002/14651858.CD007909.pub3.
- Wald ER, Applegate KE, Bordley C, et al. Clinical practice guideline for the diagnosis and management of acute bacterial sinusitis in children aged 1 to 18 years. *Pediatrics*. 2013;132(1):e262–e280.

CODES

ICD10

- J32.9 Chronic sinusitis, unspecified
- J01.90 Acute sinusitis, unspecified
- J01.10 Acute frontal sinusitis, unspecified

FAQ

- Q: Are all of the sinuses present at birth?
- A: No. The maxillary and ethmoid sinuses form during the 3rd and 4th gestational months and are present at birth. They continue to enlarge until the preteen years. The sphenoid sinuses are pneumatized by 5 years; isolated sphenoid sinusitis is rare. The frontal sinuses are present at age 7–8 years and are not completely developed until late adolescence.
- Q: Does the nasal discharge seen with sinusitis have to be purulent and thick?
- A: No. Although the nasal discharge is often described as purulent and thick, it may also be clear or mucoid or thick or thin. Multiple studies have shown that a change in color or consistency is not a specific sign of a bacterial infection.
- Q: Are radiographic studies useful in the diagnosis of sinusitis?
- A: There is evidence to suggest that plain radiographs (x-rays) have limited value in the diagnosis of sinusitis and are not recommended in cases of uncomplicated sinusitis. Mucosal thickening may be seen with viral URIs and allergic rhinitis. Studies have shown that x-rays do not correlate well with CT scans in the diagnosis of chronic sinusitis.
- Q: Can one make the diagnosis of sinusitis based on CT scan results alone?
- A: No. Up to 50% of patients who had CT scans performed for other reasons had soft tissue changes in their sinuses. Mucosal thickening and opacification on CT imaging have been seen in large numbers of asymptomatic patients. These findings seem to occur more frequently in infants younger than 12 months of age. Given the poor specificity of CT imaging of the paranasal sinuses, results must be used in the context of the patient's clinical presentation.

SLEEP APNEA–OBSTRUCTIVE SLEEP APNEA SYNDROME

Akinyemi O. Ajayi

BASICS

DESCRIPTION

- Sleep-disordered breathing encompasses a range of breathing disorders occurring during sleep. These conditions include primary snoring (PS), respiratory events related to arousals (RERA), and obstructive sleep apnea syndrome (OSAS).
- Obstructive apnea is defined as the cessation of airflow at the nose and mouth despite respiratory effort, associated with some gas exchange abnormality and/or loss of regular sleep patterns.

PHYSIOLOGY

- OSAS may be subdivided into mild, moderate, and severe forms.
- Many children with OSAS exhibit partial airway obstruction. This is known as obstructive hypoventilation or hypopnea and is more commonly seen in children than is complete obstruction.
- OSAS is distinct from central apnea (cessation of airflow that is not accompanied by respiratory effort), which indicates brain immaturity or dysfunction.
- Upper airway resistance syndrome is a respiratory disorder characterized by partial airway obstruction and arousals leading to sleep fragmentation and is not associated with gas exchange abnormalities.
- Central apnea up to 20 seconds may be a normal finding in premature or newborn infants during the 1st month of life.
- Periodic breathing: 3 or more episodes of central apnea lasting at least 3 seconds each, separated by <20 seconds. Periodic breathing may be found in the newborn; however, it should not exceed >4% of sleep time (from a sleep study) and is not associated with bradycardia or hypoxemia.

RISK FACTORS

- In infants, OSAS is uncommon; however, it may exist with craniofacial anomalies, neurologic disorders associated with low muscle tone, laryngomalacia or tracheomalacia, and gastroesophageal reflux.
- Impaired arousal mechanisms also contribute to abnormalities seen in OSAS.
- In older children, OSAS may be associated with obesity. This form may resemble the adult type of OSAS.
- PS or habitual snoring implies snoring that does not lead to abnormalities in gas exchange or sleep fragmentation; however, 20–50% of children with habitual snoring may have OSAS.

Genetics

- Several genetic disorders with associated craniofacial anomalies, hypotonia, and obesity may lead to OSAS. These include the following:
  - Pierre Robin syndrome
  - Treacher Collins syndrome
  - Down syndrome
  - Mucopolysaccharide disorders
  - Arnold-Chiari malformations
  - Prader-Willi syndrome
  - Hereditary neuromuscular disorders

COMMONLY ASSOCIATED CONDITIONS

- Adenotonsillar hypertrophy
- Craniofacial anomalies including midfacial hypoplasia and mandibular hypoplasia
- Laryngomalacia
- Neurologic and neuromuscular disorders that cause hypotonia may underlie poor ventilation during sleep.
- Gastroesophageal reflux
- Obesity
- Metabolic disorders
- Allergic rhinitis, nasal septum deviation, nasal polyps
- Sedatives, seizure medications, and anesthesia

DIAGNOSIS

HISTORY

- Nocturnal symptoms include difficulty breathing when asleep, snoring, apnea, and restless sleep with frequent arousals.
- Daytime symptoms: excessive sleepiness, frequent upper respiratory/ear infections, conductive hearing loss, mouth breathing, poor appetite, and a hyponasal voice
- Other concerns: attention-deficit/hyperactivity disorder (ADHD), gastroesophageal reflux, poor school performance, and headaches (especially in the morning and upon awakening)
  - OSAS rarely produces these symptoms acutely but tends to occur over weeks to months.
  - Parents may notice that symptoms worsen with upper respiratory infections.
- The possibility of sleep-disordered breathing or a primary sleep disorder should be considered in children evaluated for ADHD.

PHYSICAL EXAM

- Assessment of the child's growth. In severe cases of OSAS, failure to thrive has been reported.
- Obesity remains a risk factor, especially in older children.
- Assessment of tonsillar size

ALERT

Normal-sized tonsils do not exclude OSAS.

- Presence of mouth breathing, hyponasal speech, adenoidal facies, midfacial hypoplasia, retrognathia, micrognathia, or other craniofacial anomalies may be present at times and may suggest the diagnosis.
- Nasal obstruction due to polyps, nasal septum deviation, turbinate hypertrophy, or congestion
- Tongue size
- Mobility and elevation of the soft palate; hard palate integrity
- In extreme cases, cardiac involvement may lead to cor pulmonale and heart failure. Examination may suggest signs of pulmonary hypertension or congestive heart failure, such as an increased second heart sound.
- A neurologic examination to evaluate general muscle strength, tone, and developmental status, especially in infants and children who do not improve after adenotonsillectomy

DIAGNOSTIC TESTS & INTERPRETATION

Lab

- Polysomnography
  - The gold standard for the diagnosis of OSAS is nocturnal polysomnography to differentiate the type of sleep apnea and to assess severity.
  - Polysomnography is an 8–10-hour-long multichannel study performed in a controlled setting to assess respiratory and/or sleep abnormalities.
  - Indices such as oxygenation, ventilation, apnea index (AI), apnea–hypopnea index (AHI), arousal index, arousal awakening index, and periodic limb movements index are determined along with sleep efficiency and sleep stages.
  - Monitoring includes electroencephalogram, electrooculogram, electromyogram, arterial oxygen saturation, end tidal CO_2 tension, airflow, respiratory effort, and electrocardiogram.
  - Normative respiratory and sleep variables for children have recently been published and include an AHI of <1 being normal.
  - Scoring for pediatric polysomnography differs from that of adults. This includes using 2 respiratory cycles to define both obstructive apnea and central apnea or 2 respiratory cycles associated with a 30% decline in airflow and a >4% decline in oxygen level to define hypopnea. Lower AHI values are considered significant in children compared with adults.
- Other studies
  - Validated questionnaires are helpful to screen for OSAS in the office.
  - Routine blood work is generally noncontributory; in severe forms, polycythemia, hypercarbia, and elevated bicarbonate may be noted.
  - Evaluation for gastroesophageal reflux may include pH monitoring during sleep, barium swallow, or radionuclide studies (milk scan).
  - Home testing is not approved for use in children with suspected OSAS.

Imaging

- Lateral neck x-ray is easy to perform to assess adenoid and tonsillar size as well as patency of the nasopharyngeal airway.
- Nocturnal audio- and videotaping, as well as abbreviated nap polysomnography, are useful studies if the results are positive but generally have a poor negative predictive value.
- Upper airway endoscopy as well as bronchoscopy may be performed to evaluate anatomic or dynamic causes for airway obstruction (pharyngeal hypotonia, pharyngeal stenosis, laryngotracheomalacia, vocal cord polyps, papilloma).
- Head or neck computed tomography or magnetic resonance imaging (MRI) should be considered for complex craniofacial anomalies. If central apnea is noted, then MRI studies should also evaluate the brainstem to evaluate for an Arnold-Chiari malformation.
- In severe cases of OSAS, a cardiac evaluation, including electrocardiogram, chest x-ray, and echocardiogram, may be indicated.

DIFFERENTIAL DIAGNOSIS
- PS or habitual snoring
- Upper airway resistance syndrome: This condition is associated with sleep fragmentation and daytime sleepiness.
- Obesity–hypoventilation syndrome: a variant of OSAS
- Central apnea and periodic breathing
- Congenital central hypoventilation syndrome
- Other causes of excessive daytime sleepiness include the following:
  - Disorganized home environment, emotional stress
  - Substance abuse/drug intoxication: psychotropic medications, antihistamines, anticonvulsants, narcotics
  - Narcolepsy: Onset typically around adolescence, but cataplexy may occur later and delay the diagnosis.
  - Epilepsy: absence spells of unresponsiveness, electroencephalogram changes
- Causes of obstructive apnea include any cause of lymphoidal hypertrophy in the upper airway (allergies, viral/bacterial tonsillitis, neoplasm, epiglottitis, retropharyngeal abscess), chronic phenytoin exposure, and excessive storage material in upper airway submucosa.
- Causes of abnormal laxity of upper airway soft tissues: Down syndrome, acute polyneuropathy (Guillain-Barré syndrome), chronic neuromuscular disease, Prader-Willi syndrome, myasthenia gravis
- Causes of abnormal control/coordination of upper airway musculature: almost any cause of diffuse CNS dysfunction, including cerebral palsy and acquired lesions of the CNS such as stroke and head trauma
- Causes of central apnea: beyond infancy, most commonly due to drugs that suppress ventilatory drive; in premature infants, may be due to nonspecific immaturity of neural ventilatory control mechanism; sepsis, seizures, brainstem compression, brain tumors, Arnold-Chiari type 2 (although increasingly seen with type 1)
- Gastroesophageal reflux may potentiate central apnea and should be investigated.
- Androgen steroids may cause central apnea in adults.

TREATMENT

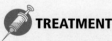

INITIAL STABILIZATION
- Severe cases may require urgent intervention.
- Severe cases of upper airway obstruction are usually diagnosed during polysomnography or during procedures involving sedation or anesthesia.
  - Ensure adequate ventilation and oxygenation, with quick assessment of the cause.
  - Temporary relief of the obstruction should be undertaken by an experienced team.
  - Transfer to an intensive care unit where the airway can be monitored carefully
  - Following relief of airway obstruction, pulmonary and airway edema, as well as copious secretion production, may develop.
  - Modalities of care should include placement of a nasopharyngeal airway, noninvasive ventilation with continuous positive airway pressure/bilevel positive airway pressure (CPAP/BiPAP), or placement of an endotracheal tube for mechanical ventilation.
- Risk factors for postoperative complications in children with OSAS include age <3 years, severe OSAS, pulmonary hypertension, obesity, prematurity, failure to thrive, craniofacial or neuromuscular disorders, and/or upper respiratory tract infection.

GENERAL MEASURES
- In most cases, adenotonsillectomy is 1st-line therapy. However, some patients continue to have significant postoperative OSAS that requires further evaluation.
- Noninvasive ventilatory support with CPAP or BiPAP may be helpful.
- Intranasal steroids and leukotriene modifiers have been shown to have a positive effect in children with mild sleep apnea. Duration of use and long-term outcomes remain unclear.
- In complicated cases, when craniofacial malformations are involved, surgical procedures such as tongue reduction, uvulopalatopharyngoplasty, or mandibular or maxillary advancement may be indicated.
- When there is evidence of gastroesophageal reflux, treatment with acid-suppression agents and chalasia precautions are indicated.
- Weight loss may be useful in obese children.
- Laser surgery and dental appliances may be useful in adults with mild OSAS, but there is no experience with these approaches in children.
- In extreme cases, a tracheostomy may be indicated, especially when significant craniofacial abnormalities exist.

ALERT
Treatment of gastroesophageal reflux in infants with obstructive apnea may be helpful even in the absence of obvious symptoms of reflux.

ONGOING CARE

COMPLICATIONS
Complications are due to chronic hypoxemia, hypercarbia, acidosis, as well as impaired sleep and include the following:
- Pulmonary hypertension, later cor pulmonale (rare)
- Systemic hypertension has been reported in adults and a few pediatric cases.
- Congestive heart failure; arrhythmias are common in adults with underlying coronary artery disease.
- Neurodevelopmental complications: daytime somnolence, poor school performance, hyperactivity, and social withdrawal
- Poor growth and failure to thrive
- Postanesthesia respiratory failure and death have been reported in children with OSAS.

FOLLOW-UP
- Clinical improvement is expected soon after adenotonsillectomy. In children <1 year of age with severe forms of OSAS, underlying craniofacial anomalies, or neurologic disorders, repeat overnight polysomnography is indicated 6–8 weeks after surgery.
- Regrowth of adenoid tissue may occur months to years after adenoidectomy. Therefore, if clinical symptoms, such as snoring, difficulty breathing while asleep, or a decline in school performance recur, a reevaluation is indicated.

ADDITIONAL READING

- American Academy of Sleep Medicine. *International Classification of Sleep Disorders*. 2nd ed. Westchester, IL: American Academy of Sleep Medicine; 2005:56–60.
- American Sleep Apnea Association. http://www.sleepapnea.org.
- D'Andrea LA. Diagnostic studies in the assessment of pediatric sleep-disordered breathing: techniques and indications. *Pediatr Clin North Am*. 2004;51(1):169–186.
- Marcus CL, Brooks LJ, Draper KA, et al. Diagnosis and management of childhood obstructive sleep apnea syndrome. *Pediatrics*. 2012;130(3):576–584.
- Pandit C, Fitzgerald DA. Respiratory problems in children with Down syndrome. *J Paediatr Child Health*. 2011;48(3):E147–E152.
- Rosen CL. Obstructive sleep apnea syndrome in children: controversies in diagnosis and treatment. *Pediatr Clin North Am*. 2004;51(1):153–167.
- Witmans M, Young R. Update on pediatric sleep disordered breathing. *Pediatr Clin North Am*. 2011;58(3):571–589.

CODES

ICD10
- G47.30 Sleep apnea, unspecified
- G47.33 Obstructive sleep apnea (adult) (pediatric)
- G47.36 Sleep related hypoventilation in conditions classd elswhr

FAQ
- Q: Can my child still have OSAS after adenotonsillectomy?
- A: Yes. At times, the adenoid tissue can grow back again. In addition, some cases of OSAS are related to a small upper airway that is restricted by anatomic or neurologic conditions. In these cases, adenotonsillectomy will not always resolve OSAS.
- Q: Does OSAS cause neurologic problems?
- A: Several studies suggest neurocognitive deficits in children with OSAS. The most common findings include reduced school performance and ADHD.

SLIPPED CAPITAL FEMORAL EPIPHYSIS

David D. Sherry

BASICS

DESCRIPTION

Slipped capital femoral epiphysis (SCFE) is displacement of the epiphysis of the head of the femur.

EPIDEMIOLOGY

- Males > females (3:2)
- Left hip twice as often as right, 25% bilateral
- Associated with obesity, increased height, genital underdevelopment, pituitary tumors, growth hormone therapy

Incidence

- 1–5 per 100,000
- Age of onset: boys, 14–16 years; girls, 11–13 years (essentially, premenarche)

RISK FACTORS

Genetics

5% of children affected have a parent with SCFE.

PATHOPHYSIOLOGY

- Unclear: abnormal stress on normal physeal plate versus a process that weakens the plate
- The femoral head slips posteriorly and inferiorly, exposing the anterior and superior aspects of the metaphysis of the femoral neck.

COMMONLY ASSOCIATED CONDITIONS

- Obesity
- Endocrine dysfunction
- Primary hypothyroidism
- Pituitary dysfunction
- Hypogonadism
- Cryptorchidism
- Chemotherapy
- Pelvic radiotherapy
- Renal rickets

DIAGNOSIS

HISTORY

Pain in hip or knee

ALERT

Hip pain may be absent; there may be no pain, or only thigh or knee pain due to referred pain.

- Occasional history of trauma; however, usually not sufficient to explain the findings
- 3 patterns
  - Chronic: most common, onset of symptoms >3 weeks, lack of full internal rotation of hip
  - Acute: sudden onset with inability to walk or severe pain and difficulty walking
  - Acute-on-chronic: sudden exacerbation of symptoms that have been present for a while

PHYSICAL EXAM

- Limp if unilateral or waddling gait if bilateral
- Positive Trendelenburg sign
- Tenderness and occasional palpable thickening over hip
- Thigh atrophy
- Lack of full internal rotation of hip and decreased motion in all planes secondary to mechanical limitation due to the slip
- Maneuver: When the hip is flexed, the thigh is forced into external rotation.

DIAGNOSTIC TESTS & INTERPRETATION

Imaging

- Anteroposterior and lateral view (frog leg or Lowenstein)
- Measure degree of displacement.
  - Minimal: alteration in plane of epiphysis relative to femoral neck; significant if angle <82 degrees
  - Mild: displacement <1 cm
  - Moderate: displacement >1 cm, <2/3 diameter of femoral neck
- Epiphyseal plate widened and irregular
- Decreased height of physis
- "Blanch sign": dense area in femoral neck
- A "Klein line" drawn along the superior femoral neck on the anteroposterior view should transect the epiphysis but not on the slipped side.
- Hormonal evaluation if suspected

Pathologic Findings
Histologic findings include widening of the epiphyseal plate, large clefts, and necrotic debris in the cartilage and synovitis.

DIFFERENTIAL DIAGNOSIS
- Septic arthritis of the hip
- Ischemic necrosis (Legg-Calve-Perthes)
- Tuberculosis of the hip; however, pain is associated with movement in all directions, and there should be other evidence of disease.
- Renal rickets
- Achondroplasia
- Shwachman syndrome: metaphyseal chondrodysplasia with pancreatic insufficiency

TREATMENT

ADDITIONAL TREATMENT
General Measures
- Designed to prevent complications and further slipping; urgent orthopedic consultation mandatory
- Conservative: bed rest with traction; probably does not reduce slipping; temporizing until surgery can be scheduled
- Manipulative reduction: risk of damage to epiphyseal vessels or breakdown of callus, probably only to be considered if within 24 hours of acute slip
- Epiphyseal fixation: risk of damage to articular surface or growth plate
- Intertrochanteric osteotomy
- Salvage: hip fusion

ONGOING CARE

FOLLOW-UP RECOMMENDATIONS
Patient Monitoring
Chondrolysis and avascular necrosis are uncommon side effects of slipped capital femoral epiphysis.

COMPLICATIONS
- Ischemic necrosis of epiphysis
  - Usually due to manipulative reduction of the slippage
  - More common in males
  - Radiographs reveal increased density, irregularity, and ultimately collapse of epiphysis.
- Chondrolysis (acute cartilage necrosis)
  - Seen in 1–40%
  - More common in females and blacks
  - Etiology unclear
  - Radiographs reveal narrowed joint space, sclerosis of acetabular rim, and osteoporosis of femoral head.

PROGNOSIS
- Most patients with SCFE can return to activities 3–6 months postoperatively.
- Compared to chronic SCFE, acute SCFE has higher likelihood of poor outcome.
- Satisfactory outcomes associated with in situ fixation of chronic SCFE

ADDITIONAL READING

- Larson AN, Sierra RJ, Yu EM, et al. Outcomes of slipped capital femoral epiphysis treated with in situ pinning. *J Pediatr Orthop*. 2012;32(2):125–130.
- Lehmann CL, Arons RR, Loder RT, et al. The epidemiology of slipped capital femoral epiphysis: an update. *J Pediatr Orthop*. 2006;26(3):286–290.
- Loder RT. Controversies in slipped capital femoral epiphysis. *Orthop Clin North Am*. 2006;37(2): 211–221, vii.
- Peck D. Slipped capital femoral epiphysis: diagnosis and management. *Am Fam Physician*. 2010;82(3): 258–262.
- Tosounidis T, Stengel D, Kontakis G, et al. Prognostic significance of stability in slipped upper femoral epiphysis: a systematic review and meta-analysis. *J Pediatr*. 2010;157(4):674–680, 680.e1.
- Wensaas A, Svenningsen S, Terjesen T. Long-term outcome of slipped capital femoral epiphysis: a 38-year follow-up of 66 patients. *J Child Orthop*. 2011;5(2):75–82.

CODES

ICD10
- M93.003 Unspecified slipped upper femoral epiphysis (nontraumatic), unspecified hip
- M93.023 Chronic slipped upper femoral epiphysis (nontraumatic), unspecified hip
- M93.033 Acute on chronic slipped upper femoral epiphysis (nontraumatic), unspecified hip

SMALLPOX (VARIOLA VIRUS)

Hamid Bassiri

BASICS

DESCRIPTION

- Smallpox is a life-threatening, acute, eruptive, contagious disease caused by variola virus.
- The disease is characterized by a febrile prodrome followed by the development of rash.
- Rash evolves in a characteristic fashion: macules → papules → vesicles → pustules; scabs form and fall off, leaving scars called pockmarks.
- There are 2 clinical forms of smallpox:
  - Variola minor is a less common and less severe form of disease.
  - There are 5 types of variola major, the more common and serious form of disease.
    - Ordinary smallpox
    - Modified smallpox
    - Flat smallpox
    - Hemorrhagic smallpox
    - Variola sine eruptione

EPIDEMIOLOGY

- The last documented case of endemic smallpox was in Somalia in 1977.
- The last case in the United States was in the late 1940s.
- Smallpox was declared eradicated by the World Health Organization in 1979.
- Historically in unvaccinated individuals, ordinary smallpox accounted for 90% of cases, hemorrhagic smallpox for 7% of cases, and flat and modified smallpox for the remainder.
- Modified smallpox was rare in unvaccinated individuals but accounted for 25% of cases of disease in vaccinated individuals.

GENERAL PREVENTION

- Prior to 1972, all U.S. children were vaccinated.
- Vaccines were produced from the vaccinia virus, a closely related orthopoxvirus to variola.
- Historically, the vaccine was prepared from virus grown on the skin of animals, and in some cases, the vaccine was contaminated with animal proteins, bacteria, and other viruses.
- Newer smallpox vaccines are developed from vaccinia clones grown in tissue culture and therefore are free of contamination from bacteria and other viruses.
- Only laboratories in the United States and Russia currently have stockpiles of smallpox virus.
- Due to concern for use of smallpox as an agent of bioterrorism, the U.S. Strategic National Stockpile still stores smallpox vaccine.
- The only currently FDA-licensed smallpox vaccine, ACAM2000 (which replaced Dryvax), is used for active immunization of persons determined to be at highest risk for infection.
- The Advisory Committee on Immunization Practices recommends smallpox vaccination for the following:
  - Public health response teams responsible for investigating suspected smallpox cases
  - Hospital-based health care teams responsible for assessing and caring for suspected smallpox cases
- Vaccine efficacy
  - 95% efficacious in preventing disease if given prior to exposure
  - May prevent smallpox or decrease severity if given 1–3 days after exposure
  - May decrease severity of disease if given 4–7 days after exposure
- Vaccination is estimated to provide protective immunity for 3–10 years but may decrease the severity of disease for 10–20 years.
- Vaccine administration
  - A skin abrasion is created using a bifurcated needle dipped in vaccine.
  - The vaccine site should be loosely covered to prevent the spread of virus to others.
  - After 3–4 days, a red pruritic papule appears at the vaccination site, which evolves into a vesicle followed by a pustule; after a few weeks, a scab forms, then falls off leaving a scar.
- Contraindications to vaccine:
  - Atopic dermatitis or exfoliative skin disorder
  - Immunosuppression
  - Pregnancy or breastfeeding
  - Close contact of someone who is pregnant, immunosuppressed, or has skin disease
  - Allergy to vaccine component
  - Moderate or severe acute illness
  - Inflammatory eye disease
  - Heart disease (myocardial infarction, stroke, cardiomyopathy, heart failure, or angina) or ≥3 risk factors for heart disease
  - Age <1 year
  - These contraindications may be reevaluated if smallpox is reintroduced into the population.
- Common adverse reactions to vaccination:
  - Fever, swelling, lymphadenitis, and headache are seen in 2–16% of adults receiving the vaccine for the first time.
  - A mild rash occurs in ~8% of cases.
- Less common vaccine reactions:
  - Vaccinia keratitis and/or vision loss
  - Accidental inoculation with blister formation
  - Moderate to severe generalized rash
  - Eczema vaccinatum
  - Encephalitis
  - Congenital or generalized vaccinia
  - Myopericarditis
  - Progressive vaccinia/vaccinia gangrenosum
  - Bacterial superinfection

PATHOPHYSIOLOGY

- The virus infects the upper respiratory tract and replicates; rarely, primary infections can occur via skin, conjunctival, or placental routes.
- The virus enters the bloodstream (primary viremia) and is taken up by macrophages.
  - Patient is asymptomatic during this time.
- Next, the virus enters the reticuloendothelial system where it continues to replicate.
- Secondary viremia occurs as the virus reenters the bloodstream and infects organs.
  - Can cause epidermal necrosis and swelling
  - Infections of the bone marrow, kidneys, liver, lymph nodes, spleen, and other organs result in coagulopathy and multiorgan system failure.
- Exact mechanisms of viral toxicity are not understood but may involve both viral cytopathic effects and inflammatory pathology.

ETIOLOGY

- Variola virus is a member of the poxvirus family and (*Orthopox* genus).
- Variola is a double-stranded DNA virus most commonly transmitted during face-to-face contact via respiratory aerosols or direct contact with infected skin lesions.
- Transmission of the virus via air in enclosed settings or via infected fomites is uncommon.
- Humans are the only vectors.

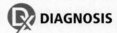

DIAGNOSIS

- Ordinary smallpox
  - Incubation period lasts 7–17 days, followed by a 1–4 day febrile prodrome characterized by high fever, headache, back pain, chills, abdominal pain, and emesis.
  - Eruptive phase begins with lesions of the mouth, tongue, and oropharynx.
  - The rash
    - Often starts on face and spreads to rest of body within 24–48 hours
    - On day 1, rash is macular.
    - On day 2, rash becomes papular.
    - On days 4 and 5, rash becomes vesicular.
    - By day 7, rash becomes pustular.
    - By 2–3 weeks, scabs form.
    - Scabs fall off and leave pockmarks.
- Modified smallpox
  - Milder than ordinary smallpox
  - Accelerated course
  - Lesions are not as deep
- Flat smallpox
  - Characterized by soft, flat, semiconfluent or confluent rash that does not evolve to pustules but can still result in significant skin loss
- Hemorrhagic smallpox
  - Shorter incubation time
  - Skin becomes dusky
  - Bleeding in skin and mucous membranes
  - Can be difficult to diagnose unless exposure to variola virus is known
- Variola sine eruptione
  - May be asymptomatic or cause an influenza-like illness
  - Noncontagious
  - Seen in infants with protective maternal antibodies and in vaccinated individuals

- If there has not been a release or circulation of smallpox, the CDC protocol for evaluating patients for smallpox can be used to guide the assessment of a suspicious rash illness.
- The CDC risk evaluation tool can be found at http://www.bt.cdc.gov/agent/smallpox/diagnosis/riskalgorithm/
  - If a patient has an acute, generalized rash on the body with vesicles or pustules, use the major and minor criteria to assess the likelihood of smallpox.
  - Major criteria
    - Febrile prodrome: 1–4 days prior to rash onset, including a temperature ≥101°F and 1 or more of the following: prostration, headache, backache, chills, vomiting, or severe abdominal pain
    - Classic smallpox lesions are deep-seated, firm/hard, round, well-circumscribed vesicles or pustules that can become umbilicated or confluent as they evolve on any one part of the body (e.g., the face or arm); all the lesions are in the same stage of development.
  - Minor criteria
    - Centrifugal distribution with greatest concentration of lesions on face and extremities
    - First lesions appear on the oral mucosa, palate, face, or forearms.
    - Patient appears toxic or moribund
    - Slow evolution: Lesions evolve from macules to papules to pustules over days (each stage lasts 1–2 days).
    - Lesions on the palms and soles
  - High risk of smallpox
    - Febrile prodrome and classic lesions in same stage of development
  - Moderate risk of smallpox
    - Febrile prodrome and either 1 other major criterion or ≥4 minor criteria
  - Low risk of smallpox
    - No febrile prodrome, or febrile prodrome and <4 minor criteria

DIAGNOSTIC TESTS & INTERPRETATION

Diagnostic Procedures/Other

- Use the CDC smallpox evaluation protocol to guide testing.
  - If high risk of smallpox:
    - Consult infectious disease and/or dermatology.
    - Public health agency will advise on management and collection of samples.
    - Testing will be performed at an approved laboratory prior to other tests.
  - If moderate risk of smallpox:
    - Consult infectious disease and/or dermatology.
    - Perform testing for varicella and other disorders including herpes simplex virus as indicated.
    - If no diagnosis is made after testing, ensure adequacy of specimen and have consultants reevaluate.
    - If smallpox still cannot be ruled out, then classify case as high-risk case.
  - If low risk of smallpox, and history and physical exam are highly suggestive of varicella, then varicella testing is optional.
  - If low risk of smallpox and diagnosis is uncertain, then testing should be done for varicella and other disorders as indicated.
- Variola testing
  - Should not be performed in low- and moderate-risk cases because of risk of false positives
  - Should only be performed in designated high-containment facilities
  - Lesion specimens (fluid, cells, and scabs) are preferred for testing, but blood, tonsillar swabs, and biopsy specimens may be used.
  - Serologic studies and electron microscopy cannot distinguish between the variola virus and other orthopoxviruses.
  - Polymerase chain reaction (PCR) assays can distinguish variola virus from other orthopoxviruses.
  - Variola virus can be cultured.

DIFFERENTIAL DIAGNOSIS

- Multiple rash illnesses, including the following, can be confused with smallpox:
  - Varicella and herpes zoster
  - Herpes simplex virus
  - Measles
  - Rubella
  - Monkeypox, cowpox, and tanapox
  - Viral exanthema including enterovirus
  - Disseminated molluscum contagiosum
  - Impetigo, insect bites, or scabies
  - Post-smallpox vaccine rash (vaccinia)
  - Secondary syphilis
  - Acne and contact dermatitis
  - Drug reactions including erythema multiforme
  - Meningococcemia can be confused with hemorrhagic smallpox.

ALERT

- Varicella can be confused with smallpox.
- Varicella lesions present in different stages, are superficial, and concentrate on the trunk and face, sparing the palms and soles.
- Smallpox lesions all present in the same stage, are deep, and concentrated on the face and limbs, often involving the palms and soles.

TREATMENT

MEDICATION

- Patients suspected of having smallpox should be vaccinated against smallpox, especially if they are in the early stages of the disease.
- The efficacy of antiviral drugs are not known; however, cidofovir has shown efficacy in reducing smallpox virus replication in vitro and in animal studies, and tecovirimat (ST-246) shows promise and is currently in clinical trials.
- The use of vaccinia immune globulin (VIG) can be considered for complications from vaccinia immunization but not for smallpox therapy or postexposure prophylaxis.
- Cidofovir or VIG are available through the Strategic National Stockpile.

ADDITIONAL TREATMENT

General Measures

- Suspected cases of smallpox require notification of state and local authorities, who should then notify the CDC.
- For patients with acute, generalized vesicular or pustular rash, institute airborne and contact precautions and alert infection control.
  - If high risk, report to state and local public health agency immediately.
- Individuals recently exposed (within 3–4 days) to someone with contagious smallpox (e.g., someone with oral or skin lesions) should receive postexposure vaccination, as this offers the potential to limit disease and also provides significant protection from death.
- Individuals with smallpox may be contagious during the febrile prodrome, are contagious during the early rash phase, and remain contagious until all the scabs have fallen off.

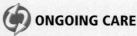

ONGOING CARE

PROGNOSIS

- The mortality rate for variola minor was <1%.
- Historically, the overall mortality rate for variola major was 30% but was close to 100% for the flat and hemorrhagic forms of the disease.
- The highest mortality rates occurred among young children, pregnant women, elderly individuals, and those with immunodeficiency.
- Long-term sequelae include pockmarks, vision loss, and limb deformities.

COMPLICATIONS

- Dehydration and electrolyte abnormalities can occur during the vesicular and pustular stages and should be corrected.
- Secondary bacterial superinfections may require antibiotic treatment.
- Corneal ulcers or keratitis, arthritis, or encephalitis may develop.

ADDITIONAL READING

- Besser JM, Crouch NA, Sullivan M. Laboratory diagnosis to differentiate smallpox, vaccinia, and other vesicular/pustular illnesses. *J Lab Clin Med*. 2003;142(4):246–251.
- Breman JG, Henderson DA. Diagnosis and management of smallpox. *N Engl J Med*. 2002;346(17):1300–1308.
- Moore ZS, Seward JF, Lane JM. Smallpox. *Lancet*. 2006;367(9508):425–435.

CODES

ICD10

B03 Smallpox

SNAKE AND INSECT BITES

Payal K. Gala • Jill C. Posner

BASICS

DESCRIPTION

- Injury to the human skin and/or subcutaneous tissues caused by bite, envenomation, or sting, causing local but sometimes systemic effects
- Snake bites
  - Crotalinae (pit vipers: cottonmouths, copperheads, and rattlesnakes)
  - Elapidae (coral snakes)
- Spider bites
  - Black widow (*Latrodectus mactans*)
  - Brown recluse (*Loxosceles reclusa*)
- Insect stings: Hymenoptera, fire ants (*Solenopsis*), wasps (including hornets and yellow jackets), bees

EPIDEMIOLOGY

- Only 15% of all snake bites are from poisonous snakes, and only ~2/3 of those involve true envenomation. Crotaline snakes are the most common cause of venomous snake bites in the United States. Almost 3,500 Crotaline exposures were reported to U.S. poison control centers in 2010. Coral snake bites constitute <1% of all snake bites.
- The black widow spider is found in most areas of North America but especially in southern New England. The brown recluse spider is found in southern and midwestern states.
- 1–4% of the U.S. population is at risk for anaphylaxis from Hymenoptera stings.

Incidence

- Annually, ~8,000 people sustain a poisonous snake bite in the United States, 99% of which are from crotaline snakes, and 5–6 fatalities occur.
- The incidences of black widow and brown recluse spider bites are unknown.
- 50–150 people die each year from sting anaphylaxis.

PATHOPHYSIOLOGY

- Snake bites
  - Snake venom consists of numerous enzymes and polypeptides that are neurotoxic, cytotoxic, and/or hemotoxic.
  - Pit viper venom produces significant local inflammation and injury to vascular endothelium and may lead to coagulopathy, thrombocytopenia, and shock.
  - The venom of the coral snake is primarily neurotoxic and may produce neuromuscular paralysis and respiratory depression.
- Spider bites
  - Most of the 20,000 species of predominantly venomous spiders in the United States lack fangs capable of penetrating human skin or toxin strong enough to produce more than a mild reaction. However, the black widow and brown recluse spiders can cause significant harm.
  - The black widow venom, α-latrotoxin, is a neurotoxin that stimulates myoneural junctions and nerve terminals by increasing synaptic release of acetylcholine and by initiating a massive influx of calcium, causing severe skeletal muscle pain and cramping and autonomic disturbances such as hypertension, tachycardia, and diaphoresis. Pediatric patients are more severely inflicted given the ratio of milligram of venom to kilogram of body weight.
  - The brown recluse venom, mainly sphingomyelinase D and hyaluronidase, acts on erythrocyte membranes, platelets, endothelial cells, and other cells, resulting in tissue infarction and necrosis. Systemic symptoms are more likely to occur in children, presumably because of a smaller ratio of body weight to venom volume. Hemolysis, hemoglobinuria, renal failure, DIC, shock, seizures, and death may occur.
- Insect stings
  - The fire ant bites with its jaws and then swings its head around to inflict multiple stings. The venom has a direct toxic effect on mast cell membranes, causing an immediate urticarial reaction at the bite site.
  - The venoms of the bee and wasp (hornet and yellow jacket) contain antigens that trigger an IgE antibody response, resulting in allergic reactions that vary in severity from mild local effects to anaphylaxis.
  - Cross reaction between Hymenoptera species occurs. Those who react to fire ants may also react to bees and wasps.

DIAGNOSIS

HISTORY

ALERT

- If the snake is brought in for identification, use caution! The head of a dead snake can deliver a venomous bite for up to 1 hour after death/decapitation.
- Snake bites
  - Poisonous snakes have triangular-shaped heads, a pit (heat sensor in front of each eye), fangs, slit-like pupils, and a single row of subcaudal plates and may have a rattle:
    - The corals have oval heads and round pupils yet are still poisonous.
  - Nonpoisonous snakes have oval heads, no pits, rows of small teeth, round pupils, a double row of subcaudal plates, and no rattles.
  - In the Elapidae family, the coral snake can be differentiated from the benign king snake by the pattern of the colored bands: "Red on yellow, kill a fellow; red on black, venom lack."
- Spider bites: identification of spider (rare): The black widow is about the size of a quarter, glossy black, gray, or brown, with a red, orange, or yellow hourglass-shaped marking on the ventral surface. A single bite can deliver a lethal dose of venom. The brown recluse is small (1–1.5 cm), gray, or reddish/brown, with a violin-shaped mark on the dorsum of the cephalothorax.
- Insect bites
  - Identify type of insect (bee, wasp, ant).
  - Assess for history of insect bite allergy.

PHYSICAL EXAM

- Crotalinae (pit viper) bites
  - Intense local pain/burning occur in the 1st few minutes, followed by edema and perioral numbness that may extend to the scalp and periphery. Paresthesias may be accompanied by a metallic taste.
  - Local ecchymosis and vesicles appear within the 1st few hours, and by 24 hours, hemorrhagic blebs are present.
  - Without treatment, edema and tissue necrosis through the bitten extremity may occur. Compartment syndrome is rare.
  - Nausea, vomiting, weakness, chills, and sweating can also occur with systemic absorption of venom.
  - Neuromuscular involvement (e.g., diplopia, dysphagia, lethargy) can develop within several hours.
  - Signs of hypovolemic shock, hemorrhagic diathesis, coagulopathy, and neuromuscular dysfunction may occur in life-threatening envenomations.
- Elapidae (coral snake) bites
  - Mild, often unimpressive local signs and symptoms (pain, swelling) but significant neurologic effects that include extremity paresthesias, weakness, fasciculations, and bulbar dysfunction that can progress to flaccid paralysis and respiratory failure
  - Inspect bite wound for fang punctures.
  - Carefully assess neurovascular integrity, and consider compartment pressures if severe edema.
- Black widow spider bites
  - No local symptoms associated with bite
  - Within 8 hours after bite, regional or generalized pain and muscle cramping, fasciculations; abdominal rigidity without tenderness is a hallmark sign.
  - Children often have nausea and vomiting.
  - Respiratory difficulty may occur.
  - Hypertension, tachycardia, and cholinergic effects (diaphoresis, salivation, lacrimation, and bronchorrhea)
  - Death may occur from respiratory or cardiovascular collapse.
  - Syndrome can last 3–6 days.
- Brown recluse spider bites
  - Spectrum from minor local reaction to severe necrosis
  - Local reaction: pain, erythema, swelling, and pruritus; classic "bull's eye" lesion or "red-white-and-blue" sign
  - Ischemia and skin necrosis: A bright red papule appears within a few hours of the bite and can evolve within 48–72 hours into a hemorrhagic vesicle surrounded by blue discoloration (necrosis) or white blanching (vasospasm), the bull's eye. Shortly after, a firm, purple necrotic lesion appears, and within 7–14 days, black eschar is visible. Ulcer healing can take weeks to months, leaving a deep scar.
- Insect bites
  - Small local reactions: painful, pruritic, urticarial lesion at the sting site
  - Large local reaction: edema and erythema, may be several centimeters in diameter
  - Anaphylaxis is rare with fire ants but occurs more frequently with bee stings.

DIAGNOSTIC TESTS & INTERPRETATION

Lab

- Snake bites: CBC, platelet count, PT/PTT, fibrinogen, fibrin split products, electrolytes, creatine kinase, creatinine, urinalysis
- Spider bites: CBC, PT/PTT, fibrinogen, electrolytes, creatinine, creatine kinase, urinalysis, Coombs test
- Insect bites: no tests done routinely

DIFFERENTIAL DIAGNOSIS

- Black widow spider bites: acute abdomen, renal colic, opioid withdrawal, tetanus
- Poisonous snake bites: nonpoisonous snake bite (leaves scratches, not punctures), rodent bites, thorn wounds
- Brown recluse spider bite: other spider bites, insect bites and stings (including Lyme), cellulitis, poison ivy/oak, Stevens-Johnson syndrome, toxic epidermal necrolysis, erythema nodosum, chronic herpes simplex, purpura fulminans, diabetic ulcer, gonococcal hemorrhagic lesion, pyoderma

TREATMENT

- Crotalinae (pit vipers) bites
  - Remove constrictive items (jewelry or clothing) and immobilize extremity at or below level of heart. Cryotherapy, arterial tourniquets, ice immersion, incision, excision, and oral suctioning are not recommended!
  - Focus on rapid transport to medical facility.
  - Address airway, breathing, and circulation.
  - The use of a constrictive band is controversial. Main indication is for cases of prolonged transport time to a medical facility or rapid progression of systemic symptoms. A flat band is placed 5–10 cm proximal to the bite, with enough pressure to impede lymphatic and superficial venous flow but not arterial flow. 1–2 fingers should fit easily between the band and patient's extremity. Be careful of progressive edema leading to tightening of constrictive band if applied. Also remember that these bands can worsen local cytotoxic effects.
  - Another option is a compression bandage alone with immobilization of the involved extremity (pressure-immobilization method). This is thought to delay systemic absorption of venom.
- Elapidae (coral snakes)
  - Constriction band, suction, and drainage do not prevent coral snake venom absorption.

ADDITIONAL TREATMENT

General Measures

Consider contacting your local poison control center to assist with diagnosis and management. The national phone number for all centers is 1-800-222-1222.

- Crotalinae (pit vipers) bites
  - Wound care: irrigation and dressing
  - Determine if envenomation has occurred via serial examinations (q30min) and laboratory studies (q4h).
  - Antivenom: Administration of antivenom should be made in consultation with a toxicologist and/or herpetologist. General indications include progressive local swelling, pain or ecchymosis, and any systemic signs or symptoms.
  - Crotalidae Polyvalent Immune Fab (CroFab) is the Crotalinae antivenom product approved by the FDA. Antivenin (Crotalidae) Polyvalent (ACP) was often associated with serum sickness and anaphylaxis and is no longer manufactured.
  - Data suggest that the use of CroFab is safe and effective and is associated with fewer immediate and delayed hypersensitivity reactions than ACP, although they do occur and must be monitored.
  - Some hospitals (in endemic areas) and many zoos stock antivenoms. In addition, the regional poison control center may have access to the Antivenom Index and will be able to help locate the nearest supply.
  - Early administration of Fab within 6 hours is advised. Initial dose is 4–6 vials of Fab diluted in 250 mL normal saline infused over 1 hour. Dosing is based on amount of venom injected, not weight of patient.
  - Supportive care: volume replacement, packed red blood cells, platelets, fresh frozen plasma, cryoprecipitate as indicated for hypovolemia and bleeding diathesis. Observe for respiratory and renal failure.
  - Frequent assessment of tissue perfusion and measurement of compartment pressure; fasciotomy only for elevated compartment pressures
  - Empiric antibiotics are controversial but may be indicated in cases of extensive tissue involvement.
  - Analgesia and tetanus prophylaxis
- Elapidae (coral snakes)
  - Crotalinae antivenom is ineffective in treating Elapidae envenomation. Antivenom formerly manufactured by Wyeth Laboratories is no longer in production. Currently, there are only 2 lots of FDA-approved Elapidae antivenom in the United States, both of which have expired on October 2014. It is not known at this time when more will be manufactured.
  - Any degree of neurotoxicity or systemic symptoms is an indication for antivenom therapy. Prophylactic therapy should be avoided due to limited supply and need to preserve antivenom.
  - Local wound care, supportive care, analgesia, and tetanus vaccination
- Black widow spider bites
  - To alleviate muscle pain and cramping, parenteral opioids and benzodiazepines can be administered.
  - Calcium infusions had been used anecdotally but have not proven to be effective.
  - Latrodectus-specific antivenom is available for more severe envenomations given via IV infusion. Specific indications include young age, pregnancy, life-threatening hypertension and tachycardia, respiratory difficulties, or severe symptoms refractory to other treatment measures. Administration of an equine serum preparation has been associated with hypersensitivity reactions and occasionally death. 1 vial is generally sufficient.
- Brown recluse spider bites
  - Most bites can be treated on an outpatient basis with local wound care with Burow solution or hydrogen peroxide and symptom treatment for pain and pruritus.
  - No antivenom is available in the United States.
  - Patients with systemic symptoms, serious infection, or extensive necrosis warrant hospitalization, IV fluids, and aggressive supportive care.
  - Skin grafting or debridement may be warranted for wound management. Surgical excision is no longer indicated.
  - Neither dapsone nor hyperbaric oxygen therapy has proved to be effective; dapsone in children is associated with methemoglobinemia.
- Insect bites or stings
  - Rarely require more than ice and antihistamine for pruritus
  - If stinger remains in skin, remove by pinching with forceps or scraping. Emphasis should be on quick removal to decrease exposure to venom. Do not squeeze venom gland.
  - Life-threatening anaphylaxis should be treated with subcutaneous epinephrine (0.01 mL/kg 1:1,000 or 1 mg/mL, max 0.3 mL), methylprednisolone IV/IM (2 mg/kg), and/or diphenhydramine IV/IM (1.25 mg/kg).
- Bacterial superinfection is rare but, if present, can usually be treated with oral and/or topical antibiotics.

ONGOING CARE

PROGNOSIS

- Snake bites: Because the majority of snake bites are from nonvenomous snakes, and ~1/3 of bites from venomous snakes do not involve envenomation, the majority of bites cause only local injury. However, once serious injury is established, prognosis becomes unclear.
- Spider bites: Children have severe reactions and rare fatalities.
- Insect bites: Most bites and stings cause minimal local effects, although some cause serious systemic reactions and, rarely, death. For those patients with severe anaphylactic reactions, discharge the patient with a subcutaneous epinephrine autoinjector.

ADDITIONAL READING

- Anz AW, Schweppe M, Halvorson J, et al. Management of venomous snakebite injury to the extremities. *J Am Acad Orthop Surg*. 2010;18(12):749–759.
- Goto CS, Feng SY. Crotalidae polyvalent immune Fab for the treatment of pediatric crotaline envenomation. *Pediatr Emerg Care*. 2009;25(4):273–282.
- Quan D. North American poisonous bites and stings. *Crit Care Clin*. 2012;28(4):633–659.
- Schmidt JM. Antivenom therapy for snakebites in children: is there evidence? *Curr Opin Pediatr*. 2005;17(2):234–238.
- Walker JP, Morrison R, Stewart R, et al. Venomous bites and stings. *Curr Probl Surg*. 2013;50(1):9–44.
- Warrell DA. Venomous bites, stings, and poisoning. *Infect Dis Clin North Am*. 2012;26(2):207–223.

CODES

ICD10

- T63.481A Toxic effect of venom of arthropod, accidental, init
- T63.001A Toxic effect of unsp snake venom, accidental, init
- T63.301A Toxic effect of unsp spider venom, accidental, init

S

SOCIAL ANXIETY DISORDER

David Becker • Anna E. Ordóñez

BASICS

DESCRIPTION

- Social anxiety disorder, also known as social phobia, is a psychological condition with developmental underpinnings.
- The disorder is characterized by marked and persistent fear of social situations in which the person is exposed to unfamiliar people or possible scrutiny by others.
- *DSM-5* criteria:
  - Marked fear or anxiety of one or more social situations in which the individual is exposed to possible scrutiny by others (In children: anxiety must occur in peer situations, not just in interactions with adults)
  - The individual fears that he or she will act in a way or show anxiety symptoms that will be negatively evaluated.
  - The social situations almost always provoke fear or anxiety and are avoided or endured with intense fear or anxiety.
  - The fear/anxiety is out of proportion to the actual threat posed by the situation/context and is persistent, typically lasting 6 months or more.
  - The fear/anxiety or avoidance causes significant distress or impairment in social, occupational, or other areas of functioning.
  - The fear/anxiety is not attributable to psychological effects of substances, a medical condition, or by another psychiatric diagnosis.
  - Specify if performance only (fear/anxiety restricted to speaking/performing in public)

EPIDEMIOLOGY

- Approximately 7% of youths suffer from social anxiety disorder.
- The prevalence is somewhat higher in girls than in boys.

RISK FACTORS

- Preexisting shyness or social inhibition
- Avoidant temperament
- Behavioral inhibition
- Family history: 1st-degree relatives have 2–6 times greater chance of having the disorder.
- Moderate genetic component based on twin studies

COMMONLY ASSOCIATED CONDITIONS

- Anxiety disorders
  - Generalized anxiety disorder
  - Specific phobia
  - Selective mutism
  - Obsessive-compulsive disorder
  - Panic disorder
- ADHD
- Depression

DIAGNOSIS

HISTORY

- The diagnostic evaluation should entail gathering of data through separate interviews with the child/adolescent and the parents.
- Current symptoms should be elicited with attention to severity, duration, and level of functional impairment.
- Core symptoms of marked anxiety in social situations, fear of negative scrutiny by others, and avoidance of these situations should be present.
- Distress can be manifested by physical symptoms such as
  - Blushing
  - Palpitations
  - Trembling
  - Gastrointestinal (GI) upset
- Younger children may exhibit periods of selective mutism in social situations while having the ability to talk freely while at home.
- Older children may appear oppositional and exhibit school refusal.
- Symptoms may be exacerbated by environmental transitions such as a new school or the family moving.

PHYSICAL EXAM

There are no pertinent findings on physical exam.

DIAGNOSTIC TESTS & INTERPRETATION

Lab

Consider additional screening if symptoms are more pervasive than just social situations.

Diagnostic Procedures/Other

- Diagnostic scales:
  - Multidimensional Anxiety Scale for Children (MASC): broad anxiety scale (ages 8–18 years), self-report
  - Social Phobia and Anxiety Inventory for Children (SPAI-C) (ages 8–17 years), self-report
  - Social Anxiety Scale for Children-Revised (SASC-R) (ages 8–14 years) and Adolescents (SAS-A) (ages 13–18 years), self-administered
  - Liebowitz Social Anxiety Scale for Children and Adolescents (LSAS-CA) (ages 13–17 years), clinician-administered

DIFFERENTIAL DIAGNOSIS

- Normative shyness (personality trait without significant adverse impact on functioning)
- Anxiety disorders
- Depression
- Autistic spectrum disorders

TREATMENT

GENERAL MEASURES

- Potential pitfalls
  - Incomplete assessment of the comorbid psychiatric illnesses
  - Parental accommodation of the child's avoidant patterns

- Both psychotherapy and medications have roles in core treatment and symptom alleviation.
- Additional therapies such as group therapy, individual and family psychoeducation, and/or self-regulation strategies can be considered first line in mild cases or adjuncts for more clinically impairing cases.
- Combination treatment with SSRIs and CBT may be superior to either treatment alone.

ADDITIONAL THERAPIES

- The most studied and most supported by structured clinical trials is cognitive behavioral therapy (CBT).
  - Exposure to a hierarchy of avoided situations with concomitant cognitive reframing is core to CBT.
- Other psychotherapeutic approaches such as play therapy, interpersonal, or psychodynamic therapy may be better suited in some cases.
- Supportive psychosocial treatments can include mind–body strategies to support self-regulation skills. These may include the following:
  - Biofeedback
  - Progressive muscle relaxation
  - Self-hypnosis
  - Mindfulness techniques
- Group therapy may also be helpful.
- Family therapy or collaborative work with parents may be important to decrease parental accommodation or help with other dysfunctional dynamics.

MEDICATION

- Selective serotonin reuptake inhibitors (SSRIs)
  - First line for symptom control and adjunctive psychopharmacologic support.
  - Begin half the recommended starting dose for children with anxiety disorders.
  - Side effects include GI upset, headaches, dizziness, and agitation.
  - There is a black box warning by the FDA indicating that all antidepressants may increase suicidal thinking and behavior in children and adolescents. It is not clear how this warning may apply to treatment of social anxiety disorder that presents without depression.
  - Close monitoring is important following initiation of treatment.
    - Fluoxetine (Prozac) (10–60 mg)
    - Sertraline (Zoloft) (25–200 mg)
    - Paroxetine (Paxil) (10–40 mg)
    - Citalopram (Celexa) (10–40 mg)
    - Escitalopram (Lexapro) (10–20 mg)
    - Fluvoxamine (Luvox) (25–200 mg)
- Serotonin-norepinephrine reuptake inhibitor (SNRI)
  - Second-line
  - Side effects include somnolence, insomnia, dizziness, anxiety, headache, sweating, and tremor.
  - There is a black box warning by the FDA indicating that all antidepressants may increase suicidal thinking and behavior in children and adolescents.
  - Venlafaxine extended release (Effexor XR) (25–225 mg)
- Benzodiazepines
  - May be considered for short-term symptomatic relief in rare circumstances
  - Not appropriate for long-term therapy
  - Side effects include sedation, dizziness, and weakness.

ONGOING CARE

FOLLOW-UP RECOMMENDATIONS

Patient Monitoring

- Psychotherapy on a weekly or twice-weekly regimen
- If medication is initiated, close monitoring on a weekly basis is recommended for the first 4 weeks followed by monthly monitoring.
- The primary care provider should monitor the response to the chosen treatment plan at least every 2–3 months.
- Monitoring of any emerging comorbidities is suggested.

PROGNOSIS

- Among patients who come to the attention of clinicians, social anxiety disorder is generally considered a chronic condition that does not significantly improve without intervention.
- Significant comorbidities may develop in adulthood, such as depression and alcohol dependence.

ADDITIONAL READING

- American Psychiatric Association. *Diagnostic and Statistical Manual of Mental Disorder*. 5th ed. Arlington, VA: American Psychiatric Association; 2013.
- Beesdo K, Knappe S, Pine D. Anxiety and anxiety disorder in children and adolescents: developmental issues and implications for DSM-V. *Psychiatr Clin North Am*. 2009;32(3):483–524.
- Beesdo-Baum K, Knappe S, Fehm L, et al. The natural course of social anxiety disorder among adolescents and young adults. *Acta Psychiatr Scand*. 2012;126(6):411–425.
- Beidel DC, Ferrell C, Alfano CA, et al. The treatment of childhood social anxiety disorder. *Psychiatr Clin North Am*. 2001;24(4):831–846.
- Khalid-Khan S, Santibanez MP, McMicken C, et al. Social anxiety disorder in children and adolescents: epidemiology, diagnosis, and treatment. *Paediatr Drugs*. 2007;9(4):227–237.
- Masi G, Pfanner C, Mucci M, et al. Pediatric social anxiety disorder: predictors of response to pharmacological treatment. *J Child Adolesc Psychopharmacol*. 2012;22(6):410–414.
- Walkup JT, Albano AM, Piacentini J, et al. Cognitive behavior therapy, sertraline, or a combination in childhood anxiety. *N Engl J Med*. 2008;359:1–14.

CODES

ICD10

- F40.10 Social phobia, unspecified
- F41.8 Other specified anxiety disorders
- F40.11 Social phobia, generalized

S

SORE THROAT

Daniel E. Felten

BASICS

DESCRIPTION

Throat pain with swallowing (odynophagia) or without swallowing may be a lone complaint or accompanied by a variety of other complaints. The most likely etiologies are self-limited but must rule out potentially life-threatening causes.

EPIDEMIOLOGY

- Sore throat is a common complaint year-round, but etiology depends on season and age of patient.
- In winter months, viral agents are more active.
- In spring and fall, postnasal drip from allergic rhinitis is a common cause of throat irritation.

GENERAL PREVENTION

- Careful hand washing and avoidance of respiratory secretions are key to minimizing spread of most infectious agents.
- Noninfectious etiology often triggered by specific exposure, so avoidance of that trigger would limit symptoms

ETIOLOGY

- Infectious
  - Urgent/emergent: epiglottitis, peritonsillar cellulitis/abscess, retropharyngeal abscess, Lemierre syndrome
  - Viral: adenovirus, influenza, coxsackie, parainfluenza, Epstein-Barr virus (EBV), cytomegalovirus (CMV), herpes simplex virus (HSV), human immunodeficiency virus
  - Bacterial: group A β-hemolytic *Streptococcus* (GAS, *Streptococcus pyogenes*), *Mycoplasma pneumoniae*, groups C and G streptococci, diphtheria, *Neisseria gonorrhoeae*, anaerobic bacteria, tularemia, *Arcanobacterium haemolyticum*
  - Fungal: *Candida*
- Environmental
  - Tobacco smoke or aerosolized irritant
- Trauma
  - Foreign body: either retained or causing laceration to posterior pharynx
  - Burns: hot liquids/foods
  - Caustic ingestion
  - Voice overuse
- Tumor
  - Acute lymphocytic leukemia or T-cell lymphoma can rarely present as sore throat and fever.
- Allergic/inflammatory
  - Postnasal drip from allergic rhinitis
- Miscellaneous
  - Kawasaki disease
  - PFAPA: periodic fever, aphthous stomatitis, pharyngitis, adenitis
  - GERD
  - Eosinophilic esophagitis
  - Psychogenic pain
  - Referred pain

DIAGNOSIS

HISTORY

- Drooling, inability to swallow, rapid progression of symptoms, or respiratory distress may suggest more urgent/emergent problem: epiglottitis, peritonsillar abscess (especially with unilateral symptoms), or retropharyngeal abscess.
- Exposures, ingestions, foreign bodies: need to elicit whether patient was exposed to agent that could cause progression of symptoms
  - Caustic ingestion burns may progress rapidly and require transfer to higher level of care.
  - Foreign body ingestion may require removal or endoscopic visualization.
- Outbreaks in child care setting or school: GAS, influenza, and coxsackie can spread rapidly.
- Sexual activity or concern for sexual abuse: oral sex a risk factor for development of pharyngitis due to *N. gonorrhoeae*
- Children who are immunocompromised or children on chronic inhaled corticosteroids who are otherwise immune competent are at risk for esophageal candidiasis. Throat pain is often chronic and not responsive to other treatments.
- Associated symptoms
  - Fever, headache (HA), stomach pain: Consider GAS.
  - Fever, HA, rhinorrhea myalgias, fatigue: Consider influenza.
  - Rhinorrhea, cough, conjunctivitis: more likely viral
  - Runny nose, itchy nose, congestion: Consider postnasal drip from allergic rhinitis.

PHYSICAL EXAM

ALERT

- Although rare since the introduction of the vaccine for *Haemophilus influenzae* type b, patients may present with epiglottitis.
- Caution approaching a febrile, toxic-appearing patient who is unable to control secretions and exhibiting any respiratory distress. Defer exam or imaging until patient is in a setting where an emergent airway could be established if epiglottitis is suspected.

- General
  - Ill appearing, respiratory distress: epiglottitis, retropharyngeal abscess
- Pharynx and oral cavity
  - Exudative tonsillitis: usually GAS but also present in EBV, *N. gonorrhoeae*, *Arcanobacterium*, HSV, adenovirus
  - Vesicles or ulceration on tonsils, tonsillar pillars, or buccal mucosa; inflammation of gums: HSV, coxsackievirus, echovirus
  - Posterior pharyngeal cobblestoning: postnasal drip from allergic rhinitis
  - Asymmetry in tonsil size or deviation of uvula: peritonsillar abscess
  - Burns on lips or tongue: hot liquid or caustic ingestion
- Eyes, ears, nose
  - Conjunctivitis with sore throat: adenovirus
  - Rhinorrhea: viral etiology most likely
  - Boggy nasal turbinates, allergic shiners: postnasal drip from allergic rhinitis
- Lymph nodes
  - Tender anterior cervical lymph nodes: classic for GAS
  - Diffuse lymphadenopathy +/− splenomegaly: EBV, less likely CMV
- Skin
  - Scarlatiniform rash (diffuse, erythematous, fine-papular, "sand-papery" rash): scarlet fever from GAS pharyngitis but can be seen with infections due to *A. haemolyticum* and in Kawasaki disease
  - Vesicular rash, particularly on palms, soles, and/or buttocks: coxsackievirus

DIAGNOSTIC TESTS & INTERPRETATION

Lab

- Rapid antigen detection test
  - Initial test of choice if GAS pharyngitis suspected
  - High specificity ($\geq$95%), variable sensitivity (55–90%)
  - Need to confirm negatives with culture or DNA probe for GAS
- Heterophile antibody test (Monospot)
  - Can be used to confirm EBV infection
  - Not reliable under age 4 years
- Cultures for other bacteria (e.g., *N. gonorrhoeae*, *A. haemolyticum*) require special handling and specific medium for growth.

Imaging

- Lateral neck x-ray
  - Thumb print sign: enlarged epiglottis. Do not get x-ray in unstable patient.
  - Widened prevertebral soft tissue space suggestive of retropharyngeal abscess

- Chest x-ray if foreign body is suspected
  - Must ensure object passes out of esophagus
  - Look for free air indicating perforation
- CT scan of neck
  - For diagnosis of retropharyngeal abscess in setting of suggestive lateral neck x-ray or peritonsillar abscess if suggested by physical exam

TREATMENT

The treatment of sore throat is primarily supportive, including fluids and pain control. Additional treatment depends on underlying etiology.

MEDICATION

- Pain relievers such as ibuprofen or acetaminophen are generally sufficient to manage pain.
  - Rarely, addition of codeine or other opioid may be warranted in patients who are unable to maintain sufficient PO intake.
  - Use codeine with caution due to variability in metabolism by cytochrome P450 CYP2D6. Patients who are "ultra-rapid metabolizers" of codeine convert up to 15% (vs. 3%) of the drug to morphine, which can lead to toxicity.
  - Alternatively, for less severe pain, topical treatments such as throat lozenges or throat sprays may provide additional comfort with fewer potential side effects.
- GAS pharyngitis: penicillin G benzathine IM (600,000 U <27 kg, 1.2 million U >27 kg) or penicillin V potassium PO (250 mg b.i.d. <27 kg, 500 mg b.i.d. >27 kg × 10 days) or amoxicillin (50 mg/kg/day; max 1,000 mg) first line
  - 1st-generation cephalosporin for penicillin-allergic patients with nonanaphylactic reactions
  - Clindamycin for patients with type I hypersensitivity to penicillin
  - Macrolides are also acceptable alternatives.
- Some studies have shown steroids (oral or IM) to be of benefit to patients with severe symptoms. However, they should be used only in limited circumstances due to side effects.
- Esophageal candidiasis: fluconazole (6 mg/kg × 1, then 3 mg/kg daily; max 400 mg/day) or itraconazole (5–10 mg/kg/day divided daily or b.i.d.; max 600 mg/day) × 14–21 days after resolution of symptoms

ISSUES FOR REFERRAL

- Epiglottitis: Exam, airway stabilization, and ongoing management must be done in controlled setting.
- Peritonsillar abscess: often requires drainage either by needle aspiration, incision and drainage, or tonsillectomy
- Presence of foreign body: may need removal

INPATIENT CONSIDERATIONS

Initial Stabilization

- Patients with signs of airway compromise or respiratory distress may require emergent airway management.
  - Patients suspected to have epiglottitis must have airway stabilized prior to any other treatment or diagnostic testing.
  - If no impending airway obstruction, can undertake diagnostic and therapeutic interventions, including IV placement for administration of IV fluids if patient is not tolerating PO, antibiotics for treatment of abscess or cellulitis, or anesthetic agents if endotracheal intubation becomes necessary
  - Supplemental O_2 as needed
  - Make NPO if surgical intervention is required.

Admission Criteria

- Patients with conditions causing airway compromise require monitoring until they demonstrate response to treatment.
- Pain control or hydration: Patients with uncontrolled throat pain may be unable to take adequate PO to maintain hydration at home.

ADDITIONAL READING

- Galioto N. Peritonsillar abscess. *Am Fam Physician*. 2008;77(2):199–202.
- Madadi P, Koren G. Pharmacogenetic insights into codeine analgesia: implications to pediatric codeine use. *Pharmacogenomics*. 2008;9(9):1267–1284.
- Sadowitz PD, Page NE, Crowley K. Adverse effects of steroid therapy in children with pharyngitis with unsuspected malignancy. *Pediatr Emerg Care*. 2012;28(8):807–809.
- Schwartz B, Marcy SM, Phillips WR, et al. Pharyngitis—principles of judicious use of antimicrobial agents. *Pediatrics*. 1998;101:171–174.
- Wing A, Villa-Roel C, Yeh B, et al. Effectiveness of corticosteroid treatment in acute pharyngitis: a systematic review of the literature. *Acad Emerg Med*. 2010;17(5):476–483.

CODES

ICD10

- J02.9 Acute pharyngitis, unspecified
- R07.0 Pain in throat
- J02.0 Streptococcal pharyngitis

FAQ

- Q: Are steroids effective adjuvant therapy for sore throat?
- A: There have been a number of good studies that have shown that giving steroids to patients with GAS pharyngitis has decreased time to improvement in symptoms on average about 5.2 hours. However, there was no significant difference in pain at 24 hours. In patients with non–GAS-associated sore throat, the results are more mixed. One study did show significant decrease in time to improvement in symptoms in patients with severe symptoms.
- Q: What is the risk of giving steroids to a patient with sore throat?
- A: None of the studies of steroid use in treatment of acute throat pain reported any significant side effects in the treatment groups. There were some reports of GI upset that often were attributed to concurrent use of antibiotics. However, sore throat and fever is rarely the presentation of acute lymphocytic leukemia (ALL), and it has been shown that steroid administration prior to the diagnosis of ALL has a significant adverse effect of the chance a patient will achieve complete remission. Current COG protocol may assign children with ALL who have received steroids prior to diagnosis to more intensive treatment groups depending on time of steroid administration.
- Q: Should antibiotics be given to children with sore throat based on physical exam findings that suggest GAS pharyngitis?
- A: No. Most cases of sore throat in children are due to viruses, and the rapid antigen detection test (RADT) is a widely available screening test that is easy to administer. The test has an excellent specificity, and patients with a positive RADT should be treated. Negative results should be sent for culture or DNA probe, which may delay treatment by 24–48 hours. However, the primary reason for treating GAS pharyngitis with antibiotics is to prevent rheumatic fever, which can be accomplished as long as antibiotics are administered within 10 days of onset of symptoms.

S

SPEECH DELAY

Maureen C. McMahon

BASICS

DESCRIPTION

- Speech delay is delay in the acquisition of spoken language.
- Language is a system of symbols through which humans communicate thoughts, feelings, and ideas. It has 3 components—receptive, expressive, and visual language.
  - Receptive language is the ability to process and understand language.
  - Expressive language is the ability to communicate through speech, written, or formal sign language.
  - Visual elements include eye contact, pointing, and gestures.
- Speech delay can be primary as in specific language impairment (SLI) or developmental language disorder (DLD), or secondary to another condition such as a syndrome or neurologic disorder. SLI is impaired speech/language in an otherwise normally developing child who lacks signs or stigmata of other conditions.
- Constitutional language delay, a retrospective diagnosis, is language delay associated with eventual achievement of normal speech and language milestones by school age. There are no subsequent difficulties with learning to read or write.
- Expressive language disorders include the following:
  - Verbal dyspraxia: little speech produced with great effort, very dysfluent, single words most commonly
  - Speech programming deficit disorder: poorly organized, difficult-to-understand speech
- Mixed receptive and expressive disorders
  - Verbal auditory agnosia: impaired ability to decode speech, resulting in a severe expressive impairment. Can often learn language visually
  - Phonologic/syntactic deficit disorder: most common type of DLD. Comprehension exceeds spoken ability. Speech is dysfluent, grammatically incorrect with short utterances.
  - Most frequent causes of speech delay:
    - Hearing loss
    - SLI
    - Autism spectrum disorder
    - Intellectual disability (formerly mental retardation)

EPIDEMIOLOGY

- Up to 15% of 2-year-old have speech and language delays.
- 5% of school-aged children have speech and language delays.
- 3:1 male-to-female ratio in DLD

RISK FACTORS

- Family history of speech/language delay or disorder
- Male gender
- Low maternal education
- Maternal depression
- Prematurity
- Birth weight <1,000 g

DIAGNOSIS

DIFFERENTIAL DIAGNOSIS

- Hearing loss
  - Isolated genetic hearing loss
  - Hearing loss secondary to in utero cytomegalovirus (CMV) infection: full syndrome at birth or asymptomatic infection with delayed onset of progressive hearing loss
  - Acquired hearing loss: following head trauma, tumor-associated, complication of bacterial meningitis, end result of frequent acute otitis media or chronic otitis media with effusion
- Intellectual disability
- Autism spectrum disorder
- SLI
- Constitutional language delay
- Selective mutism
- Environmental
  - Lack of stimulation and/or poor linguistic environment
  - Child abuse or neglect
  - Lead poisoning
- Congenital
  - Cerebral palsy
  - Hydrocephalus
  - Down syndrome
  - Fragile X syndrome
  - 22q11 microdeletion syndrome
  - Fetal alcohol syndrome
  - Turner syndrome
  - Klinefelter syndrome
  - Prader-Willi syndrome
  - Angelman syndrome
  - Muscular dystrophy
  - Tuberous sclerosis
  - Neurofibromatosis
  - Williams syndrome
  - Branchio-oto-renal (BOR) syndrome
  - Craniofacial anomalies such as Treacher Collins and Goldenhar syndromes
- Nutritional
  - Malnutrition
  - Iron deficiency
- Infectious
  - HIV encephalopathy
  - Other in utero viral infection
  - Congenital toxoplasmosis
  - Congenital syphilis

ALERT

- Avoid late referral of congenital hearing loss: Amplification and therapy by 6 months of age can result in near-normal rate of speech/language acquisition.
- Constitutional language delay is a retrospective diagnosis. Do not miss a language disorder if assuming a delayed toddler is a "late bloomer."
- Avoid overlooking fine or gross motor delays.
- Avoid missing a genetic or neurologic diagnosis.

HISTORY

Does the family note a concern about speech delay or hearing impairment?

- **Question:** Perinatal history?
- *Significance:* prenatal care, maternal illness, NICU admission, hyperbilirubinemia requiring exchange transfusion, treatment with ototoxic drugs such as gentamicin, newborn hearing screen results
- **Question:** Full developmental history?
- *Significance:* to determine if global delay or isolated speech and language delay
- **Question:** Parental concern about delayed expressive language?
- *Significance:* often the presentation of autism
- **Question:** History of feeding, swallowing difficulties, or poor acceptance of textured foods?
- *Significance:* signs of oromotor dysfunction which may indicate a neurologic problem
- **Question:** Family history of speech delay, hearing loss, neurologic disorder, or syndrome?
- *Significance:* may direct further evaluation
- **Question:** Any regression or loss of language milestones?
- *Significance:* should prompt a neurologic and metabolic workup
- **Question:** What is the social interaction of the child?
- *Significance:* Lack of interest in playing is a red flag for autism.
- **Question:** Any concern regarding child abuse or neglect or psychosocial deprivation?
- *Significance:* may have occurred as the result of a parental, genetic, or developmental disorder; drug or alcohol abuse; poverty; child malnutrition; or environmental toxins such as lead
- **Question:** History of frequent acute otitis media or otitis media with effusion and conductive hearing loss?
- *Significance:* may precede speech delay
- **Question:** Visual impairments?
- *Significance:* may impact speech development because interpretation of facial expressions and gestures is a component of infant receptive language development
- **Question:** History of traumatic brain injury?
- *Significance:* Speech delay may occur with a seizure disorder.

PHYSICAL EXAM

Complete examination looking for signs that may be associated with speech delay.

- **Finding:** Microcephaly?
- *Significance*: associated with intellectual disability, in utero CMV infection, or dysmorphic features
- **Finding:** Macrocephaly?
- *Significance*: associated with hydrocephalus, various syndromes
- **Finding:** Dysmorphic features?
- *Significance*: suggestive of a syndrome

- **Finding:** Excess drooling and open-mouth posture?
- *Significance:* signs of poor oral motor control of muscles used for speech production
- **Finding:** Craniofacial abnormalities?
- *Significance:* Articulation difficulty may be due to velopalatal insufficiency (VPI) seen with unrepaired cleft lip or palate.
- **Finding:** Scarred tympanic membranes or middle ear fluid?
- *Significance:* may be clue to acquired intermittent or chronic conductive hearing loss
- **Finding:** Macroorchidism?
- *Significance:* fragile X syndrome
- **Finding:** Neurologic exam—hypertonia or hypotonia, abnormal reflexes, other focal findings?
- *Significance:* suggestive of neurologic impairment
- **Finding:** Café au lait spots, hypopigmented macules, shagreen patch, axillary or inguinal freckling?
- *Significance:* skin findings suggestive of a neurocutaneous syndrome

DIAGNOSTIC TESTS & INTERPRETATION

- The American Academy of Pediatrics recommends a specific development screening tool be administered at the 9, 18, and 24 or 30-month well-child care visits and an autism-specific tool be administered at the 18- and 24-month visits.
- Office development screening tools
  - Denver Developmental Assessment II
- Early Language Milestone Scale (ELMS)
- Clinical Linguistic and Auditory Milestone Scale (CLAMS)
- Hearing evaluation
  - Most states have mandated Universal Newborn Hearing Screening Programs.
  - Screening tests: automated auditory brainstem response (AABR) and transient evoked otoacoustic emissions (OAEs)
  - Hearing should be tested in all speech-delayed children, even if the newborn hearing screen was normal.
  - <6 months of age: The definitive test is brainstem auditory evoked response (BAER).
  - >6 months of age in a neurologically normal child: The definitive test is behavioral audiometry, such as visual reinforcement audiometry (VRA), performed by a trained audiologist.
- Selected speech/language milestones
  - 2 months: cooing, response to voice
  - 6 months: babbling
  - 4–9 months: turns to sound, responds to name
  - 9 months: dada/mama nonspecific, begins to understand "no"
  - 9–12 months: jargon
  - 12 months: dada, mama specific, 1 additional word, jargon is complex, points to gesture, follows 1-step command
  - 18 months: 10 words, knows body parts
  - 2 years: 50 words, 2-word phrases, 50% intelligible by strangers, pronouns, can point to specific objects in a picture, may know 1 color, follows 2-step commands
  - 3 years: 300–500 words, tells stories, 75% intelligible by strangers
  - 4 years: grammatically correct sentences, 100% intelligible by strangers
- Routine cranial imaging or screening tests for metabolic diseases are not recommended.
- **Test:** Full speech and language evaluation
- *Significance:* To delineate the disorder and determine therapy
- **Test:** Individuals with Disabilities Education Act (IDEA) mandates early intervention services from birth to 3 years.
- *Significance:* Children can get a full developmental evaluation and appropriate therapy if sufficient delays are demonstrated.
- **Test:** EEG
- *Significance:* Indicated if there is concern for seizures
- **Test:** Genetics evaluation
- *Significance:* Should be obtained for congenital hearing loss or if there is concern for a syndrome or genetic diagnosis
- **Test:** Prolonged sleep EEG
- *Significance:* Indicated with loss of language milestones (consider the diagnosis of Landau–Kleffner syndrome)

TREATMENT

GENERAL MEASURES

- Congenital hearing loss is managed by a team consisting of an otolaryngologist, audiologist, and speech/language therapist who individualize management. Options are amplification, cochlear implant for the severely impaired, or use of sign language.
- Speech and language therapy can be provided through physician referral or parent-generated referral to early intervention programs.
- Sign language can be used as a bridge to promote communication while the child learns verbal skills. It will not preclude or delay the development of speech.
- Augmentative communication devices such as picture boards or programmed computers with voice synthesizers can be used by children with physical impairments such as cerebral palsy.
- Children with DLD usually speak adequately by school age. Some percentage will go on to have difficulty reading and writing.
- Children with constitutional language delay will achieve normal milestones by school entrance without reading disability or other learning problem.

ADDITIONAL READING

- Agin M. The "late talker"—when silence isn't golden. *Contemp Pediatr*. 2004;21:22–32.
- Campbell T, Dollaghan C, Rockette H, et al. Risk factors for speech delay of unknown origin in 3-year old children. *Child Dev*. 2003;74(2):346–357.
- Coplan J. Normal speech and language development: an overview. *Pediatr Rev*. 1995;16(3):91–100.
- Feldman H. Evaluation and management of language and speech disorders in preschool children. *Pediatr Rev*. 2005;26(4):131–140.
- Rapin I. Practitioner review: developmental language disorders: a clinical update. *J Child Psychol Psychiatry*. 1996;37(6):643–655.
- Sokol J, Hyde M. Hearing screening. *Pediatr Rev*. 2002;23(5):155–162.

CODES

ICD10

- F80.9 Developmental disorder of speech and language, unspecified
- F80.4 Speech and language development delay due to hearing loss
- F80.1 Expressive language disorder

FAQ

- Q: Do 2nd- and 3rd-born children speak later than 1st-born children?
- A: No. The norms for expected speech/language development are the same regardless of birth order. 2nd- and 3rd-born children should have the same degree of motivation to speak as their 1st-born sibling.
- Q: When should I refer a child for speech/language evaluation?
- A: If the parents or physician have any concern for speech delay, then referral for evaluation is wise. Some speech-delayed children will eventually normalize and meet all milestones. It is difficult to distinguish who is constitutionally delayed from those who have another disorder. There are several indications for a prompt referral: no pointing or babbling by 1 year, no single words by 16 months, no 2-word spontaneous phrases by 2 years, no sentences by 3 years, poor intelligibility for age, child has behavioral "melt downs" or tantrums with efforts to communicate, or any regression in language skills.
- Q: Do children raised in bilingual households have expressive language delay?
- A: No. Living in a bilingual household is not a cause of expressive language delay. However, toddlers who are learning 2 languages may interchange words in both languages. Total vocabulary and phrase length are typically normal in these children by 2–3 years of age.

SPEECH PROBLEMS

Helen M. Sharp • Kathryn Hillenbrand

BASICS

DESCRIPTION

- Communication is the exchange of ideas between two or more individuals.
- Language is a systematic means of communication that relies on a socially agreed upon set of symbols and rules for combining those symbols. Language includes comprehension, expression, and social-pragmatic rules (e.g., eye contact and turn-taking).
- Speech is produced through vocal and articulatory movements using neuromotor control of respiration, phonation (vocalization), and articulation to shape airflow and vocal sounds into strings of speech sounds (phonemes) to form words and word combinations.
- Articulation refers to the use of oral and pharyngeal structures (lips, tongue, palate, teeth) to shape vocal sounds and airflow into recognizable speech.
- Hearing is the process of transferring sound from the environment to the brain via the outer, middle, and inner ear systems.
- Speech disorders have three general points of origin: (1) neurologic, (2) structural, or (3) functional. Functional disorders are those that are unrelated to neurologic or structural disorders. More than one of these causes may be present in the same child.
- Speech disorders can be classified and are described as follows:
  - Articulation or phonologic disorders
    - Disrupt the way a child says one or more speech sounds
    - Simplifications of complex adult speech are often normal very early in speech development but should be evaluated if these changes linger or are atypical.
  - Fluency disorders
    - Disrupt the easy flow of speech production and include the conditions of stuttering and cluttering.
    - Examples of stuttering include repetitions of sounds, syllables, words, or phrases, pauses, blocks, or hesitations.
    - Easy repetitions are common in children ages 2–4 years and typically resolve quickly. Persistence, visible struggle, or avoidance of talking warrant referral.
  - Motor speech disorders
    - Disrupt timing, coordination, or the execution of the motor plan for speech
    - Divided into two major categories: (1) dysarthrias, which are most often related to neuromotor weakness or paralysis, and (2) apraxia, a motor planning disorder in the absence of neuromotor weakness or paralysis
  - Voice disorders
    - Heard as atypical laryngeal quality such as hoarseness (dysphonia) or completely absent voice (aphonia)
  - Resonance disorders
    - Describe speech quality usually described as nasality
    - Hypernasality (excessively nasal quality) is associated with velopharyngeal dysfunction and is atypical.
    - Hyponasality (inadequate nasality) is common in young children in association with acute upper respiratory infection or adenoid hypertrophy.
- Language disorders may occur in receptive, expressive, pragmatic, or some combination of these domains. Language disorders may occur in conjunction with other developmental, sensory, neurologic, or structural concerns but may also be isolated as an area of delay (see "Language Delay" and "Autism" chapters).

EPIDEMIOLOGY

- The American Speech-Language Hearing Association states that communication disorders occur in 1 of every 8 people in the population.
  - Newborn screening identifies hearing loss or deafness in 1–6 per 1,000 newborns, with higher rates in neonatal intensive care.
- Speech sound disorders including articulation, phonologic, and developmental apraxia of speech are considered the most prevalent communication problem diagnosed in 10–15% of preschoolers and 6% of school-aged children.
  - Fluency disorders affect 11% of children by age 4 years. Boys are nearly three times more likely to persist in stuttering beyond age 4 years.
- Cerebral palsy affects 1 in 500 children born each year and may include mild to severe motor speech disorders and risk of other communication disorders.
- Voice disorders such as chronic hoarseness are reported in 6–23% of children.

DIAGNOSIS

HISTORY

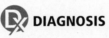

- Prenatal history
  - Prenatal exposures to alcohol, prescription or nonprescription medications, or infections are known to relate to developmental delay and/or hearing loss.
- Medical history
  - Prematurity, trauma, seizure disorders, major surgeries, and systemic infections are all risk factors for communication disorders.
  - Multiple anomalies may relate to an underlying syndrome.
- Feeding history
  - Neuromotor and structural disorders may be noted in early feeding history
  - Ask about failure to thrive, frequent pneumonia, prolonged feeding time, or chronic nasal regurgitation.
- Family history
  - Heredity may be a factor associated with stuttering, specific language impairment, autism spectrum disorders, cleft palate, developmental apraxia of speech, hearing loss, deafness, and other speech-language disorders.
- Social history
  - Evaluate for history of abuse, trauma, or neglect.
  - Smoking in the home is a known risk for middle ear infections.
  - Frequent verbal interaction and reading promote speech and language skills.
- Speech and language history
  - Routine screening for speech and language milestones aid early identification.
  - Duration of symptoms for voice and resonance disorders will separate acute infection from true disorders.
  - Regression of speech or language skills may be associated with autism spectrum disorders or trauma.
- Key milestones
  - By 1 year of age
    - Points to (or gazes toward) known person or object name (Where's mama?)
    - Produces at least *one* true word; may not be recognized by all but is consistent
  - By 2 years of age
    - Identifies body parts, follows one-element commands (Get your book.)
    - Uses about 50 expressive words and starts to *combine 2 words* together (up dada)
  - By 3 years of age
    - Follows *2–3 element commands*, combines *3-word phrases*, and uses short questions (e.g., Why?)
    - Speech is understood by familiar listeners the majority of the time.
  - By 4 years of age
    - Uses longer sentences and tells short stories/sequences of events
    - Answers who, what, where, and when questions
    - Speech is understood by an unfamiliar listener nearly all the time.
- Physical and social development
  - Missed physical or social milestones are indicative of overall delay. Delayed or absent social milestones may aid in early identification of autism spectrum disorders.

PHYSICAL EXAM

- Face. Evaluate for facial symmetry at rest (structural) and during movement (neurologic). Drooling is typical during early infancy and teething but should resolve by 18–24 months.
- *Eye color*. Iris heterotropia together with white forelock frequently associate with hearing loss in Waardenburg syndrome.
- *Skin*. Café au lait spots are associated with neurofibromatosis and hearing loss.
- *Head shape and size*. Microcephaly, macrocephaly, or plagiocephaly or other skull asymmetries may be associated with developmental delay, hypotonia, or craniosynostosis conditions.
- *Symmetry, structure, and height of ears*. Ear tags, atresia, and low-set ears have high association with hearing loss and should prompt audiologic and otolaryngology evaluation.
- *Intraoral* exam. Dental health, palatal shape, and jaw relationships should be noted. Soft palate (velar) elevation should be symmetric on "ah." Bifid uvula, bluish color of velum, or V-shaped notch at the border of the hard and soft palate are indicative of a submucous cleft palate. Absent gag response is not a contraindication to feeding but should be noted.
- *Phonation*. Listen to vocal quality on sustained "ah." Wet voice may indicate swallowing disorder. Rough, hoarse, or strained vocal quality is atypical and requires evaluation.

DIAGNOSTIC TESTS & INTERPRETATION

Screening Procedures

- Speech-language screening
  - Brief check on domains of communication designed to determine whether to refer child for full speech-language evaluation
  - Results often reported as "Pass/Refer" with minimal or no interpretation.
  - May be conducted by speech-language pathologist, audiologist, teacher, or other professional
- Hearing screening
  - Brief assessment that may be conducted for newborns or older children to detect presence or absence of response to sound at a set hearing level across frequencies
  - Results often reported as "Pass/Refer" with minimal or no interpretation.
  - Screening may be conducted by an audiologist, speech-language pathologist, nurse, or trained paraprofessional.

Diagnostic Procedures/Other

- Speech-language evaluation
  - Measurement of receptive, expressive, and/or pragmatic language skills; articulatory/phonologic development; and oral structural and physiologic examination with interpretation of findings and recommendations
  - Conducted by speech-language pathologist
- Hearing evaluation
  - Testing to obtain auditory thresholds (in decibels, dB) across sound frequencies (in Hertz, Hz) in both ears
  - If hearing loss is identified, further testing to determine if the source is middle ear (conductive) or inner ear (sensorineural) or mixed (both conductive and sensorineural)
  - Very young children may be tested using auditory brainstem response (ABR) or otoacoustic emissions (OAE).
  - Conducted by an audiologist
- Cognitive evaluation
  - Testing to assess overall cognitive development across verbal and nonverbal domains with results interpreted together with recommendations for interventions and/or school placement
  - Typically conducted by a psychologist
- Genetics evaluation and testing
  - Comprehensive family history, physical exam, metabolic, and/or cytogenetic testing often to identify or rule out specific diagnoses (e.g., fragile X, 22q deletion syndrome, neurofibromatosis, or genes associated with hereditary hearing impairment)
  - Interpretation of findings includes explanation to family of carrier status and recurrence risk.
  - Typically conducted by clinical geneticist or interdisciplinary genetics clinic
- Radiologic or other imaging studies: rarely used to assess underlying cause of speech or language disorders but may be used to rule out or identify related conditions such as intraventricular hemorrhage or swallowing and resonance disorders

DIFFERENTIAL DIAGNOSIS

Communication disorders may be associated with other underlying conditions. A diagnosis of speech or language delay should include a process of evaluating the child for underlying causes, which alter the treatment approach:

- Hearing loss. Evaluate for familial or congenital loss; chronic middle ear infection; or acquired loss (e.g., ototoxic medications, systemic infection, underlying syndrome, or noise exposure).
- Developmental delay or autism spectrum disorders. Failure to develop verbal language in the absence of hearing loss should yield examination of physical and social–behavioral milestones to rule out overall delay and/or autism spectrum disorders.
- Neuromotor disorders. Neuromotor disorders may yield low facial/oral tone, weakness, or paralysis that may reduce speech intelligibility. Developmental apraxia of speech requires assessment and may coincide with limb apraxia.
- Vocal overuse or trauma. Evaluate for overuse patterns from habitual screaming, poor singing technique, and cheerleading.
- Structural and dental changes. Dental malocclusion or oral structural anomalies may reduce speech intelligibility for particular speech sounds.
- Sleep apnea. Poor sleep may be the cause of behavioral and learning concerns.
- Selective mutism. Specific situations in which the child will not speak in the absence of evident speech or language disorder. May coincide with social withdrawal, shyness, social anxiety
- Social isolation, neglect, or malnutrition should be ruled out, as these may associate with delays or losses of communication skills.
- Seizure disorders such as Landau-Kleffner syndrome can be associated with loss of language skills.

TREATMENT

- Direct service
  - In-home services
    - Evaluation and treatment for high-risk infants and toddlers in family-centered, natural environment, with minimal or no expense to family
  - Clinic-based services. Evaluation and individual or group treatment through a hospital, private, or university speech–language–hearing clinic
    - May be needed for specialized services
  - School-based services
    - Evaluation, individual or group treatment usually through special education services that yield an Individualized Education Plan (IEP)
    - Service delivery is often limited to conditions that impact the child's educational performance.
- Related services
  - Interdisciplinary team care
    - Children with complex medical needs should be served by an interdisciplinary team such as a cleft palate/craniofacial, spina bifida, autism, feeding, or multiple disability clinic.
    - Provides comprehensive physical, functional, and psychosocial care of the child and family in collaboration with primary care providers
  - Otolaryngology. Detailed examination of laryngeal structures, airway, palatal structures, enlarged tonsils, and/or management of otologic concerns

ONGOING CARE

- Early identification of hearing, speech, or language problems is critical and leads to better outcomes.
- Children who have untreated hearing, speech sound, and language disorders are at risk for academic difficulties.
- Many speech problems can be resolved with short-term treatment. Some conditions may require longer term management extending through adolescence.
- Adenoid removal is usually contraindicated for children with cleft palate, including submucous cleft palate. Airway and apnea management may be an exception that requires interdisciplinary decision making.

S

ADDITIONAL READING

- American Speech-Language-Hearing Association (ASHA). http://www.asha.org.
- Graham SA, Fisher SE. Decoding the genetics of speech and language. *Curr Opinion Neurobiol*. 2013;23(1):43–51.
- Possamai V, Hartley B. Voice disorders in children. *Pediatr Clin North Am*. 2013;60(4):879–892.
- Sharp HM, Hillenbrand K. Speech and language development and disorders in children. *Pediatr Clin North Am*. 2008;55(5):1159–1173.

CODES

ICD10

- R47.9 Unspecified speech disturbances
- F80.81 Childhood onset fluency disorder
- R48.2 Apraxia

FAQ

- Q: Does ankyloglossia negatively affect speech production?
- A: The tongue tip is used for speech sounds /t, d, n, l, s, z/. If the child can make one or more of these sounds, then ankyloglossia can go untreated.
- Q: Does "baby sign" help or delay the acquisition of speech and language?
- A: Evidence suggests teaching gestural communication is associated with slightly advanced auditory–verbal language skills before 24 months of age and may decrease toddler–parent frustration. By 30–36 months of age, no significant differences are observed between children who used baby sign and those who did not.
- Q: Does chronic otitis media slow the acquisition of speech or language?
- A: Early speech and language may be delayed in the presence of otitis media. If treated, differences in language skills typically resolve by school age.

SPINAL MUSCULAR ATROPHY

Jennifer A. Markowitz

BASICS

DESCRIPTION

- Spinal muscular atrophy (SMA) is a progressive disorder of motor neurons in the spinal cord and brainstem.
- Major symptom is proximal weakness.
- 3 forms are described based on clinical features:
  - Type I, also known as Werdnig-Hoffman disease, typically presents by 6 months of age; these children never sit.
  - Type II typically presents between 6 and 18 months of age; these children sit independently but never walk.
  - Type III, also known as Kugelberg-Welander disease, may be diagnosed later; these children stand and walk at some point.
- There appears to be a spectrum of severity within and between each type.

EPIDEMIOLOGY

The most common genetic cause of infant mortality

Incidence

Incidence estimated at 1 in 6,000–10,000 live births; carrier frequency 1 in 40–50, although some variation between populations seems to exist.

RISK FACTORS

Genetics

- Genetic testing is recommended in all cases, even when the diagnosis appears clear.
- Genetic counseling is critical for all families with children affected by SMA, as the chance of recurrence is 25%.
- *SMN2* copy number varies among the general population and is loosely correlated with SMA type (type I likely to have fewer copies); however, all copies of *SMN2* are not equal (some make more SMN protein than others), and an individual patient's *SMN2* copy number should not be used for prognostic purposes.
- Universal newborn screening is strongly recommended by some but is controversial; a pilot study has been approved in limited states.

ETIOLOGY

- All 3 types of proximal SMA follow an autosomal recessive inheritance and are caused by mutations in the survival motor neuron (*SMN*) gene on 5q11.2 to 13.3.
- 2 copies of *SMN* on each chromosome. *SMN1* (SMNt), the telomeric copy, produces stable SMN protein. *SMN2* (SMNc), the centromeric copy, is an inverted duplication of *SMN1* with a single nucleotide change in an exonic splice enhancer, which produces mostly an unstable, truncated protein product and a smaller percentage of stable, full-length SMN protein.
- Individuals with SMA harbor homozygous deletions of exon 7 in the *SMN1* gene, which renders it nonfunctional. The presence of *SMN2* essentially "rescues" individuals with *SMN1* deletions because complete absence of SMN protein appears to be embryonically lethal. The level of SMN protein roughly correlates with the severity of disease, making this a target of therapeutics development.
- The SMN protein plays a role in RNA processing; it is unclear why motor neurons (anterior horn cells) are selectively vulnerable to this defect, although a role in axonal mRNA trafficking and splicing is being explored.
- SMA appears to affect other organ systems, especially in those with the most severe form; cardiovascular, autonomic, and metabolic abnormalities are reported.

COMMONLY ASSOCIATED CONDITIONS

Other anterior horn cell diseases:

- SMA with respiratory distress (SMARD) or diaphragmatic SMA due to mutations in the *IGHMBP2* gene on chromosome 11q
- Distal SMAs, a group of disorders with distal weakness, genetically heterogeneous
- Other variants are associated with arthrogryposis, pontocerebellar hypoplasia, congenital fractures, and congenital heart disease. Few such cases have been shown to have *SMN* mutations.
- Fazio-Londe disease: rare degeneration of anterior horn cells in the brainstem, childhood onset
- Kennedy disease, or X-linked spinal and bulbar muscular atrophy: anterior horn cell disease with adult onset; affected men have gynecomastia, bulbar weakness, and reduced fertility.

DIAGNOSIS

HISTORY

- Hypotonia and weakness are the primary features. Infants with SMA I will be floppy and less active and have delayed motor milestones, with preserved language/social interaction (a bright, alert demeanor is often remarked upon).
- Some babies with type I present with feeding problems and failure to thrive.
- History of reduced vigor of prenatal movements

PHYSICAL EXAM

- Weakness and absent or reduced reflexes suggest a neuromuscular rather than central etiology for hypotonia. A proximal pattern of weakness is consistent with SMA, myopathies, and muscular dystrophies; a distal pattern usually suggests polyneuropathies.
- Weakness is almost universally symmetric, but occasional cases of asymmetric weakness have been reported in SMA III.
- Extraocular movements remain intact in SMA.
- Facial strength diminishes in children with type I over time, and jaw contractures may be present in type II.
- Dysmorphic features, or involvement of other organs, may point to alternative diagnoses. Occasionally, SMA presents with contractures (spectrum of arthrogryposis multiplex congenita).
- Tongue fasciculations strongly suggest SMA, but their absence does not exclude the diagnosis.
- Tremor of a specific type, polyminimyoclonus, is often present in type II.

DIAGNOSTIC TESTS & INTERPRETATION

Lab

- Initial screening tests: Serum creatinine kinase may be mildly elevated.
- Genetic testing
  - Genetic testing of DNA extracted from blood (*SMN* deletions): now the gold standard in diagnosis, may be done prenatally, >95% sensitive
  - Genetic testing for Prader-Willi syndrome (fluorescence in situ hybridization and methylation) may be indicated if there is no *SMN* gene deletion and electromyography (EMG) is normal in an infant who appears to have SMA.
- Other testing
  - EMG may be helpful if the clinical presentation is atypical for SMA or if genetic testing is negative. EMG shows high-amplitude, long-duration motor units with a reduced recruitment pattern.
  - With the advent of molecular testing, muscle biopsy is rarely performed. Use when genetic testing is unrevealing. The characteristic findings are fiber-type grouping with generalized atrophy of muscle fibers.
  - If the entire evaluation is negative, MRI of the spine may be indicated to evaluate for an anomaly or mass lesion.

DIFFERENTIAL DIAGNOSIS

- Other genetic neuromuscular disorders include congenital muscular dystrophy, congenital myopathy, glycogen storage disorders (Pompe disease), myotonic dystrophy, mitochondrial disease, congenital myasthenia gravis, and Prader-Willi syndrome.
- More acute course may suggest infant botulism or Guillain-Barré syndrome, although the latter is rare in this age group.
- Systemic disorders: sepsis, meningitis, acute bowel syndromes
- SMA II differential: congenital muscular dystrophy, congenital myopathy, and congenital myasthenia gravis
- SMA III differential includes Duchenne, Becker, and the limb girdle muscular dystrophies; Lambert-Eaton myasthenic syndrome; and limb girdle congenital myasthenic syndromes.
- Spinal cord mass lesions may rarely resemble SMA.

TREATMENT

ALERT

An apparently minor respiratory infection may carry a higher risk of respiratory failure in SMA I and later stages of SMA II and III. Depending on family/patient wishes regarding respiratory support, consider admitting such a patient to the hospital for observation. Infants with SMA may be exquisitely sensitive to postural shifts—watch for hypoventilation, for example, with forward truncal flexion associated with some seating arrangements.

ADDITIONAL TREATMENT

General Measures

- A multidisciplinary approach to care is recommended, with early and proactive involvement of orthopedics, nutrition, pulmonary, and physical and occupational therapy as well as social work and psychological support for families and patients.
- Physical therapy is appropriate for all 3 types; although it may not affect the course in SMA I, it can lessen discomfort and make care easier by improving range of motion and preventing contractures.
- A wheelchair provides mobility in SMA II. Children as young as age 2 years may be considered for a motorized wheelchair, depending on developmental level. Adults with SMA III may require the use of a wheelchair later in their course.
- Bracing of ankles, wrists, and back can help reduce contractures and slow progression of scoliosis.
- Spinal fusion surgery may preserve respiratory function.
- Low threshold for empiric antibiotics for respiratory infection is appropriate.
- Chest physiotherapy and early implementation of cough-assist device can help prevent pneumonia and atelectasis.
- Be wary of symptoms of hypoventilation (disturbed sleep, daytime fatigue, moodiness, morning headaches), which may occur prior to other symptoms of respiratory insufficiency.
- Low threshold to order a sleep study if hypoventilation is suspected
- In acute respiratory illness, supplemental oxygen is appropriate as long as the patient is also evaluated and treated for hypercarbia.
- Noninvasive positive pressure ventilation (bilevel positive airway pressure [BiPAP] and other regimens) may improve quality of life and life expectancy in patients with decreased respiratory function. More aggressive respiratory management is becoming more common and accepted among families and physicians, but the extent of interventions varies widely. Start discussions about family/patient preferences early, as respiratory decompensation can occur very quickly.
- Avoid catabolic state with proactive nutritional support, including tube feeding.
- However, note that type II patients may have increased adiposity, and overweight is also a risk.
- Monitor for osteopenia, which is almost universal in types I and II, and ensure adequate calcium and vitamin D intake.
- Social and psychological support for caregivers and patients

ONGOING CARE

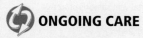

PATIENT EDUCATION

- Families of SMA: http://www.curesma.org
- Fight SMA: http://www.fightsma.org
- Muscular Dystrophy Association: http://www.mdausa.org
- Spinal Muscular Atrophy Foundation: http://www.smafoundation.org

PROGNOSIS

- Survival in all 3 forms has been increasing with improved supportive care and, in type I, ventilatory support.
- Most children with SMA type I die by 2 years without major pulmonary interventions. With ventilatory support, patients may survive several years longer; survival as long as 2 decades has been observed with tracheostomy and full mechanical ventilation.
- Children with SMA type II typically survive into late adolescence or early adulthood; this life expectancy is increasing with more aggressive pulmonary management.
- Individuals with SMA type III survive well into adulthood and often have a normal life expectancy. In 1 study of patients with SMA type III with onset <3 years, 50% could not walk 20 years later; for those with onset >3 years, 30% could not walk 20 years later.
- Intelligence is generally preserved.
- Death typically ensues from respiratory complications. Discuss the level of respiratory interventions, including resuscitation, early in SMA I and in the advanced stages of SMA II and III.

COMPLICATIONS

- Recurrent pneumonias, hypoventilation
- Swallowing difficulties may require tube feeding.
- Scoliosis may require surgery.

ADDITIONAL READING

- Arnold WD, Burghes AH. Spinal muscular atrophy: development and implementation of potential treatments. *Ann Neurol*. 2013;74(3):348–362.
- Chung BH, Wong VC, Ip P. Spinal muscular atrophy: survival pattern and functional status. *Pediatrics*. 2004;114(5):e548–e553.
- Hardart MK, Truog RD. Spinal muscular atrophy—type I. *Arch Dis Child*. 2003;88(10):848–850.
- Iannaccone ST, Burghes A. Spinal muscular atrophies. *Adv Neurol*. 2002;88:83–98.
- Khirani S, Colella M, Caldarelli V, et al. Longitudinal course of lung function and respiratory muscle strength in spinal muscular atrophy type 2 and 3. *Eur J Paediatr Neurol* 2013;17(6):552–560.
- Kolb SJ, Kissel JT. Spinal muscular atrophy: a timely review. *Arch Neurol*. 2011;68(8):979–984.
- Lunn MR, Wang CH. Spinal muscular atrophy. *Lancet*. 2008;371(9630):2120–2133.
- Messina S, Pane M, De Rose P, et al. Feeding problems and malnutrition in spinal muscular atrophy type II. *Neuromuscul Disord*. 2008;18(5):389–393.
- Ogino S, Leonard DG, Rennert H, et al. Genetic risk assessment in carrier testing for spinal muscular atrophy. *Am J Med Genet*. 2002;110(4):301–307.
- Petit F, Cuisset JM, Rouaix-Emery N, et al. Insights into genotype-phenotype correlations in spinal muscular atrophy: a retrospective study of 103 patients. *Muscle Nerve*. 2011;43(1):26–30.
- Prasad AN, Prasad C. The floppy infant: contribution of genetic and metabolic disorders. *Brain Dev*. 2003;25(7):457–476.
- Prior TW, Snyder PJ, Rink BD, et al. Newborn and carrier screening for spinal muscular atrophy. *Am J Med Genet Part A*. 2010;152A(7):1608–1616.
- Shababi M, Lorson CL, Rudnik-Schoneborn SS. Spinal muscular atrophy: a motor neuron disorder or a multi-organ disease? *J Anat*. 2013;224(1):15–28.
- Wang CH, Finkel RS, Bertini ES, et al. Participants of the International Conference on SMA Standard of Care. Consensus statement for standard of care in spinal muscular atrophy. *J Child Neurol*. 2007;22(8):1027–1049.
- Zerres K, Rudnik-Schoneborn S. Natural history in proximal spinal muscular atrophy. Clinical analysis of 445 patients and suggestions for a modification of existing classifications. *Arch Neurol*. 1995;52(5):518–523.

CODES

ICD10

- G12.9 Spinal muscular atrophy, unspecified
- G12.0 Infantile spinal muscular atrophy, type I [Werdnig-Hoffman]
- G12.1 Other inherited spinal muscular atrophy

FAQ

- Q: Can routine vaccinations be given to children with SMA?
- A: Yes. In addition to routine vaccinations, yearly influenza and respiratory syncytial virus (RSV) vaccinations are recommended.
- Q: How much respiratory support should a child with SMA receive?
- A: Standards of care are evolving rapidly, and a consensus remains elusive. Noninvasive respiratory interventions are becoming more widely accepted. Noninvasive respiratory options should be offered to all patients with SMA I and those in the later stages of SMA II. Tracheostomy is more controversial.
- Q: Are more effective therapies for SMA being developed?
- A: There are ongoing studies in animal models and on humans, involving both pharmacologic and gene-based therapies. Patients and families should be informed about clinical trials that may be available to them. Families of SMA, the Muscular Dystrophy Association, and other groups, as well as Clinicaltrials.gov, are sources of information on such research.

SPLENOMEGALY

Matthew J. Ryan

BASICS

DESCRIPTION

- A palpable spleen is found in most premature infants and in 30% of term infants. A spleen tip is still palpable in 10% of infants at 1 year of age and in 1% of children at 10 years of age.
- Normal spleens are not greater than 6 cm at 3 months, 7 cm at 12 months, 9.5 cm at 6 years, 11.5 cm at 12 years, and not greater than 13 cm for adolescents.
- Splenomegaly can also be a spleen width >4 cm or diameter >7 cm.
- Normal spleen size varies but is typically less than 250 g.
- The clinical significance of splenomegaly found on radiologic study, but not palpable on physical exam, is unclear in the absence of other laboratory or clinical data.
- Normal spleens are soft at the midclavicular line, nontender, and often palpable only on deep inspiration.
- Dullness on percussion beyond the 11th intercostal space suggests splenomegaly.
- A spleen edge palpated >2 cm below the costal margin is always an abnormal finding.
- Splenic tenderness is always abnormal.

PATHOPHYSIOLOGY

- The spleen is a hematopoietic organ with 2 main parts:
  - White pulp is the lymphoid tissue.
  - Red pulp is the red cell mass.
- Splenic sinusoids are lined with macrophages that destroy abnormal red cells.
- The spleen also serves as a reservoir for platelets. A normal-sized spleen can hold 1/3 of the circulating platelets; an enlarged spleen can hold up to 90% of the circulating platelet mass.
- Normal splenic volume by CT scan is 214.6 cm^3 (range, 107.2 cm^3–314.5 cm^3).
- Splenic size does correlate with height.

DIAGNOSIS

HISTORY

- **Question:** History of acute illness?
- *Significance*: Suggests infection
- **Question:** History of GI bleeding with splenomegaly?
- *Significance*: Suggests portal hypertension
- **Question:** Familial history of hematologic or immune disease?
- *Significance*: Suggests genetic etiology
- **Question:** An enlarged liver, developmental delay, or neurologic findings?
- *Significance*: May suggest a storage disease or metabolic disorder

PHYSICAL EXAM

Begin the abdominal examination in the lower left quadrant because an enlarged spleen may be missed in the upper quadrant exam. Stand to the right of the patient; use the right hand to palpate and the left hand to support the patient's left lower rib cage. Flexing the legs at the knees may help to relax the abdominal musculature.

- **Finding:** Auscultate for rub or bruit?
- *Significance*: Vascular malformation
- **Finding:** Look for signs of storage disease?
- *Significance*: Retinal exam, coarse facies
- **Finding:** Complete evaluation of lymph nodes?
- *Significance*: Enlargement suggests infection or neoplasia.
- **Finding:** Palpate for ascites or hepatomegaly?
- *Significance*: Suggests underlying hepatic disease
- **Finding:** Prominent abdominal veins or hemorrhoids?
- *Significance*: Suggest increased portal venous pressure
- **Finding:** Pain/tenderness?
- *Significance*: Suggests capsular distention secondary to perisplenitis or trauma; also raises the question of splenic infarct
- **Finding:** Asthmatic patients may have palpable spleen?
- *Significance*: Secondary to overinflation of lungs with a depressed diaphragm

DIAGNOSTIC TESTS & INTERPRETATION

Lab

- **Test:** Blood culture, thick smear of blood for malaria, viral testing
- *Significance:* evaluate for infection
- **Test:** CBC with manual differential and smear
- *Significance*: For sickle cell disease, hemolytic anemia, leukemia
- **Test:** Decreased WBC count and platelets
- *Significance*: Often seen with splenic sequestration or portal hypertension
- **Test:** Reticulocyte count
- *Significance*: For hemolytic anemia
- **Test:** Hepatic function panel (liver enzymes, albumin, bilirubin) and prothrombin time (PT)/international normalized ratio (INR), partial thromboplastin time (PTT)
- *Significance*: For cirrhosis, hepatic obstruction
- **Test:** Serum lactate dehydrogenase (LDH)
- *Significance*: For hemolysis or tumor screen

Imaging

- If no hemolytic disease, no sign of infection, no sign of congestion:
  - Ultrasound with Doppler
  - Liver spleen scan
- If no hemolytic disease, no sign of infection but signs of congestion:
  - Ultrasound with Doppler
  - MRI; consider MRA/MRV

Diagnostic Procedures/Other

Biopsy of lymph node, liver, or other tissue, depending on findings

DIFFERENTIAL DIAGNOSIS

- Infectious
  - Bacterial
    - Bacteremia
    - Pneumonia
    - Sepsis
    - Subacute bacterial endocarditis
    - Salmonellosis
    - Tuberculosis
    - Brucellosis
    - Staphylococcal shunt infections
    - Tularemia
    - Syphilis
    - Leptospirosis
  - Viral
    - Epstein-Barr virus (mononucleosis)
    - Cytomegalovirus
    - HIV
    - Rubella
    - Herpes
    - Hepatitis A, B, C
  - Rickettsial/protozoan
    - Rocky Mountain spotted fever
    - Malaria
    - Toxoplasmosis
    - Trypanosomiasis
    - Babesiosis
    - Schistosomiasis
    - Visceral larval migrans
    - Kala azar
  - Fungal
    - Histoplasmosis
    - Coccidioidomycosis
- Hematologic disorders
  - Hereditary spherocytosis
  - Sickle cell disease in early childhood or during splenic sequestration crisis
  - Hemoglobin C disease
  - Thalassemia major
  - Autoimmune hemolytic anemia
  - Glucose-6-phosphate dehydrogenase deficiency
  - Isoimmunization disorders
  - Infantile pyknocytosis
  - Iron deficiency anemia (rare)
  - Thrombocytopenic purpura
- Vascular disorders
  - Cavernous transformation of the portal vein
  - Budd-Chiari syndrome
  - Splenic vein thrombosis
  - Congenital portal vein stenosis or atresia
  - Splenic hematoma
  - Splenic hemangioma

- Liver disease/cirrhosis (examples include, but are not limited to)
  - Biliary atresia
  - Wilson disease
  - Cystic fibrosis
  - α-1-Antitrypsin deficiency
  - Hereditary hemochromatosis
  - Congenital hepatic fibrosis
  - Autoimmune hepatitis
  - Primary sclerosing cholangitis
- Metabolic diseases (storage)
  - Gangliosidoses
  - Mucolipidoses
  - Metachromatic leukodystrophy
  - Wolman disease
  - Gaucher disease
  - Niemann-Pick disease
  - Amyloidosis
- Neoplastic diseases
  - Leukemia
  - Lymphoma
  - Lymphosarcoma
  - Neuroblastoma
  - Histiocytosis X
  - Familial hemophagocytic lymphohistiocytosis
- Miscellaneous
  - Serum sickness
  - Connective tissue disorders
  - Juvenile rheumatoid arthritis
  - Systemic lupus erythematosus
  - Sarcoidosis
  - Splenic hamartoma
  - Splenic cysts: congenital and posttraumatic
  - Trauma: subcapsular hematoma
- Nonsplenic upper left quadrant abdominal masses
  - Large kidney
  - Retroperitoneal tumor
  - Adrenal neoplasm
  - Ovarian cyst
  - Pancreatic cyst
  - Mesenteric cyst
  - Rib anomaly

ALERT

- Life-threatening causes: sepsis, severe hemolytic anemia, trauma, splenic sequestration
- A large-bore IV access route should be rapidly placed when a life-threatening cause is suspected.

TREATMENT

GENERAL MEASURES

- Treatment depends on underlying etiology.
- Spleen guards can be used to protect from traumatic splenic rupture.

ISSUES FOR REFERRAL

- Increasing size over serial examinations (hepatology, hematology/oncology)
- Unexplained lymphadenopathy (oncology)
- Liver dysfunction and or ascites (hepatology)
- Signs of storage or metabolic disease (metabolism, GI)
- Howell-Jolly bodies on peripheral smear, suggesting splenic dysfunction (hematology)

SURGERY/OTHER PROCEDURES

Splenectomy indicated in certain situations including symptomatic hematologic disorders, abscess, and neoplasms.

ONGOING CARE

General goal is to determine the etiology of the large spleen.

- Establish the presence of enlarged spleen, not a palpable spleen that is pushed down by inflated lungs.
- Rule out common causes such as a viral infection, bacterial infection, or anemia.
- Rule out malignancy or storage disease or other rare causes of large spleen.
- Ensure proper immunizations or antibiotic prophylaxis.
- Ongoing care depends on the underlying etiology of the splenomegaly.

ADDITIONAL READING

- Benter T, Klühs L, Teichgräber U. Sonography of the spleen. *J Ultrasound Med*. 2011;30(9):1281–1293.
- Donnelly LF, Foss JN, Frush DP, et al. Heterogeneous splenic enhancement patterns on spiral CT images in children: minimizing misinterpretation. *Radiology*. 1999;210(2):493–497.
- McCormick PA, Murphy KM. Splenomegaly, hypersplenism and coagulation abnormalities in liver disease. *Best Pract Res Clin Gastroenterol*. 2000;14(6):1009–1031.
- Pozo AL, Godfrey EM, Bowles KM. Splenomegaly: investigation, diagnosis and management. *Blood Rev*. 2009;23(3):105–111.
- Prassopoulos P, Daskalogiannaki M, Raissaki M, et al. Determination of normal splenic volume on computed tomography in relation to age, gender and body habitus. *Eur Radiol*. 1997;7(2):246–248.
- Rosenberg HK, Markowitz RI, Kolberg H, et al. Normal splenic size in infants and children: sonographic measurements. *AJR Am J Roentgenol*. 1991;157(1):119–121.

CODES

ICD10

- R16.1 Splenomegaly, not elsewhere classified
- D73.5 Infarction of spleen
- D18.03 Hemangioma of intra-abdominal structures

FAQ

- Q: How long will the enlarged spleen secondary to a viral infection be present?
- A: The enlarged spleen may persist for several months.
- Q: Should patients with decreased splenic function due to splenomegaly be immunized?
- A: Immunization with a pneumococcal conjugate and/or polysaccharide vaccine should be carried out in all patients with compromised splenic function. In those patients who will be undergoing a scheduled splenectomy, the *Streptococcus pneumoniae*, meningococcus, and *Haemophilus influenzae* type B vaccines should be given at least 14 days prior to the operation.
- Q: Should a child with an enlarged spleen refrain from sports?
- A: Contact sports should be avoided for a child with an enlarged spleen. An enlarged spleen is engorged with blood, and a splenic rupture would be a catastrophic event. Children with persistent splenomegaly should be considered for a spleen guard.

SPONDYLOARTHROPATHY

Melissa L. Mannion • Randy Q. Cron

BASICS

DESCRIPTION

A group of inflammatory arthritides associated with enthesitis (inflammation at the bony insertion of tendons and ligaments) and axial involvement, typically sacroiliitis

- Enthesitis-related arthritis
- Ankylosing spondylitis (AS)
- Psoriatic arthritis
- Inflammatory bowel disease–associated arthropathy

EPIDEMIOLOGY

- Spondyloarthritis accounts for 15–20% of juvenile arthritis.
- AS typically affects adolescent boys. Much less common in blacks:
  - HLA-B27 occurs in 70–90% of patients and is present in 8% of whites and 6% of blacks in the general population.

Prevalence

~1/10,000 white boys

RISK FACTORS

Genetics

- HLA-B27 associated
- Usually a family history of a male relative with disease

PATHOPHYSIOLOGY

Inflammatory synovitis of joints and inflammation at sites of ligament and tendon attachment (entheses). Progression to ankylosis is a result of calcification of the anterior and posterior longitudinal ligaments of the spine.

ETIOLOGY

Autoimmune or autoinflammatory arthritis of unknown etiology, microbiome may play a role in disease

DIAGNOSIS

- Inflammatory back pain (better with exercise, not relieved by rest) of insidious onset that has been present for at least 6 weeks
- Inactivity stiffness resulting in gelling of peripheral joints and back

HISTORY

- Back pain and joint pain/swelling
- Family history

PHYSICAL EXAM

- Sacroiliac (SI) tenderness
  - Indicates site of inflammation
- Pain on direct palpation at insertion of Achilles tendon and plantar fascia at calcaneal insertion (location of entheses)
  - Indicates site of inflammation
- Patrick test (FABER)
  - FABER stands for "Flexion, ABduction and External Rotation"
  - A series of maneuvers to screen for issues with the sacroiliac and hip joints
- Psoriasis, nail pitting, or dactylitis

DIAGNOSTIC TESTS & INTERPRETATION

- Schober test of lumbar spine flexibility
  - Mark 15-cm vertical span at mid-lower back at level of iliac crest while patient is standing.
  - Have patient bend forward at the waist as far as possible without bending knees.
  - Remeasure span.
  - Abnormal if <5 cm increase in span

Lab

CBC, erythrocyte sedimentation rate (ESR), HLA-B27, rheumatoid factor (RF), and antinuclear antibody (ANA) tests

- ESR is occasionally not elevated.
- RF and ANA are typically negative.

Imaging

Sacroiliac views

- Demonstrate evidence of pseudowidening, erosions, and/or sclerosis, with fusion being a late finding.
- Because x-ray findings may take years to develop in the presence of disease, MRI is supplanting x-ray as the initial modality to assess SI involvement in some centers.

DIFFERENTIAL DIAGNOSIS

- Caution
  - Overdiagnosis in HLA-B27–positive individuals in whom other causes for joint swelling should be considered
- Infection
  - Reactive arthritis caused by enteric pathogens or *Chlamydia* species
  - Whipple disease
  - Intestinal bypass–associated arthritis
  - Discitis
  - Pott disease (vertebral tuberculosis)
- Tumors
  - Osteoid osteoma
- Trauma
  - Traumatic injury causing lower back pain/spasm
  - Herniated disc
- Metabolic
  - Ochronosis
- Congenital
  - Kyphosis
- Immunologic
  - Oligoarticular juvenile idiopathic arthritis
- Psychological
  - Feigning lower back pain/stiffness
- Miscellaneous
  - Fibromyalgia

TREATMENT

MEDICATION

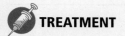

- NSAIDs
  - Naproxen
  - Indomethacin
  - Diclofenac
- Disease-modifying drugs
  - Sulfasalazine
  - Methotrexate
  - Leflunomide
  - Tumor necrosis factor (TNF) inhibitors

ADDITIONAL TREATMENT

General Measures

- Therapy may need to be lifelong.
- After initiation of therapy, should see some improvement in stiffness, synovitis, and range of motion over weeks to several months
- Only TNF inhibitors are effective for axial involvement.

ADDITIONAL THERAPIES

Physical therapy

- Physical therapy is an essential component of treatment.
- Must encourage range-of-motion exercises and avoid prolonged neck flexion

SURGERY/OTHER PROCEDURES

In advanced cases, total hip replacement, C-spine fusion, and/or spinal wedge osteotomy (the latter if posture is severely affected)

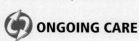

ONGOING CARE

DIET

- Ensure food intake with NSAIDs.
- Ensure folate intake with methotrexate.

PATIENT EDUCATION

Activity

- As tolerated. In cases of severe/advanced disease, modify behaviors accordingly in consideration of reduced spine flexibility and subsequent risk of serious injury.

PROGNOSIS

Poor if disease remains active for 10 years or more.

COMPLICATIONS

- Acute anterior uveitis
- Aortic insufficiency
- Worsening stiffness
- Ankylosis with risk of vertebral subluxation, fracture, and nerve damage, including cauda equina syndrome
- Acute or chronic eye pain
- Chest pain or shortness of breath

ALERT

A red, painful eye in a patient with HLA-B27–positive spondyloarthropathy should not be assumed to be infectious conjunctivitis. Slit-lamp exam is required to diagnose acute anterior uveitis.

ADDITIONAL READING

- Colbert RA. Classification of juvenile spondyloarthritis: enthesitis-related arthritis and beyond. *Nat Rev Rheumatol*. 2010;6(8):477–485.
- Colbert RA. Early axial spondyloarthritis. *Curr Opin Rheumatol*. 2010;22(5):603–607.
- Homeff G, Burgos-Vargas R. TNF-alpha antagonists for the treatment of juvenile-onset spondyloarthritides. *Clin Exp Rheumatol*. 2002;20(6)(Suppl 28):S137–S142.
- Sherry DD, Sapp LR. Enthesalgia in childhood: site-specific tenderness in healthy subjects and in patients with seronegative enthesopathic arthropathy. *J Rheumatol*. 2003;30(6):1335–1340.
- Stoll ML, Lio P, Sundel RP, et al. Comparison of Vancouver and International League of Associations for rheumatology classification criteria for juvenile psoriatic arthritis. *Arthritis Rheum*. 2008;59(1):51–58.
- Tse SM, Laxer RM. New advances in juvenile spondyloarthritis. *Nat Rev Rheumatol*. 2012;8(5):269–279.
- Tse SM, Laxer RM, Babyn PS, et al. Radiologic improvement of juvenile idiopathic arthritis-enthesitis-related arthritis following anti-tumor necrosis factor-alpha blockade with etanercept. *J Rheumatol*. 2006;33(6):1186–1188.

CODES

ICD10

- M12.88 Oth specific arthropathies, NEC, vertebrae
- M46.1 Sacroiliitis, not elsewhere classified
- M45.9 Ankylosing spondylitis of unspecified sites in spine

FAQ

- Q: Should HLA-B27 be checked routinely in boys with back pain?
- A: Inflammatory back, joint, or entheseal pain; family history; and exam findings should increase your suspicion for HLA-B27–positive disease. Detection of HLA-B27 alone should not precipitate an extensive workup because it is so common in the normal healthy population. However, the risk for developing a spondyloarthropathy is 16 times greater than in HLA-B27–negative individuals.
- Q: Can affected individuals play contact sports?
- A: This is probably not a good idea in patients with ankylosis because as the spine fuses, the risk for fracture of the spine (especially the cervical spine) increases. However, children with milder forms of disease, such as enthesitis-related arthritis, should not be discouraged.

STAPHYLOCOCCAL SCALDED SKIN SYNDROME

Lauren G. Solan • Craig H. Gosdin

BASICS

DESCRIPTION

- A spectrum of generalized exfoliative skin disease with blistering of the upper layer of skin caused by an epidermolytic toxin produced by certain strains of *Staphylococcus aureus*
- In neonates and young infants, also known as Ritter disease or pemphigus neonatorum
- Classically described as skin tenderness and erythema, with bullae formation and desquamation
- Severity of the disease ranges from
  - Few blisters localized to site of infection
  - Mild illness with desquamation of skinfolds following impetigo
  - Generalized severe exfoliation involving much of the body (typically seen in neonates)
  - Classic staphylococcal scalded skin syndrome (SSSS): tenderness, erythema, desquamation, or bullae formation. May resemble scalding injury
- Pitfalls
  - Failure to differentiate from streptococcal disease, as SSSS requires treatment with penicillinase-resistant antibiotic therapy (e.g., nafcillin)
  - Late recognition leading to delayed therapy and shock
  - Not appreciating increased fluid losses through affected skin
  - Differentiation from toxic epidermal necrolysis (TEN) is critical, as therapy is very different.

EPIDEMIOLOGY

- Most cases occur in neonates and children.
  - 62% of affected children are <2 years of age.
  - 98% of affected children are <6 years of age.
- Rare in adults due to increased circulating antibodies and adult kidney excretion of the toxin

Incidence

- No differences in incidence based on gender in children; however, in adults, the male-to-female ratio is 2:1.

RISK FACTORS

- Immunocompromised state (in children or adults)
  - Maternal antibodies transferred via breast milk are partially protective, but neonatal cases can still occur.
- Increased *S. aureus* carriage and susceptibility to toxin (usually in adults)
- Renal impairment either due to immature renal clearance of toxin in children or underlying renal disease

GENERAL PREVENTION

- Good hand hygiene practices, including adherence to contact precautions in hospitalized patients, to prevent spread from asymptomatic carriers
- Prevent skin from becoming overly moist or macerated.
- Isolation of hospitalized patient
  - Suspected or documented cases should be placed in contact isolation.

PATHOPHYSIOLOGY

- Exfoliative toxins circulate throughout the body, causing blisters at sites distant from the infection.
- Destruction of protein desmoglein 1 (attachment protein found only in the superficial epidermis) by exfoliative toxin A (ETA) and exfoliative toxin B (ETB) cause intraepidermal splitting leading to bullae development and skin desquamation.

ETIOLOGY

- Exfoliative toxin released by *S. aureus*:
  - 2 major serotypes of the toxin: ETA and ETB
  - Mostly caused by *S. aureus* belonging to phage group II, types 71 and 55

COMMONLY ASSOCIATED CONDITIONS

- Skin and soft tissue infections or abscesses
- Bullous impetigo

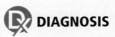

DIAGNOSIS

ALERT

- **Diagnosis is primarily clinical; do not delay treatment.** Cultures and other diagnostic tests are largely confirmatory.
- Confusion with TEN may lead to use of corticosteroids or discontinuation of antibiotics, resulting in worsening infection from prolonged toxin production.

HISTORY

- Nonspecific virus-like prodrome with irritability, sore throat, conjunctivitis, and upper respiratory infection is typical.
- Usual onset of fever within 48 hours after prodrome
- Rash typically begins periorally, then extends to the trunk and extremities, and finally desquamates.
- Recent localized extracutaneous infection is common.
  - Infections involving the nasopharynx, middle ear, conjunctivae, pharynx, tonsils, umbilicus, or urinary tract are frequently recalled.
- A history of recent drug use suggests other etiology such as TEN.

PHYSICAL EXAM

- Erythroderma: red, painful skin
- Large flaccid bullae that leave behind denuded skin resembling a burn after rupturing appear within 1–2 days
  - Bullae often appear in areas of trauma or in areas that are rubbed or touched, including intertriginous zones.
- Nikolsky sign (gentle friction applied to apparently healthy skin will cause blistering and sloughing) appears within 1–2 days.
- Distribution of lesions: most commonly face, neck, axilla, perineum
- Facial edema with perioral and periocular crustiness is typical and may be the primary clinical features.
- Conjunctivitis with or without periorbital edema may also be present.

ALERT

- Nikolsky sign can be seen in both TEN and SSSS, but in SSSS, it is often noted over areas of unaffected skin as well.
- SSSS does NOT involve the mucous membranes, but TEN does.

DIAGNOSTIC TESTS & INTERPRETATION

Lab

- General: CBC may be normal; erythrocyte sedimentation rate (ESR) typically elevated; electrolytes and renal function should be followed closely in severe cases and cases with dehydration.
- Microbiologic diagnosis: Culture of the original infected site, other involved sites/abnormal skin, blood, urine, nasopharynx, and umbilicus should be performed to determine the organism and antibiotic susceptibility.
  - Typically isolate phage group II *S. aureus*
  - Some immunologic methods exists to specifically identify the exfoliative exotoxins.
  - Intact bullae are sterile.
  - Blood cultures are typically negative.
- Histologic diagnosis: Skin biopsy can be used to differentiate SSSS from TEN; SSSS demonstrates separation of the epidermis at the granular layer, whereas with TEN, there is necrosis of the entire epidermis with a deeper plane of separation at the basement membrane.

DIFFERENTIAL DIAGNOSIS
- TEN
- Kawasaki disease
- Bullous impetigo
- Erythema multiforme bullosum
- Erythema multiforme major (Stevens-Johnson syndrome)
- Streptococcal scarlet fever
- Streptococcal or staphylococcal toxic shock syndrome (TSS)
- Bullous varicella
- Burns, including inflicted burns in suspected child abuse
- Primary bullous disorders (e.g., bullous mastocytosis)
- Chronic bullous disease of childhood
- Pemphigus vulgaris or foliaceus
- Epidermolysis bullosa

TREATMENT

GENERAL MEASURES
- Hospitalization is necessary for antibiotic therapy and supportive care.
- Consider consultation with infectious disease and/or dermatology.
- Apply principles of good burn care in severe cases, including the following:
  - Consideration of management in a critical care setting
  - Aggressive and early fluid and electrolyte management including daily maintenance requirements in addition to replacement of increased insensible skin losses
  - Petrolatum gauze should cover eroded areas to prevent further skin trauma.
  - Blisters should be left intact.
  - Children should be allowed to rest unclothed on clean linens, and handling of the child should be kept to a minimum.
  - Use of pressure-relieving mattresses

MEDICATION
- 1st-line agent: parenteral antistaphylococcal antibiotics: nafcillin, oxacillin, or 1st-generation cephalosporin (e.g., cefazolin)
- Some experts add clindamycin to inhibit exotoxin production.
- Clindamycin or vancomycin can be used for penicillin-allergic patients (severe allergies).
- 2nd-line agent: vancomycin for severe cases with toxic-appearing patient or concern for methicillin-resistant *Staphylococcus aureus* (MRSA)
- MRSA is rare but can occur.
- Antibiotic therapy can be tailored once sensitivities are known.
- Topical antibiotics are of no benefit.
- Oral antibiotics are not effective initially, but once a clear response has been noted with parenteral antibiotics, an oral antibiotic active against *S. aureus* can be used to complete the course of therapy.
- Corticosteroids have been shown to be detrimental both in experimental animal models as well as clinical trials.
- Adequate pain management is essential.

ALERT

Avoid nonsteroidal anti-inflammatories due to potential for renal impairment,

ONGOING CARE

PROGNOSIS
- Usually complete recovery within 10–14 days **without** scarring if treated
- Prognosis is more guarded in infants and those with underlying illness.
- Childhood mortality approximately 4%, whereas adult mortality reportedly >60%
- Does not tend to recur

COMPLICATIONS
- Occasional shedding of hair and nails
- Fungal or bacterial superinfection following desquamation
- Serious fluid and electrolyte disturbances may occur in cases involving large surface areas, which may lead to poor temperature control, sepsis, shock, and death.
- Neonates are particularly susceptible.

ADDITIONAL READING

- Braunstein I, Wanat KA, Abuabara K, et al. Antibiotic sensitivity and resistance patterns in pediatric staphylococcal scalded skin syndrome. *Pediatr Dermatol*. 2014;31(3):305–308. doi:10.1111/pde.12195.
- Li MY, Hua Y, Wei GH, et al. Staphylococcal scalded skin syndrome in neonates: an 8-year retrospective study in a single institution. *Pediatr Dermatol*. 2013;31(1):43–47. doi:10.1111/pde.12114.
- Patel GK, Finlay AY. Staphylococcal scalded skin syndrome: diagnosis and management. *Am J Clin Dermatol*. 2003;4(3):165–175.
- Schenfeld LA. Images in clinical medicine. Staphylococcal scalded skin syndrome. *N Engl J Med*. 2000;342(16):1178.
- Stanley JR, Amagai M. Pemphigus, bullous impetigo, and the staphylococcal scalded-skin syndrome. *N Engl J Med*. 2006;355(17):1800–1810.

CODES

ICD10
L00 Staphylococcal scalded skin syndrome

FAQ
- Q: Can SSSS recur?
- A: Yes, although it is uncommon.
- Q: Is SSSS contagious?
- A: Yes. The staphylococci are spread primarily from person to person (familial clusters have been reported), even from mother to fetus, most efficiently by someone with lesions, but asymptomatic carriers may also spread infection. Spread of organisms does not necessarily lead to signs of toxin production in those acquiring infection.
- Q: How can one distinguish TEN from SSSS?
- A: TEN is frequently confused with SSSS and may be differentiated by skin biopsy showing cleavage plane at the dermal–epidermal junction. TEN is more common in older children and adults and is usually secondary to drug hypersensitivity (e.g., sulfonamides, barbiturates, pyrazolone derivatives).
- Q: Can *Staphylococcus* be isolated from the bullae?
- A: SSSS bullae are sterile, although organisms may be found in a distant focus, such as the nares or conjunctivae. In bullous impetigo, however, staphylococci may be isolated from the bullae.

S

STATUS EPILEPTICUS

Heather Olson • Tobias Loddenkemper

BASICS

DESCRIPTION

- Status epilepticus (SE) is defined as continuous seizure activity >30 minutes or recurrent seizures in 30 minutes without return to baseline. In practice, an operational definition of convulsive seizures >5 minutes is treated as presumed SE.
- SE presents in several forms:
  - Generalized SE: continuous or repeated generalized convulsion(s) with persistent loss of consciousness and neurologic function
  - Nonconvulsive SE, myoclonic SE, or absence SE: persistent encephalopathy, often with variable subtle motor signs such as myoclonus or nystagmus
  - Repeated partial seizures with alteration of consciousness (focal SE) or preserved consciousness (epilepsia partialis continua)
- Systemic complications of SE:
  - Hyperthermia, rhabdomyolysis
  - Tachycardia, hypertension early → hypotension late
  - Hypoxia, hypercapnia, aspiration pneumonia
  - Impaired cerebral autoregulation
  - Rare: cardiac arrhythmias, neurogenic pulmonary edema, bone fractures

ALERT

- Neuromuscular blockers used in intubation may obscure ongoing seizures. EEG monitoring is mandatory for all patients who have had any pharmacologic paralysis during SE.
- Continued encephalopathy after convulsions have ended may indicate continued electrographic seizures (nonconvulsive SE).
- Nonepileptic seizures can be mistaken for SE. EEG establishes the diagnosis.

EPIDEMIOLOGY

- Incidence in pediatric patients is 17–23/100,000. In children <1 year old, incidence is 135–156/100,000.
- ~40–70% of children have no history of seizures.

RISK FACTORS

- Known epilepsy
- Remote or acute central nervous system insult
- History of previous SE
- Low anticonvulsant drug levels
- Younger age

GENERAL PREVENTION

- Adherence to the anticonvulsant medication regimen and clinical follow-up in patients with epilepsy
- Refrain from rapid changes in anticonvulsants unless urgently needed.
- Prompt treatment of convulsive seizures

PATHOPHYSIOLOGY

SE may be related to acute or chronic factors or frequently of unknown etiology.

- Common acute factors:
  - Fever
  - Infectious meningoencephalitis
  - Metabolic: electrolyte abnormalities, hypoglycemia
  - Intoxications
  - Trauma or hemorrhage
  - Ischemic stroke, hypoxic–ischemic injury
  - Medications: low anticonvulsant drug levels or abrupt withdrawal of anticonvulsants, inappropriate anticonvulsants (e.g., absence SE with phenytoin or carbamazepine use in generalized epilepsy)
- Subacute or chronic factors:
  - Epilepsy of any cause
  - Brain tumors
  - Brain malformations (e.g., lissencephaly, polymicrogyria hemimegalencephaly, neurocutaneous syndromes—tuberous sclerosis complex, Sturge-Weber syndrome)
  - Other structural brain abnormalities such as strokes hypoxic–ischemic encephalopathy (HIE), or periventricular leukomalacia (PVL)
  - Genetic epilepsies: Dravet syndrome (febrile SE), Angelman syndrome (myoclonic SE), progressive myoclonic epilepsy syndromes
  - Inflammatory disorders (e.g., Rasmussen encephalitis, *N*-methyl-D-aspartate [NMDA] receptor antibody syndrome)

DIAGNOSIS

HISTORY

- Ask about prior seizures, treatment with antiepileptic drugs (AEDs), and other neurologic abnormality, including previous neurologic workup such as MRI brain or EEG.
- Ask specifically about precipitating factors: fever, preceding illness, head trauma, change in antiepileptic medication, and family history of seizures

PHYSICAL EXAM

- Vital signs: fever, respiratory rate/O_2 sats (adequacy of air exchange and abnormal breathing patterns), heart rate, BP (hypertension suggests intracranial hypertension)
- Signs of head trauma: retinal hemorrhages, excess bruising, bone fractures, evidence of intracranial hypertension such as bulging fontanelle
- Meningismus signals CNS infection, intracranial hemorrhage, or spine trauma. May be absent in young infants with meningitis
- Signs of systemic infection: fever (also potentiates seizure activity), petechiae, rash, mucosal lesions, lymphadenopathy
- Skin examination: Check for evidence of neurocutaneous disorders (e.g., café au lait spots, ash leaf spots, shagreen patches).
- Observe clinical presentation, specifically focal features or asymmetry.
- Postictal exam: Transient neurologic abnormalities (e.g., pupillary asymmetries, eye deviation, focal motor weakness [Todd paresis], aphasia) may not correlate with the underlying structural lesion. After seizure has stopped, a neurologic examination should be performed, with attention to mental status, focal weakness, tone, or sensation.

DIAGNOSTIC TESTS & INTERPRETATION

Lab

Initial:

- STAT glucose, electrolytes, calcium, magnesium, and arterial blood gas
- Anticonvulsant levels if indicated
- CBC, liver function tests
- Toxicology screen, urinalysis

Imaging

Neuroimaging, CT, or MRI: indicated for SE, especially with partial-onset seizures (including aura), focally abnormal EEG, focal neurologic signs, or history of head trauma. MRI is the preferred neuroimaging test, but CT may be more appropriate for urgent imaging or if the patient is medically unstable.

Diagnostic Procedures/Other

- EEG: recommended to determine continued electrographic seizures and to identify focal versus generalized abnormalities. Urgent EEG recommended in patients with persistent SE or encephalopathy and in those with concern for nonconvulsive SE and nonepileptic SE.
- Lumbar puncture (LP): indicated to evaluate CNS infection in cases with suspected meningitis of encephalitis. Contraindications include intracranial hypertension known or suspected from exam or CT scan, cerebral mass lesion, and obstructive hydrocephalus. Lumbar puncture may be deferred if suspicion of CNS infection is low, that is, patient is afebrile, and an alternate etiology is present

DIFFERENTIAL DIAGNOSIS

- Nonepileptic SE: clinically suspected with eye closure; asynchronous, thrashing limb movements; pelvic thrusting, fluctuating responsiveness, head side to side movements, purposeful resistance to passive movement; and normal concurrent EEG. Induction of a seizure by suggestion further supports this diagnosis.
- Movement disorders (including dystonia, chorea, and very frequent tics) can be mistaken for persistent seizure activity.
- Postanoxic myoclonus: status after prolonged cardiopulmonary arrest. These movements are usually nonrhythmic and segmental but can appear rhythmic at times. EEG is recommended for diagnosis.

TREATMENT

INITIAL STABILIZATION

- ABCs (stabilization of airway, supporting respiration, maintaining BP, and gaining intravascular access)
- Assess for hypoxia, hemodynamics, hyperthermia, hypoglycemia, hyponatremia.
- BP, EKG, and respiratory function should be monitored.
- Airway control may be maintained by head positioning, and oral airway placement and oxygen supplementation provided via nasal cannula, mask, or bag–valve–mask ventilation. If the need for respiratory assistance persists, endotracheal intubation may be required.
- For hypoglycemia: 2–4 mL/kg of D25
- Rectal acetaminophen and a cooling blanket for fever

MEDICATION

Anticonvulsant administration should be initiated when continuous seizure activity persists for >5 minutes. The most important modifiable treatment parameter is timing to treatment, and sooner treatment provides better seizure control.

ALERT

- 1st line: benzodiazepines
  - Lorazepam 0.05–0.1 mg/kg IV (max 5 mg over 1–4 minutes)
  - If no IV: diazepam 0.2–0.5 mg/kg/dose PR (max 20 mg/dose) or nasal or buccal midazolam
- 2nd line
  - Fosphenytoin 20 mg PE/kg IV
  - If fosphenytoin unavailable: phenytoin 20 mg/kg IV
- 3rd line
  - Phenobarbital 20 mg/kg IV; can give additional 10 mg/kg if needed
  - Alternatives: valproic acid 20–40 mg/kg over 5–10 minutes, levetiracetam, or others
- 4th line: refractory SE
  - Midazolam or pentobarbital continuous infusion to seizure control or burst suppression
  - Alternatives: propofol (beware of propofol infusion syndrome with prolonged use), inhalational anesthetics

GENERAL MEASURES

- Attempt to establish IV access, but do not waste time on IV access. Consider IM midazolam, IN midazolam, or IO access or rectal diazepam immediately. The most important modifiable treatment parameter is timing to treatment.
- Consider bedside EEG monitoring in any patient who needs more than the listed second line treatment.

ONGOING CARE

PATIENT MONITORING

- Cardiorespiratory monitoring, level of care as appropriate for clinical status
- Monitor hydration and creatine kinase (CK) levels in case of convulsive SE.
- Consider need for continued video-EEG monitoring and medication titration.

PATIENT EDUCATION

- Need for long-term anticonvulsant drug therapy after SE depends on the etiology, patient's age, and circumstances in which SE occurred.
  - Chronic anticonvulsant therapy is indicated when SE is caused by structural brain lesions and in other patients with a clear predisposition toward seizures.
  - Chronic anticonvulsant therapy is generally not needed in children who have SE from transient metabolic disturbances (e.g., hyponatremia, intoxication, fever).
- Educate family members regarding first aid for seizures. Discuss potential risks of seizure recurrence even if the child is taking an anticonvulsant drug. Review risks of climbing, swimming, bathing, and head protection for wheeled toys (bikes, skateboards, scooters).
- Provide caregivers with rectal diazepam with instructions for its use for seizure ≥ 5 minutes in duration.
- For patients with known epilepsy, counsel families regarding importance of medication compliance.

PROGNOSIS

The morbidity and mortality of SE reflect etiology and are lower in children than in adults. Recent mortality estimates in children range from 1 to 3%, with risk of new neurologic sequelae estimated at 15% and subsequent epilepsy at 30%. Refractory SE, however, has a morbidity estimated at 32% and a mortality of 17%. Factors associated with outcome include duration of SE, patient age, and underlying cause.

ADDITIONAL READING

- Appleton R, Macleod S, Martland T. Drug management for acute tonic-clonic convulsions including convulsive status epilepticus in children. *Cochrane Database Syst Rev*. 2008;(3):CD001905.
- Chin RF, Neville BG, Peckham C, et al. Treatment of community-onset, childhood convulsive status epilepticus: a prospective, population-based study. *Lancet Neurol*. 2008;7(8):696–703.
- Hirsch LJ, Gaspard N. Status epilepticus. *Continuum (Minneap Minn)*. 2013;19(3):767–794.
- Loddenkemper T, Goodkin HP. Treatment of pediatric status epilepticus. *Curr Treat Options Neurol*. 2011;13(6):560–573.
- Ostrowsky K, Arzimanoglou A. Outcome and prognosis of status epilepticus in children. *Semin Pediatr Neurol*. 2010;17(3):195–200.
- Riviello JJ Jr., Ashwal S, Hirtz D, et al. Practice parameter: diagnostic assessment of the child with status epilepticus (an evidence-based review). *Neurology*. 2006;67(9):1542–1550.
- Singh RK, Stephens S, Berl MM, et al. Prospective study of new-onset seizures presenting as status epilepticus in childhood. *Neurology*. 2010;74(8):636.
- Trinka E, Höfler J, Zerbs A. Causes of status epilepticus. *Epilepsia*. 2012;53(Suppl 4):127–138.

CODES

ICD10

- G40.901 Epilepsy, unsp, not intractable, with status epilepticus
- G40.401 Oth generalized epilepsy, not intractable, w stat epi
- G40.411 Oth generalized epilepsy, intractable, w status epilepticus

FAQ

- Q: Does SE cause brain injury?
- A: Research suggests that neuronal loss may occur with prolonged SE. This illness represents a neurologic emergency. Other determinants of outcome are hypoxic brain injury due to hypoventilation during a seizure and brain injury because of an identifiable underlying cause of SE such as encephalitis. Outcome in children with idiopathic SE without hypoxia is usually very good. Outcome of SE due to other brain injury (e.g., hypoxia, encephalitis, trauma) depends on the severity of the inciting process.
- Q: How safe is administration of rectal diazepam for clusters of seizures?
- A: Studies suggest that when dosing guidelines are followed, this agent is safe and effective in terminating clusters of seizures, obviating a trip to the emergency room. Respiratory depression is very rare but can occur.
- Q: How likely is SE to recur?
- A: It is estimated at 17% in the 1st year and predominantly in children with other neurologic conditions.

STEVENS-JOHNSON SYNDROME AND TOXIC EPIDERMAL NECROLYSIS

Lara Wine Lee • James R. Treat

BASICS

DESCRIPTION
- Stevens-Johnson syndrome (SJS) and toxic epidermal necrolysis (TEN) are severe, potentially fatal, mucocutaneous drug reactions characterized by epidermal necrosis involving skin and at least 2 mucous membranes.
- The cutaneous necrosis leads to widespread epidermal detachment and loss of skin barrier function.
- Given the potential risk for infection and fluid and electrolyte imbalances with widespread denudation, SJS and TEN are considered medical emergencies.

EPIDEMIOLOGY
Incidence
- Overall annual risk of 0.5–1.9 per million in the general population
- The precise incidence in children is unknown.
- Patients with HIV have a 1,000-fold increased risk.

RISK FACTORS
- Exposure to inciting medications
- Infection with *Mycoplasma pneumoniae*, HIV
- Genetic background
- Coexistence of cancer
- Concomitant radiotherapy

Genetics
- Recently, strong associations have been made between HLA alleles and SJS/TEN.
- Associations are ethnic population–specific and therefore universal screening of HLA alleles is rarely recommended.
- The FDA recommends checking for HLA-B*1502 in Asian populations where this HLA subtype is highly prevalent before prescribing carbamazepine.

GENERAL PREVENTION
Once SJS/TEN has occurred, the inciting medication and any cross-reacting medications should be avoided.

PATHOPHYSIOLOGY
- Widespread keratinocyte and mucosal cell death occurs secondary to CD8+ T-cell–mediated apoptosis via Fas and Fas ligand pathways and/or direct granulysin secretion. Fas receptors are located on keratinocytes and, when activated with Fas ligand, induce apoptosis and therefore necrosis of epidermal cells. Granulysin is released from cytotoxic T cells and induces apoptosis by creating holes in target cell membranes.
- The exact mechanism by which the implicated drug or infection triggers activation of cytotoxic T cells and the upregulation of the Fas/FasL pathway is unknown.
- Soluble Fas ligand is increased in patients with SJS/TEN.
- IVIG theoretically acts to block the Fas–FasL connection, thereby interrupting keratinocyte death and epidermal necrosis. Trials that show a benefit of IVIG use demonstrate improvement of disease severity but not complete abolition of symptoms; this incomplete effect may be due to IVIG being started too late in the disease progression or due to a potential alternative pathway to keratinocyte destruction.

ETIOLOGY
- <5% of cases have no known cause.
- Medications
  - Over 100 medications have been implicated in causing SJS/TEN.
  - High-risk drugs include aromatic amine anticonvulsants such as carbamazepine, phenobarbital and phenytoin, lamotrigine, β-lactam antibiotics, sulfa medications (including trimethoprim-sulfamethoxazole and sulfasalazine), minocycline, cephalosporins, quinolones, NSAIDs (especially peroxicam and meloxicam), allopurinol, and nevirapine.
- Acetaminophen (very rare)
  - Recently, the FDA issued a warning about the risk of acetaminophen-related SJS/TEN.
  - Although SJS/TEN is a very rare occurrence in patients taking acetaminophen, the ubiquity of acetaminophen in prescription and OTC products prompted the requirement for new labeling.
- A greater risk of developing SJS/TEN is seen in the first 8 weeks of treatment with these medications, with the highest risk being 1–3 weeks after exposure.
- *M. pneumoniae*
  - A well-established nondrug cause of SJS/TEN
  - More commonly implicated in children and adolescents
- There is scant evidence that vaccines, neoplastic syndromes, and autoimmune disease such as SLE may play a role in etiology.
- Herpes simplex virus–associated erythema multiforme (EM) was historically categorized on the spectrum with SJS and TEN, but new classification schemes place it as a separate entity.

DIAGNOSIS

HISTORY
- Prodromal period for 1–7 days of low-grade fever, sore throat or upper respiratory infection or dysphagia, and general malaise; patient may also complain of pain or stinging in the eyes.
- Subsequent development of targetoid red papules and plaques with dusky, blistered, or eroded center as well as mucosal (lip, intraoral, conjunctival, urethral, anal) pain with blistering and erosions
- Recent initiation of high-risk agent (see earlier list) or upper respiratory symptoms such as cough indicative of *Mycoplasma* infection

PHYSICAL EXAM
- Acute phase
  - Early skin lesions are erythematous targetoid macules and patches with a dusky center that then vesiculate.
  - The eruption usually starts on the face, presternal area of chest, and palms and soles. >90% of patients also have ocular and/or genital mucosa involvement consisting of erythema and erosions as well as hemorrhaging, crusting, and blisters.
  - Skin and mucosal lesions are very tender.
- Intraoral lesions may precede the cutaneous findings.
- Ocular involvement at the onset of disease is common. Early ocular disease ranges from acute conjunctivitis, eyelid edema, and ocular discharge to pseudomembrane formation and corneal erosion.
- Secondary phase
  - Over hours to days, necrosis, blistering, and sloughing cause large areas of epidermal detachment.
  - Lesions are characterized by a positive Nikolsky sign (epidermal detachment upon mechanical stress).
- Extensive mucosal involvement may include the esophagus, distal gastrointestinal (GI) tract, and respiratory epithelium.
- Occasionally *Mycoplasma*-induced SJS can involve only the mucosal surfaces with little or no cutaneous involvement.

ALERT
- The progression of disease to sheets of widespread epidermal necrosis and sloughing may be hours. This is a medical emergency.
- The systemic severity of SJS and TEN is often underestimated based on the severity of skin disease.
- Ocular involvement is often early and severe.

DIAGNOSTIC TESTS & INTERPRETATION
Lab
Initial lab tests
- CBC with differential, metabolic panel, hepatic function test, coagulation studies, urinalysis, mycoplasma serology, or PCR if indicated
- Anemia and lymphocytopenia are common and portend a poor prognosis.

Imaging

Symptom-directed imaging may be indicated depending on the extent of mucosal and systemic involvement.

Clinical Diagnosis

- The diagnosis of SJS and TEN is largely clinical based on history and physical exam.
- By definition, <10% affected body surface area (BSA) is SJS; 10–30% affected BSA is SJS/TEN overlap; >30% affected BSA is TEN.

Diagnostic Procedures/Other

- Skin biopsy with cryosection can be performed to confirm the clinical diagnosis if in doubt.
- Histologic examination with direct immunofluorescence (DIF) can be performed to rule out other autoimmune blistering diseases such as paraneoplastic pemphigus if in doubt.

Pathologic and Diagnostic Findings

- Skin biopsy shows full-thickness epidermal necrosis and few inflammatory cells; the skin biopsy may additionally show separation at the subepidermal level.
- DIF shows no immunoglobulin or complement deposition in the epidermis or in the epidermal–dermal zone.

DIFFERENTIAL DIAGNOSIS

- Staphylococcal scalded skin syndrome (SSSS)
- Linear IgA dermatosis
- Paraneoplastic pemphigus, pemphigus vulgaris, and bullous pemphigoid
- Acute generalized exanthematous pustulosis
- Disseminated fixed bullous drug eruption
- Drug-induced hypersensitivity syndrome (drug reaction with eosinophilia and systemic symptoms [DRESS])

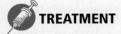

TREATMENT

MEDICATION

First Line

- Stop all potentially offending medications.
- Early admission to burn unit or pediatric intensive care unit for initial stabilization and management of fluid, electrolytes, and nutrition; airway stability; and eye care
- Prompt ophthalmology and dermatology consultation
- Otolaryngology, urology, or gynecology consultation may be needed based on extent of mucosal involvement.
- Meticulous wound care with bland emollients; avoid silver sulfadiazine as it may cause SJS owing to its sulfa moiety.
- Topical antibiotics should be used in areas of superinfection. The prophylactic use of topical antibiotics is somewhat controversial. Most agree that they should be applied to areas with a higher risk of superinfection, such as the perioral, periocular, and intertriginous areas.
- IVIG: 0.5–1 g/kg/dose given in 2–4 doses for a total of 2–3 g/kg total
- There have been variable results from a limited number of quality studies looking at the effects of IVIG. Multiple studies have demonstrated a beneficial effect especially if started early in the course.
- Adverse effects of IVIG include acute renal failure, DIC, osmotic nephrosis, anaphylaxis, serum sickness, aseptic meningitis, and thrombosis, among others.
- Steroids (prednisolone, dexamethasone, methylprednisolone) were the mainstay of therapy in the 1990s but now are less commonly used because of the increased risk of sepsis, infection, and other complications especially when used in TEN with widespread epidermal loss.
- Thalidomide, cyclosporine, TNF antagonists, plasmapheresis, and cyclophosphamide have been studied in the treatment of SJS/TEN, primarily in adults and some limited data may support their use.
- Prophylactic systemic antibiotics are not recommended, as they place the patient at an increased risk of candidemia and resistant infections.

ADDITIONAL TREATMENT

- Pain control is key to patient comfort.
- Good oral care using agents such as "magic mouthwash" helps debride dead skin and provide oral anesthesia.

SURGERY/OTHER PROCEDURES

- Surgical debridement. Studies have shown that surgical debridement of wounds prior to wound care yielded no additional benefit.
- Lysis of synechiae and vaginal adhesion
- Ocular amniotic membrane transplantation

Discharge Criteria

When afebrile, the loss of skin is clearly done, and reepithelialization has occurred; cleavage of synechiae in the eyes is no longer needed; and the patient can eat and drink appropriately

ONGOING CARE

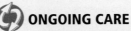

FOLLOW-UP RECOMMENDATIONS

Follow-up with a dermatologist and/or wound care specialist. Reepithelialization often starts within days and may take up to 3 weeks to be completed.

Patient Monitoring

- SCORTEN is a well-validated, widely used scoring system in adults used for its predictive value, which is best at day 3. Variables include age, percentage BSA affected, BUN, serum glucose, HR, serum bicarbonate, and associated malignancy.
- Monitor for skin, urinary tract, and pulmonary infections; synechiae in the eyes; and vaginal and urethral adhesions.

PROGNOSIS

- Mortality is 1–5% in SJS and up to 25–35% in TEN (although most of this data is from the adult literature and likely the mortality is lower in children).
- Prognosis depends on BSA affected, time to cessation of offending medication, and time to initiation of supportive care.

COMPLICATIONS

- Mucosal complications occur in >70% of patients with acute-phase mucosal involvement. Ocular complications occur in 50% of patients with TEN.
- Systemic: sepsis, multiorgan failure, major metabolic dysregulation
- Mucosal: respiratory failure, pneumonia, pulmonary embolus, UTI, GI hemorrhage, obstruction, and perforation
- Cutaneous: skin infections, scarring, hypo-/hyperpigmentation, nail dystrophies
- Ocular: synechiae, dry eyes, bacterial conjunctivitis, suppurative keratitis, endophthalmitis, impaired tear ducts, corneal ulcers, vision loss

ADDITIONAL READING

- Bastuji-Garin S, Rzany B, Stern RS, et al. Clinical classification of cases of toxic epidermal necrolysis, Stevens-Johnson syndrome, and erythema multiforme. *Arch Dermatol*. 1993;129(1):92–96.
- Del Pozzo-Magana BR, Lazo-Langner A, Carleton B, et al. A systematic review of treatment of drug-induced Stevens-Johnson syndrome and toxic epidermal necrolysis in children. *J Popul Ther Clin Pharmacol*. 2011;18:e121–e133.
- Ferrandiz-Pulido C, Garcia-Patos V. A review of causes of Stevens-Johnson syndrome and toxic epidermal necrolysis in children. *Arch Dis Child*. 2013;98(12):998–1003.
- Karlin E, Phillips E. Genotyping for severe drug hypersensitivity. *Curr Allergy Asthma Rep*. 2014;14(3):418.
- Levi N, Bastuji-Garin S, Mockenhaupt M, et al. Medications as risk factors of Stevens-Johnson syndrome and toxic epidermal necrolysis in children: a pooled analysis. *Pediatrics*. 2009;123(2):e297–e304.
- Treat J. Stevens-Johnson syndrome and toxic epidermal necrolysis. *Pediatr Ann*. 2010;39(10):667–674.

CODES

ICD10

- L51.1 Stevens-Johnson syndrome
- L51.3 Stevens-Johnson synd-tox epdrml necrolysis overlap syndrome
- L51.2 Toxic epidermal necrolysis [Lyell]

STOMATITIS

Cara L. Biddle

BASICS

DESCRIPTION

- Inflammation of the mucous membranes of the mouth including the buccal mucosa, gingiva, tongue, lips, hard palate, and soft palate
- Also called gingivostomatitis when the gums are specifically involved
- Enteroviruses (causing herpangina and hand-foot-and-mouth disease) and herpes simplex virus type 1 are the most common infectious causes of stomatitis.
- Recurrent aphthous stomatitis (or canker sores) is also common in children. Etiology is unknown.

EPIDEMIOLOGY

- Enteroviruses (including coxsackie viruses)
  - More common in the summer and fall months in temperate climates but occur year-round in the tropics
  - Herpangina and hand-foot-and-mouth disease are most common in infants, toddlers, and young children.
- Herpes simplex virus type 1 (HSV-1)
  - Infections occur throughout the year.
  - Most primary HSV infections in childhood after the neonatal period are asymptomatic.
  - Primary herpetic gingivostomatitis is most common in infants, toddlers, and young children.
  - Recurrent HSV-1 infections can occur any time after the primary infection.
  - Seroprevalence of HSV-1 in the United States: more than 25% by age 7 years; more than 40% by age 21 years
- Recurrent aphthous stomatitis is most common in older children and adolescents.

GENERAL PREVENTION

- Wash hands after contact with infected individuals to help prevent spread of viral stomatitis.
- Disinfect surfaces, toys, and other objects used by an infected child to decrease spread. Enteroviruses can survive on surfaces long enough to allow transmission of infection.
- Use contact precautions for hospitalized patients with viral stomatitis.

PATHOPHYSIOLOGY

- Enteroviral infections
  - Spread by fecal–oral and respiratory routes. Can also be passed from mother to infant prenatally, in the peripartum period, and possibly via breast milk
  - Result in viremia which spreads virus to target organs
- HSV-1 infections
  - Spread via contact with mucous membranes or open skin
  - Travel from the skin to the trigeminal sensory ganglion where infection persists for life. Reactivation causes recurrent symptoms.

ETIOLOGY

- Herpangina: most often coxsackie A viruses; also caused by other enteroviruses
- Hand-foot-and-mouth disease: most often coxsackie A viruses; also coxsackie B, enterovirus 71, and echoviruses
- Primary herpetic gingivostomatitis: typically HSV-1; can also be caused by HSV-2
- Recurrent aphthous stomatitis: possible causative factors: physical and chemical trauma, foods, nutrient deficiencies, immunodeficiency, systemic illness, infections, genetic predisposition, smoking, stress, medications

DIAGNOSIS

HISTORY

- History of present illness
  - Onset and duration
  - Mouth pain or sores in mouth
  - Drooling
  - Fever
  - Intake of liquids and food
  - Urine output
  - Activity level
  - Close contact with similar symptoms
- Review of systems
  - Vomiting, diarrhea, abdominal pain
  - Rash on body
  - Headache, mental status changes
  - Respiratory symptoms
  - Previous history of oral lesions
- Chronic health issues and family history: immunodeficiency (including HIV infection), inflammatory bowel disease, gluten enteropathy, anemia, neutropenia, rheumatologic disease
- Include recent medication history to assess risk for Stevens-Johnson syndrome.

PHYSICAL EXAM

- Exam of lips and oral cavity
  - Mucous membranes: Moist? Erythematous? Swollen? Friable?
  - Oral lesions: Color? Location? Number? Ulceration?
- Additional physical exam
  - General appearance
  - Hydration status
  - Respiratory, cardiovascular, and abdominal exam
  - Skin exam for additional rash
  - Lymphadenopathy
- Typical physical findings
  - Herpangina: vesicles and ulcers surrounded by erythematous ring on tonsillar pillars, soft palate, uvula, tonsils, and/or posterior pharynx
  - Hand-foot-and-mouth: inflamed oropharynx with scattered vesicles and ulcers with an erythematous ring on buccal mucosa, tongue, gingiva, hard and soft palate, and/or posterior pharynx. Maculopapular, vesicular, and/or pustular lesions on hands and fingers, feet, and buttocks. Hand and foot lesions most commonly on dorsal surface but can also be on palms and soles.
  - Primary herpetic gingivostomatitis (herpes labialis): inflamed gingiva with mucosal hemorrhages. Clusters of vesicles throughout the mouth including the lip's mucocutaneous margin and perioral skin
  - Recurrent herpes labialis: cluster of vesicles on lip or mucocutaneous margin
  - Aphthous stomatitis: shallow round or ovoid ulcers with gray base and surrounding erythema
- Also consider the following:
  - Varicella: grouped vesicles or ulcers on hard palate, buccal mucosa, tongue, or gingiva. Diffuse vesicles in various stages of healing on skin of body
  - Stevens-Johnson syndrome: erythema and edema of lips. Painful intraoral bullae that rupture, leaving erosions. Rash on body includes urticaria, target lesions, and bullae.
  - Behçet syndrome: oral ulcers accompanied by genital ulcers, uveitis, rash, and other systemic symptoms
  - Periodic fever with aphthous stomatitis, pharyngitis, and adenitis (PFAPA syndrome): prodrome of systemic symptoms, sore throat, and aphthous ulcers on lips or buccal mucosa followed by abrupt onset of fever and chills

DIAGNOSTIC TESTS & INTERPRETATION

Lab

- Diagnosis of stomatitis is typically made by history, location and characteristics of oral lesions, and additional physical findings.
- Confirmatory lab tests are available if needed:
  - Enterovirus can be identified by polymerase chain reaction (PCR) assay or culture of stool, throat, blood, urine, tracheal aspirate, or conjunctiva or by tissue biopsy.
  - HSV can be detected by viral culture, PCR, direct fluorescent antibody (DFA) staining, or enzyme immunoassay (EIA).
  - For HSV culture: Unroof a vesicle with scalpel or sterile needle, and use swab to soak up fluid and scrape the base. Use appropriate viral transport media.

DIFFERENTIAL DIAGNOSIS

- Infectious
  - Enteroviruses (coxsackievirus and others)
  - HSV
  - Varicella
  - HIV infection
  - Syphilis
  - Candida
- Recurrent aphthous stomatitis
- Trauma
- Burn
- Other
  - Chemotherapy-associated stomatitis
  - Stevens-Johnson syndrome
  - Behçet syndrome
  - Reiter syndrome
  - PFAPA syndrome
  - Geographic tongue

TREATMENT

MEDICATION

- Pain control
  - Acetaminophen or ibuprofen
  - Acetaminophen with codeine in severe cases. Use caution due to risk of sedation and constipation. Do not use in combination with regular acetaminophen.
  - Use codeine with caution due to variability in metabolism by cytochrome P450 CYP2D6. Patients who are "ultra-rapid metabolizers" of codeine convert up to 15% (vs. 3%) of the drug to morphine, which can lead to toxicity.
- Antivirals
  - Oral acyclovir can be used for immunocompetent children with herpetic gingivostomatitis if started within the first 72–96 hours of illness. May shorten the duration of symptoms and viral shedding
  - Topical acyclovir is not recommended for primary herpetic gingivostomatitis.
- Topical therapy: "magic mouthwash"
  - 1:1 mixture of diphenhydramine and calcium carbonate or bismuth subsalicylate (plus viscous lidocaine in severe cases)
  - Use with caution. Many young children cannot "swish and spit" and will swallow the medication. Applying magic mouthwash to ulcers with a swab may cause additional irritation to friable mucosa. Use of viscous lidocaine can result in systemic toxicity (e.g., arrhythmias), anesthesia of the oral mucosa leading to mechanical trauma, and anesthesia of the posterior pharynx leading to choking or aspiration.

ADDITIONAL TREATMENT

General Measures

- Maintain hydration. Offer small amounts of cool, nonacidic liquids frequently. Use a syringe to continue giving liquids when children are refusing to drink. Try popsicles as another source of liquids.
- Offer soft, cool foods such as ice cream, yogurt, and Jell-O. Avoid foods that are salty, spicy, hard, or acidic, as they are likely to irritate the mouth sores and cause more pain.
- Apply petroleum jelly or other barrier ointment to the lips to limit cracking and prevent adhesions in herpetic gingivostomatitis.

ONGOING CARE

FOLLOW-UP RECOMMENDATIONS

Patient Monitoring

- Most children with stomatitis can be cared for at home with pain control and maintenance of hydration.
- Providers should ensure that parents and caregivers are familiar with signs and symptoms of dehydration.
- Children with poor oral intake due to pain may be unable to maintain hydration at home and require admission for intravenous fluids.

PROGNOSIS

- Primary herpetic gingivostomatitis results in permanent HSV infection. Recurrent infection can be triggered by stress, fever, trauma, sun exposure, immunosuppression, or extremes in temperature. Children may have tingling, pain, itching, or paresthesias before the appearance of recurrent lesions.
- Recurrent aphthous stomatitis causes significant morbidity due to recurrences of painful oral lesions.

COMPLICATIONS

- Enteroviral infection
  - Respiratory: bronchiolitis, pneumonia, pleurodynia
  - Neurologic: viral meningitis, encephalitis, motor paralysis
  - Gastrointestinal: vomiting, diarrhea, abdominal pain, pancreatitis, hepatitis
  - Genitourinary: orchitis
  - Ophthalmologic: uveitis, acute hemorrhagic conjunctivitis
  - Cardiac: myocarditis, pericarditis
  - Muscular: myositis

ALERT

Enterovirus 71 (EV71) can cause both hand-foot-and-mouth disease and herpangina and can also cause children to develop severe neurologic disease (including brainstem encephalomyelitis and acute paralysis) followed by secondary pulmonary edema/hemorrhage and cardiopulmonary collapse.

- HSV infection
  - Herpetic keratitis: herpetic eye infection due to autoinoculation from mouth lesions
  - Herpetic whitlow: development of herpetic lesions on the extremities (typically fingers) due to direct contact with mouth lesions
  - Eczema herpeticum: extensive herpes infection of the skin in children with atopic dermatitis or other chronic skin disease
  - HSV encephalitis

ADDITIONAL READING

- Chattopadhyay A, Shetty K. Recurrent aphthous stomatitis. *Otolaryngol Clin North Am*. 2011;44(1):79–88.
- Faden H. Management of primary herpetic gingivostomatitis in young children. *Pediatr Emerg Care*. 2006;22(4):268–269.
- Gibson AM, Sommerkamp SK. Evaluation and management of oral lesions in the emergency department. *Emerg Med Clin North Am*. 2013;31(2):455–463.
- Madadi P, Koren G. Pharmacogenetic insights into codeine analgesia: implications to pediatric codeine use. *Pharmacogenomics*. 2008;9(9):1267–1284.
- Usatine RP, Tinitigan R. Nongenital herpes simplex virus. *Am Fam Physician*. 2010;82(9):1075–1082.

CODES

ICD10

- K12.1 Other forms of stomatitis
- B00.2 Herpesviral gingivostomatitis and pharyngotonsillitis
- B08.4 Enteroviral vesicular stomatitis with exanthem

FAQ

- Q: My child is refusing to drink any liquids. How can I keep her hydrated?
- A: Mouth sores can be very painful. Even if your child is not having fever, give regularly scheduled doses of ibuprofen or acetaminophen around the clock for pain control. Offer cool, nonacidic liquids and foods, which will be less likely to irritate the mouth sores. Use a syringe to put small amounts of liquids in her mouth every few minutes if she refuses to drink anything.
- Q: What should I do at home to prevent spread of the infection?
- A: Frequent hand washing is the most important way to prevent the spread of infection. Avoid sharing contaminated toys, utensils, and other objects until they have been cleaned, and wipe down surfaces to disinfect. For enteroviral infections, it is particularly important to do careful hand washing after diaper changes because the virus is shed in the stool.
- Q: When can my child return to school or daycare?
- A: Viral stomatitis is contagious. Children who drool are the most contagious and should not return to school until the mouth sores heal. Children with aphthous ulcers or recurrent herpes labialis should not be excluded from school.

STRABISMUS

Leah G. Reznick

BASICS

DESCRIPTION

- Strabismus is defined as any form of ocular misalignment. It derives from the Greek word *strabismos* (to squint).
- Strabismus can be intermittent or constant.
- There are many types of strabismus, which are defined by the direction of misalignment.
  - Exotropia: out-turning of eyes
  - Esotropia: in-turning of eyes
  - Hypertropia: one eye higher than the other eye
- Strabismus can be comitant (amount of misalignment is the same in all directions of gaze) or incomitant (variable angle of deviation, which is dependent on the direction of gaze).
  - Comitant strabismus is the most common form of strabismus. These children are typically developmentally normal.
  - Incomitant strabismus is less common. It is caused by paralytic strabismus such as cranial nerve palsies or restrictive strabismus such as Brown syndrome.
- Strabismus may cause permanent loss of three-dimensional vision, amblyopia (visual acuity loss), and/or ocular torticollis.
- Strabismus can result in significant psychosocial problems for children, which warrant attention.
- Patients with intermittent strabismus can also develop lifelong loss of depth perception and visual acuity. These children should be evaluated and potentially treated for their strabismus.

EPIDEMIOLOGY

Prevalence

For children younger than 6 years of age, the prevalence of strabismus is 4–5%.

RISK FACTORS

- Low birth weight
- Maternal cigarette smoking
- Retinopathy of prematurity
- Refractive errors: high hyperopia and anisometropia
- Congenital or acquired vision loss
- Cerebral palsy
- Craniofacial syndromes
- Seizure disorders
- Developmental delays
- Hydrocephalus

Genetics

- There is a 4-fold increase in the risk of strabismus for a child with an affected family member.
- There is limited knowledge of the genetic inheritance patterns of common strabismus. There appears to be polygenic pattern, but the *STBMS1* gene has been isolated as a specific locus for a few individuals.

PATHOPHYSIOLOGY

- There is a limited understanding of the pathophysiology of the most common comitant strabismus. There is no specific pathologic abnormality of the cranial nerves, extraocular muscles, or orbits. Therefore, a "tight" or "weak" muscle is not the cause of the strabismus problem.
- Accommodative esotropia is a common form of strabismus in young children. It is associated with high hyperopia (farsightedness) and anisometropia (see "Refractive Error"). When a child with high hyperopia attempts to focus at any distance, he or she needs to focus his or her intraocular lens (accommodation). This focusing can trigger overconvergence of the eyes (esotropia).
- Paretic strabismus is caused by weakness of cranial nerves and their associated extraocular muscles. Examples of this type of pathology include cranial nerve palsies—III, IV, and VI; Möbius syndrome; or Duane syndrome.
- Neuromuscular diseases such as myasthenia gravis can cause strabismus with decreased extraocular muscle function.
- Restrictive strabismus is a result of muscle tightness causing a limitation in eye movement. Examples include Graves disease, Brown syndrome, or trauma to extraocular muscles.
- Sensory strabismus results from poor visual acuity in one eye.

COMMONLY ASSOCIATED CONDITIONS

- Strabismus can be a sign of a vision- or life-threatening neurologic problem.
  - A physician needs to consider that retinoblastoma, brain tumor, cataract, and other conditions may initially present with ocular misalignment.
- Other ocular problems often coexist with strabismus including amblyopia, nystagmus, and refractive error.

DIAGNOSIS

- It is normal for infants younger than 2 months of age to have intermittent strabismus but not constant strabismus.
- After 4 months of age, any strabismus is abnormal and warrants an ophthalmologic exam.
- Children do not commonly "grow out" of strabismus.
- A delay in diagnosis and treatment can lead to a worse prognosis for normal visual development.

SIGNS AND SYMPTOMS

- Children are typically asymptomatic. Because the brain suppresses one eye in childhood strabismus, the patient has no diplopia and is not aware of ocular misalignment.
- Strabismus needs to be screened for and identified by primary care providers and family members.

HISTORY

- Onset of misalignment
- Frequency, duration, and direction of deviation
- Torticollis
- History of eye or head trauma
- Birth and developmental history focusing on prematurity, seizure disorder, or neurologic abnormality
- History of glasses, patching, or other vision therapy
- Family history of strabismus, amblyopia, refractive error, or childhood vision problems

PHYSICAL EXAM

- Patient's visual acuity should be evaluated in an age-appropriate manner individually for each eye (see "Amblyopia" and "Refractive Error").
- The presence of torticollis may indicate strabismus.
- Ocular alignment
  - Corneal light reflex (Hirschberg test): With a patient looking at a light, look for the location of the corneal light reflex. The light reflex should be focused at the center of each pupil symmetrically. If the reflex is located outside of the pupillary center and asymmetric, the child likely has strabismus. If it is positioned laterally, the child has esotropia, and if it is positioned medially, the child has exotropia.
  - Red reflex test (Brückner): With dimmed room lights, an examiner uses a direct ophthalmoscope to look at the red reflex of both eyes simultaneously from 2–3 feet. Normally, the pupils should be red and the pupils should symmetrically fill with light. If there is asymmetry to the brightness, a dulled reflex, or a black or white area within the reflex, there is likely an ocular problem, which could be strabismus.
  - Alternate cover test: The examiner should get the patient to focus on a single target. While they are holding fixation, the examiner should occlude each eye for a brief period of time. The examiner should watch for movement of the eye to pick up fixation. If the eyes remain still while you alternately occlude each eye, then there is no strabismus. If the eyes move from inward to outward, the child has esotropia. If the eyes move from outward to inward, the child has exotropia.
- Ocular rotations
  - Each eye should be evaluated for full movement in horizontal and vertical directions. If the eye has limited movement in a particular direction, then there may be paralytic or restrictive strabismus. If there is limited movement, a patient should be evaluated by an ophthalmologist urgently.
- Complete ophthalmic examination is indicated whenever there is suspicion of strabismus or abnormal vision based on history, screening tests, or examination.

DIAGNOSTIC TESTS & INTERPRETATION

Serologic or radiologic testing is rarely performed to work up the etiology of routine strabismus.

Lab

In select patients, a physician may order antiacetylcholine receptor antibodies testing to test for myasthenia gravis or thyroid function studies to test for thyroid eye disease.

Imaging

If orbital or neurologic pathology is suspected, an MRI or CT scan may be performed to evaluate for a restrictive or paralytic strabismus.

DIFFERENTIAL DIAGNOSIS

- In the initial evaluation, one needs to differentiate between true strabismus and pseudostrabismus.
  - Children with wide epicanthal folds often give the false appearance of esotropia due to minimal amount of conjunctiva showing in the medial canthal region.
  - Rather than looking at the amount of "whites" showing, a practitioner can use the corneal light reflex (Hirschberg test) to see if the light reflex lies in the central pupil and perform a cover test.
  - If there is any doubt about the presence of strabismus, a referral to an ophthalmologist is warranted.
- In children with abnormal eye movements (incomitant strabismus), the differential diagnosis includes the following:
  - Cranial nerve palsies (III, IV, or VI)
  - Craniofacial anomalies
  - Orbital fracture
  - Systemic or localized motor abnormalities such as myasthenia gravis
  - Orbital pseudotumor
  - Thyroid eye disease (Graves)
  - Strabismus syndromes
- Strabismus syndromes include the following:
  - Duane syndrome: congenital aberrant innervation of cranial nerve III
  - Möbius syndrome: congenital absence of cranial nerve VI and VII
  - Brown syndrome: an abnormality of the trochlear-superior oblique tendon causing a monocular elevation deficit
- Sensory strabismus is caused by any form of vision loss. The strabismus can be either esotropia or exotropia. If a child has sensory strabismus, it is crucial to identify the cause of vision loss because it can be life threatening (such as retinoblastoma or intracranial tumor).

ADDITIONAL TREATMENT

General Measures

- If a child remains strabismic for a prolonged period, it can result in irreversible loss of depth perception and vision loss (amblyopia). Therefore, it is imperative that a child receives prompt evaluation and treatment.
- Treatment options can include glasses, occlusion therapy, orthoptic exercises, surgery, or a combination of these therapies.
- Glasses are primary treatment for a common form of strabismus—accommodative esotropia.
- Occlusion therapy is typically used for amblyopia rather than strabismus. If occlusion therapy improves vision, occasionally, the strabismus may improve, but more importantly, better vision improves prognosis for strabismus treatment.
- Eye exercises (orthoptic exercises) are useful in patients with convergence insufficiency. There is no evidence that they improve typical childhood esotropia and exotropia.

SURGERY/OTHER PROCEDURES

- If patching and glasses do not improve strabismus, then surgery is often recommended to improve binocular vision.
- In strabismus surgery, the eye muscles are either weakened by moving the muscle's insertion or tightened (strengthened) by removing a small piece of muscle tissue.
- For most patients, strabismus surgery is performed in an outpatient setting with minimal risk or morbidity.
- In large-case series, there is ~80% success rate for surgery and a ~20% reoperation risk.

ONGOING CARE

Long-term follow-up is important for children to monitor their vision development until at least 10 years of age. There is a risk for amblyopia and strabismus recurrence even after a successful surgical correction.

ADDITIONAL READING

- American Academy of Ophthalmology Pediatric Ophthalmology/Strabismus Panel. *Preferred Practice Pattern® Guidelines. Esotropia and Exotropia*. San Francisco: American Academy of Ophthalmology; 2012. http://www.aao.org/ppp. Accessed March 17, 2015.
- American Academy of Ophthalmology Pediatric Ophthalmology/Strabismus Panel. *Preferred Practice Pattern® Guidelines: Pediatric Eye Evaluations*. San Francisco: American Academy of Ophthalmology; 2012. http://www.aao.org/ppp. Accessed March 17, 2015.
- Handler S, Fierson WM, Section on Ophthalmology, et al. Learning disabilities, dyslexia, and vision. *Pediatrics*. 2011;127(3):e818–e856.

CODES

ICD10

- H50.9 Unspecified strabismus
- H50.10 Unspecified exotropia
- H50.00 Unspecified esotropia

FAQ

- Q: Will a child's strabismus resolve on its own?
- A: In most cases, children do not outgrow strabismus. Diagnosis and treatment should not be delayed.
- Q: Should a child wait to have surgery until he or she is older?
- A: When a child has strabismus, there are anatomic changes to the brain to prevent diplopia. The longer a child spends strabismic, the more adaptation occurs and the harder it is to regain normal depth perception. Therefore, it is important not to delay diagnosis and treatment. There is improved prognosis with prompt treatment.
- Q: Does strabismus cause learning difficulties?
- A: There is no proven association between strabismus and learning disabilities. If a child has learning difficulties and has strabismus, the learning issues should be evaluated outside of the strabismus.
- Q: How does loss of depth perception affect a child?
- A: A child may demonstrate subtle changes in fine motor skills, visual–spatial tasks, and athletic capabilities.
- Q: Will surgery in older children and adults improve their ocular function?
- A: With surgery, older children and adults may expand their visual fields and restore binocularity. The psychosocial effects of strabismus can significantly affect a person's sense of self and social interaction. For this reason, strabismus surgery can dramatically improve quality of life.
- Q: When is vision therapy prescribed for strabismus?
- A: Vision therapy has limited use for patients with strabismus. Eye exercises have been proven effective for one type of exotropia called convergence insufficiency. For most childhood strabismus, there is no evidence that vision therapy successfully treats ocular misalignment.

S

STREP INFECTION: INVASIVE GROUP A β-HEMOLYTIC STREPTOCOCCUS

Maribeth Chitkara

BASICS

DESCRIPTION

Infection associated with isolation of group A β-hemolytic streptococci (GABHS) from a normally sterile body site; includes 3 clinical syndromes:

- GABHS toxic shock syndrome (STSS)
- GABHS necrotizing fasciitis (NF)
  - Infection characterized by extensive local necrosis of skin and subcutaneous soft tissues
- Isolation of GABHS from normally sterile sites in patients not meeting criteria for STSS or NF (e.g., meningitis, osteomyelitis, septic arthritis, myositis, surgical wound infections) with or without bacteremia

Diagnostic criteria for STSS:

- (I) Isolation of GABHS
  - A: From a normally sterile site (e.g., blood, CSF, tissue, peritoneal fluid)
  - B: From a nonsterile site (e.g., throat, vagina, sputum, open surgical wound)
- (II) Clinical signs of severity
  - A: Hypotension
  - B: Two or more of the following signs:
    - Renal impairment
    - Coagulopathy
    - Hepatic involvement
    - Adult respiratory distress syndrome
    - A generalized erythematous macular rash that may desquamate
    - Soft tissue necrosis, including NF or myositis, or gangrene
- A *definite* case fulfills criteria IA and II (A and B). A *probable* case fulfills criteria IB and II (A and B) and no other identifiable cause.

EPIDEMIOLOGY

- Overall mortality rates for invasive GABHS infections are lower in children (5–15%) than in adults (30–80%).
- Most cases occur in winter and early spring.

Incidence

- It is estimated that the annual incidence in the United States is 1.5–5.9 cases per 100,000 persons.
- Incidence is highest in infants and the elderly.
- 85% of cases are sporadic, 10% hospital-acquired, 4% in chronic care facilities, 1% in cases with a close index contact.

RISK FACTORS

- Risk factors for invasive GABHS infections include injuries resulting in bruising or muscle strain, surgical procedures, and viral infections such as varicella.
- High-risk groups include patients with diabetes mellitus, chronic cardiac or pulmonary disease, HIV infection or AIDS, and those with a history of IV drug use.

GENERAL PREVENTION

- Routine immunization against varicella
- Isolation of hospitalized patients
  - In addition to standard precautions, droplet precautions for children with pneumonia
  - Contact precautions should be used for at least 24 hours after the start of antimicrobial therapy in children with extensive or draining cutaneous infections.
- Several GABHS vaccine candidates are in varying stages of development. A 26-valent recombinant M protein vaccine is the only vaccine to have entered into clinical trials.

PATHOPHYSIOLOGY

- The pathogenic mechanism has not been fully defined; however, an association with streptococcal pyrogenic exotoxins (SPE) has been suggested.
- SPE A, B, and C (responsible for rash of scarlet fever) along with streptococcal exotoxins, mitogen factor, and superantigen stimulate activation of T lymphocytes and macrophages to produce large quantities of cytokines resulting in shock and tissue damage.
- There may be no identifiable focus of infection.

ETIOLOGY

Streptococcus pyogenes is the only species of β-hemolytic streptococci to be associated with invasive infections.

DIAGNOSIS

HISTORY

- Historic features vary depending on the GABHS syndrome.
- May have preceding soft tissue infection such as cellulitis
- A preceding clinical pharyngitis is not common.
- Consider GABHS infection in any child with varicella who has any of the following:
  - Localized skin findings of erythema, warmth, swelling, or induration
  - Return of fever after having been afebrile
  - A temperature of ≥39°C (102.7°F) beyond the 3rd day of illness
  - Any fever persisting beyond the 4th day of illness
- In children without varicella, presentation can mimic influenza infection (fever, chills, myalgias). Abrupt onset of localized or severe pain and absence of respiratory symptoms or a contact history are clues to help distinguish STSS from influenza.
- Incubation period for STSS is unknown.

PHYSICAL EXAM

- Vital signs
  - Elevated temperature
  - Tachycardia
  - Hypotension (late sign)
- Toxic appearance is common but may not be present, especially early in the disease course.
- Skin exam varies:
  - Often, there are no cutaneous findings.
  - With varicella infection, vesicular lesions may have underlying erythema, warmth, or induration but can also appear normal.
  - NF should be suspected in child who presents with diffuse swelling of an extremity followed by the development of bullae with fluid that rapidly evolves from clear to violaceous in color.
  - Erythroderma, a generalized macular exfoliative and erythematous rash, is sometimes observed with STSS.
- Deep infections will have exam findings consistent with the specific focus (e.g., joint pain and limitation of mobility in septic arthritis, respiratory symptoms in GABHS pneumonia).
- Pain and/or hyperesthesias out of proportion to clinical findings may be noted.

DIAGNOSTIC TESTS & INTERPRETATION

Lab

- CBC (leukocytosis with immature neutrophils may be noted but WBC can also be normal)
- Electrolytes, BUN, creatinine, and glucose
- Liver function tests
- Screen for disseminated intravascular coagulation
- Creatine kinase level (may be elevated in NF)
- Blood culture
- Culture of wound and tissue aspirates
- Throat culture
  - If culture negative, a rise in antibody titers to streptolysin O, deoxyribonuclease B, or other streptococcal extracellular products 4–6 weeks after infection may help confirm the diagnosis.
  - These antibodies may remain elevated for several months and indicate an infection in the recent past.

Imaging

In cases of NF: Consider MRI to confirm diagnosis and extent of infection.

DIFFERENTIAL DIAGNOSIS

- Bacterial sepsis
- Toxic shock syndrome from *Staphylococcus aureus*
- Other soft tissue infections
  - Cellulitis
  - Erysipelas
  - Clostridial or mixed anaerobic and aerobic fasciitis/gangrene

ALERT

- Diagnosis is primarily clinical and requires a high degree of suspicion because of the rapid progression of infection.
- Diagnosis should be considered even in suspect cases with absence of rash, cellulitis, or superinfected varicella lesions.
- In cases of NF, extent of involvement in subcutaneous tissues may be underestimated. Infection may be more widespread than what is apparent on physical exam.
- In STSS cases, care should be taken to search for a localized infection as a possible source of toxin production.

TREATMENT

MEDICATION

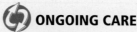

- Parenteral therapy at maximum doses for both GABHS and *S. aureus* should be instituted promptly with the capacity to do both of the following:
  - Kill organism with bactericidal cell wall inhibitor.
  - Decrease enzyme, toxin, or cytokine production with protein synthesis inhibitor.
- Recommended regimens:
  - Oxacillin (150 mg/kg/24 h divided q6h) or nafcillin (200 mg/kg/24 h divided q4–6h; maximum 12 g/24 h) *plus* clindamycin (25–40 mg/kg/24 h divided q6h or q8h)
  - In penicillin-allergic patients, consider vancomycin (40 mg/kg/24 h divided q6h) *plus* clindamycin.
  - In areas with high prevalence of community-acquired methicillin-resistant *S. aureus* vancomycin should be used in place of β-lactamase–resistant penicillins.
- Once GABHS has been identified, antibiotic regimen should be changed to high-dose penicillin G (200,000–400,000 U/kg/24 h in 4–6 divided doses) *plus* clindamycin.
  - No penicillin G–resistant isolates of GABHS have been reported.
  - There are strains resistant to clindamycin, so it should not be used alone until shown to be sensitive.
- Antibiotics should be continued for a minimum of 14 days in patients with bacteremia and for 14 days after last positive culture obtained during surgical debridement for patients with deep soft tissue infections.
- The use of IV immunoglobulin may be considered in cases refractory to aggressive therapy, for infection in an area that precludes drainage, or persistent oliguria with pulmonary edema. Various regimens have been used: 150–400 mg/kg/24 h for 5 days or 1–2 g/kg as single dose.

ADDITIONAL TREATMENT

General Measures

- Volume resuscitation
- Replete electrolytes as indicated
- Inotropes as indicated
- Blood products as indicated for anemia or thrombocytopenia
- Airway support for severe depression of level of consciousness or respiratory insufficiency

SURGERY/OTHER PROCEDURES

Consider surgical consult early in management of NF. Extensive debridement of necrotic tissue is often indicated. Fasciotomy may be required to relieve compartment syndrome.

ONGOING CARE

PROGNOSIS

- Fulminant course with rapid deterioration is characteristic of invasive GABHS infections.
- Prognosis is improved with early recognition and aggressive management.
- Case fatality rate for invasive GABHS infections is 13.7% (36% for STSS and 24% for NF).
- Increased morbidity and mortality reported in cases of coinfection with H1N1 influenza
- Poor prognostic factors:
  - Emm/M strain types 1, 3, or 12
  - Increased age
  - Occurrence in winter/early spring
  - Development of GI symptoms

COMPLICATIONS

- From deep and systemic infections:
  - Sepsis syndrome
  - Hematologic seeding and development of focal infection
  - Infection site–specific complications (e.g., meningitis, neurologic impairment; septic arthritis, joint destruction)
- From NF:
  - Severe tissue necrosis usually requires extensive surgical debridement and may require amputation of involved extremities.
  - Compartment syndrome
  - Functional disabilities
  - Cosmetic sequelae
- From STSS:
  - Multiorgan system failure
  - Acute respiratory distress syndrome
  - Disseminated intravascular coagulation
  - Acute tubular necrosis and renal failure
  - Hepatic failure
  - Cardiac insufficiency
  - Cerebral ischemia and edema
  - Metabolic derangements

ADDITIONAL READING

- American Academy of Pediatrics. Group A streptococcal infections. In: Pickering LK, Baker CJ, Kimberlin DW, et al, eds. *Red Book: 2012 Report of the Committee on Infectious Diseases*. 29th ed. Elk Gove Village, IL: American Academy of Pediatrics; 2012:668–680.
- American Academy of Pediatrics Committee on Infectious Diseases. Severe invasive group A streptococcal infections: a subject review. *Pediatrics*. 1998;101(1, Pt 1):136–140.
- Burnett AM, Domachowske JB. Therapeutic considerations for children with invasive group A streptococcal infections: a case series report and review of the literature. *Clin Pediatr*. 2007;46(6):550–555.
- Lamagni TL, Neal S, Keshishian C, et al. Predictors of death after severe *Streptococcus pyogenes* infection. *Emerg Infect Dis*. 2009;15(8):1304–1307.
- Langlois DM, Andreae M. Group A streptococcal infections. *Pediatr Rev*. 2011;32(10):423–430.
- Martin JM, Green M. Group A *Streptococcus*. *Semin Pediatr Infect Dis*. 2006;17(3):140–148.
- O'Loughlin RE, Roberson A, Cieslak PR, et al. The epidemiology of invasive group A streptococcal infection and potential vaccine implications: United States, 2000-2004. *Clin Infect Dis*. 2007;45(7):853–862.

CODES

ICD10

- B95.0 Streptococcus, group A, causing diseases classd elswhr
- B95.1 Streptococcus, group B, causing diseases classd elswhr
- A48.3 Toxic shock syndrome

S

FAQ

- Q: For whom should the diagnosis of invasive GABHS be entertained?
- A: Consider GABHS in any child with varicella who experiences recrudescence of fever, fever ≥39°C (102.2°F) beyond the 3rd day of illness, or any fever beyond the 4th day of illness. A high index of suspicion should be maintained in patients with septicemia and in febrile patients with pain and hyperesthesia out of proportion to the clinical findings.
- Q: Is NSAID use in patients with varicella associated with GABHS?
- A: There are reports suggesting an association between the use of NSAIDs and the development of invasive GABHS diseases, but a causal relationship has not been established. There is evidence that NSAIDs impair granulocyte function and enhance production of cytokines. Additionally, they may mask signs of disease by suppressing the pain and fever that might encourage a patient with invasive GABHS infection to seek medical attention. No formal recommendations for restricting the use of NSAIDs are being made at this time.
- Q: Should close contacts of patients with invasive GABHS infections receive chemoprophylaxis?
- A: Although the risk of developing disease for household contacts is elevated in comparison to the general population, the risk is not sufficiently high to warrant routine testing or treatment for GABHS colonization. No clearly effective chemoprophylactic regimen has been identified. However, in high-risk populations (people >65 years or those with HIV, varicella, or diabetes mellitus), targeted chemoprophylaxis may be considered. Chemoprophylaxis is not recommended in schools or child care facilities.

STROKE

Melissa G. Chung • Warren Lo

BASICS

DESCRIPTION

Acute CNS insult that causes objective evidence (e.g., radiographic, pathologic) of neurologic damage in a vascular territory and clinical symptoms lasting more than 24 hours. A stroke can be ischemic due to decreased arterial blood flow (acute ischemic stroke [AIS]), venous thrombotic (cerebral sinovenous thrombosis [CSVT]), or hemorrhagic. Acute neurologic dysfunction lasting less than 24 hours and not causing evidence of brain injury is a transient ischemic attack (TIA). Acute neurologic dysfunction lasting less than 24 hours with diffusion changes on MRI is an ischemic stroke. Acute hemiparesis, sensory loss, aphasia, cranial nerve deficits, or altered consciousness (especially if occurring together) should prompt rapid evaluation for possible stroke to prevent delays in diagnosis.

EPIDEMIOLOGY

Incidence

- The neonatal period is the highest risk period for pediatric stroke. Neonatal stroke occurs in approximately 1 in 4,000 live births.
- Incidence of AIS is 1.2–7.9 per 100,000 per year in children over a month of age.
- Hemorrhagic stroke incidence is estimated to be 0.5–5.1 per 100,000 children per year.
- CSVT occurs in 0.67 per 100,000 children per year.

RISK FACTORS

Genetics

Pediatric stroke occurs secondary to a plethora of etiologies as noted below. Some risk factors are genetic:

- Hemoglobin SS (Hgb SS, sickle cell disease): autosomal recessive (AR)
- Factor V Leiden mutation
- Prothrombin G20210A gene mutation
- Classic homocystinuria: *CBS* gene, AR
- Mitochondrial encephalomyopathy, lactic acidosis and stroke-like symptoms (MELAS): maternal inheritance
- Cerebral autosomal dominant arteriopathy with subcortical infarcts and leukoencephalopathy (CADISIL): *NOTCH-3*, autosomal dominant (AD)
- Fabry disease: *GLA* gene, X-linked
- Ehlers-Danlos type IV: *COL3A1* gene, AD
- Marfan syndrome: *FBN1* gene, AD

ETIOLOGY

- Cardiac
  - Congenital heart defects
  - Cardiac rhabdomyoma or myxoma
  - Infectious endocarditis
  - Rheumatic heart disease
  - Prosthetic heart valves
  - Cardiomyopathy/myocarditis
- Vascular
  - Congenital/genetic vasculopathies including Ehlers-Danlos type 4, Marfan syndrome, Sturge-Weber syndrome, PHACES, neurofibromatosis type I
  - Fibromuscular dysplasia, moyamoya disease, postradiation vasculopathy, intracranial aneurysm, arterial agenesis or hypoplasia, traumatic dissection, transient cerebral arteriopathy, focal arteriopathy, arteriovenous malformation
- Vasculitis, inflammatory
  - Systemic: systemic infections, varicella, lupus, hemolytic uremic syndrome, AIDS, Takayasu arteritis, drug abuse, Behçet disease
  - Primary angiitis of the CNS
  - Cranial or cervical infections
- Hematologic/coagulation disorders
  - Severe anemia, polycythemia, or thrombocytosis
  - Hemoglobinopathies especially Hgb SS
  - Primary thrombophilia: antithrombin III deficiency, factor V Leiden homozygous mutation, protein S and C deficiencies, prothrombin G20210A homozygous mutation, hemophilia A and B
  - Acquired thrombophilia: disseminated intravascular coagulation, leukemia or other neoplasm, L-asparaginase treatment, anticardiolipin/antiphospholipid syndrome, oral contraceptives, nephrotic syndrome, pregnancy/postpartum period, inflammatory bowel disease, thrombotic thrombocytopenic purpura, warfarin/heparin use
- Trauma
  - Blunt cervical or intraoral trauma
  - Carotid ligation (e.g., with extracorporeal membrane oxygenation [ECMO])
  - Fat, air, foreign body, amniotic fluid embolism
  - Catheter angiography
  - Chiropractic manipulation
- Metabolic disorders
  - Hyperhomocysteinemia
  - Mitochondrial disorders
  - Fabry disease
- Miscellaneous
  - Migraine
  - Severe hypotension or hypertension
  - Reversible vasoconstriction syndrome
  - Cervical vessel compression

DIAGNOSIS

HISTORY

- Timing and progression of symptoms, including last known time when patient was normal.
- *Analysis of risk factors/etiology*: Inquire about history of trauma, recent medication/drug use, cardiac history, infectious history, skin lesions (acute and chronic), other symptoms/signs of inflammatory disorders, and personal and family history of excessive bleeding or clotting.

ALERT

Acute stroke may present with stuttering symptoms rather than abrupt onset of maximal deficits.

PHYSICAL EXAM

- Note level of alertness, vital signs, presence of cough/gag and respiratory pattern as signs of possible increased intracranial pressure (ICP), and/or need for respiratory support/intubation.
- Age-appropriate neurologic examination including special attention to mental status, funduscopic exam for papilledema, cranial nerve abnormalities, and focal motor deficits. Pediatric National Institutes of Health (NIH) stroke scale use is encouraged.
- General examination: careful cardiac exam for murmurs or dysrhythmias; evaluate for neurocutaneous syndromes or connective tissue disorders

DIAGNOSTIC TESTS & INTERPRETATION

Lab

- Blood chemistry, particularly glucose
- CBC, prothrombin (PT), partial thromboplastin time (PTT), and fibrinogen
- Fasting lipid panel
- Thrombophilia screening (best to consult hematology): antithrombin III, protein C and S levels, factor V Leiden mutation, prothrombin G20210A mutation, and antiphospholipid screen
- More extensive testing in unexplained cases should be tailored to the individual patient and may include the following:
  - Homocysteine
  - Mitochondrial disorder: blood +/− CSF lactate, genetic testing, muscle biopsy
  - Connective tissue disorder gene testing
  - Testing for systemic inflammatory disease (best done in consultation with rheumatology) such as erythrocyte sedimentation rate (ESR), C-reactive protein (CRP), antiphospholipid antibodies, antinuclear antibody, etc.
  - Intracranial infection: lumbar puncture (after imaging) with opening pressure, cell counts, glucose and protein, viral studies, and cultures; blood cultures
  - Consider drug screen.

Imaging

- After stabilization, prompt neuroimaging:
  - Non–contrast-enhanced images to look for possible hemorrhage
  - Gold standard for diagnosis of AIS is MRI with diffusion-weighted imaging.
  - Contrast images (CT or MR) should be obtained if there is concern for infection.
  - Consider vascular imaging (MR or CT) of the head and neck to evaluate for focal stenosis/thrombosis, dissection, vasculopathy, or congenital malformation.
  - Perfusion imaging (CT or MRI) may be helpful in defining the penumbra to evaluate the possible benefit of endovascular procedures.

- More extensive testing in undiagnosed cases may include the following:
  - ECG to assess for rhythm dysfunction
  - Echocardiography with bubble study
  - Conventional catheter angiography

ALERT
CT scan may be normal in the first 24 hours after nonhemorrhagic stroke.

DIFFERENTIAL DIAGNOSIS
Several disorders may mimic an acute stroke:
- Hypoglycemia
- Complicated migraine (hemiplegic, basilar)
- Postepileptic paralysis (Todd paralysis)
- Alternating hemiplegia of childhood
- Posterior reversible encephalopathy syndrome
- Brain tumor
- Conversion disorder
- Metabolic encephalopathies
- Intoxication/toxins
- Syncope
- Acute vestibular disease

TREATMENT
Recommendations are extrapolated from adult stroke literature and expert opinion, as randomized control trials in pediatric stroke have only been conducted in sickle cell patients.

MEDICATION
- Hyperacute treatment with tissue plasminogen activator (tPA) is recommended only in the setting of a clinical trial per American Heart Association (AHA) guidelines.
- Consider low-molecular-weight heparin or unfractioned heparin for CSVT, craniocervical dissection, or cardioembolic stroke.
  - Avoid anticoagulation for intracranial dissection due to increased risk of subarachnoid hemorrhage.
  - Avoid anticoagulation in large hemispheric strokes due to risk of hemorrhagic conversion.
- Antiplatelet therapy, such as aspirin 3–5 mg/kg/day, is reasonable in children whose strokes are not secondary to sickle cell disease, dissection, or cardioembolism.

ADDITIONAL TREATMENT
General Measures
- Admit patients with acute stroke to the hospital for close monitoring for clinical deterioration and for workup for underlying etiology.
- Patients with diminished or fluctuating level of alertness, large hemispheric strokes, or posterior fossa strokes may require monitoring in an intensive care unit for respiratory deterioration or signs of increased ICP.
- Consultation with neurology, hematology, and other pediatric subspecialists as clinically indicated (e.g., rheumatology, genetics)

ALERT
- Obtain urgent hematology consult for children with sickle cell disease and AIS for exchange transfusion.
- Urgent neurosurgical evaluation is indicated for large hemispheric stroke, intracranial hemorrhage, or posterior fossa stroke for possible surgical decompression.

INPATIENT CONSIDERATIONS
Initial Stabilization
- Immediately attend to airway, breathing, and circulation to avoid hypoxia and hypotension, which may cause secondary brain injury.
- Start empiric antibiotics if there is clinical concern for acute CNS infection.
- Maintain adequate hydration particularly in patients with CSVT.
- Avoid hypoglycemia.
- Aggressively treat fevers to avoid increased cerebral metabolic demand.
- Up to 25% of children have seizures with an acute stroke (may be the presenting sign). Treat seizures aggressively.
- Bedrest for at least the first 24 hours is recommended for patients with large territory strokes, stuttering symptoms, or increased ICP.

IV Fluids
Isotonic-based fluids, preferably 0.9 NS, should be used to avoid hyponatremia and brain edema.

ONGOING CARE

FOLLOW-UP RECOMMENDATIONS
Patient Monitoring
- Follow serial neurologic examinations.
- Initiate rehabilitation (physical, occupational, speech therapies) early.
- For patients with significant neurologic deficits, consider discharge to inpatient rehabilitation.

DIET
Strongly consider a swallow study in patients with facial weakness or cranial nerve involvement before allowing oral intake.

PROGNOSIS
- More than half of children with AIS have residual neurologic deficits.
- Predictors of poor outcome after hemorrhagic stroke include Glasgow Coma Scale score ≤7 at admission, infratentorial hemorrhage, age <3 years, or large hemorrhage volume (Appendix, Tables 5 and 6).

COMPLICATIONS
- Acute complications include increased ICP/cerebral edema, seizures, dysphagia resulting in aspiration, and respiratory failure.
- Mortality from AIS is estimated to be 5–18% and from hemorrhagic stroke 7–54%.

ADDITIONAL READING

- DeVeber G, Andrew M, Bjornson B, et al. Cerebral sinovenous thrombosis in children. *N Engl J Med*. 2001;345(6):417–423.
- Jordan LC, Hillis AE. Challenges in the diagnosis and treatment of pediatric stroke. *Nat Rev Neurol*. 2011;7(4):199–208.
- Roach ES, Golomb MR, Adams R, et al. Management of stroke in infants and children: a scientific statement from a Special Writing Group of the American Heart Association. Stroke Council and the Council on Cardiovascular Disease in the Young. *Stroke*. 2008;39(9):264–291.

CODES

ICD10
- I63.9 Cerebral infarction, unspecified
- I63.50 Cereb infrc due to unsp occls or stenos of unsp cereb artery
- I61.9 Nontraumatic intracerebral hemorrhage, unspecified

FAQ
- Q: Will my child have another stroke?
- A: Overall risk of recurrence is estimated to be about 6.6–25%, but the risk primarily depends on the cause of the stroke. Children with Hgb SS and congenital heart defects have a higher risk for recurrence. Children with neonatal strokes without an identified risk factor are unlikely to have a second stroke.
- Q: Which therapies will help my child the most?
- A: Significant research is being conducted in rehabilitation after pediatric stroke, but there is no consensus on the best approach. Constraint-induced therapy has shown promising results. Therapies should not focus on just motor deficits but include cognitive and behavioral difficulties as well.

STUTTERING

Gary A. Emmett

BASICS

DESCRIPTION

Stuttering (also referred to as stammering or dysfluency) is an involuntary disturbance in the normal fluency and timing of speech that is not appropriate for the age of the speaker. Various patterns are seen:

- Prolongation of sounds or syllables
- Repetition of sounds, syllables, or even whole words
- Pauses in the middle of words
- Blocking—either silence or pauses filled with nonsense sounds in the middle of words as if considering what to say next
- Avoidance—word substitutions that are used to skip known problem words; also called circumlocution
- Overemphasis of some syllables or words; also called tension
- Stuttering is significant when it interferes with the patient's life in academic, occupational, or social arenas. Many children with developmental delays have dysfluencies of speech, but it is not considered stuttering unless the dysfluencies are present more frequently than expected for the level of disability.

EPIDEMIOLOGY

- At least 1% of all studied populations affected
- Males stutter 3 times more often than females.
- Stuttering is found in every culture and language. The language spoken in the home does not increase or decrease the amount of stuttering.
- Stuttering begins between 2 and 7 years of age, with 98% of cases presenting by age 10 years.
- Girls start stuttering several months earlier on average than boys; however, they also speak, in general, earlier than boys do.

RISK FACTORS

Genetics

Stuttering does cluster in families:

- Monozygotic twins have a higher concordance for stuttering than dizygotic twins.
- The more closely related one is to a stutterer, the more likely one is to stutter.
- Identical twins have a concordance for stuttering of ≥30%.
- In specific families with a high propensity for stuttering, Lee et al. (and others) have shown single gene defects that correlate highly with dysfluency.

GENERAL PREVENTION

There is no known prevention strategy for stuttering.

PATHOPHYSIOLOGY

Stuttering appears to be associated with an excessive amount of dopamine, or closely related vasoactive compounds, in the brain:

- Patients with Parkinson disease often develop adult-onset stuttering.
- PET scans show increased vasoactive substances in the brains of those who stutter.
- Medications that increase brain dopamine (antidepressants) or are dopaminergic (major tranquilizers) can induce stuttering in nonstutterers; medications that lower dopamine (e.g., clomipramine) may stop stuttering.
- Many differences exist between the brains of stutterers and nonstutterers in glucose uptake, dopamine release, and metabolic activity of the basal ganglia, but no single physiologic process has been well defined as the cause of stuttering.

ETIOLOGY

- Specific etiology is not known, but many factors contribute. Stuttering may be more pronounced when a child is fatigued, excited, upset, rushed, or exposed to some other stressor.
- Environmental factors are thought to have a role. Children adopted by a parent who stutters are more likely to stutter than children adopted by a parent who does not stutter.

COMMONLY ASSOCIATED CONDITIONS

- Other language problems: articulation disorders, phonologic disorders, learning disabilities, dyslexia, ADHD
- Students with developmental delay or intellectual impairment are found to stutter up to 25% of the time.

DIAGNOSIS

HISTORY

- Stuttering runs in families by both nature and nurture.
- Age of onset and length of persistence
  - Onset is insidious, with the child often unaware of the problem.
  - If stuttering starts after the 10th birthday, suspect an intracranial mass or brain ischemia.
- Physiologic stuttering is rarely present during oral reading, singing, acting, and reciting in rhythm or while talking to pets or inanimate objects.
- Medications, especially those that increase dopamine, may activate stuttering.
- Increased intracranial pressure from disease or trauma may lead to stuttering.

PHYSICAL EXAM

- There are no specific physical exam findings of stuttering. Observations of children improve the ability to make this diagnosis. Stuttering is 2 or more repetitions of a speech unit.
- Stutterers often improve in one-to-one situations with familiar people, so ask the parents to bring in a video recording of the child in a variety of situations: when talking in public, singing, and talking to a pet or infant.
- Observations that may be made in the office and correlate strongly with the diagnosis of stuttering include the following:
  - Multiple repetitions and/or prolongations
  - Rising pitch with difficult words
  - Grimacing or other physical tension such as taking deep breaths or jerking the head back when speaking
  - Inappropriate emphasis of words not normally emphasized, extremely slow speech, or speech without intonation
- Although unwillingness to speak to the examiner is normal, unwillingness to speak to the parent is not.

DIAGNOSTIC TESTS & INTERPRETATION

Diagnostic Procedures/Other

- None currently available, but PET scan may be a useful modality in the future
- If stuttering begins after the age of 10 years, or if the patient has additional neurologic or developmental problems, a workup for brain abnormalities should be considered.

DIFFERENTIAL DIAGNOSIS

- Developmental
  - Normal development: dysfluencies associated with rapid onset of full speech capabilities that will usually resolve very quickly
  - Transitory dysfluency is an ill-defined term but generally means stuttering in preschool-aged children that lasts <1 year.
  - Cluttering: Patients with extremely rapid speech will have dysfluencies that resolve with slowing down of speech.
  - Pervasive developmental disorder (autism spectrum disorder): may also have echolalia, tonelessness, and poor eye contact
- Neurologic
  - Tics/Tourette syndrome: similar time of onset, initially somewhat similar symptoms. Stuttering is usually not associated with simultaneous physical movement.
  - Trauma, tumor, or major CNS disease, such as Parkinson disease, may cause late-onset stuttering.

- Medications
  - Any medication that increases the presence of dopamine may worsen (or cause) stuttering. Examples are SSRI-type antidepressants or major tranquilizers.

TREATMENT

GENERAL MEASURES

- Therapy must work on improving the child's fluency and increasing acceptance and tolerance of this problem by the patient and his or her family.
- In a multicultural learning atmosphere, sensitivity to the learning styles of each social group is paramount in achieving successful results.
- Current evidence-based analysis suggests that early intervention by a certified speech pathologist is always indicated.

ADDITIONAL THERAPIES

- Speech therapy
  - Stuttering in young children can be resolved with very short courses of therapy, often ≤3 months. Stuttering remains resolved in ≥95% of these early treatment cases. The younger the patient is at the time of referral to speech therapy, the shorter the course of therapy needed, and the more likely that the therapy will be successful.
  - Many experts in dysfluency believe that early intervention is more likely to be successful than waiting to start therapy if the stuttering has not spontaneously resolved by the 7th birthday.
  - Among the more successful new programs for young children who stutter is the Lidcombe Program of Early Stuttering Intervention, an intense behavioral therapy program that centers on the belief that stuttering is physical in nature. The program teaches parents and caregivers to praise the child for speaking fluently and to correct them occasionally when they stutter. Parents are supported throughout the process by the clinician. The therapy ultimately enables the child to speak fluently and to monitor his or her own speech.
- Other therapies
  - A successful new therapy for adolescents and adults is a hearing-aid type device (SpeechEasy, www.speecheasy.com) that feeds the individual's speech directly back into an earpiece.
  - Devices that make hearing monaural or provide a white noise background in the ear also improve stuttering.
  - Information for families is available through organizations such as The Stuttering Foundation, a nonprofit organization (www.stutteringhelp.org).

ALERT

- Because stuttering waxes and wanes with time, temporary improvement does not equal cure.
- Any behavioral therapy must be done under the guidance of a well-trained professional because inappropriate criticism may worsen stuttering.
- Waiting to see if stuttering goes away by age 7 years is not the best strategy for young children, as was often taught in the past.
- The literature does not give a clear time frame for how long stuttering in preschool children should last before requiring evaluation and treatment, but a significant stutter that lasts for >1 year should be referred to a speech therapist.
- No medications are known to reduce stuttering safely. Acupuncture, hypnosis, and yoga have been used with some success but not in controlled studies.

ONGOING CARE

FOLLOW-UP RECOMMENDATIONS

If stuttering is reported by the parents in a preschool-aged child, follow up in 1–2 months to see if it was only a transitory dysfluency that has resolved. If not, obtain a speech therapy consult for evaluation.

Patient Monitoring

- Periodic follow-up to ensure that speech therapy is in place and that progress is being made
- Reassessment to ensure that child is adapting to social situations and interacting with others

PATIENT EDUCATION

- The following suggestions, although helpful to parents, should be recommended in conjunction with, but not in place of, speech therapy. Parents may be too critical of their own children.
  - Take time out of each day to speak with the child one-on-one.
  - Model slow speech.
  - Wait for the child to speak. Take turns speaking.
  - Allow for transition time between activities and tasks.
  - Keep a notebook of things that help make speech better and things that elicit stuttering.

PROGNOSIS

- Up to 80% of stuttering cases spontaneously regress by age 16 years.
- Severity of stuttering does not relate to persistence of stuttering.
- The longer stuttering exists, the more likely it will persist.

COMPLICATIONS

- Anxiety and depression, often far out of proportion to the degree of dysfluency
- Blocking and hesitation, giving an impression of delayed intellectual development
- Voluntary withdrawal from social interaction to avoid embarrassment

ADDITIONAL READING

- Craig A, Hancock K, Tran Y, et al. Epidemiology of stuttering in the community across the entire life span. *J Speech Lang Hear Res*. 2002;45(6):1097–1105.
- Jones M, Onslow M, Packman A, et al. Randomised controlled trial of the Lidcombe programme of early stuttering intervention. *BMJ*. 2005;331(7518):659–661.
- Lee W, Kang C, Drayna D, et al. Analysis of mannose 6-phosphate uncovering enzyme mutations associated with persistent stuttering. *J Biol Chem*. 2011;286(46):39786–39793.
- Onslow M, O'Brian S. Management of childhood stuttering. *J Paediatr Child Health*. 2013;49(2):E112–E115.
- Rosenfield DB, Viswanath NS. Neuroscience of stuttering. *Science*. 2002;295(5557):973–974.
- The Stuttering Foundation. Videotape No. 70: Stuttering and the preschool child. Help for families. Memphis, TN: Stuttering Foundation of America; 2000. http://www.stutteringhelp.org.
- van Beijsterveldt CE, Felsenfeld S, Boomsma DI. Bivariate genetic analyses of stuttering and nonfluency in a large sample of 5-year-old twins. *J Speech Lang Hear Res*. 2010;53(3):609–619.
- Ward D. The aetiology and treatment of developmental stammering in childhood. *Arch Dis Child*. 2008;93(1):68–71.
- Yairi E, Ambrose N. Epidemiology of stuttering: 21st century advances. *J Fluency Disord*. 2013;38(2):66–87.

CODES

ICD10

F80.81 Childhood onset fluency disorder

FAQ

- Q: Are some children more prone to stuttering?
- A: Yes. "Sensitive" children (many different definitions in many different studies) are more likely to stutter as are the children of highly critical parents.
- Q: Should family and friends complete the sentences of children who stutter?
- A: No. Children who cannot complete a thought should be gently asked to slow down and try again with no time limit set; others should simply wait until the child has completed his or her sentence. Children with a stuttering problem should also be praised when they do not stutter.

S

SUBDURAL HEMATOMA

Daphne M. Hasbani • Sabrina E. Smith

BASICS

DESCRIPTION

A subdural hematoma (SDH) is a collection of blood between the outer pial and inner dural meningeal layers. The bleeding is usually venous in origin, although either cortical arteries or bridging veins may be torn.

EPIDEMIOLOGY

- Heterogeneous causes; occur in all age groups
- Incidence in infants <1 year old estimated at 20–25/100,000.

RISK FACTORS

- In infants and young children, SDHs are frequently the result of abusive head trauma.
- In older children, SDHs are often the result of motor vehicle collisions.
- Neonatal SDHs occur with spontaneous deliveries but may be more frequent following deliveries with forceps or vacuum extraction. SDHs related to birth usually resolve.
- Risk factors for abusive head trauma include disability or prematurity of the child, unstable family situations, parents of young age, and low socioeconomic status.
- 1 study found that fathers were the most frequent perpetrators, followed by boyfriends, female babysitters, and mothers, in descending order of frequency.
- Accidental trauma

Genetics

There is no clear genetic predisposition except when hereditary coagulopathy or metabolic disease is implicated.

GENERAL PREVENTION

- Parents should be counseled about appropriate methods to channel frustration and anger toward infants and children. Shaking an infant when the parent is angry is never appropriate.
- Bicycle helmets, car seats, and seat belts are all valuable in preventing head injuries in children.

PATHOPHYSIOLOGY

- SDHs may be acute or chronic:
  - Arterial SDHs grow quickly, whereas venous SDHs may accumulate slowly, remaining undetected for weeks or months.
  - Acute SDHs contain blood, whereas chronic SDHs contain proteinaceous exudate and blood-breakdown products.
  - Rebleeding may be the underlying cause of many chronic SDHs.
- Significant force is usually required for SDH unless there are predisposing circumstances; SDH is only rarely due to trivial or minor trauma. However, SDH can occur with relatively minor trauma in individuals with bleeding disorders, children on chronic dialysis, and those with enlarged extracerebral spaces or cortical atrophy.
- SDHs in abusive head trauma may be due to the striking of the infant's head against a surface (such as a mattress):
  - The sudden deceleration associated with the impact may tear bridging veins traveling in the subdural space.
- The term shaking-impact syndrome may be more accurate than shaken baby syndrome.

ETIOLOGY

- See "Risk Factors."
- SDHs can also occur after ventricular shunting and extracorporeal membrane oxygenation (ECMO).

COMMONLY ASSOCIATED CONDITIONS

- Some metabolic disorders, such as glutaric aciduria type I and Menkes disease, can be associated with both acute and chronic SDHs.
- Victims of motor vehicle collisions with SDH may have other intracranial injuries such as diffuse axonal injury.
- Traumatic SDHs are often associated with cerebral contusions. Other associated injuries include skull fractures, diffuse axonal injury, and penetrating injuries.
- Sequelae: epilepsy, developmental delay, cerebral palsy

DIAGNOSIS

A careful history and detailed physical exam are essential to explore possible causes of the SDH, assess the child's neurologic status, and look for evidence of other injuries. Prompt neuroimaging is critical.

HISTORY

- Newborns: SDHs due to birth trauma may present with lethargy, pallor, poor feeding, apnea, and seizures. However, many term newborns with small SDHs are asymptomatic.
- Infants and young children: SDHs may also present with a nonspecific history of lethargy, irritability, vomiting, poor feeding, apnea, and seizures.
- Older children: present with a history of trauma and alteration of consciousness
- Caution
  - Be suspicious if the stated history does not fit with the pattern or severity of the injury.
  - Physicians and other health care professionals with experience in child abuse should be consulted early if abuse is suspected.

PHYSICAL EXAM

- Newborns may present with decreased responsiveness, a bulging fontanelle, hypotonia, or hypertonia. Retinal hemorrhages are not specific at this age because they are seen in up to 40% of newborns following a vaginal delivery.
- Infants and young children may also present with nonspecific physical signs, but focal neurologic signs may be present. Retinal hemorrhages are most often associated with abusive head trauma, but they have been reported after accidental trauma leading to SDH. Bilateral retinal hemorrhages with retinal folds or detachments are particularly associated with abusive head trauma.
- Other signs of child abuse include burns, lacerations, and bruises in various stages of healing and belt marks, choke marks, and multiple fractures of different ages.
- Older children present with signs of external head trauma, decreased responsiveness, and focal neurologic signs.
- SDHs present with nonspecific signs such as vomiting, irritability, lethargy, failure to thrive, anemia, and seizures.

DIAGNOSTIC TESTS & INTERPRETATION

Imaging

- CT scan is the imaging study of choice in acute head trauma with neurologic signs:
  - SDH appears as an extra-axial area of increased density, crescentic in shape, and often associated with cerebral contusion or mass effect.
  - CT also may show evidence of cerebral edema, with loss of gray matter/white matter differentiation and small ventricles.
  - Subacute SDHs may be difficult to distinguish from adjacent gray matter on CT scan.
  - Loss of gray/white matter differentiation may occur.
  - Chronic SDHs appear as areas of low density on CT scan, often bilateral.
- MRI is helpful to clarify subacute and chronic SDHs and to identify small SDHs missed by CT.
- Ultrasound is less helpful because it may be difficult to distinguish the subdural space from the subarachnoid space.
- If child abuse is suspected, a skeletal survey or bone scan is useful to look for fractures of different ages.
- Incidental SDH may be found on neuroimaging studies in newborns; frequently, no intervention is required other than close follow-up.

DIFFERENTIAL DIAGNOSIS

- SDHs are usually traumatic, but separating accidental from abusive head trauma may be difficult: Falls in infants may cause linear skull fractures but rarely SDHs. On noncontrast head CT, homogeneous hyperdense SDH is more common following accidental trauma, whereas mixed-density SDH is more common following abusive head trauma.
- Macrocephaly or other signs/symptoms since birth may help to date the origin of the SDH to the perinatal or neonatal period.
- Epidural hematomas, subarachnoid hemorrhages, and acute SDHs cannot be distinguished clinically:
  - The lucid interval sometimes seen with epidural hematomas in adults is not a reliable sign.
  - A head CT should differentiate the different entities.

- Chronic SDHs must be differentiated from benign enlargement of the subarachnoid spaces, a self-limited condition characterized by progressive macrocrania and extra-axial fluid collections with the density of spinal fluid:
  - MRI can differentiate benign enlargement of the subarachnoid spaces from SDH.
  - Rarely, SDH can also occur in children with benign enlargement of the subarachnoid spaces.

TREATMENT

MEDICATION

Seizures

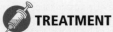

- Phenytoin and levetiracetam are good choices if IV medication is needed, with phenobarbital as a reasonable alternative, especially in neonates.
- Prophylactic anticonvulsants given for a few weeks are effective in reducing early posttraumatic seizures but may not affect long-term risk of epilepsy.

ADDITIONAL TREATMENT

General Measures

- The treatment of choice for large, acute SDHs is surgical evacuation. Smaller SDHs may be managed conservatively, with careful monitoring for signs of neurologic deterioration.
- While awaiting surgery, attention to airway, breathing, and circulation (ABCs) is critical. Tracheal intubation should be performed if the child's Glasgow Coma Scale score is <8 or if airway protective reflexes are impaired.
- Measures to control intracranial pressure (ICP) include elevating the head of the bed 30 degrees to promote venous drainage and osmotic therapy with mannitol:
  - ICP monitoring should be considered.
  - Mild hyperventilation (Pco_2 30–35 mm Hg) may be helpful but should not be instituted prophylactically.
  - The efficacy of these measures in improving long-term outcome following large SDHs has not been established. Mild hypothermia and hypertonic saline have been used in some cases of traumatic brain injury in adults, but these are not proven therapies in children.
- Seizures should be treated promptly.
- Treatment of chronic SDHs is more controversial:
  - If there are no signs of elevated ICP, conservative treatment is reasonable, and most collections will resolve.
  - Subdural taps are indicated if ICP rises.
  - If taps are not successful, a subdural peritoneal shunt may be placed.
- Treatment of SDHs that develop after ventricular shunting is particularly challenging.

ISSUES FOR REFERRAL

Social work services should be consulted in cases of known or suspected child abuse.

SURGERY/OTHER PROCEDURES

The treatment of choice for large, acute SDHs is surgical evacuation.

INPATIENT CONSIDERATIONS

Initial Stabilization

- Children with SDHs may be critically ill on presentation.
- The aggressiveness of acute therapy depends on the child's clinical condition.
- Neuroimaging studies and, if necessary, prompt neurosurgical consultation should be performed.

IV Fluids

Isotonic fluids should be given because hypotonic fluids may worsen cerebral edema.

ONGOING CARE

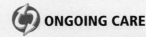

FOLLOW-UP RECOMMENDATIONS

Children with neurologic sequelae from head injury may benefit from admission to a rehabilitation hospital.

PROGNOSIS

- In general, long-term outcome is related to the condition of the child at time of presentation. Prolonged elevation of ICP, concomitant ischemic brain injury, or significant cerebral edema before treatment is worrisome and indicates a poor prognosis.
- Children typically have a better outcome from head injury than do adults, but children <7 years of age often do worse than older children, especially if the SDH is the result of abusive head trauma.

COMPLICATIONS

- SDHs may result in mass effect, focal neurologic signs, and coma.
- Increased ICP and seizures are other serious complications.
- Neurologic sequelae of SDHs are more severe than epidural hematomas because of associated cerebral contusions.
- Long-term problems include headache, seizures, hydrocephalus, cerebral palsy, difficulty concentrating, poor school performance, fixed neurologic deficits, and neurobehavioral problems.
- Epilepsy eventually develops in ~10–15% of patients after severe head injury: This risk generally does not warrant the use of prophylactic anticonvulsants.

ADDITIONAL READING

- Foerster BR, Petrou M, Lin D, et al. Neuroimaging evaluation of non-accidental head trauma with correlation to clinical outcomes: a review of 57 cases. *J Pediatr*. 2009;154(4):573–577.
- Matschke J, Voss J, Obi N, et al. Nonaccidental head injury is the most common cause of subdural bleeding in infants <1 year of age. *Pediatrics*. 2009;124(6):1587–1594.
- McNeely PD, Atkinson JD, Saigal G, et al. Subdural hematomas in infants with benign enlargement of the subarachnoid spaces are not pathognomonic for child abuse. *AJNR Am J Neuroradiol*. 2006;27(8):1725–1728.
- Swift DM, McBride L. Chronic subdural hematoma in children. *Neurosurg Clin North Am*. 2000;11(3):439–446.
- Tung GA, Kumar M, Richardson RC, et al. Comparison of accidental and nonaccidental traumatic head injury in children on noncontrast computed tomography. *Pediatrics*. 2006;118(2):626–633.

CODES

ICD10

- S06.5X0A Traum subdr hem w/o loss of consciousness, init
- P52.8 Other intracranial (nontraumatic) hemorrhages of newborn
- P10.0 Subdural hemorrhage due to birth injury

FAQ

- Q: When did the bleed occur?
- A: With chronic SDHs, the time and type of injury may be difficult to establish because no trauma may be reported and the trauma may have occurred weeks or months before. Neuroimaging can give some indication of the injury's timing.
- Q: What limitations should be imposed after an acute SDH?
- A: Because SDH may recur with minor trauma, it is prudent to avoid any activities that have significant risk of fall or a blow to the head for weeks to months or until neuroradiologic resolution of the hematoma.
- Q: Why are anticonvulsants not used to prevent seizures following SDHs?
- A: Seizure medications may be given for a few weeks to prevent early seizures following an SDH. After a few weeks, the risks and side effects of the medications outweigh the risk of developing seizures. If seizures begin at a time remote from the injury, then seizure medications can be restarted.
- Q: My baby twisted out of my arms, fell head first onto a tile floor, and suffered a head injury. Will I be reported for child abuse?
- A: Not if the injuries fit with the stated history. In this case, the most likely injury would be a linear skull fracture. If more serious intracranial injuries occur, they will probably not be associated with retinal hemorrhages or other injuries such as older fractures in multiple stages of healing.

SUBSTANCE USE DISORDERS

Sara M. Buckelew

BASICS

DESCRIPTION

- In adolescence, substance use tends to occur along a continuum from abstinence to experimentation to nonproblematic use to problematic use to substance use disorder.
- *DSM-5* defines substance use disorder as a maladaptive pattern of use leading to clinical impairment or distress, which is based on presence of specific criterion including the following:
  – Substance use resulting in failure to fulfill obligations (such as school or work)
  – Substance use in situations that are hazardous (such as driving)
  – Continued use despite interpersonal problems exacerbated by use
  – Development of tolerance
  – Development of withdrawal
  – Craving for the substance
  – Persistent desire or unsuccessful efforts to curb/cut down usage
  – Significant time and energy spent obtaining substances
  – Continued use despite recognition of associated psychological or physical consequences of continued use (with or without physiologic dependence)
- Substance use disorder combines the previous diagnoses of substance abuse and substance dependence from the *DSM-IV*.
- Substance use disorder exists along a continuum from mild to severe depending on the number of criterion met.

EPIDEMIOLOGY

- Substance use estimates vary by substance, age of youth, and geographical location. Up to date, epidemiologic data can be found online at www.monitoringthefuture.org which includes data for cigarette, alcohol, and other illicit drug use among 8th,10th, and 12th graders. Another source of substance abuse data includes the Youth Risk Behavior Survey (YRBS) conducted by the Centers for Disease Control and Prevention.
- Although rates of overall use over time have remained relatively stable, rates for each individual substance have varied.
- Adolescent substance use has been associated with increased morbidity and mortality including depression, suicide, motor vehicle accidents, unintentional injuries, teenage pregnancy, high-risk sexual activity, and sexually transmitted infections (STIs).

RISK FACTORS

- Early initiation: Adolescents who begin using alcohol or drugs at an early age have an increased risk of developing an addictive disorder later in life. Later initiation of use may be a protective factor.
- Individual factors such as low self-esteem and impulsivity
- Social factors such as peer use
- Family factors such as a negative parent–child/adolescent relationship, permissive or authoritarian parenting style, parental divorce during adolescence
- Other environmental factors such as school failure and availability of substances within the community
- Individual and family factors may be protective as well such as positive self-esteem and positive, open and supportive relationships with family.

GENETICS

Research demonstrates a genetic predisposition to alcohol dependence. Children of alcoholic parents are 4–6 times more prone to developing alcohol dependence.

COMMONLY ASSOCIATED CONDITIONS

- Mood disorders
- Anxiety disorders, including posttraumatic stress disorder
- Eating disorders (specifically bulimia nervosa)
- Attention deficit disorder
- Learning disorders
- Conduct disorders
- Psychotic disorders

DIAGNOSIS

HISTORY

- Adolescent-appropriate screening using a validated measure should be administered at least annually at every adolescent preventive care visit and appropriate urgent/acute care visits.
- Screening should be performed confidentially and with the adolescent alone (without parents).
- SBIRT Model recommended for adolescents. Includes the following steps: Screening, Brief Intervention, and Referral to Treatment. The Brief Intervention is based in principles of motivational interviewing in addressing behavior change.
- The CRAFFT (an acronym for key components in the questions: car, relax, alone, forget, family/friends, trouble) screen is one of several tools validated for adolescent.
- All patients who screen positive warrant a more complete assessment including more in-depth substance use history. Questions should include what substances are used, frequency of use, mode of use (nasal, ingestions, smoking, intravenous), how they are obtaining the substances, and peer group usage.
- The 5 A's was developed to address smoking cessation and includes Asking about use; Advising all smokers to quit; Assessing a patients willingness to quit; Assisting the patient with smoking cessation; and Arranging follow-up.

PHYSICAL EXAM

- Vital signs: increased blood pressure and increased pulse seen in stimulants (such as cocaine, amphetamines), cannabis, phencyclidine (PCP)
- General: odor of alcohol, marijuana, or tobacco; poor personal hygiene; slurred speech; intoxicated appearance
- HEENT: rhinitis and/or nasal mucosa irritation if snorting substances
- Eyes: injected conjunctiva with cannabis; nystagmus with PCP; pupillary constriction with opiates; pupillary dilatation with cocaine, PCP, and opiate withdrawal
- Respiratory depression with opiates, overdose on depressants (such as alcohol and benzodiazepines)
- Respiratory: wheezing/abnormal breath sounds due to smoking substances (tobacco, cannabis, other substances)
- Skin: needle marks in injection users

DIAGNOSTIC TESTS & INTERPRETATION

Lab

- Urine drug screens are most commonly used. Their use in the emergency situation is critical when overdose or acute intoxication is suspected. They can be used effectively as part of a drug treatment program. With limited exceptions, random and routine drug screening is not recommended by the American Academy of Pediatrics and is of limited value.
- Urine drug screens typically include
  – Cannabinoids
  – Cocaine
  – Amphetamines
  – Opiates
  – PCP

Diagnostic Procedures/Other

Screening for STIs including HIV (particularly in IV drug users) and hepatitis B and C is recommended as part of a risk reduction program.

DIFFERENTIAL DIAGNOSIS

- Mood disorders
- Attention deficit disorder
- Psychotic disorders

TREATMENT

MEDICATION

- Cigarette/nicotine dependence
  – Nicotine replacement available in number of different forms including nicotine replacement patch, lozenge, inhaler, and gum
  – Bupropion may be recommended in those who have failed with nicotine replacement alone.
  – Varenicline is not approved in those <18 years of age.

- Alcohol dependence
  - Medications available for adults such as naltrexone, disulfiram, and acamprosate are not approved for adolescents.
- Buprenorphine (partial agonist of the mu opioid receptor) for treatment of opioid dependence. Approved in those aged 16 years and older and may be used for maintenance. Methadone has been used for short-term detoxification but not typically used for maintenance due to poor adherence.
- Comorbid and associated psychiatric illnesses such as mood disorders, anxiety disorders, and ADHD should be medicated appropriately.

ADDITIONAL TREATMENT

General Measures

- Treatment can be provided in a number of different settings both outpatient and inpatient with varying intensity, including the following:
  - Outpatient treatment: typically 1 hour weekly, may be individual therapy or family therapy
  - Intensive outpatient program or partial hospitalization program: more intensive outpatient program where teen lives at home but may be participating in individual and group therapy multiple hours per day and multiple days per week
  - Residential treatment/therapeutic boarding school: where teen is no longer living at home and receiving more intensive services

ISSUES FOR REFERRAL

- Rates of treatment are low, with only 6–10% of those adolescents with substance use disorders receiving treatment.
- All youth with a concern for substance abuse or comorbid disease should be referred to an experienced mental health professional or addiction specialist.

ADDITIONAL THERAPIES

Strongest body of evidence in the treatment of adolescent substance use disorders is therapy.

- Cognitive behavioral therapy: structured and goal-oriented therapy designed to assist teen in identifying behavioral strategies to address distorted thoughts and subsequent emotions
- Family therapy: Some research demonstrates that family treatments are superior to individual therapy.
- 12-step programs such as Alcoholics Anonymous (AA) and Narcotics Anonymous (NA): typically small group format where participants may provide support for each other
- Brief intervention/brief advice/motivational interviewing: a counseling style that is patient-focused, aimed at exploring benefits and cons of usage in order to direct the patient toward behavior change

INPATIENT CONSIDERATIONS

- Detoxification should be considered for youth when there is concern for withdrawal. Includes medical management of withdrawal symptoms.
- Residential treatment is an intensive, structured program for adolescents who may require this particularly acutely. For those who require 24-hour care and support

ONGOING CARE

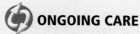

FOLLOW-UP RECOMMENDATIONS

Patient Monitoring

- Patients should be screened annually at all preventive visits.
- When an action plan is created or in those receiving brief advice or brief interventions, patients should be followed closely.
- The pediatrician may play an important role in monitoring for relapse in those who have undergone treatment.

PATIENT EDUCATION

All youth who have not initiated substance use should be given positive reinforcement about their behaviors and encouraged to discuss the topic in the future.

PROGNOSIS

- Youth who receive treatment do better than those who do not.
- Approximately 1/3–½ of youth who receive treatment will relapse within 12 months following treatment completion.
- Factors associated with relapse include psychiatric comorbidity, poor coping skills, poor familial relationships, and return to prior peer groups.
- Continued involvement in therapy and ongoing support helps to protect against relapse.

COMPLICATIONS

Acute intoxication/overdose can have significant associated morbidity and mortality.

ADDITIONAL READING

- Adger H Jr, Saha S. Alcohol use disorders in adolescents. *Pediatr Rev*. 2013;34(3):103–114.
- Committee on Substance Abuse, Levy SJ, Kokotailo PK. Substance use screening, brief intervention, and referral to treatment for pediatricians. *Pediatrics*. 2011;128(5):e1330–e1340.
- Howlett KD, Williams H, Subramaniam G. Understanding and treating adolescent substance abuse: a preliminary review. *Focus*. 2012;10:293–299.
- Kaplan G, Ivanov I. Pharmacotherapy for substance abuse disorders in adolescence. *Pediatr Clin North Am*. 2011;58(1):243–258.
- Sanchez-Samper X, Knight J. Drug abuse by adolescents: general considerations. *Pediatr Rev*. 2009;30(3):83–93.
- Winters KC, Botzet AM, Fahnhorst T. Advances in adolescent substance abuse treatment. *Curr Psychiatry Rep*. 2011;13(5):416–421.

CODES

ICD10

- F19.10 Other psychoactive substance abuse, uncomplicated
- F10.10 Alcohol abuse, uncomplicated
- F12.10 Cannabis abuse, uncomplicated

S

FAQ

- Q: Should I screen adolescents who use substances for suicide risk?
- A: Yes. All adolescents with a history of substance misuse should be screened for suicide risk and suicidal ideations. Adolescents who use substances have a higher percentage of psychiatric comorbidity and a higher risk of suicide.
- Q: What do I tell parents about their teen's substance use?
- A: The laws about confidentiality pertaining to adolescent substance use and disclosure to parents depend on the state. It is important to know the laws in your state.
- Q: What symptoms would you expect to see based on a patient's blood alcohol level?
- A: Blood alcohol levels (BAL) can be indicative of the severity and may vary due to metabolism and body weight. A BAL of 0.05% is associated with slowing reaction time and altered cognition; 0.1–0.2%: intoxication, drowsiness, and loss of balance; 0.2–0.3% may lead to vomiting and stupor; 0.3–0.4% may lead to hypothermia and coma; and >0.4% may lead to death.

SUDDEN INFANT DEATH SYNDROME

Katherine Deye • Rachel Moon

BASICS

DESCRIPTION

- Sudden infant death syndrome (SIDS) is the sudden and unexpected death of an infant younger than 1 year of age, with onset of the lethal episode apparently occurring during sleep, which remains unexplained after a thorough investigation, including the performance of a complete autopsy, review of the circumstances of death, and review of the clinical history.
- SIDS is a subcategory of deaths described as "sudden unexpected deaths in infancy" (SUDI) or "sudden unexpected infant deaths" (SUID). SUID can include both explained deaths, including suffocation, asphyxia, entrapment, trauma (accidental or nonaccidental), cardiac arrhythmia, infection, and metabolic disorders, and unexplained deaths, including SIDS and those with an undetermined/ill-defined cause of death.

EPIDEMIOLOGY

- Most common cause of death in postneonatal (>1 month old) infants
- Peak age of incidence: 2–4 months; uncommon before 2 weeks or after 6 months
- Incidence has been decreasing:
  - 1970s: ~2.5 SIDS deaths per 1,000 live births: SIDS defined somewhat loosely
  - 1980s: ~1.4 per 1,000 live births
  - 1990s: ~1.2 per 1,000 (1992)–0.7 per 1,000 live births (1999): "Back to Sleep" campaign encouraging supine positioning during sleep in 1994 is associated with steady decline in deaths.
  - 2000s: Since 2001, SIDS rate has remained constant (~0.5/1000 live births).
- The rate of SUID (suffocation, asphyxia) or other undetermined or unspecified causes of death has risen.
  - For example, the death rate from accidental suffocation and strangulation in bed (ASSB) has more than quadrupled in recent years.
  - Largely because of improved death scene investigations, many deaths that previously would have been classified as SIDS are now being classified as having resulted from these other causes of death.

RISK FACTORS

- Male sex
- Premature birth or low birth weight
- Inadequate prenatal care
- Poverty
- Lower maternal educational level
- Exposure to prenatal, gestational, and postnatal tobacco smoke
- Alcohol and illicit drug use in utero and after infant's birth
- Maternal substance abuse
- Young maternal age
- Prone and side sleeping position
- Overheating and overbundling
- African American or American Indian/Alaska Native heritage
- Soft sleep surface
- Soft and loose bedding
- Bed sharing, particularly if sharing bed with one or more smokers; if the infant is <11 weeks of age (even if neither parent is a smoker); if sleeping on a surface with soft bedding; if bed sharing adults have consumed alcohol or drugs; if bed sharing with people who are not the infant's parents; and if the sleep surface is very soft (couches, armchairs, waterbeds)

Potential protective factors include the following:

- Breastfeeding
- Pacifier use at bedtime and naptime
- Regular prenatal care
- Immunizations
- Room sharing without bed sharing

Genetics

- Most likely represents a heterogeneous group of causes of death
- Genetic factors may play a role in some of these deaths. Candidate genes include those encoding ion channel proteins, serotonin transporters, nicotine-metabolizing enzymes and those regulating autonomic nervous system development, inflammation, energy production, hypoglycemia, and thermal regulation.
- There appears to be a complex gene and environment interaction.
- Parents should be reassured that the chance of recurrence in future siblings is small and will be examined during the investigation of the SIDS death.

GENERAL PREVENTION

- Place infants on their backs for every sleep until 1 year of life.
- Use a firm sleep surface.
- Do not use blankets, pillows, bumper pads, sheepskins, or comforters in the infant's sleep area.
- Avoid tobacco smoke exposure during pregnancy and after birth.
- Room sharing without bed sharing is recommended.
- Breastfeed as much and as long as possible.
- Consider offering a pacifier at naptime and bedtime. If breastfeeding, wait until breastfeeding is well established (3–4 weeks) before introducing a pacifier.
- Do not use alcohol or illicit drugs during pregnancy or after birth.
- Avoid overheating.
- Do not cover infant's head during sleep.
- Immunize your infant.
- Do not use home cardiorespiratory monitors as a strategy to reduce the risk of SIDS.

PATHOPHYSIOLOGY

- The "triple risk" model of SIDS describes the interplay of three factors thought to contribute to these deaths: a vulnerable infant, a critical period of development, and stressful environmental challenges.
  - Individual traits that influence an infant's vulnerability to SIDS are characterized as intrinsic risk factors. Examples include serotonin receptor abnormalities noted in the ventral medulla of SIDS infants at autopsy, suggesting derangements in the neural circuits responsible for arousal and cardiorespiratory functioning. Autopsy studies have also revealed changes in the serotonin transporter gene (*5-HTT*) that ultimately reduce serotonin concentration at these nerve synapses.
  - The period from birth to age 6 months is one of rapid brain growth and maturation, as well as motor skill acquisition, such as the ability to lift and turn the head in the event of life-threatening rebreathing or asphyxia.
  - Exogenous risk factors such as soft bedding, tobacco smoke, side or prone positioning, and overheating place these vulnerable infants at risk for asphyxia or other physiologic disturbances.
- Failure of arousal in the face of asphyxia or other physiologic disturbances likely contributes to the final pathway leading to these infants' deaths. Known risk factors for SIDS have been linked to arousal and cardiorespiratory responses. For example:
  - Prematurely born infants have immature central respiratory responses.
  - When compared with supine-sleeping infants, prone-sleeping infants have increased arousal thresholds.
  - Prenatal and postnatal nicotine exposure blunts arousal responses to hypoxia.

DIAGNOSIS

HISTORY

- SIDS is a diagnosis of exclusion.
  - A thorough postmortem evaluation, including death scene investigation, complete autopsy, and review of the infant's clinical history, should be done.
  - Standardized forms developed by the Centers for Disease Control and Prevention for the collection of the circumstances and factors contributing to these deaths and reporting of cases of SUID are available online at www.cdc.gov/sids/SUIDRFdownload.htm.
- Parents and other caregivers should be interviewed in a sensitive manner so as not to imply that parents or caregivers are blamed for the death. Specifically, the following should be ascertained:
  - Signs and symptoms (such as fever, cough, irritability, easy fatigability, and lethargy) that may be suggestive of an acute or chronic medical condition that may have caused or contributed to the death
  - Family history of sudden death, condition associated with cardiac arrhythmia, epilepsy, metabolic or genetic disease
  - Known risk factors for SIDS and other SUID, including sleep position when placed and found, sleep environment, bed sharing, prematurity, parental smoking history, and history of maternal substance abuse
  - Evidence suggestive of accidental suffocation, strangulation, or entrapment

– Evidence suggestive of nonaccidental traumatic injury and other forms of abuse (including medical child abuse, also known as "Munchausen syndrome by proxy")

PHYSICAL EXAM

- Normal-appearing infant without obvious reason for death
- May have postmortem lividity and/or a pink, frothy discharge from the mouth or nose
- May have signs of terminal motor activity (clenched fists, trismus, or anal dilation)
- Lack of signs of injury or neglect (malnourishment, dehydration, wasting)
- Care must be taken with the deceased body; only medical examiners and coroners have legal authority to establish the cause of death.

Manipulation or examination of body after the declaration of death may violate applicable laws. All medical paraphernalia used during resuscitation must be left in place.

DIAGNOSTIC TESTS & INTERPRETATION

Lab

- A full autopsy, including the cranium and cranial contents, must be performed on all infants who die suddenly and unexpectedly.
- A toxicology screen; microbiologic evaluation for bacterial, viral, and fungal infections; and urine and serum chemistries to evaluate for metabolic disease should be performed—whether these are performed at the hospital or by the medical examiner is dictated by local resources and protocols.

Imaging

- Skeletal survey
  – Whether this is performed at the hospital or by the medical examiner is dictated by local resources and protocols.

Pathologic Findings

- After a review of a thorough death scene investigation, clinical history, and complete autopsy, pathologists are able to make the diagnosis of SIDS when no other specific cause of death has been identified.
- There are no pathologic findings that are pathognomonic. Approximately 80–85% of SIDS infants are noted to have intrathoracic petechiae on examination. Additional common autopsy findings include pulmonary congestion and edema as well as minor airway inflammation.

DIFFERENTIAL DIAGNOSIS

- In approximately 10–15% of cases of suspected SIDS, an alternate cause of death is identified. These include the following:
  – Environmental: asphyxia (due to such causes as overlaying, wedging, choking, obstruction of nose or mouth, rebreathing, neck compression, immersion in water); hyperthermia, hypothermia, toxic exposures
  – Infectious: sepsis (bacterial, viral), pneumonia, bronchiolitis, meningitis, myocarditis, pertussis
  – Trauma: accidental and nonaccidental trauma (cranial injuries, abdominal trauma, nonaccidental suffocation, and drowning)
  – Metabolic: electrolyte disturbances, inborn errors of metabolism, especially involving energy production or toxic metabolites (e.g., medium chain acyl-CoA dehydrogenase deficiency, defects in glycogenolysis, defects in oxidative phosphorylation, urea cycle defects, aminoacidopathies, glycogen storage disease)
  – Congenital/anatomic: congenital heart disease, Arnold-Chiari malformation, malrotation, volvulus
  – Miscellaneous: adrenal insufficiency, cardiac arrhythmias (channelopathies)

TREATMENT

ADDITIONAL TREATMENT

General Measures

- Prevention rather than treatment is the goal. All caregivers of infants should be educated about SIDS risk reduction strategies, ideally before the infant's birth.
- For families who have experienced a SIDS death, grief counseling may be helpful.
- Families who are contemplating a subsequent pregnancy should be offered genetic and metabolic screening to rule out any hereditary conditions that may mimic SIDS. Avoidance of risk factors should be stressed. However, this discussion should be done with sensitivity, as discussion of risk factors may incur feelings of guilt, particularly if risk factors were associated with the infant's death.

ADDITIONAL READING

- American Academy of Pediatrics; Committee on Child Abuse and Neglect. Addendum: distinguishing sudden infant death syndrome from child abuse fatalities. *Pediatrics*. 2001;108(3):812.
- Hymel KP, American Academy of Pediatrics; Committee on Child Abuse and Neglect; National Association of Medical Examiners. Distinguishing sudden infant death syndrome from child abuse fatalities. *Pediatrics*. 2006;118(1):421–427.
- Jaafar SH, Jahanfar S, Angolkar M, et al. Effect of restricted pacifier use in breastfeeding term infants for increasing duration of breastfeeding. *Cochrane Database Syst Rev*. 2012;7:CD007202. doi:10.1002/14651858.CD007202.pub3.
- Kinney HC, Thach BT. The sudden infant death syndrome. *N Engl J Med*. 2009;361(8):795–805.
- Moon RY, Fu L. Sudden infant death syndrome: an update. *Pediatr Rev*. 2012;33(7):314–320.
- Moon RY, Task Force on Sudden Infant Death Syndrome. SIDS and other sleep-related infant deaths: expansion of recommendations for a safe infant sleeping environment. *Pediatrics*. 2011;128(5):1030–1039.
- Weese-Mayer DE, Ackerman MJ, Marazita ML, et al. Sudden infant death syndrome: review of implicated genetic factors. *Am J Med Genet A*. 2007;143A(8):771–788.
- Willinger M, James LS, Catz C. Defining the sudden infant death syndrome (SIDS): deliberations of an expert panel convened by the National Institute of Child Health and Human Development. *Pediatr Pathol*. 1991;11(5):677–684.

CODES

ICD10

R99 Ill-defined and unknown cause of mortality

FAQ

- Q. What is the difference between SIDS and an undetermined cause of death?
- A. SIDS, which is a subcategory of SUID, is most commonly defined as "the sudden death of an infant under 1 year of age, which remains unexplained after a thorough case investigation, including performance of a complete autopsy, examination of the death scene, and a review of the clinical history" (Willinger et al, 1991). When the cause of death cannot be clearly established (e.g., appears to be SIDS, but death occurred in a sleep environment where accidental suffocation cannot be ruled out), cause of death may be "ill-defined" or "undetermined."
- Q. Won't giving a baby a pacifier interfere with breastfeeding?
- A: If a baby is breastfed, there is a theoretical risk of "nipple confusion." A recent Cochrane Collaboration review on the topic (2012) concluded that "for mothers who are motivated to breastfeed their infants, pacifier use before or after breastfeeding was established did not significantly affect the prevalence or duration of exclusive and partial breastfeeding up to 4 months of age." However, long-term data beyond 4 months of age are lacking. If concerned, parents can wait until breastfeeding is well established, usually about 3–4 weeks, before introducing a pacifier.
- Q: Is it okay for a baby to take a nap while lying prone on the parent's chest?
- A. No. Parents often fall asleep unintentionally, which can result in a hazardous situation. Falling asleep with the baby while on a couch or sofa is particularly dangerous.

SUICIDE

Leonard J. Levine • Jonathan R. Pletcher

BASICS

DESCRIPTION
- Suicidal behavior is a voluntary self-harming act with the intent of ending one's own life.
- Attempted suicide occurs when the act does not result in death (also, failed or near-suicide).
- Suicidal ideation is any thought, with or without a specific plan, to end one's life.
- Suicidality can include suicidal ideation, preparatory acts, and/or attempts.

EPIDEMIOLOGY
- Suicide is the 3rd leading cause of death for adolescents and emerging young adults (10–26 years), whereas it is the 10th overall cause of death for Americans.
- Adolescent mortality from suicide tripled between the 1950s and the 1990s and has remained overall stable since, after declining in 1990s then rising over the past decade.
- Females attempt suicide at a rate 2–4 times that of males and are most likely to attempt suicide through ingestion.
- Males 15–24 years old are 5 times as likely to die by suicide as females and are most likely to use more lethal methods.
- Completed suicide rates are highest in non-Hispanic white (13.9/100,000) and Native American (10.6/100,000) adolescents. Suicide rates for black males 10–19 years old doubled between the years 1980 and 1995.
- Gay, lesbian, bisexual, transgender, and questioning youth report significantly higher rates of suicide thoughts and attempts than their heterosexual peers.
- More than half of all deaths by suicide in the United States involve a firearm.

Incidence
- Annually in the United States, ~2,000 adolescents die from suicide and over a million suicide attempts come to medical attention; there were as many as 11 times the number of attempts as completed suicides.
- Overall, suicide accounted for 10.9 deaths per 100,000 persons aged 15–24 years in 2011.
- In 2013, 17% of youth surveyed in grades 9–12 reported seriously considering suicide at some point in the preceding year: >8% reported attempting suicide in the previous year.

RISK FACTORS
- Previous suicide attempt(s)
- Social isolation
- Substance/alcohol abuse
- Family history of suicide
- Family history of severe mental illness or substance abuse
- Past or present sexual or physical abuse
- Family conflict or disruption
- Presence of firearms in the home

GENERAL PREVENTION
- Universal screening of all adolescents for suicidality should occur in primary and acute care settings.
- Brief, validated screening tools are available for medical settings.
- There is ample evidence that direct inquiry, paper-and-pencil questionnaires, and computer-assisted screening enhance identification.
- Warning signs, aside from obvious emotional distress, can include the following:
  - Chronic physical symptoms, with or without discrete physiologic etiology (e.g., chronic headache, abdominal pain)
  - Change in level of functioning in school, work, or home
  - Changes in mood or affect
- If suicidal ideation is reported, components of risk assessment include the following:
  - Frequency and timing of suicidal thoughts
  - Active planning
  - Access to lethal means such as firearms
  - History of past suicide attempt(s)
  - History of mental health problems, including substance abuse, and treatment
  - Acute or anticipated psychosocial stressor
  - Family history of suicide
  - Family violence
  - Exploration of coping strategies and social support systems
- Referral or consultation with a psychiatrist or mental health professional is indicated with any question or risk for suicide attempt.

PATHOPHYSIOLOGY
- Decreased central serotonergic activity may result in aggressive or impulsive behaviors, which may be aimed at oneself.
- An underlying psychiatric or personality disorder acutely worsened by a stressful life event may trigger a suicidal act.
- Feelings of isolation and lack of external support can result in hopelessness and limit opportunities for care.
- Suicide may be an impulsive act to express frustration or rage.

ETIOLOGY
Suicidal behavior in adolescents results from the interaction of long-standing individual and family factors, social environment, and acute stressors:
- Diagnostic criteria for psychiatric disorders such as major depressive episode and borderline personality disorder include suicidality (*DSM-5*).
- Intense emotional state, in particular shame or humiliation, can be "trigger events" for a suicidal act.
- Personality and social factors, such as antisocial behavior, aggressive or impulsive proclivities, and social isolation, can also contribute.

DIAGNOSIS

HISTORY
- The provider should establish a quiet environment with clear discussion of confidentiality and limitations before inquiring about suicidal ideation or attempt.
- If positive, a comprehensive history should always be obtained or reviewed by a trained mental health worker. Components include the following:
  - Sensitively ascertain any planning, including method and timing.
  - Ask factors that could increase lethality of attempt (e.g., number of pills ingested).
  - Circumstances of attempt (e.g., remote site, public display)
  - History of prior attempts
  - Current psychological status (e.g., feelings and/or level of depression, hopelessness, impulsivity, self-esteem)
  - Family consistency and dynamics
  - Pharmaceuticals available at home; what is missing
  - History of interpersonal conflict or loss
  - Family history of suicide
  - History of substance use
  - History of psychological disorder
  - History of abuse, neglect, or incest
  - Social supports and coping strategies
  - Feelings of regret or continued desire for self-harm

PHYSICAL EXAM
- Regardless of ingestion history, closely observe vital signs, skin, mucous membranes, and pupils for evidence of toxidrome.
- Examine skin for signs of physical abuse or self-mutilation, including extremities and torso.
- A complete neurologic examination is essential for the evaluation of intracranial processes, acute mental status changes, and ingestions.

DIAGNOSTIC TESTS & INTERPRETATION
Different laboratories offer different spectra and sensitivities in their toxicology screens.

Lab
- Serum and urine toxicology screens
- Urine pregnancy test: Pregnancy status could be a precipitating factor and, if positive, could affect treatment options.
- Acetaminophen level, as it is highly hepatotoxic and is used frequently by teenagers
- EKG is indicated for ingestions, including antidepressants and benzodiazepines.

Imaging

Abdominal plain film: if history of iron or vitamin ingestion or severe trauma

TREATMENT

MEDICATION

- For recent ingestions, GI decontamination with activated charcoal may be appropriate, as is the administration of pertinent antidotes (e.g., naloxone for opioids, *N*-acetylcysteine for acetaminophen).
- Although psychotherapy is an essential component to the care of the suicidal ideation, pharmacotherapy with antidepressants can also play a role.
- SSRIs (fluoxetine, sertraline, and citalopram) have been shown to be effective in treating depressive disorders in adolescents. Use of SSRIs in patients with the potential for suicidal behavior requires close monitoring. In general, SSRIs may cause a short-term increase from 1 to 2% in the risk of suicidality in depressed teens.
- Tricyclic antidepressants (TCAs) have high lethality potential. TCAs are not indicated in treating depression in children and adolescents.

ADDITIONAL TREATMENT

General Measures

- Parents and professionals should avoid minimizing attempts as "not serious" or as "just seeking attention."
- Psychiatric disposition should be determined by, or in conjunction with, a mental health professional. Considerations for admission:
  - Historical factors indicating high risk for repeated attempt
  - Ongoing suicidal ideation and/or planning
  - Family instability and lack of support
  - Altered mental status
  - Lack of alternative interventions (e.g., intensive psychiatric follow-up, day treatment program)
  - Medication initiation that has risk for increasing suicidal thoughts (e.g., SSRIs)
- When discharge to a caregiver is being considered, the following minimal criteria should be in place at the time of discharge:
  - The patient reliably expresses regret and denies ongoing suicidal thoughts.
  - The patient is medically stable.
  - The patient's adult caregiver reports understanding of the seriousness of the attempt and importance of follow-up.
  - The patient and parents agree to contact a health professional or go to the emergency department if suicidal intent recurs. The patient and family should have 24-hour access to mental health or physical health professionals.
  - The patient must not have impaired mental status (e.g., psychoses, delirium).
  - Lethal methods of self-harm are not immediately available to the patient.
  - Follow-up for underlying mental health disorders have been arranged, including a transfer of key information and clear communication of follow-up locations and times with a behavioral health provider accessible to the patient.
  - Acute precipitants and crises have been addressed.
  - Caregivers and patients are in agreement with the discharge plan.
  - Barriers to obtaining follow-up treatment, in particular insurance and social stigma, have been addressed and will not preclude the next step toward ongoing treatment.

ADDITIONAL THERAPIES

In addition to medication, important psychiatric interventions include acute, short-term, inpatient psychiatric hospitalization, partial hospitalization (with intensive treatment and support), and outpatient therapy.

INPATIENT CONSIDERATIONS

Initial Stabilization

- Airway, breathing, circulation (ABCs)
- One-to-one monitoring is typically indicated until formal mental health evaluation is obtained.
- Decontamination of GI tract and circulation is rarely indicated.
- When available, a poison control center or toxicologist will be helpful with evaluation and treatment of most drug ingestions.

ONGOING CARE

FOLLOW-UP RECOMMENDATIONS

Long-term psychotherapy (individual and family therapy) is often needed for adolescents who attempt suicide. Improvement may be slow and punctuated by setbacks.

PROGNOSIS

- 20–50% of those attempting suicide will try again.
- Multiple reports show that a majority of adolescents and young adults who attempt suicide disengage with treatment after a few visits due to a multitude of systemic and societal factors.

COMPLICATIONS

- Long-term organ damage or physical disability, depending on the method used
- Long-lasting emotional sequelae in survivors, resulting from frustration, anger, and guilt
- Repeat suicide attempt or completion

ADDITIONAL READING

- Centers for Disease Control and Prevention. Suicide and self-inflicted injury. http://www.cdc.gov/nchs/fastats/suicide.htm. Accessed June 22, 2014.
- Cooper WO, Callahan ST, Shintani A, et al. Antidepressants and suicide attempts in children. *Pediatrics*. 2014;133(2):204–210.
- National Institute of Mental Health. Statistics. http://www.nimh.nih.gov/health/publications/suicide-in-the-us-statistics-and-prevention/index.shtml#intro. Accessed February 29, 2011.
- Shain BN; American Academy of Pediatrics Committee on Adolescence and the American Academy of Child and Adolescent Psychiatry. Suicide and suicide attempts in adolescents. *Pediatrics*. 2007;120(3):669–676.
- Williams SB, O'Connor EA, Eder M, et al. Screening for child and adolescent depression in primary care settings: a systemic evidence review for the US Preventive Services Task Force. *Pediatrics*. 2009;123(4):e716–e735.

CODES

ICD10

- R45.851 Suicidal ideations
- T14.91 Suicide attempt
- Z91.5 Personal history of self-harm

FAQ

- Q: Should I ever keep suicide attempts or plans confidential?
- A: No. The limits of confidentiality should be clearly outlined to patients and families at the first visit or early in the patient's adolescence. These limits include anything that will directly place the patient's life in danger such as suicidal intent, ongoing or recent abuse, or homicidal intentions.
- Q: If I directly question my patients about suicide, won't that put the idea in their head?
- A: No. In the majority of cases, patients will be relieved by having a professional who wants to talk about suicide. There is only risk in asking if nothing is done with the answer. Appropriate referral to mental health services or counseling will save patients' lives.
- Q: Is a patient who is engaging in self-injurious behavior but denies suicidal ideation actually suicidal?
- A: Any adolescent who is practicing self-mutilation to cope with emotional distress is at risk of developing additional unhealthy coping behaviors. Furthermore, they are likely suffering from a mood disorder that places them at risk for developing suicidality. There is no evidence to support management of self-injurious behavior as if the patient has a secret agenda.

SUPERIOR MESENTERIC ARTERY SYNDROME

Eric H. Chiou • Kristin L. Van Buren

BASICS

DESCRIPTION

- Superior mesenteric artery (SMA) syndrome is extrinsic compression of the third portion of the duodenum between the SMA and aorta.
- It is also called Wilkie syndrome, cast syndrome, or aortomesenteric duodenal compression syndrome.
- The diagnosis is somewhat controversial because symptoms do not always correlate with radiologic findings and do not always improve following treatment.

EPIDEMIOLOGY

- Rare
- More common in adolescents
- Also seen following corrective scoliosis surgery with a rate of 0.5–2.4%

ETIOLOGY

- The SMA arises from the aorta at the L1 vertebral body level and forms an acute downward aortomesenteric angle that is normally between 35–65 degrees, due in part to the mesenteric fat pad.
- The third portion of the duodenum lies within the aortomesenteric angle, and narrowing of the angle (<25 degrees) can lead to duodenal compression by the SMA anteriorly and the L3 vertebral body posteriorly.
- Any factor that narrows the aortomesenteric angle can cause duodenal compression. Common conditions that predispose to narrowing of this angle are as follows:
  - Illnesses associated with significant weight loss leading to loss of the mesenteric fat pad:
    - Anorexia nervosa, malignancy, spinal cord injury, trauma, or burns
  - Rapid linear growth in children
  - Increase in lordosis of the back such as from immobilization by body cast, scoliosis surgery, or prolonged bed rest in a supine position
    - Weight percentile for height of <5% is a risk factor for development of SMA syndrome following scoliosis surgery.
  - Variations of the ligament of Treitz: A short ligament lifts the third or fourth part of the duodenum into the narrower segment in the aortomesenteric angle.
- If the left renal vein is also compressed, this can lead to microscopic hematuria, also known as nutcracker syndrome.

DIAGNOSIS

HISTORY

- Clinical presentation can be acute or chronic with gradual, progressive symptoms.
- Symptoms are generally consistent with proximal small bowel obstruction, including the following:
  - Nausea
  - Vomiting (bilious and nonbilious, postprandial)
  - Gastroesophageal reflux
  - Epigastric abdominal pain
  - Eructation
  - Weight loss
  - Early satiety
  - Dehydration
  - Bloating
  - Failure to thrive
- Symptoms may be relieved when patient is lying prone, in left lateral decubitus, or in knee-chest positions.

PHYSICAL EXAM

- Nonspecific findings of small bowel obstruction include the following:
  - Abdominal distension
  - Succussion splash
  - High-pitched bowel sounds
- No pathognomonic signs or symptoms, but a history of weight loss, immobilization, or back surgery followed by symptoms of early satiety, bloating, and vomiting after meals would suggest the diagnosis.

DIAGNOSTIC TESTS & INTERPRETATION

Imaging

- Imaging should show duodenal obstruction with dilated stomach and proximal duodenum, active peristalsis, and a narrow angle between the aorta and the SMA.
- Abdominal radiograph is usually the initial diagnostic imaging test.
  - Findings can be nonspecific but may also reveal suggestive findings of obstruction, including a distended stomach or a dilated proximal duodenum with a sharp cutoff of the third portion of the duodenum where the SMA crosses the duodenum.
- Additional evaluation with upper gastrointestinal (GI) series:
  - Passage of contrast is typically delayed and often stops at the third portion of the duodenum. Contrast passes when the patient is moved to a prone position, where gravity will increase the aortomesenteric angle.
  - Similar findings can be seen with CT.
- Additional imaging may be required if the diagnosis remains unclear.
  - Superior mesenteric arteriography with simultaneous barium contrast radiography to show SMA superimposed on duodenum
  - CT and MR angiography have now replaced superior mesenteric arteriography.
- An aortomesenteric angle <25 degrees is the most useful diagnostic marker, especially if the aortomesenteric distance is <8 mm.
- Determination of the aortomesenteric angle in severe cases may help with decision for surgery.

DIFFERENTIAL DIAGNOSIS

- Causes of small bowel obstruction:
  - Luminal obstruction: foreign body
  - Intramural obstruction: duplication cyst, web, tumor, bezoar, stricture
  - Extramural obstruction: tumor, annular pancreas, bands, adhesions, volvulus, intussusception

- Duodenal dysmotility
  - Intrinsic neuronal disorder
  - Muscular weakness (holovisceral myopathy, diabetes)
  - Fibrosis (scleroderma, lupus retroperitoneal fibrosis)
  - Collagen vascular diseases
  - Chronic idiopathic intestinal pseudo-obstruction
- Anorexia nervosa/bulimia

TREATMENT

GENERAL MEASURES

- Correct fluid and electrolyte imbalances.
- Decompress obstruction.
  - Insert nasogastric tube to decompress stomach and proximal duodenum.
- Definitive treatment is aimed at correcting the precipitating factor.
- Feed to improve nutrition and weight gain.
  - Feeding in a prone or left lateral decubitus position can help relieve pain but may require a jejunal tube to bypass the obstruction.
  - Total parenteral nutrition may be needed if cannot tolerate enteral nutrition.
- If a patient had recent spinal surgery:
  - Frequent repositioning of patients in body casts
  - Reversal of back surgery may be necessary in some patients.
- Surgery is typically unnecessary.
  - Surgery is indicated only if supportive care is ineffective.
  - Usually performed in patients with a prolonged history of weight loss or pronounced duodenal dilation
  - Surgical options include duodenojejunostomy, gastrojejunostomy, or Strong procedure (mobilization of duodenum by dividing the ligament of Treitz).
- Consider psychiatric evaluation if eating disorder suspected.

ONGOING CARE

PROGNOSIS

- Delay in diagnosis of SMA syndrome can result in the following:
  - Electrolyte disturbances
  - Dehydration and malnutrition
  - In severe cases, possible GI pneumatosis, perforation, formation of a duodenal bezoar, or death
- Most patients do not require surgery and improve with supportive care alone.

ADDITIONAL READING

- Agrawal GA, Johnson PT, Fishman EK. Multidetector row CT of superior mesenteric artery syndrome. *J Clin Gastroenterol*. 2007;41(1):62–65.
- Jain R. Superior mesenteric artery syndrome. *Curr Treat Options Gastroenterol*. 2007;10(1):24–27.
- Kadji M, Naouri A, Bernard P. Superior mesenteric artery syndrome: a case report. *Ann Chir*. 2006;131(6–7):389–392.
- Kim IY, Cho NC, Kim DS, et al. Laparoscopic duodenojejunostomy for management of superior mesenteric artery syndrome: two case reports and a review of the literature. *Yonsei Med J*. 2003;44(3):526–529.
- Kurbegov A, Grabb B, Bealer J. Superior mesenteric artery syndrome in a 16-year-old with bilious emesis. *Curr Opin Pediatr*. 2010;22(5):664–667.
- Merrett ND, Wilson RB, Cosman P, et al. Superior mesenteric artery syndrome: diagnosis and treatment strategies. *J Gastrointest Surg*. 2009;13(2):287–292.
- Okugawa Y, Inoue M, Uchida K, et al. Superior mesenteric artery syndrome in an infant: case report and literature review. *J Pediatr Surg*. 2007;42(10):E5–E8.
- Schwartz A. Scoliosis, superior mesenteric artery syndrome, and adolescents. *Orthop Nurs*. 2007;26(1):19–24.
- Vulliamy P, Hariharan V, Gutmann J, et al. Superior mesenteric artery syndrome and the "nutcracker phenomenon." *BMJ Case Rep*. 2013;21:2013.
- Welsch T, Büchler MW, Kienle P. Recalling superior mesenteric artery syndrome. *Dig Surg*. 2007;24(3):149–156.

CODES

ICD10

K55.1 Chronic vascular disorders of intestine

FAQ

- Q: When the diagnosis of SMA syndrome is suspected, what are the next steps in management?
- A: The general sequence is to confirm the diagnosis with an imaging study such as an upper GI contrast study and also to initiate supportive care of refeeding and mobilization.
- Q: The following treatment modalities are known to be useful in treatment of SMA syndrome: do nothing, or feed with a jejunal tube, a liquid diet, prone feeding, or total parenteral nutrition. Which program works?
- A: All of the above have been used in SMA syndrome. Weight gain has also been accomplished with total parenteral nutrition.
- Q: Does radiographic testing or a feeding clinical trial help in confirming the diagnosis?
- A: Yes. It may be helpful to confirm the diagnosis and look at the aortomesenteric angle with a CT or MR angiography. In addition, a clinical trial of feeding and weight gain often becomes the criterion for confirmation of the diagnosis.

S

SUPRAVENTRICULAR TACHYCARDIA

Francesca A. Byrne

BASICS

DESCRIPTION

- The term supraventricular tachycardia (SVT) is generally used to refer to atrioventricular nodal reentry tachycardia (AVNRT), atrioventricular reciprocating tachycardia (AVRT), and atrial tachycardia (AT) but includes any tachycardia originating at or above the atrioventricular (AV) node.
- The heart rate in SVT in infants generally ranges from 220 to 320 beats per minute (bpm) and in older children from 150 to 250 bpm.

EPIDEMIOLOGY

- SVT is the most common arrhythmia in childhood.
- Incidence of SVT is 35 per 100,000 per year.
- Incidence of SVT among patients with Wolff-Parkinson-White syndrome (WPW) is about 1% per year.
- Prevalence of SVT is 1 in 250–25,000 children.
- AVRT is the most common type of SVT in children, occurring in ~75% of cases.
- AVNRT rarely occurs before age 2 years.
- 50–60% of pediatric patients with SVT present in the 1st year of life.

RISK FACTORS

- Most children with SVT have structurally normal hearts; however, children with congenital heart disease (CHD) have an increased risk of SVT.
- SVT is commonly observed in patients who have undergone surgery for CHD, for example, after the Mustard/Senning procedure, the Fontan operation, and repair of an atrial septal defect.

Genetics

- WPW syndrome has been noted in several families, and an autosomal dominant (AD) mode of inheritance has been demonstrated:
  - ~20% of cases of WPW have associated CHD, such as Ebstein anomaly, L-looped transposition of the great arteries, and hypertrophic cardiomyopathy.
  - Many patients with the WPW pattern on electrocardiogram (ECG) do not develop SVT; when episodes of SVT do occur, the patient has WPW *syndrome*.
- ~50% of the cases of junctional ectopic tachycardia (JET) occur in a familial setting with an AD mode of inheritance.

PATHOPHYSIOLOGY

There are 2 major mechanisms for SVT:

- Reentry tachycardia: This is the most common mechanism for SVT. It involves a circuit rhythm within the atria (atrial flutter), within the AV node (AVNRT), or using an accessory pathway (AVRT); characterized by sudden onset and termination, regular rate, and responsiveness to pacing maneuvers and DC cardioversion
- Automatic tachycardia: Automaticity refers to a group of cell's enhanced ability to spontaneously depolarize, which can overdrive suppress the sinus node. Examples are ectopic atrial tachycardia, multifocal atrial tachycardia, and JET; characterized by warm-up and cool-down phases, an irregular rate that is sensitive to catecholamine states, and lack of responsiveness to pacing and cardioversion

ETIOLOGY

SVT can frequently be precipitated by exercise, infection, fever, or drug exposure.

DIAGNOSIS

HISTORY

- Infants manifest signs and symptoms of low cardiac output and congestive heart failure (CHF) with prolonged SVT (>48 hours): tachypnea, retractions, irritability, decreased feeding, excessive sweating, hypotension, poor perfusion, and decreased urine output.
- A toddler or older child may experience palpitations, shortness of breath, chest pain, anxiety, and dizziness or syncope:
  - It is important to know what the child was doing at the time the arrhythmia started and whether there is an abrupt onset and termination.
  - Older children often report being able to terminate episodes of tachycardia by performing a vagal maneuver.

PHYSICAL EXAM

The following need to be assessed in all patients presenting with SVT:

- Heart rate and regularity
- Respiratory rate
- Blood pressure
- Hydration status
- Peripheral perfusion
- Liver size
- Mental status
- Presence of gallop rhythm

DIAGNOSTIC TESTS & INTERPRETATION

Imaging

Initial approach

- Chest radiograph to assess for pulmonary edema and cardiomegaly
- Echocardiogram to assess underlying cardiac anatomy and ventricular function

Follow-Up Tests & Special Considerations

Repeat imaging may be warranted if there are initial abnormalities.

Diagnostic Procedures/Other

- Outpatient: Diagnosis can be made with a 24-hour or transtelephonic event monitor.
- Inpatient
  - 15-lead ECG during SVT if patient is hemodynamically stable
  - Continuous ECG monitoring during therapeutic maneuvers can aid in diagnosis.
- Patients with WPW pattern have ventricular preexcitation (short PR interval and a delta wave) on the ECG during sinus rhythm.
- An exercise stress test may be indicated in older patients with exercise-induced SVT or those with WPW syndrome to help determine the risk of rapid conduction through the accessory pathway.
- Electrophysiologic study is often performed to evaluate drug effect or to map in conjunction with catheter ablation.
- Nonpharmacologic maneuvers (ice, vagal) and pharmacologic maneuvers (IV adenosine) may distinguish tachycardias that involve the AV node from other types of SVT.

DIFFERENTIAL DIAGNOSIS

- Narrow-complex SVT needs to be distinguished from sinus rhythm and sick sinus syndrome with tachyarrhythmia.
- Structural heart disease should be excluded in all cases of newly diagnosed SVT.
- Wide-complex tachycardia can occur in the setting of SVT with bundle branch block or aberrant conduction, antegrade conduction down an accessory pathway, or preexcited atrial flutter/fibrillation in WPW. This can be difficult to distinguish from ventricular tachycardia. Unless it is known that the patient has SVT, wide-complex tachycardia should always be interpreted as ventricular tachycardia until proven otherwise.
- Differentiating between types of SVT can be accomplished by evaluating the regularity of the rate, modes of onset/termination, and the responsiveness to pacing and cardioversion.

TREATMENT

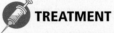

GENERAL MEASURES

- Short-term treatment goals are to terminate the tachycardia.
  - Nonpharmacologic vagal maneuvers; for example, ice to the face for 15–30 seconds, rectal stimulation, Valsalva, gag, and headstand may be helpful. In younger children, Valsalva can be achieved by having the child blow into an obstructed straw or thumb. Pacing maneuvers via an esophageal catheter may also be used. Carotid massage and orbital pressure should not be performed in children.
  - In a stable child, adenosine (rapid IV bolus, 0.1 mg/kg and increase by 0.1 mg/kg to a maximum of 0.3 mg/kg up to 12 mg) may be used to block the AV node for reentrant SVT that requires the AV node. The half-life of the drug is <10 seconds. Because of the risk of atrial fibrillation, DC cardioversion should be available. Use adenosine with caution in asthmatic patients, as it can cause acute bronchospasm.
  - IV verapamil is an effective therapy in older children with SVT but should be avoided in children <12 months of age because of its vasodilatory and negative inotropic effect.
  - Unstable patients with hemodynamic compromise warrant termination with synchronized DC cardioversion (0.5–2.0 J/kg).

- Long-term treatment goals are to reduce the frequency of episodes of SVT. Long-term treatment may not be necessary when the episodes are infrequent, self-terminating, or produce minimal symptoms.
- Catheter ablation using radiofrequency energy or cryoenergy is an alternative to long-term drug therapy and is 1st-line therapy in the following scenarios:
  - SVT refractory to medical therapy
  - Side effects from the medical regimen
  - Patient choice due to frequency, duration, or poor quality of life
  - Life-threatening arrhythmias (syncope)
  - Rapid conduction properties of an accessory pathway (e.g., WPW)
  - Congenital or acquired heart disease

MEDICATION

- Long-term preventive pharmacotherapy is an alternative approach in some patients
- Reentrant SVT
  - β-Blockers (propranolol or atenolol) are 1st-line treatment in individuals with WPW and patients with exercise-induced SVT.
  - Procainamide and amiodarone may be used in cases that are more resistant.
  - Oral digoxin is an option in patients with hemodynamically stable SVT. Digoxin is contraindicated in patients with WPW.
  - Atrial flutter may be treated with digoxin, procainamide, sotalol, or amiodarone as a single agent or in combination.
- Automatic SVT: Automatic tachycardias may be responsive to antiarrhythmics such as procainamide, flecainide (avoid if the patient has structural heart disease), amiodarone, or β-blockers either alone or in different combinations.

INPATIENT CONSIDERATIONS

Initial Stabilization

- Always assess the child's ABCs (airway, breathing, and circulation).
- Initial management of SVT depends on the child's hemodynamic condition.

Admission Criteria

- Hemodynamically unstable SVT requiring electrical cardioversion
- Tachycardia-induced cardiomyopathy

ONGOING CARE

PROGNOSIS

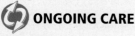

- Of patients who present in infancy, 30–70% will be asymptomatic by 1 year of age. However, ~1/3 of these patients may experience a reappearance of their tachycardia at an average age of 8 years.
- Most older children who present with SVT will have persistent recurrence of SVT.

FOLLOW-UP RECOMMENDATIONS

- As SVT may recur, neonates and infants have historically received maintenance therapy for the 1st year of life and then been observed off medications if they are not having breakthrough episodes of SVT. This approach has recently been challenged, and studies evaluating the ideal duration for maintenance therapy in the neonate and infant are being proposed.
- In children who present beyond infancy, spontaneous resolution of the tachycardia substrate is less likely, and treatment may need to be continued into adulthood. These patients may be considered for catheter ablation therapy.
- Over-the-counter sympathomimetic cold medications and caffeine should be avoided, as they may increase the likelihood of SVT.

COMPLICATIONS

Complications from SVT can arise from 1 of 3 causes:

- Persistent tachycardia can lead to CHF, tachycardia-induced cardiomyopathy, and cardiovascular collapse. This is especially true of the infant whose symptoms go unrecognized for 24–48 hours.
- Some patients with WPW syndrome (<5%) can have rapid conduction through the accessory pathway. A rapid ventricular response to atrial flutter/fibrillation can potentially cause ventricular fibrillation and sudden death. Therefore, digoxin and verapamil should not be used in patients with WPW syndrome.
- Side effects of pharmacologic agents used to treat SVT include bradycardia, other arrhythmias due to proarrhythmic effects (digoxin, procainamide, amiodarone, flecainide), and noncardiac side effects (GI, liver, pulmonary, and thyroid dysfunction).

ADDITIONAL READING

- Cohen MI, Triedman JK, Cannon BC, et al. PACES/HRS expert consensus statement on the management of the asymptomatic young patient with a Wolff-Parkinson-White (WPW, ventricular preexcitation) electrocardiographic pattern. *Heart Rhythm*. 2012;9:1006–1024.
- Drago F. Paediatric catheter cryoablation: techniques, successes and failures. *Curr Opin Cardiol*. 2008;23(2):81–84.
- Fox DJ, Tischenko A, Krahn AD, et al. SVT: diagnosis and management. *Mayo Clin Proc*. 2008;83(12):1400–1411.
- Friedman RA, Walsh EP, Silka MJ, et al. Radiofrequency catheter ablation in children with and without CHD. *Pacing Clin Electrophysiol*. 2002;25(6):1000–1017.
- Manole E, Saladino RA. Emergency department management of the pediatric patient with supraventricular tachycardia. *Pediatr Emerg Care*. 2007;23(3):176–185.
- Paul T, Bertram H, Bökenkamp R, et al. Supraventricular tachycardia in infants, children and adolescents: diagnosis, and pharmacological and interventional therapy. *Paediatr Drugs*. 2000;2(3):171–181.
- Sanatani S, Potts, Reed JH, et al. The study of antiarrhythmic medications in infants (SAMIS): a multicenter, randomized controlled trial comparing the efficacy and safety of digoxin versus propranolol for prophylaxis of supraventricular tachycardia in infants. *Circ Arrhythm Electrophysiol*. 2012;5(5):984–991.

CODES

ICD10

I47.1 Supraventricular tachycardia

FAQ

- Q: How should infants on chronic therapy be monitored?
- A: Parents with infants on chronic therapy for SVT should be educated about counting the heart rate by palpation or auscultation at least 1 or 2 times daily. This method of surveillance is just as effective as apnea/bradycardia monitors. Because alarm monitors can increase parental anxiety with frequent false alarms, they are generally not recommended. Patients on amiodarone should be monitored with liver function tests and thyroid function tests at baseline and every 3–6 months.
- Q: What is the concern with verapamil?
- A: Verapamil is an L-type calcium channel blocker that blocks conduction in the AV node and is very effective in treating SVT in adults. Because myocardial contractility in infants depends mostly on the trans-sarcolemmal L-type calcium channels, hypotension and cardiovascular collapse have been reported in children <1 year of age.
- Q: What are success rates and risks of catheter ablation?
- A: The success rate of radiofrequency catheter ablation varies from 80 to 97%, depending on the location of the bypass tract or ectopic focus. The incidence of major complications is <2%, with the most common being heart block requiring a pacemaker, cardiac perforation, brachial plexus injury, and embolization. The risk of complete heart block is greater in patients whose accessory pathway is located close to the AV node. In such patients, cryoablation is a safer ablation technique because of its potentially reversible electrical and thermal effect.

SYMPATHOMIMETIC POISONING

Robert J. Hoffman • Richard Loffhagen

BASICS

DESCRIPTION

- Excess autonomic stimulation by adrenergic agents produces the clinical syndrome typically described as "sympathomimetic."
- Overdose from sympathomimetic agents occurs secondary to the use of prescription drugs, nonprescription drugs such as OTC cold medicine (e.g., pseudoephedrine), dietary supplements (e.g., ephedra, synephrine), and illicit drugs such as cocaine, amphetamine, and methamphetamine.
- A more recent trend is the use of mephedrone and methylenedioxypyrovalerone (MDPV) among others are sold legally under the guise of "bath salts."
- The sequelae of sympathomimetic overdose are generally related to the neurologic and cardiovascular systems.
- Severe problems may include agitation-induced hyperthermia, cardiac dysrhythmia, hypertension, myocardial ischemia, and infarction; CVA; seizure; and cardiovascular collapse.
- Bath salts appear to be associated with a much higher incidence of psychotic events than other sympathomimetics.
- A number of potent amphetamine analogs, such as paramethoxymethamphetamine (PMA), which have a high incidence of morbidity and mortality, are increasingly common components of tablets sold as MDMA.

EPIDEMIOLOGY

- Cocaine, methamphetamine, and MDMA (commonly called "Molly" or "ecstasy") are the 3 most common illicit stimulant drugs causing emergency visits in the United States.
- Prescription stimulants such as methylphenidate and albuterol are often frequent causes of intentional as well as unintentional poisoning.

PATHOPHYSIOLOGY

- Relevant pathophysiology is based on the adrenergic receptor type stimulated by the drug in question. The adrenergic receptors of relevance include $\alpha 1$, $\beta 1$, and $\beta 2$ receptors.
- Ephedrine and pseudoephedrine stimulate both α and β receptors:
  - Excessive cardiovascular stimulation results in symptoms qualitatively similar to those that occur with catecholamines.
  - Ephedrine and pseudoephedrine have weaker penetration of the CNS relative to drugs of abuse.
  - As a result, users may suffer from systemic complications of the relatively larger doses necessary to achieve the CNS "high" of other stimulants.
- Nonelective β-adrenergic agonists
- Isoproterenol, rarely used, is the prototypical nonselective β-agonist causing the following:
  - Tachycardia, hypotension, tachydysrhythmia, myocardial ischemia, and flushing due to its cardiostimulatory and vasodilatory properties
  - Commonly, CNS effects of anxiety, fear, and headache occur.
- Selective $\beta 2$-adrenergic agonists are commonly used, and these include albuterol, levalbuterol, salmeterol, terbutaline, and others.
- Common adverse effects include the following:
  - Tachycardia, palpitations, and tremor
  - Hypotension, often with widened pulse pressure
  - Nausea, vomiting, and sometimes diarrhea
  - Hyperglycemia and hypokalemia
  - Elevation of CPK as well as troponin, although myocardial infarction is never expected to occur in otherwise healthy children with selective $\beta 2$ agonist exposure
  - Anxiety, fear, and headache also may occur.
- $\alpha 1$ Selective agonists include phenylephrine and phenylpropanolamine, although the latter is no longer commercially produced in any meaningful quantity in the United States.
  - Hypertension due to direct vasoconstrictive effects is the most common effect.
  - Reflex bradycardia may occur, particularly with phenylpropanolamine.
  - Headache due to elevated BP and even CVA may occur.

ETIOLOGY

Causative agents:

- Agents with combined α- and β-adrenergic activity: epinephrine, norepinephrine, dopamine, ephedrine, and pseudoephedrine
- $\alpha 1$-Adrenergic agonists: phenylephrine, phenylpropanolamine
- β-adrenergic agonists: nonselective β-agonist isoproterenol
- Selective $\beta 1$ agonists: dobutamine
- Selective $\beta 2$ agonists: albuterol, salmeterol, terbutaline, ritodrine
- OTC agents: ephedrine-containing cold medicine, ephedra, Ma Huang
- Illicit drugs: cocaine, amphetamine, methamphetamine, MDMA (ecstasy), MDPV (bath salts)
- Theophylline and caffeine may cause a clinical syndrome of sympathomimetic poisoning.

COMMONLY ASSOCIATED CONDITIONS

- Many sympathomimetic agents are capable of producing psychiatric symptoms, particularly psychosis.
- This psychosis is similar to or indistinguishable from schizophrenia.
- 2 rare results of MDMA use include serotonin syndrome and SIADH with symptomatic hyponatremia.

DIAGNOSIS

SIGNS AND SYMPTOMS

- The clinical effects of these agents' overdose vary based on their receptor selectivity.
- Most agents have some degree of combined α- and β-adrenergic activity (ephedrine, pseudoephedrine).
  - Hypertension, tachycardia, dysrhythmia, acute coronary syndromes, pulmonary edema and cerebrovascular injury, anxiety, a sense of impending doom, apprehension, fear, and headache may occur.
  - At very high doses, agents cross the blood–brain barrier, which results in CNS symptoms, such as headache, seizures, and intracranial hemorrhage.

HISTORY

- History of exposure may be helpful but is often unavailable or deliberately concealed, particularly use of illicit drugs such as cocaine, methamphetamine, and ecstasy.
- Use of OTC medicines, such as multisymptom cold preparations or dietary supplements
- High suspicion of sympathomimetic overdose especially in patients with the sympathomimetic toxidrome
- The onset of symptoms usually occurs within 1 hour.
  - Typically, prescription and OTC sympathomimetic agents are inhaled or orally administered.
  - Inhalation or injection results in immediate symptoms.
  - Cocaine, amphetamine, and methamphetamine or the sympathomimetics are most commonly used in this manner.
  - Sympathomimetic toxicity following ingestion typically peaks 1–4 hours and last 4–8 hours, but sustained-release preparations may alter this time course.
- Chest pain due to dysrhythmia, myocardial ischemia, infarction, etc. may be a complaint.
- Headache, visual changes, epistaxis

PHYSICAL EXAM

Sympathomimetic toxicity is a clinical diagnosis.

- Vital sign derangement is the most common and most reliable indicator of toxicity.
- Mental status changes are also common although less reliable as they do not occur with the same regularity and may be the result of toxicologic or psychiatric phenomenon.
- The patient's general appearance (e.g., agitation, diaphoretic, delirium, psychotic) is often suggestive of toxicity.
- HEENT: mydriasis, visual changes, epistaxis, poor dentition
- Tachycardia and hypertension are the most common vital sign abnormalities.
- Skin: diaphoresis, flushing, the track marks associated with IV drug use
- CNS: Focal neurologic findings may occur. Focal cranial nerve abnormalities are particularly concerning for the possibility of CVA. CNS stimulation or agitation is very common.

DIAGNOSTIC TESTS & INTERPRETATION

- Sympathomimetic overdose is a clinical diagnosis and assays are only adjunctive.

- Unless there are specific forensic indications, such as malicious poisoning or child abuse, drugs of abuse screening is not recommended and is not useful.
- Serum acetaminophen level should be considered in patients with ingestion with intent of self-harm.
- The measurement of electrolytes, BUN, creatinine, and blood sugar may be useful.
- Cardiac markers (e.g., CPK-MB, troponin) are appropriate to screen for cardiac injury.
- An EKG should be obtained to assess for ischemia as well as dysrhythmias.

Imaging

A noncontrast head CT should be obtained in unresponsive patients or those with focal neurologic deficits.

DIFFERENTIAL DIAGNOSIS

- Hyperthyroidism/thyroid storm
- Anticholinergic syndrome
- Pheochromocytoma
- Withdrawal syndromes
- Mania
- Subarachnoid hemorrhage
- Serotonin syndrome
- Neuroleptic malignant syndrome
- Other situations of increased endogenous catecholamine release

TREATMENT

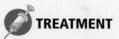

INITIAL STABILIZATION

Managing ABCs should be addressed first, but sympathomimetic toxicity usually does not result in illness requiring any specific airway, breathing, or circulation issues.

GENERAL MEASURES

Maintaining vital signs within acceptable limits and controlling patient agitation are commonly required.

- Managing ABCs is paramount.
- If protocol permits, sedation of agitated patients with a benzodiazepine may be appropriate.
- Use of benzodiazepines is helpful to address both cardiovascular stimulation as well as psychomotor agitation.
- Use of specific cardiovascular medications may be needed.
- Use of antipsychotics, such as haloperidol or droperidol, is relatively contraindicated both because these medications may lower seizure threshold, impair heat dissipation, and increase risk of cardiac dysrhythmia.

SPECIAL THERAPY

- Severe hyperthermia should be treated with active cooling.
- Patients with core temperature of ≥107°F should be placed in an ice bath and have core temperature monitored.

IV Fluids

- Unless there is a contraindication, at least maintenance IV fluid should be administered.
- IV fluids may protect against rhabdomyolysis as well as potential dehydration that may occur with stimulant exposure.

MEDICATION

Agitation, vasoconstrictive effects, chronotropic and inotropic effects, and psychomotor agitation are the most common issues requiring mediation therapy for sympathomimetic toxicity.

First Line

- Psychomotor agitation may be managed with benzodiazepines.
- The quantity of benzodiazepine required will directly depend on degree of adrenergic stimulation.
- In some cases, large doses may be required for sedation.
  - Lorazepam in doses of 0.1 mg/kg IV q15min titrated to effect is preferred due to predictable duration of action.
  - Diazepam 0.1 mg/kg IV q15min titrated to effect may also be used.
- Vasoconstrictive effects may be managed with a variety of medications.
  - Phentolamine 0.1 mg/kg/dose (up to 5 mg/dose) IV repeated q10min PRN
  - A dihydropyridine calcium channel blocker, such as nifedipine or amlodipine, may be used.
  - Sodium nitroprusside 0.3–10 mcg/kg/min IV, titrated to effect
- Chronotropic and inotropic effects may be managed with conduction-modulating calcium channel blockers such as diltiazem or verapamil.

Second Line

- A β-blocker may be used only if an α-adrenergic antagonist is concomitantly administered.
- Use of a β-blocker without α-adrenergic blockade may result in paradoxical increase in BP and death.
  - Labetalol has some α-adrenergic blockade and may be used alone as a 2nd-line agent: 0.2–0.5 mg/kg/dose IV, maximal dose 20 mg, followed by infusion of 0.25–1 mg/kg/h
  - Esmolol 500 mcg/kg IV bolus over 1 minute followed by infusion 50 mcg/kg/min titrated to effect up to 500 mcg/kg/min
- Severe cardiovascular symptoms resulting from β-agonists or methylxanthines such as theophylline or caffeine may be treated with a β-blocker.
  - This treatment may seem counterintuitive in the management of hypotension.
  - Severe $\beta 2$ agonist effects resulting in hypotension may be counteracted by using a β-blocker.
  - Such therapy should only be undertaken under the direction of a medical toxicologist, intensivist, or other clinician familiar with and experienced with use of such cardiovascular medications.

ONGOING CARE

Admission Criteria

Any patient with severely deranged vital signs, end organ manifestations such as chest pain, severe headache, focal neurologic deficit, or agitation should be admitted.

Discharge Criteria

Any patient with vital signs within safe limits, normal mental status, and no evidence of end organ damage or manifestations may be discharged from the emergency department or inpatient unit.

PROGNOSIS

If end organ damage such as myocardial infarction or CVA are prevented, prognosis for full recovery to premorbid status is excellent.

COMPLICATIONS

The most common catastrophic complications are cardiovascular, including dysrhythmia, myocardial infarction, and CVA.

S

ADDITIONAL READING

- Carr BC. Efficacy, abuse, and toxicity of over-the-counter cough and cold medicines in the pediatric population. *Curr Opin Pediatr*. 2006;18(2): 184–188.
- Haller CA, Meier KH, Olson KR. Seizures reported in association with use of dietary supplements. *Clin Toxicol*. 2005;43(1):23–30.
- Haynes JF Jr. Medical management of adolescent drug overdoses. *Adolesc Med Clin*. 2006;17(2):353–379.
- Kuehn BM. Citing serious risks, FDA recommends no cold and cough medicines for infants. *JAMA*. 2008;299(8):887–888.
- Thirthalli J, Benegal V. Psychosis among substance users. *Curr Opin Psychiatry*. 2006;19(3):239–245.

CODES

ICD10

- T44.901A Poisn by unsp drugs aff the autonm nervous sys, acc, init
- T44.991A Poisoning by oth drug aff the autonm nervous sys, acc, init
- T48.5X1A Poisoning by oth anti-cmn-cold drugs, accidental, init

SYNCOPE

Nancy Drucker

BASICS

DESCRIPTION

Transient loss of consciousness, typically lasting no longer than 1–2 minutes, due to a transient drop in cerebral perfusion pressure

GENERAL PREVENTION

- Avoiding circumstances predisposing to the most common form of syncope (vasovagal)
- Sitting or lying down when warning signs occur
- Maintaining adequate hydration, especially during illness/exertion

PATHOPHYSIOLOGY

Most common mechanism is vasovagal or neurocardiogenic, in which a variety of stimuli and conditions—pain, dehydrated state, emotional upset, carotid pressure—trigger increased vagal tone, leading to slowed heart rate, peripheral vasodilatation, and decreased cerebral perfusion.

DIAGNOSIS

DIFFERENTIAL DIAGNOSIS

- Cardiac
  - Congenital heart defect, myocarditis, cardiomyopathy, coronary artery anomaly, heart block (congenital or acquired complete heart block, status post cardiac surgery), arrhythmia secondary to long QT syndrome, Brugada syndrome, arrhythmogenic right ventricular dysplasia, catecholaminergic polymorphic ventricular tachycardia, Wolff-Parkinson-White syndrome. Syncope due to an arrhythmia may be familial and may occur as unprovoked syncope or as exercise-induced syncope that may resemble an epileptic convulsion.
- Neurologic
  - Migraines (predisposed to orthostatic intolerance); arteriovenous malformation; pulmonary hypertension; intracranial hypertension due to hydrocephalus, mass, pseudotumor
- Pulmonary
  - Pulmonary hypertension
- Other
  - Medications/toxins
- Other causes of syncope by age group include the following:
  - Toddlers
    - Pallid or cyanotic breath-holding spells; these occur in response to pain, fear, excitement, or frustration, begin with a deep inspiration or exhalation, although the precipitating "gasp" may not be apparent (iron deficiency may be associated). A history of pallid breath-holding spells is not uncommon in adolescents with vasovagal syncope.
  - Older children
    - Situational syncope: venipuncture, defecation, hair brushing, stretching
    - Dysautonomia, orthostatic hypotension
    - Dehydration
    - Adrenal insufficiency
- Syncopal spells in children may be accompanied by a convulsion (nonepileptic) that usually lasts <1 minute (EEG shows normal findings or slowing, not epileptiform activity).
- Alternative causes of loss of consciousness not due to syncope include the following:
  - Head trauma
  - Epilepsy ("temporal lobe syncope")
  - Psychogenic
  - Stroke
  - Hypoglycemia (rare except in certain metabolic disorders)

HISTORY

- **Question:** Detailed history of the spell (focus on signs/symptoms prior to the event)?
- *Significance*: Most important information used to distinguish syncope from seizure or head trauma
- **Question:** The child or observers may recall "presyncopal" signs?
- *Significance*: Often present in patients with benign syncope—such as warmth, diaphoresis, lightheadedness, nausea, palpitations, auditory, or visual changes—all lasting only a few seconds before loss of consciousness
- **Question:** Family history?
- *Significance*: Obtaining a careful history is essential. Family history of sudden unexpected death, seizures, syncope, cardiomyopathy, or arrhythmias especially at younger ages or requiring pacemaker/implantable defibrillator should trigger further testing and investigation.
- **Question:** Syncope during exercise or without warning?
- *Significance*: May indicate an underlying arrhythmia
- **Question:** Generalized tonic–clonic movements?
- *Significance*: May occur with syncope—presyncopal signs point to the nonepileptic nature of the event
- **Question:** Increasing duration of unconsciousness?
- *Significance*: Suggests increasing probability that the event is epileptic rather than syncope
  - Caution: Syncope may be associated with a convulsion in a patient with epilepsy.
  - Epilepsy may rarely mimic a syncopal episode or recurrent presyncopal symptoms; temporal lobe syncope seems to occur principally in adults or adolescents.
- **Question:** Details of body position, eye movements, and respiratory pattern?
- *Significance*: May help determine etiology
- **Question:** Carbon monoxide poisoning?
- *Significance*: May cause syncope-like spells; ask about potential exposure

PHYSICAL EXAM

Key findings to document include the following:

- Vital signs with orthostatic pulse and BP changes
- 4-extremity BP
- Pulses in arm and leg
- Funduscopy: possible papilledema
- Cranial bruits
- Precordial thrill
- Heart sounds (gallop, click, rub, significant murmur)

DIAGNOSTIC TESTS & INTERPRETATION

Often, only a thorough physical exam, detailed history, and family history are needed if findings are consistent with vasovagal syncope.

- **Test:** EKG and cardiac consultation
- *Significance*: If the event is suspected to be symptomatic of a heart condition or there is a concerning history/family history, an EKG and cardiac consultation may be indicated.

- **Test:** Treadmill EKG, Holter monitoring, echocardiogram, EEG, MRI (Chiari malformation)
- *Significance*: Children with unexplained syncope may undergo more extensive testing.
- **Test:** Glucose, CBC, blood gases, spinal tap
- *Significance*: Laboratory testing may be appropriate based on clinical suspicion of underlying causes.

ALERT
Pitfall: Recurrent syncope due to prolonged QT interval may be missed on routine EKG; prolongation of QT interval may only be noted on treadmill testing or cardiac monitoring.

TREATMENT

MEDICATION

- Medications are not usually necessary; however, in more extreme clinical presentation, patients may benefit from:
- Midodrine (midodrine hydrochloride): Adult dosing is 10 mg orally, 3 times daily. Dosing should take place during the daytime hours when the patient needs to be upright, pursuing the activities of daily living. A suggested dosing schedule of approximately 4-hour intervals is as follows: shortly before or upon arising in the morning, midday, and late afternoon (not later than 6 p.m.).

ADDITIONAL TREATMENT

General Measures

- Clinical intervention is aimed primarily at training the patient in prevention/anticipation:
  - Avoiding circumstances predisposing to the most common form of syncope (vasovagal)
  - Sitting or lying down when warning signs occur
  - Maintaining adequate hydration, especially during illness/exertion
  - Support stockings may be beneficial.
- Therapy is otherwise addressed to underlying causes, in the unusual circumstance that one is found.
- Syncope during exercise always warrants a cardiovascular evaluation, with EKG as initial step.

ONGOING CARE

- Many children experience a developmental stage in which for unknown reasons they have frequent vasovagal episodes. Most common age group is adolescents; however, syncopal spells may continue through adulthood.
- Persistent and frequent spells may prompt more extensive laboratory testing, as described earlier.

ADDITIONAL READING

- Batra AS, Hohn AR. Consultation with the specialist: palpitations, syncope, and sudden cardiac death in children: who's at risk? *Pediatr Rev*. 2003;24(8):269–275.
- DiVasta AD, Alexander ME. Fainting freshmen and sinking sophomores: cardiovascular issues of the adolescent. *Curr Opin Pediatr*. 2004;16(4):350–356.
- Driscoll DJ, Jacobsen SJ, Porter CJ, et al. Syncope in children and adolescents. *J Am Coll Cardiol*. 1997;29(5):1039–1045.
- Friedman MJ, Mull CC, Sharieff GQ, et al. Prolonged QT syndrome in children: an uncommon but potentially fatal entity. *J Emerg Med*. 2003;24(2):173–179.
- Kapoor WN. Syncope. *N Engl J Med*. 2000;343(25):1856–1862.
- McVicar K. Seizure-like states. *Pediatr Rev*. 2006;27(5):e42–e44.
- Sapin SO. Autonomic syncope in pediatrics: a practice-oriented approach to classification, pathophysiology, diagnosis, and management. *Clin Pediatr*. 2004;43(1):17–23.
- Strickberger SA, Benson DW, Biaggioni I, et al. AHA/ACCF scientific statement on the evaluation of syncope. *Circulation*. 2006;113(2):316–327.
- Strieper MJ. Distinguishing benign syncope from life-threatening cardiac causes of syncope. *Semin Pediatr Neurol*. 2005;12(1):32–38.
- Task Force for the Diagnosis and Management of Syncope, European Society of Cardiology, European Heart Rhythm Association, et al. Guidelines for the diagnosis and management of syncope (version 2009). *Eur Heart J*. 2009;30(21):2631–2671.
- Willis J. Syncope. *Pediatr Rev*. 2000;21(6):201–204.

CODES

ICD10
R55 Syncope and collapse

FAQ

- Q: What limitations in activity are appropriate for children with recurrent syncope who have normal heart structure and function?
- A: Precautions should be taken similar to those for children of similar age who have epilepsy—closely monitored water recreation and restrictions on climbing; however, most children with recurrent syncope do not experience spells in the midst of vigorous activity and do warrant activity restrictions.
- Q: Do breath-holding spells cause brain damage?
- A: Pallid breath-holding spells appear to be uniformly benign; in rare cases, older children with cyanotic breath-holding spells have had neurologic sequelae of recurrent hypoxemia.

S

SYNDROME OF INAPPROPRIATE ANTIDIURETIC HORMONE SECRETION

Todd D. Nebesio

BASICS

DESCRIPTION

Inappropriate secretion of antidiuretic hormone (ADH) or ADH-like peptide in the presence of low serum sodium, low serum osmolality, and high urine osmolality and in the absence of renal, adrenal, or thyroid pathology

EPIDEMIOLOGY

Incidence

The syndrome of inappropriate antidiuretic hormone secretion (SIADH) can occur at any age. Its incidence depends on the various possible etiologies.

RISK FACTORS

Genetics

Genetic causes of SIADH are exceedingly rare. However, rare cases have been described with gain-of-function mutations in the vasopressin-2 receptor contributing to SIADH and undetectable serum ADH levels.

PATHOPHYSIOLOGY

- ADH is synthesized within the neurons of the hypothalamus, transported in conjunction with neurophysin down the supraopticohypophyseal tract, and stored in the posterior pituitary.
- ADH acts on the renal collecting ducts.
- Interaction of ADH with its receptors forms intracellular cyclic AMP (cAMP), which increases water permeability through insertion of aquaporins (water channels) in renal collecting ducts and consequently enhances reabsorption of free water.
- SIADH results when elevated concentrations of ADH or ADH-like peptides cause free water retention and hypervolemia, leading to hyponatremia. Three possible mechanisms include
  - Increased hypothalamic production of ADH (e.g., CNS disorders such as stroke or meningitis)
  - Independent production of ADH or ADH-like substances from ectopic sources (e.g., lung oat cell carcinoma or olfactory neuroblastoma)
  - Decreased venous return that stimulates atrial volume receptors and thereby leads to ADH release (e.g., heart failure, cirrhosis, pulmonary and intrathoracic diseases, such as tuberculosis).

ETIOLOGY

- Idiopathic
- CNS pathology, causing increased secretion of ADH or ADH-like peptides: meningitis, head trauma, neurosurgical procedures, encephalitis, brain tumor, brain abscess, hydrocephalus, hypoxia, subarachnoid hemorrhage, cerebral venous thrombosis
- Ectopic production of ADH or ADH-like peptides: oat cell carcinoma of the lung, bronchogenic carcinoma, olfactory neuroblastoma, and pancreatic carcinoma
- Pulmonary disease (leading to secondary elevation in ADH secretion or ADH-like peptides): tuberculosis, viral or bacterial pneumonia, asthma, cystic fibrosis, pneumothorax, positive pressure ventilation
- Drugs (which mimic ADH or stimulate its release): vincristine, cyclophosphamide, carbamazepine, chlorpropamide, phenothiazines, clofibrate, nicotine, SSRIs
- Iatrogenic exogenous administration of ADH: vasopressin infusion for treatment of diabetes insipidus, excess desmopressin (DDAVP) in conjunction with fluid intake
- Severe, prolonged nausea
- Postoperative patient (e.g., as part of triple-phase response after hypothalamic-pituitary surgery, after transsphenoidal pituitary surgery)
- Rocky Mountain spotted fever

DIAGNOSIS

HISTORY

- Unusual water intake (suspicious for psychogenic polydipsia)
- Review of intake and output for inpatients
- Decreased urine output
- Anorexia, lethargy
- Weight gain or weight loss
- Renal disease
- Vomiting
- Diarrhea
- Use of diuretics
- Burns
- Heart disease
- Liver disease
- Brain injury: trauma, surgery, hypoxia, toxin

PHYSICAL EXAM

- A complete neurologic and physical exam must be performed. Classically, patients with SIADH manifest subtle signs of hypervolemia but without increased urine output.
- With or without edema
- No signs of dehydration
- Signs of fluid overload
- Absent hyperpigmentation of skin creases/gums (presence suggests Addison disease)
- Hyponatremia; may cause lethargy or irritability and muscle cramps. In severe cases, patients may lose deep tendon reflexes, seize, or be comatose.

ALERT

- Pitfall: Failure to distinguish SIADH from other causes of hyponatremia such as adrenal insufficiency, hypothyroidism, or cerebral salt wasting (CSW) can result in erroneous medical management and lead to worsening hyponatremia.
- Patients with SIADH are still capable of producing urine; basing the diagnosis on urine volume alone can be misleading.

DIAGNOSTIC TESTS & INTERPRETATION

Lab

- Specific tests
  - Simultaneous urinary osmolality, serum osmolality, and serum sodium (order a basic metabolic panel)
  - Urine sodium: usually >30 mmol/L (but not usually >100 mmol/L)
  - Serum uric acid: sometimes low in SIADH
  - Presence of hyponatremia (serum sodium <130 mEq/L), decreased serum osmolality (<260 mOsm/kg), with an inappropriately elevated urinary osmolality (>260 mOsm/L)
  - Plasma ADH concentration: diagnostic but not helpful for rapid diagnosis
- Nonspecific tests
  - Fractional renal excretion of sodium: Net sodium loss is normal or elevated and depends on sodium intake.
  - Urinary specific gravity: helpful but not as specific as urine osmolality
  - Blood glucose: Hyperglycemia results in hypertonic hypernatremia (benign).
  - Triglycerides: Hyperlipidemia causes hypertonic hypernatremia (benign).

Imaging

Head MRI with special cuts of the pituitary and hypothalamus if concern of CNS etiology.

DIFFERENTIAL DIAGNOSIS

- Hypovolemic hyponatremia (e.g., hyponatremic dehydration, seen after running a marathon)
- Euvolemic hyponatremia (e.g., hypothyroidism, adrenal insufficiency)
- Hypervolemic hyponatremia (e.g., CHF, cirrhosis, nephrotic syndrome)
- Diuretics
- Total body sodium loss through vomiting, nasogastric suction, diarrhea, or increased intestinal secretions
- Renal failure
- Severe potassium depletion
- Water intoxication
- CSW: excess production or effects of atrial and/or brain natriuretic peptide hormones
- Reset hypothalamic osmostat
- Rocky Mountain spotted fever
- Hypertonic hyponatremia (sometimes called "pseudohyponatremia," although blood sodium is low with normal total body sodium stores) with hyperglycemia (diabetic ketoacidosis), severe hyperlipidemia, or after administration of mannitol

TREATMENT

MEDICATION

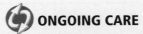

- For emergency use only: hypertonic saline (1.5–3% NaCl)
- Diuretics should be avoided because they worsen hyponatremia.
- ADH antagonists, such as tolvaptan, have been shown to be effective for treatment of SIADH in research trials for adults.
- Demeclocycline (for chronic SIADH)
- Oral urea (for chronic SIADH)

ADDITIONAL TREATMENT

General Measures

- The most important aspects of therapy for SIADH are diagnosis and treatment of the underlying cause.
- If hyponatremic and Na >120 mEq/L and no neurologic signs, first step in management is fluid restriction.
- Hyponatremia may result in seizure, which requires immediate treatment with 3% hypertonic saline until the seizure activity stabilizes. Despite the urgent need for correction of hyponatremia to address the severe neurologic symptoms, the rate of sodium correction should not exceed 12 mEq/L in 24 hours.

INPATIENT CONSIDERATIONS

Admission Criteria

Patients with severe hyponatremia and/or neurologic manifestations will need to be admitted for correction of hyponatremia under close medical supervision.

IV Fluids

- Fluid restriction is essential to treat and prevent worsening hyponatremia. Thus, IV fluids, in general, are not recommended for patients with SIADH. If IV fluids are clinically necessary, a rate comparable to insensible losses (1/3 daily maintenance) is recommended with close attention to serum sodium levels.
- The hyponatremia in SIADH is due to free water retention and not due to decreased total body sodium content. For this reason, changing IV fluids from hypotonic solutions to hypertonic (normal saline) without restriction of the IV fluid rate will still result in worsening hyponatremia.

Discharge Criteria

- Depends on the primary etiology causing SIADH
- Generally, when the serum sodium is stabilized and the patient is neurologically stable

ONGOING CARE

FOLLOW-UP RECOMMENDATIONS

Patient Monitoring

- When to expect improvement: usually during the first 48–72 hours
- Signs to watch for: changes in neurologic status

DIET

Fluid restriction is the most important aspect in the treatment of SIADH. Generally, only fluids for insensible losses (1/3 daily maintenance) are recommended.

PROGNOSIS

Based on the primary cause

COMPLICATIONS

- Severe hyponatremia can cause seizures and, rarely, brain damage. Correcting hyponatremia too quickly can lead to central pontine myelinolysis (CPM), a devastating demyelinating disease that impairs vital functions such as breathing.
- Susceptibility to CPM due to correction of hyponatremia is strongly influenced by the severity and preexisting duration of hyponatremia in the patient.
- Serum sodium should not be increased >12 mEq/L in 24 hours.

ADDITIONAL READING

- Ellison DH, Berl T. Clinical practice. The syndrome of inappropriate antidiuresis. *N Engl J Med*. 2007;356(20):2064–2072.
- Feldman BJ, Rosenthal SM, Vargas GA, et al. Nephrogenic syndrome of inappropriate antidiuresis. *N Engl J Med*. 2005;352(18):1884–1890.
- Fenske W, Allolio B. The syndrome of inappropriate secretion of antidiuretic hormone: diagnostic and therapeutic advances. *Horm Metab Res*. 2010;42(10):691–702.
- Palmer BF. Hyponatremia in patients with central nervous system disease: SIADH versus CSW. *Trends Endocrinol Metab*. 2003;14(4):182–187.
- Rivkees SA. Differentiating appropriate antidiuretic hormone secretion, inappropriate antidiuretic hormone secretion and cerebral salt wasting: the common, uncommon, and misnamed. *Curr Opin Pediatr*. 2008;20(4):448–452.

CODES

ICD10

E22.2 Syndrome of inappropriate secretion of antidiuretic hormone

FAQ

- Q: Is the use of diuretics beneficial in treating SIADH?
- A: No. Although diuretics may relieve the effects of volume overload, they can also worsen hyponatremia. Overall, diuretics usually cause more detriment than benefit.
- Q: What distinguishes SIADH from CSW?
- A: CSW occurs because of increased natriuresis from increased plasma and CSF levels of atrial natriuretic peptide (ANP) after neurologic insults (e.g., subarachnoid hemorrhage). Owing to the natriuresis, these patients become dehydrated with notable decreased plasma volume and elevated BUN. In contrast, patients with SIADH have free water overload, causing hyponatremia. CSW is associated with high urine output, in contrast to SIADH, which has low urine output. However, patients with SIADH who are treated with excess solute (3% saline) may exhibit a natural natriuresis and high urine output. Thus, polyuria alone should never be used to distinguish between CSW and SIADH. Net sodium loss is very high in CSW (>100 mmol/L), but SIADH has normal to slightly elevated net sodium loss; thus, urinary sodium levels are often not specific in distinguishing CSW from SIADH. Laboratory features of CSW include suppressed plasma aldosterone and often normal serum uric acid concentration. Note that plasma ADH concentration is high in SIADH and initially in CSW as well. However, in CSW, after the intravascular volume has been restored, ADH will decrease again, and patients may not exhibit elevated urine osmolality. In these patients, persistent hyponatremia with elevated urine osmolality is more suggestive of SIADH, which is far more common than CSW.
- Q: Why is it important to distinguish SIADH from CSW?
- A: Therapies differ dramatically for these conditions. Unlike the water restriction used to treat SIADH, treatment of dehydration in CSW requires replacement of ongoing salt and water losses. However, CSW is much less common than SIADH and appropriate diagnosis of each condition is necessary to avoid worsening of the hyponatremia by the treatment regimen.

S

SYNOVITIS–TRANSIENT

David D. Sherry

BASICS

DESCRIPTION
Transient inflammatory process resulting in arthralgia and arthritis (especially affecting the hip) and occasionally rash precipitated by an exposure to an infectious agent

EPIDEMIOLOGY
- Any age at risk
- Common in ages 3–10 years
- Males affected 1.5 times more commonly

RISK FACTORS
Genetics
No specific associations

PATHOPHYSIOLOGY
A type III hypersensitivity reaction mediated by immune complex deposition within the skin and joint spaces

ETIOLOGY
Usually viral (especially upper respiratory but also enterovirus)

DIAGNOSIS

HISTORY
- Preceding viral syndromes
- Day care
- Relatively rapid onset of symptoms, with refusal to bear weight, in a non–toxic-appearing child
- Recent nonspecific upper respiratory or GI infection

PHYSICAL EXAM
- General examination usually benign
- Occasional low-grade fever
- Child refuses to bear weight but may tolerate limited ranging of joint.
- Effusions in peripheral joints are rare and usually small and evanescent.
- Pitfalls
  - Distinctions between transient synovitis and a septic joint may be impossible.
  - Extreme pain and guarding on passive ranging raises suspicion for septic joint.

DIAGNOSTIC TESTS & INTERPRETATION
Lab
- CBC
  - Usually mild leukocytosis
- Erythrocyte sedimentation rate (ESR)
  - Usually midrange elevation (35–50 mm/h)

Imaging
- Radiography
  - Usually normal findings or demonstrates small effusion
  - No evidence of periosteal changes
- Ultrasound
  - Affected hip joints may have demonstrable effusions.
- MRI
  - Normal signal intensity may help differentiate transient synovitis from septic hip.

Diagnostic Procedures/Other
- Joint aspirate culture is usually not needed.
- Be wary of contaminated joint aspiration cultures.
- Up to 50% of infected joints are negative on culture.

DIFFERENTIAL DIAGNOSIS
- Infection
  - Lyme disease
  - Septic arthritis
  - Tuberculosis
  - Gonorrhea
- Environment
- Trauma (fracture or soft tissue injury)
  - Slipped capital femoral epiphysis
  - Avascular necrosis
- Tumors
  - Osteoid osteoma
- Immunologic
  - Juvenile idiopathic arthritis
  - Spondyloarthropathy
- Psychological
  - Psychogenic limp
  - Imitative limp
- Miscellaneous
  - Hypothyroidism

TREATMENT

MEDICATION

- Usually responsive to NSAIDs such as ibuprofen (up to 10 mg/kg/dose q.i.d.)
- Very rarely, a short course of oral steroids is necessary.
  - Usually, 1–3 weeks of a tapering course of NSAIDs are effective.

ADDITIONAL TREATMENT

General Measures

Pitfalls

- Missing a septic hip or, alternatively, overinvestigating transient synovitis with invasive procedures
- Avoid initiation of therapy until septic joint has been ruled out.

ONGOING CARE

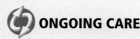

FOLLOW-UP RECOMMENDATIONS

Usually significant improvement in 24–48 hours

Patient Monitoring

Ongoing synovitis despite therapeutic levels of NSAIDs or any bony change indicates need to change diagnosis.

PROGNOSIS

Excellent, although on occasion, patients will experience recurrence of symptoms with subsequent viral syndromes or if there is an underlying spondyloarthropathy.

COMPLICATIONS

Questionably associated with subsequent avascular necrosis of femoral head and coxa magna

ADDITIONAL READING

- Del Baccaro MA, Champoux AN, Bockers T, et al. Septic arthritis versus transient synovitis of the hip: the value of screening laboratory tests. *Ann Emerg Med*. 1992;21(12):1418–1422.
- Do TT. Transient synovitis as a cause of painful limps in children. *Curr Opin Pediatr*. 2000;12(1):48–51.
- Luhmann SJ, Jones A, Schootman M, et al. Differentiation between septic arthritis and transient synovitis of the hip in children with clinical prediction algorithms. *J Bone Joint Surg Am*. 2004;86-A(5): 956–962.
- Taekema HC, Landham PR, Maconochie I. Towards evidence based medicine for paediatricians: distinguishing between transient synovitis and septic arthritis in the limping child—how useful are clinical prediction tools? *Arch Dis Child*. 2009;94(2):167–168.
- Uziel Y, Butbul-Aviel Y, Barash J, et al. Recurrent transient synovitis of the hip in childhood: long-term outcome among 39 patients. *J Rheumatol*. 2006;33(4):810–811.

CODES

ICD10

- M67.30 Transient synovitis, unspecified site
- M67.359 Transient synovitis, unspecified hip
- M67.351 Transient synovitis, right hip

FAQ

- Q: Are there any chronic sequelae from transient synovitis?
- A: Not usually. This is generally a benign disease, but there is a questionable association with avascular necrosis of the femoral head.
- Q: Is there an association with chronic arthritis?
- A: No. There is no known increased risk for chronic arthritis in affected children unless this is the first manifestation of a spondyloarthropathy.

SYPHILIS

Joseph B. Cantey • Pablo J. Sanchez

BASICS

DESCRIPTION

- Systemic infection caused by the spirochete, *Treponema pallidum*
- Can be congenital or acquired
- Consider sexual abuse when syphilis is diagnosed in young children.

EPIDEMIOLOGY

- Congenital syphilis is defined as transmission from an infected mother to her unborn or newborn baby.
- Infection transmitted to the fetus at any stage of disease; during primary and secondary syphilis, rate of transmission is 60–100%.
- ~10.8 cases per 100,000 live births in 2008
- Acquired syphilis is sexually transmitted from an infected to an uninfected individual.
- Nasal secretions are highly infectious in congenital syphilis, and open, moist skin lesions are infectious in congenital and acquired syphilis.

RISK FACTORS

- Lack of prenatal care
- Maternal use of illicit drugs
- Sexual abuse
- Infection with HIV

DIAGNOSIS

SIGNS AND SYMPTOMS

- Congenital syphilis
  - Clinical manifestations range from clinically inapparent to stillbirth.
  - Clinical signs include hepatosplenomegaly, periostitis, osteochondritis, persistent rhinorrhea, or maculopapular rash.
- Acquired syphilis
  - Primary stage: painless, indurated ulcers (chancres), single or multiple, at the site of inoculation ~3 weeks after exposure (range 10–90 days); lesions usually resolve without treatment in 3–6 weeks.
  - Secondary stage: generalized rash, which is often maculopapular and involves the palms and soles; condyloma lata, hypertrophic papular lesions; fever, malaise, lymphadenopathy; signs appear 3–6 weeks after initial chancre and may last 2–10 weeks.
  - Relapse: Symptoms of secondary syphilis may recur 1 or more times before the latent period.
  - Latent period: Untreated, illness may enter a latent stage; patients are asymptomatic, not contagious; lasts 1–40 years or more; patients seroreactive but without other evidence of disease.
    - Early latent period: 1st year of latent period
    - Late latent period: subsequent years
  - Tertiary stage: Up to 1/3 of untreated secondary syphilis cases progress to tertiary or late disease; can occur many years after the primary infection; may see gummatous changes of the skin, bone, and/or viscera or cardiovascular syphilis
  - Neurosyphilis: CNS involvement in 3–7% of untreated cases; can develop at any stage of disease; signs include changes in mood/behavior, hyperactive reflexes, impaired memory and/or judgment, and Argyll-Robertson pupils

HISTORY

- Newborn/infants
  - Obtain a detailed prenatal history; inquire about all syphilis testing done on the mother; if mother has a history of syphilis, ensure documented treatment. The local department of health should have detailed records that include titers and treatment on all cases of syphilis.
  - Newborns should be evaluated for congenital syphilis if the mother is not adequately treated for syphilis (treated with nonpenicillin regimen, such as erythromycin), mother treated adequately but less than 4 weeks before delivery, maternal syphilis treated prior to pregnancy with insufficient follow-up to assess serologic response to treatment, if the infant's titer is 4-fold greater than the mother's titer, or if the infant has clinical signs of infection.
- Older children/adolescents
  - Ask about possible sexual abuse in children.
  - Ask about sexual activity in adolescents, including experience, number of lifetime partners, ages of partners, history of other STDs, and use of barrier contraception.
  - Ask about other risk behaviors.
  - Ask about risk factors for HIV exposure.

PHYSICAL EXAM

- Early congenital syphilis
  - Intrauterine growth restriction; irritability, bulging fontanel, if neurosyphilis is present
  - Alopecia (scalp and eyebrows)
  - Fissures in the lips, nares, anus (rhagades); mucocutaneous lesions
  - Rhinitis ("snuffles") may occur at one to several weeks of age and may be blood-tinged and purulent.
  - Lymphadenopathy
  - Pneumonia alba: Check for tachypnea and/or respiratory distress.
  - Myocarditis
  - Hepatosplenomegaly with or without jaundice
  - Pseudoparalysis of an extremity
  - Rash: bullous ("syphilitic pemphigus") and/or maculopapular ("blueberry muffin") lesions symmetrically distributed on palms, soles, and other parts of the body
  - Condyloma lata: flat, wartlike, moist lesions around the anus/vagina; chancres
- Late congenital syphilis
  - Bony deformities, such as short maxilla, high-arched palate, saddle nose, mulberry molars, Higoumenakis sign (enlargement of the sterno-clavicular portion of the clavicle), protuberance of the mandible, saber shins, scaphoid scapulae
  - Rhagades, neurologic involvement
- Acquired syphilis
  - Primary syphilis
    - Chancre (painless ulcer), single, most commonly located on the genitalia, and/or
    - Painless inguinal adenopathy
  - Secondary syphilis: flulike illness with fever, headache, sore throat, nasal discharge, generalized arthralgias and myalgias, malaise, generalized painless and mobile lymphadenopathy; hepatosplenomegaly; maculopapular rash involving the palms and soles that may involve mucous membranes; condyloma lata (moist, papular lesions); alopecia; signs of meningitis, hepatitis, nephropathy, ocular involvement

DIAGNOSTIC TESTS & INTERPRETATION

- Pitfalls:
  - False-positive nontreponemal test (e.g., rapid plasma reagin [RPR]) results may be seen with lab error, autoimmune disease, tuberculosis, lymphoma, viral infections (including Epstein-Barr, hepatitis, varicella, HIV, and measles viruses), endocarditis, malaria, and IV drug abuse.
  - False-positive treponemal tests may be seen in other spirochetal diseases (i.e., Lyme disease, leptospirosis) and rarely in autoimmune disease (i.e., systemic lupus erythematosus) and viral infections.
  - False-negative nontreponemal test (e.g., RPR) results may be seen with prozone phenomenon if titers are high.
  - Mothers of infants with congenital syphilis should also be tested for gonorrhea, chlamydia, HIV, and hepatitis B virus infection.
  - In newborns, cord blood testing may result in false-positive and false-negative results; therefore, serum from the infant is the preferred source of testing.
  - Infants should not be discharged from the nursery until the results of maternal syphilis tests are known.
  - "Reverse screening" algorithm refers to using treponemal test first, then confirming a positive result with nontreponemal test.
  - Discordant results should be confirmed with a second, different treponemal test
  - Unclear how to manage well-appearing infants born to mothers identified by reverse screening who have positive treponemal tests but nonreactive RPR (most experts recommend single IM dose of penicillin G, 50,000 U/kg)

Lab

- Nontreponemal tests
  - VDRL (Venereal Disease Research Laboratory) or RPR test to measure nontreponemal antibodies
  - Used for routine screening; quantitative serum titers generally correlate with disease activity; need to confirm positive results with a treponemal antibody test. 4-fold titer change (e.g., from 1:8 to 1:32) necessary to document clinically significant change. Titers for different nontreponemal tests are not equivalent; therefore, use same test (and preferably same lab) when following serial titers.
  - VDRL (not RPR) is used on CSF to evaluate for neurosyphilis.
- Treponemal antibody tests
  - Used for confirmation of positive nontreponemal test
  - FTA-ABS (fluorescent treponemal antibody-absorption), TPPA (*T. pallidum* particle agglutination), MHA-TP (microhemagglutination assay for *T. pallidum* antibodies), or EIA (enzyme immunoassay for antitreponemal IgG)
  - Treponemal tests usually remain positive for life once infected; not useful for measuring treatment effectiveness
- Dark-field microscopy

- CSF analysis
  - Findings include mononuclear pleocytosis, moderately elevated protein, and normal glucose.
  - Should be performed in all patients with acquired syphilis of >1 year's duration
  - Perform on infants when congenital syphilis suspected, if the physical examination is consistent with syphilis, if infant's titer is 4-fold greater than that of mother, or if dark-field or fluorescent antibody test positive on body fluids
  - Remember that CSF protein levels in normal newborns are higher than in older children; some are as high as 150–200 mg/dL.

Imaging

Long bone plain films: Rule out metaphyseal osteochondritis and/or diaphyseal periostitis.

DIFFERENTIAL DIAGNOSIS

- Congenital syphilis
  - Herpes simplex virus (HSV)
  - Toxoplasmosis
  - Cytomegalovirus
  - Rubella
  - Neonatal hepatitis
  - Osteomyelitis
- Acquired syphilis
  - Chancroid (*Haemophilus ducreyi*)
  - Granuloma inguinale
  - Calymmatobacterium granulomatis
  - Lymphogranuloma venereum (*Chlamydia trachomatis*)
  - Scabies
  - Mycotic infections
  - Genital herpes (HSV)
  - Venereal warts (human papillomavirus [HPV])
  - Viral exanthem (e.g., enteroviruses may cause a maculopapular rash involving the palms and soles)

TREATMENT

MEDICATION

- Infants <28 days of age
  - Aqueous crystalline penicillin G (50,000 U/kg/dose) IV q12h for first 7 days of life, then q8h for a total of 10 days *or* procaine penicillin G (50,000 U/kg/dose) IM daily for 10 days
  - If >1 day of treatment is missed, restart 10-day course.
- Infants >28 days of age
  - Aqueous crystalline penicillin G (50,000 U/kg/dose) IV q4–6h for 10 days
- Primary, secondary, and early latent (<1 year duration) syphilis
  - Infant/child: penicillin G benzathine 50,000 U/kg IM (maximum, 2.4 million units), single dose
  - Adolescent/adult: doxycycline 100 mg PO b.i.d. or tetracycline 500 mg PO q.i.d. for 14 days for nonpregnant, penicillin-allergic patients
- Late latent syphilis (>1 year duration) or disease of unknown duration
  - Infant/child: penicillin G benzathine, 50,000 U/kg IM (maximum 2.4 million U) weekly for 3 consecutive weeks
  - Adolescent/adult: doxycycline 100 mg PO b.i.d. or tetracycline 500 mg PO q.i.d. for 4 weeks for nonpregnant, penicillin-allergic patients
- Pregnant women with penicillin allergy who require therapy for syphilis should be desensitized
- Alternative therapy can be found at www.cdc.gov/nchstp/dstd/penicillinG.htm.

ONGOING CARE

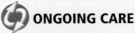

ISSUES FOR REFERRAL

All cases should be reported to the local department of (public) health.

PROGNOSIS

- The prognosis is better the earlier syphilis is detected and treated.
- Following appropriate therapy, the disease usually is totally arrested.
- With late findings of syphilis involving the nervous and/or cardiovascular systems, there may not be clinical improvement.
- Untreated infection in the neonate progresses to neurosyphilis within 1 year.
- Osteochondritis and periostitis in the newborn are usually self-limited and heal in the first 3–6 months of life.
- Hemolytic anemia seen in congenital syphilis may persist for weeks.

COMPLICATIONS

- Stillbirth or spontaneous abortion
- Perinatal death in 40% of pregnancies in mothers with untreated early syphilis
- Prematurity
- Hydrops fetalis
- Nephrosis
- Pneumonia alba
- Intrauterine growth restriction and failure to thrive
- Disseminated intravascular coagulation
- Pseudoparalysis of Parrot: paralysis of one of the limbs of an infant affected by congenital syphilis; usually unilateral
- Acute syphilitic leptomeningitis
- Cranial nerve palsies
- Interstitial keratitis: 5–20 years after birth
- Cerebral infarction
- Seizure disorder, mental retardation
- Rhagades: cluster of scars radiating around the mouth
- Mulberry molars: maldevelopment of the cusps in the first molars
- Clutton joints: painless arthritis of the knees and, rarely, other joints
- Hutchinson triad: Hutchinson teeth (notched upper central incisors), interstitial keratitis, 8th-nerve deafness
- Saber shins: anterior bowing of the midportion of the tibia

PATIENT MONITORING

- Congenital syphilis:
  - Clinical follow-up and serial nontreponemal serologic testing every 2–3 months until titer decreases 4-fold or test is nonreactive
  - After adequate treatment, nontreponemal tests should be nonreactive after 6 months; infants with a history of abnormal CSF findings need serial CSF analyses every 6 months until CSF is normal.
  - Treated infants, follow-up at 1, 2, 4, 6, and 12 months of age; serologic tests should be performed 2, 4, 6, and 12 months after therapy until they become nonreactive or the titer has decreased 4-fold.
  - If titers have not shown a decline by 6–12 months, require reevaluation and treatment.
- Primary and secondary syphilis
  - Clinical follow-up and serial nontreponemal titers at 6 and 12 months after treatment (more often, if at high risk for reinfection or treatment failure): Nontreponemal titers should drop 4-fold within 6 months of treatment of primary or secondary syphilis and within 12–24 months after treatment of latent or tertiary syphilis.

ADDITIONAL READING

- American Academy of Pediatrics. Syphilis. In: Pickering LK, Baker CJ, Kimberlin DW, et al, eds. *Red Book: 2012 Report of the Committee on Infectious Diseases*. 29th ed. Elk Grove Village, IL: American Academy of Pediatrics; 2012:690–703.
- Binniker MJ. Which algorithm should be used to screen for syphilis? *Curr Opin Infect Dis*. 2012;25(1): 79–85.
- Centers for Disease Control and Prevention. Congenital syphilis—United States, 2003–2008. *MMWR Morb Mortal Wkly Rep*. 2010;59(14): 413–417.
- Centers for Disease Control and Prevention. Primary and secondary syphilis—United States, 2003–2004. *MMWR Morb Mortal Wkly Rep*. 2006;55(10): 269–273.
- Chakraborty R, Luck S. Managing congenital syphilis again? The more things change. *Curr Opin Infect Dis*. 2007;20(3):247–252.
- Chakraborty R, Luck S. Syphilis is on the increase. *Arch Dis Child*. 2008;93(2):105–109.
- Hyman EL. Syphilis. *Pediatr Rev*. 2006;2791):37–39.
- Tobian AA, Serwadda D, Quinn TC, et al. Male circumcision for the prevention of HSV-2 and HPV infections and syphilis. *N Engl J Med*. 2009;360(13): 1298–1309.
- Wendel GD, Stark BJ, Jamison RB, et al. Penicillin allergy and desensitization in serious infections during pregnancy. *N Engl J Med*. 1985;312(19): 1229–1232.

CODES

ICD10

- A53.9 Syphilis, unspecified
- A50.9 Congenital syphilis, unspecified
- A51.5 Early syphilis, latent

FAQ

- Q: Can an infant have congenital syphilis if the mother had a negative RPR during pregnancy?
- A: A mother with a negative RPR during pregnancy may have acquired syphilis late in pregnancy and transmitted it to her fetus. If the mother was not tested at delivery, then the diagnosis may have been missed.
- Q: What is the prozone phenomenon?
- A: When a nontreponemal test is falsely negative due to high concentrations of antibody to *T. pallidum*; diluting the serum will result in positive test results.

TAPEWORM

Karen E. Jerardi • Samir S. Shah

BASICS

DESCRIPTION

- Tapeworms cause 2 major types of zoonotic disease syndromes, depending on whether humans are the definitive or intermediate host.
- When humans serve as definitive hosts, adult tapeworms infect the GI tract and interfere with nutrition; patients may be asymptomatic.
- When humans serve as intermediate hosts for the larval cestode, serious pathology results.
- Causative organisms include the following:
  - *Taenia saginata* (beef tapeworm)
  - *Taenia solium* (pork tapeworm)
  - *Diphyllobothrium latum* (fish tapeworm)
  - *Dipylidium caninum* (dog tapeworm)
  - *Echinococcus granulosus*

EPIDEMIOLOGY

- Beef tapeworm
  - Estimated 77 million people infested worldwide
  - Widespread in cattle-breeding areas of the world, endemic in Asia, Latin America, Eastern Europe
- Pork tapeworm
  - Estimated >50 million people infested worldwide
  - Taeniasis: typically asymptomatic infection with adult tapeworm (from undercooked pork)
  - Cysticercosis: infection with larval parasite (fecal–oral transmission from carriers).
  - High prevalence in developing areas of Asia, Central and South America
  - 1,000 new cases of neurocysticercosis in United States annually
- Fish tapeworm
  - Infection is most prevalent in temperate climates of Europe (Finland, Estonia, Sweden most common), and Canada.
  - Persons who prepare or eat raw freshwater fish are most at risk.
  - In the United States, infected salmon have been implicated in most cases.
- Dog tapeworm
  - Found in dogs and cats worldwide
- Echinococcosis
  - Associated with the practice of feeding sheep viscera to dogs
  - It is hyperendemic in sheep-raising areas of South America, Australia, areas of Africa, China, Central Asia, and the Western United States.

GENERAL PREVENTION

- Adult tapeworms
  - Proper cooking prevents transmission of beef, pork, and fish tapeworms.
- Pork tapeworm
  - Refrigeration of pork infested with cysticerci at temperatures >0°C (32°F) does not affect parasite survival. However, storage of pork for 4 days at −5°C (21.2°F) or 1 day at −24°C (−11.2°F) kills most cysticerci.
- Fish tapeworm
  - Brief cooking (at >56°C [132.8°F] for 5 minutes) or freezing (−18°C [−0.4°F] for 24–48 hours) renders the fish safe to consume.
- Dog tapeworm
  - Periodic deworming of pets
- Echinococcosis
  - Careful disposal of sheep viscera and mass chemotherapy of dogs can interrupt the life cycle of *E. granulosus* as the cestode moves between sheep and carnivore hosts.

PATHOPHYSIOLOGY

- Beef tapeworm
  - Cattle (intermediate host) ingest the eggs of *T. saginata* in contaminated feeds. The eggs hatch, releasing embryos which penetrate intestinal mucosa, enter the bloodstream, and settle in skeletal muscle, where they develop into larvae. Larvae in undercooked meat are consumed by humans and mature into adult tapeworms within the human (definitive host) GI tract. They grow up to 25-m long.
- Pork tapeworm: Humans are the only definitive host for the adult pork tapeworm. Both humans and pigs are intermediate hosts for its embryonic form, cysticercosis.
  - Pigs ingest *T. solium* eggs. In the intestine, the eggs release embryos that penetrate the mucosa, enter the bloodstream, and settle in various tissues to differentiate into cysticerci (infective larvae). Cysticerci are ingested by humans (definitive host) who consume undercooked pork.
  - Humans ingest food contaminated with human feces containing *T. solium* eggs. The eggs hatch, liberating embryos which penetrate the intestinal mucosa leading to blood-borne distribution to the brain, subcutaneous tissues, muscle, and eye, where they develop into cysticerci.
- Fish tapeworm
  - When sewage containing *D. latum* eggs contaminates freshwater lakes and streams, eggs hatch into the water becoming embryos. Embryos are eaten by crustaceans and then passed on to fresh water fish. Humans are infected when they consume these undercooked fish. The larvae mature into adult tapeworms in the intestines of humans in 3–5 weeks' time and can survive up to 10 years. Rarely, the tapeworm migrates thru intestinal wall to other tissues (sparganosis).
- Dog tapeworm
  - Larvae develop in fleas (intermediate host) after ingestion of the eggs; humans are infected through accidental ingestion of infected fleas.
- Echinococcosis (hydatid disease)
  - Humans ingest eggs of *E. granulosus* through contaminated dog feces. After ingestion, the eggs hatch and release embryos (oncospheres) in the small intestine. Penetration through the mucosa leads to blood-borne distribution to the liver, lungs, and other sites, where development of cysts begins. Within the cysts, new larvae (scolices) develop, accumulate fluid, and encroach on surrounding structures.

DIAGNOSIS

HISTORY

- Recent travel or immigration
- GI tract
  - Nausea, weight loss, diarrhea, abdominal tenderness or distention
  - Fish and, rarely, dog tapeworm infections can be complicated by intestinal obstruction.
  - May observe proglottids that resemble rice or seeds in stool from dog tapeworm
- Jaundice
  - Hepatic cysts from echinococcosis may be palpable in the right upper quadrant.
  - Biliary tree extension can lead to obstructive jaundice and cholangitis.
- Respiratory tract
  - Pulmonary hydatid cyst due to *E. granulosus* causes cough, dyspnea, and hemoptysis; rupture of a cyst can cause anaphylaxis.
- Hematologic
  - Anemia from vitamin B_{12} deficiency occurs in 2% of fish tapeworm infections due to competition for absorption in ileum. Other signs of pernicious anemia include glossitis, peripheral neuropathy, decreased vibration sense, and ataxia.
- CNS
  - New-onset seizures (partial or generalized) occur with neurocysticercosis and some species of *Echinococcus*.
  - Neurocysticercosis may present with alteration in mental status, signs of elevated intracranial pressure (headache, vomiting, visual changes), or meningitis.
  - Neurocysticercosis and vitamin B_{12} deficiency due to fish tapeworm can mimic psychotic illness with delirium or hallucinations.
  - CNS symptoms in neurocysticercosis typically appear 5–7 years after initial infection (range: 6 months to 30 years).
- Note: For echinococcosis, a presymptomatic stage may last for years before the enlarging cysts cause symptoms. The variability of signs and symptoms depends on the target organ.

DIAGNOSTIC TESTS & INTERPRETATION

Lab

- Beef tapeworm
  - Ziehl–Neelsen stain of stool identifies eggs.
  - Proglottids or eggs in stool with microscopic examination (62% sensitivity)
  - ELISA test detects *Taenia* antigens in stool (85% sensitivity, 95% specificity).
- Pork tapeworm
  - Serum enzyme-linked immunoelectrotransfer blot (most sensitive) and ELISA of serum and/or CSF
  - Stool samples for intestinal worms
- Fish tapeworm
  - Stool samples for eggs and proglottids are diagnostic, collect multiple specimens.
  - Mild eosinophilia (5–15%)
  - Low vitamin B_{12} levels (50%)
  - Megaloblastic anemia 2%

- Dog tapeworm
  - Characteristic egg packets (loose membrane containing up to 20 eggs) or proglottids may be identified in stool.
- Echinococcosis
  - IgE levels are elevated. Eosinophilia is present in <25% of infected persons.
  - Polymerase chain reaction (PCR) of stool
  - Mild elevation of hepatic enzymes may be present with hepatic hydatid cysts.
  - The Casoni skin test (injection of hydatid fluid into the dermis) yields an erythematous papule in <60 minutes in 50–80% of infected patients. False-positive rate is 30% in uninfected patients.
  - Serologic testing is falsely negative in 10–50% of cases. False-negative results are more likely in patients with pulmonary hydatid cysts and in children. No serologic test excludes the diagnosis of hydatid cysts.

Imaging

- Pork tapeworm
  - Contrast-enhanced CT or MRI of the brain may reveal cysticerci; ring-enhancing lesions with surrounding edema represent a dying parasite; calcification represents a resolved infection.
  - Imaging is usually diagnostic.
- Echinococcosis
  - On x-ray, pulmonary cysts demonstrate a sharply demarcated, smooth-bordered cyst; there is a crescent-shaped air level after cyst rupture. Liver and spleen lesions may calcify over time.
  - Hydatid cysts: Internal septa or daughter cysts after cyst rupture are detected by CT, MRI, or ultrasound; present in ~50% of patients with unilocular liver cysts

Diagnostic Procedures/Other

Echinococcosis: In seronegative persons, a presumptive diagnosis can be confirmed by demonstrating protoscolices or hydatid membranes in liquid obtained by ultrasound-guided percutaneous cyst aspiration. This procedure is controversial because anaphylaxis may occur with cyst rupture.

DIFFERENTIAL DIAGNOSIS

- Non–tapeworm gastroenteritis
- Inflammatory bowel disease
- Cholecystitis or biliary obstruction (i.e., gallstones, neoplasms, or liver disease)
- B_{12} deficiency from dietary deficiency or pancreatic insufficiency
- Idiopathic epilepsy
- Echinococcal cysts must be differentiated from benign cysts, cavitary tuberculosis, abscesses, and neoplasms.

TREATMENT

MEDICATION

- Beef, pork, fish, and dog tapeworm (and most other intestinal cestodes)
  - Praziquantel: 5–10 mg/kg as a single dose; no safety profile exists for children <4 years of age.
  - Niclosamide (second line for beef tapeworm): children 11–34 kg, 1 g as a single dose; children >34 kg, 1.5 g as a single dose (not available in the United States)
  - Supplement with vitamin B_{12} for fish tapeworm.
- Neurocysticercosis
  - Treatment should be individualized based on number, location, and viability of cysticerci on MRI or CT scan.
  - Treatment may not be indicated for single degenerating cysts, calcifications, or encephalitis. Most experts recommend therapy for patients with nonenhancing or multiple cysticerci.
  - Albendazole: 15 mg/kg/24 h (maximum, 800 mg/24 h) in 2 divided doses for 8–30 days or praziquantel 50–100 mg/kg/24 h in 3 divided doses for 30 days
  - Steroids (1 mg/kg/day of prednisone or 0.5 mg/kg/day of dexamethasone), in combination with albendazole, decrease seizure frequency and number of CNS cysts.
  - Antiepileptic drugs are recommended and shunt placement, and/or mannitol should be considered for treatment of hydrocephalus.
  - Antiparasitic therapy is contraindicated in patients with diffuse cerebral edema ("cysticercal encephalitis") because the inflammatory response that follows treatment may worsen cerebral edema.
  - No definite recommendations exist regarding the use of corticosteroids alone.
- Echinococcosis
  - Albendazole 15 mg/kg/24 h (max 800 mg/24 h) in 2 divided doses for 1–6 months
  - May require 3 courses of therapy with drug-free intervals of 14 days between courses
- Note: The benzimidazoles, including albendazole, are contraindicated in patients with blood dyscrasia, leukopenia, and liver disease. Prolonged courses require monitoring of liver function and hematopoiesis.

SURGERY/OTHER PROCEDURES

- Echinococcosis: surgical resection of intact hydatid cysts, especially if >10 cm, secondarily infected, or causing symptoms
- Subcutaneous sparganosis: surgical resection or ethanol injection

ONGOING CARE

FOLLOW-UP RECOMMENDATIONS

Patient Monitoring

- Beef tapeworm
  - Stool should be checked for eggs and proglottids 1 month after therapy.
- Pork tapeworm
  - Repeat CNS imaging studies at 2-month intervals (with continued therapy) until successful elimination of parenchymal brain cysticerci.
- Fish tapeworm
  - Perform stool examination 12 weeks after therapy to test for cure.
- Dog tapeworm
  - No follow-up stool examination required, but the appearance of proglottids >1 week after therapy indicates treatment failure.
- Echinococcosis
  - Requires prolonged follow-up with ultrasound or other imaging procedures

COMPLICATIONS

- Cysticercosis
  - Cysticerci can develop in the brain, muscle, eye, or other organs. Ophthalmologic exam is warranted in cases of neurocysticercosis.
- Echinococcosis
  - Cysts grow slowly, causing symptoms only when relatively large.
  - They frequently develop in the liver (50–70%) and lung (20–30%); 5–10% of cysts involve other organs, including the eye, brain, spleen, heart, bone, and kidneys.
  - Rupture of cysts can cause anaphylaxis.
  - Bone involvement can cause pathologic fractures, and renal involvement can cause pain or hematuria.

ADDITIONAL READING

- Baird RA, Wiebe S, Zunt JR, et al. Evidence-based guideline: treatment of parenchymal neurocysticercosis. *Neurology*. 2013;80(15):1424–1429.
- García HH, Gonzalez AE, Evans CA, et al. *Taenia solium* cysticercosis. *Lancet*. 2003;362(9383):547–556.
- Moon TD, Oberhelman RA. Antiparasitic therapy in children. *Pediatr Clin North Am*. 2005;52(3):917–948.
- Schantz PM. Tapeworms (cestodiasis). *Gastroenterol Clin North Am*. 1996;25(3):637–653.

CODES

ICD10

- B71.9 Cestode infection, unspecified
- B68.1 Taenia saginata taeniasis
- B68.0 Taenia solium taeniasis

FAQ

- Q: Can vegetarians develop neurocysticercosis?
- A: Yes, because neurocysticercosis results from ingestion of *T. solium* eggs in products contaminated with infected fecal matter. GI symptoms result from eating infected pork.
- Q: Is treatment for neurocysticercosis always indicated?
- A: The findings are controversial. In many children, the lesion disappears spontaneously within 2–3 months. Guidelines for treatment depend on the number and location of lesions, as well as the viability of the parasites within the nervous system. A growing parasite deserves active management, either with antiparasitic drugs or surgical excision.

TEETHING

Karen R. Fratantoni • Anupama R. Tate

BASICS

DESCRIPTION

Teething is the normal developmental process of primary tooth eruption whereby the tooth moves from its position in the alveolar bone through the mucosa into the mouth. Parents/caregivers, physicians, and dentists often associate many localized and systemic symptoms with the teething process, including mouthing/biting, drooling, changes in appetite, and fever.

DIAGNOSIS

Consider the following diagnostic approach when evaluating an infant or toddler who presents with chief complaint of teething:

- Careful history and physical exam
- Evaluation of signs/symptoms inconsistent with teething (fever >102°F/38.8°C, irritability, diarrhea) and treatment of possible illness
- If teething is suspected or confirmed and serious illness ruled out, offer education and advice for parents/caregivers around the management of teething symptoms.

HISTORY

Teething is a normal developmental process for which anticipatory guidance should be offered at appropriate well visits. The following questions will be helpful for providers in determining if teething should be considered in the differential diagnosis.

- Is teething likely to be occurring at the child's age?
  - First tooth appears by 6 months of age; however, 1% of children will get their first tooth before 4 months old and 1% after 12 months old.
  - Completion of a set of 20 deciduous/primary teeth by 30 months of age
  - Teeth emerge in pairs, with lower central incisors usually appearing first.
  - Rule of thumb: age (in months) − 6 = average number of teeth (until 24 months old)
- Has the child had fever?
  - General consensus is that temperature >102°F or 38.8°C should not be attributed to teething.
  - One prospective longitudinal study showed an association between mild tympanic temperature elevations (with maximum 36.8°F) and day of tooth eruption.
  - Another study showed mild temperature elevation in the 8-day teething period.
- Does the child have one or more symptoms often attributed to teething?
  - Common symptoms parents often attributed to teething include biting, drooling, gum rubbing, irritability, sucking, wakefulness, ear rubbing, facial rash, and decrease in appetite for solids.
  - One prospective study showed an increase of the above symptoms in the period from 4 days prior to 3 days after tooth eruption, considered to be the 8-day window of teething.
  - There is no consensus in the medical literature about the association of teething and these minor symptoms.
- Is the child irritable?
  - Irritability with an inability to console is concerning and must not be attributed to teething.

> **ALERT**
> Fever >38.8°C/102°F, irritability, or diarrhea should NOT be attributed to teething and should prompt a careful history, physical exam, and investigation for possible etiology, including otitis media, meningitis, serious bacterial illness, or viral infection.

- Is the child exhibiting changes in sleep pattern?
  - Teething should not cause significant sleep disturbances.
  - Further history should be obtained regarding the nature of the sleep changes, some of which are common in children between 6 and 12 months old.
- Are there changes in the mouth which make the parent think the child may be teething?
  - Swelling of the gums may be noted prior to tooth eruption.
  - An area of gum swelling with discoloration may represent an eruption cyst for which no treatment is required.

DIFFERENTIAL DIAGNOSIS

- Infectious
  - Gingivostomatitis causing pain or drooling
  - Viral or bacterial illnesses causing pain, fever, fussiness, or change in behavior
- Toxic ingestion causing drooling
- Trauma or burn to the mouth
- Normal developmental behaviors: Drooling, gum rubbing, and finger sucking may be consistent with typical development.

PHYSICAL EXAM

- Often, there are no pertinent findings on physical exam.
- Gum swelling and eruption cysts are both normal findings.

DIAGNOSTIC TESTS & INTERPRETATION

No laboratory tests are indicated in the otherwise healthy child with teething.

TREATMENT

GENERAL MEASURES

- Nonpharmacologic
  - Application of cold/frozen objects onto the gums causes vasoconstriction and reduces inflammation.
  - Biting on teething rings or other objects can offer relief by applying pressure to the gums.
  - Objects used for this purpose include teething rings, pacifiers, cold spoons, frozen bagels or bananas, or a cold washcloth.
    - Teething rings can be placed in the refrigerator but not the freezer, which could disrupt the integrity of the plastic cover.
    - Discard teething rings made prior to 1998, as they may contain diisononyl phthalate, a plastic softening agent which was later found to be toxic and potentially carcinogenic.
    - Do not attach a teething ring to a tether around the child's neck, as that may cause strangulation.
    - Care should be taken to not give the child an object which could be a potential choking hazard.

- Pharmacologic management
  - Acetaminophen (15 mg/kg PO q 4–6 hours) or ibuprofen (10 mg/kg PO q 6–8 hours) may be used for pain relief as needed but should not be given around-the-clock so as not to mask fever.
  - Over-the-counter teething preparations containing benzocaine have been associated with methemoglobinemia and are not recommended. The FDA released a Drug Safety Communication in 2011 to inform the public of this potentially fatal adverse effect.
  - Homeopathic remedies include belladonna, clove oil, olive oil, fennel, green onion, ginger, vanilla, and chamomile. Depending on the amount ingested and the size of the child, toxicity may be a concern.
  - Remedies used in the past that are no longer recommended include alcoholic liquors, honey, emetics, purgatives, and lancing of the gums.

ISSUES FOR REFERRAL

- Children should have a dental home by the age of 12 months.
- Children who have delayed eruption of their first primary tooth beyond 15 months should be evaluated. The following conditions have been associated with delayed eruption: anodontia, impacted teeth, hypothyroidism, hypopituitarism, calcium/phosphorus metabolism problems, ectodermal dysplasias, Gaucher disease, osteopetrosis, Apert syndrome, cleidocranial dysplasia, and Down syndrome.
- Referral to a dentist should be considered for children with significant variation in eruption caused by dental infections, additional teeth in the path of eruption, insufficient space in the dental arch, and/or ectopic placement of teeth.
- Presence of or risk for dental caries at an early age should prompt a dental evaluation.
- Natal teeth should be evaluated only if they are loose and pose an aspiration risk or if they interfere with breastfeeding.

PATIENT EDUCATION

- Information available at http://www.ada.org/en/Home-MouthHealthy/aztopics/t/teething
- Parent handout available at http://patiented.solutions.aap.org/handout.aspx?resultClick=1&gbosid=166311

ADDITIONAL READING

- American Academy of Pediatrics. A pediatric guide to children's oral health. http://www2.aap.org/oralhealth/docs/oralhealthfcpagesf2_2_1.pdf. Accessed March 15, 2015.
- Anderson J. "Nothing but the tooth": dispelling myths about teething. *Contemp Pediatr*. 2004;21:75–87.
- Ashley MP. It's only teething . . . a report of the myths and modern approaches to teething. *Br Dent J*. 2001;191(1):4–8.
- Lehr J, Masters A, Pollack B. Benzocaine-induced methemoglobinemia in the pediatric population. *J Pediatr Nurs*. 2012; 27(5):583–588.
- Macknin ML, Piedmonte M, Jacobs J, et al. Symptoms associated with infant teething: a prospective study. *Pediatrics*. 2000;105(4, Pt 1):747–752.
- Markman L. Teething: facts and fiction. *Pediatr Rev*. 2009;30(8):e59–e64.
- Ramos-Jorge J, Pordeus I, Ramos-Jorge M, et al. Prospective longitudinal study of signs and symptoms associated with primary tooth eruption. *Pediatrics*. 2011;128(3):471–476.
- Sood S, Sood M. Teething: myths and facts. *J Clin Pediatr Dent*. 2010;35(1):9–14.
- Wake M, Hesketh K, Lucas J. Teething and tooth eruption in infants: a cohort study. *Pediatrics*. 2000;106(6):1374–1379.

CODES

ICD10

K00.7 Teething syndrome

FAQ

- Q: When does a child need to see the dentist?
- A: Every infant should receive an oral health assessment from the primary care provider by 6 months of age to assess the patient's risk for oral disease or caries. Parents should be provided education on infant oral health and evaluation of fluoride supplementation. The AAP and the AAPD recommend that the patient establish a dental home by 1 year of age or sooner if with concern for dental caries, trauma, teeth staining, or family history of early dental caries.
- Q: What is the proper care of newly erupted teeth?
- A: Brushing with a toothbrush helps reduce bacterial colonization and should be done by a parent twice daily using a soft toothbrush of age-appropriate size. Never put the baby to bed with a bottle due to increased risk for early childhood dental caries.
- Q: Will thumb sucking affect my baby's teeth?
- A: Thumb sucking is a normal part of infancy but, if allowed to continue into early childhood, can cause problems with the child's bite. If it continues past the age of 3 years, the primary care or dental provider should counsel parents on strategies to reduce the behavior.
- Q: Is there a cluster of symptoms that can predict when teeth will emerge?
- A: Studies have failed to show a group of symptoms which is predictive of tooth eruption.
- Q: What are natal and neonatal teeth?
- A: Natal teeth are teeth present at birth, most often representing the premature eruption of primary teeth but occasionally can be a third set of teeth. They are usually left in place unless they cause difficulty with nursing or are loose and pose an aspiration risk. Neonatal teeth, however, erupt in the 1st month of life. Occurring in approximately 1 in 2,000 children, natal and neonatal teeth are not usually pathologic but have been associated with various syndromes, including Hallermann-Streiff syndrome, Ellis-van Creveld syndrome, craniofacial dysostosis, congenital pachyonychia, Pierre Robin, adrenogenital syndrome, and Sotos syndrome.

TENDONITIS

David D. Sherry

BASICS

DESCRIPTION
Inflammation of a tendon or along the tendon sheath

EPIDEMIOLOGY
- Increases with age and at time of puberty
- May be slightly more common in girls

RISK FACTORS
Genetics
Hypermobile individuals may be prone to tendonitis.

PATHOPHYSIOLOGY
Inflammation and microtearing may be present.

ETIOLOGY
Frequently associated with repetitive motion/overuse activities

DIAGNOSIS

HISTORY
- Trauma or overuse
  - Verify acute nature of injury.
- Signs and symptoms
  - Pain
  - Tenderness

PHYSICAL EXAM
- Evidence of hematoma
  - Palpate around and about affected areas, detecting point tenderness especially at tendon insertions as well as over bony prominences.
- Evidence of bursitis or arthritis
  - Systemic conditions, such as spondyloarthropathy, can lead to inflammation of tendons, bursa, and joints, and bursitis can mimic the pain of tendonitis.
- Pop or snap felt at the time of the event
  - Sometimes this is felt when tendons and ligaments are torn or avulsed.
- Caution: false positives
  - Patients may have torn ligaments, fractures, or arthritis and not just tendonitis on examination.
- Pitfalls
  - Overdiagnosis in young children, in whom overuse is rare and other diagnoses should be considered
  - Underdiagnosis in older children in whom repetitive activities are likely to occur

DIAGNOSTIC TESTS & INTERPRETATION
Lab
Erythrocyte sedimentation rate (ESR): occasionally helpful to rule out inflammatory conditions if history and/or physical exam are suggestive

Imaging
Plain radiograph: Affected area may be indicated to rule out a fracture or avulsion or identify a bone spur.

DIFFERENTIAL DIAGNOSIS
- Infection
  - Especially gonococcal disease, septic arthritis, or osteomyelitis; rarely, tuberculosis
- Environmental
  - Fracture
- Metabolic
  - Homocystinuria
- Congenital
  - Generalized hypermobility
  - Marfan syndrome
  - Ehlers-Danlos
- Immunologic
  - Ankylosing spondylitis and the reactive spondyloarthropathies (inflammatory bowel disease, reactive arthritis)
  - Juvenile idiopathic arthritis
- Psychological or neuropathic
  - Amplified musculoskeletal pain

TREATMENT

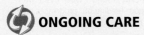

MEDICATION
- NSAIDs initially
- Rarely, if ever, do soft tissue steroid injections have a role in children.

ADDITIONAL TREATMENT
General Measures
- Rest/reduced use of the affected tendon/muscle group is essential, occasionally requiring splinting.
- Duration of therapy
  - 1–4 weeks

ADDITIONAL THERAPIES
- Physical or occupational therapy for eccentric muscle strengthening
- Either self-directed or formal help with resumption of desired activity to improve biomechanics

ONGOING CARE

FOLLOW-UP RECOMMENDATIONS
Improvement often takes 2–6 weeks.

Patient Monitoring
If the provocative activity is resumed too soon, the irritation will recur.

PROGNOSIS
Usually good for children; however, many will suffer recurrences if proper exercises before desired activity are not continued.

COMPLICATIONS
Ongoing pain and predisposition for recurrence

ADDITIONAL READING

- Almekinders LC, Temple JD. Etiology, diagnosis, and treatment of tendonitis: an analysis of the literature. *Med Sci Sports Exerc.* 1998;30(8):1183–1190.
- Jonsson P, Alfredson H. Superior results with eccentric compared to concentric quadriceps training in patients with jumper's knee: a prospective randomised study. *Br J Sports Med.* 2005;39(11):847–850.
- Marsh JS, Daigneault JP. Ankle injuries in the pediatric population. *Curr Opin Pediatr.* 2000;12(1):52–60.
- Pommering TL, Kluchurosky L. Overuse injuries in adolescents. *Adolesc Med State Art Rev.* 2007;18(1):95–120.

CODES

ICD10
M77.9 Enthesopathy, unspecified

FAQ
- Q: Which activities can result in overuse syndromes and tendonitis?
- A: Virtually any repetitive activity in which children engage can cause tendonitis. For example, pain in the tendons of the thumb has occurred in children overusing video games.

T

TETANUS

Hamid Bassiri

BASICS

DESCRIPTION

- Tetanus is characterized by muscle rigidity and spasms due to production of a neurotoxin in infected wounds by *Clostridium tetani*.
- There are four clinical forms of tetanus: generalized, neonatal, localized, and cephalic.

EPIDEMIOLOGY

- Tetanus remains a problem in certain countries but is rare in countries with widespread immunization (in the United States <40 cases/year).
- Rare cases have been reported in patients with protective levels of antitetanus antibodies.
- Generalized tetanus is the most common form of disease.
- Neonatal tetanus is rare in the United States but is seen in countries in which mothers are not immunized and nonsterile care of the umbilical cord is practiced.

RISK FACTORS

- Inadequate immunization
- Neonate born to unimmunized mother
- Elderly with declining immune status
- Injection drug use
- Chronic wounds
- Acute traumatic injury
- Foreign bodies
- Nonsterile delivery conditions and practice of applying mud or feces to umbilical cord

GENERAL PREVENTION

- All wounds should be cleaned with soap and water and foreign bodies should be removed.
- Universal immunization with tetanus toxoid (for details and information on catch-up schedules, refer to CDC Web site)
- Tetanus postexposure prophylaxis should be initiated at the time of injury:
  - For clean minor wounds:
    - If patient has had ≥3 prior doses of tetanus toxoid (DTaP, Tdap, or Td) and it has been <10 years since the last dose, no prophylaxis is indicated; if it has been ≥10 years since last dose, give tetanus toxoid.
    - If patient has had <3 prior doses of tetanus toxoids, give tetanus toxoid.
  - For all other wounds:
    - If patient has had ≥3 prior doses of tetanus toxoid and it has been <5 years since the last dose, no prophylaxis is indicated; if it has been ≥5 years since the last dose, give tetanus toxoid.
    - Patients with <3 prior doses of tetanus toxoid should receive tetanus immune globulin (TIG) and tetanus toxoid at separate sites.
    - Patients with HIV or severe immunodeficiency should receive TIG regardless of prior immunization history.
  - In neonates or infants <6 months of age who have not received 3 doses of DTaP, the decision to use TIG should be based on mother's tetanus immunization status; if unknown or inadequate, should give TIG
  - Type of tetanus toxoid to use for prophylaxis:
    - For children <7 years old, use DTaP; if pertussis vaccine is contraindicated, use DT.
    - For a child 7–10 years old, use Tdap.
    - For an adolescent 11–18 years old who has not received Tdap, use Tdap; for those who have received Tdap or for those whom pertussis is contraindicated, use Td.
  - TIG dose is 250 U IM (regardless of age or weight); if TIG is unavailable, use IV immunoglobulin (IVIG) or tetanus antitoxin (TAT).
    - Because TAT is equine in origin, test patient for sensitivity prior to use.
    - TAT is no longer available in the United States.

PATHOPHYSIOLOGY

- *C. tetani* produces tetanospasmin, a powerful metalloprotease neurotoxin.
- Tetanospasmin can be absorbed directly into skeletal muscles adjacent to the injury.
- Tetanospasmin can travel to the CNS via retrograde axonal transport through peripheral nerves or via lymphocytes.
  - In the CNS, tetanospasmin prevents the release of gamma-aminobutyric acid (GABA) and glycine in inhibitory nerve terminals, resulting in sustained excitatory discharges (motor spasms and increased muscle tone) and autonomic instability; tetanospasmin does not directly affect cognitive processes.
  - In the peripheral nervous system, tetanospasmin may block inhibitory impulses to motor neurons.
  - Loss of regulation of adrenal catecholamine release precipitates tachycardia, hypertension, and sweating.
- Infection does not confer immunity, and all patients need to be immunized during recovery.

ETIOLOGY

- Tetanus is caused by *C. tetani*, a spore-forming, anaerobic Gram-positive bacillus.
- *C. tetani* is found in soil, animal and human feces, house dust, and salt and fresh water.
- Under anaerobic conditions, spores become vegetative and produce tetanospasmin; anaerobic conditions in wounds are promoted by extensive necrosis, foreign bodies, or other suppurative infections.

DIAGNOSIS

HISTORY

- Incubation period is 3–21 days (usually 10 days) but varies, as inoculations distal to CNS are associated with longer incubation periods.
- Generalized tetanus
  - "Lockjaw" or trismus is initial symptom in 50–75% of cases.
  - Other early complaints include dysphagia, neck pain and stiffness, stiffness and pain in other muscle groups, urinary retention, restlessness, irritability, and headache.
  - More muscle groups involved as disease progresses
  - Noise, light, touch, and other stimuli can trigger painful spasms.
- Neonatal tetanus (generalized tetanus during neonatal period)
  - Occurs following vaginal delivery to unimmunized mothers
  - Usually due to umbilical stump infections
  - Typically presents at around 1 week of life with irritability and poor feeding but progresses rapidly to generalized tetanic spasms
- Local tetanus
  - Painful muscle contractions and stiffness limited to the area near the wound
  - Can persist for several weeks
  - Can progress to generalized tetanus
- Cephalic tetanus (local tetanus of head/neck affecting cranial nerves)
  - Caused by *C. tetani* infections of head/neck including chronic infections of the head/neck (e.g., chronic otitis media)
  - Unlike generalized tetanus, flaccid CN palsies (especially CN VII) predominate; trismus may develop, however; if trismus is absent, could be confused with Bell palsy due to other etiologies

PHYSICAL EXAM

- Vital sign abnormalities
  - Severe, labile episodes of hypertension and tachycardia; hypotension is a late feature.
  - Initially, patients are afebrile but may develop hyperthermia with sustained contractions or from superinfections.
- Trismus is often initial presenting sign.
- Persistent trismus causes *risus sardonicus*, wrinkling of the forehead, and distortion of the eyebrows and the corners of the mouth.
- With disease progression, other muscle groups develop tetanic contractions and spasms:
  - Can lead to a severe opisthotonic posture
  - Can mimic seizures
  - Can be extremely painful
  - Can be associated with laryngospasm and tetany of respiratory musculature
  - The anxiety and pain associated with these spasms may precipitate additional spasms.
- Sweating can occur from autonomic instability.
- Normal mental status is the norm.
- In cephalic tetanus, CN palsies can be seen.
  - Look for underlying wounds or chronic infections of the face, scalp, neck, or ear.

DIAGNOSTIC TESTS & INTERPRETATION

Diagnostic Procedures/Other

- Lab tests often yield little information; WBC is usually normal or mildly elevated and CSF studies are unremarkable, but serum calcium levels may help exclude hypocalcemic tetany.
- Gram stain and anaerobic wound cultures yield *C. tetani* in <1/3 of cases.
- Presence of protective tetanus antibody titer does not exclude possibility of disease.
- EEG and EMG findings are nonspecific.

DIFFERENTIAL DIAGNOSIS

- Infections
  - Dental infections, retropharyngeal and peritonsillar abscesses, poliomyelitis, viral encephalitis, and meningoencephalitis may present with trismus and/or CN findings.
- Toxins and medications
  - Dystonic reactions to phenothiazine medications may resemble tetanus.
  - Strychnine poisoning may mimic generalized tetanus.
  - Malignant neuroleptic syndrome causes increased muscular rigidity resembling tetanic spasms.
- Metabolic
  - Hypocalcemic tetany is usually not as severe as that seen in tetanus.
- Stiff-man syndrome can result in fluctuating tonic contractions resembling tetanic spasms.
- Bell palsy may resemble cephalic tetanus.

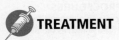

TREATMENT

MEDICATION

First Line

- Neutralization of unbound neurotoxin:
  - Human TIG 3,000–6,000 U IM as a single dose; part of the dose may be infiltrated around the wound.
  - Administer prior to antibiotics and wound manipulation.
- Tetanus toxoid should be administered IM at a site contralateral to where TIG is given.
- Antibiotics can decrease burden of vegetative *C. tetani* that produce tetanospasmin:
  - First line: metronidazole 30 mg/kg/24 h PO or IV in 4–6 divided doses; maximum 4 g/24 h
  - Alternative: parenteral penicillin G 1–200,000 U/kg/24 h IV in 4–6 divided doses; maximum 12,000,000 U/24 h
  - Treat for 10–14 days
  - Cephalosporins are not effective.
- Sedation and muscle relaxation
  - Diazepam 0.1–0.2 mg/kg IV q4–6h
  - Phenothiazines, especially chlorpromazine, may be helpful.
  - Titrate sedation to desired effect and monitor for respiratory depression.
- Nondepolarizing neuromuscular blockade and mechanical ventilation:
  - Use if spasms cannot be adequately controlled or if spasm of airway and respiratory musculature compromises ventilation:
  - Vecuronium 0.08–0.1 mg/kg IV followed by continuous infusion or hourly dosing
  - Avoid succinylcholine due to increased risk of hyperkalemia and arrhythmia.
- Management of autonomic dysfunction
  - Beta-blockers (e.g., labetalol 0.4–1 mg/kg/h) can control hypertension or arrhythmias.
  - Magnesium sulfate can significantly reduce cardiovascular instability and act as an adjunctive agent to control muscle spasms.

Second Line

If TIG is not available:

- IVIG 200–400 mg/kg may be used (not FDA approved for this use)
- TAT can be given in doses of 1,500–3,000 U IM or IV (to achieve a serum concentration of 0.1 IU/mL) but only after a negative skin test or desensitization:
  - TAT is not available in the United States.
  - Anaphylactic reactions can occur with varying severity in up to 20% of patients.

ADDITIONAL TREATMENT

General Measures

- Tetanus is not a transmissible disease.
- Keep patient in a quiet, darkened room with minimum stimulus.
- Monitor cardiac and respiratory status closely.
- Be prepared to perform a tracheotomy to prevent fatal laryngospasm.
- Monitor for and treat urinary retention and constipation.
- Parenteral nutrition is usually required to maintain adequate nutrition and hydration.
- Monitor for and correct electrolyte abnormalities, especially hyperkalemia.

SURGERY/OTHER PROCEDURES

Aggressive surgical debridement of wounds and removal of foreign bodies is critical.

INPATIENT CONSIDERATIONS

Initial stabilization

- Prompt recognition of clinical signs of tetanus and initiation of emergency care are crucial.
- All suspected cases of tetanus should be rapidly transferred to a tertiary care center capable of providing ventilatory and cardiovascular support in an intensive care setting.
- In the emergency department, treatment with TIG should be initiated to neutralize unbound neurotoxin; however, supportive care including aggressive airway management, ventilatory support, and pharmacologic interventions (sedation, muscle relaxation) are also critical to ameliorate the effects of bound neurotoxin.

ONGOING CARE

PROGNOSIS

- Signs and symptoms usually progress for ~1 week, then plateau for ~1 week, and gradually improve over the next 2–6 weeks.
- Overall mortality rates have decreased with advances in the ability to provide respiratory support in an intensive care setting.
- Mortality rates vary from 1–18% for localized tetanus, 15–30% for cephalic tetanus, 45–55% for generalized tetanus, to 50–100% for neonatal tetanus.
- Children and young adults have a better prognosis than older individuals or neonates.
- A more rapid onset and progression of disease from trismus to generalized spasms is associated with a more severe course.
- In the absence of complications, survivors usually recover fully without sequelae.

COMPLICATIONS

- Most complications are related to the severe tetanic muscle contractions:
  - Rhabdomyolysis and hyperkalemia
  - Vertebral body and other fractures
  - Muscle hemorrhages
- Respiratory failure from spasms of the upper airway or diaphragm is the most common cause of death in acute phase, whereas arrhythmia and myocardial infarction are most common cause of death later in disease.
- Cerebrovascular hemorrhages may be seen in rare cases, especially in neonatal tetanus.
- Pneumonia, including aspiration, can occur.

ADDITIONAL READING

- Brook I. Tetanus in children. *Pediatr Emerg Care*. 2004;20(1):48–51.
- Hassel B. Tetanus: pathophysiology, treatment, and the possibility of using botulinum toxin against tetanus-induced rigidity and spasms. *Toxins*. 2013; 5(1):73–83.
- Rhee P, Nunley MK, Demetriades D, et al. Tetanus and trauma: a review and recommendations. *J Trauma*. 2005;58(5):1082–1088.
- Thwaites CL, Farrar JJ. Preventing and treating tetanus. *BMJ*. 2003;326(7381):117–118.

CODES

ICD10

- A35 Other tetanus
- A33 Tetanus neonatorum

FAQ

- Q: What types of wounds are tetanus-prone?
- A: Punctures, avulsion wounds, crush injuries, burns, wounds from frostbite or missiles, and wounds contaminated with saliva, soil, or feces

T

TETRALOGY OF FALLOT

Aarti Dalal • Christopher Petit

BASICS

DESCRIPTION

Anatomic hallmark is anterior malalignment of infundibular (outlet) septum which results in

- A large and unrestrictive ventricular septal defect (VSD)
- Various degrees of right ventricular outflow tract obstruction (RVOTO)
- Overriding aorta
- Right ventricular hypertrophy (RVH) secondary to exposure to systemic pressure

EPIDEMIOLOGY

- The most common cyanotic congenital heart disease
- 3.5–10% of all congenital heart disease

RISK FACTORS

Genetics

Some cases of tetralogy of Fallot are associated with a chromosome 22q11 microdeletion.

PATHOPHYSIOLOGY

- Severity of clinical signs and symptoms depends on the degree of RVOTO and related right-to-left shunt at the VSD.
- Physiology is a spectrum ranging from too little pulmonary blood flow due to severe RVOTO ("blue tet") to moderate pulmonary overcirculation ("pink tet").

COMMONLY ASSOCIATED CONDITIONS

- May be associated with other syndromes including trisomy 21, Alagille syndrome, fetal alcohol syndrome, and those involving a variety of limb abnormalities.
- Tetralogy of Fallot may also be associated with midline abdominal defects (e.g., omphalocele) as in the pentalogy of Cantrell.

DIAGNOSIS

SIGNS AND SYMPTOMS

- Heart murmur in the newborn period
- Various degrees of progressive cyanosis
- Paroxysmal cyanosis, especially when crying or during and after physical activity

PHYSICAL EXAM

- Cyanosis may be present at birth or may appear later during infancy or childhood as a result of progressive RVOTO.
- Normal S_1 and single loud S_2 secondary to a more anteriorly located aorta
- Systolic ejection murmur at left upper sternal border secondary to RVOTO

DIAGNOSTIC TESTS & INTERPRETATION

- Electrocardiography
  - Right axis deviation (+90–180 degrees)
  - RVH
- Chest radiograph
  - Right aortic arch (30%)
  - Decreased pulmonary vascular markings
  - Boot-shaped heart (*coeur en sabot*) with concave main pulmonary artery segment
- Echocardiogram
  - Anterior malalignment VSD
  - Presence of additional VSDs
  - Degree of infundibular stenosis
  - Presence of valvar pulmonary stenosis and/or branch pulmonary artery stenosis
  - Overriding aorta, arch sidedness
  - Coronary artery anatomy
- Cardiac catheterization
  - Generally not indicated unless there is concern regarding the branch pulmonary artery anatomy, coronary anatomy, or additional VSDs that need to be defined before surgery

DIFFERENTIAL DIAGNOSIS

- Tetralogy of Fallot should be considered in all infants with a heart murmur and/or various degrees of cyanosis as well as acyanotic infants or children with a history of hypercyanotic episodes.
- Other forms of cyanotic congenital heart disease should be considered, including the following:
  - Double outlet right ventricle (DORV),
  - Transposition of the great arteries (TGAs)
  - Pulmonary atresia with a VSD (PA-VSD).

TREATMENT

MEDICATION

- Hypercyanotic episodes ("tet spells")
  - The goal is to increase preload and promote pulmonary blood flow.
  - Knee-chest position
  - Intravenous fluid bolus
  - $NaHCO_3$
  - Oxygen
  - Morphine sulfate (0.1 mg/kg IV or IM)
  - Beta-blocker (esmolol infusion for immediate therapy, propranolol for long-term prophylaxis)
  - Phenylephrine (0.02 mg/kg IV)
  - Polycythemia: oral iron supplement to prevent iron deficiency and microcytosis
  - Subacute bacterial endocarditis (SBE) prophylaxis

SURGERY/OTHER PROCEDURES

- Palliative surgery: Blalock-Taussig systemic-to-pulmonary artery shunt (also known as the Blalock-Taussig-Thomas shunt)
- Corrective surgery: VSD patch closure and right ventricular outflow tract reconstruction

ONGOING CARE

PROGNOSIS

- 35-year survival is approximately 85%.
- More than 90% of children with tetralogy of Fallot are expected to survive to adulthood.
- Higher risk of adverse outcomes in patients with repair at age >3 years.
- There is a higher risk of developmental delay in children with tetralogy of Fallot (as with all congenital heart disease).
- Residual hemodynamic abnormalities are common:
  - Pulmonary insufficiency (with transannular patch repair)
  - Residual RVOTO
  - Right ventricular dysfunction in adulthood due to chronic volume overload
  - Left pulmonary artery stenosis is particularly common in tetralogy of Fallot.
  - Residual VSD
- Conduction abnormalities (e.g., complete heart block, atrial and ventricular tachyarrhythmias)
  - Incidence of sudden death is 2.5% per decade of follow-up and is generally attributed to ventricular arrhythmias
- The need for reintervention (pulmonary valve insertion) increases after the 2nd decade of life.
  - Right ventricular end-diastolic volume >150 mL/m^2, QRS > 180 ms, history of tachyarrhythmias, RVOTO, exercise intolerance, syncope
  - Surgical versus transcatheter intervention (Melody valve)

COMPLICATIONS

Preoperatively

- Paroxysmal hypoxic episodes (i.e., hypercyanotic episodes, also called tet spell)
- Bacterial endocarditis
- Cerebrovascular accident secondary to cyanosis, polycythemia, and microcytic anemia

Postoperatively

- Right ventricular dysfunction
- Ventricular arrhythmias
- Sudden death (ventricular arrhythmias and/or complete heart block)

ADDITIONAL READING

- Apitz C, Webb G, Redington A. Tetralogy of Fallot. *Lancet*. 2009;374(9699):1462–1471.
- Cobanoglu A, Schultz JM. Total correction of tetralogy of Fallot in the first year of life: late results. *Ann Thorac Surg*. 2005;74(1):133–138.
- Geva T. Indications for pulmonary valve replacement in repaired tetralogy of Fallot: the quest continues. *Circulation*. 2013;128(17):1855–1857.
- Hirsch JC, Bove EL. Tetralogy of Fallot. In: Mavroudis C, Backer CL, eds. *Pediatric Cardiac Surgery*. 3rd ed. Philadelphia: Mosby; 2003:383–397.
- Martinez RM, Ringewald J, Fontanet HL, et al. Management of adults with Tetralogy of Fallot. *Cardiol Young*. 2013;23(6):921–932.
- Murphy AM, Cameron DE. The Blalock-Taussig-Thomas collaboration. A model for medical progress. *JAMA*. 2008;300(3):328–330.
- Siwik ES. *Moss and Adams Heart Diseases in Infants, Children and Adolescents*. 5th ed. Baltimore: Williams & Wilkins; 2001:880–902.
- Walker WT, Temple IK, Gnanapragasam JP, et al. Quality of life after repair of tetralogy of Fallot. *Cardiol Young*. 2002;12(6):549–553.
- Warnes CA, Williams RG, Bashore TM, et al. ACC/AHA 2008 guidelines for the management of adults with congenital heart disease: a report of the American College of Cardiology/American Heart Association Task Force on Practice Guidelines (writing committee to develop guidelines on the management of adults with congenital heart disease). *Circulation*. 2008;118(23):e714–e833.

CODES

ICD10-CM

Q21.3 Tetralogy of Fallot

FAQ

- Q: What is the etiology of the tet spell?
- A: There is an increase in resistance to flow through the right ventricular outflow tract and/or pulmonary vascular bed that leads to a dramatic decrease in pulmonary blood flow and increased right-to-left shunt at the level of the VSD. Therefore, treatment should be aimed at increasing pulmonary blood flow either by decreasing pulmonary vascular resistance (e.g., oxygen, morphine), increasing systemic vascular resistance (e.g., knee-chest position, phenylephrine), or decreasing dynamic obstruction by decreasing heart rate and thus increasing right ventricular preload (e.g., beta-blockers).
- Q: When is an optimal time for surgical repair of tetralogy of Fallot?
- A: Surgical correction should be guided by symptoms. Progressive hypoxemia or recurrent tet spells indicate a need for surgical intervention. A "pink tet" can be referred for elective repair in early infancy (3–6 months) and before the end of the 1st year of life.

THALASSEMIA

Irina Pateva • Peter de Blank

BASICS

DESCRIPTION

- Thalassemia syndromes are hereditary microcytic anemias that result from mutations that quantitatively reduce globin synthesis.
- Normal hemoglobin is a tetramer of 2 α and 2 β chains:
  - α-Thalassemia: reduced or absent α-globin production
  - β-Thalassemia: reduced or absent β-globin production

GENERAL PREVENTION

Thalassemia can be prevented by identifying and counseling potential parents who can have children with thalassemia. Diagnosis can be made in early pregnancy by chorionic villus sampling.

EPIDEMIOLOGY

- α-Thalassemia: predominantly in Chinese subcontinent, Malaysia, Indochina, and Africa and in African Americans
- β-Thalassemia: Mediterranean countries, Africa, India, Pakistan, Middle East, and China

Genetics

- α-Thalassemia
  - Normally, there are 4 α-globin genes, 2 on each chromosome 16.
  - Most mutations in α-thalassemia are large deletions.
  - Deletions may be in *trans* conformation (1 deletion on each chromosome, common in African Americans) or *cis* conformation (2 genes deleted on same chromosome, common in Asians).
  - Hemoglobin Constant Spring is an α-globin gene mutation caused by a point mutation that reduces or eliminates production of α-globin, leading to a more severe phenotype.
  - The 4 α-thalassemia syndromes reflect the inheritance of molecular defects affecting the output of 1, 2, 3, or 4 α genes.
- β-Thalassemia
  - Normally, there are 2 β-globin genes, 1 on each chromosome 11.
  - Most mutations in β-thalassemia are point mutations.
  - Many mutations abolish the expression completely (β^0), whereas others variably decrease quantitative expression (β^+).
  - Heterozygous state for β-globin mutation produces β-thalassemia trait.
  - Homozygous state produces β-thalassemia major or β-thalassemia intermedia.
  - NOTE: Rare dominant β-thalassemia mutations exist, causing ineffective erythropoiesis with a single mutation (due to creation of unstable β-globin variants).

Genotype	Name	Degree of anemia
α-thalassemia		
$\alpha\alpha$ / α –	Silent carrier	Asymptomatic
α–/α– or $\alpha\alpha$/– –	α-thalassemia trait	Asymptomatic
α –/– –	α-thalassemia intermedia, HbH disease	Moderate to severe
– –/– –	α-thalassemia major	Hydrops fetalis
β-thalassemia		
$\beta/\beta+$ or β/β^0	β-thalassemia trait	Asymptomatic
β/β^0 or $\beta+/\beta+$	β-thalassemia intermedia	Variable, intermittent, or chronic transfusions
$\beta^0/\beta+$ or β^0/β^0	β-thalassemia major	Severe, chronic transfusions

PATHOPHYSIOLOGY

- Decrease in either α- or β-globin synthesis leads to fewer completed α_2–β_2 tetramers produced per RBC, which results in a decrease in intracellular hemoglobin and microcytosis.
- Unpaired globin chains precipitate, resulting in apoptosis of red cell precursors (ineffective erythropoiesis) and damage to the RBC membrane leading to hemolysis.
- Ineffective erythropoiesis causes hepatosplenomegaly and osseous changes.
- The erythrocyte's lifespan is shortened by hemolysis and splenic trapping.
- Degree of anemia varies depending on the specific gene defect.
- Chronic transfusion therapy and, to a lesser degree, increased absorption of dietary iron in thalassemia major lead to iron accumulation.
- Increased absorption of dietary iron and intermittent transfusions in thalassemia intermedia lead to iron accumulation.
- Iron overload leads to cardiac arrhythmias and congestive heart failure (CHF) that can be fatal, liver inflammation and fibrosis, and endocrinopathies (e.g., diabetes mellitus, hypothyroidism, gonadal failure, osteoporosis).

DIAGNOSIS

HISTORY

- Severe α-thalassemia (4 gene deletion) presents prenatally by ultrasound or at birth with hydrops fetalis and severe anemia.
- Severe β-thalassemia usually presents between 3 and 12 months old, as production of the normal fetal hemoglobin decreases.
- α-Thalassemia syndromes will present with microcytosis in infancy. Hemoglobin H disease may present later, with mild to moderate anemia on screening or after worsening hemolysis related to intercurrent infection.
- Mediterranean, African, or Asian ethnic backgrounds are common in patients with thalassemia.
- Familial history of anemia, long-term transfusions, recurrent iron therapy for presumed iron deficiency anemia, or splenectomy
- Newborn screening varies by state but can contribute to a presumptive diagnosis of α-thalassemia or β-thalassemia major. Abnormal patterns include presence of Hb Barts (consistent with α-thalassemia) or isolated HbF (consistent with β-thalassemia major). Extreme prematurity and previous blood transfusions can obscure results, and confirmatory testing is required.

PHYSICAL EXAM

- Pallor indicates anemia.
- Heart murmur: Flow murmurs are often heard in significant anemia. Patients with severe anemia may present with CHF.
- Variable degrees of icterus: Hemolysis leads to increased bilirubin production.
- Abnormal facies (frontal bossing and maxillary hyperplasia): facial bone expansion by hypertrophic marrow in poorly transfused patients with β-thalassemia
- Failure to thrive: Related to anemia and energy expended in ineffective erythropoiesis
- Variable degrees of hepatosplenomegaly (or CHF) due to extramedullary hematopoiesis

DIAGNOSTIC TESTS & INTERPRETATION

Lab

- CBC with RBC indices
  - Mean cell volume (MCV), mean cell hemoglobin (MCH), and mean cell hemoglobin concentration (MCHC) are all decreased in α- and β-thalassemia.
  - RBC volume distribution width (RDW) is usually normal.
  - Peripheral smear may reveal microcytosis, hypochromia, anisocytosis, poikilocytosis, target cells, nucleated RBCs, and/or polychromasia.
  - Hemoglobin 9–12 g/dL in α- or β-thalassemia trait
  - Hemoglobin usually 7–10 g/dL in HbH disease
  - Hemoglobin usually 7–10 g/dL in β-thalassemia intermedia
  - Hemoglobin $<$7 g/dL in thalassemia major (without transfusions)
- Reticulocyte count: usually mildly elevated in HbH and β-thalassemia intermedia and major
- Indirect bilirubin: may be elevated in severe thalassemia where there is significant red cell destruction

- Hemoglobin electrophoresis
  - α-Thalassemia trait (2 defective genes) will have 5–10% Hb Barts (a tetramer of 4 γ chains) at birth, which should be detected on the newborn's screen. This disappears in 1–2 months, after which time the electrophoresis will be normal in α-thalassemia trait.
  - β-Thalassemia trait: HbF 1–5%, HbA2 3.5–8%, remainder HbA. The elevated HbA2 will distinguish α- from β-thalassemia trait.
  - HbH disease (3 defective α genes): 5–30% HbH (β_4), remainder HbA
  - Hydrops fetalis (4 defective α genes): mainly Hb Barts(γ_4)
  - β-Thalassemia major (2 defective β genes): HbF 20–100%, HbA2 2–7%. In most cases, little or no HbA is detected, unless recently transfused.
- Iron studies, serum ferritin: useful to help distinguish thalassemia from iron deficiency
- Mentzer Index: MCV/RBC <13 is more likely thalassemia, >13 more likely iron deficiency

DIFFERENTIAL DIAGNOSIS

- Iron deficiency anemia can be distinguished with iron studies.
- Anemia of chronic inflammation (can be distinguished with soluble transferrin receptor assay)
- Lead poisoning

TREATMENT

- Silent carriers (single α gene deletion) and α- and β-thalassemia trait
  - Genetic counseling only
  - Distinguish from iron deficiency microcytosis to avoid excess iron supplementation
- For HbH disease:
  - Folic acid daily
  - Transfusions whenever necessary (aplastic episode, infection)
  - Splenectomy if with evidence of hypersplenism
  - Cholecystectomy if necessary
- For β-thalassemia intermedia:
  - Folic acid daily
  - No iron supplements
  - Transfusions whenever necessary (aplastic episode, infection, acute complication)
  - Splenectomy is less commonly performed due to increased risk of thrombosis and pulmonary hypertension.
  - Cholecystectomy if necessary
  - HbF-inducing agents such as hydroxyurea may be beneficial.
  - Monitoring and treatment of iron overload
- β-Thalassemia major
  - Stem cell transplantation (umbilical cord blood or bone marrow) using histocompatible sibling donor can cure the disease and is being used more frequently.
  - Regular transfusions of RBCs every 3–4 weeks to maintain hemoglobin at 9–10 g/dL
  - Chelation therapy: It is important to balance the treatment of iron overload with the dangers of overchelation (toxicity to ears, eyes, bone).
  - Chelation options include the following:
    - Deferoxamine (SC or IV infusion over 8–24 hours)
    - Deferasirox (once daily PO chelator). Side effects include GI discomfort, rash, renal failure +/− proteinuria, hepatic failure
    - Deferiprone (t.i.d. PO chelator), FDA approved for iron overload in thalassemia syndromes. Especially useful for cardiac iron removal. Side effects include arthropathy, GI upset, and agranulocytosis.
  - Folic acid daily
  - Penicillin V potassium oral prophylaxis (125–250 mg b.i.d.) for splenectomized patients
  - *Pneumococcus*, *Meningococcus*, and *Haemophilus influenzae* vaccines before splenectomy and annual influenza A vaccination
  - Cholecystectomy if indicated
  - No iron supplements
  - Genetic counseling for those with any thalassemia syndrome

ALERT

Thalassemia trait is often treated incorrectly as presumptive iron deficiency anemia. Iron studies should be performed to confirm the diagnosis if there is no improvement in hemoglobin level after a few weeks of iron therapy.

ONGOING CARE

For patients with thalassemia major and intermedia:

- Serum ferritin, blood chemistries, and liver function tests should be monitored.
- Annual monitoring for cardiac complications (echocardiogram, EKG) and endocrine function is recommended.
- Liver iron quantitation by biopsy, MRI, or other techniques are necessary intermittently to quantitate the status of iron overload accurately.
- Newer cardiac T_2* MRI techniques to assess the degree of cardiac iron loading, which correlates with risk of cardiac complications
- Annual audiologic and ophthalmologic screening is recommended for persons receiving chelation therapy (to monitor for chelator toxicity).
- Dual-energy x-ray absorptiometry (DEXA) scan or bone peripheral quantitative computed tomography (PQCT) annually

PROGNOSIS

- Life expectancy for patients with β-thalassemia major has improved over the years because of regular transfusions and chelation therapy.
- Bone marrow transplant from a histocompatible sibling donor may be curative.

COMPLICATIONS

Most complications occur in patients with β-thalassemia intermedia or major and can be divided into 2 categories:

- Complications related to anemia/ineffective erythropoiesis and hemolysis (seen mostly in thalassemia intermedia):
  - Skeletal abnormalities secondary to hyperplastic marrow
  - Osteopenia, osteoporosis, and fractures
  - Growth retardation
  - Extramedullary hematopoiesis
  - Leg ulcers
  - CHF owing to severe anemia
  - Thrombophilia, particularly in thalassemia intermedia after splenectomy
  - Hypercoagulability: DVT, PE
  - Gallstones from hemolysis
  - Pulmonary hypertension
  - Allo- or autoimmunization with RBC antibodies
- Complications of iron overload:
  - Cardiac abnormalities: pericarditis, arrhythmias, CHF
  - Hepatic abnormalities: cirrhosis and liver failure (onset usually after 2nd decade)
  - Endocrine disturbances: delayed puberty, growth retardation, diabetes mellitus, hypothyroidism, hypoparathyroidism
  - Infection: particularly *Yersinia* species

ADDITIONAL READING

- Higgs DR, Engel JD, Stamatoyannopoulos G. Thalassaemia. *Lancet*. 2012;379(9813):373–83.
- Olivieri NF, Brittenham GM. Management of the thalassemias. *Cold Spring Harb Perspect Med*. 2013;3(6):a011767.
- Peters M, Heijboer H, Smiers F, et al. Diagnosis and management of thalassaemia, *BMJ*. 2012;344:e228.
- Rachmilewitz EA, Giardina P. How I treat thalassemia. *Blood*. 2011;118(13):3479–3488.
- Rund D, Rachmilewitz E. Beta-thalassemia. *N Engl J Med*. 2005;353(11):1135–1146.

CODES

ICD10

- D56.9 Thalassemia, unspecified
- D56.0 Alpha thalassemia
- D56.1 Beta thalassemia

FAQ

- Q: Is prenatal testing available?
- A: Yes.
- Q: In a transfused patient, when does iron overload become a problem and when is chelation started?
- A: Usually after the age of 3–4 years.
- Q: At what age should monitoring for cardiac iron overload begin in β-thalassemia major?
- A: 6–10 years of age.

T

THORACIC INSUFFICIENCY SYNDROME

Stamatia Alexiou • Robert Campbell • Oscar H. Mayer

BASICS

DESCRIPTION

- Thoracic insufficiency syndrome (TIS) is the inability of the thorax to support normal respiration or lung growth.
- Patients are skeletally immature with varied anatomic deformities that often include the following:
  - Flail chest syndrome: rib absence due to a congenital malformation or chest wall tumor resection, rib instability in cerebrocostomandibular syndrome, and others
  - Constrictive chest wall syndrome, including rib fusion and scoliosis: VACTERL association, chest wall scarring from radiation treatment, windswept deformity of the chest from progressive scoliosis, and others
  - Hypoplastic thorax syndrome including Jeune syndrome, Ellis–van Creveld syndrome, Jarcho-Levin syndrome, or spondylothoracic dysplasia (STD)
  - Scoliosis (without rib anomaly) or neuromuscular scoliosis
- The recognizable anatomic abnormalities often occur before respiratory insufficiency, with patients compensating for low lung volumes and poor respiratory mechanics by increasing their respiratory rate.
- Subsequently decreased activity and chronic respiratory insufficiency

PATHOPHYSIOLOGY

- The thorax is the respiratory pump, requiring adequate diaphragm (abdominal) and chest wall movement. Limitation in resting lung volume (functional residual capacity [FRC]) and/or the ability of the rib cage to expand during respiration can significantly alter respiratory function and cause TIS.
- The window of rapid lung growth and alveolar development is during the first 3 years of life.
  - Although alveolar development is felt to continue up until 5 or 8 years of age, recent evidence suggests that it can occur through childhood and adolescence.
  - Without concurrent thoracic growth, however, the lung cannot grow normally.
- Growth of the thoracic pump is also necessary so that the respiratory system can continue to meet a patient's metabolic demands.
  - Thoracic spinal height (TSH) directly contributes to thoracic volume and lung volume.
  - At birth, the TSH is 13 cm normally, then during the first 5 years of life, thoracic spinal growth is 1.4 cm/year, 0.6 cm/year from 5 to 10 years, and 1.2 cm/year from 10 to 18 years of age.
  - A thoracic length of 22 cm at skeletal maturity, the normal TSH of a 10-year-old, appears to be the minimum height necessary for normal respiration.
- Complex scoliosis with spinal rotation and lordosis into the convex hemithorax, the "windswept" deformity of the thorax, can further restrict lung volume.
- In neuromuscular disorders, unilateral caudal rotation of the ribs, the "collapsing parasol deformity," typically occurs on the convex side of the scoliosis and may also severely narrow the thorax, worsen thoracic mechanics, and further increase work of breathing.

ETIOLOGY

- The etiologies of TIS can be grouped into unilateral or bilateral volume depletion deformities (VDDs) of the thorax that reduce the volume available for the lungs in certain subsets of patients with rare syndromes. This causes primary TIS or deformity of the chest from scoliosis.
  - Type I: absent ribs and scoliosis
  - Type II: fused ribs and scoliosis
  - Type III: hypoplastic thorax
  - Type IIIa: foreshortening (Jarcho-Levin)
  - Type IIIb: narrowed (Jeune)
- In addition, progressive congenital scoliosis without rib anomalies can result in TIS from a variant of type II VDD of the thorax.
- Type IIIB VDD of the thorax can also develop in neurogenic scoliosis, as in spinal muscular atrophy with marked intercostal muscle weakness.
- Spinal deformity, such as lumbar kyphosis in spina bifida, collapses the torso into the pelvis, raising abdominal pressure blocking diaphragm excursion, and causing secondary TIS.

COMMONLY ASSOCIATED CONDITIONS

- Congenital renal abnormalities can occur in 25–30% of congenital scoliosis.
- Cervical spine abnormalities, causing stenosis and proximal instability
- Spinal cord abnormalities, including spinal cord syrinx and tethered cord, which are especially prevalent in meningomyelocele
- Jeune syndrome
  - Congenital renal abnormalities
  - Hepatic fibrosis
  - Cervical spinal stenosis in 60% of cases
  - Retinal dystrophy
- Ellis–van Creveld syndrome: tracheomalacia
- STD: congenital diaphragmatic hernia
- Cerebrocostomandibular syndrome, Pierre Robin sequence: micrognathia
- Severe tracheal compression and narrowing can occur in advanced scoliosis or severe anteroposterior narrowing.

DIAGNOSIS

HISTORY

- Prenatal ultrasound showing a hypoplastic thorax
- Onset of clinical scoliosis
- Onset of respiratory symptoms:
  - Relative exertional intolerance
  - Ineffective cough resulting in recurrent respiratory infections
  - Need for supplemental oxygen or noninvasive ventilatory support (bilevel positive airway pressure [BLPAP] or continuous positive airway pressure [CPAP])
- Progression of the spinal or chest wall deformity
- Signs and symptoms:
  - Exertional limitation relative to age and gross motor capability
  - Recurrent respiratory illnesses
  - Balance problems
  - Back pain

PHYSICAL EXAM

- Comprehensive respiratory examination:
  - Assessment of work of breathing including accessory muscle use and thoracoabdominal asynchrony
  - Qualitative assessment of chest wall compliance and motion
  - Symmetry of aeration during auscultation
- Thoracic circumference is usually found to be <75% of head circumference at birth.
- Thumb excursion test: The palms of each hand are loosely positioned posteriorly over each side of the chest with the thumbs aligned on either side of the spinal column, and relative excursion is assessed by the amount of lateral thumb movement.
- Assessment for rib hump by having the patient bend forward while standing upright.
- Measure of liver size to evaluate for hepatomegaly and possible cor pulmonale

DIAGNOSTIC TESTS & INTERPRETATION

Lab

- Serum bicarbonate as an indirect assessment for chronic hypoventilation
- Arterial blood gas if there is a concern for acute respiratory failure
- Liver function testing to assess for coincident liver failure
- Brain-type natriuretic peptide to help assess for progressive heart strain or failure
- Genetic testing as indicated based on suspected underlying condition

Imaging
- Standing anteroposterior and lateral radiographs to establish severity of scoliosis in the sagittal and coronal planes; bending films to establish the flexibility of the curve
- Chest CT scan with 5-mm cuts noncontrast with optimal pediatric settings to minimize radiation, with spinal and chest wall reconstruction to assess 3-dimensional anatomy
- MRI of spine and spinal cord to look for spinal cord abnormality
- Dynamic MRI to assess motion of chest wall, diaphragm, and abdomen
- Additional radiologic testing may be employed in certain cases (e.g., ventilation–perfusion scan of the lungs to quantify right vs. left functional perfusion asymmetry)
- Echocardiogram to evaluate for cor pulmonale and pulmonary hypertension

Diagnostic Procedures/Other
- Pulmonary assessment: baseline and subsequent pulmonary function testing at each clinic visit
  - Dynamic lung volumes and flows
    - Forced vital capacity (FVC)
    - Timed expiratory volume (forced expiratory volume in 0.5 or 1 second) and the ratio to FVC
    - Forced expiratory flow between 25% and 75% of vital capacity (FEF25–75%)
  - Static lung volume measurements
    - Total lung capacity (TLC), functional residual capacity (FRC), residual volume (RV), and RV/TLC
    - Maximal inspiratory (MIP) and maximal expiratory pressure (MEP) measurements
- Specialized measurements of respiratory system compliance (stiffness) and partitioned measurements of chest wall and lung compliance
- Pulse oximetry and end-tidal carbon dioxide measurement
- Overnight polysomnography to assess the degree of underlying respiratory insufficiency and need for supplemental oxygen or noninvasive ventilation
- Exercise testing adapted for the capabilities of the patient (6-minute walk test) can be used to assess for exertional limitation.
- If there is significant thoracospinal abnormality and certainly if there is other dysmorphology, a genetics assessment is very helpful to comprehensively assess for other comorbidities and help anticipate future problems.

TREATMENT

ADDITIONAL TREATMENT
General Measures
- Bracing and halo-gravity traction can be used as a temporizing procedure and at best has been shown to control some forms of scoliosis or partially improve, but not correct, scoliosis.
- Physical and occupational therapy

SURGERY/OTHER PROCEDURES
- The goal of surgical treatment is to stabilize the chest and spine in order to support normal growth until skeletal maturity is attained, at which point procedures such as a spinal fusion can be considered.
- Vertical expandable prosthetic titanium rib (VEPTR) expansion thoracoplasty techniques enable 5 types of acute thoracic reconstructions to handle each of the subtypes of TIS.
  - The procedure can be performed as early as 4–6 months of age to exploit the growth potential of the developing lungs and provide additional thoracic volume and compensatory lung growth.
  - After implantation to stabilize the initial thoracospinal reconstruction, it can then be expanded about every 6 months commensurate with patient growth until skeletal maturity.

ONGOING CARE

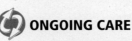

FOLLOW-UP RECOMMENDATIONS
- After TIS surgery, patients are followed with radiographs at regular intervals.
- Pulmonary follow-up should include careful assessment for respiratory insufficiency.
- Longitudinal measure of lung function and growth to demonstrate an improvement in respiratory status or lung function, or at the very least a decrease in the rate of decline, in the most severely affected patients

PROGNOSIS
- Prognosis will vary depending on the underlying cause of TIS, severity of respiratory insufficiency, and the age of the patient at surgery.
  - In infants and toddlers, however, there may be preservation of lung growth, but there has not been evidence to support regaining lung function that has been lost.
  - The expectation in infancy would be for growth preservation and an increase in lung volume above the preoperative value as a percent of predicted. There does appear to be an inverse relationship between the age of the patient at the time of surgery and the level of positive impact of VEPTR insertion on lung function.
  - In school-aged and older children, lung volume remains stable.
  - For older patients near skeletal maturity, the focus is chest wall reconstruction, spinal stabilization, and stabilization in pulmonary function.
- Jeune syndrome is one of the more severe forms of TIS, with 60–70% mortality in early infancy from respiratory failure. However, after VEPTR insertion, there has been a 50% decrease in mortality.
- Of those patients with TIS due to an STD, 47% die in infancy from respiratory complications and pulmonary hypertension. VEPTR treatment of STD remains controversial.
- Improved quality of life following VEPTR insertion

COMPLICATIONS
- In the immediate postoperative period—wound infection, skin slough, and bleeding
- Implant-related complication such as device breakage or dislodgement is uncommon.
- Decreased chest wall compliance
- Neurologic complications are rare.

T

ADDITIONAL READING

- Campbell RM Jr. VEPTR: past experience and the future of VEPTR principles. *Eur Spine J*. 2013;22(Suppl 2):S106–S117.
- Gadepalli SK, Hirschl RB, Tsai WC, et al. Vertical expandable prosthetic titanium rib device insertion: does it improve pulmonary function? *J Pediatr Surg*. 2011;46(1):77–80.
- Mayer OH. Management of thoracic insufficiency syndrome. *Curr Opin Pediatr*. 2009;21(3):333.

CODES

ICD10
- Q76.8 Other congenital malformations of bony thorax
- Q76.6 Other congenital malformations of ribs
- Q77.2 Short rib syndrome

THROMBOSIS

Char Witmer

BASICS

DESCRIPTION

Pathologic arterial or venous intravascular occlusion secondary to abnormal thrombus formation.

The following are common thrombotic events:

- Deep venous thrombosis (DVT): involves large systemic veins outside the central nervous system (CNS)
- Cerebral sinovenous thrombosis (CSVT): involves intracranial venous sinuses
- Ischemic stroke: CNS arterial occlusion with infarction of brain tissue
- Intracardiac thrombosis: mural, valvular, or foreign body associated
- Femoral artery thrombosis: can be associated with vessel catheterization
- Renal vein thrombosis: commonly in the neonatal period; may be unilateral or bilateral
- Myocardial infarction: Kawasaki disease, antiphospholipid antibody syndrome or with severe familial hypercholesterolemia
- Budd-Chiari syndrome: thrombosis of the hepatic vein
- Portal vein thrombosis

EPIDEMIOLOGY

- Incidence of venous thrombosis in children is estimated at 4.9 per 100,000 per year.
- Age distribution is bimodal; peak rates are found in the neonatal and adolescent age groups.
- Idiopathic thrombosis is rare in children.
- >90% of pediatric venous thrombosis is associated with additional risk factors.
- Central venous lines are the most common risk factor for venous thrombosis in children.

RISK FACTORS

- Neonatal
  - Prematurity
  - Maternal diabetes
  - Umbilical catheters or other central lines
  - Sepsis
  - Polycythemia
  - Perinatal asphyxia
- Malignancy/bone marrow disorders
  - Leukemia (hyperleukocytosis, acute promyelocytic leukemia)
  - Myeloproliferative disorders
  - Paroxysmal nocturnal hemoglobinuria
- Medications
  - L-Asparaginase
  - Oral contraceptives (with estrogen)
  - Heparin-induced thrombocytopenia
  - Steroids
- Anatomic
  - Indwelling catheters
  - Congenital heart disease
  - Prosthetic heart valves
  - Intracardiac baffles
  - Tumor compression
  - Atresia of the inferior vena cava
  - Thoracic outlet obstruction (Paget-Schroetter syndrome)
  - May-Thurner syndrome (compression of the left iliac vein by the right iliac artery)
- Miscellaneous
  - Infection
  - Trauma
  - Surgery
  - Obesity
  - Prolonged immobilization or paralysis
  - Dehydration
  - Antiphospholipid syndrome
  - Inherited prothrombotic state
- Risk factors/conditions specific for arterial disease
  - Kawasaki disease
  - Takayasu arteritis
  - Hyperlipidemia
  - Antiphospholipid syndrome

COMMONLY ASSOCIATED CONDITIONS

- Nephrotic syndrome
- Inflammatory disorders
- Liver disease
- Sickle cell disease
- Diabetes mellitus

DIAGNOSIS

DIFFERENTIAL DIAGNOSIS

- Other disorders that cause extremity swelling:
  - Low albumin
  - Obstruction of venous flow by a catheter without thrombus formation
  - Hemihypertrophy
- A high hematocrit in neonates can make the cerebral veins appear "dense" on a head CT and be misinterpreted as thrombosis.
- Arterial stroke mimics: complex migraine, demyelinating disease, metabolic disease, tumor

ALERT

- Normal ranges for coagulation tests are age dependent: Diagnosing an inherited deficiency in any of the anticoagulant proteins can be difficult in the neonatal period. Repeat testing at 6–12 months of age is necessary.
- Consumption can occur during acute thrombosis; therefore, low levels of the anticoagulant proteins must be repeated.
- Warfarin will decrease the levels of protein C, protein S, and clotting factors II, VII, IX, and X.

APPROACH TO THE PATIENT

- Phase 1
  - Perform complete history and physical exam.
  - Establish diagnosis using the appropriate radiographic study.
- Phase 2
  - Send initial laboratory studies (CBC, PT/aPTT, D-dimer, β-hCG testing in postmenarchal females).
  - If deemed safe, begin anticoagulation therapy with unfractionated heparin or low-molecular-weight heparin.
  - *Patients with life- or limb-threatening thrombosis may require thrombolysis.*
- Phase 3
  - If appropriate, consider sending a complete lab workup for a hypercoagulable state; outpatient anticoagulation; follow thrombosis radiologically.

HISTORY

- Presence of risk factors previously listed
- Family history of thrombosis
- Personal history of thrombosis
- Neonatal seizure: common and often the only presenting sign for CSVT or arterial ischemic stroke in neonates

PHYSICAL EXAM

- Extremity DVT: unilateral swelling/edema of a limb
- Thrombosis of the inferior vena cava: bilateral lower extremity edema of a limb
- Superior vena cava syndrome: plethoric, swollen head and neck
- Arterial thrombosis: pale extremity with decreased perfusion/pulses
- Renal vein thrombosis: abdominal mass in neonate with hematuria
- Pulmonary embolism: tachypnea, shallow respirations
- Peripheral venous collateral formation: superficial dilated cutaneous veins
- Postthrombotic syndrome: chronic discoloration (darkening) of the skin, ulcerations, pain, intermittent swelling

DIAGNOSTIC TESTS & INTERPRETATION

- The following tests can be used to investigate for a prothrombotic state:
  - Factor V Leiden mutation analysis
  - Prothrombin 20210A mutation analysis
  - Lupus anticoagulant screen (dilute Russell viper venom time, aPTT)
  - Anticardiolipin antibodies (IgG, IgM)
  - Anti-β2-glycoprotein antibodies (IgG, IgM)
  - Protein C activity
  - Protein S activity
  - Antithrombin activity
  - Homocysteine
  - Lipoprotein(a)
  - Factor VIII activity

Imaging

Radiologists should be consulted for choosing the best imaging study for diagnosis and follow-up.

- Contrast angiography: gold standard, but invasive and sometimes technically difficult to perform in small children
- Ultrasound: most commonly used imaging study because of noninvasiveness, absence of radiation, and ability to be performed at the bedside
- In the diagnosis of upper extremity–related DVT, often a combination of ultrasound and venography is necessary:
  - Compression ultrasound of the upper central veins may be impeded by the distal end of the clavicle.
  - Venography has poor sensitivity for diagnosing thrombosis of the internal jugular veins.
  - Recommended approach for diagnosis of an upper extremity thrombosis is to start with ultrasound and proceed to venography if the ultrasound is normal and there is a high clinical suspicion for thrombosis.
- Echocardiogram may be useful in evaluating atrial thrombi, which may result from central venous catheters.
- Pulmonary angiography, ventilation–perfusion scans, and spiral CT scans are the imaging studies used for the diagnosis of pulmonary embolism, although none of these have been studied in children.
- In patients with a pulmonary embolism, it is important to look for a source of thrombosis in the upper and lower extremities.
- Other diagnostic imaging options include CT or MRV:
  - Noninvasive
  - Sensitivity and specificity not known
  - May be helpful in evaluating proximal thrombosis
- For diagnosis of CSVT, the most sensitive imaging study is a brain MRI with venography.

TREATMENT

- Unfractionated heparin:
  - Given as a bolus followed by an infusion, adjusted to maintain the aPTT at 1.5–2.5 times baseline
  - Younger children require higher doses of heparin to achieve a therapeutic level secondary to physiologically decreased antithrombin levels.
- Low-molecular-weight heparin
  - More predictable dose response
  - Given subcutaneously twice a day
  - Equivalent in efficacy to unfractionated heparin in the acute management of uncomplicated DVT
  - Renal clearance
- Thrombolytic therapy
  - Recombinant tissue plasminogen activator
  - May be given systemically or locally
  - High risk of bleeding
- Warfarin
  - Oral anticoagulant
  - Initially started when a patient is already receiving a form of heparin. The heparin is discontinued when the warfarin is in the therapeutic range.
  - Warfarin is adjusted to maintain an international normalized ratio (INR) of 2–3 for treatment of DVT.
  - Used for outpatient management
- Aspirin
  - Beneficial in stroke and other arterial events
  - Irreversibly inhibits platelet function

GENERAL MEASURES

- Therapy for acute thrombosis and long-term management is individualized.
- Consult a pediatric hematologist or someone with expertise in pediatric anticoagulant therapy.

ONGOING CARE

COMPLICATIONS

- Inferior vena cava filters are used to prevent pulmonary embolism. There are limited pediatric studies. They should only be considered in the setting of a lower extremity DVT with a contraindication to anticoagulation (i.e., recent extensive surgery or active bleeding) or if a patient experiences a pulmonary embolism while on therapeutic anticoagulation. Temporary filters should be placed and removed as soon as possible, as they are a nidus for further thrombosis formation. The risk/benefit ratio needs to be considered individually.
- Vary depending on the location and severity of the thrombosis
- In acute DVT, pulmonary embolism is the most significant complication.
- Recurrent thrombosis and postthrombotic syndrome are common chronic complications.
- In arterial thromboembolic disease, the ischemic injury to the involved organ determines the acute and long-term complications.

ALERT

- Central venous catheter–related thrombosis may be subtle despite extensive damage to the venous system. Recurrent line infection, line occlusion, and prominent venous collaterals on the chest suggest upper extremity DVT. The long-term consequences of this are not known.
- Warfarin can cause purpura fulminans if started in a nonheparinized patient.

ADDITIONAL READING

- Goldenber N, Bernard T. Venous thromboembolism in children. *Pediatr Clin North Am*. 2008;55(2):305–322.
- Monagle P, Chan AK, Goldenberg NA, et al. Antithrombotic therapy in neonates and children: Antithrombotic therapy and prevention of thrombosis, 9th ed: American College of Chest Physicians Evidence-Based Clinical Practice Guidelines. *Chest*. 2012;141(2)(Suppl):e737s–e801s.
- Raffini L. Thrombolysis for intravascular thrombosis in neonates and children. *Curr Opin Pediatr*. 2009;21(1):9–14.
- Witmer CM, Ichord R. Crossing the blood brain barrier: clinical interactions between neurologists and hematologists in pediatrics—advances in childhood arterial ischemic stroke and cerebral venous thrombosis. *Curr Opin Pediatr*. 2010;22(1):20–27.

CODES

ICD10

- I82.90 Acute embolism and thrombosis of unspecified vein
- I82.409 Acute embolism and thrombosis of unspecified deep veins of unspecified lower extremity
- G08 Intracranial and intraspinal phlebitis and thrombophlebitis

FAQ

- Q: When is it appropriate to use low-molecular-weight heparin rather than unfractionated heparin?
- A: There are several advantages to low-molecular-weight heparin. The pharmacokinetics is predictable, and frequent monitoring is not necessary. It is administered subcutaneously, not intravenously. Alternatively, low-molecular-weight heparin cannot be completely reversed with protamine and it is renally cleared.
- Q: When is it appropriate to use thrombolytic therapy?
- A: If a thrombus is high risk (i.e., limb-threatening), thrombolytic therapy can be used. Intracranial bleeding, other active bleeding, and surgery within 7 days are contraindications to thrombolytic therapy. For arterial thrombotic events, thrombolytic therapy is often the treatment of choice because of the rapid resolution of the clot and restoration of blood flow.
- Q: What precautions should be taken for invasive procedures and for athletics when a patient is on anticoagulant therapy?
- A: Lumbar punctures, arterial punctures, and surgical procedures should be avoided. If they are necessary, then the anticoagulant should be reversed or held prior to the procedure. While on anticoagulation, participation in contact sports such as football, karate, and boxing is discouraged.

TICK FEVER

Gordon E. Schutze

BASICS

DESCRIPTION

- Tick-borne relapsing fever (TBRF) and Colorado tick fever (CTF) will be discussed in this chapter.
- TBRF is a vector-borne infection characterized by recurrent fevers caused by several species of spirochetes of the genus *Borrelia*. In the United States, the vector for TBRF is the soft-bodied tick of the genus *Ornithodoros*.
- CTF is a febrile, usually benign, systemic illness caused by coltivirus in the family Reoviridae and transmitted by a tick bite. Although *the primary* reservoir for infection is the *Dermacentor andersoni* tick (wood tick), the causative organism has been *isolated* from many other ticks.

EPIDEMIOLOGY

- TBRF
  - Reported in almost all western states up to and including Texas
  - Sites of high exposure include limestone caves and forested areas.
  - Most cases present during June through September; ~450 cases were reported in the United States between 1977 and 2000.
- CTF
  - Human infections typically occur in areas where *D. andersoni* is found: Western United States and southwestern Canada at elevations of 4,000–10,000 feet
  - Cases usually occur between May and June when adult ticks are most active.
  - There are only a very small number of cases reported annually the United States.
  - Infection is more common in males and the median age of those infected is 43 years, but 25% of cases occur in those younger than 20 years.
- Transfusion-related and laboratory-associated infection are rare but have been reported.

GENERAL PREVENTION

- Both of these infections can be prevented by avoidance or protection from the tick vector.
- Light-colored, long-sleeved shirts and pants should be worn when tick-infested areas cannot be avoided.
- Permethrin should be applied to clothing and diethyltoluamide (DEET) and picaridin applied to exposed skin to help repel ticks.
- Persons who enter endemic areas should inspect themselves and each other frequently for adherent ticks.
- Avoid rodent-infested homes in endemic areas. If necessary, rodent-nesting materials should be removed with protective gloves.
- Confirmed cases should be reported to health authorities so that control measures can be instituted.

PATHOPHYSIOLOGY

- TBRF
  - Ornithodoros ticks typically feed at night and for short periods.
  - When an Ornithodoros tick feeds on a natural host (e.g., squirrels, chipmunks, and rodents), *Borrelia* subsequently invade all tissues of the tick including the salivary glands. Ticks in the larval stage are unlikely to be infectious.
  - *Borrelia* is transmitted to humans when the tick takes a blood meal and then detaches itself. Transmission is possible within minutes of the start of a blood meal. After transmission, spirochetemia develops, resulting in systemic symptoms.
  - Between episodes of spirochetemia, organisms likely persist in the CNS, bone marrow, liver, and spleen.
  - Pathologic findings in humans include petechial hemorrhages on visceral surfaces, hepatosplenomegaly, and a histiocytic myocarditis.
- CTF
  - Ticks are infected during their larval stage when they feed on viremic, intermediate hosts such as chipmunks, ground squirrels, and porcupines.
  - Once infected, ticks remain infected for life (as long as 3 years).
  - Human infection typically takes place when the adult *D. andersoni* wood tick attaches and ingests a blood meal from an incidental human host.
  - CTF virus is thought to infect hematopoietic cells, causing leukopenia and prolonged viremia for up to 3–4 months.

ETIOLOGY

- TBRF is caused by several species of spirochetes in the genus *Borrelia*. *Borrelia hermsii*, *Borrelia turicatae* and *Borrelia parkeri* are the most common species found in the United States.
- CTF is caused by CTF virus, a double-stranded RNA coltivirus in the family Reoviridae.

DIAGNOSIS

HISTORY

- Both TBRF and CTF most commonly present with high fever, headache, myalgias, and chills. A thorough history documenting recent travel and a description of the fever curve are necessary to help direct the clinician to either diagnosis.
- TBRF
  - Fevers present after a mean incubation period of 5–7 days (range 4–18 days). Symptoms resolve after 3–6 days but then recur within 7 days. Relapses may be less severe than the initial episode with prolonged asymptomatic intervals. Average number of relapses is 3–5 in untreated patients.
  - Patients commonly complain of headache, myalgia, nausea, vomiting, arthralgias, and abdominal pain. Less commonly, patients are symptomatic with confusion, dry cough, diarrhea, photophobia, rash, dysuria, or hepatosplenomegaly.
  - Patients rarely are aware of a recent tick bite.
- CTF
  - CTF has a usual incubation period of 3–4 days (range 0–14 days):
    - In ~50% of patients, fever will present in a "saddleback" pattern. The fever persists for 2–3 days with resolution for 2–3 days. Fever then recurs and lasts for another 2–3 days. Some patients will have a 3rd febrile period.
    - Patients may complain of lethargy, photophobia, retro-orbital pain, and conjunctival injection.
    - Less commonly, patients will have gastrointestinal symptoms, pharyngitis, nuchal rigidity, and a rash.
    - Unlike TBRF, 90% of patients presenting with CTF will have a previous history of tick exposure.

PHYSICAL EXAM

The presentation for TBRF and CTF are varied. High fevers (39–41°C) are common to both. Additional findings for each may include the following:

- TBRF
  - Elevated pulse and BP are common.
  - Tender hepatosplenomegaly with jaundice
  - Nuchal rigidity suggesting meningitis.
  - Gallop on cardiac auscultation suggesting underlying myocarditis
  - A macular rash starting on the trunk that becomes generalized and or petechial in nature
  - Neurologic deficits are less common but can include delirium, cranial nerve deficits (7th or 8th nerve palsy), and visual impairment from iridocyclitis.
- CTF
  - A small, red painless papule may be seen.
  - A maculopapular rash with petechial lesions has been reported in ~10% of cases.
  - Pharyngitis is reported in 20% of cases.
  - Hepatosplenomegaly has been found in some patients.
  - Nuchal rigidity and delirium are rare but, if present, suggest meningitis or encephalitis.

DIAGNOSTIC TESTS & INTERPRETATION

- TBRF
  - The diagnosis can be readily made by identification of loosely coiled spirochetes on thick and thin smears of the peripheral blood. Blood samples taken at the time of fever have the highest yield.
  - Increased sensitivity can be obtained by examining acridine orange–stained preparations of dehemoglobinized thick smears or buffy coat preparations.

- The organism can only be cultured on special culture medium. Intraperitoneal inoculation of mice with the patient's blood can lead to spirochetemia in the mice.
- Multiple serologic antibody studies exist, including direct and indirect immunofluorescence, ELISA, and immunoblot analysis:
  - A 4-fold rise in titers between acute and convalescent studies is considered confirmatory.
  - These studies may have false-positive reactions in patients with prior spirochete infections such as Lyme disease.
- Polymerase chain reaction (PCR) analysis can be useful in identifying the causative organism but is not readily available.
- Other nonspecific laboratory findings may include leukocytosis, anemia, thrombocytopenia, unconjugated hyperbilirubinemia, elevated hepatic transaminases, and proteinuria.
- If myocarditis is present, an electrocardiogram can reveal abnormalities such as a prolonged corrected QT interval.
- In cases complicated by meningitis, the CSF will typically have moderately elevated protein and a mononuclear pleocytosis.

- CTF
  - Leukopenia is a hallmark of this illness.
  - Direct immunofluorescent examination of blood smears for intraerythrocytic viral antigen is a rapid approach to the diagnosis.
  - PCR testing and viral cultures are available in certain laboratories. PCR testing is the most sensitive and timely approach for diagnosing acute infection.
  - Various techniques (e.g., complement fixation, indirect immunofluorescence, EIA, and Western blot) have been used to establish a serologic diagnosis:
    - Serologic testing for antibody presence is not diagnostic in the acute phase because antibodies are slow to rise. Presence of a 4-fold rise in neutralizing antibody titers at >2 weeks after onset can be confirmatory.
    - Associated laboratory findings include leukopenia and thrombocytopenia.
- In patients with meningitis or encephalitis, CSF studies may also reveal elevated protein and a lymphocytic pleocytosis.

DIFFERENTIAL DIAGNOSIS

- TBRF and CTF are similar clinically. The presence of biphasic or relapsing fever along with a history of travel to an area where appropriate vectors are found are helpful clues in diagnosing either disease. Leukopenia and a history of a tick bite may differentiate CTF from TBRF. TBRF and CTF may be misdiagnosed as influenza or enteroviral infections, especially with the 1st febrile episode.
- Other infectious illnesses that may present with recurrent fevers include yellow fever, dengue fever, lymphocytic choriomeningitis, brucellosis, malaria, leptospirosis, rat bite fever, and chronic meningococcemia. The patient's travel history and animal exposure should help differentiate among some of these diagnoses.

TREATMENT

MEDICATION

- TBRF
  - The treatment of choice is oral tetracycline/doxycycline for 7–10 days. Children <8 years of age and pregnant women should receive erythromycin or penicillin.
  - Newer macrolides may be effective but are not routinely recommended.
  - In >50% of cases, treatment results in a Jarisch-Herxheimer reaction (severe fevers, rigors, diaphoresis, and hypotension) related to rapid clearing of the spirochetemia. Close observation, IV fluids, and good supportive care are important in treating possible reactions.
  - Some experts support the use of an initial single dose of oral penicillin V potassium (7.5 mg/kg) or IV penicillin G (10,000 U/kg given over 30 minutes) in patients presenting with systemic symptoms. It is thought that this initial dose of penicillin leads to gradual clearance of spirochetes, decreasing the risk of the Jarisch-Herxheimer reaction. These patients should then receive a 10-day course of tetracycline or erythromycin because penicillin has been associated with an increased rate of relapse.
  - Single-dose tetracycline or erythromycin has been successful for the treatment of louse-borne epidemic relapsing fever in Ethiopia.
- CTF
  - There is no specific therapy for patients with CTF, as the treatment is primarily supportive.

ONGOING CARE

PROGNOSIS

- TBRF
  - Generally responds rapidly to appropriate antibiotic therapy
  - Mortality in patients treated appropriately is thought to be <1%.
- CTF
  - Usually a self-limiting illness without sequelae
  - Death is rare but has been reported in children with generalized bleeding likely secondary to thrombocytopenia; thus, thrombocytopenia should be monitored closely.
  - Prolonged weakness may persist for ≥3 weeks and is more likely in those patients >30 years old.

COMPLICATIONS

- TBRF
  - May be associated with splenic rupture, diffuse histiocytic interstitial myocarditis, hepatitis, pneumonia, ARDS, and iridocyclitis
  - CNS complications include meningitis, meningoencephalitis, and focal deficits such as cranial nerve palsy.
  - In utero infection may result in fetal loss or severe neonatal infection.
- CTF
  - Complications are rare but most commonly occur in children.
  - May lead to aseptic meningitis, encephalitis, myocarditis, pneumonitis, hepatitis, hemorrhage, and epididymo-orchitis

ADDITIONAL READING

- Badger MS. Tick talk: unusually severe case of tick-borne relapsing fever with acute respiratory distress syndrome—case report and review of the literature. *Wilderness Environ Med*. 2008;19(4):280–286.
- Brackney MM, Marfin AA, Staples JE, et al. Epidemiology of Colorado tick fever in Montana, Utah, and Wyoming, 1995–2003. *Vector Borne Zoonotic Dis*. 2010;10(4):381–385.
- Cutler SJ. Relapsing fever—a forgotten disease revealed. *J Appl Microbiol*. 2010;108(4):1115–1122.
- Dworkin MS, Schwan TG, Anderson DE Jr, et al. Tick-borne relapsing fever. *Infect Dis Clin N Am*. 2008;22(3):449–468.
- Larsson C, Andersson M, Bergstrom S. Current issues in relapsing fever. *Curr Opin Infect Dis*. 2009;22(5):443–449.
- Romero JR, Simonsen KA. Powassan encephalitis and Colorado tick fever. *Infect Dis Clin North Am*. 2008;22(3):545–559.
- Roscoe C, Epperly T. Tick-borne relapsing fever. *Am Fam Physician*. 2005;72(10):2039–2044.

CODES

ICD10

- A68.1 Tick-borne relapsing fever
- A93.2 Colorado tick fever

FAQ

- Q: When should a clinician suspect tick fever?
- A: A history of recurring or relapsing fever in the appropriate epidemiologic setting (such as travel history to the western parts of the United States, summertime illness, history of tick exposure) should raise the possibility of a tick fever.

T

TICS

Rebecca K. Lehman

BASICS

DESCRIPTION

- A tic is a sudden, repetitive, stereotyped, involuntary movement (e.g., blinking, grimacing) or vocalization (e.g., throat clearing, sniffing). Tics can be further classified as simple (e.g., nose twitching, grunting) or complex (e.g., hand gestures, jumping, echolalia). Tics characteristically change in anatomic location, frequency, type, complexity, and severity over time, although each tic has a stable appearance from one occurrence to the next. Most individuals are able to suppress their tics for brief periods of time, and some endorse having premonitory sensory urges that precede their tics. Tics typically abate during sleep but can persist in some cases.
- *DSM-5* classification of tic disorders:
  - *Tourette syndrome (TS)*: Both ≥2 motor and ≥1 vocal tics have been present at some time, although not necessarily concurrently; tics have been present for >1 year since first tic onset (regardless of the duration of tic-free periods); onset <18 years
  - *Persistent (chronic) motor or vocal tic disorder*: ≥1 motor or vocal tics but not both; tics have been present for >1 year since first tic onset; onset <18 years
  - *Provisional tic disorder*: ≥1 motor and/or vocal tics; tics have been present for <1 year since first tic onset; onset <18 years
  - *Other specified tic disorder*: tics causing clinically significant distress or impairment but not meeting the full criteria for a tic disorder. Provider should specify the atypical feature(s), for example, "with onset after age 18 years."
  - *Unspecified tic disorder*: as above, but provider chooses *not* to specify the reason that full criteria for a tic disorder are not met (e.g., there is insufficient information to make a more specific diagnosis)
  - When there is evidence of an underlying organic etiology, a diagnosis of "other specified tic disorder" should be used.
- Pediatric autoimmune neuropsychiatric disorder associated with *Streptococcus* (PANDAS): a controversial entity first described in 1998. In theory, group A β-hemolytic streptococcal (GABHS) infection triggers antibodies that cross-react with the basal ganglia and cause obsessive-compulsive disorder (OCD) symptoms and/or tics in some individuals. The National Institute of Mental Health defines PANDAS as follows:
  - Presence of OCD and/or a tic disorder
  - Prepubertal onset
  - Sudden, explosive onset of symptoms and a course of dramatic exacerbations and remission
  - Temporal relationship between symptom onset and exacerbations and GABHS infections
  - Presence of neurologic abnormalities (hyperactivity, choreiform movements, tics) during exacerbations
  - These diagnostic criteria do not always prove helpful in distinguishing PANDAS from other "standard" tic disorders. The high incidence of GABHS infections and high prevalence of asymptomatic carriers make it difficult to prove a link between GABHS infection and tics.
- Other autoimmune neuropsychiatric conditions with less restrictive diagnostic criteria have been proposed, including Pediatric Acute-Onset Neuropsychiatric Syndrome (PANS) and Childhood Acute Neuropsychiatric Symptoms (CANS).

EPIDEMIOLOGY

- Described in almost all ethnic groups
- Affects males > females
- Typical onset is between ages 5 and 7 years.

Prevalence

- The prevalence of chronic tics and TS in school-age children is 3–6% and 0.1–1%, respectively.
- Transient tics occur in 20–25% of children.

RISK FACTORS

Genetics

No single gene has been associated with tics or TS; however, the family history is often positive for tics. The prevalence of TS in 1st-degree relatives is 10 times that in the general population.

GENERAL PREVENTION

Tics cannot be prevented, but educating patients, families, and school personnel about tics can minimize their impact. Aggressive management of comorbid conditions strongly influences patient outcomes.

PATHOPHYSIOLOGY

The pathophysiology underlying tics and TS is not completely understood but is thought to involve abnormal dopamine neurotransmission within the basal ganglia. Evidence also implicates problems with serotonin, norepinephrine, and acetylcholine.

ETIOLOGY

Theory: Environmental or hormonal perturbations trigger tics in genetically susceptible individuals.

COMMONLY ASSOCIATED CONDITIONS

- ~50% of children with chronic motor tics or TS meet diagnostic criteria for attention-deficit/hyperactivity disorder (ADHD), and ~50% have OCD or obsessive-compulsive traits.
- Anxiety, learning disabilities (LD), oppositional defiant disorder, conduct disorder, and rage episodes are also associated with TS.

DIAGNOSIS

The diagnosis of tics is clinical. Physical examination and ancillary studies are typically normal.

HISTORY

- Document a description of the patient's past and current tics, including age of onset, type, anatomic location(s), duration, number, frequency, complexity, severity, and exacerbating or alleviating factor(s).
- Determine the degree to which the tics are causing interference and/or impairment.
- Assess for commonly associated conditions.
- In prepubertal patients with severe, sudden-onset OCD symptoms and/or tics, inquire about recent GABHS infections.

PHYSICAL EXAM

Physical examination is usually normal. Tics may not be seen; thus, it may be necessary to depend on history. Having the child intentionally reproduce the sound(s) and/or movement(s) of concern and/or having the parents provide video can aid in differentiating tics from other movement disorders.

DIAGNOSTIC TESTS & INTERPRETATION

Lab

There is little evidence to support routine testing for GABHS in children suspected of having PANDAS. Throat cultures should be obtained in children with symptoms of pharyngitis.

Diagnostic Procedures/Other

Diagnosis depends largely on history. Diagnostic tests are unnecessary. Psychological testing may elucidate comorbid conditions (ADHD, OCD, LD).

DIFFERENTIAL DIAGNOSIS

- Certain simple tics (eye blinking, sniffing, throat clearing) may be mistaken for allergy symptoms, whereas complex tics may be mistaken for purposeful, voluntary movements.
- Stereotypies are patterned, episodic, repetitive, purposeless, rhythmic movements. The movements are constant in pattern and location, without variation over time.
- Chorea is characterized by rapid, random, purposeless movements that often have a "dance-like" quality. Unlike tics, chorea is not stereotyped.
- Dystonia is characterized by repetitive, sustained muscle contractions that cause abnormal postures and movements, often with a twisting quality. Dystonic tics result in sustained postures and can be difficult to distinguish from dystonia; however, the presence of a premonitory urge suggests the former diagnosis.
- Myoclonus is a sudden, brief, shock-like movement. It is not suppressible and is not associated with a premonitory sensation.

- Automatisms, seen in some forms of epilepsy, may look like tics but are neither associated with premonitory sensations nor under partial voluntary control. EEG is normal in children with tics but may be abnormal in those with seizures.
- Hemifacial spasm (HFS) is a rare condition that results in frequent, involuntary muscle contractions involving one side of the face. Early cases of HFS may be difficult to distinguish from motor tics, but HFS is limited to one side of the face, and the spasms last longer than tics.

TREATMENT

Many tics do not interfere with children's lives and therefore do not require specific treatment. Educating the child and family about tics is often sufficient. Clinical decisions must take comorbid symptoms into account, and treatments must target the most impairing symptoms first. The waxing and waning nature of tics confounds treatment; it may take weeks to identify whether an intervention is helping.

MEDICATION

- Mild/occasional tics: Medication is not needed.
- Moderate or severe: α-2 Agonist or dopamine antagonist may reduce severity/frequency.
- With OCD: Selective serotonin reuptake inhibitors can be helpful. Fluoxetine, fluvoxamine, and sertraline appear to be equally effective.
- With ADHD: α-2 Agonist may help hyperactivity/impulsivity. Consider addition of a stimulant if symptoms are refractory or if inattention is the primary complaint.
- PANDAS: As above. There is insufficient evidence to support the use of long-term antibiotics and/or immunomodulation.

First Line

- Clonidine and guanfacine are used off-label as 1st-line treatments for tics. Both are available in immediate- and extended-release forms.
  - Clonidine: Start 0.05 mg at bedtime. Increase by 0.05 mg/week to effect, side effects, or a maximum of 0.4 mg/day, divided 3 or 4 times/day. Available as a tablet and transdermal patch.
  - Guanfacine: Start 0.5 mg at bedtime. Increase by 0.5–1 mg/week to effect, side effects, or a maximum of 3 mg/day, divided twice a day.
- Sedation and orthostatic hypotension are common initial adverse effects, more so with clonidine than guanfacine.
- Avoid abrupt discontinuation, which can cause rebound hypertension.

Second Line

- Antipsychotic medications are considered 2nd-line treatments. Weight gain is common with all antipsychotic medications, but the atypical agents are generally preferred because they are better tolerated overall and are less likely to cause extrapyramidal side effects.
- Commonly used atypical agents include risperidone, aripiprazole, ziprasidone, and olanzapine.
- Typical antipsychotics (haloperidol, pimozide) are potent but are associated with troublesome side effects; therefore, they should only be used for those with refractory, disabling tics. Common side effects: sedation, weight gain, metabolic syndrome, and galactorrhea. Serious side effects: extrapyramidal reactions, neuroleptic malignant syndrome, and tardive dyskinesia.

ALERT

Poor metabolizers of pimozide may be at increased risk for QT prolongation and cardiac arrhythmias; therefore, the FDA has stated that CYP2D6 genotyping should be performed before exceeding 4 mg of pimozide in adults or 0.05 mg/kg/day in children and that the dose of pimozide should not be increased earlier than 14 days in patients who are known CYP2D6 poor metabolizers.

ADDITIONAL TREATMENT

General Measures

There is no evidence that lifestyle changes or restriction of activities modify the course of tic disorders.

ADDITIONAL THERAPIES

- A recent randomized controlled trial of children and adolescents with TS and chronic tic disorder demonstrated that a comprehensive behavioral intervention—consisting of awareness training, competing response training, relaxation training, and social support—resulted in greater improvement in tic severity than supportive therapy and education alone. The effect size of the intervention was on par with that of medication.
- Focal motor (or vocal) tics, especially those that are dystonic, may be treated with botulinum toxin injections to the affected muscles.

SURGERY/OTHER PROCEDURES

Recent experimental data have shown deep brain stimulation (DBS) as a potential treatment for adults with severe and refractory tics.

ONGOING CARE

DIET

There is no evidence that dietary modifications alter the course of tic disorders.

PATIENT EDUCATION

The Tourette Syndrome Association (www.tsa-usa.org) is a valuable resource for information. There are many local chapters.

PROGNOSIS

Although common, tics cause impairment in a minority of children. Peak severity occurs in preadolescence. Most patients have partial or complete resolution of tics as adults. Long-term outcome depends on associated comorbidities.

COMPLICATIONS

Tics can be emotionally distressing and can result in social disability. Injuries—due to complex tics, compulsions, impulsivity, inattention, and other factors—may be more common in patients with TS than in the general population. Chronic, repetitive, and forceful tics can cause musculoskeletal problems (e.g., cervical spine arthritis, disc herniation) or other neurologic problems (e.g., cervical myelopathy, stroke secondary to vertebral artery dissection).

ADDITIONAL READING

- Mink JW, Walkup J, Frey KA, et al. Patient selection and assessment recommendations for deep brain stimulation in Tourette syndrome. *Mov Disord*. 2006;21(11):1831–1838.
- Piacentini J, Woods DW, Scahill L, et al. Behavior therapy for children with Tourette disorder: a randomized controlled trial. *JAMA*. 2010;303(19):1929–1937.
- Shprecher D, Kurlan R. The management of tics. *Mov Disord*. 2009;24(1):15–24.
- Snider LA, Seligman LD, Ketchen BR, et al. Tics and problem behaviors in schoolchildren: prevalence, characterization, and associations. *Pediatrics*. 2002;110(2, Pt 1):331–336.
- Tourette's Syndrome Study Group. Treatment of ADHD in children with tics: a randomized controlled trial. *Neurology*. 2002;58(4):527–536.

CODES

ICD10

- F95.9 Tic disorder, unspecified
- F95.2 Tourette's disorder
- F95.0 Transient tic disorder

FAQ

- Q: Can a child with tics and ADHD be treated with stimulant medication?
- A: Although there have been concerns of stimulants making tics worse, there is no evidence that stimulants cause chronic tics. Furthermore, several recent studies have shown that treatment of ADHD with stimulants does not worsen tics and may lead to improvement.
- Q: Should mild tics be treated if they lead to teasing?
- A: The best approach is to educate the child, parents, and teacher about tics. The child can be armed with a response to questions, such as "Those are tics. They are just something I do, and I can't help it."

TOXIC ALCOHOLS

Richard Loffhagen • Robert J. Hoffman

BASICS

DESCRIPTION

- Toxic alcohols discussed here include ethylene glycol, isopropyl alcohol, and methanol.
- Ethylene glycol is a sweet, odorless, colorless liquid, commonly used as automobile antifreeze solution as well as for other uses.
- Isopropyl alcohol is used as rubbing alcohol, as well as in liquid soaps and for other uses.
- Methanol is wood alcohol used in windshield wiper fluid, Sterno, and other products.

GENERAL PREVENTION

Poison proofing homes and giving parents poison prevention advice is the most effective way to prevent toxic alcohol exposures in children.

RISK FACTORS

Toxicity via dermal absorption can occur in infants or young children with permeable skin.

PATHOPHYSIOLOGY

All toxic alcohols have direct effects as intoxicants. More importantly, ethylene glycol and methanol are metabolized to toxic by-products that result in severe morbidity or mortality.

- All toxic alcohols may result in altered mental status or coma similar to ethanol. CNS depression may result in respiratory depression requiring ventilatory support.
- Ethylene glycol is metabolized to oxalic acid and glycolic acid, ultimately forming calcium oxalate crystals, which may precipitate in the renal tubules and cause renal failure.
- Methanol is metabolized to formaldehyde and then formic acid, which may damage the retina and cause visual impairment or blindness.
- The metabolism of ethylene glycol and methanol to their toxic metabolites may be prevented by competitively inhibiting alcohol dehydrogenase with either fomepizole or ethanol.
- Therapy to inhibit alcohol dehydrogenase is used for ethylene glycol and methanol exposure.
- Isopropyl alcohol is metabolized to acetone.
- Inhalational absorption of isopropyl alcohol may rarely occur.

DIAGNOSIS

- Signs and symptoms:
  - Inebriation may occur after exposure.
  - Isopropyl alcohol may cause severe gastrointestinal irritation or hemorrhage.

HISTORY

- Typically, a history of exposure is available.
- In absence of this history, and osmolal gap or anion gap with metabolic acidemia is suggestive of toxic alcohol exposure.

PHYSICAL EXAM

- Tachycardia and hypotension are the most frequent vital sign abnormalities that occur.
- Hyperpnea or tachypnea often accompanies metabolic acidemia.
- Cardiovascular effects may include hypocalcemic QT prolongation and myocarditis.
- Neurologic abnormalities may include ataxia, CNS depression, coma, dysarthria, focal neurologic changes, hyporeflexia, hypotonia, nystagmus, or seizure.
- Gastrointestinal effects may include gastritis emesis, hematemesis, pain, or pancreatitis.
- Ophthalmologic findings may include blurred vision, diplopia, hazy vision, or nystagmus.
- Constricted visual fields, hyperemic optic disks with retinal edema, and transient or permanent blindness may result from methanol exposure.
- Hematuria, renal insufficiency, or renal failure may occur, particularly from ethylene glycol.
- Fluid and electrolyte abnormalities from ethylene glycol or methanol may include hypokalemia, hypocalcemia, hypomagnesemia, and elevated anion gap metabolic acidosis.
- Acetonemia and ketonemia may result from isopropyl alcohol ingestion.
- Hypoglycemia may be associated with toxic alcohol exposure as well as with ethanol therapy.
- Respiratory irritation from isopropyl alcohol inhalation or respiratory depression from any toxic alcohol ingestion may occur.

DIAGNOSTIC TESTS & INTERPRETATION

- Check serum electrolytes, BUN, creatinine, and glucose.
  - As metabolism occurs, an increased anion gap metabolic acidemia results with ethylene glycol or methanol toxicity.
  - Absence of this gap early after ingestion is expected and does not rule out ingestion.
  - Elevated anion gap metabolic acidemia supports the diagnosis of ethylene glycol or methanol exposure.
  - Acidemia is an indication for use of fomepizole or ethanol as well as potential indication for hemodialysis.
  - Fomepizole treatment should not be delayed waiting to determine if acidemia will develop.
  - Anion gap metabolic acidemia does not result from isopropyl alcohol poisoning.
- Blood gas analysis should be performed to assess for degree of metabolic acidemia in any patient with low serum bicarbonate.
  - Initial use of venous blood gas to screen for abnormality is acceptable.
  - Repeated blood gas analysis should occur every 1–2 hours if acidemia results.
- Serum level of ethylene glycol, isopropyl alcohol, or methanol should be obtained.
  - An ethylene glycol or methanol level greater than 20 mg/dL is an indication for fomepizole or ethanol infusion.
  - An ethylene glycol or methanol level greater than 50 mg/dL is an indication for hemodialysis.
- Serum ionized calcium is useful in managing ethylene glycol toxicity.
- Urinalysis with microscopic examination is recommended with ethylene glycol exposure.
  - Presence of oxalate crystals corroborates poisoning.
  - Absence of crystals does not exclude the possibility of ethylene glycol toxicity.
  - Fluorescence of urine is unreliable and is neither sensitive nor specific for exposure.
- A spurious rise in creatinine may occur.
- Proteinuria and hematuria may be present with ethylene glycol or isopropyl alcohol exposure.
- Serum osmolality or osmolarity may be useful in predicting the level of ethylene glycol, isopropyl alcohol, or methanol if rapid laboratory quantification cannot be performed.
- Serum ethanol level should simultaneously be performed to determine quantity of ethanol contribution to osmolal gap.
- An elevated osmolal gap can be used to rule in, but not exclude, toxic alcohol exposure.
- An elevated osmolal gap indicates the presence of unmeasured solute such as ethanol, ethylene glycol, isopropyl alcohol, or methanol.
- Absence of an osmolal gap does not exclude the possibility of toxic alcohol exposure.
- Osmolal gap is calculated as follows: Osmolal gap = (calculated serum osmolality − measured osmolality).
- The measured osmolality is determined by the laboratory.
- The calculated osmolality is determined as follows: $2 \times$ [Na (mEq/L)] + [BUN (mg/dL)/2.8] + [glucose (mg/dL)/18].
- Normal osmolal gap is less than 15 mEq/L.
- Any patient with increased osmolal gap should be presumed to have toxic alcohol exposure.
- Additional tests may include ECG to detect cardiac conduction disturbance or serum acetaminophen and salicylate levels in patients with intentional ingestion or with presumed intent of self-harm.
- Tests necessary to rule out differential diagnoses should be obtained when appropriate.

DIFFERENTIAL DIAGNOSIS

Drugs and disorders that may alter lab values include acetone, diethylene glycol, ethanol, iron, isoniazid, lactic acidemia, mannitol, methanol, propylene glycol, renal failure, salicylates, toluene, and various forms of ketoacidosis.

Imaging

Neuroimaging to rule out intracranial pathology may rarely be indicated.

TREATMENT

INITIAL STABILIZATION

- Prompt evaluation of airway, breathing, circulation, serum glucose, and ECG (A,B,C,D,E) is critical.
- Consultation with a medical toxicologist or poison center is recommended.

General Measures

Supportive care is the most important general principle. The illness is managed with intent of close monitoring and addressing issues as they arise.

- For ingestion less than 1 hour previously, an attempt to aspirate gastric contents with a nasogastric tube is reasonable.
- Treatment for ethylene glycol or methanol exposure should focus on acid-base correction and preventing organ damage.
- Hemodialysis should be considered for the following:
  - Any patient with severe metabolic acidemia from ethylene glycol or methanol
  - Any patient with evidence of end organ damage, particularly if metabolic acidemia is present
  - Any patient with profound hypotension or life-threatening symptoms resulting from isopropyl alcohol toxicity

Nursing

- Protect inebriated patients from falls.
- For the duration of inebriation or therapy with ethanol, vigilance for detection of hypoglycemia should be maintained.

IV Fluids

- IV fluid to maintain adequate blood pressure may be necessary.
- Maintenance IV fluid may be required in patients who are unable to take PO.
- IV fluid may be necessary to aid in prevention of calcium oxalate crystals in the urine.
- IV fluid may be helpful to prevent renal injury if rhabdomyolysis occurs.
- 8.4% sodium bicarbonate may be used in resistant acidosis and should be given via a central line if available.

MEDICATION

- For ethylene glycol or methanol poisoning (but NOT isopropyl alcohol), either fomepizole or ethanol are used to competitively inhibit alcohol dehydrogenase.
- Fomepizole is highly preferable to ethanol for this purpose, as ethanol has many severe, adverse side effects and fomepizole does not.
- Indications for fomepizole or ethanol include the following:
  - Serum level of ethylene glycol or methanol greater than 20 mg/dL
  - Metabolic acidemia with any quantity of detectable ethylene glycol or methanol
- Use of fomepizole or ethanol will prolong the half-life of ethylene glycol and methanol.
  - Without therapy, the ethylene glycol half-life is 3–4 hours, and methanol 14–20 hours.
  - With fomepizole or ethanol, the ethylene glycol half-life is 12 hours, and methanol 30–50 hours.
- Some clinicians consider a necessary duration of therapy longer than several days to be an indication for hemodialysis. Successful use of prolonged therapy with fomepizole to avoid hemodialysis has been reported.
- Fomepizole is contraindicated in patients with documented allergic reaction to the drug.
- Ethanol should be used with extreme caution in Asians, as aldehyde dehydrogenase deficiency may result in severe illness and hypotension.
- The loading dose of fomepizole is dose of 15 mg/kg IV.
- Initial maintenance dosing is 10 mg/kg q12h for 4 doses. Because fomepizole induces its own metabolism, the subsequent maintenance dose is increased to 15 mg/kg q12h thereafter.
- Each dose is diluted into normal saline or D5W (<25 mg/mL) and infused over 30 minutes.
- Each time after hemodialysis is performed, a loading dose must be readministered.
- Ethanol is administered as a 10% solution in D5W. This dilution requirement often results in a very large quantity of free water administration.
- The ethanol loading dose is 10 mL/kg (max 200 mL) of a 10% solution infused IV over 1 hour.
- A maintenance dose of 1–2 mL/kg of 10% ethanol is then given IV.
- Target blood ethanol level is 100–125 mg/dL.
- Patients receiving ethanol should have the ethanol level and serum glucose checked hourly.
- Oral ethanol may be used when IV is not available or if the patient is willing and capable of drinking. This is possibly feasible in adolescents.
- Adjunctive treatment with folate or leucovorin for methanol, and thiamine and pyridoxine for ethylene glycol may be given:
  - This continues until methanol or ethylene glycol levels are undetectable.
  - Folate or tetrahydrofolate (leucovorin) may hasten the elimination of formic acid resulting from methanol exposure.
  - Leucovorin 1–2 mg/kg may be administered IV every 6 hours.
  - Pyridoxine and thiamine hasten elimination of ethylene glycol metabolites.

FOLLOW-UP RECOMMENDATIONS

- Asymptomatic patients with undetectable ethylene glycol or methanol levels and no metabolic acidemia may be safely discharged.
- Most exposures for which ethylene glycol or methanol levels cannot be obtained should be followed for 12–24 hours to detect development of metabolic acidemia or other symptoms.
- From the hospital, patients with ethylene glycol or methanol level less than 20 mg/dL, no anion gap, no metabolic acidemia, and stable renal function and vision may be discharged.
  - Patients with isopropyl alcohol exposure who develop no symptoms or have only mild symptoms may be discharged within 4–6 hours.

Admission Criteria

- Any patient requiring therapy with fomepizole, ethanol, or hemodialysis
- Any patient with renal impairment, visual impairment, or other organ effect
- Any patient for whom consequential ingestion is suspected and ethylene glycol or methanol levels are unavailable

Discharge Criteria

- Inpatients who have received therapy with fomepizole, ethanol, or hemodialysis must be medically and metabolically stable for at least 12–24 hours prior to discharge.
- Patients with ethylene glycol or methanol exposure who have not developed symptoms or metabolic derangement may be discharged within 24 hours.

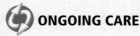

ONGOING CARE

PROGNOSIS

- For ethylene glycol and methanol exposure, prognosis depends on the degree of toxin metabolism, as well as adequacy of care.
- Speed and adequacy of therapy with fomepizole or ethanol, as well as prompt hemodialysis when indicated is critical.
- For isopropyl alcohol, prognosis depends on severity of intoxication and adequacy of supportive care.

COMPLICATIONS

Blindness, coma, hepatic injury, hypertension or hypotension, myocarditis, temporary or permanent neurologic injury, pancreatitis, renal failure, respiratory depression, rhabdomyolysis, seizure may occur as a result of toxic alcohol exposure.

Patient Monitoring

Symptomatic exposure to ethylene glycol or methanol may warrant intensive care monitoring.

ADDITIONAL READINGS

- Brent J. Fomepizole for the treatment of pediatric ethylene and diethylene glycol, butoxyethanol, and methanol poisonings. *Clin Toxicol*. 2010;48(5): 401–406.
- Howland MA. Antidotes in depth: ethanol. In: Goldfrank LR, Flomenbaum NE, Lewin NA, et al, eds. *Goldfrank's Toxicologic Emergencies*. 8th ed. Stamford, CT: Appleton & Lange; 2006.
- Weiner S. Toxic alcohols. In: Goldfrank LR, Flomenbaum NE, Lewin NA, et al, eds. *Goldfrank's Toxicologic Emergencies*. 8th ed. Stamford, CT: Appleton & Lange; 2006.

CODES

ICD-10

- T52.8X1A Toxic effect of organic solvents, accidental, init
- T51.2X1A Toxic effect of 2-Propanol, accidental (unintentional), initial encounter
- T51.1X1A Toxic effect of methanol, accidental (unintentional), initial encounter

T

TOXIC SHOCK SYNDROME

Amanda C. Schondelmeyer • Erin E. Shaughnessy

BASICS

DESCRIPTION

Toxic shock syndrome is an acute febrile illness characterized by hypotension and gastrointestinal and respiratory distress progressing to multisystem organ failure. The clinical syndrome is caused by bacterial exotoxins produced most commonly by the following:

- TSS toxin-1 (TSST-1)–producing strains of *Staphylococcus aureus*—referred to as TSS
- Group A β-hemolytic streptococci (GAS or *Streptococcus pyogenes*), referred to as streptococcal toxic shock–like syndrome (STSS)
- Cases have also been reported in association with groups B, C, and G1 streptococci and *Streptococcus mitis*.

EPIDEMIOLOGY

- In the 1980s, most cases were associated with superabsorbent tampon use; subsequently, these products have been removed from the market, resulting in a decline in menstrual-related staphylococcal TSS.
- Developing countries bear a much higher burden for STSS.
- Currently, ~50% of cases are non–menstrual related.

Incidence

- TSS: 3.4 cases per 100,000 in 2003
- Current incidence of menses-related TSS: 1–5 per 100,000 women of menstrual age per year
- STSS: 2–4 cases per 100,000 in developed countries with >10 per 100,000 per year in developing countries
- STSS incidence is highest among young children and associated with focal infections, pneumonia, or bacteremia.

RISK FACTORS

- Use of superabsorbent tampon, diaphragm, or contraceptive sponge; local or invasive staphylococcal or streptococcal infection
- Recent gynecologic procedure
- Focal infections including surgical and postpartum wounds, sinus, soft tissue, and musculoskeletal infections and respiratory infections
- STSS most often occurs with skin and soft tissue infections.
  - Preceding varicella infection increases risk.

GENERAL PREVENTION

- Scrupulous wound care
- Limitation of intravaginal foreign body use (e.g., tampon, sponge) and strict adherence to manufacturer's directions
- Early recognition and appropriate treatment of infections

PATHOPHYSIOLOGY

- Both *Staphylococcus aureus* and *Streptococcus pyogenes* can produce exotoxins.
- Some exotoxins function as superantigens, interacting with immune cells to induce massive cytokine production leading to the predominant symptoms.
- Cytokines result in fever, capillary leak, hypotension, and end-organ dysfunction.

DIAGNOSIS

HISTORY

- Patients may report use of tampons, contraceptive sponge, or diaphragm.
  - TSS may occur at any time during menses.
- Inquire about recent wounds or surgical procedures including catheters (e.g., intravenous, peritoneal dialysis).
  - Incubation period for postoperative TSS may be as short as 12 hours.
- Patient may report recent childbirth or abortion.
- Patients may report abrupt onset of high fever, chills, malaise, headache, pharyngitis, erythroderma fatigue, and dizziness or syncope.
- Gastrointestinal symptoms including profuse watery diarrhea, vomiting, abdominal pain

PHYSICAL EXAM

- Initial exam should evaluate for soft tissue or musculoskeletal focus of infection or retained foreign body.
- Patients are typically ill appearing and may have general erythroderma.
  - Skin findings may be less prominent with severe hypotension.
- Vitals signs: fever, tachycardia, tachypnea, orthostasis, or frank hypotension
  - Tachycardia with normotension may occur early in disease.
- Skin: erythroderma, peripheral cyanosis, and edema
  - Desquamation: begins on trunk and extremities 5–7 days after symptom onset
  - There may be vesicle or bullae formation or presence of violaceous hue.
- Mucosa: bulbar conjunctival injection and oral mucosal hyperemia
- Mental status: may be altered, somnolent, agitated, disoriented, or obtunded
  - Mental status changes may worsen as disease progresses.
- Caveats for physical exam
  - Patients may not have all symptoms upon presentation.

DIAGNOSTIC TESTS & INTERPRETATION

- U.S. Centers for Disease Control and Prevention (CDC) criteria for diagnosis of staphylococcal TSS requires 6 criteria for confirmed cases and 5 for probable:
  - Fever 38.9°C (102.0°F) or higher
  - Diffuse macular erythroderma
  - Desquamation 1–2 weeks after onset, particularly affecting palms and soles
  - Hypotension defined as systolic blood pressure below 5th percentile for children, orthostatic changes >15 mm Hg, or orthostatic syncope or dizziness
  - Involvement of three or more organ systems: gastrointestinal, muscular, mucous membrane, renal, hepatic, hematologic, or neurologic
  - Negative blood (may be positive for *S. aureus*), throat, or CSF cultures and/or negative titers for Rocky Mountain spotted fever (RMSF), leptospirosis, or measles
- U.S. CDC criteria for diagnosis of streptococcal TSS. Confirmed cases meet clinical definition in addition to isolation of GAS from normally sterile site; probable cases meet clinical definition with isolation of GAS from nonsterile site:
  - Hypotension as defined above
  - Any 2 of the following: renal impairment, coagulopathy, hepatic impairment, acute respiratory distress syndrome (ARDS), erythematous macular rash that may desquamate, or soft tissue necrosis

Lab

Initial laboratory evaluation should be aimed at diagnosing organ dysfunction to guide supportive therapy and identifying potential source and pathogen to guide antimicrobial therapy.

- Cultures
  - Blood cultures: ideally obtained prior to antimicrobial therapy but still helpful if patient has been on outpatient therapy prior to presentation
    - Positive in 60% of STSS but <5% of staphylococcal TSS
  - Other cultures
    - Culture of other fluids (abscess, pleural, cerebrospinal) should be guided by clinical presentation.
    - *S. aureus* may be isolated from vagina or cervix in menstrual TSS, although asymptomatic carriage can occur.
    - Culture of GAS from the throat or other nonsterile site may be helpful although does not confirm STSS.
- Antibodies (Ab)
  - TSST-1 Ab are available for informational purposes/research only.
  - Antistreptolysin O (ASO), antideoxyribonuclease B, or other streptococcal extracellular products
    - May increase 4–6 weeks after infection in streptococcal-mediated disease
    - May not be helpful in acute phases of disease
- Arterial blood gas
  - Helpful in cases of respiratory distress and poor perfusion to help guide ventilation strategies
- Complete blood count
  - Leukocytosis with left shift (neutropenia is an ominous sign)
  - Thrombocytopenia may indicate ongoing disseminated intravascular coagulation (DIC).
- Renal profile: may reflect acute kidney injury with elevated creatinine
- Hepatic profile: may have elevations in liver enzymes and evidence of synthetic dysfunction with decreased fibrinogen and coagulation factor levels
- Coagulation studies
  - May reveal prolonged prothrombin and partial thromboplastin times (PT/PTT) with or without evidence of DIC; low fibrinogen, elevated fibrin degradation products.
- Urinalysis
  - May reveal sterile pyuria
- Lumbar puncture
  - May reveal CSF pleocytosis
  - Gram stain positive for organisms or overt abnormalities indicating meningitis argue against STSS or TSS.
- Creatine phosphokinase (CPK)
  - May be elevated, reflecting skeletal muscle involvement

Imaging

Chest x-ray should be obtained if there is evidence of respiratory distress or oxygen requirement.

- May show diffuse bilateral infiltrates in ARDS

DIFFERENTIAL DIAGNOSIS

- Septic shock from other bacterial or viral
- Streptococcal scarlatiniform eruption
- Leptospirosis
- RMSF or ehrlichiosis if travel to or living in endemic areas
- Kawasaki disease:
  - TSS may present simultaneously with Kawasaki disease.
  - Coronary artery dilatation has been reported in cases presenting as TSS.
- Toxic epidermal necrolysis (TEN)
- Drug-induced hypersensitivity reaction

TREATMENT

SPECIAL THERAPY

- Remove all foreign bodies.
- Incision and drainage and or surgical debridement for abscess, myositis, and necrotizing fasciitis

MEDICATION

First-line therapy should be broad initially and guided by local rates of methicillin-resistant *Staphylococcus* aureus (MRSA).

- Vancomycin IV (15 mg/kg every 6 hours, max daily dose 4,000 mg) should be administered as first line if MRSA is a consideration.
  - Renal toxicity is a known adverse effect.
  - Dose should be adjusted for renal impairment and serum creatinine followed.
  - Trough levels (before 4th dose) should be used to adjust dose under the guidance of an experienced pharmacist.
- Clindamycin IV (40 mg/kg divided every 6–8 hours, max daily dose 2,700 mg) should be administered in addition to 1st-line therapy to end production of toxins.
- Ceftriaxone (100 mg/kg divided every 12–24 hours, max daily dose 2,000 mg) should be added empirically for gram-negative coverage until organism or diagnosis is confirmed.
- Antistaphylococcal penicillins (i.e., nafcillin, oxacillin, dicloxacillin) may be considered in place of vancomycin if local MRSA rates are low.
- IVIG is commonly used as adjunct therapy to antibiotics, but its efficacy is unclear.
  - Proposed mechanism is by providing neutralizing antibodies to exotoxins and inhibiting T-cell activation.
- Continue antibiotic therapy for at least 10–14 days; total treatment length should be guided by initial focus of infection if present.
- Consultation with infectious disease specialist is recommended in cases where the diagnosis is unclear.
- Therapy can be changed to oral when patient is tolerating oral nutrition.

INITIAL STABILIZATION

Treatment of suspected TSS or STSS should occur ideally at a tertiary care center with close access to a pediatric intensive care unit.

- Initial resuscitation should proceed rapidly to support adequate tissue perfusion and oxygenation.
  - IV isotonic fluid bolus should be given initially with further fluid boluses and pressor therapy guided by perfusion and vital signs
    - Be mindful of potential cardiac dysfunction when providing fluid resuscitation.
  - Stabilize airway if respiratory distress
- Antibiotic therapy should be administered as soon as possible.

ONGOING CARE

Aside from antimicrobial therapy, the mainstays of treatment are supportive care for organ dysfunction.

- Temperature usually returns to normal within 2 days if on effective therapy.
- Gastrointestinal, hepatic, and musculoskeletal changes resolve rapidly with rare permanent sequelae except for muscle weakness.
- Full-thickness desquamation of fingers, toes, palms, and soles begins 10–12 days after onset.
  - Hair and nail loss may occur 4–16 weeks after illness onset; should resolve within 5–6 months.
- Encephalopathy is common but rarely causes seizures; usually resolves within 4–5 days.
- Poor prognosis is often heralded by development of pulmonary edema and worsening cardiac function.
  - Cardiac and pulmonary failure are the most common causes of death.
  - Toxin-mediated cardiomyopathy should resolve with effective treatment.

PROGNOSIS

- Nonmenstrual TSS has a case fatality rate of 5%; menstrual TSS case fatality rate was approximately 1.8% between 1987 and 1996.
- STSS case fatality rate exceeds 50%.
- Recurrences are associated with inadequate treatment or persistent focus.
- Death usually occurs within the first few days but may occur as late as 2 weeks following onset.

COMPLICATIONS

Multisystem organ failure secondary to distributive shock/hypotension, including the following:

- Pulmonary edema
- DIC
- Acute renal failure (oliguric and nonoliguric)
- Hepatic failure
- Myocardial dysfunction; may have arrhythmias
- Cerebral edema with toxic or ischemic encephalopathy
- Metabolic disturbances
- Tissue death and potentially limb amputation
- Neuropsychological disturbances including memory loss; abnormal electroencephalograms (EEGs) are rare

ADDITIONAL READING

- Bisno AL, Stevens DC. Streptococcal infection of skin and soft-tissues. *N Engl J Med*. 1996;334(4):240–245.
- Byer RL, Bachur RG. Clinical deterioration among patients with fever and erythroderma. *Pediatrics*. 2006;118(6):2450–2460.
- Low DE. Toxic shock syndrome: major advances in pathogenesis, but not treatment. *Crit Care Clin*. 2013;29(3):651–675.
- O'Loughlin RE, Roberson A, Cieslak PR, et al. The epidemiology of invasive group A streptococcal infection and potential vaccine implications: United States, 2000–2004. *Clin Infect Dis*. 2007;45(7):853–862.
- Shah SS, Hall M, Srivastava R, et al. Intravenous immunoglobulin in children with streptococcal toxic shock syndrome. *Clinical Infect Dis*. 2009;49(9):1369–1376.

CODES

ICD10

- A48.3 Toxic shock syndrome
- B95.61 Methicillin suscep staph infct causing dis classd elswhr
- B95.0 Streptococcus, group A, causing diseases classd elswhr

FAQ

- Q: Can TSS recur?
- A: Yes. Inadequate eradication of the nidus of infection or inadequate treatment may result in recurrence. Poor immune function may also contribute to recurrence.
- Q: Can TSS be diagnosed in patients who have no risk factors?
- A: Yes. There have been reports meeting the case definition where none of the known associated factors was present.
- Q: Should I wait for confirmation of the diagnosis prior to treating with antibiotics?
- A: No. Antibiotic therapy should be initiated immediately in any patient suspected of having TSS.

TOXOPLASMOSIS

Caitlin Messner • Rebecca Schein

BASICS

DESCRIPTION

Toxoplasmosis is caused by *Toxoplasma gondii*, an obligate intracellular protozoan parasite with a complex life cycle, which can cause a wide range of clinical symptoms depending on individual strain virulence and the host immune system.

- Primary infection is often asymptomatic and may result in fever, lymphadenopathy, and eye disease.
- Congenital infection classically presents with triad of chorioretinitis, hydrocephalus, and brain calcifications.
- Reactivation of disease may develop after either primary or congenital infection and most commonly presents as chorioretinitis.
- Patients with immune deficiency can develop brain abscesses, encephalitis, fever of unknown origin, or pneumonia.

EPIDEMIOLOGY

- Toxoplasmosis is the leading cause of death due to foodborne illness in the United States.
- *T. gondii* is found worldwide and can infect most warm-blooded animals.
- Cats are the definitive hosts, and the parasite replicates sexually in the feline small intestine.
- Vertical transmission is more common with primary infection during pregnancy or within 3 months prior to conception. Treatment of primary maternal infection can decrease fetal transmission rate by half from 50–60% to 25–30%.

Incidence

Congenital infection in the United States occurs in an estimated 1 per 10,000 live births or 400 new cases annually.

Prevalence

- Worldwide, the rate of infection varies greatly and ranges from 7% to 80%.
- In the United States, overall seroprevalence is 11% but may be as high as 40% in areas with lower socioeconomic status.

GENERAL PREVENTION

- Main risk factors for *T. gondii* infection are eating raw or rare meat, consuming local cured or smoked meat, working with meat, drinking unpasteurized goat milk, or having more than 3 kittens.
- Untreated or contaminated water is also a risk factor and has been responsible for outbreaks of toxoplasmosis.
- Pregnant women should be counseled to avoid cat feces exposure including gardening, landscaping, and changing litter boxes and to avoid consuming undercooked meat.

PATHOPHYSIOLOGY

- Cats shed oocysts in feces, which then sporulate and become infectious.
- Humans are infected by eating raw or undercooked meat infested with oocytes; accidental ingestion of contaminated soil, food, or water; contaminated blood transfusion or organ donation; or via transplacental transmission from mother to fetus.
- In the human host, tissue cysts are formed in skeletal muscle, myocardium, brain, and eyes.
- Tissue cysts persist for the life of the host.
- Reactivation can occur when the immune system is compromised particularly due to T-cell deficiency.

DIAGNOSIS

HISTORY

- Exposure to raw meat, unfiltered water, cats or kittens
- Immune deficiency disease
- Maternal illness during pregnancy

PHYSICAL EXAM

- Primary infection may be asymptomatic.
- Symptoms are nonspecific and include lymphadenopathy, fever, headache, sore throat, malaise, myalgia, or arthralgia. A mononucleosis-like syndrome with rash and hepatosplenomegaly is seen occasionally.
- Congenital infection is asymptomatic at birth in 70–90% of patients. Visual impairment, learning disabilities, or mental retardation commonly develop over time.
- Signs of symptomatic congenital infection include rash, generalized lymphadenopathy, hepatosplenomegaly, jaundice, pericarditis, thrombocytopenia, meningoencephalitis, hydrocephalus, microcephaly, and brain calcifications.
- The classic triad of toxoplasmosis in neonates is chorioretinitis, hydrocephalus, and brain calcifications.
- Ocular toxoplasmosis commonly is due to reactivation of chronic infection.
- In persons with secondary immunodeficiency, reactivation disease can result encephalitis, pneumonia, or systemic toxoplasmosis.

DIAGNOSTIC TESTS & INTERPRETATION

Lab

- Serology testing for *T. gondii*–specific antibodies is the primary means of diagnosis.
- The presence of immunoglobulin G (IgG) determines if a person has ever been infected, whereas immunoglobulin M (IgM) or IgG avidity test detect primary infection.
- Pregnant women in high-prevalence area should be screened with both IgM to detect acute infection and IgG for latency. If IgG is present, an avidity test will determine if infection occurred within the last 3–4 months.
- Infants suspected of congenital toxoplasmosis should be tested for the presence of *T. gondii* immunoglobulin A (IgA) in addition to IgG and IgM due to higher sensitivity in this age group.
- As serology testing can vary, any positive tests should be confirmed by a reference laboratory.
- Amniotic fluid may tested for *T. gondii* DNA.
- Diagnosis can be made by direct observation of the parasite in tissue specimens, cerebral spinal fluid, or biopsy material.
- Immunocompromised patients including those with HIV should be tested for *T. gondii*–specific IgG, prior to starting therapy.

Imaging

- Prenatal ultrasound is useful to detect signs of congenital infection including hydrocephalus, brain calcifications, or pericarditis.
- Head CT or MRI will detect calcifications and hydrocephalus.

Diagnostic Procedures/Other

- Ophthalmologic examinations for characteristic retinal lesions
- Hearing exams, as hearing loss may be absent in infancy and develop over time

DIFFERENTIAL DIAGNOSIS

- Primary infection
  - Epstein-Barr virus (EBV)
  - Cytomegalovirus (CMV)
  - HIV
  - Lymphoma
- Congenital infection
  - CMV (calcifications are periventricular)
  - Herpes simplex virus (HSV)
  - Rubella
  - Syphilis

TREATMENT

MEDICATION

- Most cases of acute infection do not require treatment.
- Persons with eye disease, severe organ damage, pregnant women, congenital infection (symptomatic or asymptomatic), and immunocompromised hosts should be treated.
- Therapy is a combination of pyrimethamine and sulfadiazine.
- Folinic acid is also given to protect against the hematologic side effects of pyrimethamine.
- Spiramycin treatment of pregnant women may reduce congenital transmission.
- Treatment is prolonged and congenital infection is treated for 1 year.
- Trimethoprim/sulfamethoxazole should be used for prophylaxis to prevent disease in those with HIV infection and CD4 count less than 100/μL or severe immunosuppression with known IgG antibody to toxoplasma.

ONGOING CARE

FOLLOW-UP RECOMMENDATIONS

- Children with congenital infection should be monitored for neurologic manifestations, including hearing loss and chorioretinitis that may develop over time.
- Ophthalmologic exams and audiometry should be performed periodically for at least the first 10 years of life after congenital infection.
- Head circumference should be monitored due to development of hydrocephalus in congenital infections.

PROGNOSIS

- Congenital infections are also mostly asymptomatic at birth; however, hearing loss, vision loss, and seizures may present months to years later.
- Bad neurologic outcomes are associated with early maternal infection, lack of prenatal treatment, presence of chorioretinitis, and clinical signs noted at birth.
- Treatment improves clinical outcomes, including cognitive function.
- Immunocompromised patients require chronic suppressive therapy until demonstrated immune recovery.
- Appropriately treated patients typically due well.

COMPLICATIONS

- Congenital infection
  - Chorioretinitis
  - Hydrocephalus
  - Seizures
  - Intellectual delay
  - Seizures
  - Sensorineural hearing loss
  - Microcephaly
- Primary infection: Rare complications are myocarditis, pericarditis, pneumonia, meningitis, or encephalitis.

ADDITIONAL READING

- Berrébi A, Assouline C, Bessieres MH, et al. Long-term outcome of children with congenital toxoplasmosis. *Am J Obstet Gynecol*. 2010;203(6):552.e1–e6.
- Del Pizzo J. Focus on diagnosis: congenital infections (TORCH). *Pediatr Rev*. 2011;32(12):537–542.
- McLeod R, Boyer K, Karrison, T, et al. Outcome of treatment for congenital toxoplasmosis, 1981-2004: the National Collaborative Chicago-Based, Congenital Toxoplasmosis Study. *Clin Infect Dis*. 2006;42(10):1383–1394.
- Rober-Gangneux F, Darde M. Epidemiology of and diagnostic strategies for toxoplasmosis. *Clin Microbiol Rev*. 2012;25(2):264–296.

CODES

ICD10

- B58.9 Toxoplasmosis, unspecified
- P37.1 Congenital toxoplasmosis
- B58.3 Pulmonary toxoplasmosis

FAQ

- Q: What newborns require evaluation for congenital toxoplasmosis?
- A: Newborns with known maternal disease or concerning exposure and those with hydrocephalus, intracranial calcifications, strabismus, intrauterine growth restriction, or other concern for congenital infection should have serologic testing for *T. gondii* specific IgG, IgM, and IgA.
- Q: How do people get toxoplasmosis?
- A: By ingesting oocytes from undercooked meat, drinking unpasteurized milk, or by exposure to cat feces in litter or soil.
- Q: Who is at risk developing severe toxoplasmosis?
- A: Infants born to mother infected with *T. gondii* during pregnancy and persons with immune suppression due to acquired immune deficiency syndrome (AIDS), chemotherapy, or organ transplantation.
- Q: How can I prevent toxoplasmosis?
- A: Thoroughly cook meat, wash all fruits and vegetables well, eat only pasteurized dairy products, and wash hands well after contact with sand or soil.

TRACHEITIS

Charles A. Pohl

BASICS

DESCRIPTION

Infection of the trachea associated with airway inflammation and obstruction

- Acute tracheitis: sudden onset; higher morbidity and mortality
- Subacute tracheitis: indolent presentation and course; more common among children with prolonged intubation, tracheostomy, and/or underlying respiratory or neurologic conditions

EPIDEMIOLOGY

- Viral prodrome common
- Increased incidence during viral respiratory season (fall and winter): up to 75% coinfected with influenza A
- Gender predisposition unclear (2:1 male-to-female ratio has been reported)
- 3% mortality rate

GENERAL PREVENTION

- Routine childhood immunization with *Haemophilus influenzae* type b, influenza, measles, and pneumococcal vaccines
- Avoid overaggressive suctioning of children with artificial airways.

PATHOPHYSIOLOGY

- Epithelial damage from a viral infection or mechanical trauma (e.g., endotracheal intubation, surgical procedure) occurs in the trachea at the level of the cricoid cartilage. As a result, the damaged tissue is more susceptible to bacterial superinfection.
- Mucosal damage characterized by marked subglottic edema, copious purulent secretions, and a pseudomembrane (mucosal lining, inflammatory products, and bacteria). These changes lead to marked airway obstruction.
- Toxic shock syndrome may be a consequence if the infection is associated with toxin-producing strains of *Staphylococcus aureus* or *Streptococcus pyogenes*.

ETIOLOGY

- Bacteria
  - *Staphylococcus aureus* (most common), group A β-hemolytic *Streptococcus*, *Moraxella catarrhalis*, nontypeable *H. influenzae*, *Streptococcus pneumoniae*
  - *Pseudomonas aeruginosa* and other gram-negative enteric bacteria have been associated with nosocomial infections.
  - *Mycobacterium tuberculosis*, *Mycoplasma pneumoniae*, *Corynebacterium diphtheriae*, *H. influenzae* type b, and respiratory anaerobic bacteria are uncommon pathogens.
- Viruses: Influenza, parainfluenza, respiratory syncytial, herpes simplex, and measles viruses have been found with bacterial pathogen(s).
- Fungi: seen with underlying immunodeficiency disorders or chronic steroid use

DIAGNOSIS

HISTORY

- Hyperpyrexia; nonpainful, brassy cough; noisy respirations; lethargy; dyspnea; rapid progression of airway occlusion (hours to a few days)
- Hoarseness, dysphagia, neck pain, drooling, and croupy cough are less common with bacterial tracheitis.
- Presence of upper airway infection
- Lack of clinical improvement with racemic epinephrine should raise the suspicion for tracheitis.
- An indolent progression of symptoms, including increase of supplemental oxygen requirement and tracheal secretions (thicker and color changes), may be seen in subacute tracheitis.
- Affects any age (peak age 1–6 years)

PHYSICAL EXAM

- Toxic appearance; anxious, agitated, or lethargic; labored breathing with signs of severe respiratory distress (e.g., air hunger posture, retractions); pallor or cyanosis; severe stridor; concomitant signs of pneumonia
- Deviated uvula suggests a peritonsillar abscess.
- Asymmetric lung sounds are often found in patients with foreign bodies in the airway.
- Generalized lymphadenopathy and splenomegaly are clues for infectious mononucleosis.

DIAGNOSTIC TESTS & INTERPRETATION

Imaging

- Radiographs must be completed in controlled settings by personnel who are trained in airway management.
- Lateral and anteroposterior neck films: Findings include distention of the hypopharynx, subglottic narrowing, and irregularity of the tracheal wall owing to mucosal sloughing or the presence of a pseudomembrane.
- Chest radiograph: Obtain if pneumonia, which may be concurrent, is suspected.

Diagnostic Procedures/Other

- Laryngoscopy or bronchoscopy
  - Direct visualization and suctioning of obstructed airway is both diagnostic and therapeutic.
  - Findings include a red, edematous, and/or eroded trachea and bronchi with purulent secretions and pseudomembrane.
  - Consider in an ill-appearing child with an unclear diagnosis or when the child's condition does not respond to current management
- Tracheal bacterial culture (for aerobic and anaerobic bacteria): the gold standard for diagnosis
- Tracheal Gram stain for pathogens and white blood cells (especially polymorphonuclear leukocytes): helps differentiate bacterial infection from colonization
- Blood culture: rarely helpful in diagnosis ($<$50% positive)
- CBC: little diagnostic value but may show leukocytosis with a left shift
- ESR and/or C-reactive protein: may be elevated

DIFFERENTIAL DIAGNOSIS

- Infectious
  - Epiglottitis/supraglottitis (presence of supraglottic inflammation)
  - Laryngotracheitis (croup)
  - Peritonsillar and parapharyngeal abscesses
  - Retropharyngeal abscess
  - Infectious mononucleosis (Epstein-Barr virus)
  - Diphtheria (rare)
- Environmental
  - Aspiration or inhalation of a caustic substance, including alkali products (e.g., oven cleaner) or smoke
  - Foreign body aspiration
  - Generalized allergic reaction or anaphylaxis leading to angioedema
- Tumors (rare)
  - Papillomas secondary to human papillomavirus
  - Hamartoma and inflammatory pseudotumor
  - Laryngeal tumors

- Trauma
  - Posttraumatic tracheal stenosis
  - Blunt trauma to neck
- Congenital
  - Tracheal stenosis
  - Vascular ring and slings
  - Laryngotracheal web and clefts
  - Laryngotracheomalacia
  - Vocal cord paralysis
  - Arnold-Chiari malformation

ALERT
- Watch for sudden deterioration from tracheal inflammation and secretions. Continuous monitoring is necessary.
- Bacterial tracheitis must be considered in all children with sudden upper respiratory distress and hyperpyrexia.

TREATMENT

MEDICATION

Select antibiotic therapy based on Gram stain and culture results of tracheal secretions and the most likely pathogens. Also consider known prior colonization and institutional pathogens in children with preexisting artificial airway and hospital-acquired infections:

- Mild illness
  - Empiric therapy with amoxicillin-clavulanic acid or a 2nd-generation cephalosporin for 10–14 days (50 mg/kg/24 h depending on the antibiotic used)
  - Consider a semisynthetic penicillin such as dicloxacillin (40 mg/kg/24 h) if *H. influenzae* type b vaccine completed and clindamycin (10–30 mg/kg/24 h) if presence of a penicillin allergy or MRSA suspected
- Moderate to severe illness
  - Empiric therapy with an antistaphylococcal agent such as clindamycin plus a 3rd-generation cephalosporin or with ampicillin-sulbactam
  - Consider vancomycin IV (60–80 mg/kg/24 h) if a hospital-acquired infection (MRSA) is present or in cases of toxic shock pending culture results.
- Anaerobic, pseudomonas, and other gram-negative coverage should be considered in children not responding to initial therapy or having preexisting artificial airways.
- In contrast to croup, nebulized racemic epinephrine and steroids do not provide significant relief.
- Duration: based on clinical response; usually 10–14 days

ADDITIONAL TREATMENT

General Measures

- Support by stabilizing circulation, airway, breathing (ABCs).
- Maintain airway.
- Initiate IV, oxygen, and monitor.
- Rapid assessment of ABCs is essential with emphasis on airway control.
- Supplemental oxygen is usually needed.
- Pediatric ICU care is initially recommended.
- Anticipate and prepare for emergent endotracheal intubation and tracheostomy.
- Endoscopy with suctioning and debridement is often necessary for diagnosis and therapy.
- Subsequent airway suctioning and monitoring prevents adverse outcomes.
- Increased ventilatory support is often required for children with preexisting artificial airways.

ONGOING CARE

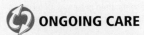

FOLLOW-UP RECOMMENDATIONS

- Routine surveillance cultures in children with artificial airways are not recommended. They usually represent colonization in an asymptomatic patient.
- Signs to watch for:
  - Toxic appearance, excessive secretions, persistent fever, or worsening respiratory distress after introducing antibiotics suggest a resistant organism, an unusual pathogen, or a different diagnosis.
  - Recurrent respiratory distress, especially stridor, with subsequent respiratory tract infections suggests underlying tracheal stenosis.
  - Sudden deterioration on a ventilator may indicate endotracheal tube obstruction, pneumothorax, or mechanical problems.

DIET

NPO until the airway is stabilized and the patient is able to tolerate oral foods

PROGNOSIS

- Most children recover without any sequelae.
- Younger patients are more likely to require intubations and longer hospital stays.
- Children at risk for subacute tracheitis are more likely to have recurrent episodes.

COMPLICATIONS

- Atelectasis
- Pulmonary edema and pneumonia
- Septicemia
- Staphylococcal toxin syndromes (e.g., toxic shock syndrome)
- Prolonged mechanical ventilation with associated complications (including air leak, infection, pneumothorax, and tracheal stenosis)
- Subglottic stenosis
- Respiratory failure and arrest
- Death (<3.7%)

ADDITIONAL READING

- Hopkins A, Lahiri T, Salerno R, et al. Changing epidemiology of life-threatening upper airway infections: the reemergence of bacterial tracheitis. *Pediatrics*. 2006;118(4):1418–1421.
- Salamone FN, Bobbit DB, Myer CM, et al. Bacterial tracheitis reexamined: is there a less severe manifestation. *Otolaryngol Head Neck Surg*. 2004;131(6):871–876.
- Tebruegge M, Pantazidou A, Thorburn K, et al. Bacterial tracheitis: a multi-centre perspective. *Scand J Infect Dis*. 2009;41(8):548–557.
- Tebruegge M, Pantazidou A, Yau C. Bacterial tracheitis—tremendously rare, but truly important: a systemic review. *J Pediatr Infect Dis*. 2009;4:199–209.

CODES

ICD10

- J04.10 Acute tracheitis without obstruction
- J04.11 Acute tracheitis with obstruction
- J05.10 Acute epiglottitis without obstruction

FAQ

- Q: How can you differentiate a child with severe croup from one with tracheitis?
- A: Infectious croup and tracheitis can present with similar features of fever, toxic appearance, respiratory distress, and stridor. Direct endoscopic visualization and culture of the upper airway is the test of choice to distinguish these medical conditions. Croup is commonly associated with parainfluenza virus and a "steeple sign" of the upper trachea on an anteroposterior neck radiograph.
- Q: Is influenza A virus a common pathogen of tracheitis?
- A: This subject is controversial. Influenza A virus is frequently recovered from tracheal cultures in children who present with tracheitis. It remains unclear, though, whether this virus is a pathogen or predisposing factor in tracheitis.
- Q: Is the supraglottic area usually involved in tracheitis?
- A: No. Unlike with epiglottitis, the supraglottic region is usually spared in tracheitis. Lack of supraglottic involvement suggests bacterial tracheitis rather than epiglottitis.

TRACHEOESOPHAGEAL FISTULA AND ESOPHAGEAL ATRESIA

Kimberly M. Lumpkins • F. Dylan Stewart

BASICS

DESCRIPTION

- Esophageal atresia with tracheoesophageal fistula (EA-TEF) is a congenital condition of incomplete formation of the esophagus. In most cases, the atretic (blind-ending) esophagus has an aberrant fistula to the trachea (TEF).
- Five types are described:
  – EA with distal TEF is the most common (Gross type C, 85%).
  – Pure EA without TEF occurs in 10% (Gross type A).
  – EA with proximal TEF and EA with both distal and proximal TEFs are quite rare (1% each, gross types B and D).
  – Pure TEF without EA occurs in 3–4% ("H type fistula", Gross type E).

EPIDEMIOLOGY

- The prevalence of EA-TEF is 1 in 2,500–4,000 live births. This appears to be consistent worldwide.
- Slight male predominance (1.2:1)

RISK FACTORS

- Many maternal exposures have been postulated to contribute, but none are well established.
  – Maternal diabetes (nongestational) during 1st trimester, older age, maternal diethylstilbestrol (DES) exposure, horticultural work, alcohol, and smoking have all been implicated.

Genetics

- No specific genetic cause of EA-TEF has been established.
- Twin concordance is only 2.5%.

ETIOLOGY

- The foregut diverticulum separates into the trachea and esophagus at approximately 4–5 weeks of gestation.
- In EA-TEF, it is postulated that the lateral folds that fuse to separate the trachea and esophagus fail to form. Disruption of signalling in the *Wnt* and *Bmp* pathways has been implicated in this chain of development. This theory remains controversial, and the exact nature of the defect is unresolved.

COMMONLY ASSOCIATED CONDITIONS

- EA-TEF is associated with the VACTERL (vertebral defects, anal atresia, cardiac defects, TEF, radial or renal anomalies, and limb anomalies) sequence of congenital anomalies (10–25% of EA-TEF infants).
- Can be found in association with trisomies 13, 18, and 21 as well as CHARGE (coloboma, heart disease, choanal atresia, retarded growth, genital hypoplasia, and ear anomalies with deafness) syndrome, Feingold syndrome, DiGeorge syndrome, and others

DIAGNOSIS

HISTORY

- Prenatal ultrasound may demonstrate features suggestive of EA-TEF such as absence of a stomach bubble, a dilated proximal pouch, or polyhydramnios.
  – Only a minority of patients are prenatally identified, and the positive predictive value of these signs is low.
  – Prenatal diagnosis most common in cases of pure EA without TEF
- In patients without a prenatal suspicion of EA-TEF, the diagnosis is usually first entertained when a newborn has excessive secretions and repeated bouts of choking and spitting up during attempts at feeding.
- In patients with an H-type fistula, diagnosis may be delayed. These patients often present with recurrent respiratory infections or aspiration events later in childhood.

PHYSICAL EXAM

- Infants with EA-TEF are frequently normal in physical appearance.
- Failure of passage of a stiff 10F or 12F nasogastric tube at 10–12 cm is the major diagnostic test.
- Exam should focus on evidence of VACTERL anomalies.
- Careful cardiac auscultation
- Respiratory auscultation may reveal crackles or other signs of aspiration.
- Documentation of patent anus
- Examination of limbs for skeletal abnormalities (absent radii or thumbs)
- Observation of other congenital anomalies consistent with genetic syndromes

DIAGNOSTIC TESTS & INTERPRETATION

Lab

- There are no specific laboratory findings associated with EA-TEF.
- Underlying pathology may lead to expected laboratory findings (e.g., electrolyte derangement with severe renal anomalies).

Imaging

- CXR/abdominal XR: first recommended test
  – NG tube coiled in the proximal pouch in the upper chest or neck
  – Bowel gas present distally (type C)
  – No bowel gas with pure atresia (type A)
  – Possible vertebral and rib anomalies
  – Rule out "double bubble" of coincident duodenal atresia.
- Additional required imaging studies include a renal ultrasound, echocardiogram, and spinal ultrasound to rule out other VACTERL anomalies. Limb radiographs are indicated if abnormalities are seen on physical exam.
- Echocardiogram is crucial for operative planning as well as to assess for cardiac defects. Ask the cardiologist to comment specifically on the sidedness of the aortic arch.
- Esophagram
  – For a suspected H-type fistula: Prone pressure esophagram may demonstrate the communication between the trachea and esophagus; however, the finding can be subtle and repeated studies may be necessary.
  – Esophagram is otherwise contraindicated in patients with EA-TEF because of high risk of aspiration.

DIFFERENTIAL DIAGNOSIS

- Congenital esophageal stricture
- Severe gastroesophageal reflux disease (GERD)
- Vascular ring
- Tracheal bronchus (H-type fistula)
- Laryngotracheoesophageal cleft (H-type fistula)

TREATMENT

GENERAL MEASURES

Preoperative management

- Strict NPO until surgical correction is undertaken
- Maintain a Replogle suction tube in the proximal pouch to decrease aspiration from pooled secretions.
- Initiate acid suppression therapy.
- Maintain head of bed (HOB) elevated to 45 degrees.

ADDITIONAL TREATMENT

Complete workup for VACTERL anomalies as described above

SURGERY/OTHER PROCEDURES

- Surgical repair is required for all forms of EA-TEF.
- Repair is performed as early as feasible in the newborn period to avoid ongoing lung damage from repeated aspiration events.
- Extremely premature or ill infants can undergo fistula ligation without esophageal repair. The esophagus can be reconstructed at a later date when the infant is more stable.
- Bronchoscopy at time of repair is controversial. It may identify the rare case of dual TEF or laryngotracheoesophageal cleft.
- Repair via thoracotomy or thoracoscopy at the surgeon's discretion through the right chest (except in cases of a right-sided arch on echocardiogram, where a left-sided approach may be preferable).
- The fistula is ligated by sutures or clips; the proximal esophageal pouch is mobilized and the esophagus brought together with a sutured anastomosis.

- In a long-gap atresia (esophageal ends separated by more than 3 vertebral bodies) where the esophageal ends do not meet, a gastric pull-up or esophageal growth induction (Foker) process may be used. Alternately, a gastrostomy tube can be placed for nutrition and esophageal anastomosis performed in delayed fashion.
- Most surgeons place a feeding tube across the esophageal anastomosis to act as a stent and allow early enteral feeding.
- Chest tube placement is at the discretion of the surgeon.
- Postoperative paralysis and prolonged intubation are sometimes employed to reduce tension on the repair, but there is no strong evidence in favor of this practice.
- Pure H-type TEF can often be repaired by a cervical incision, avoiding entry into the chest.

ONGOING CARE

FOLLOW-UP RECOMMENDATIONS

EA-TEF patients require long-term follow-up for GERD, dysphagia, and esophageal motility issues. Surveillance endoscopy may be considered in young adulthood for risk of esophageal cancer, but this strategy is not yet established.

PROGNOSIS

Survival depends predominantly on the presence or absence of cardiac anomalies. Overall survival is approximately 95%. Survival of babies >1.5 kg without cardiac anomalies is 98%.

COMPLICATIONS

- Esophageal leak
  - Early complication of EA-TEF repair
  - Seen on contrast esophagram
  - Will usually resolve with conservative management (NPO, TPN, and chest tube drainage of any collection)
  - Predisposes to the subsequent development of esophageal stricture and recurrent TEF
- Esophageal stricture
  - Common complication of EA-TEF repair
  - Symptoms include coughing and choking during feeds.
  - An esophagram is diagnostic.
  - Serial esophageal dilations may relieve symptoms.
  - Acid suppression can improve response to dilation and fundoplication may be required in refractory cases.
- Tracheomalacia
  - Symptomatic tracheomalacia occurs in 20% of patients with EA-TEF.
  - Diagnose by rigid or flexible bronchoscopy.
  - Presents at 2–3 months of age with barking cough or stridor
  - Although children will outgrow tracheomalacia, the occurrence of "death spells" may mandate a surgical aortopexy to reduce severity of symptoms.
- GERD
  - Very common in EA-TEF patients due to disordered esophageal motility and anatomic alteration of the lower esophageal sphincter (LES) by esophageal traction
  - Unlike typical pediatric patients, reflux does not improve with age.
  - 15–70% of TEF patients eventually require fundoplication.
  - Predisposes the patient to Barrett esophagus, and recent data suggest that the lifetime risk of esophageal carcinoma may be 50 times higher than average
- Recurrent TEF is a difficult problem requiring endoscopic or operative correction.
- As most complications of EA-TEF present with choking, coughing, and cyanosis, it can be hard to distinguish between potential etiologies. A rational strategy of esophagram and bronchoscopy is needed to determine the appropriate treatment plan.

ALERT

- Positive pressure ventilation (PPV) preoperatively may lead to preferential ventilation of the fistula. Avoidance of PPV is preferred when feasible.
- If intubation is required, placement of the endotracheal tube past the fistula is the textbook recommendation. However, the fistula is frequently at the carina, which can render this process impossible.
- In case of dislodgement, the postoperative nasogastric feeding tube should not be replaced without consultation with the surgeon to avoid disruption of the esophageal repair.
- If a postoperative EA-TEF infant requires urgent reintubation, mask-ventilate as gently as possible during induction to avoid disruption of the esophageal anastomosis. Maximize visualization of the vocal cords, as inadvertent esophageal intubation can be catastrophic.

ADDITIONAL READING

- Burge DM, Shah K, Spark P, et al. Contemporary management and outcomes for infants born with oesophageal atresia. *Br J Surg*. 2013;100(4):515–521.
- De Jong Em, Felix JF, de Klein A, et al. Etiology of esophageal atresia and tracheoesophageal fistula: "mind the gap." *Curr Gastroenterol Rep*. 2010; 12(3):215–222.
- Jacobs IJ, Que J. Genetic and cellular mechanisms of the formation of esophageal atresia and tracheoesophageal fistula. *Dis Esophagus*. 2013;26(4): 356–358.
- Kunisaki SM, Foker JE. Surgical advances in the fetus and neonate: esophageal atresia. *Clin Perinatol*. 2012;39(2):349–361.
- Tovar JA, Fragoso AC. Gastroesophageal reflux after esophageal atresia repair. *Eur J Paediatr Surg*. 2013;23(3):175–181.

CODES

ICD10

- Q39.1 Atresia of esophagus with tracheo-esophageal fistula
- Q39.2 Congenital tracheo-esophageal fistula without atresia
- Q39.0 Atresia of esophagus without fistula

FAQ

- Q: What is the diagnostic workup for suspected TEF?
- A: A chest radiograph with gentle forward pressure held on the nasogastric tube is the preferred diagnostic study. Without pressure, the film may imply a falsely high level of the cervical pouch. Once TEF is confirmed, the recommended evaluation includes echocardiogram, spinal and renal ultrasounds, and a surveillance radiograph of the spine.
- Q: What is the prognosis for babies with TEF?
- A: Overall survival is approximately 95%, with most mortalities occurring in very preterm babies and those with congenital cardiac defects. Reflux is common and may require fundoplication in some cases. Esophageal dysmotility is nearly universal, but the long-term implications of this are unclear.

TRACHEOMALACIA/LARYNGOMALACIA

Thomas G. Saba • Amy G. Filbrun

BASICS

DESCRIPTION

- Malacia refers to "softness" of airway structures.
- Laryngomalacia
  - Dynamic collapse of the supraglottic structures of the larynx resulting in airway obstruction
  - Most common congenital anomaly of the larynx
  - Most common noninfectious cause of stridor in children
- Tracheomalacia
  - Dynamic collapse of the trachea resulting in airway obstruction
  - Common cause of chronic wheezing in infants and children
  - Clinical manifestations depend on if lesion is part of the intrathoracic or extrathoracic portions of the trachea.

ETIOLOGY

- Laryngomalacia
  - Anatomic abnormalities:
    - Short aryepiglottic folds
    - Elongated, flaccid, omega-shaped epiglottis prolapses posteriorly.
    - Redundant arytenoid mucosa
  - Neurologic abnormalities:
    - Immaturity of neuromuscular control results in hypotonia of pharyngeal muscles.
- Tracheomalacia
  - Weakness of the tracheal wall secondary to softening of the anterior cartilaginous rings and/or decreased tone of the posterior membranous wall
  - Classified as primary or secondary
    - Primary: congenital; results from immature development of the tracheal structures; may occur with other congenital anomalies such as tracheoesophageal fistula, laryngomalacia, and facial anomalies
    - Secondary: acquired in a normally developed trachea after some insult such as prolonged positive pressure ventilation, recurrent infection or aspiration, or external compression
  - During exhalation, increased collapsing pressure across a compliant airway wall causes invagination of the posterior membrane.
  - With increasing age, the length, area, thickness, and amount of cartilage increases in the anterior rings as well as the size and contractility of the membranous wall.

DIAGNOSIS

HISTORY

- Laryngomalacia
  - Symptoms may be present at birth or delayed until 1–2 months of age.
  - Inspiratory stridor
  - May be asymptomatic during sleep or quiet breathing
  - Worsens with crying, agitation, feeding, upper respiratory infections, supine positioning
- Tracheomalacia
  - Primary: Symptoms may be delayed until 2–3 months of age.
  - Secondary: Symptoms delayed until after causative insult occurs.
  - Expiratory wheeze, if intrathoracic portion of trachea involved
  - Inspiratory stridor, if extrathoracic portion of trachea involved
  - Harsh barking cough
  - Symptoms worsen with crying, agitation, feeding, and infections.
  - Impaired mucus clearance, frequent infections
  - Rarely, cyanosis, hyperextension of neck, breath-holding spells, feeding difficulties

PHYSICAL EXAM

- Laryngomalacia
  - High-pitched or vibratory, inspiratory stridor
  - Suprasternal retractions
  - Positional changes noted: usually worsens with flexion of neck, supine position
  - Stridor transmitted throughout the chest on auscultation
- Tracheomalacia
  - Homophonous expiratory wheeze (intrathoracic malacia)
  - High-pitched inspiratory stridor (extrathoracic malacia)
  - Intercostal retractions, worse during activity, and acute respiratory infections

DIAGNOSTIC TESTS & INTERPRETATION

Diagnostic Procedures/Other

- Flexible fiberoptic laryngo/bronchoscopy
  - Gold standard for diagnosis of dynamic airway collapse
  - Performed during spontaneous breathing
  - Visualize the degree, extent, and location of laryngomalacia and/or tracheomalacia.
  - Evaluate for other airway lesions in the differential diagnosis.
- Barium esophagography
  - Used to evaluate for external vascular compression of the esophagus
  - Might help to identify gastroesophageal reflux
- Chest radiograph
  - Usually normal in both laryngomalacia and tracheomalacia
  - Important to rule out other causes of chronic cough or abnormalities that may cause external airway compression
- Airway fluoroscopy
  - Insensitive except in severe cases; unable to visualize AP and lateral caliber simultaneously
- MRI
  - Useful to evaluate for extrinsic vascular airway compression
- CT
  - Paired end-inspiratory and dynamic expiratory multidetector CT, free-breathing cine CT—both sensitive and specific
  - Exposure to radiation
- Pulmonary function tests
  - Might show flow limitation, typical notching in expiratory portion of flow-volume loop

DIFFERENTIAL DIAGNOSIS

- Laryngomalacia: differential diagnosis of chronic stridor
  - Vocal cord abnormalities: vocal cord paralysis/paresis
  - Laryngeal abnormalities: laryngeal cleft, laryngeal web, subglottic hemangioma, papilloma
  - Subglottic stenosis (biphasic stridor)
- Tracheomalacia: differential diagnosis of chronic homophonous wheeze
  - Structural abnormalities: vascular compression/ring, tracheal stenosis/web, cystic lesion, mass/tumor
  - Nonstructural abnormalities: gastroesophageal reflux disease (GERD), retained foreign body, persistent bacterial bronchitis

ALERT
- The differential diagnosis for stridor in children includes life-threatening causes.
- If history or clinical course deviates from expected pattern, consider comorbidities (asthma, GERD) or investigating for alternative diagnosis.
- Investigate lower airways in more severe cases of laryngomalacia for other airway anomalies.
- The use of $beta_2$ agonists may increase the tracheal wall collapsibility by decreasing muscular tone, thereby making the symptoms worse.
- Bronchoscopy should ideally be done under conscious sedation during spontaneous breathing to avoid altering vocal cord movement and airway dynamics.
- The use of rigid bronchoscopy may stent open the trachea, making tracheomalacia more difficult to identify; flexible bronchoscopy is a more appropriate test.

TREATMENT

GENERAL MEASURES
- Laryngomalacia
  - Most cases resolve spontaneously by 15–18 months of age.
  - Observation and reassurance
  - Consider feeding modifications (pacing, positioning, texture change).
  - Strong association with GERD. Treat if symptomatic; empiric treatment is controversial.
- Tracheomalacia
  - Usually resolves spontaneously by 18–24 months of age
  - Observation and reassurance, chest physiotherapy for mucus clearance
  - Treatment of exacerbating factors, such as upper respiratory infections, asthma, or GERD

Surgery
- Laryngomalacia
  - 10% of cases of laryngomalacia are severe (apnea, cyanosis, severe retractions, failure to thrive, feeding difficulty, obstructive apnea), and require further investigation and treatment.
    - Supraglottoplasty: excision of redundant arytenoid mucosa, trimming of epiglottis, division of tight aryepiglottic folds
    - Tracheostomy
  - Postoperative complications: scarring, dysphagia
- Tracheomalacia
  - For severe cases, little evidence supporting noninvasive and surgical therapies
  - Tracheostomy may be needed in severe cases to bypass lesion or to provide continuous positive airway pressure.
  - Consider aortopexy (suspending the anterior trachea to widen the airway) in severe cases refractory to more conservative management.
  - Airway stents are associated with significant complications; reserved for children with otherwise poor prognosis
  - External airway splints currently under investigation

ONGOING CARE

FOLLOW-UP RECOMMENDATIONS
Monitor for recurrent respiratory symptoms, poor growth, and other exacerbating conditions (asthma, GERD).

PROGNOSIS
- In cases of isolated laryngomalacia and/or tracheomalacia, prognosis is usually excellent.
- In patients with history of tracheoesophageal fistula, vascular ring, or other airway anomalies, tracheal dysfunction may persist after corrective surgery.

ADDITIONAL READING

- Ambrosio A, Brigger MT. Pediatric supraglottopasty. *Adv Otorhinolaryngol*. 2012;73:101–104.
- Carden KA, Boiselle PM, Waltz DA, et al. Tracheomalacia and tracheobronchomalacia in children and adults: an in-depth review. *Chest*. 2005;127(3):984–1005.
- Kugler C, Stanzel F. Tracheomalacia. *Thorac Surg Clin*. 2014;24(1):51–58.
- Masters IB. Congenital airway lesions and lung disease. *Pediatr Clin North Am*. 2009;56(1):227–242.
- Masters IB, Chang AB. Tracheobronchomalacia in children. *Expert Rev Respir Med*. 2009;3(4):425–439.

CODES

ICD10
- Q32.0 Congenital tracheomalacia
- Q31.5 Congenital laryngomalacia

FAQ
- Q: When will the symptoms improve?
- A: As anatomic structures mature with age, laryngomalacia symptoms may improve by 6 months of age, with usual resolution by 18 months of age. Primary tracheomalacia may last longer, but in both entities symptoms usually resolve completely by age 2 years. Natural history of secondary tracheomalacia is dependent on cause.
- Q: Should all patients have an endoscopic evaluation?
- A: No. Diagnosis is usually made based on the history and physical examination. Infants with mild to moderate typical presentation need only careful monitoring for recurrence or worsening of symptoms and for poor growth. However, airway evaluation should be performed in all cases where a different pathology is considered or when symptoms worsen or persist past the expected age of resolution.

TRANSFUSION REACTION

Kristin A. Shimano

BASICS

DESCRIPTION

- Any acute or subacute adverse reaction that develops as a consequence of the administration of blood components
- Types include the following:
  - Acute reactions: hemolytic, febrile, allergic, anaphylactic, septic, transfusion-related acute lung injury (TRALI), transfusion-associated circulatory overload (TACO)
  - Delayed reactions: delayed hemolytic, transfusion-associated graft-versus-host disease (TA-GVHD)
  - Late complications of transfusion: infection, alloimmunization, iron overload

EPIDEMIOLOGY

1% of pediatric blood product recipients develop some type of transfusion reaction.

PATHOPHYSIOLOGY

- Acute hemolytic transfusion reaction
  - Antigen–antibody interaction leads to complement activation on the surface of the transfused RBCs, resulting in acute intravascular hemolysis and vasomotor instability.
  - Usually ABO blood group incompatibility
  - Most commonly due to medical error
- Febrile nonhemolytic transfusion reaction (FNHTR)
  - Cytokines released by leukocytes in the product
  - 40% of patients with one febrile reaction will have a subsequent one.
- Urticarial (allergic)
  - IgE-mediated
  - Recipient allergic response to donor plasma proteins or other constituents of plasma
  - Sporadic and donor dependent
- Anaphylactic
  - Overwhelming acute allergic reaction. Can be mediated by anti-IgA formed by a recipient who is IgA deficient and receives blood products containing IgA
- Bacterial sepsis
  - Intravascular infusion of viable bacteria and endotoxins leads to fever, chills, and/or acute septic shock.
  - Contaminated blood product; most commonly a platelet product near the end of shelf life
- Delayed hemolytic transfusion reaction (DHTR)
  - Previously transfused patients who are sensitized to a minor blood group antigen, especially Jk^a or Jk^b (Kidd antigen), develop an anamnestic response on reexposure.
  - Antibody is below detectable levels in antibody screen and crossmatch; after transfusion, titers rise (usually within 2–10 days) and extravascular hemolysis occurs.
- TRALI
  - Antileukocyte antibodies or neutrophil-activating factors in transfused product interact with recipient neutrophils, causing leukocyte aggregates that deposit in the lung.
  - Multiparous female donors with HLA sensitization often are implicated.
- TACO
  - Circulatory overload leading to heart failure
  - Administration of an excessive volume of a blood product or infusion at an excessive rate
- TA-GVHD
  - Patients with inherited or acquired T-cell immunodeficiency can develop TA-GVHD from transfused immunocompetent T cells.
  - Can also occur if the donor and recipient are related and share HLA types

DIAGNOSIS

HISTORY

- Acute hemolytic
  - Fever/chills
  - Abdominal or flank pain
  - Pink or tea-colored urine
  - Tachycardia
  - Hypotension
  - Oliguria
- FNHTR
  - Fever, chills 1–6 hours after transfusion
- Urticarial
  - Urticaria
  - Flushing
  - Pruritus
- Anaphylactic
  - Urticaria
  - Bronchospasm
  - Hypotension
- Bacterial sepsis
  - Fever
  - Chills
  - Hypotension
- DHTR
  - Fever
  - Malaise
  - Dark urine
  - Jaundice
  - Shock (rarely)
  - Renal failure 2–10 days after transfusion
- TRALI
  - Acute dyspnea, tachypnea, rales, decreased oxygenation within 6 hours of transfusion
- TACO
  - Hypertension
  - Dyspnea
  - Rales
  - Cardiac arrhythmia
- TA-GVHD
  - Fever
  - Rash
  - Diarrhea
  - Cough 4–30 days after transfusion

DIAGNOSTIC TESTS & INTERPRETATION

Lab

- Acute hemolytic
  - Direct Coombs test: positive
  - CBC: anemia
  - Urinalysis: hemoglobinuria
  - Prothrombin time (PT), partial thromboplastin time (PTT), fibrinogen, fibrin split products: disseminated intravascular coagulation (DIC)
- FNHTR
  - Direct Coombs test: negative or no change from pretransfusion
  - Immediate Gram stain of the product
  - Blood culture of the patient and product
  - All results should be negative; a diagnosis of exclusion.
- Urticarial
  - No specific testing
- Anaphylactic
  - IgA level in recipient. If undetectable, test for anti-IgA antibody (of the IgE class).
- Bacterial sepsis
  - Immediate Gram stain and blood culture of the transfused product: result positive for bacteria
- DHTR
  - CBC: anemia
  - Bilirubin: elevated
  - Indirect Coombs test (antibody screen): positive
  - Direct Coombs test: positive (mixed field) if done early
- TRALI
  - Leukocyte antibody testing in the implicated donor(s)

Imaging

- Chest radiograph: increased pulmonary vascular markings or infiltrates for hypervolemia (TACO) and TRALI

TREATMENT

GENERAL PREVENTION

- Acute hemolytic
  - Proper labeling of blood specimens and products and adherence to procedures for correct identification of product and recipient will eliminate most acute hemolytic transfusion reactions.
- FNHTR
  - Administration of leukodepleted products, especially for long-term transfused patients who have a high incidence of febrile transfusion reactions
  - No evidence to support premedication with Tylenol or Benadryl to prevent FNHTR
- Urticarial
  - Administration of washed erythrocyte products (in patients with repeated or severe allergic reactions)
  - No conclusive evidence to support premedication with antihistamines
- Anaphylactic
  - If due to anti-IgA in an IgA-deficient recipient, provision of IgA deficient products may be possible.
- Bacterial sepsis
  - Sterile technique in blood collection, storage, and administration; inspection of product before transfusion
  - Bacterial screening of platelet products before they are transfused
- DHTR
  - Appropriately performed antibody screen and crossmatch as pretransfusion testing
  - Check blood bank records for previous antibodies.
- TRALI
  - Deferral of donors is implicated in proven TRALI cases.
- TACO
  - Administer appropriate volumes (typically 10–15 mL/kg) at appropriate rate, usually over 3–4 hours unless hypovolemic or actively bleeding.
  - Patients with chronic anemia are euvolemic and should be transfused with smaller volumes over longer time periods.
- TA-GVHD
  - Patients at risk (immunocompromised, neonates) must receive irradiated blood products.

ADDITIONAL TREATMENT

General Measures

- Acute hemolytic
  - Stop transfusion immediately.
  - Supportive care with hydration, pressors, and diuretics to maintain circulation and urine output
- FNHTR
  - Stop transfusion.
  - Antipyretics (acetaminophen)
  - Demerol for severe chills and rigors
  - May resume transfusion if patient is stable and acute hemolytic transfusion reaction and bacterial sepsis are ruled out
- Urticarial
  - Stop transfusion.
  - Antihistamine (diphenhydramine)
  - Steroids or epinephrine in severe reactions
  - Transfusion may be resumed if mild reaction
- Anaphylactic
  - Epinephrine
  - IV fluids, pressors
  - Respiratory support
- Bacterial sepsis
  - Stop transfusion.
  - Fluids if hypotensive
  - Antibiotics to eradicate *Staphylococcus* and Gram negatives including *Yersinia* species
- DHTR
  - Depends on degree of hemolysis; if profound, management as acute hemolytic reaction. If mild, no therapy may be needed.
- TRALI
  - Supportive care, usually resolves in 12–24 hours
- TACO: diuretics (furosemide)
- TA-GVHD: no treatment, almost always fatal

ONGOING CARE

COMPLICATIONS

- Posttransfusion hepatitis: caused by hepatitis B or C viruses, others
- AIDS: caused by HIV
- Cytomegalovirus (CMV)
  - Symptomatic infection in patients with inherited or acquired immunodeficiency states, premature neonates
  - These individuals should receive CMV-safe products.
- Other transfusion-transmissible infections
  - Epstein-Barr virus, syphilis, malaria, toxoplasmosis, human T-lymphotropic virus I (HTLV-I), Chagas disease, babesiosis, filariasis, West Nile virus, parvovirus B19
- Alloimmunization
  - Formation of antibodies to erythrocyte, platelet, and HLA antigens can develop in some multiply transfused patients; may cause delays in pretransfusion testing, febrile transfusion reactions, delayed hemolytic transfusion reactions, and platelet transfusion refractoriness.
  - HLA alloimmunization may also affect eligibility and organ procurement for solid organ transplantation.
- Iron overload
  - Long-term transfusion recipients will accumulate iron as a by-product of erythrocyte breakdown.
  - An iron-chelating drug will enhance its excretion.

ADDITIONAL READING

- Lindholm PF, Annen K, Ramsey G. Approaches to minimize infection risk in blood banking and transfusion practice. *Infect Disord Drug Targets*. 2011;11(1):45–56.
- Slonim AD, Joseph JG, Turenne WM, et al. Blood transfusions in children: a multi-institutional analysis of practices and complications. *Transfusion*. 2008;48(1):73–80.
- Tobian AA, King KE, Ness PM. Transfusion premedications: a growing practice not based on evidence. *Transfusion*. 2007;47(6):1089–1096.
- Vamvakas EC, Blajchman MA. Transfusion-related mortality: the ongoing risks of allogeneic blood transfusion and the available strategies for their prevention. *Blood*. 2009;113(15):3406–3417.

CODES

ICD10

- T80.92XA Unspecified transfusion reaction, initial encounter
- T80.919A Hemolytic transfusion reaction, unspecified incompatibility, unspecified as acute or delayed, initial encounter
- R50.84 Febrile nonhemolytic transfusion reaction

FAQ

- Q: What is the risk of acquiring certain viral infections?
- A: Hepatitis B: 1:300,000 transfused units; hepatitis C: 1:1,800,000 transfused units; HIV: 1:2,300,000 transfused units
- Q: What is the risk of developing bacterial sepsis?
- A: 1:1,000,000 red cell units; 1:13,000–100,000 platelet units
- Q: Is directed donor blood safer?
- A: No. There is no evidence that the infection risk is lower, and some studies suggest that the infection risk may be higher.
- Q: Is it safe to give a transfusion to a patient with fever?
- A: Yes. However, if the temperature rises during the transfusion or if symptoms such as chills or hypotension develop, the transfusion should be stopped and the patient evaluated for a transfusion reaction.

T

TRANSIENT ERYTHROBLASTOPENIA OF CHILDHOOD

Julie W. Stern

BASICS

DESCRIPTION
An acquired, self-limited suppression of red cell production in an otherwise healthy child

EPIDEMIOLOGY
- Mean age at diagnosis is 26 months.
- $<$10% are $>$3 years of age at diagnosis.
- Slight male predominance (male:female ~5:3)
- No seasonal predominance

RISK FACTORS
Genetics
- There is no simple genetic pattern.
- Familial transient erythroblastopenia of childhood has been reported (rarely), suggesting a combination of environmental factors and genetic propensity.

GENERAL PREVENTION
There is no known way to prevent transient erythroblastopenia of childhood.

ETIOLOGY
- Unknown
- Possible viral causes include parvovirus B19 and human herpesvirus 6 (HHV-6), but this remains hypothetical.
- A serum inhibitor, such as an IgG directed at the committed erythroid stem cell progenitor, has also been proposed but not yet proven.

DIAGNOSIS

HISTORY
- Pallor
  - Typically slow in onset and therefore often missed by parents
  - Often noted by an adult who sees the child less frequently
- Activity level
  - Often preserved because of slow onset of anemia
  - An extremely anemic child may be irritable, sleepy, and/or lethargic.
- History of fever, easy bruisability, or frequent/severe infections (especially bacterial): should alert the clinician to consider other diagnoses such as leukemia and bone marrow failure syndromes

PHYSICAL EXAM
- Child is generally well appearing and not chronically ill.
- Pallor
- Tachycardia secondary to anemia
- Usually no organomegaly, ecchymosis, petechiae, or jaundice

DIAGNOSTIC TESTS & INTERPRETATION
Diagnostic Procedures/Other
- CBC
  - Low hemoglobin, normal mean corpuscular volume (MCV), normal RBC morphology
  - Total WBC count/morphology and platelet count should be normal; if not, consider leukemias.
  - Absolute neutrophil count may be decreased (rarely $<$500/μL), but morphology must be normal.
  - Red cell distribution width may be elevated during recovery.
- Reticulocyte count
  - Low to zero during anemic phase
  - Should be high during recovery
- Chemistry/blood bank:
  - Bilirubin, lactate dehydrogenase, ferritin, iron levels, and direct and indirect Coombs testing should be normal to rule out iron deficiency anemia and immune hemolysis.
- Parvovirus titers, parvovirus polymerase chain reaction (PCR) testing
- Immunoglobulin (Ig) levels in some cases
- Hemoglobin electrophoresis with quantitative fetal hemoglobin
  - Should be normal in transient erythroblastopenia of childhood
  - Fetal Hgb elevated in Diamond-Blackfan anemia
- Chest radiograph: to determine degree of cardiomegaly
- Bone marrow aspiration
  - Not mandatory to make diagnosis
  - May be necessary to rule in transient erythroblastopenia of childhood and rule out other diagnoses such as Diamond-Blackfan or leukemia
  - Presence or absence of early RBC precursors may help predict time to recovery.
  - Maturation of megakaryocytes and the myeloid cell line must be normal, especially if neutropenia is present.

DIFFERENTIAL DIAGNOSIS
- Environmental: iron deficiency anemia
- Metabolic: hypothyroidism
- Diamond-Blackfan anemia (this diagnosis usually made within 1st year of life)
- Neoplasm
  - Leukemia
  - Myelodysplastic syndromes
- Miscellaneous
  - Renal disease
  - Anemia of chronic disease
  - Blood loss (usually GI)

TREATMENT

MEDICATION
- No role for prednisone, iron supplements, anabolic steroids, or other immunosuppressive agents
- Short-term folic acid may be indicated during reticulocytosis.

ADDITIONAL TREATMENT
General Measures
- Initial inpatient observation for complications of severe anemia; daily CBC at least initially to gauge rate of fall of hemoglobin/rise of reticulocyte count and to estimate time to recovery

- Packed RBC transfusion
  - If there is evidence of cardiovascular compromise
  - If a transfusion is needed, transfuse slowly to prevent fluid overload. A good rule of thumb is to transfuse the same number of mL/kg as the patient's hemoglobin over 3–4 hours. Should a 2nd transfusion be needed, attempt to use a 2nd aliquot of the same unit to decrease donor exposure.
- Normal activity and diet for age, as tolerated
- Instruct family on signs and symptoms of severe anemia.

ONGOING CARE

FOLLOW-UP RECOMMENDATIONS

- Clinic visits weekly to monitor hemoglobin and reticulocytes. These visits may need to be more frequent in the beginning of the illness and less frequent as recovery becomes evident.
- Elevation of reticulocyte count is the first sign of recovery.

PROGNOSIS

- All children recover usually within 1–2 months from diagnosis (may take up to 8–12 months for full recovery).
- Prognosis is excellent.
- Recurrence is rare.

COMPLICATIONS

- Cardiovascular compromise secondary to severe anemia is often less than expected given the level of anemia. High-output CHF is unusual.
- Neurologic symptoms including confusion and transient hemiparesis have been reported but are rare.
- A significant number of patients also have neutropenia (absolute neutrophil count $\leq$1,500/μL) during either the acute or recovery phase of the illness.

ALERT

- Isolation is necessary because of possible teratogenicity of parvovirus 19 and contagion within the hospital.
- Transient erythroblastopenia of childhood must be an isolated normocytic, normochromic anemia. If the other cell lines are affected (except for mild neutropenia) or if the anemia is macrocytic, consider bone marrow failure syndromes.
- Iron therapy has no place in the treatment of transient erythroblastopenia of childhood. Be sure to check RBC indices and reticulocyte count prior to instituting iron therapy for anemia.

ADDITIONAL READING

- Bhambhani K, Inoue S, Sarnaik SA. Seasonal clustering of transient erythroblastopenia of childhood. *Am J Child Dis*. 1988;142(2):175–177.
- Shaw J, Meeder R. Transient erythroblastopenia of childhood in siblings: case report and review of the literature. *J Pediatr Hematol Oncol*. 2007;29(9): 659–660.
- Skeppner G, Kreuger A, Elinder G. Transient erythroblastopenia of childhood: prospective study of 10 patients with special reference to viral infections. *J Pediatr Hematol Oncol*. 2002;24(4):294–298.

CODES

ICD10

D60.1 Transient acquired pure red cell aplasia

FAQ

- Q: Can other children in a family get this illness?
- A: The cause(s) of this illness in otherwise normal children is unknown. It is very rare for other family members to be affected. It is appropriate to reassure parents regarding this issue.
- Q: Are transfusions always necessary?
- A: No. Only in cases of heart failure is a transfusion necessary. Most often, children can be managed with watchful waiting.
- Q: How can transient erythroblastopenia of childhood be distinguished from Diamond-Blackfan syndrome?
- A: Children with Diamond-Blackfan syndrome are usually <1 year old and can have elevated hemoglobin F levels. If a bone marrow aspirate is obtained during the recovery phase of transient erythroblastopenia of childhood, the diagnosis will be clear. Often, however, only time will tell. Children with transient erythroblastopenia of childhood always recover; those with Diamond-Blackfan syndrome do not.
- Q: Is transient erythroblastopenia of childhood a precursor to leukemia?
- A: No. However, if recovery does not occur in a timely manner, or if neutropenia worsens, a bone marrow aspirate may be indicated if not previously completed.

TRANSIENT TACHYPNEA OF THE NEWBORN

Colleen A. Hughes Driscoll • Bernadette A. Hillman

BASICS

DESCRIPTION

- Early onset of tachypnea (respiratory rate >60 breaths/minute) in the newborn following an uneventful delivery
- Symptoms of respiratory distress including mild retractions, expiratory grunting, and nasal flaring may occur. Cyanosis is rarely involved.

EPIDEMIOLOGY

Incidence

- Estimated 4–6 per 1,000 live births
- Incidence is likely underestimated.
- Most common cause of respiratory distress in newborns
- Higher in males

RISK FACTORS

- Early gestation
- Cesarean section delivery (with or without preceding labor)
- Male gender
- Maternal diabetes
- Macrosomia
- Low birth weight
- Maternal history of asthma
- Unexplained transient tachypnea of the newborn (TTN) in individuals belonging to the same family suggests a genetic predisposition.

GENERAL PREVENTION

- Vaginal delivery should be recommended in the absence of maternal or fetal indications for cesarean section.
- Elective cesarean section before 39 weeks' gestation should be avoided.

ETIOLOGY

- During fetal life, pulmonary epithelial cells are secretory, delivering chloride into the alveolar space.
- Sodium and water follow chloride into the alveoli, establishing and maintaining fetal lung fluid.
- During labor and delivery, fetal lung fluid is absorbed through a variety of proposed mechanisms:
  - Epithelial cells transition from secretory cells to absorptive cells in response to circulating epinephrine levels, which trigger opening of epithelial sodium channels (ENaC).
  - Compression of the fetal thorax from uterine contractions and passage through the vaginal canal contributes to removal of fluid from the lungs through the pulmonary circulation.
  - Prostaglandin-mediated dilation of lymphatic vessels occurs with resultant absorption of interstitial lung fluid into the lymphatic system.
- TTN occurs when there is inadequate fluid clearance from the lungs.
- It is believed that this excess interstitial lung fluid contributes to decreased lung compliance.

DIAGNOSIS

HISTORY

- Tachypnea presenting within the first few hours of life
- Presence of familial risk factors
  - Maternal diabetes
  - Maternal asthma
  - Family history of unexplained TTN
- Birth-related risk factors
  - Perinatal depression
- Absence of risk factors that suggest an infectious, metabolic, or anatomic disease process such as the following:
  - Maternal chorioamnionitis or other untreated maternal infections
  - Meconium or blood-stained amniotic fluid
  - Prolonged rupture of membranes
  - Long-standing oligohydramnios or anhydramnios
  - Advanced resuscitation at delivery
- Presence of risk factors for other conditions should prompt additional investigations.

PHYSICAL EXAM

- Respiratory rate >60 breaths/minute
- Grunting, nasal flaring, mild to moderate retractions; rarely, cyanosis
- Symmetric breath sounds on auscultation
- Symmetry of thoracic cavity, possibly with barrel-shaped chest appearance due to lung hyperinflation
- Lungs are generally clear on auscultation, but crackles may be present.
- Absence of stridor
- Absence of signs, symptoms, or other abnormalities in one or more additional organ systems

DIAGNOSTIC TESTS & INTERPRETATION

- TTN is a diagnosis of exclusion.
- Degree of diagnostic workup will vary and will depend on risk factors and clinical manifestations of the mother and baby.
- Risk factors or physical findings consistent with other disease processes should prompt diagnostic testing as clinically indicated.
- CBC
  - Leukopenia or leukocytosis with increased immature to total neutrophil count suggests infection.
- C-reactive protein
  - May be elevated within the first 24 hours with infectious etiology
- If abnormalities exist on these laboratory evaluations, a workup for infection is warranted and should minimally include a blood culture and chest radiograph.
- Arterial blood gas
  - Respiratory acidosis (particularly for P_{CO_2} >60 mmHg), metabolic acidosis, or metabolic alkalosis suggest alternative etiologies for respiratory distress.
  - A significantly elevated A–a gradient may suggest an extrapulmonary or intrapulmonary right-to-left shunt.
- Pulse oximetry
  - Typically, preductal saturations will be greater than 95% on room air.
  - Supplemental oxygen is rarely required; oxygen supplementation of more than 40% FiO_2 suggests an alternative etiology.
- Echocardiogram
  - Respiratory distress and cyanosis may be a manifestation of congenital heart disease.

Imaging

- Chest radiograph
  - Findings are variable but generally include pronounced perihilar vascular marking and fluid opacity in the interlobar spaces.
  - Slight flattening of the diaphragms and increase in the intercostals spaces can be present if air trapping occurs.
- Of note, there may be poor concordance between the clinical diagnosis of TTN and the presence of radiographic findings of TTN, as radiographic interpretation in cases of TTN is relatively variable.

DIFFERENTIAL DIAGNOSIS

- Respiratory
  - Delayed adaption of the newborn
  - Meconium/blood/amniotic fluid aspiration
  - Respiratory distress syndrome
  - Pulmonary hypoplasia
  - Persistent pulmonary hypertension of the newborn
  - Pneumothorax
  - Pneumomediastinum

- Infection
  - Pneumonia
  - Sepsis
- Neurologic
  - Hypoxic brain injury
  - Conditions that present with central hypotonia
- Cardiac
  - Congenital cyanotic heart disease
  - Cardiovascular anatomy that contributes to pulmonary overcirculation
- Metabolic
  - Conditions that present with metabolic acidosis or hyperammonemia
- Miscellaneous
  - Disorders related to abnormal embryonic pulmonary development (e.g., congenital diaphragmatic hernia, congenital cystic adenomatous malformation, congenital emphysema)
  - Congenital airway abnormalities (e.g., Pierre Robin sequence, choanal atresia)

ALERT

TTN is a diagnosis of exclusion. A thorough review of the maternal history, birth history, and physical examination is essential in determining the degree of workup needed to exclude more severe etiologies.

TREATMENT

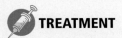

GENERAL MEASURES

- Resolution of symptoms will occur in time, most often within the first 2 days of life.
- Initial management
  - Direct observation under radiant heat for signs of worsening tachypnea/distress or other abnormal vital signs
  - NPO for initial observation period
  - Monitoring for hypoglycemia
  - Continuous cardiorespiratory monitoring and pulse oximeter monitoring—preductal saturation goal of >95% as the infant transitions to extrauterine circulation
  - Administration of antibiotics and appropriate diagnostic workup if infection or metabolic condition is suspected

ONGOING CARE

FOLLOW-UP RECOMMENDATIONS

Patient Monitoring

- Admission to a Special Care Nursery or Neonatal Intensive Care Unit and chest radiography are indicated for the following:
  - Symptoms persisting beyond 2 hours from onset
  - Worsening of symptoms or onset of additional symptoms
  - Infection is suspected.
  - Persistent need for oxygen
  - Chest radiograph is abnormal.
  - IV fluids are required to maintain nutrition/hydration.

PATIENT EDUCATION

Infant can transition to routine care when

- There has been steady improvement in symptoms during the observation period.
- The respiratory rate permits adequate oral nutrition.
- When oxygen is no longer required to maintain normal oxygen saturations

PROGNOSIS

- TTN is typically self-resolved and few, if any, long-term sequelae exist.
- Recent studies have shown an association between TTN and developing wheezing symptoms at school age.

COMPLICATIONS

- Hypoxia requiring oxygen administration
- Occasionally, mechanical ventilation is necessary, and rarely, extracorporeal membrane oxygenation is needed if persistent pulmonary hypertension develops.

ADDITIONAL READING

- Abughalwa M, Taha S, Sharaf N, et al. Antibiotics therapy in classic transient tachypnea of the newborn: a necessary treatment or not? A prospective study. *Neonatology Today*. 2010;7(6):3–8.
- American College of Obstetricians and Gynecologists. ACOG Committee opinion no. 559: cesarean delivery on maternal request. *Obstet Gynecol*. 2013: 121(4);904–907.
- Consortium on Safe Labor, Hibbard JU, Wilkins I, et al. Respiratory morbidity in late preterm births. *JAMA*. 2010;304(4):419–425.
- Costa S, Rocha G, Leitão A, et al. Transient tachypnea of the newborn and congenital pneumonia: a comparative study. *J Matern Fetal Neonatal Med*. 2012:25(7):992–994.
- Guglani LG, Lakshminrusimha S, Ryan R. Transient tachypnea of the newborn. *Pediatr Rev*. 2008; 29(11):e59–e65.
- Hermansen CL, Lorah KN. Respiratory distress in the newborn. *Am Fam Physician*. 2007:76(7):987–994.
- Liem JJ, Hug SI, Ekuma O, et al. Transient tachypnea of the newborn may be an early clinical manifestation of wheezing symptoms. *J Pediatr*. 2001:151(1): 29–33.
- Mendola P, Männiatö TI, Leishear K, et al. Neonatal health of infants born to mothers with asthma. *J Allergy Clin Immunol*. 2014;133(1):85–90.
- Silasi M, Coonrod DV, Kim M, et al. Transient tachypnea of the newborn: is labor prior to cesarean delivery protective? *Am J Perinatol*. 2010:27(10): 797–802.
- Yurdakok M. Transient tachypnea of the newborn: what is new? *J Matern Fetal Neonatal Med*. 2010; 23(Suppl 3):24–26.

CODES

ICD10

P22.1 Transient tachypnea of newborn

FAQ

- Q: For how long does the tachypnea generally occur?
- A: Most babies' respiratory rates improve within 72 hours; in persistent cases, it may last longer.
- Q: What respiratory rate is safe for trial of PO feeds?
- A: <70 breaths/minute without an exaggerated respiratory effort.
- Q: What respiratory rate is safe for hospital discharge?
- A: <60 breaths/minute for greater than 12 hours to ensure resolution of symptoms and confirm the diagnosis of TTN.

TRANSPOSITION OF THE GREAT ARTERIES

Bradley S. Marino • Pirouz Shamszad

BASICS

DESCRIPTION

Abnormal anatomic relationship between the great arteries and the ventricles in which the aorta arises from the anatomic right ventricle and the pulmonary artery arises from the anatomic left ventricle

Incidence

Incidence is 20–30 per 100,000 live births, with a 60–70% male predilection.

Prevalence

Transposition of the great arteries represents up to 7% of all cases of congenital heart disease.

PATHOPHYSIOLOGY

- Systemic and pulmonary circulations are separated and function in parallel.
- Desaturated systemic venous blood is ejected from the right heart to the aorta, whereas the oxygenated pulmonary venous blood is ejected from the left ventricle into the lungs.
- Degree of hypoxemia depends on amount of intercirculatory mixing (patent ductus arteriosus [PDA], patent foramen ovale [PFO], ventricular septal defect [VSD]).
  - Degree of left-to-right shunting is the effective systemic blood flow, whereas right-to-left shunting determines effective pulmonary flow.

COMMONLY ASSOCIATED CONDITIONS

- PDA and PFO with intact ventricular septum (50%)
- VSD (40%)
- Posterior malalignment VSD with left ventricular outflow tract obstruction (e.g., subpulmonic stenosis, pulmonary stenosis, pulmonary atresia) (10%)
- Anterior malalignment VSD with right ventricular outflow tract obstruction (e.g., subaortic stenosis, aortic stenosis, coarctation of the aorta or interruption of the aortic arch) (10%)
- Leftward juxtaposition of the atrial appendages (5%)
- Straddling of the atrioventricular valve

DIAGNOSIS

HISTORY

- Infants are of normal birth weight or sometimes large for gestational age.
- Cyanosis
- Tachypnea often without retractions
- Poor feeding

PHYSICAL EXAM

- General
  - Moderate to severe cyanosis
- Cardiovascular
  - Heart sounds: Single loud S_2, but no heart murmur is heard in infants with intact ventricular septum; soft systolic murmur in those infants with a VSD and a systolic ejection murmur of valvar or subvalvar aortic or pulmonic stenosis may be heard.
- Respiratory
  - Generally, dyspnea and tachypnea present without retractions in a neonate without a VSD; with a large VSD and congestive heart failure (CHF), retractions may be present.
- Abdomen
  - Hepatomegaly may occur with a large VSD and CHF.

DIAGNOSTIC TESTS & INTERPRETATION

Lab

Arterial blood gas

- Hypoxemia (Po_2 often in low 30s) unchanged in 100% FiO_2. Infants with inadequate mixing have Po_2 <25 torr with metabolic acidosis.

Imaging

- Chest radiograph
  - Mild cardiomegaly with an egg-shaped heart with narrow superior mediastinum (so-called egg on a string) and increased pulmonary vascular markings
- ECG
  - Initially normal, progressing to right ventricular hypertrophy and right axis deviation
- Echocardiogram
  - 2D ECHO and color-flow Doppler studies usually provide all anatomic and functional information required for management of infants with D-transposition of the great arteries (D-TGA). The study should focus on the alignment of the great arteries and other associated anomalies, specifically defects that promote intercirculatory mixing, the presence of left or right ventricular outflow tract obstruction, and the coronary anatomy.

Pathologic Findings

- In D-TGA, the aorta is oriented anteriorly and rightward from the pulmonary artery and originates from the right ventricle, carrying desaturated blood to the body. The pulmonary artery originates posteriorly from the left ventricle and carries oxygenated blood to the lungs. There is fibrous continuity between the pulmonary and mitral valves; subaortic conus (infundibulum) is present. In the normal heart, the aorta arises posteriorly from the left ventricle and carries oxygenated blood to the body, there is fibrous continuity between the aortic and mitral valves, and subpulmonary conus is present.
- TGA types
  - The most common type of TGA, known as D-TGA, has transposed great arteries with cardiac segments S, D, and D: situs solitus of the atria and viscera (S), dextroventricular segment situs (D), aortic valve annulus to the right of the pulmonary artery (D). There is atrioventricular concordance and ventriculoarterial discordance.
  - L-TGA, or "corrected transposition," has transposed great arteries with cardiac segments S, L, and L: situs solitus of the atria and viscera (S), levoventricular segment situs (L), and the aortic valve annulus is to the left of the pulmonary artery (L). There is atrioventricular discordance and ventriculoarterial discordance.
- Abnormal coronary artery (CA) branching occurs in 33%.
  - Circumflex artery off the right CA (16%), single right CA (4%), single left CA (2%)

DIFFERENTIAL DIAGNOSIS

The differential diagnosis for the neonate with TGA is that for the cyanotic neonate.

- Cardiac
  - Lesions with ductal-dependent pulmonary blood flow
    - Tricuspid atresia with normally related great arteries
    - Tetralogy of Fallot
    - Tetralogy of Fallot with pulmonic atresia
    - Critical pulmonic stenosis
    - Pulmonary atresia with intact ventricular septum
    - Ebstein anomaly
    - Heterotaxy (most forms)
  - Ductal-independent mixing lesions
    - Total anomalous pulmonary venous connection without obstruction
    - Truncus arteriosus
  - Lesions with ductal-dependent systemic blood flow
    - Hypoplastic left heart syndrome
    - Interrupted aortic arch
    - Critical coarctation of the aorta
    - Critical aortic stenosis
- Pulmonary
  - Primary lung disease
  - Airway obstruction
  - Extrinsic compression of the lungs
- Neurologic
  - CNS dysfunction
  - Respiratory neuromuscular dysfunction
- Hematologic
  - Methemoglobinemia
  - Polycythemia

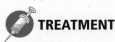

TREATMENT

MEDICATION

- Correction of metabolic acidosis, hypoglycemia, and hypocalcemia improves myocardial function.
- Prostaglandin E1 (PGE1) is used for severe cyanosis to promote left (aorta) to right (pulmonary artery) shunting at the ductus arteriosus, thereby increasing pulmonary blood flow, distention of the left atrium, and improved mixing at the atrial level. Side effects of PGE1 include apnea, fever, and hypotension.

SURGERY/OTHER PROCEDURES

- Interventional catheterization
  - Balloon atrial septostomy (Rashkind procedure) is used in the severely hypoxemic infant with an intact or restrictive atrial septum to promote intercirculatory mixing at the atrial level and stabilize the neonate before definitive or palliative surgery.
- Definitive surgery for D-TGA includes procedures that redirect the pulmonary and systemic venous return at the atrial, ventricular, and great artery levels.
  - Atrial inversion: Atrial inversion procedures involve baffling the pulmonary venous blood flow to the tricuspid valve (systemic circulation) and the systemic venous blood flow to the mitral valve (pulmonary circulation). The 2 atrial inversion operations include the Mustard procedure, in which prosthetic or pericardial baffles are used to redirect the blood, and the Senning procedure, in which the baffles are composed of an atrial septal flap and the right atrial free wall. The Senning or Mustard procedures may be used in the following infants:
    - Infants with D-TGA with intact ventricular septum who have not had surgical repair within the 1st month of life
    - Neonates with D-TGA with intact ventricular septum and severe pulmonic stenosis. Most centers would perform a Rastelli procedure for this anatomic variant (see subsequent list items).
    - Neonates with D-TGA with "unswitchable coronaries" (<1% of cases)
  - Ventricular inversion
    - D-TGA with a VSD and severe pulmonic stenosis: The Rastelli operation may be used to redirect blood flow at the ventricular level. In this operation, the proximal main pulmonary artery is divided and oversewn, and the left ventricular blood flow is baffled to the aorta by creating an intraventricular tunnel between the VSD and the aortic valve. A conduit is placed from the right ventricle to the pulmonary artery to redirect the right ventricular blood flow.
  - Arterial switch
    - D-TGA with intact ventricular septum and "switchable" coronaries: The arterial switch operation (ASO) is performed in which the great arteries are transected above their respective semilunar valves and switched with reimplantation of the CAs into the neoaortic root (native pulmonary valve root).
    - D-TGA with anterior malalignment VSD with severe aortic stenosis: ASO with VSD patch closure and transannular patch of the right ventricular outflow tract

ONGOING CARE

PROGNOSIS

- Without treatment, mortality is 30% within the 1st week of life, 50% within the 1st month, 70% within the first 6 months, and 90% within the 1st year.
- In most centers, the mortality rate after ASO for D-TGA with intact ventricular septum or D-TGA with a VSD is <3%. Factors that have been shown to increase the mortality risk include an intramural course of the left CA, retropulmonary course of the left CA, complex arch abnormalities, right ventricular hypoplasia, multiple VSDs, and straddling atrioventricular valves.

COMPLICATIONS

- Complications of intra-atrial surgeries include absence of sinus rhythm (>50% of cases), supraventricular arrhythmias (50%), moderately to severely depressed right ventricular function (20%), residual intra-atrial baffle shunt (20% of cases), tricuspid regurgitation (5–10% of cases), obstruction of systemic venous return (5% of cases), and obstruction of pulmonary venous return (<2% of cases). Follow-up observation is recommended every 12 months to detect arrhythmias, tricuspid regurgitation, or depressed right ventricular function that generally occurs years after surgery. Arrhythmias include sinus node dysfunction (e.g., marked sinus bradycardia, ectopic atrial rhythm, junctional rhythm, or junctional bradycardia) and supraventricular tachycardia, especially atrial flutter.
- Complications after the Rastelli operation include left ventricular outflow tract obstruction, conduit obstruction, and complete heart block. Follow-up observation is recommended every 12 months to monitor for conduit obstruction, left ventricular outflow tract obstruction, and heart block.
- The most common complication after the ASO is neoaortic root dilation with or without neoaortic insufficiency. Other rarer complications include supravalvar pulmonary stenosis at the anastomotic site (5% of cases), supravalvar aortic stenosis at the anastomotic site (5% of cases), and CA obstruction, which may lead to ischemia and infarction. These complications are uncommon and usually hemodynamically insignificant. Mortality varies depending on the period of time being assessed:
  - Early mortality is usually related to kinking or obstruction of the CAs during transfer to the neoaorta, an "unprepared" left ventricle, or hemorrhage from the multiple suture lines.
  - Late mortality (i.e., 1–2%) usually results from myocardial ischemia, pulmonary vascular obstructive disease, or during reoperation for supravalvar stenosis.
- Follow-up observation is recommended every 12 months to monitor for neoaortic root dilation, neoaortic valve insufficiency, supravalvar aortic or pulmonic stenosis, and CA ischemia.

ADDITIONAL READING

- Bellinger DC, Wypij D, Du Plessis AJ, et al. Neurodevelopmental status at eight years in children with dextro-transposition of the great arteries: the Boston Circulatory Arrest Trial. *J Thorac Cardiovasc Surg*. 2003;126(5):1385–1396.
- Culbert EL, Ashburn DA, Cullen-Dean G, et al. Congenital Heart Surgeons Society. Quality of life of children after repair of transposition of the great arteries. *Circulation*. 2003;108(7):857–862.
- Formigari R, Toscano A, Giardini A, et al. Prevalence and predictors of neoaortic regurgitation after arterial switch operation for transposition of the great arteries. *J Thorac Cardiovasc Surg*. 2003;126(6):1753–1759.
- Langley SM, Winlaw DS, Stumper O, et al. Midterm results after restoration of the morphologically left ventricle to the systemic circulation in patients with congenitally corrected transposition of the great arteries. *J Thorac Cardiovasc Surg*. 2003;125(6):1229–1241.
- Marino BS, Wernovsky G, McElhinney D, et al. Neo-aortic valvar function after the arterial switch. *Cardiol Young*. 2006;16(5):481–489.
- Mavroudis C, Backer CL. Physiologic versus anatomic repair of congenitally corrected transposition of the great arteries. *Semin Thorac Cardiovasc Surg Pediatr Card Surg Annu*. 2003;6:16–26.
- Pasquali SK, Hasselblad V, Li JS, et al. Coronary artery pattern and outcome of arterial switch operation for transposition of the great arteries: a meta-analysis. *Circulation*. 2002;106(20):2575–2580.
- Warnes CA. Transposition of the great arteries. *Circulation*. 2006;114(24);2699–2709.
- Williams WG, McCrindle BW, Ashburn DA, et al; Congenital Heart Surgeon's Society. Outcomes of 829 neonates with complete transposition of the great arteries 12–17 years after repair. *Eur J Cardiothorac Surg*. 2003;24(1):1–9.

CODES

ICD10

- Q20.3 Discordant ventriculoarterial connection
- Q20.5 Discordant atrioventricular connection

T

TRANSVERSE MYELITIS

Paul R. Lee • Avindra Nath

BASICS

DESCRIPTION

An acute or subacute inflammatory lesion of the spinal cord manifesting with the appearance of new autonomic, motor, and sensory symptoms. The "transverse" descriptor is a reference to the classic symptom presentation with an identifiable sensory level traversing the midline. Transverse myelitis (TM) is associated with cerebrospinal fluid (CSF) or radiographic abnormalities consistent with an inflammatory spinal cord lesion. TM is usually monophasic but can be a manifestation of a chronic disease.

EPIDEMIOLOGY

- Incidence: Estimated 1–8/million cases per year in the United States (20% children) or approximately 300 affected children annually. There are two incidence distributions in children—a peak between 0 and 2 years of age and another broader distribution from 5 to 17 years of age.
- Prevalence: estimated 34,000 in the United States with disabilities due to TM
- The female-to-male ratio is approximately 1:1 for <10 years, with a female predominance observed after age 10 years (2.6:1) in a North American cohort.

RISK FACTORS

- Fever, findings consistent with infection, or vaccinations in the preceding weeks are reported in the majority (>50%) of children with TM, but specific infections are rarely diagnosed.
- Mild trauma and obesity are associated with an increased risk of TM.

ETIOLOGY

Unknown. Several infectious and autoimmune conditions have been associated with TM without a clear unifying immunopathogenesis.

COMMONLY ASSOCIATED CONDITIONS

- TM in children is predominantly idiopathic.
- TM can be a manifestation of the acquired demyelinating syndromes, for example, acute disseminated encephalomyelitis (ADEM), multiple sclerosis (MS), or neuromyelitis optica (NMO).
- The enteroviruses (coxsackie A7, 9, 23, and B strains) and other viruses (dengue fever, hepatitis, human herpes, influenza, polio, and West Nile virus) have been reported in association with acute TM.
- TM can occur during acute mycoplasma, spirochete, or parasitic infections.
- TM has been reported in combination with Guillain-Barré syndrome (GBS).
- TM can occur as part of a systemic autoimmune inflammatory disease (mixed connective tissue disease, systemic sclerosis, systemic lupus erythematosus, sarcoidosis, Sjögren syndrome, Behçet disease, juvenile rheumatoid arthritis, autoimmune thyroid disease, or antiphospholipid syndrome).
- Metabolic deficiencies and mitochondrial disease can cause TM-like presentations.

DIAGNOSIS

HISTORY

- Children with TM most commonly (~60%) report pain (in neck, back, and lower extremities) as their initial symptom, followed by motor deficits (~30%) and sensory loss (~10%). Loss of bladder/bowel control, gait disturbances, and visual loss are also noted.
- Pediatric TM is often postinfectious and can be found after vaccinations. A history within the past 30 days of vaccination, fever, upper respiratory symptoms, leukocytosis, or other indications of a recent infection is noted in the majority of cases.
- A sudden precipitous onset or acute total sensory/motor/reflex loss below a spinal level should provoke an emergent exploration of potential obstructive, vascular, or traumatic etiologies, as TM symptoms evolve over hours to days, not minutes.
- A prior history of paroxysmal neurologic symptoms such as transient sensory deficits, weakness, trigeminal neuralgia, or visual loss may suggest this TM presentation is a relapse of a neuroimmune disease.
- A prior history of known/suspected systemic autoimmune disease or coagulopathy should be used to guide subsequent evaluation.
- Radiation exposure can cause a TM-like presentation with a latency of up to 10 years.

PHYSICAL EXAM

- A complete neurologic examination is imperative. Typical examination findings include a bandlike sensory level with distal sensory loss, weakness of the lower extremities, ataxia, and urinary retention. Reflexes may be increased or diminished, and abnormal extensor response of the great toe (Babinski sign) is often present.
- Findings are usually bilateral and symmetric and referable to a spinal level (usually thoracic) but can be relatively asymmetric or in rare instances exclusively unilateral.
- Closely monitor heart rate and blood pressure. TM lesions anywhere from the brainstem to the upper thoracic cord could disrupt sympathetic–parasympathetic balance, resulting in bradycardia and hypotension. In lesions of the thoracic cord, autonomic dysreflexia can occur as a late complication.
- Follow patient respiratory status because lesions of the cervical cord at or above level C5 could impair diaphragm function. Brainstem lesions can involve the nucleus of spinal accessory nerve, causing pharyngeal muscle weakness and loss of airway patency. Respiratory decompensation is less common in TM than in GBS.
- Also observe for deficits of proprioception and vibration sense indicating involvement of the posterior columns (suggesting syphilis, B_{12} deficiency.)
- Concurrent diminished visual acuity, blindness, loss of color vision, or optic nerve pallor indicates optic neuritis. Rapid vision loss with TM is likely NMO and mandates aggressive treatment.
- Spinal shock, characterized by suspension of spinal cord function and areflexia below a spinal level, may occur early in TM. Loss of reflexes also raises concern for GBS.
- Fever and neck pain are common findings in TM but when present with other indications of meningeal irritation increases importance of evaluation for meningitis.
- Excessive irritability, stupor, altered awareness, or neurocognitive problems suggest encephalopathy due to ADEM.
- The examination of the infant with TM is challenging. Lack of spontaneous movement or resistance to examination, asymmetric movements, absent response to painful stimuli, bladder distension or abdominal fullness, or priapism can be presenting signs in infants. Muscle, bone, or joint pain may cause refusal to ambulate/bear weight without spinal cord pathology.

DIAGNOSTIC TESTS AND INTERPRETATION

Lab

- Complete blood cell count and differential to assess for acute infection
- Serum aquaporin-4 IgG. Consider repeating if prior negative result for recurrence of TM (~80% of children seropositive in relapsing NMO vs. 13% in initial TM), if optic neuritis also present, or MRI findings suggestive of NMO. CSF aquaporin-4 IgG may be more sensitive than serum assay.
- Lumbar puncture (if no risk of herniation) and CSF analysis
  - Cell count (mean ~200 WBCs/μL in TM; cell counts >30–50 more likely to have NMO than MS)
  - Protein (elevated in 20–50% of TM cases; elevated protein and low CSF cell count is more typical of GBS)
  - Glucose (if low consider infectious etiology)
  - CSF Gram stain and culture
  - IgG index (elevated in MS)
  - Oligoclonal bands (present in 90% of MS and 30% of NMO cases)

If history, examination findings, or endemic likelihood, consider these additional studies:

- CSF: Enterovirus, human herpesvirus (HHV) 1/2/6, varicella-zoster virus (VZV), Epstein-Barr virus (EBV), cytomegalovirus (CMV), dengue, or West Nile viral DNA polymerase chain reaction (PCR); paraneoplastic panel, lactate, pyruvate
- *Mycoplasma pneumoniae* IgM/IgG with throat swab PCR, *Bartonella henselae* IgM/IgG titer, *Borrelia burgdorferi* IgM/IgG, rapid plasma reagin (RPR), hepatitis A/B/C, or influenza testing

- If chronic myelopathy is present, evaluate for mumps, measles, HIV, human T-lymphotropic virus (HTLV) I/II
- Purified protein derivative (PPD) with anergy panel, tuberculosis culture
- Schistosomiasis stool or urine examination
- Autoimmune disease: antinuclear antibody (ANA), rheumatoid factor (RF), anti-dsDNA antibody, antiphospholipid antibodies, angiotensin-converting enzyme (with chest radiography) antithyroid antibodies, rheumatologic or paraneoplastic panel
- Prothrombin time (PT), partial thromboplastin time (PTT), international normalized ratio (INR), and coagulopathy panel
- Copper or B_{12} serum levels
- Mitochondrial function serum testing

Imaging

- Inflammation of the spinal cord identified by imaging or CSF findings is required for a diagnosis of TM. Acute neurologic deficits referring to the spinal cord mandate emergent spinal imaging. An MRI scan with gadolinium enhancement of the whole spine is preferred; short inversion time inversion recovery (STIR) sequences are sensitive for identifying abnormalities. If patient cannot tolerate lengthy scan, or there is a time-critical concern, scanning segments where symptoms localize can suffice. Full spine and brain should be imaged later to establish presence of clinically silent lesions or baseline imaging.
- Longitudinally extensive TM (T2 hyperintense lesion spanning ≥3 segments) is typical of idiopathic TM or NMO, not MS.
- Selective enhancement of the nerve roots without cord involvement suggests GBS.
- All patients presenting with acute TM should have an ophthalmologic examination with ocular coherence tomography and visual-evoked potentials. Subclinical optic neuritis suggests a diagnosis of MS or NMO.
- MRI of the brain with contrast or dedicated optic nerve imaging is needed with encephalopathy/brain lesions or optic nerve involvement. Lesions in subcortical white matter suggest ADEM or MS.

Diagnostic Procedures/Other

An electromyogram and nerve conduction studies can be used in clinically ambiguous cases to differentiate GBS from TM.

DIFFERENTIAL DIAGNOSIS

- Infectious myelitis
- Postradiation myelopathy
- Compressive myelopathy
  - Trauma
  - Extramedullary: arteriovenous malformation, discitis, epidural abscess, vertebral osteomyelitis, tumor
  - Intramedullary: arteriovenous malformation, tumor
- Ischemic myelopathy
  - Spinal cord infarct, angiitis/vasculitis, fibrocartilaginous embolism
- Autoimmune
  - Acquired demyelination syndromes
  - Systemic autoimmune disease
  - Paraneoplastic syndrome

TREATMENT

MEDICATION

First Line

Methylprednisolone IV (dose: 30 mg/kg/day or a maximum dose of 1 g/day) or an oral equivalent is recommended initial treatment for noninfectious TM. Strong evidence exists in adults (*not children*) for efficacy in TM. Typical treatment length is 5–7 days followed by oral corticosteroid taper starting at dose of 1 mg/kg/day (maximum 60 mg/day prednisone equivalent) over 3–4 weeks.

Second Line

- If steroids are not effective or contraindicated, plasmapheresis is an alternative. Evidence exists for efficacy of plasmapheresis treatment in children. Typically, 5–7 exchanges are performed. Consider for NMO with progressive visual loss.
- Intravenous immunoglobulin G (IVIG; dose: 2 g/kg divided over 2–5 days) is an alternative or add-on treatment.
- Cyclophosphamide (dose: 500–750 mg/m^2) administered once is reportedly effective in refractory TM cases.
- Immunomodulatory therapies for MS can begin after acute treatment. Rituximab is an option for TM due to NMO.

GENERAL MEASURES

- Most patients will have urinary retention and constipation, so appropriate bowel/bladder regimen should be implemented proactively.
- Short-term and long-term pain management plans are needed in almost all TM patients.

ADDITIONAL THERAPIES

- Physical, occupational, or speech/language therapists should be engaged as soon as possible to maintain function during hospitalization and assess needs for possible longer duration placement.
- Long-term neurologic follow-up (1–3 years) is necessary to assess for new symptoms, recurrence, and zenith of recovery.

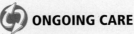

ONGOING CARE

PROGNOSIS

- Complete recovery in 33–50% of pediatric cases. Up to 20% can have significant residual disabilities (not ambulatory, severe sensory loss, lack of sphincter control).
- Mortality due to acute TM is <5%.
- Infants may have extensive lesions and worse outcomes. Other factors associated with a poorer prognosis: rapid onset of symptoms (<24 hours to nadir), more sensory loss/weakness or length of time spent at symptom nadir, need for ventilation, longitudinal extent of lesion, higher sensory level, or diminished/absent reflexes at onset

ADDITIONAL READING

- Banwell B, Kennedy J, Sadovnick D, et al. Incidence of acquired demyelination of the CNS in Canadian children. *Neurology*. 2009;72(3):232–239.
- Defresne P, Hollenberg H, Husson B, et al. Acute transverse myelitis in children: clinical course and prognostic factors. *J Child Neurol*. 2003;18(6):401–406.
- Pidcock FS, Krishnan C, Crawford TO, et al. Acute transverse myelitis in childhood: center-based analysis of 47 cases. *Neurology*. 2007;68(18):1474–1480.
- Scott TF, Frohman EM, De Seze J, et al. Evidence-based guideline: clinical evaluation and treatment of transverse myelitis. *Neurology*. 2011;77(24):2128–2134.
- Thomas T, Branson HM, Verhey LH, et al. The demographic, clinical, and magnetic resonance imaging (MRI) features of transverse myelitis in children. *J Child Neurol*. 2012;27(1):11–21.

CODES

ICD10

- G37.3 Acute transverse myelitis in demyelinating disease of central nervous system
- A89 Unspecified viral infection of central nervous system

FAQ

- Q: What is the typical clinical timeline of TM?
- A: TM symptoms typically begin over 2–3 days. Functional nadir can occur within hours to 1 month of onset. This nadir averages 7 days before recovery. Patient recovery can be rapid (within weeks) or span years.
- Q: What is the likelihood of recurrence?
- A: 60–80% of pediatric TM is monophasic. Approximately 15% of patients with TM will be diagnosed with MS or NMO and therefore would be at risk for a relapse.

TRICHINOSIS

Carolyn A. Paris • George Anthony Woodward

BASICS

DESCRIPTION

- Infection caused by ingestion of undercooked meat containing nematode (roundworm) larval cysts of the *Trichinella* genus
- Clinical disease in humans characterized by an intestinal phase followed by a muscular phase
- Extremely wide host range and geographic distribution

EPIDEMIOLOGY

- Historically, most U.S. infections are due to *Trichinella spiralis* in commercial pork.
- Currently, more U.S. infections are associated with wild game meat (especially bear) or through spillover to domestic animals.
- Occasional grouped outbreaks (e.g., families and communities with common exposure)
- Reservoir hosts include rodents, domesticated animals (e.g., dogs, cats), raccoons, opossums, and skunks.

Incidence

- Estimated 10,000 cases per year worldwide, with a mortality rate of 0.2% in main 55 countries reporting
- Between 2002 and 2007 in the United States, average of 11 cases annually
- Decreasing reported case numbers attributed to decline in prevalence of *Trichinella* in commercial swine (1.41% in 1900, 0.125% in 1966, and 0.013% in 1995), federal regulation preventing uncooked meat consumption by commercial swine, and increased public awareness regarding proper meat handling and preparation
- Likely underreported, particularly in developing countries with modest health controls

Prevalence

- ~4% of cadavers in 1970 study with evidence of previous infection (additional estimates range from 10 to 20% prevalence)

RISK FACTORS

- Consumption of inadequately cooked meat, even in small quantities
- Consumption of foreign meat (e.g., horse in France, dog in China) or wild game (e.g., bear, cougar, hyena, lion, panther, fox, horse, seal, walrus)
- Exposure to adulterated food (e.g., pork mixed in beef product)
- Traveling to underdeveloped countries
- Compromised immune status of host

GENERAL PREVENTION

- Consume only fully cooked meat, pork, and wild game; meat should reach >145°F internally, no pink color
- Freezing kills *T. spiralis* in pork (<6 inches thick) at −20°F for 6 days, −10°F for 10 days, and −5°F for 20 days.
- Freezing may not kill other *Trichinella* species, particularly in wild game.
- Curing, smoking, salting, and drying meat (including jerky) are not reliable sterilization methods.
- Routinely clean meat processing equipment.
- Irradiation may not kill *Trichinella* but should prevent replication.
- Avoid feeding swine uncooked meat scraps.
- Actively control reservoir hosts (e.g., rodents).

PATHOPHYSIOLOGY

- *Trichinella* are obligate intracellular parasites capable of infecting warm-blooded animals
- At least 8 *Trichinella* species identified: *Trichinella spiralis* (most common), *Trichinella britovi*, *Trichinella pseudospiralis*, *Trichinella papuae*, *Trichinella nativa*, *Trichinella nelsoni*, *Trichinella murrelli*, and *Trichinella zimbabwensis*
- Life cycle of all species comprises 2 generations in the same host (broad range of species—mammal, birds, and reptiles), but only humans become clinically affected.
- Disease not transmissible person to person
- Larvae in undercooked meat eaten by the patient are released after cyst wall digestion by gastric enzymes, pass to the small intestine, invade mucosa, then develop into adult worms.
- Incubation period is 1–2 weeks.
- Fertilized females release larvae (~500) over 2–3 weeks; adult worms do not multiply in human host and are expelled in feces.
- Newborn larvae travel the bloodstream to seed skeletal muscles, where they grow 10-fold, coil, encyst, and cause muscle fibers to enlarge and become edematous. Nonskeletal muscle may have granulomatous reactions, but larvae are found only in skeletal muscle.
- Cysts (hyaline capsules) may calcify over several months to years.
- Growing body of research on the ability of parasites to modulate the immune system and implications of this for immune-mediated diseases

ETIOLOGY

T. spiralis is the organism that causes trichinosis and is acquired by the consumption of raw or undercooked, infected meat.

COMMONLY ASSOCIATED CONDITIONS

- Rheumatic syndromes: polyarteritis nodosa–like systemic necrotizing vasculitis, symmetric polyarteritis, glomerulonephritis
- Immunocompromised hosts are at risk for more serious or prolonged infection.

DIAGNOSIS

HISTORY

- Ingestion of inadequately cooked meat (commercial and noncommercial pork, game animals, foreign meat)
- Others with similar symptoms and same dietary exposure
- Signs and symptoms
  - Clinical severity varies, from asymptomatic (most common) to fatal (rare); depends on *Trichinella* species and inoculum size
  - Children often have fewer and milder symptoms than adults.
  - Many signs and symptoms (i.e., periorbital and muscle edema, eosinophilia) due to allergic reaction to parasite antigens
  - Nonspecific signs and symptoms may mimic other illnesses
  - Enteral phase (24 hours–7 days after infection): symptoms due to intestinal ulceration from mucosal invasion by adult worms
    - Diarrhea, abdominal pain, nausea, vomiting, anorexia
    - May persist for weeks
  - Parenteral phase (1–8 weeks after infection): symptoms due to systemic invasion
    - General: fever (begins at 2 weeks, peaks after 4 weeks, night spikes to 40–41°C), weakness, malaise, myalgias
    - Ocular: periorbital edema, subconjunctival hemorrhage, conjunctivitis, disturbed vision, ocular pain, chemosis
    - Muscular: myalgias, myositis (usually in extraocular muscles, then masseters, tongue, neck, limb flexors, lumbar muscles, intercostals, and diaphragm) with dyspnea, cough, hoarseness
    - Neurologic: headache, focal paralysis, delirium, psychosis
    - Skin: urticarial rash, subungual hemorrhages
    - Parenteral phase symptoms typically peak 2–3 weeks after infection.
    - Malaise and weakness may persist for weeks.
    - Cardiac: myocarditis, arrhythmias secondary to myocarditis
  - Convalescent phase (begins 2nd month, may last months to years): myalgias, weakness

PHYSICAL EXAM

Fever, periorbital and generalized edema, muscular tenderness, urticaria, plus findings related to neurologic or cardiac involvement mentioned in "History" section

DIAGNOSTIC TESTS & INTERPRETATION

Lab

- Stool ova and parasite examination
- CBC and differential: leukocytosis (moderate) with eosinophilia (up to 70%, peaks 10–21 days postinoculation but prior to clinical symptoms)

- Elevation of muscle enzymes (lactate dehydrogenase [LDH], creatinine phosphokinase [CPK], aldolase)
- Specific anti-*Trichinella* antibody detection
- Serologic tests are available through the U.S. Centers for Disease Control and Prevention or state and some private labs.
- Detection of *Trichinella*-specific DNA by polymerase chain reaction (availability limited)
- *Trichinella* serology
  - 2 tests required to ensure accurate diagnosis: first to detect antigen (enzyme-linked immunosorbent assay [ELISA]) and the second to detect antibodies to parasite surface antigens (FA)
  - Bentonite flocculation (1:5- or 4-fold increase), latex flocculation test, ELISA, or immunofluorescence

Imaging

- X-ray: may show calcified cysts in muscle (6–24 months postinfection) or enlarged heart
- EKG: myocarditis may cause premature contractions, prolonged PR interval, small QRS with intraventricular block, and/or T wave flattening or inversion
- CT: small CNS lesions, IV enhancing ring calcifications
- Electromyography: Results resemble those of polymyositis and inflammatory myopathies.

Diagnostic Procedures/Other

- Skeletal muscle biopsy (especially deltoid or gastrocnemius muscle from the patient at least 17 days after infection)
  - Inflammatory cells surround encysted larvae in necrotic muscle fibers.
  - Granulomatous reaction present in nonskeletal muscle but not encysted larvae.
  - Usually unnecessary, negative result possible in infected patient due to sampling error
- Can test suspected meat if available

DIFFERENTIAL DIAGNOSIS

- Infection: viral syndromes, parasitic, spirochete, gastroenteritis, influenza, sinusitis, typhoid fever, measles, scarlet fever, meningitis, rheumatic fever, encephalitis, encephalomyelitis, poliomyelitis, tetanus, schistosomiasis, hookworm, strongyloides, or helminthic infection
- Miscellaneous: fever of unknown origin, dermatomyositis, myocarditis, inflammatory bowel disease, angioneurotic edema, rheumatoid arthritis, glomerulonephritis, polyneuritis, eosinophilic leukemia, polyarteritis nodosa, nonabsorption syndromes

TREATMENT

MEDICATION

First Line

- Systemic corticosteroids for severe symptoms (not recommended as monotherapy, may prolong adult worm survival in intestines) *plus*
- Albendazole (Albenza)
  - 15 mg/kg/day divided b.i.d for 15 days
  - Max dose 800 mg/day
  - Teratogenic/embryotoxic in rats
  - Approved <2 years
- Mebendazole and albendazole are most efficacious during the enteral phase (active against intestinal worms, little effect on muscle-embedded larvae).

Second Line

Pyrantel pamoate (Antiminth)

- Used during pregnancy; not approved <2 years
- Effective only against adult worms, not encysted larvae

ADDITIONAL TREATMENT

General Measures

- Most patients recover without specific therapy.
- Symptomatic treatment: acetaminophen or NSAIDs, bed rest

ISSUES FOR REFERRAL

Cardiac, neurologic, pulmonary complications

INPATIENT CONSIDERATIONS

Admission Criteria

Cardiac, neurologic, or pulmonary complications indicate more severe disease

Discharge Criteria

Resolution of cardiac symptoms

ONGOING CARE

FOLLOW-UP RECOMMENDATIONS

- Expect improvement over several weeks.
- At 3–4 weeks, retreatment may be indicated if symptoms persist or there are ova in the feces.

Patient Monitoring

Cardiopulmonary monitoring

DIET

- Avoid further exposures.
- Breastfeeding may continue; the single case report of cessation of milk production was associated with parenteral mebendazole.

PATIENT EDUCATION

If concern for trichinosis exposure or symptoms, seek medical care early. Treatment is most efficacious the 1st week after exposure.

PROGNOSIS

- Mild to moderate illness usually resolves spontaneously with minimal sequelae. Muscle swelling and weakness may persist.
- Poorer prognosis (can be fulminant and fatal) with cardiac, CNS, or pulmonary involvement
- Children usually are less symptomatic, have fewer complications, and recover more quickly.

COMPLICATIONS

- Cardiac: myocarditis (may result in death 4–8 weeks after infection), secondary arrhythmias, hypotension, pericardial effusion
- Neurologic: meningoencephalitis, CNS granulomas, headaches
- Pulmonary: pneumonia, pneumonitis, pleural effusion, pulmonary embolism or infarct
- Renal: glomerulonephritis
- Hepatic: fatty change
- Muscular: prolonged myalgias
- Ocular: retinal hemorrhages
- Complications rarely are permanent.

ADDITIONAL READING

- American Academy of Pediatrics. Trichinellosis. In: Pickering LK, Baker CJ, Kimberlin DW, et al, eds. *Red Book: 2012 Report of the Committee on Infectious Diseases*. 29th ed. Elk Grove Village, IL: American Academy of Pediatrics. 2012;728–729.
- Bruschi F. Trichinellosis in developing countries: is it neglected? *J Infect Dev Ctries*. 2012;6(3):216–222.
- Gottstein B, Pozio E, Nockler K. Epidemiology, diagnosis, treatment, and control of trichinellosis. *Clin Microbiol Rev*. 2009;22(1):127–145.
- Ilic N, Gruden-Movsesijan A, Sofronic-Milosavljevic L. *Trichinella spiralis*: shaping the immune response. *Immunol Res*. 2012;52(1–2):111–119.
- Ozdemir D, Ozkan H, Akkoc N, et al. Acute trichinellosis in children compared with adults. *Pediatr Infect Dis J*. 2005;24(10):897–900.
- Roy SL, Lopez AS, Schantz PM. Trichinellosis surveillance—United States, 1997–2001. *MMWR Surveill Summ*. 2003;52(6):1–8.

CODES

ICD10

- B75 Trichinellosis
- M63.80 Disorders of muscle in diseases classd elswhr, unsp site

FAQ

- Q: Is trichinosis contagious from person to person?
- A: No, except through infected breast milk.
- Q: Do special precautions need to be taken when treating a patient with presumed trichinosis?
- A: Only thorough hand washing. No isolation required.
- Q: What should we recommend for a patient who has eaten contaminated meat?
- A: Treatment with mebendazole or thiabendazole should be considered.
- Q: What are the classic hallmark signs of trichinosis?
- A: Diarrhea, abdominal pain, periorbital edema, myositis, fever, and eosinophilia, especially when combined with history of ingestion of potentially poorly cooked meat.

TRICHOTILLOMANIA

Ilse A. Larson, MD • Carol A. Mathews, MD

BASICS

DESCRIPTION

Trichotillomania (TTM) is the recurrent pulling out of one's hair resulting in hair loss. Pulling causes clinically significant distress or functional impairment, is accompanied by repeated efforts to stop, and is not due to another mental disorder or a general medical condition.

- Hair pulling can occur in any region of the body, but the most common sites are the scalp, eyelashes, and eyebrows. Other relatively common sites include the axilla, face, and pubic area. Sites may vary over time.
- Pulling can occur in brief episodes throughout the day or in sustained bouts.
- Automatic pulling is outside the patient's awareness.
- Focused pulling is in response to identifiable affective triggers.
- Some patients experience tension immediately before pulling or when attempting to resist the behavior, whereas others experience pleasure or relief when pulling.
- Patients may search for and pull hairs with specific qualities (e.g., thick hairs or short hairs).
- More than half of patients engage in a "ritual" with the hair before discarding it.
- TTM does not include habitual hair twirling.

EPIDEMIOLOGY

- Typical onset in childhood or adolescence: often coincides with the onset of puberty
- In childhood, girls and boys are equally affected.
- In adulthood, the ratio of affected females to males is 10:1.

Prevalence

1–3% lifetime prevalence

RISK FACTORS

TTM is more common in individuals with obsessive-compulsive disorder (OCD) and in their 1st-degree relatives.

Genetics

- One study of 34 twin pairs showed concordance in 38% of monozygotic and 0% of dizygotic twins, suggesting heritability.
- No specific genes implicated, although animal models of TTM exist.

COMMONLY ASSOCIATED CONDITIONS

- Trichophagia (ingesting hair), which can lead to trichobezoar. It is estimated that between 5 and 18% of patients with TTM ingest their hair.
- Psychiatric comorbidity is common (seen in 1/3–2/3 of children with TTM) and includes autism, pervasive developmental disorder (PDD), anxiety, mood, attention deficit, substance use, and eating disorders.
- Patients may also engage in nail-biting, skin-picking, or other pathologic grooming behaviors.

DIAGNOSIS

HISTORY

Patients may present with a complaint of hair loss or with concern regarding pulling behavior.

PHYSICAL EXAM

- Areas of hair loss do not show complete alopecia; instead, they contain hairs of different lengths, hairs with blunt ends, and remnants of hair bulbs. Hair density is normal in other areas.
- In some cases, pulling is widely distributed and hair loss may not be readily apparent.
- In children, patches of loss may be more prevalent on the side of the patient's dominant hand.

DIAGNOSTIC TESTS & INTERPRETATION

Diagnostic Procedures/Other

Several instruments are available for clinical use; the Massachusetts General Hospital Hair Pulling Scale is one tool commonly used to monitor symptom severity and response to treatment.

DIFFERENTIAL DIAGNOSIS

- Alopecia areata
- Tinea capitis
- Dermatologic conditions causing pruritus; normative hair removal (e.g., for cosmetic reasons)
- Other obsessive-compulsive or related disorders where pulling is part of a symmetry or other ritual
- Body dysmorphic disorder

TREATMENT

MEDICATION

- Few placebo-controlled randomized trials have included children or adolescents.
- *N*-acetylcysteine
  - A randomized controlled trial (RCT) of 50 adults demonstrated efficacy of *N*-acetylcysteine (56% of patients responded to treatment compared to 16% of patients on placebo).
  - A similarly designed study of 34 children showed no effect, with clinically modest but statistically significant improvements in symptoms in both treatment and control groups.

- Olanzapine
  - Has been shown to be efficacious in a study of 25 adults (85% of treatment group responded as compared to 17% of placebo group)
  - However, 84% of treatment group reported undesirable side effects.
- SSRIs do not reduce hairpulling but are efficacious for treating comorbid conditions and are used in some adults with TTM.

ADDITIONAL THERAPIES

- For mild cases in young children, reward systems or "home remedies" like a hat or Band-Aids on fingers may help.
- Behavior modification programs, habit reversal training methods, and cognitive behavioral therapy have all been used.
- One RCT of 24 children showed sustained effect of behavioral therapy (75% in behavioral therapy group were responders as compared with 0% in minimal attention control group at 8 weeks; effect sustained over 8-week maintenance period).

GENERAL MEASURES

- Triggers should be identified and minimized with a focus on stress management strategies.
- Parent and family education about TTM and associated conditions is essential.
- The Trichotillomania Learning Center (www.trich.org) has valuable educational materials for patients, parents, and clinicians as well as a list of mental health providers with experience treating TTM.

ONGOING CARE

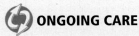

FOLLOW-UP RECOMMENDATIONS

Patients with TTM should be referred to a mental health professional with training in behavioral therapy and, ideally, with experience treating patients with TTM.

PROGNOSIS

TTM often waxes and wanes, with symptoms reemerging at times of stress or transition.

COMPLICATIONS

- TTM can lead to significant academic, social, and developmental impairment.
  - 55% of children reported that TTM made it more difficult to study and 35% reported academic impairment as a direct result of pulling.
  - 55% of parents of children with TTM reported that their child avoided social events as a direct result of pulling.
  - 80% of parents of children with TTM felt that their child's pulling contributed to another psychiatric problem.
- Trichobezoar resulting from trichophagia can cause serious gastrointestinal complications including obstruction and perforation.

ADDITIONAL READING

- American Psychiatric Association. *Diagnostic and Statistical Manual of Mental Disorders*. 5th ed. Washington, DC: American Psychiatric Association; 2013.
- Bloch MH, Landeros-Weisenberger A, Dombrowski P, et al. Systematic review: pharmacological and behavioral treatment for trichotillomania. *Biol Psychiatry*. 2007;62(8):839–846.
- Bloch MH, Panza KE, Grant JE, et al. N-acetylcysteine in the treatment of pediatric trichotillomania: a randomized, double-blind, placebo-controlled add-on trial. *J Am Acad Child Adolesc Psychiatry*. 2013;52(3):231–240.
- Duke DC, Keeley ML, Geffken GR, et al. Trichotillomania: a current review. *Clin Psychol Rev*. 2010;30(2):181–193.
- Franklin ME, Flessner CA, Woods DW, et al. The child and adolescent trichotillomania impact project: descriptive psychopathology, comorbidity, functional impairment, and treatment utilization. *J Dev Behav Pediatr*. 2008;29(6):493–500.
- Franklin ME, Zagrabbe K, Benavides KL. Trichotillomania and its treatment: a review and recommendations. *Expert Rev Neurother*. 2011;11(8):1165–1174.
- Grant JE, Odlaug BL, Kim SW. N-acetylcysteine, a glutamate modulator, in the treatment of trichotillomania. *Arch Gen Psychiatry*. 2009;66(7):756–763.
- Novak CE, Keuthen NJ, Stewart SE, et al. A twin concordance study of trichotillomania. *Am J Med Genet B Neuropsychiatr Genet*. 2009;150B(7):944–949.
- Van Ameringen M, Mancini C, Patterson B, et al. A randomized, double-blind, placebo-controlled trial of olanzapine in the treatment of trichotillomania. *J Clin Psychiatry*. 2010;71(10):1336–1343.

CODES

ICD10

- F63.3 Trichotillomania
- F50.8 Other eating disorders

FAQ

- Q: What are signs and symptoms of trichobezoar?
- A: Patients can present with abdominal pain, nausea, vomiting, weight loss, or gastrointestinal bleeding. X-ray shows a characteristic abdominal mass, and hair may be present in the patient's stool.
- Q: Which patients with hairpulling behaviors should be referred for evaluation and treatment?
- A: Patients with patches of alopecia, distress related to their alopecia or pulling behavior, and those with deliberate pulling should be referred.
- Q: To whom should I refer patients with suspected or diagnosed TTM?
- A: Ideally, a psychologist or other mental health professional with training in behavioral therapy, cognitive behavioral therapy, or exposure-response management therapy.

TUBERCULOSIS

Andrew P. Steenhoff

BASICS

DESCRIPTION

- Pediatric tuberculosis (TB) is the disease state caused by *Mycobacterium tuberculosis*, an acid-fast bacillus (AFB). Pediatric TB should be regarded as a spectrum of exposure through infection to disease because progression from an infected person (exposure) to infection and disease can occur much faster (within 3–6 months) in children <2 years of age (occurring within the incubation of the disease stated below).
- Progression through this spectrum depends on age; such disease progression being 40–50% for children up to 2 years old, ~20% for those 2–4 years old, and 10–15% for those ≥5 years old. 5–10-year-old children are the most protected age group. Adolescence is another vulnerable age group.

EPIDEMIOLOGY

- Most common route of infection is via the respiratory tract. TB is spread from a person with disease by droplet nuclei that are inhaled by other people. Infection occurs after close and prolonged contact with an adult or adolescent who has active untreated infectious disease, usually pulmonary TB, in a poorly ventilated space. However, there are people who develop TB without knowledge of an infectious contact.
- Congenital infection occurs, although rarely, in the setting of an untreated mother in the last trimester of pregnancy.
- Infection with the tubercle bacillus needs to be differentiated from disease (i.e., TB).
- The interval between onset of infection and disease is usually 10–12 weeks.
- The greatest chance of disease occurring (i.e., of developing a positive result in tests using purified protein derivative [PPD], now renamed tuberculin skin test [TST]) is within the 1st 2 years after infection. However, for infants and children <5 years of age, progression through the spectrum of pediatric TB (exposure–infection–disease) is age dependent (see "Description").
- Postpubertal adolescents and immunosuppressed people including people with diabetes, with chronic renal failure, the malnourished, and those taking steroids for any reason have higher risks for progression of infection to disease.

GENERAL PREVENTION

- There are now several treatment regimens available for the treatment of latent TB infection. The reader is referred to the Centers for Disease Control and Prevention (CDC) Web site in the "Additional Reading" section.
- Preferred regimen is isoniazid (isonicotinic acid hydrazide-INH), 10–20 mg/kg/day PO for 9 months or, if compliance is not anticipated, 2 times a week as direct observed therapy at 20–30 mg/kg, with a maximum dose of 900 mg usually administered by a school nurse, child care worker, or the local TB control program, ideally without breaks in treatment, although the patient has 12 months to complete the course. If a break occurs near the end of treatment, it need not be restarted because such treatment is ~90% effective against development of active TB for 20 years in nonimmunosuppressed children. This recommendation prevents disease in the treated patient and, as a public health measure, interrupts transmission to contacts of that infected person with 90% efficacy.
- Other drugs for latent TB when INH cannot be tolerated or case-patient has INH-resistant but rifampicin-susceptible TB include 6 months of INH 10–20 mg/kg by direct observed therapy (for a total of 72 doses).
- For adults and children 12 years and older, a once-weekly 3-month course of INH and rifapentine can be considered via direct observed therapy (12 doses total).
- Bacille Calmette-Guérin (BCG) vaccine is recommended in the United States only for infants and children who test negative to PPD and who are continually exposed to contagious adults or to adults with TB that is resistant to both INH and rifampin and who cannot be kept away from the contagious adult.

COMMONLY ASSOCIATED CONDITIONS

- HIV infection
- Lymphoma
- Diabetes
- Chronic renal failure
- Malnutrition
- Immunosuppression, including chronic daily steroid use, high-dose steroid use or tumor necrosis factor-α (TNF-α) agonists, cancer chemotherapy
- Social issues: incarcerated adolescents, infants, and children in homeless shelters

DIAGNOSIS

HISTORY

- Exposure: family member with TB or positive skin test
- Migrant farm workers
- Immigration from a TB-endemic geographic area (e.g., Haiti, Southeast Asia, Africa, South and Central America, Russia, and elsewhere in Eastern Europe, where greater concern about drug-resistant strains ought to be exercised); visit by individuals from those countries; or visited the above countries
- Higher incidence in Native Americans
- Contact with adults who have active TB
- HIV-positive people
- Immunosuppressed state
- Incarcerated adolescents and their relatives who visit
- Homeless people
- Poor people in urban areas
- Exposure to milk from untested herds
- Malnutrition
- Long-term steroid usage

PHYSICAL EXAM

- Cervical and/or axillary adenopathy
- May reflect underlying disease or state (e.g., HIV, malnutrition, long-term steroid use)
- Pulmonary rales or clear chest
- Enlarged liver or spleen
- Site-specific findings (e.g., gibbus [vertebral TB]) or focal neurologic signs (TB meningitis)
- Signs and symptoms:
  - Failure to thrive
  - Cervical or axillary lymphadenopathy without any other cause or that is prolonged
  - Cough >2 weeks
  - Weight loss
  - Change in sensorium
  - Fever in infants and adolescents, rarely in children 5–10 years of age
  - Decreased energy levels/playfulness >2 weeks

DIAGNOSTIC TESTS & INTERPRETATION

Lab

- Culture for TB: sputum, 3 gastric washings (early morning), pleural fluid, CSF, urine
- Culture may take 2–3 weeks by the radiometric method.
- Positive cultures are found in <50% of children.

Imaging

Chest radiographs may show hilar adenopathy with or without atelectasis. However, any infiltrate or pleural effusion in a child with a positive TST result and a risk factor for TB should be considered a TB suspect until proven otherwise. Infiltrates from bacterial or viral pathogens generally clear within 6–8 weeks; TB infiltrates tend not to clear so rapidly.

Diagnostic Procedures/Other

- Skin testing: TST
  - The Mantoux test comprises 5 tuberculin units with PPD administered intradermally. Details may be found at http://www.cdc.gov/tb.
  - The CDC does not recommend routine skin testing in low-risk groups in communities with low prevalence of TB.
  - Children at high risk should be tested annually:
    - Those in contact with adults from regions with high TB prevalence
    - Children who spend time in homeless shelters
  - Those in contact with adults with TB, HIV, and other disease-producing immunosuppressed states: A skin test result may become positive 3–6 weeks after exposure; however, most commonly, it does not turn positive for 2–3 months—hence the rationale for treating an exposed child with INH and retesting with a PPD in 3 months.
  - A positive TST is a SENTINEL public health event indicating TB transmission in a community even if all other tests and examinations are negative.
  - Interferon gamma release assays (IGRA) are being used with more frequency to diagnose TB exposure in children. These tests can be used as an alternative to TST in screening high-risk children; they are most helpful in children who

have received BCG vaccine in the past, as these tests are more specific for TB. There are limited data on the use of these tests in children younger than 4 years of age.
- A promising new molecular diagnostic test, Xpert MTB/RIF, is both simple and accurate but performs less well in children compared to adults.

DIFFERENTIAL DIAGNOSIS

- Malignancy
- Cervical or axillary adenopathy
- Pulmonary infiltrate: other chronic organisms, disorders, and conditions (e.g., *Nocardia*, histoplasmosis). Infiltrates owing to bacterial or viral pathogens resolve faster than TB; thus, reevaluation of a suspect in 8–12 weeks clarifies this differential.
- Hilar adenopathy: In TB is usually unilateral, but Epstein-Barr virus, adenovirus, pertussis, and malignancy may possibly mimic symptoms.
- GI disease: Most common differential diagnosis is Crohn disease.
- Meningitis: fungal meningitis, partially treated bacterial meningitis (rarely)

TREATMENT

MEDICATION

- Initial treatment in areas with multidrug-resistant TB >4%: Until sensitivities are known, a 4-drug regimen should be started: INH, 10–15 mg/kg/day; rifampin, 10–20 mg/kg/day; pyrazinamide (PZA), 15–30 mg/kg/day; and either ethambutol, 15–20 mg/kg/day, or streptomycin, 20–40 mg/kg/day (depending on whether diagnosis is meningitis or miliary TB, for which a bactericide is desired); however, many cases in children of foreign-born parents are increasingly streptomycin resistant, making ethambutol a better choice.
- If the organism is sensitive to therapy, treatment with the initial 4 primary drugs should continue for the first 2 months; by then, all sputum specimens should have a negative result on culture, followed by 4 months of INH and rifampin. When this regimen is adhered to, prognosis and a complete cure are achieved in 97–98% of patients.
- If sputum specimens continue to test positive, the initiation phase is longer. For meningeal TB, the duration of treatment is always longer (12 months).

ADDITIONAL TREATMENT

General Measures

- Hospitalization (if the patient has disease)
  - In cases of extensive disease (e.g., miliary TB or meningitis), and when an adult source case is not known, aggressive attempts should be made to obtain an organism from gastric aspirates, sputum induction, bronchoalveolar lavage, CSF, pleural or joint aspirate, bone aspirate, liver or tissue biopsy, and, in some cases, blood cultures.
- Isolation policies
  - Unless the clinician can verify that the parent or any adult visitors are not themselves contagious, many infection control units require isolation of the child because the family members' state of contagion remains unknown at admission.
  - Nonpulmonary TB (e.g., GI TB, meningitis, bone TB, and TB with joint involvement) does not require isolation.
  - Children >8 years of age and adolescents should be isolated until they have completed 10 days of therapy. Occasionally, immunocompromised children <8 years old also have cavitary disease and hence they, too, should be isolated.

ONGOING CARE

FOLLOW-UP RECOMMENDATIONS

Patient Monitoring

Follow-up and contact tracing are key to making TB preventable.

PROGNOSIS

- Mortality for untreated TB is 40% over 4 years.
- For miliary TB and meningeal TB, prognosis depends on the stage of presentation as already discussed.
- For outbreaks of multidrug-resistant TB, death rates range from 70 to 90% within 4 months of diagnosis.

COMPLICATIONS

- Missed diagnosis: failure to consider TB in a child who is failing to thrive and whose TST is negative
- TB meningitis: Outcome depends on the stage at which anti-TB medication starts:
  - If pharmacotherapy is started at stage I, complete recovery occurs in 94%, with neurologic sequelae in 6%.
  - If delayed until stage II, complete recovery occurs in 51%, with neurologic sequelae in 40% and death in 7%.
  - If delayed until stage III, complete recovery occurs in 18%, with neurologic sequelae in 61% and death in 20%.
- Miliary TB: at least 2 organ systems involved
- Bone TB: most commonly spinal manifestation
- Renal TB: presents as a fever of undetermined origin (FUO), with or without urinary symptoms
- Congenital TB manifests with hepatosplenomegaly; may have CSF abnormalities and abnormalities on CSF testing and chest radiograph. Patients are too young for TST to be useful.
- Drug toxicity: Pediatric patients are much more tolerant of anti-TB medications than adults; thus, regular monitoring of liver function test results is not routinely required, although clinical monitoring for symptoms such as abdominal pain and loss of appetite on a monthly basis remains the cornerstone for identifying any toxicity.
- Hepatitis with INH, rifampin, and PZA; neurologic and hematologic complications with INH; skin rashes predominantly with rifampin and INH, but reports have occurred with all anti-TB medications; ototoxicity with streptomycin; but ocular toxicity with ethambutol in the pediatric age group has not been documented, and therefore it is a safe drug to use. Management of common side effects and drug interactions may be found in the 2006 American Thoracic Society/CDC/Infectious Disease Society of America statements (see "Additional Reading").

ADDITIONAL READING

- American Thoracic Society/Centers for Disease Control and Prevention/Infectious Disease Society of America. Treatment of tuberculosis recommendations. *Am J Respir Crit Care Med*. 2006;147:935–952.
- Boehme CC, Nabeta P, Hillemann D, et al. Rapid molecular detection of tuberculosis and rifampin resistance. *N Engl J Med*. 2010;363(11):1005–1015.
- Centers for Disease Control and Prevention. Latent tuberculosis infection: a guide for primary health care providers. www.cdc.gov/tb/publications/ltbi/treatment.htm. Accessed March 24, 2015.
- Cruz AT, Starke JR, Lobato MN. Old and new approaches to diagnosing and treating latent tuberculosis in children in low-incidence countries. *Curr Opin Pediatr*. 2014;26(1):106–113.
- MMWR trends in TB 2004. Global incidence of multidrug-resistant tuberculosis. *MMWR Recomm Rep*. 2004;53:1–24.
- Perez-Velez CM, Marais BJ. Tuberculosis in children. *N Engl J Med*. 2012;367(4):348–361.
- Targeted tuberculin testing and treatment of latent tuberculosis infection. American Thoracic Society. *MMWR Recomm Rep*. 2000;49(RR-6):1–51.

CODES

ICD10

- A15.9 Respiratory tuberculosis unspecified
- P37.0 Congenital tuberculosis
- A15.0 Tuberculosis of lung

FAQ

- Q: Should all children in close proximity to inner city areas with a prevalence of TB be screened annually with PPD?
- A: The AAP and CDC encourage targeted screening based on risk factors indicated earlier. The targeted screening questionnaire should be administered at every visit until age 2 years then annually thereafter. See tools at http://www.cdc.gov/tb.
- Q: Can the whole blood assay, IGRA (e.g. "QuantiFERON-TB Gold"), be used instead of the TST to differentiate children who were born in other countries and had BCG?
- A: Yes. The IGRA tests can be used as an alternative to TST, although additional larger studies are needed to evaluate the test characteristics of IGRAs in children. See www.cdc.gov/mmwr/pdf/rr/rr5905.pdf and Cruz et al. in the section "Additional Reading."

TUBEROUS SCLEROSIS COMPLEX

Garrick A. Applebee

BASICS

DESCRIPTION

- Tuberous sclerosis complex (TSC) is a neurocutaneous syndrome characterized by a spectrum of signs and symptoms that present over a patient's lifetime, including neurologic disorders, multisystem tumor growth, and dermatologic manifestations.
- First described by Bourneville in 1880, the classic diagnostic triad of adenoma sebaceum, intellectual disability, and seizures has been revised to include other manifestations because many patients with tuberous sclerosis do not exhibit this triad.

EPIDEMIOLOGY

Incidence

Current estimates suggest an incidence of 1 in 5,000 to 1 in 15,000 births. 60–70% of cases reflect sporadic mutation; 30–40% of cases are familial.

RISK FACTORS

Genetics

- 2 clearly identified loci for familial and sporadic cases based on linkage analyses are 9q34 and 16p13, corresponding to *TSC1* and *TSC2* genes, respectively. *TSC1* encodes the protein hamartin and *TSC2* encodes the protein tuberin. Together, hamartin and tuberin join to form a regulatory complex of mTOR (the serine-threonine kinase, mammalian target of rapamycin). Permanent activation of mTOR through mutations in the genes coding for these proteins causes dysregulation of cellular growth, differentiation, and migration, leading to the clinical symptoms and multisystem cellular overgrowth seen in TSC.
- >1,000 mutations in these genes are known to exist, leading to highly variable phenotypes in this disorder.
- *TSC2* mutations: more common in sporadic cases, associated with more severe phenotypes
- 10–15% of cases meeting clinical criteria have no identifiable gene mutations.

ETIOLOGY

Tuberous sclerosis is either inherited in an autosomal dominant pattern or results from a spontaneous/sporadic mutation.

DIAGNOSIS

HISTORY

- Primary symptoms include seizures, intellectual disability, and skin lesions.
- All types of seizures are seen in TSC. Seizures may begin at any time and are present in 70–80% of patients. In infancy, infantile spasms are a common presenting seizure; 1/3 of patients develop infantile spasms.
- Intellectual disability and neurobehavioral abnormalities (e.g., autism, which is present in 25% of patients) may manifest as developmental delay, but some patients are without cognitive defect.
- Skin lesions may appear in infancy or during early childhood.
- It is important to obtain a full family history, reviewing involved systems.
- Inquire about history of seizures, mental retardation, skin lesions, and cardiac or renal disease/cancers.
- Screening for symptoms of hydrocephalus (headache, vomiting) is important: 10% of patients develop CSF obstruction from subependymal giant cell tumors.
- Women are primarily affected by pulmonary lymphangiomyomatosis, which may manifest as dyspnea or pneumothorax in early adulthood.

PHYSICAL EXAM

- Maintain a high level of suspicion for tuberous sclerosis in any patient presenting with the following:
  - Infantile spasms or childhood seizures
  - Autism
  - Intellectual impairment/developmental delay
  - Peculiar skin lesions
  - Ash leaf and café au lait spots are small (often <5 mm) but may be found anywhere on skin and are often present at birth. Examination with a Wood lamp may help to identify hypopigmented lesions (e.g., ash leaf spots).
  - Cardiac rhabdomyomas (however, not all these patients will ultimately be diagnosed with TSC)
- Facial angiofibromas are typically found around the nose and cheeks and look like acne; they develop in later childhood to adolescence. They neither itch nor suppurate.
- Ungual fibromas appear around the nail bed.
- Shagreen patches are brownish, leathery skin patches near the sacrum.
- Funduscopic examination may reveal whitish-yellow areas in epipapillary and peripapillary regions around the optic nerve head. They rarely impair vision. Papilledema may be seen with hydrocephalus.
- Signs of heart failure or tachyarrhythmia may be seen in infants with cardiac tumors.
- Flank pain, nausea, vomiting, and hematuria may suggest renal involvement.
- Procedures: Dilated funduscopic examination may also aid in full visualization of the optic nerve head.
- Definite diagnosis requires 2 major or 1 major plus 2 minor features:
  - Major criteria: facial angiofibroma, ungual fibroma, shagreen patch, hypomelanotic papule (ash leaf spot), cortical tuber, subependymal giant cell tumor, retinal hamartoma, cardiac rhabdomyoma, renal angiomyolipoma, lymphangiomyomatosis
  - Minor criteria: pitting in tooth enamel, hamartomatous rectal polyps, bone cysts, cerebral white matter radial migration lines, gingival fibromas, retinal achromic patch, "confetti" skin lesions (grouped lightly pigmented spots), multiple renal cysts
- As with other dominant, multisystem conditions, the findings in TSC have variable penetrance, and clinical manifestations may appear at different developmental points.
- Although seizures and intellectual disability are common in TSC, they vary, are nonspecific, and so are not considered in the diagnostic criteria.

DIAGNOSTIC TESTS & INTERPRETATION

Lab

- Blood and CSF lab test results are typically normal unless renal function is significantly compromised by renal cysts or renal angiomyolipomas.
- ECG may reveal cardiac dysrhythmias, present in 47% of persons with cardiac rhabdomyomas.
- In patients with intellectual disability or seizures, EEG helps to evaluate cerebral activity.
- In infants with suggestive history, an EEG may help diagnose infantile spasms, which are associated on EEG with a highly disorganized pattern of large-amplitude, asynchronous, sharp waves termed *hypsarrhythmia*.
- Later in childhood, patients with tuberous sclerosis may develop Lennox-Gastaut syndrome, which consists of developmental delays, seizures, and a characteristic EEG pattern of slow (i.e., ≤2.5 Hz), generalized spike-wave complexes.

Imaging

- Subependymal or other cerebral calcifications on CT, often found in the course of emergent evaluation of new seizures, suggest TSC—consider MRI.
- Guidelines suggest MRI of the brain with gadolinium administration yearly or in alternate years until age 21 years and every 2–3 years thereafter. Imaging will identify tubers, subependymal nodules, hydrocephalus, and giant cell tumors. These appear hyperintense on T-weighted images and may enhance with gadolinium.
- Echocardiogram can detect cardiac rhabdomyomas in infants with tuberous sclerosis; prenatal ultrasound commonly identifies these tumors.
- CT of the lungs is indicated in women with TSC to screen for lymphangiomyomatosis.
- Renal ultrasound (every 1–2 years) or CT will demonstrate renal lesions.

Pathologic Findings

Findings reflect the primary tissue in which lesions are identified:

- Brain
  - 3 characteristic lesions are cortical tubers, subependymal nodules, and subependymal giant cell tumors.
  - In tubers, the cerebral cortical architecture is disrupted, and these regions may undergo calcification, which can be visible on skull radiographs or brain CT.
  - Subependymal nodules consist of large abnormal astrocytes emanating from the lateral ventricular surface.
  - Subependymal giant cell tumors are low-grade benign astrocytic neoplasms.
- Skin
  - Facial angiofibromas may be mistaken for acne and are highly suggestive of tuberous sclerosis; they appear as pinkish-yellow plaques on the malar regions and nasolabial folds.
  - Ash leaf spots are hypopigmented hypomelanotic macules occurring anywhere on the body.
  - Ungual fibromas are fleshy growths along the lateral borders of the nail bed.
  - Shagreen patches are areas of shaggy leathery skin typically in the lumbosacral area.
- Retina
  - Whitish-yellow angiomyolipomas or hamartomas occur near the optic nerve head or the retinal periphery and may calcify.
- Heart
  - Rhabdomyomas in the ventricular wall occur in infancy and contain abundant nodules of large eosinophilic cells; this is the most common type of cardiac tumor of infancy and early childhood which 4% of the time will occur in the absence of TSC.
- Kidney
  - Renal cysts, polycystic kidneys, angiomyolipomas, and, more rarely, renal carcinomas
- Other organ systems
  - Less commonly affected are the lungs, GI tract, spleen, vascular bed, and lymphatic system.

DIFFERENTIAL DIAGNOSIS

Neurocutaneous syndromes in which skin lesions, intellectual disability, and seizures are characteristic features should be considered:

- Neurofibromatosis
- Sturge-Weber syndrome
- von Hippel-Lindau disease
- Neurocutaneous melanosis
- Albright syndrome
- Incontinentia pigmenti
- Linear sebaceous nevus

TREATMENT

MEDICATION

- Everolimus (a rapamycin analog) is an immunosuppressant agent that inhibits mTOR, thereby inhibiting the cellular proliferation seen in tuberous sclerosis patients. It has been approved by FDA for management of subependymal giant cell tumors, and its use in targeting other tuberous sclerosis complications is under investigation.
- Anticonvulsant therapy as needed. Infantile spasms may be treated with adrenocorticotropic hormone or vigabatrin.
- Medical management of heart failure or cardiac dysrhythmias is indicated in tuberous sclerosis patients with cardiac rhabdomyomas.

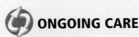

ONGOING CARE

PROGNOSIS

Cognitive disability unfortunately will not improve unless the cognitive impairment results from uncontrolled seizures. Seizure control is medically refractory in up to 40% of cases, and some children require epilepsy surgery to remove cortical tubers or subependymal nodules. Cardiac tumors may also require surgical intervention. Renal angiomyolipomas can be embolized angiographically or surgically corrected. Subependymal giant cell astrocytomas that cause hydrocephalus may require resection.

ADDITIONAL READING

- Au KS, Ward CH, Northrup H. Tuberous sclerosis complex: disease modifiers and treatments. *Curr Opin Pediatr*. 2008;20(6):628–633.
- Crino PB. The pathophysiology of tuberous sclerosis complex. *Epilepsia*. 2010;51(Suppl 1):27–29.
- Curatolo P, Bombardieri R, Jozwiak S. Tuberous sclerosis. *Lancet*. 2008;372(9639):657–668.
- Franz DN, Bissler JJ, McCormack FX. Tuberous sclerosis complex: neurological, renal and pulmonary manifestations. *Neuropediatrics*. 2010;41(5): 199–208.
- Krueger DA, Care MM, Holland K, et al. Everolimus for subependymal giant-cell astrocytomas in tuberous sclerosis. *N Engl J Med*. 2010;363(19): 1801–1811.

CODES

ICD10

Q85.1 Tuberous sclerosis

FAQ

- Q: Can tuberous sclerosis be transmitted in subsequent pregnancies?
- A: An affected patient with the tuberous sclerosis gene mutation has a 50% chance of transmitting the mutation to his or her children.
- Q: Is genetic testing available?
- A: Molecular genetic testing for mutations at the *TSC1* and *TSC2* loci are available but are not required for diagnosis because not all clinical cases of TSC have identifiable mutations.
- Q: Will my child need brain surgery?
- A: In the event of refractory seizures, removal of cortical tubers may help seizure control. Surgery may also be indicated in cases of obstructive hydrocephalus. If a brain tumor is detected by MRI, neurosurgical evaluation is indicated.

T

TULAREMIA

Gordon E. Schutze

BASICS

DESCRIPTION

Tularemia is an infection caused by *Francisella tularensis*, a small, fastidious, nonmotile, gram-negative coccobacillus; 4 distinct subspecies have been described:

- *tularensis* (type A): found primarily in North America; causes the most severe cases of tularemia in humans
- *holarctica* (type B): subspecies found primarily in Europe and Asia; less virulent than *tularensis*
- *novicida*: rarely isolated but can be found worldwide
- *mediasiatica*: recovered from ticks and animals in Central Asia; not associated with disease in immunocompetent humans
- An additional species, *Francisella philomiragia* (formerly *Yersinia philomiragia*), has also been reported. This is a rare cause of human disease and is possibly associated with salt water exposure.
- Tularemia typically presents with fever, myalgias, and headache 3–6 days after initial exposure. The extent of the illness depends on infecting dose, subspecies, and route of entry.
- 6 clinical forms are typically described:
  - Ulceroglandular tularemia
    - Constitutes 75% of all cases
    - A papule, which ruptures and ulcerates, occurs at the site of entry.
  - Glandular tularemia
    - Identical to the ulceroglandular form
    - However, does not have an identified primary skin lesion
  - Oculoglandular tularemia
    - Occurs when the organism gains access via the conjunctival sac
    - Usually from the patient rubbing the eyes with contaminated fingers
    - Yellow nodules and ulcers may appear on the palpebral conjunctiva associated with enlarged preauricular nodes.
  - Oropharyngeal tularemia
    - Occurs after the ingestion of contaminated food or water
    - An ulcerative or membranous tonsillitis accompanies a painful sore throat.
    - Lower GI tract involvement with vomiting, diarrhea, and abdominal pain may be associated.
  - Typhoidal tularemia
    - Presents with fever of unknown origin, without localizing lymphadenopathy or skin findings
    - Shock, pleuropulmonary findings, odynophagia, diarrhea, and bowel necrosis are often associated.
  - Pneumonic tularemia
    - Occurs after inhalation of the organism
    - It can also be present in association with ulceroglandular and typhoidal tularemia.
    - Pulmonary tularemia is the most fulminant and lethal form.
    - Symptoms include fever, dry cough, and pleuritic chest pain.
    - Tularemia in this form is a feared potential biologic weapon because an exposure to only 1–10 colony-forming units can result in infection. Although not transmitted person to person, laboratory workers working with organism on an agar plate are at risk for this form of disease.

ALERT

- *F. tularensis* is currently listed as a class A bioterrorism agent because of its potential ease for dissemination and infection as well as potential for high case fatality rates.
- In the past, resistant forms of *F. tularensis* have been engineered, but the actual use of this organism as a bioterrorism agent has not been documented.
- The diagnosis of inhalation tularemia should raise the suspicion of bioterrorism.

EPIDEMIOLOGY

- *F. tularensis* is found primarily in the Northern hemisphere from the 30–70-degree latitudes. Wild mammals (e.g., rabbits, hares, squirrels, beavers, deer, and rodents) may be infected as well as invertebrates (e.g., ticks, deerflies, horseflies, and mosquitoes).
- Humans acquire tularemia after a bite by an infected arthropod or through contact with tissues or body fluids of an infected animal. The subspecies *holarctica* has been shown to persist in various water sources, and waterborne transmission to humans has been reported.
- Inhalational exposure can happen in the laboratory setting or after the organism is aerosolized during meat preparation.
- Most commonly reported during the summer months in children between 5 and 9 years of age and those >75 years old

RISK FACTORS

- Most frequently infected groups include hunters, trappers, farmers, and veterinarians.
- Activities involving wild animals or exposure to various arthropod vectors
- Infection has been linked to landscapers using lawn mowers and brush cutters.
- Laboratory personnel working with samples known to be or potentially infected with *Francisella*

GENERAL PREVENTION

- Isolation of the hospitalized patient
  - Standard precautions are recommended for protection against secretions. Human-to-human transmission has not been reported.
- Control measures
  - Protective clothing and insect repellent should be used to minimize insect bites.
  - Inspection for ticks and their immediate removal should be routine after outdoor activity in endemic areas.
  - Rubber gloves should be worn while handling or cooking wild animals (e.g., rabbits, lemmings) possibly contaminated with *Francisella*.
  - Laboratory workers should wear rubber gloves and masks in a biosafety level 3 environment when working with specimens potentially containing *Francisella*.
- Vaccine
  - Significant research into various vaccine techniques continues to evolve given concerns of *F. tularemia* as an agent of bioterrorism.

PATHOPHYSIOLOGY

- Entry into the human is via skin, mucous membranes, or inhalational.
- A primary lesion develops at the site of exposure.
- Local tender lymph node swelling ensues.
- After skin inoculation or inhalation, the organism can spread via the bloodstream to various organs.

ETIOLOGY

Human infection can result from various modes of entry:

- Skin contact with infected animals
- Vector-borne infection described after the bite of a tick, mosquito, horsefly, or deerfly

- Inhalation of aerosolized organism seen in laboratory workers, crop harvesting, disturbance of contaminated hay, and grass cutting
- Ingestion of contaminated food products or water

DIAGNOSIS

HISTORY

- In the right clinical setting, a history that elicits any occupational exposure or recreational activity previously noted as risk factors should raise suspicion for tularemia.
- History of a recent tick or fly bite may be recalled among affected patients.
- A history of a papule that became ulcerated is classic for the ulceroglandular form.
- Fever >101°F for 2–3 weeks is common, with associated weight loss.

PHYSICAL EXAM

- A papule or ulcer may be seen at the inoculation site.
- Skin lesions should be sought, especially when lymphadenopathy is present.
- Lymph node swelling is typically tender with overlying erythema.
- After a 3–6-day incubation period, symptoms may include fever, myalgias, and headache.
- Hepatosplenomegaly, purulent conjunctivitis, adenopathy, an ulcerative skin lesion, and tonsillitis are other localized findings.

DIAGNOSTIC TESTS & INTERPRETATION

Lab

- Serum tube agglutination titers of 1:160 or greater are generally considered positive.
- A 4-fold rise in titers over a 2-week period is necessary to define a current infection.
- Cultures of blood, skin, ulcers, lymph nodes, gastric washings, and respiratory secretions require special media containing cysteine.
- Laboratory personnel should be made aware of the infection risk from specimens. Growth of the organism requires a biosafety level 3 laboratory.
- Polymerase chain reaction (PCR) tests are available in some laboratories. They are more sensitive than culture and can be performed on tissue samples. Current PCR techniques do not differentiate subspecies, but such techniques are under development.
- Fluorescent in situ hybridization techniques have been used in the research setting to differentiate subspecies and may be clinically useful in the future.

DIFFERENTIAL DIAGNOSIS

Depending on the form of tularemia, the infection can mimic other illnesses such as streptococcal or staphylococcal infection, cat-scratch disease, mononucleosis, cutaneous anthrax, pasteurellosis, Q fever, legionellosis, typhoid fever, or mycobacterial disease. In general, tularemia should be considered in the following differential diagnoses:

- Fever of unknown origin
- Fever with purulent conjunctivitis
- Fever with hepatosplenomegaly
- Fever with skin ulcer

TREATMENT

MEDICATION

- IV/IM antibiotic therapy with gentamicin is considered 1st-line therapy.
- 2nd-line therapeutic options include streptomycin, ciprofloxacin, or doxycycline. Relapses have been associated with the latter two, and they are generally only used in adults or in specific situations.
- Duration of treatment is typically 7–10 days. In severe disease, some experts recommend combination therapy such as gentamicin with ciprofloxacin or doxycycline.

INPATIENT CONSIDERATIONS

Initial Stabilization

- If respiratory compromise is present, oxygen supplementation and/or assisted ventilation must be rapidly addressed.
- Recognition and prompt aggressive treatment of shock should be a major priority.

PROGNOSIS

- When recognized and treated with appropriate antibiotics, the course is generally <1 month.
- Mortality is low, except in cases of fulminant disease or are otherwise immunocompromised.
- The subspecies *tularensis* is thought to be more virulent than the others.
- Both typhoidal and pneumonic forms of tularemia are associated with the highest risk for mortality.

COMPLICATIONS

- Lymph node suppuration, meningitis, endocarditis, hepatitis, and renal failure have all been associated with tularemia. Lymph node suppuration despite adequate therapy may occur in up to 25% of patients with ulceroglandular or glandular disease.
- Infection with *F. tularensis* may be complicated by necrotic and granulomatous lesions in the liver and spleen as well as parenchymal degeneration.
- A sepsis syndrome with shock, fever, myalgias, and severe headache can be seen. Recognition and prompt aggressive treatment of shock should be a major priority.
- Skin manifestations, including vesiculopapular rash, erythema nodosum, and erythema multiforme have been associated with tularemia.

ADDITIONAL READING

- Barry EM, Cole LE, Santiago AE. Vaccines against tularemia. *Hum Vaccin*. 2009;5(12):832–838.
- Cross JT Jr, Schutze GE, Jacobs RF. Treatment of tularemia with gentamicin in pediatric patients. *Pediatr Infect Dis J*. 1995;14(2):151–152.
- Eliasson H, Broman T, Forsman M, et al. Tularemia: current epidemiology and disease management. *Infect Dis Clin N Am*. 2006;20(2):289–311.
- Nigrovic LE, Wingerter SL. Tularemia. *Infect Dis Clin North Am*. 2008;22(3):489–504.
- Snowden J, Stovall S. Tularemia: retrospective review of 10 years' experience in Arkansas. *Clin Pediatr (Phila)*. 2011;50(1):64–68.
- Tarnvik A, Chu MC. New approaches to diagnosis and therapy of tularemia. *Ann N Y Acad Sci*. 2007; 1105:378–404.

CODES

ICD10

- A21.9 Tularemia, unspecified
- A21.0 Ulceroglandular tularemia
- A21.1 Oculoglandular tularemia

FAQ

- Q: If a tick is removed from my child, should antibiotics be started?
- A: No. Empiric antimicrobial therapy will not prevent tularemia.
- Q: Can my child get tularemia again?
- A: No. It appears once infection has occurred, the patient is protected from further new infections.

T

TURNER SYNDROME

John S. Fuqua

BASICS

DESCRIPTION

Presence of typical findings in a phenotypic female with complete or partial absence of the second sex chromosome

EPIDEMIOLOGY

Prevalence: 1:2,000–5,000 liveborn females

Genetics

- Frequency of genotypes
  - 45,X 55%
  - 46,Xi(Xq) 17%
  - 45,X/46,XX 13%
  - 46,Xr(X) 5%
  - 45,X/46,XY 5%
  - Other 5%
- Recurrence risk is low in subsequent pregnancies in the absence of familial defects of the X chromosome.

PATHOPHYSIOLOGY

Deletion of the *SHOX* gene at Xp22.33 is responsible for the majority of the height deficit in affected patients. Fetuses with Turner syndrome have accelerated loss of germ cells from the second half of gestation through the first few years of life, with eventual gonadal failure.

ASSOCIATED CONDITIONS

- Short stature (~100%)
- Hypogonadism (90%)
- ADHD (24%)
- Strabismus/hyperopia (17%)
- Conductive hearing loss (21%)
- Sensorineural hearing loss in adults (60%)
- Autoimmune thyroiditis (27%)
- Coarctation of the aorta (11%)
- Bicuspid aortic valve (16%)
- Hypertension (50%)
- Horseshoe kidney (10%)
- Renal collecting system abnormalities (20%)
- Celiac disease (6%)
- Glucose intolerance in adults (40–50%)

DIAGNOSIS

HISTORY

- Intrauterine growth retardation
- Slow postnatal growth, beginning in infancy
  - Eventual short stature
- Lymphedema, especially in infancy
- Frequent otitis media and middle ear effusions
- Normal overall intelligence, with performance IQ less than verbal IQ
  - Focused difficulties in math, visuospatial skills, executive functioning
- Decreased social cognition, with problems reading facial expressions, body language, and other nonverbal cues
- Lack of pubertal maturation for age

PHYSICAL EXAM

- HEENT
  - Down slanting palpebral fissures, ptosis, epicanthal folds
  - Low set, posteriorly rotated ears
  - Arched palate
  - Micrognathia
  - Neck webbing (pterygium colli)
  - Low set posterior hairline
- Musculoskeletal
  - Short stature
  - Wide carrying angle (cubitus valgus)
  - Short 4th metacarpals
  - Broad chest relative to height
  - Scoliosis
  - Genu valgum
  - Madelung deformity of wrist
- Other:
  - Increased number of pigmented nevi
  - Absent breast development, normal pubic hair for age
  - Edema of feet and/or hands
  - Hyperconvex fingernails, dystrophic toenails

DIAGNOSTIC TESTS & INTERPRETATION

Laboratory diagnosis of Turner syndrome is based on karyotype. Once the diagnosis is established, additional tests should be performed to identify associated conditions or complications.

Lab

- If older than 4 years old: TSH, free T_4, screening for celiac disease
- If older than 10 years old: TSH, free T_4, celiac disease serologic screening, LFTs, fasting lipids, CBC, renal function, LH, FSH

Imaging

In all patients, regardless of age: renal ultrasonography and 2-D echocardiography with color Doppler or cardiac MRI

Diagnostic Procedures/Other

- EKG
- Audiologic evaluation
- Orthodontic assessment
- Educational/psychosocial evaluation
- Scoliosis screening

TREATMENT

GENERAL MEASURES

- Treatment of girls with Turner syndrome focuses on promoting linear growth and pubertal maturation as well as screening for and managing other associated conditions.
- Spontaneous puberty, manifested as breast development, occurs in 14% of girls with a 45,X karyotype and 32% of girls with other Turner syndrome karyotypes. Up to 50% of those with spontaneous puberty may go on to have menses that persist into late adolescence or early adulthood.
- Nearly all girls with Turner syndrome eventually have ovarian failure.

MEDICATION

- Growth hormone administration is part of standard care for girls with Turner syndrome.
  - Treatment should start when growth failure is recognized.
  - Recommended dose for girls with Turner syndrome is 54 mcg/kg/24 h or 0.375 mg/kg/week.
- Addition of oxandrolone, a nonaromatizable androgen, may be considered in girls older than age 9 years to help promote growth.
  - This treatment may accelerate pubic and axillary hair growth, so oxandrolone is generally reserved for peripubertal patients.
  - The recommended dose is 0.05 mg/kg/24 h or less.

- Estrogen is required for pubertal-aged girls without spontaneous breast development who have elevated FSH levels.
  - Induction of puberty may be delayed to accrue additional linear growth, but early diagnosis and treatment with growth hormone may normalize height and allow for estrogen treatment at a physiologic age.
  - There are many estrogen treatment regimens available, including oral and transdermal routes. Treatment is usually initiated at doses that are 1/8–1/10 of the adult doses.
  - Doses are gradually increased to adult values over 2–4 years. After 2–4 years, intermittent progestin treatment is given to induce menstrual bleeding.

ADDITIONAL TREATMENT

Associated conditions may require treatment, including antihypertensives, SBE prophylaxis, levothyroxine, gluten-free diet, myringotomy tubes, and strabismus care.

ONGOING CARE

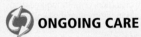

FOLLOW-UP RECOMMENDATIONS

- Age 4–5 years
  - Assessment of social skills, psychoeducational evaluation prior to school entry
- Age 5–12 years
  - Every year: BP, TSH, LFTs, educational and social progress
  - Every 1–5 years: audiology and ENT
  - Every 2–5 years: celiac disease screening
  - As needed: dental and orthodontic evaluations
- Age 12 years–adult
  - Every year: BP, TSH, LFTs, fasting lipids, blood glucose
  - Every 1–5 years: audiology and ENT
  - Assessment of pubertal development and psychosexual adjustment
  - Every 5–10 years: cardiac MRI
  - As needed: celiac disease screening

PROGNOSIS

- Height percentile at diagnosis is highly predictive of adult height if not treated with growth hormone or estrogen, with a correlation coefficient of 0.95.
- Height loss in untreated girls with Turner syndrome is approximately 20 cm compared to the midparental target height.
- Mean adult height in untreated girls is 144 cm.
- The presence of webbed neck (pterygium colli) on physical exam is predictive of both aortic coarctation and ovarian failure.
- 90% of women with Turner syndrome have ovarian failure.
- 40–50% of adults with Turner syndrome have insulin resistance or abnormal glucose tolerance.
- Girls and women with Turner syndrome have an increased risk for depression, anxiety, and social withdrawal.

ALERT

Girls and women with Turner syndrome are at increased risk for aortic dissection, manifested as chest or back pain. Those with a bicuspid aortic valve or with an ascending aortic size index >2.5 cm/m^2 are at highest risk.

ADDITIONAL READING

- Bondy CA; Turner Syndrome Study Group. Care of girls and women with Turner syndrome: a guideline of the Turner Syndrome Study Group. *J Clin Endocrinol Metab*. 2007;92(1):10–25.
- Carlson M, Airhart N, Lopez L, et al. Moderate aortic enlargement and bicuspid aortic valve are associated with aortic dissection in Turner syndrome: report of the international Turner syndrome aortic dissection registry. *Circulation*. 2012;126(18):2220–2226.
- Davenport ML. Approach to the patient with Turner syndrome. *J Clin Endocrinol Metab*. 2010;95(4):1487–1495.
- Davenport ML, Crowe BJ, Travers SH, et al. Growth hormone treatment of early growth failure in toddlers with Turner syndrome: a randomized, controlled, multicenter trial. *J Clin Endocrinol Metab*. 2007;92(9):3406–3416.
- Devernay M, Ecosse E, Coste J, et al. Determinants of medical care for young women with Turner syndrome. *J Clin Endocrinol Metab*. 2009;94(9):3408–3413.
- Donaldson MD, Gault EJ, Tan KW, et al. Optimising management in Turner syndrome: from infancy to adult transfer. *Arch Dis Child*. 2006;91(6):513–520.
- Gault EJ, Perry RJ, Cole TJ, et al; British Society for Paediatric Endocrinology and Diabetes. Effect of oxandrolone and timing of pubertal induction on final height in Turner's syndrome: randomised, double blind, placebo controlled trial. *BMJ*. 2011;342:d1980.
- Kim HK, Gottliebson W, Hor K, et al. Cardiovascular anomalies in Turner syndrome: spectrum, prevalence, and cardiac MRI findings in a pediatric and young adult population. *Am J Roentgenol*. 2011;96(2):454–460.
- Pinsker JE. Clinical review: Turner syndrome: updating the paradigm of clinical care. *J Clin Endocrinol Metab*. 2012;97(6):E994–E1003.
- Ross JL, Quigley CA, Cao D, et al. Growth hormone plus childhood low-dose estrogen in Turner's syndrome. *N Engl J Med*. 2011;364(13):1230–1242.
- Schoemaker MJ, Swerdlow AJ, Higgins CD, et al; United Kingdom Clinical Cytogenetics Group. Mortality in women with Turner syndrome in Great Britain: a national cohort study. *J Clin Endocrinol Metab*. 2008;93(12):4735–4742.

CODES

ICD10

- Q96.9 Turner's syndrome, unspecified
- Q96.0 Karyotype 45, X
- Q96.1 Karyotype 46, X iso (Xq)

FAQ

- Q: Are older parents at increased risk to have a child with Turner syndrome?
- A: No. Turner syndrome is not associated with either advanced maternal or paternal age.
- Q: Are there special precautions for girls with bicuspid aortic valve?
- A: Affected patients with bicuspid aortic valves should receive SBE prophylaxis.
- Q: Can assisted reproductive technology allow women with Turner syndrome to carry a pregnancy?
- A: In vitro fertilization of donor oocytes has been performed in women with Turner syndrome. However, pregnant women with Turner syndrome have a significantly increased risk for hypertension and gestational diabetes. Importantly, they also are at high risk for aortic dissection. Thus, pregnancy is controversial and usually discouraged at this time.

ULCERATIVE COLITIS

Naamah Zitomersky

BASICS

DESCRIPTION

Ulcerative colitis (UC) is a chronic, relapsing, inflammatory disease of the colon, which extends continuously from the rectum proximally to a varying extent. UC is categorized as an inflammatory bowel disease (IBD), along with Crohn disease (CD). Unlike CD, UC does not affect the small bowel.

EPIDEMIOLOGY

- The incidence of pediatric-onset UC is between 1 and 4/100,000 children/year in most North American and European regions.
- Roughly 15–20% of patients with UC develop the disease before the age of 18 years.
- Incidence peaks between 15 and 30 years of age.

ETIOLOGY

The precise cause of UC, as with IBD in general, is unknown, but is thought to involve both genetic predisposition and environmental triggers.

RISK FACTORS

Genetics

- Family history of IBD in ~15–20% of patients with UC
- There is an increased incidence of family history in patients diagnosed prior to 20 years of age.
- Higher concordance in monozygotic than in dizygotic twins
- Genome-wide association studies (GWAS) have identified multiple loci associated with UC. Mutations in genes involving intestinal barrier functions are seen in UC more often than healthy controls.
- Recent studies identified five new IBD susceptibility loci that are associated with early-onset disease.

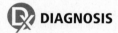

DIAGNOSIS

Patients with UC typically present with bloody diarrhea, tenesmus, and lower quadrant abdominal pain. When symptoms become severe, weight loss, fatigue, and vomiting can be seen. Colonoscopy with histopathologic review of biopsies is the gold standard in diagnosis of UC.

HISTORY

A detailed history is important in making the diagnosis:

- Rectal bleeding (90%)
- Abdominal pain (90%)
- Diarrhea (50%)
- Weight loss (10%)
- Growth failure
- Recent travel (enteric infections)
- Antibiotic use (*Clostridium difficile*)
- Family history of IBD

PHYSICAL EXAM

- Fever, tachycardia
- Evidence of weight loss or poor growth
- Signs of anemia
- Uveitis
- Mouth sores
- Arthritis
- Abdominal tenderness typically in lower quadrants or abdominal distention
- Perianal/rectal examination (UC is not typically associated with perianal disease, but hemorrhoids or erythema can be seen.)

DIAGNOSTIC TESTS & INTERPRETATION

Lab

- CBC
  - Iron deficiency anemia and anemia of chronic disease can be seen.
  - Thrombocytosis is another frequent finding.
- Iron studies (iron deficiency)
- ESR, CRP; disease activity
- Electrolytes (hydration), CMP. Serum albumin may be low, hypoalbuminemia may be present in fulminant colitis.
- Liver panel (hepatobiliary disease)
- Perinuclear antineutrophil cytoplasmic antibody (pANCA; positive in 80% of UC patients, 20% of CD patients)
- Stool for blood, white cells (colitis)
- Fecal calprotectin and fecal lactoferrin: may be elevated during times of active inflammation
- Stool cultures:
  - *C. difficile*, *Salmonella*, *Shigella*, *Campylobacter*, *Yersinia*, *Escherichia coli* (enterohemorrhagic), *Aeromonas*, amebiasis, cytomegalovirus

Imaging

- Plain abdominal radiograph
  - Important in diagnosing perforation, ileus, obstruction, and toxic megacolon
  - In toxic megacolon, the colon is dilated, and there are multiple air–fluid levels indicative of ileus. Serial x-rays are mandatory.
- An upper GI with small bowel follow-through (UGI/SBFT) may help to exclude small intestinal inflammation indicative of CD.
- New imaging modalities, such as MR enterography (MRE), CT enterography, are currently being performed in place of UGI/SBFT. MRE has the advantage of avoiding radiation exposure.
- MRI may have a role in differentiating transmural and mucosal inflammation and is useful for demonstrating perianal fistulas more consistent with CD than UC.
- Right upper quadrant ultrasound may be useful for evaluating associated hepatobiliary disease if it is suspected.
- Endoscopic retrograde cholangiopancreatography (ERCP) or MRCP are also useful in diagnosing primary sclerosing cholangitis (3% of UC patients).

Diagnostic Procedures/Other

- Colonoscopy (with biopsies) is the gold standard and is necessary to confirm the diagnosis of UC. It is critical to visualize and biopsy the entire colon, including terminal ileum, to differentiate CD from UC.
- Upper endoscopy may increase chances of detecting CD and may detect chronic gastritis sometimes seen with UC.
- Video capsule endoscopy (VCE) is more sensitive than UGI/SBFT for diagnosing small bowel disease indicative of CD rather than UC.
- Pitfalls:
  - Infectious colitis (especially *C. difficile*) can mimic the findings of UC so this should first be ruled out with stool culture. Recurrent *C. difficile* occurs frequently in UC.
  - Differentiating Crohn colitis from UC: Small intestinal inflammation and perianal disease (fistula, abscess) are more indicative of CD.
  - Serum inflammatory markers and CBC may be normal in children with active colitis especially with mild disease.
  - The combination of positive pANCA and negative anti–*Saccharomyces cerevisiae* antibody (ASCA) has a reported sensitivity of 60–70% and a specificity of 95–97% for UC in adults. The sensitivity and specificity are lower for pediatric patients.
  - Toxic megacolon is a surgical emergency. It is characterized by a dilated colon at risk for breakdown of its barrier to toxins entering the systemic circulation. Signs and symptoms include peritonitis, mental status changes, and fluid and electrolyte imbalance. Plain abdominal radiograph shows a segment or total colonic dilatation. Risk factors include new diagnosis of UC, pancolitis, concurrent use of opiates and/or anticholinergics, and recent colonoscopy.

Pathologic Findings

- Chronic or chronic active colitis, with continuous inflammation limited to the mucosa
- Crypt architectural distortion, cryptitis (aggregation of inflammatory cells in the crypt epithelium), crypt abscesses
- Site of colon affected:
  - Rectum (virtually 100%)
  - Left side (50–60%)
  - Pancolitis (10%)
- Small intestine is technically not involved, but occasionally the terminal ileum of patients with UC can be found to have mild inflammation on radiologic or histologic examination. This is thought to be from refluxed colonic contents (backwash ileitis).
- Skip lesions are not seen in UC.
- Chronic gastritis may be present in patients with UC.

DIFFERENTIAL DIAGNOSIS

- Infectious colitis: *C. difficile*, *Salmonella*, *Shigella*, *Campylobacter*, *Yersinia*, *E. coli* (enterohemorrhagic), *Aeromonas*, cytomegalovirus
- Crohn disease
- Congenital Hirschsprung enterocolitis
- Bleeding juvenile polyps
- Milk protein allergy especially in infants
- Immunodeficiency states (rare) onset of colitis within the first 2 years of life, often with perianal involvement; skin folliculitis, or eczema; other fungal or bacterial infections
- Eosinophilic colitis
- Autoimmune enteropathy
- Hemolytic-uremic syndrome
- Henoch-Schönlein purpura
- Trauma due to anal sex or sexual abuse

TREATMENT

MEDICATION

- Mild disease can be treated with oral mesalamine, topical corticosteroid enema or foam, or mesalamine enema/suppositories.
- For mild to moderate disease, Budesonide MMX is a once-daily, extended-release budesonide, which has been shown to induce remission in adults with mild to moderate UC and has fewer side effects than systemic corticosteroids.
- For moderate disease, mesalamine, a short course of oral corticosteroid and the addition of an immunomodulators such as azathioprine or 6-mercaptopurine may help to maintain disease remission and minimize the need for recurrent steroid use.

- Antibodies against tumor necrosis factor (TNF)-α include infliximab and adalimumab; both are used in the treatment of moderate to severe UC or steroid-resistant UC.
- Vedolizumab is an anti-integrin, which is a steroid-sparing agent used for induction and maintenance of moderate to severe UC in adults. $\alpha 4\beta 7$ integrins are expressed on B and T lymphocytes and facilitate binding to intestinal vasculature. Vedolizumab is a gut-selective antibody that blocks gut lymphocyte recruitment by blocking its interaction with mucosal addressin cell adhesion molecule-1.
- Fulminant disease: hospitalization, if concern for toxic megacolon—complete bowel rest with total parenteral nutrition, broad-spectrum antibiotics, discontinuation of anticholinergics and narcotics, avoidance of endoscopy, IV corticosteroids, serial abdominal radiographs, frequent examinations, stool monitoring (frequency, amount of blood, and volume of stool output); early surgical consult
- If treatment of acute symptoms with IV steroids fails (after 3–5 days), therapy with tacrolimus, cyclosporine, or infliximab can be started.
- Pediatric Ulcerative Colitis Activity Index (PUCAI): obtained on day 3–5; may identify patients with severe UC who will require escalation of therapy. Prevents unnecessary prolonged exposure to corticosteroids
- Short-term medications for severe colitis should be used as a bridge to surgery or to transition to another steroid-sparing agent, such as an immunomodulator or biologic.
- Tacrolimus (PO) 0.1 mg/kg/dose every 12 hours with goal trough levels of 10–15 ng/mL after 2 days.
- Cyclosporine (IV): 4 mg/kg/24 h for 2 weeks (therapeutic levels vary depending on the technique used in the laboratory)
- Cyclosporine (PO): 6–8 mg/kg/24 h for 6–8 months
- Tacrolimus and cyclosporine are both nephrotoxic. Should only be used by experienced clinicians
- Trimethoprim/sulfamethoxazole should be given for *Pneumocystis carinii* prophylaxis.
- 5-aminosalycilates:
  - Mesalamine (PO): 40–60 mg/kg/24 h (maximum 4.8 g/day)
  - Mesalamine (enema): 4 g at bedtime (for proctitis or isolated left-sided disease)
  - Mesalamine (suppository): 500 mg b.i.d.
- Corticosteroids:
  - Methylprednisolone (IV): 1–2 mg/kg/24 h (equivalent to prednisone 60 mg maximum)
  - Prednisone (PO): 1–2 mg/kg/24 h oral (up to maximum 60 mg/day)
  - For proctitis and isolated left-sided disease
  - Hydrocortisone enema: 100 mg once to twice daily
  - Hydrocortisone foam: 80 mg once to twice daily
  - Budesonide multimatrix system 9 mg/24 h orally
- Immunomodulators:
  - Mercaptopurine (6-MP) (PO): 1–1.5 mg/kg/24 h or azathioprine (PO): 2 mg/kg/24 h
  - Check thiopurine methyltransferase genetics or activity prior to initiation to avoid pancytopenia in those who lack this enzyme. Also monitor CBC and lipase every 2 weeks on initiation and with dosing changes to look for cytopenias or pancreatitis.
- Biologics:
  - Infliximab (IV): 5 mg/kg weeks 0, 2, 6, then every 8 weeks, dose and frequency can be increased to capture symptoms
  - Adalimumab (IM): for patients weighing 40 kg and greater, 160 mg on week 0, 80 mg on week 2, followed by 20 or 40 mg every 2 weeks starting on week 4. Reduce dosage by 50% for patients <40 kg.
- Anti-integrin
  - Vedolizumab (adult dosage) 300 mg IV weeks 0, 2, 6 weeks then every 8 weeks and can be increased to every 4 weeks to capture symptoms.

SURGERY/OTHER PROCEDURES

- Patients with fulminant disease who fail medical therapy should be referred for colectomy.
- Patients with chronically active disease unresponsive to medication, growth failure, or with corticosteroid dependence should also consider colectomy.
- Because UC is limited to the colon, colectomy is considered a curative procedure. It also eliminates the elevated colon cancer risk.
- Sometimes surgery is urgently required for perforation, significant and persistent bleeding, toxic megacolon, and failure of medical treatment.
- Can be electively performed for chronic incapacitating disease, growth failure, corticosteroid dependence, dysplastic changes in the colon, or long-standing disease (usually after 10 years).
- Ileoanal anastomosis and pouch construction is surgery of choice for most pediatric patients and usually is performed in 3 stages over 6 months. 10% of cases are subsequently found to have Crohn disease after colectomy.

ONGOING CARE

FOLLOW-UP RECOMMENDATIONS

- Outpatient follow-up with a pediatric gastroenterologist should be arranged.
- Important parameters to follow routinely include abdominal symptoms, rectal bleeding, stool frequency/consistency, height/weight, hemoglobin, WBC count (for patients on immunosuppressives), ESR, albumin, bilirubin, and liver enzymes.
- There is ongoing debate about monitoring for mucosal healing in UC. Adult studies have shown better outcomes, reduction in disease progression, and fewer complications in individuals who achieve mucosal healing.
- Colon cancer screening with colonoscopy should be performed within 10 years of diagnosis.

COMPLICATIONS

- Bleeding
- Anemia
- Toxic megacolon
- Extraintestinal manifestations include hepatobiliary disease (3–5%), uveitis (up to 4%), arthritis affecting large joints (10%), spondylitis (6%), erythema nodosum (>5%), pyoderma gangrenosum (>1%), renal calculi (5%).
- Malignancy risk is 8% 10–25 years after colitis is diagnosed and it increases ~10% for every subsequent decade.
- Colonic stricture
- Thrombosis: Patients with IBD have a 3-fold higher risk of thrombosis compared to individuals without IBD. This risk rises further to 15-fold with disease flares. Presentation with calf pain or shortness of breath should prompt evaluation for deep vein thrombosis or pulmonary embolism.

ADDITIONAL READING

- Bousvaros A, Antonioli DA, Colletti RB, et al. Differentiating ulcerative colitis from Crohn disease in children and young adults: a report of a working group of the North American Society for Pediatric Gastroenterology, Hepatology, and Nutrition and the Crohn's and Colitis Foundation of America. *J Ped Gastroenterol Nutr*. 2007;44(5):653–674.
- Bousvaros A, Kirschner BS, Werlin SL, et al. Oral tacrolimus treatment of severe colitis in children. *J Pediatr*. 2000;137(6):794–799.
- Feagan BG, Rutgeerts P, Sands BE, et al. Vedolizumab as induction and maintenance therapy for ulcerative colitis. *N Engl J Med*. 2013;369(8):699–710.
- Hyams JS, Lerer T, Griffiths A, et al. Outcome following infliximab therapy in children with ulcerative colitis. *Am J Gastroenterol*. 2010;105(6):1430–1436.
- Lees CW, Barrett JC, Parkes M, et al. New IBD genetics: common pathways with other diseases. *Gut*. 2011;60(12):1739–1753.
- Loftus EV Jr. Epidemiology and risk factors for colorectal dysplasia and cancer in ulcerative colitis. *Gastroenterol Clin North Am*. 2006;35(3):517–531.
- Shikhare G, Kugathasan S. Inflammatory bowel disease in children: current trends. *J Gastroenterol*. 2010;45(7):673–682.
- Turner D, Levine A, Escher JA, et al. Management of pediatric ulcerative colitis: joint ECCO and ESPGHAN evidence-based consensus guidelines. *J Pediatr Gastroenterol Nutr*. 2012;55(3):340–361.
- Zitomersky NL, Verhave M, Trenor CC III. Thrombosis and inflammatory bowel disease: a call for improved awareness and prevention. *Inflamm Bowel Dis*. 2011;17(1):458–470.

CODES

ICD10

- K51.90 Ulcerative colitis, unspecified, without complications
- K51.80 Other ulcerative colitis without complications
- K51.311 Ulcerative (chronic) rectosigmoiditis with rectal bleeding

FAQ

- Q: Will my child have this disease forever?
- A: Some people will have only the initial attack and then be symptom-free, but usually and more often in pediatrics, individuals will have episodes of recurrences and remissions. Surgical removal of the colon represents a curative procedure, although some patients may develop inflammation in the pouch created out of the remaining bowel (pouchitis).
- Q: What is the cause of UC?
- A: Both genetic and environmental factors are important in the development of UC.
- Q: Where can I learn more about UC?
- A: The North American Society for Pediatric Gastroenterology, Hepatology and Nutrition provides a Web site for children with IBD and their families (www.gastrokids.org). The Crohn's and Colitis Foundation of America (www.CCFA.org) is a nonprofit organization dedicated to the care and education of people with CD and UC.

UPPER GASTROINTESTINAL BLEEDING

Michael A. Manfredi

BASICS

DESCRIPTION

- Upper gastrointestinal bleeding (UGIB) is defined as bleeding in the GI tract that occurs proximal to the ligament of Treitz.
- The classic clinical symptom of UGIB is hematemesis, consisting of either bright red or "coffee grounds"-appearing blood.
- Other symptoms of UGIB include melena, occult blood loss, as well as hematochezia with rapid, severe bleeds.
- When hematemesis is suspected, a clinician must exclude non-GI causes, including hemoptysis (coughing up blood), nose bleeds, and bleeding from the mouth and pharynx.

EPIDEMIOLOGY

- Most large, prospective studies of UGIB in children have assessed the incidence in pediatric critical care settings to range from 6.4 to 25% of admissions.
- 80% of UGIB resolve spontaneously.

ETIOLOGY

- Neonatal period (birth to 1 month)
  - Swallowed maternal blood
  - Necrotizing enterocolitis
  - Duodenal or antral webs
  - Hemorrhagic disease of the newborn
  - Esophagitis
  - Gastritis
  - Stress ulcer
  - Foreign body irritation
  - Vascular malformation
  - GI malformation
- Infancy (1 month to 2 years)
  - Esophagitis/gastritis
  - Stress ulcer
  - Mallory-Weiss tear
  - Pyloric stenosis
  - Vascular malformation
  - Duplication cysts
  - Metabolic disease
- Preschool age (2–5 years)
  - Esophageal varices
  - Esophagitis/gastritis/ulcer
  - Foreign body/bezoar
  - Mallory-Weiss tear
  - Vascular malformation
  - Meckel diverticulum
- School age (>5 years)
  - Esophageal varices
  - Infection
  - Esophagitis/gastritis/ulcer
  - Mallory-Weiss tear
  - Inflammatory bowel disease
  - Drugs: NSAIDS, α-adrenergic antagonists
  - *Helicobacter pylori*
- All ages: liver failure—coagulopathy, Henoch-Schönlein purpura

RISK FACTORS

- Liver disease may cause portal hypertension and/or coagulopathy.
- Renal disease may cause gastritis or angiodysplasia.
- Renal failure or cirrhosis may cause gastric antral vascular ectasia.
- Recent trauma or stress (e.g., burns, head trauma, surgery) may be associated with a stress ulcer or gastritis.

GENERAL PREVENTION

- Avoid or minimize the use of drugs that can lead to peptic ulcers, for example, NSAIDs and aspirin.
- In patients with chronic GI conditions, optimize therapy and monitoring.
- Correct coagulopathy.
- Prophylactic medical or endoscopic therapy is beneficial for patients with known variceal bleeding.

DIAGNOSIS

APPROACH TO THE PATIENT

- The initial evaluation of patients presenting with GI bleeding should focus on assessing vital signs, obtaining a history of present illness, as well as pertinent medical history, performing a physical examination, and lab testing.
- General goals: Determine location of the bleeding and etiology, begin stabilization, and start treatment.
  - **Phase 1:** Determine whether the emesis contains blood versus nonblood substances. Red food coloring, fruit-flavored drinks, juices, vegetables, and some medicines may resemble blood. A pH-buffered Gastroccult test can be used to identify blood in the vomitus.
  - **Phase 2:** Assess severity of bleeding. Is there a change in vital signs, hematocrit, BP, capillary filling, pulse?
  - **Phase 3:** Stabilize patient, and decide if emergency treatment or referral is needed.

HISTORY

- GI symptoms:
  - Emesis prior to hematemesis may suggest Mallory-Weiss tear.
  - Odynophagia and GERD may suggest esophageal ulcer.
  - Epigastric pain may suggest peptic ulcer.
- Characteristics of UGIB:
  - Color of blood: may help determine whether bleeding is active
  - Emesis: bright red blood versus coffee ground
  - Stool: melena versus maroon colored versus hematochezia
- Amount of blood
  - May indicate severity of bleeding (i.e., drops vs. 1 teaspoon vs. 1 tablespoon)
- Duration of symptoms
  - May help determine if this is an acute or chronic issue
- Medication history:
  - The patient's current or recently used medications may help determine the cause.
  - Gastrotoxic medications, such as NSAIDs and aspirin, as well as anticoagulant medication use may be implicated.
  - In addition, a history of medications in the house should also be obtained due to possible accidental ingestion in younger children.
- Prior history of UGIB
  - May help determine the location of current bleed
  - If the prior bleed was recent, this may facilitate timely specialty consultation with gastroenterology, surgery, and/or interventional radiology.
- Prior GI history
  - Gastroesophageal reflux, peptic ulcer disease, and/or previous GI surgery are risk factors for UGIB. May suggest symptoms are due to recurrence of disease
- Social history
  - A history of alcohol use could be associated with gastritis or Mallory-Weiss tear

PHYSICAL EXAM

- Immediately assess hemodynamic stability:
  - Heart rate: Tachycardia may be an early sign of intravascular volume depletion.
  - Blood pressure: Hypotension is a late sign of volume depletion and may not be present even with significant blood loss, as vasoconstriction maintains BP until decompensation occurs.
  - In the setting of normal blood pressure, obtain orthostatic BP.
  - Capillary refill: Delayed capillary refill suggests intravascular volume depletion.
  - Oxygen saturation: Decreased arterial saturation values may be due to decreased oxygen-carrying capacity.
  - Evaluate for signs of shock:
    - Vital sign derangement (as listed earlier)
    - Cool clammy extremities
    - Poor mentation
- Abdomen
  - Evaluate bowel sounds for evidence of possible bowel obstruction.
  - Assess for abdominal tenderness, which may suggest peptic disease.
  - Evaluate for ascites, which may suggest liver disease.
  - Evaluate for signs of chronic liver disease of portal hypertension:
    - Hepatomegaly
    - Splenomegaly
    - Spider angioma
    - Caput medusa
    - Palmar erythema
    - Ascites

- Rectal examination
  - Heme-positive stool may or may not be present. If positive, supports diagnosis of UGIB
- Skin
  - Petechiae, ecchymosis, or hemangiomas may suggest a coagulopathy or a vascular anomaly.
- HEENT
  - Evaluate for nasopharyngeal source of bleeding.
  - Evaluate the buccal mucosa for syndromic findings: freckles (Peutz-Jeghers syndrome) and telangiectasias (Osler-Weber-Rendu syndrome).

DIAGNOSTIC TESTS & INTERPRETATION

- NG tube lavage
  - No longer recommended in patients with suspected UGIB for diagnosis, prognosis, visualization, or therapeutic effect
- Gastroccult test for blood
  - If possible, confirm red substances are blood.
  - In neonates, may need to check for fetal hemoglobin with the Apt test, which identifies fetal hemoglobin versus swallowed maternal blood.
- CBC
  - Initial hemoglobin values may be unreliable because a time delay between blood loss and hemodilution may occur and falsely produce near-normal values. Therefore, hemoglobin should be measured serially.
  - If leukopenia or thrombocytopenia is present, consider chronic liver disease and portal hypertension.
  - If anemia is present with normal erythrocyte indices, there is truly an acute cause for bleeding. If erythrocyte indices indicate iron deficiency anemia, consider varices or a mucosal lesion (i.e., chronic blood loss).
- Coagulation profile
  - If PT or PTT is abnormal, consider liver disease or disseminated intravascular coagulation (DIC) with sepsis.
  - If DIC screen is negative, consider liver disease. Important to avoid contamination of blood sample with heparin.
- Liver function test results may be abnormal in chronic liver disease.

Imaging

- Barium tests
  - Not useful in the acute setting
  - Barium can obscure view when performing esophagogastroduodenoscopy (EGD).
- Abdominal x-ray
  - If small bowel obstruction or foreign body is suspected
- Ultrasound
  - If portal hypertension is suspected
- Bleeding scan
  - Useful in the patient with significant bleeding that precludes endoscopy or in whom endoscopy is nondiagnostic
  - Technetium-99m–tagged erythrocyte scan detects rapid bleeding at a rate of 0.1–0.5 mL/min. Can be performed at 30-minute intervals for up to 24 hours
  - Meckel scan: Technetium-99m pertechnetate-tagged can detect a Meckel diverticulum that contains gastric mucosa.
- Angiography
  - Requires bleeding rate of 0.5–1 mL/min to detect location. Useful in detecting vascular causes of upper GI bleeding
  - Can also be therapeutic (i.e., injection of coils into a vascular malformation)
- Upper endoscopy
  - Upper endoscopy is the prime diagnostic and therapeutic tool for evaluating UGIB in pediatric patients.
  - 90–95% sensitive at locating bleeding site

TREATMENT

GENERAL MEASURES

- Initial management:
  - Make patient NPO.
  - Obtain stable IV access.
  - Blood type and cross-match for PRBCs should be obtained.
  - Stabilize the patient with IV fluids and blood products as necessary (target hemoglobin ≥7 g/dL).
  - Target INR <2.5
- Disease-specific therapy:
  - Peptic ulcer disease (medical therapy)
    - Proton pump inhibitors
    - H_2 blockers
    - Sucralfate
    - Prokinetic agents
    - *H. pylori* eradication
  - Peptic ulcer disease (endoscopic therapy)
    - Hemoclip
    - Thermal therapy (i.e., bipolar vs. argon plasma coagulation)
    - Injection therapy (i.e., 1:10,000 epinephrine)
  - Esophageal varices:
    - Octreotide infusion
    - Esophageal band ligation
    - Sclerotherapy
    - Sengstaken-Blakemore tube
    - Portosystemic shunts

ISSUES FOR REFERRAL

- Immediate referral if bleeding is profuse, if patient is hemodynamically unstable, or if bleeding will not stop
- Refer any patient with evidence of chronic iron deficiency anemia and heme-positive stools.

SURGERY/OTHER PROCEDURES

- Patients with significant UGIB should generally undergo endoscopy within 24 h of admission, following resuscitative efforts to optimize hemodynamic parameters.
- If rebleeding occurs after endoscopy or if endoscopy is unable to achieve initial hemostasis, then surgery or angiography should be considered.

ONGOING CARE

- Monitor hemoglobin in the hospital until patient's condition is stable.
- If bleeding has stopped, endoscopy should still be strongly considered to determine source of bleeding.
- Once patient is discharged, monitor patient's hemoglobin and stool for occult blood weekly until stable.
- More specific follow-up depends on the underlying condition.

ADDITIONAL READING

- Chawla S, Seth D, Mahajan P, et al. Upper gastrointestinal bleeding in children. *Clin Pediatr*. 2007;46(1):16–21.
- Kato S, Sherman P. What is new related to *Helicobacter pylori* infection in children and teenager? *Arch Pediatric Adolsc Med*. 2005;159(5):415–421.
- Kim SJ, Kim KM. Recent trends in the endoscopic management of variceal bleeding in children. *Pediatr Gastroenterol Hepatol Nutr*. 2013;16(1): 1–9.
- Pai N, Manfredi MA. Endoscopic management of gastrointestinal bleeding in pediatrics. *Tech Gastrointest Endosc*. 2013;15(1):18–24.
- Uppal K, Tubbs RS, Matusz P, et al. Meckel's diverticulum: a review. *Clin Anat*. 2011;24(4):416–422.

CODES

ICD10

- K92.2 Gastrointestinal hemorrhage, unspecified
- K92.0 Hematemesis
- K92.1 Melena

FAQ

- Q: When should you refer a patient for UGIB?
- A: You should refer patients immediately if there is evidence of significant and/or active bleeding, and or the patient is hemodynamically unstable. Patients with evidence of chronic iron deficiency anemia and heme-positive stools should be referred for elective, but timely evaluation.

URETEROPELVIC JUNCTION OBSTRUCTION

J. Christopher Austin • Michael C. Carr

BASICS

DESCRIPTION

Ureteropelvic junction (UPJ) obstruction is a partial blockage of the kidney at the point where the renal pelvis transitions into the proximal ureter.

EPIDEMIOLOGY

- 45% of all cases of significant prenatal hydronephrosis are due to UPJ obstruction.
- Occurs more commonly in males (M/F 2:1)
- Left-sided lesion more common (66%)
- Bilateral in 10–40%
- 50% of patients have an additional genitourinary malformation, most commonly
  - Vesicoureteral reflux
  - Contralateral UPJ obstruction
  - Multicystic dysplastic kidney
  - Renal agenesis
- Of patients with VATER association, 21% have UPJ obstruction and thus should be screened with renal ultrasound. (VATER stands for vertebral defects, anal atresia, tracheoesophageal fistula with esophageal atresia, and radial and renal anomalies.)

PATHOPHYSIOLOGY

- The obstruction can cause varying degrees of hydronephrosis.
- Mild forms of UPJ obstruction result in dilation of the renal pelvis without loss of function.
- More severe forms result in dilation of the renal pelvis and calyces with loss of renal parenchyma and decreased function.
- In the most severe cases, the kidney may have cystic dysplasia and very poor function.
- Congenital hydronephrosis owing to an intrinsic narrowing is nearly always asymptomatic.
- When the obstruction is intermittent owing to a crossing vessel, the renal pelvis becomes distended (most commonly owing to a transient increase in urine output), which drapes it over the vessel and kinks the ureter, resulting in an acute obstruction. The acute distention of the renal pelvis results in pain (renal colic).

ETIOLOGY

- Intrinsic: a congenital narrowing of the UPJ, which is most commonly owing to abnormal musculature and fibrosis of this area, resulting in an adynamic segment
- Extrinsic: kinking at the UPJ, which is most commonly owing to the renal pelvis draping over a lower pole crossing vessel. This type of obstruction can be intermittent.

DIAGNOSIS

HISTORY

- Antenatal
  - If unilateral, timing and severity of hydronephrosis and status of the contralateral kidney are factors.
  - When bilateral or affecting a solitary kidney, renal insufficiency is a concern.
  - The presence of oligohydramnios, increased renal echogenicity, and cystic changes are indicators of poor renal function and dysplasia.
- Postnatal
  - Feeding intolerance/respiratory distress (very rarely caused by UPJ obstruction)
- Older children
  - History of episodic abdominal (may not lateralize well), flank, or back pain
  - Length of episodes (usually 30 minutes to several hours); associated nausea and vomiting
  - Relation of episodes to fluid intake; history of urinary tract infections or gross hematuria

PHYSICAL EXAM

- Newborn
  - Palpate kidneys.
  - Affected kidney may feel enlarged but should not be tense.
  - A tense mass can indicate a severe obstruction and should be imaged promptly.
- Older child
  - Careful abdominal exam for enlarged kidney and tenderness
  - Costovertebral angle tenderness

DIAGNOSTIC TESTS & INTERPRETATION

Lab

- Newborn
  - If bilateral or a solitary kidney, serial assessments of renal function are necessary (serum electrolytes and creatinine), starting at 24–48 hours of age.
  - With a normal contralateral kidney, no immediate laboratory testing is necessary.
- Older children
  - Urinalysis to detect hematuria or pyuria. Culture if infection is suspected

Imaging

Antenatally detected hydronephrosis: Infants with moderate to severe unilateral or bilateral antenatally detected hydronephrosis typically are evaluated with 3 imaging studies—renal/bladder ultrasound, voiding cystourethrogram (VCUG), and renal scan:

- Renal/bladder ultrasound: In most cases, immediate imaging is not necessary. Because of a period of relative oliguria of a newborn in the first 24–48 hours of life, an ultrasound may underestimate the degree of hydronephrosis. This should not preclude evaluating an infant during this time as long as any normal study is followed up with a repeat study in 4–6 weeks. Evaluation should reveal the severity of dilation of the renal pelvis and calyces, changes in the amount and echogenicity of the parenchyma, and the presence of cortical cysts:
  - The evaluation of the full bladder is important for excluding dilated distal ureters, thickening of the bladder wall owing to outlet obstruction, and ureteroceles.
  - In cases of bilateral hydronephrosis, a solitary hydronephrotic kidney, or a tense kidney on physical examination, imaging should be promptly performed.
- VCUG: This study will detect the presence of vesicoureteral reflux as well as exclude the presence of posterior urethral valves and other abnormalities of the bladder:
  - The test can be delayed until after discharge from the nursery unless there is concern about posterior urethral valves, in which case it should be performed early.
  - The presence of ureteral dilation on ultrasound strengthens the argument to perform a VCUG. The detection of vesicoureteral reflux, particularly in a circumcised male patient, may not confer benefit in their clinical management.
- Renal scan: This study can quantify the differential renal function or the amount each kidney contributes to overall renal function (the normal differential is 50% ± 5% for each kidney):
  - The 2 most commonly used radionuclides are mercaptoacetyltriglycine (MAG-3) and diethylenetriamine penta-acetic acid (DTPA). In addition to the ability to detect diminished function, if there is poor drainage of the affected kidney, furosemide is given to wash out the radiotracer.
  - The time for washing out half of the accumulated radiotracer (T1/2) is often given in the report.
  - A prompt T1/2 (<10 minutes) is indicative of a nonobstructed kidney.
  - A slower T1/2 may be indicative of obstruction when it is >20 minutes. An intermediate T1/2 (10–20 minutes) is indeterminate for obstruction. Owing to effects of hydration, the amount of hydronephrosis, and variables in the timing of the diuretic administration, the T1/2 may be unreliable.

- Intravenous pyelogram (IVP): This study is most useful for evaluating the anatomy of the kidney and the ureters:
  - It can also be used for evaluating an older child with intermittent symptoms if it can be done during a symptomatic episode.
  - A normal study during a symptomatic episode of abdominal or flank pain excludes an intermittent UPJ obstruction as the cause of the child's pain.
  - If a normal study is obtained while the child is asymptomatic, an intermittent UPJ obstruction remains a possible cause.
- Magnetic resonance urography (MRU): A new technique being studied that provides both anatomic and functional detail. Dynamic contrast-enhanced MRI requires sedation and placement of a bladder catheter. The images are obtained following infusion of gadolinium-DTPA. Furosemide is given 15 minutes before the start of the study. This technique is being studied for use instead of ultrasound and renal scans in the hope that it will be a more precise tool in deciding whether or not the child requires surgical repair.

DIFFERENTIAL DIAGNOSIS

- Vesicoureteral reflux: Higher grades of reflux will result in the dilation of the upper urinary tract.
- Distal ureteral obstruction: obstruction at the level of the bladder owing to ureterovesical junction obstruction, ureterocele, or an ectopic ureter
- Bladder outlet obstruction: dilation of the upper urinary tract secondary to obstruction of the lower urinary tract owing to posterior urethral valves, urethral atresia, or stricture
- Megacalycosis: congenital dilation and increased numbers of calyces without significant renal pelvis dilation or obstruction
- Multicystic dysplastic kidney: can be difficult to differentiate severe hydronephrosis from cysts by ultrasound. Renal scan will demonstrate no function in multicystic dysplastic kidneys.
- Triad syndrome: a triad of hypoplastic abdominal wall musculature, bilateral undescended testes, and dilation of the urinary tract (also known as prune belly syndrome or Eagle-Barrett syndrome)

TREATMENT

GENERAL MEASURES

- The decision to observe or surgically correct a UPJ obstruction depends on several factors. One must consider the age and overall health of the neonate, the amount of functional impairment of the kidney, whether it is a unilateral or bilateral process, the drainage pattern on renal scan, and whether or not it is symptomatic. There is no strict rule for who should be observed and who should undergo surgery. This decision should be made on an individual basis.
- Antibiotic prophylaxis
  - Newborns should be started on a once-a-day daily dose of amoxicillin or cephalexin at 1/4–1/2 the normal therapeutic dose.
  - The antibiotic can be switched to trimethoprim, trimethoprim/sulfamethoxazole, or nitrofurantoin at 2 months of age.
  - The duration that infants should be left on antibiotics is controversial among practicing pediatric urologists. Almost all agree that infants should be started on prophylactic antibiotics at birth.
  - They should be continued at least until the infant undergoes a VCUG to exclude reflux. Several factors including age, sex, and degree of hydronephrosis are taken into account when deciding whether or not to stop the prophylaxis.
- Observation
  - Infants with the hydronephrosis thought to be owing to a narrowing at the UPJ are typically observed when there is preserved function (>40%) in the affected kidney, and the contralateral kidney is normal.
  - The pattern of drainage is taken into account, and if there is prompt drainage and normal differential function (50% ± 5%), these patients are followed with less frequent follow-up studies than those with less function or poor drainage.
  - Most patients have follow-up imaging studies done at 3–6-month intervals during their 1st year of life, and they are gradually spaced out as time goes by if the hydronephrosis remains stable or improves.
- Older children with hydronephrosis owing to a UPJ obstruction are often detected during a symptomatic episode. If the UPJ obstruction is asymptomatic and the function of the kidney is preserved, the child may be observed as well.

SURGERY/OTHER PROCEDURES

- The gold standard for the repair of the UPJ obstruction has been a pyeloplasty:
  - During the procedure, the narrowed UPJ is most commonly excised, and the ureter is reanastomosed to the renal pelvis.
  - This procedure is successful 95% of the time.
- Less invasive approaches include endoscopically incising the narrowing (endopyelotomy) or balloon dilation:
  - These approaches have been used in adults with rates of success in the 50–70% range but are considerably less invasive.
  - Endoscopic procedures have not been routinely offered as a 1st-line therapy for the treatment of UPJ obstructions because of their limited experience in children and the lower rates of success.
- Laparoscopic pyeloplasty is being performed in older children and adolescents and will likely be more common in the next several years. Robotically assisted procedures are now being done, further enhancing the minimally invasive approach. Both offer a similar rate of success to a traditional pyeloplasty with decreased perioperative morbidity because of the small incisions for the laparoscopic instruments.

ADDITIONAL READING

- Carr MC, Casale P. Anomalies in surgery of the ureter in children. In: Wein AJ, Kavoussi LR, Novick AC, et al, eds. *Campbell-Walsh Urology*. 10th ed. Philadelphia: W.B. Saunders; 2012.
- Darge K, Higgins M, Hwang TJ, et al. Magnetic resonance and computed tomography in pediatric urology: an imagining overview for current and future daily practice. *Radiol Clin North Am*. 2013;51(4):583–598.

CODES

ICD10

- Q62.39 Other obstructive defects of renal pelvis and ureter
- Q62.11 Congenital occlusion of ureteropelvic junction
- N13.8 Other obstructive and reflux uropathy

FAQ

- Q: My unborn baby has hydronephrosis. My obstetrician told me that it is most likely a UPJ obstruction. Is my baby going to need surgery to correct this?
- A: Not necessarily; only ~1/3 of babies with significant hydronephrosis ultimately require surgical correction.
- Q: Will my child's kidney look normal after the surgery to fix it?
- A: Often the kidney has less dilation and an improved appearance but not completely normal. Of greater importance is that there is no longer obstruction and the function is preserved or improved.

URINARY TRACT INFECTION

Mercedes M. Blackstone

BASICS

DESCRIPTION

- Urinary tract infection (UTI) is defined by having pyuria and ≥50,000 CFUs/mL of a single urinary tract pathogen from an appropriately collected specimen.
- Upper tract infection or pyelonephritis: infection of the renal parenchyma; most febrile babies with a positive culture have upper tract infection
- Lower tract infection or cystitis: infection limited to the bladder, not involving the kidneys; occurs more in older children and adolescents; usually no fever

EPIDEMIOLOGY

- Bimodal age distribution with peak incidence in infants <1 year of age (40 per 1,000)
- 2nd peak in adolescent females
- Overall prevalence of about 7% in febrile infants and young children; varies according to risk factors below
- Higher prevalence in Caucasian girls

RISK FACTORS

- Sex/age: Boys are most at risk for UTI during 1st year of life; girls until school age and again in adolescence.
- Circumcision status: Uncircumcised males <1 year of age have increased risk of UTI; prevalence is 10 times higher for uncircumcised males versus circumcised males <3 months of age.
- Race/ethnicity: Caucasian children are 2–4 times more likely than African-American children to have UTI:
  - May be due in part to differences in blood group antigens on the surfaces of uroepithelial cells, which affect bacterial adherence
- Abnormal urinary tract: Children with vesicoureteral reflux (VUR) and obstruction are at higher risk for UTI.
- Bowel and bladder dysfunction
- Requiring frequent catheterization
- Sexual activity
- Clinical decision rule in febrile girls 2–24 months of age. Consider testing if ≥3 of following are present:
  - Temperature ≥39°C, fever for ≥2 days, non-African-American race, age <1 year, absence of another potential source of fever

GENERAL PREVENTION

- Teach correct wiping—front to back—to young children.
- Consider prophylactic antibiotics for select children with recurrent infection, high-grade VUR, and urologic anomalies:
  - Existing evidence with 1-year follow-up does not support antibiotic prophylaxis for patients with low-grade VUR.
- Attention to good voiding and stooling habits; treat constipation
- Consider single-dose postcoital antibiotics for adolescents with recurrent UTI.
- Cranberry juice has not been shown to help.

PATHOPHYSIOLOGY

- Bacterial invasion of the urinary tract from ascending flora from skin or gut
- Shorter urethra in females puts them at increased risk.
- Poor bladder emptying (neurogenic bladder, obstructive uropathies) facilitates movement of pathogens into the upper tract.
- In young infants, can be from hematogenous spread

ETIOLOGY

Urinary tract pathogens

- *Escherichia coli* is responsible for about >80% of UTIs in children.
- Other fairly common microbes include *Klebsiella* species, *Enterococcus*, and *Proteus mirabilis*.
- Less common: *Enterobacter cloacae*, group B hemolytic streptococci, *Citrobacter*, *Pseudomonas* species, *Staphylococcus aureus*, *Serratia* species, and *Staphylococcus saprophyticus* (teenage girls)
  - Can also have viral or fungal causes of UTI

COMMONLY ASSOCIATED CONDITIONS

- ~5–10% of babies with febrile UTIs (pyelonephritis) are bacteremic, but the clinical course is likely unchanged.
- VUR, urinary abnormalities, bowel and bladder dysfunction

DIAGNOSIS

HISTORY

- Babies
  - Nonspecific symptoms, often fever alone
  - Can have vomiting, irritability, poor feeding, and lethargy
  - Rarely, failure to thrive or jaundice
- Older children
  - Classic symptoms of the lower tract include urgency, frequency, dysuria, hesitancy, suprapubic discomfort, hematuria, and malodorous urine. Classic symptoms of the upper tract include fever, chills, nausea, and flank pain.
  - May have history of constipation
  - Can also present with secondary enuresis
  - Ask older children about sexual activity.
- Special question
  - Has the young child had a history of UTI, unexplained fevers, or urinary tract anomaly?

PHYSICAL EXAM

- Temperature and blood pressure should be documented.
- Babies and toddlers: often no physical findings or fever alone
  - Less common: abdominal pain or distention, poor growth or weight gain, malodorous urine
  - Associated findings: may see evidence of foreign body, phimosis, labial adhesions, or midline abnormality of the lower back, which could indicate a neurogenic bladder
- Older children
  - Lower tract: suprapubic tenderness; may see evidence of constipation
  - Upper tract: fever; costovertebral angle tenderness to percussion
  - Evaluation for sexually transmitted infections

DIAGNOSTIC TESTS & INTERPRETATION

Lab

- Urine culture collected sterilely is the gold standard for diagnosis:
  - Bladder catheterization in young children (or less commonly, suprapubic aspirate)
  - Midstream clean-catch method for older cooperative children
  - A specimen should not be obtained by applying a bag to the perineum; contamination rates are too high.
- False positives
  - Contaminated urine by perineum or stool organisms
- Cultures take 24–48 hours, so several rapid screening tests are available:
  - Conventional urinalysis: ≥5 WBC/HPF (uses centrifuged urine) and bacteria suggests UTI.
  - Enhanced urinalysis (combines microscopy on uncentrifuged urine with Gram stain): ≥10 WBC/mm^3 and positive Gram stain consistent with infection
    - High sensitivity and specificity; helpful in neonates
  - Urine dipstick alone equivalent to conventional microscopy
    - Leukocyte esterase (LE) indicates presence of urinary leukocytes.
    - Remember that conditions other than UTI may also present with pyuria.
    - Nitrites are formed by nitrate-splitting bacteria (high rate of false negatives because urine has to sit in the bladder for ≥4 hours for nitrites to be detected).
    - Moderate or large LE and nitrites alone suggest UTI; together they are highly specific.
- Serum testing is not routinely indicated in the patient with suspected UTI.
  - Blood culture: not indicated in the well-appearing patient ≥2 months because bacteremia does not alter management
  - Inflammatory markers: White blood cell (WBC) count, C-reactive protein (CRP), erythrocyte sedimentation rate (ESR), and procalcitonin (PCT) may all be elevated in UTIs but are not particularly helpful in predicting diagnosis or distinguishing between upper and lower tract disease.
  - Serum creatinine: not necessary for routine UTI but should be obtained in patients with recurrent disease or renal anomalies

ALERT

Pitfalls

- 10–25% of infants will have a negative urinalysis despite culture- or nuclear scan–documented UTI, so a culture should always be obtained in this population.
- Conversely, there are very high rates of asymptomatic bacteriuria in the pediatric population, so a mildly positive urinalysis should be weighed in the context of the pretest probability for UTI.
- Failure to culture by sterile means: leads to a contaminated culture that is difficult to interpret
- Failure to screen a young child with another possible source of fever; children with otitis media, upper respiratory infections, and gastroenteritis can have a concurrent UTI.

Imaging

- There is controversy surrounding indications for imaging in routine febrile UTIs. UTI without fever does not require radiologic evaluation.
- Ultrasound (US): identifies hydronephrosis, congenital anomalies, and abscesses. Not good at detecting scars or VUR:
  - Recommended by the American Academy of Pediatrics (AAP) clinical practice guideline for febrile children 2–24 months of age with first UTI; however, use of US in females with first febrile UTI has been questioned.
  - Normal prenatal US beyond 32 weeks' gestation substantially reduces the likelihood of an abnormal US.
- Voiding cystourethrogram (VCUG): test of choice to detect and characterize VUR
  - No longer routinely recommended by the AAP after first febrile UTI
  - Indicated for young children with recurrent febrile UTIs or an abnormal renal US
- In addition to the children covered by the AAP parameter, consider imaging for UTIs in boys, children with recurrent infections, and children with persistent voiding dysfunction, urinary abnormalities, poor growth, hypertension, or concerning family history.
- Renal cortical scan: detects acute pyelonephritis and renal scarring. Unclear use in clinical setting; consider in febrile children if diagnosis is unclear.

DIFFERENTIAL DIAGNOSIS

- True UTI can easily be confused with asymptomatic bacteriuria.
- The differential diagnosis of isolated or prolonged fever is very broad.
- Infants: gastroenteritis, occult bacteremia, occult pneumonia, meningitis, viral syndrome
- Older children and adolescents
  - Common: vaginal foreign body, vulvovaginitis/urethritis, epididymitis, gastroenteritis, sexually transmitted infection, pelvic inflammatory disease
  - Less common: excessive drinking, urinary calculi, diabetes mellitus or insipidus, appendicitis, Kawasaki disease, tubo-ovarian abscess, ovarian torsion, group A streptococcal infection
  - Rare: mass adjacent to bladder, spinal cord process (tumor, abscess), hypercalcemia

TREATMENT

MEDICATION

First Line

- Empiric antibiotic therapy should be initiated in febrile children with suspected UTI in order to prevent scarring.
- *E. coli* is the most common pathogen associated with first UTI; it is typically sensitive to multiple antimicrobials.
- Gram staining, when available, can help guide empiric therapy as can local patterns of susceptibility.
- Empiric inpatient therapy: IV therapy with a 3rd-generation cephalosporin such as cefotaxime (120 mg/kg/day divided t.i.d.) or ceftriaxone (75 mg/kg/day) or the combination of ampicillin (100 mg/kg/day divided q.i.d.) and gentamicin (7.5 mg/kg/day divided t.i.d.)
  - High-risk patients who are immunocompromised, have indwelling catheters, or have recurrent UTIs should initially receive broad-spectrum antibiotics that cover the organisms involved in prior infections.
- Empiric outpatient therapy: Options include cefixime (8 mg/kg/day once daily), cefdinir (14 mg/kg once daily), amoxicillin-clavulanate (45 mg/kg of amoxicillin component per day divided b.i.d.), co-trimoxazole (6–12 mg TMP/kg/day divided b.i.d.), or cephalexin (50–100 mg/kg/day divided q6–8h).
  - Many communities have high rates of resistance to amoxicillin and co-trimoxazole; resistance to amoxicillin-clavulanate and cephalexin is also on the rise.
- Antibiotic duration (IV/oral)
  - Children ≤2 years of age with a febrile UTI, UTI, or urinary tract abnormalities should receive a total of 7–14 days of antibiotic therapy.
  - Older children without fever or significant history likely have an uncomplicated cystitis are eligible for a short course of antibiotics (5–7 days).
- Antibiotic prophylaxis after UTI
  - Benefit somewhat unclear; AAP no longer recommends prophylactic antibiotics after first febrile UTI
  - Consider prophylaxis for patients with high-grade VUR in consultation with an urologist.

INPATIENT CONSIDERATIONS

ADMISSION CRITERIA

- The majority of patients with UTI can receive outpatient therapy with close follow-up.
- Consider hospitalization for young infants (consider hospitalization under 6 months, hospitalize under 2 months).
  - Ill patients with concern for development of urosepsis
  - Complex or immunocompromised host
  - Concern for dehydration or inability to tolerate medications
  - Social concerns, lack of follow-up
  - Failed outpatient management

ONGOING CARE

FOLLOW-UP RECOMMENDATIONS

Patient Monitoring

- Consider a repeat urine culture after 2 days of therapy if the patient is not improving on an appropriate antibiotic regimen.
- Such patients should also receive imaging.
- Urinalysis and urine culture for subsequent febrile illnesses

PROGNOSIS

Prompt treatment of febrile UTIs reduces the risk for scarring and its sequelae. These children generally have a very good prognosis.

COMPLICATIONS

- Repeated febrile UTIs in young children may lead to renal scarring.
- Renal scarring in childhood carries a risk of hypertension, preeclampsia, and end-stage renal disease as an adult.

ADDITIONAL READING

- Gorelick MH, Shaw KN. Clinical decision rule to identify young febrile children at risk for urinary tract infection. *Arch Pediatr Adolesc Med*. 2000;154(4):386–390.
- McGillivray D, Mok E, Mulrooney E, et al. A head-to-head comparison: "clean-void" bag versus catheter urinalysis in the diagnosis of urinary tract infection in young children. *J Pediatr*. 2005;147(4):451–456.
- Montini G, Rigon L, Zucchetta P, et al. Prophylaxis after first febrile urinary tract infection in children? A multicenter, randomized, controlled noninferiority trial. *Pediatrics*. 2008;122(5):1064–1071.
- Montini G, Tullus K, Hewitt I. Febrile urinary tract infections in children. *N Engl J Med*. 2011;365(3):239–250.
- Shaikh N, Morone NE, Bost JE, et al. Prevalence of urinary tract infection in childhood: a meta-analysis. *Pediatr Infect Dis J*. 2008;27(4):302–308.
- Shaikh N, Morone NE, Lopez J, et al. Does this child have a urinary tract infection? *JAMA*. 2007;298(24):2895–2904.
- Roberts KB, Subcommittee on Urinary Tract Infection, Steering Committee on Quality Improvement and Management, Urinary tract infection: clinical practice guideline for the diagnosis and management of the initial UTI in febrile infants and children 2 to 24 months. *Pediatrics*. 2011;128(3):595–610.

CODES

ICD10

- N39.0 Urinary tract infection, site not specified
- N12 Tubulo-interstitial nephritis, not spcf as acute or chronic
- N30.90 Cystitis, unspecified without hematuria

FAQ

- Q: Which children should have a radiologic evaluation after a UTI?
- A: Boys. Febrile children younger than age 2 years, and anyone with recurrent febrile UTIs, hypertension, or family history of urinary tract abnormalities.
- Q: Does a urine culture need to be done if the catheterized dipstick or urinalysis is negative?
- A: >10% of febrile infants with pyelonephritis will have a false-negative screening test (dipstick, urinalysis). A sterile urine culture should be done in these young patients.

UROLITHIASIS

Kara N. Saperston • Michael DiSandro

BASICS

DESCRIPTION
- Urolithiasis is the occurrence of calculi (stones) within the urinary tract, including the kidney, ureter, or bladder.
- Stones may be composed of calcium oxalate, calcium phosphate, uric acid, cystine, magnesium ammonium phosphate, xanthine, indinavir, and triamterene.

EPIDEMIOLOGY
The incidence of stones in children of both sexes has increased over the last 25 years.

RISK FACTORS
- Poor fluid intake
- Immobility
- Urinary tract obstruction
- Urinary tract infection (*Proteus mirabilis or Escherichia coli*)
- Bladder augmentation
- Dumping syndrome
- In children, 50% have a metabolic syndrome associated with urolithiasis.
- 75% have a metabolic predisposition to forming stones.

PATHOPHYSIOLOGY
- The urine contains multiple solutes; some help prevent crystallization and some contribute to crystal formation.
- The likelihood of a solute crystalizing varies with the pH of the urine (e.g., uric acid crystal formation is more likely at lower pH).
- When enough crystals form in the urine and urine flow out of the kidney is slow or obstructed
- Crystals then coalesce into a small nidus upon which more crystals will form. This process then leads to stone formation.

COMMONLY ASSOCIATED CONDITIONS
Children who present with urolithiasis younger than age 6 years are more likely to develop hypertension (HTN) and diabetes mellitus (DM) later in life.

DIAGNOSIS

HISTORY
- Sudden or gradual onset of flank pain
- Location of stone is guided by the pain.
  - Midabdominal or suprapubic pain may indicate ureteral location of stone.
  - Testicular or labial pain indicates the stone is near the ureteral orifice.
  - Younger children are more likely to have nonspecific and/or nonlocalized pain.
- Nausea and/or vomiting
- Vague midabdominal pain
- Gross or microscopic hematuria is seen in only 50% of patients.
- Urinary tract infection (UTI) or fever
- Recent furosemide exposure
- Immobilization (postsurgical, wheelchair use)

PHYSICAL EXAM
- +/− Costovertebral angle (CVA) tenderness
- Abdominal tenderness, without rebound tenderness. Patient will have peritonitis only if a stone is accompanied by severe pyelonephritis.
- +/− Restless and unable to find a comfortable position
- +/− Blood in the urine

DIAGNOSTIC TESTS & INTERPRETATION

Lab
- Urinalysis and urine culture
- 24-hour urine collection for calcium, citrate, creatinine, magnesium, oxalate, pH, phosphate, and uric acid
- Basic metabolic panel including calcium, phosphorus, and uric acid
- If hypercalcuria, then obtain vitamin D and PTH levels.
- CBC: if infection suspected

Imaging
- Renal ultrasound: limited ability to visualize ureteral stones
- Plain abdominal radiograph
- CT scan of abdomen and pelvis, only if absolutely necessary
  - Remember radiation ALARA goal (as low as reasonably achievable).

DIFFERENTIAL DIAGNOSIS
- UTI, upper or lower tract
- Appendicitis
- Gastroenteritis
- Congenital ureteropelvic junction (UPJ) obstruction
- Henoch-Schönlein purpura
- Tumor
- Papillary necrosis
- Trauma
- Renal artery/vein thrombosis
- Nutcracker phenomenon

ALERT
A stone causing urinary obstruction with an associated urinary tract infection is high risk and a surgical emergency.

TREATMENT

MEDICATION
- Fluid
- Watchful waiting
- Consider expulsion therapy.
  - Alpha-blockers: Flomax (may cause headache and hypotension) (not FDA approved)

ADDITIONAL THERAPIES
- Surgical removal
  - Ureteroscopy
  - Extracorporeal shock wave lithotripsy (ESWL)
  - Percutaneous nephrolithotomy (PCNL)

GENERAL MEASURES
- After diagnosis, referral to pediatric urology for surgical management and to pediatric urology or pediatric nephrology for complete metabolic evaluation and treatment
- Stones <3 mm may pass without surgical intervention.
- Regardless of the size, further metabolic evaluation by a specialist should occur.

ONGOING CARE

FOLLOW-UP RECOMMENDATIONS
- All stones passed should be sent for chemical analysis.
- Increase fluid intake: Urine should be clear.
- Avoid vitamin D and C supplementation until metabolic workup is complete.
- Avoid high cranberry intake.
- Minimize sodium intake and reduce animal protein intake.
- Targeted reduction of specific foods such as oxalate-containing foods if with hyperoxaluria

PROGNOSIS
- 1/2–1/3 of children with metabolic abnormality will form another stone.
- Severe hyperoxaluria is associated with primary hyperoxaluria that can cause early renal failure and may require kidney transplant to correct renal failure and simultaneous liver transplant to correct the hereditary metabolic defect.
- Cystinuria: Treatment with Thiola and D-penicillamine can be associated with myelosuppression.

ADDITIONAL READING

- Dave S, Khoury AE, Braga L, et al. Single-institutional study on role of ureteroscopy and retrograde intra-renal surgery in treatment of pediatric renal calculi. *Urology*. 2008;72(5):1018.
- Dwyer ME, Krambeck AE, Bergstralh EJ, et al. Temporal trends in incidence of kidney stones among children: a 25-year population based study. *J Urol*. 2012;188(1):247.
- Erturhan S, Bayrak O, Sarica K, et al. Efficacy of medical expulsive treatment with doxazosin in pediatric patients. *Urology*. 2013;81(3):640.

CODES

ICD10
- N20.9 Urinary calculus unspecified
- N20.0 Calculus of kidney
- N20.1 Calculus of ureter

FAQ
- Q: When should a child with a stone be admitted for management?
- A: If the stone has obstructed a solitary kidney, if the child has an elevated white blood cell count or UTI in the setting of obstruction, and if the child is immunocompromised and shows signs of a UTI.

URTICARIA

Christopher P. Raab

BASICS

DESCRIPTION

- Urticarial lesions are best described as raised, pruritic, circumscribed erythematous papules.
  - Single lesions may coalesce as they enlarge, forming generalized, raised, erythematous areas.
  - Transient, typically lasting several hours
  - Also known as "hives" or "nettle rash"
  - Acute: <6 weeks' duration
  - Chronic: >6 weeks' duration
- Other similar but non-urticarial entities:
  - Angioedema
    - Urticarial-like lesions
    - Form in the deep dermal, subcutaneous, and submucosal layers
  - Anaphylaxis
    - Hypersensitivity reaction after exposure to an antigen
    - Producing respiratory compromise secondary to airway edema, urticarial rash, pruritus, and hypotension; can lead to shock

EPIDEMIOLOGY

- Female-to-male ratio of 3:2
- No variation in race

Incidence

Lifetime incidence of 15–25%

GENERAL PREVENTION

When a trigger is identified, avoidance is the main preventive measure.

PATHOPHYSIOLOGY

- Immune mediated
  - Antigen is cross-linked to IgE on a mast cell.
  - This causes mast cell activation, leading to the release of vasoactive mediators, such as histamine, leukotrienes, prostaglandin D2, platelet-activating factor, and other vasoactive mediators.
  - These vasoactive mediators cause pruritus, vasodilatation, and capillary leak, which lead to the characteristic findings.
  - Common triggers include some medications such as penicillins, foods such as milk or eggs, and envenomations.
- Non–immune mediated
  - Degranulation of mast cells secondary to other non-IgE reactions such as physical changes, chemicals, some medications such as beta-lactams and sulfa-containing drugs, and some foods
- Autoimmune mediated
  - Degranulation of mast cells caused by cross-linking of IgE by IgG or IgG binding to the high-affinity IgE (FcεRI) receptor on mast cells

ETIOLOGY

Acute urticaria

- Viral infections are thought to make up ~80% of all cases of acute urticaria in children. Most commonly isolated causes include the following viruses:
  - Epstein-Barr
  - Coxsackievirus A and B
  - Hepatitis A, B, and C
- Parasitic infections
- Bacterial infections (especially group A strep)
- Medications: most frequently reported include the following:
  - NSAIDs
  - Opiates
  - Vancomycin
- Radiocontrast
- Foods
- Transfusion of blood products
- Food additives and dyes
- Natural remedies including cranberry, feverfew, glucosamine, and ginger
- Insect venom including bees, wasps, hornets

Chronic urticaria

- Idiopathic: Most have an unknown cause, but many feel that an association with an autoimmune mechanism is likely.
- Physical (~20–30%)
  - Dermatographism (9%): Stroking of skin using mild to moderate pressure with fingernail or hard object causes linear urticaria at site of contact.
  - Cholinergic (5%): diffuse erythema and elevated but pale urticarial lesions; intense pruritus; associated with sweating reflex, so often associated with overheating or exertion; may be worsened in combination with other triggers in specific combinations
  - Cold (3%): Urticarial lesions present at areas of skin exposed to low temperatures; familial and nonhereditary forms
  - Aquagenic: Urticarial lesions arise when the patient is exposed to water (e.g., bathtub, swimming pool).
  - Delayed pressure/vibratory: Deep or prolonged pressure on skin produces significant urticaria and often angioedema. Vibratory urticaria is a form of delayed pressure urticaria caused by repetitive vibration (e.g., use of a jackhammer).
- Mast cell disease
  - Urticaria pigmentosa: excessive number of mast cells in skin, bone marrow, lymph nodes, and other tissues; flares characterized by pruritus, flushing, tachycardia, nausea, and vomiting
  - Systemic mastocytosis
- Systemic disease
  - Rheumatologic
    - Urticarial vasculitis: erythematous wheals that resemble urticaria but histologically appear as leukocytoclastic vasculitis; often presents with systemic symptoms and lasts >24 hours
    - Cryopyrin-associated periodic syndromes can present with urticaria, such as Muckle-Wells syndrome: chronic recurrent urticaria, deafness, amyloidosis, and arthritis.
  - Neoplasms
  - Infections: parasites especially noted to cause chronic urticaria
  - Autoimmune: antibodies to IgE or IgE receptor (FcεRI)

DIAGNOSIS

HISTORY

- Description of rash: Lesions may not be present at time of exam due to transient nature. Digital photos are often useful.
- Duration of symptoms, acute versus chronic:
  - If acute (<6 weeks), ask about
    - Viral symptoms including rhinorrhea, cough, fever, congestion, malaise
    - Any medications (prescription or over the counter) or any herbal remedies
    - Any new foods or beverages
    - Any new exposures to perfumes, chemicals, or other skin products
  - If chronic (>6 weeks)
    - History of previous episodes including timing, exposures, any past history of urticaria or angioedema
    - Other symptoms or variations in presentation
    - Symptoms of systemic diseases, such as hyperthyroidism, systemic lupus erythematosus (SLE), juvenile idiopathic arthritis, myositis, amyloidosis, infections, and lymphoma
    - Duration of lesions

PHYSICAL EXAM

- Appearance of rash: classic wheal and flare appearance
- Respiratory: Look for evidence of stridor, wheezing, or dyspnea. If present, be concerned for airway compromise or lower airway edema from an anaphylactic reaction.
- Facial or neck swelling: concern for possible airway compromise
- A full physical exam should be performed to look for signs of systemic disease or malignancy, such as
  - Upper respiratory tract infections
  - Thyromegaly
  - Lymphadenopathy or splenomegaly to suggest lymphoma
  - Joint examination for any evidence of connective tissue disease, arthritis, or SLE

DIAGNOSTIC TESTS & INTERPRETATION

Lab

- Testing is often fruitless unless indicated by history and physical examination.
- Skin testing may be performed if the causative agent is thought to be 1 of several food items.
- If symptoms are difficult to handle or persist >3 months, consider
  – CBC with differential
  – ESR
  – Thyroid studies (thyroid-stimulating hormone [TSH], free T_4, antithyroglobulin, and antiperoxisomal antibody)
- If symptoms are atypical, last >1 year, or are suggestive of urticarial vasculitis
  – Complement studies
  – ANA titer
  – Liver function tests
  – Skin punch biopsy

DIFFERENTIAL DIAGNOSIS

- Viral exanthema
- Atopic dermatitis
- Contact dermatitis
- Insect bites
- Maculopapular drug rash
- Erythema multiforme
- Plant-induced eruptions
- Henoch-Schönlein purpura
- SLE
- Autoinflammatory disease
  – Systemic onset juvenile idiopathic arthritis
  – Cryopyrin-associated periodic syndromes: familial cold autoinflammatory syndrome, Muckle-Wells syndrome, neonatal onset multisystem inflammatory disease (NOMID)
  – Mevalonate kinase deficiency
  – Tumor necrosis factor-receptor–associated periodic syndrome (TRAPS)

TREATMENT

Emergent treatment: If with any difficulty breathing, stridor or wheezing, or other signs of anaphylaxis, give epinephrine 0.01 mL/kg of the 1:1,000 solution SC/IM.

MEDICATION

- Acute urticaria
  – Usually self-resolving but can treat with 2nd-generation nonsedating antihistamines
  – 1st-generation antihistamines: diphenhydramine 1 mg/kg/dose or total 5 mg/kg/d divided PO q6h or hydroxyzine 2 mg/kg/day PO divided q6h for pruritus
- Chronic urticaria: See below.

First Line

- Antihistamines/H_1 antagonists:
- Less sedating, longer acting, and should be mainstay of therapy
  – Cetirizine (Zyrtec): Dosing varies by age from 2.5 to 10 mg daily.
  – Loratadine (Claritin): 5 mg daily
- Fexofenadine (Allegra): 6 months to <2 years of age, 15 mg twice daily; 2–11 years of age, 30 mg twice daily; and >12 years of age, 60 mg twice daily. 1st-generation antihistamines are effective but more sedating:
  – Diphenhydramine (Benadryl): 5 mg/kg/day divided q6h
  – Hydroxyzine (Atarax): 0.5 mg/kg/dose q6h
  – Cyproheptadine (Periactin): 2 mg up to 3 times a day: primary treatment for cold urticaria

Second Line

Increase 2nd-generation H_1 antagonist dose to maximum for age. In adult guidelines, increasing the dose up to 4-fold is more effective.

Third Line

- Addition of a second nonsedating 2nd-generation H_1 antihistamine
- Leukotriene inhibitors: minimal additive response noted in clinical studies
  – Montelukast (Singulair): 5 mg daily
- Combined H_1 and H_2 antagonists
  – H_2 antagonists: added as 2nd agent because skin cells have both H_1 and H_2 receptors and a synergistic effect can be achieved by addition of an H_2 blocker
  – Ranitidine (Zantac): 2–4 mg/kg/day divided twice daily
- Doxepin (Sinequan): a tricyclic antidepressant. >12 years of age, 10–50 mg/day and can slowly titer up to 100 mg/day; potent antihistamine but poorly tolerated due to sedation, hypotension, anticholinergic side effects, and massive weight gain
- Other immune-modifying agents used in chronic urticaria:
  – Other nonstandard therapies have been tried in small case studies: cyclosporine, colchicine, dapsone, IV immunoglobulin (IVIG), plasmapheresis, methotrexate, cyclophosphamide, calcium channel blockers, ephedrine
  – Corticosteroids: Titer to lowest effective dose. Start with standard dose of 0.5–1 mg/kg/day of prednisone; often poorly tolerated secondary to substantial side effects including hypertension, immunosuppression, hyperglycemia, physical changes
  – Omalizumab: Anti-IgE antibody has been shown to reduce signs and symptoms of chronic urticaria in those at maximum standard therapies.

ONGOING CARE

FOLLOW-UP RECOMMENDATIONS

Patient Monitoring

- Watch for signs and symptoms of anaphylaxis; this is the major complication.
- Patients with chronic urticaria should follow up with their physician on a regular basis to monitor symptoms and response to therapies.

PROGNOSIS

- Chronic urticaria
- Resolution in 50% by 12 months
- Another 20% resolve by 5 years
- 10–20% >20 years; many of those who continue to have symptoms are felt to have an autoimmune etiology.
- May have recurrences; physical urticaria subtypes are more likely to recur.

COMPLICATIONS

Anaphylaxis with resulting edema of the upper airway is the major life-threatening complication. The patient should seek immediate medical attention.

ADDITIONAL READING

- Bailey E, Shaker M. An update on childhood urticaria and angioedema. *Curr Opin Pediatr*. 2008;20(4): 425–430.
- Dibbern DA Jr. Urticaria: selected highlights and recent advances. *Med Clin North Am*. 2006;90(1): 187–209.
- Dibbern DA Jr, Dreskin S. Urticaria and angioedema: an overview. *Immunol Allergy Clin North Am*. 2004; 24(2):141–162.
- Kaplan A, Ledford D, Ashby M, et al. Omalizumab in patients with symptomatic chronic idiopathic/spontaneous urticaria despite standard combination therapy. *J Allergy Clin Immunol*. 2013;132(1): 101–109.
- Krause K, Grattan CE, Bindslev-Jensen C, et al. How not to miss autoinflammatory disease masquerading as urticarial. *Allergy*. 2012;67(12);1465–1474.
- Powell RJ, Du Toit GL, Siddique N, et al. BSACI guidelines for the management of chronic urticaria and angio-oedema. *Clin Exp Allergy*. 2007;37(5): 631–650.
- Sheikh J. Advances in the treatment of chronic urticaria. *Immunol Allergy Clin North Am*. 2004;24(2): 317–334.
- Zuberbier T, Asero R, Bindslev-Jensen C, et al. EAACI/GA(2)LEN/EDF/WAO guideline: management of urticaria. *Allergy*. 2009;64(10):1427–1443.

CODES

ICD10

- L50.9 Urticaria, unspecified
- L50.0 Allergic urticaria
- L50.6 Contact urticaria

FAQ

- Q: When should I refer patients to a specialist, and to what specialty should I send them?
- A: Often, referral is made when a trigger cannot be identified, if it is felt to be a food or medication trigger, and/or the symptoms persist for >6 weeks. Refer to a dermatologist or allergist–immunologist experienced in the evaluation and workup of urticaria.
- Q: When should treatment with corticosteroids or other nonstandard therapies be used to treat chronic urticaria?
- A: Typically, these medications carry significant side effects and should be reserved for those patients in whom the urticaria is causing significant alterations in activities of daily living.
- Q: When does a patient need to be hospitalized or observed during an episode of urticaria?
- A: Concerning signs include extensive angioedema, respiratory symptoms such as stridor or wheezing, or nausea/vomiting. Symptoms of anaphylaxis should be treated with epinephrine and the patient observed for several hours to ensure that symptoms do not recur.

VACCINE ADVERSE EVENTS

Kristen A. Feemster

BASICS

ALERT

Adverse events after immunization may be a true vaccine-associated event or may be a coincidental event that would happen without immunization. Epidemiologic studies are important to establish causation.

DESCRIPTION

- A clinically significant event that occurs after administration of a vaccine and has been causally related to the vaccine
- All suspected adverse events should be reported; however, reporting does not imply causation.
- Contraindication to immunization: condition that increases risk of a serious adverse reaction
- Precaution for immunization: condition that might increase risk of an adverse event or may decrease effectiveness of vaccine to mount an immune response
  - Usually a temporary condition
  - Immunization indicated with a precaution if benefits outweigh risk

EPIDEMIOLOGY

- Adverse events monitored prelicensure to establish safety and postlicensure to identify rare adverse events that would not be detected in prelicensure studies. Reporting is guided by the following:
  - National Childhood Vaccine Injury Compensation Program
    - Established by National Childhood Vaccine Injury Act of 1986 to establish a no-fault mechanism to manage claims of vaccine injury outside of the civil law system and provide compensation
    - Petitioners can file claims based on the Vaccine Injury Table (see "Patient Education") created by the program or can attempt to prove causation for an injury that is not listed.
    - Program also mandates reporting of adverse events by health care professionals and creation of vaccine information materials.
  - Vaccine Adverse Event Reporting System (VAERS)
    - Passive surveillance system to monitor all vaccines licensed in the United States
    - All reports reviewed by FDA medical officers.
    - Can detect possible unrecognized adverse events but limited ability to determine true causal relationships
    - Reporting to VAERS mandated by the National Childhood Vaccine Injury Compensation Program
  - Vaccine Safety Datalink
    - Active surveillance system formed by CDC in partnership with managed care organizations covering 9 million people
    - Can perform better observational studies to help determine causation
  - Clinical Immunization Safety Assessment (CISA) Network
    - Network of 7 academic centers established by CDC in 2001 to develop research protocols to diagnose, evaluate, and manage adverse events
    - Develops evidence-based guidelines for immunizing people at risk for serious adverse events after vaccination

Incidence

- Difficult to measure incidence owing to current reporting systems for adverse events
- There are ~30,000 reports each year to VAERS.
  - 13% considered serious adverse events.
- As of July 2013, ~15,000 claims filed under the National Childhood Vaccine Injury Compensation Act since 1988, and ~3,400 families compensated.

DIAGNOSIS

HISTORY

- Common mild adverse events after vaccination include the following:
  - Fever
  - Local erythema, swelling, and/or tenderness
  - Sleepiness and decreased appetite
  - Increased fussiness
  - Mild rash: occurs in 1 of 25 people up to 1 month after varicella vaccination
- Moderate to serious adverse events to currently recommended vaccines are rare but include the following:
  - Syncope, particularly among adolescents
  - Febrile seizures (MMR, varicella, and DTaP vaccines)
  - Temporary joint pain or stiffness (MMR)
  - Temporary thrombocytopenia (MMR)
  - High fever
  - Shoulder injury related to vaccination
- To minimize the possibility of vaccine adverse events and to maximize the effectiveness of vaccination, the following contraindications and precautions should be followed.

DIFFERENTIAL DIAGNOSIS

Allergic reaction to an unrelated exposure

Intercurrent illness

ONGOING CARE

APPROACH

- Before vaccination
  - Discuss benefits and potential adverse events so that families know what to expect.
  - Actively review vaccine information sheets.
  - Solicit concerns so that they can be addressed.

General **contraindications** for vaccination include the following:

- History of an **anaphylactic** reaction to a vaccine component
  - History of egg allergy no longer contraindication to influenza vaccination unless documented history of anaphylaxis.
- Pregnancy for **live virus vaccines** unless mother is at high risk for the vaccine-preventable condition
- Primary T-cell immunodeficiencies (i.e., severe combined immunodeficiency)
  - No live vaccines
  - Inactivated vaccines can be safely administered but may not generate an adequate immune response.
- Primary B-cell immunodeficiencies
  - If severe (i.e., X-linked agammaglobulinemia), no live bacterial vaccines, live-attenuated influenza vaccine (LAIV), or yellow fever vaccine
  - Less severe antibody deficiencies can receive live vaccines except for OPV.
- Phagocyte dysfunction
  - No live bacterial vaccines
  - All live virus and inactivated vaccines probably safe and effective
- Secondary immunosuppression (transplant, malignancy, autoimmune disease)
  - No live vaccines depending on degree of immunosuppression
  - Can achieve adequate response to vaccination within 3 months to 1 year after stopping immunosuppressive therapy
- HIV/AIDS
  - Can give MMR and varicella vaccine unless severely immunocompromised
  - No OPV or LAIV
- High-dose corticosteroids >14 days
  - No live virus vaccines until therapy discontinued for at least 1 month
- Vaccine-specific contraindications
  - DTaP/Tdap:
    - Encephalopathy within 7 days of previous DTP, DTaP, or Tdap dose not attributable to another cause
  - Rotavirus
    - Severe combined immunodeficiency
    - Previous history of intussusception
  - Hib conjugate vaccine should not be given to infants <6 weeks of age.
  - LAIV: Advisory Committee on Immunization Practices (ACIP) recommends against use in multiple groups (please see "Influenza" chapter).

General **precautions** for receiving a vaccine include moderate to severe acute illness with or without fever. Vaccine-specific **precautions** include the following:

- DTaP/DTP
  - Fever ≥104°F or shock-like state within 48 hours of previous DTaP/DTP dose
  - Persistent, inconsolable crying >3 hours within 48 hours of previous DTaP/DTP dose
  - Seizure within 3 days of previous DTaP/DTP dose

- Any tetanus toxoid–containing vaccine
  - Guillain-Barré within 6 weeks of a previous tetanus toxoid–containing vaccine dose
  - Progressive neurologic disorder (infantile spasms, poorly controlled epilepsy)
  - Children with stable neurologic conditions can be vaccinated.
  - History of Arthus hypersensitivity reaction after previous tetanus toxoid–containing dose
    - Wait 10 years between doses of tetanus toxoid–containing vaccines.
- Hepatitis B
  - Infants <2,000 g in weight
- Hepatitis A, IPV, and HPV vaccines
  - Pregnancy
- Inactivated influenza and LAIV
  - Guillain-Barré within 6 weeks of a previous tetanus toxoid–containing vaccine dose
  - LAIV only: antiviral receipt within 48 hours of vaccination (avoid antivirals for 14 days)
- Varicella
  - Receipt of antibody-containing blood product within past 11 months
  - Immunocompromised household contacts are not a contraindication or precaution, but if rash develops 7–25 days after vaccination, should avoid direct contact with immunocompromised individual.
  - Antiviral receipt within 24 hours of vaccination (avoid antivirals for 14 days)
- MMR
  - Receipt of antibody-containing blood product within past 11 months
  - History of thrombocytopenic purpura
  - Need for tuberculin skin test
- Rotavirus
  - Immunosuppression
  - Receipt of antibody-containing blood product within 6 weeks
  - Chronic gastrointestinal disease
  - Previous history of intussusception
- The following are NOT precautions or contraindications to vaccine receipt:
  - Mild or recent illness
  - History of a mild to moderate local reaction to a vaccine
  - Concurrent antimicrobial therapy
  - Recent exposure to an infectious disease
  - Breastfeeding
  - History of other nonvaccine allergies
  - Stable neurologic conditions (e.g., cerebral palsy, developmental delay)

MANAGEMENT

- If a patient presents with a potential adverse event:
  - Take thorough history and perform exam to characterize symptoms and determine timing of symptom onset.
  - Evaluate for other potential causes of symptoms.
  - Determine likelihood of causality.
  - Report all adverse events to VAERS.
  - If the family would like to file a claim, refer to National Childhood Vaccine Injury Compensation Program.
- Addressing safety concerns
  - >10% of parents delay or refuse certain vaccines for their children.
  - Growing prevalence of misinformation about vaccines challenge provider–parent communication.
  - Despite increasing vaccine safety concerns, health care professionals are one of the most trusted sources of information regarding vaccines.
  - Provide tailored information emphasizing benefits of vaccination and potential consequences of not accepting vaccination.
  - Apply principles of risk communication.
  - Actively solicit concerns before vaccination.
  - If parents have specific concerns, refer to additional sources for reliable and accurate information (see references in "Patient Education").
  - Document vaccine discussions.
- Reporting adverse events
  - VAERS is the primary reporting site for suspected adverse events. Health care providers, vaccine recipients, or parents of vaccine recipients and vaccine manufacturers can all report.
  - Health care providers are required to report
    - Any adverse event listed by vaccine manufacturer as a contraindication for the receipt of additional doses of the vaccine
    - Any adverse event included on the VAERS reportable event table that occurred within the specified time period
- Vaccine Injury Compensation Program
  - Covers all vaccines recommended for routine administration for children by the ACIP
  - To qualify for compensation, must prove there was an injury listed in the Vaccine Injury Table that occurred within prescribed time period, prove that a vaccine caused an injury not listed on the Table, or prove that a vaccine aggravated a preexisting condition
  - Effects of injury must last >6 months after vaccination and result in hospitalization, surgery, or death.

PATIENT EDUCATION

- Vaccine Adverse Event Reporting System: http://vaers.hhs.gov
- Vaccine Safety Datalink Project: www.cdc.gov/od/science/iso/vsd
- Clinical Immunization Safety Assessment Network: http://www.cdc.gov/vaccinesafety/Activities/CISA.html
- Vaccine Injury Compensation Program: http://www.hrsa.gov/vaccinecompensation/
- Vaccine Injury Table: http://www.hrsa.gov/vaccinecompensation/vaccinetable.html
- Vaccine Education Center at the Children's Hospital of Philadelphia: http://www.chop.edu/service/vaccine-education-center/home.html
- National Network for Immunization Information: www.immunizationinfo.org
  - Resources for communicating with families
- Immunization Action Coalition: www.immunize.org
- Parents of Kids with Infectious Diseases: www.pkids.org
- AAP Immunization Initiatives Web site: https://www2.aap.org/immunization/
  - Refusal to vaccinate waivers

ADDITIONAL READING

- Cook KM, Evans G. The National Vaccine Injury Compensation Program. *Pediatrics*. 2011;127(Suppl 1):S74–S77.
- Glanz JM, Newcomer SR, Narwaney KJ, et al. A population-based cohort study of undervaccination in 8 managed care organizations across the United States. *JAMA Pediatr*. 2013;167(3):274–281.
- Halsey NA, Edwards KM, Dekker CL, et al. Algorithm to assess causality after individual adverse events following immunizations. *Vaccine*. 2012;30(39):5791–5798.
- Institute of Medicine. *Adverse Effects of Vaccines: Evidence and Causality*. Washington, DC: National Academy Press, 2012.
- Sadaf A, Richards JL, Glanz J, et al. A systematic review of interventions for reducing parental vaccine refusal and vaccine hesitancy. *Vaccine*. 2013;31(40):4293–4304.

CODES

ICD10

- T88.1XXA Oth complications following immunization, NEC, init
- T80.62XA Other serum reaction due to vaccination, initial encounter
- T80.52XA Anaphylactic reaction due to vaccination, initial encounter

FAQ

- Q: Many parents request spacing vaccines. Is there evidence that giving multiple vaccines at a time is too much for a child's immune system?
- A: Recommended vaccines have a very small amount of antigen compared to natural infection, and they activate a small proportion of immune system memory. Additionally, all vaccines given together have been tested when given at the same time to make sure they remain safe and effective.
- Q: What is the bottom line regarding autism and vaccines?
- A: Multiple studies including a recent Institute of Medicine (IOM) report have not shown any causal relationship between thimerosal-containing vaccines and autism or MMR and autism. Additionally, the U.S. court system through the Omnibus Autism Proceeding has recently ruled that there is insufficient evidence to show any causal relationship between thimerosal-containing vaccines or MMR and autism.

VAGINITIS

Sara M. Buckelew

BASICS

DESCRIPTION

- Vaginitis is inflammation or irritation of the vagina causing typical symptoms of vaginal discharge, burning, and itching.
  - May be due to infection such as trichomoniasis, candidiasis, or bacterial vaginosis (BV); see Appendix, Table 7.
  - Noninfectious causes include foreign body or exposure to an irritant or allergen.
- Vulvovaginitis is irritation or inflammation of both the vulva and the vagina; most often due to *Candida albicans*
- In postpubertal females, BV is the most prevalent cause of vaginal discharge and typically causes a fishy odor.
- Physiologic leukorrhea (i.e., "physiologic discharge") is usually associated with pubertal onset and frequently precedes menarche. It is typically thin, white, and mucoid.

EPIDEMIOLOGY

- Vaginitis affects females of all ages.
- In prepubescent girls, 25–75% of vaginitis is non-specific in etiology.
- Approximately 75% of women have had at least one episode of vulvovaginitis due to candida in their lifetime.
- The most common causes of postpubertal vaginitis are as follows:
  - BV (22–50%)
  - Vulvovaginal candidiasis (17–39%)
  - *Trichomonas vaginalis* (4–35%)

RISK FACTORS

- For prepubertal females, poor hygiene is a common risk factor.
- For BV: vaginal douching, smoking, intrauterine device usage, non-white race, prior pregnancy, unprotected sexual intercourse, usage of spermicide, homosexual relationships
- For trichomoniasis: multiple sexual partners, other sexually transmitted infections, lack of condom usage, smoking
- For vulvovaginal candidiasis: use of systemic antibiotics, uncontrolled diabetes mellitus, diet high in refined sugars
- Irritant risk factors often include soaps, tampons, topical products and medications, extreme cleansing, clothing, and douching.

PATHOPHYSIOLOGY

- In prepubescent female, with prepubertal hormones, the vagina has a neutral pH, atrophic mucosa, and a warm environment that easily allow for bacterial overgrowth.
- Physiologic leukorrhea
  - Estrogen levels; the volume of discharge varies with the menstrual cycle and is especially heavy at the time of ovulation.
- Candida vulvovaginitis
  - Use of antibiotics increases the occurrence of candidiasis by eliminating competitive organisms.
- BV
  - Caused by shift in vaginal flora
  - Normal *Lactobacillus* species decrease and overgrowth of bacteria, including *Gardnerella vaginalis*, *Mycoplasma hominis*, and anaerobes such as *Prevotella* and *Mobiluncus* species

ETIOLOGY

- All ages:
  - Chemical, irritant, allergy
  - Nonspecific vaginitis (may be associated with hygiene)
  - Foreign body or material such as rolled up toilet paper
  - Candidiasis associated with antibiotic use
  - Trauma, mechanical irritation
  - Sexual abuse
- More common in prepubertal females:
  - Group A β-hemolytic *Streptococcus*
  - *Haemophilus influenzae*
  - *Shigella*
  - Pinworms or scabies
  - Congenital abnormalities
- More common in postpubertal females:
  - Physiologic leukorrhea (may cause discharge but not irritation)
  - BV
  - Trichomoniasis
  - STIs such as gonorrhea and chlamydia
  - Pubic lice

DIAGNOSIS

HISTORY

- For many adolescent girls, vaginal symptoms may be uncomfortable to talk about. Important to meet alone with an adolescent.
- Symptoms alone cannot distinguish between the different causes of vaginitis but can assist the clinician.
- Describe the discharge including color (white, green-yellow, gray?), consistency (frothy? thick?), amount, odor, and duration of symptoms.
- Is there pain? Pain with intercourse? Burning?
- Bladder symptoms: Is there dysuria? Frequency? Urgency?
- Is there itching? Is it worse at night? Is it present in other family members?
- Exposure to any new possible irritants (e.g., new soap, spermicides, douching)
- Anything that makes symptoms better or worse?
- Prior history of similar symptoms? Prior treatment for past vaginitis?
- Sexual history including number of partners, use of barrier methods, history of STI
- Any medications, such as systemic antibiotics
- STI risk factors
- Any chronic diseases such as diabetes or other immunocompromised conditions

PHYSICAL EXAM

- Vital signs, including height, weight, BMI, and temperature
- Inspect pubic hair for sexual maturity rating (tanner scores) and also evidence of infection or irritation.
- External genital or vaginal evidence of erythema, excoriation, and discharge. In younger children, this can be done in the "frog-leg" position.
- Discharge should be sampled.
- Examination of other evidence for irritation or inflammation such as warts, injury, and ulceration
- Consistency, color of discharge
- If patient is sexually active, speculum exam may need to be performed to evaluate the cervix. "Strawberry cervix" can be a sign of inflammation seen in trichomoniasis.
- Bimanual exam also should be considered if symptoms suggest risk for pelvic inflammatory disease.

DIAGNOSTIC TESTS & INTERPRETATION

Lab

In order to best evaluate etiology, a sample of discharge should be collected. The sample can be obtained by the clinician or by the patient typically using a cotton-tipped applicator.

- Odor/"whiff" or "amine" test:
  - Slide prepared with drop of 10% KOH
  - The examiner should whiff the slide for presence of a fishy odor suggestive of BV, also seen in trichomoniasis, negative in candida.
- Wet mount of the vaginal discharge mixed with saline for microscopy
  - This slide is examined for evidence of trichomonads, clue cells, and yeast.
  - Clue cells are vaginal epithelial cells with adherent coccobacilli seen on wet mount and when >20% of epithelial cells suggestive of BV.
- Wet mount with 10% KO
  - May demonstrate budding yeast ("spaghetti with meatballs" appearance) suggestive of candida
- Nitrazine paper
  - Measures pH of sample
  - Vaginal pH >5 seen in BV, >5.4 seen in trichomoniasis, <4.9 candidiasis
- Urinalysis may be helpful if patient complains of dysuria.

- STI testing as warranted based on risk factors. Chlamydia PCR can be obtained by cervical or vaginal swab or urine; gonorrhea PCR or culture (cervical or vaginal swab)
- Consider a pregnancy test as indicated.

DIFFERENTIAL DIAGNOSIS

- Physiologic leukorrhea
- Candidiasis
- BV
- Trichomonas
- Other STIs including chlamydia, gonorrhea, herpes simplex virus infection, HPV
- Skin conditions including psoriasis.
- Lichen sclerosis (hypotrophic dystrophy of the vulva)
- Congenital abnormalities, such as ectopic ureter
- Sexual abuse
- Mechanical irritation from lack of lubrication, trauma
- Pinworm infection

TREATMENT

MEDICATION

- Medication management depends on the etiology.
- Vulvovaginal candidiasis
  - Topical antifungals such as clotrimazole, butoconazole, miconazole, or terconazole are available over the counter.
  - Oral fluconazole 6 mg/kg up to a maximum of 150 mg as a single dose can also be given.
  - Longer treatments may be necessary for recurrent or severe infections.
- BV
  - Antibiotics are treatment of choice.
  - Oral metronidazole 500 mg twice daily for 7 days or intravaginal metronidazole gel for 5 days or clindamycin cream (7 days) or suppository (100 mg ovules for 3 days)
  - Higher rates of recurrence are seen with single-dose therapy for BV.
  - Relapse may require longer courses of treatment.
- Trichomonas
  - Metronidazole 2 g orally in a single-dose
  - Sexual partners should be treated simultaneously if possible to avoid reinfection.
- Chlamydia
  - Azithromycin 1 g orally for 1 dose or doxycycline 100 mg orally twice daily for 7 days
- Gonorrhea
  - Ceftriaxone 125 mg intramuscular for one dose
  - PLUS azithromycin 1 g orally for 1 dose or doxycycline 100 mg orally twice daily for 7 days
- HSV
  - For initial outbreak: acyclovir 400 mg orally 3 times daily for 7–10 days or 200 mg 5 times daily for 7–10 days; can use valacyclovir or famciclovir alternatively
  - Suppressive therapy for recurrent infections can use acyclovir, valacyclovir, or famciclovir.
- Lichen sclerosus
  - Mild pruritus consider mild emollient
  - More severe symptoms consider topical steroids
- Group A β-hemolytic *Streptococcus* and *H. influenzae*
  - Amoxicillin 40 mg/kg/day to max 500 mg divided twice daily for 7 days
- Shigella
  - Trimethoprim/sulfamethoxazole
- Pinworm infestations
  - Mebendazole 100 mg orally, repeat dosage 2 weeks later
  - Consider treatment of entire family

ADDITIONAL TREATMENT

General Measures

- Good hygiene and avoidance/removal of irritants includes hand washing following toileting, encourage wiping from front to back, clean with a mild non-scented soaps or lotions, wear cotton underwear, and avoid bubble baths and douching.
- Warm bath/Sitz baths followed by air-drying
- Use of topical emollients, zinc creams, or topical low-potency steroids to assist with itching and/or inflammation

COMPLEMENTARY & ALTERNATIVE TREATMENTS

Probiotics may be helpful in preventing recurrence in BV and candida vulvovaginitis.

ONGOING CARE

FOLLOW-UP RECOMMENDATIONS

Patient Monitoring

- If symptoms persist following over the counter or other treatment, patients need to be reevaluated by a clinician as may be another etiology.
- Patients with an STI such as trichomonas, gonorrhea, or chlamydia should make certain that all sexual partners receive treatment in order to prevent reinfection.

ALERT

Patients taking metronidazole for trichomonas or BV should be told explicitly to avoid alcohol.

PATIENT EDUCATION

- In prepubescent females: Encourage good hygiene to prevent recurrence.
- In sexually active adolescents: Encourage regular condom usage. Consider discussion of contraceptive options.

PROGNOSIS

With treatment, vaginitis typically resolves quickly with no complications.

COMPLICATIONS

- BV is associated with premature labor and preterm birth, premature rupture of membranes, and increased risk of acquiring STIs.
- Trichomonas
- Gonorrhea and chlamydial infections that are not treated can lead to pelvic inflammatory disease.

ADDITIONAL READING

- Freeto JP, Jay MS. "What's really going on down there?" A practical approach to the adolescent who has gynecologic complaints. *Pediatr Clin North Am*. 2006;53(3):529–545.
- Hainer BL, Gibson MV. Vaginitis. *Am Fam Physician*. 2011;83(7):807–815.
- Jasper JM. Vulvovaginitis in the prepubertal child. *Clin Ped Emerg Med*. 2009;10:10–13.
- Sharma B, Preston J, Greenwood P. Management of vulvovaginitis and vaginal discharge in prepubertal girls. *Rev Gynaecol Pract*. 2004;4:111–120.
- Sobel JD. Vaginitis. *N Engl J Med*. 1997;337(26):1896–1903.
- Syed T, Braverman P. Vaginitis in adolescents. *Adolesc Med Clin*. 2004;15(2):235–251.

CODES

ICD10

- N76.0 Acute vaginitis
- N89.8 Other specified noninflammatory disorders of vagina
- B37.3 Candidiasis of vulva and vagina

FAQ

- Q: How do you diagnose BV?
- A: BV is a clinical diagnosis based on having 3 out of 4 Amsel Criteria:
  - Thin, homogenous discharge
  - Vaginal pH >4.5
  - Positive "whiff" test
  - >20% clue cells on wet mount or Gram stain
- Q: Should sex partners of patients with vaginitis be treated?
- A: Depends on the etiology of the vaginitis. For BV and candida, there are no treatment recommendations for sex partners. For patients with trichomonas, partners should be treated, and to reduce recurrence, partners should avoid sexual intercourse until both have been treated and are asymptomatic.
- Q: In prepubescent females, is a positive culture definitive for infection?
- A: One common issue in prepubertal females is how to distinguish between normal vaginal flora and potential pathogens. Growth of normal pathogens even in girls who are symptomatic are not diagnostic.

VARICOCELE

Sophia D. Delpe • Adam B. Hittelman

BASICS

DESCRIPTION

A varicocele is an abnormal tortuosity and dilation of the testicular veins and the pampiniform venous plexus of the spermatic cord.

EPIDEMIOLOGY

Incidence

- Rare in prepubertal boys, increases with age to approximately 15% in late adolescence and healthy adult population
  - 2–10 years old, <1%
  - 11–14 years old, 7.8%
  - 15–19 years old, 14.1%
- Based on World Health Organization observational study (1992), 15–20% of adult varicocele patients have fertility problems.
  - Varicocele presents in 25% of men with abnormal semen analysis and 12% of men with normal semen parameters.
  - Present in 35–40% of males with primary infertility
- Left-sided predominance, 90%
- No racial predilection

RISK FACTORS

- Exact mechanisms have not been fully elucidated.
- May be related to physiologic changes in puberty, such as rapid testicular growth and increased testicular blood flow
- Associated with increased height and low body mass index
- Increased risk in 1st-degree relatives of patients with a varicocele

PATHOPHYSIOLOGY

- Association between varicocele and testicular dysfunction/fertility compromise
  - Impaired spermatogenesis: decreased motility, decreased density, and increased number of pathologic sperm forms
- Ipsilateral testicular hypotrophy
  - Recent data demonstrates correlation between varicocele grade and testicular hypotrophy, although not observed in prior studies.
  - Testicular "catch-up growth" after varicocelectomy
  - Catch-up growth in 30–50% of patients managed conservatively
- Potential field defect, affecting growth of bilateral testicles
- Exact mechanisms not clearly elucidated—multiple theories:
  - Hyperthermia: Varicocele increases intratesticular temperature, likely by interfering with the pampiniform plexus' ability to provide countercurrent cooling system.
  - Potential reflux of renal and adrenal metabolites, causing testicular damage
  - Increased production of nitric oxide and reactive oxygen species correlate with severity of varicocele.
  - Endocrine abnormalities are found in subset of patients with varicocele, including low testosterone, abnormal response to gonadotropin-releasing hormone (GnRH), and impaired Leydig cell function.

ETIOLOGY

- Associated with anatomy of left testicular vein
  - Inserts into renal vein at right angle (right testicular vein drains into vena cava)
  - Incompetent or absent valves
  - Left testicular vein 8–10 cm longer than right, with increased pressure
  - Increased venous pressure from "nutcracker phenomenon": compression of left renal vein as it passes between aorta and superior mesenteric artery

DIAGNOSIS

HISTORY

- Often asymptomatic and incidentally noted on routine physical exam
  - Infertility not common issue in adolescent population
  - Associated pain/heaviness/dull ache in 2–11% of cases
- Laterality
- Age of onset
- When and how testicular abnormality first detected
- Change in size of varicocele with positioning or Valsalva
- Prior surgery or trauma
- Prior imaging

PHYSICAL EXAM

- Examine in warm room when patient is supine and standing.
- Palpate at rest and with Valsalva.
- Para- and supratesticular mass; feels like a "bag of worms"
- Assess size and consistency.
- Estimate testicular volume with orchidometer, calipers, or color Doppler ultrasound.
  - Right testicle serves as control for left.
  - >2 mL or >20% size discrepancy, right > left, is significant.

- Varicocele grade
  - Grade 1 (small): palpable only with Valsalva
  - Grade 2 (medium): easily palpable but not visible
  - Grade 3 (large): visible through scrotal skin
- Varicocele should decompress in supine position.
- Solitary right varicocele or failure of vessels to decompress in supine position raises concern for potential retroperitoneal or abdominal mass.

DIAGNOSTIC TESTS & INTERPRETATION

- Color Doppler scrotal ultrasound to diagnose varicocele and estimate testicular volume
- Semen analysis in age-appropriate patients
- GnRH simulation test leads to increased FSH and LH response.
  - Has not conclusively been shown to be good predictor of postsurgical improvement in adolescents

DIFFERENTIAL DIAGNOSIS

- Epididymal cyst/spermatocele
- Testicular mass
- Epididymal mass
- Paratesticular mass
- Inguinal hernia
- Hydrocele
- Cord lipoma

ALERT

Secondary varicocele, especially right-sided, can be a clinical indicator of retroperitoneal mass or venous obstruction. It is important to do physical exam standing and in supine position to assess for decompression of varicocele in supine position.

TREATMENT

- Treatment is not indicated in all children/adolescents with varicocele.
- Annual ultrasound assessment of testicular volume recommended.
  - Potential for interobserver variability for imaging
  - Spontaneous catch-up growth in some patients managed conservatively.
- 80–85% of men with varicocele do not exhibit effect on fertility.
- Definitive treatment is recommended for the following:
  - Size discrepancy between right and left testicle of >2 mL or 20%
  - Adolescents with abnormal semen analysis and high-grade varicocele
  - Adolescents with symptoms: pain, heaviness
  - Adolescents with bilateral varicocele
- Treatment options
  - Surgical ligation and division of testicular veins (laparoscopic vs. subinguinal approach)
    - Testicular artery- and lymphatic-sparing reduces risk of secondary hydrocele.
  - Intravenous embolization of testicular veins

ONGOING CARE

FOLLOW-UP RECOMMENDATIONS

- Persistence should be assessed by surveillance ultrasound 6 months after repair.
- Trans-scrotal US to assess for testicular catch-up growth
- Semen analysis to see if improvement in semen parameters

PROGNOSIS

After repair, recurrence can occur in 1–16% of patients (depending on surgical technique).

COMPLICATIONS

- Recurrent/persistent varicocele
- Secondary hydrocele
  - May require surgery if symptomatic
- Testicular hypotrophy/atrophy
- Persistent fertility compromise

ADDITIONAL READING

- Evers JH, Collins J, Clarke J. Surgery or embolisation for varicoceles in subfertile men. *Cochrane Database Syst Rev*. 2009;(3):CD000479.
- Preston MA, Carnat T, Flood T, et al. Conservative management of adolescent varicoceles: a retrospective review. *Urology*. 2008;72(1):77–80.
- Robinson SP, Hampton LJ, Koo HP. Treatment strategy for the adolescent varicocele. *Urol Clin North Am*. 2010;37(2):269–278.
- Serefoglu EC, Saitz TR, La Nasa JA Jr, et al. Adolescent varicocoele management controversies. *Andrology*. 2013;1(1):109–115.
- Stahl P, Schlegel PN. Standardization and documentation of varicocele evaluation. *Curr Opin Neurol*. 2011;21(6):500–505.

CODES

ICD10

I86.1 Scrotal varices

FAQ

- Q: What are long-term benefits of surgical repair of varicoceles?
- A: If varicocele is corrected, testicular catch-up growth can occur when performed in adolescents, as well as decreased risk for infertility. In adult population, 2/3 of patients will have improvement in semen analysis, and 40% of their partners will become pregnant.
- Q: Is there benefit of surgical repair of varicocele after puberty? Will this improve fertility?
- A: Testicular hypotrophy does not improve after adult varicocelectomy. Although it appears to be a progressive process, studies have not clearly demonstrated clear benefit in fertility improvement if corrected in adolescence versus when fertility compromise is diagnosed.
- Q: What happens if a varicocele is left untreated?
- A: There is good evidence to show that when left untreated, a varicocele will continue to affect testicular growth with loss of volume and progressive deterioration in semen analysis.
- Q: What is the risk of recurrence after repair?
- A: Recurrence can occur in 1–16% of adolescents, depending on surgical technique.

VASCULAR BRAIN LESIONS (CONGENITAL)

Daphne M. Hasbani • Sabrina E. Smith

BASICS

DESCRIPTION

- Developmental venous anomalies (DVAs) are the most common vascular malformation of the brain, representing 60% of all central nervous system vascular malformations. Also known as venous angiomas, DVAs are made up of a cluster of venous radicles that drain into a collecting vein. They occur in 2.5–3% of the general population.
- DVAs are associated with cavernous malformations (see below) in 8–40% of cases, and 20% of patients with mucocutaneous venous malformations of the head and neck have DVAs. They are also associated with sinus pericranii, a communication between intracranial and extracranial venous drainage pathways in which blood may circulate bidirectionally.
- Cavernous malformations (CMs), also known as cavernous hemangiomas or cavernomas, are multilobulated, low-pressure, and slow-flow vascular structures filled with blood, thrombus, or both. They do not contain elastin or smooth muscle. There is no intervening brain tissue except at the periphery of the lesion.
- Arteriovenous malformations (AVMs) are abnormal clusters of vessels that connect arteries and veins without a true capillary bed and have intervening gliotic brain tissue.
- Vein of Galen malformations (VOGMs) are a specific type of congenital AVM that involves the vein of Galen, which flows into the straight sinus after draining the internal cerebral veins and basal veins.
- Sturge-Weber syndrome (SWS), also known as encephalotrigeminal angiomatosis, is characterized by leptomeningeal angiomatosis, facial port-wine stain (capillary malformation), and glaucoma. Some patients have all 3 findings, although others have just 1 or 2 features.

PATHOPHYSIOLOGY

- DVAs are an extreme variation of normal venous development. Typically, venous drainage in the brain occurs through a superficial system and a deep system. DVAs result when a deep venous territory drains toward the surface or when a superficial territory drains to the deep venous system instead of draining in the expected direction. Intervening brain tissue is normal. The mechanism responsible for DVA formation is unknown.
- The pathogenesis of CMs is unknown, although the report of cases of new cavernoma development adjacent to a DVA suggests that DVAs may lead to CM formation. Most CMs occur sporadically, although familial syndromes exist. Several genes have been associated with familial CMs.
- The cause of AVM formation is unknown. A failure of normal capillary development with dysplastic vessels forming between primordial arteriovenous connections has been suggested.
- VOGMs are embryonic AVMs consisting of choroidal arteries draining into the precursor of the vein of Galen. They develop between weeks 6 and 11 of fetal life.
- SWS occurs sporadically in 1/40,000–50,000 births and is associated with a somatic mosaic mutation in guanine nucleotide–binding protein G(q) subunit alpha. The pathophysiology is thought to be venous dysplasia, in which the primordial venous plexus that is normally present at 5–8 weeks of gestation fails to regress. The location of this plexus around the cephalic end of the neural tube and under the ectoderm destined to form the facial skin accounts for the clinical features. Venous stasis occurs due to the absence of normal cortical venous structures, and hypoperfusion of brain tissue occurs. These findings are unilateral in the majority but can be bilateral in up to 20% of cases.

DIAGNOSIS

HISTORY

- DVAs are usually benign and asymptomatic, coming to clinical attention as an incidental finding on a neuroimaging study.
- Headache, seizure, and intracerebral hemorrhage are common in patients with CMs and AVMs. Focal neurologic deficits may result from intracerebral hemorrhage or compression of underlying brain structures by the vascular malformation.
- 95% of newborns with VOGMs present with CHF. Others present with hydrocephalus, subarachnoid hemorrhage, intraventricular hemorrhage, or failure to thrive.
- Infants and older children usually present with hydrocephalus, headache, seizures, exercise-induced syncope, or subarachnoid hemorrhage.
- Facial port-wine stain, seizures, and glaucoma are common in SWS. Other neurologic symptoms include hemiparesis, developmental delay, mental retardation, and strokelike episodes presenting with hemiparesis and visual field defects.

PHYSICAL EXAM

- Physical exam is normal in children with DVAs and children with CMs or AVMs that have not ruptured. Focal neurologic deficits may persist following intracerebral hemorrhage associated with CMs or AVMs.
- In newborns with VOGMs, signs of congestive heart failure such as tachycardia, respiratory distress, and hepatomegaly may occur. A continuous cranial bruit heard may be heard over the posterior skull, and bounding carotid pulses and peripheral pulses may be present. Scalp veins may be dilated.
- Older infants and children with VOGMs also may present with CHF but more often demonstrate increased head circumference, focal neurologic signs, and failure to thrive. Proptosis may be noted.
- Children with SWS often have a facial port-wine stain, most often in the V1 distribution. Glaucoma is also common. Hemiparesis or seizures may develop.

DIAGNOSTIC TESTS & INTERPRETATION

Routine blood studies are usually normal. Chest x-ray studies and electrocardiogram may reveal typical changes of high-output CHF in patients with VOGMs.

Imaging

- Neuroimaging studies are required for definitive diagnosis.
- DVAs can be visualized on contrast-enhanced CT or MRI. Diagnosis is made by visualization of the typical "caput medusa" appearance of the radially arranged veins draining into a collecting vein, seen as a linear or curvilinear focus of enhancement. They can also be visualized with conventional angiography, although this is not required unless a patient presents with an acute hemorrhage.
- MRI is better than CT at demonstrating CMs, which have a mulberry appearance. On MRI, they are well-circumscribed lesions of mixed signal intensity on T1- and T2-weighted sequences. Contrast enhancement is variable. They are best seen on gradient-echo T2-weighted images or susceptibility-weighted images, which are sensitive to hemosiderin or deoxyhemoglobin.
- AVMs can be seen with CT/CTA, MR/MRA, and conventional angiography. Dynamic sequences are required to characterize the anatomy of feeding and draining vessels. Conventional angiography is the gold standard.
- VOGMs can be diagnosed on fetal ultrasound or MRI. In newborns, cranial ultrasound shows a large, hypoechoic structure in the region of the vein of Galen. CT shows a high-density mass that enhances with contrast. MRI shows an area of decreased signal intensity or signal void because of high flow within the malformation. CT and MRI also show areas of cerebral ischemia or hemorrhage. Conventional angiography is required before intervention.
- In SWS, CT may show calcifications or atrophy. Gadolinium-enhanced MRI is the most sensitive study, showing leptomeningeal enhancement due to pial angiomatosis. Initial CT and MRI are often normal in the newborn period, so follow-up imaging is required.

DIFFERENTIAL DIAGNOSIS

- The differential diagnosis for headaches and seizures, common presenting symptoms of brain vascular malformations, is broad. CNS infection, vascular malformation, hydrocephalus, and mass lesion can result in both. Other causes of seizure include dysplasia and remote brain injury, both genetic and idiopathic. Other causes of headache include benign conditions such as migraine and tension headaches and structural abnormalities such as Chiari I malformations.
- VOGMs must be considered in any newborn with unexplained CHF (especially high-output failure), hydrocephalus, or intracranial hemorrhage. Other causes of high-output CHF in the newborn include anemia, hyperthyroidism, and other AVMs.
- Intracranial hemorrhage may result from AVMs, CMs, aneurysms, bleeding diatheses, hypertension, or trauma in neonates and children. In older children, sickle cell disease, vasculopathies including moyamoya syndrome and vasculitis also can lead to hemorrhage.

TREATMENT

GENERAL MEASURES

- DVAs do not typically require treatment.
- Anticonvulsants should be used to treat seizures.
- Surgical resection is the only treatment option for CMs, although conservative management may be indicated if the risk of surgery outweighs the potential benefit.
- Treatment options for AVMs include resection via microsurgery, embolization, stereotactic radiosurgery, and conservative management. Risk of hemorrhage ranges 0.9–34% per year, so decisions about treatment should be guided by symptoms at presentation and structural features of the AVM.
- Treatment of choice for VOGMs in all ages is endovascular embolization. Direct surgical intervention has unacceptable risks and is no longer recommended. Radiosurgery has been used in a small number of clinically stable older patients. Refractory CHF prompts intervention in neonates. Treatment in older infants and children is indicated to prevent cerebral ischemia (from arterial steal or from venous infarction) and to prevent hydrocephalus. Embolization can be completed in stages over a few months after CHF is controlled.
- Ventriculoperitoneal shunts may be required in patients who develop hydrocephalus following intracerebral hemorrhage related to CM or AVM or in patients with VOGMs.
- Treatment in SWS is targeted to symptoms, using anticonvulsants for seizures and eye drops or ocular shunts for glaucoma. Low-dose aspirin is recommended at the time of diagnosis to prevent further brain injury due to impaired cerebral blood flow. Seizures can lead to ongoing brain injury by increasing metabolic demand in brain tissue that has abnormal perfusion at baseline, so aggressive seizure management is recommended. Some children with intractable epilepsy may be good candidates for epilepsy surgery.

ONGOING CARE

- Generally, no specific follow-up is required for patients with DVAs.
- Follow-up with a neurologist is indicated for patients with CMs, AVMs, VOGMs, and SWS.
- Neurosurgical consultation is indicated for patients with CMs, AVMs, and VOGMs.
- A follow-up CT or MRI is indicated to evaluate patients with new neurologic signs or symptoms.
- Ophthalmologic follow-up is indicated for patients with SWS and most patients with VOGMs, especially prior to treatment when hydrocephalus may develop.

PROGNOSIS

- Prognosis is excellent for patients with isolated DVAs.
- Prognosis for patients with CMs and AVMs depends on the size, location, presenting symptoms, and specific characteristics of the lesion. Patients who have experienced an intracerebral hemorrhage have worse prognosis than those who have not.
- For patients with VOGMs, earlier age of symptoms is associated with worse prognosis. Mortality in neonates with symptomatic lesions is 36%. In a recent meta-analysis of 337 patients treated with endovascular embolization between 2001 and 2010, 84% had a good or fair clinical outcome, and mortality was 16%.
- Prognosis in patients with SWS depends on the extent and location of involvement. Seizures occur in the majority (~85%), with low normal intelligence or mental retardation in ~35%.

COMPLICATIONS

- Death can occur in patients with intracerebral hemorrhage due to CMs or AVMs.
- Mortality approaches 100% in untreated patients with VOGMs.
- In severe case of VOGMs, 80% of cardiac output may be delivered to the head because of the low vascular resistance within the malformation. Cardiac ischemia may occur because of decreased coronary artery blood flow.
- Intracerebral hemorrhage may occur as a result of CMs, AVMs, and VOGMs or as a complication of treatment.
- Longer term complications from CMs, AVMs, and VOGMs include mental retardation, seizures, hydrocephalus, and chronic motor impairment.
- In patients with SWS, visual impairment can result if glaucoma is difficult to control. Persistent hemiparesis can develop.

PATIENT MONITORING

- Serial neuroimaging should be performed in patients with CMs, AVMs, and VOGMs to guide the timing of treatment and to assess for recurrence.
- Head circumference should be monitored in patients with VOGMs as a marker of hydrocephalus.

ADDITIONAL READING

- Geibprasert S, Pongpech S, Jiarakongmun P, et al. Radiologic assessment of brain arteriovenous malformations: what clinicians need to know. *Radiographics*. 2010;30(2):483–501.
- Khullar D, Andeejani AMI, Bulsara KR. Evolution of treatment options for vein of Galen malformations: a review *J Neurosurg Pediatr*. 2010;6(5):444–451.
- Niazi TN, Klimo P Jr, Anderson RC, et al. Diagnosis and management of arteriovenous malformations in children. *Neurosurg Clin N Am*. 2010;21(3): 443–456.
- Puttgen KB, Lin DDM. Neurocutaneous vascular syndromes. *Childs Nerv Syst*. 2010;26(10):1407–1415.
- Rammos SK, Maina R, Lanzino G. Developmental venous anomalies: current concepts and implications for management. *Neurosurgery*. 2009;65(1):20–30.
- Ruiz DSM, Yilmaz H, Gailloud P. Cerebral developmental venous anomalies: current concepts. *Ann Neurol*. 2009;66(3):271–283.

CODES

ICD10

- Q28.3 Other malformations of cerebral vessels
- Q85.8 Other phakomatoses, not elsewhere classified
- D18.02 Hemangioma of intracranial structures

FAQ

- Q: Can the AVM recur after treatment?
- A: AVMs have a propensity to recur. Imaging studies give a good indication of the likelihood of recurrence.
- Q: How does a vascular malformation cause seizures?
- A: Seizures can result from ischemia, hemorrhage, or acute hydrocephalus associated with the malformation.

V

VENTRICULAR SEPTAL DEFECT

Shabnam Peyvandi

BASICS

DESCRIPTION

- A ventricular septal defect (VSD) is an opening in the ventricular septum, resulting in a communication between the left ventricle (LV) and the right ventricle (RV). The ventricular septum can be divided into 4 major areas:
  - Inlet/canal septum
  - Membranous/conoventricular septum
  - Muscular septum (largest)
  - Conal/infundibular/outlet septum (includes conal septal hypoplasia and malalignment types)
- There are several corresponding types of VSDs that have different natural histories and associated problems:
  - Inlet/canal VSDs: usually part of an atrioventricular (AV) canal defect, 5–7% of all VSDs
  - Membranous/conoventricular VSDs: 80% of all VSDs by classic teaching; fewer than muscular VSDs by echo data
  - Muscular VSDs: usually single and small but can be multiple and of variable size; 5–20% of all VSDs by classic teaching, but a large percentage are inaudible
  - Conal septal hypoplasia VSDs: usually large and unrestrictive; associated with aortic valve (AoV) cusp prolapse and aortic insufficiency
  - Anterior malalignment VSDs: usually associated with RV outflow tract obstruction. Paradigms: tetralogy of Fallot, double outlet RV
  - Posterior malalignment VSDs: usually associated with LV outflow tract obstruction. Paradigms: subaortic stenosis with coarctation or interrupted aortic arch
- There may also be multiple VSDs of different types in a single patient. Many complex forms of congenital heart disease include a VSD.

EPIDEMIOLOGY

- VSDs are the most common form of congenital heart disease.
  - ~1.5–5.7 per 1,000 term births
  - ~4.5–7.0 per 1,000 preterm births, by classic teaching
- Echo data show a higher incidence of ~50 per 1,000 live births, mostly asymptomatic muscular VSDs.

RISK FACTORS

Genetics

- Sibling and offspring recurrence risk for VSDs is estimated to be ~3–4%.
- VSD is the most common lesion in trisomies 21, 13, and 18, but >95% of children with VSDs have normal chromosomes.

COMMONLY ASSOCIATED CONDITIONS

- Congenital heart disease that includes a conal septal malalignment VSD (e.g., tetralogy of Fallot) or VSD with a conotruncal malformation (e.g., truncus arteriosus or interrupted aortic arch type B) has a 13–50% incidence of microdeletion of chromosome 22 (22q11.2 deletion syndrome).
- In a recent series, 7% of patients with an isolated membranous/conoventricular VSD had a 22q11.2 deletion.

PATHOPHYSIOLOGY

- Both the size of the VSD and the ratio of pulmonary vascular resistance (PVR) to systemic vascular resistance (SVR) determine the direction and amount of shunting.
  - Small VSD: The VSD imposes high resistance to flow with a large LV-to-RV pressure gradient, usually resulting in normal RV pressures. The restrictive size results in a small left-to-right shunt. The VSD size is usually ≤1/4 the size of the AoV annulus. The workload of the ventricles is normal.
  - Moderate VSD: The VSD imposes modest resistance to flow, usually resulting in mildly elevated RV pressures. The amount of shunting can still be large and is determined by the PVR/SVR ratio. The VSD size is usually 1/3–2/3 the size of the AoV annulus. The workload of the ventricles is increased.
  - Large VSD: The VSD imposes no resistance to flow and is unrestrictive, resulting in systemic RV pressures and RV hypertension. The workload of the ventricles is markedly increased.
- The lower the PVR/SVR ratio, the greater the degree of left-to-right shunting. A large left-to-right shunt leads to pulmonary vascular congestion, tachypnea, tachycardia, and hepatomegaly, all signs of congestive heart failure (CHF). The amount of CHF correlates directly with shunt size and usually peaks at 6–8 weeks of age, timed with the nadir of PVR and physiologic anemia. Lack of significant CHF in patients with a large VSD signifies elevated PVR and requires careful evaluation. Cardiac catheterization may be required in these patients to provide additional data.
- If a large VSD is left untreated, pulmonary vascular obstructive disease will eventually develop, leading to reversal of the shunt, cyanosis, and RV failure (Eisenmenger syndrome).

DIAGNOSIS

HISTORY

- Small VSD: The child is usually asymptomatic, with normal growth and development. Most commonly, a murmur is detected at 1–6 weeks of age.
- Moderate VSD: The child is usually symptomatic with slow weight gain and sparing of longitudinal growth. There is often an increased incidence of respiratory infections. Sweating and fatigue with feeding may be present.
- Large VSD: The child is usually quite symptomatic, especially with a larger shunt, showing signs of CHF and marked failure to thrive.
- Children with Eisenmenger syndrome have cyanosis, fatigue, and symptoms of right heart failure.

PHYSICAL EXAM

- Small VSD
  - The child usually appears healthy with normal growth.
  - The heart action is quiet, but there is often an associated systolic thrill along the left sternal border with a membranous VSD, in contrast to a small muscular VSD.
  - Heart sounds are normal. A high-frequency, pansystolic murmur is present in membranous VSDs, whereas in muscular VSDs, the murmur is not pansystolic.
  - The murmur is loudest over the region of the VSD.
- Moderate VSD
  - The child usually appears in mild distress with tachycardia and tachypnea.
  - The heart action is increased and there is often still an associated thrill.
  - The P_2 component of S_2 may be normal or accentuated.
  - A medium frequency, pansystolic murmur is present over the location of the VSD.
  - A mid-diastolic rumble is present over the mitral listening area (apex) as a result of a significant shunt and indicates ≥2:1 pulmonary-to-systemic flow ratio. Hepatomegaly may be present.
- Large VSD
  - The child usually appears ill with marked distress and marked tachycardia and tachypnea, proportional to the size of the left-to-right shunt.
  - The heart action is markedly increased without a thrill. The P_2 component of S_2 is loud and narrowly split as a result of pulmonary hypertension.
  - A soft, low-frequency pansystolic murmur is present over the VSD.
  - The loudness of the mid-diastolic rumble is proportional to the size of the left-to-right shunt.
  - CHF physical exam signs are proportional to the size of the left-to-right shunt but are usually present to a significant degree.
- If significant aortic insufficiency develops, a high-frequency, early diastolic murmur is heard along the left sternal border.
- In newborns whose PVR has not yet fallen, the increased heart action remains the key to diagnosis, as auscultation may be unimpressive.

- Likewise, in children with elevated PVR, the increased heart action remains the key to diagnosis. Auscultation shows a narrowly split S_2 with a loud P_2. The murmur loudness depends on VSD size and shunt but often is soft or absent and unimpressive.
- Once Eisenmenger syndrome develops (secondary to pulmonary vascular obstructive changes), patients manifest cyanosis, clubbing, an increased RV impulse, a narrowly split S_2 with a loud P_2 component and a soft or absent VSD murmur. There may be a systolic murmur of tricuspid insufficiency at the left lower sternal border (LLSB), a high-frequency early diastolic murmur of pulmonary insufficiency, or an S_3 at the LLSB. There is usually associated jugular venous distention and hepatomegaly, indicating high right-sided filling pressures.

DIAGNOSTIC TESTS & INTERPRETATION

Lab

- ECG
  - Small VSD: normal
  - Moderate VSD: left ventricular hypertrophy (LVH)
  - Large VSD: biventricular hypertrophy (BVH) and left atrial enlargement (LAE)
  - Eisenmenger syndrome: right ventricular hypertrophy (RVH) and right atrial enlargement (RAE)
- Cardiac catheterization
  - Generally reserved for patients with difficult VSD anatomy, associated lesions, or for the assessment of the ratio of pulmonary to systemic flow and pulmonary vascular reactivity

Imaging

- Chest radiograph
  - Small VSD: normal
  - Moderate VSD: hyperinflation, cardiomegaly, increased pulmonary vascular markings
  - Large VSD: cardiomegaly, markedly increased pulmonary vascular markings, Kerley B lines
  - Eisenmenger syndrome: normal heart size, prominent central pulmonary arteries, and decreased peripheral vascular markings
- Echocardiogram
  - All children with a murmur consistent with a VSD should undergo an echocardiogram to define the location, size, and number of VSDs and any associated defects. Color/spectral Doppler allows visualization of the shunt direction and the amount of restriction to the VSD, if any.

TREATMENT

GENERAL MEASURES

- Small VSD: no intervention; continued observation
- Moderate VSD: If signs of CHF develop, digoxin, diuretics, afterload reduction, and increased caloric intake are indicated.
- Large VSD: CHF often develops and requires aggressive therapy as noted above.
- Membranous and muscular VSDs often become smaller or close spontaneously. Generally, observation and/or medical therapy is indicated for a few months.
- Conoseptal hypoplasia and malalignment VSDs do not close spontaneously and therefore require surgical closure, often in infancy.
- After 1 year of life, a significant left-to-right shunt (Qp:Qs $\geq$2:1) or elevated pulmonary artery pressures are an indication for surgery.
- Children with elevated pulmonary artery pressures ($\geq$½ systemic) should undergo repair before 2 years of age, even if CHF symptoms are controlled.
- Development of complications, including aortic insufficiency, subaortic membrane, and double-chamber RV, is usually an indication for surgical repair.
- Surgical correction may be contraindicated if the PVR is >8 Wood units/m^2.
- Recent series of surgical VSD closure report a mortality of 0.6–2.3%.
- Complete heart block occurs in <2% of patients postoperatively but requires pacemaker therapy when it occurs.

ONGOING CARE

PROGNOSIS

- Spontaneous closure: usually by age 2 years; 90% of small muscular VSDs and 8–35% of small conoventricular VSDs
- Prognosis with surgical closure is excellent.
- The risk of Eisenmenger syndrome is considered minimal if large VSDs are surgically closed by 2 years of age.
- Caveat: Despite timely VSD surgical closure, a very small percentage of patients still go on to develop Eisenmenger syndrome.

COMPLICATIONS

- All VSDs: endocarditis—overall rate of 15 cases per 10,000 person-years of follow-up
- Moderate-to-large VSDs: LV volume overload, left atrial hypertension, CHF, poor growth, Eisenmenger syndrome
- Specific types
  - Inlet/canal VSDs: often associated with cleft mitral valve with possible AV valve insufficiency
  - Membranous/conoventricular VSDs: risk for development of aortic insufficiency typically due to prolapse of the right aortic cusp, subaortic membrane, or double-chamber RV
  - Muscular VSDs: isolated—near-zero risk for the development of subsequent lesions
  - Conal septal hypoplasia VSDs: risk for development of aortic insufficiency
  - Malalignment VSDs: usually associated with outflow tract obstruction and distal great artery hypoplasia/obstruction

PATIENT MONITORING

Subacute bacterial endocarditis (SBE) prophylaxis is recommended for 6 months after complete closure (surgical or catheter based) of a VSD.

ADDITIONAL READING

- Aquilar NE, Eugenio Lopez J. Ventricular septal defects. *Bol Asoc Med P R*. 2009;101(4):23–29.
- Hoffman JI, Kaplan S. The incidence of congenital heart disease. *J Am Coll Cardiol*. 2002;39(12): 1890–1900.
- Kidd L, Driscoll DJ, Gersony WM, et al. Second natural history study of congenital heart defects. Results of treatment of patients with ventricular septal defects. *Circulation*. 1993;87(2)(Suppl):I38–I51.
- McDaniel NL. Ventricular and atrial septal defects. *Pediatr Rev*. 2001;22(8):265–270.
- Penny DJ, Vick GW III. Ventricular septal defect. *Lancet*. 2011;377(9771):1103–1112.

CODES

ICD10

- Q21.0 Ventricular septal defect
- Q24.8 Other specified congenital malformations of heart

FAQ

- Q: Should children with a murmur consistent with a VSD undergo echocardiogram?
- A: Yes, to define the location, size, and number of VSDs and any associated lesions.
- Q: Should children with VSD have SBE prophylaxis?
- A: Based on the revised 2007 American Heart Association Guidelines, isolated VSD does not warrant SBE prophylaxis. However, SBE prophylaxis is recommended for 6 months following complete surgical or interventional catheterization closure (no residual defect) of a VSD.
- Q: Should asymptomatic children with a small VSD have activity restrictions?
- A: No, if there are no other problems.

VENTRICULAR TACHYCARDIA

Arvind Hoskoppal

BASICS

DESCRIPTION

- Ventricular tachycardia (VT) is a series of 3 or more repetitive beats originating from the ventricle at a rate faster than the upper limit of normal for age. It usually is a wide complex rhythm but can appear narrow in infants, and the QRS complex is always different from sinus rhythm. VT may, but not always, have atrioventricular (AV) dissociation.
- Sustained VT: lasts >30 seconds
- Nonsustained VT: lasts from 3 beats to 30 seconds
- VT may be monomorphic or polymorphic.
- Torsades de pointes: a polymorphic variant
  - The QRS complexes gradually change shape and axis throughout the tachycardia.
  - Associated with congenital long QT syndrome, acquired long QT, and Brugada syndrome
- Premature ventricular contractions (PVCs) have been reported in 0.8–2.2% of otherwise healthy children.

Genetics

- Long QT syndrome may be inherited in an autosomal recessive or autosomal dominant pattern. It is related to a variety of cardiac ion channel defects and may be associated with hearing loss and/or a family history of sudden death.
- Brugada syndrome is most commonly related to a defect in the cardiac sodium channel (SCN 5A) and appears to be inherited in an autosomal dominant pattern.

PATHOPHYSIOLOGY

VT may result from a reentrant mechanism, triggered mechanism, or abnormal automaticity.

ETIOLOGY

- Diverse and often overlapping
- Idiopathic
- Myocarditis or dilated cardiomyopathy
- Long QT syndrome (LQTS)
- Right ventricular dysplasia
- Brugada syndrome
- Before and after surgery for congenital heart disease (e.g., tetralogy of Fallot, transposition of the great arteries, aortic stenosis, hypertrophic cardiomyopathy, myocardial tumors, Ebstein anomaly, and pulmonary vascular occlusive disease)
- Metabolic disturbances (hypoxia, acidosis, hypo/hyperkalemia, hypomagnesemia, hypothermia)
- Drug toxicity (e.g., digitalis toxicity, antiarrhythmic agents)
- Substance abuse (cocaine, methamphetamine)
- Myocardial ischemia (e.g., Kawasaki disease, congenital coronary anomalies)
- Trauma
- Invasive lines or catheters
- Pericardial effusion
- Catecholaminergic polymorphic VT

DIAGNOSIS

Based on electrocardiogram (ECG), rhythm strip, Holter, or event monitor

HISTORY

- Varies widely, ranging from asymptomatic to sudden cardiac arrest/death
- Other symptoms include palpitations, presyncope or syncope, exercise intolerance, and dizziness.

PHYSICAL EXAM

- Can be normal; occasional heart rhythm irregularity secondary to frequent PVCs
- Acute, sustained VT may have signs of hemodynamic compromise, including lack of pulse.
- Signs of underlying heart disease, if any, are present.

DIAGNOSTIC TESTS & INTERPRETATION

Lab

- Serum electrolytes, including magnesium and potassium levels, blood gas, and serum drug levels as appropriate
- Urine toxicology screen
- ECG
  - ≥3 consecutive ventricular complexes faster than the upper limit of normal for age
  - Bundle branch morphology (right or left) may indicate the site of origin of the VT. May have AV dissociation
  - Typically, repolarization (T-wave) abnormalities are present.
  - The QTc interval should be measured in lead II during sinus rhythm.
  - Evaluate for Brugada syndrome in leads V_1 and V_2 (right bundle branch block, coved-type ST elevation, and T-wave inversion in the right precordial leads). Brugada syndrome ECG findings may be more obvious when the patient is febrile.
- Echocardiogram
  - Rule out congenital heart disease (CHD), pericardial and pleural effusions, tumors, and hypertrophic cardiomyopathy and assess ventricular function.
  - Cardiac magnetic resonance imaging may be helpful in addressing abnormalities that are beyond the resolution of echocardiography.
- Ambulatory Holter monitor
  - Quantitative assessment of ventricular ectopy, and frequency of VT
  - Less frequent episodes may need an event monitor or loop recorder.
- Exercise stress test (>5 years old)
  - Benign PVCs are characteristically suppressed with exercise and return in the immediate recovery period.
  - Exacerbation or worsening of ventricular arrhythmias is concerning.
- Cardiac catheterization: assessment of hemodynamics, endomyocardial biopsy, and coronary artery angiography
- Electrophysiologic study indications
  - Confirm diagnosis and mechanism of a wide complex rhythm.
  - Evaluate suspected VT in the setting of structural or functional heart disease, syncope, or cardiac arrest.

– Evaluate nonsustained VT in patients with CHD.
– Determine appropriate medical therapy in a patient with inducible VT.
– Evaluate syncope in the setting of palpitations (SVT vs. VT).
– Characterize VT with consideration for catheter ablation.
  ○ *Note*: Electrophysiologic studies are generally not helpful in individuals with LQTS.

DIFFERENTIAL DIAGNOSIS

Wide complex tachyarrhythmia

- Should always suspect VT until proven otherwise
- Supraventricular tachycardia (SVT) with aberrancy
- Antidromic tachycardia (antegrade conduction down an accessory pathway during an AV reciprocating tachycardia (e.g., Wolff-Parkinson-White syndrome)
- Atrial flutter or fibrillation with rapid antegrade conduction over an accessory pathway

TREATMENT

- **Acute**
  - If the patient is hemodynamically compromised, prompt synchronized direct-current (1–2 joules/kg; adult, 100–400 joules) cardioversion is indicated.
  - Asynchronous cardioversion for ventricular fibrillation or pulseless VT
  - Cardiopulmonary resuscitation as necessary
  - Lidocaine (1 mg/kg bolus over 1 minute, followed by an infusion at 20–50 μg/kg/minute, assuming normal liver and kidney function)
  - If torsades de pointes, $MgSO_4$ may be given
  - Overdrive ventricular pacing may terminate the tachycardia; however, pacing may accelerate the VT or induce ventricular fibrillation.
  - IV amiodarone (side effect: hypotension, responds to volume)
- **Chronic**
  - Medications
    - Class IB (mexiletine and phenytoin). β-Blockers (propranolol, atenolol, nadolol) are used in LQTS and may be effective in exercise-induced VT and postoperative CHD.
    - Class III agents (amiodarone and sotalol) should be avoided in patients with LQTS.
    - Class IC agents (flecainide) may be proarrhythmic, and sudden death has been reported in patients with structural heart disease who were taking class IC agents.
    - Verapamil for right ventricular outflow tract VT and verapamil-sensitive left ventricular VT
  - Atrial pacing at rates slightly faster than VT rates may suppress tachycardia.
  - Catheter ablation using radiofrequency energy or cryoenergy
  - Implantable cardioverter defibrillators

ONGOING CARE

PROGNOSIS

- Generally very good in patients with idiopathic VT and a structurally normal heart.
- Suppression of ventricular ectopy with exercise has a favorable prognosis.
- In patients with heart disease (congenital or acquired) or LQTS, VT may increase the risk of presyncope, syncope, and possibly sudden death.

COMPLICATIONS

- Cardiovascular compromise (sudden death)
- Acquired cardiomyopathy (from long-standing VT and a lack of AV synchrony)

PATIENT MONITORING

- Depends on the underlying cause
- ECG, Holter monitor, and exercise stress test

ADDITIONAL READING

- Gilbert-Barness E, Barness LA. Pathogenesis of cardiac conduction disorders in children: genetic and histopathologic aspects. *Am J Med Genet A*. 2006;140(19):1993–2006.
- Hebbar AK, Hueston WJ. Management of common arrhythmias: part II. Ventricular arrhythmias and arrhythmias in special populations. *Am Fam Physician*. 2002;65(12):2491–2496.
- Kleinman ME, Chameides L, Schexnayder SM, et al. Part 14: pediatric advanced life support: 2010 American Heart Association Guidelines for Cardiopulmonary Resuscitation and Emergency Cardiovascular Care. *Circulation*. 2010;122(18)(Suppl 3):S876–S908.
- Sarubbi B. The Wolff-Parkinson-White electrocardiogram pattern in athletes: how and when to evaluate the risk for dangerous arrhythmias. The opinion of the paediatric cardiologist. *J Cardiovasc Med (Hagerstown)*. 2006;7(4):271–278.
- Wren C. Cardiac arrhythmias in the fetus and newborn. *Semin Fetal Neonatal Med*. 2006;11(3): 182–190.
- Yabek SM. Ventricular arrhythmias in children with an apparently normal heart. *J Pediatr*. 1991;119 (1, Pt 1):1–11.

CODES

ICD10

- I47.2 Ventricular tachycardia
- I45.81 Long QT syndrome
- Q24.8 Other specified congenital malformations of heart

FAQ

- Q: Do frequent single PVCs require treatment?
- A: In an otherwise healthy child with a structurally normal heart, normal QT interval, and PVCs that suppress with exercise, no treatment is indicated.
- Q: Should siblings of patients with LQTS be evaluated?
- A: Yes. Siblings and parents (even if asymptomatic) should have an ECG, Holter monitor, and exercise stress test for definitive evaluation of the QT interval. Commercial genetic testing is currently available to detect mutations in some of the most common genes that cause the LQTS. The test will positively identify ~75% of patients with the LQTS. Genetic testing may be considered in patients in whom there is a high suspicion of LQTS.

VESICOURETERAL REFLUX

Michael H. Hsieh

BASICS

DESCRIPTION

Vesicoureteral reflux (VUR) occurs when urine passes backward from the bladder to the ureters or kidneys.

EPIDEMIOLOGY

Prevalence

VUR occurs in ~1% of children. There are 2 different groups of patients:

- Those who were detected prenatally without any history of urinary tract infection (UTI)
  - ~20–30% of patients with prenatal hydronephrosis have VUR. Screening this population for VUR is controversial.
  - The ratio of males to females in this group is 3:1. This ratio is believed to be caused by a period of high-pressure voiding in boys, which resolves by 18 months.
- Those who were detected after an acute UTI
  - ~30–50% of children with a febrile UTI will have VUR.

RISK FACTORS

Genetics

- 30% of siblings will have VUR (usually low-grade), and the great majority will have been asymptomatic with only rare renal scarring.
- Parents with VUR have a 60% chance of having children with VUR:
  - Whether or not to screen siblings is controversial as low-grade VUR usually resolves without treatment or sequelae.
  - One may elect to screen siblings with a history of recurrent febrile illnesses even in the absence of definitely diagnosed UTIs.

PATHOPHYSIOLOGY

- VUR in combination with UTI can lead to pyelonephritis, renal scarring, and possibly end-stage renal disease.
- Primary VUR is classified into 5 grades by the International Reflux Study based on the voiding cystourethrogram (VCUG):
  - Grade I: reflux into ureter
  - Grade II: reflux into renal pelvis without dilation of calyces
  - Grade III: blunting of calyces, mild dilation of ureter
  - Grade IV: grossly dilated ureter, moderate calyceal dilation with maintained papillary impressions
  - Grade V: grossly dilated ureter with loss of papillary impressions
- The grading scale is important because spontaneous resolution rates are very different between grades I–III and grades IV–V.

ETIOLOGY

- A combination of abnormal anatomy and abnormal voiding pressure:
  - Primary VUR results from either a short ureteral tunnel through the bladder wall or transient high-pressure voiding, which occurs normally in the first 18 months of life.
  - Patients with primary low-grade VUR can expect improvement and even resolution of the VUR with time as the ureteral tunnel grows or when bladder pressures decrease.
- Secondary VUR occurs when there is an associated lesion responsible for the abnormal anatomy or increased intravesical (bladder) pressure:
  - Patients with secondary reflux require treatment of their primary problem and still may require surgery to treat their secondary reflux.
  - Secondary reflux may occur in neurologically normal patients with bladder and bowel dysfunction, ureteroceles, posterior ureteral valves, and prune belly syndrome or in neurologically abnormal patients with spina bifida.
  - The distinction between primary and secondary reflux is important because large prospective trials have been conducted on patients with primary reflux and it is not appropriate to extend those findings to patients with secondary reflux.
  - Another important distinction is whether the diagnosis of VUR was made as a result of a prenatal diagnosis of hydronephrosis or whether the child presented with UTI.

DIAGNOSIS

HISTORY

- Prenatal dilation of the urinary tract or UTI as presentation
- Family or sibling history of VUR
- Family history of UTI, suggestive of infection-susceptible uroepithelium
- Family history of renal failure
- Voiding history: age at toilet training
- Daytime or nighttime incontinence
- Frequency of urination
- Sensation of emptying the bladder completely
- Signs of bladder and bowel dysfunction:
  - Urgency
  - Frequency
  - Damp underwear
  - Associated constipation: frequency of bowel movements, suggestive of pelvic floor immaturity
- Evidence of holding urine during a bladder contraction:
  - Squatting, crossing legs
  - Compressing urethra with heel (Vincent curtsy)

PHYSICAL EXAM

- Abdominal palpation (primarily to check for hard stool)
- Check for labial adhesions in girls
- Phimosis in boys
- Inspection and palpation of spine (possible neurogenic bladder)
- Blood pressure

DIAGNOSTIC TESTS & INTERPRETATION

Lab

A serum creatinine and urinalysis for proteinuria may be obtained if the renal ultrasound suggests significant renal scarring or in severe bilateral VUR.

Imaging

- Renal/bladder ultrasound
  - Ultrasound is usually obtained following a febrile UTI, or if the patient had a prenatal diagnosis of hydronephrosis, between the 2nd day and 1st week of life. The ultrasound is not as sensitive as dimercaptosuccinic acid (DMSA) scan for renal scarring.
  - The lack of hydronephrosis does not mean that the patient does not have VUR. However, renal bladder ultrasound is a useful tool for following renal growth.
- VCUG
  - A contrast study is necessary for the 1st VCUG to delineate the urethral anatomy in boys and to accurately grade the reflux in both sexes.
  - An age-appropriate volume should be instilled in the bladder. The voiding portion of the study is important because ~20% of VUR can be missed if voiding is not observed.
  - Follow-up VCUGs can be performed using radionuclide to decrease the radiation dose to the child.
  - Whether to routinely perform a VCUG for a "first" febrile UTI in children aged 2 months to 2 years is controversial
- DMSA renal scan
  - The most accurate way to diagnose pyelonephritis and renal scarring
  - It is not possible to predict which patients will develop scarring after an acute episode (unless they have prior scarring, which is a risk factor for future scarring).
  - If the diagnosis of upper tract infection versus cystitis is important, then the DMSA scan during an acute episode is useful.
  - DMSA is not usually helpful with afebrile UTI.
  - Some advocate using DMSA to identify high-risk patients requiring VCUG.

DIFFERENTIAL DIAGNOSIS

In the prenatally detected group, hydronephrosis can also be due to ureteropelvic or ureterovesical junction obstruction. The important task is to differentiate primary from secondary VUR so that the parents can be appropriately counseled.

TREATMENT

GENERAL MEASURES

- Four randomized controlled trials suggest that medical management (prophylactic antibiotics) and surgery have essentially equal outcomes in regard to hypertension, growth, and renal scarring. Surgery was more effective at preventing pyelonephritis.
- The rate of renal scarring was equal in the medical and surgical arms of the International Reflux Study. However, the timing of renal scarring was different: In the medically treated arm, new renal

scars continued to form during 5 years of follow-up, whereas in the surgical arm, the renal scars stopped within 10 months of surgery. Surgery was 95% successful in correcting reflux with a 4% complication rate. Surgery involves creation of a longer muscular backing for the ureter to create a flap-valve mechanism.

- Patients with low-grade reflux should be maintained on prophylactic antibiotics and surgery delayed because grades I–III have a significant rate of spontaneous resolution. Patients with high-grade reflux (grades IV–V) should be initially maintained on prophylactic antibiotics, but earlier consideration for surgical correction should be given due to the lower rate of spontaneous resolution. Likewise, patients with reflux and renal scarring should be considered for earlier surgery because they have already shown a propensity toward UTI and renal damage.
- Antibiotic prophylaxis does not mean treatment-dose antibiotics. The antibiotics chosen are highly concentrated in the urine, and the use of high doses only selects out resistant organisms and leads to complications such as yeast infections. Amoxicillin at 10–15 mg/kg/24 h is used for the first 2 months of life, then trimethoprim/sulfamethoxazole (40 mg/200 mg/5 mL) at 0.25 mL/kg/24 h (equivalent to 2–3 mg/kg daily of trimethoprim) or nitrofurantoin at 1–2 mg/kg/24 h.
- Patients who are detected with VUR in infancy should probably have a contrast VCUG at 18 months to 2 years to determine if VUR has resolved.
- In toilet-trained children, maintenance of a regular voiding pattern and regular bowel movements decreases the risk of febrile UTI and increases the chance of VUR resolution.
- Patients being managed on antibiotic prophylaxis undergo annual follow-up nuclear VCUG to document improvement or resolution of VUR. Grading is less precise with nuclear VCUG, but the radiation dose is lower. A renal ultrasound is also obtained to follow renal growth and check for gross renal scars.
- Indications for crossing over to surgery are as follows:
  - Patient or parent wishes
  - Nonadherence with medical therapy
  - Breakthrough infections while on medical therapy if a careful review of voiding habits demonstrates that bladder and bowel dysfunction is not responsible for the UTI. Lack of new renal scarring may also suggest that continued medical management is appropriate.
  - New renal scarring
  - Persistence of grades IV or V reflux after an appropriate period of antibiotic prophylaxis
- The use of injectable bulking agents has a 80–85% success 1 year after 1 treatment of low-grade VUR, with progressively decreasing success rate as the grade of VUR increases. Centers with more experience with injection have higher success rates. The minimally invasive nature of these treatments is balanced with a lower success rate. Deflux (dextranomer/hyaluronic acid) is the most commonly used injectable in the United States and is widely used in treating grades I–III VUR. Deflux treatment in higher grades of VUR and robotic and laparoscopic ureteral reimplantation are being explored in select patients.
- The use of continuous antibiotic prophylaxis has been questioned because although it decreases the risk of UTI for higher grade VUR, it has not been shown to decrease renal scarring compared to placebo. An NIH multi-institutional trial to determine the benefits of continuous prophylaxis versus placebo treatment is ongoing. The Swedish Reflux Trial showed a decreased rate of febrile UTI in girls with grades III–IV VUR who underwent injection therapy or prophylaxis, compared to those on surveillance. New renal scarring was less frequent in girls on prophylaxis compared to those on surveillance.
- The management of patients who continue to have VUR after several years of prophylactic antibiotics is controversial. Although most feel comfortable discontinuing antibiotics for boys with VUR after age 6 years because the risk of renal scarring is decreased and boys are at low risk for UTI, the adolescent girl is at increased risk for complications during pregnancy if she has a past history of UTI. The few studies on this subject seem to indicate that the patients with VUR and recurrent UTI are at risk for pregnancy-related complications whether or not the VUR has been surgically corrected, suggesting that the propensity toward UTI plays a more important role.

ONGOING CARE

FOLLOW-UP RECOMMENDATIONS

Patient Monitoring

Patients with renal scarring should have annual BP checks and urinalysis for proteinuria through adolescence.

PROGNOSIS

- In primary VUR, 80–90% of grades I and II reflux, 70% of grade III, 40% of grade IV, and 25% of grade V resolve over a 5-year period.
- The annual rate of spontaneous resolution is between 15% and 20% for grades I–III.
- Bilateral reflux is less likely to resolve than unilateral reflux.
- Patients age 5 years or older at presentation are less likely to resolve than those who present at <5 years of age.
- Reflux that appears in the filling phase of VCUG ("passive reflux") may be less likely to resolve than reflux that only appears during voiding phase.
- Ultimately, the goal is prevention of renal scarring rather than resolution of the reflux because low-pressure sterile reflux does not lead to renal scarring.
- Chronic kidney disease is very unlikely in the absence of bilateral grade III or higher VUR.

ADDITIONAL READING

- Brandstrom P, Neveus T, Sixt R, et al. The Swedish reflux trial: IV renal damage. *J Urol*. 2010;184(1):292–297.
- Elder JS, Diaz M, Caldamone AA, et al. Endoscopic therapy for vesicoureteral reflux: a meta-analysis. I. Reflux resolution and urinary tract infection. *J Urol*. 2006;175(2):716–722.
- Keren R, Carpenter M, Greenfield S, et al. Is antibiotic prophylaxis in children with vesicoureteral reflux effective in preventing pyelonephritis and renal scars? A randomized, controlled trial. *Pediatrics*. 2008;122(6):1409–1410.
- Pennesi M, Travan L, Peratoner L, et al. Is antibiotic prophylaxis in children with vesicoureteral reflux effective in preventing pyelonephritis and renal scars? A randomized, controlled trial. *Pediatrics*. 2008; 121(6):e1489–e1494.
- Peters C, Skoog S, Arant B Jr, et al. Summary of the AUA guideline on management of primary vesicoureteral reflux in children. *J Urol*. 2010;184(3):1134–1144.
- Subcommittee on Urinary Tract Infection. Urinary tract infection: clinical practice guideline for the diagnosis and management of the initial UTI in febrile infants and children 2 to 24 months. *Pediatrics*. 2011;128(3):595–610.

CODES

ICD10

- N13.70 Vesicoureteral-reflux, unspecified
- Q62.7 Congenital vesico-uretero-renal reflux
- N13.71 Vesicoureteral-reflux without reflux nephropathy

FAQ

- Q: How soon after a UTI should the VCUG be performed?
- A: Once the patient is clinically stable and afebrile and sterile urine has been documented, the VCUG can be performed.
- Q: Why not operate immediately to repair the reflux when it is diagnosed?
- A: Depending on the grade of reflux, many cases will resolve in time.

VIRAL HEPATITIS

Scott Elisofon

BASICS

DESCRIPTION
- Viral hepatitis is defined as a systemic viral infection, in which the predominant manifestation is that of hepatic injury and dysfunction.
- It is primarily caused by hepatotropic viruses, which include hepatitis A–E.
- 10% of cases are caused by other viruses, such as Epstein-Barr virus (EBV), cytomegalovirus (CMV), herpes simplex virus (HSV), varicella-zoster virus (VZV), rubella, parvovirus, adenovirus, enteroviruses, and others.

EPIDEMIOLOGY
Incidence
- Hepatitis A: ~17,000 cases per year in the United States. 8% occur in day care centers.
- Hepatitis B: 140,000–320,000 infections per year worldwide. ~40,000 U.S. cases per year
- Hepatitis C: 20,000 infections per year in the United States
- Hepatitis E: Common in poorly developed countries but rare in the United States.

Prevalence
- Hepatitis B: United States has a low prevalence with <1% of the population infected; higher rates in certain subgroups such as immigrants from endemic areas, homosexuals, and parenteral drug users
- Hepatitis C: United States has prevalence of 1.8%, representing ~3.9 million people (85% chronically infected).

RISK FACTORS
- Hepatitis A (transmission: fecal–oral)
  - Day care attendance, household exposure, travel to endemic areas, men who have sex with men
  - Maximum infectivity 2 weeks before jaundice
- Hepatitis B and C (transmission: blood, body fluids, and sexual contact)
  - Recipients of blood or blood products
  - IV drug users
  - Multiple sexual partners
  - Homosexual males
  - Body piercing and tattoos
  - HIV-positive status
  - Infants born to a mother with hepatitis B or C
  - Household contacts with hepatitis B or C

GENERAL PREVENTION
- Good sanitation, hygiene, vaccination, screening blood products, condom use, safe disposal of needles
- Hepatitis A
  - Vaccination of all children between the ages of 1 and 18 years, especially those travelling to endemic regions or those with liver disease
  - Vaccine (Havrix, Vaqta): 0.5-mL dose IM and 2nd dose 6–12 months later
  - Prior to travel to an endemic region, immune globulin 0.02 mL/kg should be given to children younger than 1 year of age and considered for children who are immunocompromised or have liver disease.
  - Infected patients should avoid return to day care center for 2 weeks after illness subsides.
  - Postexposure prophylaxis for children >1 year of age: hepatitis A vaccine
  - Postexposure prophylaxis for <1 year of age and immunocompromised individuals: immune globulin 0.02 mL/kg IM
- Hepatitis B
  - Screen all pregnant women.
  - Hepatitis B vaccine to all infants at birth; complete 3-vaccine series 0.5-mL dose IM during infancy.
  - Vaccine and hepatitis B immunoglobulin to high-risk infants
  - Mother's with previous vertical transmission should consult a high-risk obstetrician and hepatitis B expert at least 3–6 months prior to delivery of another infant.
- Hepatitis C
  - Elective C-section has not been shown to reduce vertical transmission.
  - During vaginal delivery, avoid fetal scalp monitoring and prolonged rupture of membranes >8 hours.
  - Avoid sharing of toothbrushes, nail clippers, and razors.
  - Breastfeeding is allowed, unless the mother has active bleeding from nipples.

PATHOPHYSIOLOGY
- Acute viral hepatitis tends to affect the liver parenchyma, whereas chronic viral hepatitis affects portal and periportal areas.
- Chronic viral hepatitis (B or C) is defined by continuing viral replication and inflammation of the liver for >6 months.
- Worsening injury leads to extensive fibrosis that occurs between portal tracts (portal bridging), nodular changes, and finally, cirrhosis.

DIAGNOSIS

HISTORY
- History should focus on risk factors for viral exposure, sick contacts, travel history, and high-risk behaviors.
- Family history of liver or autoimmune disease, medications, or drug and alcohol use should also be explored.

PHYSICAL EXAM
- Jaundice, hepatomegaly, or tenderness over the liver may or may not be present during acute infection.
- Signs and symptoms during acute infection:
  - Fever
  - Malaise and fatigue
  - Nausea and vomiting, anorexia
  - Jaundice: in hepatitis A, seen in 88% of adults but only 65% of children
  - Hepatomegaly
  - Right upper quadrant (RUQ) abdominal pain
  - Dark urine and pale stools
  - Arthralgias/arthritis
  - The vast majority of affected patients are minimally symptomatic or asymptomatic, especially with chronic infection.

DIAGNOSTIC TESTS & INTERPRETATION
Lab
- Liver tests
  - Marked elevation of aspartate aminotransferase/alanine aminotransferase (AST/ALT) during acute infection
  - May be normal to mildly elevated in chronically infected individuals
  - Bilirubin from mild to marked elevation
  - In severe hepatitis, monitor PT/INR, albumin, electrolytes, glucose, and CBC.
- Biochemical markers for each virus for diagnosis, management, and monitoring
  - Hepatitis A
    - Virus (HAV) IgM: recent infection
    - Anti-HAV IgG: past exposure or immunization-acquired
  - Hepatitis B
    - Surface antigen (HBsAg): current infection, acute or chronic
    - Surface antibody (HBsAb): immunized or resolved infection
    - "e" antigen (HBeAg): active viral replication; "infectious"
    - "e" antibody (HBeAb): end of severe infectivity (except in precore mutants). End point for many hepatitis B therapies and studies
    - Core antigen (HBcore) IgM: early phase of acute infection, not present in chronic HBV
    - Core total Ab: exposed to HBV
    - HBV DNA: quantification useful to assess viral load
    - HBV mutations: useful to assess resistance to treatment
    - HBV genotyping can sometimes be helpful in determining if interferon therapy would be beneficial (genotype D unfavorable for interferon use).
  - Hepatitis C
    - HCV Ab: exposure to HCV
    - HCV RNA: Quantitative, assess viral load; qualitative, assess presence/absence of virus.
    - HCV genotype: useful to determine duration of treatment and likelihood of response
  - Hepatitis D
    - HDV Ab: exposure to hepatitis D

Diagnostic Procedures/Other
Liver biopsy is often needed to determine type and extent of liver damage. It is usually indicated prior to initiation of antiviral therapy in children with hepatitis B or C.

Pathologic Findings
A wide array of histologic features is possible on liver biopsy, including inflammation, necrosis, and fibrosis, based on the severity and chronicity of disease.

DIFFERENTIAL DIAGNOSIS
- Many disorders give rise to elevated transaminases, and clues to a viral origin are based on the history, serology, and histologic findings.
- The diagnosis of "non A–E hepatitis" is often used when the cause is almost certainly viral, but no virus is isolated.
- Other possibilities include drug-induced, ischemic, alcoholic, autoimmune hepatitis, as well as Wilson disease or α_1-antitrypsin deficiency.

TREATMENT

MEDICATION

- Hepatitis A
  - No specific therapy is necessary for previously immunized or infected patients.
  - Postexposure prophylaxis is recommended for nonimmunized patients household contacts, intimate exposure contacts, and children and staff in nursery or day care centers with outbreaks.
  - Hepatitis A vaccine for children >1 year of age. Children <1 year of age or immunocompromised individuals should receive immune globulin 0.02 mL/kg IM × 1.
- Hepatitis B
  - Postexposure prophylaxis with hepatitis B vaccine and hepatitis B immunoglobulin (HBIG) is indicated for neonates born to mothers who are hepatitis B carriers and for unvaccinated individuals after sexual contact with carriers or accidental exposure to infected blood products.
  - Persons previously vaccinated with known titer >10 mIU/mL do not require any intervention, and children vaccinated with low titer need only a booster HBV vaccine.
  - There is no treatment for acute hepatitis B, although lamivudine is reported to be effective in fulminant HBV hepatitis.
  - Treatment is not usually considered when patients are immune tolerant (normal ALT, (HBeAg)-positive, with high HBV DNA).
  - Children should be monitored every 6–12 months with ALT, HBeAg, and HBeAb. When ALT is elevated, treatment is considered by hepatitis B experts.
  - Some pediatric studies suggest that antiviral therapy hastens but does not increase the rate of HBeAg seroconversion.
  - Medications that have been used for chronic hepatitis B include the following: interferon, peginterferon, lamivudine, adefovir, tenofovir, or entecavir.
  - Lamivudine is no longer routinely recommended in chronic HBV due to a high rate of resistance with prolonged treatment.
  - Adefovir dipivoxil and tenofovir are approved for children >12 years of age and entecavir for children >16 years of age.
  - The factor most predictive of treatment response in children with chronic hepatitis B is an elevated pretreatment ALT.
  - Each year, approximately 5% of children spontaneously clear HBeAg, at which point the disease usually becomes inactive, although a few will later reactivate.
- Hepatitis C
  - For acute hepatitis C, treatment with interferon in first 3 months after acquiring infection has been quite successful in adults and should be considered in children.
  - Antiviral therapy for chronic infection can be initiated at any time after 3 years of age, and is indicated for children with progressive or advanced disease
  - Pegylated interferon and ribavirin is currently the treatment of choice for chronic hepatitis C in children >3 years of age.
  - Treatment duration depends on genotype:
    - Genotypes 1 and 4: 1 year (type 1 most common in United States)
    - Genotypes 2 and 3: 6 months (types more likely to respond to therapy)
  - Several protease inhibitors, telaprevir and boceprevir, have recently been approved for treatment of chronic HCV in adults in combination with peginterferon and ribavirin.

General Measures

- Most cases of acute hepatitis do not require hospitalization.
- Dehydration, coagulopathy, or severe cases need inpatient care; monitor and correct coagulation defects and fluid, electrolyte, and acid–base imbalances.
- Report acute cases to public health department.
- Patients with acute liver failure should be transferred to a pediatric transplant center.

ONGOING CARE

FOLLOW-UP RECOMMENDATIONS

- For hepatitis B and C, serial measurement of serum AST/ALT, viral markers, α-fetoprotein, and ultrasound of the liver
- Liver biopsy pretreatment and for evaluation of disease progression

PROGNOSIS

- Hepatitis A
  - Mild disease usual
  - Rarely results in relapsing, fulminant, or cholestatic disease
  - No chronic liver disease
  - Mortality <1%
  - Protective antibodies develop in response to infection and persist for life.
- Hepatitis B
  - Fulminant hepatitis 1–2%
  - Mortality 0.8%
  - Chronic sequelae: Rate of chronicity is inversely proportional to age of acquisition: 90% in infants, 25% in ages 1–5 years, and 6–10% in older children; cirrhosis <5%, hepatocellular carcinoma
- Hepatitis C
  - Fulminant hepatitis 1%
  - Chronic sequelae: Infants infected via vertical transmission have 60–80% chance of chronic infection. Cirrhosis is uncommon, and hepatocellular carcinoma is rare in children and adolescents. If untreated, HCV can lead to advanced liver disease in adults.
  - HCV is the most common indication for liver transplantation in adults.

COMPLICATIONS

- Patients with advanced liver disease due to chronic hepatitis B or C are at risk of complications associated with cirrhosis and portal hypertension.
- Patients with chronic hepatitis B or with cirrhosis due to hepatitis C are at increased risk of hepatocellular carcinoma.
- Hepatitis B
  - Hepatitis D coinfection: Acute hepatitis B and D virus infection occur simultaneously.
  - Hepatitis D superinfection: Acute hepatitis D occurs in a chronic carrier of hepatitis B.

Pregnancy Considerations

Hepatitis E: mortality of 20% caused by acute liver failure in pregnant women

ADDITIONAL READING

- Daniels D, Grytdal S, Wasley A; Centers for Disease Control and Prevention. Surveillance for acute viral hepatitis—United States, 2007. *MMWR Surveill Summ*. 2009;58(3):1–27.
- Haber BA, Block JM, Jonas MM, et al. Recommendations for screening, monitoring, and referral of pediatric chronic hepatitis B. *Pediatrics*. 2009;124(5):e1007–e1013.
- Mack CL, Gonzalez-Peralta RP, Gupta N, et al. NASPGHAN practice guidelines: diagnosis and management of hepatitis C infection in infants, children, and adolescents. *J Pediatr Gastroenterol Nutr*. 2012;54(6):838–855.
- Mohan N, González-Peralta RP, Fujisawa T, et al. Chronic hepatitis C infection in children. *J Pediatr Gastroenterol Nutr*. 2010;50(2):123–131.
- Murray KF, Shah U, Mohan N, et al. Chronic hepatitis. *J Pediatr Gastroenterol Nutr*. 2010;47(2): 225–233.

CODES

ICD10

- B19.9 Unspecified viral hepatitis without hepatic coma
- B19.10 Unspecified viral hepatitis B without hepatic coma
- B19.20 Unspecified viral hepatitis C without hepatic coma

FAQ

- Q: Why do infants who acquire HBV at birth have a higher incidence of chronicity?
- A: The immaturity of the neonatal immune system contributes to the higher incidence of chronicity in this population.
- Q: Should a mother with HCV positivity breastfeed?
- A: Transmission of HCV via breast milk is unlikely.

VOLVULUS

Jeffrey R. Lukish

BASICS

DESCRIPTION

Volvulus represents an abnormal rotation (torsion) of the viscera that results in ischemia. Gastric, cecal, and midgut volvulus can occur. Midgut volvulus is the most common form in infants and children.

EPIDEMIOLOGY

- Malrotation with midgut volvulus occurs in 1 in 6,000 live births.
- Slightly more common in boys
- Most children with midgut volvulus present in the 1st month of life.

RISK FACTORS

- Children with malrotation have a narrow mesenteric vascular pedicle and are predisposed to volvulus.
- Familial associations can occur.
- The risk of volvulus in patients with malrotation does not decrease with age.

ETIOLOGY

Volvulus occurs due to failure of the fetal gut to undergo normal in utero rotation and fixation (malrotation), resulting in a narrow mesenteric vascular pedicle.

COMMONLY ASSOCIATED CONDITIONS

Up to 30% of children with malrotation have congenital heart disease. Additionally, 30–60% of patients with other congenital gastrointestinal (GI) malformations (gastroschisis, omphalocele, intestinal atresia, Hirschsprung disease) have malrotation.

DIAGNOSIS

HISTORY

- The primary presenting sign is the sudden onset of bilious vomiting.

ALERT

Infants and children with bilious emesis require evaluation to rule out malrotation and volvulus.

- Recurrent colicky abdominal pain
- Feeding intolerance
- Chylous ascites and/or protein-losing enteropathy due to lymphatic congestion and bacterial overgrowth
- In older children, recurrent abdominal pain and emesis and constipation
- Bloody stools or blood-tinged mucus per rectum can occur and can be late manifestations of ischemic bowel.

PHYSICAL EXAM

- Infants with volvulus may manifest complaints of severe pain without significant physical exam findings (out of proportion to physical exam).
- Abdominal tenderness (mild to severe)
- Irritability, lethargy
- Palpable abdominal mass
- Edema of abdominal wall (late finding)
- Flexion of legs
- Tachypnea and tachycardia
- Hypotension (late finding)

ALERT

Pitfalls in management include the following:

- Delay in diagnosis
- Failure to recognize the key sign of bilious emesis
- Failure to recognize colicky pain (in infants) or cyclic bilious emesis (in older children) as possible manifestations of malrotation
- Failure to order the diagnostic study (a limited upper gastrointestinal series ["upper GI"]) to evaluate the duodenal sweep

DIAGNOSTIC TESTS & INTERPRETATION

Lab

Laboratory analysis is unpredictable. May see elevated acute phase reactants, leukocytosis, metabolic acidosis, and thrombocytopenia

Imaging

- No imaging modality is 100% sensitive.
  - The goal is to delineate whether the duodenum follows a normal sweep to the right of the vertebral bodies before transition to the jejunum.
  - The 3rd portion of the duodenum crosses behind the superior mesenteric artery to the left of the vertebral body at L1 and rises to the level of the pyloric bulb before transition into the jejunum.
- Plain radiographs
  - Can be normal or show a paucity of bowel gas
  - A dilated stomach and duodenum (double bubble) can be present.
- Abdominal ultrasound
  - May show inversion of normal position of superior mesenteric artery (SMA) and superior mesenteric vein (SMV)
  - If SMA is to the right of the SMV, malrotation may be present.
  - The ultrasound has a sensitivity of 80%.
- Upper GI tract (contrast) radiography
  - May show abnormal position of the ligament of Treitz and, if volvulus is present, a corkscrew appearance of the midgut
  - The upper GI is approximately 95% sensitive for identifying malrotation.
  - False positives may occur in children with a distended stomach or ileus. In these cases, the ligament of Treitz is then pushed into an abnormal position.
- Barium enema (BE)
  - Can be useful in evaluating the position of the colon and cecum
  - The sensitivity of BE for diagnosing malrotation and volvulus is 75%.
  - In cases of cecal, sigmoid, or transverse colonic volvulus, contrast enema shows a beak deformity at site of volvulus.

DIFFERENTIAL DIAGNOSIS

- Ileus
- Intestinal atresia
- Perforated viscus
- Necrotizing enterocolitis
- Meconium ileus or meconium plug syndrome
- Hirschsprung enterocolitis
- Appendicitis
- Intussusception
- Pyelonephritis

TREATMENT

GENERAL MEASURES

- Any child who presents with bilious emesis and an acute abdomen may require emergent surgical exploration. The concern for midgut volvulus is paramount, and delays for further workup may not be warranted.

- Intravenous fluid resuscitation is indicated, until normal urine output is established.
- Nasogastric decompression and intravenous antibiotics are indicated.

SURGERY/OTHER PROCEDURES

- Laparotomy with reduction of the torsion and inspection of the bowel for necrosis or ischemia
- The Ladd procedure consists of 4 components:
  - Reduction and untwisting of the volvulus by a 360-degree counterclockwise rotation of the midgut
  - Division of abnormal adhesions extending over the duodenum (Ladd bands) that are transfixing the cecum in the right upper quadrant
  - Division and opening of the mesenteric attachments to provide a wider vascular base to the midgut and appendectomy
  - Removal of the appendix: The appendix is removed because it is in a highly unusual place and would result in a diagnostic dilemma should the child develop appendicitis.
- Many surgeons can perform the Ladd procedure laparoscopically.
- Second-look operations may be indicated if a large portion of the midgut is ischemic; the volvulus may be reduced with reexploration in 12–24 hours.
- On rare occasions, bowel resection and ostomy may be necessary.

ONGOING CARE

FOLLOW-UP RECOMMENDATIONS

Patient Monitoring

- Prognosis depends on extent of involvement and degree of bowel ischemia.
- A majority of these children develop a profound ileus and require TPN for days or potentially weeks postoperatively.
- Third-space volume loss is common postoperatively. Monitoring of intake/output is critical to maintain euvolemia.
- Postoperative small bowel obstruction and even recurrent volvulus can occur.

COMPLICATIONS

- Recurrent volvulus (occurs in 2% of patients)
- Short gut syndrome
- Adhesive bowel obstruction
- Wound infection and abdominal abscess

ADDITIONAL READING

- Draus JM Jr, Foley DS, Bond SJ. Laparoscopic Ladd procedure: a minimally invasive approach to malrotation without midgut volvulus. *Am Surg.* 2007;73(7):693–696.
- El-Gohary Y, Alagtal M, Gillick J. Long-term complications following operative intervention for intestinal malrotation: a 10-year review. *Pediatr Surg Int.* 2010;26(2):203–206.
- Fonio P, Coppolino F, Russo A. Ultrasonography (US) in the assessment of pediatric non traumatic gastrointestinal emergencies. *Crit Ultrasound J.* 2013;5(Suppl 1):S12.
- Ladd WE. Surgical diseases of the alimentary tract in infants. *N Engl J Med.* 1936;215:705–708.
- Malek MM, Burd RS. Surgical treatment of malrotation after infancy: a population-based study. *J Pediatr Surg.* 2005;40(1):285–289.
- Nagdeve NG, Qureshi AM, Bhingare PD, et al. Malrotation beyond infancy. *J Pediatr Surg.* 2012; 47(11):2026–2032.
- Sizemore A, Rabbani K, Ladd A, et al. Diagnostic performance of the upper gastrointestinal series in the evaluation of children with clinically suspected malrotation. *Pediatr Radiol.* 2008;38(5):518–528.
- Stephens LR, Donoghue V, Gillick J. Radiological versus clinical evidence of malrotation, a tortuous tale—10-year review. *Eur J Pediatr Surg.* 2012; 22(3):238–242.

CODES

ICD10

- K56.2 Volvulus
- K31.89 Other diseases of stomach and duodenum
- Q43.8 Other specified congenital malformations of intestine

FAQ

- Q: When should workup for volvulus be initiated?
- A: In any child with bilious vomiting.
- Q: What is the best diagnostic study to confirm the diagnosis?
- A: Limited upper GI to evaluate the duodenal sweep and position of the ligament of Treitz.
- Q: What is the most common age of presentation of volvulus?
- A: In the 1st month of life; however, it can occur in any age.
- Q: What are the other types of volvulus that have been reported in children?
- A: Gastric, small bowel, and colonic volvulus can occur in children. Gastric volvulus presents with abdominal pain and retching. Two types occur: meso-axial (rotation about the lesser and greater curvature) and organo-axial (rotation around the longitudinal axis of the stomach). A majority of these children have structural abnormality of the stomach such as asplenia or abnormal fixation to the esophagus. Both small bowel and colonic volvulus present similarly to midgut volvulus, with high-grade bowel obstruction, abdominal pain, and bilious vomiting.
- Q: Can volvulus occur in teenagers and young adults?
- A: Yes. Age is not a determinant of presentation of volvulus, which may occur in older children and adults. As in infants, catastrophic consequences can occur, including entire midgut loss.
- Q: Who developed the Ladd procedure?
- A: William Edwards Ladd, MD (1880–1967) first described the procedure in 1936. He was a pioneer in the field of pediatric surgery. He was the first surgeon-in-chief at Boston Children's Hospital and coauthored the first pediatric surgical textbook.

VOMITING

Peter D. Ngo

BASICS

DESCRIPTION

- Vomiting is the forceful expulsion of gastric contents through the mouth.
  - Vomiting is a prominent feature of many disorders of infancy and childhood.
  - It is often the only presenting symptom of many diseases.
- Regurgitation is defined as small, effortless mouthfuls of food or stomach contents.
- Retching is contraction of the abdominal musculature against a closed glottis, restricting expulsion of stomach contents (also referred to as "dry heaves").

PATHOPHYSIOLOGY

- Vomiting can be:
  - A defense mechanism to expel ingested toxins
  - An abnormality of, or damage to, the postrema area of the brain (a.k.a. the chemoreceptor trigger zone or vomiting center), which is located at the base of the fourth ventricle
  - A result of intestinal obstruction or anatomic abnormalities
  - Due to chronic gastrointestinal mucosal disease
  - The result of a generalized metabolic disease
  - A result of increased intracranial pressure

DIAGNOSIS

HISTORY

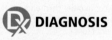

- A full history should include medication and drug use, trauma, family history of migraines and chronic gastrointestinal diseases, and travel history.
- Special attention should be directed to the timing of the emesis, relationship to meals, position and time of day, as well as to the chronicity of symptoms.
- Fever: may suggest an infectious etiology
- Abdominal pain and frequent, forceful, or bilious emesis
  - Often associated with anatomic or obstructive intestinal disorder
  - For example, obstruction of a lumen (i.e., common bile duct stone or ureteropelvic junction [UPJ] obstruction) can present as vomiting.
- Age of patient
  - Some etiologies of vomiting may be aged-based.
  - For example, pyloric stenosis or inborn errors of metabolism should be considered in infants with vomiting, dehydration, and biochemical abnormalities.
  - In adolescents, disordered eating patterns (bulimia) and the possibility of pregnancy should be considered.
- Mental retardation, pica, and patchy baldness: indicate foreign body or hair ingestion and the development of a gastric bezoar
- Nausea and epigastric pain related to meals: often indicate gastritis, gastric emptying delay, or gallbladder disease
- Symptoms alleviated by meals: may signify gastroesophageal reflux or gastric ulcer
- Alternating vomiting and lethargy: may indicate intussusception
- Chronic headaches, fatigue, weakness, weight loss, and early morning vomiting: neurologic causes of vomiting secondary to increased intracranial pressure
- Right- or left-sided abdominal pain: may indicate renal disease
- Recurrent, intermittent episodes of vomiting interspersed with periods of wellness may suggest cyclic vomiting syndrome (CVS).
- Recurrent vomiting and other gastrointestinal symptoms are commonly seen with mucosal diseases such as celiac disease, eosinophilic esophagitis, and inflammatory bowel disease.

PHYSICAL EXAM

A careful and complete physical examination can often contribute to determining the cause of vomiting in children:

- Visible bowel loops: obstruction
- Palpation for bowel loops and tenderness and auscultation for evidence of absent bowel sounds or borborygmi (rumbling bowel sounds): intestinal obstruction
- Rectal examination: testing the stool for occult blood
- Discoloration of skin and sclera: jaundice (liver/gallbladder or metabolic disease)
- Orange tint of sclera or skin: hypervitaminosis A
- Unusual odor: metabolic disease, diabetic ketoacidosis
- Chronic vomiting: evidence of neurologic dysfunction, including nystagmus, head tilt, papilledema, abnormal reflexes, and weakness
- Tense anterior fontanelle: may indicate meningitis, hydrocephalus, or vitamin A toxicity
- Enlarged parotid glands and hypersalivation: bulimia and other feeding disorders
- Pelvic examination: pregnancy, pelvic inflammatory disease, or ovarian disease

DIAGNOSTIC TESTS & INTERPRETATION

Lab

- CBC
  - Anemia and iron deficiency can occur with gastritis/esophagitis, inflammatory bowel disease, celiac disease, and ulcer disease.
- Blood chemistry
  - Electrolyte abnormalities are found in pyloric stenosis and metabolic disease.
  - An elevated alanine aminotransferase, conjugated bilirubin, and gamma-glutamyl transferase (GGT) can indicate liver, gallbladder, or metabolic disease.
- Urinalysis: pyelonephritis, nephrolithiasis
- Lipase/amylase: pancreatitis
- BUN/creatinine: Elevated levels can occur with renal disease.
- Urine culture: UTI
- Stool studies: occult blood, infection, *Helicobacter pylori* antigen
- If chronic vomiting history
  - Tissue transglutaminase IgA, endomysial antibody, or deamidated gliadin IgA and serum IgA (celiac disease)
  - Erythrocyte sedimentation rate and/or C-reactive protein (inflammatory bowel disease but can also be elevated in acute infection/illness)

Imaging

- Plain abdominal radiographic study
  - Can detect ileus and/or obstruction
  - May also need upright or left lateral decubitus films
- Abdominal ultrasound
  - Liver, gallbladder, renal, pancreatic, ovarian, or uterine disease
  - In infants, abdominal ultrasound is the test of choice for pyloric stenosis.
  - Useful when considering abdominal abscess and appendicitis
  - Can detect intussusception
- Contrast radiography
  - Intestinal anatomic abnormalities (e.g., malrotation, intussusception, volvulus, hiatal hernia), gastric bezoar, achalasia
- Gastric scintigraphy (gastric emptying study)
  - Evaluate rate of gastric emptying; assess for gastroparesis.
- Abdominal CT
  - Not generally indicated for evaluation of vomiting, although it is an effective tool when more anatomic abdominal detail is required (abscess, tumor).
- Head CT
  - Can be helpful in evaluation of acute neurologic causes of vomiting (i.e., cerebrovascular insult; hydrocephalus)
- Brain MRI
  - Provides superior imaging of the brain stem, where the vomiting center is located, without radiation exposure
  - Test of choice if considering intracranial mass

Diagnostic Procedures/Surgery

- Upper endoscopy
  - Can identify esophageal, gastric, and duodenal inflammation (reflux esophagitis, eosinophilic esophagitis, gastritis, ulcer disease, celiac disease)
  - Provides means to obtain biopsies or cultures for infections (*H. pylori*, duodenal *Giardia*, cytomegalovirus gastritis)
- Gastroesophageal and antroduodenal manometry: can be used to evaluate for primary or secondary motility disorders, evaluation of suspected rumination syndrome

DIFFERENTIAL DIAGNOSIS
- Disorders of gastrointestinal tract:
  - Anatomic
    - Esophageal: stricture, web, ring, atresia
    - Stomach: pyloric stenosis, web, hiatal hernia
    - Intestine: duodenal atresia, malrotation, duplication
    - Colon: Hirschsprung disease, imperforate anus
  - Motility
    - Achalasia
    - Gastroesophageal reflux
    - Intestinal pseudoobstruction
    - Gastroparesis
    - Ileus
  - Obstruction
    - Foreign body/bezoar
    - Intussusception
    - Stricturing Crohn disease
    - Volvulus
    - Incarcerated hernia
  - Eosinophilic esophagitis
  - Hepatobiliary disease
  - Appendicitis
  - Necrotizing enterocolitis
  - Peritonitis
  - Celiac disease
  - Peptic ulcer
  - Trauma
    - Duodenal hematoma
    - Pancreatitis (pseudocyst)
- Neurologic
  - Intracranial mass lesions:
    - Tumor
    - Cyst
    - Subdural hematoma
  - Cerebral edema
  - Hydrocephalus
  - Pseudotumor cerebri
  - Arnold-Chiari malformation
  - Migraine (head, abdominal)
  - Seizures
  - Postconcussion syndrome
- Renal
  - Obstructive uropathy
    - UPJ obstruction
    - Hydronephrosis
    - Nephrolithiasis
  - Renal insufficiency
  - Glomerulonephritis
  - Renal tubular acidosis
- Metabolic
  - Inborn errors of metabolism:
    - Galactosemia
    - Fructose intolerance
    - Hereditary fructose intolerance
    - Amino acid or organic acid metabolism
    - Urea cycle defects
    - Fatty acid oxidation disorders
    - Lactic acidosis
- Infection
  - Sepsis
  - Meningitis
  - UTI
  - *H. pylori*
  - Parasites
  - *Giardia*
  - Viral/bacterial gastroenteritis
  - Viral hepatitis (A, B, C)
  - Pneumonia
  - *Bordetella pertussis*
  - Streptococcal pharyngitis
- Endocrine
  - Diabetes
    - Diabetic ketoacidosis
    - Diabetic gastroparesis
  - Adrenal insufficiency
- Respiratory
  - Sinusitis
  - Laryngitis
- Immunologic
  - Food allergy
  - Anaphylaxis
  - Graft-versus-host disease
  - Chronic granulomatous disease
- Other:
  - Pregnancy
  - Rumination
  - Bulimia
  - Motion sickness
  - CVS
  - Overfeeding
  - Pain
  - Cannabinoid hyperemesis
  - Medications:
    - Drugs (chemotherapy)
    - Vitamin toxicity
  - Vascular (superior mesenteric artery syndrome)
  - Porphyria
  - Familial dysautonomia

ALERT
Vomiting accompanied by hematemesis, intestinal obstruction (bilious vomiting), dehydration, neurologic dysfunction, or an acute abdomen should be treated as a medical emergency, and hospitalization should be considered.

TREATMENT
- Potential therapeutic interventions are broad, and therapy should be directed toward the underlying etiology.
- Historically, empiric antiemetic medications were contraindicated in cases of acute vomiting, although more recent studies suggest ondansetron may reduce frequency of admission.
- Oral rehydration therapy is typically the first line of treatment. IV fluids are appropriate if oral rehydration therapy fails or are contraindicated.
- Neurotransmitters involved in vomiting include dopamine, acetylcholine, histamine, endorphins, serotonin, and neurokinins. The mechanism of many antiemetic medications is blockade of these neurotransmitters.

ISSUES FOR REFERRAL
- Chronic vomiting (2–3 weeks)
- Weight loss
- Severe abdominal pain or irritability
- Gastrointestinal bleeding
- Bilious emesis
- Evidence of intestinal obstruction
- Serum electrolyte abnormalities
- Abnormal neurologic examination
- Dehydration
- Signs of acute abdomen
- Lethargy

ADDITIONAL READING

- Fedorowicz Z, Jagannath VA, Carter B. Antiemetics for reducing vomiting related to acute gastroenteritis in children and adolescents. *Cochrane Database Syst Rev*. 2011;(9):CD005506.
- Freedman SB, Adler M, Seshadri R, et al. Oral ondansetron for gastroenteritis in a pediatric emergency department. *N Engl J Med*. 2006;354(16):1698–1705.
- Li B, Misiewicz L. Cyclic vomiting syndrome: a brain-gut disorder. *Gastroenterol Clin North Am*. 2003;32(3):997–1019.
- Li BK, Sunku BK. Vomiting and nausea. In: Wyllie R, Hyams JS, eds. *Pediatric Gastrointestinal and Liver Disease*. 4th ed. Philadelphia: Saunders; 2011.

CODES
ICD10
- R11.10 Vomiting, unspecified
- P92.1 Regurgitation and rumination of newborn

FAQ
- Q: What are the most common causes of nonbilious vomiting in an infant?
- A: Gastroesophageal reflux and milk protein allergy, although hypertrophic pyloric stenosis, sepsis, and malrotation must be considered.
- Q: What is appropriate management of a 6-month-old presenting with an episode of bilious emesis and lethargy?
- A: Referral for emergent abdominal ultrasound and surgical consult for possible intussusception
- Q: Is bilious emesis always associated with small bowel obstruction?
- A: Repeated episodes of vomiting can cause duodenal contents to reflux into the stomach resulting in bile-stained emesis without small bowel obstruction. Nevertheless, evaluation should include high suspicion and workup for possible obstruction.

VON WILLEBRAND DISEASE

Char Witmer

BASICS

DESCRIPTION

- An inherited bleeding disorder caused by either a quantitative or qualitative defect of the von Willebrand protein
- Characterized by mucocutaneous bleeding or bleeding after surgical procedures

EPIDEMIOLOGY

Prevalence

The prevalence of von Willebrand disease in the general pediatric population is estimated to be ~1%.

RISK FACTORS

Genetics

- The gene for von Willebrand factor is found on chromosome 12.
- Type 1 (see "Pathophysiology") follows an autosomal dominant inheritance pattern with variable penetrance.
- Type 2 can be autosomal dominant or recessive.
- Type 3 follows an autosomal recessive inheritance pattern.

GENERAL PREVENTION

- Avoid contact sports.
- For patients with recurrent epistaxis, measures should be taken to avoid drying of the mucosa by applying petroleum jelly, humidifying the air, and reducing trauma to the nasal mucosa by keeping the fingernails short and discouraging nose picking.
- It may be advisable for patients to wear an emergency ID bracelet indicating that they have von Willebrand disease in the event they are involved in an accident that renders them unconscious.
- Avoid medications that negatively affect platelet function (i.e., ibuprofen, aspirin).
- Combination oral contraceptive pills are very effective for some patients with menorrhagia.
- Appropriate hemostatic therapy is needed prior to dental or surgical procedures to prevent bleeding.

PATHOPHYSIOLOGY

- Von Willebrand factor is a large multimeric protein that allows platelets to adhere to sites of endothelial injury, initiating the primary step in hemostasis—formation of the platelet plug.
- Von Willebrand factor also serves as a carrier for factor VIII in the peripheral circulation, protecting it from degradation. Deficiency of von Willebrand factor results in a shorter factor VIII half-life, causing a lower level of circulating factor VIII.
- When von Willebrand factor is either deficient or defective, primary hemostasis is compromised, resulting in a bleeding diathesis characterized by easy bruising, frequent epistaxis, menorrhagia, and prolonged bleeding following surgical or dental procedures.
- Acquired forms of von Willebrand disease have been described in association with hypothyroidism, Wilms tumor, other neoplasms, cardiovascular disorders with increased shear stress (aortic stenosis), myeloproliferative disorders, uremia, and medications, including ciprofloxacin, griseofulvin, and valproate therapy.
- Classification: There are three major categories of von Willebrand disease:
  - Type 1
    - Mild to moderate quantitative deficiency
    - The most common type, accounting for 70–80% of patients
    - Generally a mild bleeding disorder
  - Type 2
    - Qualitative deficiency of von Willebrand factor
    - Diagnosed in 15–20% of patients
    - Tend to have more significant bleeding symptoms than in type 1
    - Type 2 von Willebrand disease is further classified into four subtypes.
    - Type 2A: loss of the intermediate- and high-molecular-weight multimers. The loss is secondary to either abnormal assembly or secretion of multimers or increased proteolytic degradation. The multimer deficiency results in decreased platelet binding.
    - Type 2B: an abnormal von Willebrand factor that spontaneously binds to normal platelets, resulting in accelerated clearance of these platelets and loss of high-molecular-weight multimers. This can result in mild thrombocytopenia.
    - Type 2N: The abnormal von Willebrand factor does not bind factor VIII optimally. This decrease in binding results in a shorter plasma half-life of factor VIII, resulting in reduced plasma factor VIII levels. Type 2N can be confused with mild hemophilia.
    - Type 2M: The abnormal von Willebrand factor fails to bind normally to platelets. Normal multimers
  - Type 3
    - Near-complete quantitative deficiency of von Willebrand factor, which also results in a secondary deficiency of factor VIII
    - Accounts for <5% of patients and results in a severe bleeding disorder

DIAGNOSIS

HISTORY

- A family history of von Willebrand disease or bleeding tendency is an important question in the evaluation for von Willebrand disease. However, be aware that variation in frequency and severity of bleeding symptoms can occur from person to person, even within an affected family.
- Bruising is common, with increased quantity, increased size (>5 cm), and often in unusual locations with minimal trauma.
- Recurrent and/or prolonged epistaxis
- Menorrhagia occurs in 70–90% of women with von Willebrand disease.
- Excessive posttraumatic or postsurgical bleeding

PHYSICAL EXAM

- Bruises: increased number, size, and/or unusual location
- May be entirely normal

DIAGNOSTIC TESTS & INTERPRETATION

Lab

- Screening tests for a bleeding disorder:
  - Prothrombin time (PT) is normal in von Willebrand disease.
  - Activated partial thromboplastin time (aPTT) may be prolonged if there is a decrease in factor VIII levels but can be normal.
  - Platelet count is normal except in type 2B patients, who may have mild thrombocytopenia.
  - Bleeding time is usually prolonged but may be normal in patients with mild type 1 von Willebrand disease (not recommended as a screening test).
  - Platelet function assay (PFA)-100 is usually prolonged but may be normal in mild type 1 von Willebrand disease (not recommended as a screening test).
- Specific tests for von Willebrand disease include the following:
  - Von Willebrand factor antigen: quantitation of von Willebrand factor by immunoassay
  - Von Willebrand factor activity (ristocetin cofactor): assesses the function of von Willebrand factor using the antibiotic ristocetin, which induces platelet aggregation in the presence of von Willebrand factor
  - Factor VIII: factor VIII clotting activity
  - Von Willebrand factor multimers: multiple molecular forms of von Willebrand factor evaluated on agarose gel
    - Multimer analysis is important in delineating the type of von Willebrand disease. Do not send as part of the initial screening for von Willebrand disease.

DIFFERENTIAL DIAGNOSIS

- Primary hemostatic disorders
  - Platelet function abnormalities, congenital thrombocytopenia
  - Mild inherited coagulation factor deficiencies
  - Hemophilia A
- Acquired and secondary hemostatic disorders
  - Liver disease
  - Uremia
  - Acquired thrombocytopenia
  - Drugs that affect platelet function
  - Acquired factor inhibitors (extremely rare in children)
- Connective tissue disorders
  - Ehlers-Danlos syndrome
  - Scurvy
- Prolonged aPTT but no bleeding symptoms
  - Inhibitor
  - Factor XII deficiency

ALERT

- The diagnosis of von Willebrand disease is not always straightforward.
- Because of normal physiologic variation in plasma levels of von Willebrand factor, repeated measurements over time may be necessary to establish the diagnosis.
- Conditions that may increase von Willebrand factor levels:
  - The newborn period
  - Surgery
  - Liver disease
  - Hyperthyroidism
  - High-stress states
  - Pregnancy
  - Inflammatory or infectious disease
  - Steroids
  - Oral contraceptives (high dose)
  - Other estrogens

TREATMENT

GENERAL MEASURES

- There are several options for the management of bleeding in patients with von Willebrand disease. Superficial bleeding can usually be stopped by applying local pressure, ice, or topical thrombin, particularly in type 1.
- There are two main approaches to systemic therapy in von Willebrand disease: increasing the release of endogenous von Willebrand factor or exogenous replacement of von Willebrand factor. The appropriate therapy depends on the type of von Willebrand disease and the clinical scenario.

MEDICATION

- Desmopressin (DDAVP) is a synthetic analog of vasopressin that stimulates endothelial cell release of von Willebrand factor. It is effective in patients who have a functional von Willebrand factor, as in type 1 von Willebrand disease. It may be used for some patients with type 2 von Willebrand disease but is ineffective in type 3:
  - Available in intravenous and intranasal formulations
  - An infusion of 0.3 μg/kg results in a 3–5-fold increase in von Willebrand factor and factor VIII; nasal administration is slightly less effective.
  - Side effects include facial flushing, lightheadedness, or nausea.
  - Prior to use in a surgical setting, patients should have a trial to demonstrate an appropriate response (10% of patients do not respond).
  - May worsen thrombocytopenia in type 2B; it is not recommended
  - DDAVP may not be useful when prolonged hemostasis is required. After 24–48 hours, there is depletion of stored von Willebrand factor, causing it to be ineffective (tachyphylaxis).
  - It is important to remember that DDAVP will also cause fluid retention and, in some cases, hyponatremia. This can be avoided with fluid restriction for 24 hours following treatment.
- Factor concentrates
  - Humate-P or Alphanate
  - Plasma-derived, intermediate-purity factor VIII concentrate products with adequate levels (especially large multimers) of von Willebrand factor
  - Therapy of choice for some patients with type 2 von Willebrand disease and all patients with type 3 von Willebrand disease
  - Useful in type 1 von Willebrand disease when prolonged hemostasis is necessary
- Antifibrinolytics: aminocaproic acid or tranexamic acid
  - Stabilize the fibrin clot by inhibiting the physiologic process of clot lysis
  - Best for oral mucosal bleeding

ONGOING CARE

PROGNOSIS

- Von Willebrand disease type 1 is often a very mild bleeding disorder and may go undetected.
- Most patients with von Willebrand disease have a normal life expectancy and, with proper education and treatment, minimal risk for permanent disability.
- Type 3 von Willebrand disease is a severe bleeding disorder, and life-threatening hemorrhage can occur.

COMPLICATIONS

- Significant perioperative bleeding can occur, especially with tonsillectomy, but the most common complications are recurrent epistaxis, prolonged bleeding with cuts and abrasions, and menorrhagia.
- Patients with type 3 von Willebrand disease have a more severe bleeding disorder and can have bleeding complications similar to those seen in hemophilia such as hemarthroses and intracranial hemorrhage.

ADDITIONAL READING

- Cox Gill J. Diagnosis and treatment of von Willebrand disease. *Hematol Oncol Clin North Am*. 2004;18(6):1277–1299.
- Mannucci PM. Treatment of von Willebrand's Disease. *N Engl J Med*. 2004;351(7):683–694.
- Mohri H. Acquired von Willebrand syndrome: features and management. *Am J Hematol*. 2006;81(8):616–623.
- Pruthi RK. A practical approach to genetic testing for von Willebrand disease. *Mayo Clin Proc*. 2006; 81(5):679–691.
- Robertson J, Lillicrap D, James PD. Von Willebrand disease. *Pediatr Clin North Am*. 2008;55(2):377–392.

CODES

ICD10

D68.0 Von Willebrand's disease

FAQ

- Q: What sports activities can a person with von Willebrand disease participate in safely?
- A: People with type 1 von Willebrand disease can participate in most activities, although it is usually advised to avoid situations in which significant trauma takes place, like contact sports such as football or boxing. Patients with type 3 von Willebrand disease should avoid activities with moderate trauma. For type 2 patients, the risk of bleeding varies.
- Q: Is life expectancy lower in people with von Willebrand disease?
- A: For most patients with von Willebrand disease, their life expectancy and quality of life will be normal.
- Q: Are there any medications contraindicated in a patient with von Willebrand disease?
- A: Aspirin should not be given, as it interferes with platelet function. Nonsteroidal anti-inflammatory agents cause a milder effect on platelets and should also be avoided when possible. Patients should use acetaminophen for fever or pain.

WARTS

Prina P. Amin • Erika Abramson

BASICS

DESCRIPTION

- Warts (verrucae) are common, benign, and frequently self-limited epithelial growths caused by human papillomavirus (HPV) infection of keratinocytes.
- Types of warts
  - Cutaneous
    - Common warts (verruca vulgaris)
    - Flat warts (verruca plana)
    - Plantar warts (weight-bearing)
  - Anogenital
  - Laryngeal (laryngeal papillomatosis)

EPIDEMIOLOGY

Prevalence

- Cutaneous warts
  - Mostly affect children and young adults
  - Affect girls more than boys
  - 5.3% prevalence from age 6 to 15 years of age
  - Up to 1/3 of school-aged children have had warts.
- Anogenital warts
  - Exact prevalence in children and adolescents is unknown.
  - Approximately 1% of sexually active adults have external genital warts.
- Laryngeal warts
  - Rare with no known cure; transmission occurs in utero or through birth canal

RISK FACTORS

- Direct or indirect contact
- Autoinoculation can cause persistent infection and spread.
- Use of communal pool surfaces, bathrooms, and shower rooms increases risk.
- Areas of skin trauma and breakdown have increased susceptibility to HPV infection.
- Regularly walking barefoot outside also increases risk.
- Excessive foot perspiration
- Immunosuppressed patients, particularly transplant patients, are highly vulnerable.
- Individual susceptibility factors related to developing warts after exposure to HPV are less clear.

GENERAL PREVENTION

- Cutaneous warts
  - Use protective footwear in warm, moist environments and communal areas.
  - Wear cotton socks and change twice a day, especially if significant perspiration.
  - Avoid sharing nail files.
  - Avoid scratching and nail-biting to prevent autoinoculation.
- Anogenital warts
  - Avoid sexual contact with multiple partners.
  - Condoms may be protective.
  - Quadrivalent HPV vaccine protects against HPV subtypes 6, 11, 16, and 18.
  - Recommended universally for males and females, ages 9–26 years

PATHOPHYSIOLOGY

- Warts are caused by HPV infection of the epithelium.
- HPV replication leads to cell proliferation and formation of characteristic lesions.

ETIOLOGY

- Over 150 subtypes of HPV exist.
- Certain subtypes have a predilection for particular body sites and produce characteristic lesions:
  - Plantar and common palmar warts often caused by HPV 1 and 2
  - Anogenital warts commonly caused by HPV 6, 11, 16, 18, 31, and 45
  - Laryngeal papillomatosis is associated with HPV 6 and 11.

DIAGNOSIS

HISTORY

- Ask about risk factors for warts.
- Assess history of warts in close contacts (caregiver).
- Assess for immunosuppression.
- For anogenital warts: Take detailed sexual history and assess risk for sexual abuse.
- Assess symptoms: Warts are usually asymptomatic with the exception of plantar warts or warts near nails, which may be painful.
- Assess duration: Warts may be present for months to years without intervention.

PHYSICAL EXAM

- Common warts (verruca vulgaris)
  - Rough keratotic papules and nodules that can be single or grouped
  - Often dome-shaped
  - Appear anywhere but most often affect fingers, hands, knees, and elbows
- Flat warts (verruca plana)
  - Generally 2–4 mm, slightly elevated, flat-topped lesions with minimal scale
- Plantar warts (weight-bearing warts)
  - Thick, hyperkeratotic lesions that may be tender to palpation
  - Tend to occur at pressure points on soles of feet
  - May have punctate black dots representing thrombosed capillaries
  - Disrupt normal skin markings
- Anogenital warts
  - Usually multiple, clustered soft lesions that are pink or gray
  - 4 morphologic types: condyloma acuminata (cauliflower-shaped), smooth papules (dome-shaped, flesh-colored), keratotic papules (resemble common warts), flat warts
- Laryngeal warts (laryngeal papillomatosis)
  - Visible only under direct airway examination
  - Children may present with stridor, hoarseness, and signs of airway obstruction.
  - In children, laryngeal warts are diagnosed most often between 2 and 3 years, with most children presenting before age 5 years.

DIAGNOSTIC TESTS & INTERPRETATION

- Diagnosis is based on visual identification.
- Biopsy may be indicated when the diagnosis is uncertain or warts are resistant to treatment.
- In anogenital warts, testing for other sexually transmitted infections is recommended.

DIFFERENTIAL DIAGNOSIS

- Common warts
  - Molluscum contagiosum
  - Moles
  - Skin tag
  - Squamous cell carcinoma or melanoma
- Flat warts
  - Lichen planus
  - Lichenoid keratosis
- Plantar warts
  - Callus
  - Corns
  - Squamous cell carcinoma or melanoma
  - Foreign body
- Anogenital warts
  - Pearly penile papules
  - Molluscum contagiosum
  - Condylomata lata (secondary syphilis lesions)
  - Vulvar carcinoma
  - Lichen planus
  - Squamous cell carcinoma

ALERT

- Any child or adolescent with anogenital warts should prompt consideration for sexual abuse and consultation with a child abuse specialist as necessary.
- Testing for other sexually transmitted infections should occur in any pediatric patient with anogenital warts.
- In any patient with extensive HPV infection, consideration must be given to underlying immunodeficiencies including HIV.

TREATMENT

- General
  - Warts are often self-limited and resolve without treatment.
  - 2/3 of warts will resolve within 2 years with no treatment.
  - Earlier treatment may be warranted for warts that are painful or cause significant social stigma.
- Cutaneous warts
  - Salicylic acid
    - 1st-line therapy for cutaneous warts
    - Over-the-counter (OTC) formulations contain 5–27% salicylic acid and are applied topically 1–2× daily for up to 12 weeks.
    - Prescription strength 40% adhesive plaster is available to be applied for 24–48 hours and are particularly useful for plantar warts.
    - Repetitive filing of the wart with either an emery board, pumice stone, or metal file and soaking the wart for 10–20 minutes prior to treatment may improve response to topical salicylic acid.
    - Applying a thin layer of petrolatum around the wart to protect the surrounding healthy tissue may prevent pain during treatment.
  - Duct tape or moleskin
    - Used as 1st-line therapy
    - May be helpful, although studies on effectiveness are mixed
    - To use, cut tape or moleskin approximately ¼ inch larger than wart and cover for 6 days.
    - After 6 days, remove, soak wart, and file with an emery board, pumice stone, or metal file; leave uncovered overnight.
    - Reapply duct tape in 6 day cycles until resolution.
  - Cryotherapy
    - 2nd-line therapy
    - Involves freezing the wart using one of several methods, the most commonly used being liquid nitrogen
    - Can be painful and is more expensive than 1st-line agents
    - Fewer data support its efficacy as compared to salicylic acid.
    - Most commonly used in the office although newer OTC cryotherapy products are available.
  - 3rd-line therapies are generally performed in conjunction with a pediatric dermatologist.
    - Phototherapy
    - Immunotherapies
    - Intralesional therapies
    - Antimitotic therapies
    - Curettage
    - Laser ablation
- Anogenital warts
  - Treatment issues
    - Main goal of treatment is to remove symptomatic warts.
    - Most warts will clear within 3 months after initiation of therapy.
    - Treatment does not eradicate HPV, prevent recurrence, or reduce cancer risk.
  - Podofilox (0.5% gel) or imiquimod (5% cream) are 1st-line therapy (avoid in pregnancy).
    - Podofilox gel is applied topically q12h for 3 days; no treatment for 4 days; then repeat cycles until warts disappear; avoid unprotected sexual activity during treatment due to possible irritant effect.
    - Imiquimod: for patients aged 12 years and older; apply 3×/week at bedtime; wash off 6–10 hours later; treat until resolution
  - Cryotherapy for anogenital warts is an option for experienced providers.
  - 2nd-line options include podophyllin resin, intralesion treatments, trichloroacetic acid, surgical removal, laser therapy, and photodynamic therapy.

ONGOING CARE

FOLLOW-UP RECOMMENDATIONS

Patient Monitoring

Patients should be seen at regular intervals to assess clearance of the lesions and monitor for side effects.

Issues for Referral

Consider referral to pediatric dermatology if

- Lesions are atypical or extensive.
- Lesions progress during therapy.
- Multiple failed treatment occurs.
- Lesions are located on the face.
- Frequent or prompt recurrence occurs.
- Warts are pigmented, indurated, ulcerated, or fixed to underlying structures.
- Individual warts are greater than 1 cm.
- Patients are immunocompromised.

Consider referral to a child abuse specialist if anogenital warts are present AND

- Caregivers suspect sexual abuse.
- A sexual predator has access to the child.
- Child discloses abuse.
- Child is older than 48 months of age.
- Any other sexually transmitted infection is detected.
- Physical exam suggests any type of abuse.
- Provider is uncomfortable with evaluating for sexual abuse.

PROGNOSIS

- 2/3 of warts clear without treatment within 2 years.
- However, early treatment is recommended while warts are small and few in number to prevent enlargement and spread.

COMPLICATIONS

- Bacterial infection such as cellulitis or abscess can occur if patients pick at warts.
- Other complications are generally related to treatment and can include pain and scarring.
- Malignant transformation to squamous cell carcinoma can rarely occur for both cutaneous and anogenital warts; this is most problematic in immunosuppressed patients.

ADDITIONAL READING

- Boull C, Groth D. Update: treatment of cutaneous viral warts in children. *Pediatr Dermatol*. 2011;28(3):217–229.
- Kwok C, Holland R, Gibbs S. Efficacy of topical treatments for cutaneous warts: a meta-analysis and pooled analysis of randomized controlled trials. *Brit J Dermatol*. 2011;165(2):233–246.
- Kwok CS, Gibbs S, Bennett C, et al. Topical treatments for cutaneous warts. *Cochrane Database Syst Rev*. 2012;9:CD001781.
- Mulhem E, Pinelis S. Treatment of nongenital cutaneous warts. *Am Fam Physician*. 2011;84(3):288–293.
- Sinclair K, Woods C, Sinal S. Venereal warts in children. *Pediatr Rev*. 2011;32(3):115–121.

CODES

ICD10

- B07.9 Viral wart, unspecified
- B07.0 Plantar wart
- A63.0 Anogenital (venereal) warts

FAQ

- Q: Do condoms protect against HPV?
- A: Condoms lower the risk of HPV; however, HPV can infect areas not covered by the condom and so condoms are not fully protective.
- Q: Does a patient with cutaneous warts need to be excluded from school or sports?
- A: No. Exclusion is not fully effective because asymptomatic transmission can occur. In addition, risk of transmission is low.
- Q: How can a callous and wart be differentiated?
- A: Careful paring with a #15 scalpel of a callous shows preserved skin markings and no bleeding. Paring of a wart often reveals black dots, which are thrombosed blood vessels.

WEIGHT LOSS

Mark F. Ditmar

BASICS

DESCRIPTION

Documented decrease in weight from a previous measurement. Outside of newborn period (weight loss in the first 2 weeks is common), acute illnesses resulting in fluid losses, and obese children voluntarily on a designed weight reduction program, weight loss is an unusual and worrisome symptom, regardless of the percentage decline.

DIAGNOSIS

HISTORY

Determine that weight loss is real and not due to scale error, different scales, different technique (e.g., clothed vs. unclothed).

- **Question:** Child's diet?
- *Significance*: A prospective 3-day dietary record can be useful for demonstrating insufficient caloric intake.
- **Question:** Age?
- *Significance*: The patient's age can very much indicate the most likely causes of weight loss to which questions about the history can be directed.
  - Patient <2 weeks old: physiologic weight loss, underfeeding, inappropriate feeding, inborn error of metabolism, congenital heart disease, gastroesophageal reflux
  - Patient <4 months old: malnutrition, improper formula preparation, cystic fibrosis, gastroesophageal reflux, pyloric stenosis, congenital heart disease, congenital adrenal hyperplasia, inborn error of metabolism
  - Patient 4 months–8 years old: chronic infection, cystic fibrosis, malabsorption, neglect/abuse, renal disease, liver disease, diabetes mellitus
  - Patient >8 years old: eating disorder, chronic infection, neoplasm, renal disease, liver disease, substance abuse, diabetes mellitus, inflammatory bowel disease, collagen vascular disease
- **Question:** Vomiting, especially projectile?
- *Significance*: suggestive of intestinal obstruction, gastroesophageal reflux, inborn error of metabolism
- **Question:** Cramping, bloating, or abnormally greasy, voluminous stools?
- *Significance*: possible malabsorption
- **Question:** Tiring during feeding or difficulty feeding due to cough and dyspnea?
- *Significance*: suggests congestive heart failure in newborn/infant, hypothyroidism
- **Question:** Altered mental status, seizures, unusual body/fluid odors?
- *Significance*: possible inborn error of metabolism
- **Question:** Maternal history of multiple miscarriages, neonatal deaths, or consanguinity?
- *Significance*: possible inborn error of metabolism
- **Question:** Foreign travel?
- *Significance*: possible chronic infection (e.g., tuberculosis, parasitic disease)
- **Question:** History of severe infections, persistent candidal infections?
- *Significance*: possible immunodeficiency, congenital or acquired
- **Question:** Headaches, especially early morning?
- *Significance*: possible increased intracranial pressure, CNS malignancy
- **Question:** Increased appetite with weight loss?
- *Significance*: suggests hyperthyroidism, cystic fibrosis, pheochromocytoma
- **Question:** Polyuria, polydipsia, and polyphagia?
- *Significance*: possible new-onset diabetes
- **Question:** Concomitant delayed puberty?
- *Significance*: suggests chronic severe weight loss, pituitary abnormalities, anorexia nervosa
- **Question:** Fear of fatness, preoccupation with food, distorted body image, and/or amenorrhea?
- *Significance*: possible eating disorder
- **Question:** Chronic sadness or irritability, insomnia or hypersomnia?
- *Significance*: possible depression/affective disorder

PHYSICAL EXAM

- **Finding:** Hypothermia, bradycardia?
- *Significance*: suggests anorexia nervosa, hypothyroidism
- **Finding:** Tachycardia, resting?
- *Significance*: hyperthyroidism, pheochromocytoma, anemia, acute weight loss
- **Finding:** Orthostatic changes?
- *Significance*: significant weight loss, possibly acute
- **Finding:** Hypotension, resting?
- *Significance*: Addison disease, anorexia nervosa, significant acute dehydration
- **Finding:** Visual field abnormalities?
- *Significance*: suggests possible CNS malignancy
- **Finding:** Clubbing?
- *Significance*: suggests chronic cardiac, pulmonary, or intestinal disease
- **Finding:** Swollen joint?
- *Significance*: juvenile idiopathic arthritis, inflammatory bowel disease
- **Finding:** Significant abdominal distension?
- *Significance*: suggests celiac disease
- **Finding:** Enlarged liver and/or spleen?
- *Significance*: suggests malignancy, chronic infection, storage disease, inborn error of metabolism
- **Finding:** Muscle weakness?
- *Significance*: connective tissue disorder, electrolyte abnormality, muscular dystrophy

ALERT

- Be certain that the weight loss is real. In some studies, up to 25% of weight loss is artifactual, resulting from measurement errors (e.g., excessive movement of scale, dressed vs. undressed patient).
- Newborns with weight loss, especially at the 2-week visit, may manifest passivity and paradoxical lack of interest in feeding, although the reason for their problem is malnourishment due to inadequate intake (often from improper positioning or too infrequent feedings). They may not act "hungry." Observation of the feeding technique (by a practitioner with expertise or a lactation consultant for breastfed babies) is vital.

DIAGNOSTIC TESTS & INTERPRETATION

- **Test:** CBC for evidence of the following:
- *Significance:*
  - Anemia—macrocytic associated with folate/B_{12} deficiency, microcytic with iron deficiency or chronic infection
  - Polycythemia—suggestive of chronic pulmonary or cardiac disease
  - Neutropenia—suggestive of hematologic malignancy, Shwachman syndrome, immunodeficiency
  - Lymphopenia—suggestive of immunodeficiency
  - Eosinophilia—suggestive of parasitic disease
  - Leukocytosis—suggestive of infection
  - Lymphoblasts—suggestive of leukemia
  - Thrombocytosis—suggestive of chronic infection, malignancy
- **Test:** serum electrolytes
- *Significance*: abnormalities in dehydration, adrenal insufficiency (low sodium, high potassium), renal disease, anorexia nervosa
- **Test:** BUN, creatinine
- *Significance*: abnormal in renal disease, dehydration
- **Test:** erythrocyte sedimentation rate
- *Significance*: may be elevated in inflammatory bowel disease, chronic infections, rheumatoid diseases
- **Test:** stool for occult blood and pH, reducing substances (Clinitest)
- *Significance*:
  - Occult blood suggests inflammatory bowel disease.
  - Low pH and positive reducing substances suggest malabsorption.
- **Test:** Urinalysis
- *Significance*:
  - Hematuria and/or proteinuria suggest renal disease.
  - Glycosuria suggests diabetes mellitus.
  - Very low specific gravity suggests diabetes insipidus, chronic renal failure, hypercalcemia.
  - Pyuria suggests UTI.
  - pH >6 suggests renal tubular acidosis (type I).
- **Test:** urine culture
- *Significance*: Evaluation for UTI
- **Test:** serum protein levels
- *Significance*: Very low levels imply impaired liver function, severe chronic weight loss, or protein malabsorption.
- **Test:** tuberculosis skin test
- *Significance*: possible chronic infection
- **Test:** liver function tests
- *Significance*: evaluation for hepatitis, chronic liver disease
- **Other tests:** Depending on age and clinical findings, other tests to consider include the following: thyroid function tests (TSH), sweat test, tests for malabsorption (e.g., lactose breath test, stool fat, stool for trypsin), tests for metabolic disease (e.g., plasma ammonia, lactate, serum/urine amino acids, urine organic acids), imaging studies (e.g., CT, MRI, bone scan), immunologic studies.

DIFFERENTIAL DIAGNOSIS

- Nutritional
  - Malnutrition
  - Dieting
  - Iron deficiency/zinc deficiency
  - Postoperative recovery
  - Inability to eat (new orthodontic appliances, loss of teeth, chronic mouth ulcerations)
- Congenital/anatomic
  - Congenital heart disease
  - Pyloric stenosis
  - GI malformation (duodenal atresia, annular pancreas, and volvulus)
  - Short bowel syndrome
  - Lymphangiectasia
  - Superior mesenteric artery syndrome
  - Gastroesophageal reflux
  - Immunodeficiency disorders
  - Hirschsprung disease
- Infectious
  - UTI
  - Tuberculosis
  - Stomatitis
  - Osteomyelitis
  - HIV
  - Hepatitis
  - Parasitic disease
  - Abscess, intraabdominal
  - Gastroenteritis
  - Postinfectious malabsorption
  - Pericarditis
  - Histoplasmosis
  - Acute severe febrile illness (pyelonephritis, pneumonia, septic arthritis)
- Tumor
  - Diencephalic syndrome
  - Leukemia
  - Lymphoma
  - Pheochromocytoma
  - Other neoplasms
- Endocrine
  - Diabetes mellitus
  - Diabetes insipidus
  - Hyperthyroidism
  - Adrenal insufficiency
  - Congenital adrenal hyperplasia
  - Hypopituitarism
  - Hypercalcemia
- Genetic/metabolic
  - Cystic fibrosis
  - Shwachman-Diamond syndrome
  - Lactose intolerance
  - Renal tubular acidosis
  - Chronic renal failure
  - Inborn errors of metabolism
  - Storage diseases
  - Muscular dystrophy
  - Lipodystrophy
- Allergic/inflammatory
  - Inflammatory bowel disease
  - Juvenile idiopathic arthritis
  - Systemic lupus erythematosus
  - Sarcoidosis
  - Pancreatitis
  - Hepatitis
  - Celiac disease (gluten enteropathy)
- Psychiatric
  - Rumination syndrome
  - Depression/affective disorders
  - Anorexia nervosa/bulimia nervosa
- Toxic, environmental, drugs
  - Lead poisoning
  - Mercury poisoning
  - Vitamin A poisoning
  - Chronic methylphenidate, dextroamphetamine, or valproic acid use
  - Substance abuse, especially amphetamines and crack cocaine
- Trauma
  - Chronic subdural hematomas
- Miscellaneous
  - Child abuse
  - Chronic illness (e.g., pulmonary disease, renal disease)
  - Cerebral palsy
  - Factitious (e.g., scale error)

ALERT

Emergency care is indicated for the following:

- Significant dehydration
  - Abnormal vital signs with orthostasis, decreased urine output, decreased skin turgor, delayed capillary refill (>3 seconds)
  - Mandates cardiovascular support (IV hydration) and a more urgent diagnosis (e.g., inborn error of metabolism, obstructive GI disease, congenital adrenal hyperplasia, diabetic ketoacidosis)
- Abnormal mental status or significant lethargy which may be seen in the following:
  - Severe dehydration
  - Adrenal insufficiency
  - Hypoxic states
  - Toxic ingestions
  - Renal or respiratory failure
  - Increased intracranial pressure
  - Severe electrolyte abnormalities
- Increasing vomiting in the setting of known weight loss in infants
  - High risk for dehydration, hypoglycemia, and electrolyte abnormalities
  - Need to evaluate for treatable conditions (e.g., obstructive GI disease, inborn errors of metabolism, congenital adrenal hyperplasia, congenital heart disease) in which a delay is life-threatening
- Severe malnutrition (weight loss >20% of ideal body weight)
  - High risk for metabolic derangements, including dysrhythmias secondary to electrolyte abnormalities
- Aggressive evaluation is warranted.

TREATMENT

APPROACH TO THE PATIENT

- Establish if the weight loss is voluntary or involuntary.
- Determine the acuity or chronicity and severity of weight loss, and the need for hospitalization.
- Attempt to narrow the diagnostic possibilities by history and physical exam, particularly by assessing if the loss might be attributable to diminished intake, diminished absorption, or increased requirements.
- Treatment is then based on the most likely diagnosis following evaluation.

ADDITIONAL READING

- Klein-Gitelman M. An adolescent girl with weight loss and syncope. *Pediatr Ann*. 2012;41(3):e1–e5.
- Macdonald PD, Ross SRM, Grant L, et al. Neonatal weight loss in breast and formula fed infants. *Arch Dis Child Fetal Neonatal Ed*. 2003;88(6):F472–F476.
- Schechter M. Weight loss/failure to thrive. *Pediatr Rev*. 2000;21(7):238–239.

CODES

ICD10

- R63.4 Abnormal weight loss
- K21.9 Gastro-esophageal reflux disease without esophagitis
- E46 Unspecified protein-calorie malnutrition

FAQ

- Q: How common is weight loss in the first 2 weeks of life?
- A: Formula-fed babies may lose up to 7% of birth weight and breastfed newborns up to 10% before regaining their birth weight by 2 weeks of age. An infant who has not regained his or her birth weight by 2 weeks requires evaluation and intervention.
- Q: How important a finding is weight loss?
- A: Involuntary weight loss is a *diagnostic exigency*—a cause must be found or the loss self-resolved. If a diagnosis is not uncovered in the setting of continued weight loss, referral to a pediatric diagnostic center is indicated.

W

WEST NILE VIRUS (AND OTHER ARBOVIRUS ENCEPHALITIS)

Jessica Newman • Jason Newland

BASICS

DESCRIPTION

- Viruses transmitted by an arthropod vector that can cause CNS infections, undifferentiated febrile illness, acute polyarthropathy, and hemorrhagic fevers
- Most arboviral infections are asymptomatic.
- West Nile virus (WNV) is an arbovirus in the flavivirus family.
- WNV was first recognized in the United States in 1999 during an outbreak of encephalitis in New York City.
- More than 150 arboviruses are known to cause human disease.
- Other arboviruses can produce similar syndromes or acute hemorrhagic fevers.

EPIDEMIOLOGY

- Arboviruses are spread by mosquitoes, ticks, and sand flies. The major vector for WNV in the United States is the Culex mosquito. WNV has been spread through blood transfusions, transplanted organs, and, rarely, intrauterine.
- Arboviruses are maintained in nature through cycles of transmission among birds, horses, and small animals. Humans and domestic animals are infected incidentally as "dead-end" hosts.
- Disease among birds has been a hallmark of WNV in the United States and has served as a sensitive surveillance indicator of WNV activity.
- Each North American arbovirus has specific geographic distributions and is associated with a different ratio of asymptomatic to clinical infections. These agents cause disease of variable severity and have distinct age-dependent effects. WNV has now been identified throughout the United States and is also found in Europe, Africa, and Asia.

Incidence

- The peak incidence of arboviral encephalitis occurs during the late summer and early fall. Seasonality depends on the breeding and feeding seasons of the arthropod host.
- WNV is the leading cause of arboviral CNS disease. Encephalitis is most commonly seen in older adults, generally aged >60 years. Cases of WNV in children are unusual.
- Fewer than 10 cases each of Eastern equine encephalitis and Western equine encephalitis are reported nationally each year. Eastern equine encephalitis tends to produce a more fulminant illness than LaCrosse or Western equine encephalitis.

GENERAL PREVENTION

- Public health department efforts focus on surveillance of viral activity to predict and prevent outbreaks:
  - Active bird surveillance to detect the presence of WNV activity
  - Active mosquito surveillance to detect viral activity in mosquito populations
  - Passive surveillance by veterinarians and human health care professionals to detect neurologic illnesses consistent with encephalitis
  - Screening of blood and organ donors
- Personal precautions to avoid mosquito bites including use of repellents, protective clothing, and screens; avoiding peak feeding times (dawn and dusk); and installation of air conditioners
- Coordination of mosquito control programs in endemic infection areas
- Vaccines for prevention of most arbovirus infections are not available. A vaccine is available for Japanese encephalitis and yellow fever (YF) for travelers to endemic areas who are planning prolonged stays.
- Infection control measures
  - Standard precautions are recommended for the hospitalized patient.
  - Respiratory precautions are recommended when vector mosquitoes are present.
  - Patients with dengue and YF can be viremic and should be protected against vector mosquitoes to avoid potential transmission.

PATHOPHYSIOLOGY

- The incubation period for WNV and other arboviral encephalitis agents is 2–14 days (up to 21 days in immunocompromised hosts).
- The incubation period reflects the time necessary for viral replication, viremia, and subsequent invasion of the CNS.
- Virus replication begins locally at the site of the insect bite; transient viremia leads to spread of virus to liver, spleen, and lymph nodes. With continued viral replication and viremia, seeding of other organs including the CNS occurs.
- Virus can rarely be recovered from blood within the 1st week of onset of illness but not after neurologic symptoms have developed.

ETIOLOGY

- Arboviruses can be divided into 2 groups based on the predominant clinical syndrome.
- In the United States, 7 arboviruses are important causes of encephalitis: WNV, California encephalitis virus (LaCrosse strain), Eastern equine encephalitis, Western equine encephalitis, St. Louis encephalitis, Powassan encephalitis virus, and Venezuelan equine encephalitis virus.
- Arboviruses such as YF, dengue fever, and Colorado tick fever typically cause acute febrile diseases and hemorrhagic fevers and are not characterized by encephalitis.
- Clinical manifestations of WNV
  - Asymptomatic: most common
  - Self-limited febrile illness: 67% of symptomatic cases
  - Neuroinvasive disease: aseptic meningitis, encephalitis, or flaccid paralysis—<1% cases

DIAGNOSIS

HISTORY

- The diagnosis of arboviral infections of the CNS is difficult.
- Characteristic epidemiology that suggests a specific etiology is an important part of the history.
- The season of disease, prevalent diseases within the community, and animal exposures may provide clues to the diagnosis:
  - Enteroviral infections are seen in the warmer months (summer and early fall) in temperate climates.
  - Mosquito propagation in damp climates or standing water during the summer months may increase the likelihood of arthropod-borne viruses.
  - History of an animal bite or bat exposure may suggest the possibility of rabies.
- WNV (symptomatic infection) is characterized by sudden onset of fever, headache, myalgias, muscle weakness, and GI symptoms (nausea, vomiting, or diarrhea).
- Neuroinvasive WNV can be characterized by neck stiffness and headache, mental status changes, movement disorders, or flaccid paralysis.
- Encephalitis caused by arboviruses is characterized by acute onset of fever and headache in almost all patients. Associated symptoms may include seizures, altered consciousness, disorientation, and behavioral disturbances.

PHYSICAL EXAM

- Neurologic signs are more commonly diffuse but may be focal. These clinical findings can help to distinguish patients with meningitis, which is characterized by nuchal rigidity and fever usually without an altered sensorium.
- Other signs possibly observed in WNV infection:
  - A rash is seen in ~50% of patients and is described as nonpruritic, roseolar, or maculopapular on the chest, back, and arms, which lasts 1 week.
  - Diffuse lymphadenopathy is also common.
- Neurologic examination in WNV infection may reveal motor weakness or flaccid paralysis, increased deep tendon reflexes and extensor plantar responses, and tremor or abnormal movement of extremities.

DIAGNOSTIC TESTS & INTERPRETATION

The diagnosis of arboviral encephalitis depends on the recognition of epidemiologic risk factors and typical signs and symptoms with the aid of laboratory and radiographic studies.

Lab

- Routine laboratory tests
  - CBC typically reveals a mild leukocytosis.
  - Mild increase in erythrocyte sedimentation rate (ESR)
  - Mild to moderate CSF pleocytosis, predominately mononuclear cells
  - Elevated CSF protein
  - Normal CSF glucose
- Serology
  - IgM and IgG enzyme-linked immunosorbent assay (ELISA) or indirect fluorescent antibody (IFA) for WNV and other arboviruses
  - The diagnosis of arbovirus encephalitis is made by 1 of the following:
    - Detection of virus-specific IgM antibodies in the CSF is confirmatory.
    - A 4-fold rise in serum antibody titers is confirmatory. Acute-phase titers should be collected 0–8 days after onset of symptoms. Convalescent phase titers should be collected 14–21 days after acute specimen. A single negative acute-phase specimen is inadequate for diagnosis, but a positive test can provide evidence of recent infection.
  - Isolation of the virus from tissue, blood, or CSF
  - Polymerase chain reaction (PCR) to detect viral RNA

Imaging

- Imaging studies such as MRI or CT can assist in ruling out other potential causes of encephalopathy or encephalitis.
- MRI has proved useful in differentiating postinfectious encephalomyelitis from acute viral encephalitis. The former is characterized by enhancement of multifocal white matter lesions.

Diagnostic Procedures/Other

- EEG
  - Diffuse generalized slowing of brain waves
  - Periodic high-voltage spike waves originating in the temporal lobe region and slow-wave complexes at 2–3-second intervals are suggestive of herpes simplex virus infection.

DIFFERENTIAL DIAGNOSIS

Infectious

- Viral
  - Herpes simplex virus
  - Enterovirus
  - HIV
  - HHV-6
  - Epstein-Barr virus
  - Cytomegalovirus
  - Lymphocytic choriomeningitis virus
  - Rabies
  - Mumps
  - Influenza
  - Adenovirus
- Nonviral
  - Cat-scratch disease (*Bartonella henselae*)
  - *Mycoplasma pneumoniae*
  - Postinfectious encephalomyelitis: generally follows a vague viral syndrome, usually upper respiratory tract, by days to weeks
  - Abscess/subdural empyema
  - Meningitis
    - Tuberculous
    - Cryptococcal or other fungal (histoplasmosis, coccidioidomycoses, blastomycoses)
    - Bacterial
    - Listeria
  - Toxoplasmosis
  - *Plasmodium falciparum* infection (malaria)
  - Parasites (cysticercosis, echinococcus, amebiasis, trypanosomiasis)

Noninfectious: tumor, carcinomatous meningitis, systemic lupus erythematosus, sarcoidosis, vasculitis, hemorrhage, toxic encephalopathy, metabolic disorders

TREATMENT

GENERAL MEASURES

- No specific antiviral therapy is available.
- Supportive therapy including cardiorespiratory function, fluid and electrolyte balance, seizure control, and reduction of intracranial pressure is important.
- Consider intravenous immunoglobulin (IVIG)/plasmapheresis for associated Guillain-Barré syndrome; IVIG has been used in cases of flaccid paralysis with some response.
- Recovery can be seen after prolonged periods of coma.

ONGOING CARE

FOLLOW-UP RECOMMENDATIONS

Patient Monitoring

- Neurobehavioral follow-up should be considered in children with severe or complicated disease.
- If WNV is diagnosed during pregnancy, detailed fetal ultrasound (US) should be considered 2–4 weeks after illness onset with evaluation for congenital anomalies and neurologic deficits.
- Infant serum should be tested for WNV IgM at birth and 6 months with IgG at 6 months.

PROGNOSIS

- Prognosis for recovery depends on the specific infecting agent and host factors such as age and underlying illness.
- Eastern equine and Japanese encephalitis have the worst prognoses, with mortality occurring in 30% of cases.

COMPLICATIONS

- Optic neuritis
- Seizures
- Coma
- Death
- Guillain-Barré syndrome
- Severe neurologic sequelae
- Myocarditis
- Pancreatitis
- Hepatitis

ADDITIONAL READING

- Asnis DS, Conetta R, Teixeira AA, et al. The West Nile virus outbreak of 1999 in New York: the Flushing Hospital experience. *Clin Infect Dis*. 2000;30(3):413–418.
- Hayes EB. West Nile virus disease in children. *Pediatr Infect Dis J*. 2006;25(11):1065–1066.
- Lindsey NP, Hayes EB, Staples JE, et al. West Nile virus disease in children, United States, 1999-2007. *Pediatrics*. 2009;123(6):e1084–e1089.
- Rizzo C, Esposito S, Azzari S, et al. West Nile virus infections in children: a disease pediatricians should think about. *Pediatr Infect Dis J*. 2011;30(1):65–66.
- Romero JR, Newland JG. Viral meningitis and encephalitis: traditional and emerging viral agents. *Semin Pediatr Infect Dis*. 2003;14(2):72–82.

CODES

ICD10

- A92.30 West Nile virus infection, unspecified
- A92.31 West Nile virus infection with encephalitis
- A85.2 Arthropod-borne viral encephalitis, unspecified

FAQ

- Q: Should testing for arboviruses, including WNV, be performed on all patients with encephalitis?
- A: Diagnostic testing for arboviruses is not recommended for all patients with encephalitis. The prevalence of these diseases is low, and the diagnosis of more common causes of childhood encephalitis (e.g., herpes simplex virus) should be pursued initially. Patients with no other identifiable cause of encephalitis who have epidemiologic risk factors such as geographic location, season, and exposure history suggestive of arbovirus encephalitis should be evaluated. Testing of patients with aseptic meningitis or Guillain-Barré syndrome is low yield.

WHEEZING

Samuel B. Goldfarb • Lee J. Brooks

BASICS

DESCRIPTION

Wheezing is a continuous sound that is caused by turbulent airflow through an obstructed airway.

- Often described as musical in nature and with a variable pitch
- Wheezing is an expiratory sound; stridor is an inspiratory sound.
- Wheezing occurs from obstruction in the intrathoracic airway, whereas stridor is caused by an obstruction in the extrathoracic airway.
- If heard in both inspiration and expiration, there may be a fixed obstruction or separate lesions in both the intrathoracic and extrathoracic airways.

DIAGNOSIS

DIFFERENTIAL DIAGNOSIS

Extrathoracic (usually results in stridor or stertor rather than wheezing)

- Nasal/nasopharynx
  - Acute: nasal turbinate edema or secretions, foreign body
  - Chronic: adenoidal enlargement, nasal polyps, choanal stenosis, midface hypoplasia
- Oropharynx
  - Acute: peritonsillar abscess, retropharyngeal abscess, palatine tonsillitis
  - Chronic: adenotonsillar hypertrophy, macroglossia, micrognathia
- Hypopharynx
  - Acute: acute nasal, nasopharyngeal, or oropharyngeal obstruction
  - Chronic: hypopharyngeal hypotonia, glossoptosis, obesity, neoplasia
- Larynx
  - Acute: laryngospasm, laryngotracheobronchitis (croup), epiglottitis, foreign body (large and irregular)
  - Chronic: laryngomalacia, papillomatosis, hemangioma, granuloma, congenital cyst or web, laryngocele
- Glottis
  - Acute: vocal cord paralysis or paresis, vocal cord inflammation or polyp, psychogenic wheezing
  - Chronic: paradoxical vocal cord motion (vocal cord dysfunction); psychogenic wheezing; brainstem compression; injury to the vagus, glossopharyngeal, or recurrent laryngeal nerves; papillomatosis
- Subglottis/extrathoracic trachea
  - Acute: laryngotracheobronchitis (croup), bacterial, rachitic, recent endotracheal extubation
  - Chronic: subglottic stenosis (congenital or after prolonged intubation), papillomatosis

Intrathoracic

- Trachea (extrinsic compression)
  - Acute: uncommon
  - Chronic
    - Vascular: vascular ring/sling, compression by an aberrant pulmonary artery
    - Cardiac: left main bronchus compression, recurrent laryngeal nerve compression "cardiovocal syndrome"
    - Anterior mediastinum: lymphoma, thymoma, teratoma
    - Middle mediastinum: lymphoma, lymphadenopathy (tuberculosis, mycotic infection, sarcoidosis)
    - Posterior mediastinum: neurogenic tumors, esophageal duplication or cyst, bronchogenic cyst
- Trachea (intramural lesions)
  - Acute: uncommon
  - Chronic: tracheomalacia
    - Congenital: cartilaginous defect (Campbell-Williams syndrome), muscular defect (Mounier-Kuhn syndrome), s/p tracheoesophageal fistula (TEF) repair, external compression/distortion, complete tracheal rings
    - Acquired: chronic inflammation (recurrent infection, gastroesophageal reflux, recurrent aspiration), prolonged positive pressure ventilation, external compression
- Trachea (intraluminal lesions)
  - Acute: foreign body (irregularly shaped and elongated), bacterial tracheitis (with chronic tracheostomy tube usage)
  - Chronic: tracheal granulomas, hemangioma, papillomatosis, tracheal web
- Bronchi/bronchioles
  - Acute: viral bronchiolitis, bronchopneumonia, foreign body (small, smooth shape), immune defect (transient hypogammaglobulinemia of the newborn is most common), granuloma, neoplasia
  - Chronic: asthma, bronchopulmonary dysplasia, bronchomalacia, carcinoid, adenoma

APPROACH TO THE PATIENT

- Phase 1: Determine the severity of the patient's general status and degree of respiratory distress and triage accordingly.
- Phase 2: Construct a differential diagnosis.
- Phase 3: Initiate appropriate therapies.

HISTORY

- **Question:** Pattern of the wheezing?
- *Significance*:
  - A rapid onset suggests a foreign body or a post-exposure exacerbation of asthma.
  - A slow onset suggests an infection.
  - Periods of recurrent wheezing suggest asthma.
  - Nocturnal and early morning wheezing or coughing are consistent with gastroesophageal reflux, sinusitis, and/or sensitivity to common bedroom allergens.
  - Wheezing in association with or soon after a meal can be seen in swallowing dysfunction, gastroesophageal reflux, or, less commonly, tracheoesophageal fistula.
  - Wheezing that worsens with crying is suggestive of tracheomalacia and/or bronchomalacia or a fixed intraluminal or extraluminal obstruction.
- **Question:** Wheezing correlated with exertion?
- *Significance*: Suggests asthma triggered by exercise
- **Question:** Multiple exacerbations with recurrent or chronic symptoms?
- *Significance*:
  - Recurrent cycles of exacerbations, with clearing in between, suggest a process such as asthma, cystic fibrosis, ciliary dyskinesia, and bronchopulmonary dysplasia.
  - Chronic or persistent wheezing is more common with fixed anatomic abnormalities.
- **Question:** Common triggers?
- *Significance*: Could be
  - Smoke
  - Dust
  - Animal dander
  - Change in humidity or temperature
  - Change in seasons (pollens, grasses, molds)
  - Exercise
  - Infections (usually viral)
  - Inflammation of any sort
  - meals (aspiration, GERD, TEF)
- **Question:** Family history?
- *Significance*: A family history of wheezing, asthma, allergic rhinitis, or atopy suggests a diagnosis of asthma.
- **Question:** An episode of choking preceding the first onset of wheezing?
- *Significance*: Suggests foreign body aspiration

PHYSICAL EXAM

- **Finding:** Patient's degree of respiratory difficulty?
- *Significance*:
  - Tachypnea
  - Accessory muscle usage: Use of intercostal and sternocleidomastoid muscles and abdominal musculature indicates increased expiratory effort to overcome airway obstruction.
  - Nasal flaring: With increasing respiratory difficulty, the nares will be dilated to decrease the resistance to air flow.
- **Finding:** Auscultate: Assess airflow, adventitious sounds, and the inspiratory-to-expiratory ratio. Is the wheezing diffuse or localized?
- *Significance*:
  - Aeration: Decreased aeration is much worse prognostically than wheezing because it is directly related to the amount of aeration and ventilation. With decreased aeration, wheezing may not be audible.

- Ratio of inspiration to exhalation: With increased intrathoracic airway obstruction, the time needed to exhale will become greater because of a greater decrease in airway caliber during exhalation. Normal ratio is 1:3.
- Localized wheezing may suggest a foreign body.

- **Finding:** Presence of nasal crease, the "allergic salute" (i.e., rubbing the nose with the palm of the hand), atopic dermatitis, boggy nasal turbinates, clear postnasal drainage, allergic shiners, or Dennie lines?
- *Significance*: Suggestive of allergic rhinitis or atopic disease including asthma
- **Finding:** Patients with first-time, persistent, or atypical episodes of wheezing?
- *Significance*: "All that wheezes is not asthma": Although most episodes of wheezing will represent viral infections or asthma, clinicians need to be mindful of alternative diagnoses.
- **Finding:** The 3 *R*'s of asthma?
- *Significance*:
  - Recurrence: symptoms that recur multiple times with full resolution in between episodes
  - Reactivity: symptoms that can be triggered during exposures (temperature extremes, smoke, dust, humid or dry air, aromas, etc.)
  - Reversibility: symptoms that resolve with bronchodilator therapy

DIAGNOSTIC TESTS & INTERPRETATION

- **Test:** Bronchodilator responsiveness
- *Significance*:
  - A postbronchodilator improvement in wheezing indicates a reversible process such as asthma.
  - A bronchodilator may worsen wheezing in disorders of airway wall rigidity such as bronchomalacia or tracheomalacia.
  - There may be no change following a bronchodilator in situations with foreign bodies, fixed airway obstruction due to significant inflammation (i.e., status asthmaticus), or airway remodeling.
- **Test:** Pulmonary function testing (spirometry)
- *Significance*:
  - Spirometry remains the standard and most helpful measure of pulmonary function.
  - Normative data have been described in children >6 years of age.
  - Normal spirometry does not rule out asthma.
  - Methacholine challenge test is a provocative test to evaluate for asthma.
  - Exercise test with spirometry to evaluate for exercise-induced asthma
- **Test:** Pulse oximetry measurement of oxygen saturation (Spo_2)
- *Significance*: Pulse oximetry is an insensitive measure of mild to moderate respiratory difficulty during wheezing, but oxyhemoglobin saturation <92% may be seen in severe compromise.
- **Test:** Arterial blood gas
- *Significance*:
  - Arterial blood gases provide a direct measure of oxygenation (Pao_2) and ventilation ($Paco_2$) and can also help to determine severity.
  - A normal or high normal $Paco_2$ in a tachypneic patient (when it should be low) may be a sign of impending respiratory failure.

Lab

- **Test:** Microbiologic studies
- *Significance*:
  - Positive bacterial culture of sputum is helpful in directing or focusing antibiotic therapy. A Gram stain showing sheets of polymorphonuclear leukocytes and a predominant organism is helpful to differentiate a potentially causative organism from the multitude of normal flora.
  - Positive respiratory virus screen or culture (often within 12 hours) can prevent needless antibiotic therapy and may be helpful in predicting future disease.
- **Test:** Tuberculosis skin test
- *Significance*: Mantoux purified protein derivative—tuberculosis. May be falsely positive in a patient who received BCG vaccine. May be falsely negative in a patient who is anergic
- **Test:** CBC including eosinophil count, quantitative immunoglobulins, IgE, complement, HIV testing, allergy skin testing
- Significance: Screening for immune defects, atopy

Imaging

- Chest radiography (posteroanterior and lateral views)
  - Should be strongly considered in all patients with new-onset wheezing or an asymmetric lung exam
  - Can show findings suggestive of airway obstruction (hyperinflation, hyperlucency, flattening of the diaphragms)
  - Asymmetry in aeration on right and left lateral decubitus films suggests foreign body or other obstructing lesions on the side having the greatest air trapping.

TREATMENT

ADDITIONAL TREATMENT

General Measures

- A trial of bronchodilator therapy (e.g., albuterol) may be both therapeutic and diagnostic of the reversible airway obstruction characteristic of asthma.
- For acute asthma exacerbation: corticosteroids PO or IV
- Ipratropium bromide may be helpful in reducing airway secretions and reducing airway obstruction, but it is not FDA approved for treatment of asthma. May be helpful in tracheomalacia as might bethanechol.
- Inhaled corticosteroids, antileukotriene agents, and, less, frequently methylxanthines (aminophylline and theophylline) are used as maintenance medications.
- Antibiotics should be used in patients with suspected pneumonia.
- In emergency setting epinephrine, terbutaline, and magnesium sulfate can be used along with supportive care such as supplemental oxygen.

ALERT

Factors that may indicate a respiratory emergency:

- Signs of mild to moderate respiratory difficulty: tachypnea, intercostal and suprasternal retractions, nasal flaring, head bobbing and exaggerated shoulder movement during breathing, abdominal breathing and subcostal retractions (may be normal in infants, especially during active [REM] sleep), relative difficulty speaking in complete sentences, significant wheezing, prolonged exhalation, and low $Paco_2$ in the face of tachypnea
- Signs of impending respiratory failure: cyanosis, fatigue, inability to speak in >1- or 2-word phrases, altered mental status (e.g., confusion, agitation), decreased respiratory drive, inadequate ventilation (poor air flow), no audible wheezing, high normal or rising $Paco_2$ in the face of tachypnea or respiratory distress
- Determine which patients require assisted ventilation (e.g., bag-mask ventilation, noninvasive [nasal] ventilation, or endotracheal intubation)
- Lack of response to aggressive bronchodilator therapy, without a history of asthma or recurrent wheeze, or biphasic adventitious sounds should immediately raise the suspicion of a fixed lesion.

ADDITIONAL READING

- Castro-Rodriguez JA, Rodrigo GJ. Efficacy of inhaled corticosteroids in infants and preschoolers with recurrent wheezing and asthma: a systemic review with meta-analysis *Pediatrics*. 2009;123(3): e519–e525.
- Cowan K, Guilbert TW. Pediatric asthma phenotypes. *Curr Opin Pediatr*. 2012;24(3):344–351.
- Nelson KA, Zorc JJ. Asthma update. *Pediatr Clin North Am*. 2013;60(5):1035–1048.
- Piippo-Savolainen E, Korppi M. Long-term outcomes of early childhood wheezing. *Curr Opin Allergy Clin Immunol*. 2009;9(3):190–196.

CODES

ICD10

R06.2 Wheezing

FAQ

- Q: What percentage of recurrent wheezing resolves by school age?
- A: Roughly 40% of children with ≥1 episode of wheezing before 3 years clear by 6 years of age.
- Q: Should chest radiographs be routinely obtained in children experiencing their first episodes of wheezing?
- A: For a child with new-onset asymmetric wheezing, a chest radiograph should be obtained. For a child with symmetric wheezing, chest radiography may not be helpful and should be ordered judiciously.

WILMS TUMOR

David T. Teachey

BASICS

DESCRIPTION

Wilms tumor is a malignant tumor of the kidney occurring in the pediatric age group. It is also called nephroblastoma.

EPIDEMIOLOGY

More common in girls than boys

Incidence

- 1 in 10,000 live births
- Increased incidence in children with neurofibromatosis

Prevalence

- Most common primary malignant renal tumor of childhood
- 5–6% of all childhood cancers

RISK FACTORS

Genetics

- 15–20% are presumed hereditary.
- Familial cases are more often bilateral and occur at an earlier age.
- A tumor suppressor gene related to Wilms tumor (*WT1*) has been localized to chromosome 11p13. Mutations in this gene occur in ~20% of Wilms tumors.
- Another tumor suppressor gene, *WT2*, has been localized on 11p15.

ETIOLOGY

- 20% of Wilms tumors have a mutation in the *WT1* tumor suppressor gene.
- Causes in the remaining 80% of patients are unknown.

COMMONLY ASSOCIATED CONDITIONS

- 12–15% of patients have other congenital anomalies.
- May be associated with aniridia, hemihypertrophy, and cryptorchidism
- Associated syndromes
  - WAGR (Wilms tumor, aniridia, genitourinary abnormalities, mental retardation)
  - Beckwith-Wiedemann syndrome (macroglossia, omphalocele, visceromegaly, hemihypertrophy)
  - Denys-Drash syndrome (ambiguous genitalia, progressive renal failure, and increased risk of Wilms tumor)

DIAGNOSIS

HISTORY

- Abdominal distention
- Abdominal pain (20–30% of cases)
- Hematuria (20–30% of cases)
- Fever, anorexia, vomiting
- Family history of Wilms tumor
- Rapid increase in abdominal size (suggestive of hemorrhage in the tumor)

PHYSICAL EXAM

- Asymptomatic abdominal mass extending from flank toward midline (most common presentation)
- Anemia (secondary to hemorrhage in the tumor)
- Fever
- Hypertension (owing to increased renin production in 25% of cases)
- Varicocele (indicates obstruction to spermatic vein owing to tumor thrombus in renal vein or inferior vena cava)
- Aniridia, hemihypertrophy, cryptorchidism, hypospadias
- Signs of Beckwith-Wiedemann and neurofibromatosis

DIAGNOSTIC TESTS & INTERPRETATION

Lab

- CBC
- Electrolytes
- Urine analysis: for microscopic hematuria
- Liver and kidney function tests
- Coagulation factors

Imaging

- Ultrasound of abdomen
  - Diagnostic of mass of renal origin
  - Evaluate for extension of tumor into inferior vena cava.
- CT scan of abdomen, chest radiograph, and chest CT: to evaluate for metastatic disease
- Bone scan: only if clear cell sarcoma, renal cell carcinoma, or rhabdoid tumor on pathology
- MRI of head: only for clear cell sarcoma and rhabdoid tumors
- EKG and echocardiogram in patients who will receive anthracycline chemotherapy

Pathologic Findings

- Gross pathology
  - Often cystic with hemorrhages and necrosis
  - Usually no calcification (useful in differentiating from neuroblastoma, which is calcified on plain radiograph)
  - May extend into the inferior vena cava
- Histology
  - Triphasic pattern blastemal, epithelial, and stromal cell
  - Blastemal cells aggregate into nodules like primitive glomeruli; the presence of diffuse anaplasia indicates a poor prognosis.
- Clinicopathologic staging
  - Stage I: Tumor is restricted to one kidney and completely resected. The renal capsule is intact.
  - Stage II: Tumor extends beyond the kidney but is completely excised.
  - Stage III: Residual nonhematogenous tumor is confined to the abdomen.
  - Stage IV: There is hematogenous spread to lungs, liver, bone, or brain.
  - Stage V: Bilateral disease

DIFFERENTIAL DIAGNOSIS
- Polycystic kidney
- Renal hematoma
- Renal abscess
- Neuroblastoma
- Other neoplasms of kidney: clear cell carcinoma, rhabdoid tumor

ALERT
Rarely, Wilms tumor may present with polycythemia. It can present as fever of unknown origin without any other signs or symptoms.

TREATMENT

SPECIAL THERAPY
Radiotherapy
- Not required for stage I and II patients unless anaplastic, clear cell, or rhabdoid
- Radiotherapy to tumor bed with 1,080 cGy for stages III and IV. If gross tumor spillage or peritoneal seeding, treat whole abdomen
- Whole-lung radiation (1,200 cGy) for pulmonary metastasis

MEDICATION
- Chemotherapy
  - For stages I and II favorable histology: vincristine and actinomycin D every 3 weeks for 6 months
  - For stages III and IV favorable histology, stage I–III focal anaplasia, and stage I diffuse anaplasia: vincristine, actinomycin D, and doxorubicin for 6–15 months
  - Add cyclophosphamide and/or etoposide for higher stage anaplastic tumors (stage IV focal or II–IV diffuse).
- Side effects of therapy
  - Temporary loss of hair
  - Peripheral neuropathy
  - Impaired function of the remaining kidney over years following radiation
  - Cardiac toxicity with doxorubicin
  - Second malignant neoplasms in few cases

SURGERY/OTHER PROCEDURES
- Nephrectomy
  - Preoperative chemotherapy in case of very large tumors with inferior vena cava extension
  - For bilateral disease, nephrectomy of more affected side and partial nephrectomy of the other side, followed by chemotherapy and radiation

ONGOING CARE

PROGNOSIS
- Stages I and II: >90% cured
- Stage III: 85% cured
- Stage IV: 70% cured
- Favorable prognostic factors
  - Tumor weight <250 g
  - Age at presentation <24 months
  - Stage I disease
  - Favorable histology
- Poor prognostic factors
  - Diffuse anaplastic pathology
  - Clear cell sarcoma variant
  - Rhabdoid tumor variant
  - Lymph node involvement
  - Distant metastasis
  - Tumors with loss of heterozygosity (LOH) of chromosomes 1p and/or 16q

COMPLICATIONS
- Extension into inferior vena cava
- Metastasis to lungs and liver
- Cardiac toxicity secondary to doxorubicin
- Liver dysfunction secondary to actinomycin D and radiation therapy

FOLLOW-UP RECOMMENDATIONS
Patient Monitoring
- Every 3 months for 18 months, every 6 months for 1year, and then yearly
- Chest radiograph, urinalysis, and abdominal ultrasound at regular intervals

ADDITIONAL READING

- Blakely ML, Ritchey ML. Controversies in the management of Wilms' tumor. *Semin Pediatr Surg*. 2001;10(3):127–131.
- Davidoff AM. Wilms tumor. *Adv Pediatr*. 2012; 59(1):247–267.
- Hohenstein P, Hastie ND. The many facets of the Wilms' tumour gene, WT1. *Hum Mol Genet*. 2006;15(Spec No 2):R196–R201.
- Martinez CH, Dave S, Izawa J. Wilms' tumor. *Adv Exp Med Biol*. 2010;685:196–209.
- McLean TW, Buckley KS. Pediatric genitourinary tumors. *Curr Opin Oncol*. 2010;22(3):268–273.

CODES

ICD10
- C64.9 Malignant neoplasm of unsp kidney, except renal pelvis
- C64.1 Malignant neoplasm of right kidney, except renal pelvis
- C64.2 Malignant neoplasm of left kidney, except renal pelvis

FAQ
- Q: What should be done to protect the remaining kidney during sports?
- A: Children should wear a kidney guard to protect the unaffected kidney during contact sports.
- Q: Can a child grow and live normally with 1 kidney?
- A: Yes.

W

WILSON DISEASE

Waqar Waheed

BASICS

DESCRIPTION

Wilson disease (WD), also known as hepatolenticular degeneration, is an autosomal recessive disorder of copper metabolism affecting several organs, most notably the liver, brain, and cornea.

EPIDEMIOLOGY

Children usually present with hepatic manifestations; adolescents and young adults may present with neurologic symptoms.

- Worldwide carrier rate is 1:100.
- Prevalence is 1:30,000.
- Most cases present between ages 5 and 35 years.
- Worldwide distribution

RISK FACTORS

Genetics

- Autosomal recessive inheritance with 1 of >500 known defects of the WD gene (*ATP7B*) on chromosome 13q14.3 membrane (ATPase)
- The affected protein facilitates biliary excretion of excess copper; incorporates copper into apoceruloplasmin for transport
- Heterozygotes are generally asymptomatic.
- Siblings have 25% risk of disease, 50% chance of being an asymptomatic carrier, and a 25% chance of being unaffected and not a carrier.
- Clinical phenotype of WD is modified by mutations in other genes, including *MTHFR, COMMD1, ATOX1*, and *XIAP*.
- Use of direct mutational analysis to phenotype WD is limited by the high number of mutations.

PATHOPHYSIOLOGY

- Loss of ATP7b function causes; a) impaired biliary copper excretion (the only route for elimination of copper) and b) failure to incorporate copper to apoceruloplasmin during ceruloplasmin biosynthesis, leading to ceruloplasmin deficiency
- Copper accumulates preferentially in the liver, leading to cirrhosis.
- After liver is saturated, copper overflows and settles in the brain (primarily in the basal ganglia leading to impaired motor control), as well as other tissues including kidneys, heart, blood, and cornea.
- Excess copper damages mitochondria, causing oxidative damage to cells. In addition, toxic intracellular copper deposition promotes apoptotic cell death by the inhibition of IAPs (inhibitor of apoptosis proteins).

DIAGNOSIS

HISTORY

- Hepatic
  - In children, symptoms of hepatic disease predominate, ranging from asymptomatic hepatomegaly and elevated transaminases to chronic hepatitis and even fulminant hepatic failure.
  - Mean age for onset of hepatic symptoms ~10 years
  - Fulminant liver failure is associated with hemolysis and coagulopathy unresponsive to vitamin K.
- Neurologic
  - Neurologic symptoms are rare before age 10 years.
  - Neurologic signs in children: behavior change, decline in school performance, poor hand–eye coordination, motor abnormalities—dystonia, tremors, dysphagia, dysarthria, chorea, ataxia, and parkinsonism
  - Other manifestations include seizures, myoclonus, and dysautonomia.
- Psychiatric: develop depression, anxiety, psychosis, and/or obsessive-compulsive disorder
- Other: Nonspecific complaints are common—abdominal pain, nausea, anorexia, and fatigue.
- Signs and symptoms:
  - 45% of all patients present with liver disease, 35% with neurologic symptoms and 10% psychiatric.
  - Remaining 10%: hemolytic anemia, jaundice, cardiomyopathy, other
  - Consider WD in all cases of liver abnormality in which viral and autoimmune causes have been excluded.
  - Also consider WD in every young patient with unexplained neuropsychiatric symptoms including with a movement disorder.

PHYSICAL EXAM

- Ophthalmologic
  - Kayser-Fleischer (KF) rings: copper deposits on Descemet membrane of cornea (at limbus)
    - Not pathognomonic for WD; may be seen in cholestatic liver disease
    - May require slit-lamp examination to detect
  - 95% with neurologic signs have KF rings.
  - 50–65% with hepatic presentation has KF rings.
- Cardiovascular: signs of cardiomyopathy, dysrhythmia, congestive heart failure
- Abdominal
  - Hepatomegaly, ascites
  - Splenomegaly from portal hypertension
- Skin
  - Jaundice due to hemolysis
  - Bleeding diathesis from liver disease
  - Edema
- Neurologic
  - Movement disorders
  - Neurologic deficits

DIAGNOSTIC TESTS & INTERPRETATION

Lab

- Serum ceruloplasmin
  - An acute-phase reactant; increased with inflammation, infection, or trauma; level may increase to reference range.
  - Made mostly in the liver; it is the major carrier of copper in blood.
  - Low serum ceruloplasmin can be helpful in diagnosing WD.
    - Very low (<50 mg/L): strong evidence for WD
    - Low (<200 mg/L) plus symptoms and KF rings: diagnostic of WD
  - Ceruloplasmin levels also low in renal or GI protein loss, Menkes disease, and end-stage liver disease
- Serum copper
  - Low total serum copper (<80 mcg/dL) in WD
  - Level is decreased in proportion to decreased ceruloplasmin in circulation.
  - In acute fulminant liver failure, serum copper is increased owing to sudden release of stores (most is not bound to ceruloplasmin).
- Free copper estimation
  - Measure of nonceruloplasmin toxic copper in the blood; normal values 1.3–1.9 μmol/L (8–12 mcg/dL), in WD >3.9 μmol/L (25 mcg/dL).
  - Useful in cases where false elevation of ceruloplasmin is suspected; when a measurement of urinary copper is difficult to obtain, as well to monitor chelators efficacy during maintenance phase of therapy (goal <25 mcg/dL)
  - Calculated by the formula: total serum copper in mcg/mL × 100 − (ceruloplasmin in mg/dL × 3) = free copper
- Urinary copper excretion
  - Reflects unbound copper in blood
  - Level is high in WD: >100 mcg/24 h in symptomatic patient is diagnostic.
  - In equivocal cases, marked increase in urinary copper output after initiation of chelation therapy may help in diagnosis.
- Other:
  - Mutational analysis if familial mutation is known

Imaging

- Abdominal ultrasound for liver size and pathology
- MRI of the brain/basal ganglia should be obtained prior to initiation of therapy.
- "Face of the giant panda" sign that is characteristic of Wilson disease (red nuclei, substantia nigra, tegmentum)

Diagnostic Procedures/Other

- Liver biopsy is the definitive procedure for tissue diagnosis and hepatic disease staging.
- Biopsy should be obtained when diagnosis is not straightforward and in younger patients.
- Hepatic parenchymal copper concentration >250 mcg/g dry weight
- Hepatic copper level <50 mcg/g dry weight excludes WD.

DIFFERENTIAL DIAGNOSIS

- Liver disease
  - Viral hepatitis
  - Autoimmune hepatitis/primary biliary cirrhosis
  - Menkes disease (low ceruloplasmin)
  - Cholestatic disease from parenteral nutrition (KF rings)
- Neurologic disease
  - Essential tremor
  - Sydenham or Huntington chorea
  - Hereditary dystonia
  - Other neurodegenerative diseases
- Psychiatric disease: depression, psychoses
- Protein loss from GI or renal abnormalities

TREATMENT

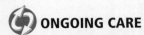

- Lifetime therapy aimed at treating copper overload
- Consists of two phases
  - (1) Removing or detoxifying the tissue copper (achieved by chelators)
  - (2) Preventing reaccumulation (low-dose chelators, dosages reduced by about 33% from original induction dose and/or by use of zinc salts)
- Successful therapy is measured in terms of a restoration of normal levels of free serum copper and its excretion in the urine.

MEDICATION (DRUGS)

- Penicillamine
  - Mode of action (MOA)
    - Chelates copper and promotes renal excretion
    - Also induces metallothionein (which forms a nontoxic combination with copper)
    - Efficacy: Improvement in clinical features noted after 2–3 months, continuing over a period of 1–2 years.
  - Dosages and monitoring:
    - Initial dose: 1–1.5 g/24 h in 2–4 divided doses PO, maximum total daily dose 20 mg/kg, taken 1 or 2 hours after food (absorption decreased by approximately 50% when taken with food).
    - May start at a lower dose (250–500 mg/day) with gradual escalation over a few weeks
    - Monitoring: clinical assessment + hematologic, biochemical (transaminases), and urinary parameters every week for 1 month, then every month for 6 months, and subsequently q6mo.
    - While on therapy, 24-hour urine copper exceeds ≥2,000 mcg/day, with gradual decline over 6–12 months to values below ≤200–500 mcg/day.
    - Once this level achieved and free serum copper <15 mcg/dL, the maintenance dose can be lowered to 0.5–1 g/24 h in divided doses (usually after 4–6 months).
    - At this point, a zinc salt could be added to the treatment regimen, preferably before meals to avoid any interaction with penicillamine.
    - The goal of treatment is a 24-hour urine copper excretion of 50–100 mcg
  - Side effects in 20–30%
    - Acute neurologic deterioration caused by rapid mobilization of hepatic copper stores leading to increased brain copper deposition, or from the development of intracellular copper complexes
    - Reduce dose to 250 mg/24 h or switch to trientine or zinc.
    - Pyridoxine deficiency, risk factors include intercurrent infection or a growth spurt. B_6 supplementation 25–50 mg/24 h
    - Skin complications due to interference with collagen and elastin formation
    - Hypersensitivity reactions (rash, fever, lymphadenopathy), bone marrow suppression, myasthenia gravis, optic neuritis, nephritis, lupuslike syndrome
    - Discontinue if the total white blood cell count <3,000 cells per mm^3, neutrophils <2,000 cells per mm^3, platelets <120,000 per mm^3, or if a steady decline over three successive tests even if the values are above the earlier mentioned parameters for discontinuation.
    - Discontinue also if >2+ proteinuria on a dipstick, red cell or white casts or >10 red cells seen per high-power field on urine microscopy.
- Trientine
  - MOA: chelates copper/promotes renal excretion
  - Dosages and monitoring:
    - Has become initial drug of choice
    - Used in combination with zinc
  - Dosages: pediatric dose 20 mg/kg/24 h PO divided 2–3×/24 h up to a maximum of 1,500 mg/24 h. Round dose to the nearest 250 mg.
  - Maintenance therapy: 750–1,000 mg/24 2–3×/day, avoid taking with food.
  - Monitoring: same as penicillamine
  - Side effects: fewer than penicillamine
    - Risk of sideroblastic anemia (drug's effects on mitochondrial iron metabolism), hemorrhagic gastritis, nephritis, arthritis, worsened neurologic signs
    - Serum copper increases during treatment.
    - Also chelates iron, creating toxic complex; do not give supplemental Fe (if iron supplementation required, administer Fe in short courses, separated by trientine by at least 2 hours).
- Zinc
  - Routinely combined with trientine
  - Also used alone as maintenance therapy
  - Used successfully in asymptomatic or presymptomatic affected family members of individuals with Wilson disease
  - MOA
    - Interferes with absorption from GI tract by inducing metallothionein in enterocytes, which chelates metals. Copper is bound within the enterocyte and not absorbed into the portal circulation. It is shed in stool along with normal shedding of enterocytes.
    - Also induces copper-binding metallothionein in the liver
    - May create a negative copper balance, removing all extra copper stores, resulting in improvement of hepatic and brain function, and loss of KF rings
  - Dosage: 50 mg t.i.d. PO, empty stomach
  - Side effects:
    - Few side effects: gastric irritation, nausea
    - Overtreatment may result in anemia, decreased wound healing, or neuromyelopathy from copper deficiency.
  - No altered dose needed for surgery.
  - Compliance with overall therapy monitored by urine zinc levels, which should be above 2 mg
  - After chelation for 4–6 months, with normal labs, usually OK to change to zinc for maintenance
- Ammonium tetrathiomolybdate
  - Not FDA-approved
  - Complex with copper in the intestinal tract, preventing absorption.
  - Absorbed drug forms a complex with copper and albumin in blood, which is metabolized by liver and excreted in bile.
  - Particularly suited for treatment of neurologic manifestation in Wilson disease, as it is not associated with exacerbation on initiation of treatment.
  - S/E: bone marrow suppression, elevated aminotransferases
- Antioxidants and experimental therapies
  - Antioxidants (vitamin E/*N*-acetylcysteine) may protect against oxidative damage.

ADDITIONAL TREATMENT

General Measures

- Immunize for hepatitis A, B.
- Avoid excess alcohol.
- Well water or water via copper pipes needs to be tested: If >0.1 ppm Cu, find alternative source.

SURGERY/OTHER PROCEDURES

- Orthotopic liver transplant required for fulminant liver failure or end-stage liver cirrhosis, which is resistant to chelation therapy.
- Uncertain indication for therapy-resistant neurologic symptoms. Several case reports suggest improved neurologic symptoms after transplantation.
- 5% with WD need liver transplants.

ONGOING CARE

FOLLOW-UP RECOMMENDATIONS

Patient Monitoring

- Patients require lifelong dietary copper restriction and chelation therapy.
- Continual monitoring for compliance and side effects of medications is crucial.
- Sudden discontinuation of therapy may precipitate fulminant hepatic failure.
- 1st-degree relatives >age 3 years should be screened with history, physical exam, LFTs, CBC, serum ceruloplasmin, 24-hour urine copper, and ophthalmologic examination for KF rings.
- Reproductive and genetic counseling for carriers should be offered. Prenatal testing

DIET

Low-copper diet for life: Avoid liver and other organ meats, shellfish, nuts, mushrooms, and chocolate.

COMPLICATIONS

- Renal: Copper accumulation leads to Fanconi syndrome (tubular dysfunction, glycosuria, hypophosphatemia, and low uric acid).
- Hematologic: Coombs-negative hemolytic anemia, coagulopathy from liver failure
- Cardiac: cardiomyopathy/dysrhythmias
- Rare associations include renal stones, gallstones, osteomalacia, osteoporosis, arthralgias, pancreatitis, hypoparathyroidism, skin pigmentation, and a bluish discoloration at the base of the fingernails (azure lunulae)

PROGNOSIS

- If WD is recognized early and treated, most patients experience complete recovery.
- Progression to hepatocellular carcinoma is rare, unlike hemochromatosis.

ADDITIONAL READING

- Ala A, Walker P, Ashkan K, et al. Wilson's disease. *Lancet*. 2007;369(9559):397–408.
- Brewer GJ, Askari F, Dick Rb, et al. Treatment of Wilson's disease with tetrathiomolybdate: V. Control of free copper by tetrathiomolybdate and comparison with trientine. *Transl Res*. 2009;154(2):70–77.
- Das SK, Ray K. Wilson's disease: an update. *Nat Clin Pract Neurol*. 2006;2(9):482–493.
- European Association for Study of Liver. EASL clinical practice guidelines: Wilson's disease. *J Hepatol*. 2012;56(3):671.

CODES

ICD10

E83.01 Wilson's disease

WISKOTT-ALDRICH SYNDROME

Elena Elizabeth Perez

BASICS

DESCRIPTION

- An X-linked primary immunodeficiency caused by a mutation in the Wiskott-Aldrich syndrome (*WAS*) gene
- Originally described as clinical triad of thrombocytopenia with small platelets, eczema, and recurrent infections with opportunistic and pyogenic organisms
- Increased bleeding tendency secondary to thrombocytopenia likely results from impaired platelet production, increased turnover, and defective function.
- Disease variants also resulting from *WAS* gene mutations include X-linked thrombocytopenia (XLT) and X-linked neutropenia (XLN).
- Classic WAS is characterized by broad immunodeficiency, decreased number and function of T cells, disturbed marginal B-cell homeostasis, and skewed immunoglobulin isotypes, with defective antibody responses to vaccinations, impaired NK-cell cytotoxicity, and abnormal regulatory T-cell function as well as reduced phagocyte chemotaxis.

EPIDEMIOLOGY

- Presents in infancy with serious bleeding episodes secondary to thrombocytopenia (such as circumcision with increased bleeding, bloody diarrhea, ecchymoses)
- Recurrent infections usually start after 6 months of age:
  - Bacterial: otitis media, sinusitis, meningitis, sepsis, and pneumonia
  - Viral infections: herpes simplex virus, varicella with systemic complications
- Milder phenotypes may lack history of recurrent infections.
- Decline in T- and B-cell numbers with time
- Eczema is usually present by 1 year of age (may be resistant to therapy, sometimes requiring systemic antibiotics).

Incidence

- For WAS/XLT, estimate is 10 in 1 million live births.
- Prevalence of XLT equal to WAS

RISK FACTORS

Genetics

- X-linked recessive disease
- Defective Wiskott-Aldrich syndrome protein gene located on X p11.22p–11.23
- ~60% of cases will have a positive family history for WAS.
- XLT without the other findings is caused by mutations of the same gene.
- Genotype/phenotype correlation
  - Lack of Wiskott-Aldrich syndrome protein (WASP) expression: increased infections, severe eczema, intestinal hemorrhage, death from intracranial bleeding, and malignancies
  - Survival rate significantly lower in WASP-negative patients

ETIOLOGY

- Mutations in the gene for the WASP
- WASP is involved in the reorganization of the actin cytoskeleton in hematopoietic cells:
  - Following activation of WASP, reorganization of actin cytoskeleton results in polarization of cells (e.g., polarized actin mesh in platelets for clotting and in macrophages for phagocytosis, and polarization of T or B cells to form immunologic synapses).
- WASP is a cytoplasmic protein involved in cell mobility, immune regulation, cell signaling, cell-to-cell interactions, signaling, and cytotoxicity.
- Defects in WASP can lead to dysfunction in adaptive and innate immunity, immune surveillance, and platelet homeostasis and function as well as neutropenia.
- "Classic" WAS and XLT result from loss-of-function mutations.
- XLT can be misdiagnosed as idiopathic thrombocytopenic purpura (ITP) that does not carry increased risk of malignancy, so testing for WASP expression and *WAS* gene mutation is important in any male with thrombocytopenia and small platelets.
- XLN results from "activating" mutations in WAS that lead to increased actin polymerization; profound neutropenia, with or without associated lymphopenia; decreased T-cell proliferation in vitro; and increased risk of myelodysplastic changes in bone marrow.
- WASP is also important for regulatory T-cell function.

COMMONLY ASSOCIATED CONDITIONS

Associated with IgA nephropathy, autoimmune disorders, and an increased incidence of B-cell lymphomas

DIAGNOSIS

- Diagnosis should be considered in any boy who has congenital or early-onset thrombocytopenia with small platelets.
- Definitive diagnosis
  - Male patient
  - Congenital thrombocytopenia (<70,000/mm^3)
  - Small platelets (mean platelet volume <0.5 fL)
  - Mutation in the *WASP* gene or absent WASP mRNA

HISTORY

- Persistent or severe bleeding in infancy due to thrombocytopenia
- Recurrent infections, especially by bacteria with capsular polysaccharides (e.g., *pneumococcus*)
- Eczema can be of variable severity:
  - "Acute or chronic"
  - 80% of cases associated with eczema
  - May result from imbalance of cytokines skewed toward Th2
- Older patients may report recurrent viral infections.
- Most common autoimmune features include autoimmune hemolytic anemia, cutaneous vasculitis, arthritis, and nephropathy.
- Less common autoimmune features include inflammatory bowel disease, ITP, and neutropenia.
- Autoimmune features are poor prognostic indicators and can occur simultaneously.
- Maternal family history of WAS or XLT

PHYSICAL EXAM

- Evaluation should focus on presence of infection.
- Dermatologic examination is significant for the extent of eczema and the presence of petechiae or ecchymoses.
- Splenomegaly

DIAGNOSTIC TESTS & INTERPRETATION

Lab

- CBC with differential
- Small platelets, decreased mean platelet volume, decreased platelet count
- Normal IgG, decreased IgM, increased IgA and IgE (reflecting immune dysregulation)
- Reduced or absent responses to polysaccharide antigens and isohemagglutinins to ABO antigens
- T- and B-lymphocyte enumeration and mitogen stimulation studies may progressively deteriorate with increasing age.

Diagnostic Procedures/Other

- WAS disease scoring system useful for defining clinical phenotypes associated with WAS mutations (XLN, XLT vs. classic WAS)
- Sequencing of WAS gene
- Lymph node biopsy in suspected malignancy
- Bone marrow aspirate to evaluate thrombocytopenia

DIFFERENTIAL DIAGNOSIS

- Other causes of thrombocytopenia such as ITP
- In 1 cohort, approximately 7% of patients diagnosed as having ITP actually had WAS as an underlying cause of thrombocytopenia.
- Severe atopic disease with dermatitis and secondary skin infections
- HIV infection
- Hyper-IgE syndrome

TREATMENT

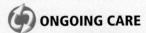

GENERAL MEASURES

- Antibiotics for acute infections and prophylactically in postsplenectomy patients
- Splenectomy may be helpful for persistent severe thrombocytopenia in select patients. However, this may greatly increase the risk of overwhelming infections with encapsulated organisms.
- Splenectomy should be reserved for emergencies in classic WAS patients who are candidates for hematopoietic stem cell transplantation (HSCT) because it is a risk factor for death. Splenectomy in XLT with severe bleeding may increase platelet counts, but risk of severe infection requires lifelong antibiotic prophylaxis.
- Thrombocytopenia precautions: No aspirin and avoidance of situations in which trauma (especially head trauma) is likely to occur, such as contact sports.
- Platelet transfusions may be necessary for severe bleeding. Use irradiated blood products to avoid graft versus host disease and cytomegalovirus-negative products in case of bone marrow transplantation.
- Immunoglobulin replacement therapy is helpful in managing recurrent infections in some patients:
  - HSCT is the treatment of choice for the classic WAS phenotype.
  - Allogeneic stem cell transplant from human leukocyte antigen (HLA) genotypically identical sibling or 9/10 or 10/10 allele matched unrelated donor for any WAS patient with disease score 3–5 (see "Additional Reading") or with absent WASP expression
  - Outcomes are improving with 5-year survival rates >80% for matched sibling donors and similar for matched unrelated donor grafts <5 years of age. Transplant outcomes for patients >5 years of age with matched sibling or matched unrelated are also improving over time.
- Consider food allergy as exacerbating factor for eczema.
- First retroviral-based gene therapy trial in WAS recently completed in Germany with good immune reconstitution and increase in platelet counts in 9/10 patients. Lentiviral-based gene therapy trials are starting in the near future.
- XLT patients have excellent long-term survival with supportive treatment, but HLA-matched sibling transplant can be considered owing to morbidity.

ONGOING CARE

FOLLOW-UP RECOMMENDATIONS

Patient Monitoring

- Signs and symptoms of malignancy should be evaluated expeditiously.
- As patients age, a progressive increase in infectious and autoimmune complications may occur.

COMPLICATIONS

- Progressive decline in immunologic function with an increase in infections. Humoral and cellular immune systems are affected.
- Increased frequency of autoimmune phenomena such as arthritis and vasculitis. The most common is hemolytic anemia. Vasculitis, Henoch-Schönlein purpura, inflammatory polyarthritis, and inflammatory bowel disease are also observed.
- ~100-fold increased risk of malignancy compared with the general pediatric population. Malignancy is more common in adolescents. Associated with Epstein-Barr virus
- Bleeding episodes can be life threatening.
- Immune reconstitution via stem cell transplant or gene therapy needed to prevent autoimmune disorders, lymphoma, and other malignancy
- Success of bone marrow transplant in last 10 years significantly improved.
- Splenectomy not recommended for classic WAS but may have role in XLT.

ADDITIONAL READING

- Albert MH, Notarangelo LD, Ochs HD. Clinical spectrum, pathophysiology and treatment of the Wiskott-Aldrich syndrome. *Curr Opin Hematol*. 2011;18(1):42–48.
- Auiti A, Biasco L, Scaramuzza S, et al. Lentiviral hematopoietic stem cell gene therapy in patients with Wiskott-Aldrich syndrome. *Science*. 2013; 341(6148):1233151.
- Binder V, Albert M, Kabus M, et al. The genotype of the original Wiskott phenotype. *N Engl J Med*. 2006;355(17):1790–1793.
- Bosticardo M, Marangoni F, Aiuti A, et al. Recent advances in understanding the pathophysiology of Wiskott-Aldrich syndrome. *Blood*. 2009;113(25): 6288–6295.
- Bryant N, Watts R. Thrombocytopenic syndromes masquerading as childhood immune thrombocytopenic purpura. *Clin Pediatr*. 2011;50(3):225–230.
- Charrier S, Dupre L, Scaramuzza S, et al. Lentiviral vectors targeting WASp expression to hematopoietic cells, efficiently transduce and correct cells from WAS patients. *Gene Ther*. 2007;14(5):415–428.
- Imai K, Morio T, Zhu Y, et al. Clinical course of patients with WASP gene mutations. *Blood*. 2004; 103(2):456–464.
- Jin Y, Mazza C, Christie J, et al. Mutations of the Wiskott-Aldrich syndrome protein (WASP): hotspots, effect on transcription, and translation and phenotype/genotype correlation. *Blood*. 2004;104(13): 4010–4019.
- Massaad MJ, Ramesh N, Geha RS. Wiskott-Aldrich syndrome: a comprehensive review. *Ann N Y Acad Sci*. 2013;1285:26–43.
- Ochs HD. The Wiskott-Aldrich syndrome. *Clin Rev Allergy Immunol*. 2001;20(1):61–86.
- Schurman SH, Candotti F. Autoimmunity in Wiskott-Aldrich syndrome. *Curr Opin Rheumatol*. 2003;15(4):446–453.
- Shcherbina A, Candotti F, Rosen F, et al. High incidence of lymphomas in a subgroup of Wiskott-Aldrich syndrome patients. *Br J Haematol*. 2003;121(3):529–530.
- Simon KL, Anderson SM, Garabedian EK, et al. Molecular and phenotypic abnormalities of B lymphocytes in patients with Wiskott-Aldrich syndrome. *J Allergy Clin Immunol*. 2014;133(3):896–9.e4

CODES

ICD10

D82.0 Wiskott-Aldrich syndrome

FAQ

- Q: What is the life expectancy for patients with Wiskott-Aldrich syndrome?
- A: Before currently available therapies, most affected patients died in childhood. Currently, many patients live into their 3rd and 4th decades, even without bone marrow transplantation. Major causes of mortality are infections (44%), bleeding (23%), and malignancies (26%). Incidence of malignancy increases in 3rd decade of life. Successfully transplanted patients have a prolonged life expectancy. Patients with no gene expression have a poorer outcome.
- Q: Should patients with Wiskott-Aldrich syndrome receive live viral vaccines?
- A: These vaccines should be avoided because of the variable cellular immune defects associated with Wiskott-Aldrich syndrome. In general, patients receiving IV immunoglobulin do not require vaccinations.
- Q: What is the chance of a sibling having Wiskott-Aldrich syndrome?
- A: As with any X-linked disease, there is a 50% chance of another affected male child or asymptomatic carrier female. Genetic counseling should be offered to carrier females.
- Q: Can Wiskott-Aldrich syndrome be diagnosed prenatally?
- A: In families with affected males, fetal blood sampling can be performed in male fetuses to assess the size of the platelets. Small platelet size and family history of Wiskott-Aldrich syndrome suggest an affected infant.

YERSINIA ENTEROCOLITICA

Julia Shaklee Sammons

BASICS

DESCRIPTION

Yersinia enterocolitica is a gram-negative bacillus that produces an enteric infection characterized by fever, diarrhea, and abdominal pain that may mimic acute appendicitis.

EPIDEMIOLOGY

- *Y. enterocolitica* is estimated to cause 116,716 infections in the United States annually.
  - According to surveillance by the Foodborne Diseases Active Surveillance Network (FoodNet) from 1996 to 2009, the overall annual incidence of *Y. enterocolitica* infections was 0.5 per 100,000 persons but significantly declined over the time period.
  - Most infections occurred in young children; 47% were in children <5 years, and 32% were in infants <1 year.
  - Among subgroups, the highest annual incidence was among infants <1 year at 12.3 per 100,000 persons.
- Transmission of *Y. enterocolitica*
  - Occurs through ingestion of contaminated food or water (particularly raw or undercooked pork or unpasteurized milk products) or contact with infected animals (swine are the principal reservoir)
  - Fecal–oral and person-to-person transmission are also possible.
  - In the United States, most epidemics have been related to the improper handling of raw pork intestine (chitterlings), most often during winter holiday festivities among African American households in the South.
  - Transmission to young children occurs through contact with adult caregivers preparing the chitterlings.
- Transmission through transfusion of contaminated blood products is also possible. The FDA has reported that contamination of the U.S. blood supply by bacteria, although rare, is most frequently due to *Y. enterocolitica*.
- The incubation period is ~1–14 days (average 4–6). The mean duration of organism excretion is 42 days; however, asymptomatic carriage can persist even longer.
- Systemic disease or bacteremia occurs more commonly in young infants or those with predisposing conditions, including a clinical state of iron overload or deferoxamine therapy, immunosuppression, diabetes mellitus, malnutrition, and cirrhosis or other liver diseases.

GENERAL PREVENTION

- Infection control
  - Contact precautions are indicated for patients with enterocolitis until diarrhea resolves.
- General measures
  - Attempts to eliminate reservoirs and reduce frequency of ingesting contaminated foods and beverages are necessary.
  - Ingestion of undercooked meats, especially pork and unpasteurized milk, should be avoided.
  - Meticulous hand hygiene before and after handling uncooked meat products and avoidance of preparation of meats near or during preparation of infant bottles for feeding are essential.

PATHOPHYSIOLOGY

- The portal of entry for *Y. enterocolitica* is the gastrointestinal tract.
- *Y. enterocolitica* adheres to epithelial cells and mucus, producing heat-stable enterotoxins, which play a role in the development of watery diarrhea.
  - Another cytotoxin then directly injures the distal small and large bowel, producing stools characterized by blood and mucus.
  - Release of these toxins leads to the development of an enterocolitis, most commonly in younger age groups.
- Mesenteric adenitis and/or terminal ileitis may lead to a pseudoappendicitis syndrome, typically in the older child or young adult.
- Bacteremia may lead to focal abscesses in a variety of organs, including the lung, liver, spleen, and kidney.

ETIOLOGY

- The genus *Yersinia* consists of 11 species, of which *Yersinia enterocolitica*, *Yersinia pseudotuberculosis*, and *Yersinia pestis* are the 3 most commonly encountered pathogens.
- *Y. enterocolitica* is a facultative, non–lactose-fermenting, urease-positive, gram-negative bacillus.
- Over 60 serotypes and 6 biotypes of *Y. enterocolitica* have been identified. Serotypes O:3, O:5.27, O:8, and O:9 and biotypes 2, 3, and 4 are most commonly isolated from patients. Serotype O:3 is the most common type in the United States.

DIAGNOSIS

Diagnosis depends on elucidation of the pertinent exposure history as well as recognition of typical symptoms and laboratory testing.

HISTORY

- Enterocolitis is the most common manifestation of *Y. enterocolitica* infection in young children and is characterized by fever, abdominal pain, and diarrhea with blood or mucus.
  - 25% of patients have hematochezia.
  - Typical duration of illness is 1–3 weeks but may be longer (up to several months).
  - The history taking should include questions regarding exposure to unpasteurized milk products and raw pork or poultry, especially the preparation of pork chitterlings.
- A pseudoappendicitis syndrome due to mesenteric adenitis and/or terminal ileitis predominates in older children and adults and is associated with fever, right lower quadrant abdominal pain, and leukocytosis.
- *Yersinia* bacteremia is found most commonly in infants <1 year of age or those with predisposing conditions, particularly states of iron overload (e.g., sickle cell disease, thalassemia).
- Extraintestinal manifestations of *Y. enterocolitica* infection are uncommon and include pharyngitis, suppurative lymphadenitis, pyomyositis, osteomyelitis, abscess, UTI, pneumonia, endocarditis, meningitis, peritonitis, panophthalmitis, conjunctivitis, and septic arthritis.

PHYSICAL EXAM

Because of the wide range of clinical symptoms, including extraintestinal manifestations, the physical exam is nonspecific for this infection.

DIAGNOSTIC TESTS & INTERPRETATION

Lab

- *Y. enterocolitica* can be isolated from blood, sputum, CSF, urine, and bile; these specimens do not require selective culture media techniques.
  - Stool samples should be plated on selective media such as cefsulodin-triclosan-novobiocin agar.
  - If routine enteric media (MacConkey) are used, a cold enrichment technique will increase recovery of the organism.
  - The laboratory should be notified that *Yersinia* is suspected if not routinely sought.

- Serologic methods (tube agglutination assay, enzyme-linked immunosorbent assay [ELISA]) are available with a rise in titers noted 1 week after onset of symptoms and peak titers observed by the 2nd week of illness. These tests identify IgM, IgG, and IgA antibodies against *Y. enterocolitica*.
- Cross-reactivity between *Y. enterocolitica* and *Brucella abortus*, *Rickettsia* species, *Morganella morganii*, *Salmonella* species, and thyroid tissue antigen make serodiagnosis of limited usefulness.

Imaging

Abdominal ultrasound can be used to distinguish pseudoappendicitis from acute appendicitis through demonstration of bowel wall edema in the terminal ileum and cecum.

DIFFERENTIAL DIAGNOSIS

- *Y. enterocolitica* should be considered in all patients with fever, abdominal pain, and stools with blood or mucus as well as in patients with the extraintestinal manifestations described earlier.
- Pitfalls
  - Not all bacterial colitis presents with bloody or mucus-appearing diarrhea. Therefore, suspicion should exist if the diarrhea is prolonged or environmental exposures pose a risk for developing infection.
  - The possibility of *Y. enterocolitica* bacteremia should be considered in blood transfusion–related illnesses, thalassemia, or prior history of liver disease.

TREATMENT

GENERAL MEASURES

- The benefit of treatment of uncomplicated enterocolitis, mesenteric adenitis, or pseudoappendicitis has not been established in immunocompetent hosts.
- Antimicrobial therapy has been shown to benefit patients with systemic infections, focal extraintestinal infections, and enterocolitis in an immunocompromised host.
- For most isolates, trimethoprim/sulfamethoxazole, chloramphenicol, aminoglycosides, tetracycline or doxycycline, fluoroquinolones, and 3rd-generation cephalosporins are effective treatment options.
- *Y. enterocolitica* is usually resistant to most penicillins and 1st-generation cephalosporins.

ONGOING CARE

FOLLOW-UP RECOMMENDATIONS

- Symptoms of enterocolitis usually abate within 2 weeks of the onset of illness.
- Shedding of the organism in stool can last more than 6 weeks after diagnosis.
- For extraintestinal manifestations, the expected course depends on the specific organ system involved.

PROGNOSIS

- The prognosis is usually quite good, as most infections are gastrointestinal.
- Systemic disease (i.e., septicemia with subsequent secondary spread) has higher morbidity and mortality. Mortality related to septicemia can be as high as 50%.

COMPLICATIONS

- Postinfectious sequelae may occur 1–2 weeks after gastrointestinal symptoms and include erythema nodosum as well as reactive arthritis involving weight-bearing joints. These complications are seen most often in adults, particularly those with HLA-B27 antigen.
- Reactive arthritis syndrome, myocarditis, glomerulonephritis, erysipelas, chronic diarrhea persisting for months, and hemolytic anemia have also been reported.
- Intestinal perforation and ileocolic intussusception are possible.

ADDITIONAL READING

- Abdel-Haq NM, Asmar BI, Abuhammour WM, et al. *Yersinia enterocolitica* infection in children. *Pediatr Infect Dis J*. 2000;19(10):954–958.
- Guinet F, Carniel E, Leclercq A, et al. Transfusion-transmitted *Yersinia enterocolitica* sepsis. *Clin Infect Dis*. 2011;53(6):583–591.
- Natkin J, Beavis KG. *Yersinia enterocolitica* and *Yersinia pseudotuberculosis*. *Clin Lab Med*. 1999; 19(3):523–536.
- Ong KL, Gould LH, Chen DL, et al. Changing epidemiology of *Yersinia enterocolitica* infections: markedly decreased rates in young black children, Foodborne Diseases Active Surveillance Network (FoodNet), 1996–2009. *Clin Infect Dis*. 2012; 54(Suppl 5):S385–S390.
- Scallan E, Hoekstra RM, Angulo FJ, et al. Foodborne illness acquired in the United States—major pathogens. *Emerg Infect Dis*. 2011;17(1):7–15. doi:10.3201/eid1701.091101p1.

CODES

ICD10

- A04.6 Enteritis due to Yersinia enterocolitica
- A05.8 Other specified bacterial foodborne intoxications

FAQ

- Q: How long is a child considered infectious with *Y. enterocolitica*?
- A: Although the typical course of enterocolitis is ~14 days, shedding of the organism in the stool can last 6 weeks or longer. Strict adherence to hand hygiene should be discussed with the child's parent or caregiver, particularly for those with incontinent or diapered children, to ensure infection control.
- Q: If there is no history of stools with blood or mucus, can you exclude *Y. enterocolitica* as the likely infectious agent in a child with diarrhea?
- A: No. In fact, early in the course of illness, the diarrhea is more likely to be watery owing to the enterotoxins produced (see "Pathophysiology").
- Q: How is the diagnosis of *Y. enterocolitica* determined if you are unable to isolate the organism from a clinical specimen?
- A: When a diagnosis cannot be made during acute infection or in the clinical setting of postinfectious complications, a serologic titer of >1:128 is suggestive of previous infection of *Y. enterocolitica*. Keep in mind the possibility of cross-reactivity with *Brucella*, *Rickettsia*, *Morganella*, and *Salmonella* species as well as thyroid antigens.

Appendix I
The 5-Minute Educator

Terry Kind

Part 1: Precepting
Part 2: Direct Observation
Part 3: Feedback
Part 4: Clinical Reasoning

PART 1: PRECEPTING

Cara Lichtenstein

DESCRIPTION

Precepting is the education and teaching of learners in a clinical care setting.

TECHNIQUES USED BEFORE THE VISIT

Orient the learner at the start of the rotation:

- Gather information on background, strengths, and weaknesses of the learner.
- Communicate goals and set expectations for the rotation.
- Discuss your style of feedback and how frequently it will be given.
- Introduce trainee to office staff they will work with during the rotation.
- Familiarize trainee with recordkeeping (electronic medical record, paper charts).

Wave Scheduling

- Build in preceptor teaching time without reducing overall number of patients.

Time (a.m.)	Room 1	Room 2
8:30–8:50	Patient A seen by student	Patient B seen by preceptor
8:50–9:10	Patient A seen by preceptor and student	—
9:10–9:30	Student charts on patient A	Patient C seen by preceptor
9:30–9:50	Patient D seen by student	Patient E seen by preceptor
9:50–10:10	Patient D seen by preceptor and student	—
10:10–10:30	Student charts on patient D	Patient F seen by preceptor

Prime learners before they go in to room:

- Prompt learner to retrieve stored information and prepare for immediate use.
- Orient the learner to the patient or possible medical problem.
  - For example: cc ear tugging: What will help you determine what the origin of the ear tugging is?
  - For example: cc speech delay: What is the typical speech of a 2-year-old like?
  - For example: cc 2-week well-child visit: What do you think the purpose(s) of this visit is?
- Give the learner a task and goal.
  - For example: cc "1st-time wheeze": The task may be to gather a focused history, and the goal may be to formulate a broad differential diagnosis of causes of wheezing.
- Make a plan for when to meet back and discuss the case.

TECHNIQUES USED DURING THE VISIT

Reflective Modeling

- Allows learners to observe the preceptor interacting with and examining the patient
- Preceptor talks aloud during the visit explaining to patient AND to learner what's going on, what they think the diagnosis or next steps are, and why they don't think something else is going on.

Activated Demonstration

- Goal is for trainee to learn by observing preceptor's interaction with a patient.
- Briefly prime them in advance for what to look for.
- Set up the observation.
  - Determine student's relevant knowledge.
  - Identify what student should learn from observation.
    - Watch the technique the preceptor use for examining the ear, exposing the oropharynx, etc.
    - Watch how the preceptor enlist the help of the parent.
    - Watch how the preceptor navigates, excusing the parent from the room so the preceptor can talk with the teen (patient) privately.
  - Provide clear guidelines for what student should do while observing.
    - For example: Quietly observe; jot notes with what you are observing.

Student Clinical Observation of Preceptor (SCOOP)

- Allows learner to observe preceptor's interaction with patient and family
- Learner uses a tool or writes 3 things they observed.
- Items discussed together afterwards

Brief Structured Clinical Observation (SCO)

- Allows assessment of learners skill level through direct observation
- Preceptor spends short period of time (5 minutes) observing part of visit (can be history, physical, or information giving).
- Uses a tool to give immediate feedback to learner on directly observed performance

Presenting in the Room

- After confirming there are no sensitive issues, learner presents in front of family.
- Saves time, as preceptor can examine patient while learner is presenting
- Family can correct any misinformation or clarify questions on the spot.
- Patients perceive increased time spent with doctor, better care, and more adequate explanation of problems.

TECHNIQUES USED AFTER THE VISIT

One-Minute Preceptor

- A structure allowing preceptors to assess learners effectively, teach key points of a case, and provide feedback efficiently, using 5 "microskills"
  - **Get a commitment** about diagnosis or treatment.
  - **Probe for supporting evidence** for that diagnosis or treatment.
  - **Teach general rules** about the case or diagnosis.
  - **Reinforce what was correct** with positive feedback.
  - **Correct mistakes** with suggestions for future improvements.

SNAPPS

- Method of presentation that focuses on clinical reasoning and self-directed learning that is learner-driven
- Preceptor sets expectation that learner will present using SNAPPS:
  - **Summarize** the history and findings.
  - **Narrow** the differential.
  - **Analyze** the differential diagnosis by comparing/contrasting possibilities.
  - **Probe** (student probes the preceptor) for further understanding, with questions about areas of uncertainty.
  - **Plan** for patient management.
  - **Self**-directed learning: **Select** an issue to learn more about.

GENERAL TEACHING TIPS

- Wait 3 seconds after asking a question.
- Focus only on 1–2 teaching points per encounter.
- If you don't know, say you don't know.
- Examples speak louder than words.

PITFALLS TO AVOID

- "Taking over" the case by providing answers instead of questions
- Inappropriately long, esoteric, or noninteractive lectures
- Not waiting long enough to get an answer
- Preprogrammed answers
- Not appreciating the level of the learners and teaching beyond their ability

ADDITIONAL READING

- Allevi AM, Lane JL. Microskills in office teaching. *Pediatr Ann*. 2010;39(2):72–77.
- Ferenchick G, Simpson D, Blackman J, et al. Strategies for efficient and effective teaching in the ambulatory care setting. *Acad Med*. 1997;72(4):277–280.
- Neher JO, Stevene NG. The one-minute preceptor: shaping the teaching conversation. *Fam Med*. 2003;35(6):391–393.
- Strategies in Clinical Teaching: a community-based faculty development Web site from the University of Kansas School of Medicine–Wichita: http://wichita.kumc.edu/strategies/index.html.

PART 2: DIRECT OBSERVATION

Sandra Cuzzi

BASICS

- **Definition**: the process of observing a learner (e.g., student, resident) during an actual patient encounter for the purpose of assessing clinical skills
- **Aim**: to help preceptors gather accurate information about a learner's performance in real-life clinical scenarios
- **Assessment:** communication skills, history taking, physical exam techniques, information giving, professionalism, and evaluation of competence

GETTING STARTED

Primary Purpose

Defining the primary purpose of direct observation is important in choosing the tool, setting, scope, and skills to be observed.

- **Formative**: timely feedback given to initiate discussion and promote reflection, with the goal of improving clinical skills and modifying behavior
- **Summative**: scheduled summary evaluation to "grade" or rank, with the goal of assessing global performance
- **Documentation of competency**: Direct observation is required by the accrediting bodies for both medical student and resident education.

Using an Observation Tool

- Advantages of using a tool are that it:
  - Clarifies expectations for all involved
  - Standardizes what preceptors watch for
  - Guides feedback to make it more specific
  - Fulfills documentation requirements
- Formative assessment: Primary focus of tool is to facilitate feedback so proven reliability and validity is not as important.
- Summative assessment: critical for the tool to be well-studied, valid, and reliable
- Use an existing tool for direct observation that fits the primary purpose.
- Mini-clinical evaluation exercise (mini-CEX)
  - Best studied tool with excellent validity
  - For formative or summative assessment
  - Requires observation over 10–20 minutes, which can make it difficult to incorporate into a busy clinical setting
- Structured clinical observation (SCO)
  - Most commonly used tool in pediatrics for formative assessment
  - Divided into 3–4 specific sections, 1 for each part of the clinical encounter, with a behavioral checklist to guide feedback
  - Used for 3–5-minute observations; complete only the section of patient encounter that is observed.

Determine Setting, Scope, and Skills

- Look for opportunities where an observer is already present during a clinical encounter.
- For example, a physician working in the newborn nursery may be present to observe learner's newborn physical exam skills or a social worker present at family meetings where learners are leading the discussion can engage in direct observation.
- Opportunities can lend themselves to shorter observation (e.g., inpatient or outpatient visit) or longer ones (e.g., counseling session).
- Shorter observations tend to work best as formative feedback; longer ones can be used for summative evaluations.

IMPLEMENTATION

Potential Barriers to Direct Observation

- Lack of time
- Inadequate training, discomfort, or difficulty in observation and/or feedback
- Hawthorne effect: Presence of observer changes behavior of those observed.
- Family perception regarding observation
- Logistical barriers (scheduling, patient flow, space configuration)

Orienting the Preceptor and Learner

- Clearly state expectations once setting, scope, and, skills are defined.
- Understand preceptor and learner attitudes, experience, and knowledge regarding direct observation.
- If setting up a direct observation program institution-wide, then determine what content areas need to be covered and provide preceptor faculty development.
- Orient all to the process and logistics.

Number of Observations

- When paired with feedback, every observation has value to the learner as formative assessment.
- 4–5 observations will probably identify an "outlier" in terms of minimal competency.
- Ideally, 10–12 observations are needed over time to be reliable in assessing competency for summative assessment.

Practical Tips

- Multiple short observations allow for less time commitment, observation in a variety of clinical scenarios, and can monitor improvement over time.
- A preceptor may want to routinely set up direct observation with the first patient in a clinical session (e.g., first afternoon patient).
- Set up the specific observation beforehand with the learner and family.
- Brief 3–5-minute observations
- Take notes while observing: Set up 2 columns, 1 for "things done well", the other for "things to improve," or consider filling out the tool's checklist as you observe.
- Be a "fly on the wall": Sit away from line of sight of the patient, avoid the temptation to interrupt.
- At times, the preceptor can get involved at a certain predetermined stage of the process (e.g., after physical exam, preceptor confirms findings and advises on technique).
- Provide timely focused feedback right after observing.

Creating a Culture of Observation

- Goal: Create a culture in which observation is understood, expected, nonthreatening, and routine for everyone including patients, parents, learners, and preceptors.
- Orient the participants and set expectations.
- Make it a joint responsibility between learner and preceptor to arrange.
- Observe at regular intervals so it becomes routine.
- Consistently give feedback after observing.
- Identify "champions" of direct observation as role models and mentors.
- Encourage opportunities for preceptors to be observed by learners too.

ADDITIONAL READING

- Hanson JL, Bannister SL, Clark A, et al. Oh, what can you see: the role of observation in medical student education. *Pediatrics*. 2010;126(5):843–845.
- Hamburger EK, Cuzzi S, Coddington DA, et al. Observation of resident clinical skills: outcomes of a program of direct observation in the continuity clinic setting. *Acad Pediatr*. 2011;11(5):394–402.
- Hauer KE, Holmboe ES, Kogan JR. Twelve tips for implementing tools for direct observation of medical trainees' clinical skills during patient encounters. *Med Teach*. 2011;33(1):27–33.
- Holmboe ES. Faculty and the observation of trainees' clinical skills: problems and opportunities. *Acad Med*. 2004;79(1):16–22.
- Lane JL, Gottlieb RP. Structured clinical observations a method to teach clinical skills with limited time and financial resources. *Pediatrics*. 2000;105(4):973–977.

PART 3: FEEDBACK

Terry Kind • Dewesh Agrawal

BASICS

Description

Feedback

- Formative, nonevaluative, objective appraisal of performance aimed at modifying and improving clinical skills, correcting deficits, and improving future performance
- Targeted to specific (observed) behaviors the trainee already does well and those in need of improvement
- Immediate and *formative*, not summative
- Presents information, not judgment
- Can be positive (reinforcing) or negative (constructive or corrective) or both
- Feedback involves a specific event or occurrence versus compliment/criticism, which are more vague and general.
- Like evaluation, should ideally be based on objective observations

Evaluation

- Summative judgment
- Equivalent to grading and/or assigning a final grade for the rotation
- Intent is to tell learners how they performed.
- Like feedback, should ideally be based on objective observations

Compliment and Criticism

- COMPLIMENT: a polite expression of praise or admiration
- CRITICISM: an expression of disapproval based on perceived faults or mistakes
- These are typically general, judgmental, and are not goal-based or not based on specific observations.

BARRIERS

- Potential barriers to providing effective feedback:
  - Insufficient time; competing demands
  - Insufficient observation; gathering essential information is difficult.
  - Don't have the necessary skills; didn't have good role models
  - Difficult to give negative feedback; want to be "popular"
  - Fears of student reprisals or failure to recruit into specialty
  - Not my responsibility; unimportant
  - Don't know where to start
  - Lack of sufficient structure
  - Defensive learner or one who lacks insight into his or her deficiencies
  - Lack of well-defined, mutually agreed upon goals established
- Conditions that promote appropriate feedback
  - Feedback is part of the institutional culture and is given frequently.
  - Adequate time and timing (promptly)
  - Private setting
  - Learner knows when/where it will happen.
  - Based on specific, observed, and potentially modifiable behaviors
  - Based on objective observations, not on interpretations of the learner's motives
  - Matches with well-defined learning goals
  - Nonjudgmental language

ALERT
Remember that the GOAL of feedback is to improve performance.

MODELS

Fast

- **F** = frequently given and in digestible chunks
- **A** = accurate, based on observation
- **S** = specific, focused on modifiable behaviors
- **T** = timely

Insight

- **I** = INQUIRY: How does the resident/student/learner think it went?
- **N** = NEEDS: What learning needs does the resident/student/learner identify?
- **S** = SPECIFIC: Was your feedback specific?
- **I** = INTERCHANGE: Was there a discussion?
- **G** = GOALS: What are the next steps?
- **H** = HELP: Are there ways you can help?
- **T** = TIMING: When will follow-up occur?

Feedback Grid (Walsh, 2006)

- **Continue:** Comment on aspects of performance that were effective and should be done in the future.
- **Start or do more:** Comment on behaviors that the student knows how to do and should start doing or do so more often.
- **Consider:** Comment on "doable challenges" for the future growth of the student.
- **Stop, or do less:** Comment on observed actions that were not helpful and/or could be harmful.

Pearls (Milan, 2006)

- **P** = partnership for joint problem solving
- **E** = empathic understanding
- **A** = apology for barriers to the learner's success
- **R** = respect for learner's values and choices
- **L** = legitimation of feelings and intentions
- **S** = support for efforts at correction

Sandwich

- Provide a compliment or some reinforcing feedback, then provide some constructive feedback, then close with another compliment or additional reinforcing feedback.
- The negative feedback is sandwiched between 2 positive statements.

SOAP Format

- **S** = subjective self-assessment by learner; ask learner how he or she thinks it went.
- **O** = objective balanced; descriptive feedback is provided.
- **A** = assess and summarize; ask learner to summarize 2 "take-home" points.
- **P** = plan for next steps incorporating new strategies.

ADDITIONAL READING

- Branch WT Jr, Paranjape A. Feedback and reflection: teaching methods for clinical settings. *Acad Med*. 2002;77(12):1185–1188.
- Ende J. Feedback in clinical medical education. *JAMA*. 1983;250(6):777–781.
- Hewson MG, Little ML. Giving feedback in medical education: verification of recommended techniques. *J Gen Intern Med*. 1998;13(2):111–116.
- Milan FB, Parish SJ, Reichgott MJ. A model for educational feedback based on clinical communication skills strategies: beyond the "feedback sandwich." *Teach Learn Med*. 2006;18(1):42–47.
- Ramani S, Krackov SK. Twelve tips for giving feedback effectively in the clinical environment. *Med Teach*. 2012;34(10):787–791.
- Richardson BK. Feedback. *Acad Emerg Med*. 2004;11(12):e1–e5.
- Walsh A. Working with IMGs: delivering effective feedback. In: Walsh A, ed. *A faculty development program for teachers of international medical graduates*. London, Ontario, Canada: The Association of Faculties of Medicine of Canada; 2006. http://www.afmc.ca/img. Accessed March 3, 2015.

FAQ

- Q: Is there anything wrong with just using the "feedback sandwich"?
- A: It can either confuse or dilute the real message. It may be perceived as insulting or condescending by the learner. Sometimes the learner only focuses on positives or negatives and fails to understand the big picture.
- Q: Is it ever okay to say "good job"?
- A: Compliments are best used when paired with reinforcing feedback that is more specific and based on observed behavior.

PART 4: CLINICAL REASONING

Mary Ottolini • Terry Kind

BASICS

Description

- The process of acquiring and interpreting clinical data to determine the etiology of a patient's presenting complaint
- Involves having a framework for storing and organizing medical knowledge effectively, which is critical for avoiding diagnostic error
- The experienced clinician uses problem representation, searches through "illness scripts" to make a diagnosis and employs strategies to avoid cognitive biases.

Developmental Progression

Clinical educators simultaneously diagnose the patient and diagnose the learner's developmental level of clinical reasoning.

- **Analytic reasoning:** Through basic pathophysiology, differential diagnoses are considered in "silos" or "disembodied" unrelated to patient's specific findings.
- **Development of illness scripts:** linking signs and symptoms of current patient to patterns of signs and symptoms seen in previous patients, filtering and grouping the data gathered into illness scripts
- **Problem representation:** creating a nuanced illness script for a current patient by synthesizing information into "semantic qualifiers," reflecting cognitive processing based on prior experience

The Clinical Reasoning Process

PATIENT STORY

↑↓

DATA ACQUISITION

↓

PROBLEM REPRESENTATION

↓

HYPOTHESIS GENERATION

↓

SEARCH FOR ILLNESS SCRIPT

↓

DIAGNOSIS

Problem Representation

SUMMARY statement of mental model of patient

- Key features of HPI/PE +
- Semantic qualifiers (adjectives)

Illness Scripts

Prototypical disease presentations based on the following:

- Epidemiology: Who gets the illness? (age, exposure, travel, etc.)
- Timing: onset and progression
- Classic/exclusionary findings
- Pathophysiology/anatomic explanation

Problem representation and illness scripts promote the "CHUNKING" of data or compiling information into a clinical syndrome, based on patterns and experience.

"Vertical Versus Horizontal Reading"

Deliberately compare/contrast illness scripts for 2–3 diagnoses for a clinical syndrome (vertically), rather than 1 diagnosis at a time (horizontally).

Type 1 Versus Type 2 Reasoning

Experts move back and forth between types (i.e., dual-processing) depending on prior experience with illness presentation:

- **Type 1:** heuristics or "rules of thumb" as mental shortcuts if a pattern of signs and symptoms or illness script is recognized
- **Type 2:** analytical/deductive reasoning used when the presentation is unusual; slow and deliberate process

FACTORS LEADING TO DIAGNOSTIC ERRORS

Cognitive Biases

- Predictable errors in reasoning occurring particularly with TYPE 1 (heuristic) processing; can make gathering essential information and clinical reasoning difficult
- COMMON BIASES
  - Premature closure: relying on initial diagnostic impression despite subsequent information to the contrary
  - Anchoring bias: relying too heavily on 1 piece of information
  - Confirmation bias: searching for, interpreting, and remembering information in a way that confirms one's preconceptions
  - Diagnostic momentum: sticking with one diagnostic label due to frequent repetition

ALERT

Diagnostic error is currently a leading cause of serious medical errors. Improved clinical reasoning can be taught as a strategy to decrease diagnostic errors.

  - Availability bias: overreliance on what easily comes to mind
  - Base-rate neglect: ignoring the true prevalence of a disease

Strategies to Overcome Biases

- Metacognition: deliberately reflecting "in-action" and thinking about thinking
  - Did the diagnosis come too easily?
  - Is there any data that doesn't fit?
  - Am I investing too much in one finding?
  - Do I dislike the patient/parent?
- Take a "diagnostic time-out"
  - Recognize when time pressure may lead to premature closure on the wrong diagnosis.

Oral Presentation Framework

Encourage students to include clinical reasoning in their presentations:

P: PROBLEM REPRESENTATION: assessment-driven presentation

BE: BACKGROUND EVIDENCE: Focus on pertinent positives and negatives.

A: ANALYSIS: Compare and contrast 2 likely illness scripts.

R: RECOMMENDATION: plan based on a problem rather than system

ADDITIONAL READING

- Bowen J. Educational strategies to promote clinical diagnostic reasoning. *N Engl J Med*. 2006;355(21):2217–2225.
- Croskerry P. "Achieving quality in clinical decision making: cognitive strategies and detection of bias." *Acad Emerg Med*. 2002;9(11):1184–1204.
- Newman-Toker DE, Pronovost PJ. Diagnostic errors—the next frontier for patient safety. *JAMA*. 2009;301(10):1060–1062.
- Schmidt HG, Norman GR, Boshuizen HP. A cognitive perspective on medical expertise: theory and implication. *Acad Med*. 1990;65(10):611–621.
- Schmidt HG, Rikers RM. How expertise develops in medicine: knowledge encapsulation and illness script formation. *Med Educ*. 2007;41(12):1133–1139.
- Thammasitboon S, Cutrer WB, Thammasitboon S, et al. Diagnostic error and strategies to minimize them. *Curr Probl Pediatr Adolesc Health Care*. 2013;43(9):225–257.

FAQ

- Q: Can the clinical reasoning process be taught?
- A: Yes, promoting "problem representation" and comparing and contrasting the differentiating features using illness scripts helps trainees to organize and store their patient experiences so that they can recall them in future similar situations.
- Q: Can one overcome cognitive errors?
- A: Yes. Using metacognition, or "thinking about your thinking," a form of situational awareness, one can develop a habit of taking a "diagnostic time-out."

Appendix II
Cardiology Laboratory

Gurumurthy Hiremath • Laura Robertson

BLOOD PRESSURE MEASUREMENT

- **All children >3 years old should have their blood pressure (BP) measured as part of their physical exam.**
- If <3 years old, measure BP if there are comorbidities present that predispose them to hypertension.
- **Measure BP in right upper arm** for purposes of consistency, comparability to standard tables and to avoid a spurious value in cases of coarctation.
- BP by auscultation is the preferred method.
- Abnormal BP obtained by oscillometry should be confirmed by auscultation.
- **Optimal BP cuff size (Table 1)**
  - Bladder length covers 80–100% of the circumference of the arm.
  - Bladder width covers 40% of the upper arm circumference.
- **Refer to BP standards based on gender, age, and height** that now include 50th, 90th, 95th, and 99th percentiles **(Tables 2 and 3)**.
- **Hypertension** is defined as average systolic BP (SBP) and/or diastolic BP (DBP) that are ≥95th percentile for gender, age, and height on 3 occasions.
- **Prehypertension:** If the SBP or DBP is ≥90th percentile and <95th percentile, it is called "prehypertension."
- **Aortic coarctation:** An upper extremity BP >10 mm Hg higher than the lower extremity BP is pathologic and suggests the presence of aortic coarctation, aortic arch hypoplasia, or interrupted aortic arch. If suspected, check BP in all 4 extremities.

PULSE OXIMETRY

Systemic arterial blood oxygen content is a combination of oxygen bound to hemoglobin (Hgb) plus dissolved oxygen. The calculation:

- **Oxygen Content = (Hgb** in gm/dL × **1.36** in mL O_2/g of Hgb × **% O_2 saturation)** + (Pao_2 × 0.003 O_2/dL per mm Hg)
- Decreased arterial oxygen content is called **"hypoxemia,"** which can result in **"hypoxia"** which is failure to oxygenate at tissue level (manifesting as metabolic acidosis). **"Cyanosis"** is the clinical manifestation of bluish discoloration of skin or mucosa resulting from hypoxemia.
- **Etiologies of systemic arterial desaturation:**
  - Pulmonary venous desaturation (lung disease).
  - Right-to-left shunting (cardiac disease)
  - Hgb disorders

Visible central cyanosis occurs when the deoxygenated Hgb is >3 g/dL.

- **Polycythemic neonate** (Hgb = 20 g/dL) with an arterial saturation of 80% *will have 4 g/dL of deoxygenated Hgb and will appear cyanotic.*
- **Anemic neonate** (Hgb = 10 g/dL) with an arterial saturation of 80% *will have only 2 g/dL of deoxygenated Hgb and will not appear cyanotic.*

How to Measure Saturations Properly

- **Pulse oximetry is an established screening tool to detect critical congenital heart disease in newborns.** See **Figure 1**.
  - **Preductal:** Measure saturation in the right ear lobe or right arm.
  - **Postductal:** Measure saturation in either leg.

Differential Saturation Interpretation

- **Lower postductal saturation** suggests coarctation of aorta, pulmonary hypertension, critical left-sided obstructive lesions, or infradiaphragmatic total anomalous pulmonary venous return.
- **Higher postductal saturation** suggests transposition or supracardiac total anomalous pulmonary venous return.

Table 1. Recommended Dimensions for BP Cuff Bladders

Age Range	Width, cm	Length, cm	Maximum Arm Circumference, cm*
Newborn	4	8	10
Infant	6	12	15
Child	9	18	22
Small adult	10	24	26
Adult	13	30	34
Large adult	16	38	44
Thigh	20	42	52

BP, blood pressure.
*Calculated so that the largest arm would still allow the bladder to encircle arm by at least 80%.
From National High Blood Pressure Education Program Working Group on High Blood Pressure in Children and Adolescents. The fourth report on the diagnosis, evaluation, and treatment of high blood pressure in children and adolescents. *Pediatrics*. 2004;114(2)(Suppl):555–576.

Table 2. BP Levels for Boys by Age and Height Percentile

Age, y	BP Percentile	SBP, mm Hg							DBP, mm Hg						
		Percentile of Height							Percentile of Height						
		5th	10th	25th	50th	75th	90th	95th	5th	10th	25th	50th	75th	90th	95th
1	50th	80	81	83	85	87	88	89	34	35	36	37	38	39	39
	90th	94	95	97	99	100	102	103	49	50	51	52	53	53	54
	95th	98	99	101	103	104	106	106	54	54	55	56	57	58	58
	99th	105	106	108	110	112	113	114	61	62	63	64	65	66	66
2	50th	84	85	87	88	90	92	92	39	40	41	42	43	44	44
	90th	97	99	100	102	104	105	106	54	55	56	57	58	58	59
	95th	101	102	104	106	108	109	110	59	59	60	61	62	63	63
	99th	109	110	111	113	115	117	117	66	67	68	69	70	71	71
3	50th	86	87	89	91	93	94	95	44	44	45	46	47	48	48
	90th	100	101	103	105	107	108	109	59	59	60	61	62	63	63
	95th	104	105	107	109	110	112	113	63	63	64	65	66	67	67
	99th	111	112	114	116	118	119	120	71	71	72	73	74	75	75
4	50th	88	89	91	93	95	96	97	47	48	49	50	51	51	52
	90th	102	103	105	107	109	110	111	62	63	64	65	66	66	67
	95th	106	107	109	111	112	114	115	66	67	68	69	70	71	71
	99th	113	114	116	118	120	121	122	74	75	76	77	78	78	79
5	50th	90	91	93	95	96	98	98	50	51	52	53	54	55	55
	90th	104	105	106	108	110	111	112	65	66	67	68	69	69	70
	95th	108	109	110	112	114	115	116	69	70	71	72	73	74	74
	99th	115	116	118	120	121	123	123	77	78	79	80	81	81	82
6	50th	91	92	94	96	98	99	100	53	53	54	55	56	57	57
	90th	105	106	108	110	111	113	113	68	68	69	70	71	72	72
	95th	109	110	112	114	115	117	117	72	72	73	74	75	76	76
	99th	116	117	119	121	123	124	125	80	80	81	82	83	84	84
7	50th	92	94	95	97	99	100	101	55	55	56	57	58	59	59
	90th	106	107	109	111	113	114	115	70	70	71	72	73	74	74
	95th	110	111	113	115	117	118	119	74	74	75	76	77	78	78
	99th	117	118	120	122	124	125	126	82	82	83	84	85	86	86
8	50th	94	95	97	99	100	102	102	56	57	58	59	60	60	61
	90th	107	109	110	112	114	115	116	71	72	72	73	74	75	76
	95th	111	112	114	116	118	119	120	75	76	77	78	79	79	80
	99th	119	120	122	123	125	127	127	83	84	85	86	87	87	88
9	50th	95	96	98	100	102	103	104	57	58	59	60	61	61	62
	90th	109	110	112	114	115	117	118	72	73	74	75	76	76	77
	95th	113	114	116	118	119	121	121	76	77	78	79	80	81	81
	99th	120	121	123	125	127	128	129	84	85	86	87	88	88	89
10	50th	97	98	100	102	103	105	106	58	59	60	61	61	62	63
	90th	111	112	114	115	117	119	119	73	73	74	75	76	77	78
	95th	115	116	117	119	121	122	123	77	78	79	80	81	81	82
	99th	122	123	125	127	128	130	130	85	86	86	88	88	89	90
11	50th	99	100	102	104	105	107	107	59	59	60	61	62	63	63
	90th	113	114	115	117	119	120	121	74	74	75	76	77	78	78
	95th	117	118	119	121	123	124	125	78	78	79	80	81	82	82
	99th	124	125	127	129	130	132	132	86	86	87	88	89	90	90

Table 2. BP Levels for Boys by Age and Height Percentile *(continued)*

Age, y	BP Percentile	SBP, mm Hg							DBP, mm Hg						
		Percentile of Height							Percentile of Height						
		5th	10th	25th	50th	75th	90th	95th	5th	10th	25th	50th	75th	90th	95th
12	50th	101	102	104	106	108	109	110	59	60	61	62	63	63	64
	90th	115	116	118	120	121	123	123	74	75	75	76	77	78	79
	95th	119	120	122	123	125	127	127	78	79	80	81	82	82	83
	99th	126	127	129	131	133	134	135	86	87	88	89	90	90	91
13	50th	104	105	106	108	110	111	112	60	60	61	62	63	64	64
	90th	117	118	120	122	124	125	126	75	75	76	77	78	79	79
	95th	121	122	124	126	128	129	130	79	79	80	81	82	83	83
	99th	128	130	131	133	135	136	137	87	87	88	89	90	91	91
14	50th	106	107	109	111	113	114	115	60	61	62	63	64	65	65
	90th	120	121	123	125	126	128	128	75	76	77	78	79	79	80
	95th	124	125	127	128	130	132	132	80	80	81	82	83	84	84
	99th	131	132	134	136	138	139	140	87	88	89	90	91	92	92
15	50th	109	110	112	113	115	117	117	61	62	63	64	65	66	66
	90th	122	124	125	127	129	130	131	76	77	78	79	80	80	81
	95th	126	127	129	131	133	134	135	81	81	82	83	84	85	85
	99th	134	135	136	138	140	142	142	88	89	90	91	92	93	93
16	50th	111	112	114	116	118	119	120	63	63	64	65	66	67	67
	90th	125	126	128	130	131	133	134	78	78	79	80	81	82	82
	95th	129	130	132	134	135	137	137	82	83	83	84	85	86	87
	99th	136	137	139	141	143	144	145	90	90	91	92	93	94	94
17	50th	114	115	116	118	120	121	122	65	66	66	67	68	69	70
	90th	127	128	130	132	134	135	136	80	80	81	82	83	84	84
	95th	131	132	134	136	138	139	140	84	85	86	87	87	88	89
	99th	139	140	141	143	145	146	147	92	93	93	94	95	96	97

BP, blood pressure; DBP, diastolic blood pressure; SBP, systolic blood pressure.
From National High Blood Pressure Education Program Working Group on High Blood Pressure in Children and Adolescents. The fourth report on the diagnosis, evaluation, and treatment of high blood pressure in children and adolescents. *Pediatrics*. 2004;114(2)(Suppl):555–576.

Table 3. BP Levels for Girls by Age and Height Percentile

Age, y	BP Percentile	SBP, mm Hg							DBP, mm Hg						
		Percentile of Height							Percentile of Height						
		5th	10th	25th	50th	75th	90th	95th	5th	10th	25th	50th	75th	90th	95th
1	50th	83	84	85	86	88	89	90	38	39	39	40	41	41	42
	90th	97	97	98	100	101	102	103	52	53	53	54	55	55	56
	95th	100	101	102	104	105	106	107	56	57	57	58	59	59	60
	99th	108	108	109	111	112	113	114	64	64	65	65	66	67	67
2	50th	85	85	87	88	89	91	91	43	44	44	45	46	46	47
	90th	98	99	100	101	103	104	105	57	58	58	59	60	61	61
	95th	102	103	104	105	107	108	109	61	62	62	63	64	65	65
	99th	109	110	111	112	114	115	116	69	69	70	70	71	72	72
3	50th	86	87	88	89	91	92	93	47	48	48	49	50	50	51
	90th	100	100	102	103	104	106	106	61	62	62	63	64	64	65
	95th	104	104	105	107	108	109	110	65	66	66	67	68	68	69
	99th	111	111	113	114	115	116	117	73	73	74	74	75	76	76
4	50th	88	88	90	91	92	94	94	50	50	51	52	52	53	54
	90th	101	102	103	104	106	107	108	64	64	65	66	67	67	68
	95th	105	106	107	108	110	111	112	68	68	69	70	71	71	72
	99th	112	113	114	115	117	118	119	76	76	76	77	78	79	79
5	50th	89	90	91	93	94	95	96	52	53	53	54	55	55	56
	90th	103	103	105	106	107	109	109	66	67	67	68	69	69	70
	95th	107	107	108	110	111	112	113	70	71	71	72	73	73	74
	99th	114	114	116	117	118	120	120	78	78	79	79	80	81	81
6	50th	91	92	93	94	96	97	98	54	54	55	56	56	57	58
	90th	104	105	106	108	109	110	111	68	68	69	70	70	71	72
	95th	108	109	110	111	113	114	115	72	72	73	74	74	75	76
	99th	115	116	117	119	120	121	122	80	80	80	81	82	83	83
7	50th	93	93	95	96	97	99	99	55	56	56	57	58	58	59
	90th	106	107	108	109	111	112	113	69	70	70	71	72	72	73
	95th	110	111	112	113	115	116	116	73	74	74	75	76	76	77
	99th	117	118	119	120	122	123	124	81	81	82	82	83	84	84
8	50th	95	95	96	98	99	100	101	57	57	57	58	59	60	60
	90th	108	109	110	111	113	114	114	71	71	71	72	73	74	74
	95th	112	112	114	115	116	118	118	75	75	75	76	77	78	78
	99th	119	120	121	122	123	125	125	82	82	83	83	84	85	86
9	50th	96	97	98	100	101	102	103	58	58	58	59	60	61	61
	90th	110	110	112	113	114	116	116	72	72	72	73	74	75	75
	95th	114	114	115	117	118	119	120	76	76	76	77	78	79	79
	99th	121	121	123	124	125	127	127	83	83	84	84	85	86	87
10	50th	98	99	100	102	103	104	105	59	59	59	60	61	62	62
	90th	112	112	114	115	116	118	118	73	73	73	74	75	76	76
	95th	116	116	117	119	120	121	122	77	77	77	78	79	80	80
	99th	123	123	125	126	127	129	129	84	84	85	86	86	87	88
11	50th	100	101	102	103	105	106	107	60	60	60	61	62	63	63
	90th	114	114	116	117	118	119	120	74	74	74	75	76	77	77
	95th	118	118	119	121	122	123	124	78	78	78	79	80	81	81
	99th	125	125	126	128	129	130	131	85	85	86	87	87	88	89

Table 3. BP Levels for Girls by Age and Height Percentile *(continued)*

Age, y	BP Percentile	SBP, mm Hg							DBP, mm Hg						
		Percentile of Height							Percentile of Height						
		5th	10th	25th	50th	75th	90th	95th	5th	10th	25th	50th	75th	90th	95th
12	50th	102	103	104	105	107	108	109	61	61	61	62	63	64	64
	90th	116	116	117	119	120	121	122	75	75	75	76	77	78	78
	95th	119	120	121	123	124	125	126	79	79	79	80	81	82	82
	99th	127	127	128	130	131	132	133	86	86	87	88	88	89	90
13	50th	104	105	106	107	109	110	110	62	62	62	63	64	65	65
	90th	117	118	119	121	122	123	124	76	76	76	77	78	79	79
	95th	121	122	123	124	126	127	128	80	80	80	81	82	83	83
	99th	128	129	130	132	133	134	135	87	87	88	89	89	90	91
14	50th	106	106	107	109	110	111	112	63	63	63	64	65	66	66
	90th	119	120	121	122	124	125	125	77	77	77	78	79	80	80
	95th	123	123	125	126	127	129	129	81	81	81	82	83	84	84
	99th	130	131	132	133	135	136	136	88	88	89	90	90	91	92
15	50th	107	108	109	110	111	113	113	64	64	64	65	66	67	67
	90th	120	121	122	123	125	126	127	78	78	78	79	80	81	81
	95th	124	125	126	127	129	130	131	82	82	82	83	84	85	85
	99th	131	132	133	134	136	137	138	89	89	90	91	91	92	93
16	50th	108	108	110	111	112	114	114	64	64	65	66	66	67	68
	90th	121	122	123	124	126	127	128	78	78	79	80	81	81	82
	95th	125	126	127	128	130	131	132	82	82	83	84	85	85	86
	99th	132	133	134	135	137	138	139	90	90	90	91	92	93	93
17	50th	108	109	110	111	113	114	115	64	65	65	66	67	67	68
	90th	122	122	123	125	126	127	128	78	79	79	80	81	81	82
	95th	125	126	127	129	130	131	132	82	83	83	84	85	85	86
	99th	133	133	134	136	137	138	139	90	90	91	91	92	93	93

BP, blood pressure; DBP, diastolic blood pressure; SBP, systolic blood pressure; y, year.
From National High Blood Pressure Education Program Working Group on High Blood Pressure in Children and Adolescents. The fourth report on the diagnosis, evaluation, and treatment of high blood pressure in children and adolescents. *Pediatrics*. 2004;114(2)(Suppl):555–576.

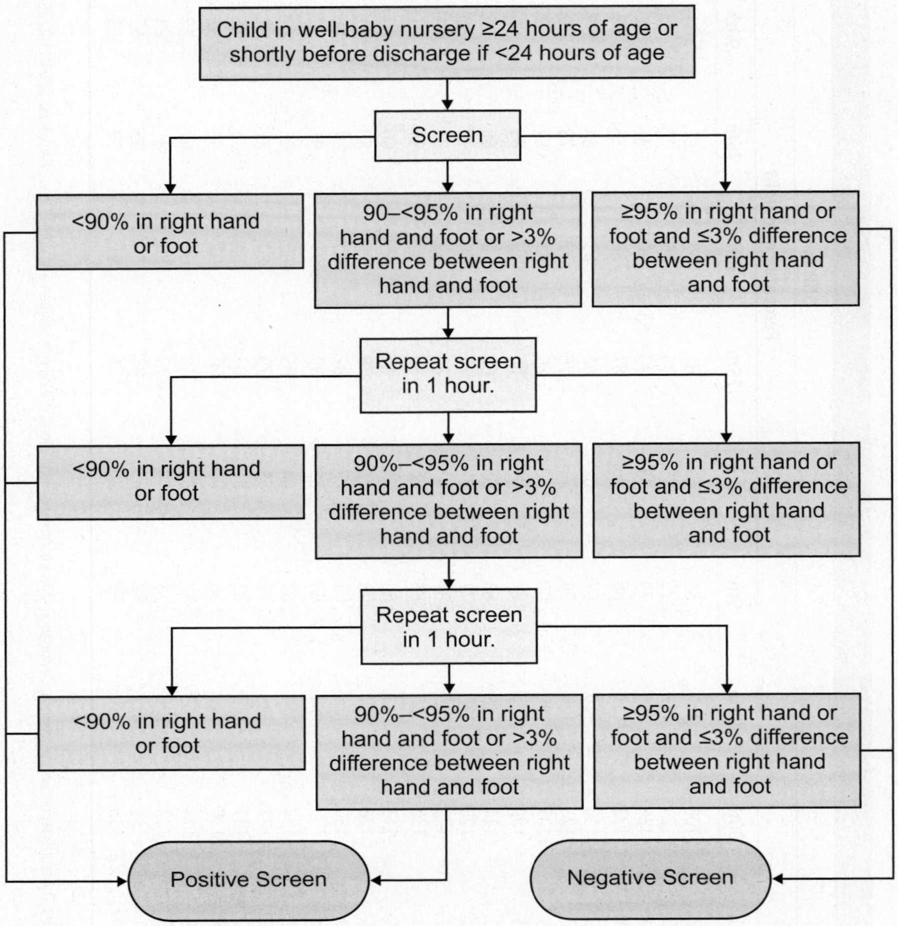

FIGURE 1. The proposed pulse-oximetry monitoring protocol based on results from the right hand and either foot. From Kemper AR, Mahle WT, Martin GR, et al. Strategies for implementing screening for critical congenital heart disease. *Pediatrics.* 2011;128(5):e1259–e1267.

Hyperoxia Test

- In infants with cyanosis, a hyperoxia test using arterial blood gas is performed to differentiate cyanotic congenital heart disease from other etiologies of hypoxia. If a right radial arterial PaO_2 on 100% FiO_2 is <150 mm Hg, cyanotic congenital heart disease is likely **(Table 4)**.

ELECTROCARDIOGRAPHY

- The standard ECG consists of 12 leads that include 3 limb leads (I, II, III), 3 augmented limb leads (aVR, aVL, aVF), and 6 precordial leads (V_1–V_6). In children, additional precordial leads are often used, making it a 15-lead ECG (V3R, V4R, and V_7).
- The standard ECG paper speed is 25 mm/s with amplitude of 0.1 mV/mm **(Fig. 2)**. Each small box is 40 ms, and each large box is 200 ms.
- **Pediatric ECG parameters are age-dependent**. See **Table 5** for comprehensive standards of normal ECG in children.

Rate and Rhythm

- **Heart rate is calculated by dividing 60,000 ms/min by the measured cycle length**. The rhythm is considered sinus if each QRS is preceded by a P wave, and the P wave is upright in I, II, and aVF.

Axes

- Axes can be calculated in a hexaxial reference plane for all three waves of the ECG.
- **P-wave axis** indicates whether the rhythm begins in the sinus node or an alternative pacemaker.
- **QRS axis changes with age**. In the newborn period, the mean vector of depolarization is rightward, reflecting the dominance of the right ventricle in early infancy. As the left ventricular mass increases relative to the right side, the QRS axis shifts more leftward.
- **A superior QRS (northwest axis) suggests an endocardial cushion defect or tricuspid atresia**.
- The **T wave** represents ventricular repolarization. Within the first 72 hours of life, the T wave should invert in lead V_1. Persistence of upright T wave beyond 7 days of age until adolescence is a sensitive indicator of increased right ventricular pressure. As the left ventricle becomes progressively more dominant, the T-wave axis parallels the QRS axis. Thus, during adolescence, the T wave becomes upright in lead V_1 and the T-wave axis becomes leftward.
- The **QRS-T angle** should be ≤90 degrees. Abnormally wide QRS-T angle may be a result of ventricular hypertrophy with strain pattern or ventricular conduction disturbance.

Atrioventricular Conduction and Intervals

- The PR interval is measured from the onset of the P wave to the beginning of the QRS complex and reflects the time for atrial depolarization and delay through the AV node. In general, with age, the heart rate is slower and the PR interval is longer.
- A **short PR interval** occurs when there is Wolff-Parkinson-White syndrome, Lown-Ganong-Levine syndrome, glycogen storage disease, or low atrial pacemaker.

Table 4. Diagnostic Testing in Cyanosis

Test	Pulmonary Parenchymal Disease	Intra- or Extrapulmonary Right to Left Shunt	Central Hypoventilation	Transposition Physiology	Hemoglobin Disorders
Respiratory distress	Present; may have fever	No	No; apnea/hypoventilation	Mild distress, usually tachypnea due to increased PBF	No
Cardiac exam	Normal	May have single S_2, RV heave, thrill and murmurs	Normal	Single S_2, flow murmur, RV heave	Normal
Chest x-ray	Pulmonary pathology	Variable cardiac silhouette; usually clear lung fields	Normal	Egg-on-end appearance, pulmonary venous congestion ±	Normal
Differential saturation (preductal vs. postductal)	Absent	Present if right-to-left shunt at ductus; postductal < preductal	Absent	Postductal > preductal	Absent
CBC	Elevated white cell count	Polycythemia if chronic	Normal	Polycythemia if chronic	Normal
Arterial blood gas on 100% FiO_2	Pao_2 >150 mm Hg $Paco_2$ variable	Pao_2 <150 mm Hg Normal $Paco_2$	Pao_2 >150 mm Hg, usually much higher; elevated $Paco_2$	Pao_2 <150 mm Hg, usually <50 mm Hg; normal $Paco_2$	Normal Pao_2 and $Paco_2$

CBC, complete blood count; FiO_2, fraction of inspired oxygen; PBF, pulmonary blood flow; RV, right ventricle.
Adapted from Hiremath G, Kamat D. Diagnostic considerations in infants and children with cyanosis. *Pediatr Ann*. 2015;44(2):76–80.

Abnormal Atrioventricular Conduction

- **First-degree AV block** is PR prolongation for age and heart rate.
- **Second-degree AV block** can be Mobitz Type I (Wenckebach), where there is progressive PR prolongation before a dropped beat or Mobitz Type II, where there is abrupt failure of AV conduction without previous PR prolongation.
- **Third-degree AV block** involves no conduction of atrial impulses to the ventricle.
- **QRS widening** is seen with a bundle branch block, preexcitation (e.g., Wolff-Parkinson-White syndrome), intraventricular block, ventricular arrhythmias, and ventricular-paced rhythms.
- **Left bundle branch block** is diagnosed when there is slurred R wave in left precordial leads (V_6) and slurred S wave in right precordial leads (V_1).
- **Right bundle branch block** is diagnosed when there is a wide and slurred S wave in leads V_1 and V_6, slurred R (rSR' pattern or M shaped QRS complex) in lead V_1. Left anterior hemiblock can be diagnosed in the setting of left axis deviation associated with right bundle branch block.
- **QT interval** represents the time it takes for ventricular depolarization and repolarization and is measured from the onset of the Q wave to the termination of the T wave. Given that the QT interval should shorten with increasing heart rates, the QT measurement should be adjusted for heart rate using **Bazett formula**:

$$QTc = \frac{\text{measured QT}}{\text{square root of the R-R interval}}$$

- **The QTc interval is less than 0.45 seconds for infants younger than 6 months, and less than 0.44 seconds for children.**
- The QTc is prolonged in **long QT syndrome** wherein there are genetic abnormalities of either the cardiac potassium or sodium channels. Other conditions that prolong the QTc interval include head injury, myocarditis, medications (such as, procainamide, amiodarone, quinidine) and electrolyte abnormalities (e.g., hypocalcemia, hypomagnesemia, hypokalemia).

Waveforms

- When the P-wave amplitude is greater than 3 mm in lead II or lead V_1, **right atrial enlargement** is present. If the P wave has duration greater than 0.1 seconds in lead II or is biphasic with a prominent negative component in lead V_1, **left atrial enlargement** is present.
- Abnormally, tall R waves in lead V_1 or deep S waves in V_5 and V_6 represent **right ventricular hypertrophy**. Similarly, tall R waves in leads V_5 and V_6 or deep S waves in lead V_1 **represent left ventricular hypertrophy**.
- Low-voltage QRS complexes suggest myocarditis, pericarditis, pericardial effusion, or hypothyroidism.
- Tall, peaked T waves can be seen with ventricular hypertrophy associated with strain, myocardial infarction, or hyperkalemia.

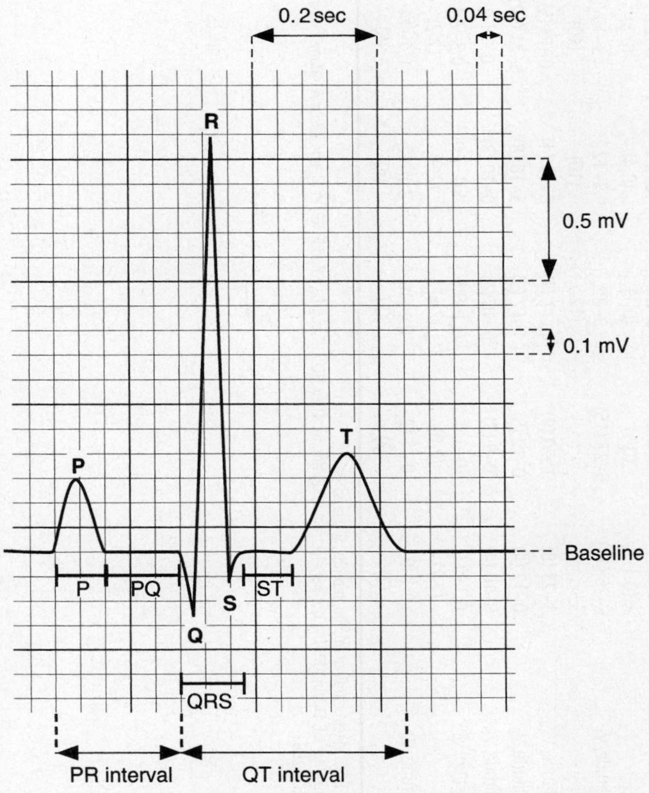

FIGURE 2. A normal electrocardiogram showing waveforms and intervals. The standard paper speed is 25 mm/s; therefore, a single 1-mm box equals 0.04 seconds, and a large (5-mm) box equals 0.20 seconds.

Table 5. Normal ECG Standards for Children by Age

	0–1 d	1–3 d	3–7 d	7–30 d	1–3 mo	3–6 mo	6–12 mo	1–3 y	3–5 y	5–8 y	8–12 y	12–16 y
Heart rate per minute	94–155 (122)	91–158 (122)	90–166 (128)	06–182 1 (149)	120–179 (149)	105–185 (141)	108–169 (131)	89–152 (119)	73–137 (109)	65–133 (100)	62–130 (91)	60–120 (80)
Frontal plane QRS axis (degrees)	59–189 (135)	64–197 (134)	76–191 (133)	0–160 7 (109)	30–115 (75)	7–105 (60)	6–98 (55)	7–102 (55)	6–104 (56)	10–139 (65)	6–116 (60)	9–128 (59)
PR lead II (s)	0.08–0.16 (0.107)	0.08–0.14 (0.108)	0.07–0.15 (0.102)	0.07–0.14 (0.100)	0.07–0.13 (0.098)	0.07–0.15 (0.105)	0.07–0.16 (0.106)	0.08–0.15 (0.113)	0.08–0.16 (0.119)	0.09–0.16 (0.123)	0.09–0.17 (0.128)	0.09–0.18 (0.135)
QRS duration, V_5 (s)	0.02–0.07 (0.05)	0.02–0.07 (0.05)	0.02–0.07 (0.05)	0.02–0.08 (0.05)	0.02–0.08 (0.05)	0.02–0.08 (0.05)	0.03–0.08 (0.05)	0.03–0.08 (0.06)	0.03–0.07 (0.06)	0.03–0.08 (0.06)	0.04–0.09 (0.06)	0.04–0.09 (0.07)
P-wave amplitude lead II	0.5–2.8 (1.6)	0.3–2.8 (1.6)	0.7–2.9 (1.7)	0.7–3.0 (1.9)	0.7–2.6 (1.5)	0.4–2.7 (1.6)	0.6–2.5 (1.6)	0.7–2.5 (1.5)	0.3–2.5 (1.4)	0.4–2.5 (1.4)	0.3–2.5 (1.4)	0.3–2.5 (1.4)
Q-wave amplitude, aVF	0.1–3.4 (1.0)	0.1–3.3 (1.0)	0.1–3.5 (1.1)	0.1–3.5 (1.2)	0.1–3.4 (0.9)	0–3.2 (0.9)	0–3.3 (1.0)	0–3.2 (0.9)	0–2.9 (0.6)	0–2.5 (00.6)	0–2.7 (0.5)	0–2.4 (0.4)
Q-wave amplitude, V_6	0–1.7 (0.1)	0–2.2 (0.1)	0–2.8 (0.1)	0–2.8 (0.4)	0–2.6 (0.3)	0–2.6 (0.3)	0–3.0 (0.4)	0–2.8 (0.6)	0.1–3.3 (0.8)	0.1–4.6 (0.8)	0.1–2.8 (0.6)	0–2.9 0.4
R amplitude, V_1	5–26 (13)	5–27 (15)	3–25 (12)	3–12 (10)	3–19 (10)	3–20 (10)	2–20 (9)	2–18 (8)	1–18 (8)	1–14 (7)	1–12 (5)	1-10 (4)
S amplitude, V_1	1–23 (8)	1–20 (9)	1–17 (7)	0–11 (4)	0–13 (5)	0–17 (6)	1–18 (7)	1–21 (8)	2–22 (10)	3–23 (12)	3–25 (12)	3–22 (11)
R amplitude, V_6	0–12 (4)	0–12 (5)	1–12 (5)	3–16 (8)	5–21 (12)	6–22 (13)	6–23 (13)	6–23 (13)	8–25 (15)	8–26 (16)	9–25 (16)	7–23 (14)
S amplitude, V_6	0–10 (4)	0–9 (3)	0–10 (4)	0–10 (3)	0–7 (3)	0–10 (3)	0–8 (2)	0–7 (2)	0–6 (2)	0–4 (1)	0–4 (1)	0–4 (1)
R-to-S ratio, V_1	0.1–9.9 (2.2)	0–1.6 (2.0)	0.1–9.8 (2.8)	1.0–7.0 (2.9)	0.3–7.4 (2.2)	0.1–6.0 (2.3)	0.1–4.0 (1.8)	0.1–4.3 (1.4)	0.03–2.7 (0.9)	0.02–2.0 (0.8)	0.02–1.9 (0.6)	0.02–1.8 (.5)
R-to-S ratio, V_6	0.1–9 (2)	0.1–12 (3)	0.1–10 (2)	0.1–12 (4)	0.2–14 (5)	0.2–18 (7)	0.2–22 (8)	0.3–27 (10)	0.6–30 (11)	0.9–30 (12)	1.5–33 (14)	1.4–39 (15)

d, days; ECG, electrocardiogram; mo, months; y, years.
From Van Hare GF, Dubin AM. The normal electrocardiogram. In: Allen HD, Driscoll DJ, Shaddy RE, et al, eds. *Moss & Adams' Heart Disease in Infants, Children, and Adolescents: Including the Fetus and Young Adult*. 7th ed. Philadelphia: Lippincott Williams & Wilkins; 2008:253–268.

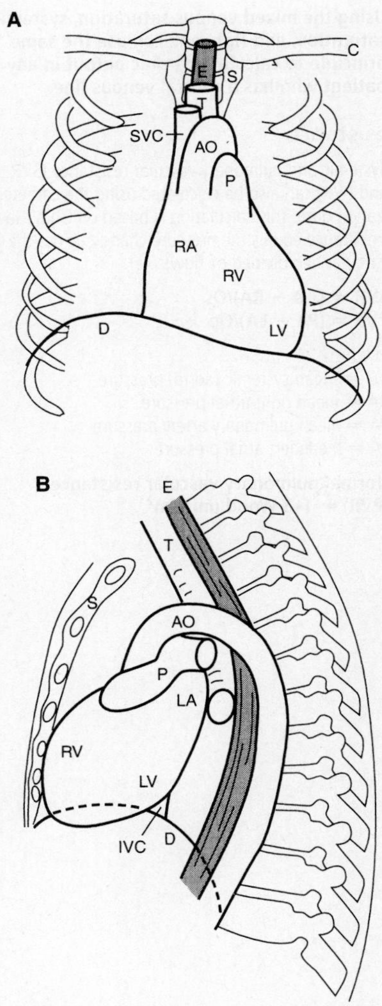

FIGURE 3. Normal cardiac silhouette. (Modified from Sapire DW. *Understanding and Diagnosing Pediatric Heart Disease*. East Norwalk, CT: Appleton & Lange; 1991:64, with permission.)

- Low voltage, flat T waves are associated with electrolyte abnormalities (hypokalemia, hypoglycemia), hypothyroidism, myocarditis, pericarditis, ischemia, or medications (i.e., digitalis).

CHEST ROENTGENOGRAM

The plain chest roentgenogram is inexpensive, expedient, readily available, and continues to provide important information to the clinician when cardiac disease is suspected. The normal cardiac silhouette in the anteroposterior and lateral views are shown in **Figure 3**.

Heart Size

- **Cardiomegaly** can be due to dilated cardiac chambers or pericardial effusion. A quantitative assessment of cardiac size should be made on the inspiratory film, when 9–10 ribs are visualized above the level of the diaphragm.
- **The cardiothoracic ratio** is then determined by comparing the transverse dimension of the heart relative to the width of the thoracic cavity. **The heart is considered enlarged if the cardiothoracic ratio exceeds 60%**.

Pulmonary Vascularity

- When there is a suspicion of congenital heart disease, the appearance of the pulmonary vascular markings plays an important role in understanding the pathophysiology.
- **Increased vascularity** is seen when a large left-to-right shunt is present (as in atrial septal defect, ventricular septal defect, patent ductus arteriosus). Increased pulmonary arterial flow makes the vessels appear sharp and prominent.
- **Decreased vascularity** is seen in right-sided obstructive lesion that result in decreased pulmonary blood flow or in Eisenmenger syndrome.
- **Pulmonary venous congestion** indicated by bronchial cuffing, and Kerley B lines (horizontal lines seen at periphery of lung fields suggesting fluid-filled interlobar septa), suggest pulmonary venous obstructive disease or congestive heart failure.

Specific Cardiac Lesions

- Distinctive radiographic configurations of the cardiac silhouette have been associated with specific cardiac lesions as listed below:
  - **Tetralogy of Fallot:** "boot-shaped" heart
  - **Total anomalous pulmonary venous return (supracardiac type):** "snowman" or "figure of 8"
  - **Coarctation of aorta:** "figure 3"
  - **D-transposition of great arteries**: "egg on a string"
  - **L-transposition of great arteries**: "box-shaped heart"
  - **Ebstein anomaly**: "wall-to-wall" heart

ECHOCARDIOGRAPHY

- Echocardiography involves the use of ultrasound technology to image the heart. It is an invaluable tool that provides details of the cardiac anatomy, function, and physiology.
- Echocardiography can be done bedside and is very valuable in emergently ruling out pericardial effusions and checking ventricular function.
- **Transesophageal echo** is done when more detailed information is needed or to guide cardiac surgery or catheterization procedures, using a probe inserted through the esophagus.
- **Normal values for valve and chamber dimensions vary with age/size and are available in the literature for comparison**.
- **Ejection fraction (EF)** is calculated by using left ventricular end-diastolic and end-systolic volumes in 2 planes. **Normal left ventricular EF: 56–75%**
- **Shortening fraction (SF)** is also a measure of left ventricular contractility and is measured in M-mode. **Normal left ventricular SF: 28–38%**

CARDIAC CATHETERIZATION

- **Diagnostic cardiac catheterization** measures direct oximetry and hemodynamics. In conjunction with angiography, it provides complete data on cardiac anatomy and physiology.
- **The normal pressures and oxygen saturations for children are shown in Figure 4.**

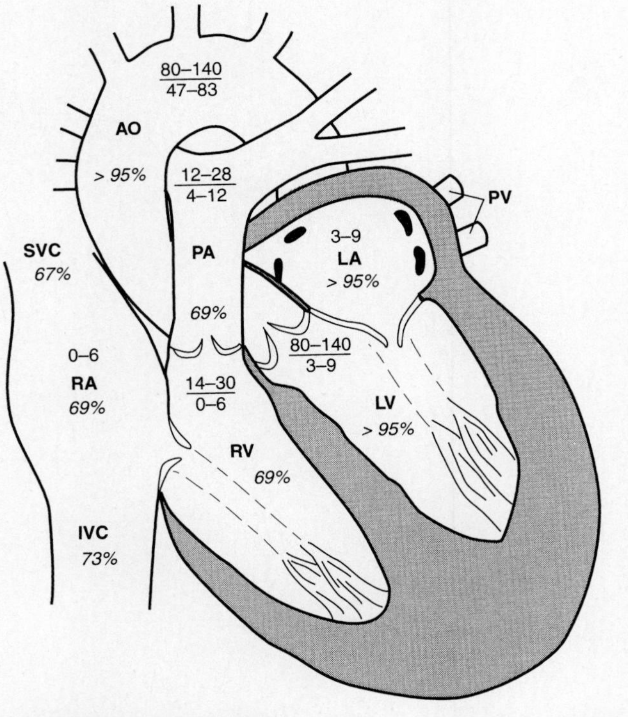

FIGURE 4. Normal pressures (systolic over diastolic, in mm Hg), mean pressures, and oxygen saturations for children during cardiac catheterization. The data are based on information compiled from healthy patients between the ages of 2 months and 20 years. AO, aorta; IVC, inferior vena cava; LA, left atrium; LV, left ventricle; PA, pulmonary artery; PV, pulmonary vein; RA, right atrium; RV, right ventricle; SVC, superior vena cava.

- **Interventional catheterization** has therapeutic applications including device closure of atrial septal defects, ventricular septal defects, and patent ductus arteriosus; performance of pulmonary artery angioplasty and stent placement; balloon dilation of valvar aortic and pulmonary stenosis; balloon angioplasty and stent repair of coarctation; and transcatheter replacement of pulmonary valves.

Calculation of Flows, Shunts, and Resistances

- **Cardiac output** can be calculated using thermodilution or Fick principle. When using Fick principle, oxygen is used as an indicator and blood flow can be calculated using oxygen consumption (measured or assumed) divided by the arteriovenous oxygen content difference.

$$\textbf{Qs (cardiac output)} = \frac{\textbf{(oxygen consumption)}}{\textbf{(systemic arterial oxygen content} - \textbf{systemic venous oxygen content)}}$$

- In most instances, the fraction of dissolved oxygen as a percentage of total oxygen content is negligible and can be ignored. That makes the equation for cardiac output simpler as shown below:

$$\textbf{Qs (systemic blood flow in L/min)} = \frac{\mathbf{O_2}\textbf{ consumption (L/min)}}{\textbf{(1.36)} \times \textbf{(10)} \times \textbf{(Hgb g/dL)} \times \textbf{(aorta sat} - \textbf{superior vena cava sat)}}$$

Similarly,

$$\textbf{Qp (pulmonary blood flow in L/min)} = \frac{\mathbf{O_2}\textbf{ consumption (L/min)}}{\textbf{(1.36)} \times \textbf{(10)} \times \textbf{(Hgb in g/dL)} \times \textbf{(pulmonary vein sat} - \textbf{pulmonary artery sat)}}$$

- **Normal cardiac output** = **3–4.5 L/min/m^2**
- Mathematically, the ratio of pulmonary blood flow to systemic blood flow is easier to calculate and is expressed as:

$$\textbf{Qp/Qs} = \frac{\textbf{aortic sat} - \textbf{SVC sat}}{\textbf{pulmonary venous sat} - \textbf{pulmonary arterial sat}}$$

- **Using the mixed venous saturation, systemic saturation, and Hgb, one can use the same principle to calculate cardiac output in any patient who has a central venous line.**

Resistance

- Systemic and pulmonary vascular resistance (SVR and PVR) can also be calculated using the catheterization data. This calculation is based on Ohm's law (resistance equals the pressure change across the vascular bed divided by flow):

SVR = (AO − RA)/Qs
PVR = (PA − LA)/Qp

in which
AO = mean systemic (aorta) pressure
RA = mean right atrial pressure
PA = mean pulmonary artery pressure
LA = mean left atrial pressure

- **Normal pulmonary vascular resistance (PVR) = 1–3 Wood units/m^2**

Appendix III
Syndromes Glossary

Angela Scheuerle

4p– syndrome (Wolf-Hirschhorn syndrome; deletion 4p; monosomy 4p)—characterized by growth failure of prenatal onset, microcephaly, "Greek helmet" facies (high forehead, prominent glabella, arched eyebrows, straight nose): hypertelorism, hypotonia, neurocognitive impairment, seizures; scoliosis

5p– syndrome (Cri du chat syndrome; deletion 5p; monosomy 5p)—characterized by catlike cry in infancy due to an abnormal larynx, growth failure of prenatal onset, microcephaly, neurocognitive impairment, hypotonia, round face, hypertelorism

13q– syndrome (deletion 13q; 13q monosomy)—characterized by growth deficiency of prenatal onset, microcephaly, and typically involves malformations of the brain, heart, kidneys, and digits; usually lethal, but severity varies with the size of the deletion. If the deletion involves the retinoblastoma gene, there is a high risk of cancer

22q11.2 deletion syndrome (microdeletion of 22q11.21)—phenotype varies widely from isolated mild learning disabilities and speech problems to complete DiGeorge syndrome. Common abnormalities include cleft soft palate or velopharyngeal incompetence, conotruncal heart defects, renal malformations, short stature, long fingers, and characteristic facies. Complete DiGeorge syndrome includes thymic aplasia, cellular immunodeficiency, parathyroid abnormalities, hypocalcemia, and interrupted aortic arch.

Aagenaes syndrome—autosomal recessive; characterized by recurrent intrahepatic cholestasis, which decreases with age and with lymphedema. Higher incidence in Norwegians

Aarskog syndrome—X-linked recessive; mutations in *FGD1*; characterized by short stature, mild to moderate mental deficiency in 1/3 of patients, musculoskeletal and genital anomalies; hypertelorism, small nose with anteverted nares, broad philtrum and nasal bridge, abnormal auricles and widow's peak, brachyclinodactyly, broad thumbs, broad feet with bulbous toes, simian crease, ptosis, syndactyly, "shawl" scrotum (penoscrotal transposition), cryptorchidism, inguinal hernia, hyperopic astigmatism, large corneas, ophthalmoplegia, strabismus, delayed puberty, mild pectus excavatum, prominent umbilicus; delayed bone age

Abetalipoproteinemia—autosomal recessive; mutations in *MTTP*; characterized by hypocholesterolemia and malabsorption of lipid-soluble vitamins. Secondary effects include retinal degeneration, neuropathy, and coagulopathy; early signs include failure to thrive, diarrhea, and acanthocytosis (star-shaped RBCs); childhood features include poor muscle control, ataxia, progressive pigmentary degeneration of the retina; by adulthood, there is significant cerebellar ataxia; absent or reduced lipoproteins and low carotene, vitamin A, and cholesterol levels. Higher incidence in Ashkenazi Jews

Achondroplasia—autosomal dominant; mutations in *FGFR3;* 90% of cases result from new mutations, usually paternal in origin; characterized by disproportionate short stature with rhizomelia, macrocephaly, small foramen magnum (risk of cord compression), caudal narrowing of spinal canal, mild hypotonia, normal intelligence, and relative glucose intolerance

Acrodermatitis enteropathica—autosomal recessive; mutations in *SLC39A4;* characterized by abnormal intestinal absorption of zinc, resulting in zinc deficiency. Secondary effects include vesicobullous and eczematous skin lesions in the perioral and perineal areas, cheeks, knees, and elbows; photophobia, conjunctivitis, and corneal dystrophy; chronic diarrhea; glossitis; nail dystrophy; growth retardation; superinfections and candidal infections; treatment requires lifelong zinc supplementation.

Agenesis of corpus callosum—multifactorial; complete or partial absence of the major tracts connecting the right and left hemispheres. Can be associated with hydrocephalus, seizures, developmental delay, spasticity, and hypertelorism; can be isolated or found with other brain malformations, and in many multiple anomaly and chromosomal syndromes

Aicardi syndrome—X-linked dominant, gene remains unknown; lethal in males; characterized by microcephaly, various brain malformations including cysts and heterotopias, infantile spasms, chorioretinal lacunae, and costovertebral skeletal abnormalities

Alagille syndrome (arteriohepatic dysplasia)—autosomal dominant; mutations in *JAG1*; characterized by paucity or absence of intrahepatic bile ducts with progressive destruction of bile ducts and 5 clinical abnormalities: cholestasis, cardiac disease characteristic facies (broad forehead, deep-set eyes that are widely spaced and underdeveloped, a small, pointed mandible), skeletal defects, and eye abnormalities. 39% of cases also have renal involvement.

Albright syndrome—see "McCune-Albright syndrome."

Alexander disease—autosomal dominant; mutations in *GFAP*; 3 subtypes: infantile, juvenile, adult; characterized by megalencephaly in infants, neurocognitive delay, and, spasticity; seizures in childhood; older patients show bulbar or pseudobulbar symptoms and spasticity. Subpial and subependymal astrocyte footplates have hyaline eosinophilic inclusions; progressive, degenerative disease with death with most patients dying within 10 years of onset; features similar to Canavan syndrome

Alport syndrome—X-linked, mutations in *COL4A5*: there are less common autosomal dominant and recessive forms; characterized by renal failure due to glomerulonephropathy, sensorineural hearing loss, and variable eye anomalies. Usually presents in infancy with hematuria, with proteinuria and hearing loss being later findings. Carrier mothers may show microscopic hematuria.

Andermann syndrome (Charlevoix disease)—autosomal recessive; mutations in *SLC12A6*; characterized by agenesis of the corpus callosum, progressive motor and sensory neuropathy, and neurocognitive defects. There are characteristic facies.

Andersen disease—see "glycogen storage disease IV."

Angelman syndrome—absence of maternal alleles of 15q11.2 that include the *UBE3A* gene. Mechanisms include deletion on the maternal chromosome, or paternal uniparental disomy. Rarely, mutations in the gene itself. Ataxic gait (wide-based, arms held upward) seizures, paroxysmal laughter, mental deficiency, absent or severely reduced speech, microcephaly; blonde hair and blue eyes in the deletion cases, characteristic facies with maxillary hypoplasia, large mouth, tongue protrusion and prognathia.

Apert syndrome (acrocephalosyndactyly type I)—autosomal dominant; mutations in *FGFR2*; characterized by craniosynostosis (typically coronal), turribrachycephaly, underdevelopment of the middle 3rd of the face, hypertelorism and proptosis; a narrow, high, arched palate; a short, beaked nose; variable but pronounced syndactyly. Other anomalies include malrotation and gastrointestinal atresias. Neurocognitive delays are present, but intelligence can be normal.

Ataxia telangiectasia syndrome—autosomal recessive; mutations in *ATM*; characterized by progressive ataxia within the first year, telangiectasias by age 8 years are a later finding. Degenerative central nervous system function, lymphopenia, immune deficit (low to absent IgA and IgE), growth deficiency, and mental deficits. Increased risk of lymphomas and leukemias in patients and carrier parents. Increased sensitivity to the effects of radiation exposure, including medical x-rays. Individuals have increased serum alpha-fetoprotein (AFP) levels.

Autosomal dominant epidermolysis bullosa dystrophica (Bart syndrome)—mutations in *COL7A1*; characterized by congenital aplasia of the skin on the lower legs and feet; nail defects and recurrent blistering of the skin and mucous membranes

Axenfeld-Rieger syndrome—autosomal dominant; mutations in *PITX2*; characterized by Rieger anomaly of the eye (anterior segment dysgenesis), glaucoma, hypodontia, maxillary hypoplasia, and umbilical abnormalities

Bardet-Biedl syndrome—autosomal recessive; mutations in various genes; this is a condition caused by abnormalities in nonmotile cilia (the ciliopathies); characterized by mental retardation, retinitis pigmentosa, obesity, polydactyly, renal anomalies, hypogonadism, and neurocognitive impairments (presentation can resemble Prader-Willi syndrome with polydactyly)

Bart syndrome—see "autosomal dominant epidermolysis bullosa dystrophica."

Bartter syndrome—autosomal recessive group of disorders of impaired renal salt reabsorption, salt wasting, hypokalemic metabolic alkalosis and hypercalciuria. Multiple related genes. Patients have normal blood pressure, but the renin level is elevated; generalized muscle weakness

Basal cell nevus syndrome—autosomal dominant; mutations in *PTCH1*, *PTCH2*, or *SUFU*; characterized by basal cell carcinomas, macrocephaly, odontogenic keratocysts of jaws, bifid ribs, pits in the palms and soles, and calcification of the falx cerebri

Beckwith-Wiedemann syndrome (exomphalos-macroglossia-gigantism syndrome)—sporadic imprinting disorder of chromosome 11 or autosomal dominant due to mutations in *CDKN1C*; characterized by overgrowth of prenatal onset, omphalocele, macroglossia, hemihypertrophy, and characteristic facies. Significant increased risk of Wilms tumor and hepatoblastoma with higher risk in patients with hemihyperplasia. Neurocognitive impairment if neonatal hypoglycemia is unrecognized or uncontrolled

Behçet syndrome—presumed autosomal dominant; gene unidentified; disease mechanism unknown.

Recurrent inflammatory lesions: oral and genital ulcers, various skin and eye lesions

Bloch-Sulzberger syndrome—see "incontinentia pigmenti."

Bloom syndrome—autosomal recessive; mutations in *BLM*; characterized by growth deficiency of prenatal onset, high risk of malignancy, microcephaly with dolichocephaly, facial telangiectatic erythema in a butterfly pattern, skin pigmentation changes, mild neurocognitive impairment, and characteristic facies increased prevalence in Ashkenazi Jews; chromosome instability syndrome

Blue diaper syndrome—probably autosomal recessive; gene unidentified; defect in intestinal transport of tryptophan; bacterial degradation of the tryptophan form water-soluble metabolites that turn blue on exposure to oxygen. Only two brothers have been documented with the transport defect. Other causes of blue or discolored urine should be investigated.

Byler disease—see "progressive familial intrahepatic cholestasis."

Canavan syndrome—autosomal recessive; mutations in *ASPA*; progressive, degenerative demyelination and leukodystrophy. Usually beginning in infancy with macrocephaly, hypotonia, and developmental regression. Features similar to Alexander disease. Increased prevalence in Ashkenazi Jews

Caroli disease—inheritance pattern unclear; gene unidentified; overlaps significantly with the polycystic kidney syndromes and may not represent a separate entity; characterized by cystic dilatation of the intrahepatic bile ducts; recurrent bouts of cholangitis and biliary abscesses secondary to bile stasis and gallstones

Cat-eye syndrome (tetrasomy 22)—presence of an extra chromosome comprising two identical segments of chromosome 22 (i.e., the patient has 4 total copies of chromosome 22); characterized by coloboma of iris, down-slanting palpebral fissures, anal atresia, cardiac defects, renal agenesis; mild neurocognitive impairment. Growth is usually normal.

Charcot-Marie-Tooth disease (hereditary motor and sensory neuropathy [HMSN] or peroneal muscular atrophy)—a group of sensorineural peripheral polyneuropathies with various inheritance patterns and a wide range of clinical presentation; most common cause of chronic peripheral neuropathy; characterized by insidious onset and slowly progressive weakness and atrophy of distal limb muscles, impaired sensation

CHARGE syndrome—autosomal dominant; mutations in *CHD7*; characterized by Coloboma, Heart disease, choanal Atresia, Retarded growth and development and/or CNS anomalies, Genital anomalies and/or hypogonadism, and Ear anomalies and/or deafness. The ear malformation is a characteristic. Mondini defect and hypoplastic semicircular canals of the inner ear in the presence of other typical malformations is diagnostic for CHARGE.

Chédiak-Higashi syndrome—autosomal recessive; mutations in *LYST*; characterized by oculocutaneous albinism, lack of natural killer cells, decreased neutrophil and monocyte migration, anemia, neurodegeneration, hepatomegaly, and splenomegaly

Cockayne syndrome—autosomal recessive; mutations in *ERCC6* and *ERCC8*; characterized by postnatal growth deficiency, microcephaly, neurocognitive impairment, ataxia, hearing loss, seizures, characteristic facies, hypertension, renal dysfunction, and photosensitivity

Congenital rubella syndrome—see "fetal rubella syndrome."

Cornelia de Lange syndrome (Brachmann-De Lange syndrome, de Lange syndrome)—autosomal dominant; mutations in *NIPBL* cause most cases; characterized by growth failure of prenatal onset microcephaly, hirsutism, limb reduction defects—particularly ulnar ray defects—gastroesophageal reflux, congenital heart defects, neurocognitive impairment, and characteristic facies

Crigler-Najjar syndrome, type I (glucuronyl transferase deficiency)—autosomal recessive; mutations in *UGT1A1*; absence of hepatic uridine 5′-diphospho-glucuronosyltransferase activity leading to unconjugated hyperbilirubinemia on 1st day of life without evidence of hemolysis; requires phototherapy to prevent kernicterus. Patients do not respond to phenobarbital treatment to lower serum bilirubin.

Crigler-Najjar syndrome, type II—autosomal recessive; mutations in *UGT1A1*; less severe unconjugated hyperbilirubinemia due to partial activity of uridine 5′-diphospho-glucuronosyltransferase; kernicterus is less common than in type I. Patients respond to phenobarbital treatment to lower serum bilirubin.

Crouzon syndrome (craniofacial dysostosis)—autosomal dominant; mutations in *FGFR2*; characterized by craniosynostosis (most often coronal), exophthalmos due to shallow orbits, hypertelorism, high palate, and hypoplasia of maxilla; obstructive sleep apnea is common.

Cyclic neutropenia—autosomal dominant; mutations in *ELANE*; *lack* of granulocyte macrophage colony-stimulating factor (GM-CSF); characterized by fever, mouth lesions, cervical adenitis, and gastroenteritis; underlying regular 21-day cyclic fluctuation in number of blood leukocytes

De Sanctis-Cacchione syndrome—see "xeroderma pigmentosum.".

Diamond-Blackfan syndrome (congenital pure red cell aplasia)—autosomal dominant; mutations in *RPS19*; failure of erythropoiesis; characterized by normochromic macrocytic anemia, postnatal growth retardation, craniofacial, limb heart, and urinary system malformations in 30–50%. One of the ribosomopathies

DiGeorge syndrome—see "22q11.2 deletion syndrome."

Down syndrome—see "trisomy 21."

Dubin-Johnson syndrome—autosomal recessive; mutations in *ABCC2*; characterized by elevated conjugated bilirubin, large amounts of coproporphyrin I in urine, and deposits of melanin like pigment in hepatocellular lysosomes, there is otherwise normal liver function.

Dubowitz syndrome—autosomal recessive; gene unidentified; growth failure of prenatal onset, microcephaly, eczema-like skin disorder, brachydactyly, various ocular abnormalities, neurocognitive impairment, characteristic facies that resemble fetal alcohol syndrome

Eagle-Barrett syndrome—see "prune belly sequence."

Ectodermal dysplasia—variable inheritance; a category of disease rather than a single condition; characterized by poor development or absence of teeth, nails, hair, and sweat glands

Edwards syndrome—see "trisomy 18."

Ehlers-Danlos syndrome—autosomal dominant group of conditions classified by type; hypermobile joints and hyperextensible or fragile skin are characteristic features across the types, but the specific phenotypes vary. Classic type (type I) is caused my mutations in *COL5A1* or *COL5A2*. Abnormalities of the vasculature and hollow organs are characteristic of vascular type (type IV) caused by mutations in *COL3A1*.

Fabry disease—X-linked; mutations in *GLA*; deficiency alpha-galactosidase A leading to lysosomal storage of glycosphingolipids; involvement of blood vessels leads to tingling and burning in the hands and feet; small, red maculopapular angiofibromata on the buttocks, inguinal area, fingernails, and lips; and an inability to perspire; renal involvement including proteinuria, progressing to renal failure; increased risk of cardiovascular disease and stroke; carrier females frequently manifest symptoms. Treated with replacement enzyme

Familial adenomatous polyposis—autosomal dominant; mutations in *APC*; characterized by multiple GI polyps with malignant transformation, skin cysts, supernumerary teeth, and multiple osteoma. Gardner syndrome is a variant in which desmoid tumors and other neoplasms occur along with the colon and rectum adenomata.

Familial dysautonomia (hereditary sensory and autonomic neuropathy)—autosomal recessive; mutations in *IKBKAP*; characterized by aberrant sensory and autonomic functions; progressive course of poor growth, alacrima, decreased taste sense, postural hypotension, episodic hyperhidrosis, hypotonia, and decreased pain sensation. Higher prevalence in Ashkenazi Jews

Farber lipogranulomatosis—autosomal recessive; mutations in *ASAH1*; deficiency of acid ceramidase; characterized by subcutaneous nodules, painful and progressively deformed joints, and laryngeal involvement with hoarseness

Fetal alcohol spectrum disorder (FASD)—characterized by growth deficiency of prenatal onset, microcephaly, cardiac septal defect; delayed development; and neurocognitive impairment with a history of or suspicion for maternal alcohol use during pregnancy. Characteristic facies have been defined. Wide ranging effects that include neurocognitive problems (specifically abnormalities in executive function) even in the absence of physical features. The most severe end of the spectrum constitutes fetal alcohol syndrome. The CDC publishes specific diagnostic guidance.

Fetal alcohol syndrome—see "fetal alcohol spectrum disorder."

Fetal hydantoin syndrome—characterized by growth deficiency of prenatal onset; characteristic facies, neurocognitive impairment, and nail hypoplasia/aplasia may have cleft lip and palate, and cardiac defects

Fetal rubella syndrome—in utero rubella exposure (especially in the 1st trimester); characterized by mental deficiency, microcephaly, deafness, cataract, glaucoma, patent ductus arteriosus, cardiac septal defects, hepatosplenomegaly, anemia, and thrombocytopenia

Fetal valproate syndrome—characterized by neurocognitive impairments, neural tube defects, cardiovascular anomalies, and characteristic facies

Fetal warfarin syndrome—6–9 week exposure characterized by defects associated with aberrant cartilage: nasal hypoplasia, stippled epiphyses, hypoplastic distal phalanges. 14–20 week exposure characterized by central nervous system defects, eye anomalies, and intrauterine growth retardation. Exposure in the 3rd trimester is less concerning.

Fibrodysplasia ossificans progressiva (FOP)—autosomal dominant; mutations in *ACVR1*; characterized by short hallux, progressive ossification of muscles and subcutaneous tissues, and hearing loss; any trauma (including iatrogenic) can cause ectopic ossification.

Focal dermal hypoplasia—X-linked dominant; mutations in *PORCN*; characterized by linear atrophy of the skin with fat herniation through the dermis, linear pigmentation abnormalities, and papillomata; may have eye, oral, or digit abnormalities

Fragile X syndrome—X-linked; triplet repeat mutations in *FMR1*; characterized by mental deficiency, autism spectrum disorders, macrocephaly, prognathism, large ears, mild connective tissue dysplasia, and macroorchidism after puberty. Female full mutation carriers can manifest the phenotype. Female carriers of premutations have increased risk of premature ovarian insufficiency. Male and female permutation carriers have increased risk of fragile X–associated tremor ataxia syndrome as adults.

Friedreich ataxia—autosomal recessive; triplet repeat mutations in *FXN*; progressive loss of large myelinated axons in peripheral nerves, with symptoms usually appearing in late childhood or adolescence; characterized by progressive cerebellar and spinal cord dysfunction; patients have high-arched foot, hammer toes, and cardiac failure

Gardner syndrome—see "familial adenomatous polyposis."

Gaucher disease—autosomal recessive; mutations in *GBA*; deficiency of glucocerebrosidase, leading to accumulation and storage of glucocerebroside in the reticuloendothelial system; 3 types: (a) adult, or chronic, (b) acute neuropathic, or infantile, (c) subacute neuropathic, or juvenile; characterized by splenomegaly, hepatomegaly, delayed development, strabismus, swallowing difficulties, laryngeal spasm, opisthotonos, and bone pain

Gilbert syndrome—typically autosomal recessive, but carriers can manifest symptoms; mutations in *UGT1A1*; reduced activity of glucuronyltransferase activity leading to mild unconjugated hyperbilirubinemia that worsens with stresses on the body, such as fasting

Gilles de la Tourette syndrome—Evidence suggests that mutations in one or more genes may be involved. Neurobehavioral disorder characterized by multiple motor and vocal tics that begin before the age of 18 years; difficulties, including obsessive-compulsive disorder, ADHD, anger control problems, and poor social skills

Glanzmann thrombasthenia—autosomal recessive; mutations in *ITGA2B* and *ITGB3*; involves defective primary platelet aggregation (size and survival of platelets is normal). Presents as bleeding dyscrasias

Glycogen storage disease 1A (GSD1A; von Gierke)—autosomal recessive; mutations in *G6PC*; inherited defect in glucose-6-phosphatase resulting in accumulation of glycogen and defective gluconeogenesis; characterized by fasting hypoglycemia, growth retardation, hepatomegaly, lactic acidosis, hyperlipidemia, and hyperuricemia

Glycogen storage disease IV (GSD4; Andersen disease)—autosomal recessive; mutations in *GBE1*; defect of glycogen branching enzyme; classic form characterized by hepatomegaly and failure to thrive in the 1st few months of life, progressing to liver cirrhosis and splenomegaly. Neuromuscular forms can present at any age.

Goldenhar syndrome—see "oculo-auriculo-vertebral spectrum."

Goltz syndrome—see "focal dermal hypoplasia."

Gorlin syndrome—see "basal cell nevus syndrome."

Hand-Schüller-Christian disease—see "histiocytosis X."

Hartnup disorder—autosomal recessive; mutations in *SLC6A19*; defect in transport of monoamine monocarboxylic amino acids by intestinal mucosa and renal tubules; characterized by photosensitivity and a pellagra-like skin rash, cerebellar ataxia, emotional instability, and amino aciduria

Hereditary fructose intolerance—autosomal recessive; mutations in *ALDOB*; involves deficiency of fructose-1-phosphate aldolase or fructose 1,6-diphosphatase; characterized by vomiting, diarrhea, hypoglycemic seizures, and jaundice upon exposure to fructose or sucrose

Holt-Oram syndrome—autosomal dominant; mutations in *TBX5*; characterized by upper limb defects, typically radial ray defects, and cardiac anomalies. Most common combination is a missing or hypoplastic thumb and atrial septal defect.

Homocystinuria—autosomal recessive; mutations in *CBS*; deficient cystathionine synthetase activity leading to marfanoid habitus and neurocognitive impairment, also thrombotic events, generalized hypopigmentation, and, with progression, seizures

Hunter syndrome—see "mucopolysaccharidosis II."

Hurler syndrome—see "mucopolysaccharidosis I."

Hutchinson-Gilford progeria syndrome—autosomal dominant; mutations in *LMNA*; all cases to date have been de novo mutations; characterized by the appearance of premature aging, severe growth failure, atherosclerosis, lipodystrophy, alopecia, and decreased joint mobility. Cognitive development is normal.

Hyper-IgE (Job syndrome)—autosomal dominant; mutations in *STAT3*; characterized by recurrent deep tissue and skin staphylococcal infections; patients have eosinophilia and IgE levels that are 10 times greater than normal.

Hypogonadotropic hypogonadism with or without anosmia—X-linked or autosomal dominant; some digenic inheritance; multiple genes involved; all have some degree of hypogonadism and altered or absent sense of smell due to olfactory lobe agenesis; bimanual synkinesis; not all affected persons are infertile.

Incontinentia pigmenti (IP)—X-linked dominant; mutations in *IKBKG*; characterized by 4-stage, evolving skin lesions and abnormalities of skin appendages; eosinophilia; high risk of neonatal stroke; neurocognitive problems in patients with stroke or CNS anomalies, but majority of patients are neurocognitively normal. Malformations of internal organs are not characteristic of IP.

Jeune thoracic dystrophy—see "short-rib thoracic dysplasia with or without polydactyly."

Job syndrome—see "Hyper-IgE."

Kabuki syndrome—autosomal dominant; mutations in *KMT2D*; characterized by growth deficiency of postnatal onset, mental deficiency, hypotonia, characteristic facies resembling Kabuki dance makeup (long palpebral fissures with lateral ectropion, ptosis, arching eyebrows), skeletal anomalies, cardiac defects, and neurocognitive impairment

Kallmann syndrome—see "hypogonadotropic hypogonadism with or without anosmia."

Kartagener syndrome—see "primary ciliary dyskinesia."

Kleine-Levin hibernation syndrome—characterized by episodes of compulsive megaphagia, somnolence, and abnormal behavior predominantly in males

Klinefelter syndrome—47 XXY karyotype; paternal meiosis error; hypogonadism, tall stature with long limbs, mild neurocognitive impairments, although many are cognitively normal. Infertility is not universal.

Klippel-Feil anomaly—sporadic; multifactorial; cervical spine fusion of varying degrees; characterized by a short neck, limited neck motion, and low occipital hairline; isolated defect or can appear as part of a multisystem syndrome.

Krabbe leukodystrophy—autosomal recessive; mutations in *GALC*; deficiency in galactocerebrosidase; lysosomal storage disorder primarily affecting white matter of the central and peripheral nervous systems; characterized classically by early, severe neurodegeneration leading, in the infantile form, to death by 2 years of age. There are late-onset forms.

Larsen syndrome—autosomal recessive; mutations in *B3GAT3*; characterized by hyperlaxity, multiple congenital dislocations, short stature, heart defects, and characteristic facies

Laurence-Moon-Biedl syndrome—see "Bardet-Biedl syndrome."

LEOPARD syndrome—autosomal dominant; mutations in *PTPN11*, *RAF1*, or *BRAF*; characterized by Lentigines, EKG abnormalities, Ocular hypertelorism, Pulmonic stenosis, Abnormalities of genitalia, Retardation of growth, and sensorineural Deafness

Lesch-Nyhan syndrome—X-linked recessive; mutations in *HPRT1*; defect in purine metabolism; diminished or absent hypoxanthine guanine phosphoribosyl transferase (HPRT) activity leading to hyperuricemia; spastic cerebral palsy, choreoathetosis, uric acid urinary stones; compulsive self-mutilation, and neurocognitive impairment

Letterer-Siwe disease—see "histiocytosis X."

Lowe syndrome (oculocerebrorenal syndrome)—X-linked recessive; mutations in *OCRL*; characterized by congenital cataracts, and hydrophthalmia, vitamin D–resistant rickets, amino aciduria, hyporeflexia, hypotonia, renal Fanconi syndrome, and neurocognitive impairment

Lysosomal acid lipase deficiency (Wolman disease)—autosomal recessive; mutations in *LIPA*; lysosomal storage disease leading to cholesteryl ester and triglyceride deposition in visceral organs; fatal in infancy; characterized by intractable vomiting, failure to thrive, abdominal distention, steatorrhea, hepatosplenomegaly, and adrenal calcification

Maffucci syndrome—see "multiple enchondromatosis, Maffucci type."

Marfan syndrome—autosomal dominant; mutations in *FBN1*; characterized by ectopia lentis, dilatation of the aorta, scoliosis, pneumothorax, pectus deformities, and long, thin extremities. Diagnostic criteria have been published.

McCune-Albright syndrome—autosomal dominant; mutations in *GNAS*; surviving cases are somatic mosaics as the nonmosaic state is presumed to be an embryonic lethal; characterized by polyostotic fibrous dysplasia; café au lait skin pigmentation, and peripheral precocious puberty. Note: Diagnosis requires biopsy of affected tissue.

MELAS syndrome—mitochondrial or autosomal recessive inheritance; mutations in any of a number of genes active in mitochondria most commonly *MTTL1*; characterized by Mitochondrial myopathy, Encephalopathy, Lactic Acidosis, and Strokelike episodes; causes seizures, hemiparesis, hemianopsia, or cortical blindness, and episodic vomiting

Menkes disease (kinky hair disease)—X-linked recessive; mutations in *ATP7A*; impaired GI transport of copper results in copper deficiency; characterized by low serum copper and ceruloplasmin, short, friable, colorless scalp hair, growth failure of postnatal onset, microcephaly, progressive neurocognitive impairment. Death usually by 3 years of age

Mismatch repair cancer syndrome—heritable cancer syndrome; dominant inheritance of one mutated allele, with somatic mutation of the other; mutations in any of 4 separate genes; characterized by adenomatous colonic polyposis associated with malignant brain tumors, especially medulloblastoma and glioblastoma

Möbius syndrome—sporadic; classically characterized by cranial nerve dysfunction causing bilateral facial weakness, feeding difficulties, and impairment of ocular abduction; the term has come to include any condition that includes congenital CN VII palsy.

Morquio syndrome—see "mucopolysaccharidosis IV."

Mucopolysaccharidosis I (Hurler, Scheie)—autosomal recessive; mutations in *IDUA*; involves an accumulation of heparan sulfate and dermatan sulfate, and enzyme deficiency of α-L-iduronidase; characterized by coarse facial features, growth arrest, dysostosis multiplex, glaucoma, arthritis, cardiac valvular disease, and neurocognitive impairment. There is a spectrum of involvement from severe (Hurler phenotype) to mild (Sheie phenotype) and both may be found in the same family. Enzyme replacement therapy is available.

Mucopolysaccharidosis II (Hunter syndrome)—X-linked recessive; mutations in *IDS*; involves an accumulation of heparan sulfate and dermatan sulfate, and enzyme deficiency of l-iduronate sulfatase; characterized by macrocephaly, coarse facial features, hypertrophy of internal organs, dysostosis multiplex, and neurocognitive impairment. Enzyme replacement therapy is available.

Mucopolysaccharidosis III (Sanfilippo)—autosomal recessive; caused by a deficiency in 1 of 4 enzymes with clinically similar manifestations; lysosomal storage disease characterized by accumulation of heparan sulfate, and progressive neurocognitive impairment with mild somatic features.

Type A—mutations in *SGSH* and deficiency of heparin *N*-sulfatase

Type B—mutations in *NAGLU* and deficiency of alpha-*N*-acetylglucosaminidase

Type C—mutations in *HGSNAT* and deficiency of acetyl CoA:alpha-glucosaminide *N*-acetyltransferase

Type D—mutations in *GNS* and deficiency of *N*-acetylglucosamine-6-sulfatase

Mucopolysaccharidosis IV (Morquio syndrome)—autosomal recessive; mutations in *GALNS*; involves an accumulation of keratin sulfate and chondroitin-6-sulfate and enzyme deficiency of galactosamine-6-sulfate sulfatase; characterized by skeletal dysplasia with short-trunk dwarfism corneal clouding, small joint hyperlaxity, and cardiac valve disease; patients have laxity of the odontoid processes and are at risk for life-threatening atlantoaxial subluxation. Enzyme replacement therapy is available.

Multiple enchondromatosis, Maffucci type—all cases to date have been sporadic; presumed to be somatic mosaicism for mutations in currently unidentified gene; characterized by multiple enchondroma of the bone and soft tissue hemangiomas; patients have short stature, skeletal deformities, scoliosis, and high risk of malignant transformation.

Multiple exostoses, type I—autosomal dominant; mutations in *EXT1*; characterized by presence of multiple osteochondromas (exostosis) occurring most commonly on the metaphysis of long bones, but any bone can be involved, except the skull. Secondary deformity of legs, forearms, and hands typically occur.

Multiple hereditary exostosis—see "multiple exostoses, type I."

Nail-patella syndrome—autosomal dominant; mutations in *LMX1B*; characterized by dystrophic and hypoplastic nails, hypoplastic patellae, iliac horns, malformed radial heads, and nephrotic syndrome

Niemann-Pick disease—autosomal recessive; types A and B result from mutations in *SMPD1*; deficiency of acid sphingomyelinase resulting in accumulation of sphingomyelin in RES and other cells; characterized by failure to thrive, organomegaly, macular cherry red spot, and rapidly progressive neurodegeneration; in its most severe form, patients are normal at birth but by 6 months, experience delayed development and loss of developmental milestones with death by 3 years; increased prevalence in Ashkenazi Jews

Noonan syndrome—autosomal dominant; mutations in any of a number of genes, the most common is *PTPN11*; clinical features similar to Turner syndrome (but Noonan affects both sexes equally); characterized by short stature, heart defects (most commonly pulmonic stenosis and hypertrophic cardiomyopathy), bleeding diathesis, and characteristic facies. Neurocognitive function varies and is often average.

Oculo-Auriculo-Vertebral spectrum (OAV, Hemifacial microsomia, Goldenhar)—sporadic; multifactorial; characterized by craniofacial malformations—typically unilateral—starting with microtia and involving ipsilateral skull and face bones, eyeball, and facial soft tissue structures. Severe cases may also involve vertebrae. Cognitive function tends to be normal.

Osler-Weber-Rendu syndrome (hereditary hemorrhagic telangiectasia)—autosomal dominant; mutations in *ENG*; vascular dysplasia; characterized by telangiectases and arteriovenous malformation of the skin, mucosa, and viscera (lung, liver, brain)

Osteogenesis imperfecta—autosomal dominant; types I–IV caused by mutations in *COL1A1* or *COL1A2*; types differentiated by clinical presentation, all involving soft or fragile bones and consequences thereof; other features are conductive hearing loss (due to ossicle fracture), thin sclerae (which appear blue or grey), and dentinogenesis imperfecta.

Type I—frequent fractures with secondary deformation; normal lifespan

Type II—all new mutation or born to unaffected mosaic parent; severe prenatal-onset fractures; typically lethal in infancy

Type III—intermediate between types I and II

Type IV—bone deformation with less tendency to frank fractures

Osteopetrosis—various inheritance patterns. Multiple genes involved. Widely varying phenotypes. Patients have dense bones that are prone to fractures and have mild anemia and craniofacial disproportion; radiologic changes include increased cortical bone density, longitudinal and transverse dense striations at the ends of the long bones, lucent and dense bands in the vertebrae, and thickening at the base of the skull.

Patau syndrome—see "trisomy 13."

Pelizaeus-Merzbacher disease—X-linked recessive; mutations in *PLP1*; characterized by failure of normal CNS myelination; nystagmus, spastic quadriplegia, ataxia and neurocognitive impairment; patients may also have optic atrophy and seizures; infantile and adult onset subtypes

Peutz-Jeghers syndrome—autosomal dominant; mutations in *STK11*; characterized by melanotic macules on the lips and mucous membranes, intestinal polyposis, and increased risk of malignancy

Pierre Robin sequence—characterized by micrognathia, glossoptosis, and cleft soft palate. May be found as an isolated entity or a component of multisystem syndromes, most commonly 22q11.2 deletion syndrome and Stickler syndrome

Poland anomaly—characterized by a unilateral absence or hypoplasia of the pectoralis muscle with ipsilateral breast hypoplasia and sometimes associated upper limb abnormalities. May be found as an isolated entity or a component of multisystem syndromes

Prader-Willi syndrome—absence of paternal alleles of 15q11.2 that include the *SNRPN* gene. Mechanisms include deletion on the paternal chromosome, or maternal uniparental disomy. Rarely, mutations in the gene itself; characterized by hypotonia and initial failure to thrive, followed by marked obesity due to an insatiable appetite; other features include mental retardation, hypogonadism, small hands and feet, and short stature. Appropriate treatment with growth hormone and diet control ameliorates the obesity, increased lean muscle mass, and raises height.

Primary ciliary dyskinesia—autosomal recessive; multiple genes involved; characterized by mucociliary function abnormalities in the respiratory tract, male infertility due to immotile sperm, and hydrocephalus. Kartagener syndrome includes heterotaxy and is caused by mutations in *DNAI1*.

Progeria syndrome—see "Hutchinson-Gilford progeria syndrome."

Progressive Familial Intrahepatic Cholestasis (Byler disease)—autosomal recessive; mutations in *ATP8B1*, *PFIC2*, and *PFIC3*; characterized by intrahepatic cholestasis leading to cirrhosis and end-stage liver disease before adulthood and anticipated secondary effects of liver failure; short stature, failure to thrive, splenomegaly

Prune belly sequence—characterized by deficiency of the abdominal musculature; most commonly in association with a grossly distended urinary system due to bladder outlet obstruction. The primary defect is variable, even within the urinary system. Obstruction and dilation of other viscera, or presence of a mass can lead to prune belly as a secondary feature. There are some cases described that appear to be primary failure of the muscle to form.

Rieger syndrome—see "Axenfeld-Rieger syndrome."

Riley-Day syndrome—see "familial dysautonomia."

Rotor syndrome—autosomal recessive; digenic inheritance of homozygous mutations in *SLCO1B1* and *SLCO1B3*; characterized by mild conjugated bilirubinemia and jaundice that may be exacerbated by infection, surgery, pregnancy, or drugs; usually asymptomatic with normal life expectancy; clinically, similar to Dubin-Johnson; however, patients with Rotor have normal-appearing hepatocytes.

Rubinstein-Taybi syndrome—autosomal dominant; mutations in *CREBBP*; characterized by growth deficiency of postnatal onset, microcephaly, broad thumbs and halluces, neurocognitive impairment, and characteristic facies; increased risk of neoplasia

Russell-Silver syndrome—20–60% caused by imprinting abnormalities of chromosome 11, 10% by maternal uniparental disomy of chromosome 7; characterized by growth failure and short stature of prenatal onset with head sparing (relative but not absolute macrocephaly) and characteristic facies. Can have 5th finger clinodactyly, hemihypertrophy, and hyperpigmented macules

Sandhoff disease (GM2-gangliosidosis type II)—autosomal recessive; mutations in *HEXB*; deficiency of hexosaminidase B leading to accumulation of GM2 gangliosides, particularly in neurons; progressive neurodegenerative disorder; hypotonia in the first 6 months of life, startle reaction, macular cherry-red spots, macrocephaly, organomegaly, and progressive neurocognitive impairment; manifestations similar to Tay-Sachs disease. No ethnic predilection

Sanfilippo syndrome, types A, B, C, and D—see "mucopolysaccharidosis III."

Scheie syndrome—see "mucopolysaccharidosis I."

Seckel syndrome—autosomal recessive; multiple subtypes differentiated by gene involved; characterized by growth failure of prenatal onset, extreme short stature, microcephaly, neurocognitive impairment, and characteristic facies

Short-rib thoracic dysplasia with or without polydactyly)—autosomal recessive; mutations in various genes; this is a set of conditions caused by abnormalities in nonmotile cilia (the ciliopathies); characterized by skeletal dysplasia; short ribs; polydactyly; orofacial clefts; and abnormalities of the brain, eye, heart, kidneys, liver, pancreas, intestines, and genitalia. Includes Jeune, Ellis-van Creveld, Hydrolethalus, and others

Shwachman-Diamond syndrome—autosomal recessive; mutations in *SBDS*; characterized by exocrine pancreatic dysfunction, bone marrow dysfunction with risk of malignant transformation, and skeletal abnormalities with disproportionate short stature

Smith-Lemli-Opitz syndrome—autosomal recessive; mutations in *DHCR7*; disorder of cholesterol synthesis; characterized by growth retardation, microcephaly, hypospadias with cryptorchidism, characteristic 2–3 toe Y-shaped syndactyly, photosensitivity, neurocognitive impairment, and characteristic facies. Dietary cholesterol supplementation may result in clinical improvement of neurocognitive status.

Sotos syndrome (cerebral gigantism)—autosomal dominant; mutations in *NSD1*; characterized by macrocephaly, rapid somatic growth (final height is usually the average for the family) large hands and feet, neurocognitive impairment that may be mild, and characteristic facies.

Stickler syndrome—autosomal dominant; mutations in *COL2A1*, *COL11A1*, or *COL11A2*; characterized by Pierre Robin anomaly at birth and mild skeletal features with more obvious problems later; characteristic vitreous and retinal abnormalities, high-frequency hearing loss, osteoarthritis before age 40 years; cognition usually normal

Sturge-Weber syndrome—multifactorial, can be caused by autosomal dominant somatic mutation of *GNAQ*; characterized by a port-wine stain on the face at the 1st branch of the trigeminal nerve; patients have ipsilateral leptomeningeal angiomatosis with intracranial calcifications leading to seizures and mental retardation and may also have ocular complications, such as glaucoma.

Tay-Sachs disease (GM2-gangliosidosis type I)—autosomal recessive; mutations in *HEXA*; characterized by deficient hexosaminidase activity which leads to accumulation of GM2 gangliosides in the CNS; patients have loss of motor milestones, seizures, macular cherry-red spot, and progressive neurodegeneration leading to blindness, paralysis, and death within the 2nd or 3rd year of life. Highest prevalence in Ashkenazi Jews

Testicular regression syndrome—characterized by bilateral gonadal absence in a person with 46 XY karyotype; phenotype depends on the amount of early testicular tissue present and active; ranges from phenotypic female to anorchic phenotypic male

Tetrasomy 22—see "cat eye syndrome."

Tourette syndrome—see "Gilles de la Tourette syndrome."

Treacher Collins syndrome—autosomal dominant; mutations in *TCOF1*; characterized by mandibulofacial dysostosis; characteristic finding of hypoplastic zygomatic arches and mandibles, micrognathia, downward slanting palpebral fissures, coloboma of the lower eyelid, microtia with associated conductive hearing deficits, and a cleft palate with or without cleft lip; cognitive function is normal.

Trisomy 13 (Patau syndrome)—characterized by holoprosencephaly, aplasia cutis congenita, cleft lip and/or cleft palate, microphthalmia, postaxial polydactyly; cardiovascular anomalies in 80%; majority abort spontaneously; median survival is 7 days.

Trisomy 18 (Edwards syndrome)—characterized by severe neurocognitive impairment, growth failure of prenatal onset, and characteristic facies with prominent occiput, micrognathia; other common features are clenched hands with overriding fingers, a short sternum, and rocker bottom feet; cardiac and renal anomalies in up to 50% of cases; the majority abort spontaneously; median survival is 2 weeks.

Trisomy 21 (Down syndrome)—characterized by neurocognitive impairment and characteristic facies; 40% have congenital heart disease (particularly atrioventricular canal defects); other common findings are GI disorders (Hirschsprung disease, duodenal atresia), musculoskeletal abnormalities, leukemia, hearing loss, and thyroid disease. The majority of cases abort spontaneously. Survival past infancy depends on the specific defect(s) present.

Tuberous sclerosis—autosomal dominant; mutations in *TSC1* or *TSC2*, also a contiguous gene deletion syndrome involving *TSC2*; characterized by hamartoma in brain, skin, heart, kidneys, and lung with secondary effects; seizures, neurocognitive impairment, renal and pulmonary compromise; pathognomonic skin lesions include hypopigmented macules (ash leaf spots), connective tissue nevi (shagreen patch), adenoma sebaceum, and subungual or periungual fibromas.

Turcot syndrome—see "mismatch repair cancer syndrome."

Turner syndrome (monosomy X)—45 X karyotype; paternal meiosis error; characterized by gonadal dysgenesis with sterility and primary amenorrhea, and short stature; may have cardiac malformations, congenital lymphedema of the extremities, and characteristic facial and body features

Usher syndrome—autosomal recessive; mutations in any of a number of genes; characterized by early retinitis pigmentosa, vestibular dysfunction, and sensorineural deafness

Vanishing testes syndrome—see "testicular regression syndrome."

VATER association—characterized by Vertebral defects, Anal atresia, Tracheoesophageal fistula with Esophageal atresia, and Radial and/or renal anomalies; may be expanded to VACTERL to include Congenital heart defects or other Limb defects; at least two noncardiac components must be present for the diagnosis; overlaps with diagnosable genetic conditions which must be considered; VATER is a diagnosis of exclusion rather than a primary diagnosis.

von Gierke disease—see "glycogen storage disease."

von Hippel—Lindau disease—autosomal dominant; mutations in *VHL* or *CCND1*; familial cancer syndrome; benign and malignant tumors, most frequently retinal, cerebellar and spinal hemangioblastoma, renal cell carcinoma, pheochromocytoma, and pancreatic tumors

Waardenburg syndrome—autosomal dominant; multiple types and subtypes; mutations most commonly in *PAX3*; pigmentary abnormalities of the hair, skin, and eyes (white forelock, heterochromia iridis, premature graying of hair) congenital sensorineural hearing loss, and characteristic facies

Wegener granulomatosis—complex genetics; necrotizing granulomatous vasculitis involving (a) the airways, leading to rhinorrhea, chronic sinusitis, nasal ulceration; (b) the lungs, causing hemoptysis, dyspnea, and cough; (c) the kidneys, manifested as hematuria and/or proteinuria due to glomerulonephritis; other symptoms include fever, malaise, weight loss, myalgias, arthralgias, ophthalmic involvement, neuropathies, and cutaneous nodules or ulcers.

Werner syndrome—autosomal recessive; mutations in *RECQL2*; characterized by scleroderma-like skin changes, premature arteriosclerosis, diabetes mellitus, and an appearance of premature aging; short stature, slender limbs, and a stocky trunk

Williams syndrome—autosomal dominant; deletion in 7q11.23; characterized by hypercalcemia in infants, supravalvular aortic stenosis, peripheral pulmonary artery stenosis, short stature, neurocognitive impairment, particularly in math, hypersocial with affinity for music, hyperacusis, characteristic facies

Wiskott-Aldrich syndrome—X-linked recessive; mutations in *WAS*; characterized by immunodeficiency, thrombocytopenia, severe eczema, and recurrent infections

Wolff-Parkinson-White syndrome—accessory conduction pathway found in 25% of patients with supraventricular tachycardia; typical electrocardiographic findings include a short PR interval and slow upstroke of the QRS (delta wave); may be an isolated finding, or related to structural cardiac defects; genetic or acquired

Wolman disease—see "lysosomal acid lipase deficiency."

Xeroderma pigmentosum—autosomal recessive; characterized by extreme sunlight sensitivity, slowly progressive neurocognitive impairment, photophobia, and cutaneous and ocular malignancies; skin is unable to repair itself after exposure to ultraviolet light; patients may have freckling, progressive skin atrophy, erythema, scaling bullae and crusting, telangiectasia.

Zellweger syndrome (cerebrohepatorenal syndrome)—autosomal recessive; mutations in *PEX1*; disorder of peroxisome biogenesis (absence of peroxisomes); characterized by severe neurologic dysfunction, hepatic cirrhosis and characteristic facies. The vast majority of patients die within the 1st year of life.

Appendix IV
Tables and Figures

Michael D. Cabana

Table 1. Developmental Milestones from Birth to 5 Years

Age (mo)	Adaptive/Fine Motor	Language	Gross Motor	Personal–Social
1	Grasp reflex (hands fisted)	Facial response to sounds	Lifts head in prone position	Stares at face
2	Follows object with eyes past midline	Coos (vowel sounds)	Lifts head in prone position to 45 degrees	Smiles in response to others
4	Hands open Brings objects to mouth	Laughs and squeals Turns toward voice	Sits: head steady Rolls to supine	Smiles spontaneously
6	Palmar grasp of objects	Babbles (consonant sounds)	Sits independently Stands, hands held	Reaches for toys Recognizes strangers
9	Pincer grasp	Says "mama," "dada" nonspecifically, comprehends "no"	Pulls to stand	Feeds self Waves bye-bye
12	Helps turn pages of book	2–4 words Follows command with gesture	Stands independently Walks, one hand held	Points to indicate wants
15	Scribbles	4–6 words Follows command no gesture	Walks independently	Drinks from cup Imitates activities
18	Turns pages of book	10–20 words Points to 4 body parts	Walks up steps	Feeds self with spoon
24	Solves single-piece puzzles	Combines 2–3 words Uses "I" and "you"	Jumps Kicks ball	Removes coat Verbalizes wants
30	Imitates horizontal and vertical lines	Names all body parts	Rides tricycle using pedals	Pulls up pants Washes, dries hands
36	Copies circle Draws person with 3 parts	Gives full name, age, and sex Names 2 colors	Throws ball overhand Walks up stairs (alternating feet)	Toilet-trained Puts on shirt, knows front from back
42	Copies cross	Understands "cold," "tired," "hungry"	Stands on 1 foot for 2–3 s	Engages in associative play
48	Counts 4 objects Identifies some numbers and letters	Understands prepositions (under, on, behind, in front of) Asks "how" and "why"	Hops on 1 foot	Dresses with little assistance Shoes on correct feet
54	Copies square Draws person with 6 parts	Understands opposites	Broad-jumps 24 inches	Bosses and criticizes Shows off
60	Prints first name Counts 10 objects	Asks meaning of words	Skips (alternating feet)	Ties shoes

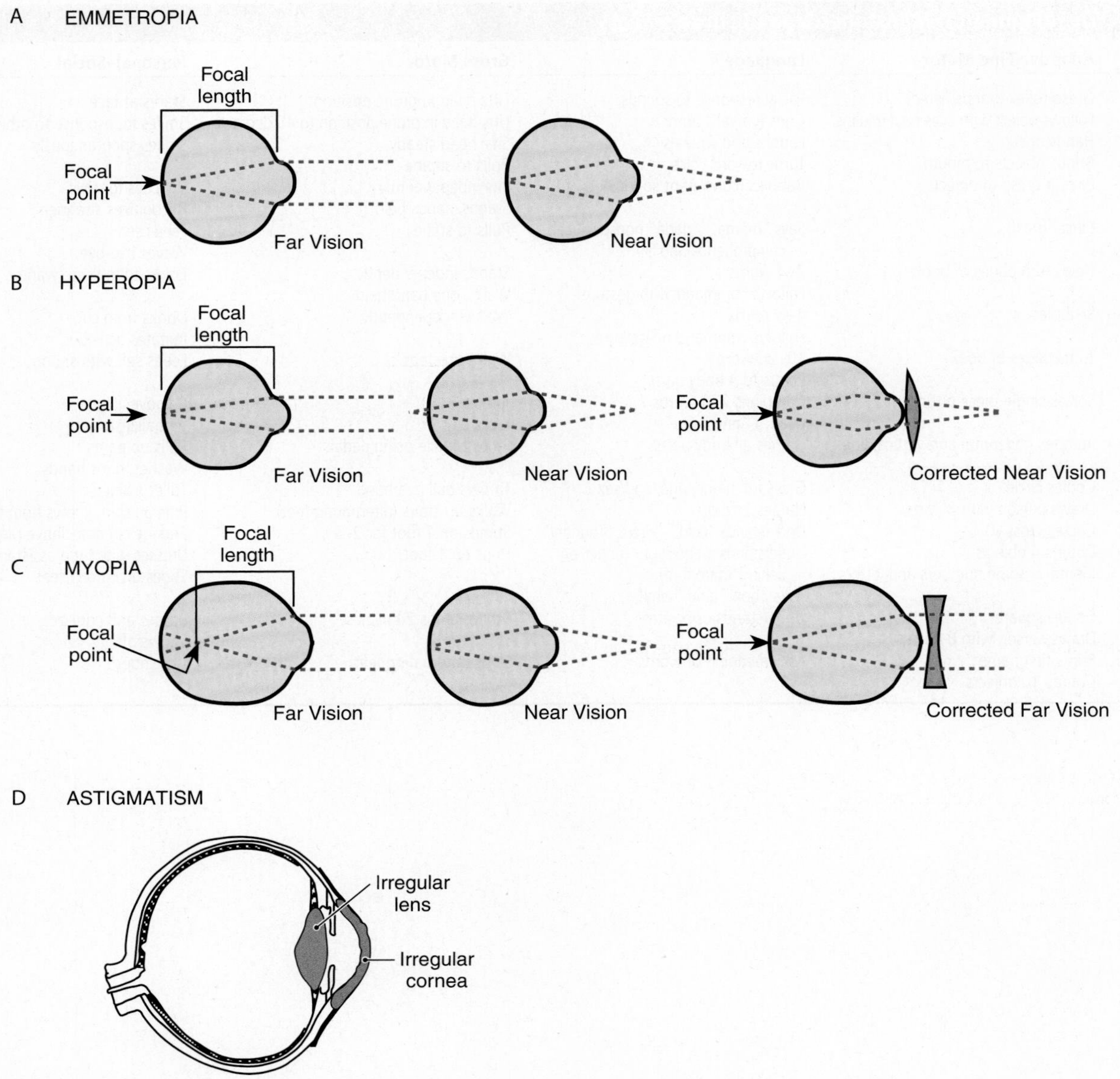

FIGURE 1. The normally refractive eye, common refractive errors, and their corrections. **A:** In a normal (emmetropic) eye, light rays from a near or far object are adequately refracted so that the rays converge directly on the retina, enabling formation of a clear image. **B:** In a farsighted (hypermetropic, hyperopic) eye, an image from a near point is focused behind the retina. The resulting condition can be corrected with convex lenses. **C:** In a nearsighted (myopic) eye, an image from a far point is focused in front of the retina. This refractive condition can be corrected with concave lenses. **D:** Refractive errors of astigmatism result from irregular curvatures of the cornea, lens, or both. Consequently, horizontal and vertical points from various visual fields are focused at two different focal points on the retina, resulting in distorted vision. (From Bhatnagar SC. *Neuroscience for the Study of Communicative Disorders*. 4th ed. Philadelphia: Lippincott Williams & Wilkins; 2012.)

PRIMARY AND PERMANENT DENTITION

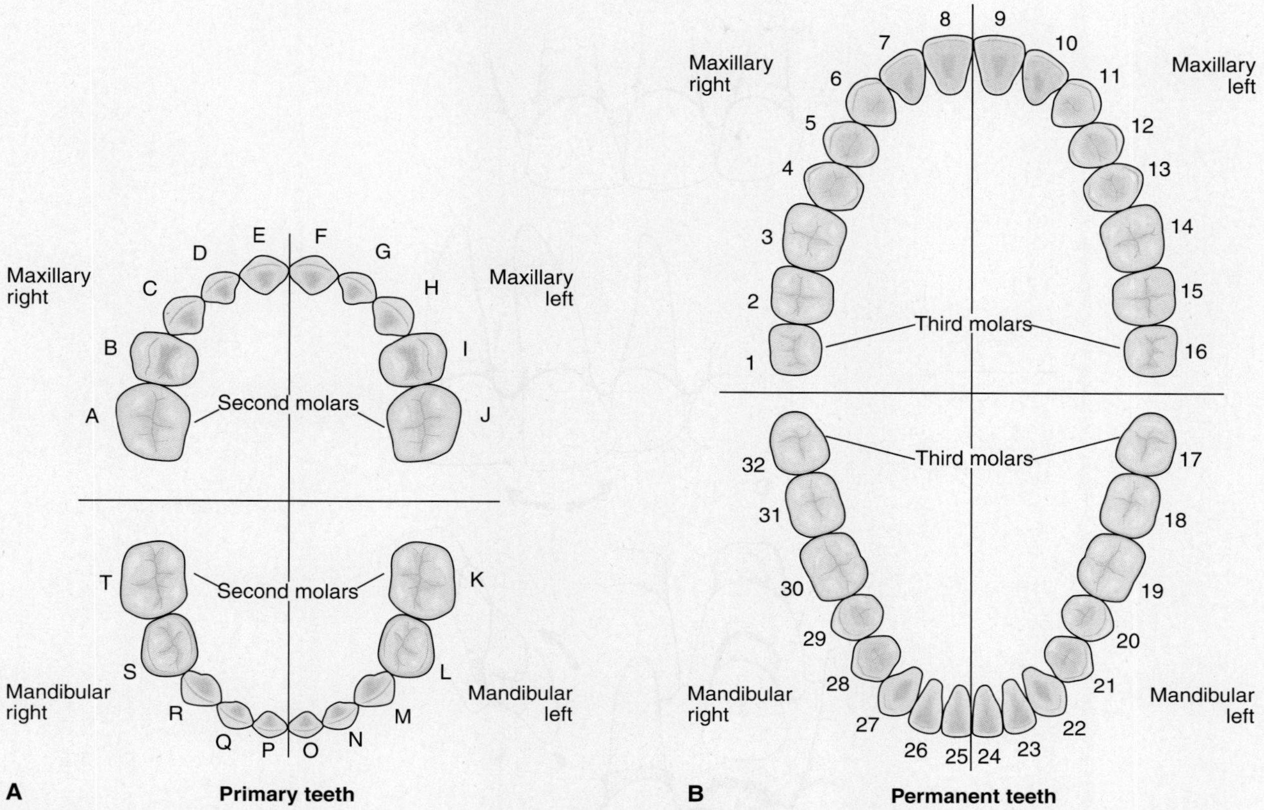

FIGURE 2. The Universal Numbering System. **A:** Primary teeth. **B:** Permanent teeth. (From Lippincott Williams & Wilkins. *Lippincott Williams & Wilkins' Comprehensive Dental Assisting.* Philadelphia: Lippincott Williams & Wilkins; 2011.)

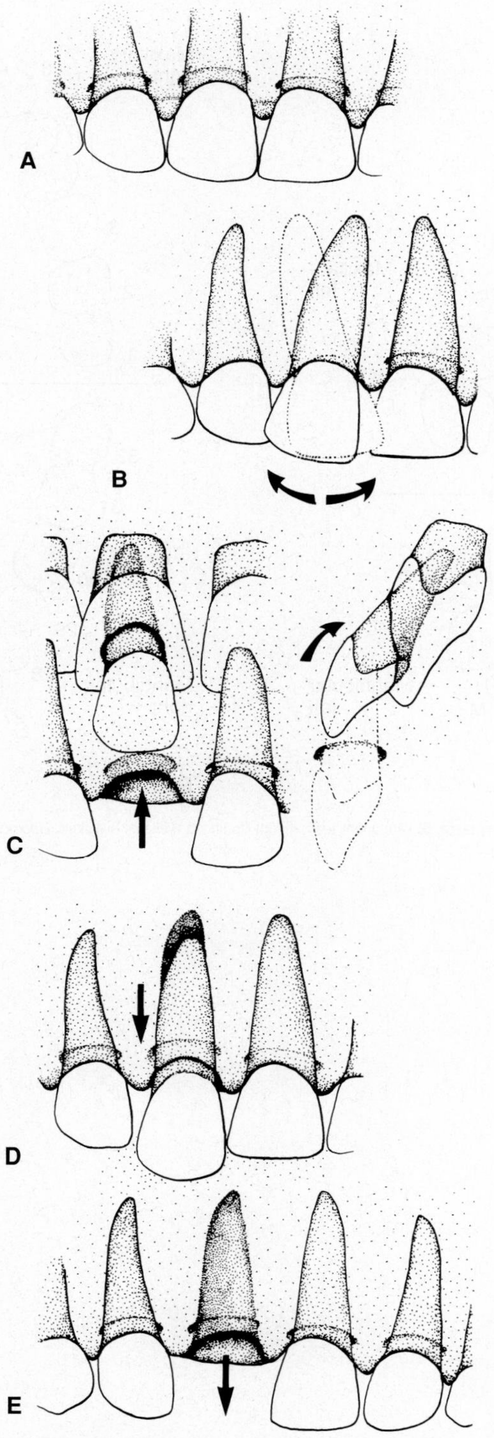

FIGURE 3. The various types of trauma to the periodontal structures: concussion/subluxation **(A)**, lateral luxation **(B)**, intrusion (if primary tooth is intruded note location of developing permanent tooth bud) **(C)**, extrusion **(D)**, and avulsion **(E)**. Refer emergencies B through E to the dental staff as soon as possible. (From Fleisher GR, Ludwig S, Henretig FM, et al. *Textbook of Pediatric Emergency Medicine*. 5th ed. Philadelphia: Lippincott Williams & Wilkins; 2005.)

Table 2. Clinical Signs of Dehydration in Children

Parameter	Mild	Moderate	Severe
Activity	Normal	Lethargic	Lethargic to comatose
Color	Pale	Gray	Mottled
Urine output	Decreased (<2–3 mL/kg/hr)	Oliguric (<1 mL/kg/hr)	Anuric
Fontanelle	Flat	Depressed	Sunken
Mucous membranes	Dry	Very dry	Cracked
Skin turgor	Slightly decreased	Markedly decreased	Tenting
Pulse	Normal to increased	Increased	Grossly tachycardic
Blood pressure	Normal	Normal	Decreased
Weight loss	5%	10%	15%

Hypernatremic dehydration may be accompanied by moderate clinical signs.
Reprinted with permission from Rogers MC. Shock. In: Rogers MC, Helfaer MA, eds. *Handbook of Pediatric Intensive Care*. 2nd ed. Baltimore: Williams Wilkins; 1994:140.

Table 3. Characteristics of the Three Stages of Parapneumonic Pleural Effusions

	Exudative Stage	Fibrinolytic Stage	Organizing Stage (Empyema)
Appearance	Nonpurulent, not turbid	Nonpurulent, not turbid	Purulent, turbid
Fluid consistency	Free-flowing	Loculated	Organized
Gram stain and culture results	Negative	Transitional	Positive (before antibiotic treatment)
Glucose	>100 mg/dL	<50 mg/dL	<50 mg/dL
Protein	<3 g/dL	>3 g/dL	>3 g/dL
pH	>7.30	<7.30	<7.30
WBCs	Few	PMNs	PMNs

PMNs, polymorphonuclear neutrophils; WBCs, white blood cells.

Table 4. Pleural Fluid Diagnostic Studies

Study	Transudate	Exudate
Biochemical		
Pleural LDH	<200 IU	≥200 IU
Pleural fluid/serum LDH ratio[a]	<0.6	≥0.6
Pleural fluid/serum protein ratio[a]	<0.5	≥0.5
Specific gravity	<1.016	≥1.016
Protein level	<3.0 g/dL	≥3.0 g/dL
Other studies		
Glucose	Usually >40 mg/dL	Typically <40 mg/dL
Amylase	May be elevated in some neoplasms, GI trauma, or surgery	
Rheumatoid factor, LE prep, ANA	Are occasionally helpful if collagen vascular disorders are within the differential	
Hematologic		
WBC count	Although high counts (>100/mm^3) are suggestive of an exudate, the results are quite variable	
WBC differential	May actually provide more useful information	
Lymphocyte count	May be elevated in neoplasms, tuberculosis, and some fungal infections	
Segmented neutrophils	May be elevated in bacterial infections, connective tissue disease, pancreatitis, or pulmonary infarction	
Eosinophil count	May be elevated in bacterial infections, neoplasms, and connective tissue diseases	
RBC count	If >100,000/mm^3, is suggestive of trauma, neoplasms, or pulmonary infarction	
Cytology and chromosomal studies	May show evidence of malignant cells or chromosomal abnormalities	
Microbiology		
Gram stain		
Fluid culture for aerobes and anaerobes		
Acid-fast stain (if tuberculosis is in the differential)		
Fungal culture		
Viral culture		
Counterimmune electrophoresis may aid in the detection of a bacterial infection)		

ANA, antinuclear antibody; LDH, lactate dehydrogenase; LE prep, lupus erythematosus cell preparation; WBC, white blood cell.
[a]These tests are more reliable in differentiating transudate from exudate than specific gravity or protein level.

Table 5. Glasgow Coma Scale

Eyes open		Best motor response	
Spontaneously	4	Obey commands	6
To speech	3	Localize pain	5
To pain	2	Withdrawal	4
None	1	Flexion to pain	3
Best verbal response		Extension to pain	2
Oriented	5	None	1
Confused	4		
Inappropriate	3		
Incomprehensible	2		
None	1		

Adapted from Fleisher G, Ludwig S, eds. *Textbook of Pediatric Emergency Medicine*. 3rd ed. Baltimore: Williams Wilkins; 1993:272.

Table 6. Glasgow Coma Scale for Adults and Children and Modified Score for Infants

	Glasgow Coma Score (Adults/Older Children)		**Modified Glasgow Coma Score (Infants)**
Eye opening	Spontaneous	4	Spontaneous
	To verbal stimuli	3	To speech
	To pain	2	To pain
	None	1	None
Best verbal response	Oriented	5	Coos and babbles
	Confused speech	4	Irritable, cries
	Inappropriate words	3	Cries to pain
	Nonspecific sounds	2	Moans to pain
	None	1	None
Best motor response	Follows commands	6	Normal spontaneous movements
	Localizes pain	5	Withdraws to touch
	Withdraws to pain	4	Withdraws to pain
	Flexes to pain	3	Abnormal flexion
	Extends to pain	2	Abnormal extension
	None	1	None

Table 7. Key Characteristics of Vaginal Discharges

	Presenting Symptoms	Discharge	Nonmenstrual pH	Amine/ Whiff Test	Vaginal Smear	Treatment
Nonspecific vaginitis	Foul-smelling discharge Itching	Scant to copious Brown to green in color	Variable	Negative	Leukocytes Bacteria and other debris	Improved perineal hygiene
Physiologic leukorrhea	None	Variable Scant to moderate Clear to white	<4.5	Negative	Normal epithelial cells Lactobacilli predominate	None
Bacterial vaginosis	Foul-smelling discharge	Gray-white	>4.7	Positive	Epithelial cells with bacteria ("clue cells") Gram-negative rods	Metronidazole Clindamycin
Candidiasis	Severe itching Vulvar inflammation	White, "curd-like"	<4.5	Negative	Fungal hyphae and buds	Topical or intra-vaginal imidazoles, triazoles Oral ketoconazole
Trichomonal vaginitis	Copious discharge Itching	Profuse Yellow to green	5.0–6.0	Occasionally present	Motile flagellated organisms	Metronidazole
Foreign body	Foul-smelling discharge	Foul-smelling Purulent Dark brown	Variable (usually >4.7)	Occasionally present	Leukocytes Epithelial cells with bacteria and debris	Remove foreign body. Irrigate vagina.
Contact vulvovaginitis	Vulvar inflammation Itching Edema	Scant White to yellow	Variable (usually <4.5)	Negative	Leukocytes Epithelial cells	Remove irritant. Topical steroids

FOOD POISONING OR FOODBORNE ILLNESS

Table 8. Epidemiologic Aspects of Food Poisoning

Organism	Pathogenesis	Source	Prevention
Salmonella	Infection	Meats, poultry, eggs, dairy products	Proper cooking and food handling, pasteurization
Staphylococcus	Preformed enterotoxin	Meats, poultry, potato salad, cream-filled pastry, cheese, sausage	Careful food handling, rapid refrigeration
Clostridium perfringens	Enterotoxin	Meats, poultry	Avoid delay in serving foods, avoid cooling and rewarming foods.
Clostridium botulinum	Preformed neurotoxin	Honey, home-canned foods, uncooked foods	Proper refrigeration (see text)
Vibrio parahaemolyticus	Infection enterotoxin	Sea fish, seawater, shellfish	Proper refrigeration
Bacillus cereus			
Diarrheal type	Sporulation enterotoxin	Many prepared foods	Proper refrigeration
Vomiting type	Preformed toxin	Cooked or fried rice, vegetables, meats, cereal, puddings	Proper refrigeration of cooked rice and other foods
Enterohemorrhagic including STEC 0157-H7	Cytotoxins	Milk, beef	Thorough cooking of beef, consumption of pasteurized milk products
Enterotoxigenic *Escherichia coli* (traveler's diarrhea)	Enterotoxin	Food or water	Travelers should drink only bottled or canned beverages and water, and avoid ice, raw produce including salads, and peeled fruit. Cooked foods should be eaten hot.

STEC, Shiga toxin–producing *Escherichia coli*.

Table 9. Clinical Aspects of Food Poisoning

Organism	Incubation	Symptoms	Duration
Bacillus cereus	Vomiting toxin 1–6 h Diarrhea toxin 6–24 h	Vomiting ± diarrhea; fever uncommon	8–24 h
Brucella	Several days to months; usually >30 d	Weakness, fever, headache chills, arthralgia, weight loss; splenomegaly	
Campylobacter	2–10 d; usually 2–5 d	Diarrhea (often bloody), abdominal pain, fever	
Clostridium botulinum	2 h to 8 d; usually 12–48 h	Poor feeding, weak cry, constipation, diplopia, blurred vision, respiratory weakness; symmetric descending paralysis	
Clostridium perfringens	6–24 h	Diarrhea, abdominal cramps, vomiting and fever uncommon	<24 h
Escherichia coli	→	→	
E. coli 0157:H7	1–10 d; usually 3–4 d	Diarrhea (often bloody), abdominal cramps, little or no fever. Can cause HUS	5–10 d
ETEC	6–48 h	Diarrhea, abdominal cramps, nausea, fever, and vomiting; uncommon	5–10 d
Listeria monocytogenes	2–6 wk	Meningitis, neonatal sepsis, fever	Variable
Nontyphoidal *Salmonella*	6–72 h	Diarrhea often with fever and abdominal cramps	<7 d
Salmonella typhi	3–60 d; usually 7–14 d	Fever, anorexia, malaise, headache, myalgias ± diarrhea or constipation	3–4 wk
Shigella	12 h to 6 d; usually 2–4 d	Diarrhea (often bloody), frequently fever, abdominal cramps	1 d to 1 mo
Staphylococcus aureus	30 min to 8 h; usually 2–4 h	Vomiting, diarrhea	<24 h
Vibrio	4–30 h	Diarrhea, cramps, nausea, vomiting	Self-limited
Yersinia enterocolitica	1–10 d; usually 4–6 d	Diarrhea, abdominal pain (often severe), mesenteric adenitis, pseudoappendicular syndrome	1–3 wk

ETEC, enterotoxigenic *Escherichia coli*; HUS, hemolytic uremic syndrome.

Table 10. U.S. Food and Drug Administration Pharmaceutical Pregnancy Categories

Pregnancy Category A	Adequate and well-controlled human studies have failed to demonstrate a risk to the fetus in the 1st trimester of pregnancy (and there is no evidence of risk in later trimesters).
Pregnancy Category B	Animal reproduction studies have failed to demonstrate a risk to the fetus and there are no adequate and well-controlled studies in pregnant women OR animal studies have shown an adverse effect, but adequate and well-controlled studies in pregnant women have failed to demonstrate a risk to the fetus in any trimester.
Pregnancy Category C	Animal reproduction studies have shown an adverse effect on the fetus and there are no adequate and well-controlled studies in humans, but potential benefits may warrant use of the drug in pregnant women despite potential risks.
Pregnancy Category D	There is positive evidence of human fetal risk based on adverse reaction data from investigational or marketing experience or studies in humans, but potential benefits may warrant use of the drug in pregnant women despite potential risks.
Pregnancy Category X	Studies in animals or humans have demonstrated fetal abnormalities and/or there is positive evidence of human fetal risk based on adverse reaction data from investigational or marketing experience, and the risks involved in use of the drug in pregnant women clearly outweigh potential benefits.

Table 11. Assessment of Etiology of Rickets Based on Laboratory Results

	Ca	Phos	Alk phos	iPTH	25-(OH)D	1,25-$(OH)_2$D	Urine Ca/ Cr	TRP
Nutritional/insufficient sunlight	N or ↓	↓	↑	↑	↓	↑	↓	↑
Malabsorption	N or ↓	↓	↑	↑	↓	↑	↓	↑
Renal tubular defects	N or ↓	↓	↑	↑	N	↑	↑	N or ↓
Altered vitamin D metabolism	N or ↓	↓	↑	↑	↓	↑	↓	↑
Genetic forms of rickets								
X-linked, AD, and AR hypophosphatemic rickets	N	↓	↑	N or ↑	N	N or ↑	N or ↓	↓
1α-hydroxylase deficiency	↓	↓	↑	↑	N	↓	↓	↑
Vitamin D receptor mutations (vitamin D resistance)	↓	↓	↑	↑	N	↑	↓	↑
Hereditary hypophosphatemic rickets with hypercalciuria	N or ↓	↓	↑	↑	N	↑	↑	↓
Hypophosphatasia	N or ↑	N or ↑	↓	N or ↓	N	N or ↓	N or ↑	N

AD, autosomal dominant; alk phos, alkaline phosphatase; AR, autosomal recessive; Ca, calcium; Ca/Cr, calcium/creatinine ratio; iPTH, intact parathyroid hormone; N, normal; 1,25-(OH)2-D, 1,25-dihydroxy vitamin D; phos, phosphorus; TRP, tubular reabsorption of phosphorus ([1 − (U phos × P Cr/U Cr × S Phos)] × 100, normal 85–95%); 25-(OH)-D, 25-hydroxy vitamin D.

Table 12. Dietary Reference Intake for Calcium and Vitamin D

	Calcium			Vitamin D		
Age	Estimated Average Requirement (mg/d)	Recommended Dietary Allowance (mg/d)	Upper Level Intake (mg/d)	Estimated Average Requirement (IU/d)	Recommended Dietary Allowance (IU/d)	Upper Level Intake (IU/d)
0–6 mo	200	200	1,000	400	400	1,000
6–12 mo	260	260	1,500	400	400	1,500
1–3 y	500	700	2,500	400	600	2,500
4–8 y	800	1,000	2,500	400	600	3,000
9–18 y	1,100	1,300	3,000	400	600	4,000
19–30 y	800	1,000	2,500	400	600	4,000

Adapted from Ross AC, Abrams SA, Aloia JF, et al. Dietary reference intakes for calcium and vitamin D. http://www.iom.edu/~/media/Files/Report%20Files/2010/Dietary-Reference-Intakes-for-Calcium-and-Vitamin-D/Vitamin%20D%20and%20Calcium%202010%20Report%20Brief.pdf. Accessed March 1, 2015.

Table 13. Clinical and Biochemical Features of Congenital Adrenal Hyperplasia

Enzyme Defect	Sexual Ambiguity: Female	Sexual Ambiguity: Male	Additional Clinical Manifestations	Predominant Steroids
Desmolase	−	+	Salt wasting	—
3β-hydroxysteroid dehydrogenase	+	+	Salt wasting	17-OH-pregnenolone, DHEA
21-hydroxylase	+	−	Salt wasting	17-OH-progestone, androstenedione
11-hydroxylase	+	−	Hypertension	11-deoxycortisol
17-hydroxylase	−	+	Hypertension	DOC, corticosterone

DHEA, dehydroepiandrosterone; DOC, deoxycorticosterone.

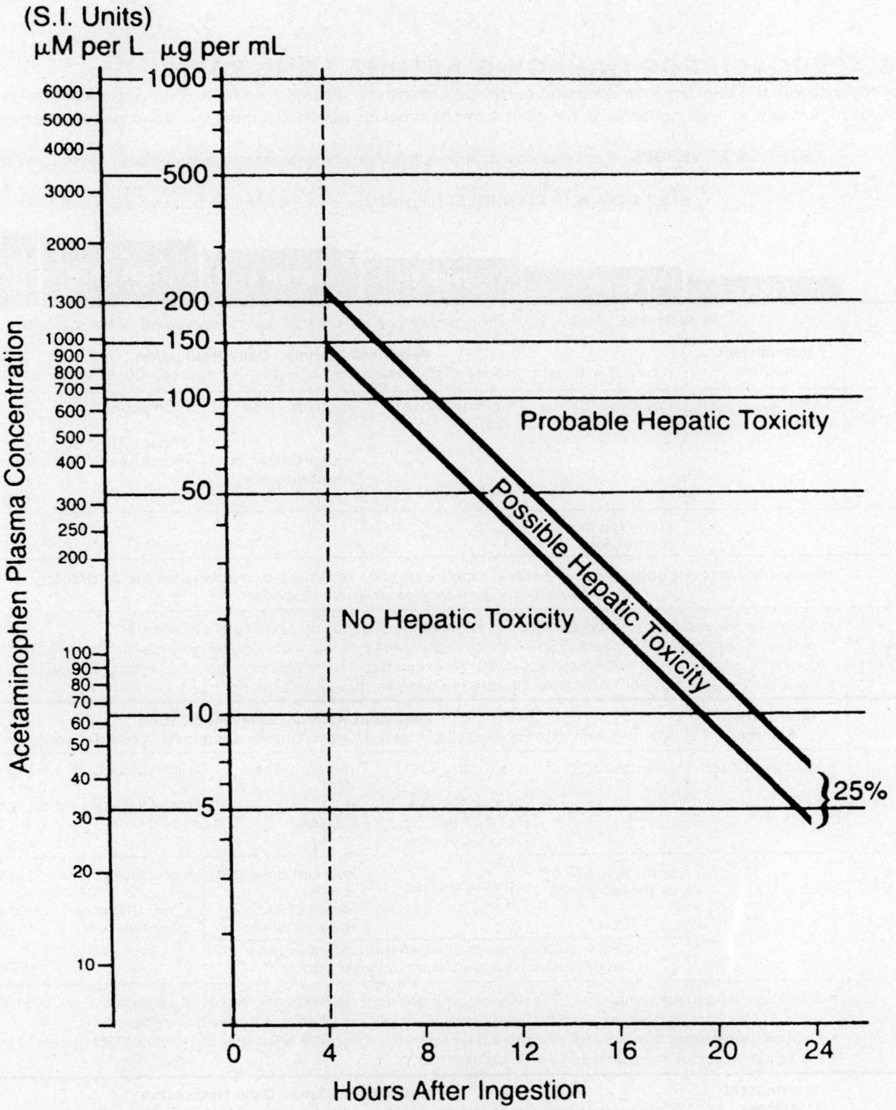

FIGURE 4. Nomogram for estimating severity of acute poisoning. (Reprinted with permission from Rumack BH, Matthew H. Acetaminophen poisoning and toxicity. *Pediatrics*. 1975;55(6):871–876.)

STEPWISE APPROACH FOR MANAGING ASTHMA LONG TERM

The stepwise approach tailors the selection of medication to the level of asthma severity (see page 5) or asthma control (see page 6). The stepwise approach is meant to help, not replace, the clinical decisionmaking needed to meet individual patient needs.

ASSESS CONTROL:

STEP UP IF NEEDED (first, check medication adherence, inhaler technique, environmental control, and comorbidities)

STEP DOWN IF POSSIBLE (and asthma is well controlled for at least 3 months)

		STEP 1	**STEP 2**	**STEP 3**	**STEP 4**	**STEP 5**	**STEP 6**
		At each step: Patient education, environmental control, and management of comorbidities					
0–4 years of age		**Intermittent Asthma**	**Persistent Asthma: Daily Medication** Consult with asthma specialist if step 3 care or higher is required. Consider consultation at step 2.				
	Preferred Treatment†	SABA* as needed	low-dose ICS*	medium-dose ICS*	medium-dose ICS* + either LABA* or montelukast	high-dose ICS* + either LABA* or montelukast	high-dose ICS* + either LABA* or montelukast + oral corticosteroids
	Alternative Treatment†,‡		cromolyn or montelukast				
		If clear benefit is not observed in 4–6 weeks, and medication technique and adherence are satisfactory, consider adjusting therapy or alternate diagnoses.					
	Quick-Relief Medication	▪ SABA* as needed for symptoms; intensity of treatment depends on severity of symptoms. ▪ With viral respiratory symptoms: SABA every 4–6 hours up to 24 hours (longer with physician consult). Consider short course of oral systemic corticosteroids if asthma exacerbation is severe or patient has history of severe exacerbations. ▪ Caution: Frequent use of SABA may indicate the need to step up treatment.					
5–11 years of age		**Intermittent Asthma**	**Persistent Asthma: Daily Medication** Consult with asthma specialist if step 4 care or higher is required. Consider consultation at step 3.				
	Preferred Treatment†	SABA* as needed	low-dose ICS*	low-dose ICS* + either LABA,* LTRA,* or theophylline(b)	medium-dose ICS* + LABA*	high-dose ICS* + LABA*	high-dose ICS* + LABA* + oral corticosteroids
	Alternative Treatment†,‡		cromolyn, LTRA,* or theophylline§	**OR** medium-dose ICS	medium-dose ICS* + either LTRA* or theophylline§	high-dose ICS* + either LTRA* or theophylline§	high-dose ICS* + either LTRA* or theophylline§ + oral corticosteroids
			Consider subcutaneous allergen immunotherapy for patients who have persistent, allergic asthma.**				
	Quick-Relief Medication	▪ SABA* as needed for symptoms. The intensity of treatment depends on severity of symptoms: up to 3 treatments every 20 minutes as needed. Short course of oral systemic corticosteroids may be needed. ▪ Caution: Increasing use of SABA or use >2 days/week for symptom relief (not to prevent EIB*) generally indicates inadequate control and the need to step up treatment.					
≥12 years of age		**Intermittent Asthma**	**Persistent Asthma: Daily Medication** Consult with asthma specialist if step 4 care or higher is required. Consider consultation at step 3.				
	Preferred Treatment†	SABA* as needed	low-dose ICS*	low-dose ICS* + LABA* **OR** medium-dose ICS*	medium-dose ICS* + LABA*	high-dose ICS* + LABA* **AND** consider omalizumab for patients who have allergies††	high-dose ICS* + LABA* + oral corticosteroid§§ **AND** consider omalizumab for patients who have allergies††
	Alternative Treatment†,‡		cromolyn, LTRA,* or theophylline§	low-dose ICS* + either LTRA,* theophylline,§ or zileuton‡‡	medium-dose ICS* + either LTRA,* theophylline,§ or zileuton‡‡		
			Consider subcutaneous allergen immunotherapy for patients who have persistent, allergic asthma.**				
	Quick-Relief Medication	▪ SABA* as needed for symptoms. The intensity of treatment depends on severity of symptoms: up to 3 treatments every 20 minutes as needed. Short course of oral systemic corticosteroids may be needed. ▪ Caution: Use of SABA >2 days/week for symptom relief (not to prevent EIB*) generally indicates inadequate control and the need to step up treatment.					

* **Abbreviations:** EIB, exercise-induced bronchospasm; ICS, inhaled corticosteroid; LABA, inhaled long-acting beta$_2$-agonist; LTRA, leukotriene receptor antagonist; SABA, inhaled short-acting beta$_2$-agonist.

† Treatment options are listed in alphabetical order, if more than one.

‡ If alternative treatment is used and response is inadequate, discontinue and use preferred treatment before stepping up.

§ Theophylline is a less desirable alternative because of the need to monitor serum concentration levels.

** Based on evidence for dust mites, animal dander, and pollen; evidence is weak or lacking for molds and cockroaches. Evidence is strongest for immunotherapy with single allergens. The role of allergy in asthma is greater in children than in adults.

†† Clinicians who administer immunotherapy or omalizumab should be prepared to treat anaphylaxis that may occur.

‡‡ Zileuton is less desirable because of limited studies as adjunctive therapy and the need to monitor liver function.

§§ Before oral corticosteroids are introduced, a trial of high-dose ICS + LABA + either LTRA, theophylline, or zileuton, may be considered, although this approach has not been studied in clinical trials.

FIGURE 5. National Heart, Lung, and Blood Institute, National Institutes of Health. Asthma care quick reference: http://www.nhlbi.nih.gov/files/docs/guidelines/asthma_qrg.pdf. Accessed March 1, 2015.

Table 14. Estimated Comparative Daily Dosages: Inhaled Corticosteroids for Long-Term Asthma Control

	0–4 years of age			5–11 years of age			≥ 12 years of age		
Daily Dose	**Low**	**Meduim***	**High***	**Low**	**Meduim***	**High***	**Low**	**Meduim***	**High***
MEDICATION									
Beclomethasone MDI†	N/A	N/A	N/A	80–160 mcg	>160–320 mcg	>320 mcg	80–240 mcg	>240–480 mcg	>480 mcg
40 mcg/puff				1–2 puffs 2×/day	3–4 puffs 2×/day		1–3 puffs 2×/day	4–6 puffs 2×/day	
80 mcg/puff				1 puff 2×/day	2 puffs 2×/day	≥3 puffs 2×/day	1 puff am, 2 puffs pm	2–3 puffs 2×/day	≥4 puffs 2×/day
Budesonide DPI†	N/A	N/A	N/A	180–360 mcg	>360–720mcg	>720mcg	180–540 mcg	>540–1,080 mcg	>1,080 mcg
90 mcg/inhalation				1–2 inhs† 2×/day	3–4 inhs† 2×/day		1–3 inhs† 2×/day		
180 mcg/inhalation					2 inhs† 2×/day	≥3 inhs† 2×/day	1 inh† am, 2 inhs† pm	2-3 inhs† 2×/day	≥4 inhs† 2×/day
Budesonide Nebules	0.25–0.5 mg	>0.5–1.0 mg	>1.0 mg	0.5 mg	1.0 mg	2.0 mg	N/A	N/A	N/A
0.25 mg	1–2 nebs†/day			1 neb† 2×/day					
0.25 mg	1 neb†/day	2 nebs†/day	3 nebs†/day	1 neb†/day	1 neb† 2×/day				
1.0 mg		1 neb†/day	2 nebs†/day		1 neb†/day	1 neb† 2×/day			
Ciclesonide MDI†	N/A	N/A	N/A	80–160 mcg	>160–320 mcg	>320 mcg	160–320 mcg	>320–640 mcg	>640 mcg
80 mcg/puff				1–2 puffs/day	1 puff am, 2 puffs pm– 2 puffs 2×/day	≥3 puffs 2×/day	1–2 puffs 2×/day	3–4 puffs 2×/day	
160 mcg/puff				1 puff/day	1 puff 2×/day	≥2 puffs 2×/day		2 puffs 2×/day	≥3 puffs 2×/day
Flunisolide MDI†	N/A	N/A	N/A	160 mcg	320–480 mcg	≥480 mcg	320 mcg	>320–640 mcg	>640 mcg
80 mcg/puff				1 puff 2×/day	2–3 puffs 2×/day	≥4 puffs 2×/day	2 puffs 2×/day	3–4 puffs 2×/day	≥5 puffs 2×/day
Fluticasone MDI†	176 mcg	>176–352 mcg	>352 mcg	88–176 mcg	>176–352 mcg	>352 mcg	88–264 mcg	>264–440 mcg	>440 mcg
44 mcg/puff	2 puffs 2×/day	3–4 puffs 2×/day		1–2 puffs 2×/day	3–4 puffs 2×/day		1–3 puffs 2×/day		
110 mcg/puff		1 puff 2×/day	≥2 puffs 2×/day		1 puff 2×/day	≥2 puffs 2×/day		2 puffs 2×/day	3 puffs 2×/day
220 mcg/puff								1 puff 2×/day	≥2 puffs 2×/day
Fluticasone DPI†	N/A	N/A	N/A	100–200 mcg	>200–400 mcg	>400 mcg	100–300 mcg	>300–500 mcg	>500 mcg
50 mcg/inhalation				1–2 inhs† 2×/day	3–4 inhs† 2×/day		1–3 inhs† 2×/day		
100 mcg/inhalation				1 inh† 2×/day	2 inhs† 2×/day	>2 inhs† 2×/day		2 inhs† 2×/day	≥3 inhs† 2×/day
250 mcg/inhalation						1 inh† 2×/day		1 inh† 2×/day	≥2 inhs† 2×/day
Mometasone DPI†	N/A	N/A	N/A	110 mcg	220–440 mcg	>440 mcg	110–220 mcg	>220–440 mcg	>440 mcg
110 mcg/inhalation				1 inh†/day	1–2 inhs† 2×/day	≥3 inhs† 2×/day	1–2 inhs† pm	3–4 inhs† pm or 2 inhs† 2×/day	≥3 inhs† 2×/day
220 mcg/inhalation					1–2 inhs†/day	≥3 inhs† divided in 2 doses	1 inh† pm	1 inh† 2×/day or 2 inhs† pm	≥3 inhs† divided in 2 doses

*It is preferable to use a higher mcg/puff or mcg/inhalation formulation to achive as low a number of puffs or inhalations as possible.

†**Abbreviations:** DPI, dry power inhaler (requires deep, fast inhalation); inh, inhalation; MDI, metered dose inhaler (releases a puff of medication); neb, nebule.

National Heart, Lung, and Blood Institute, National Institutes of Health. Asthma care quick reference: http://www.nhlbi.nih.gov/files/docs/guidelines/asthma_qrg.pdf. Accessed March 1, 2015.

INDEX

B